PRINCIPLES AND PRACTICE OF GYNECOLOGIC ONCOLOGY

EIGHTH EDITION

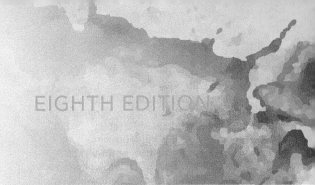

EIGHTH EDITION

PRINCIPLES
AND PRACTICE
OF GYNECOLOGIC
ONCOLOGY

Dennis S. Chi, MD
Ronald O. Perelman Chair in Gynecologic
   Surgery
Deputy Chief, Gynecology Service
Head, Ovarian Cancer Surgery
Department of Surgery
Memorial Sloan Kettering Cancer Center
New York, New York

Don S. Dizon, MD, FACP
Professor of Medicine and Professor of Surgery
Brown University
Director, The Pelvic Malignancies Program
Lifespan Cancer Institute
Director of Medical Oncology
Rhode Island Hospital
Associate Director, Community Outreach and
   Engagement
Legorreta Cancer Center at Brown University
Providence, Rhode Island

Catheryn Yashar, MD, FACRO,
   FACR, FABS, FASTRO
Professor and Vice-Chair of Clinical Affairs,
   Radiation Medicine
Chief Medical Officer, UC San Diego Health
University of California, San Diego
San Diego, California

Dineo Khabele, MD,
   FACOG, FACS
Mitchell and Elaine Yanow Professor
Chair, Department of Obstetrics and Gynecology
Washington University School of
   Medicine in St Louis
St Louis, Missouri

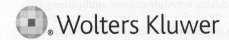

Philadelphia • Baltimore • New York • London
Buenos Aires • Hong Kong • Sydney • Tokyo

Acquisitions Editor: Joe Cho
Development Editor: Barton Dudlick
Editorial Coordinator: Venugopal Loganathan
Editorial Assistant: Kristen Kardoley
Marketing Manager: Phyllis Hittner
Production Project Manager: Justin Wright
Manager, Graphic Arts & Design: Stephen Druding
Manufacturing Coordinator: Lisa Bowling
Prepress Vendor: S4Carlisle Publishing Services

Eighth Edition

9 8 7 6 5 4 3 2 1

Printed in the United States of America

Library of Congress Cataloging-in-Publication Data

Names: Chi, Dennis S., editor. | Dizon, Don S., editor. | Yashar, Catheryn M., editor. | Khabele, Dineo, editor.
Title: Principles and practice of gynecologic oncology / [edited by] Dennis S. Chi, Don S. Dizon, Catheryn Yashar, Dineo Khabele.
Description: Eighth edition. | Philadelphia: Lippincott Williams & Wilkins, [2025] | Includes bibliographical references and index.
Identifiers: LCCN 2023028582 (print) | LCCN 2023028583 (ebook) | ISBN 9781975183271 (hardback) | ISBN 9781975183288 (ebook)
Subjects: MESH: Genital Neoplasms, Female | BISAC: MEDICAL / Oncology / General | MEDICAL / Gynecology & Obstetrics
Classification: LCC RC280.G5 (print) | LCC RC280.G5 (ebook) | NLM WP 145 | DDC 616.99/465—dc23/eng/20230929
LC record available at https://lccn.loc.gov/2023028582
LC ebook record available at https://lccn.loc.gov/2023028583

Dedication

This book is dedicated to our families: Hae-Young Chi and children Jessica, Stephanie, and Andrew Chi; Henry Stoll and children Isabelle, Harrison, and Sophia Dizon-Stoll; Arnold Yashar and children William, Jacob, and Drew Yashar. Their patience, good humor, encouragement, and love have inspired us throughout our careers. In this regard, they have each made significant contributions to this book.

We would also like to express our gratitude to our own esteemed professors who guided and mentored us, and to all of the colleagues we have worked alongside, learned from, and taught us over the years. The Gynecologic Oncology community that the readers of this book belong to is dedicated to the advancement of knowledge in the field and its application to outstanding patient care. The considerable progress we have achieved together in the understanding, diagnosis, treatment, and prevention of these cancers is presented in this book. On behalf of the Gynecologic Oncology community, we dedicate this edition of *Principles and Practice of Gynecologic Oncology* to the brave and courageous patients we all serve, and take inspiration in the oath we all share.

HIPPOCRATIC OATH

I swear to fulfill, to the best of my ability and judgment, this covenant:

❖ I will respect the hard-won scientific gains of those physicians in whose steps I walk, and gladly share such knowledge as is mine with those who are to follow.

❖ I will apply, for the benefit of the sick, all measures which are required, avoiding those twin traps of overtreatment and therapeutic nihilism.

❖ I will remember that there is art to medicine as well as science, and that warmth, sympathy, and understanding may outweigh the surgeon's knife or the chemist's drug.

❖ I will not be ashamed to say "I know not," nor will I fail to call in my colleagues when the skills of another are needed for a patient's recovery.

❖ I will respect the privacy of my patients, for their problems are not disclosed to me that the world may know. Most especially must I tread with care in matters of life and death. Above all, I must not play at God.

❖ I will remember that I do not treat a fever chart, a cancerous growth, but a sick human being, whose illness may affect the person's family and economic stability. My responsibility includes these related problems, if I am to care adequately for the sick.

❖ I will prevent disease whenever I can, for prevention is preferable to cure.

❖ I will remember that I remain a member of society, with special obligations to all my fellow human beings, those sound of mind and body as well as the infirm.

❖ If I do not violate this oath, may I enjoy life and art, respected while I live and remembered with affection thereafter. May I always act so as to preserve the finest traditions of my calling and may I long experience the joy of healing those who seek my help.

Preface

The publication in 2017 of the seventh edition of *Principles and Practice of Gynecologic Oncology* marked the 25th anniversary of the creation of this textbook. The founding editors, William J. Hoskins, Carlos A. Perez, and Robert C. Young, represented the disciplines of Gynecologic Oncology, Radiation Oncology, and Medical Oncology. They created the first multidisciplinary textbook in the field and, in their words, "strove to produce a definitive reference written at the expert level." The focus on multidisciplinary approaches to treatment and a detailed presentation of the literature on which clinical care is based continue to be a guiding principle.

The second set of editors, Richard R. Barakat, Maurie Markman, Marcus Randall, and for two editions Andrew Berchuck, also represented Gynecologic, Medical, and Radiation Oncology. Over the course of several editions, they incorporated new chapters that reflected dramatic progress in the understanding and treatment of women's cancers. Simultaneously, advances in technology facilitated the use of full color throughout the book as well as increasingly user-friendly online versions that allow access to cutting-edge information at the point of care.

As the editors of *Principles and Practice of Gynecologic Oncology*, we owe a debt of gratitude to our predecessors. We are proud to continue their tradition of bringing together multidisciplinary expertise that also includes Pathology, Radiology, and Basic/Translational Science colleagues. Given the pace of discovery and change within the field, we strove to ensure that this new edition reflects the many advances in the field. To this end, this edition includes updates on the numerous advances in molecular, immunologic, and targeted therapies. With an overwhelming amount of information on gynecologic cancers available on the internet combined with limited time to read, study, and digest all the new studies and approaches, we worked to reorganize the book to make it more reader-friendly and focused on disease sites. Rather than having the sections of the book devoted to general oncologic principles and then one section dedicated specifically to a dozen or so disease sites, in this eighth edition each disease site is its own section. The sections are divided into separate chapters specific to the disease site such as surgery for cervical cancer, treatment of persistent and recurrent endometrial cancer, and new therapeutics for ovarian cancer. We hope these changes will decrease redundancy, focus the key aspects of each disease site, and provide the reader with a more expeditious reference source.

We have given considerable thought to the issue of how best to maintain the relevance of the book between printed editions in an era of instant access to new information on the internet. Solutions include smartphone access to the content of the textbook with enhanced search capabilities, as well as more frequent online updates as new studies are reported. We also now include online access to a comprehensive library of surgical videos to ensure that surgical techniques are not only read but also visualized.

The planning and organization of this eighth edition began just before the lockdowns of the COVID pandemic. With fear and uncertainty about global, national, and personal health, our contributors persevered in taking care of patients, their families, and their communities. We are so thankful for their dedication and thoroughness. They volunteered their downtime to help us revamp this eighth edition and now, with the COVID pandemic hopefully behind us, we can all focus on our shared passion to cure and eradicate gynecologic cancers worldwide.

Dennis S. Chi, MD, FACOG, FACS
Don S. Dizon, MD, FACP, FASCO
Catheryn Yashar, MD, FACRO, FACR,
*   FABS, FASTRO*
Dineo Khabele, MD, FACOG, FACS

Acknowledgments

The editors acknowledge the contributions of numerous individuals without whom this book would not have been possible. The talented staff of Wolters Kluwer, specifically production manager Justin Wright, editorial coordinator Venugopal Loganathan, and development editor Barton Dudlick, provided invaluable encouragement, direction, and guidance during the creative process and in technical execution. Bharathi Sanjeev provided outstanding production services. From the Academic Office of the Gynecology Service, Department of Surgery, Memorial Sloan Kettering Cancer Center, we acknowledge the invaluable contributions of editors George Monemvasitis and Jenifer Levin. Their attention to detail, patience, and communication skills were of the utmost importance throughout the publication process. Our appreciation for all their efforts cannot be adequately expressed, but we hope they know how much we value their contributions.

Section Editors

Sushil Beriwal, MD, MBA, FASTRO, FABS
Academic Chief and Professor
Allegheny Health Network
Pittsburgh, Pennsylvania

Ross S. Berkowitz, MD
William H. Baker Professor of Gynecology
Harvard Medical School
Director of Gynecologic Oncology
Brigham and Women's Hospital
Dana-Farber Cancer Institute
Director of New England Trophoblastic Disease Center
Boston, Massachusetts

Jubilee Brown, MD
Professor, Wake Forest University
Division Director of Gynecologic Oncology
Atrium Health Levine Cancer Institute
Charlotte, North Carolina

Andrew R. Bruggeman, MD
Assistant Professor
Radiation Medicine and Applied Sciences
UC San Diego Health
La Jolla, California

Marcela G. del Carmen, MD, MPH
Professor of Obstetrics, Gynecology and Reproductive Biology
Division of Gynecologic Oncology
Department of Obstetrics and Gynecology
Massachusetts General Hospital
Harvard Medical School
Boston, Massachusetts

Sean C. Dowdy, MD, FACS, FACOG
Professor and Vice-Chair
Department of Obstetrics and Gynecology
Mayo Clinic College of Medicine
Rochester, Minnesota

Ramez N. Eskander, MD
Professor of Gynecologic Oncology
Division of Gynecologic Oncology
Department of Obstetrics, Gynecology and Reproductive Sciences
Moores Cancer Center
University of California, San Diego
La Jolla, California

Amanda Nickles Fader, MD
Professor of Gynecology and Obstetrics
Professor of Oncology
Vice-Chair, Gynecologic Surgical Operations
Baltimore, Maryland

Katherine Fuh, MD, PhD
Associate Professor of Obstetrics and Gynecology
Washington University
St Louis, Missouri

Theresa A. Graves, MD, FACS
Clinical Director
Lifespan Cancer Institute Breast Center
Director, Center for Breast Care
Brown Surgical Associates
Associate Professor of Surgery
The Warren Alpert Medical School of Brown University
Providence, Rhode Island

Laura J. Havrilesky, MD, MHSc
Professor of Obstetrics and Gynecology
Gynecologic Oncology
Duke University
Durham, North Carolina

Mario M. Leitao Jr, MD
Attending Surgeon
Department of Surgery/Gynecologic Oncology
Memorial Sloan Kettering Cancer Center
New York, New York

Ernst Lengyel, MD, PhD
Professor and Chairman
Section of Gynecologic Oncology
Department of Obstetrics and Gynecology
University of Chicago
Chicago, Illinois

Contributors

Sunil J. Advani, MD
Professor
Radiation Medicine and Applied Sciences
Co-Leader
Cancer Biology and Signaling Program. Moores Cancer Center
University of California, San Diego
La Jolla, California

Ebtesam Ahmed, PharmD
Clinical Professor
Clinical Health Professions
St. John's University College of Pharmacy
Queens, New York

Shannon Dawn Armbruster, MD, MPH
Assistant Professor
Division of Gynecologic Oncology
Virginia Tech Carilion School of Medicine
Roanoke, Virginia

Emeline M. Aviki, MD, MBA
Assistant Attending, Gynecologic Surgery
Department of Surgery
Memorial Sloan Kettering Cancer Center
New York, New York

Rani Bansal, MD, BA
Oncology Fellow
Division of Hematology/Oncology
Brown University
Providence, Rhode Island

Meena Bedi, MD
Radiation Oncologist
Department of Radiation Oncology
Medical College of Wisconsin
Milwaukee, Wisconsin

Andrew Berchuck, MD
Director, Division of Gynecologic Oncology
Obstetrics and Gynecology
Duke University
Durham, North Carolina

Sushil Beriwal, MD, MBA, FASTRO, FABS
Academic Chief and Professor
Allegheny Health Network
Pittsburgh, Pennsylvania

Priya Bhosale, MD
Professor
Department of Diagnostic Radiology
Division of Diagnostic Imaging
The University of Texas MD Anderson Cancer Center
Houston, Texas

Agnes Julia Bilecz, MD, PhD
Pathologist
Department of Pathology
University of Chicago
Chicago, Illinois
2nd Department of Pathology
Semmelweis University
Budapest, Hungary

Deborah Billmire, MD
Professor of Surgery
Department of Surgery, Division of Pediatric Surgery
Indiana University School of Medicine
Indianapolis, Indiana

Teresa K. L. Boitano, MD
Assistant Professor, Division of Gynecologic Oncology
Department of Obstetrics and Gynecology
University of Alabama,
Birmingham, Alabama

Antonio Braga, MD, PhD
Director of Rio de Janeiro Trophoblastic Disease Center
Department of Obstetrics and Gynecology
Associated Professor, Rio de Janeiro Federal University and Fluminense
    Federal University
Maternity School of Rio de Janeiro Federal University and Antonio Pedro
    University Hospital of Fluminense Federal University
Full Professor, Vassouras University
Rio de Janeiro, RJ, Brazil

Amy Bregar, MD
Instructor of Obstetrics and Gynecology
Division of Gynecologic Oncology
Department of Obstetrics and Gynecology
Massachusetts General Hospital
Harvard Medical School
Boston, Massachusetts

James J. Burke, II, MD, FACOG, FACS
The Donald G. Gallup Scholar of Gynecologic Oncology
Professor and Director, Gynecologic Oncology
Mercer University School of Medicine, Savannah Campus
Savannah, Georgia

Robert Tucker Burks, MD
Professor
Department of Pathology and Laboratory Medicine
Indiana University School of Medicine
Indianapolis, Indiana

Susana M. Campos, MD, MPH
Medical Oncologist
Director of Clinical Pathways, Division of Gynecologic Oncology
Director of Educational Initiatives, Division of Gynecologic Oncology
Institute Physician
Assistant Professor of Medicine
Harvard Medical School
Brigham and Women's Hospital
Dana Farber Cancer Institute
Boston, Massachusetts

Fernanda Freitas Oliveira Cardoso, MD, PhD
Rio de Janeiro Trophoblastic Disease Center
Department of Obstetrics and Gynecology
Affiliated Professor, Rio de Janeiro Federal University
Maternity School of Rio de Janeiro Federal University
Rio de Janeiro, RJ, Brazil

Marcela G. del Carmen, MD, MPH
Professor of Obstetrics, Gynecology and Reproductive Biology
Division of Gynecologic Oncology
Department of Obstetrics and Gynecology
Massachusetts General Hospital
Harvard Medical School
Boston, Massachusetts

Christine Chin, MD
Assistant Professor of Radiation Oncology
Columbia Irving Medical Center
Vagelos College of Physicians and Surgeons
New York, New York

Rani Chudasama, MD, BA
Oncology Fellow
Division of Hematology/Oncology
Brown University
Providence, Rhode Island

David E. Cohn, MD, MBA, FACHE
Chief Executive Officer (Interim), Chief Medical Officer,
  and Professor
Division of Gynecologic Oncology
The James Cancer Hospital
Columbus, Ohio

Bradley R. Corr, MD
Assistant Professor
Division of Gynecologic Oncology
Department Obstetrics and Gynecology
University of Colorado
Aurora, Colorado

Allan Covens, MD, FRCSC
Chair, Gynecologic Oncology
Department of Obstetrics and Gynaecology
University of Toronto
Toronto, Ontario, Canada

Don S. Dizon, MD, FACP
Professor of Medicine and Professor of Surgery
Brown University
Director, The Pelvic Malignancies Program
Lifespan Cancer Institute
Director of Medical Oncology
Rhode Island Hospital
Associate Director, Community Outreach and Engagement
Legorreta Cancer Center at Brown University
Providence, Rhode Island

Christine Duffy, MD, MPH
Director of Adult Cancer Survivorship Program
Lifespan Cancer Institute
Providence, Rhode Island

Kevin M. Elias, MD, FACOG
Assistant Professor
Division of Gynecologic Oncology
Department of Obstetrics and Gynecology
New England Trophoblastic Disease Center
Brigham and Women's Hospital
Dana-Farber Cancer Institute
Harvard Medical School
Boston, Massachusetts

Lora Hedrick Ellenson, MD
Attending Physician
Department of Pathology and Laboratory Medicine
Memorial Sloan Kettering Cancer Center
New York, New York

Beth A. Erickson, MD
Professor
Department of Radiation Oncology
Medical College of Wisconsin
Milwaukee, Wisconsin

Elizabeth Euscher, MD
Professor
Department of Pathology
The University of Texas MD Anderson Cancer Center
Houston, Texas

Mary Anne Fenton, MD
Clinical Associate Professor
Lifespan Cancer Institute
The Warren Alpert Medical School of Brown University
Providence, Rhode Island

Gini F. Fleming, MD
Professor of Medicine
Section of Hematology/Oncology
University of Chicago Medicine
Chicago, Illinois

Lindsay Frazier
Professor of Pediatrics, Harvard Medical School
Institute Physician, Pediatric Hematology/Oncology
Dana-Farber Cancer Institute/Boston Children's Hospital
Boston, Massachusetts

Katherine Fuh, MD, PhD
Associate Professor
Department of Obstetrics and Gynecology
Washington University School of Medicine in St Louis
St Louis, Missouri

David M. Gershenson, MD
Professor
Department of Gynecologic Oncology and Reproductive Medicine
The University of Texas MD Anderson Cancer Center
Houston, Texas

Allison Gockley, MD
Assistant Professor
Harvard Medical School
Gynecologic Oncologist
Massachusetts General Hospital
Boston, Massachusetts

Charlie Gourley, BSc, MB ChB, PhD, FRCP
Professor and Honorary Consultant in Medical Oncology
CRUK Scotland Centre
University of Edinburgh
Edinburgh, Scotland, United Kingdom

Stephanie L. Graff, MD
Director of Breast Oncology
Assistant Professor of Medicine
Division of Medical Oncology and Hematology
Lifespan Cancer Institute
The Warren Alpert Medical School of Brown University
Providence, Rhode Island

Theresa A. Graves, MD, FACS
Clinical Director
Lifespan Cancer Institute Breast Center
Director, Center for Breast Care
Brown Surgical Associates
Associate Professor of Surgery
The Warren Alpert Medical School of Brown University
Providence, Rhode Island

Andrea R. Hagemann, MD, MSCI
Associate Professor of Obstetrics and Gynecology
Division of Gynecologic Oncology
Department of Obstetrics and Gynecology
Washington University in St Louis School of Medicine
St Louis, Missouri

Matthew M. Harkenrider, MD
Associate Professor
Department of Radiation Oncology
Stritch School of Medicine, Loyola University Medical Center
Maywood, Illinois

Laura J. Havrilesky, MD, MHSc
Professor of Obstetrics and Gynecology
Gynecologic Oncology
Duke University
Durham, North Carolina

Jaroslaw T. Hepel, MD, FACRO
Associate Professor
Department of Radiation Oncology
Lifespan Cancer Institute
The Warren Alpert Medical School of Brown University
Providence, Rhode Island

R. Tyler Hillman, MD, PhD
Assistant Professor and CPRIT Scholar in Cancer Research
Department of Gynecologic Oncology and Reproductive Medicine
Department of Genomic Medicine
The University of Texas MD Anderson Cancer Center
Houston, Texas

Neil S. Horowitz, MD
Associate Professor of Obstetrics, Gynecology, and
    Reproductive Biology
Harvard Medical School
Co-Director, New England Trophoblastic Disease Center
Brigham and Women's Hospital
Dana-Farber Cancer Institute
Boston, Massachusetts

Elizabeth L. Jewell, MD, MHSc, FACOG, FACS
Associate Professor of Surgery
Department of Surgery
Weill Cornell Medical Center
Vice-Chair, Regional Network and Affiliates
Director of Surgery, MSK Monmouth and Basking Ridge
Director of MSK Monmouth ORs
Interim Associate Deputy Physician-in-Chief, Strategic Partnerships
Medical Director, Department of Surgery
Memorial Sloan Kettering Cancer Center
New York, New York

Jenna Kahn, MD
Assistant Professor
Department of Radiation Medicine
Oregon Health and Science University
Portland, Oregon

Josephine Kang, MD, PhD
Assistant Professor
Department of Radiation Oncology
New York Presbyterian
Weill Cornell Medical Center
New York, New York

Emily M. Ko, MD, MSCR
Assistant Professor
Division of Gynecologic Oncology
Department of Obstetrics and Gynecology
University of Pennsylvania
Philadelphia, Pennsylvania

Shalini L. Kulasingam, PhD
Professor
Division of Epidemiology and Community Health
University of Minnesota School of Public Health
Minneapolis, Minnesota

Charles A. Kunos, MD, PhD
Professor
Radiation Medicine
University of Kentucky
Lexington, Kentucky

Katherine C. Kurnit, MD, MPH
Assistant Professor
Section of Gynecologic Oncology
Department of Obstetrics and Gynecology
University of Chicago
Chicago, Illinois

Charles N. Landen Jr, MD, MS
Associate Professor
Department of Obstetrics and Gynecology
University of Virginia
Charlottesville, Virginia

Carrie Langstraat, MD
Associate Professor
Department of Obstetrics and Gynecology
Mayo Clinic
Rochester, Minnesota

Ricardo R. Lastra, MD
Associate Professor of Pathology
Department of Pathology
University of Chicago Medical Center
Chicago, Illinois

Barrett Lawson, MD
Assistant Professor
Department of Pathology
The University of Texas MD Anderson Cancer Center
Houston, Texas

Charles A. Leath III, MD, MSPH
Direction, Division of Gynecologic Oncology
Ellen Gregg Shook Culverhouse Endowed Chair
Department of Obstetrics and Gynecology
University of Alabama at Birmingham
Birmingham, Alabama

Mario M. Leitao Jr, MD
Attending Surgeon
Department of Surgery/Gynecologic Oncology
Memorial Sloan Kettering Cancer Center
New York, New York

Ernst Lengyel, MD, PhD
Professor and Chairman
Section of Gynecologic Oncology
Department of Obstetrics and Gynecology
University of Chicago
Chicago, Illinois

Margaret I. Liang, MD, MS
Assistant Professor
Division of Gynecologic Oncology
Department of Obstetrics and Gynecology
Cedars-Sinai Medical Center
Los Angeles, California

Diane C. Ling, MD
Assistant Professor of Radiation Oncology
Department of Radiation Oncology
University of Southern California
Los Angeles, California

Sanjana Luther, MD
Fellow
Department of Gastroenterology
Mount Sinai
New York, New York

Izildinha Maestá, MD, PhD
Director of Botucatu Trophoblastic Disease Center
Department of Obstetrics and Gynecology
Associated Professor, São Paulo State University
Botucatu, SP, Brazil

Martha B. Mainiero, MD
Director of Breast Imaging
Professor of Diagnostic Imaging
Rhode Island Hospital
The Warren Alpert Medical School of Brown University
Providence, Rhode Island

Giorgia Mangili, MD
Senior Physician
Gynaecology, Obstetric Unit
IRCCS San Raffaele Scientific Institute
Milan, Italy

Emily J. Martin, MD, MS
Assistant Clinical Professor
Department of Medicine
David Geffen School of Medicine at UCLA
Los Angeles, California

Koji Matsuo, MD, PhD, FACOG
Associate Professor, Chief in Oncology Research
Division of Gynecologic Oncology
University of Southern California
Los Angeles, California

Jyoti Mayadev, MD
Professor of Radiation Medicine and Applied Sciences
University of California, San Diego
La Jolla, California

Katherine M. McBride, MD, FACS
Assistant Professor General Surgery
Associate Program Director Surgical Critical Care Fellowship
Mercer University School of Medicine, Savannah Campus
Savannah, Georgia

Diana Miao, MD
Department of Gynecology and Obstetrics
Johns Hopkins Hospital
Baltimore, Maryland

Jeffrey C. Miecznikowski, PhD
Associate Professor
Department of Biostatistics
SUNY University at Buffalo
Buffalo, New York

Austin Miller, PhD
Clinical Trials Development Division
Director of Biostatistics
Biostatistics and Bioinformatics
Roswell Park Comprehensive Cancer Center
Buffalo, New York

Chelsea Miller, MD
Radiation Oncologist
Department of Radiation Oncology
Lifespan Cancer Institute
The Warren Alpert Medical School of Brown University
Providence, Rhode Island

Kathryn M. Miller, MD
Fellow
Department of Surgery
Memorial Sloan Kettering Cancer Center
New York, New York

Kathryn A. Mills, MD
Assistant Professor
Department of Obstetrics and Gynecology
University of Chicago
Chicago, Illinois

Amir Momeni-Boroujeni, MD
Gynecologic and Molecular Pathologist
Department of Pathology and Laboratory Medicine
Memorial Sloan Kettering Cancer Center
New York, New York

Firas Mourtada, PhD, MSE, DABR, FAAPM, FABS, FASTRO
Professor & Enterprise Medical Physics Director
Department of Radiation Oncology, Sidney Kimmel Cancer Center
Thomas Jefferson University Hospital
Philadelphia, Pennsylvania

Dimitrios Nasioudis, MD
Fellow
Division of Gynecologic Oncology
Department of Obstetrics and Gynecology
University of Pennsylvania
Philadelphia, Pennsylvania

Natsai C. Nyakudarika, MD
Clinical Assistant Professor
Division of Gynecologic Oncology
Department of Obstetrics and Gynecology
Los Angeles (UCLA) Medical Center
Harbor-University of California
Torrance, California

Roisin E. O'Cearbhaill, MD
Associate Professor Medicine
Memorial Sloan Kettering Cancer Center
Weill Cornell College of Medicine
New York, New York

M. H. M. Oonk, MD
Gynecologic Oncologist
Department of Obstetrics and Gynecology
University Medical Center Groningen
Groningen, The Netherlands

Gabriela Paiva, MD
Rio de Janeiro Trophoblastic Disease Center
Department of Obstetrics and Gynecology
Affiliated Professor, Rio de Janeiro Federal University
Maternity School of Rio de Janeiro Federal University
Rio de Janeiro, RJ, Brazil

Russell K. Portenoy, MD
Executive Director
MJHS Institute for Innovation in Palliative Care
New York, New York
Professor of Neurology and Family and Social Medicine
Albert Einstein College of Medicine
Bronx, New York

Allison M. Puechl, MD
Assistant Professor of Gynecologic Oncology
Atrium Health Levine Cancer Institute
Charlotte, North Carolina

Isabelle Ray-Coquard, PhD
PU-PH
Léon Bérard Center
Lyon, France

Laura Salama, MD
Hematology Oncology Fellow
Department of Hematology and Oncology
Lifespan Cancer Institute
The Warren Alpert Medical School of Brown University
Providence, Rhode Island

Angeles Alvarez Secord, MD, MHSc
Professor
Division of Gynecologic Oncology
Department of Obstetrics and Gynecology
Duke Health
Durham, North Carolina

Tiffany Y. Sia, MD
Gynecologic Oncology Fellow
Department of Surgery
Memorial Sloan Kettering Cancer Center
New York, New York

Michael W. Sill, PhD
Senior Biostatistician
Clinical Trials Development Division
Roswell Park Comprehensive Cancer Center
Buffalo, New York

Priya K. Simoes, MD, CNSC
Assistant Professor
Division of Gastroenterology
Department of Medicine
Mount Sinai West and Mount Sinai Morningside
New York, New York

Olesya Solheim, MD, PhD
Consultant in Gynaecology and Obstetrics
Department of Gynaecological Oncology
The Norwegian Radium Hospital
Oslo University Hospital
Oslo, Norway

Anil K. Sood, MD
Professor
Department of Gynecologic Oncology and Reproductive Medicine
The University of Texas MD Anderson Cancer Center
Houston, Texas

Sara Stoneham, MBBCh, FCPaeds SA, MRCPCH
Paediatric and TYA Oncology Consultant
Children's and Young People Cancer Services,
University College London Hospital,
London, United Kingdom

Sue Yazaki Sun, MD, PhD
Director of São Paulo Hospital Trophoblastic Disease Center
Department of Obstetrics
Associated Professor, Universidade Federal de São Paulo
São Paulo, SP, Brazil

Brenna E. Swift, MD, MASc
Gynecologic Oncology Fellow
University of Toronto
Toronto, Ontario, Canada

Charu Taneja, MD
Clinical Assistant Professor of Surgery
Department of Surgery
Rhode Island Hospital
The Warren Alpert Medical School of Brown University
Providence, Rhode Island

Julia Tassinari, BS, MD
Clinical Instructor of Surgery
Department of Surgery
The Warren Alpert Medical School of Brown University
Providence, Rhode Island

Ashley Valenzula, DO, MBA
Assistant Professor
Department of Gynecologic Oncology
Mercer University School of Medicine
Memorial Health University Medical Center
Savannah, Georgia

Willemijn L. van der Kolk, BSc
PhD Candidate
Department of Obstetrics and Gynaecology
Cancer Research Center Groningen
University Medical Center Groningen
Groningen, The Netherlands

Akila N. Viswanathan, MD, MPH
Professor and Director
Radiation Oncology and Molecular Radiation Sciences
Johns Hopkins University School of Medicine
Baltimore, Maryland

Michelle E. Wakeley, MD
Resident Physician
Department of Surgery
The Warren Alpert Medical School of Brown University
Providence, Rhode Island

Dan Wang, MD
Fellow
Department of Obstetrics and Gynecology
Peking Union Medical College Hospital
Chinese Academy of Medical Science and Peking Union Medical College
National Clinical Research Center for Obstetric and Gynecologic Diseases
Beijing, People's Republic of China

Yihong Wang, MD, PhD
Associate Professor
Department of Pathology and Laboratory Medicine
The Warren Alpert Medical School of Brown University
Pathologist
Department of Pathology
Rhode Island Hospital
Providence, Rhode Island

Robert C. Ward, MD
Assistant Professor of Diagnostic Imaging
Department of Diagnostic Imaging
The Warren Alpert Medical School of Brown University
Providence, Rhode Island

Catherine Watson, MD
Assistant Professor
Department of Obstetrics and Gynecology
Vanderbilt University Medical Center
Nashville, Tennessee

Doreen L. Wiggins, MD, MHL
Breast Surgery
Associate Professor of Surgery Clinician Education
The Warren Alpert Medical School of Brown University
Providence, Rhode Island

Casey W. Williamson, MD, MAS
Assistant Professor
Radiation Medicine
Oregon Health and Science University
Portland, Oregon

Evgeny Yakirevich, MD, DSc
Professor
Department of Pathology and Laboratory Medicine
The Warren Alpert Medical School of Brown University
Pathologist
Department of Pathology
Rhode Island Hospital
Providence, Rhode Island

Robert H. Young, MD
Robert E. Scully Professor of Pathology
Massachusetts General Hospital
Harvard Medical School
Department of Pathology
Massachusetts General Hospital
Boston, Massachusetts

Dmitriy Zamarin, MD, PhD
Translational Research Director, Gynecologic Medical Oncology
Department of Medicine
Memorial Sloan Kettering Cancer Center
New York, New York

Oliver Zivanovic, MD
Assisting Attending
Gynecology Surgery
Memorial Sloan Kettering Cancer Center
New York, New York

Video List

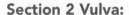

Section 2 Vulva:

Video 1 Sentinel inguinofemoral lymph node identification in vulvar cancer and the use of near-infrared imaging for sentinel lymph node detection

Section 3 Cervix:

Video 2 Radical abdominal trachelectomy
Video 3 Extraperitoneal lymph node dissection
Video 4 Robotic-assisted supralevator total pelvic exenteration
Video 5 Total pelvic infralevator exenteration using Ligasure
Video 6 Urinary reconstruction following cystectomy: the ileal conduit
Video 7 Urinary reconstruction after pelvic exenteration: modified Indiana pouch
Video 8 Modified rectus abdominis myocutaneous (RAM) flap for neovagina creation after exenteration

Section 4 Uterine Corpus:

Video 9 Sentinel lymph node mapping for uterine cancer: a practical illustration of injection and mapping techniques
Video 10 Sentinel lymph node (SNL) mapping using robotic-assisted fluorescence imaging

Section 5 Ovary:

Video 11 Robotic Xi infrarenal aortic node dissection with lower pelvic port placement
Video 12 Retroperitoneal lymph node dissection (RPLND) for primary ovarian cancer
Video 13 Surgical vascular anatomy on the upper abdomen
Video 14 Vascular and ligamentous attachments
Video 15 How to approach suspicious lymph nodes on the upper abdomen
Video 16 Resection of tumor from the supragastric lesser sac with peritonectomy
Video 17 Morison pouch peritonectomy in cytoreductive surgery
Video 18 Diaphragm peritonectomy with resection of Glisson capsule for advanced ovarian cancer
Video 19 Diaphragm peritonectomy with full-thickness resection for advanced ovarian cancer
Video 20 Liver mobilization with diaphragm peritonectomy and liver wedge resection
Video 21 Excision of tumor along ligamentum venosum
Video 22 Excision of tumor along ligamentum teres
Video 23 Mobilization of right liver with wedge resection segments 6 and 7

Video List

Contents

SECTION 11

BREAST CANCER 473

SECTION 12

SPECIAL TOPICS 551

OVERVIEW OF BASIC BIOLOGY

Overview of Basic Biology

Katherine Fuh, Angeles Alvarez Secord, Charles Gourley, and Andrew Berchuck

INTRODUCTION

The basic biology of gynecologic cancers shares similarities as well as differences with other solid tumors. This chapter aims to provide a background to these basic concepts in order to better understand the potential causes, persistence, or progression of gynecologic cancers. We will focus on key concepts on tumor initiation as well as metastasis, persistence, treatment resistance, and recurrence. In particular, once a tumor has initiated and begins to proliferate, tumor cells will metastasize and interact with tumor microenvironment cells (mesothelial cells, fibroblasts, adipocytes, and immune cells) and promote angiogenesis with endothelial cells (1). A common occurrence in gynecologic cancers is treatment resistance, and we will discuss the biology of how this may occur.

Tumor Initiation: Biology of Oncogenes and Tumor Suppressors

The initiating events in human cancers are diverse, but malignant transformation is invariably caused by the development of genetic and epigenetic alterations that disrupt normal cell growth, senescence, and death. Several classes of genetic alterations are involved in carcinogenesis, including changes in the sequence (mutations) of genes or their promoters, gains (amplifications) or losses (deletions) in the number of copies of genes, and rearrangement and translocation of genes from their normal chromosomal locations that sometimes create new proteins by fusing the reading frames of genes. These alterations result in activation of genes that promote oncogenic processes such as cell proliferation or migration (oncogenes) or inactivation of genes that inhibit proliferation or result in cell senescence or cell death (tumor suppressor genes). DNA repair genes also function as tumor suppressors because they inhibit accumulation of cancer-causing genetic alterations. Inherited mutations in DNA repair genes are among the most common causes of hereditary cancer syndromes (eg, *BRCA*-related breast and ovarian cancer syndrome and Lynch syndrome) **(Tables 1.1 and 1.2).**

Gene alterations that stimulate cellular growth can also cause malignant transformation. Oncogenes may become overactive when affected by gain-of-function point mutations. In some cancers, amplification of oncogenes occurs with resultant overexpression of the corresponding protein. Instead of two copies of one of these genes, there may be many additional copies. Most mutations in oncogenes that cause cancer alter a single amino acid at specific codons that produce overactive protein products (eg, *KRAS*, *BRAF*), and only one allele needs to be mutated. In contrast, inactivation of tumor suppressors (eg, *RB1*, *BRCA1*, *BRCA2*, *MLH1*) requires loss of both copies of the gene (two hits) (2). Mutations in tumor suppressors may occur throughout the gene or in the promoter, and are usually small insertions, deletions, or base substitutions that alter the reading frame and thereby result in nonfunctional truncated protein products. Loss of the second non-mutated allele generally occurs because of chromosomal deletion, leading to abrogation of tumor suppressor activity. Some tumor suppressors (eg, MLH1) are inactivated by methylation of their promoters, which prevents transcription of the gene into messenger RNA. Cancers may have several genetic alterations, but only a small fraction of these are "driver" mutations that are directly responsible for malignant transformation. The majority of mutations are "passenger" events that arise because of genetic instability and do not contribute to tumor growth. Loss of tumor suppressor gene function is a frequent event in the development of most cancers.

Mutation of the *TP53* tumor suppressor gene is the most frequent genetic event described thus far in human cancers and is a ubiquitous feature of some tumor types, such as high-grade serous ovarian cancers (3). The *TP53* gene encodes a 393-amino-acid protein that plays a central role in the regulation of both proliferation and apoptosis. In normal cells, p53 protein resides in the nucleus and exerts its tumor suppressor activity by binding to transcriptional regulatory elements of genes, such as the CDK inhibitor p21, that act to arrest cells in G1. The *MDM2* gene product degrades p53 protein when appropriate, whereas p14ARF downregulates *MDM2* when upregulation of p53 is needed to initiate cell cycle arrest (4).

Many cancers have missense mutations in one copy of the *TP53* gene that result in substitution of a single amino acid, most commonly in exons 5 through 8, which encode the DNA binding domains that are involved in regulating transcription. Although these mutant *TP53* genes encode full-length proteins, they are unable to bind to DNA and regulate transcription of other genes. Mutation of one copy of the *TP53* gene often is accompanied by deletion of the other copy, leaving the cancer cell with only mutant p53 protein. If the cancer cell retains one normal copy of the *TP53* gene, mutant p53 protein can complex with wild-type p53 protein and prevent it from oligomerizing and interacting with DNA. Because inactivation of both *TP53* alleles is not required for loss of p53 function, mutant p53 is said to act in a "dominant negative" fashion. Normal cells have low levels of p53 protein because it is rapidly degraded by E3 ubiquitin ligase MDM2. There are missense mutations that encode protein products that are resistant to degradation. This results in gain-of-function activities and overaccumulation of mutant p53 protein in the nucleus, as detected immunohistochemically. A smaller fraction of cancers have mutations in the *TP53* gene that encode truncated protein products leading to loss of function. In these cases, loss of the other allele occurs as the second event is seen with other tumor suppressor genes. Beyond simply inhibiting proliferation, wild-type (wt) p53 is thought to play a role in preventing cancer by stimulating apoptosis of cells that have undergone excessive genetic damage. In this regard, p53wt has been described as the "guardian of the genome" because it delays entry into S phase until the genome has been cleansed of mutations. If DNA repair is inadequate, p53wt may initiate apoptosis, thereby eliminating cells with genetic damage.

Human papillomavirus (HPV) E6 and E7 viral oncoproteins play a pivotal role in cervical cancer. There is a requirement for E6 and E7 persistence to produce HPV-mediated cancer. Both E6 and E7 contribute to uncontrolled proliferation through deregulation of growth suppressors. E6 targets p53, whereas retinoblastoma (Rb) is one of the major targets of E7. Together, these oncoproteins

■ TABLE 1.1. Molecular Alterations Involved in Cancer Pathogenesis

Genetic Changes

Mutations

- Mutations in oncogenes change a single amino acid and lead to gain of activity that stimulates proliferation. These mutations are dominant and not dependent on changes in the other copy of the gene.
- Mutations in tumor suppressor genes and DNA repair genes generally are small base insertions/deletions or single base changes that cause stop codons. These lead to truncated protein products that are nonfunctional. Loss of tumor suppressor activity is usually dependent on deletion of the other copy of the gene.
- Driver mutations play a critical role in the process of malignant transformation, whereas passenger mutations are simply bystander damage caused by genomic instability.

DNA copy number changes
Deletion of one or both copies of a tumor suppressor gene because of genomic instability leads to loss of a gene product.
Gain of additional copies of an oncogene leads to increased activity.
Aneuploidy with gain or loss of complete chromosomes is common in many cancers.

Gene rearrangements and translocations
When a gene is moved from its normal location to another chromosomal location, its expression may be increased because of proximity to a gene promoter or because of fusion of two genes.

Clonal evolution
The genomic landscape of most cancers continues to evolve over time and space and the alterations observed in most cancers are often not present in all of the malignant cells.

Other Biological Processes

Epigenetic alterations

- Hypermethylation of CpG islands in the promoter regions of tumor suppressor genes may lead to their inactivation.
- Loss of promoter methylation in genes that stimulate proliferation may provide an oncogenic stimulus.
- Changes in acetylation of histone proteins that coat DNA may play a role in carcinogenesis.

Aberrant gene splicing
Alternative splice forms of genes may produce messenger RNAs and proteins with altered activity.

Noncoding RNAs
Noncoding RNAs regulate gene expression and their aberrant expression likely plays a role in the development and behavior of some cancers.

stimulate proliferation, delay differentiation, inhibit apoptosis, and evade immune detection.

The Cancer Genome Atlas (TCGA) project performed a comprehensive genomic and transcriptomic characterization of most forms of human cancer. Ovarian and endometrial cancers were among the first to be studied by TCGA, with cervical cancer added later (3,5). The International Cancer Genome Consortium (ICGC) performed similar genomic analyses of human cancers. Both TCGA and ICGC have deposited their data online in the public domain to stimulate

further research (6). Next-generation DNA sequencing has allowed mutational analysis of complete cancer genomes across tumor types from which tumor mutational burden (TMB) can be defined. This is defined as the total number of somatic mutations per coding area of a tumor genome. TMB is a clinical biomarker associated with response to immune checkpoint inhibitor (ICI) therapy in some cancers (7). Other than POLE-mutated and microsatellite instability (MSI) endometrial cancers (8-10), most all other gynecologic cancers have TMB below the biomarker selection cutoff of less than 10 mut/Mb.

■ TABLE 1.2. Origins of Genetic Damage in Human Cancers

Type of Genetic Damage	Examples
Germline alterations	
High-penetrance genes	BRCA1, BRCA2 (breast, ovarian cancers) MLH1, MSH2 (Lynch syndrome)
Moderate-penetrance genes	RAD51C/D, BRIP1 (ovarian cancer)
Low-penetrance genes	SNPs associated with various cancers
Exogenous carcinogens	
Ultraviolet radiation	TP53 mutations in skin cancers
Tobacco	TP53 mutations in lung cancers
Viruses	HPV inactivation of RB and TP53 in cervical cancer
Endogenous DNA damage	
Cytosine methylation and deamination	TP53 mutations in many cancer types
DNA hydrolysis	Various genes
Spontaneous errors in DNA synthesis	Various genes
Free radical production because of oxidative stress	Various gene

HPV, human papillomavirus; SNP, single-nucleotide polymorphism.

Clinical Implications of Understanding the Molecular Pathogenesis of Cancer

An understanding of the molecular pathogenesis of cancer provides the opportunity to better define subgroups within a given type of cancer that may differ with respect to clinical behavior and survival (11). Monoclonal antibodies and small molecules targeting aberrantly expressed cellular proteins that are true drivers of malignancy have been successful in treating some cancers. The evolution of Food and Drug Administration (FDA)-approved targeted therapies is generally accompanied by the requirement for companion diagnostic tests that demonstrate the presence of the targeted alteration (eg, *HER-2/neu* amplification/overexpression by immunohistochemistry [IHC] guides the use of the monoclonal antibody trastuzumab, and mismatch repair [MMR] deficiency guides the use of anti-PD1 inhibitor, pembrolizumab) (12,13).

Peptide Growth Factors and Receptor Tyrosine Kinases

Peptide growth factors produced by tumor, immune, or microenvironmental cells and secreted into the circulation or the local environment, such as those of the vascular endothelial growth factor (VEGF), epidermal growth factor (EGF), platelet-derived growth factor (PDGF), and fibroblast growth factor (FGF) families, upon binding to their receptor stimulate a cascade of events that can lead to proliferation, invasion, immune activation, and microenvironmental remodeling. Growth factors are involved in normal cellular processes such as stromal-epithelial communication, tissue regeneration, and wound healing. The concept that autocrine growth stimulation might be a key strategy by which cancer cell proliferation becomes autonomous has received considerable attention. In this model, it is postulated that cancers secrete stimulatory growth factors that then interact with receptors on the same cell. Although peptide growth factors provide a growth stimulatory signal, there is little evidence to suggest that overproduction of growth factors is a precipitating event in the development of most cancers. Increased expression of peptide growth factors likely facilitates, rather than drives, malignant transformation.

Cell membrane receptors that bind peptide growth factors are composed of an extracellular ligand binding domain, a membrane spanning region, and a cytoplasmic activation domain; intracellular receptor activation is frequently mediated by phosphorylation events. Binding of a growth factor to the extracellular domain often results in dimerization and conformational shifts in the receptors and activation of the tyrosine kinase moiety. The kinase may autophosphorylate and/or phosphorylate next-step molecular targets leading to activation of secondary signals that stimulate proliferation. Growth of some cancers is driven by overexpression of receptor tyrosine kinases (RTKs). The epidermal growth factor receptor (EGFR) family of RTKs plays a significant role in the development of several types of cancers, such as non–small cell lung cancer (NSCLC), and includes *ErbB-1* (EGFR), *ErbB-2* (HER-2/*neu*), *ErbB-3*, and *ErbB-4*. These receptors are activated by binding of ligands, including EGF, transforming growth factor-α, amphiregulin, and the neuregulins.

RTKs located on the cell surface can be appealing therapeutic targets. A number of agents that target the EGFR family have been developed and translated into clinical practice. Trastuzumab is a monoclonal antibody that binds to HER-2/*neu*, blocking downstream signaling, and is widely used in the treatment of breast and uterine serous cancers that overexpress this receptor (12).

Deoxyribonucleic Acid Repair

Targeting DNA repair has become a critical aspect of therapeutic development. DNA damage occurs naturally with thousands of mutations on a daily basis, leading mammalian cells to have evolved complex DNA repair systems to maintain the integrity of the genome. A series of cell cycle checkpoints exist that allow cell replication to pause for successful DNA repair, or alternatively for cell death if repair cannot be accomplished. DNA damage checkpoints occur at the boundaries between G1/S and G2/M and during S phase and mitotic spindle assembly. There are several repair mechanisms that operate on specific types of DNA damage during these checkpoints, including MMR, nucleotide excision repair (NER), base excision repair (BER), homologous recombination repair (HRR), and nonhomologous end joining (NHEJ). Loss of DNA repair activity increases the likelihood of mutations accumulating and propagating in the genome with deleterious effect. Once a cancer develops, these pathways are utilized to promote repair and thus lead to cell survival.

Double-strand break repair: HRR and classical NHEJ (C-NHEJ) or intrinsically mutagenic: alternative end joining (alt-EJ) and single-strand annealing (SSA)

Double-stranded DNA (dsDNA) damage can be caused by exogenous factors such as ionizing radiation, ultraviolet rays, alkylating agents, chemotherapeutic drugs or by endogenous factors such as reactive oxygen species or errors in cellular DNA metabolism. This dsDNA damage leads to the need for double-strand break repair in which cells employ two main mechanisms to repair double-strand breaks: high-fidelity HRR or error-prone NHEJ. HRR is a process that provides high-fidelity, template-dependent repair of complex DNA damage such as DNA cross-links, double-strand breaks, single-strand DNA gaps, and DNA interstrand cross-links. Because HR pathway is mediated by BRCA1 and BRCA2, patients with epithelial ovarian cancer and germline or somatic BRCA1 or BRCA2 mutations demonstrate impaired ability to repair ds breaks through HRR. This in part explains the increased sensitivity to platinum agents given the impairment to repair through HRR (14,15). If double-stranded breaks are not repaired precisely, this can cause deletions, translocations, and fusions in the DNA, producing genomic rearrangements. In contrast, repair by NHEJ involves direct resealing of the two broken ends independent of sequence homology. NHEJ represents the simplest and fastest mechanism to deal with a double-strand break. In terms of additional repair pathways, there are two that are repaired by mutagenic repair pathways, namely, SSA or alt-EJ. Alt-EJ can join double-strand breaks on different chromosomes, thus generating mutagenic rearrangements. SSA mediates end joining between interspersed nucleotide repeats in the genome and involves reannealing of Replication Protein A (RPA)-covered ssDNA by the RAD52 protein (16).

Deoxyribonucleic Acid Mismatch Repair

About 3% of endometrial cancers arise because of inherited germline mutations in MMR genes, defined as Lynch syndrome. Most cases are due to alterations in *MSH2* and *MLH1*, but *MSH6*, *PMS1*, *PMS2*, and *MSH3* mutations also occur. More frequently, in up to 22% sporadic endometrioid cancers of the endometrium, the *MLH1* MMR gene is inactivated because of promoter methylation, leading to MSI. MMR gene mutations are also a feature in 5% of clear cell ovarian cancer and 18% of endometrioid ovarian cancer (17,18). MMR deficiency detected by IHC is reported in 25% of endometrial cancers, which is higher than the 15% in sporadic colorectal cancers (19,20). MMR proteins excise nucleotides that are incorrectly paired with a corresponding nucleotide on the opposite DNA strand. It involves recognition of a base pair mismatch, recruitment of a separate cadre of repair enzymes, excision of the incorrect sequence, and resynthesis by DNA polymerase using the parental strand as a template. The recognition of small loops generated by insertion or deletion of nucleotides, as well as single base mismatches is primarily accomplished by a complex called MUTSα, which is a heterodimer of MSH2 and MSH6. MLH1 and

PMS2 are recruited to the site to initiate the subsequent steps of repair, including excision, DNA synthesis, and ligation.

Loss of MMR leads to a "mutator phenotype" in which there is accumulation of genetic mutations throughout the genome, particularly in repetitive DNA microsatellite sequences. Examples of microsatellite sequences include mono (AAAA), di (CACACACA), and tri (CAGCAGCAGCAG) nucleotide repeats. Replication errors in these repetitive sequences are common and their inefficient repair leads to the propensity to accumulate mutations; this is referred to as MSI. Some microsatellite sequences are in noncoding areas of the genome, whereas others are within genes. It is thought that accumulation of mutations in microsatellite sequences of tumor suppressor genes may inactivate them and accelerate the process of malignant transformation. Another consequence of MSI causing many mutations is that some of these encode protein products with new antigenic epitopes. This may result in a more immunogenic profile, making the cancer susceptible to treatment with ICI drugs such as anti-PD1/PDL1 inhibitors (13,21,22).

Epigenetic Regulation of Gynecologic Cancers

DNA methylation is one of the most extensively studied mechanisms of epigenetic modifications. DNA methylation is regulated by specific enzymes and these methylation patterns affect gene transcription. The DNA methylation process is catalyzed by enzymes of the DNA methyltransferase (DNMT, referred to as the writers) family because these enzymes transfer methyl groups from S-adenosyl-L-methionine (SAM) to cytosine residues to form 5-mC. The majority of DNA methylation occurs in CpG islands. Approximately 70% of CpG islands in the human genome are present in gene promoters where methylation of these sites most often leads to transcription repression. DNA methylation has been a widely studied epigenetic alteration in endometrial cancer and ovarian cancer (23-29). There are ongoing studies on how to modulate DNA damage repair and enhance therapeutics through epigenetic regulation.

Metastasis

The first region for metastasis of most gynecologic tumors is local, intraperitoneally and in the pelvis. Hematogenous metastases may be concurrent or occur much later (1,30-32). Hematogenous spread is the common mechanism for parenchymal spread, such as to the lung, liver, bone, and brain (31). In 1889, Sir James Paget stated that the microenvironment of each organ, *the soil*, influences the survival and growth of tumor cells, *the seed*. For example, the omentum is a common site for ovarian and endometrial tumor cells to metastasize. The rich background of pluripotent adipocytes, fibroblasts, mesothelial cells, and immune cells creates a dynamic and active permissive environment (1,33-39). The mesothelial cell, the single-cell layer of the peritoneum and outer serosal layer of organs, is a pluripotent mesenchymal cell that responds to changes in its surroundings (37,40). There have been a number of studies that have provided evidence for active crosstalk between ovarian cancer cells and several types of stromal cells in the omental metastatic tumor microenvironment (41-43).

Energy Metabolism

Cancer cells require increased glucose to satisfy their metabolic demands. This is the basis of fluorodeoxyglucose (FDG)-positron emission tomography (PET) imaging. Normal tissues generate energy using mitochondrial oxidative phosphorylation and only switch to breaking down glucose to derive energy in the absence of oxygen, which leads to the accumulation of lactate. In contrast, glycolysis of glucose to lactate occurs in cancers even in the presence of oxygen, a phenomenon called "aerobic glycolysis" or the Warburg effect, in honor of its discoverer (44,45). Because cancers often outgrow their blood supply and become hypoxic, the ability to survive using aerobic glycolysis instead of oxidative phosphorylation may be selected for during malignant transformation. Lactate production by cancers may also promote invasion and metastasis by acidifying the microenvironment (46). Omental adipocytes have been identified to act as an energy source for cancer cells and have been found to increase the metastatic potential in ovarian cancer (35,47).

Angiogenesis

Angiogenesis, a key process to maintain the supply of nutrients and oxygen in tissues, is the generation of new blood vessels from preexisting ones. It is regulated by multiple systems including growth factors of which VEGF is the most widely studied. Tumor, stromal, and immune cells secrete VEGF mainly in response to hypoxia and low nutrient content, and activation of selected oncogenes (48,49). Secreted VEGF promotes angiogenesis through its receptors expressed predominantly on endothelial cells. Tumor angiogenesis takes place by dysregulated proliferation and organization of endothelial cells leading to disorganized and leaky vessels within tumors, differing from the normal vasculature (50,51). Along with endothelial cells, fibroblasts build and remodel new extracellular matrix that increases stiffness and induces further angiogenesis (52-54).

SUMMARY

Gynecologic cancers have distinct features particular to each tumor type. However, the underlying biology of the process of metastasis and treatment resistance shares similarities. By understanding these processes, future treatment can be more rationally developed.

REFERENCES

1. Lengyel E. Ovarian cancer development and metastasis. *Am J Pathol*. 2010;177:1053-1064.

2. Sowter HM, Ashworth A. BRCA1 and BRCA2 as ovarian cancer susceptibility genes. *Carcinogenesis*. 2005;26:1651-1656.

3. Cancer Genome Atlas Research Network. Integrated genomic analyses of ovarian carcinoma. *Nature*. 2011;474:609-615.

4. Kung CP, Weber JD. It's getting complicated—a fresh look at p53-MDM2-ARF triangle in tumorigenesis and cancer therapy. *Front Cell Dev Biol*. 2022;10:818744.

5. Cancer Genome Atlas Research Network; Kandoth C, Schultz N, et al. Integrated genomic characterization of endometrial carcinoma. *Nature*. 2013;497:67-73.

6. ICGC/TCGA Pan-Cancer Analysis of Whole Genomes Consortium. Pan-cancer analysis of whole genomes. *Nature*. 2020;578:82-93.

7. McGrail DJ, Pilie PG, Rashid NU, et al. High tumor mutation burden fails to predict immune checkpoint blockade response across all cancer types. *Ann Oncol*. 2021;32:661-672.

8. Leon-Castillo A, Britton H, McConechy MK, et al. Interpretation of somatic POLE mutations in endometrial carcinoma. *J Pathol*. 2020;250:323-335.

9. Leon-Castillo A, Gilvazquez E, Nout R, et al. Clinicopathological and molecular characterisation of 'multiple-classifier' endometrial carcinomas. *J Pathol*. 2020;250:312-322.

10. McAlpine J, Leon-Castillo A, Bosse T. The rise of a novel classification system for endometrial carcinoma; integration of molecular subclasses. *J Pathol*. 2018;244:538-549.

11. Bowtell DD, Bohm S, Ahmed AA, et al. Rethinking ovarian cancer II: reducing mortality from high-grade serous ovarian cancer. *Nat Rev Cancer*. 2015;15:668-679.

12. Fader AN, Roque DM, Siegel E, et al. Randomized phase II trial of carboplatin-paclitaxel versus carboplatin-paclitaxel-trastuzumab in uterine serous carcinomas that overexpress human epidermal growth factor receptor 2/neu. *J Clin Oncol*. 2018;36:2044-2051.

13. Le DT, Durham JN, Smith KN, et al. Mismatch repair deficiency predicts response of solid tumors to PD-1 blockade. *Science*. 2017;357:409-413.

14. Kristeleit RS, Miller RE, Kohn EC. Gynecologic cancers: emerging novel strategies for targeting DNA repair deficiency. *Am Soc Clin Oncol Educ Book*. 2016;35:e259-e268.

15. Ledermann JA, Drew Y, Kristeleit RS. Homologous recombination deficiency and ovarian cancer. *Eur J Cancer*. 2016;60:49-58.

16. Ceccaldi R, Rondinelli B, D'Andrea AD. Repair pathway choices and consequences at the double-strand break. *Trends Cell Biol.* 2016;26:52-64.

17. Heong V, Tan TZ, Miwa M, et al. A multi-ethnic analysis of immune-related gene expression signatures in patients with ovarian clear cell carcinoma. *J Pathol.* 2021;255:285-295.

18. Hollis RL, Thomson JP, Stanley B, et al. Molecular stratification of endometrioid ovarian carcinoma predicts clinical outcome. *Nat Commun.* 2020;11:4995.

19. Backes FJ, Leon ME, Ivanov I, et al. Prospective evaluation of DNA mismatch repair protein expression in primary endometrial cancer. *Gynecol Oncol.* 2009;114:486-490.

20. McMeekin DS, Tritchler DL, Cohn DE, et al. Clinicopathologic significance of mismatch repair defects in endometrial cancer: an NRG Oncology/Gynecologic Oncology Group study. *J Clin Oncol.* 2016;34:3062-3068.

21. Le DT, Uram JN, Wang H, et al. PD-1 blockade in tumors with mismatch-repair deficiency. *N Engl J Med.* 2015;372:2509-2520.

22. O'Malley DM, Bariani GM, Cassier PA, et al. Pembrolizumab in patients with microsatellite instability-high advanced endometrial cancer: results from the KEYNOTE-158 study. *J Clin Oncol.* 2022;40:752-761.

23. Khabele D, Son DS, Parl AK, et al. Drug-induced inactivation or gene silencing of class I histone deacetylases suppresses ovarian cancer cell growth: implications for therapy. *Cancer Biol Ther.* 2007;6:795-801.

24. Caplakova V, Babusikova E, Blahovcova E, Balharek T, Zelieskova M, Hatok J. DNA methylation machinery in the endometrium and endometrial cancer. *Anticancer Res.* 2016;36:4407-4420.

25. Smith HJ, Straughn JM, Buchsbaum DJ, Arend RC. Epigenetic therapy for the treatment of epithelial ovarian cancer: a clinical review. *Gynecol Oncol Rep.* 2017;20:81-86.

26. Turner TB, Meza-Perez S, Londono A, et al. Epigenetic modifiers upregulate MHC II and impede ovarian cancer tumor growth. *Oncotarget.* 2017;8:44159-44170.

27. Gupta VG, Hirst J, Petersen S, et al. Entinostat, a selective HDAC1/2 inhibitor, potentiates the effects of olaparib in homologous recombination proficient ovarian cancer. *Gynecol Oncol.* 2021;162:163-172.

28. Matei D, Nephew KP. Epigenetic attire in ovarian cancer: the emperor's new clothes. *Cancer Res.* 2020;80:3775-3785.

29. Oza AM, Matulonis UA, Alvarez Secord A, et al. A randomized phase II trial of epigenetic priming with guadecitabine and carboplatin in platinum-resistant, recurrent ovarian cancer. *Clin Cancer Res.* 2020;26:1009-1016.

30. Pradeep S, Kim SW, Wu SY, et al. Hematogenous metastasis of ovarian cancer: rethinking mode of spread. *Cancer Cell.* 2014;26:77-91.

31. Mariani A, Webb MJ, Keeney GL, Calori G, Podratz KC. Hematogenous dissemination in corpus cancer. *Gynecol Oncol.* 2001;80:233-238.

32. Liu FY, Yen TC, Chen MY, et al. Detection of hematogenous bone metastasis in cervical cancer: 18F-fluorodeoxyglucose-positron emission tomography versus computed tomography and magnetic resonance imaging. *Cancer.* 2009;115:5470-5480.

33. Joyce JA, Pollard JW. Microenvironmental regulation of metastasis. *Nat Rev Cancer.* 2009;9:239-252.

34. Klopp AH, Zhang Y, Solley T, et al. Omental adipose tissue-derived stromal cells promote vascularization and growth of endometrial tumors. *Clin Cancer Res.* 2012;18:771-782.

35. Nieman KM, Kenny HA, Penicka CV, et al. Adipocytes promote ovarian cancer metastasis and provide energy for rapid tumor growth. *Nat Med.* 2011;17:1498-1503.

36. Nowicka A, Marini FC, Solley TN, et al. Human omental-derived adipose stem cells increase ovarian cancer proliferation, migration, and chemoresistance. *PLoS One.* 2013;8:e81859.

37. Grither WR, Longmore GD. Inhibition of tumor-microenvironment interaction and tumor invasion by small-molecule allosteric inhibitor of DDR2 extracellular domain. *Proc Natl Acad Sci USA.* 2018;115:E7786-E7794.

38. Friedl P, Alexander S. Cancer invasion and the microenvironment: plasticity and reciprocity. *Cell.* 2011;147:992-1009.

39. Jung HY, Fattet L, Yang J. Molecular pathways: linking tumor microenvironment to epithelial-mesenchymal transition in metastasis. *Clin Cancer Res.* 2015;21:962-968.

40. Kenny HA, Chiang CY, White EA, et al. Mesothelial cells promote early ovarian cancer metastasis through fibronectin secretion. *J Clin Invest.* 2014;124:4614-4628.

41. Meza-Perez S, Randall TD. Immunological functions of the omentum. *Trends Immunol.* 2017;38:526-536.

42. Thibault B, Castells M, Delord JP, Couderc B. Ovarian cancer microenvironment: implications for cancer dissemination and chemoresistance acquisition. *Cancer Metastasis Rev.* 2014;33:17-39.

43. Yeung TL, Leung CS, Yip KP, Au Yeung CL, Wong ST, Mok SC. Cellular and molecular processes in ovarian cancer metastasis. A review in the theme: cell and molecular processes in cancer metastasis. *Am J Physiol Cell Physiol.* 2015;309:C444-C456.

44. Warburg O. On respiratory impairment in cancer cells. *Science.* 1956;124:269-270.

45. Warburg O. On the origin of cancer cells. *Science.* 1956;123:309-314.

46. Wang ZH, Peng WB, Zhang P, Yang XP, Zhou Q. Lactate in the tumour microenvironment: from immune modulation to therapy. *EBioMedicine.* 2021;73:103627.

47. Gharpure KM, Pradeep S, Sans M, et al. FABP4 as a key determinant of metastatic potential of ovarian cancer. *Nat Commun.* 2018;9:2923.

48. Krock BL, Skuli N, Simon MC. Hypoxia-induced angiogenesis: good and evil. *Genes Cancer.* 2011;2:1117-1133.

49. Shweiki D, Itin A, Soffer D, Keshet E. Vascular endothelial growth factor induced by hypoxia may mediate hypoxia-initiated angiogenesis. *Nature.* 1992;359:843-845.

50. Baluk P, Hashizume H, McDonald DM. Cellular abnormalities of blood vessels as targets in cancer. *Curr Opin Genet Dev.* 2005;15:102-111.

51. Kastelein AW, Vos LMC, van Baal JOAM, et al. Poor perfusion of the microvasculature in peritoneal metastases of ovarian cancer. *Clin Exp Metastasis.* 2020;37:293-304.

52. Bielenberg DR, Zetter BR. The contribution of angiogenesis to the process of metastasis. *Cancer J.* 2015;21:267-273.

53. Paku S, Paweletz N. First steps of tumor-related angiogenesis. *Lab Invest.* 1991;65:334-346.

54. Hanahan D, Weinberg RA. Hallmarks of cancer: the next generation. *Cell.* 2011;144:646-674.

2

VULVAR CANCER

CHAPTER **2.1**

Epidemiology of Vulvar Cancer

Willemijn L. van der Kolk and M. H. M. Oonk

Vulvar cancer is a rare disease that accounts for nearly 6% of all gynecologic malignancies and for 0.7% of all cancers in women (1). According to the American Cancer Society, an estimated 6,470 women will be diagnosed with vulvar cancer in the United States in 2023, and an estimated 1,670 will die of the disease (1). Vulvar squamous cell carcinoma (SCC) accounts for more than 90% of the cases (2). The median age at diagnosis is 68 years, and most cases occur in postmenopausal women in the sixth or seventh decade (2). An increase in incidence in younger women has been observed, which is probably because of an increased prevalence of high-risk human papillomavirus (HPV)-related cases (3). Other types of

vulvar cancer, such as basal cell carcinoma, melanoma, and adenocarcinoma, are extremely rare.

REFERENCES

1. Siegel RL, Miller KD, Fuchs HE, Jemal A. Cancer statistics, 2023. *CA Cancer J Clin*. 2023;73(1):17-48.
2. Weinberg D, Gomez-Martinez RA. Vulvar cancer. *Obstet Gynecol Clin North Am*. 2019;46(1):125-135.
3. Bray F, Laversanne M, Weiderpass E, Arbyn M. Geographic and temporal variations in the incidence of vulvar and vaginal cancers. *Int J Cancer*. 2020;147(10):2764-2771.

CHAPTER **2.2**

Vulvar Cancer: Anatomy, Natural History, and Patterns of Spread

Willemijn L. van der Kolk and M. H. M. Oonk

ANATOMY

The vulva, meaning covering or wrapping, encompasses all external female genital organs. These include the mons pubis, clitoris, labia minora and majora, vulvar vestibule, vestibular bulbs, Bartholin glands and Skene glands, and the perineal body. The vulva is bordered superiorly by the anterior abdominal wall, laterally by the labiocrural fold at the medial thigh, and inferiorly by the anus. The mons pubis is a prominent mound of hair-bearing skin and subcutaneous adipose and connective tissue that is located anterior to the pubic symphysis. The labia majora are two elongated skin folds that course posterior from the mons pubis and blend into the perineal body. The labia minora are a smaller pair of skin folds medial and parallel to the labia majora that extend inferiorly to form the margin of the vulvar vestibule.

Superiorly, the labia minora separate into two components that course above and below the clitoris, fusing with those of the opposite side to form the prepuce and frenulum, respectively. The skin of the labia minora contains sebaceous glands near its junction with the labia majora, but it is not hair-bearing and it has little or no underlying adipose tissue. The clitoris is supported externally by the fusion of the labia minora (prepuce and frenulum) and is approximately 2 to 3 cm anterior to the urethral meatus. It is

composed of erectile tissue organized into the glans, body, and two crura. Two loosely fused corpora cavernosa form the body of the clitoris and extend superiorly from the glans, ultimately dividing into the two crura. The crura course laterally beneath the ischiocavernosus muscles and attach to the ischial rami.

The vulvar vestibule is the area between the labia minora. Hart's line is a demarcation between the vulvar vestibule and the labia minor and represents the area of change from nonkeratinized squamous mucosal epithelium of the vulvar vestibule to keratinized epithelium on the labia minora. The vagina, urethra, periurethral glands, minor vestibular glands (also known as Skene glands), and the Bartholin glands open onto the vestibule. Anteriorly, the minor vestibular glands are located beneath the vestibular mucosa and open predominantly onto the more anterior vestibule. The Bartholin glands, two small, mucus-secreting glands situated within the subcutaneous tissue of the posterior labia majora, have ducts opening onto the posterolateral portion of the vestibule. The vestibular bulbs are two loosely connected erectile organs located lateral to the vulva vestibule. They lie beneath the bulbocavernosus muscle and medial to the body of the clitoris. The perineal body is a 3- to 4-cm band of skin and subcutaneous tissue located between the posterior extensions of the labia majora. It separates the vulva vestibule from the anus and forms the posterior margin of the vulva.

Vascular Anatomy and Neurologic Innervation

The vulva has a rich blood supply derived primarily from the internal pudendal artery, which arises from the anterior division of the internal iliac (hypogastric) artery, and the superficial and deep external pudendal arteries, which arise from the femoral artery. The internal pudendal artery exits the pelvis and passes behind the ischial spine to reach the posterolateral vulva, where it divides into several small branches to the ischiocavernosus and bulbocavernosus muscles, the perineal artery, artery of the bulb, urethral artery, and dorsal and deep arteries of the clitoris. Both external pudendal arteries travel medially to supply the labia majora and their deep structures. These vessels anastomose freely with branches from the internal pudendal artery.

Multiple spinal cord levels are involved in the innervation of the vulva. The ilioinguinal nerve from L1 and the genital branch of the genitofemoral nerve (L1-2) innervate the mons pubis and the anterior part of the labia majora. Either of these nerves may be easily injured during pelvic lymph node (LN) dissection, with resulting paresthesias. The pudendal nerve (S2-4) enters the vulva parallel to the internal pudendal artery and gives rise to several branches that innervate the lower vagina, labia, clitoris, perineal body, and their supporting structures.

Groin Anatomy and Lymphatic Drainage

The femoral triangle is bordered superiorly by the inguinal ligament, laterally by the medial border of the sartorius muscle, and medially by the adductor longus muscle. The roof of the femoral canal is the fascia lata, and the floor consists of the pectineus, iliopsoas, and adductor longus muscles. The femoral triangle encompasses several structures: the femoral artery and vein, the femoral nerve, and the femoral canal. The fascia lata has a crescent-shaped opening called the fossa ovalis or the saphenous opening, which is covered by the cribriform fascia. The great saphenous vein pierces through the cribriform fascia, accompanied by several superficial branches from the femoral artery and lymphatics. The femoral artery and vein and the femoral canal are contained within the femoral sheath.

The lymphatics of the vulva run anteriorly through the labia majora, turn laterally at the mons pubis, and drain primarily into the superficial inguinal LNs. The clitoris and the perineal body

have bilateral lymph drainage. Dye studies have demonstrated that vulvar lymphatic channels do not extend laterally to the labiocrural folds and do not cross the midline, unless the site of dye injection is at the clitoris or perineal body (1). However, under specific circumstances (eg, blockage of lymph channels, prior vulvar or groin surgery, or large groin metastases), contralateral lymphatic drainage may occur (2,3).

The inguinal nodes are subdivided into the superficial and deep inguinal nodes. The superficial inguinal LNs are located anteriorly within the femoral triangle along the saphenous vein and its branches (**Figure 2.2-1A-C**). They drain the perineal genitalia, anus, perianal skin, anterior abdominal wall below the umbilicus level, and round ligament of the uterus. The deep inguinal LNs are located in the femoral canal, medial to the femoral vein. They drain the lower extremity and also receive drainage from the superficial inguinal nodes and clitoris. Both the superficial and deep inguinal nodes drain into the external iliac nodes.

The first LN to receive drainage from the vulva is called the sentinel lymph node (SLN). It can be identified by lymphatic mapping techniques, for example, the lymphoscintigram. The sentinel node is frequently found on the medial side of the femoral vein and superior to the adductor muscle. The lymphatics can drain from the sentinel node and other inguinofemoral LNs into the external iliac, common iliac, and aortic LNs.

NATURAL HISTORY (PATTERNS OF SPREAD)

Vulvar cancer can spread in three ways: by local growth and direct invasion of adjacent organs (eg, vagina, anus, or urethra), by lymphatic spread to the inguinofemoral LNs, and by hematogenous spread to distant sites (eg, lung or liver). Risk factors for inguinofemoral LN metastases include tumor size, tumor stage, grading, depth of stromal invasion (DOI), and vascular and lymphovascular space invasion (4). Nodal metastases are rare if DOI is less than 1 mm, but the risk rises sharply with DOI greater than 1 mm. In addition, Dabi et al found that the presence of lichen sclerosus (LS) is a risk factor (5). HPV is widely accepted as a positive prognostic factor and seems to be associated with less groin involvement, but evidence for the latter is scarce (6-8). Pelvic LN metastases are observed in 18.5% of patients with inguinofemoral metastases (9). In the absence of inguinofemoral metastases and/or

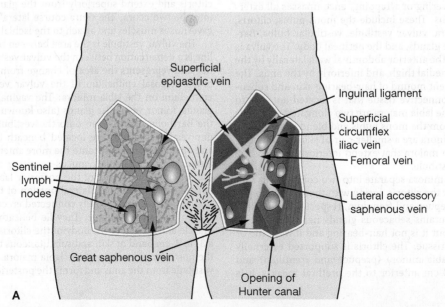

Superficial epigastric vein

Inguinal ligament

Superficial circumflex iliac vein

Femoral vein

Sentinel lymph nodes

Lateral accessory saphenous vein

Great saphenous vein

Opening of Hunter canal

A

■ **Figure 2.2-1.** Lymphatic anatomy in the groin. **A** Some possible locations of sentinel nodes.

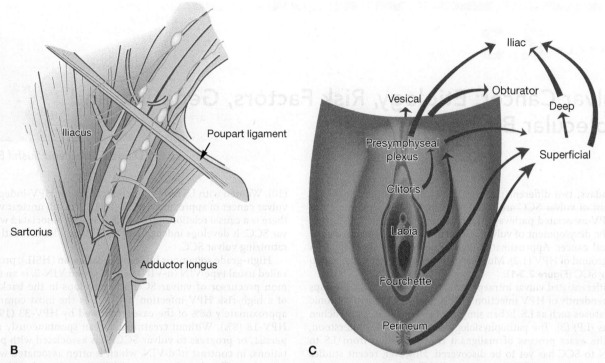

Figure 2.2-1. (*continued*) **B** Nodes between the femoral artery and the vein. Lymph nodes between the vessels are common in the pelvis but not in the groin. **C** Direct drainage from the clitoral area of the vulva to both groin and pelvic lymph nodes.

a negative SLN procedure, the risk of pelvic LN metastases or distant metastases is low (9,10). Rodríguez-Trujillo et al found that only one patient (1/93; 1.1%) had a distant metastasis after a negative SLN or inguinofemoral dissection (11).

In lateralized vulvar cancer (medial border of the tumor >1 cm from the virtual midline), LN metastases are usually located in the ipsilateral groin. Contralateral metastases in patients with lateralized vulvar cancer are rare and occur mainly in tumors greater than 4 cm (12). They have also been described in 0% to 6.5% of patients with early-stage vulvar SCC (tumors ≤4 cm). In these patients, isolated contralateral LN metastases are only found when the tumor is located 1 cm or less from the midline (13,14). Midline tumors (tumors within 1 cm of the midline) have bilateral lymphatic flow and more often give rise to bilateral groin LN metastases (15).

Distant metastases are rare. Approximately 2% to 7% of patients with vulvar cancer present with distant metastases at some point, but at presentation a risk close to zero is observed (16). Distant metastases can occur because of further lymphatic spread and/or hematogenous dissemination. Prieske et al found that distant metastases are unilocal in 65% of the cases (16). The most common sites for distant metastases are lung, liver, and bone (16). Spread beyond the inguinofemoral LNs is considered stage IVB.

REFERENCES

1. Plentl AA, Friedman EA. Lymphatic system of the female genitalia: the morphologic basis of oncologic diagnosis and therapy. *Major Probl Obstet Gynecol*. 1971;2:1-223.

2. Iversen T, Aas M. Lymph drainage from the vulva. *Gynecol Oncol*. 1983;16(2):179-189.

3. De Hullu J, Oonk MH, Ansink AC, et al. Pitfalls in the sentinel lymph node procedure in vulvar cancer. *Gynecol Oncol*. 2004;94(1):10-15.

4. Klapdor R, Wölber L, Hanker L, et al. Predictive factors for lymph node metastases in vulvar cancer. An analysis of the AGO-CaRE-1 multicenter study. *Gynecol Oncol*. 2019;154(3):565-570.

5. Dabi, Y., Gosset, M., Bastuji-Garin, S., Mitri-Frangieh, R., Bendifallah, S., Darai, E., Paniel, B. J., Rouzier, R., Haddad, B., & Touboul, C. (2020). Associated Lichen Sclerosis Increases the Risk of Lymph Node Metastases of Vulvar Cancer. *J Clin Med*, 9(1). https://doi.org/10.3390/JCM9010250

6. Rasmussen CL, Sand FL, Hoffmann Frederiksen M, Kaae Andersen K, Kjær SK. Does HPV status influence survival after vulvar cancer? *Int J Cancer*. 2018;142(6):1158-1165.

7. Wakeham K, Kavanagh K, Cuschieri K, et al. HPV status and favourable outcome in vulvar squamous cancer. *Int J Cancer*. 2017;140(5):1134-1146.

8. Hinten F, Molijn A, Eckhardt L, et al. Vulvar cancer: two pathways with different localization and prognosis. *Gynecol Oncol*. 2018;149(2):310-317.

9. Woelber L, Hampl M, Eulenburg CZ, et al. Risk for pelvic metastasis and role of pelvic lymphadenectomy in node-positive vulvar cancer-results from the AGO-VOP.2 QS vulva study. *Cancers (Basel)*. 2022;14(2):418.

10. Woelber L, Bommert M, Prieske K, et al. Pelvic lymphadenectomy in vulvar cancer—does it make sense? *Geburtshilfe Frauenheilkd*. 2020;80(12):1221-1228.

11. Rodríguez-Trujillo A, Fusté P, Paredes P, et al. Long-term oncological outcomes of patients with negative sentinel lymph node in vulvar cancer. Comparative study with conventional lymphadenectomy. *Acta Obstet Gynecol Scand*. 2018;97(12):1427-1437.

12. Nica A, Covens A, Vicus D, et al. Sentinel lymph nodes in vulvar cancer: management dilemmas in patients with positive nodes and larger tumors. *Gynecol Oncol*. 2019;152(1):94-100.

13. Winarno AS, Mondal A, Martignoni FC, Fehm TN, Hampl M. The potential risk of contralateral non-sentinel groin node metastasis in women with early primary vulvar cancer following unilateral sentinel node metastasis: a single center evaluation in University Hospital of Düsseldorf. *BMC Womens Health*. 2021;21(1):23.

14. Ignatov T, Gaßner J, Bozukova M, et al. Contralateral lymph node metastases in patients with vulvar cancer and unilateral sentinel lymph node metastases of Nordic Federation of Societies of Obstetrics and Gynecology (NFOG). *Acta Obstet Gynecol Scand*. 2021;100(8):1520-1525.

15. Coleman RL, Ali S, Levenback CF, et al. Is bilateral lymphadenectomy for midline squamous carcinoma of the vulva always necessary? An analysis from Gynecologic Oncology Group (GOG) 173. *Gynecol Oncol*. 2013;128(2):155-159.

16. Prieske K, Haeringer N, Grimm D, et al. Patterns of distant metastases in vulvar cancer. *Gynecol Oncol*. 2016;142(3):427-434.

CHAPTER **2.3**

Vulvar Cancer: Etiology, Risk Factors, Genetics, and Molecular Biology

Diane C. Ling and Sushil Beriwal

Nowadays, two different pathways that play a role in the development of vulvar SCC are recognized: an HPV-independent and an HPV-associated pathway. The relation between HPV infection and the development of vulvar SCC is not as straightforward as in cervical cancer. Approximately 18% of vulvar SCC develops in a background of HPV (1,2). Multiple pathways can eventually lead to vulvar SCC (**Figure 2.3-1**).

Differentiated vulvar intraepithelial neoplasia (d-VIN) develops independently of HPV infection. d-VIN is associated with chronic dermatoses such as LS, lichen simplex chronicus (LSC), and lichen planus (LP) (3). The pathophysiology remains poorly understood, and the exact process of malignant transformation from LS to d-VIN to SCC has yet to be discovered. However, recent studies show a relation with TP53 mutations (3). The absolute cancer risk of d-VIN is not yet determined, and studies show a risk ranging from 33% to 86% (4). A recent cohort study by Thuijs et al shows a risk of 58.3% (5).

Two other types of HPV-independent vulvar lesions have been described: the vulvar acanthosis with altered differentiation (VAAD), described by Nascimento et al in 2004, and the differentiated exophytic vulvar intraepithelial lesion (DEVIL), described by Watkins et al in 2017 (6,7). These lesions are closely related to d-VIN, and the three entities may even coexist. This suggests that they exist on a spectrum (8). There is a significant morphologic overlap between DEVIL and VAAD and only subtle histologic differences can be found, but these are often subjective (9). DEVIL and VAAD differentiate themselves from d-VIN in lacking a p53 mutation. Although data are limited, VAAD and DEVIL have proven to be precancerous lesions, preceding verrucous carcinoma and low-grade SCC, respectively (8).

The etiology of LS is still unclear, but evidence suggests that it is an autoimmune disorder with genetic susceptibility factors. It mostly develops in prepubertal girls and postmenopausal women but can occur in women of all ages. The first-line treatment is with topical corticosteroids, but LS is considered an incurable disease

(10). Women with LS have an increased risk for HPV-independent vulvar cancer of approximately 5% (9,11). It is still unclear whether there is a causal relationship or if LS is merely associated with vulvar SCC. It develops independent of HPV and leads mostly to keratinizing vulvar SCC.

High-grade squamous intraepithelial lesion (HSIL), previously called usual type VIN (u-VIN) or VIN-2 and VIN-3, is an uncommon precursor of vulvar SCC and develops in the background of a high-risk HPV infection. HPV-16 is the most common, in approximately 68% of the cases, followed by HPV-33 (19%) and HPV-18 (8%). Without treatment, it can spontaneously resolve, persist, or progress to vulvar SCC. It is associated with p16 mutations, in contrast to d-VIN, which is often associated with p53 mutations. The absolute cancer risk is approximately 10% according to a recent cohort study by Thuijs and colleagues (5). When treated, percentages drop to 3% to 5% (11). Smoking and immunosuppression are cofactors for the development of vulvar SCC in a background of HSIL.

Several vulvar dermatoses have been associated with vulvar SCC. LSC is a risk factor for vulvar SCC, but no direct association has been identified (9,12). The relationship between LP and vulvar SCC has not been well established yet. So far, there is insufficient evidence to determine whether LP is a precursor lesion (13).

Although HPV DNA is associated with most high-grade intraepithelial lesions (80%), it is much less commonly seen in association with invasive lesions (~20%-50%) (14). Vulvar SCC with HPV positivity is more common in younger age groups, whereas vulvar SCC with HPV negativity is more common in older women. However, in older women, the incidence of HPV-associated vulvar SCC is rising and now accounts for half of vulvar SCC, especially in women over 50 (15).

Distinct genomic signatures of HPV-positive and HPV-negative vulvar SCC have been identified. HPV-positive vulvar SCC tends to have genomic alterations in the PI3K/mTOR pathway and higher tumor mutational burden (TMB) (16). On the other hand, HPV-negative vulvar SCC has been associated with genomic alterations in TP53, TERTp, CDKN2A, CCND1, FAT1, NOTCH1, and epidermal growth factor receptor (EGFR) (17).

REFERENCES

1. Kortekaas KE, Bastiaannet E, van Doorn HC, et al. Vulvar cancer subclassification by HPV and p53 status results in three clinically distinct subtypes. *Gynecol Oncol.* 2020;159(3):649-656.
2. Hinten F, Molijn A, Eckhardt L, et al. Vulvar cancer: two pathways with different localization and prognosis. *Gynecol Oncol.* 2018;149(2):310-317.
3. Jin C, Liang S. Differentiated vulvar intraepithelial neoplasia: a brief review of clinicopathologic features. *Arch Pathol Lab Med.* 2019;143(6):768-771.
4. Voss FO, Thuijs NB, Vermeulen RFM, Wilthagen EA, van Beurden M, Bleeker MCG. The vulvar cancer risk in differentiated vulvar intraepithelial neoplasia: a systematic review. *Cancers (Basel).* 2021;13(24):6170.
5. Thuijs NB, van Beurden M, Bruggink AH, Steenbergen RDM, Berkhof J, Bleeker MCG. Vulvar intraepithelial neoplasia: incidence and long-term risk of vulvar squamous cell carcinoma. *Int J Cancer.* 2021;148(1):90-98.

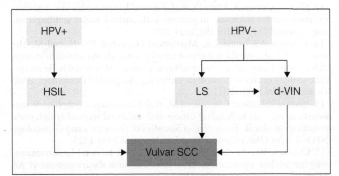

Figure 2.3-1. Pathways leading to vulvar SCC. d-VIN, differentiated vulvar intraepithelial neoplasia; HPV, human papillomavirus; HSIL, high-grade squamous intraepithelial lesion; LS, lichen sclerosus; SCC, squamous cell carcinoma.

6. Nascimento AF, Granter SR, Cviko A, Yuan L, Hecht JL, Crum CP. Vulvar acanthosis with altered differentiation: a precursor to verrucous carcinoma? *Am J Surg Pathol.* 2004;28(5):638-643.

7. Watkins JC, Howitt BE, Horowitz NS, et al. Differentiated exophytic vulvar intraepithelial lesions are genetically distinct from keratinizing squamous cell carcinomas and contain mutations in PIK3CA. *Mod Pathol.* 2017;30(3):448-458.

8. Singh N, Gilks CB. Vulval squamous cell carcinoma and its precursors. *Histopathology.* 2020;76(1):128-138.

9. Jenkins TM, Mills AM. Putative precancerous lesions of vulvar squamous cell carcinoma. *Semin Diagn Pathol.* 2021;38(1):27-36.

10. Krapf JM, Mitchell L, Holton MA, Goldstein AT. Vulvar lichen sclerosus: current perspectives. *Int J Womens Health.* 2020;12:11-20.

11. van de Nieuwenhof HP, van der Avoort IA, de Hullu JA. Review of squamous premalignant vulvar lesions. *Crit Rev Oncol Hematol.* 2008;68(2):131-156.

12. Prieske K, Woelber L, Muallem MZ, et al. Age, treatment and prognosis of patients with squamous cell vulvar cancer (VSCC)—analysis of the AGO-CaRE-1 study. *Gynecol Oncol.* 2021;161(2):442-448.

13. Halonen P, Jakobsson M, Heikinheimo O, Riska A, Gissler M, Pukkala E. Lichen sclerosus and risk of cancer. *Int J Cancer.* 2017;140(9):1998-2002.

14. Brusen Villadsen A, Bundgaard-Nielsen C, Ambuhl L, et al. Prevalence and type distribution of human papillomavirus infections in Danish patients diagnosed with vulvar squamous cell tumors and precursors. *Gynecol Oncol Rep.* 2021;37:100828.

15. Eva LJ, Sadler L, Fong KL, Sahota S, Jones RW, Bigby SM. Trends in HPV-dependent and HPV-independent vulvar cancers: the changing face of vulvar squamous cell carcinoma. *Gynecol Oncol.* 2020;157(2):450-455.

16. Williams EA, Werth AJ, Sharaf R, et al. Vulvar squamous cell carcinoma: comprehensive genomic profiling of HPV+ versus HPV− forms reveals distinct sets of potentially actionable molecular targets. *JCO Precis Oncol.* 2020;4:PO.19.00406.

17. Carlson JA, Amin S, Malfetano J, et al. Concordant p53 and mdm-2 protein expression in vulvar squamous cell carcinoma and adjacent lichen sclerosus. *Appl Immunohistochem Mol Morphol.* 2001;9(2):150-163.

CHAPTER **2.4**

Vulvar Cancer: Preinvasive Disease

Willemijn L. van der Kolk

The nomenclature for vulvar squamous intraepithelial lesions has changed numerous times over the years, which may lead to confusion when reviewing older literature. The term "vulvar intraepithelial neoplasia" (VIN) was first adopted by the International Society for the Vulvovaginal Disease (ISSVD) in 1986. It was subdivided into squamous subtype, which included VIN-1, VIN-2, and VIN-3; and nonsquamous subtype, which included Paget disease and melanoma in situ (1). In 2004, the ISSVD proposed a revised classification that consisted of two VIN groups, "u-VIN, HPV related," which was subtyped into warty, basaloid, and mixed; and "d-VIN, HPV unrelated." The term VIN-1 was discarded as it was felt to represent only benign HPV infection and reactive changes (2).

In 2012, the lower anogenital squamous terminology (LAST) for HPV-related squamous intraepithelial lesions was proposed (3). This terminology was applied to any HPV-related male or female genital tract or anal/perianal lesion and was not specific to vulvar lesions. Lesions were categorized into a two-tier system consisting of HSIL or low-grade squamous intraepithelial lesion (LSIL), and the old terminology of VIN-1, VIN-2, or VIN-3 was discarded.

In 2015, the ISSVD proposed the following terminology: LSIL, HSIL, and d-VIN (4). The term LSIL encompasses flat condyloma, or HPV effect, and was previously referred to as VIN-1. LSIL is not precancerous and does not require treatment unless symptomatic. HSIL was previously called u-VIN in the 2004 ISSVD terminology, and prior to that it was referred to as VIN-2 and VIN-3. D-VIN was previously known as VIN simplex type. LSIL is often associated with low-risk HPV subtypes (6 and 11), whereas HSIL is associated with high-risk HPV subtypes (5-7), and d-VIN is not HPV-associated.

In the 2020 World Health Organization (WHO) classification of female genital tumors, there is a focus on the distinction between HPV-associated and HPV-independent VIN (8). HPV-associated VIN corresponds to LSIL (VIN-1) and HSIL (u-VIN; VIN-2 and VIN-3). The term "HPV-independent VIN" was introduced and includes d-VIN, DEVIL, and VAAD. d-VIN is a precursor lesion to more aggressive SCC, DEVIL is a precursor to less aggressive keratinizing SCC, and VAAD is a precursor/risk lesion to verrucous carcinoma. Vulvar aberrant maturation (VAM) is an umbrella term that is not included in the WHO classification and is sometimes used to describe lesions such as DEVIL and VAAD that have aberrant maturation and arise from lichenoid dermatitis, but lack the basal atypia required for the diagnosis of d-VIN.

According to the ISSVD, the histologic definition of d-VIN requires basal atypia combined with negative or nonblock-positive p16 and basal overexpressed, aberrant negative, or wild-type p53 (9). It usually shows keratinizing morphology with acanthosis, aberrant rete ridge pattern, and premature maturation, often arising in a background of LS. On the other hand, HSIL usually shows warty-basaloid morphology and is nonkeratinizing.

Distinguishing between HPV-associated and HPV-independent precursors has important implications for treatment and prognosis. d-VIN and steroid-resistant VAM (HPV independent) are treated with excision, whereas HSIL (HPV dependent) may be treated with imiquimod, light amplification by stimulated emission of radiation (LASER), and excision (9). d-VIN has a higher likelihood of progressing to invasive SCC, and HPV-independent SCC is less radiosensitive and has worse prognosis than HPV-associated SCC (10-15).

REFERENCES

1. Klapdor R, Wölber L, Hanker L, et al. Predictive factors for lymph node metastases in vulvar cancer. An analysis of the AGO-CaRE-1 multicenter study. *Gynecol Oncol.* 2019;154(3):565-570.

2. Sideri M, Jones RW, Wilkinson EJ, et al. Squamous vulvar intraepithelial neoplasia: 2004 modified terminology, ISSVD vulvar oncology subcommittee. *J Reprod Med.* 2005;50:807-810.

3. Darragh TM, Colgan TJ, Cox JT, et al; Members of the LAST Project Work Groups. The lower anogenital squamous terminology standardization

project for HPV-associated lesions: background and consensus recommendations from the college of American pathologists and the American society for colposcopy and cervical pathology. *Int J Gynecol Pathol.* 2013;32:76-115.

4. Bornstein J, Bogliatto F, Haefner HK, et al. The 2015 International Society for the Study of Vulvovaginal Disease (ISSVD) terminology of vulvar squamous intraepithelial lesions. *J Low Genit Tract Dis.* 2016;20:11-14.

5. Fergus KB, Lee AW, Baradaran N, et al. Pathophysiology, clinical manifestations, and treatment of lichen sclerosus: a systematic review. *Urology.* 2020;135:11-19.

6. Krapf JM, Mitchell L, Holton MA, Goldstein AT. Vulvar lichen sclerosus: current perspectives. *Int J Womens Health.* 2020;12:11-20.

7. Woelber L, Bommert M, Prieske K, et al. Pelvic lymphadenectomy in vulvar cancer—does it make sense? *Geburtshilfe Frauenheilkd.* 2020;80(12):1221-1228.

8. Höhn AK, Brambs CE, Hiller GGR, et al. 2020 WHO classification of female genital tumors. *Geburtshilfe Frauenheilkd.* 2021;81(10):1145-1153.

9. Heller DS, Day T, Allbritton JI, et al. Diagnostic criteria for differentiated vulvar intraepithelial neoplasia and vulvar aberrant maturation. *J Low Genit Tract Dis.* 2021;25(1):57-70.

10. Hinten F, Molijn A, Eckhardt L, et al. Vulvar cancer: two pathways with different localization and prognosis. *Gynecol Oncol.* 2018;149(2):310-317.

11. Eva LJ, Sadler L, Fong KL, Sahota S, Jones RW, Bigby SM. Trends in HPV-dependent and HPV-independent vulvar cancers: the changing face of vulvar squamous cell carcinoma. *Gynecol Oncol.* 2020;157(2):450-455.

12. Eva LJ, Ganesan R, Chan KK, et al. Differentiated-type vulval intraepithelial neoplasia has a high-risk association with vulval squamous cell carcinoma. *Int J Gynecol Cancer.* 2009;19:741-744.

13. McAlpine JN, Kim SY, Akbari A, et al. HPV-independent differentiated vulvar intraepithelial neoplasia (dVIN) is associated with an aggressive clinical course. *Int J Gynecol Pathol.* 2017;36:507-516.

14. McAlpine JN, Leung SCY, Cheng A, et al. Human papillomavirus (HPV)-independent vulvar squamous cell carcinoma has a worse prognosis than HPV-associated disease: a retrospective cohort study. *Histopathology.* 2017;71:238-246.

15. Horne ZD, Dohopolski MJ, Pradhan D, et al. Human papillomavirus infection mediates response and outcome of vulvar squamous cell carcinomas treated with radiation therapy. *Gynecol Oncol.* 2018;151:96-101.

CHAPTER **2.5**

Vulvar Cancer: Clinical Presentation, Diagnostic Evaluation, and Workup

Willemijn L. van der Kolk and M. H. M. Oonk

CLINICAL PRESENTATION

Women with VIN may present with pruritus, burning sensation, or dysuria, especially in the setting of a periurethral lesion, although up to 40% of VIN are asymptomatic. Women with invasive vulvar SCC often present with pruritus and/or discomfort in the vulvar region as well as a vulvar mass. Often, a recognizable exophytic or endophytic lesion is present, and ulceration is not uncommon. About 5% of patients present with multifocal disease (1). Most women present with an early-stage vulvar SCC (Figure 2.5-1A). Advanced-stage vulvar SCC (**Figure 2.5-1B,C**) is more often seen in older women.

There is often a delay in diagnosis, which can be multifactorial. Women can delay visiting their general physician because they feel embarrassed. It is not uncommon that women are prescribed empiric topical therapies for several months, without proper examination of the vulva. Lanneau et al showed that among young patients with vulvar cancer (age below 45 years), almost half had symptoms for more than a year prior to diagnosis (2). Vandborg et al reported that patients with vulvar cancer had the longest delay in diagnosis of all patients with gynecologic cancer. They also showed that in the absence of blood loss, general practitioners were less likely to perform gynecologic examination, although the length of delay was shortened when examination was performed (3). A recent German study showed the potential mean delay of vulvar cancer diagnosis ranged from 186 to 328 days (4).

DIAGNOSTIC EVALUATION

The diagnostic evaluation starts with a thorough history and physical examination. Attention should be paid to coexisting morbidities and clinical extent of the disease. Initial evaluation should include bimanual pelvic examination and rectovaginal examination, measurements of the primary tumor, assessment for extension to adjacent mucosal or bony structures, and palpation of the inguinal LNs. It is helpful to record the distance from vital structures such as the clitoris, urethral meatus, and anus, because these structures limit the ability to obtain adequate surgical margins. Because vulvar cancers may be related to HPV, clinical examination of the vagina, cervix, and anus should also be performed as HPV may be multifocal. If no recent cervical Papanicolaou (Pap) smear has been taken, this should be performed as well (5). Patients with large or fixed tumors, and those who are difficult to examine in the clinic, may benefit from an exam under anesthesia, with cystourethroscopy and proctosigmoidoscopy for tumors near the urethra or anus, respectively.

Diagnosis must always be confirmed by taking a punch biopsy under local anesthesia. Selecting the most appropriate site for a biopsy can be difficult, because of coexisting premalignancies or precursors. In such cases, multiple biopsies are often required. Because VIN can present in different forms and can be multifocal, any new lesion should be biopsied. If a nonbiopsied or noninvasive vulvar lesion does not completely resolve or is refractory to therapy, it should be biopsied to obtain a definitive diagnosis. Tissue biopsies should include the cutaneous lesion in question and representative contiguous underlying stroma, so that the presence and DOI can be accurately assessed. Because DOI is a central issue in the management of vulvar cancer, punch biopsies are encouraged and shave biopsies are generally discouraged. If invasion is suspected and a punch biopsy fails to confirm the clinical suspicion, then an incisional or excisional biopsy should be performed. However, complete excisional biopsies should be avoided if possible, because it may complicate a subsequent SN procedure.

When the diagnosis of vulvar SCC is confirmed, further diagnostic imaging depends on the extent of disease. In patients with microinvasive vulvar SCC, no imaging is required, because chances of LN metastasis are close to zero (6). In patients with unifocal

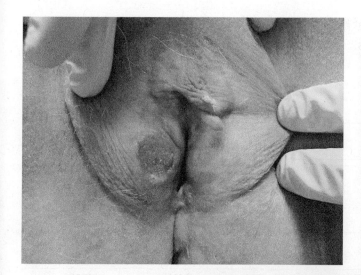
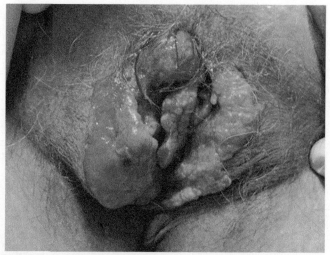
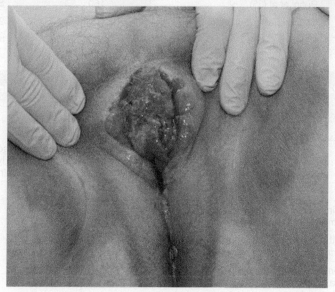

Figure 2.5-1. A: Early-stage VSCC. B, C: Advanced-stage VSCC. VSCC, vulvar squamous cell carcinoma.

tumors less than 4 cm and clinically nonsuspicious LNs, imaging of the groins is recommended to rule out gross nodal involvement prior to the SN procedure.

Different imaging techniques have been studied for their ability to rule out groin node metastases (**Table 2.5-1**). The combination of ultrasound-guided fine needle aspiration (FNA) biopsy and ultrasound has shown an excellent sensitivity and specificity at 80% to 93% and 82% to 100%, respectively. An advantage of ultrasound is its minimally invasive nature, although a disadvantage is that the accuracy is highly operator dependent. Nowadays, pelvic magnetic resonance imaging (MRI) with vaginal gel and contrast is increasingly being utilized to evaluate the relationship of the disease to adjacent structures as well as for staging of the inguinal and pelvic LNs. Computed tomography (CT) and positron emission tomography (PET) CT can be used in the assessment of distant disease. However, the sensitivity of CT and MRI is not sufficient to omit a lymphadenectomy based on imaging results (**Table 2.5-1**). Fluorodeoxyglucose (FDG)-PET-CT shows promising values of sensitivity and specificity for the distinction between negative nodes and metastatic

nodes (**Table 2.5-1**), but more research is needed for consensus. Suspicious LNs should be biopsied if the findings would alter the surgical plan.

Staging

The International Federation of Gynecology and Obstetrics (FIGO) adopted a modified surgical staging system for vulvar cancer in 1989, which was revised in 1995, 2009, and more recently in 2021 (7) (**Table 2.5-2**).

The 2021 staging revision was formulated in collaboration with the U.S. National Cancer Database and is the first from FIGO to incorporate data analyses to validate prognostics. The 2021 revision includes a new definition for depth of invasion (see Pathology section), allows findings from cross-sectional imaging to be incorporated, and now uses the same definition for LN metastases utilized in cervical cancer. Just as with the recently updated FIGO 2018 cervical cancer staging, LNs with isolated tumor cells (ITCs) will be staged as node negative, whereas micrometastases or macrometastases will be staged as node positive, or stage III.

■ TABLE 2.5-1. Sensitivity and Specificity of Different Imaging Techniques

Imaging Technique	Author	Number of Patients	Sensitivity	Specificity
Ultrasound	Garganese et al.(45)	144	90%	78%
	De Gregorio et al.(46)	60	76%	91%
	Pouwer et al.(47)	76	100%	92%
Ultrasound FNA	Angelico et al.(48)	43	77%	100%
	Land et al.(49)	44	80%	100%
MRI	Kataoka et al.(50)	49	87%	81%
	Bipat et al.(51)	60	52%	85-89%
	Hawnaur et al.(52)	10	89%	91%
	Singh et al.(53)	39	86%	82%
CT	Bohlin et al.(54)	134	43%	96%
	Land et al.(49)	44	58%	75%
18F-FDG-PET/CT	Rufini et al.(55)	160	86%	66%
	Collarino et al.(56)	33	95%	75%
	Oldan et al.(57)	21	100%	89%

■ TABLE 2.5-2. Integrated 2021 FIGO and AJCC Staging System for Squamous Cell Carcinoma of the Vulva

FIGO		AJCC 8th Edition		
		T	**N**	**M**
		T0: No evidence of primary tumor (not in FIGO system)	N0(i+): Isolated tumor cells in regional lymph node no greater than 0.2 mm (not in FIGO system)	
I: Tumor confined to the vulva				
IA	Lesions ≤2 cm in size, confined to vulva or perineum and with stromal invasion ≤1 mm, with negative nodes	T1a	N0	M0
IB	Lesions >2 cm in size or with stromal invasion >1 mm, confined to the vulva or perineum, with negative nodes	T1b	N0	M0
II	Tumor of any size with extension to adjacent perineal structures (lower 1/3 urethra, lower 1/3 lower vagina, lower 1/3 anus), with negative nodes	T2	N0	M0
IIIA	Tumor of any size with extension to upper 2/3 urethra, upper 2/3 vagina, bladder mucosa, rectal mucosa, or regional lymph node metastases ≤5 mm	T1, T2, or T3; T3 = upper 2/3 urethra, upper 2/3 vagina, bladder mucosa, rectal mucosa	N1a = 1-2 lymph nodes each <5 mm) N2a = ≥3 lymph nodes each <5 mm	M0
IIIB	Regional lymph node metastases >5 mm	T1, T2, or T3	N1b = 1 lymph node ≥5 mm N2b = ≥2 lymph nodes ≥5 mm	M0
IIIC	Regional lymph node metastases with extracapsular spread	T1, T2, or T3	N2c	M0
IVA	Tumor of any size fixed to bone, OR fixed or ulcerated regional lymph node metastases	T1, T2, or T3; fixed to pelvic bone = T3	N3 = inguinal skin ulceration or fixed nodes	M0
IVB	Distant metastasis: includes pelvic nodes	Any	Any	M1

AJCC 8th Edition Prognostic Stage Groupings

Stage	T, N, M combination
IA	T1a, N0, M0
IB	T1b, N0, M0
II	T2, N0, M0
IIIA	T1 or T2, N1, M0
IIIB	T1 or T2, N2a or N2b, M0
IIIC	T1 or T2, N2c, M0
IVA	Either T1 or T2, N3, M0 or T3, any N, M0
IVB	any T, any N, M1

From Rogers LJ, Cuello MA, Olawaiye AB. Cancer of the vulva: 2021 update. *Int J Gynecol Obstet*. 2021;155 suppl 1 (suppl 1):7-18, John Wiley and Sons.

REFERENCES

1. Kim KW, Shinagare AB, Krajewski KM, et al. Update on imaging of vulvar squamous cell carcinoma. *AJR Am J Roentgenol.* 2013;201(1):W147-W157. https://pubmed.ncbi.nlm.nih.gov/23789687/

2. Lanneau GS, Argenta PA, Lanneau MS, et al. Vulvar cancer in young women: demographic features and outcome evaluation. *Am J Obstet Gynecol.* 2009;200(6):645.e1-645.e5.

3. Vandborg MP, Christensen RD, Kragstrup J, et al. Reasons for diagnostic delay in gynecological malignancies. *Int J Gynecol Cancer.* 2011;21(6):967-974.

4. Muigai J, Jacob L, Dinas K, Kostev K, Kalder M. Potential delay in the diagnosis of vulvar cancer and associated risk factors in women treated in German gynecological practices. *Oncotarget.* 2018;9(9):8725-8730.

5. de Bie RP, van de Nieuwenhof HP, Bekkers RL, et al. Patients with usual vulvar intraepithelial neoplasia-related vulvar cancer have an increased risk of cervical abnormalities. *Br J Cancer.* 2009;101(1):27-31.

6. Expert Panel on GYN and OB Imaging, Lakhman Y, Vargas HA, et al. ACR Appropriateness Criteria® staging and follow-up of vulvar cancer. *J Am Coll Radiol.* 2021;18(5S):S212-S228.

7. Olawaiye AB, Cotler J, Cuello MA, et al. FIGO staging for carcinoma of the vulva: 2021 revision. *Int J Gynaecol Obstet.* 2021;155(1):43-47.

CHAPTER **2.6**

Therapy for Vulvar Cancer: Radiation, Systemic Therapy, and Treatment of Persistent and Recurrent Disease

Diane C. Ling and Sushil Beriwal

GENERAL MANAGEMENT

High-Grade Vulvar Intraepithelial Neoplasia

Vulvar LSILs (previously called VIN-1) are not precancerous lesions and do not require treatment unless symptomatic. HSIL (HPV dependent by definition according to 2020 WHO classification; previously called u-VIN, or VIN-2 and VIN-3) and d-VIN (HPV independent) both require treatment, and the goal of treatment is both symptom relief and prevention of progression into invasive disease.

Distinguishing between HPV-associated and HPV-independent lesions has important implications for treatment and prognosis. d-VIN and steroid-resistant VAM are treated with excision, whereas HSIL may be treated with topical imiquimod, ablation, or excision (1). In general, excision is preferred because of the risk for occult invasive disease, especially in the setting of prior vulvar HSIL, d-VIN, LS, or immunosuppression. Careful assessment of surgical margins is imperative given the high risk of recurrence following positive margins. Extensive or diffuse HSIL may require a wider excision and is sometimes treated with partial vulvectomy of the superficial skin. Vulvar skin should be sutured primarily if possible, but sometimes a split-thickness skin graft is required.

In the setting of extensive multifocal disease, CO_2 laser ablation or argon beam coagulation can be considered after extensive sampling to rule out invasive disease. This can also be considered for lesions that involve the clitoris, urethra, anus, or vaginal introitus. These methods may spare the patient a morbid surgery, but do not yield a specimen for histology.

Topical treatments such as imiquimod or 5-fluorouracil (5-FU) cream can be used in select cases. Imiquimod is an immune modulator that is believed to affect the function of the Toll-like receptor (Tlr) as a costimulatory molecule for T-cell-mediated immune response to malignant cells. It has well-documented activity for treatment of genital warts as well as vulvar dysplasia. It is often the initial treatment for recurrent vulvar HSIL (2). It is typically applied 3 to 5 times per week for a total duration of 16 weeks. Side effects include local inflammation at the application site resulting in mild-to-moderate erythema or erosions. Although 5-FU cream is very effective, it is used rarely because of significant side effects (3).

Invasive Vulvar Squamous Cell Carcinoma: Management of the Primary Tumor

Early-Stage Tumors

Tumors demonstrating a DOI of 1 mm or less have minimal risk for lymphatic dissemination (4-6). Excisional procedures that incorporate a 1-cm normal tissue margin are likely to provide curative results. Patients in this category represent the only subset for whom surgical evaluation of the inguinal LNs can be omitted. These superficially invasive carcinomas tend to arise in younger patients with HSIL/VIN lesions that are commonly associated with oncogenic HPV infections. Occult invasion in lesions thought to be intraepithelial is common (132,133,7,8). Consequently, the entire lower genital tract and vulva should be carefully evaluated before surgical resection of these lesions is attempted. The risk of vulvar recurrence or development of a new lesion at another vulvar site is significant. After primary therapy, these patients should undergo frequent follow-up examinations.

Management of clinical stage I and II vulvar cancer includes wide radical excision of the primary tumor with unilateral or bilateral sentinel lymph node biopsy (SLNB), with or without inguinofemoral lymphadenectomy. SLNB should be offered as an alternative to inguinofemoral lymphadenectomy for women with tumors of size 4 cm or less, with no suspicious LNs on physical examination or imaging and no prior groin surgery or radiation that might interfere with lymphatic drainage pathways.

The primary tumor is removed with a wide radial margin of normal skin (2 cm), along with a deep margin to the deep perineal fascia; thus, the vulvar specimen will contain tumor, skin, subcutaneous fat, vascular perforators, and dermal lymphatics. This approach provides excellent long-term survival and local control in approximately 88% of patients (9). Every attempt should be made to preserve structures such as the clitoris and urethral meatus. Deep margins are rarely a problem except on the perineum, where there is little or no subcutaneous fat. In this case, removal of the capsule of the anus or some of the sphincter muscle itself can be performed without loss of anal function.

Vulvar defects for small primary tumors can usually be closed with simple mobilization of the skin and fat surrounding the vulva. In cases where primary closure is not possible, any one of a number of plastic closures is useful (discussed later). Consultation with a plastic surgeon in such cases can be invaluable.

Overall survival (OS) for women following an adequate resection of a primary squamous carcinoma limited to the vulva and with uninvolved inguinal LNs is greater than 90%. Patients with stage II who have negative margins and uninvolved nodes but involvement of the lower vagina or urethra should obtain similar results.

Locally Advanced Tumors

Locally advanced disease is defined as such by either disease extent (eg, T3-T4, or LNs fixed to vessel/muscle) or location (eg, T1 tumor abutting anal verge or urethra), making upfront surgical resection not feasible. Many locally advanced vulvar tumors are bulky; however, some are of modest size but are considered high risk because of proximity to critical midline structures. Some primary tumors can be curatively excised by radical vulvectomy. Surgical resection of 1 to 1.5 cm of the distal urethra to achieve a negative surgical margin does not appear to compromise bladder continence (10). Although radical surgery is an option for patients with locally advanced tumors, contemporary therapeutic strategies have centered on sequenced radiation therapy (RT) or chemoradiation (CRT) followed by radical surgery as a means to preserve either urinary or fecal continence or both. Vulvar cancers are sufficiently sensitive to therapeutic radiation such that function-sparing operations are feasible in selected patients with advanced disease who receive combined modality treatment (11). For patients with stage IVA tumors, similar experiences have been reported; ultraradical (exenterative) resections may also be considered for select patients.

Invasive Vulvar Squamous Cell Carcinoma: Management of Lymph Nodes

Clinically Node-Negative Patients

In the pre-SLNB era, it was determined from Gynecologic Oncology Group (GOG) 37 that patients who undergo bilateral inguinofemoral lymphadenectomy as initial therapy and are found to have positive nodes—especially those with more than one positive node—benefit from postoperative irradiation to the bilateral groin and lower pelvis (12). RT in this situation is superior to pelvic node dissection. However, the morbidity of combining inguinofemoral lymphadenectomy with radiation can be substantial and includes chronic groin and extremity complications, primarily lymphedema (12).

Nowadays, SLNB is standard of care for patients with early-stage clinically node-negative vulvar cancer (13). The ideal management of patients with a microscopically positive SLN who do not undergo inguinofemoral LN dissection was investigated in the Groningen International Study on Sentinel Nodes in Vulvar Cancer (GROINSS)-VII/GOG 270 trial (14). In this trial, women with a negative SLN were observed; women with SLN micrometastases (≤2 mm) received postoperative RT, and women with SLN macrometastases (>2 mm) were managed with inguinofemoral lymphadenectomy and RT. Concurrent radiosensitizing cisplatin was optional. The GROINSS-VII study found that patients with a micrometastasis or ITCs could safely omit inguinofemoral LN dissection and undergo adjuvant RT alone. However, patients with macrometastases had suboptimal outcomes with adjuvant RT alone (20% groin recurrence rate), resulting in a protocol modification to require inguinofemoral lymphadenectomy in addition to RT in these patients. Therefore, at this time, patients with macrometastases on SLNB require completion inguinofemoral LN dissection, followed by adjuvant RT with consideration of concurrent chemotherapy in those with higher risk disease such as two or more involved nodes or extracapsular extension.

Clinically Node-Positive Patients

Some women have LN metastases detected by preoperative physical examination or diagnostic imaging, or at the time of their primary surgery. An optimal management strategy for clinically apparent node-positive patients is yet to be defined. Surgical resection of bulky nodal disease improves regional control and probably enhances the curative potential of RT. In multivariate analysis, Hyde et al (15) found that, for patients with clinically positive groin nodes who underwent surgery followed by RT, the method of surgical groin node dissection (nodal "debulking" vs full groin dissection) had no prognostic significance. On the other hand, some patients present with extensive, unresectable nodal disease. There is increasing early data suggesting a role for upfront chemoradiation for patients with unresectable locally advanced disease (discussed later in Radiation section).

Management of Distant Metastatic Disease

Treatment for stage IVB vulvar cancer is generally palliative, although a subset of these patients with pelvic LN metastases as their only site of distant metastases is potentially curable with aggressive locoregional treatment based on retrospective studies (16).

Management of Recurrent Squamous Vulvar Cancers

Vulvar cancer recurrences can be categorized into three clinical groups: local (vulva), groin, and distant. Historically, it was thought that most localized vulvar recurrences were salvageable, with one study showing recurrence-free survival (RFS) in up to 75% of cases when the recurrence is limited to the vulva and can be excised with a gross clinical margin (17). However, more recent data suggest lower salvage rates than previously thought (13,18). For instance, long-term follow-up of the GROINSSV study showed a 10-year vulva recurrence of 40%, and 10-year disease-specific survival decreased from 90% to 69% for patients without versus with a local recurrence (13). In addition, a recent subset analysis of the AGO-CARE-1 study showed that 30% of patients who developed isolated vulvar recurrence had a second recurrence (18). The observation that many of these recurrences arise at sites remote from the initial primary tumor or that they occur years after apparently successful primary treatment suggests that some recurrences probably represent new primary tumors rather than the development of new disease. Salvage therapy is individualized based on patient comorbidities and extent of disease but generally consists of multimodality management, with some combination of resection of bulky disease and local radiation, perhaps using intensity-modulated RT (IMRT), with or without systemic therapy. Recurrences in the groin, on the other hand, are almost universally fatal. Patients who develop distant metastases are candidates for palliative systemic cytotoxic or targeted therapy or transition to comfort care.

Management of Nonsquamous Vulvar Cancers

Malignant Melanoma

The primary treatment modality for vulvar melanoma is surgical excision. Radical vulvectomy with bilateral inguinofemoral lymphadenectomy was the historical treatment of choice (19). However, because most failures are distant, radical local resection does not appear to enhance survival. Furthermore, many patients with vulvar melanoma are elderly, with coexisting medical problems, making less radical and morbid surgery compelling. More recent reviews recommend some form of hemivulvectomy or wide local excision along with inguinal lymphadenectomy or SLN mapping (20,21). DOI, mitotic activity, and the presence of ulceration are prognostically significant and should be considered in treatment planning. Based on information derived from large series of patients with cutaneous melanomas at nongenital sites, regional lymphadenectomy should probably be considered a prognostic rather than a therapeutic procedure. In a multivariate analysis of 644 patients with vulvar melanoma, Sugiyama et al (22) reported 5-year disease-specific survival rates of 68%, 29%, and 19% for patients with zero, one, and two or more positive LNs, respectively. Lymphadenectomy can be avoided in patients with superficial melanomas (<1 mm), for whom the risk of metastatic disease is negligible. SLN identification and biopsy have been increasingly applied to the surgical management of cutaneous malignant melanomas, and multiple authors assert that for those surgeons who are competent with the technique, SLN mapping and biopsy should be considered a standard practice (20,21).

Historically, systemic therapy for high-risk localized or metastatic melanoma was considered strictly palliative; durable responses were rare, and adverse effects were considerable. Interferon α-2b, dacarbazine, temozolomide, and platinum-based cytotoxic therapies have shown activity in patients with small-volume tumor burden; however, toxicities are considerable, with limited improvements in survival (20). More recently, with improved molecular characterization of cutaneous (nonvulvar) melanomas and the development of multiple targeted inhibitors that have dramatically improved survival for this disease, systemic therapies for high-risk localized as well as metastatic and recurrent melanoma follow the evolving treatment paradigms of nonvulvar malignant melanoma. Examples of such targets with associated inhibitors are B-Raf (vemurafenib), c-Kit (imatinib), and CTLA-4 (ipilimumab) (23). A more involved discussion of systemic therapy for melanoma is beyond the scope of this chapter. For those gynecologic oncologists without considerable experience in the treatment of patients with melanoma, we recommend early referral for patients with high-risk localized vulvar or metastatic melanoma to a medical oncologist or gynecologic oncology center that specializes in the systemic care of patients with malignant melanoma.

Patients with superficial lesions have an excellent chance for cure after surgical resection; however, patients with deeper lesions, or metastases at the time of diagnosis, have a worse prognosis. These patients are good candidates for investigational trials.

Basal Cell Carcinoma

Basal cell carcinomas (BCCs) should be removed by excisional biopsy using a minimum surgical margin of 1 cm. Lymphatic or distant spread is exceedingly rare (24). Local recurrence may happen, particularly in tumors removed with suboptimal resection margins.

Adenocarcinoma

Patients presenting with vulvar adenocarcinoma should first undergo a clinical evaluation to determine whether the lesion in question is a vulvar cancer or a metastasis. Despite the paucity of data regarding the evaluation and treatment of vulvar adenocarcinoma, resection of localized disease with a radical margin is recommended by radical wide excision, and hemivulvectomy or radical vulvectomy seems appropriate (25). Some form of inguinal lymphadenectomy should be included with primary surgical resection. RT may have a role in enhancing local control for women with large primary tumors or inguinal metastases.

Paget Disease

Paget disease is associated with a concurrent underlying invasive adenocarcinoma component in approximately 15% of cases (26). As many as 20% to 30% of these patients will have or will later develop an adenocarcinoma at another nonvulvar location (27,28), although some more recent series suggest a lower incidence of secondary malignancies (29). Observed sites of nonvulvar malignancies developing in patients with extramammary Paget disease include breast, lung, colorectum, gastric area, pancreas, and upper female genital tract. Screening and surveillance for tumors at these sites should be considered in patients with Paget disease.

Paget disease should be resected with at least a 1-cm margin. If underlying invasion is suspected, the deep margins should be extended to the perineal fascia. Black et al (30) showed that patients with microscopically positive margins had a significantly higher rate of recurrence; however, with extended follow-up, all patients eventually recurred. Others have shown that despite surgical efforts to the contrary, microscopically positive margins are frequent, and disease recurrence is common regardless of margin status. Repeat local excision of recurrent disease is usually effective in the absence of invasion (28). Reportedly, topical imiquimod also has activity in extramammary Paget disease. In several small case series, complete response (CR) rates of as much as 92% have been reported (31,32). There are case reports of Paget disease treated with either adjuvant RT or definitive RT for medically inoperable or recurrent disease. A Cochrane review in 2019 reported use of RT as primary modality in 14 patients, although radiation treatment regimens and doses were not consistently reported (33). Some authors have suggested that when Paget disease is treated with RT, a dose of 40 to 50 Gy is recommended for intraepithelial Paget and 55 to 65 Gy for invasive Paget disease (34).

RADIATION THERAPY

Early accounts of poor survival rates after primary RT of vulvar carcinomas led some investigators to surmise that RT had a narrow therapeutic role in the curative management of patients with vulvar cancer (35). The use of high doses of radiation alone, delivered with low-energy cobalt-60 photons and en face electron boosts, in patients who were mostly poor surgical candidates resulted in a suboptimal therapeutic benefit between tumor control probability and normal tissue complications (36). More modern-day practices, such as incorporating consecutive daily fractionation, attention to dosimetric planning detail, and appreciation of vulvar and low pelvic radiation tissue tolerance limits, have undoubtedly shown that relatively high doses of radiation can be delivered safely. RT is now accepted as an important element in the multidisciplinary management of patients with vulvar cancer both as adjuvant therapy for early-stage disease and as preoperative or definitive therapy for locally advanced disease.

Adjuvant Radiotherapy to the Vulva

Standard of care for early-stage vulvar cancer includes surgical resection where possible without causing excess morbidity or disfigurement. Following initial resection of a vulvar primary tumor, various surgicopathologic features are associated with a higher risk of local recurrence, including tumor margins less than 8 mm after tissue fixation (deep or at the skin surface), lymphovascular space invasion (LVSI), and deep tumor penetration (37,38). Avoidance of local recurrence is critical given poor salvage rates, particularly among those with nodal relapse.

Although no prospective trials of postoperative vulvar site RT have been completed, adjuvant radiation of the primary tumor bed in selected patients with close/positive margins or multiple other high-risk features (LVSI, depth >1 cm, or size >4 cm with high-grade histology) does improve vulvar tumor control (39-41). For example, in a retrospective series by Faul et al (40), patients with positive surgical margins had a significant reduction (33% vs 69%) in the risk of locoregional recurrence, if receiving adjuvant RT. A similar benefit was seen for patients with close surgical margins (5% vs 31%).

More recent data indicate a potential dose-response relationship for patients with close (≤5 mm) or positive margins, where patients receiving 56 Gy or more had lower rates of vulvar recurrence compared with 50.4 Gy or less (21% vs 34%, P = .046) (41). A large national database study furthermore showed a survival advantage for patients with positive margins treated with RT dose of 54 Gy or more, with no benefit to doses above 60 Gy compared with 54.0 to 59.9 Gy (42). In combination, the data suggest that patients with close/positive margins benefit from adjuvant RT to the vulva to reduce risk of relapse. Nonetheless, after RT, the rates of locoregional relapse remain elevated, suggesting that reexcision, when feasible, may be appropriate (40,41).

Of note, when adjuvant RT is delivered to the pelvic LNs for nodal indications, the vulvar primary site should be included in the treatment field as well. This is in contrast with historical practice, where attempts were made to avoid irradiation of the vulva in order to lessen treatment morbidity and because vulvar recurrences were thought to be salvageable. For instance, GOG 37 used a central block to avoid the vulva. However, more recent data suggest lower salvage rates than previously thought. For instance, long-term follow-up of the GROINSS-V study showed a 10-year vulva recurrence of 40%, and 10-year disease-specific survival decreased from 90% to 69% for patients without versus with a local recurrence (13). In addition, a recent subset analysis of the AGO-CARE-1 study showed that 30% of patients who developed isolated vulvar recurrence had a second recurrence (18). Subsequently, the AGO-CARE-1 study showed that adjuvant RT to the vulva reduces the risk of local recurrence in node-positive patients irrespective of local risk factors. This benefit was greatest in patients positive for HPV, suggesting HPV status may be predictive in addition to prognostic (43). Finally, overall treatment time greater than 15 weeks from the date of initial surgery to completion of RT has been shown to correlate with worse OS (44).

Adjuvant Regional Radiotherapy

Prophylactic Regional Radiotherapy for Clinically Node-Negative Patients

The biggest predictor of mortality from vulvar cancer is inguinal nodal recurrence, as such recurrences are rarely salvageable (13). The two most important predictors of inguinal LN involvement are DOI (6), followed by clinical tumor size (45). In general, well-lateralized T1a lesions (<2 cm in size with ≤1 mm stromal invasion) have a low probability of nodal involvement, and for these patients surgical nodal evaluation may be omitted.

Traditionally, the standard of care for nodal management in early-stage vulvar cancer with DOI greater than 1 mm was inguinofemoral LN dissection. In this procedure, removal of both superficial and deep inguinal LNs was recommended given higher inguinal recurrence rates with limited superficial inguinal lymphadenectomy. Significant perioperative complications associated with inguinofemoral LN dissection include wound dehiscence, infection, and long-term lymphedema.

The GOG 88 study explored the question of whether groin radiation could replace inguinofemoral dissection as a less morbid treatment for patients with clinically negative inguinal nodes (46). This study randomized patients with stage IB-III, node-negative vulvar cancer status post radical vulvectomy to either bilateral inguinal RT (50 Gy in 25 fractions) or bilateral inguinofemoral dissection followed by adjuvant RT to the pelvic and inguinal nodes in case of pathologically positive nodes. This study was closed after the entry of only 58 patients when there appeared to be a higher rate of groin recurrence in the RT arm (0% vs 18.5%).

However, significant criticisms of this study include inadequate imaging assessment of the LNs and suboptimal RT technique resulting in inadequate radiation dose delivered to the target. As this study was performed in the two-dimensional (2D) RT era, CT-based planning was not used, and target volumes were not defined. Although the dose was prescribed to 3 cm depth in GOG 88, subsequent studies found that the median depth of inguinal nodes is greater than 5 cm (47). Review of GOG 88 treatment delivery revealed that all five patients who failed in the groin had inadequate tumor doses delivered (<47 Gy), and the mean depth of the inguinal vessels was 6.1 cm (48). Furthermore, 50 Gy is likely not an adequate dose for macroscopic nodal disease.

By contrast, retrospective studies have shown that with careful RT planning using modern techniques such as IMRT delivering 40 to 50 Gy prophylactically to the inguinal-pelvic LNs, regional recurrences are rare (49-52). In a large single-institution retrospective analysis, Katz et al (49) reported no differences in the inguinal relapse rates for patients treated with prophylactic groin

irradiation compared with those undergoing LN dissection. Combined across retrospective series, the incidence of groin recurrence following treatment of the undissected nodal region appears to be 0% to 12%. Improved pretreatment radiographic staging may further contribute to lower inguinal recurrence rates.

Adjuvant Regional Radiotherapy for Involved Lymph Nodes

Although the role of prophylactic RT in the undissected but high-risk groin remains controversial, there is strong evidence that adjuvant RT after surgical assessment improves regional tumor control and survival in patients who have documented nodal metastases following inguinal node dissection. This was established by the prospective GOG 37 trial (12,53), following which postoperative RT became standard for most patients with inguinal LN metastases.

In GOG 37, 114 patients underwent radical vulvectomy and inguinal lymphadenectomy. Patients who had positive inguinal nodes were randomized intraoperatively to receive either pelvic node dissection on the side containing positive groin nodes or postoperative irradiation to the bilateral pelvic and inguinal nodes. This trial was closed before the projected accrual goal, based on interim analysis identifying a significant survival benefit with RT (68% vs 54%, $P = .03$). The difference in 2-year survival rates of patients treated with RT or pelvic dissection was most marked for patients presenting with clinically positive nodes (59% vs 31%, respectively) and for those with two or more positive groin nodes (63% vs 37%, respectively). Extended follow-up showed a nonsignificant 6-year OS benefit to the radiation arm (51% vs 41%) (12). Coupled with higher rates of inguinal failure for patients treated with surgery alone (24% vs 5%), these results emphasized the poor salvage rate seen in patients developing groin recurrences. Interestingly, 8% of patients in both treatment arms had recurrences at the primary site, even though the vulva was not included in the RT field, raising the question of whether radiation to the vulva would have further increased the benefit of radiation.

One challenge at present is whether RT should be applied to patients with a single node with an adequate dissection and without ulceration or extracapsular extension. On unplanned subset analysis in GOG 37, the survival benefit seen with radiation was maintained for those with N2/3 disease, two or more positive LNs, or inadequate nodal dissection (defined as node positivity ≥20% of dissected nodes). On the other hand, no significant difference in survival was seen for patients with one microscopically positive node; the authors later commented that the number of patients in this subset was insufficient for reliable analysis. Retrospective data suggest that patients with even a single positive inguinal nodal metastasis benefit from adjuvant radiation, particularly if the groin dissection was less extensive or if nodal positive ratio is greater than 20% (12,54-56).

Another indication that radiation may be useful in patients with a single positive inguinal LN comes from the GROINSS-V study (13). Patients with a single sentinel node metastasis larger than 2 mm had a lower disease-specific survival (69.5%) than patients with a single sentinel node metastasis 2 mm or less (94.4%, $P = .001$).

Despite nodal dissection and adjuvant radiation, outcomes are poor in node-positive patients, even in the modern era. In GOG 37, the 6-year OS was only 51%, while retrospective data show similarly suboptimal survival (12,54-56). Prospective GOG trials have demonstrated high rates of distant relapse among node-positive patients, particularly in those with multiple node involvement (11,12). Although there is growing application of concurrent chemotherapy in the preoperative setting, the role of chemotherapy postoperatively has yet to be clearly addressed. Registry-based data using the National Cancer Database (NCDB) illustrated an OS benefit with adjuvant chemotherapy for patients with node-positive vulvar cancer undergoing adjuvant RT (hazard ratio [HR], 0.62; $P < .001$) (57), although prospective data are lacking.

In summary, based on GOG 37, current indications for adjuvant nodal RT following inguinofemoral LN dissection consist of: two or more positive inguinal LNs, fixated or ulcerated LN, extranodal extension, or inadequate LN dissection (≥20% positive LNs). The role of adjuvant RT in patients with a single positive LN without extranodal extension remains controversial, but retrospective data suggest these patients should be strongly considered to receive radiation based on suboptimal outcomes.

Adjuvant Radiotherapy in the Setting of Sentinel Lymph Node Biopsy

As discussed elsewhere in the text, SLNB should be offered as standard of care for women with early-stage clinically node-negative tumors of size 4 cm or more and DOI greater than 1 mm. The application of sentinel node biopsy for this population enables avoidance of the morbidity of inguinal dissection, in addition to potential identification of unexpected LN drainage patterns because of pathologic ultrastaging otherwise missed by standard dissection, and has been validated by the prospective GROINSS-VI and GOG 173 studies (13,58).

The GROINSS-VII study was designed to determine whether adjuvant RT could be a safe alternative to completion inguinofemoral dissection in patients with a positive SLNB (14). In this study, patients with negative SLNs were observed, whereas patients with positive SLN(s) received adjuvant RT with or without chemotherapy. Interim analysis demonstrated a high rate of inguinal recurrences in patients with macrometastases, defined as LN greater than 2 mm (2% for LN ≤2 mm vs 20% for LN >2 mm). Based on these findings, the trial protocol was modified to mandate completion dissection followed by possible adjuvant RT for patients with macrometastases.

Final GROINS-VII results were recently published. Overall, 21% of patients had positive SLN, of which 50% had macrometastases and 50% had micrometastases or ITCs. Among the 162 patients with macrometastases, 31% received only RT to the groins (of which 14% also had concurrent chemotherapy), and 65% underwent completion inguinofemoral LN dissection (of which 56% also received adjuvant RT). In patients with macrometastases, 2-year isolated groin recurrence rate was 22% following RT alone versus 6.9% following inguinofemoral dissection. These results suggest suboptimal efficacy of RT for macrometastases, but significant concerns have been raised regarding inadequate contouring and target volume delineation described in the original protocol, which could lead to potential geographical miss, prompting subsequent protocol modification of RT contouring details (59). Of note, no groin recurrences were observed in seven patients who received adjuvant chemoradiation, and there was a trend toward better disease control in patients who received chemoradiation ($P = .091$), suggesting that the use of concurrent chemotherapy warrants further investigation in this population.

On the other hand, GROINSS-VII results confirmed the safety of adjuvant RT with omission of completion lymphadenectomy in patients with micrometastases (≤2 mm). Among 160 patients with micrometastases/ITCs, 79% underwent adjuvant RT, with a 2-year ipsilateral isolated groin recurrence rate of 1.6%. Among the subset of patients with only ITCs, the groin recurrence rate was 0%.

Preoperative Radiotherapy

In patients who present with more advanced primary tumors, RT may be delivered preoperatively. Advocates of this approach have listed several theoretical advantages for patients with locally advanced vulvar carcinomas:

1. Less radical resection of the vulva may be adequate to achieve local tumor control after preoperative treatment of the vulva with radiation.

2. Tumor regression during radiation may allow the surgeon to obtain adequate tumor-free surgical margins without sacrificing important pelvic structures such as the urethra, anus, and the clitoris.

3. RT alone may be sufficient to sterilize microscopic regional disease when the inguinal nodes are not radiographically determined to be involved and may mobilize fixed and matted nodes, facilitating subsequent surgical excision.

Although the published experiences with preoperative single-modality RT are small, several investigators have reported excellent responses and high local control rates after treatment of advanced tumors with relatively modest doses of radiation followed by local resection (60,61). These early reports provided evidence that radiation could significantly debulk advanced local disease and allow for more conservative, viscera-sparing surgery, while preserving good local control.

Data have since emerged supporting the therapeutic benefit of concurrent chemotherapy with radiation, typically followed by limited surgical resection, in managing locally advanced disease (11,62,63). Typical regimens have included combinations of radiation coadministered with 5-FU, and cisplatin or mitomycin C. However, randomized trials of the role of concurrent chemotherapy have not been done and are unlikely to be feasible given the small number of patients with this disease.

The most compelling data in support of concurrent chemoradiation in the management of locally advanced disease come from two large prospective phase II trials performed by the GOG. In the first study (GOG protocol 101), 71 evaluable patients with locally advanced T3 or T4 disease who were deemed not resectable by standard radical vulvectomy underwent preoperative CRT (62). Chemotherapy consisted of two cycles of 5-FU and cisplatin. Radiation was delivered to a dose of 47.6 Gy, using a planned split-course regimen, with part of the radiation given twice daily during the 5-FU infusion. Patients underwent planned resection of the residual vulvar tumor, or incisional biopsy of the original tumor site in the case of complete clinical response (cCR), 4 to 8 weeks after CRT. A cCR was noted in 33 of 71 patients (47%). Following vulvar excision or biopsy, 22 patients (31%) were found to have no residual tumor in the pathologic specimen. In all, only 2 of 71 patients (3%) had unresectable disease after CRT, and in only 3 patients was it impossible to preserve urinary and/or gastrointestinal continuity following complete resection of the primary tumor. With a median follow-up interval of 50 months, 11 patients (16%) have developed locally recurrent disease in the vulva (62). These results are all the more notable considering the relatively low dose of radiation used in these typically bulky, advanced tumors.

In GOG 101, there was also a separately reported cohort of 46 evaluable patients with N2 or N3 nodal disease who were deemed initially unresectable (64). Patients received 47.6 Gy of RT in split-course fashion, with two concurrent cycles of 5-FU and cisplatin, as described earlier. Planned inguinofemoral LN dissection was performed 3 to 8 weeks later. In only two patients (5%) did nodal disease remain unresectable, and the pCR rate was 41%. At a median follow-up of 78 months, only 1 of 37 patients (3%) who completed the fully prescribed regimen of preoperative therapy and bilateral inguinofemoral node dissection relapsed in the groin. This study, although nonrandomized, provided further evidence of the efficacy of combined CRT in the management of local regionally advanced vulvar cancer.

Building on this experience, investigators sought to study weekly cisplatin (40 mg/m^2) coadministered with radiation (GOG protocol 205). Additionally, this study eliminated the break in RT and increased RT dose to 57.6 Gy. In this trial, 58 evaluable patients with untreated locally advanced T3 or T4 disease not amenable to standard radical vulvectomy underwent preoperative radiation with concurrent chemotherapy (11). Following preoperative therapy, 64% had a cCR and 50% had a pathologic complete response (pCR), a notable improvement compared with the regimen used in GOG 101.

Following preoperative chemoradiation for locally advanced disease, it remains unclear whether surgery is necessary in those who achieve cCR. In GOG 101, approximately 70% of patients who achieved cCR were found to have no pathologic residual disease in the surgical specimen (62). In GOG 205, 34 of 37 patients (92%) underwent surgical biopsy only to assess treatment response (11). Of these 34 women, 29 (78%) had biopsies showing a pCR. Based on this 22% to 30% risk of discordant findings between CR and partial response (PR), at a minimum, an excisional biopsy of the primary site should be completed to confirm a CR to treatment.

In an attempt to further improve on the pCR rate, the ongoing GOG 279 uses concurrent gemcitabine with cisplatin, integration of IMRT, and dose escalation to 64 Gy (NCT01595061). This trial recently closed to accrual, with results pending.

Definitive Radiotherapy

Historical data evaluating the use of RT alone for vulvar cancer were generally disappointing, with a significant number of recurrences and considerable toxicity. However, integration of more modern, advanced techniques such as IMRT has resulted in more favorable results from preoperative RT (51,52). As such, some have reexplored the role of definitive RT using higher cumulative doses.

Stecklein et al published a series of 33 patients with grossly enlarged inguinal nodes treated with dose-escalated definitive RT or chemoradiation (65) at MD Anderson Cancer Center. Patients received 40 to 50 Gy to the pelvis, vulva, and groins with either three-dimensional (3D) RT or IMRT, followed by a boost to gross disease to at least 60 Gy. The 3-year actuarial vulvar, groin, and distant recurrence rates were 24.2%, 17.7%, and 30.3%, whereas the 3-year OS was 51%, consistent with other dose-escalated series. Only three major late events were deemed potentially related to irradiation, consisting of iliac artery thrombosis, femoral neck fracture, and grade 3 lymphedema.

In a series of 49 women treated with dose-escalated ($\geq$55 Gy) IMRT-based chemoradiation from 2012 to 2018 at the University of Pittsburgh Medical Center, the median vulva dose was 66 Gy for patients undergoing definitive treatment and 59.4 Gy for those undergoing preoperative therapy (66). The median dose to involved nodes was 60.6 Gy. Almost all (94%) patients received concurrent chemotherapy, consisting of weekly cisplatin for a median of five cycles, and 55% ($n = 27$) were grossly node-positive by imaging. The cCR and pCR were 76% and 70%, respectively, which was notably higher compared to both GOG 101 and GOG 205. Only 9 of the 27 patients who presented with imaging-positive LNs underwent groin assessment at the time of surgery, selected based on the presence of visible residual nodal disease on posttreatment CT, and for these patients the nodal pCR rate was 67%. Of the 27 node-positive patients, the crude isolated inguinal nodal recurrence rate was 3.7% ($n = 1$). Two-year disease-free survival for definitive and preoperative patients was 81% and 55%, respectively. Grade 3 or higher acute and late toxicities occurred in 29% and 6%, respectively.

A recent Dutch multicenter phase II study showed the feasibility of capecitabine-based CRT to 64.8 Gy for locally advanced vulvar cancer, with a local cCR rate of 62% at 12 weeks after treatment. At 2 years, 42% had persistent local cCR and 58% had regional control (67). As mentioned previously, the ongoing GOG 279 trial is examining treatment intensification with RT dose escalated to 64 Gy with concurrent gemcitabine and cisplatin, and has recently closed to accrual.

In an effort to reach higher doses when treating definitively, a few studies have assessed the role of interstitial brachytherapy, either alone or after external beam radiotherapy (EBRT) (68,69). When delivering a high dose via EBRT (mean dose, 50.4 Gy) followed by an interstitial brachytherapy boost (mean dose, 28.7 Gy), Tewari et al (69) illustrated no local failures among patients with primary advanced vulvar SCC. Hoffman et al (68) similarly evaluated patients treated with interstitial brachytherapy with or without EBRT, demonstrating disease control in 7 of 10 patients receiving 70 to 90 Gy, albeit with high rates of necrosis. The considerable hot spot at the skin achieved with brachytherapy may account for this high rate of soft tissue necrosis. Brachytherapy boost should therefore be used cautiously and possibly selectively for patients with significant vaginal extension.

In summary, given the encouraging early results, dose-escalated definitive IMRT-based chemoradiation may be an acceptable alternative to extensive surgery for locally advanced vulvar cancer, with salvage surgery reserved for persistent or recurrent disease.

Radiation Therapy Technique

Patients should undergo CT or PET-CT simulation using vacuum-bag immobilization in the supine position, with lower extremities abducted in the "frog leg" position in order to reduce the presence of skin folds, which may contribute to excess skin toxicity by an auto bolus effect. Radiopaque wire should be placed to identify the visible gross disease and any relevant postoperative scars. If there is vaginal involvement, full and empty bladder scans should be obtained for use in creation of an internal target volume (ITV) to account for organ motion.

Consensus guidelines for radiation target delineation and treatment for vulvar cancer have been published (70). For adjuvant RT, the primary tumor clinical target volume (CTV) should include the entire surgical bed. Nodal CTV should include the inguinal nodal region and entire nodal dissection bed including areas of extranodal extension, and include one echelon of LN drainage above and below the involved nodes. In case of unilateral groin involvement, the contralateral groin is typically included prophylactically as well. Although the GROINSS-VII protocol allowed ipsilateral nodal treatment if the other side was negative by SLNB, recurrence patterns according to receipt of ipsilateral versus bilateral groin RT were not reported (14). Of note, when delineating the inguinal nodal compartment, it is important to use anatomic landmarks as opposed to using fixed expansions around the vessels (71). Elective nodal CTV also includes external iliac, internal iliac, and distal common iliac LNs. Dose should be 45 to 50.4 Gy to the pelvic and inguinal nodal regions and to the primary tumor surgical bed in the case of widely negative margins. In cases of close or positive margin, higher doses of 54 to 60 Gy should be used to the area of margin concern or extracapsular extension (40,41).

For preoperative or definitive radiation, the gross tumor volume (GTV) should be delineated based on both clinical examination and imaging findings including MRI for the primary tumor and PET-CT for involved LNs. The CTV should include the entire vulva, as well as the GTV with a 1-cm margin. Additional areas may need to be included depending on involvement of adjacent structures including vagina, anus, anal canal, rectum, periurethral region, urethra, bladder, and clitoris. A brachytherapy boost to the primary tumor may be required in case of significant vaginal extension, periurethral disease, or thick perineal disease.

In preoperative cases, RT dosing typically consists of 45 Gy in 25 fractions to the primary tumor and elective nodes, 50 to 50.4 Gy in 25 to 28 fractions to the involved inguinal nodal region, 55 to 58.8 Gy in 25 to 28 fractions to grossly involved nodes, and a sequential boost to the primary vulvar tumor to 56 to 60 Gy. For bulky involved nodes greater than 2 cm, an additional sequential nodal boost of 4 to 6 Gy should be considered, with plan for surgical removal of any residual LNs that persist after chemoradiation. In addition, final dose may be adjusted based on disease location, treatment tolerance and response, and likelihood of resectability. If the disease is assessed by the surgeon as unlikely to be resectable with acceptable functional outcome, then definitive chemoradiation to a total dose of 66 Gy should be considered.

A 0.5- to 1.0-cm-thick customized bolus for the vulva should be used daily during treatment and also may be required on the groin in case of superficial involved node, skin involvement, or extracapsular extension. Separate plans should be generated with and without bolus so that once the patient develops a brisk skin reaction, one can switch to the no-bolus plan. In addition, during treatment planning, a 1- to 2-cm-thick virtual bolus is created for IMRT plan optimization, which serves to extend the isodose line beyond the skin to create flash (72). On the first few days of treatment, in vivo surface dosimetry should be checked using a device such as a thermoluminescent dosimeter in order to confirm the delivered dose. A mid-treatment replan may be needed in case of significant swelling or response to treatment.

Intensity-Modulated Radiotherapy

In modern practice, IMRT has largely replaced conventional 2D and 3D external beam approaches in the treatment of vulvar cancer (**Figure 2.6-1**) and has been incorporated in recent clinical trials (ie, GOG 279). It is an attractive approach to RT in the pelvis and groin because of its ability to escalate radiation dose while

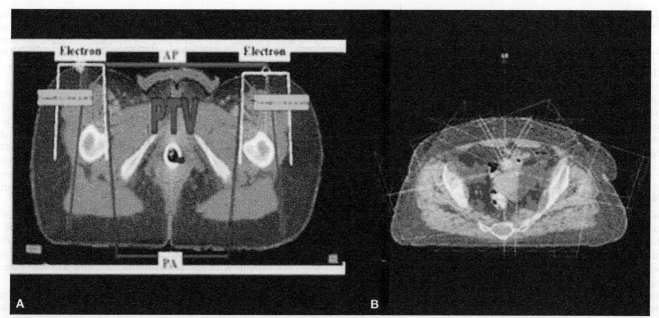

Figure 2.6-1. A: Conventional radiotherapy. B: Intensity-modulated radiation therapy in the management of vulvar cancer. (Reprinted with permission from Beriwal S, Heron D, Kim H, et al. Intensity-modulated radiotherapy for the treatment of vulvar carcinoma: a comparative dosimetric study with early clinical outcome. *Int J Radiat Oncol Biol Phys.* 2006;64:1395-1400.)

decreasing radiation dose to nearby healthy normal tissue, improving the therapeutic window for radiation. Although outcome data on IMRT for vulvar cancer remain limited to mainly single-institution series (51,52), the adoption of IMRT has been spurred by experience extrapolated from the treatment of anal carcinoma (73) and other gynecologic cancers in multi-institutional clinical trials (74,75). Prospective studies randomizing patients with cervical and endometrial cancer to postoperative pelvic RT using IMRT versus 3D technique have shown decreased acute bowel toxicity, improved patient-reported bowel quality of life, as well as decrease in both late bowel and bladder toxicities with IMRT (74,75). IMRT is also associated with improved bone marrow sparing, leading to less acute hematologic toxicity (76) and pelvic insufficiency fractures (77).

Conventional (Two- and Three-Dimensional) Radiotherapy

Historically, conventional RT approaches were based on bony anatomy as opposed to CT-based planning using anatomically defined targets. The typical plan utilized an anterior field that encompassed the inguinal regions, lower pelvic nodes, and vulva and a narrower posterior field that encompassed the lower pelvic nodes and vulva but excluded most of the femoral heads. The intent was to cover one nodal echelon proximal to the involved nodal echelon. The inferior-most borders of the fields extended 2 to 3 cm caudal to the saphenous and femoral vein junction. If the fields are evenly weighted to the midplane of the pelvis using 6 MV photons, the contribution of the anterior field to the groin nodes at a depth of 3 to 5 cm is generally 60% to 70% of the dose to the mid-pelvis. The difference would be made up by supplementing the dose to the lateral groins with anterior electron fields of appropriate energy. Some practitioners would use 6 MV from the anterior field and 15 MV from the posterior field to spare posterior organs at risk. Gross disease in the groin or vulva was boosted sequentially with en face electron fields or conformal photon RT.

Acute Complications of Radiation Therapy

Acute radiation skin reactions are brisk, and doses of 35 to 45 Gy routinely induce patchy or confluent moist desquamation. However, with adequate local care, this acute reaction usually heals within 3 to 4 weeks. Sitz baths, steroid cream, and treatment of

possible superimposed Candida infection all help to minimize the discomfort. Although most patients will develop patchy to confluent dermatitis by the fourth week of treatment, this is usually tolerated if the patient is warned in advance and assured that the discomfort will resolve after treatment is completed. Although a treatment break is occasionally required, delays should be minimized, because they may allow time for repopulation of tumor cells. IMRT helps reduce dose to uninvolved skin, especially in groin regions, which reduces dermatitis (73).

Late Complications of Radiation Therapy

Many factors contribute to the late morbidity of RT in patients with vulvar carcinoma. Patients with advanced vulvar carcinomas are often treated with RT following radical surgery, which may include extensive dissection of the inguinal and possibly pelvic nodes. Lymphedema is a chronic, disabling condition that occurs in more than 40% of patients after groin dissection as reported in the prospective GOG 244 study (78). The incidence of lower extremity edema after inguinal irradiation alone appears to be small (46). RT is likely to contribute to the cumulative incidence of peripheral leg edema following radical node dissection, but there was no significant difference evident in the GOG 37 randomized study of radiation (16%) versus pelvic node dissection (22%) (53).

Other complications include the risk of pelvic and femoral head fracture, most notably when delivering RT to the inguinal nodes (79,80). Older techniques provided substantial dose to the femoral heads, which can be decreased by techniques such as IMRT (73,81). IMRT technique has also been associated with decreased long-term bowel and bladder toxicity (74,75).

The effect of RT on the long-term cosmesis and function of the vulva is poorly understood. Although treatment with radiation or CRT and wide excision is becoming a more accepted alternative to extensive surgery for selected patients, and major complication rates appear to be acceptable, very little has been reported regarding subtler late effects of such treatment in the vulva. Possible late effects include atrophy and telangiectasias. Late effects are expected to be dose related. Better information will become available only as treating physicians record and report the late cosmetic and functional results of treatment (82). Pelvic RT is associated with late vaginal toxicity such as vaginal stenosis, which may be prevented with use of a vaginal dilator (83).

CHEMOTHERAPY

Primary Treatment of Advanced Disease

Chemotherapy monotherapy is an option for the palliative treatment of advanced disease. However, patients with advanced vulvar cancers tend to be older, with significant medical comorbidities, making them poor candidates for cytotoxic therapy because of concomitant diseases that increase the likelihood of significant adverse effects. Furthermore, recurrent vulvar cancer often occurs in the setting of extensive prior surgery and/or RT, making tolerance to cytotoxic therapy poor.

Neoadjuvant Chemotherapy

In order to reduce the morbidity of subsequent curative intent surgical therapy, a number of small studies have been performed to assess the feasibility of neoadjuvant chemotherapy in advanced primary vulvar cancer not initially amenable to surgery or RT. SCC is the only histologic type of vulvar cancer for which there are data assessing this approach. Geisler et al treated 13 patients with neoadjuvant cisplatin (50 mg/m^2) and 5-FU (1,000 mg/m^2/24 hours) q3w ($n = 10$ cisplatin and 5-FU, $n = 3$ cisplatin only). The combination achieved CRs in 100% of patients (10% CR); 9/10 patients then underwent radical vulvar resection and inguinofemoral lymphadenectomy. In all patients, preservation of anal and urethral sphincter function was achieved; 9/9 patients who completed both neoadjuvant chemotherapy and surgery remained alive and free of disease at 49 months (84).

In a more recent prospective study of 10 patients with advanced primary vulvar cancer whose only curative option was PE combined with neoadjuvant chemotherapy, patients were offered either paclitaxel (175 mg/m^2, d1) + ifosfamide (5 mg/m^2, d2) + cisplatin (70 mg/m^2, d1) [TIP], or paclitaxel (175 mg/m^2, d1) + cisplatin (70 mg/m^2, d1) [TP] at the discretion of the treating physician (TIP $n = 4$, TP $n = 5$). Overall response rate (ORR) was 80%; 9/9 patients underwent radical surgery with inguinofemoral lymphadenectomy, and all were disease-free at completion of primary combined therapy. After a median follow-up of 40 months, 56% of patients were alive and without evidence of disease (NED) (85).

A prospective multicenter trial compared four cisplatin-based regimens and one bleomycin-based regimen in 35 patients with advanced vulvar cancer; 33 of 35 patients completed chemotherapy, with PRs noted in 30 patients and stable disease noted in 3 patients; 27 patients subsequently underwent radical surgery (25 with inguinofemoral lymphadenectomy). Of 16 patients with clinically apparent nodes before treatment, 11 were found with residual nodal disease, and they then underwent CRT. At a median of 49 months of follow-up, 24 of 27 patients remained NED (86).

Before neoadjuvant therapy is considered a standard approach in advanced patients, further study involving larger numbers of patients and more controlled therapy regimens is recommended.

Systemic Treatment of Metastatic and Recurrent Vulvar Cancer

Despite the success of curative intent therapies in patients with advanced vulvar cancer, a significant proportion of patients will recur (40%-50%), and 5-year OS in this group of patients is less than 10% (62,87). Unfortunately, in view of the rarity of this disease, there is no clear standard for treatment of patients with metastatic or recurrent disease who are not amenable to surgery or RT. As a result, most patients are treated with regimens extrapolated from study of chemotherapy in metastatic SCC of the cervix or anus. Accordingly, most patients are treated with cisplatin-based combination regimens, with or without bevacizumab. Additional systemic therapy options under investigation include targeted agents and/or immunotherapy.

Early studies in vulvar cancer with single-agent cytotoxic chemotherapies such as piperazinedione, cisplatin (50 mg/m^2, q21d), and mitoxantrone were disappointing, with no responses noted (88,89). A prospective phase II study evaluated the use of cisplatin (80 mg/ m^2, q21d) + vinorelbine (25 mg/m^2, d1, d8) in 16 chemotherapy-naïve patients; 15 patients were evaluable for response, and ORR was 40%, with 4 CRs, 2 PRs, and 5 patients with stable disease. Median progression-free survival (PFS) was 10 months, with a median OS of 19 months. Toxicity was considered manageable, with nausea/ vomiting and leukopenia the primary grade 3 and 4 toxicities (90).

In HPV-negative vulvar SCC, high levels of EGFR expression are associated with advanced disease and worse outcome, which led to interest in the use of EGFR tyrosine kinase inhibitors (TKIs) in patients with advanced and recurrent vulvar cancer (91-93). A phase II prospective GOG trial using erlotinib in 41 patients with advanced or recurrent vulvar cancer described PRs in 28% and stable disease (SD) in 40% of patients. Unfortunately, responses were not durable, and grade 3 and 4 toxicities (diarrhea, dehydration, and renal failure) were notable (91).

Extrapolating from cervical cancer data showing the benefit of bevacizumab, an anti–vascular endothelial growth factor (VEGF) agent, this agent has been used in combination with cisplatin and paclitaxel for recurrent/metastatic vulvar squamous cell cancer as well (94). Patients with vulvar melanoma harboring KIT mutations may benefit from KIT or MAPK targeted agents (95).

The use of immunotherapy in vulvar cancer is an evolving area of research. A phase II study on the single-agent nivolumab for patients positive for HPV has shown promising results (96), and ongoing studies are investigating the use of pembrolizumab (97,98).

REFERENCES

1. Heller DS, Day T, Allbritton JI, et al. Diagnostic criteria for differentiated vulvar intraepithelial neoplasia and vulvar aberrant maturation. *J Low Genit Tract Dis.* 2021;25(1):57-70.
2. Tristram A, Hurt CN, Madden T, et al. Activity, safety, and feasibility of cidofovir and imiquimod for treatment of vulval intraepithelial neoplasia (RT(3)VIN): a multicentre, open-label, randomised, phase 2 trial. *Lancet Oncol.* 2014;15:1361-1368.
3. Krupp PJ, Bohm JW. 5-fluorouracil topical treatment of in situ vulvar cancer. A preliminary report. *Obstet Gynecol.* 1978;51(6):702-706.
4. Klapdor R, Wölber L, Hanker L, et al. Predictive factors for lymph node metastases in vulvar cancer. An analysis of the AGO-CaRE-1 multicenter study. *Gynecol Oncol.* 2019;154(3):565-570.
5. Yoder BJ, Rufforny I, Massoll NA, Wilkinson EJ. Stage 1A vulvar squamous cell carcinoma: an analysis of tumor invasive characteristics and risk. *Am J Surg Pathol.* 2008;32:765-772.
6. Homesley HD, Bundy BN, Sedlis A, et al. Prognostic factors for groin node metastasis in squamous cell carcinoma of the vulva (a Gynecologic Oncology Group study). *Gynecol Oncol.* 1993;49:279-283.
7. Chafe W, Richards A, Morgan L, et al. Unrecognized invasive carcinoma in vulvar intraepithelial neoplasia (VIN). *Gynecol Oncol.* 1988;31(1):154-165.
8. Modesitt SC, Waters AB, Walton L, et al. Vulvar intraepithelial neoplasia III: occult cancer and the impact of margin status on recurrence. *Obstet Gynecol.* 1998;92(6):962-966.
9. Burke TW, Levenback CF, Coleman RC. Surgical therapy of T1 and T2 vulvar carcinoma—further experience with radical wide excision and selective inguinal lymphadenectomy. *Gynecol Oncol.* 1995;57(2):215-220.
10. de Mooij Y, Burger MP, Schilthuis MS, et al. Partial urethral resection in the surgical treatment of vulvar cancer does not have a significant impact on urinary continence. A confirmation of an authority-based opinion. *Int J Gynecol Cancer.* 2007;17(1):294-297.
11. Moore DH, Ali S, Koh WJ, et al. A phase II trial of radiation therapy and weekly cisplatin chemotherapy for the treatment of locally-advanced squamous cell carcinoma of the vulva: a Gynecologic Oncology Group study. *Gynecol Oncol.* 2012;124(3):529-533.
12. Kunos C, Simpkins F, Gibbons H, et al. Radiation therapy compared with pelvic node resection for node-positive vulvar cancer: a randomized controlled trial. *Obstet Gynecol.* 2009;114(3):537-546.
13. te Grootenhuis NC, van der Zee AG, van Doorn HC, et al. Sentinel nodes in vulvar cancer: long-term follow-up of the GROningen INternational Study on Sentinel nodes in Vulvar cancer (GROINSS-V) I. *Gynecol Oncol.* 2016;140(1):8-14.
14. Oonk MHM, Slomovitz B, Baldwin PJW, et al. Radiotherapy versus inguinofemoral lymphadenectomy as treatment for vulvar cancer patients with micrometastases in the sentinel node: results of GROINSS-V II. *J Clin Oncol.* 2021;39(32):3623-3632.

15. Hyde SE, Valmadre S, Hacker NF, et al. Squamous cell carcinoma of the vulva with bulky positive groin nodes-nodal debulking versus full groin dissection prior to radiation therapy. *Int J Gynecol Cancer*. 2007;17(1):154-158.

16. Thaker NG, Klopp AH, Jhingran A, et al. Survival outcomes for patients with stage IVB vulvar cancer with grossly positive pelvic lymph nodes: time to reconsider the FIGO staging system? *Gynecol Oncol*. 2015;136(2):269-273.

17. Piura B, Masotina A, Murdoch J, et al. Recurrent squamous cell carcinoma of the vulva: a study of 73 cases. *Gynecol Oncol*. 1993;48(2):189-195.

18. Woelber L, Eulenburg C, Kosse J, et al. Predicting the course of disease in recurrent vulvar cancer—a subset analysis of the AGO-CaRE-1 study. *Gynecol Oncol*. 2019;154(3):571-576.

19. Phillips GL, Bundy BN, Okagaki T, et al. Malignant melanoma of the vulva treated by radical hemivulvectomy. A prospective study of the Gynecologic Oncology Group. *Cancer*. 1994;73(10):2626-2632.

20. Wechter ME, Reynolds RK, Haefner HK, et al. Vulvar melanoma: review of diagnosis, staging, and therapy. *J Low Genit Tract Dis*. 2004;8(1):58-69.

21. Moxley KM, Fader AN, Rose PG, et al. Malignant melanoma of the vulva: an extension of cutaneous melanoma? *Gynecol Oncol*. 2011;122(3):612-617.

22. Sugiyama VE, Chan JK, Shin JY, et al. Vulvar melanoma: a multivariable analysis of 644 patients. *Obstet Gynecol*. 2007;110(2 pt 1):296-301.

23. Janco JM, Markovic SN, Weaver AL, et al. Vulvar and vaginal melanoma: case series and review of current management options including neoadjuvant chemotherapy. *Gynecol Oncol*. 2013;129(3):533-537.

24. Lui PC, Fan YS, Lau PP, et al. Vulvar basal cell carcinoma in China: a 13-year review. *Am J Obstet Gynecol*. 2009;200(5):514.e1-514.e5.

25. Fuh KC, Berek JS. Current management of vulvar cancer. *Hematol Oncol Clin North Am*. 2012;26(1):45-62.

26. Creasman WT, Gallager HS, Rutledge F. Paget's disease of the vulva. *Gynecol Oncol*. 1975;3(2):133-148.

27. Fanning J, Lambert HC, Hale TM, et al. Paget's disease of the vulva: prevalence of associated vulvar adenocarcinoma, invasive Paget's disease, and recurrence after surgical excision. *Am J Obstet Gynecol*. 1999;180(1 pt 1):24-27.

28. Ciavattini A, Sopracordevole F, Di Giuseppe J. Surgical treatment of Paget disease of the vulva: prognostic significance of stromal invasion and surgical margin status. *J Low Genit Tract Dis*. 2016;20(3):e53-e54.

29. Niikura H, Yoshida H, Ito K, et al. Paget's disease of the vulva: clinicopathologic study of type 1 cases treated at a single institution. *Int J Gynecol Cancer*. 2006;16(3):1212-1215.

30. Black D, Tornos C, Soslow RA, et al. The outcomes of patients with positive margins after excision for intraepithelial Paget's disease of the vulva. *Gynecol Oncol*. 2007;104(3):547-550.

31. Ho SA, Aw DC. Extramammary Paget's disease treated with topical imiquimod 5% cream. *Dermatol Ther*. 2010;23(4):423-427.

32. Feldmeyer L, Kerl K, Kamarashev J, et al. Treatment of vulvar Paget disease with topical imiquimod: a case report and review of the literature. *J Dermatol Case Rep*. 2011;5(3):42-46.

33. Edey KA, Allan E, Murdoch JB, Cooper S, Byant A. Interventions for the treatment of Paget's disease of the vulva. *Cochrane Database Syst Rev*. 2019;6(6):CD009245.

34. Son S, Lee J, Kim Y, et al. The role of radiation therapy for the extramammary Paget's disease of the vulva; experience of 3 cases. *Cancer Res Treat*. 2005;37(6):365-369.

35. Helgason NM, Hass AC, Latourette HB. Radiation therapy in carcinoma of the vulva: a review of 53 patients. *Cancer*. 1972;30(4):997-1000.

36. Busch M, Wagener B, Duhmke E. Long-term results of radiotherapy alone for carcinoma of the vulva. *Adv Ther*. 1999;16(2):89-100.

37. Chan JK, Sugiyama V, Pham H, et al. Margin distance and other clinico-pathologic prognostic factors in vulvar carcinoma: a multivariate analysis. *Gynecol Oncol*. 2007;104:636-641.

38. Heaps JM, Fu YS, Montz FJ, et al. Surgical-pathologic variables predictive of local recurrence in squamous cell carcinoma of the vulva. *Gynecol Oncol*. 1990;38(3):309-314.

39. Ignatov T, Eggemann H, Burger E, et al. Adjuvant radiotherapy for vulvar cancer with close or positive surgical margins. *J Cancer Res Clin Oncol*. 2016;142:489-495.

40. Faul CM, Mirmow D, Huang Q, et al. Adjuvant radiation for vulvar carcinoma: improved local control. *Int J Radiat Oncol Biol Phys*. 1997;38(2):381-389.

41. Viswanathan AN, Pinto AP, Schultz D, et al. Relationship of margin status and radiation dose to recurrence in post-operative vulvar carcinoma. *Gynecol Oncol*. 2013;130(3):545-549.

42. Chapman BV, Gill BS, Viswanathan AN, et al. Adjuvant radiation therapy for margin-positive vulvar squamous cell carcinoma: defining the ideal dose-response using the National Cancer Data Base. *Int J Radiat Oncol Biol Phys*. 2017;97:107-117.

43. Woelber L, Prieske K, Eulenburg CZ, et al. Adjuvant radiotherapy and local recurrence in vulvar cancer—a subset analysis of the AGO-CaRE-1 study. *Gynecol Oncol*. 2022;164(1):68-75.

44. Ashmore S, Crafton SM, Miller EM, et al. Optimal overall treatment time for adjuvant therapy for women with completely resected, node-positive vulvar cancer. *Gynecol Oncol*. 2021;161:63-69.

45. Gonzalez Bosquet J, Kinney WK, Russell AH, et al. Risk of occult inguinofemoral lymph node metastasis from squamous carcinoma of the vulva. *Int J Radiat Oncol Biol Phys*. 2003;57:419-424.

46. Stehman FB, Bundy BN, Thomas G, et al. Groin dissection versus groin radiation in carcinoma of the vulva: a Gynecologic Oncology Group study. *Int J Radiat Oncol Biol Phys*. 1992;24(2):389-396.

47. McCall AR, Olson MC, Potkul RK. The variation of inguinal lymph node depth in adult women and its importance in planning elective irradiation for vulvar cancer. *Cancer*. 1995;75(9):2286-2288. doi:10.1002/1097-0142(19950501)75:9<2286::AID-CNCR2820750916>3.0.CO;2-G

48. Koh WJ, Chiu M, Stelzer KJ, et al. Femoral vessel depth and the implications for groin node radiation. *Int J Radiat Oncol Biol Phys*. 1993;27(4):969-974.

49. Katz A, Eifel PJ, Jhingran A, et al. The role of radiation therapy in preventing regional recurrences of invasive squamous carcinoma of the vulva. *Int J Radiat Oncol Biol Phys*. 2003;57(2):409-418.

50. Leiserowitz GS, Russell AH, Kinney WK, et al. Prophylactic chemoradiation of inguinofemoral lymph nodes in patients with locally extensive vulvar cancer. *Gynecol Oncol*. 1997;66(3):509-514.

51. Beriwal S, Shukla G, Shinde A, et al. Preoperative intensity modulated radiation therapy and chemotherapy for locally advanced vulvar carcinoma: analysis of pattern of relapse. *Int J Radiat Oncol Biol Phys*. 2013;85(5):1269-1274.

52. Beriwal S, Coon D, Heron DE, et al. Preoperative intensity-modulated radiotherapy and chemotherapy for locally advanced vulvar carcinoma. *Gynecol Oncol*. 2008;109(2):291-295.

53. Homesley HD, Bundy BN, Sedlis A, et al. Radiation therapy versus pelvic node resection for carcinoma of the vulva with positive groin nodes. *Obstet Gynecol*. 1986;68(6):733-740.

54. Parthasarathy A, Cheung MK, Osann K, et al. The benefit of adjuvant radiation therapy in single-node-positive squamous cell vulvar carcinoma. *Gynecol Oncol*. 2006;103(3):1095-1099.

55. Mahner S, Jueckstock J, Hilpert F, et al. Adjuvant therapy in lymph node-positive vulvar cancer: the AGO-CaRE-1 study. *J Natl Cancer Inst*. 2015;107(3):dju426.

56. Xanthopoulos E, Mitra N, Grover S, et al. Adjuvant radiation therapy in node-positive vulvar cancer. *Int J Radiat Oncol Biol Phys*. 2013;87(2):S128-S129.

57. Gill BS, Bernard ME, Lin JF, et al. Impact of adjuvant chemotherapy with radiation for node-positive vulvar cancer: a National Cancer Data Base (NCDB) analysis. *Gynecol Oncol*. 2015;137:365-372.

58. Coleman RL, Ali S, Levenback CF, et al. Is bilateral lymphadenectomy for midline squamous carcinoma of the vulva always necessary? An analysis from Gynecologic Oncology Group (GOG) 173. *Gynecol Oncol*. 2013;128(2):155-159.

59. Glaser S, Olawaiye A, Huang M, et al. Inguinal nodal region radiotherapy for vulvar cancer: are we missing the target again? *Gynecol Oncol*. 2014;135(3):583-585.

60. Hacker NF, Berek JS, Juillard GJ, et al. Preoperative radiation therapy for locally advanced vulvar cancer. *Cancer*. 1984;54(10):2056-2061.

61. Jafari K, Magalotti F, Magalotti M. Radiation therapy in carcinoma of the vulva. *Cancer*. 1981;47(4):686-691.

62. Moore DH, Thomas GM, Montana GS, et al. Preoperative chemoradiation for advanced vulvar cancer—a phase II study of the Gynecologic Oncology Group. *Int J Radiat Oncol Biol Phys*. 1998;42(1):79-85.

63. Mak RH, Halasz LM, Tanaka CK, et al. Outcomes after radiation therapy with concurrent weekly platinum-based chemotherapy or every-3-4-week 5-fluorouracil-containing regimens for squamous cell carcinoma of the vulva. *Gynecol Oncol*. 2011;120(1):101-107.

64. Montana GS, Thomas GM, Moore DH, et al. Preoperative chemoradiation for carcinoma of the vulva with N2/N3 nodes: a Gynecologic Oncology Group study. *Int J Radiat Oncol Biol Phys*. 2000;48(4):1007-1013.

65. Stecklein SR, Frumovitz M, Klopp AH, et al. Effectiveness of definitive radiotherapy for squamous cell carcinoma of the vulva with gross inguinal lymphadenopathy. *Gynecol Oncol*. 2018;148:474-479.

66. Richman AH, Vargo JA, Ling DC, et al. Dose-escalated intensity modulated radiation therapy in patients with locally-advanced vulvar cancer—does it increase response rate? *Gynecol Oncol*. 2020;159:657-662.

67. van Triest B, Rasing M, van der Velden J, et al. Phase II study of definitive chemoradiation for locally advanced squamous cell cancer of the vulva: an efficacy study. *Gynecol Oncol*. 2021;163:117-124.

68. Hoffman M, Greenberg S, Greenberg H, et al. Interstitial radiotherapy for the treatment of advanced or recurrent vulvar and distal vaginal malignancy. *Am J Obstet Gynecol.* 1990;162(5):1278-1282.

69. Tewari K, Cappuccini F, Syed AM, et al. Interstitial brachytherapy in the treatment of advanced and recurrent vulvar cancer. *Am J Obstet Gynecol.* 1999;181(1):91-98.

70. Gaffney DK, King B, Viswanathan AN, et al. Consensus recommendations for radiation therapy contouring and treatment of vulvar carcinoma. *Int J Radiat Oncol Biol Phys.* 2016;95:1191-1200.

71. Kim CH, Olson AC, Kim H, et al. Contouring inguinal and femoral nodes; how much margin is needed around the vessels? *Pract Radiat Oncol.* 2012;2(4):274-278.

72. Dyer BA, Jenshus A, Mayadev JS. Integrated skin flash planning technique for intensity-modulated radiation therapy for vulvar cancer prevents marginal misses and improves superficial dose coverage. *Med Dosim.* 2019;44:7-10.

73. Kachnic LA, Winter K, Myerson RJ, et al. RTOG 0529: a phase 2 evaluation of dose-painted intensity modulated radiation therapy in combination with 5-fluorouracil and mitomycin-C for the reduction of acute morbidity in carcinoma of the anal canal. *Int J Radiat Oncol Biol Phys.* 2013;86(1):27-33.

74. Klopp AH, Yeung AR, Deshmukh S, et al. Patient-reported toxicity during pelvic intensity-modulated radiation therapy: NRG Oncology-RTOG 1203. *J Clin Oncol.* 2018;36:2538-2544.

75. Chopra S, Gupta S, Kannan S, et al. Late toxicity after adjuvant conventional radiation versus image-guided intensity-modulated radiotherapy for cervical cancer (PARCER): a randomized controlled trial. *J Clin Oncol.* 2021;39:3682-3692.

76. Klopp AH, Moughan J, Portelance L, et al. Hematologic toxicity in RTOG 0418: a phase 2 study of postoperative IMRT for gynecologic cancer. *Int J Radiat Oncol Biol Phys.* 2013;86(1):83-90.

77. Sapienza LG, Salcedo MP, Ning MS, et al. Pelvic insufficiency fractures after external beam radiation therapy for gynecologic cancers: a meta-analysis and meta-regression of 3929 patients. *Int J Radiat Oncol Biol Phys.* 2020;106:475-484.

78. Carlson JW, Kauderer J, Hutson A, et al: GOG 244—the lymphedema and gynecologic cancer (LEG) study: incidence and risk factors in newly diagnosed patients. *Gynecol Oncol.* 2020;156:467-474.

79. Baxter NN, Habermann EB, Tepper JE, et al. Risk of pelvic fractures in older women following pelvic irradiation. *JAMA.* 2005;294(20):2587-2593.

80. Ikushima H, Osaki K, Furutani S, et al. Pelvic bone complications following radiation therapy of gynecologic malignancies: clinical evaluation of radiation-induced pelvic insufficiency fractures. *Gynecol Oncol.* 2006;103(3):1100-1104.

81. Beriwal S, Heron DE, Kim H, et al. Intensity-modulated radiotherapy for the treatment of vulvar carcinoma: a comparative dosimetric study with early clinical outcome. *Int J Radiat Oncol Biol Phys.* 2006;64(5):1395-1400.

82. Barton DP. The prevention and management of treatment related morbidity in vulval cancer. *Best Pract Res Clin Obstet Gynaecol.* 2003;17(4):683-701.

83. Damast S, Jeffery DD, Son CH, et al. Literature review of vaginal stenosis and dilator use in radiation oncology. *Pract Radiat Oncol.* 2019;9:479-491.

84. Geisler JP, Manahan KJ, Buller RE. Neoadjuvant chemotherapy in vulvar cancer: avoiding primary exenteration. *Gynecol Oncol.* 2006;100(1):53-57.

85. Raspagliesi F, Zanaboni F, Martinelli F, et al. Role of paclitaxel and cisplatin as the neoadjuvant treatment for locally advanced squamous cell carcinoma of the vulva. *J Gynecol Oncol.* 2014;25(1):22-29.

86. Aragona AM, Cuneo N, Soderini AH, et al. Tailoring the treatment of locally advanced squamous cell carcinoma of the vulva: neoadjuvant chemotherapy followed by radical surgery: results from a multicenter study. *Int J Gynecol Cancer.* 2012;22(7):1258-1263.

87. Witteveen PO, van der Velden J, Vergote I, et al. Phase II study on paclitaxel in patients with recurrent, metastatic or locally advanced vulvar cancer not amenable to surgery or radiotherapy: a study of the EORTC-GCG (European Organisation for Research and Treatment of Cancer–Gynaecological Cancer Group). *Ann Oncol.* 2009;20(9):1511-1516.

88. Thigpen JT, Blessing JA, Homesley HD, et al. Phase II trials of cisplatin and piperazinedione in advanced or recurrent squamous cell carcinoma of the vulva: a Gynecologic Oncology Group study. *Gynecol Oncol.* 1986;23(3):358-363.

89. Muss HB, Bundy BN, Christopherson WA. Mitoxantrone in the treatment of advanced vulvar and vaginal carcinoma: a Gynecologic Oncology Group study. *Am J Clin Oncol.* 1989;12(2):142-144.

90. Cormio G, Loizzi V, Gissi F, et al. Cisplatin and vinorelbine chemotherapy in recurrent vulvar carcinoma. *Oncology.* 2009;77(5):281-284.

91. Horowitz NS, Olawaiye AB, Borger DR, et al. Phase II trial of erlotinib in women with squamous cell carcinoma of the vulva. *Gynecol Oncol.* 2012;127(1):141-146.

92. Olawaiye A, Lee LM, Krasner C, et al. Treatment of squamous cell vulvar cancer with the anti-EGFR tyrosine kinase inhibitor Tarceva. *Gynecol Oncol.* 2007;106(3):628-630.

93. Bacha OM, Levesque E, Renaud MC, et al. A case of recurrent vulvar carcinoma treated with erlotinib, an EGFR inhibitor. *Eur J Gynaecol Oncol.* 2011;32(4):423-424.

94. Tewari KS, Sill MW, Long HJ III, et al. Improved survival with bevacizumab in advanced cervical cancer. *N Engl J Med.* 2014;370(8):734-743.

95. Zarei S, Voss JS, Jin L, et al. Mutational profile in vulvar, vaginal, and urethral melanomas: review of 37 cases with focus on primary tumor site. *Int J Gynecol Pathol.* 2020;39(6):587-594.

96. Naumann RW, Hollebecque A, Meyer T, et al. Safety and efficacy of nivolumab monotherapy in recurrent or metastatic cervical, vaginal, or vulvar carcinoma: results from the phase I/II checkmate 358 trial. *J Clin Oncol.* 2019;37(31):2825-2834.

97. Yeku O, Russo AL, Lee H, et al. A phase 2 study of combined chemo-immunotherapy with cisplatin-pembrolizumab and radiation for unresectable vulvar squamous cell carcinoma. *J Transl Med.* 2020;18(1):350.

98. Ott PA, Bang YJ, Piha-Paul SA, et al. T-cell-inflamed gene-expression profile, programmed death ligand 1 expression, and tumor mutational burden predict efficacy in patients treated with pembrolizumab across 20 cancers: KEYNOTE-028. *J Clin Oncol.* 2019;37(4):318-327.

CHAPTER **2.7**

Surgery for Vulvar Cancer

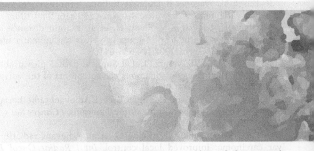

Updated by Diane C. Ling and Sushil Beriwal

In planning a surgical approach, it is important to take into account the patient's age, medical comorbidities, desire for sexual function preservation, tumor size, and disease stage. In the case of a locoregional vulvar cancer, surgery will remain the first choice of therapy (1).

Historical Background

Development of the en bloc technique of radical vulvectomy with bilateral inguinofemoral lymphadenectomy during the 1940s and 1950s was a dramatic improvement over prior surgical options, which greatly enhanced survival, particularly for women with smaller tumors and negative LNs. In this era before effective RT that could provide local and regional disease control, the ability to successfully resect vulvar tumors reduced the occurrence of terminal progression characterized by intractable pain, immobility, malodorous drainage, and bleeding. Long-term survival of 85% to 90% can be routinely obtained with radical surgery. Unfortunately, en bloc radical vulvectomy with inguinofemoral lymphadenectomy is associated with very morbid postoperative complications such as wound breakdown, lymphedema, disfigurement, and loss of sexual function. Appropriate indications for this procedure in the primary treatment of vulvar cancer are now very rare.

Presently, smaller vulvar tumors can be acceptably managed by less radical, double or triple incision surgical approaches, and many authors have proposed more limited resections for certain subsets considered to represent early or low-risk disease (2). The advantages of such approaches include retention of a significant portion of the uninvolved vulva, preservation of body image and sexual function, less operative morbidity, and fewer complications later. For women with high-risk locally advanced tumors, multimodality programs that incorporate radiation, surgery, and chemotherapy have now been validated, based on success with similar approaches in women with squamous cancers of the cervix and anus (2,3).

Wide Radical Excision

Several names have been applied to the procedures used to resect small vulvar cancers: partial deep excision, radical wide excision, radical local excision, wide local excision, modified radical vulvectomy, and hemivulvectomy. Regardless of the preferred nomenclature, the surgical procedure should be adequately defined and described. Surgical incisions are devised to allow for at least a 1- to 2-cm resection margin encompassing the primary lesion (**Figure 2.7-1**). Dissection is carried to the deep perineal fascia. Tumors located close to the anus or anal sphincter can be managed by radical wide excision with sphincter or flap repair, or they can be treated with combined modality therapy, as outlined in the RT section. Most wide radical excision sites can be closed primarily. In some patients, fasciocutaneous pedicle flaps can be used to facilitate coverage of the vulvar defect. Some form of inguinal lymphadenectomy, performed through a separate incision, is generally combined with radical wide excision.

Ambulation is begun, if possible, on the day of surgery. Perineal irrigation and air (natural or forced) drying is started within 24 hours of the surgery. The average hospital stay for patients undergoing radical wide excision is usually 1 to 2 days. Wound breakdown, usually of minor degree, is reported in at least 15% of cases (4). The incidence and severity of groin complications is proportional to the extent of the lymphadenectomy.

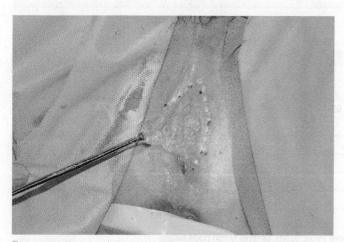

Figure 2.7-1. An early vulvar cancer identified in a background of vulvar intraepithelial neoplasia (VIN) III. A planned 2-cm margin is outlined.

Inguinofemoral Lymphadenectomy

Appropriate surgical management of the groin nodes has been evolving for many years. Original descriptions of radical vulvectomy included en bloc resection of the vulva with inguinal and pelvic LNs. The extent of lymphadenectomy was steadily reduced, first eliminating the pelvic node dissection and then reducing the extent of the groin dissection. The concept of superficial inguinal lymphadenectomy was proposed in the late 1970s; however, this approach was ultimately rejected by gynecologic oncologists owing to an unexpectedly high relapse rate (5).

The most common current approach starts with an incision parallel to and just above or below the inguinal ligament. The incision is carried through Camper fascia, and small flaps are elevated to expose the LN-bearing fat and preserve blood supply to the skin. There is no need to skeletonize the femoral artery; however, identification of the medial wall of the femoral vein helps ensure removal of the medial fat pad, where the SLN is frequently found. The dissection can usually be performed solely with electrocautery or a small vessel-sealing device. The saphenous vein is encountered at the lower medial margin of the dissection and, whenever possible, should be preserved to reduce the risk for postoperative lymphedema. The dissected specimen is removed for pathologic assessment. The skin incision can be closed with either staples or absorbable sutures. A closed-suction drain is placed and removed when output is less than 25 mL/d.

Unfortunately, historic nomenclature for performance of inguinofemoral lymphadenectomy has been inconsistent and often confusing. The authors find the terms "deep" and "superficial" especially troubling and, in the SLN era, largely meaningless. A satisfactory groin dissection has been performed when the inguinal ligament, adductor longus, saphenous vein, medial wall of the femoral vein, and the fossa ovalis have been identified, and the LNs and most adipose tissue within these boundaries are removed. Cadaver studies identify 8 to 10 LNs in the femoral triangle defined by the inguinal ligament, sartorius muscle, and adductor longus. Surgical node counts are dependent on the thoroughness of the surgeon and pathologist.

Sentinel Inguinal Lymph Node Biopsy

The SLN is defined as the first draining LN of a tumor and can be identified using a lymphatic mapping technique. This is based on the observation that peritumoral injection of a liquid-based material results in superficial cutaneous lymphatic channel absorption of this material followed quickly by transport to the SLN. Either a vital blue dye or radiocolloid, or both, can be used to facilitate SLN identification by direct visualization and/or detection of low levels of radioactivity by a handheld radiation detection device or imaging study (**Figures 2.7-2 and 2.7-3**). The modern SLN concept was first described by Morton and colleagues in patients with cutaneous melanoma; shortly thereafter, it was described in patients with vulvar cancer (6,7). Preliminary experience with both intraoperative lymphatic dye and radioisotope injections confirmed that the SLN of the vulva is always in the inguinal LN basin and can be identified in most patients (8,9). This early experience supported the concept that the successful assessment of lymphatic metastases may ultimately be accomplished with resection/biopsy of one or two SLNs.

Based on these pilot study results, two large multi-institutional trials were initiated to determine the utility of SLNB in women with vulvar cancer. The GROINSS-V trial used a prospective, observational design, enrolling 403 evaluable women with tumors of size 4 cm or less who underwent SLNB alone. Of these, 276 women had a negative SLNB and were closely observed for recurrence during a 2-year follow-up period. Eight patients (2.9%) suffered a groin relapse. When patients with multifocal primary tumors were removed from the analysis, the relapse rate was only 2.3% (10). Long-term results in 377 patients with unifocal disease from this same study were subsequently reported, detailing 36.4% and

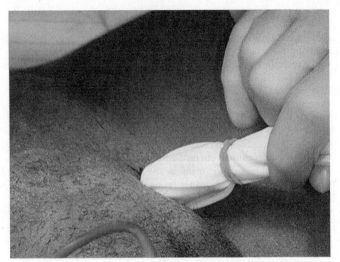

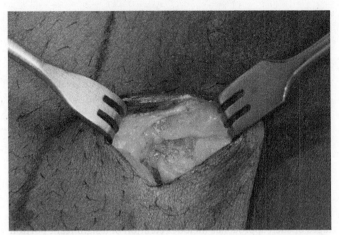

■ **Figure 2.7-2.** Transdermal localization of a sentinel node using a handheld gamma counter. The probe has a collimator and is pointed away from the primary tumor. Radioactivity will fall off rapidly until the sentinel node is encountered. Mark the site of an increase in activity.

■ **Figure 2.7-3.** A hot, blue sentinel node identified through a small incision. Frozen section is requested only if the sentinel node is grossly suspicious. Immunohistochemical staining is performed if the routine hematoxylin and eosin staining does not reveal metastatic disease. After a sentinel node is removed, the wound is explored with the gamma counter to ensure that there is no other sentinel node in the field.

46.4% (*P* = .03) 10-year local recurrence rate for sentinel node–negative and sentinel node–positive patients, respectively. In addition, they found that isolated groin recurrence rate was 2.5% for sentinel node–negative patients and 8% for sentinel node–positive patients at 5 years. The authors concluded that although survival is favorable for sentinel node-negative patients, the high rate of local recurrence in these patients is of concern (11).

The second study, GOG 173, employed a validation design. All women underwent SLNB followed by unilateral or bilateral inguinofemoral lymphadenectomy: 515 women were enrolled, and 418 were evaluable. If the primary tumor was more than 2 cm from the midline, a unilateral SLNB and inguinofemoral lymphadenectomy were performed. If the tumor was within 2 cm of the midline, or involved the midline, bilateral inguinal lymphadenectomies were performed. The false-negative rate was 8.3%, and the false-negative predictive value (FNPV) was 3.7% for the entire cohort. The FNPV is a prediction of the chance of a positive non-SLN when the SLN is free of tumor and a lymphadenectomy has not been performed. In GOG 173, the FNPV for patients with tumor 4 to 6 cm in size was 7.4%; for patients with tumors less

than 4 cm, it was 2%. This means that a patient with a tumor less than 4 cm, no palpable LNs, and a negative SLNB has a 2% chance of having a positive non-SLN (12).

The results of these studies indicate that, for appropriately selected women in the care of a surgeon experienced with this technique, the risk of groin relapse following a negative SLNB is 2% to 3% (**Table 2.7-1**). This compares favorably with superficial inguinal lymphadenectomy, as reported by Stehman et al (13) for the GOG. As with all surgical innovations, individual practitioners must use care when implementing new procedures. Gynecologic oncologists can learn the procedure from peers or from surgical oncologists treating patients with melanoma or breast cancer. Prior to adopting this as the standard, each gynecologic oncologist should determine their own false-negative rate by performing SLNB followed by inguinofemoral lymphadenectomy in approximately 10 cases. Some practices see very few patients with vulvar cancer, in which case referral is appropriate. Considered together, the GROINS-V and GOG 173 trials strongly support an assertion that, under the appropriate circumstances, SLNB should be offered to eligible women with vulvar cancer.

■ **TABLE 2.7-1. Sentinel Lymph Node Biopsy Sensitivity Analysis**

Analysis	SLNB Result	Present	Absent	Total	Sensitivity	90% CI	NPV (%)	90% CI	FNPV (%)	90% CI
By patients	Positive	121	0	121						
	Negative	11	286	297						
	Total	132	286	418	91.7	86.7-95.3	96.3	93.9-97.9	3.7	2.1-6.1
By groin	Positive	140	0	140						
	Negative	12	441	453						
	Total	152	441	593	92.1	87.5-95.4	97.4	95.7-98.5	2.7	1.5-4.3
In tumors <4 cm	Positive	67	0	67						
	Negative	4	198	202						
	Total	71	198	269					2.0	0.7-4.5
In tumors >4 cm	Positive	54	0	54						
	Negative	7	88	95						
	Total	61	88	149					7.4	3.5-13.4

CI, confidence interval; FNPV, false-negative predictive value; NPV, negative predictive value; SLNB, sentinel lymph node biopsy.

Reprinted with permission from Levenback CF, Ali S, Coleman RL, et al. Lymphatic mapping and sentinel lymph node biopsy in women with squamous cell carcinoma of the vulva: a Gynecologic Oncology Group study. *J Clin Oncol*. 2012;30(31):3786-3791.

It is important to note that the largest SLN evaluations to date have all involved pathologic ultrastaging with serial sectioning and immunohistochemical (IHC) staining if routine hematoxylin and eosin (H&E) staining does not reveal metastatic disease. In most studies, including GOG 173 and GROINS-V, approximately half of the LN metastases were detected by IHC staining. SLNB thus reduces the number of unnecessary lymphadenectomies performed in node-negative women, while at the same time identifying additional women who may benefit from adjuvant therapy.

A subanalysis of GOG 173 data also provided guidance regarding when unilateral groin evaluation is safe. GOG 173 required bilateral LN evaluation except when the tumor was more than 2 cm from a midline structure. There were 234 women enrolled in GOG 173 who had a preoperative lymphoscintigraphy (LSG), and at least one SLN was identified during surgery. There were 105 women with midline primary tumors; 32 of these women had unilateral drainage on preoperative LSG. Four of these patients had LN metastases on the side that did not have LSG drainage. There were 65 women with tumors located within 2 cm of the midline but not directly involving a midline structure; 27 women (42%) had unilateral drainage on LSG and bilateral surgical groin evaluation. None of these patients had metastases to the side without LSG drainage. These data support the time-honored oncologic surgical experience that midline tumors can have bilateral drainage and a unilateral LSG should not result in omission of one side (14). Conversely, if the tumor is lateralized (>2 cm from midline) and unilateral drainage is confirmed by LSG, unilateral SLNB is appropriate. The authors routinely obtain preoperative LSG, preferably by single-photon emission computerized tomography (SPECT)/CT (see **Figure 2.7-4**), regardless of the location of the primary tumor, because it helps confirm the location of the SLN in three dimensions as well as the lymphatic drainage pattern.

The combination of local vulvar resection and SLNB holds the promise of improved outcomes for many women with vulvar cancer. Preservation of sexual function and body image, a reduction in the risk of lymphedema, and more focused use of adjuvant therapy are all possible.

Sentinel Lymph Node Biopsy Technique

As discussed earlier, SLNB should be offered as an alternative to inguinofemoral lymphadenectomy for women with tumors of size 4 cm or less, with no suspicious LNs on physical examination or imaging and no prior groin surgery or radiation that might interfere with lymphatic drainage pathways. There is insufficient

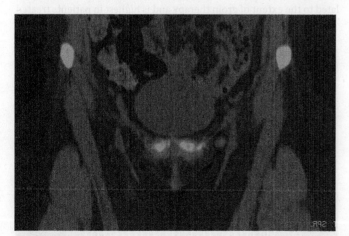

■ **Figure 2.7-4.** SPECT/CT demonstrating left sentinel lymph node just medial to the femoral vein. SPECT/CT provides superior localization of sentinel lymph nodes compared with two-dimensional lymphoscintigraphy. The number of sentinel nodes identified should correspond to the number removed at surgery. CT, computerized tomography; SPECT, single-photon emission computerized tomography.

evidence to make a recommendation regarding SLNBs in women who have tumors greater than 4 cm or multifocal disease (15,16).

The authors obtain an LSG in most patients. If possible, the surgeon should perform the injection for vulvar cancer or ensure that the nuclear medicine specialist is comfortable with injecting the vulva. The injection is painful; EMLA cream can be helpful in decreasing the associated discomfort. SLNs can be identified using a dye such as isosulfan blue, blue violet, or methylene blue or a radioactive tracer called technetium-99m (Tc-99m) with LSG; the blue dye and radiotracer can be used alone or in combination. If using Tc-99m, 0.1 to 0.5 mCi radiolabeled filtered Tc-99m is generally injected 1 day prior to surgery, followed by the performance of a preoperative scintigraphy (usually on the morning of surgery) (17).

Various techniques have been described for SLN. de Hullu et al described their technique involving a combination of Tc-99m as well as blue dye. In their protocol, 0.2 to 0.6 mL of 60 MBq Tc-99m-labeled nanocolloid is injected circumferentially around the tumor and LSG is performed, and skin sites correlating with the findings of the lymphoscintigram SLN location are marked with a pencil. On the morning of the surgery, following induction of anesthesia, 2.0 mL of patent blue dye (2.5% in aqueous solution containing 0.6% sodium chloride and 0.05% disodium hydrogen phosphate) is injected in the same locations. SLNs are then identified using a handheld gamma probe. For SLN dissections employing only blue dye, 4 mL of isosulfan blue can be injected adjacent to the primary tumor. Following injection, the tissues can be massaged to aid with dye dispersal. After approximately 5 minutes, a groin incision can be made and LN dissection carried out. In those patients with midline tumors, bilateral injections should be performed (17).

The half-life of the radiocolloid is approximately 6 hours, so a patient can be injected in the morning and operated on the same day. Frequently, this is not possible, and a second injection is necessary. If blue dye is utilized, it is visible in the SLN for only 45 minutes. The authors typically inject the radiocolloid prior to sterile prepping and draping, and inject the blue dye only when the team is prepared to make an incision. All injections are intradermal, 0.5 to 1.0 cm from the tumor itself. Intratumoral or subcutaneous injections will most likely result in a failure to identify the SLN. Transdermal localization of the SLN using a handheld gamma counter is possible in most patients. The SLN is identified using a 10-fold higher measured radiation than the basal count at the primary injection site (17).

There are pros and cons to the various methods and injection materials used in SLN dissection. If using blue dye, the color becomes visible in the nodes and lymphatic channels, quickly allowing for rapid SLN dissection (18). There is a low rate of hypersensitivity reactions to blue dye, and the dye is also inexpensive (19,20). The disadvantage of using blue dye is that it rapidly passes through the lymphatics, and so it is possible to miss the SLN (19). The advantages of LSG include the ability to determine the number and location of the SLNs preoperatively and to detect an SLN outside the nodal basin; however, the cost of equipment associated with the use of a radiotracer, as well as the involvement of nuclear medicine, requires more coordination between the operating room and radiology departments (19).

SPECT/CT is also valuable for locating the SLN in relation to the femoral vessels (**Figure 2.7-4**). A small incision is made over the location of the SLN. Although data are limited, clinical experience indicates that the SLN is commonly medial to the femoral vein and just above the adductor longus muscle. Once the SLN is removed, the wound is scanned for any residual radioactivity. It is imperative that all SLNs in the groin are removed. The gamma counter may detect second echelon nodes in the pelvis just above the inguinal ligament. If blue lymphatic channels lead to a node that is not hot or blue, it is still considered an SLN.

Studies in vulvar cancer in which SLN dissection was performed, followed by a completion inguinofemoral lymphadenectomy, suggest that the SLN is accurate in identifying LN metastasis with an NPV approaching 100% (20). A meta-analysis undertaken by Meads et al evaluated SLN detection rates between blue dye, radiotracer, and combination injection. Within this meta-analysis, combined blue dye and Tc-99m testing had the highest rate of SLN detection; pooled rates are 94.0% for Tc-99m (95% confidence interval [CI], 90.5-96.4), 68.7% for blue dye alone (95% CI, 63.1-74.0), and 97.7% for Tc-99m and blue dye combined (95% CI, 96.6-98.5) (21).

Within the pathology laboratory, the evaluation of SLNs requires detailed and systematic evaluation of the submitted specimen. The LN sample submitted requires proper identification of patient name, source, name of the surgeon submitting, node location, date, and number of nodes identified.

In sectioning SLNs, it is recognized that, to achieve close to 100% identification of all metastases, the section spacing must be one-half the diameter of the tumor to be detected (21). The LN or nodes are sliced in 1- to 2-mm slices, cutting the LN at right angles to the long axis of the node. All of the LN tissue (slices) should be submitted for study.

Once the nodal tissue is embedded in the paraffin block, the node slices can be cut at closer intervals to improve tumor detection. Although there are some variations on this sectioning method, our approach is to cut three sections from each block. After facing the block to get a full face of the sectioned nodal tissue, the first 5-μm section is cut. This section is stained with H&E. We then cut 100 μm into the block and cut another 5-μm section. This second slide is held for additional H&E staining, or IHC, if the first and last H&E sections have equivocal findings. We then cut an additional 100 μm into the block and take the third section. This slide is stained with H&E. The pathologist reviews the two H&E slides, and if the findings are equivocal, the held second slide is then studied.

Limited information is available regarding ideal surveillance following SLNB. Our preferred technique is ultrasound, because it is noninvasive and the internal architecture of the LNs can be imaged (**Figure 2.7-5A,B**). Early detection of a groin failure may help improve outcomes with multimodality treatment.

Surgical Resection for Recurrent Disease

The site and volume of recurrent vulvar lesions dictate both resectability and potential for cure. Recurrences can be categorized as local (vulvar), inguinal, or distant (pelvis, lower extremity, or beyond). Surgical therapy plays a curative or palliative role in selected subsets of patients with recurrent disease.

Wide Radical Excision

As many as 75% of patients with recurrent disease limited to the vulva can be salvaged by radical wide excision (partial deep vulvectomy) or reexcision of the tumor (22,23). Surgical principles of recurrent vulvar tumors are identical to those for primary tumors: wide excision with a measured normal tissue margin of at least 1 to 2 cm. Particular attention is also focused on obtaining a clear deep margin. Because most patients have had prior operative therapy, primary closure of the vulvar defect is frequently more difficult. More complex reconstructive efforts may be needed to restore tissue integrity.

Radical Vulvectomy

Rarely, radical vulvectomy may be indicated for recurrent vulvar cancer. The classic description of en bloc radical vulvectomy and bilateral lymphadenectomy can be based on either a "butterfly" or "longhorn" approach. The butterfly incisions use convex "wings" over the groin and around the anus to facilitate closure of the defect (**Figure 2.7-6**). The longhorn incisions were developed to limit skin resection over the groin in an attempt to reduce wound breakdown (24). The arcing superior incision is placed from the lateral margins of the groin dissection across the mons pubis. The lateral vulvar incisions are placed at the labiocrural folds, because these topographic landmarks represent the most lateral location of the superficial vulvar lymphatics. The perianal incision is placed to allow resection of the perineal body. These incisions are taken to the level of the deep inguinal and perineal fascia and permit en bloc removal of both superficial and deep groin nodes, the entire vulva, and an intervening skin bridge.

After removal of the specimen, the skin and mucosal edges are undermined to permit mobilization and primary closure with delayed absorbable suture. Some degree of tension at the suture lines is unavoidable, particularly in the perineal body and periurethral areas. Closed-suction drains are usually placed in the groin sites to remove excess lymphatic and serous fluid accumulations and are usually removed when drain output is minimal (5-14 days).

A small degree of wound breakdown is seen in approximately 50% of patients. Local wound care results in satisfactory secondary healing in most of these cases. Lymphocyst formation is relatively common and frequently presents as a tense but nontender groin mass. Percutaneous needle drainage is usually sufficient, but occasionally replacement of a groin drain may be required. Inguinal cellulitis, lower extremity lymphangitis, and lymphedema are uncommon late sequelae. The incidence of these complications is related to the extent of groin therapy and is highest in patients treated

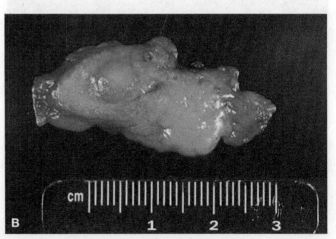

Figure 2.7-5. Close surveillance following sentinel lymph node biopsy is recommended because groin relapse is difficult to treat. Physical examination is very unreliable. A: Ultrasound can be very effective, as illustrated here. Six months after negative sentinel lymph node biopsy, ultrasound detected a 5-mm metastasis. Fine needle aspiration confirmed metastatic disease. B: The patient underwent inguinal femoral lymphadenectomy and radiation therapy. She remains disease free at 2 years.

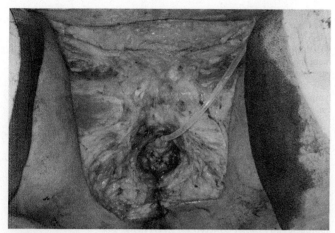

Figure 2.7-6. Butterfly incision described for a traditional radical vulvectomy with bilateral inguinal lymphadenectomy. Modern indications for radical vulvectomy are exceedingly rare. The patient shown in **Figure 18.5** was treated with concurrent chemoradiation and still had bilateral gross tumor. This figure demonstrates the field following resection.

with superficial and deep lymphadenectomy followed by inguinal RT. The three-incision concept preserves the radicality of the vulvar resection while retaining skin over the groin. Consequently, the incidence of major wound breakdown is significantly reduced to approximately 15% to 20% of cases (25). As with other techniques, the incidence and severity of groin complications such as infection, wound breakdown, or lymphocyst formation remain high (4).

Pelvic Exenteration

Curative resection may still be possible when vulvar recurrence extends to the vagina, proximal urethra, or anus. Selected patients have achieved long-term survival after PE for such recurrences (26,27). The surgical approach in these cases should be individualized to the size and location of the recurrent tumor, prior therapies, and the age and overall health of the patient. Patients considered for PE should have a thorough preoperative evaluation to exclude the presence of regional and/or distant metastases. Frequently, anterior or posterior exenteration with an extended vulvar phase will provide excellent resection margins, while allowing preservation of either urinary or fecal continence. The techniques used to perform the exenteration are identical to those routinely used for the treatment of women with recurrent cervical carcinoma. Multiple vulvar and perineal reconstructive techniques have been described for coverage of large surgical defects (28-30).

Resection of Groin Recurrence

Patients who develop isolated groin recurrence should be treated with multimodality treatment if radiotherapy is still an option. Surgical resection should be viewed with caution in the previously irradiated patient. A resection with negative margins usually requires the resection of vessels or bone with plastic reconstruction. Ultraradical surgery attempted in young patients with outstanding performance status and a small relapse in an irradiated groin that appears resectable on preoperative imaging is associated with high morbidity. Extended survival is possible for the few patients who achieve control of recurrent disease in the groin and do not later manifest distant metastasis (31). Isolated groin recurrence is a rare event, so the data to support the efficacy of this treatment are anecdotal.

Vulvar Reconstruction

With careful planning and adequate tissue mobilization, most vulvar defects can be closed primarily. When large portions of the vulva have been resected, when tissue mobility is poor, or when

RT has been administered previously, primary closure may not be feasible. Alternate tissue sources must be considered for these difficult cases. Categorically, the two types of techniques commonly employed for extensive vulvar reconstruction are fasciocutaneous flaps and myocutaneous flaps. Local advancement flaps can be used for smaller defects, and pedicled flaps harvested from the inner thigh, gluteal fold, and the abdomen are used for larger defects. The techniques referenced in the next section should be employed only by surgeons who are regularly practiced in their use.

Fasciocutaneous Advancement Flaps

A variety of fasciocutaneous advancement flaps are described for vulvar reconstruction. These flaps include skin, underlying subcutaneous tissue, and underlying fascia. Nearly all of them are based on the rich, redundant blood supply from the internal pudendal artery and subsequent superficial perineal artery perforators that approach the vulva and perineum, primarily from the posterior and lateral directions. This is significant because most vulvar fasciocutaneous flaps are designed to preserve fasciocutaneous perforators from these directions. Studies performed by John et al have evaluated approaches to perineal reconstruction following resection of large portions of the vulva and perineum. Following a wide local excision, the most common reconstructive method is the local flap. If larger amounts of tissue are removed, the next choice for reconstruction is the V-Y advancement flap, with or without incorporation of the gracilis muscle (32).

Among gynecologic oncologists, the most widely utilized pedicle flap has been the rhomboid flap; however, lotus petal flaps are also commonly used by plastic surgeons for closure of large vulvar defects. The lotus petal fasciocutaneous flap, irrespective of the specific design, is supplied primarily by perforating branches of the internal pudendal artery and also through nonperforating branches of the inferior gluteal artery. The lotus petal flap best respects a natural anatomic fold at the donor site, leading to the most cosmetic donor site closure (33). Although a detailed discussion of the techniques employed for these flaps is outside the scope of this chapter, references for multiple fasciocutaneous flaps that have been employed by these authors are referenced here (29,34,35).

Myocutaneous Flaps

Myocutaneous flaps, in comparison with fasciocutaneous advancement flaps, include a segment of muscle and usually receive their blood supply and innervation through an identifiable, named neurovascular pedicle. These are usually large, thick tissue sources that are best suited for the reconstruction of substantial defects. Each of the following listed flaps has notable advantages and disadvantages. Several types of myocutaneous flaps, namely the gracilis, gluteus maximus, tensor fascia lata, vastus lateralis, and vertical rectus abdominus flaps, have been used to repair and reconstruct large vulvar and groin defects (30). Historically, the gracilis flap was used to fill large vulvar and urogenital defects; however, in recent decades, the myocutaneous flap most commonly described for extensive vulvar reconstruction is the transverse rectus abdominis muscle (TRAM) flap based on the robust inferior epigastric pedicle. TRAM flaps are useful for repairing defects in the anterior vulvar regions (36). As with fasciocutaneous flaps, a detailed description of each flap is beyond the scope of this chapter; however, a number of techniques are referenced here (34,37).

Vulvar reconstruction with myocutaneous flaps has numerous disadvantages when compared with fasciocutaneous flaps, namely, increased intraoperative complexity, requirement for meticulous wound care postoperatively, and requirement for larger incisions. Myocutaneous flaps require the sacrifice of functional muscles. Fasciocutaneous flaps, in contrast, do not sacrifice muscle and can be performed with a more modest-sized flap thickness, resulting in less morbidity (36). Regardless of method or type of flap performed, it is important to monitor patients in the postoperative period for wound dehiscence and flap necrosis (32).

REFERENCES

1. Zweizig S, Korets S, Cain JM. Key concepts in management of vulvar cancer. *Best Pract Res Clin Obstet Gynaecol.* 2014;28(7):959-966.

2. Fuh KC, Berek JS. Current management of vulvar cancer. *Hematol Oncol Clin North Am.* 2012;26(1):45-62.

3. Moore DH, Ali S, Koh WJ, et al. A phase II trial of radiation therapy and weekly cisplatin chemotherapy for the treatment of locally-advanced squamous cell carcinoma of the vulva: a Gynecologic Oncology Group study. *Gynecol Oncol.* 2012;124(3):529-533.

4. Gaarenstroom KN, Kenter GG, Trimbos JB, et al. Postoperative complications after vulvectomy and inguinofemoral lymphadenectomy using separate groin incisions. *Int J Gynecol Cancer.* 2003;13(4):522-527.

5. Burke TW, Stringer CA, Gershenson DM, et al. Radical wide excision and selective inguinal node dissection for squamous cell carcinoma of the vulva. *Gynecol Oncol.* 1990;38(3):328-332.

6. Morton DL, Wen DR, Foshag LJ, et al. Intraoperative lymphatic mapping and selective cervical lymphadenectomy for early-stage melanomas of the head and neck. *J Clin Oncol.* 1993;11(9):1751-1756.

7. Levenback C, Burke TW, Gershenson DM, et al. Intraoperative lymphatic mapping for vulvar cancer. *Obstet Gynecol.* 1994;84(2):163-167.

8. Levenback C, Burke TW, Morris M, et al. Potential applications of intraoperative lymphatic mapping in vulvar cancer. *Gynecol Oncol.* 1995;59(2):216-220.

9. Decesare SL, Fiorica JV, Roberts WS, et al. A pilot study utilizing intraoperative lymphoscintigraphy for identification of the sentinel lymph nodes in vulvar cancer. *Gynecol Oncol.* 1997;66(3):425-428.

10. Van der Zee AG, Oonk MH, De Hullu JA, et al. Sentinel node dissection is safe in the treatment of early-stage vulvar cancer. *J Clin Oncol.* 2008;26(6):884-889.

11. te Grootenhuis NC, van der Zee AG, van Doorn HC, et al. Sentinel nodes in vulvar cancer: long-term follow-up of the GROningen INternational Study on Sentinel nodes in Vulvar cancer (GROINSS-V) I. *Gynecol Oncol.* 2016;140(1):8-14.

12. Levenback CF, Ali S, Coleman RL, et al. Lymphatic mapping and sentinel lymph node biopsy in women with squamous cell carcinoma of the vulva: a Gynecologic Oncology Group study. *J Clin Oncol.* 2012;30(31):3786-3791.

13. Stehman FB, Ali S, DiSaia PJ. Node count and groin recurrence in early vulvar cancer: a Gynecologic Oncology Group study. *Gynecol Oncol.* 2009;113(1):52-56.

14. Coleman RL, Ali S, Levenback CF, et al. Is bilateral lymphadenectomy for midline squamous carcinoma of the vulva always necessary? An analysis from Gynecologic Oncology Group (GOG) 173. *Gynecol Oncol.* 2013;128(2):155-159.

15. Slomovitz BM, Coleman RL, Oonk MH, et al. Update on sentinel lymph node biopsy for early-stage vulvar cancer. *Gynecol Oncol.* 2015;138(2):472-477.

16. Covens A, Vella ET, Kennedy EB, et al. Sentinel lymph node biopsy in vulvar cancer: systematic review, meta-analysis and guideline recommendations. *Gynecol Oncol.* 2015;137(2):351-361.

17. de Hullu JA, Hollema H, Piers DA, et al. Sentinel lymph node procedure is highly accurate in squamous cell carcinoma of the vulva. *J Clin Oncol.* 2000;18(15):2811-2816.

18. Burke TW, Levenback CF, Coleman RC. Surgical therapy of T1 and T2 vulvar carcinoma—further experience with radical wide excision and selective inguinal lymphadenectomy. *Gynecol Oncol.* 1995;57:215-219.

19. Levenback C, Coleman RL, Burke TW, et al. Intraoperative lymphatic mapping and sentinel node identification with blue dye in patients with vulvar cancer. *Gynecol Oncol.* 2001;83(2):276-281.

20. Zivanovic O, Khoury-Collado F, Abu-Rustum NR, et al. Sentinel lymph node biopsy in the management of vulvar carcinoma, cervical cancer, and endometrial cancer. *Oncologist.* 2009;14(7):695-705.

21. Meads C, Sutton AJ, Rosenthal AN, et al. Sentinel lymph node biopsy in vulval cancer: systematic review and meta-analysis. *Br J Cancer.* 2014;110(12):2837-2846.

22. Piura B, Masotina A, Murdoch J, et al. Recurrent squamous cell carcinoma of the vulva: a study of 73 cases. *Gynecol Oncol.* 1993;48(2):189-195.

23. Hopkins MP, Reid GC, Morley GW. The surgical management of recurrent squamous cell carcinoma of the vulva. *Obstet Gynecol.* 1990;75(6):1001-1005.

24. Abitbol MM. Carcinoma of the vulva: improvements in the surgical approach. *Am J Obstet Gynecol.* 1973;117(4):483-489.

25. Hacker NF, Eifel PJ, van der Velden J. Cancer of the vulva. *Int J Gynaecol Obstet.* 2012;119(suppl 2):S90-S96.

26. Miller B, Morris M, Levenback C, et al. Pelvic exenteration for primary and recurrent vulvar cancer. *Gynecol Oncol.* 1995;58(2):202-205.

27. Forner DM, Lampe B. Exenteration in the treatment of stage III/IV vulvar cancer. *Gynecol Oncol.* 2012;124(1):87-91.

28. Yii NW, Niranjan NS. Lotus petal flaps in vulvo-vaginal reconstruction. *Br J Plast Surg.* 1996;49(8):547-554.

29. Sawada M, Kimata Y, Kasamatsu T, et al. Versatile lotus petal flap for vulvoperineal reconstruction after gynecological ablative surgery. *Gynecol Oncol.* 2004;95(2):330-335.

30. McMenamin DM, Clements D, Edwards TJ, et al. Rectus abdominis myocutaneous flaps for perineal reconstruction: modifications to the technique based on a large single-centre experience. *Ann R Coll Surg Engl.* 2011;93(5):375-381.

31. Cormio G, Loizzi V, Carriero C, et al. Groin recurrence in carcinoma of the vulva: management and outcome. *Eur J Cancer Care (Engl).* 2010;19(3):302-307.

32. John HE, Jessop ZM, Di Candia M, et al. An algorithmic approach to perineal reconstruction after cancer resection—experience from two international centers. *Ann Plast Surg.* 2013;71(1):96-102.

33. Argenta PA, Lindsay R, Aldridge RB, et al. Vulvar reconstruction using the "lotus petal" fascio-cutaneous flap. *Gynecol Oncol.* 2013;131(3):726-729.

34. Franchelli S, Leone MS, Bruzzone M, et al. The gluteal fold fascio-cutaneous flap for reconstruction after radical excision of primary vulvar cancers. *Gynecol Oncol.* 2009;113(2):245-248.

35. Buda A, Confalonieri PL, Rovati LC, et al. Tunneled modified lotus petal flap for surgical reconstruction of severe introital stenosis after radical vulvectomy. *Int J Surg Case Rep.* 2012;3(7):299-301.

36. Vitale SG, Valenti G, Biondi A, et al. Recent trends in surgical and reconstructive management of vulvar cancer: review of literature. *Updates Surg.* 2015;67(4):367-371.

37. Petrie N, Branagan G, McGuiness C, et al. Reconstruction of the perineum following anorectal cancer excision. *Int J Colorectal Dis.* 2009;24(1):97-104.

CHAPTER **2.8**

Vulvar Cancer: Pathology and Prognostic Factors

Updated by Diane C. Ling and Sushil Beriwal

Most vulvar malignancies arise within squamous epithelium, most commonly on the labia majora, labia minora, clitoris, posterior fourchette, or perineal body. Within the vulvar vestibule and fourchette, squamous neoplasia may arise where keratinized stratified squamous epithelium transitions to the nonkeratinized squamous mucosa of the vestibule, also known as Hart line.

PATHOLOGY

Squamous Cell Carcinomas

SCCs constitute greater than 90% of all invasive vulvar cancers. Although the HPV status of vulvar SCC lacks therapeutic relevance at this time (1), the current 2020 WHO classification divides vulvar SCC into HPV-associated and HPV-independent SCC because of their differing pathogenesis. IHC showing strong p16 staining in the nucleus and cytoplasm (ie, "block staining") (2) is considered a reliable, although not perfect surrogate for HPV association (3).

Important pathologic features include DOI, tumor thickness, vascular space invasion, tumor growth pattern, grade, and tumor subtype. DOI is one of the most important pathologic prognostic factors and is essential for accurate staging of early-stage vulvar tumors (4). According to the updated 2021 FIGO staging, DOI is now measured from the basement membrane of the deepest, adjacent, dysplastic, tumor-free rete ridge (or nearest dysplastic rete peg) to the deepest point of invasion (5). The previous definition of DOI, from the epithelial junction of the most superficial adjacent dermal papilla to the deepest point of invasion, had been proposed in 1984 by the ISSVD and the International Society of Gynecologic Pathologists (ISGYP), but was not always found to be reproducible (6).

Tumor thickness is a separate measurement from DOI. It is measured in millimeters from the surface of the tumor or, if there is surface keratinization, from the bottom of the granular layer, to the deepest point of invasion (2,7). With large tumors, and some tumors with invasion deeper than 1 mm, thickness may be the only reliable measurement because of the lack of identifiable adjacent rete ridges or dermal papillae. However, tumor thickness is not used in the staging of vulvar cancer.

Vascular space involvement can be defined as tumor within an endothelial lined vascular space. Strict pathologic criteria require that the tumor be attached to the wall of the vessel, but this is not observed in all cases. Vascular space involvement by SCC of the vulva is associated with a higher frequency of LN metastasis and a lower OS rate (8,9).

Tumor growth pattern can be categorized as either infiltrating (or fingerlike, or spray, or diffuse) or broad and pushing (verrucous carcinoma). In some studies, infiltrating growth pattern has been associated with higher risk of LN metastasis (10). In general, tumor growth pattern influences the rate of LN metastasis and survival in tumors greater than 1 mm in DOI. In stage IA vulvar carcinomas, tumor growth pattern does not influence the risk of node involvement.

Pushing growth is squamous tumor growth that maintains continuity with the overlying epithelium and infiltrates as a well-defined and well-circumscribed tumor mass, without islands of infiltrating tumor remote from the tumor mass (**Figure 2.8-1**). Tumors with this growth pattern typically have a thickness of 5 mm or less and rarely invade vascular space. They are characteristically well differentiated, with the tumor cells resembling the squamous cells of the adjacent and overlying epithelium. There is usually minimal stromal desmoplasia, although there may be a lymphocytic inflammatory cell infiltrate (11).

Fingerlike (spray or diffuse) growth is characterized by a trabecular appearance, with small islands of poorly differentiated tumor cells found within the dermis or submucosa deeper than the bulk of the tumor mass. Tumors with this growth pattern are typically associated with a desmoplastic stromal response (**Figure 2.8-2**) and a lymphocytic inflammatory cell infiltrate. In tumors with a DOI less than 5 mm, the fingerlike pattern of growth is associated with a higher frequency of inguinal LN metastasis (11).

In some cases, a single tumor may have both compact and fingerlike growth patterns. Mixed patterns, in our experience, are more commonly encountered in frankly invasive vulvar carcinomas and are rarely seen in superficially invasive tumors. The GOG has referred to tumors with a compact pattern of growth as well

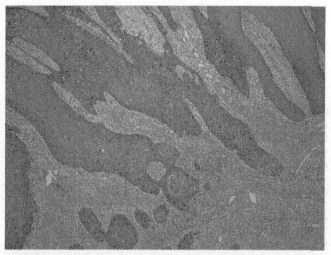

Figure 2.8-1. Confluent pattern of invasion. The tumor has a compact, pushing growth pattern with a well-defined tumor-dermal interface. The tumor diameter exceeds 1 cm and has fingerlike growth pattern, with small, variable-sized tumor nests within the adjacent dermis. The adjacent dermis has a desmoplastic, fibrotic appearance.

differentiated, and to tumors with the fingerlike pattern of growth as poorly differentiated. Using this terminology, the GOG proposed the following grading system for vulvar SCC:

- Grade 1 tumors are composed of well-differentiated tumors and contain no poorly differentiated element.
- Grade 2 tumors contain both patterns, with the poorly differentiated portions making up one-third or less of the tumor.
- Grade 3 tumors also contain both components, with the poorly differentiated portion composing more than one-third but less than one-half of the tumor.
- Grade 4 tumors have one-half or more of the tumor composed of the poorly differentiated elements.

The ISGYP Committee of Terminology for Non-neoplastic Epithelial Disorders and Tumors recommended that the following information be included in the pathology report of all excised vulvar SCCs, information also supported by the College of American Pathologists (CAP) and often used by tumor registries (12):

1. Depth of tumor invasion in millimeters
2. Thickness of the tumor in millimeters
3. Method of measurement of the DOI and thickness

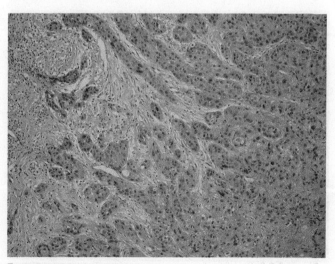

Figure 2.8-2. Fingerlike growth. The tumor forms small nests surrounded by a desmoplastic stroma.

4. Presence or absence of vascular space (lymphatic) involvement by tumor
5. Diameter of the tumor, measured from the specimen in the fresh or fixed state
6. Clinical measurement of the tumor diameter, if available

Several histopathologic types of vulvar SCC are recognized. These include SCC, keratinizing type (not related to HPV); SCC, nonkeratinizing type; basaloid carcinoma; and warty (condylomatous) carcinoma (13). Less common types include acantholytic SCC, SCC with tumor giant cells and spindle cell squamous carcinoma, SCC with sarcoma-like stroma, sebaceous carcinoma, verrucous carcinoma, and other rarer types (14,15).

Adenoid squamous carcinoma (pseudoangiosarcomatous carcinoma, acantholytic SCC, pseudoglandular SCC) refers to SCCs with pseudoglandular features. These tumors are characterized by small gland-like spaces within a tumor that otherwise appears to be a poorly differentiated SCC. It is considered a highly aggressive variant of vulvar SCC (15). This tumor should be differentiated from adenosquamous carcinomas that contain an obvious adenocarcinoma component. Adenoid squamous carcinoma does not contain sialomucin, but adenosquamous carcinoma typically does contain mucin within the adenocarcinoma component.

Sebaceous Carcinoma of the Vulva

These tumors, which arise from the sebaceous glands of the vulvar skin, may be associated with VIN. This rare tumor is aggressive. The tumor cells are relatively large, with large nuclei and prominent nucleoli with prominent cytoplasm. The cytoplasm, related to its lipid content, has a finely vacuolated appearance. The tumor may have the appearance of a SCC intermixed with sebaceous elements. Deep invasion and LN or other metastases may be present on initial presentation (16,17).

Spindle Cell Squamous Cell Carcinomas

These tumors consist of poorly differentiated neoplastic epithelial cells that have an elongated spindle shape and may mimic a spindle cell melanoma or a sarcoma (**Figure 2.8-3**) (18). SCC with spindle cell stroma is associated with a sarcoma-like stromal/dermal response that may mimic a primary sarcoma. Spindle cell SCCs can be differentiated from sarcomas by immunoperoxidase techniques. Like other SCCs, the spindle cell variant contains keratin and lacks the antigens distinctive to sarcomas of various origins. S100 antigen, HMB45, and Melan-A are usually immune-reactive in a spindle cell melanoma and lacking in a spindle cell squamous carcinoma.

Verrucous Carcinoma

Verrucous carcinoma of the vulva typically presents as an exophytic-appearing growth that can be locally destructive. Clinically, it may resemble condyloma acuminatum. The so-called Buschke-Lowenstein giant condyloma is classified as a variant of verrucous carcinoma by WHO (13). Microscopically, verrucous carcinoma is characterized by well-differentiated epithelial cells. The tumor growth pattern is characterized by a "pushing" tumor-dermal interface with minimal stroma between the acanthotic epithelium (**Figure 2.8-4**). The surface is often hyperkeratotic, and there may be parakeratosis. Observed mitoses are characteristically normal. Within the dermis, a mild lymphocytic inflammatory cell response is usually seen. Vascular space involvement by tumor is characteristically lacking. Because of its excellent prognosis, strict histologic criteria should be used in the diagnosis of verrucous carcinoma. Squamous carcinomas with focal verrucous features should not be described or diagnosed as verrucous carcinoma.

Verrucous carcinomas are characteristically diploid, unlike typical SCCs of the vulva, which are usually aneuploid by DNA analysis. The major differential diagnosis of verrucous carcinoma includes keratoacanthomas, pseudocarcinomatous hyperplasia, epithelioid sarcoma, and malignant rhabdoid tumor.

Basal Cell Carcinoma

BCC is a relatively rare tumor in the vulva, accounting for 2% to 4% of infiltrative neoplasms (19). These tumors are most commonly found in elderly women with a median age of 75 years, as compared with 67 years of age for SCCs, as noted in a recent study (20). The tumor may be a plaque or papule. Vulvar BCC most commonly arises on the labia majora and is typically relatively small, ranging from 0.2 to 2.5 cm, with a median size of 0.85 cm or less in a recent study of 35 cases (20). The surface of the tumor appears granular and is well circumscribed.

The epithelial cells composing BCC are typically small and vary in form, with small hyperchromatic nuclei that may exhibit some nuclear pleomorphism. These tumors may have a variety of growth patterns (eg, trabecular, insular), although peripheral nuclear palisading is a relatively consistent finding. BCCs often have an intraepithelial component that is contiguous with the infiltrative component, if present.

Metatypical Basal Cell Carcinoma

This is a variant of BCC that usually occurs at mucocutaneous junctions. The term *basosquamous carcinoma* is applied to these tumors because of their microscopic features, which include BCC

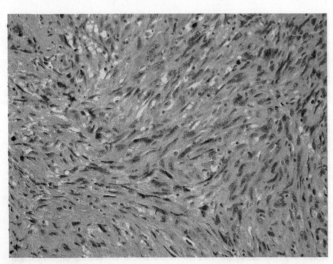

Figure 2.8-3. Spindle cell squamous carcinoma. The tumor cells have a spindle shape and poorly defined cell junctions.

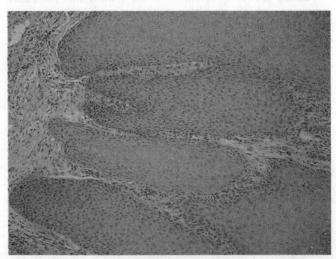

Figure 2.8-4. Verrucous carcinoma. The epithelial cells are well differentiated, and the tumor has a "pushing border" with a delicate vascular core between the epithelial elements.

intermixed with an SCC component. Nuclear pleomorphism is usually seen in metatypical BCC and in the basal cell and squamous cell components of the tumor. The deeper tumor cells, close to the underlying stroma, have the greatest degree of nuclear pleomorphism and the more prominent squamous features. These tumors have a more aggressive clinical behavior than typical BCC (11).

The differential diagnosis of metatypical BCC includes basaloid SCC, Merkel cell tumor of the skin, and metastatic small cell carcinoma. Basaloid SCC can be distinguished by its lack of characteristic basal cell growth pattern and the presence of intracellular bridges. Nuclear pleomorphism is typically much greater in basaloid SCC than in BCC. BCCs express BerEP4 on histochemical study, an antigen not expressed by basaloid SCCs (14). Basaloid SCCs are typically associated with HPV-16, which is not typically associated with BCC. Merkel cell tumors and other neuroendocrine tumors of the vulva are typically subcutaneous or dermal nodules and not intraepithelial lesions (see Neuroendocrine Tumors section).

Neuroendocrine and Neuroectodermal Tumors: Merkel Cell Tumors and Peripheral Neuroectodermal Tumor/Extraosseous Ewing Sarcoma

High-Grade Neuroendocrine Carcinoma/Merkel Cell Tumor

The WHO classifies high-grade neuroendocrine carcinoma tumors into three categories: small cell neuroendocrine carcinoma (small cell carcinoma/SCNEC); large cell neuroendocrine carcinoma; and Merkel cell tumor (21). Although SCNEC tumors are well recognized in the lung, vagina, and cervix, they are extremely rare in the vulva. The WHO recommends that the term "small cell carcinoma" be used only for high-grade neuroendocrine tumors of small cell type, which would be a very rare finding in the vulva. Most of the high-grade neuroendocrine carcinomas reported in the vulva are Merkel cell tumors of the skin that typically occur within the dermis. They are rare and may have a deceptive appearance as single or multiple cutaneous nodules. Ulceration may occur. The tumors may occur concurrently with vulvar SCC and/or VIN (21). These tumors can be divided into two major types: those composed predominantly of small, relatively uniform cells with little cytoplasm and a hyperchromatic, punctate nuclear chromatin pattern. The second type has cellular features resembling low-grade neuroendocrine tumors, with round to polygonal cells, little cytoplasm, and pale finely granular nuclear chromatin. Both types usually have a high mitotic count. Merkel cell tumors can also be subclassified as carcinoid-like (trabecular), intermediate type, and small cell (oat cell) type. By IHC, these tumors typically express neuron-specific enolase (NSE), NCAM/CD56, cytokeratin (CK) CAM 5.2, CK-20, and AE1/AE3 (21). They may also express synaptophysin and chromogranin. CK study, such as with CK-20, demonstrates a distinct perinuclear cytoplasmic dot. Dense core neurosecretory granules are seen by electron microscopy. These features differentiate it from BCC or SCC (14). Merkel cell tumors frequently have both regional LN and distant metastases and are associated with a poor prognosis.

Peripheral Neuroectodermal Tumor/ Extraosseous Ewing Sarcoma

Peripheral neuroectodermal tumor (PNET) is a rare neuroendocrine vulvar neoplasm that has been reported in children and women of reproductive age. The tumor may present as a subcutaneous or polypoid mass in the labia minora or majora, and clinically may resemble a Bartholin cyst or be ulcerated. On microscopic examination, the tumor is circumscribed, multilobulated, and contain small cells with hyperchromatic nuclei and scant cytoplasm. Some cells have small nucleoli, and mitotic figures are usually common, with mitotic counts from 3 to exceeding 10 per 10 high-power fields (HPFs). Numerous patterns of growth may be seen with highly cellular undifferentiated areas, areas with cyst formation containing eosinophilic proteinaceous material, Homer-Wright rosettes, and follicle-like structures. The cells of PNET have periodic acid-Schiff (PAS) staining cytoplasm that digests with diastase and typically express CD99 and vimentin. Although, as in Merkel cell tumors, focal reactivity for synaptophysin and NSE may be present, CK reactivity is absent but may be focally immunoreactive in some cases; dense core neurosecretory granules, as seen in Merkel cell tumor by electron microscopy, are not present (22-24).

Carcinomas Arising From Bartholin Glands

Carcinomas of Bartholin glands generally occur in older women and are rare in women younger than 50 years. Therefore, it is generally advisable to excise an enlarged Bartholin gland in women 50 years of age or older, especially if there is no known history of prior Bartholin cyst. If a cyst is drained and a palpable mass persists, excision of the gland is indicated.

Primary malignant tumors arising within Bartholin glands include SCC (88%) and adenocarcinoma (12%) (25). Most primary adenocarcinomas of the vulva arise within Bartholin glands. Adenocarcinoma may also arise from other glands or skin appendages of the vulva, including sweat glands and Skene glands (13). Invasive vulvar Paget disease has also given rise to adenocarcinoma (**Figure 2.8-5**).

Primary carcinomas within Bartholin glands are usually solid tumors and are often deeply infiltrative. A variety of histologic types of adenocarcinoma have been described within Bartholin glands, such as mucinous, papillary, and mucoepidermoid carcinoma tumor types, in addition to adenosquamous, squamous, and transitional cell carcinoma. Adenocarcinoma of Bartholin glands is typically immunoreactive for carcinoembryonic antigen (CEA). Histopathologic features that identify a carcinoma arising in Bartholin glands include a recognizable transition from a Bartholin gland to tumor. The histopathologic tumor type must be consistent with origin from a Bartholin gland, and the tumor must not appear to be metastatic to gland. These malignancies are characteristically deep and difficult to detect in their early growth. Approximately 20% of women with primary carcinoma of Bartholin glands have metastatic tumor to the inguinal LNs at the time of primary tumor diagnosis (25).

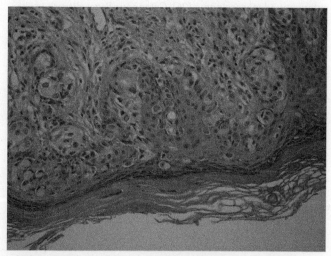

Figure 2.8-5. Paget disease. The large cells with prominent cytoplasm and large nuclei represent the intraepithelial Paget cells. A few small gland-like intraepithelial structures are formed by Paget cells.

Urothelial Cell Carcinomas

Urothelial carcinoma may be a primary tumor of the vulva, usually arising within the Bartholin glands. More commonly, urothelial carcinoma is metastatic to the vulva, having arisen within the bladder or urethra. In rare instances, the tumor presents as a Paget-like lesion of the vulva (see Paget Disease section) (26). Microscopically, urothelial carcinomas are composed of relatively uniform cells; nuclear pleomorphisms may be marked in high-grade urothelial neoplasms. The cytoplasm is eosinophilic without apparent inclusions or keratin formations, although focal keratin formation may be seen. The tumors may exhibit papillary-like growth.

Vulvar Paget Disease and Paget-Like Lesions

Vulvar Paget disease typically presents as an eczematoid, red, weeping area on the vulva, often localized to the labia majora, perineal body, clitoral area, or other sites. This disease typically occurs in older, postmenopausal Caucasian women. Because of its eczematoid, erythematous, and/or ulcerated appearance, it is not unusual for vulvar Paget disease to be misdiagnosed as eczema or contact dermatitis. Approximately 15% of women with vulvar Paget disease have underlying primary adenocarcinoma, usually arising within apocrine glands or the underlying Bartholin glands. The Wilkinson and Brown etiologic classification of vulvar Paget disease divides Paget disease into two main groups: those of cutaneous origin and those of noncutaneous origin (26). The two most common types of noncutaneous Paget disease are those associated with colorectal adenocarcinoma and those associated with bladder urothelial carcinoma. Women with Paget disease of the colorectal type usually present with a lesion that involves the perianal skin, and this lesion is a manifestation of underlying colon or rectal adenocarcinoma. Women with Paget-like disease (pagetoid urothelial intraepithelial neoplasia [PUIN]) typically present with a lesion involving the periurethral area and vulvar vestibule (26,27). In these cases, there is associated bladder and/or urethral urothelial carcinoma, with extension of the neoplastic urothelial cells to the epithelium of the vulva. In cases of PUIN, wide local excision is an acceptable surgical treatment because there is no associated underlying cutaneous adenocarcinoma. The tumor cells are from the bladder and/or urethra, representing an intraepithelial transitional cell neoplasm extending from the bladder and/or urethra (26).

Cutaneous Paget disease is most commonly a primary intraepithelial neoplasm, and in such cases, the intraepithelial Paget disease may have an associated invasive Paget disease. In rare cases, cutaneous Paget disease may be a manifestation of an underlying cutaneous adenocarcinoma (26). Cutaneous Paget disease is characterized by the presence of Paget cells found within the involved epithelium. A Paget cell is relatively large, with a prominent nucleus that typically has coarse chromatin and a prominent nucleolus. On H&E staining, the cytoplasm is distinctly pale compared with the surrounding keratinocytes. The cytoplasm may be vacuolated or appear foamy and typically is somewhat basophilic (**Figure 2.8-5**).

Paget cells of cutaneous origin are rich in CEA, which can be identified with immunoperoxidase techniques. Paget cells also express CK-7 and gross cystic disease fluid protein 15 (GCDFP-15) (26). Paget cells infrequently express CA-125, and estrogen receptor is generally negative. Immunohistochemical staining for CK-7 is useful in many cases to identify the Paget cells that are strongly CK-7 positive, whereas the adjacent epithelial cells are negative. Invasive Paget disease of size 1 mm or less in DOI has reportedly little risk for recurrence (28).

The differential diagnosis of Paget disease of cutaneous origin includes PUIN/Paget disease of urothelial origin, Paget disease of colorectal origin or other related adenocarcinoma, superficial spreading malignant melanoma, pagetoid reticulosis, and the pagetoid variant of VIN, which are keratinocytic cells resembling Paget cells. These can all be differentiated by immunoperoxidase

techniques because melanomas do not express CK but usually express S100 protein, HMB45, and Melan-A, which are absent in Paget cells (26). The Paget-like cells in PUIN express uroplakin-2 and uroplakin-3, whereas uroplakins are not expressed in Paget disease of cutaneous origin. The PUIN lesions do not express GCDFP-15. In a study of 15 cutaneous Paget disease and 3 PUIN cases, GATA-3 was found to be reactive in both lesions and did not distinguish between them (29). Adenocarcinoma cells of colonic, anal, or rectal origin express CEA, as well as caudal homeobox (CDX), whereas Paget disease of cutaneous origin does not express CDX. HSIL (VIN-3) of pagetoid type may microscopically resemble Paget disease or melanoma, but the cells of LSIL or HSIL (VIN-1, VIN-2, VIN-3) do not express CEA, S100, or melanoma antigen (26,27).

Vulvar Malignant Melanoma

Malignant melanoma is the second most common vulvar malignancy, accounting for approximately 9% of all primary malignant neoplasms on the vulva. Vulvar melanoma accounts for approximately 3% of all melanomas in women. This tumor occurs predominantly in postmenopausal Caucasian women; the mean age at diagnosis is 55 years (30). Peak frequency occurs between the sixth and seventh decades, and the highest incidence is in women 75 years of age or older, where the age-specific incidence is reported to be 1.28/100,000 (31). Typical presentations include either an asymptomatic pigmented lesion identified during a routine exam or pruritic or painful vulvar mass (**Figure 2.8-6**) (32,33). The primary site on the vulva may be the clitoris, labia minora, or labia majora. The tumor may be elevated, nodular, or ulcerated. Although tumors are usually pigmented, approximately one-fourth are amelanotic (**Figure 2.8-7**). In the clinical setting, the differential diagnosis includes pigmented condyloma acuminatum, pigmented HSIL VIN, atypical genital nevus, melanosis of the vulva, or other malignant tumors, including malignant soft tissue tumors.

A definitive diagnosis is established with a biopsy. IHC staining for melanoma-specific antigen and S100 may be helpful in uncertain cases. Melanomas may arise from existing pigmented vulvar lesions or as new isolated primary tumors. Consequently, any pigmented vulvar lesion should be considered for biopsy.

Historically, vulvar malignant melanomas have been subclassified histopathologically into three categories: superficial

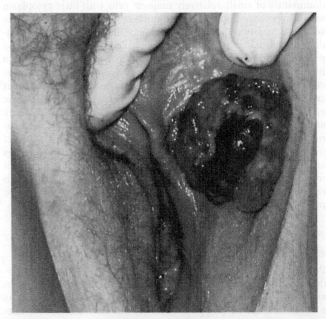

Figure 2.8-6. Nodular, darkly pigmented malignant melanoma of the left labium majus.

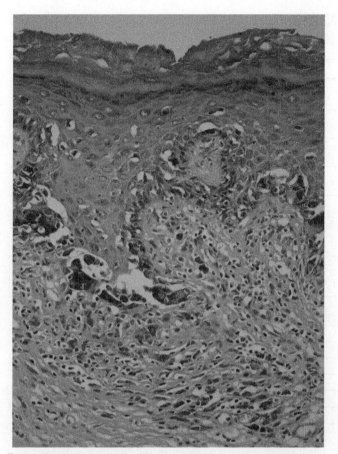

Figure 2.8-7. Malignant melanoma. The tumor is within the dermis and contains dark melanin pigment. Junctional growth is seen within the overlying epithelial-dermal junction.

spreading malignant melanoma, nodular melanoma, and mucosal lentiginous melanoma, which is also referred to as mucosal/acral lentiginous melanoma (34). Mucosal lentiginous melanomas are the type most commonly reported on the vulva, accounting for over one-half of the cases in larger series (31,34). Nodular melanomas are second in frequency, accounting for approximately one-fifth of the cases, and have the overall worst prognosis of the melanoma types, usually related to the greater thickness and deeper invasion at the time of presentation. Although it can be useful to be aware of these histopathologic categories because of persistent use in some centers, their clinical utility is limited, replaced by more objective and reproducible pathologic tumor characteristics such as DOI, ulceration, and mitotic rate.

Because of the rarity of vulvar melanoma, it has not been clear whether extrapolation of prognostic and treatment data from cutaneous nonvulvar disease is appropriate for patients with vulvar melanoma. Thus, until recently, multiple authors have described their experience with vulvar melanoma using one or more different staging systems (eg, Breslow depth, Clark levels, AJCC staging), making standardization of prognostic groups and treatment strategies difficult. Moxley et al reported a multi-institutional retrospective examination of 77 patients with vulvar melanoma. Patient stages were determined using the AJCC staging guidelines (6th edition) (2002), Breslow thickness, and Clark levels, and treatments were correlated with outcomes, specifically recurrence and OS. Among the three staging methods, only AJCC staging was significantly correlated with OS, although Breslow thickness was significantly associated with likelihood of recurrence (35). For this reason, starting with the 2009 7th edition of the Melanoma Staging and Classification, the AJCC has recommended against continued use of Clark level and Breslow thickness for management of T1

invasive melanoma lesions (36). Vulvovaginal melanoma should be staged the same as cutaneous melanoma. The current AJCC 8th edition staging system for cutaneous melanoma is shown in **Table 2.8-1**.

Melanomas arising in the vulva may metastasize to other sites within the lower female genital tract, including the cervix, vagina, urethra, and rectum. Distant metastasis is common with disseminated disease. Survival after recurrence is poor, approximately 5%.

Vulvar Sarcomas

Leiomyosarcoma

Leiomyosarcoma (LMS) is the most frequent primary vulvar sarcoma, although sarcomas of the vulva are relatively rare. It occurs in women in the fourth or fifth decade of life and most commonly arises in the labia majora or Bartholin gland area. The tumors are generally larger than 5 cm in diameter when first diagnosed, presenting as an enlarging mass. It may be deep within the subcutaneous tissue and painful in some circumstances.

On microscopic examination, these tumors are composed of interlacing spindle-shaped cells, sometimes with an epithelioid appearance. Histopathologic criteria for malignancy require at least three of the following features: size greater than 5 cm, evidence of infiltrative growth into adjacent tissue, cytologic atypia of a moderate to severe degree, and mitotic count greater than 5 mitoses per 10 HPFs. In cases with minimal pleomorphism, but with most of the other criteria, it is generally accepted that the diagnosis of LMS can be made with a mitotic count of 10 or more per 10 HPFs. Tumors that have an infiltrating border or nuclear atypia with pleomorphism and mitotic count of 5 or more per 10 HPFs are classified as LMS (37).

Malignant Fibrous Histiocytoma

Malignant fibrous histiocytoma (MFH) arises from histiocytes with fibroblastic differentiation. It is considered the second most common sarcoma of the vulva and has its peak frequency in women of middle age. MFH typically presents as a solitary mass that may appear somewhat brownish or pigmented, secondary to areas of focal hemorrhage within the tumor.

On microscopic examination, the tumor is characterized by a complex interlacing cellular growth pattern with marked nuclear pleomorphism, including multinucleated cells and large bizarre cells. Abnormal mitotic figures may be apparent. On immunoperoxidase study, these tumors contain α_1-antitrypsin and α_1-antichymotrypsin. MFH is typically infiltrative and may involve the underlying fascia. Involvement of the fascia is associated with a higher risk of local spread and distant metastasis (38).

Epithelioid Sarcoma

Epithelioid sarcoma may arise within the labia majora, subclitoral area, and clitoris. Its microscopic features may resemble squamous carcinoma, malignant melanoma, malignant rhabdoid tumor, or lymphoma. Epithelioid sarcoma is usually relatively superficial, arising in and involving the reticular dermis, but it may occur in deeper structures (39).

On microscopic examination, the tumor is nodular and may have areas of necrosis. The tumor cells have an epithelioid appearance with eosinophilic cytoplasm, but there may be metaplastic components, including cartilage and bone. On IHC, this tumor contains CK, which does not distinguish it from epithelial tumors, but is of value in differentiating it from malignant melanoma or other types of soft tissue tumors. Epithelioid sarcoma rarely metastasizes, although local recurrence is a risk. Immunoperoxidase studies are of value in differentiation, but not in differentiating epithelioid sarcoma from malignant rhabdoid tumor. The distinction of these two tumors is based primarily on microscopic features (39).

■ **TABLE 2.8-1A. TNM Staging Categories for Cutaneous Melanoma**

Classification	Thickness (mm)	Ulceration Status/Mitoses
Tis	NA	NA
T1	≤1	a: Without ulceration and mitosis <1/mm^2 b: With ulceration or mitoses ≥1/mm^2
T2	1.01-2	a: Without ulceration b: With ulceration
T3	2.01-4	a: Without ulceration b: With ulceration
T4	>4	a: Without ulceration b: With ulceration
N	**No. of metastatic nodes**	**Nodal metastatic burden**
N0	0	NA
N1	1	a: Micrometastasis[a] b: Macrometastasis[b]
N2	2-3	a: Micrometastasis[a] b: Macrometastasis[b] c: In-transit metastases/satellites without metastatic nodes
N3	4+ metastatic nodes, or matted nodes, or in-transit metastases/satellites with metastatic nodes	
M	**Site**	**Serum LDH**
M0	No distant metastases	NA
M1a	Distant skin, subcutaneous, or nodal metastases	Normal
M1b	Lung metastases	Normal
M1c	All other visceral metastases	Normal
	Any distant metastasis	Elevated

LDH, lactate dehydrogenase; NA, not applicable; TNM, tumor, node, metastasis.

[a]Micrometastases are diagnosed after sentinel lymph node biopsy.

[b]Macrometastases are defined as clinically detectable nodal metastases confirmed pathologically.

■ **TABLE 2.8-1B. TNM Stage Grouping for Cutaneous Melanoma**

Clinical Staging	T	N	M	Pathologic Staging	T	N	M
0	Tis	N0	M0	0	Tis	N0	M0
IA	T1a	N0	M0	IA	T1a	N0	M0
IB	T1b	N0	M0	IB	T1b	N0	M0
	T2a	N0	M0		T2a	N0	M0
IIA	T2b	N0	M0	IIA	T2b	N0	M0
	T3a	N0	M0		T3a	N0	M0
IIB	T3b	N0	M0	IIB	T3b	N0	M0
	T4a	N0	M0		T4a	N0	M0
IIC	T4b	N0	M0	IIC	T4b	N0	M0
III	Any T	>N0	M0	IIIA	T1-4a	N1a	M0
					T1-4a	N2a	M0
				IIIB	T1-4b	N1a	M0
					T1-4b	N2a	M0
					T1-4a	N1b	M0
					T1-4a	N2b	M0
					T1-4a	N2c	M0
				IIIC	T1-4b	N1b	M0
					T1-4b	N2b	M0
					T1-4b	N2c	M0
					Any T	N3	M0
IV	Any T	Any N	M1	IV	Any T	Any N	M1

Clinical staging includes microstaging of the primary melanoma and clinical/radiologic evaluation for metastases. By convention, it should be used after complete excision of the primary melanoma with clinical assessment for regional and distant metastases.

Reprinted with permission from Springer; from Edge SB, Byrd DR, Compton CC, et al. *AJCC Cancer Staging Manual*. Springer; 2009; Used with permission of the American College of Surgeons, Chicago, Illinois. The original source for this information is the AJCC Cancer Staging System (2023).

Malignant Rhabdoid Tumor

Malignant rhabdoid tumor has been described in the vulva and, like epithelioid sarcoma, may be relatively superficial and contain tumor cells with an epithelioid appearance with eosinophilic cytoplasm. Unlike epithelioid sarcoma, malignant rhabdoid tumors have relatively pleomorphic nuclei. Metaplastic elements are usually not present. Malignant rhabdoid tumor also has eosinophilic cytoplasmic inclusions, which are not present in epithelioid sarcoma. These inclusions give some of the cells the appearance of signet ring cells. Malignant rhabdoid tumor has a lobulated architecture but lacks necrosis or granulomatous features, which are often found in epithelioid sarcoma (37,40).

Aggressive Angiomyxoma

Aggressive angiomyxoma is a primary soft tissue tumor of the vulva and pelvis that occurs predominantly in women of reproductive age. It is locally aggressive but rarely metastatic (41). It typically presents as a deep soft tissue mass or pelvic mass, sometimes mimicking a Bartholin cyst or inguinal hernia. In the pelvis, it may displace other pelvic organs and may be best appreciated on radiologic studies.

This tumor is typically poorly circumscribed and difficult to discriminate from adjacent soft tissue. On microscopic examination, the tumor has many blood vessels. It consists predominantly of spindle- to stellate-shaped cells, with relatively small uniform nuclei representing predominantly fibroblasts and myofibroblasts. Mitotic figures are very rare. The tumor stroma varies from myxoid to densely collagenous. Nerves, small glandular structures with mucin-secreting columnar cells, and other epithelial elements may be found trapped within the tumor. The differential diagnosis is as for angiomyofibroblastoma (AMF), summarized in the next section.

Angiomyofibroblastoma

AMF is a rare, benign tumor of soft tissue origin that occurs predominantly in the female genital tract. When involving the vulva, it usually presents as a soft subcutaneous mass, but may occasionally be pedunculated (42).

On microscopic examination, the tumor usually has well-demarcated borders. Variable cellularity is present, with an edematous appearance. The cells are spindle shaped, plasmacytoid or epithelioid in appearance, and mitotic figures are rare. Cells are present in most cases and may be clustered about blood vessels. The tumor is vascular, with small- to medium-sized vessels. Some inflammatory cells, commonly lymphocytes or mast cells, may be seen around the vessels.

Tumors Metastatic to the Vulva

Metastatic tumors account for approximately 8% of all vulvar tumors, and in approximately one-half of the cases the primary tumor is in the lower genital tract, including the cervix, vagina, endometrium, and ovary. Cervical carcinoma is the most common origin of contiguous metastasis. Most metastatic tumors to the vulva involve the labia majora or Bartholin glands. In the vulva, they most often present as multiple intradermal or subcutaneous nodules but may present as a Bartholin gland mass (43-45). Cutaneous vulvar lymphatic metastases may occur as in-transit tumor emboli from anorectal tumors or as retrograde flow metastases when bulky tumors of the cervix or uterus obstruct the normal lymphatic drainage patterns (Figure 2.8-8). Local metastasis secondary to contiguous involvement of the vulva from urothelial carcinoma of the bladder or urethra, or anorectal carcinoma, may involve the vulva and present as a Paget-like lesion (see Paget Disease and Paget-Like Lesions section) or a vulvar or groin node mass. Remote metastases have been observed from tumors arising in the breast, kidney, stomach, lung, and other sites (45).

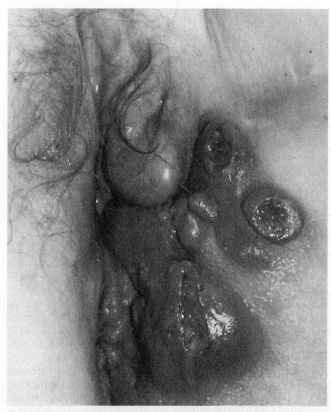

Figure 2.8-8. Multiple in-transit lymphatic metastases from a cloacogenic carcinoma of the rectum. A large constricting lesion was evident on rectal examination.

PROGNOSTIC FACTORS

Prognostic information collected during the diagnostic workup of SCCs of the vulva serves as a basis for both patient counseling and treatment decisions. Fundamental decisions regarding goals of therapy (cure vs palliation) and sequencing of primary treatment (primary surgery vs chemoradiation) should be based on four factors: (a) historical and demographic risk factors; (b) characteristics of the primary tumor, including location, laterality, size (cm), DOI, lymphovascular space invasion, and margin width; (c) clinical and/or radiographic assessment of the inguinal LNs; and (d) probability of distant metastatic disease.

After resection of the primary tumor and surgical evaluation of the inguinal LNs, additional information obtained from intraoperative observations and the final pathologic specimens serve to guide decisions regarding adjuvant therapy. The most important prognostic factors for the adjuvant management of SCC of the vulva have been incorporated into the FIGO and AJCC staging systems (**Table 2.5-2**). Among the many factors that affect recurrence risk and disease-specific mortality, nodal status, particularly the number of positive nodes, size of the largest metastasis, and the presence or absence of extracapsular extension are the most important (9). It is impossible to accurately detect LN involvement on physical exam; therefore, the FIGO staging of vulvar cancer changed from a clinical to a surgical and histopathologic approach, with evaluation of extranodal extension (ENE) also taken into account. Each of the above risk factors is discussed in relation to its temporal presentation (presurgical vs postsurgical resection). Prognostic factors associated with the resection specimen and inguinal LN evaluation following surgery are also discussed.

Presurgery

The presence of nodal involvement is the single most important determinant of disease-specific mortality. DOI, tumor size, and lymph-vascular space invasion are the primary determinants of a patient's risk for nodal metastases (46-48).

Among SCCs limited to the vulva, those with a DOI of 1 mm or less are associated with a less than 1% risk for LN metastasis. Tumors with a DOI of 1.1 to 3 mm are associated with LN metastases in 6% to 12% of patients, and approximately 15% to 20% of tumors with a DOI of 3.1 to 5 mm are associated with positive LNs (4,49,50).

Postsurgery

Following surgery, intraoperative findings and final pathologic analysis are used to estimate recurrence risk and subsequently guide decisions regarding adjuvant therapy. Among the many pathologic findings shown to affect recurrence risk, surgical nodal status is the most important (8,46,47). Metastasis to the inguinal LNs is the single most important prognostic factor for recurrence and OS in women with vulvar cancer; most recurrences happen within 2 years of primary treatment (9,47). The number of involved nodes, LN ratio of 20% or more, size of largest involved node, and extracapsular extension are all associated with PFS and disease-related death (51-54).

Aside from LN status, local recurrence has been shown to portend worse disease-free survival (55). Predictors of local recurrence include larger tumor size, multifocal disease, deep stromal invasion, presence of lichen sclerosis, close or positive margins, and perineural invasion. Surgical margin status has been strongly associated with local recurrence risk. Historically, pathologic close margins were defined as less than 8 mm, which led to the recommendation of surgical margins greater than 1 cm in fresh, unfixed tissue. This was based on the study by Heaps et al (48), which demonstrated a sharp rise in the incidence of local recurrence for tumors with microscopic margins less than 8 mm in formalin-fixed tissue specimens. A retrospective multivariate analysis by Chan et al (8) also showed that pathologic margin distance of 8 mm or less is an important predictor of local recurrence; De Hullu et al (56) reported nine local recurrences among 40 patients with tumor-free margins of 8 mm or less compared with none among 39 patients with margins greater than 8 mm. However, more recent studies have challenged this. A Dutch study recently showed no association between local recurrence and margin status when using any of three different cutoff values for margin distance: 3, 5, or 8 mm (57). However, presence of d-VIN with or without lichen sclerosis at the resection margin was associated with a significantly higher risk of local recurrence (57).

To aid the surgeon in planning surgical margins of resection, Hoffman et al (58) measured the radial occult microscopic spread of tumor in patients with invasive SCC of the vulva. They found that the gross and microscopic peripheries of most cancers were approximately the same; however, ulcerative tumors with an infiltrative pattern of invasion were more likely to extend beyond what is grossly apparent.

Finally, HPV-associated vulvar SCC is associated with a better prognosis than HPV-independent tumors. In patients managed with surgery and adjuvant radiotherapy, in-field relapses appear to be less frequent in p16-positive tumors (59,60). On the other hand, p53 mutations are associated with worse outcomes in patients with negative HPV (61).

REFERENCES

1. Barlow EL, Lambie N, Donoghoe MW, Naing Z, Hacker NF. The Clinical Relevance of p16 and p53 Status in patients with squamous cell carcinoma of the vulva. *J Oncol.* 2020;2020:3739075.
2. Darragh TM, Colgan TJ, Cox JT, et al; Members of the LAST Project Work Groups. The lower anogenital squamous terminology standardization project for HPV-associated lesions: background and consensus recommendations from the college of American Pathologists and the American Society for Colposcopy and Cervical Pathology. *Int J Gynecol Pathol.* 2013;32:76-115.
3. Heller DS, Day T, Allbritton JI, et al. Diagnostic criteria for differentiated vulvar intraepithelial neoplasia and vulvar aberrant maturation. *J Low Genit Tract Dis.* 2021;25(1):57-70.
4. Yoder BJ, Rufforny I, Massoll NA, Wilkinson EJ. Stage 1A vulvar squamous cell carcinoma: an analysis of tumor invasive characteristics and risk. *Am J Surg Pathol.* 2008;32:765-772.
5. Olawaiye AB, Cotler J, Cuello MA, et al. FIGO staging for carcinoma of the vulva: 2021 revision. *Int J Gynaecol Obstet.* 2021;155:43-47.
6. Abdel-Mesih A, Daya D, Onuma K, et al. Interobserver agreement for assessing invasion in stage 1A vulvar squamous cell carcinoma. *Am J Surg Pathol.* 2013;37:1336-1341.
7. Tavassoli FA, Devilee P, eds. *World Health Organization Classification of Tumours: Pathology and Genetics of Tumours of the Breast and Female Genital Organs.* IARC Press; 2003.
8. Chan JK, Sugiyama V, Pham H, et al. Margin distance and other clinico-pathologic prognostic factors in vulvar carcinoma: a multivariate analysis. *Gynecol Oncol.* 2007;104:636-641.
9. Raspagliesi F, Hanozet F, Ditto A, et al. Clinical and pathologic prognostic factors in squamous cell carcinoma of the vulva. *Gynecol Oncol.* 2006;102:333-337.
10. Drew PA, Al-Abbadi MA, Orlando CA, Hendricks JB, Kubilis PS, Wilkinson EJ. Prognostic factors in carcinoma of the vulva: a clinicopathologic and DNA flow cytometric study. *Int J Gynecol Pathol.* 1996;15:235-241.
11. Wilkinson EJ, Stone IK. *Atlas of Vulvar Disease.* 3rd ed. Wolters Kluwer/Lippincott Williams & Wilkins Philadelphia; 2012.
12. Wilkinson EJ. Protocol for the examination of specimens from patients with carcinomas and malignant melanomas of the vulva: a basis for checklists. Cancer committee of the American College of Pathologists. *Arch Pathol Lab Med.* 2000;124(1):51-56.
13. Crum CP, Hereington CS, McCluggage WG, et al. *Epithelial Tumors.* 4th ed. IRAC; 2014.
14. Kurman RJ, Ronnett J, Sherman ME, et al. *Tumors of the Cervix, Vagina, and Vulva.* Armed Forces Institute of Pathology; 2010.
15. Horn LC, Liebert UG, Edelmann J, et al. Adenoid squamous carcinoma (pseudoangiosarcomatous carcinoma) of the vulva: a rare but highly aggressive variant of squamous cell carcinoma-report of a case and review of the literature. *Int J Gynecol Pathol.* 2008;27(2):288-291.
16. Carlson JW, McGlennen RC, Gomez R, et al. Sebaceous carcinoma of the vulva: a case report and review of the literature. *Gynecol Oncol.* 1996;60(3):489-491.
17. Escalonilla P, Grilli R, Canamero M, et al. Sebaceous carcinoma of the vulva. *Am J Dermatopathol.* 1999;21(5):468-472.
18. Copas P, Dyer M, Comas FV, et al. Spindle cell carcinoma of the vulva. *Diagn Gynecol Obstet.* 1982;4(3):235-241.
19. de Giorgi V, Salvini C, Massi D, et al. Vulvar basal cell carcinoma: retrospective study and review of literature. *Gynecol Oncol.* 2005;97(1):192-194.
20. Sinn HP, Mayer C, Kommoss F. Clinical presentation and pathologic features of vulvar basal cell carcinomas. *J Low Genit Tract Dis.* 2015;19(3 Suppl 1):S22.
21. Crum CP, Herrington CS, McGluggage WG, et al. *Neuroendocrine Tumors.* 4th ed. IRAC; 2014.
22. Vang R, Taubenberger JK, Mannion CM, et al. Primary vulvar and vaginal extraosseous Ewing's sarcoma/peripheral neuroectodermal tumor: diagnostic confirmation with CD99 immunostaining and reverse transcriptase-polymerase chain reaction. *Int J Gynecol Pathol.* 2000;19(2):103-109.
23. Takeshima N, Tabata T, Nishida H, et al. Peripheral primitive neuroectodermal tumor of the vulva: report of a case with imprint cytology. *Acta Cytol.* 2001;45(6):1049-1052.
24. Wilkinson EJ, Crum CP, Herrington CS, et al. *Neuroectodermal Tumors.* 4th ed. IRAC; 2014.
25. Bhalwal AB, Nick AM, Dos Reis R, et al. Carcinoma of the Bartholin gland: a review of 33 cases. *Int J Gynecol Cancer.* 2016;26(4):785-789.
26. Wilkinson EJ, Brown HM. Vulvar Paget disease of urothelial origin: a report of three cases and a proposed classification of vulvar Paget disease. *Hum Pathol.* 2002;33(5):549-554.
27. Malik SN, Wilkinson EJ. Pseudo-Paget's disease of the vulva: a case report. *J Low Genit Tract Dis.* 1999;3(1):55.
28. Crawford D, Nimmo M, Clement PB, et al. Prognostic factors in Paget's disease of the vulva: a study of 21 cases. *Int J Gynecol Pathol.* 1999;18(4):351-359.
29. Newsom K, Alizadeh L, Al-Quran SZ, et al. Use of GATA-3 and uroplakin-II in differentiating primary cutaneous vulvar paget disease

from pagetoid urothelial intraepithelial neoplasia. *J Low Genit Tract Dis.* 2015;19(3 Suppl 1):S6.

30. Panizzon RG. Vulvar melanoma. *Semin Dermatol.* 1996;15(1):67-70.

31. Ragnarsson-Olding BK, Nilsson BR, Kanter-Lewensohn LR, et al. Malignant melanoma of the vulva in a nationwide, 25-year study of 219 Swedish females: predictors of survival. *Cancer.* 1999;86(7):1285-1293.

32. Raspagliesi F, Ditto A, Paladini D, et al. Prognostic indicators in melanoma of the vulva. *Ann Surg Oncol.* 2000;7(10):738-742.

33. Wechter ME, Reynolds RK, Haefner HK, et al. Vulvar melanoma: review of diagnosis, staging, and therapy. *J Low Genit Tract Dis.* 2004;8(1):58-69.

34. Benda JA, Platz CE, Anderson B. Malignant melanoma of the vulva: a clinical-pathologic review of 16 cases. *Int J Gynecol Pathol.* 1986;5(3):202-216.

35. Moxley KM, Fader AN, Rose PG, et al. Malignant melanoma of the vulva: an extension of cutaneous melanoma? *Gynecol Oncol.* 2011;122(3):612-617.

36. Balch CM, Gershenwald JE, Soong SJ, et al. Final version of 2009 AJCC melanoma staging and classification. *J Clin Oncol.* 2009;27(36):6199-6206.

37. Nucci MR, Fletcher CD. Vulvovaginal soft tissue tumours: update and review. *Histopathology.* 2000;36(2):97-108.

38. Vural B, Ozkan S, Yildiz K, et al. Malignant fibrous histiocytoma of the vulva: a case report. *Arch Gynecol Obstet.* 2005;273(2):122-125.

39. Han CH, Li X, Khanna N. Epithelioid sarcoma of the vulva and its clinical implication: a case report and review of the literature. *Gynecol Oncol Rep.* 2016;15:31-33.

40. Chokoeva AA, Tchernev G, Cardoso JC, et al. Vulvar sarcomas—short guideline for histopathological recognition and clinical management. Part 1. *Int J Immunopathol Pharmacol.* 2015;28(2):178-186.

41. Nielsen GP, Young RH. Mesenchymal tumors and tumor-like lesions of the female genital tract: a selective review with emphasis on recently described entities. *Int J Gynecol Pathol.* 2001;20(2):105-127.

42. Sims SM, Stinson K, McLean FW, et al. Angiomyofibroblastoma of the vulva: a case report of a pedunculated variant and review of the literature. *J Low Genit Tract Dis.* 2012;16(2):149-154.

43. Lerner LB, Andrews SJ, Gonzalez JL, et al. Vulvar metastases secondary to transitional cell carcinoma of the bladder: a case report. *J Reprod Med.* 1999;44(8):729-732.

44. Vang R, Medeiros LJ, Malpica A, et al. Non-Hodgkin's lymphoma involving the vulva. *Int J Gynecol Pathol.* 2000;19(3):236-242.

45. Neto AG, Deavers MT, Silva EG, et al. Metastatic tumors of the vulva: a clinicopathologic study of 66 cases. *Am J Surg Pathol.* 2003;27(6):799-804.

46. Maggino T, Landoni F, Sartori E, et al. Patterns of recurrence in patients with squamous cell carcinoma of the vulva: a multicenter CTF Study. *Cancer.* 2000;89(1):116-122.

47. Gonzalez Bosquet J, Magrina JF, Gaffey TA, et al. Long-term survival and disease recurrence in patients with primary squamous cell carcinoma of the vulva. *Gynecol Oncol.* 2005;97(3):828-833.

48. Heaps JM, Fu YS, Montz FJ, et al. Surgical-pathologic variables predictive of local recurrence in squamous cell carcinoma of the vulva. *Gynecol Oncol.* 1990;38(3):309-314.

49. Klapdor R, Wölber L, Hanker L, et al. Predictive factors for lymph node metastases in vulvar cancer. An analysis of the AGO-CaRE-1 multicenter study. *Gynecol Oncol.* 2019;154(3):565-570.

50. Homesley HD, Bundy BN, Sedlis A, et al. Prognostic factors for groin node metastasis in squamous cell carcinoma of the vulva (a Gynecologic Oncology Group study). *Gynecol Oncol.* 1993;49:279-283.

51. Homesley HD, Bundy BN, Sedlis A, et al. Assessment of current international federation of gynecology and obstetrics staging of vulvar carcinoma relative to prognostic factors for survival (a Gynecologic Oncology Group study). *Am J Obstet Gynecol.* 1991;164:997-1003; discussion 1003-1004.

52. Polterauer S, Schwameis R, Grimm C, et al. Lymph node ratio in inguinal lymphadenectomy for squamous cell vulvar cancer: results from the AGO-CaRE-1 study. *Gynecol Oncol.* 2019;153:286-291.

53. Kunos C, Simpkins F, Gibbons H, et al. Radiation therapy compared with pelvic node resection for node-positive vulvar cancer: a randomized controlled trial. *Obstet Gynecol.* 2009;114:537-546.

54. Luchini C, Nottegar A, Solmi M, et al. Prognostic implications of extranodal extension in node-positive squamous cell carcinoma of the vulva: a systematic review and meta-analysis. *Surg Oncol.* 2016;25(1):60-65.

55. te Grootenhuis NC, van der Zee AG, van Doorn HC, et al. Sentinel nodes in vulvar cancer: long-term follow-up of the GROningen INternational Study on Sentinel nodes in Vulvar cancer (GROINSS-V) I. *Gynecol Oncol.* 2016;140(1):8-14.

56. De Hullu JA, Hollema H, Lolkema S, et al. Vulvar carcinoma: the price of less radical surgery. *Cancer.* 2002;95(11):2331-2338.

57. Te Grootenhuis NC, Pouwer AW, de Bock GH, et al. Margin status revisited in vulvar squamous cell carcinoma. *Gynecol Oncol.* 2019;154:266-275.

58. Hoffman MS, Gunesakaran S, Arango H, et al. Lateral microscopic extension of squamous cell carcinoma of the vulva. *Gynecol Oncol.* 1999;73(1):72-75.

59. Dohopolski MJ, Horne ZD, Pradhan D, et al. The prognostic significance of p16 status in patients with vulvar cancer treated with vulvectomy and adjuvant radiation. *Int J Radiat Oncol Biol Phys.* 2019;103:152-160.

60. Allo G, Yap ML, Cuartero J, et al. HPV-independent vulvar squamous cell carcinoma is associated with significantly worse prognosis compared with HPV-associated tumors. *Int J Gynecol Pathol.* 2020;39:391-399.

61. Kortekaas KE, Bastiaannet E, van Doorn HC, et al. Vulvar cancer subclassification by HPV and p53 status results in three clinically distinct subtypes. *Gynecol Oncol.* 2020;159:649-656.

CHAPTER **2.9**

Vulvar Cancer: Follow-Up and Survivorship Issues

Diane C. Ling and Sushil Beriwal

RESULTS OF THERAPY

The overall results of therapy for women with squamous cancers of the vulva are excellent, largely because approximately two-thirds of patients present with early-stage tumors. Five-year survival rates for vulvar cancer have improved over the past two decades. Landrum et al used GOG data to perform an historical comparison between patients treated between 1977 and 1984 (*n* = 577) and patients treated between 1990 and 2005 (*n* = 175). Stratification into "minimal, low, intermediate, and high-risk" groups was performed to enable comparisons.

Patients treated in the era of less radical surgery and modern chemoradiation fared better than historical comparisons, with 5-year survival by risk group (minimal → high) of 100% versus 97.9%, 97% versus 87.4%, 82% versus 74.8%, and 100% versus 29.0% (1).

Several strategies to enhance survival for women with vulvar cancer are evident. High-risk patients can be educated and screened more consistently for the development of early cancer. Women with HPV infections, in situ vulvar disease, long smoking history, and other genital neoplasms are at risk for developing vulvar cancer (2). Careful screening targeted at women with these high-risk factors may lead to improvements in early diagnosis (3).

The survival rate for women with nodal spread is one-half that for women without nodal disease who have similarly sized primary tumors. Improvements in the use of molecular markers for metastatic disease and biologic aggressiveness would be helpful for triaging higher risk patients into more effective adjuvant therapies. And, of course, there is a dire need for better treatment options for node-positive patients.

SEQUELAE OF TREATMENT

Immediate complications such as wound infection and lymphocysts were common in the radical vulvectomy era. These occur much less frequently now because of the use of multimodal primary therapies, less radical surgery, and innovations such as prophylactic antibiotics and closed-suction drains. Breakdown of the vulvar incision is increased in patients who are smokers, as well as those with vasculopathy.

Lymphedema starts to appear within weeks of surgery. The severity is related to the extent of groin surgery, wound complications, postoperative RT, and preexisting conditions of the lower extremities. Lymphedema is not always limited to the lower leg and thigh. It may also include the mons, groins, and hips. The use of SLNB reduces but does not eliminate wound complications and lymphedema. Pressure stockings, sequential compression devices,

lymphedema massage, and microvascular surgery have been used to manage lower extremity lymphedema, with limited results. *Prevention* of lymphedema with the use of SLNB is the best strategy for limiting its adverse effects (4).

All gynecologic surgery, especially surgery for vulvar cancer, can have an adverse effect on body image and sexual function. Informed consent obtained for vulvar cancer surgery should include a discussion regarding these risks. No assumptions regarding a woman's sexual activity should be made on the basis of age or marital status. We have found that preoperative consultation with a sexual health expert can be invaluable for many women.

REFERENCES

1. Landrum LM, Lanneau GS, Skaggs VJ, et al. Gynecologic Oncology Group risk groups for vulvar carcinoma: improvement in survival in the modern era. *Gynecol Oncol.* 2007;106(3):521-525.
2. Clifford GM, Polesel J, Rickenbach M, et al. Cancer risk in the Swiss HIV Cohort Study: associations with immunodeficiency, smoking, and highly active antiretroviral therapy. *J Natl Cancer Inst.* 2005;97(6):425-432.
3. Santoso JT, Crigger M, English E, et al. Smoking cessation counseling in women with genital intraepithelial neoplasia. *Gynecol Oncol.* 2012;125(3):716-719.
4. Zivanovic O, Khoury-Collado F, Abu-Rustum NR, et al. Sentinel lymph node biopsy in the management of vulvar carcinoma, cervical cancer, and endometrial cancer. *Oncologist.* 2009;14(7):695-705.

CHAPTER **2.10**

Vulvar Cancer: Future Directions

Diane C. Ling and Sushil Beriwal

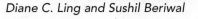

The incorporation of SLNB into the care of women with vulvar cancer raised many new questions regarding treatment of LN-positive patients. Should a woman with a microscopically positive SLN undergo full regional lymphadenectomy? How does the size of a groin metastasis impact survival, and how should it affect decisions regarding adjuvant treatment? Are ITCs clinically relevant?

The GROINS-VII/GOG 270 sought to answer some of these questions. This study showed that patients with ITCs or micrometastases can safely undergo adjuvant RT (50 Gy) in lieu of inguinofemoral lymphadenectomy. However, patients with macrometastases (>2 mm) were found to have an unacceptably high groin recurrence rate. In addition, the role of adjuvant chemotherapy is unclear. GROINS-VII/GOG 270 allowed the use of concurrent cisplatin during RT, albeit at the discretion of the treating physician.

Because of the suboptimal outcomes for patients with macrometastases in GROINS-VII, the ongoing GROINSS-VIII single-arm prospective study was opened in 2021. This trial is enrolling patients with macrometastases on SLNB and aims to evaluate whether increasing the radiation dose and adding concurrent chemotherapy can provide adequate outcomes while avoiding the morbidity of inguinofemoral nodal dissection. Patients will receive adjuvant chemoradiation using cisplatin in combination with higher RT dose (56 Gy) to the involved groin node/s using a simultaneous integrated boost technique.

Another area of significant interest will be targeted therapy. Large phase II/III trials in vulvar cancer are unlikely because of population size; however, lessons learned from squamous carcinomas of the anus, head and neck, cervix, and cutaneous melanoma

will likely provide significant insights into novel therapies for patients with vulvar cancer. In the future, different treatment protocols may be derived for HPV-positive versus HPV-negative vulvar cancers, reflecting their differences in etiology and pathogenesis.

SUMMARY

Most patients with vulvar cancer are potentially curable at the time of presentation for care. The major challenge for providers is how to balance providing curative therapy with preserving quality of life, including organ function, sexual function, and body image.

The preferred therapy for patients with early disease is surgery alone. The morbidity of surgery can be reduced with the use of SLNB as an alternative to regional lymphadenectomy. This approach has proved very successful in the treatment of patients with breast cancer and cutaneous melanoma. There is now enough clinical evidence to support routine use in patients with vulvar cancer. Further investigation is needed to determine the ideal management of patients with a positive SLN.

Women with advanced disease usually benefit from multimodality therapy. The exact combination and order of treatment rely on consultation with a team including a gynecologic oncologist, radiation oncologist, pathologist, and diagnostic imager. Vulvar cancer is sufficiently infrequent for even busy clinicians to consider referral to a high-volume center when considering the care of women with this disease.

3

VAGINAL CANCER

Vaginal Anatomy

Diana Miao, Josephine Kang, Amanda Nickles Fader, and Akila N. Viswanathan

The vagina is a fibromuscular tube that extends from the cervix down to the vestibule, or cleft, between the labia minora. The average length of the vagina is 3 to 4 inches. Superiorly, it joins the uterine cervix at an angle and, as a result, the posterior vaginal wall is longer than the anterior wall. The upper aspect of the posterior vaginal wall is separated from the rectum by a peritoneal reflection known as the pouch of Douglas. Invaginations between the vaginal mucosa and cervix form the anterior, posterior, and lateral fornices. Laterally, the vagina is adjacent to the pelvic fascia and levator ani muscles. Inferiorly, the vagina extends through the urogenital diaphragm to lie dorsal to the urethra and ventral to the rectum. The fibromuscular perineal body separates the vagina from the anal canal. At the introitus, the vagina has a perforated fold of thin connective tissue and mucous membrane known as the hymen (Figure 3.1-1).

The vaginal wall comprises the mucosa, muscularis, and adventitia. The innermost lining of the vagina is formed by a non-keratinizing, stratified squamous epithelium overlying a basement membrane. Underneath the mucosa is connective tissue composed of elastin and a thick muscularis layer composed of two layers of smooth muscle. The inner layer is arranged circularly, whereas the outer layer is arranged longitudinally. This muscular layer is covered by the third layer, a thin adventitia that merges with neighboring organs. This epithelial mucosa lacks glandular structures and instead receives lubrication from mucous secretions originating in the cervix.

The vagina has a complex pattern of lymphatic drainage, with multiple interconnections. The upper vagina drains to the obturator and hypogastric nodes, similar to the cervix. The lower vagina drains to the inguinal, femoral, and external iliac nodes, and

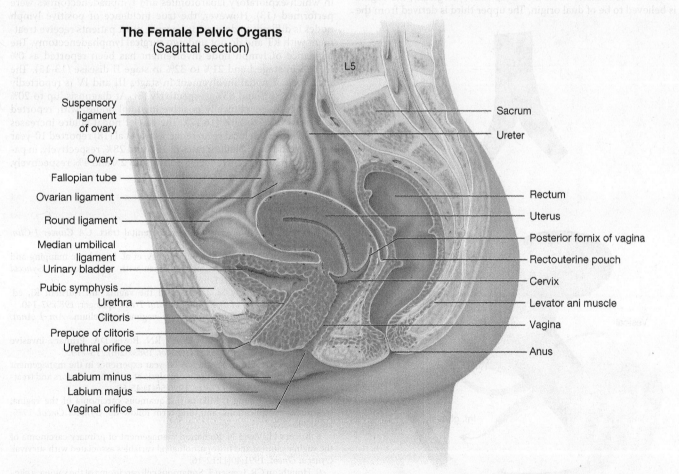

The Female Pelvic Organs
(Sagittal section)

L5

Suspensory ligament of ovary — Sacrum
— Ureter
Ovary
Fallopian tube
Ovarian ligament — Rectum
Round ligament — Uterus
Median umbilical ligament — Posterior fornix of vagina
— Rectouterine pouch
Urinary bladder
Pubic symphysis — Cervix
Urethra — Levator ani muscle
Clitoris — Vagina
Prepuce of clitoris
Urethral orifice — Anus
Labium minus
Labium majus
Vaginal orifice

Figure 3.1-1. The lower female pelvis in sagittal view. The vagina is a fibromuscular tube situated posterior to the bladder and urethra and anterior to the rectum. The anterior and posterior fornices are formed by protrusion of the cervix into the vaginal canal. Reproduced from Anatomical Chart Company. *Female Reproductive System Anatomical Chart*. Wolters Kluwer Health; 2001.

posteriorly situated lesions can drain to the inferior gluteal, presacral, or perirectal nodes. Lymphatic channels in the mucosa run parallel to networks of channels in the submucosa and muscular layer, ultimately converging to form trunks at the vaginal wall periphery, which subsequently drain to major pelvic nodal groups (**Figure 3.1-2**) (1). Lesions infiltrating the rectovaginal septum may spread to the pararectal and presacral nodes.

Because there are multiple interconnections between lymphatic channels, the pattern of drainage cannot be reliably predicted based on location of the primary tumor. Frumovitz et al (2) utilized lymphoscintigraphy to determine patterns of lymphatic drainage in 14 women diagnosed with primary vaginal cancers and found a substantial degree of anomalous drainage, resulting in a change in radiation therapy (RT) for 33% of patients. For example, among four women with lesions located in the upper third of the vagina, which is predicted to drain along the cervical lymphatic chains to the pelvis, two (50%) were found to have a sentinel node in the inguinal region. Among five women with lesions located at the vaginal introitus, a location predicted to drain along the vulvar lymphatic chains to the inguinal triangle, three (60%) were found to have a sentinel node in the pelvis.

The proximal blood supply to the vagina is by the vaginal artery, which arises from the cervical branch of the uterine artery and runs lateral to the vagina until it anastomoses with the inferior vesical and middle rectal arteries. The venous plexus runs parallel to the arteries, draining into the internal iliac vein. The vaginal vault is innervated by the lumbar plexus and pudendal nerve, with branches from sacral roots 2 to 4 (3). Embryologically, the vagina is believed to be of dual origin. The upper third is derived from the uterine canal, whereas the lower two-thirds are derived from the urogenital sinus (4).

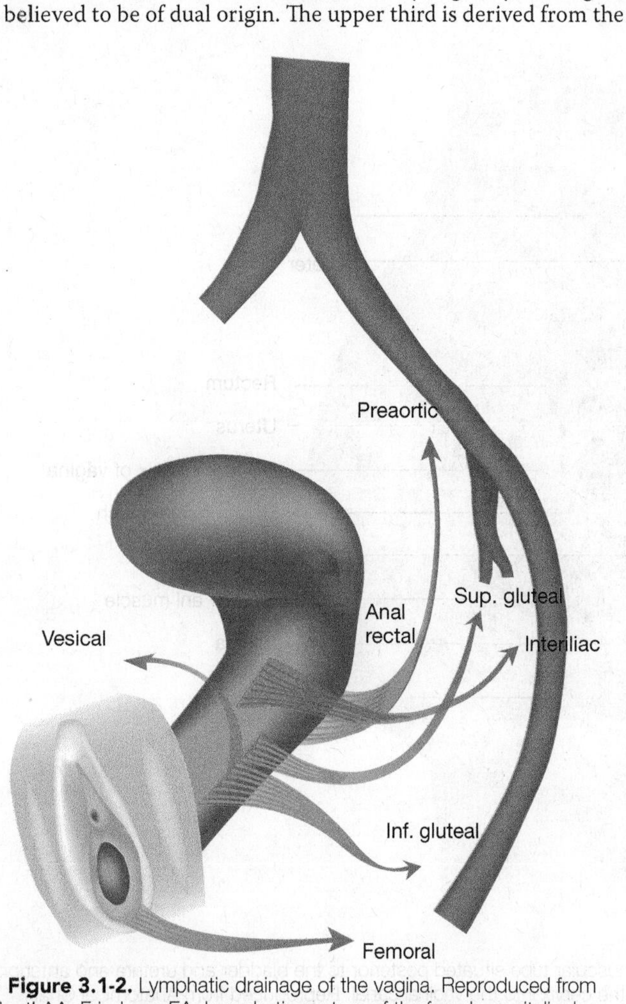

PATTERNS OF SPREAD

Vaginal cancer most frequently involves the superior one-third of the vaginal canal, with series reporting 50% to 83% of cases occurring in this region (5-11). A high proportion of patients have a history of prior hysterectomy. There is approximately equal involvement of the middle and inferior thirds (5), although some studies suggest that involvement of the lower third is more common than involvement of the middle third (7,12). The lateral walls are less frequently involved. Tumors may exhibit an exophytic or ulcerative, infiltrating growth pattern.

Vaginal tumors can spread along the vaginal walls to involve the cervix or vulva, but involvement of the cervix or vulva at the time of diagnosis excludes classification as a primary vaginal cancer. Lesions can extend radially, either into the lumen to form exophytic masses or through the vaginal wall to invade surrounding musculature and organs. Anterior wall lesions can infiltrate the vesicovaginal septum and/or urethra. Posterior wall lesions can infiltrate the rectovaginal septum and involve the rectal mucosa. Advanced disease can extend laterally toward the parametrium and paracolpal tissues, or into the urogenital diaphragm, levator ani muscles, or pelvic fascia, and eventually to the pelvic sidewall.

The risk of nodal metastasis appears to increase significantly with stage. Sparse data on nodal metastases are derived from series in which exploratory laparotomies and lymphadenectomies were performed (13). However, the true incidence of positive lymph nodes is difficult to determine because most patients receive treatment with RT and do not undergo surgical lymphadenectomy. The incidence of lymph node involvement has been reported as 0% to 14% in stage I and 21% to 32% in stage II disease (13-15). The incidence of nodal involvement in stages III and IV is reportedly as high as 78% and 83%, respectively (7). At diagnosis, up to 20% of patients have clinically positive inguinal nodes, with reported ranges of 5.3% to 20% (16,17). The risk of nodal failure increases significantly with local recurrence. Chyle et al (18) reported 10-year inguinal and pelvic failure rates of 16% and 28%, respectively, in patients with local recurrence, in contrast to 2% and 4%, respectively, in patients without local recurrence.

REFERENCES

1. Benson RC. Cancer of the female genital tract. *CA Cancer J Clin.* 1968;18(1):2-13.
2. Frumovitz M, Gayed IW, Jhingran A, et al. Lymphatic mapping and sentinel lymph node detection in women with vaginal cancer. *Gynecol Oncol.* 2008;108(3):478-481.
3. Sedlis A, Robboy SJ. Diseases of the vagina. In: Kurman RJ, ed. *Blaustein's Pathology of the Female Genital Tract.* Springer; 1987:97-140.
4. Cunha GR. The dual origin of vaginal epithelium. *Am J Anat.* 1975;143(3):387-392.
5. Benedet JL, Murphy KJ, Fairey RN, Boyes DA. Primary invasive carcinoma of the vagina. *Obstet Gynecol.* 1983;62(6):715-719.
6. Stock RG, Chen AS, Seski J. A 30-year experience in the management of primary carcinoma of the vagina: analysis of prognostic factors and treatment modalities. *Gynecol Oncol.* 1995;56(1):45-52.
7. Rubin SC, Young J, Mikuta JJ. Squamous carcinoma of the vagina: treatment, complications, and long-term follow-up. *Gynecol Oncol.* 1985; 20(3):346-353.
8. Kucera H, Vavra N. Radiation management of primary carcinoma of the vagina: clinical and histopathological variables associated with survival. *Gynecol Oncol.* 1991;40(1):12-16.
9. Houghton CR, Iversen T. Squamous cell carcinoma of the vagina: a clinical study of the location of the tumor. *Gynecol Oncol.* 1982;13(3):365-372.
10. Eddy GL, Singh KP, Gansler TS. Superficially invasive carcinoma of the vagina following treatment for cervical cancer: a report of six cases. *Gynecol Oncol.* 1990;36(3):376-379.
11. Peters WA 3rd, Kumar NB, Morley GW. Carcinoma of the vagina. Factors influencing treatment outcome. *Cancer.* 1985;55(4):892-897.

Figure 3.1-2. Lymphatic drainage of the vagina. Reproduced from Plentl AA, Friedman EA. Lymphatic system of the female genitalia. In: Plentl AA, Friedman EA, eds. *The Morphologic Basis of Oncologic Diagnosis and Therapy.* WB Saunders; 1971:55, Figure 5-2. Used with permission.

12. Gallup DG, Talledo OE, Shah KJ, Hayes C. Invasive squamous cell carcinoma of the vagina: a 14-year study. *Obstet Gynecol.* 1987;69(5):782-785.

13. Davis KP, Stanhope CR, Garton GR, Atkinson EJ, O'Brien PC. Invasive vaginal carcinoma: analysis of early-stage disease. *Gynecol Oncol.* 1991;42(2):131-136.

14. Al-Kurdi M, Monaghan JM. Thirty-two years experience in management of primary tumours of the vagina. *Br J Obstet Gynaecol.* 1981;88(11):1145-1150.

15. Senekjian EK, Frey KW, Stone C, Herbst AL. An evaluation of stage II vaginal clear cell adenocarcinoma according to substages. *Gynecol Oncol.* 1988;31(1):56-64.

16. Perez CA, Grigsby PW, Garipagaoglu M, Mutch DG, Lockett MA. Factors affecting long-term outcome of irradiation in carcinoma of the vagina. *Int J Radiat Oncol Biol Phys.* 1999;44(1):37-45.

17. Perez CA, Camel HM, Galakatos AE, et al. Definitive irradiation in carcinoma of the vagina: long-term evaluation of results. *Int J Radiat Oncol Biol Phys.* 1988;15(6):1283-1290.

18. Chyle V, Zagars GK, Wheeler JA, Wharton JT, Delclos L. Definitive radiotherapy for carcinoma of the vagina: outcome and prognostic factors. *Int J Radiat Oncol Biol Phys.* 1996;35(5):891-905.

CHAPTER **3.2**

Vaginal Cancer: Etiology, Epidemiology, Risk Factors, Genetics, and Molecular Biology

Diana Miao, Josephine Kang, Amanda Nickles Fader, and Akila N. Viswanathan

INTRODUCTION

According to the American Cancer Society estimates for 2023, there are approximately 8,470 new cases of vaginal cancer and over 1,470 deaths attributable to vaginal cancer (1). Worldwide, there were approximately 17,908 cases of vaginal cancer diagnosed in 2020 result in 8,000 deaths, with vaginal cancer accounting for about 0.1% of all cancers (2). Vaginal cancer is a rare malignancy, constituting 1% to 2% of all gynecologic malignancies (3). According to compiled data from U.S. population–based cancer registries spanning 1998 to 2003, the incidence of all vaginal cancers was 0.18 per 100,000 females for in situ cases and 0.69 per 100,000 females for invasive cases (4).

Most primary vaginal malignancies are squamous cell carcinomas (SCCs). According to a National Cancer Database (NCDB) report (5), which evaluated 4,885 patients with primary vaginal cancer registered from 1985 to 1994, approximately 92% of patients were diagnosed with in situ or invasive SCC or adenocarcinomas, 4% with melanomas, 3% with sarcomas, and 1% with other/unspecified types of cancer. Sixty-six percent of all vaginal cancers were invasive, with SCC representing 79% of all invasive cases.

The peak incidence of primary vaginal cancer is in the sixth and seventh decades of life. According to data from the Surveillance, Epidemiology and End Results (SEER) Program (6), 2,149 women in the United States were diagnosed with primary vaginal cancer from 1990 to 2004. The mean age at diagnosis was 65± 14 years, and incidence increased with age. There has been an overall decrease in the incidence of primary vaginal tumors, possibly secondary to earlier detection and to implementation of strict exclusion criteria in the International Federation of Obstetrics and Gynecology (FIGO) staging system.

At the same time, there has been a steady increase in the diagnosis of vaginal intraepithelial neoplasia (VAIN) over the past several decades, perhaps as a result of expanded cytologic screening and increased awareness. It is hypothesized that VAIN is a precursor lesion to SCC of the vagina (3,7).

Most malignant lesions in the vagina are attributable to direct spread or metastases from other gynecologic malignancies and are classified accordingly. According to the FIGO staging system, any tumor involving both the vagina and the cervix should be classified as a cervical carcinoma. Similarly, any tumor involving both the vagina and the vulva is to be classified as a vulvar carcinoma (8). A malignant vaginal lesion in a patient with a prior history of invasive cervical carcinoma within the past 5 years also excludes diagnosis as a primary vaginal cancer (9). As a result, only a minority of cancers detected in the vagina meet the criteria of a primary vaginal cancer. According to one study of 141 vaginal carcinoma cases, only 26% could be classified as such (10).

Vaginal Intraepithelial Neoplasia

Definitions/Histopathology

VAIN is defined as the presence of squamous cell atypia without evidence of invasion. Histopathologically, most lesions are epidermoid and exhibit full-thickness alterations with atypical mitoses and hyperchromatism (11). Punctation and mosaic patterns are often noted in high-grade VAIN (12). Most lesions are multifocal and can involve all surfaces of the vagina, although the superior one-third of the vagina is most common (13,14).

VAIN is further classified into low-grade (VAIN 1) and high-grade (VAIN 2-3). VAIN 1 is characterized by cytomorphologic changes limited to the upper one-third of the epithelium. Such changes include nuclear enlargement, nuclear hyperchromasia, cytoplasmic halos, and occasional binucleation. VAIN 2 and 3 are characterized by cytomorphologic changes in the basal keratinocytes, including nuclear pleomorphism, nuclear hyperchromasia and crowding, and mitotic figures (including atypical forms). VAIN 2 and 3 are distinguished by depth of cytologic change. Cytologic changes confined to the lower two-thirds of the epithelium are designated VAIN 2, whereas changes involving the full thickness of the epithelium are VAIN 3. Carcinoma in situ encompasses the full epithelial thickness and is included under VAIN 3.

Excluded from the diagnosis of VAIN is the presence of glandular intraepithelial dysplasia, or atypical vaginal adenosis; these entities are associated with in utero diethylstilbestrol (DES) exposure and are deemed to be precursors of DES-associated clear cell adenocarcinoma (15).

Epidemiology

Hummer and colleagues first reported VAIN in 1933 and defined it as atypical squamous cells without evidence of stromal invasion (7). The incidence of VAIN is estimated to be 0.2 to 0.3 per 100,000 cases, with peak incidence found in women who are between 40 and 60 years of age (3,7,16,17). VAIN is further characterized according to depth of epithelial involvement from one-third, two-thirds, and greater than two-thirds thickness as VAIN 1, 2, and 3, respectively. Several series report that the median age at diagnosis for patients with VAIN 1 or 2 is lower than that for VAIN 3 (18-20), but this has not been corroborated by other series (7,12).

Involvement of the full thickness of the epithelium is known as in situ vaginal cancer and is included as VAIN 3 (**Figure 3.2-1**). The incidence of in situ vaginal cancer is estimated to be 0.1 per 100,000 women, with peak incidence between ages 70 and 79 years, according to data from the U.S. Centers for Disease Control and Prevention's National Program of Cancer Registries, and the National Cancer Institute's SEER Program (21). These numbers are similar to data from U.S. population–based cancer registries encompassing the years from 1998 to 2003, which report incidence of in situ vaginal cancer to be 0.18 per 100,000 females (4). The peak age of in situ vaginal cancer is slightly lower than that for primary vaginal cancer.

There are multiple risk factors for VAIN; the most common are low socioeconomic level, history of genital warts, hysterectomy at an early age, history of cervical intraepithelial neoplasia (CIN), immunosuppression, prior pelvic radiation, smoking, exposure to DES, and history of sexually transmitted diseases (STDs) and/or human papillomavirus (HPV) infection (20,22-24). HPV is implicated in the development of VAIN, and the relationship between HPV and the development of intraepithelial neoplasia has also been best demonstrated for cervical lesions. HPV 16 and 18 are the most prevalent subtypes associated with VAIN (25). A review of 232 published VAIN cases documented a high prevalence of HPV using polymerase chain reaction (PCR) or hybrid capture assays for detection, with 98.5% and 92.6% of VAIN 1 and VAIN 2/3 cases positive for HPV (26). A series by Sugase and Matsukura (27) examining 71 biopsy specimens of VAIN found HPV in 100% of samples. Fifteen different known subtypes were identified (HPV 16, 18, 30, 31, 35, 40, 42, 43, 51, 52, 53, 54, 56, 58, 66). It is estimated that HPV 16/18 is identified in 40% of VAIN 1 and 60% of high-grade VAIN 2/3 cases (26).

The diagnosis of VAIN is associated with prior or concurrent neoplasia elsewhere in the lower genital tract. Multiple series suggest approximately 50% to 90% of patients with VAIN have concurrent or prior history of intraepithelial neoplasia or carcinoma of the cervix or vulva (13,16,20). Immunosuppression from human immunodeficiency virus (HIV) is also a risk factor for both VAIN and HPV, though a higher incidence of invasive vaginal cancer in infected women has not been demonstrated (28-30). The role of pelvic radiation in the development of secondary vaginal neoplasia is unclear, with conflicting data suggesting that a history of ionizing radiation may predispose to VAIN or vaginal cancer after a latency period of many years (14,31,32). In utero exposure to DES may double the risk of VAIN, thought to be due to transformation zone enlargement, increasing the risk of HPV infection (33). With widespread implementation of HPV vaccination, it is anticipated that the incidence of VAIN will start to decline. It is predicted that HPV vaccination will ultimately prevent up to 70% of VAIN cases (34,35).

Although the pathogenesis of both VAIN and CIN is attributable to HPV infection, the incidence of VAIN is notably lower. One study reported a 100-fold difference in incidence (20). It is speculated that the mature, squamous epithelium of the vagina is less vulnerable to persistent dysplasia than the metaplastic transformation zone of the cervix (7,20).

Natural History

Although the likelihood of VAIN progressing to invasive disease is difficult to predict in individual cases, multiple clinical series have demonstrated a significant overall increase in risk of invasive vaginal cancer after a diagnosis of VAIN (13,14,36,37). Similar risk factors for VAIN and invasive vaginal cancer, as well as the younger average age at presentation of VAIN compared with invasive disease, support the theory that VAIN is a precursor lesion to invasive SCC. It is believed that high-grade VAIN, in particular, is a direct precursor to invasive disease (7).

In one series, 23 patients with VAIN, with a mean age of 41 years, were followed for at least 3 years without treatment (13); the cases included multifocal lesions as well as lesions associated with CIN or vulvar dysplasia. Two cases (9%) progressed to invasive cancer; one patient had VAIN 1 and progressed to stage I vaginal carcinoma in 5 years, and the second patient had VAIN 3 and progressed to stage I vaginal carcinoma in 4 years. The overall spontaneous regression rate was 78%, all occurring in patients with VAIN 1 or VAIN 2. Similarly, several additional retrospective studies have demonstrated a range of 2% to 20% of patients with VAIN progressing to invasive vaginal cancer (13,14,36,38-40). The rate of occult invasive disease in patients with VAIN 3 is reportedly as high as 28% (41). The risk of malignant transformation in VAIN 1 and 2 is less clearly elucidated (12,22).

Malignant Tumors of the Vagina: Squamous Cell Carcinoma

Definitions/Histopathology

Grossly, SCC of the vagina can present as nodular, ulcerated, indurated, exophytic or endophytic lesions, and it is difficult to

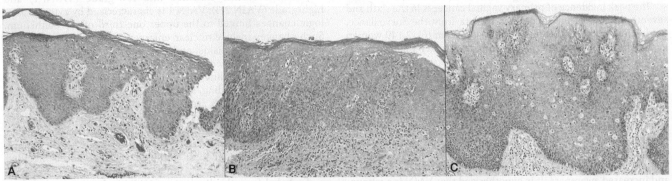

Figure 3.2-1. Vaginal intraepithelial neoplasia (VAIN). A: Low-grade squamous intraepithelial lesion of the vagina (VAIN 1) is characterized by nuclear enlargement in the upper one-third of the squamous epithelium with nuclear contour irregularities, occasional binucleation or multinucleation, and distinct cytoplasmic halos. B, C: High-grade squamous intraepithelial lesion of the vagina (VAIN 2-3) shows changes in the basal keratinocytes including nuclear pleomorphism with high N:C ratio, crowding, and hyperchromasia. In VAIN 3 lesions (C), these changes involve the full thickness of the epithelium, and frequent mitoses are usually seen. In VAIN 2 lesions (B), these changes involve less than the full thickness of the epithelium, and mitoses, when present, are confined to the lower levels of the epithelium. Images courtesy of Emily E. K. Meserve.

histologically distinguish a primary vaginal SCC from recurrent cervical or vulvar carcinoma. Histologically, tumors are graded as well, moderately, or poorly differentiated and have been described as keratinizing, nonkeratinizing, basaloid, warty, or verrucous. Most of these lesions are nonkeratinizing and moderately differentiated (42) (**Figure 3.2-2**).

Verrucous carcinoma is a distinct histologic variant of vaginal SCC (43). It commonly presents as a well-circumscribed, soft, cauliflower-like mass that is microscopically well differentiated, with a papillary growth pattern and acanthotic epithelium (**Figure 3.2-3**). There is surface maturation with parakeratosis or hyperkeratosis without koilocytosis. This variant of SCC exhibits less aggressive behavior and rarely metastasizes (43-46). Therefore, it should be considered a distinct entity from other vaginal SCC.

Sarcomatoid SCC is a rare subset of vaginal SCC, comprising 2% of all cases (**Figure 3.2-4**). It is characterized by spindle-shaped neoplastic cells that may initially be mistaken for sarcoma. However, positive stains for cytokeratin help distinguish sarcomatoid SCC as a poorly differentiated variant of vaginal SCC (47).

Epidemiology

The NCDB review by Creasman et al, for the period 1985 to 1994, revealed 3,244 cases of invasive primary vaginal carcinoma, with 24% of patients presenting with American Joint Committee on Cancer (AJCC) stage I disease, 20% AJCC stage II, 24% AJCC stages III to IV, and 32% unknown. Most tumors were moderately (28%) or poorly (28%) differentiated at presentation. Consistent with this data, a review of five series, including a total of 1,375 cases of vaginal cancer, reported the FIGO stage distribution as follows: 26% stage I, 37% stage II, 24% stage III, and 13% stage IV (48).

According to the SEER study by Shah and colleagues from 1990 to 2004 of 2,149 with primary vaginal cancer (6), most women diagnosed with primary vaginal cancer are non-Hispanic White (66%), followed by African Americans (14%), Hispanic White (12%), Asian/Pacific Islanders (7%), and others (1%). Mean age at diagnosis was 65.7 years. Incidence rates were highest for African American women (1.24/100,000 person-years) and lowest for Asian/Pacific Islanders (0.64/100,000 person-years). The greatest proportion of women (36%) presented with stage I disease, and 65% had squamous histology, consistent with other reports.

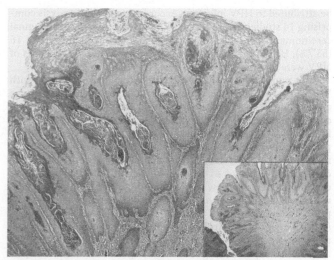

Figure 3.2-3. Verrucous squamous cell carcinoma (SCC). Verrucous SCC is a rare subtype of extremely well-differentiated SCC. Tumors are often exophytic (inset) with very bland and uniform cytologic features and often a "pushing" pattern of invasion, rather than invasion by irregular nests or single cells as seen more frequently in conventional SCC. Images courtesy of Emily E. K. Meserve.

An updated SEER analysis from 2004 to 2014 characterized 1,781 women with primary vaginal cancer. Approximately 78.4% of patients were White, 14.9% were Black, and 6.4% were Other. Most patients were of age 50 to 79 years at diagnosis (65.4%), with a minority at age 80 or older at diagnosis (20%) or between age 18 to 49 years (14.6%). Most cases were SCC (74.5%), followed by adenocarcinoma (16.7%), melanoma (3.3%), sarcoma (1.5%), and other (4.0%). Diagnosis was most common at stage I (32.8%), but many cases were also diagnosed at stages II (27.1%), III (19.6%), and IV (20.5%).

Risk factors for primary vaginal SCC are similar to those for VAIN and cervical neoplasia. Commonly cited factors include HPV infection and/or history of cervical or vulvar intraepithelial neoplasia, immunosuppression, multiple sexual partners, and early age at first intercourse. It is believed that most cases of vaginal cancer can

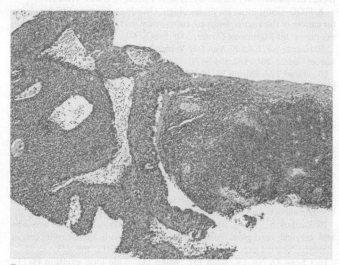

Figure 3.2-2. Moderately differentiated squamous cell carcinoma of the vagina. Invasive squamous cell carcinoma may appear as nests of atypical keratinocytes or, alternatively, may appear as complex, redundant strips of neoplastic epithelium. In moderately differentiated squamous cell carcinoma, the keratinocytes show nuclear atypia, nuclear hyperchromasia, and high N:C ratio, often with easily identifiable mitoses, and limited evidence of squamous maturation, as expected in well-differentiated examples. Images courtesy of Emily E. K. Meserve.

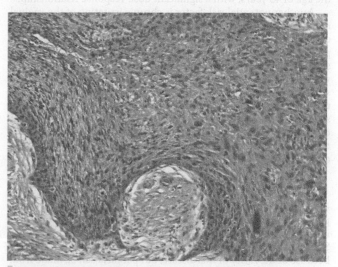

Figure 3.2-4. Sarcomatoid squamous cell carcinoma (SCC). Sarcomatoid SCC is a type of poorly differentiated SCC wherein neoplastic squamous epithelial cells exhibit a spindle cell morphology. Keratin expression is less consistent in areas of spindle cell morphology, but continuity with areas of more conventional poorly differentiated SCC, with prominent nuclear pleomorphism and necrosis, helps confirm the diagnosis of carcinoma. Images courtesy of Emily E. K. Meserve.

be attributed to HPV infection. According to a meta-analysis comprising 14 studies, the overall HPV prevalence was 70% for vaginal carcinomas, with the most common subtypes as follows: HPV 16 (53.7%), HPV 18 (7.6%), and HPV 31 (5.6%). Multiple subtypes of HPV were identified in 3.4% of cases (49).

In a population-based case-control study of 156 women with VAIN or invasive cancer, significant risk factors included early age at intercourse, increased number of lifetime sexual partners, and current smoking. HPV DNA was detectable in 80% of patients with in situ disease and in 60% of those with invasive disease; 30% of patients reported a history of treatment for invasive malignancy, most commonly cervix, or in situ anogenital neoplasia (37). A case-control study of 41 women with in situ disease or invasive carcinoma identified low socioeconomic status, history of genital warts, vaginal discharge or irritation, history of abnormal cytology, prior hysterectomy, and vaginal trauma as potential risk factors (50). A larger case-control study of 36,856 women in Sweden found an increased risk of vaginal cancer in patients with a diagnosis of alcoholism (51). This may be due to a high association with other lifestyle factors such as HPV-associated precancers and cancers, including tobacco use and having multiple sexual partners. Prior hysterectomy is not a risk factor for vaginal cancer after controlling for prior cervical dysplasia or neoplasia, and screening for vaginal cancer is unnecessary in women with a history of hysterectomy for benign disease with no prior history of CIN2 or greater and appropriate preoperative Pap smear screening (37,52,53).

Patients with a history of cervical cancer have a significantly higher risk of developing in situ as well as invasive carcinoma of the vagina. Studies suggest that 10% to 50% of patients with a history of VAIN or invasive carcinoma of the vagina have undergone treatment for in situ or invasive cervical carcinoma (14,54-61), with the interval from treatment of cervical disease to development of vaginal carcinoma averaging approximately 14 years (57,62). HIV-infected women are also at higher risk of developing vaginal carcinoma, which tends to behave more aggressively in patients who are HIV positive than who are HIV negative (63).

The role of ionizing radiation to the pelvis in the development of vaginal carcinoma is unclear, with conflicting reports. According to one study that analyzed 1,200 patients treated over a 20-year period for carcinoma of the cervix, prior RT was not shown to result in increased secondary pelvic neoplasms (32). A second study by Boice et al (31), however, reported a 14-fold increased risk of vaginal cancer in women with a history of pelvic irradiation before the age of 45 years, with a significant dose-response relationship.

Another potential risk factor is chronic irritation of the vaginal mucosa, resulting in chronic inflammation, hyperkeratosis, thickening, and acanthosis (63), with subsequent metaplastic and dysplastic changes; however, this is not proven. Although older studies showed that more vaginal cancers arise from the posterior vaginal wall, other studies report approximately equal distribution of invasive carcinomas on the anterior and posterior walls (36,57,64-66); this poses an argument against the theory that pooling of irritating substances in the posterior fornix contributes to the development of vaginal cancers, particularly on the posterior wall. Chronic irritation from the use of vaginal pessaries has also been implicated as a factor in vaginal cancer development (67,68).

Molecular Genetics

In the past decades, comprehensive genomic profiling of multiple cancer types, including gynecologic cancers, has yielded new insights into the molecular biology of gynecologic malignancies. Studies focusing specifically on vaginal cancer have been limited because of the rarity of this disease, but parallels can be made from cervical and vulvar cancers.

Comprehensive molecular characterization of 228 cervical cancers was performed in The Cancer Genome Atlas (TCGA) project (69) although not performed on vaginal cancer. The vast majority of samples were HPV positive, and these cancers demonstrated expression of E6 and E7 mRNA. The HPV-negative tumors displayed endometrial-like genomic features, including frequent mutations in *KRAS*, *ARID1A*, and *PTEN*. Amplifications in *CD274* (encoding programmed death-ligand 1 [PD-L1]) and *PDCD1LG2* (encoding PD-L2) were also seen in about 21% of samples, potentially relating to immunotherapy responsiveness. Further research specifically characterizing genomic features of HPV positive and HPV negative vaginal cancer may help to better understand and treat this rare cancer.

A study of 51 vulvovaginal melanomas (14 vaginal and 37 vulvar) has also shown that this disease is distinct from other forms of cutaneous, mucosal, and acral melanoma (70). The *BRAF* and *KIT* oncogenes were frequently mutated (26% and 22%, respectively), whereas *NRAS* mutations were rare. PD-L1 and PD-1 were also frequently expressed (56% and 75%), whereas PI3KCA pathway mutations and estrogen receptor (ER)/progesterone receptor (PR) expression were uncommon.

Further research specifically characterizing genomic features of HPV-positive and HPV-negative vaginal cancer may help to better understand and treat this rare cancer.

REFERENCES

1. Siegel RL, Miller KD, Fuchs HE, Jemal A. Cancer statistics, 2021. *CA Cancer J Clin.* 2021;71(1):7-33.
2. Sung H, Ferlay J, Siegel RL, et al. Global Cancer Statistics 2020: GLOBOCAN Estimates of Incidence and Mortality Worldwide for 36 Cancers in 185 Countries. *CA Cancer J Clin.* 2021;71(3):209-249. doi:10.3322/caac.21660.
3. Henson D, Tarone R. An epidemiologic study of cancer of the cervix, vagina, and vulva based on the third national cancer survey in the United States. *Am J Obstet Gynecol.* 1977;129(5):525-532.
4. Wu X, Matanoski G, Chen VW, et al. Descriptive epidemiology of vaginal cancer incidence and survival by race, ethnicity, and age in the United States. *Cancer.* 2008;113(10 Suppl):2873-2882.
5. Creasman WT, Phillips JL, Menck HR. The national cancer data base report on cancer of the vagina. *Cancer.* 1998;83(5):1033-1040.
6. Shah CA, Goff BA, Lowe K, Peters WA 3rd, Li CI. Factors affecting risk of mortality in women with vaginal cancer. *Obstet Gynecol.* 2009;113(5):1038-1045.
7. Gunderson CC, Nugent EK, Elfrink SH, Gold MA, Moore KN. A contemporary analysis of epidemiology and management of vaginal intraepithelial neoplasia. *Am J Obstet Gynecol.* 2013;208(5):410.e1-410.e4106.
8. FIGO Committee on Gynecologic Oncology. Current FIGO staging for cancer of the vagina, fallopian tube, ovary, and gestational trophoblastic neoplasia. *Int J Gynaecol Obstet.* 2009;105(1):3-4.
9. Hacker NF, Eifel PJ, Van Der Velden J. Cancer of the vagina. *Int J Gynaecol Obstet.* 2015;131:S84-S87.
10. Murad TM, Durant JR, Maddox WA, Dowling EA. The pathologic behavior of primary vaginal carcinoma and its relationship to cervical cancer. *Cancer.* 1975;35(3):787-794.
11. Woodruff JD. Carcinoma in situ of the vagina. *Clin Obstet Gynecol.* 1981;24(2):485-501.
12. Boonlikit S, Noinual N. Vaginal intraepithelial neoplasia: a retrospective analysis of clinical features and colpohistology. *J Obstet Gynaecol Res.* 2010;36(1):94-100.
13. Aho M, Vesterinen E, Meyer B, Purola E, Paavonen J. Natural history of vaginal intraepithelial neoplasia. *Cancer.* 1991;68(1):195-197.
14. Lenehan PM, Meffe F, Lickrish GM. Vaginal intraepithelial neoplasia: biologic aspects and management. *Obstet Gynecol.* 1986;68(3):333-337.
15. Robboy SJ, Young RH, Welch WR, et al. Atypical vaginal adenosis and cervical ectropion. Association with clear cell adenocarcinoma in diethylstilbestrol-exposed offspring. *Cancer.* 1984;54(5):869-875.
16. Cheng D, Ng TY, Ngan HY, Wong LC. Wide local excision (WLE) for vaginal intraepithelial neoplasia (VAIN). *Acta Obstet Gynecol Scand.* 1999;78(7):648-652.
17. Hampl M, Huppertz E, Schulz-Holstege O, Kok P, Schmitter S. Economic burden of vulvar and vaginal intraepithelial neoplasia: retrospective cost study at a German dysplasia centre. *BMC Infect Dis.* 2011; 11(1):73.

18. Rome RM, England PG. Management of vaginal intraepithelial neoplasia: a series of 132 cases with long-term follow-up. *Int J Gynecol Cancer.* 2000;10(5):382-390.

19. Diakomanolis E, Stefanidis K, Rodolakis A, et al. Vaginal intraepithelial neoplasia: report of 102 cases. *Eur J Gynaecol Oncol.* 2002;23(5):457-459.

20. Sillman FH, Fruchter RG, Chen YS, Camilien L, Sedlis A, McTigue E. Vaginal intraepithelial neoplasia: risk factors for persistence, recurrence, and invasion and its management. *Am J Obstet Gynecol.* 1997;176(1):93-99.

21. Watson M, Saraiya M, Wu X. Update of HPV-associated female genital cancers in the United States, 1999–2004. *J Womens Health.* 2009;18(11):1731-1738.

22. Dodge JA, Eltabbakh GH, Mount SL, Walker RP, Morgan A. Clinical features and risk of recurrence among patients with vaginal intraepithelial neoplasia. *Gynecol Oncol.* 2001;83(2):363-369.

23. González Bosquet E, Torres A, Busquets M, Esteva C, Muñoz-Almagro C, Lailla JM. Prognostic factors for the development of vaginal intraepithelial neoplasia. *Eur J Gynaecol Oncol.* 2008;29(1):43-45.

24. Jamieson DJ, Paramsothy P, Cu-Uvin S, Duerr A; HIV Epidemiology Research Study Group. Vulvar, vaginal, and perianal intraepithelial neoplasia in women with or at risk for human immunodeficiency virus. *Obstet Gynecol.* 2006;107(5):1023-1028.

25. Insinga RP, Liaw KL, Johnson LG, Madeleine MM. A systematic review of the prevalence and attribution of human papillomavirus types among cervical, vaginal, and vulvar precancers and cancers in the United States. *Cancer Epidemiol Biomarkers Prev.* 2008;17(7):1611-1622.

26. Smith JS, Backes DM, Hoots BE, Kurman RJ, Pimenta JM. Human papillomavirus type-distribution in vulvar and vaginal cancers and their associated precursors. *Obstet Gynecol.* 2009;113(4):917-924.

27. Sugase M, Matsukura T. Distinct manifestations of human papillomaviruses in the vagina. *Int J Cancer.* 1997;72(3):412-415.

28. Sillman F, Stanek A, Sedlis A, et al. The relationship between human papillomavirus and lower genital intraepithelial neoplasia in immunosuppressed women. *Am J Obstet Gynecol.* 1984;150(3):300-308.

29. Spitzer M. Lower genital tract intraepithelial neoplasia in HIV-infected women: guidelines for evaluation and management. *Obstet Gynecol Surv.* 1999;54(2):131-137.

30. Conley LJ, Ellerbrock TV, Bush TJ, Chiasson MA, Sawo D, Wright TC. HIV-1 infection and risk of vulvovaginal and perianal condylomata acuminata and intraepithelial neoplasia: a prospective cohort study. *Lancet.* 2002;359(9301):108-113.

31. Boice JD Jr, Engholm G, Kleinerman RA, et al. Radiation dose and second cancer risk in patients treated for cancer of the cervix. *Radiat Res.* 1988;116(1):3-55.

32. Lee JY, Perez CA, Ettinger N, Fineberg BB. The risk of second primaries subsequent to irradiation for cervix cancer. *Int J Radiat Oncol Biol Phys.* 1982;8(2):207-211.

33. Bornstein J, Adam E, Adler-Storthz K, Kaufman RH. Development of cervical and vaginal squamous cell neoplasia as a late consequence of in utero exposure to diethylstilbestrol. *Obstet Gynecol Surv.* 1988;43(1):15-21.

34. FUTURE I/II Study Group, Dillner J, Kjaer SK, et al. Four year efficacy of prophylactic human papillomavirus quadrivalent vaccine against low grade cervical, vulvar, and vaginal intraepithelial neoplasia and anogenital warts: randomised controlled trial. *BMJ.* 2010;341:c3493.

35. Joura EA, Leodolter S, Hernandez-Avila M, et al. Efficacy of a quadrivalent prophylactic human papillomavirus (types 6, 11, 16, and 18) L1 virus-like-particle vaccine against high-grade vulval and vaginal lesions: a combined analysis of three randomised clinical trials. *Lancet.* 2007;369(9574): 1693-1702.

36. Benedet JL, Murphy KJ, Fairey RN, Boyes DA. Primary invasive carcinoma of the vagina. *Obstet Gynecol.* 1983;62(6):715-719.

37. Daling JR, Madeleine MM, Schwartz SM, et al. A population-based study of squamous cell vaginal cancer: HPV and cofactors. *Gynecol Oncol.* 2002;84(2):263-270.

38. Liao JB, Jean S, Wilkinson-Ryan I, et al. Vaginal intraepithelial neoplasia (VAIN) after radiation therapy for gynecologic malignancies: a clinically recalcitrant entity. *Gynecol Oncol.* 2011;120(1):108-112.

39. Geelhoed GW, Henson DE, Taylor PT, Ketcham AS. Carcinoma in situ of the vagina following treatment for carcinoma of the cervix: a distinctive clinical entity. *Am J Obstet Gynecol.* 1976;124(5):510-516.

40. Choo YC, Anderson DG. Neoplasms of the vagina following cervical carcinoma. *Gynecol Oncol.* 1982;14(1):125-132.

41. Hoffman MS, DeCesare SL, Roberts WS, Fiorica JV, Finan MA, Cavanagh D. Upper vaginectomy for in situ and occult, superficially invasive carcinoma of the vagina. *Am J Obstet Gynecol.* 1992;166(1):30-33.

42. Perez CA, Arneson AN, Dehner LP, Galakatos A. Radiation therapy in carcinoma of the vagina. *Obstet Gynecol.* 1974;44(6):862-872.

43. Väyrynen M, Romppanen T, Koskela E, Castren O, Syrjänen K. Verrucous squamous cell carcinoma of the female genital tract. Report of three cases and survey of the literature. *Int J Gynaecol Obstet.* 1981;19(5):351-356.

44. Crowther ME, Lowe DG, Shepherd JH. Verrucous carcinoma of the female genital tract: a review. *Obstet Gynecol Surv.* 1988;43(5):263-280.

45. Robertson DI, Maung R, Duggan MA. Verrucous carcinoma of the genital tract: is it a distinct entity? *Can J Surg.* 1993;36(2):147-151.

46. Andersen ES, Sorensen IM. Verrucous carcinoma of the female genital tract: report of a case and review of the literature. *Gynecol Oncol.* 1988;30(3):427-434.

47. Raptis S, Haber G, Ferenczy A. Vaginal squamous cell carcinoma with sarcomatoid spindle cell features. *Gynecol Oncol.* 1993;49(1):100-106.

48. Berek JS, Hacker NF, eds. *Berek and Hacker's Gynecologic Oncology.* 5th ed. Lippincott Williams & Wilkins; 2009.

49. De Vuyst H, Clifford GM, Nascimento MC, Madeleine MM, Franceschi S. Prevalence and type distribution of human papillomavirus in carcinoma and intraepithelial neoplasia of the vulva, vagina and anus: a meta-analysis. *Int J Cancer.* 2009;124(7):1626-1636.

50. Schiffman M, Kjaer SK. Chapter 2: natural history of anogenital human papillomavirus infection and neoplasia. *J Natl Cancer Inst Monogr.* 2003;2003(31):14-19.

51. Weiderpass E, Ye W, Tamimi R, et al. Alcoholism and risk for cancer of the cervix uteri, vagina, and vulva. *Cancer Epidemiol Biomarkers Prev.* 2001;10(8):899-901.

52. Herman JM, Homesley HD, Dignan MB. Is hysterectomy a risk factor for vaginal cancer? *JAMA.* 1986;256(5):601-603.

53. Perkins RB, Guido RS, Castle PE, et al. 2019 ASCCP risk-based management consensus guidelines for abnormal cervical cancer screening tests and cancer precursors. *J Low Genit Tract Dis.* 2020;24(2):102-131.

54. Chyle V, Zagars GK, Wheeler JA, Wharton JT, Delclos L. Definitive radiotherapy for carcinoma of the vagina: outcome and prognostic factors. *Int J Radiat Oncol Biol Phys.* 1996;35(5):891-905.

55. Andersen ES. Primary carcinoma of the vagina: a study of 29 cases. *Gynecol Oncol.* 1989;33(3):317-320.

56. Ball HG, Berman ML. Management of primary vaginal carcinoma. *Gynecol Oncol.* 1982;14(2):154-163.

57. Gallup DG, Talledo OE, Shah KJ, Hayes C. Invasive squamous cell carcinoma of the vagina: a 14-year study. *Obstet Gynecol.* 1987;69(5):782-785.

58. Kirkbride P, Fyles A, Rawlings GA, et al. Carcinoma of the vagina—experience at the Princess Margaret Hospital (1974-1989). *Gynecol Oncol.* 1995;56(3):435-443.

59. Leung S, Sexton M. Radical radiation therapy for carcinoma of the vagina—impact of treatment modalities on outcome: Peter MacCallum Cancer Institute experience 1970–1990. *Int J Radiat Oncol Biol Phys.* 1993;25(3):413-418.

60. Perez CA, Camel HM, Galakatos AE, et al. Definitive irradiation in carcinoma of the vagina: long-term evaluation of results. *Int J Radiat Oncol Biol Phys.* 1988;15(6):1283-1290.

61. Spirtos NM, Doshi BP, Kapp DS, Teng N. Radiation therapy for primary squamous cell carcinoma of the vagina: Stanford University experience. *Gynecol Oncol.* 1989;35(1):20-26.

62. Davis KP, Stanhope CR, Garton GR, Atkinson EJ, O'Brien PC. Invasive vaginal carcinoma: analysis of early-stage disease. *Gynecol Oncol.* 1991;42(2):131-136.

63. Merino MJ. Vaginal cancer: the role of infectious and environmental factors. *Am J Obstet Gynecol.* 1991;165(4):1255-1262.

64. Stock RG, Mychalczak B, Armstrong JG, Curtin JP, Harrison LB. The importance of brachytherapy technique in the management of primary carcinoma of the vagina. *Int J Radiat Oncol Biol Phys.* 1992;24(4):747-753.

65. Stock RG, Chen AS, Seski J. A 30-year experience in the management of primary carcinoma of the vagina: analysis of prognostic factors and treatment modalities. *Gynecol Oncol.* 1995;56(1):45-52.

66. Rubin SC, Young J, Mikuta JJ. Squamous carcinoma of the vagina: treatment, complications, and long-term follow-up. *Gynecol Oncol.* 1985;20(3):346-353.

67. Jain A, Majoko F, Freites O. How innocent is the vaginal pessary? Two cases of vaginal cancer associated with pessary use. *J Obstet Gynaecol.* 2006;26(8):829-830.

68. Schraub S, Sun XS, Maingon P, et al. Cervical and vaginal cancer associated with pessary use. *Cancer.* 1992;69(10):2505-2509.

69. Burk RD, Chen Z, Saller C, et al. Integrated genomic and molecular characterization of cervical cancer. *Nature.* 2017;543(7645):378-384.

70. Hou JY, Baptiste C, Hombalegowda RB, et al. Vulvar and vaginal melanoma: a unique subclass of mucosal melanoma based on a comprehensive molecular analysis of 51 cases compared with 2253 cases of nongynecologic melanoma. *Cancer.* 2017;123(8):1333-1344.

Symptoms and Diagnosis of Vaginal Intraepithelial Neoplasia and Vaginal Cancer

Diana Miao, Josephine Kang, Amanda Nickles Fader, and Akila N. Viswanathan

VAGINAL INTRAEPITHELIAL NEOPLASIA

VAIN is usually asymptomatic (1) and is most commonly detected after cytologic evaluation as part of surveillance in patients with a history of CIN or invasive cervical carcinoma. Vaginal colposcopy with iodine stain is important when patients present with an abnormal Pap smear but no gross abnormality. Any colposcopically abnormal area warrants a directed biopsy. Around the vaginal vault, where occult carcinoma may be found, excisional biopsies are recommended (2). According to the 2002 American Cancer Society guidelines, surveillance cytology for VAIN in posthysterectomy patients is recommended if there is a history of cervical pathology, although it is low yield (3). The optimal incorporation of HPV testing into screening is not yet known (4). At present, evidence does not support routine surveillance in patients without a history of CIN or invasive cervical cancer.

VAGINAL CARCINOMA

Up to 65% of patients with vaginal cancer present with irregular vaginal bleeding as their primary symptom (5-7). Vaginal discharge is the second most common symptom, occurring in 10% to 15% of patients. Less frequent symptoms, associated with locally advanced disease, include the presence of a mass; pain; urinary symptoms including frequency, dysuria, or hematuria; or gastrointestinal complaints such as tenesmus, constipation, or melena. Because of the proximity of anterior wall lesions to the urethra and bladder, urinary symptoms can be seen more commonly in vaginal cancer than in cervical cancer. Up to 20% of women are asymptomatic at the time of diagnosis (5,8), with lesions detected via cytologic screening or by speculum examination.

Diagnostic Workup

The diagnostic workup should start with a thorough history and physical examination, giving careful attention to the pelvis. Complete assessment of the tumor extent and assessment of vaginal walls is facilitated by examination under anesthesia. During speculum examination, the speculum blades can obscure the anterior and posterior walls, so it is essential to rotate the speculum for visualization of all four walls from the introitus to the apex. Bimanual examination, with careful digital palpation, should be performed, assessing for parametrial and pelvic sidewall involvement and invasion of tumor to the rectal mucosa.

Inguinal nodes should be palpated for disease involvement, particularly if the primary lesion is situated in the lower portion of the vagina, because 5% to 20% of patients reportedly have involved inguinal nodes at presentation (9,10). Suspicious nodes warrant a biopsy. Laboratory tests include a complete blood count with differential and assessment of renal and hepatic function.

A definitive diagnosis is achieved with biopsy of suspected lesions, which can present as an exophytic mass, plaque, or ulcer. If a lesion is not visible in the setting of abnormal cytology, colposcopy with acetic acid, followed by Lugol iodine stain, is conducted.

Biopsies of white epithelium or atypical vascularity should be obtained after application of acetic acid. Iodine will identify Schiller-positive regions, which are nonstaining, and should correspond to areas identified following application of acetic acid. Adequate biopsies should include the cervix, if present, to rule out a cervical primary. Patients can present with multiple regions of abnormality. The differential diagnosis of a vaginal mass includes endometriosis, vaginal polyp, vaginal adenosis, or Gartner duct cyst.

Computed tomographic (CT) imaging and magnetic resonance imaging (MRI) may be used to determine FIGO stage. CT of the pelvis is obtained in place of intravenous pyelography to assess the renal parenchyma and also to obtain information on the extent of local disease and lymph node status. MRI can provide salient treatment planning information by characterizing extent of invasion and differentiating malignant tumor, which is isointense to muscle on T1 and hyperintense on T2, from normal structures and/or fibrosis (11). Advantages of MRI over other imaging modalities include superior soft tissue contrast resolution, accurate assessment of tumor volume, extent of local invasion, and accurate assessment of pelvic nodal involvement. In general, MRI is regarded as superior to CT for staging of gynecologic malignancies and should be obtained when available.

Positron emission tomography (PET) has shown efficacy in detecting the extent of primary tumor and abnormal lymph nodes in vaginal cancer with higher sensitivity than CT (**Figure 3.3-1**), as is the case in cervical carcinoma (12). Primary vaginal carcinoma and metastatic lesions demonstrate avid uptake of 2[fluorine 18]-fluoro-2-deoxy-D-glucose (FDG). In one study, 23 patients with primary vaginal carcinoma received both PET and CT during staging. CT identified the primary tumor in only 43% of patients, whereas PET identified the tumor in 100%. PET identified suspicious uptake in groin and pelvic nodes in 8 of 23 patients, compared to 4 of 23 with CT. Treatment planning was modified in 14% of patients because of findings from PET, and the authors concluded that PET detects primary tumor and abnormal lymph nodes more often than CT (12). It is important that the patient have an empty bladder before imaging, as physiologic FDG activity in a filled bladder can potentially interfere with accurate estimation of vaginal involvement. In practice, most patients planning to undergo RT are assessed with CT as well as MRI and/or PET, based on extrapolation from studies of other gynecologic malignances as well.

If imaging findings or clinical history is concerning for disease spread to the bowel or bladder, cystoscopy or proctosigmoidoscopy may be necessary in patients with symptoms suggestive of bladder or rectal infiltration.

Staging

The AJCC (13) and FIGO (14) systems are used to stage vaginal cancer (**Tables 3.3-1 and 3.3-2**). Primary vaginal melanomas and lymphomas are staged according to the AJCC staging systems for melanomas and lymphomas, respectively (13).

For patients with a prior gynecologic malignancy, a 5-year disease-free period is generally considered adequate to allow for

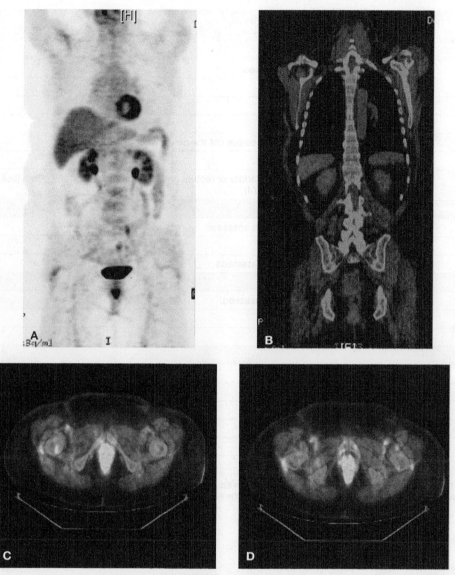

Figure 3.3-1. CT/PET fusion images of vaginal carcinoma. Coronal (A, B) and axial (C, D) images of a localized invasive vaginal carcinoma, extending into the central and lower one-third portion of the vagina above the introitus (see arrows). CT, computed tomography; PET, positron emission tomography.

■ TABLE 3.3-1. International Federation of Gynecology and Obstetrics Staging System for Carcinoma of the Vagina

Stage	Description
Stage I	Carcinoma is limited to the vaginal wall.
Stage II	Carcinoma has involved the subvaginal tissue but has not extended to the pelvic wall.[a]
Stage III	Carcinoma has extended to the pelvic wall.
Stage IV	Carcinoma has extended beyond the true pelvis or has involved the mucosa of the bladder or rectum; bullous edema as such does not permit a case to be allotted to Stage IV.
Stage IVA	Tumor invades bladder and/or rectal mucosa and/or direct extension beyond the true pelvis.

[a]Pelvic wall is defined as muscle, fascia, neurovascular structures, or skeletal portions of the bony pelvis.
From FIGO Committee on Gynecologic Oncology. Current FIGO staging for cancer of the vagina, fallopian tube, ovary, and gestational trophoblastic neoplasia. *Int J Gynaecol Obstet.* 2009;105:1.

distinction between recurrent disease and a new primary vaginal cancer. FIGO no longer recognizes carcinoma in situ as stage 0.

Stage I disease is defined as limited to the vaginal wall, and stage II disease involves subvaginal tissue without extension to the pelvic wall. Discriminating between stages I and II can be subjective; thin tumors less than 0.5 cm are generally classified as stage I, whereas thicker infiltrating tumors or those with paravaginal nodularity are classified as stage II. Perez et al proposed a modification to the FIGO system in 1973, distinguishing tumors with paravaginal submucosal extension only (stage IIA) from tumors with parametrial infiltration (stage IIB) (10). The study reported a 20% 5-year survival difference (55% vs 35%) between stages IIA and IIB. This modification has not been adopted into FIGO staging; however, some investigators consider the distinction to be prognostically relevant (9,15).

Distant metastases can occur with advanced disease at presentation or on recurrence after primary therapy. The most frequent site of hematogenous metastasis is the lung, whereas less commonly noted sites are the liver and bone (16). In a series by Perez et al (9), the incidence of distant metastasis was 16% for stage I, 31% for stage II, 46% for stage IIB, 62% for stage III, and 50% for stage IV. Some histologies may have a higher likelihood of distant

■ TABLE 3.3-2. American Joint Commission on Cancer Staging of Vaginal Cancer

Primary Tumor (T)	
Tx	Primary tumor cannot be assessed.
T0	No evidence of primary tumor
Tis/0	Carcinoma in situ
T1/I	Tumor confined to the vagina
T2/II	Tumor invades paravaginal tissues but not the pelvic wall.
T3/III	Tumor extends to the pelvic wall.
T4/IVA	Tumor invades mucosa of the bladder or rectum and/or extends beyond the pelvis (bullous edema is not sufficient to classify a tumor as T4).
Regional Lymph Nodes (N)	
Nx	Regional lymph nodes cannot be assessed.
N0	No regional lymph nodes
N1/IVB	Pelvic or inguinal lymph node metastasis
Distant Metastasis (M)	
Mx	Distant metastasis cannot be assessed.
M0	No distant metastasis
M1/IVB	Distant metastasis
Stage Groupings	
Stage 0	Tis N0 M0
Stage I	T1 N0 M0
Stage II	T2 N0 M0
Stage III	T1-3 N1 M0, T3 N0 M0
Stage IVA	T4, any N, M0
Stage IVB	Any T, any N, M1

Reprinted with permission from Springer; from *AJCC Cancer Staging Manual*. 7th Ed. Springer; 2010. www.springer.com; Used with permission of the American College of Surgeons, Chicago, Illinois. The original source for this information is the AJCC Cancer Staging System (2023).

metastases than others. Chyle et al (16) noted a higher incidence of distant metastases in patients with adenocarcinoma (48%) than in those with SCC (10%), with correspondingly lower 10-year survival rates (20% vs 50%).

REFERENCES

1. Lenehan PM, Meffe F, Lickrish GM. Vaginal intraepithelial neoplasia: biologic aspects and management. *Obstet Gynecol*. 1986;68(3):333-337.

2. Hacker NF, Eifel PJ, Van Der Velden J. Cancer of the vagina. *Int J Gynaecol Obstet*. 2015;131:S84-S87.

3. Saslow D, Runowicz CD, Solomon D, et al. American Cancer Society guideline for the early detection of cervical neoplasia and cancer. *CA Cancer J Clin*. 2002;52(6):342-362.

4. Orr JM, Barnett JC, Leath CA III. Incidence of subsequent abnormal cytology in cervical cancer patients completing five-years of post treatment surveillance without evidence of recurrence. *Gynecol Oncol*. 2011;122(3):501-504.

5. Gallup DG, Talledo OE, Shah KJ, Hayes C. Invasive squamous cell carcinoma of the vagina: a 14-year study. *Obstet Gynecol*. 1987;69(5):782-785.

6. Eddy GL, Marks RD Jr, Miller MC 3rd, Underwood PB Jr. Primary invasive vaginal carcinoma. *Am J Obstet Gynecol*. 1991;165(2):292-298.

7. Frank SJ, Jhingran A, Levenback C, Eifel PJ. Definitive radiation therapy for squamous cell carcinoma of the vagina. *Int J Radiat Oncol Biol Phys*. 2005;62(1):138-147.

8. Underwood PB, Smith RT. Carcinoma of the vagina. *JAMA*. 1971; 217(1):46-52.

9. Perez CA, Camel HM, Galakatos AE, et al. Definitive irradiation in carcinoma of the vagina: long-term evaluation of results. *Int J Radiat Oncol Biol Phys*. 1988;15(6):1283-1290.

10. Perez CA, Grigsby PW, Garipagaoglu M, Mutch DG, Lockett MA. Factors affecting long-term outcome of irradiation in carcinoma of the vagina. *Int J Radiat Oncol Biol Phys*. 1999;44(1):37-45.

11. Taylor MB, Dugar N, Davidson SE, Carrington BM. Magnetic resonance imaging of primary vaginal carcinoma. *Clin Radiol*. 2007;62(6):549-555.

12. Lamoreaux WT, Grigsby PW, Dehdashti F, et al. FDG-PET evaluation of vaginal carcinoma. *Int J Radiat Oncol Biol Phys*. 2005;62(3):733-737.

13. Edge SB, Byrd DR, Compton CC, Fritz AG, Greene FL, Trotti III A. *AJCC Cancer Staging Manual*. 7th ed. Springer; 2010.

14. FIGO Committee on Gynecologic Oncology. Current FIGO staging for cancer of the vagina, fallopian tube, ovary, and gestational trophoblastic neoplasia. *Int J Gynaecol Obstet*. 2009;105(1):3-4.

15. Prempree T, Viravathana T, Slawson RG, Wizenberg MJ, Cuccia CA. Radiation management of primary carcinoma of the vagina. *Cancer*. 1977;40(1):109-118.

16. Chyle V, Zagars GK, Wheeler JA, Wharton JT, Delclos L. Definitive radiotherapy for carcinoma of the vagina: outcome and prognostic factors. *Int J Radiat Oncol Biol Phys*. 1996;35(5):891-905.

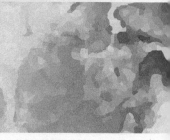

CHAPTER **3.4**

Surgery for Vaginal Intraepithelial Neoplasia and Vaginal Cancer

Diana Miao, Josephine Kang, Akila N. Viswanathan, and Amanda Nickles Fader

Surgical excision of VAIN is an option in select cases, particularly for vaginal vault lesions. Approaches include local excision, partial vaginectomy, and, in rare cases, total vaginectomy for highly extensive disease, which provides the advantage of obtaining a complete pathologic diagnosis. Most resections can be performed through a transvaginal approach. Location of VAIN in the vaginal vault or posthysterectomy suture recesses may require partial vaginectomy for complete resection, because redundancy of the vaginal mucosa makes it difficult to rule out occult disease with biopsy alone.

Excision of smaller lesions can be achieved through a cold-knife approach, electrosurgical loop excision, laser, or ultrasonic surgical aspiration (1-3). The CO_2 laser has been used for ablation of local tissue, with multiple treatments required in approximately one-third of patients (4-10). Complications include postoperative pain, scarring, and bleeding; however, the treatment is fairly well tolerated overall, with minimum impact on sexual function (11). Diakomanolis et al (12) reported that of 52 patients who underwent laser treatment or partial vaginectomy, the results favored laser ablation for multifocal disease and partial vaginectomy for unifocal disease. Ultrasonic surgical aspiration is another technique with the same efficacy as that of laser ablation; in one series of 110 patients, 1-year recurrence-free survival rates were 24% and 26%, respectively (13).

A series on surgical treatment of VAIN report recurrence rates in the range of 0% to 50%, with follow-up ranging from 3 months to 18 years (14-18). Overall, series that specifically examine upper vaginectomy report control rates of 68% to 88% (12,17,19,20). For example, Hoffman et al (17) reported that 83% of patients with VAIN 3 remained free of disease at a mean follow-up time of 38 months. Of note, 28% of all patients were found to have occult invasive disease upon upper vaginectomy. A subsequent study by Indermaur et al (13), which retrospectively reviewed 36 patients treated with upper vaginectomy for VAIN, reported 88% to be free of recurrence at a mean follow-up time of 25 months. Thirteen patients (12%) were found to have invasive cancer: eight had frank invasive disease, and five had microinvasive carcinoma. Complication rates of upper vaginectomy have been variably reported; in the series by Indermaur, there was a 9% complication rate. Potential complications from surgery depend on the extent and method of surgical resection, and range from vaginal shortening and stenosis to standard postoperative morbidity associated with abdominal procedures. It should be noted that patients with a history of RT are at a higher risk of postoperative complications, with a higher rate of fistula formation reported in one study (14).

SURGERY FOR INVASIVE CANCER

For most patients with invasive vaginal cancer, surgery has a limited role, and radiation is the treatment of choice. Owing to the rarity of these lesions, and the required individualization of treatment, it is recommended that patients be referred to a tertiary center with experienced practitioners. In general, surgery is considered useful in the following specific scenarios.

Patients with early-stage lesions (mm to less than 2 cm away from normal tissue structures) may have acceptable outcomes if a potentially curative resection can be achieved without extensive functional morbidity. Typically, amenable lesions are small, superficially invasive, well demarcated, and localized to the upper vagina. A wide local excision can be performed for in situ lesions. For more invasive lesions, a radical upper vaginectomy and pelvic lymphadenectomy can be considered; potential morbidity must be fully explained to the patient including vaginal shortening and sexual dysfunction. If the uterus is still present, a radical hysterectomy is also recommended; the goal is to achieve at least 1 cm margins (11,21).

Surgery can be considered for previously irradiated patients who cannot receive further radiation. Typically, such cases require pelvic exenteration.

Surgery is also a consideration for select patients with stage IVA disease. Extensive lesions in the proximal aspect of the vaginal canal require radical hysterectomy, upper vaginectomy, and bilateral pelvic lymphadenectomy. Older surgical series often required pelvic exenteration in 40% to 50% of cases to obtain negative margins (22,23). Anterior exenteration removes the vagina, urethra, and bladder and is often necessary to achieve negative margins for invasive anterior wall lesions. Posterior exenteration requires resection of the vagina and rectum. Deeply invasive, circumferential lesions may require a total exenteration in order to achieve clear margins. With positive margins, adjuvant radiation should be offered. Lesions that extend to the inferior vagina require a total vaginectomy with radical hysterectomy, pelvic lymphadenectomy, and possibly vulvovaginectomy and inguinofemoral lymphadenectomy (23-26). It is not uncommon for relatively small lesions to invade the rectum or urethra early in the disease course, given the close proximity of the vagina to these structures. Given the potentially devastating functional results associated with radical surgery, definitive radiation is the treatment of choice for most patients with invasive vaginal cancer, which has largely replaced surgery as the primary therapeutic modality.

Reported 5-year overall survival (OS) rates for stage I vaginal cancer treated with surgery range from 75% to 100% (Table 3.4-1) (24-29). The distinction between stage I and II disease is made clinically, based on physical examination, resulting in potential discrepancy between physicians. The NCDB review for cancers of the vagina noted superior survival rates in patients treated with surgery (27), though this likely reflects selection of healthier patients with good performance status for radical surgery. A more recent analysis utilizing the SEER database (30) found women with stage I and II disease treated with surgery only showed no statistical difference in mortality compared to have a lower risk of mortality than those treated with radiation only, combined modalities, or no treatment; however, this difference did not reach statistical significance. For patients with stage II vaginal cancer, there was a similar trend toward increased mortality in women who did not have surgery alone as their primary treatment modality, but values once again did not reach statistical significance in their multivariate adjusted model.

■ **TABLE 3.4-1. Early-Stage Vaginal Cancer Treated With Primary Surgery**

Series	Stage	# of Pts	Outcomes	Column 1	Notes
Creasman (1985-1994) (7)	I	76	5 y OS 90%		
	II	34	5 y OS 70%		
Tjalma (1974-1999) (139)	I	26	5 y OS 91%		4 pts received adjuvant RT, 5 LE, 19 htx, 2 ext
Rubin (1957-1980) (111)	I/II	9	5 y OS 75%		
Davis (1960-1987) (107)	I/II	52	5 y OS 85%		21 ext
Otton (1982-1998) (151)	I	8	5 y OS 100%		6 PV; 2 htx + removal of vaginal cuff
Stock (1962-1992) (110)	I	17	5 y DFS 56%		6 LE, 7 PV, 4 RV
	II	33	5 y DFS 68%		6 ext, 17 RV, 8 PV, 2 LE
Ball (1947-1978) (101)	I	19	5 y OS 84%		4 ext
	II	8	5 y OS 63%		1 ext

DFS, disease-free survival; ext, exenteration; htx, hysterectomy; LE, local excision; OS, overall survival; pts, patients; PV, partial vaginectomy; RT, radiation therapy; RV, radical vaginectomy.

Ling et al (31), in a small series consisting of four patients with stage I disease, report their experience using laparoscopic radical hysterectomy with vaginectomy and reconstruction of the vagina. With follow-up times ranging from 40 to 54 months, they report that all patients were free of disease, with satisfactory sexual function. The authors suggest that laparoscopic surgery may be an option for select patients with early-stage disease, with good outcomes.

Other series also report excellent results with primary surgical therapy, although authors acknowledge bias resulting from selection of healthier patients with less extensive disease for primary surgery over radiation. In a review of 100 cases by Stock et al (26), with 85 SCC cases, surgical treatment was noted to be a significantly favorable prognostic factor for disease-free survival (DFS), compared with RT alone. For patients with stage I disease treated with surgery versus RT, DFS rates were 56% and 80%, respectively. For patients with stage II disease, survival rates were 68% and 31% after surgery and RT, respectively, though this likely reflects selection bias, with patients with more extensive involvement offered RT. Overall 5-year survival was 47%. Stock et al concluded that surgery consisting of radical hysterectomy, pelvic lymphadenectomy, and upper vaginectomy could be reasonable for stage I lesions and select stage II lesions, with RT being the preferred primary modality for patients with larger lesions or more advanced disease. It should be noted, however, that 23 of 33 patients with stage II disease (70%) treated with surgery required a total vaginectomy or exenterative procedure, which carries significant morbidity and functional impairment.

Smaller series also support use of surgery in select patients with early-stage disease. Tjalma et al (28) reported on 55 cases of primary vaginal SCC. Of 27 patients with stage I disease, 26 received surgery, with 4 subsequently receiving some form of adjuvant RT. With a median follow-up time of 45 months, 5-year survival was reported to be 91%. Otton et al (29), in their retrospective review of 70 patients with stage I to II vaginal carcinoma treated at the Queensland Centre for Gynaecological Cancer Research between 1982 and 1998, report that patients treated with surgery alone, or a combination of surgery and RT, had significantly longer survival times than patients treated with radiation alone. The authors suggest that surgery may be effective in a select subset of patients with small, localized tumors that permit clear surgical margins. Peters et al (32) reviewed records of 86 patients with vaginal carcinoma, including 68 SCC cases, treated at the University of Michigan Medical Center. Twelve selected patients had surgery as primary therapy, with a 75% survival rate. Similarly, Rubin et al (23) reported on eight patients with stage I or II disease who received

surgery as primary treatment; 5-year survival was 75%, and the overall local control rate for patients with stage I disease was 80%, suggesting that highly selected patients can achieve excellent outcomes with surgery. Davis et al (22) reported on 89 patients with vaginal carcinoma, treated primarily at the Mayo Clinic from 1960 to 1987. A total of 52 patients were treated with surgery as primary therapy, with 5-year survival of 85%, compared with 65% for patients who received RT alone. In patients with stage II disease, the 5-year survival rates were 49%, 50%, and 69% for surgery, radiation, and combined treatment with surgery and RT, respectively. However, treatment modalities cannot be effectively compared using retrospective series, given selection biases.

Several series report their experience using surgery for patients with advanced stage III or IV disease, with most cases requiring radical excision, typically pelvic exenteration (23-26). Control rates, at best, are around 50%, even with highly selected patients. In practice, given the overall poor prognosis and morbidity associated with surgery, patients with advanced-stage disease should receive definitive RT, typically in combination with chemotherapy.

Another approach that has been proposed involves neoadjuvant chemotherapy followed by radical surgery (33,34). Panici et al (34) reported on 11 patients with stage II SCC of the vagina treated using three cycles of neoadjuvant paclitaxel and cisplatin followed by surgical resection. Ninety-one percent of patients obtained a partial or complete response to neoadjuvant chemotherapy; 27% achieved a complete response. All patients had disease-free resection margins after surgery, and only one patient had positive lymph nodes. At a median follow-up time of 75 months, 10 of 11 patients (91%) were alive, and of those, 8 (73%) were free of disease. Postoperative complications were mild. A case report documented the use of neoadjuvant chemotherapy consisting of bleomycin and cisplatin, followed by radical surgery, for one patient with stage II SCC of the vagina. The patient was free of disease, with satisfactory sexual function, at 30 months (33). However, it is necessary to evaluate the feasibility of this treatment in larger series of patients, with longer follow-up.

REFERENCES

1. Patsner B. Treatment of vaginal dysplasia with loop excision: report of five cases. *Am J Obstet Gynecol*. 1993;169(1):179-180.

2. Von Gruenigen VE, Gibbons HE, Gibbins K, Jenison EL, Hopkins MP. Surgical treatments for vulvar and vaginal dysplasia: a randomized controlled trial. *Obstet Gynecol*. 2007;109(4):942-947.

3. Robinson JB, Sun CC, Bodurka-Bevers D, Im DD, Rosenshein NB. Cavitational ultrasonic surgical aspiration for the treatment of vaginal intraepithelial neoplasia. *Gynecol Oncol*. 2000;78(2):235-241.

4. Audet-Lapointe P, Body G, Vauclair R, Drouin P, Ayoub J. Vaginal intraepithelial neoplasia. *Gynecol Oncol*. 1990;36(2):232-239.

5. Hoffman MS, Roberts WS, LaPolla JP, Fiorica JV, Cavanagh D. Laser vaporization of grade 3 vaginal intraepithelial neoplasia. *Am J Obstet Gynecol*. 1991;165(5):1342-1344.

6. Campagnutta E, Parin A, De Piero G, Giorda G, Gallo A, Scarabelli C. Treatment of vaginal intraepithelial neoplasia (VAIN) with the carbon dioxide laser. *Clin Exp Obstet Gynecol*. 1999;26(2):127-130.

7. Krebs HB. Treatment of vaginal intraepithelial neoplasia with laser and topical 5-fluorouracil. *Obstet Gynecol*. 1989;73(4):657-660.

8. Townsend DE, Levine RU, Crum CP, Richart RM. Treatment of vaginal carcinoma in situ with the carbon dioxide laser. *Am J Obstet Gynecol*. 1982;143(5):565-568.

9. Woodman CB, Jordan JA, Wade-Evans T. The management of vaginal intraepithelial neoplasia after hysterectomy. *Br J Obstet Gynaecol*. 1984;91(7):707-711.

10. Stuart GC, Flagler EA, Nation JG, Duggan M, Robertson DI. Laser vaporization of vaginal intraepithelial neoplasia. *Am J Obstet Gynecol*. 1988;158(2):240-243.

11. Sherman AI. Laser therapy for intraepithelial cancer of the vagina. *Am J Obstet Gynecol*. 1992;167(1):293-294.

12. Diakomanolis E, Rodolakis A, Boulgaris Z, Blachos G, Michalas S. Treatment of vaginal intraepithelial neoplasia with laser ablation and upper vaginectomy. *Gynecol Obstet Invest*. 2002;54(1):17-20.

13. Indermaur MD, Martino MA, Fiorica JV, Roberts WS, Hoffman MS. Upper vaginectomy for the treatment of vaginal intraepithelial neoplasia. *Am J Obstet Gynecol*. 2005;193(2):577-581.

14. Cheng D, Ng TY, Ngan HY, Wong LC. Wide local excision (WLE) for vaginal intraepithelial neoplasia (VAIN). *Acta Obstet Gynecol Scand*. 1999;78(7):648-652.

15. Sillman FH, Fruchter RG, Chen YS, Camilien L, Sedlis A, McTigue E. Vaginal intraepithelial neoplasia: risk factors for persistence, recurrence, and invasion and its management. *Am J Obstet Gynecol*. 1997;176(1):93-99.

16. Lenehan PM, Meffe F, Lickrish GM. Vaginal intraepithelial neoplasia: biologic aspects and management. *Obstet Gynecol*. 1986;68(3):333-337.

17. Hoffman MS, DeCesare SL, Roberts WS, Fiorica JV, Finan MA, Cavanagh D. Upper vaginectomy for in situ and occult, superficially invasive carcinoma of the vagina. *Am J Obstet Gynecol*. 1992;166(1):30-33.

18. Benedet JL, Sanders BH. Carcinoma in situ of the vagina. *Am J Obstet Gynecol*. 1984;148(5):695-700.

19. Diakomanolis E, Stefanidis K, Rodolakis A, et al. Vaginal intraepithelial neoplasia: report of 102 cases. *Eur J Gynaecol Oncol*. 2002;23(5):457-459.

20. Benedet JL, Murphy KJ, Fairey RN, Boyes DA. Primary invasive carcinoma of the vagina. *Obstet Gynecol*. 1983;62(6):715-719.

21. Hacker NF, Eifel PJ, Van Der Velden J. Cancer of the vagina. *Int J Gynaecol Obstet*. 2015;131:S84-S87.

22. Davis KP, Stanhope CR, Garton GR, Atkinson EJ, O'Brien PC. Invasive vaginal carcinoma: analysis of early-stage disease. *Gynecol Oncol*. 1991;42(2):131-136.

23. Rubin SC, Young J, Mikuta JJ. Squamous carcinoma of the vagina: treatment, complications, and long-term follow-up. *Gynecol Oncol*. 1985;20(3):346-353.

24. Ball HG, Berman ML. Management of primary vaginal carcinoma. *Gynecol Oncol*. 1982;14(2):154-163.

25. Gallup DG, Talledo OE, Shah KJ, Hayes C. Invasive squamous cell carcinoma of the vagina: a 14-year study. *Obstet Gynecol*. 1987;69(5):782-785.

26. Stock RG, Chen AS, Seski J. A 30-year experience in the management of primary carcinoma of the vagina: analysis of prognostic factors and treatment modalities. *Gynecol Oncol*. 1995;56(1):45-52.

27. Creasman WT, Phillips JL, Menck HR. The national cancer data base report on cancer of the vagina. *Cancer*. 1998;83(5):1033-1040.

28. Tjalma WA, Monaghan JM, de Barros Lopes A, Naik R, Nordin AJ, Weyler JJ. The role of surgery in invasive squamous carcinoma of the vagina. *Gynecol Oncol*. 2001;81(3):360-365.

29. Otton GR, Nicklin JL, Dickie GJ, et al. Early-stage vaginal carcinoma—an analysis of 70 patients. *Int J Gynecol Cancer*. 2004;14(2):304-310.

30. Shah CA, Goff BA, Lowe K, Peters WA 3rd, Li CI. Factors affecting risk of mortality in women with vaginal cancer. *Obstet Gynecol*. 2009;113(5):1038-1045.

31. Ling B, Gao Z, Sun M, et al. Laparoscopic radical hysterectomy with vaginectomy and reconstruction of vagina in patients with stage I of primary vaginal carcinoma. *Gynecol Oncol*. 2008;109(1):92-96.

32. Peters WA III, Kumar NB, Morley GW. Carcinoma of the vagina. Factors influencing treatment outcome. *Cancer*. 1985;55(4):892-897.

33. Lv L, Sun Y, Liu H, Lou J, Peng Z. Neoadjuvant chemotherapy followed by radical surgery and reconstruction of the vagina in a patient with stage II primary vaginal squamous carcinoma. *J Obstet Gynaecol Res*. 2010;36(6):1245-1248.

34. Panici PB, Bellati F, Plotti F, et al. Neoadjuvant chemotherapy followed by radical surgery in patients affected by vaginal carcinoma. *Gynecol Oncol*. 2008;111(2):307-311.

CHAPTER **3.5**

Prognostic Factors

Josephine Kang, Diana Miao, Amanda Nickles Fader, and Akila N. Viswanathan

A significant association between higher viral load of HPV and likelihood of persistent disease after treatment was demonstrated by So et al (1). There is also a significant association between risk of relapse in patients positive for high-risk HPV versus those who are negative (2). Of such patients, a retrospective review of 33 patients with VAIN treated at the University of Pennsylvania (3) found patients with a history of RT to be more refractory to treatment, with a significantly higher likelihood of recurrence after surgical and ablative therapy. Patients with a history of RT had an odds ratio of 3.6 for recurrent disease (95% confidence interval [CI], 1.5-9.0) compared to patients without a history of RT.

PROGNOSTIC FACTORS—VAGINAL CANCER

For vaginal cancer, stage at time of presentation is the most significant prognostic factor, according to numerous studies (4-10). The 2004 to 2014 SEER analysis demonstrated a 5-year cancer-specific survival rate of 57.8% across the entire group (11). This ranged from 76.4% for stage I, 61.9% for stage II, 53.3% for stage III, and 22.5% for stage IV disease. Univariate analysis demonstrated that age, marital status, race, pathologic grade, histology, stage, tumor size, and radiation were all related to prognosis. Specifically, older age, nonmarried status, melanoma or sarcoma histology, higher grade, larger size, and Black race were negative prognostic factors. Surgery and radiation were positive prognostic factors.

Further study of the SEER database from 1988 to 2007 has demonstrated differences in cancer outcomes between White and African American patients (12). African American patients were more likely to present with stage III or IV disease (30.4% vs 23.1%). Both groups received radiation at equal rates, but African American patients were less likely to receive surgical treatment (17.5% vs 27.7%). Overall, 5-year survival was 38.6% in African American patients versus 45% in White patients, and this survival difference persisted after controlling for age, histology, stage, grade, and treatment modality (hazard ratio [HR] 1.2).

Size of the initial lesion is a prognostic factor that has shown significance in several series. The SEER database study (4), which included 2,149 women with primary vaginal cancer, noted a significantly lower 5-year survival rate in women with tumors of size 4 cm or more than in those with tumors less than 4 cm (65% vs 84%); however, size information was missing for 52% of women. After multivariate analysis, patients with the larger tumors had an adjusted HR of 1.71 for mortality. Chyle et al (13), in their review of 301 patients treated at M.D. Anderson Cancer Center (MDACC) from 1953 to 1991, found that women with lesions larger than 5 cm in maximum diameter had a significantly higher 10-year local recurrence rate than those with smaller lesions (40% vs 20%). The series by Hellman et al (9), with 314 patients treated at the Karolinska University Hospital from 1956 to 1996, found that only three factors independently predicted poor survival on multivariate analysis: advanced age, tumor size 4 cm or more, and advanced stage. Tumors comprising two-thirds or more of the vagina and tumors growing circumferentially were associated with an extremely poor prognosis. The series by Tran et al (14), which reviewed records of 78 patients with SCC treated at Stanford University Medical Center from 1959 to 2005, also found size to be a prognostic factor for DFS on multivariate analysis, along with stage, prior hysterectomy, and pretreatment hemoglobin level. Smaller series by Tjalma et al (15) and Kirkbride et al (6) also describe adverse outcomes with larger tumor size. Other series have failed to show significance, but are likely hindered by small numbers, difficulties in accurate assessment of size, and treatment heterogeneity.

Extent of vaginal canal involvement has also been identified as significant, perhaps because it is a surrogate for tumor size. In a series by Stock et al (16) that examined 100 cases of primary vaginal carcinoma treated at Magee-Womens Hospital from 1962 to 1992, patients with involvement of one-third of the vaginal canal or less had a significantly higher 5-year DFS rate (61%) than patients with more extensive involvement (25%).

Several studies suggest HPV status is an indicator of favorable prognosis. Fuste and colleagues found a trend toward longer survival in women with HPV-positive tumors in their series of 32 patients, with median survival times of 113.9 versus 19.7 months for women with HPV-positive and HPV-negative tumors, respectively (P = .15) (17). Alonso et al (18) evaluated a total of 57 patients, of whom 70.2% had evidence of high-risk HPV. On multivariate analysis, HPV-positive status was a favorable prognostic variable for OS (HR 0.35, P = .038). Brunner et al (19) evaluated 35 patients with primary invasive SCC of the vagina. Using in situ hybridization, HPV was detected in 51.4% of cases. There was no significant influence on clinical stage, grade, or tumor size, nor did prognosis differ between HPV-positive and HPV-negative tumors. However, in a subset of patients with FIGO stage III or higher disease, HPV positivity was found to correlate with improved DFS and OS, with P values of .004 and .023, respectively.

There is conflicting evidence concerning the impact of lesion location on prognosis; it has been noted in some (13,20-23) but not all (24-26) reports. In an analysis of 110 patients by Kucera (27), 5-year survival rates were 60% for lesions of the upper third of the vagina, 37.5% for lesions of the middle third, and 37% for lesions of the lower third. Chyle et al (13) noted a 17% rate of pelvic relapse

in patients with tumors in the upper third of the vagina, 36% for patients with tumors in the middle or lower third, and 42% for patients with whole vaginal involvement. Lesions in the posterior wall were also associated with a worse prognosis than lesions involving the anterior vaginal wall (13), with 10-year recurrence rates of 32% versus 19% on univariate analysis (P < .007). The Hellman et al series (9), however, found no difference in prognosis between anterior and posterior tumors. Similarly, histologic grade has been an independent significant predictor of survival in several series (6,20,23), but not others (9). Hellman et al evaluated the impact of tumor grade and other histopathologic variables (mitotic activity, koilocytosis, growth in vessels, lymphocytic reactions) and found no correlation with survival.

Several series suggest a correlation between older age and decreased survival (9,23,28). For example, age was also noted to be a significant prognostic factor in the Urbański et al (23) series, with 5-year survival rates of 83% for patients younger than 60 compared with 25% for those 60 years of age or older (P < .0001). Age greater than 60 years was negatively associated with survival in the series by Gunderson et al (28), which examined a total of 110 patients (HR 2.16; P = .0339). Other series have failed to demonstrate the statistical significance of age (5,29).

Other possible prognostic factors include hemoglobin levels, prior hysterectomy, and smoking status. Tran et al reviewed records of 78 patients with primary SCC of the vagina treated at Stanford University Hospital and found a hemoglobin level less than 12.5 g/dL prior to definitive treatment to be prognostic for worse pelvic control and disease-specific survival (DSS); 5-year DSS rates were 55% for women with hemoglobin levels less than 12.5 g/dL and 76% for those with levels of 12.5 g/dL or more. This remained significant after multivariate analysis, along with prior hysterectomy, stage, and tumor size. The study by Tran et al (14) is the first to identify prior hysterectomy as a favorable prognostic factor on multivariate analysis. This may reflect more rigorous surveillance in posthysterectomy patients, resulting in tumors discovered at an earlier stage, or may be a reflection of less overall vaginal tissue as a substrate for tumorigenesis. Two subsequent studies have identified hysterectomy as a significant prognostic factor, but only on univariate analysis (9,13).

For patients treated with radiation, treatment time may be a significant factor impacting tumor control (31,32). Lee et al (32) found overall treatment time of 9 weeks or less to be associated with a pelvic tumor control rate of 97%, compared with 57% for treatment time of more than 9 weeks (P < .01). Pingley et al (31) also noted a correlation between treatment time and outcome; patients receiving brachytherapy within 4 weeks of external beam RT (EBRT) had a 5-year DFS rate of 60%, compared with 30% in patients who had an interval greater than 4 weeks.

A significant association between higher viral load of HPV and likelihood of persistent disease after treatment was demonstrated by So et al (1). There is also a significant association between risk of relapse in patients positive for high-risk HPV versus those who are negative (2). Of such patients, a retrospective review of 33 patients with VAIN treated at the University of Pennsylvania (3) found patients with a history of RT to be more refractory to treatment, with a significantly higher likelihood of recurrence after surgical and ablative therapy. Patients with a history of RT had an odds ratio of 3.6 for recurrent disease (95% CI, 1.5-9.0) compared to patients without a history of RT.

REFERENCES

1. So KA, Hong JH, Hwang JH, et al. The utility of the human papillomavirus DNA load for the diagnosis and prediction of persistent vaginal intraepithelial neoplasia. *J Gynecol Oncol.* 2009;20(4):232-237.

2. Jentschke M, Hoffmeister V, Soergel P, Hillemanns P. Clinical presentation, treatment and outcome of vaginal intraepithelial neoplasia. *Arch Gynecol Obstet.* 2016;293(2):415-419.

3. Liao JB, Jean S, Wilkinson-Ryan I, et al. Vaginal intraepithelial neoplasia (VAIN) after radiation therapy for gynecologic malignancies: a clinically recalcitrant entity. *Gynecol Oncol.* 2011;120(1):108-112.

4. Shah CA, Goff BA, Lowe K, Peters WA 3rd, Li CI. Factors affecting risk of mortality in women with vaginal cancer. *Obstet Gynecol.* 2009;113(5):1038-1045.

5. Perez CA, Grigsby PW, Garipagaoglu M, Mutch DG, Lockett MA. Factors affecting long-term outcome of irradiation in carcinoma of the vagina. *Int J Radiat Oncol Biol Phys.* 1999;44(1):37-45.

6. Kirkbride P, Fyles A, Rawlings GA, et al. Carcinoma of the vagina—experience at the princess margaret hospital (1974-1989). *Gynecol Oncol.* 1995;56(3):435-443.

7. Tewari KS, Cappuccini F, Puthawala AA, et al. Primary invasive carcinoma of the vagina: treatment with interstitial brachytherapy. *Cancer.* 2001;91(4):758-770.

8. Nori D, Hilaris BS, Stanimir G, Lewis JL Jr. Radiation therapy of primary vaginal carcinoma. *Int J Radiat Oncol Biol Phys.* 1983;9(10):1471-1475.

9. Hellman K, Lundell M, Silfverswärd C, Nilsson B, Hellström AC, Frankendal B. Clinical and histopathologic factors related to prognosis in primary squamous cell carcinoma of the vagina. *Int J Gynecol Cancer.* 2006;16(3):1201-1211.

10. Beller U, Benedet JL, Creasman WT, et al. Carcinoma of the vagina. *Int J Gynaecol Obstet.* 2006;95:S29-S42.

11. Huang J, Cai M, Zhu Z. Survival and prognostic factors in primary vaginal cancer: an analysis of 2004-2014 SEER data. *Transl Cancer Res.* 2020;9(11):7091-7102.

12. Mahdi H, Kumar S, Hanna RK, et al. Disparities in treatment and survival between African American and white women with vaginal cancer. *Gynecol Oncol.* 2011;122(1):38-41.

13. Chyle V, Zagars GK, Wheeler JA, Wharton JT, Delclos L. Definitive radiotherapy for carcinoma of the vagina: outcome and prognostic factors. *Int J Radiat Oncol Biol Phys.* 1996;35(5):891-905.

14. Tran PT, Su Z, Lee P, et al. Prognostic factors for outcomes and complications for primary squamous cell carcinoma of the vagina treated with radiation. *Gynecol Oncol.* 2007;105(3):641-649.

15. Tjalma WA, Monaghan JM, de Barros Lopes A, Naik R, Nordin AJ, Weyler JJ. The role of surgery in invasive squamous carcinoma of the vagina. *Gynecol Oncol.* 2001;81(3):360-365.

16. Stock RG, Chen AS, Seski J. A 30-year experience in the management of primary carcinoma of the vagina: analysis of prognostic factors and treatment modalities. *Gynecol Oncol.* 1995;56(1):45-52.

17. Fuste V, del Pino M, Perez A, et al. Primary squamous cell carcinoma of the vagina: human papillomavirus detection, p16(INK4A) overexpression and clinicopathological correlations. *Histopathology.* 2010;57(6):907-916.

18. Alonso I, Felix A, Torné A, et al. Human papillomavirus as a favorable prognostic biomarker in squamous cell carcinomas of the vagina. *Gynecol Oncol.* 2012;125(1):194-199.

19. Brunner AH, Grimm C, Polterauer S, et al. The prognostic role of human papillomavirus in patients with vaginal cancer. *Int J Gynecol Cancer.* 2011;21(5):923-929.

20. Kucera H, Vavra N. Radiation management of primary carcinoma of the vagina: clinical and histopathological variables associated with survival. *Gynecol Oncol.* 1991;40(1):12-16.

21. Ali MM, Huang DT, Goplerud DR, Howells R, Lu JD. Radiation alone for carcinoma of the vagina: variation in response related to the location of the primary tumor. *Cancer.* 1996;77(9):1934-1939.

22. Tarraza MH Jr, Muntz H, Decain M, Granai OC, Fuller A Jr. Patterns of recurrence of primary carcinoma of the vagina. *Eur J Gynaecol Oncol.* 1991;12(2):89-92.

23. Urbański K, Kojs Z, Reinfuss M, Fabisiak W. Primary invasive vaginal carcinoma treated with radiotherapy: analysis of prognostic factors. *Gynecol Oncol.* 1996;60(1):16-21.

24. Perez CA, Camel HM, Galakatos AE, et al. Definitive irradiation in carcinoma of the vagina: long-term evaluation of results. *Int J Radiat Oncol Biol Phys.* 1988;15(6):1283-1290.

25. Peters WA III, Kumar NB, Morley GW. Carcinoma of the vagina. Factors influencing treatment outcome. *Cancer.* 1985;55(4):892-897.

26. Whelton J, Kottmeier HL. Primary carcinoma of the vagina: a study of a radiumhemmet series of 145 cases. *Acta Obstet Gynecol Scand.* 1962; 41(1):22-40.

27. Kucera H, Langer M, Smekal G, Weghaupt K. Radiotherapy of primary carcinoma of the vagina: management and results of different therapy schemes. *Gynecol Oncol.* 1985;21(1):87-93.

28. Gunderson CC, Nugent EK, Elfrink SH, Gold MA, Moore KN. A contemporary analysis of epidemiology and management of vaginal intraepithelial neoplasia. *Am J Obstet Gynecol.* 2013;208(5):410.e1-410.e4106.

29. Dixit S, Singhal S, Baboo HA. Squamous cell carcinoma of the vagina: a review of 70 cases. *Gynecol Oncol.* 1993;48(1):80-87.

30. Al-Kurdi M, Monaghan JM. Thirty-two years experience in management of primary tumours of the vagina. *Br J Obstet Gynaecol.* 1981;88 (11):1145-1150.

31. Pingley S, Shrivastava SK, Sarin R, et al. Primary carcinoma of the vagina: tata memorial hospital experience. *Int J Radiat Oncol Biol Phys.* 2000;46(1):101-108.

32. Lee WR, Marcus RB Jr, Sombeck MD, et al. Radiotherapy alone for carcinoma of the vagina: the importance of overall treatment time. *Int J Radiat Oncol Biol Phys.* 1994;29(5):983-988.

CHAPTER **3.6**

Therapeutic Approach for VAIN and Invasive Vaginal Disease

Josephine Kang, Diana Miao, Amanda Nickles Fader, and Akila N. Viswanathan

VAGINAL INTRAEPITHELIAL NEOPLASIA

There is currently no consensus on the optimal treatment modality for VAIN, as reported data are generally retrospective and based on decades of experience with various treatments and patient characteristics. Thus, it is difficult to compare different therapeutic modalities (**Table 3.6-1**). Treatment approaches include local excision, partial or total vaginectomy, laser vaporization, electrocoagulation, topical 5-fluorouracil (5-FU) administration, topical 5% imiquimod, and vaginal brachytherapy (1-11). Reported success rates for different approaches range from 48% to 100% for laser vaporization (12-14), 52% to 100% for colpectomy (6,15,16),

75% to 100% for topical 5-FU (17-20), 57% to 86% for topical 5% imiquimod (11), and 83% to 100% for radiation (10,21-24). Given the breadth of available therapies, an individualized approach to patient management is advised, with consideration given to the patient's overall health, desire to preserve sexual function, candidacy for surgery, disease multifocality, and prior treatment failures.

Most patients with VAIN 1 are offered close surveillance. Lesions often regress spontaneously; in one study by Aho et al (25), 78% of patients with VAIN 1 or VAIN 2 had spontaneous regression of disease without treatment. However, over time, VAIN 1 can recur or progress. In one study by Gunderson et al (26) on 37 patients with VAIN 1, 54% of patients who were observed developed

■ **TABLE 3.6-1. Local Control of Vaginal Intraepithelial Neoplasia by Treatment Modality**

Series	Year	# Patients	% Recurrence	Follow-Up	Treatment Notes
Surgery					
Benedet and Sanders (96)	1984	136	25%	>5 yr	WLE, PV, TV
Lenehan et al (97)	1986	19	16%	5-112 mo	PV, TV
Ireland and Monaghan (98)	1988	25	4%	3 mo-11 yr	PV, TV
Hoffman et al (15)	1992	32	17%	6-73 mo	PV; 28% invasive cancer
Fanning et al (99)	1999	15	0%	22 mo	PV; 6.6% invasive cancer
Cheng et al (100)	1999	35	34%	1-124 mo	WLE
Dodge et al (5)	2001	13	0%	>7 mo	PV
Indermaur et al (6)	2005	105	12%	2-9 mo	PV, 12% invasive cancer
Terzakis et al (101)	2010	23	25%	24 mo	
Gunderson et al (26)	2013	44	27%	1-194 mo	PV, LE
Laser therapy					
Jobson and Homesley (102)	1983	24	17%	6-27 mo	
Audet-Lapointe et al (103)	1990	32	28%	7-85 mo	3.8% invasive cancer at excision 3 of 11 w/invasive cancer at recurrence
Hoffman et al (13)	1991	26	42%	2.2 yr (mean)	
Diakomanolis et al (104)	1996	25	32%	35-82 mo	
Campagnutta et al (12)	1999	39	23%	13-90 mo	
Dodge et al (5)	2001	42	38%	>7 mo	
Perrotta et al (105)	2013	21	14%	12-78 mo	
Gunderson et al (26)	2013	34	47%	1-194 mo	
Topical 5-FU					
Woodruff et al (28)	1975	9	11%	3-7 yr	1%-2% 5-FU q mo
Petrilli et al (7)	1980	15	20%	2-60 mo	BID × 5 d
Kirwan and Naftalin (29)	1985	14	7%	4-42 mo	q wk × 10 wk
Krebs (30)	1989	37	19%	12-84 mo	q wk × 10 wk
Audet-Lapointe et al (103)	1990	12	17%	9-42 mo	q d × 5 d
Dodge et al (5)	2001	22	59%	>7 mo	
Topical imiquimod					
Diakomanolis et al (31)	2002	3	See note		3 × weekly × 8 wk 3 pts with high-grade disease, therapy revealed regression to VAIN 1 (N = 2) or cure (N = 1)
Buck and Guth (32)	2003	56	14%		0.25 g q wk × 3 wk
Radiation					
Prempree et al (106)	1977	7	0%		ICB 70-80 Gy
Chyle et al (50)	1996	37	17%		ICB or orthovoltage radiation
MacLeod et al (21)	1997	14	14%	46 mo (mean)	HDR-ICB, 34-45 Gy to vaginal surface, 4-10 fx
Ogino et al (22)	1998	6	0%	13-153 mo	HDR-ICB, mean dose 23.3 Gy
Perez et al (45)	1999	20	6%		ICB 60-70 Gy
Graham et al (8)	2007	22	14%	77 mo	MDR-ICB, 48 Gy to point Z
Blanchard et al (23)	2011	28	7%	79 mo	LDR, 60 Gy to 5 mm below mucosa
Song et al (107)	2014	34	6%	48 mo	HDR-ICB, 40 Gy in 8 fx
Zolciak-Siwinska et al (108)	2015	20	10%	39 mo	HDR-ICB, 6-7.5 Gy × 3-5 fx

5-FU, 5-fluorouracil; fx, fractions; HDR, high dose rate; ICB, intracavitary brachytherapy; LDR, low dose rate; MDR, medium dose rate; PV, partial vaginectomy; TV, total vaginectomy; VAIN vaginal intraepithelial neoplasia; WLE, wide local excision.

recurrent, persistent, or progressive disease, versus 73% of patients who were treated with excision or ablation. Overall, disease recurrence/progression occurred at a median time of 17 months. Appropriate treatment for VAIN 2 should be determined on an individual basis, based on disease extent and associated patient factors. Therapy for VAIN 3 should be more aggressive, as there is a higher likelihood of progression to invasive disease, including occult invasive disease (6,15).

Topical therapies have been utilized in patients with early-stage lesions, multifocal disease, or multiple comorbidities that render them nonideal surgical candidates. Topical creams are favored in the management of young, HPV-positive women presenting with multifocal lesions (27). Topical applications have also been utilized before surgery to reduce lesion size and improve stripping of neoplastic epithelial cells from underlying stroma (1). Treatments include topical 5-FU and 5% imiquimod cream, with response rates

of up to 86% for imiquimod and 41% to 88% for 5-FU (10,18,19,28-34). Imiquimod increases levels of interferon-α, interleukin 12, and tumor necrosis factor (31), resulting in immunomodulation of the vaginal mucosa. Side effects of topical treatments include local irritation, with burning and ulceration being the most commonly reported adverse events (18,28).

Vaginal Cancer

For many patients, treatment choice will be offered based on size and location of the tumor, considerations regarding fertility preservation, and a desire for organ preservation for sexual function. A 2023 guideline for the management of patients with vaginal cancer outlines approaches by stage (35). The outcomes of retrospective series on the use of radiation for vaginal cancer are summarized in **Table 3.6-2** and in detail further.

■ TABLE 3.6-2. Outcomes for Vaginal Cancer Treated With Primary Radiation

Series	Outcome	Stage I	Stage II	Stage III	Stage IV	Treatment
Dixit et al (1985-1989) (86)	2y DSS	100%	70%	19%	0%	EBRT and/or BT
Fine et al (1963-1991) (71)	5y OS	42%	68%-	58%	0%	EBRT and/or BT
Kucera et al (1975-1984) (46)	5y OS	81%	44%	35%	32%, 0%[b]	EBRT and/or BT
Perez et al (1953-1991) (45)	PC	85%	66%, 56%[a]	65%	27%	EBRT and/or BT
	10y DFS	80%	55%, 35%[a]	38%	0%	
de Crevoisier et al (1970-2001) (109)	5y PC	79%		62%		EBRT and/or BT
Lee et al (1964-1990) (110)	5y PC	87%	88%, 68%[a]	80%	67%	EBRT and/or BT
	5y CSS	94%	80%, 39%[a]	79%	62%	
Frank et al (1970-2000) (43)	5y PC	86%	84%	71%		EBRT+BT (N = 119), EBRT (N = 63)
	5y DSS	85%	78%	58%		
Chyle et al (1953-1991) (50)	10y PC	84%	75%	60%	40%	EBRT+BT (N = 121), EBRT (N = 95), BT (N = 26)
	10y OS	55%	51%	37%	40%	Transvaginal cone (N = 2)
Stryker (1976-1994) (111)	5y DSS	78%	63%	33%	50%	EBRT+BT (N = 25), EBRT (N = 7), BT (N = 2)
Lian et al (1986-2006) (112)	5y DSS	90%	87%	32%	26%	EBRT+BT (N = 28), EBRT (N = 17), BT (N = 4), S+RT (N = 6)
Tran et al (1959-2005) (49)	5y PC	83%	76%	62%	30%	EBRT+BT (N = 43), EBRT (N = 22), BT (N = 10)
	5y DSS	92%	68%	44%	13%	
Mock et al (1986-1999) (74)	5y DSS	92%	57%	59%	0%	EBRT+BT (N = 55), EBRT (N = 5), BT (N = 26)
Urbanski et al (1965-1988) (41)	5y DFS	73%	54%	23%	0%	EBRT+BT (N = 77), BT (N = 11), EBRT (N = 15)
Beriwal et al (2000-2006) (113)	2y crude LC		100%	100%	100%	EBRT+HDR BT
Creasman et al (1985-1994) (67)	5y OS	73%	58%	36%		RT and/or S
Kirkbride et al (1974-1989) (81)	5y DSS	72%	70%	53%	42%	RT and/or S
Rubin et al (1958-1980) (66)	5y OS	75%	48%	54%	0%	RT and/or S
Stock et al (1962-1992) (57)	5y LC	72%	62%	0%	21%	RT and/or S
	5y DFS	67%	53%	0%	15%	
Shah et al (1990-2004) (48)	5y DSS	84%	75%	57%		RT and/or S
Hellman et al (1956-1996) (114)	5y DSS	75%	36%	36%	20%, 0%+	RT and/or S
Miyamoto et al (1972-2009) (115)	3y OS	56% (combined I-IV)				RT ± S

BT, brachytherapy; CSS, cause-specific survival; DFS, disease-free survival; DSS, disease-specific survival; EBRT, external beam radiation; HDR, high-dose rate; LC, local control; OS, overall survival; PC, pelvic control; RT, radiotherapy (any form); S, surgery.

[a]Outcomes for stages IIA, IIB respectively.

[b]Outcomes for stages IVA, IVB respectively.

Stage I

Though there are no randomized data comparing surgery versus radiation, surgical resection should only be considered in cases where a complete tumor resection with adequate, clear margins can be achieved in order to avoid the morbidity that occurs with adjuvant radiation (≤2 cm and away from the bladder, urethra, rectum), as reviewed in Chapter 3.4. Primary radiation incurs less morbidity and risk than surgery followed by radiation. Brachytherapy alone is an option for select patients presenting with small, superficial tumors (Treatment algorithm, **Figure 3.6-1**). Reported local control rates range from 62% to 100% (36-44). Perez et al (45) reported pelvic tumor control of 88% in patients with stage I disease who received brachytherapy, using a dose of 60 to 70 Gy, prescribed 5 mm beyond the plane of the implant or vaginal mucosa, with a vaginal surface dose of 80 to 120 Gy. Notably, tumor control in stage I vaginal carcinoma was similar to brachytherapy alone, versus brachytherapy plus EBRT. This observation is consistent with reports from some groups (45-47), but not others (43,44). Other series suggest high locoregional failure rates with brachytherapy alone. Kanayama et al (44) report three out of eight (38%) patients with stage I vaginal cancer, treated with brachytherapy alone, developed lymph node recurrence. Frank et al (43) reported on 21 patients with stage I disease who were treated with local radiation only, without regional node coverage. Nine received brachytherapy alone, 11 received EBRT with or without brachytherapy, and one received local EBRT using a transvaginal orthovoltage cone. Three of nine patients treated with brachytherapy alone developed recurrent disease in the pelvis, resulting in a 10-year pelvic disease control rate of 67%. Patients who received EBRT with or without brachytherapy did not have pelvic recurrences. A pelvic relapse rate of 18% at 10 years was noted by Frank and colleagues (43), with all pelvic failures occurring in patients treated with brachytherapy alone. Overall, results suggest caution

should be taken when brachytherapy alone is used without prophylactic lymph node irradiation, given fairly high rates of lymph node recurrence. Appropriate patient selection is critical, particularly since the distinction between stage I and II is based on clinical exam and can vary between providers.

Poorly differentiated or extensively infiltrating stage I lesions should be treated with a combination of EBRT and brachytherapy. Given possible underestimation of submucosal disease and/or nodal disease, resulting in a potentially high likelihood of recurrence with brachytherapy alone, some groups recommend incorporating EBRT into treatment of all patients with stage I disease, except for those with very small, superficial lesions (43,44). Frank et al (43), in their series of patients with vaginal cancer treated at MDACC between 1970 and 2000, noted an increased trend toward increasing use of EBRT for stage I vaginal SCC over time.

Actuarial 5-year survival rates for stage I disease range from 60% to 85% (39,43,48,49). Disease-specific survival rates for stage I disease, treated with definitive radiation, range from 75% to 95% (45,50,51). The 10-year pelvic relapse rate, comprised of local, pelvic nodal, and inguinal nodal failures, was noted to be 16% by Frank et al for patients with stage I disease (43). Most failures are locoregional. Distant metastases are uncommon and occur in about 5% of patients (36,45,52).

With low dose rate (LDR), treatment can be delivered in two applications, with the first designed to treat the entire vaginal wall and a second application to cover the tumor volume. When high-dose-rate (HDR) brachytherapy is the primary treatment, the entire length of the vagina is typically treated to a mucosal dose of 60 to 65 Gy, with an additional mucosal dose of 20 to 30 Gy delivered to the area of tumor involvement (53). Treatment can be delivered with a shielded vaginal cylinder or with a multichannel HDR cylinder to treat the tumor with a 2-cm margin and block uninvolved mucosal surfaces (54). HDR can also be used to treat superficial lesions.

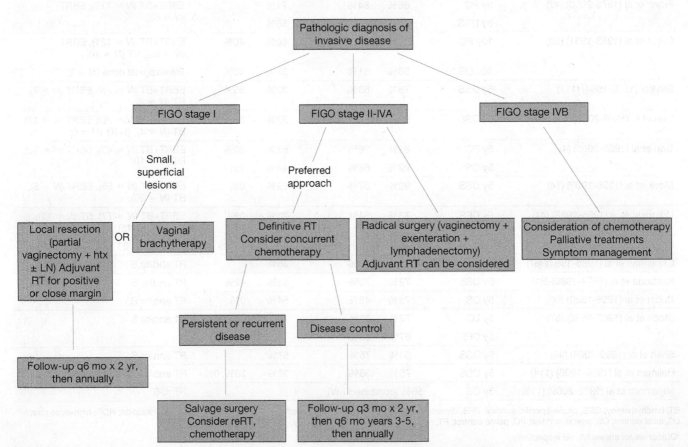

Figure 3.6-1. Proposed treatment algorithm for invasive squamous cell cancer of the vagina. htx, hysterectomy; LN, lymphadenectomy; RT, radiation treatment.

Use of a multichannel HDR cylinder is an alternative technique with favorable local control and low toxicity. The standard multichannel HDR cylinder is comprised of a central channel with 6 to 12 peripheral channels, allowing preferential dosing to the target while decreasing dose to normal structures. Vargo et al reported their outcomes for 41 patients with vaginal cancer treated with this technique to median EQD2 (equivalent dose in 2 Gy fractions) of 77.1 Gy (55). Definitive treatment consisted of EBRT followed by brachytherapy. The majority (71%) of patients had FIGO 1 disease. At 2 years, there was 93% local control, and 4% overall late grade 3 or higher toxicity, demonstrating comparable results to historical treatments. A tumor thickness cutoff of 5 mm for the apex and posterior vagina, and 7 mm for other locations, was utilized.

Guidelines from the American Brachytherapy Society recommend a cumulative D90 (dose to 90% of volume) EQD2 of 70 to 85 Gy prescribed to the vaginal tumor (56). Various regimens can be utilized to achieve this dose, with commonly utilized schedules of 45 Gy in 25 fractions of EBRT followed by HDR brachytherapy in 5 fractions of 4.5 to 5.5 Gy (EQD2 = 71.4-79.8 Gy) or 9 to 10 fractions of 3 Gy (EQD2 = 73.5-76.8 Gy).

Stage II

Stage II vaginal carcinoma involves the subvaginal tissue, but does not extend to the pelvic side wall. The primary treatment for stage II disease is radiation, most commonly as a combination of EBRT followed by vaginal brachytherapy; chemotherapy can be considered. Outcomes with brachytherapy alone have been poor; thus this approach is not recommended. With brachytherapy alone, Perez et al (45) noted a 36% pelvic tumor control rate in patients with stage II disease, compared to 67% in patients treated with a combination of EBRT and brachytherapy. The benefit of combining EBRT and brachytherapy, as opposed to using either alone, has been shown in other series as well (50,57).

During EBRT, the pelvis generally receives 45 to 50.4 Gy in 1.8 Gy fractions, with consideration of a parametrial boost if there is extensive primary infiltration or high suspicion of nodal disease. Inguinal lymph nodes are included in a modified whole-pelvic field for lesions involving the distal one-third of the vaginal canal.

Brachytherapy should be carefully delivered to ensure adequate coverage of tumor volume. An interstitial technique, ideally with three-dimensional imaging for treatment planning, is required for tumors greater than 5 mm in depth (38,58). Extensive tumors, or deeply infiltrating tumors with nondistinct margins, may be poor candidates for brachytherapy. In such cases, boosting tumors with conformal techniques or intensity-modulated radiation therapy (IMRT) may be preferred and may yield better outcomes than suboptimal brachytherapy (43). The tumor volume should receive a minimum of 75 to 80 Gy using combined EBRT and brachytherapy. Fleming et al (59) and Puthawala and colleagues (60) both report improved outcomes with higher doses of 80 to 100 Gy.

The 5-year survival rate for patients with stage II disease treated with RT alone ranges from 35% to 70% for stage IIA, and 35% to 60% for stage IIB (61). Pelvic relapse at 10 years has been reported to be 25% by Frank et al, consistent with recent series reporting 5-year pelvic control rates ranging from 76% to 84% (43,49). The likelihood of distant metastasis is higher for stage IIB lesions compared to stage IIA (39,47), with overall reported rates ranging from 22% to 46% (39,52).

Stages III and IVA

Locally advanced vaginal cancer is treated with a combined modality approach of radiation with consideration of chemotherapy, extrapolating from favorable outcomes with use of chemoradiotherapy (CRT) in patients with cervical cancer (62,63). Radiation is delivered as pelvic EBRT, followed by additional parametrial boost when warranted. If adequate tumor coverage can be achieved without undue toxicity, interstitial brachytherapy is employed to deliver a minimum tumor dose of 75 to 80 Gy. If brachytherapy is

not feasible, due to extensive tumor infiltration of the rectovaginal septum or bladder, a shrinking field technique or IMRT is used to deliver additional dose to the primary lesion (64,65). The overall cure rate for patients with stage III disease ranges from 30% to 50%. Stage IVA carries a worse prognosis. In highly selected patients with small-volume stage IV disease, pelvic exenteration can yield good long-term control; however, in practice, EBRT remains the primary treatment (41,43,45,48,57,66-69). Five-year actuarial survival rates for women with stage III disease range from 25% to 58% (48,67,70), with local failure rates of 30% to 75% (39,43,49). Outcomes for stage IV disease are worse, with survival rates of 0% to 40% (50,57,71). Despite treatment with EBRT and brachytherapy, only 20% to 30% of patients with stages III to IV disease achieve local control. Pelvic recurrences occur more often than distant recurrences (43). A combination approach utilizing chemotherapy with concurrent radiation has shown favorable outcomes. A single institution retrospective review of patients treated with RT alone, versus CRT (CRT), showed use of concurrent chemotherapy to improve DFS on multivariate analysis (HR 0.31, P = .04) (72).

Image-guided brachytherapy with CT or MRI was evaluated in a retrospective registry (EMBRACE) of 148 patients with vaginal cancer. Multivariable analysis showed that T stage, lymph node metastases, and tumor diameter (<4 cm vs ≥4 cm) were prognostic for DFS. In patients with advanced (T2-T4) tumors, improved local control was seen if the clinical target volume received more than 80 Gy EQD2α/β10 (92% vs 75% at 2 years, P-value = .036) (73).

Patients with stage IVB disease at diagnosis have poor prognosis, with a 5-year survival rate of 0% in some studies (47,74). First-line therapy often involves platinum-based chemotherapy, though efficacy may be limited (75). Treatment strategies for vaginal cancer are often extracted from data in cervical cancer given the relative rarity of vaginal cancer and the similar risk factors and relationship to HPV status.

Role of Chemotherapy and Radiation. Chemotherapy has been incorporated with radiation for the treatment of vaginal cancer, extrapolating from studies in cervical cancer showing improved progression-free survival (PFS) and OS when cisplatin is added to RT (45,62,63,72,76,77). Given the rarity of vaginal cancer, there are no randomized trials comparing radiation alone to radiation plus chemotherapy. Retrospective series are limited by small numbers or inclusion of other cancers, such as cervical and vulvar carcinomas. Nonetheless, studies suggest that a combined modality approach is feasible and may yield improved outcomes. These studies are summarized in **Table 3.6-3**.

Holleboom et al (78) published a case report documenting the use of cisplatin with EBRT and brachytherapy in a patient with advanced-stage SCC of the vagina. The patient was free of disease at 16 months. Evans et al (79) reported the use of radiation with 5-FU and mitomycin C (MMC) in seven patients with vaginal cancer. Four of the seven patients were free of disease with follow-up times ranging from 19 to 39 months. Roberts and colleagues (80) reported results for seven patients with vaginal cancer treated with concurrent 5-FU, cisplatin, and radiation. Three patients received interstitial brachytherapy after EBRT, and two patients received intracavitary brachytherapy after EBRT. Eighty-five percent of patients achieved a complete response initially. Ultimately, 61% recurred, with a median time to recurrence of 6 months. There were three local recurrences and one distant metastasis and the 5-year OS rate was 22%. Kirkbride et al (81) reported on the use of concurrent 5-FU, with or without MMC, in 26 of 153 patients with vaginal carcinoma treated at Princess Margaret Hospital. Seventy-seven percent of the patients had stage III/IV disease. Radiation was EBRT followed by interstitial or intracavitary brachytherapy to a total dose of 62 to 74 Gy. The 5-year survival rate was 50%. Dalrymple et al (82) reported results using 5-FU-based chemotherapy in combination with radiation for the treatment of primary SCC of the vagina. Thirteen of 14 patients (93%) had stage I or II disease. The median dose of radiation was 63 Gy, achieved using

■ TABLE 3.6-3. Select Series With Outcomes for Combined Chemotherapy and Radiation for Vaginal Cancer

Series	Outcomes	Stage	Notes
Miyamoto (1972-2009) (115)	3y OS 79%	St I, N = 18; St II, N = 19; St III, N = 8; St IVA, N = 6	RT+cis, 5-FU or carboplatin
Dalrymple et al (1986-1996) (82)	NED N = 9 (5-FU 74-168 mo) DOD N = 1 (12 mo) DID N = 4 (46-109 mo)	St I, N = 1; St II, N = 10; St III, N = 1	RT+5-FU, cis/5-FU or MMC
Gunderson et al (1990-2004) (84)	4y OS 64% (stage I), 40% (stage II), 12% (stage III/IV)	St I, N = 31; St II, N = 30; St III/IV, N = 69	CRT, N = 87; S+CRT, N = 43
Samant et al (1999-2004) (83)	5y OS 66%	St II, N = 6; St III, N = 4; St IVA, N = 2	RT+cis
Nashiro et al (2002-2005) (116)	DOD N = 1 (25 mo) NED N = 4 (5-FU 19-54 mo) AWD N = 1 (5-FU 19 mo)	St II, N = 2; St III, N = 1; St IVA, N = 3	RT+cis or cis/5-FU

5-FU, 5-fluorouracil; AWD, alive with disease; cis, cisplatin; CRT, chemoradiation; DID, died of intercurrent disease; DOD, died of disease; MMC, mitomycin C; NED, no evidence of disease; OS, overall survival; RT, radiotherapy (any form); S, surgery.

EBRT alone, or EBRT with intracavitary brachytherapy. The 5-year survival rate was 86% for all patients, and nine patients were free of disease with a median follow-up time of 100 months, suggesting that good local control can be achieved despite the use of lower radiation doses. There was a 31% rate of severe bowel complications reported, with two deaths as a result of bowel obstruction.

A retrospective series from MDACC by Frank and colleagues (43) included nine patients with stage II-IVA SCC of the vagina treated with radiation therapy and concurrent cisplatin-based CRT. With a mean follow-up time of 129 months, improved local control with the use of chemotherapy was noted, with 44% of patients treated with concurrent CRT remaining free of disease. Samant et al published a review of 12 patients with vaginal cancer, stage II-IVA, treated with concurrent weekly cisplatin at a dose of 40 mg/m^2 for 5 weeks (83). Patients received concurrent EBRT to a median dose of 45 Gy, with LDR interstitial or an HDR intracavitary brachytherapy boost of median dose 30 Gy. Six patients had stage II, four had stage III, and two had stage IVA disease. Ten of 12 patients (83%) had SCC; the other two had adenocarcinoma. Overall, treatment was well tolerated, with 92% of patients completing therapy as prescribed. Two of 10 patients who received interstitial brachytherapy required surgery for fistula repair. The 5-year OS, PFS, and locoregional PFS rates were 66%, 75%, and 92%, respectively, supporting use of concurrent weekly cisplatin therapy. A small series of six patients treated with CRT at the University of the Ryukyus was reported by Nashiro et al (116). All patients received EBRT to 50 Gy, followed by either a boost with shrinking fields (N = 4) or intracavitary brachytherapy (N = 2). Radiation was delivered with two to three cycles of cisplatin. Two patients had stage II, one had stage III, and three had stage IVA disease. All six achieved a complete response, and four of six patients remained free of disease at follow-up times of 18 to 55 months.

In a retrospective analysis of 71 patients with primary vaginal cancer treated from 1972 to 2009, 51 patients were treated with radiation alone and 20 were treated with CRT and RT (72). Of patients treated with chemosensitization during radiation, 85% of patients received weekly cisplatin chemotherapy, while the remainder received either carboplatin or 5-FU. Three-year actuarial OS and DFS was 56% for the RT alone group, compared to 79% for the CRT group (P = .01). Three-year DFS was 43% for the RT alone group, compared to 73% for the CRT group (P = .01). At a median follow-up of 3 years, tumor relapse was seen in 15% of patients treated with CRT compared to 45% of patients treated with radiation alone (P = .03). On multivariate analysis, the addition of chemotherapy was a significant predictor of DFS (HR 0.31).

A retrospective series by Gunderson et al examined patients treated with CRT and reported outcomes by stage (84). Of 110 patients treated between 1990 and 2004, 41 patients received CRT. Of this cohort, 4-year survival was 64% for stage I, 40% for stage II, and 12% for stage III/IV disease.

Ghia et al (85) published a retrospective patterns-of-care analysis using the SEER database, analyzing data from women with primary vaginal cancer treated with EBRT and/or brachytherapy between 1991 and 2005. Of the 326 women in the study cohort, 80.4% had SCC. It was noted that CRT was used in 7.5% of patients treated before 1999 compared to 36.1% of those treated afterward (P < .001). Cisplatin was the most frequently utilized agent, accounting for 59% of CRT treatments. Chemotherapy was significantly less likely to be used in conjunction with radiation for women older than 80 years; otherwise, there was no difference for race, stage, grade, histologic diagnosis, comorbidities, or brachytherapy use. On multivariate analysis, CRT was not found to correlate with improved cause-specific survival or OS.

Outcomes. According to SEER-based data, outcomes for vaginal cancer may be improving. A recent study by Shah et al (48) analyzed records from the SEER database of 2,149 women diagnosed with primary vaginal cancer between 1990 and 2004. The risk of mortality is noted to have decreased over time, with a 17% decrease in the risk of death for women diagnosed after 2000 relative to those diagnosed between 1990 and 1994. The authors reported 5-year disease-specific survival rates of 84% for stage I, 75% for stage II, and 57% for stages III to IV. An older study by Creasman et al (67) focused on 4,885 women diagnosed with vaginal cancer between 1985 and 1994, and reported 5-year survival rates of 96% for stage 0, 73% for stage I, 58% for stage II, and 36% for stages III to IV, with 85% of invasive cases being SCC.

In general, the rate of locoregional recurrence ranges from 10% to 20% for stage I and 30% to 40% for stage II. Patients with advanced disease often have persistent disease despite treatment. In a series by Dixit et al (86), 68% of failures in stage III patients were due to persistent disease. Most treatment failures occur within 5 years, with a median time to recurrence of 6 to 12 months (43,87), and local recurrence is the most common pattern of treatment failure in the majority of published series. Extravaginal recurrences in the pelvic lymph nodes are less common. The reported rates of distant metastasis vary, ranging from 7% to 33%, and usually occur later in the course of disease, with approximately half of all distant metastases presenting at the time of local recurrence (38,39,86,88).

For most patients with vaginal cancer, the mainstay of therapy is radiation. Patients with stage IVB disease at diagnosis have poor prognosis, with a 5-year survival rate of 0% in some studies (47,74). First-line therapy often involves platinum-based chemotherapy, though efficacy may be limited (75). Treatment strategies for vaginal cancer are often extracted from data in cervical cancer given the relative rarity of vaginal cancer and the similar risk factors and relationship to HPV status.

Recently, immune checkpoint inhibitors targeting PD-1, PD-L1, and cytotoxic T-lymphocyte-associated protein-4 (CTLA-4) have shown promise in the management of cervical cancer, as well as many other solid and hematologic malignancies. Pembrolizumab is a humanized monoclonal antibody to PD-1 that has demonstrated survival benefits in persistent, recurrent, or metastatic cervical cancer in combination with chemotherapy with or without bevacizumab. Specifically, median PFS was 10.4 months in the pembrolizumab group versus 8.2 months for placebo, and OS at 24 months was 53.0% in the pembrolizumab group versus 41.7% for placebo (89).

PD-1 inhibitors have been tested in vaginal and vulvar cancers with encouraging results, albeit with smaller sample sizes. The CHECKMATE-358 trial investigated single-agent therapy with nivolumab, another humanized monoclonal antibody to PD-1 (90). In a cohort of 24 patients with recurrent or metastatic cervical, vulvar, or vaginal cancer—including five patients with vaginal or vulvar cancer—objective response rate was 26.3% in patients with cervical cancer and 20.0% in patients with vaginal/vulvar cancer. Of note, three of the five responding patients in the cervical cancer cohort had a complete response and remained on therapy at study closure. The one responding patient in the vulvar/vaginal cancer cohort had a duration of response of 5 months. Another study of single-agent pembrolizumab including two patients with recurrent metastatic vaginal cancer showed partial response in one patient lasting 10 months until disease progression. The other patient discontinued treatment after cycle 3 due to disease progression (91). CA209-538 was a phase II trial of combination therapy with nivolumab and a monoclonal antibody to CTLA-4 called ipilimumab in rare cancers, including 41 patients with rare gynecologic cancers (92). Of these, five patients had vaginal or vulvar SCC. This trial found objective response (complete or partial response) in 11/41 patients, including patients with vaginal carcinoma.

A case report of pembrolizumab with concurrent pelvic radiation in one case of vaginal cancer refractory to carboplatin/paclitaxel demonstrated complete response (93). Further studies are ongoing in various cancer types regarding a possible synergistic effect of concurrent immunotherapy with radiotherapy (94). Local radiation therapy may initiate a local T-cell-mediated immune response. In very rare cases, this can cause an abscopal response leading to tumor regression not only at the radiation site but also distant metastatic lesions. Immune checkpoint therapy may enhance this systemic immune response to yield greater local and metastatic tumor control. However, risks and benefits of simultaneous radiation and immunotherapy have not yet been fully clinically elucidated in gynecologic cancers (95).

REFERENCES

1. Sillman FH, Fruchter RG, Chen YS, et al. Vaginal intraepithelial neoplasia: risk factors for persistence, recurrence, and invasion and its management. *Am J Obstet Gynecol.* 1997;176(1):93-99.

2. Rome R, England P. Management of vaginal intraepithelial neoplasia: a series of 132 cases with long-term follow-up. *Int J Gynecol Cancer.* 2000;10(5):382-390.

3. Diakomanolis E, Stefanidis K, Rodolakis A, et al. Vaginal intraepithelial neoplasia: report of 102 cases. *Eur J Gynaecol Oncol.* 2002;23(5):457-459.

4. Boonlikit S, Noinual N. Vaginal intraepithelial neoplasia: a retrospective analysis of clinical features and colpohistology. *J Obstet Gynaecol Res.* 2010;36(1):94-100.

5. Dodge JA, Eltabbakh GH, Mount SL, et al. Clinical features and risk of recurrence among patients with vaginal intraepithelial neoplasia. *Gynecol Oncol.* 2001;83(2):363-369.

6. Indermaur MD, Martino MA, Fiorica JV, et al. Upper vaginectomy for the treatment of vaginal intraepithelial neoplasia. *Am J Obstet Gynecol.* 2005;193(2):577-581.

7. Petrilli ES, Townsend DE, Morrow CP, et al. Vaginal intraepithelial neoplasia: biologic aspects and treatment with topical 5-fluorouracil and the carbon dioxide laser. *Am J Obstet Gynecol.* 1980;138(3):321-328.

8. Graham K, Wright K, Cadwallader B, et al. 20-year retrospective review of medium dose rate intracavitary brachytherapy in VAIN3. *Gynecol Oncol.* 2007;106(1):105-111.

9. Cardosi RJ, Bomalaski JJ, Hoffman MS. Diagnosis and management of vulvar and vaginal intraepithelial neoplasia. *Obstet Gynecol Clin North Am.* 2001;28(4):685-702.

10. Murta EF, Neves Junior MA, Sempionato LR, et al. Vaginal intraepithelial neoplasia: clinical-therapeutic analysis of 33 cases. *Arch Gynecol Obstet.* 2005;272(4):261-264.

11. De Witte C, van de Sande AJ, van Beekhuizen HJ, et al. Imiquimod in cervical, vaginal and vulvar intraepithelial neoplasia: a review. *Gynecol Oncol.* 2015;139(2):377-384.

12. Campagnutta E, Parin A, De Piero G, et al. Treatment of vaginal intraepithelial neoplasia (VAIN) with the carbon dioxide laser. *Clin Exp Obstet Gynecol.* 1999;26(2):127-130.

13. Hoffman MS, Roberts WS, LaPolla JP, et al. Laser vaporization of grade 3 vaginal intraepithelial neoplasia. *Am J Obstet Gynecol.* 1991;165 (5 pt 1):1342-1344.

14. Stuart GC, Flagler EA, Nation JG, et al. Laser vaporization of vaginal intraepithelial neoplasia. *Am J Obstet Gynecol.* 1988;158(2):240-243.

15. Hoffman MS, DeCesare SL, Roberts WS, et al. Upper vaginectomy for in situ and occult, superficially invasive carcinoma of the vagina. *Am J Obstet Gynecol.* 1992;166(1 pt 1):30-33.

16. Diakomanolis E, Rodolakis A, Boulgaris Z, et al. Treatment of vaginal intraepithelial neoplasia with laser ablation and upper vaginectomy. *Gynecol Obstet Invest.* 2002;54(1):17-20.

17. Piver MS, Barlow JJ, Tsukada Y, et al. Postirradiation squamous cell carcinoma in situ of the vagina: treatment by topical 20 percent 5-fluorouracil cream. *Am J Obstet Gynecol.* 1979;135(3):377-380.

18. Caglar H, Hertzog RW, Hreshchyshyn MM. Topical 5-fluorouracil treatment of vaginal intraepithelial neoplasia. *Obstet Gynecol.* 1981;58(5):580-583.

19. Daly JW, Ellis GF. Treatment of vaginal dysplasia and carcinoma in situ with topical 5-fluorouracil. *Obstet Gynecol.* 1980;55(3):350-352.

20. Hull M, Bowen-Simpkins P, Paintin D. Topical treatment of vaginal intraepithelial neoplasia. *Obstet Gynecol.* 1977;49(3):382.

21. MacLeod C, Fowler A, Dalrymple C, et al. High-dose-rate brachytherapy in the management of high-grade intraepithelial neoplasia of the vagina. *Gynecol Oncol.* 1997;65(1):74-77.

22. Ogino I, Kitamura T, Okajima H, et al. High-dose-rate intracavitary brachytherapy in the management of cervical and vaginal intraepithelial neoplasia. *Int J Radiat Oncol Biol Phys.* 1998;40(4):881-887.

23. Blanchard P, Monnier L, Dumas I, et al. Low-dose-rate definitive brachytherapy for high-grade vaginal intraepithelial neoplasia. *Oncologist.* 2011;16(2):182.

24. Woodman CB, Mould JJ, Jordan JA. Radiotherapy in the management of vaginal intraepithelial neoplasia after hysterectomy. *Br J Obstet Gynaecol.* 1988;95(10):976-979.

25. Aho M, Vesterinen E, Meyer B, et al. Natural history of vaginal intraepithelial neoplasia. *Cancer.* 1991;68(1):195-197.

26. Gunderson CC, Nugent EK, Elfrink SH, et al. A contemporary analysis of epidemiology and management of vaginal intraepithelial neoplasia. *Am J Obstet Gynecol.* 2013;208(5):410.e1-410.e6.

27. Haidopoulos D, Diakomanolis E, Rodolakis A, et al. Can local application of imiquimod cream be an alternative mode of therapy for patients with high-grade intraepithelial lesions of the vagina? *Int J Gynecol Cancer.* 2005;15(5):898-902.

28. Woodruff JD, Parmley T, Julian C. Topical 5-fluorouracil in the treatment of vaginal carcinoma-in-situ. *Gynecol Oncol.* 1975;3(2):124-132.

29. Kirwan P, Naftalin NJ. Topical 5-fluorouracil in the treatment of vaginal intraepithelial neoplasia. *Br J Obstet Gynaecol.* 1985;92(3):287-291.

30. Krebs HB. Treatment of vaginal intraepithelial neoplasia with laser and topical 5-fluorouracil. *Obstet Gynecol.* 1989;73(4):657-660.

31. Diakomanolis E, Haidopoulos D, Stefanidis K. Treatment of high-grade vaginal intraepithelial neoplasia with imiquimod cream. *N Engl J Med.* 2002;347(5):374.

32. Buck HW, Guth KJ. Treatment of vaginal intraepithelial neoplasia (primarily low grade) with imiquimod 5% cream. *J Low Genit Tract Dis.* 2003;7(4):290-293.

33. Iavazzo C, Pitsouni E, Athanasiou S, et al. Imiquimod for treatment of vulvar and vaginal intraepithelial neoplasia. *Int J Gynaecol Obstet.* 2008;101(1):3-10.

34. Stokes I, Sworn M, Hawthorne J. A new regimen for the treatment of vaginal carcinoma in situ using 5-fluorouracil. Case report. *Br J Obstet Gynaecol.* 1980;87(10):920-921.

35. Nout RA, Calaminus G, Planchamp F, et al. ESTRO/ESGO/SIOPe Guidelines for the management of patients with vaginal cancer. *Int J Gynecol Cancer.* 2023;33(8):1185-1202.

36. Dancuart F, Delclos L, Wharton JT, et al. Primary squamous cell carcinoma of the vagina treated by radiotherapy: a failures analysis—the M. D. Anderson Hospital experience 1955-1982. *Int J Radiat Oncol Biol Phys*. 1988;14(4):745-749.

37. Kucera H, Vavra N. Radiation management of primary carcinoma of the vagina: clinical and histopathological variables associated with survival. *Gynecol Oncol*. 1991;40(1):12-16.

38. Leung S, Sexton M. Radical radiation therapy for carcinoma of the vagina—impact of treatment modalities on outcome: Peter MacCallum Cancer Institute experience 1970-1990. *Int J Radiat Oncol Biol Phys*. 1993;25(3):413-418.

39. Perez CA, Camel HM, Galakatos AE, et al. Definitive irradiation in carcinoma of the vagina: long-term evaluation of results. *Int J Radiat Oncol Biol Phys*. 1988;15(6):1283-1290.

40. Reddy S, Saxena VS, Reddy S, et al. Results of radiotherapeutic management of primary carcinoma of the vagina. *Int J Radiat Oncol Biol Phys*. 1991;21(4):1041-1044.

41. Urbanski K, Kojs Z, Reinfuss M, et al. Primary invasive vaginal carcinoma treated with radiotherapy: analysis of prognostic factors. *Gynecol Oncol*. 1996;60(1):16-21.

42. Stock RG, Mychalczak B, Armstrong JG, et al. The importance of brachytherapy in the management of primary carcinoma of the vagina. *Int J Radiat Oncol Biol Phys*. 1992;24(4):747-753.

43. Frank SJ, Jhingran A, Levenback C, et al. Definitive radiation therapy for squamous cell carcinoma of the vagina. *Int J Radiat Oncol Biol Phys*. 2005;62(1):138-147.

44. Kanayama N, Isohashi F, Yoshioka Y, et al. Definitive radiotherapy for primary vaginal cancer: correlation between treatment patterns and recurrence rate. *J Radiat Res*. 2015;56(2):346-353.

45. Perez CA, Grigsby PW, Garipagaoglu M, et al. Factors affecting long-term outcome of irradiation in carcinoma of the vagina. *Int J Radiat Oncol Biol Phys*. 1999;44(1):37-45.

46. Kucera H, Langer M, Smekal G, et al. Radiotherapy of primary carcinoma of the vagina: management and results of different therapy schemes. *Gynecol Oncol*. 1985;21(1):87-93.

47. Prempree T, Amornmarn R. Radiation treatment of primary carcinoma of the vagina. Patterns of failures after definitive therapy. *Acta Radiol Oncol*. 1985;24(1):51-56.

48. Shah CA, Goff BA, Lowe K, et al. Factors affecting risk of mortality in women with vaginal cancer. *Obstet Gynecol*. 2009;113(5):1038-1045.

49. Tran PT, Su Z, Lee P, et al. Prognostic factors for outcomes and complications for primary squamous cell carcinoma of the vagina treated with radiation. *Gynecol Oncol*. 2007;105(3):641-649.

50. Chyle V, Zagars GK, Wheeler JA, et al. Definitive radiotherapy for carcinoma of the vagina: outcome and prognostic factors. *Int J Radiat Oncol Biol Phys*. 1996;35(5):891-905.

51. Spirtos NM, Doshi BP, Kapp DS, et al. Radiation therapy for primary squamous cell carcinoma of the vagina: Stanford University experience. *Gynecol Oncol*. 1989;35(1):20-26.

52. Davis KP, Stanhope CR, Garton GR, et al. Invasive vaginal carcinoma: analysis of early-stage disease. *Gynecol Oncol*. 1991;42(2):131-136.

53. Perez CA, Korba A, Sharma S. Dosimetric considerations in irradiation of carcinoma of the vagina. *Int J Radiat Oncol Biol Phys*. 1977;2(7-8):639-649.

54. Glaser SM, Beriwal S. Brachytherapy for malignancies of the vagina in the 3D era. *J Contemp Brachytherapy*. 2015;7(4):312-318.

55. Vargo JA, Kim H, Houser CJ, et al. Image-based multichannel vaginal cylinder brachytherapy for vaginal cancer. *Brachytherapy*. 2015;14(1):9-15.

56. Beriwal S, Demanes DJ, Erickson B, et al. American Brachytherapy Society consensus guidelines for interstitial brachytherapy for vaginal cancer. *Brachytherapy*. 2012;11(1):68-75.

57. Stock RG, Chen AS, Seski J. A 30-year experience in the management of primary carcinoma of the vagina: analysis of prognostic factors and treatment modalities. *Gynecol Oncol*. 1995;56(1):45-52.

58. Manetta A, Gutrecht EL, Berman ML, et al. Primary invasive carcinoma of the vagina. *Obstet Gynecol*. 1990;76(4):639-642.

59. Fleming P, Nisar Syed AM, Neblett D, et al. Description of an afterloading 192Ir interstitial-intracavitary technique in the treatment of carcinoma of the vagina. *Obstet Gynecol*. 1980;55(4):525-530.

60. Puthawala A, Syed AM, Nalick R, et al. Integrated external and interstitial radiation therapy for primary carcinoma of the vagina. *Obstet Gynecol*. 1983;62(3):367-372.

61. Otton GR, Nicklin JL, Dickie GJ, et al. Early-stage vaginal carcinoma—an analysis of 70 patients. *Int J Gynecol Cancer*. 2004;14(2):304-310. doi:10.1111/j.1048-891X.2004.014214.x

62. Morris M, Eifel PJ, Lu J, et al. Pelvic radiation with concurrent chemotherapy compared with pelvic and para-aortic radiation for high-risk cervical cancer. *N Engl J Med*. 1999;340(15):1137-1143.

63. Rose PG, Bundy BN, Watkins EB, et al. Concurrent cisplatin-based radiotherapy and chemotherapy for locally advanced cervical cancer. *N Engl J Med*. 1999;340(15):1144-1153.

64. Mundt AJ, Lujan AE, Rotmensch J, et al. Intensity-modulated whole pelvic radiotherapy in women with gynecologic malignancies. *Int J Radiat Oncol Biol Phys*. 2002;52(5):1330-1337.

65. Mundt AJ, Mell LK, Roeske JC. Preliminary analysis of chronic gastrointestinal toxicity in gynecology patients treated with intensity-modulated whole pelvic radiation therapy. *Int J Radiat Oncol Biol Phys*. 2003;56(5):1354-1360.

66. Rubin SC, Young J, Mikuta JJ. Squamous carcinoma of the vagina: treatment, complications, and long-term follow-up. *Gynecol Oncol*. 1985;20(3):346-353.

67. Creasman WT, Phillips JL, Menck HR. The National Cancer Data Base report on cancer of the vagina. *Cancer*. 1998;83(5):1033-1040.

68. Sinha B, Stehman F, Schilder J, et al. Indiana University experience in the management of vaginal cancer. *Int J Gynecol Cancer*. 2009;19(4):686-693.

69. Hegemann S, Schäfer U, Lellé R, et al. Long-term results of radiotherapy in primary carcinoma of the vagina. *Strahlenther Onkol*. 2009;185(3):184-189.

70. Schäfer U, Micke O, Prott FJ, et al. [The results of primary radiotherapy in vaginal carcinoma]. *Strahlenther Onkol*. 1997;173(5):272-280.

71. Fine BA, Piver MS, McAuley M, et al. The curative potential of radiation therapy in the treatment of primary vaginal carcinoma. *Am J Clin Oncol*. 1996;19(1):39-44.

72. Miyamoto DT, Viswanathan AN. Concurrent chemoradiation for vaginal cancer. *PLoS One*. 2013;8(6):e65048.

73. Westerveld H, Schmid MP, Nout RA, et al. Image-Guided Adaptive Brachytherapy (IGABT) for primary vaginal cancer: results of the International Multicenter RetroEMBRAVE cohort study. *Cancers (Basel)*. 2021;13(6):1459.

74. Mock U, Kucera H, Fellner C, et al. High-dose-rate (HDR) brachytherapy with or without external beam radiotherapy in the treatment of primary vaginal carcinoma: long-term results and side effects. *Int J Radiat Oncol Biol Phys*. 2003;56(4):950-957.

75. Thigpen JT, Blessing JA, Homesley HD, et al. Phase II trial of cisplatin in advanced or recurrent cancer of the vagina: a Gynecologic Oncology Group Study. *Gynecol Oncol*. 1986;23(1):101-104.

76. National Cancer Institute. NCI clinical announcement on cervical cancer: chemotherapy plus radiation improves survival. United States Department of Health and Human Services, Public Health Service; 1999.

77. Keys HM, Bundy BN, Stehman FB, et al. Cisplatin, radiation, and adjuvant hysterectomy compared with radiation and adjuvant hysterectomy for bulky stage IB cervical carcinoma. *N Engl J Med*. 1999;340(15):1154-1161.

78. Holleboom CA, Kock HC, Nijs AM, et al. cis-Diaminechloroplatinum in the treatment of advanced primary squamous cell carcinoma of the vaginal wall: a case report. *Gynecol Oncol*. 1987;27(1):110-115.

79. Evans LS, Kersh CR, Constable WC, et al. Concomitant 5-fluorouracil, mitomycin-C, and radiotherapy for advanced gynecologic malignancies. *Int J Radiat Oncol Biol Phys*. 1988;15(4):901-906.

80. Roberts WS, Hoffman MS, Kavanagh JJ, et al. Further experience with radiation therapy and concomitant intravenous chemotherapy in advanced carcinoma of the lower female genital tract. *Gynecol Oncol*. 1991;43(3):233-236.

81. Kirkbride P, Fyles A, Rawlings GA, et al. Carcinoma of the vagina—experience at the Princess Margaret Hospital (1974-1989). *Gynecol Oncol*. 1995;56(3):435-443.

82. Dalrymple JL, Russell AH, Lee SW, et al. Chemoradiation for primary invasive squamous carcinoma of the vagina. *Int J Gynecol Cancer*. 2004;14(1):110-117.

83. Samant R, Lau B, E C, et al. Primary vaginal cancer treated with concurrent chemoradiation using Cis-platinum. *Int J Radiat Oncol Biol Phys*. 2007;69(3):746-750.

84. Gunderson CC, Nugent EK, Yunker AC, et al. Vaginal cancer: the experience from 2 large academic centers during a 15-year period. *J Low Genit Tract Dis*. 2013;17(4):409-413.

85. Ghia AJ, Gonzalez VJ, Tward JD, et al. Primary vaginal cancer and chemoradiotherapy: a patterns-of-care analysis. *Int J Gynecol Cancer*. 2011;21(2):378-384.

86. Dixit S, Singhal S, Baboo HA. Squamous cell carcinoma of the vagina: a review of 70 cases. *Gynecol Oncol*. 1993;48(1):80-87.

87. Tabata T, Takeshima N, Nishida H, et al. Treatment failure in vaginal cancer. *Gynecol Oncol*. 2002;84(2):309-314.

88. Houghton CR, Iversen T. Squamous cell carcinoma of the vagina: a clinical study of the location of the tumor. *Gynecol Oncol*. 1982;13(3):365-372.

89. Colombo N, Dubot C, Lorusso D, et al. Pembrolizumab for persistent, recurrent, or metastatic cervical cancer. *N Engl J Med*. 2021;385(20):1856-1867.

90. Naumann RW, Hollebecque A, Meyer T, et al. Safety and efficacy of nivolumab monotherapy in recurrent or metastatic cervical, vaginal, or vulvar carcinoma: results from the phase I/II CheckMate 358 trial. *J Clin Oncol.* 2019;37(31):2825-2834.

91. How JA, Jazaeri AA, Soliman PT, et al. Pembrolizumab in vaginal and vulvar squamous cell carcinoma: a case series from a phase II basket trial. *Sci Rep.* 2021;11(1):1-7.

92. Klein O, Kee D, Gao B, et al. Combination immunotherapy with ipilimumab and nivolumab in patients with rare gynaecological malignancies. *J Clin Oncol.* 2020;38(suppl 15):6091.

93. Ansari J, Eltigani Mohmmed Y, Ghazal-Aswad S, et al. Rare case of chemotherapy-refractory metastatic vaginal squamous cell carcinoma with complete response to concurrent pembrolizumab and radiotherapy- case report and literature review. *Gynecol Oncol Rep.* 2021;38:100878.

94. Lee L, Matulonis U. Immunotherapy and radiation combinatorial trials in gynecologic cancer: a potential synergy? *Gynecol Oncol.* 2019;154(1):236-245.

95. Dyer BA, Feng CH, Eskander R, et al. Current status of clinical trials for cervical and uterine cancer using immunotherapy combined with radiation. *Int J Radiat Oncol Biol Phys.* 2021;109(2):396-412.

96. Benedet JL, Sanders BH. Carcinoma in situ of the vagina. *Am J Obstet Gynecol.* 1984;148(5):695-700.

97. Lenehan PM, Meffe F, Lickrish GM. Vaginal intraepithelial neoplasia: biologic aspects and management. *Obstet Gynecol.* 1986;68(3):333-337.

98. Ireland D, Monaghan JM. The management of the patient with abnormal vaginal cytology following hysterectomy. *Br J Obstet Gynaecol.* 1988;95(10):973-975.

99. Fanning J, Manahan KJ, McLean SA. Loop electrosurgical excision procedure for partial upper vaginectomy. *Am J Obstet Gynecol.* 1999;181(6):1382-1385.

100. Cheng D, Ng TY, Ngan HY, et al. Wide local excision (WLE) for vaginal intraepithelial neoplasia (VAIN). *Acta Obstet Gynecol Scand.* 1999;78(7):648-652.

101. Terzakis E, Androutsopoulos G, Zygouris D, et al. Loop electrosurgical excision procedure in Greek patients with vaginal intraepithelial neoplasia. *Eur J Gynaecol Oncol.* 2010;31(4):392-394.

102. Jobson VW, Homesley HD. Treatment of vaginal intraepithelial neoplasia with the carbon dioxide laser. *Obstet Gynecol.* 1983;62(1):90-93.

103. Audet-Lapointe P, Body G, Vauclair R, et al. Vaginal intraepithelial neoplasia. *Gynecol Oncol.* 1990;36(2):232-239.

104. Diakomanolis E, Rodolakis A, Sakellaropoulos G, et al. Conservative management of vaginal intraepithelial neoplasia (VAIN) by laser CO_2. *Eur J Gynaecol Oncol.* 1996;17(5):389-392.

105. Perrotta M, Marchitelli CE, Velazco AF, et al. Use of CO_2 laser vaporization for the treatment of high-grade vaginal intraepithelial neoplasia. *J Low Genit Tract Dis.* 2013;17(1):23-27.

106. Prempree T, Viravathana T, Slawson RG, et al. Radiation management of primary carcinoma of the vagina. *Cancer.* 1977;40(1):109-118.

107. Song JH, Lee JH, Lee JH, et al. High-dose-rate brachytherapy for the treatment of vaginal intraepithelial neoplasia. *Cancer Res Treat.* 2014;46(1):74-80.

108. Zolciak-Siwinska A, Gruszczynska E, Jonska-Gmyrek J, et al. Brachytherapy for vaginal intraepithelial neoplasia. *Eur J Obstet Gynecol Reprod Biol.* 2015;194:73-77.

109. de Crevoisier R, Sanfilippo N, Gerbaulet A, et al. Exclusive radiotherapy for primary squamous cell carcinoma of the vagina. *Radiother Oncol.* 2007;85(3):362-370.

110. Lee WR, Marcus RB Jr, Sombeck MD, et al. Radiotherapy alone for carcinoma of the vagina: the importance of overall treatment time. *Int J Radiat Oncol Biol Phys.* 1994;29(5):983-988.

111. Stryker JA. Radiotherapy for vaginal carcinoma: a 23-year review. *Br J Radiol.* 2000;73(875):1200-1205.

112. Lian J, Dundas G, Carlone M, et al. Twenty-year review of radiotherapy for vaginal cancer: an institutional experience. *Gynecol Oncol.* 2008;111(2):298-306.

113. Beriwal S, Heron DE, Mogus R, et al. High-dose rate brachytherapy (HDRB) for primary or recurrent cancer in the vagina. *Radiat Oncol.* 2008;3:7.

114. Hellman K, Lundell M, Silfverswärd C, et al. Clinical and histopathologic factors related to prognosis in primary squamous cell carcinoma of the vagina. *Int J Gynecol Cancer.* 2006;16(3):1201-1211.

115. Miyamoto D, Tanaka C, Viswanathan A. Concurrent chemoradiation improves survival in patients with vaginal cancer. *Int J Radiat Oncol Biol Phys.* 2010;78(3):S120-S121.

116. Nashiro T, Yagi C, Hirakawa M, et al. Concurrent chemoradiation for locally advanced squamous cell carcinoma of the vagina: case series and literature review. *Int J Clin Oncol.* 2008;13(4):335-339.

CHAPTER **3.7**

Treatment of Persistent and Recurrent Vaginal Cancer

Josephine Kang, Diana Miao, Amanda Nickles Fader, and Akila N. Viswanathan

For patients with recurrent or persistent disease, it is important to determine whether there is a reasonable chance of cure with salvage treatment or whether the primary goal is palliation. Thus, multiple factors, including extent of disease, site, extent of recurrence, disease-free interval, status of systemic disease, patient age, comorbidities, and overall performance status, must be considered.

Early-stage lesions that recur after RT can be surgically salvaged. A retrospective review of pelvic exenteration for recurrent gynecologic malignancies at the University of California Los Angeles Medical Center from 1956 to 2001 reported survival rates for patients with recurrent cervical and vaginal cancer to be 73% at 1 year and 54% at 5 years (1).

Patients with tumor persistence or recurrence after limited surgical procedures can be considered for more extensive surgery. If not, systemic chemotherapy and/or radiation can be administered.

Recurrent disease in advanced-stage patients is more challenging to treat. Most patients have received prior EBRT and thus have options limited to radical surgery or, in patients with localized disease, reirradiation. For patients with small pelvic recurrences, reirradiation with intracavitary or interstitial brachytherapy has been reported, with control rates between 50% and 75%, and grade 3 or higher complication rates between 7% and 15% (2-7). Beriwal et al (8) evaluated high dose rate (HDR) brachytherapy for primary and recurrent vaginal malignancy. In the subset of patients with a previous malignancy, crude local control rates were 100% for patients without prior RT and 67% for patients with a history of RT.

Palliative local treatment can provide symptomatic benefit for patients with advanced disease who have no curative options. Advanced disease can result in vaginal bleeding, pelvic pain, lymphedema, and visceral obstruction. Vaginal bleeding is a common symptom, which can become brisk if tumor erodes into a larger vessel. Large fractions of radiation delivered initially during the treatment course may be useful in achieving hemostasis for such cases. Other options include embolization, infusion of vasopressin, and balloon catheterization for severe hemodynamic losses.

REFERENCES

1. Berek JS, Howe C, Lagasse LD, Hacker NF. Pelvic exenteration for recurrent gynecologic malignancy: survival and morbidity analysis of the 45-year experience at UCLA. *Gynecol Oncol.* 2005;99(1):153-159.

2. Jhingran A, Salehpour M, Sam M, Levy L, Eifel PJ. Vaginal motion and bladder and rectal volumes during pelvic intensity-modulated radiation therapy after hysterectomy. *Int J Radiat Oncol Biol Phys.* 2012;82(1):256-262.

3. Xiang-E W, Shu-mo C, Ya-qin D, Ke W. Treatment of late recurrent vaginal malignancy after initial radiotherapy for carcinoma of the cervix: an analysis of 73 cases. *Gynecol Oncol.* 1998;69(2):125-129.

4. Russell AH, Koh WJ, Markette K, et al. Radical reirradiation for recurrent or second primary carcinoma of the female reproductive tract. *Gynecol Oncol.* 1987;27(2):226-232.

5. Randall ME, Barrett RJ. Interstitial irradiation in the management of recurrent carcinoma of the cervix after previous radiation therapy. *N C Med J.* 1988;49(6):306-308.

6. Gupta AK, Vicini FA, Frazier AJ, et al. Iridium-192 transperineal interstitial brachytherapy for locally advanced or recurrent gynecological malignancies. *Int J Radiat Oncol Biol Phys.* 1999;43(5):1055-1060.

7. Charra C, Roy P, Coquard R, Romestaing P, Ardiet JM, Gérard JP. Outcome of treatment of upper third vaginal recurrences of cervical and endometrial carcinomas with interstitial brachytherapy. *Int J Radiat Oncol Biol Phys.* 1998;40(2):421-426.

8. Beriwal S, Heron DE, Mogus R, Edwards RP, Kelley JL, Sukumvanich P. High-dose rate brachytherapy (HDRB) for primary or recurrent cancer in the vagina. *Radiat Oncol.* 2008;3(1):7.

CHAPTER **3.8**

Rare Histologies of Vaginal Cancer

Josephine Kang, Diana Miao, Amanda Nickles Fader, and Akila N. Viswanathan

CLEAR CELL ADENOCARCINOMA

Epidemiology

Clear cell adenocarcinoma of the vagina was first reported in 1971 by Herbst (1), who documented six cases of primary vaginal clear cell carcinoma in patients 15 to 22 years of age. Five of the six had been exposed to the synthetic estrogen DES in utero during the first trimester. This was the first report suggesting that in utero exposure to DES, prescribed during the mid-1940s to 1960s for high-risk pregnancies, could result in an increased risk of clear cell adenocarcinoma. DES-related clear cell adenocarcinoma presents at a young age, with studies documenting median age at presentation to be within the second or third decade of life (1,2). Studies suggest that there is a bimodal distribution for clear cell adenocarcinoma of the vagina, the first peak comprising young women with a mean age of 26 years, most of whom were exposed to DES in utero, and a second peak comprising women with a mean age of 71 years, not exposed to DES (1,3). Most patients present with stage I and II disease (1,4).

Risk Factors

In 45% to 95% of cases, clear cell adenocarcinoma of the vagina is associated with vaginal adenosis, defined as the abnormal presence of glandular epithelium in the vagina (5,6). Vaginal adenosis has three patterns: endocervical, tuboendometrial, and embryonic (6-8). Grossly, vaginal adenosis appears as red, velvety, grapelike clusters in the vagina. Glandular columnar epithelium of Müllerian type either appears beneath the squamous epithelium or replaces it, undergoing progressive squamous metaplasia (6).

Vaginal adenosis is believed to be a precursor lesion to clear cell adenocarcinoma of the vagina. It is a common histologic abnormality in women who have been exposed to DES in utero, presenting in up to 95% of such women (5,6). However, it is not strictly confined to this population (9).

The risk of developing clear cell adenocarcinoma in DES-exposed women is estimated to be 1 in 1,000 (4), suggesting that there are multiple factors contributing to pathogenesis. Additional factors associated with increased risk include DES exposure before the 12th week of pregnancy, a maternal history of prior miscarriage, birth in autumn, and prematurity (10).

Histopathology

Clear cell adenocarcinoma of the vagina is most often located in the upper third of the anterior vagina and may vary greatly in size. These cancers can also arise in the cervix. Grossly, they exhibit exophytic growth and are superficially invasive (11). Microscopically, they are composed of vacuolated, glycogen-rich cells, hence the term "clear cell carcinoma" (**Figure 3.8-1**). The most common histologic pattern is tubulocystic, although solid, papillary, and mixed cell patterns have also been described (12,13). Cells are cuboidal or columnar in shape, with large, atypical protruding nuclei, rimmed by a small amount of vacuolated cytoplasm.

Clinical Presentation

Patients with clear cell adenocarcinoma most often present with abnormal vaginal bleeding (1), which is found in 50% to 75% of cases. Cytology is not reliable, revealing abnormality in only 33% of cases; therefore, careful assessment of the entire vaginal vault to assess for submucosal irregularity is recommended, in addition to four-quadrant cytologic assessment (14). Abnormal discharge, urinary symptoms, and lower gastrointestinal complaints can also be noted, particularly in advanced cases. The differential diagnosis of vaginal adenocarcinoma is often challenging, because it must be distinguished from metastases from distant sites.

Prognostic Factors

For clear cell adenocarcinoma, prognostic variables associated with worse survival include advanced-stage, nontubulocystic pattern of

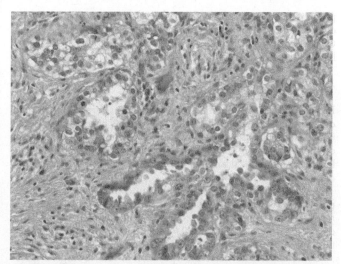

Figure 3.8-1. Clear cell carcinoma (CCC) of the vagina appears as nests and irregular glands lined by cells with characteristic clear to pale eosinophilic cytoplasm. CCC may show a mixture of architectural patterns including papillary, tubulopapillary, and tubulocystic patterns, and cytologic features may be variable from round to oval nuclei with prominent nucleoli (as seen in this example) to more significant nuclear pleomorphism and conspicuous mitoses. Images courtesy of Emily E. K. Meserve.

histology, size more than 3 cm, and depth of invasion greater than 3 mm (11). A study of 21 women with clear cell carcinoma of the vagina and cervix reported that overexpression of wild-type p53 was associated with a more favorable prognosis (15). Primary adenocarcinoma of the vagina not associated with DES exposure is extremely rare. In a review of 26 such cases by Frank et al (16), 5-year OS was 34%, significantly worse than in patients with SCC. A recent series described five cases of clear cell adenocarcinoma in patients without prior DES exposure, treated between 1990 and 2013 (17). The patients were all older than 40 years. There was high incidence of distant spread, especially to the lungs; OS at 5 years was 55%.

Treatment Options

The optimal management of clear cell adenocarcinoma is unclear. There are several published series on DES-related clear cell adenocarcinomas (11,13,18-20) using conventional treatments similar to those used for SCC of the vagina for stage I and II disease, including surgery with radical hysterectomy, vaginectomy and lymphadenectomy with construction of a neovagina, or definitive RT and consideration of radiosensitizing concurrent chemotherapy (21,22). In these series, there has been an emphasis on preservation of ovarian and vaginal function, owing to the earlier age at diagnosis in DES-exposed patients. According to data from the U.S. Registry for Research on Hormonal Transplacental Carcinogenesis, approximately one-half of all vaginal clear cell adenocarcinoma cases were treated with radical surgery alone (23).

Wharton et al (24) report the use of intracavitary or transvaginal irradiation for early-stage disease, with excellent tumor control and preservation of ovarian function. Herbst et al (25) reported on 142 cases of stage I clear cell adenocarcinoma. For the 117 patients treated with radical surgery, there was an 8% risk of recurrence and 87% OS. For patients treated with radiation, there was a 36% risk of recurrence. The authors acknowledge that it is difficult to compare surgery with radiation, as radiation was most likely used in patients with larger lesions less amenable to resection.

A series by Senekjian et al (19) reported on 219 cases of stage I clear cell vaginal adenocarcinoma. Forty-three patients received local therapy alone, consisting of vaginectomy, local excision, or local irradiation with or without excision, and the remaining patients had conventional radical surgery. At 10 years, the actuarial survival

rates were equivalent (88% vs 90%). However, the actuarial recurrence rate was significantly higher (40% vs 13%) with local excision alone. Patients who received local irradiation, with or without local excision, had decreased local recurrence compared to those treated with excision alone ($P < .03$).

A subsequent series by Senekjian et al (13) reviewed 76 cases of stage II clear cell adenocarcinoma. The 10-year OS rate was 65%. The 5-year survival rates were 80% for patients treated with surgery, 87% for patients treated with radiation, and 85% for patients treated with both. The authors advocate treatment with combination EBRT and brachytherapy for stage II disease, with surgery reserved for smaller, more easily resectable lesions in the upper vagina. The use of pelvic exenteration for primary and recurrent lesions has been reported by Senekjian and colleagues (20). Survival outcomes were comparable to those of patients treated with other modalities. Thus, to minimize morbidity and preserve quality of life, exenterative approaches are advocated only for patients with disease recurrence after RT. Herbst et al reported that a 5-year survival rate after pelvic relapse was 40% (18).

Most recurrences occur within 3 years of therapy, although recurrences 10 to 20 years after treatment have been reported (26). Most recurrences are local or locoregional, with approximately one-third detected at distant sites, most commonly in the lungs or extrapelvic lymph nodes, although there have been rare cases of central nervous system (CNS) metastases manifesting years after treatment (27). The 10-year actuarial survival rate for clear cell adenocarcinoma of the vagina is 79%. For stage I and II disease, survival rates are 90% and 80%, respectively.

OTHER ADENOCARCINOMAS

Most adenocarcinomas that present in the vagina are attributed to metastatic spread from other sites. Vaginal metastases from adenocarcinoma of the breast, kidneys, or other gynecologic primary sites have been described (28-30). Primary non–clear cell adenocarcinoma of the vagina is extremely rare and occurs predominantly in postmenopausal women. Histologic variants include endometrioid, mucinous, mesonephric, and papillary serous adenocarcinoma. Vaginal endometrioid adenocarcinoma is the most common non–clear cell subtype and presents most often in women with a history of endometriosis. Only a handful of case reports or series have been published in detail about endometrioid adenocarcinoma of the vagina (31-41). In one series of 18 cases of primary vaginal endometrioid adenocarcinoma (31), 10 cases arose from the apex; 14 of 18 cases had vaginal endometriosis, which is important in indicating a primary vaginal tumor rather than secondary spread from the endothelium. Median age at presentation was 57 years, with a range from 45 to 81 years. There have been case reports of mucinous adenocarcinoma of the vagina (32-44), with at least one arising from a focus of endocervicosis (45).

On gross examination, endometrioid adenocarcinomas can be polypoid, papillary, rough, granular, fungating, exophytic, or flat, and most arise from the superior aspect of the vagina. Microscopically, tumors display a predominant component of typical endometrioid carcinoma, with tubular glands lined by columnar cells with moderate amounts of eosinophilic cytoplasm and large elongated nuclei. Only a handful of cases of mucinous adenocarcinoma have been described (29,42-44), including rare cases arising in neovaginas (46) or arising from endocervicosis (45). Mesonephric adenocarcinoma arises from mesonephric duct remnants situated in the lateral vaginal wall (47,48). Primary papillary serous adenocarcinoma of the vagina has rarely been reported (49).

MELANOMA

According to the NCDB report by Creasman et al (50), vaginal melanomas comprise 4% of all primary vaginal cancers. Melanomas arising from the vaginal mucosa are rare, accounting for 2.8% to 5%

of all vaginal neoplasms (51-53), with just over 100 new cases reported each year in the United States. Melanomas arising from the vaginal mucosa are thought to originate from mucosal melanocytes in regions of melanosis or from atypical melanocytic hyperplasia.

The incidence of vaginal melanoma has remained stable and is reportedly 0.26 per million (54). Most reported cases are in Caucasian women; one study of 37 women with primary melanoma of the vagina reported that 84% of patients were Caucasian and only 3% African American (51). According to a report by Hu et al (55) analyzing SEER data from 1992 to 2005 on 125 cases of vaginal melanoma with known race/ethnicity, there is no significant difference in the incidence of vaginal melanoma between Caucasian and African American women, with a White/Black ratio of 1.02 after age adjustment. In the report by Creasman and colleagues, most patients were of advanced age at presentation, with only 23% of patients diagnosed before the age of 60, 28% were diagnosed between the ages of 60 and 69, 28% were diagnosed between the ages of 70 and 79, and 22% were diagnosed at age 80 or older (50).

Grossly, melanoma of the vagina tends to be pigmented and may present as a dark mass, plaque, or ulceration; multifocal presentation is also common. The most common appearance is polypoid nodular (56). The most common location at presentation is the anterior vaginal wall and lower one-third of the vagina (51,52,57).

In a case series of 37 women with primary vaginal melanoma reported by Frumovitz et al (51), median tumor size at presentation was 3 cm (range 0.4-5 cm), with median depth of invasion of 7 mm (range 1-21 mm). Twenty-one percent of patients presented with multifocal disease. Twenty-four patients (65%) presented with lesions in the distal third of the vagina or introitus.

Microscopically, tumors may be composed of epithelioid, spindle, or nevus-like cells and stain frequently positive for S-100 protein, HMB-45, and Melan A (**Figure 3.8-2**). When S-100 is negative or only focally positive, tyrosinase and MART-1 are useful markers. Poorly differentiated tumors may be difficult to distinguish from carcinomas or sarcomas. Tumor thickness correlates with prognosis and may be measured by Breslow methods (58).

Vaginal melanoma is a highly malignant disease with a propensity for early hematogenous spread. The most common presenting symptoms are slight vaginal bleeding and usually blood-tinged, foul-smelling, or purulent vaginal discharge (59). Reid et al (60) reviewed 115 patients with primary melanoma of the vagina and found depth of invasion and lesion size greater than 3 cm to be negative

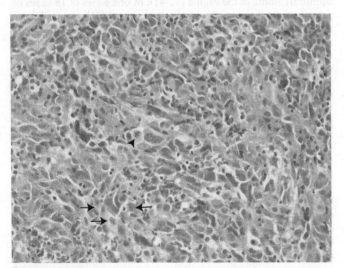

Figure 3.8-2. Vaginal melanoma. Malignant melanoma exhibits variable morphology. This example shows a vaguely nested to discohesive epithelioid neoplasm with characteristic eosinophilic nucleoli (arrows), significant nuclear pleomorphism, and mitoses (arrowhead). The presence of melanin pigment and immunohistochemistry can be helpful to confirm the diagnosis. Images courtesy of Emily E. K. Meserve.

prognostic factors. Stage was not found to be prognostic for outcome, but only 42 of the 115 patients had this information available. Compared to women with SCC, patients with vaginal melanoma have a significant 1.5-fold increased risk of mortality (61).

Treatment Options

Primary vaginal melanoma is uncommon; as a result, treatment outcomes for only a small number of patients have been reported (51,59,60,62-66), and it is difficult to make definitive treatment recommendations. Treatments used in published series include wide local excision, radical surgery, RT, chemotherapy, or a combination of modalities.

Regardless of primary treatment, outcomes have been disappointing. Overall prognosis is poor, with historic 5-year survival rates ranging from 5% to 30% regardless of treatment modality or extent of surgical resection (60,62,65). There is a high rate of distant metastases, ranging from 66% to 100% (62,67,68).

Some authors advocate incorporation of radical surgical resection into the treatment paradigm, when feasible (69-71). Surgery is favored over RT because melanoma tends to be radioresistant. Geisler et al (69) recommend primary pelvic exenteration for vaginal melanomas with invasion greater than 3 mm, reporting a 5-year survival rate of 50% if pelvic nodes are free of disease. Morrow and DiSaia (71), in their review of gynecologic melanoma, recommend radical surgery based on a review of the literature that revealed 3 out of 19 long-term survivors after exenteration with wide local excision. Chung and colleagues (62) reviewed 19 cases of primary vaginal melanoma treated between 1934 and 1976. All patients who received wide local excision developed recurrence. Five-year survival was only 21%. Miner and colleagues (72) reported on 35 patients treated at Memorial Sloan Kettering Cancer Center from 1977 to 2001: 69% underwent surgery, which was en bloc removal of the involved pelvic organs, wide excision, or total vaginectomy, with elective pelvic lymph node dissection in 74% of cases. Thirty-one percent of patients received definitive RT. Primary surgical therapy was significantly associated with a longer OS (25 vs 13 months). Recurrence-free survival was not found to correlate with surgical extent. A study by Huang et al (73) found 5-year OS to be 32%, but as high as 47% in patients who underwent surgical treatment.

Several series comparing radical surgery and local excision find equivalent outcomes (59,63,74,75). In general, treatment modality does not appear to significantly affect survival. Bonner et al (76) reported on nine cases of vaginal melanoma. Three patients were treated with wide local excision, and six underwent radical surgery. All nine patients developed locoregional recurrence. Therefore, the authors suggest adding pelvic RT to improve local control. The use of wide local excision followed by postoperative EBRT and brachytherapy has been proposed. A more recent review by Frumovitz and colleagues (51) reported that RT after wide local excision can reduce local recurrences. However, most patients develop distant metastases, most commonly in the lungs and liver.

Retrospective data suggest that RT may improve local control for vaginal melanoma (59,77). Among the few long-term survivors reported in the literature are a handful of patients who were treated with radiation. Harwood and Cummings (78) described a complete response in four patients with vaginal melanoma treated with radiation, although two subsequently relapsed. Rogo et al (79), in their series of 22 cases of vulvovaginal melanoma, reported comparable results for surgery and RT, with eight patients (36%) alive 5 years after treatment. Petru et al (77), in their series documenting 14 patients treated for primary malignant melanoma of the vagina, noted that three of nine patients treated with radiation, either as primary treatment (n = 2) or in the postoperative setting (n = 1), survived longer than 5 years. Median OS for all patients was 10 months, with a 5-year DFS rate of 14% and an OS rate of 21%.

Given the high rates of distant metastases, chemotherapy has been used, either alone or in conjunction with RT (51,80). The use of systemic chemotherapy and/or immunotherapy has not consistently been shown to improve patient outcomes thus far (80). Frumovitz et al, in their review of 37 women with stage I melanoma of the vagina treated at MDACC between 1980 and 2009, report very poor prognosis even in this group of patients with localized disease, with a 5-year OS rate of 20%. In that study, 10% of patients received nonsurgical treatment with RT, chemotherapy, or both. Patients treated surgically had significantly longer survival times compared with those treated nonsurgically. RT delivered after wide local excision reduced local recurrence and demonstrated a trend toward longer survival times, from 16.1 to 29.4 months. A study by Xia et al (66) evaluated 44 women, diagnosed and treated for vaginal melanoma between 2002 and 2011. There was no difference in OS between local excision and radical surgery. However, the authors noted increased PFS with the addition of adjuvant chemotherapy and RT (8.6 vs 16.0 months, $P = .038$). Other reports have described the use of immunotherapy after surgery and reveal that the best outcomes are achieved with this approach (73).

Based on limited but promising data suggesting an improvement in local control with the addition of adjuvant RT, treatment can be considered. However, there is no general recommendation for the treatment of primary vaginal melanoma. When RT is administered, vaginal melanoma is treated similarly to vaginal carcinoma, with volumes and doses ranging from 50 Gy for subclinical disease to 75 Gy for gross tumor.

SARCOMA

Sarcomas represent 3% of all primary vaginal cancers (50). In a report based on data from the NCDB between 1985 and 1994 (50), there were 135 cases of primary vaginal sarcoma, of heterogeneous histologies and varying age. Twenty-two percent of patients were younger than 14 years, with a median age at presentation of approximately 50 years. Consistent with this, a recent analysis of the SEER database identified 221 patients with primary vaginal sarcoma, diagnosed between 1988 and 2010, with a mean age of 54.9 years (81). Compared with other vaginal cancers, sarcomas tend to be larger, with decreased likelihood of lymph node involvement, and are more commonly treated with primary surgery without RT. It was estimated that, after adjusting for other variables, patients' vaginal sarcomas had a 69% greater risk of cancer-related mortality when compared with SCC.

Vaginal sarcoma most frequently presents as an asymptomatic vaginal mass (82). In one series, this was the most common system and was found in 35% of patients, followed by vaginal, rectal, or bladder pain (26%); bleeding or serosanguinous discharge from the vagina or rectum (18%); leukorrhea (9%); dyspareunia (7%); or difficulty in micturition (7%).

Leiomyosarcoma is the most common histology in adults, representing up to 65% of all vaginal sarcoma cases; however, overall numbers are very small, with fewer than 150 published reports in the literature (82). Vaginal leiomyosarcomas originate from the smooth muscle of the vaginal wall, but may also develop from smooth muscle cells in tissues adjacent to the vagina. Grossly, patients present with a palpable submucosal nodule, although advanced tumors may demonstrate palpable necrosis or exophytic polypoid tissue (83). Criteria to distinguish between benign leiomyoma and leiomyosarcoma include greater than five mitoses per 10 high-power field (HPF), moderate or marked cytologic atypia, and infiltrating margins (84) (**Figure 3.8-3**). In view of considerable variation in smooth muscle tumors from area to area, adequate sampling is recommended to achieve an accurate diagnosis. Microscopically, leiomyosarcomas demonstrate interlacing bundles of spindle-shaped cells, with blunt-ended nuclei and fibrillar cytoplasm (59,84). Leiomyosarcomas have a predilection for the posterior vaginal wall, with published reports suggesting approximately 43% to 45% in the posterior vagina, 17% to 21% anteriorly, and 34% to 39% laterally (82,85). Leiomyosarcomas are also aggressive; they undergo early hematogenous dissemination, frequently recur locally (50,82), and often demonstrate pulmonary metastases (86).

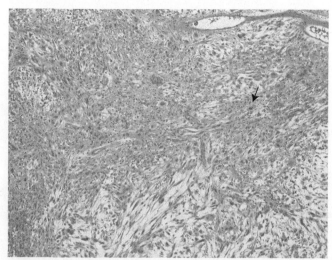

Figure 3.8-3. Leiomyosarcoma. Leiomyosarcoma of the vagina appears similar to malignant smooth muscle tumors in other anatomic sites and shows spindled to epithelioid (when morphologically higher grade) cells in a fascicular architecture. There is significant nuclear atypia with nuclear hyperchromasia and numerous mitotic figures, including atypical forms (arrow). Images courtesy of Emily E. K. Meserve.

Other less common histologies include malignant mixed Müllerian tumor (MMT), endometrial stromal sarcoma, and angiosarcoma (87,88). MMTs, also called carcinosarcomas, are highly aggressive, biphasic neoplasms composed of an epithelial component as well as a sarcomatous component. The epithelial component in vaginal MMT is most often SCC (87). The sarcomatous component may be composed of fibroblasts and smooth muscle, or include cartilage, striated muscle, bone, and other heterologous tissues. The metaplastic carcinoma theory suggests that there is a common cell of origin for MMT, with carcinoma giving rise to the sarcomatous component via metaplasia (89). The most common differential diagnosis is sarcomatoid carcinoma. The spindle and carcinomatous components are positive for cytokeratin in sarcomatous carcinoma, whereas MMT demonstrates a sarcomatous component that is positive for vimentin, with the carcinomatous component positive for cytokeratin (87).

The first case of vaginal MMT was described in 1975 by Davis et al (90), after which only 11 cases have been reported in the literature, with patients' age ranging from 57 to 74 years (87,91-95). At least one case report of MMT of the vagina detected high-risk HPV in both the carcinomatous and sarcomatous components, suggesting that some vaginal MMTs may be related to HPV (91). Fewer than 10 cases of angiosarcoma of the vagina have been reported in the literature (96,97). A history of pelvic RT is a risk factor for pelvic sarcomas, particularly angiosarcoma (88).

In the pediatric population, embryonal rhabdomyosarcoma/sarcoma botryoides is the most common histology (98), with 90% of cases occurring in children younger than 5 years.

Prognostic Factors

Review of the literature indicates that vaginal sarcomas undergo early hematogenous dissemination as well as frequent local recurrence. Pulmonary metastases are common (82,85). Adverse prognostic factors for vaginal sarcoma include high histologic grade, stage, size greater than 3 cm, infiltrative borders, and cytologic atypia (86).

Treatment Options

Despite surgery and the use of adjuvant RT in select cases, sarcoma patients sustain poor outcomes because of a high incidence of local recurrence and distant metastasis. Locoregional control is especially important for vaginal leiomyosarcoma. A series by Peters et al (99) reported on 17 cases, comprising 10 patients with leiomyosarcoma, 4 with MMT, and 3 with other types of sarcomas. There were only three patients alive and free of disease with follow-up times of 84 to 161 months. All three patients had undergone pelvic exenteration. Patients who received other forms of primary therapy all died of recurrence, with the pelvis as the first site of recurrence in all cases. In 50% of cases, the pelvis was the only site of failure, stressing the importance of local treatment. OS of 8 and 10 years following wide local excision have been reported (85).

Postoperative RT has been used to manage soft tissue sarcomas in other sites to reduce locoregional recurrence rates (100). Results from adjuvant radiation for high-grade sarcoma in other regions of the body have been extrapolated to vaginal cancer. In patients with involved margins, high doses above 62.5 Gy are generally required to achieve local control (101). Systemic treatment with doxorubicin is standard for leiomyosarcoma (102).

Outcomes

In the SEER analysis, 5-year survival was 89% for stage I and under 50% for stage II vaginal sarcomas of all types (81). Other series describe similarly poor outcomes. Five-year survival was 36% for patients with leiomyosarcoma in the Peters et al (99) series. The survival rate for patients with MMT was even lower, at 17%. There are only a few case reports and small series detailing treatment of primary vaginal MMT. Neesham and colleagues (93) published a case report of a 74-year-old patient treated with wide local excision and radiation for a 5.5-cm stage I MMT. She developed distant metastases within 6 months of local therapy. Analysis of patterns of failure suggests that local therapy does not have a significant impact on survival owing to early distant spread. Therefore, chemotherapy is typically administered after surgery for MMT in other sites and should be considered for primary vaginal lesions, along with adjuvant RT as warranted. Platinum-based chemotherapy has been used for MMT occurring elsewhere in the pelvis. It has not yet been determined whether platinum agents are best administered alone or in combination with other agents. Combination regimens include a platinum agent and/or paclitaxel and/or ifosfamide (103-106).

LYMPHOMA

Lymphomas of the female genital tract are rare, accounting for only 1% of all primary extranodal lymphomas (107). Lymphomas of the vagina are exceedingly uncommon, with fewer than 30 cases reported in the literature thus far (108-127). In one review from the Armed Forces Institute of Pathology, only 4 of 9,500 cases of lymphoma were determined to originate from the vagina (128). Diffuse large B-cell lymphoma is the most common histology, though there have also been reports of lymphoplasmacytic, Burkitt, and mucosa-associated lymphoid tissue (MALT) lymphomas (115).

On examination, the tumor is typically palpable, with infiltrative thickening and/or ulceration of the vaginal wall (123). Immunohistochemical analyses are valuable techniques for confirming diagnosis, with tumors typically expressing CD20 (116,126). The most common symptom at presentation is vaginal bleeding. Leukemic infiltrates may be difficult to distinguish from lymphoma; therefore, chloroacetate esterase or myeloperoxidase staining may be useful. Although there is no established treatment protocol for primary lymphoma of the vagina, it seems reasonable to extrapolate from results for extranodal lymphomas elsewhere in the body and to use similar chemotherapeutic and response-based RT regimens. For patients wishing to retain fertility, chemotherapy alone may be an option in select cases.

If diagnosed at an early stage, the prognosis for vaginal lymphoma is excellent, with 5-year survival rates of up to 90%. Of 10 cases reported in the literature between 1994 and 2007, all patients

except one were cured of disease after treatment with chemotherapy or a combination of RT and chemotherapy (114,116,120,122,129-132). Follow-up periods for these 10 cases ranged from 6 to 120 months, and one patient died from other causes. Eight patients had Ann Arbor stage IEA disease, one had IIEA, and one did not have stage reported. The most common chemotherapy regimen was cyclophosphamide, doxorubicin, vincristine, and prednisone (CHOP). Complete remission was also achieved using methotrexate, doxorubicin, cyclophosphamide, vincristine, prednisone, and bleomycin (MACOP-B) in one patient. Half of the patients did not receive RT because of an excellent response to chemotherapy alone.

SMALL CELL CARCINOMA OF THE VAGINA AND OTHER RARE HISTOLOGIES

Primary small cell carcinoma of the vagina is a rare entity, with fewer than 25 cases reported in the literature (133). Mean age at diagnosis is 59 years, with poor outcome because of early widespread dissemination. Eighty-five percent of patients die within 1 year of diagnosis (134,135). Neuroendocrine differentiation is often manifested by secretory granules, argyrophilia, and expression of neuroendocrine markers (136,137), staining positive for cytokeratin, neuron-specific enolase, chromogranin A, and serotonin (**Figure 3.8-4**). Thyroid transcription factor 1 can also be positive and should not be used to differentiate primary from metastatic disease. Microscopically, it is indistinguishable from that of the lung. These tumors can occur in pure form or be associated with squamous or glandular elements (134,136). Ectopic Cushing syndrome has been documented in primary small cell carcinoma of the vagina (137). Treatment typically follows general principles for small cell carcinomas of the cervix, with aggressive therapy, including combination cisplatin-based chemotherapy, RT, brachytherapy, and surgery if feasible.

Vaginal paraganglioma is a rare neuroendocrine tumor, with fewer than 10 cases reported in the literature in younger women, with median age at presentation of 31 years (138-140). It is thought to be an indolent tumor, managed surgically. The tumor can manifest with catecholamine secretion, similarly to paragangliomas elsewhere in the body (138).

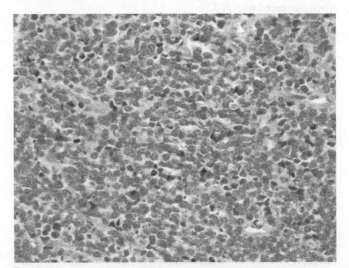

Figure 3.8-4. Neuroendocrine carcinoma of the vagina. Small cell carcinoma of the vagina is a poorly differentiated neuroendocrine carcinoma showing small blue cells with round to irregularly shaped nuclei with coarse ("salt and pepper") chromatin, very scant cytoplasm, and numerous mitotic and apoptotic figures. Importantly, designation as a primary small cell carcinoma of the vagina is possible only after exclusion of metastasis from other anatomic sites (ie, lung). Immunohistochemical markers are generally not helpful in establishing site of origin in neuroendocrine carcinomas. Images courtesy of Emily E. K. Meserve.

Adenosquamous carcinoma of the vagina is also uncommon. Microscopically, tumor cells are composed of glandular and squamous elements. One case report described adenosquamous carcinoma associated with small cell carcinoma of the endometrium in a 64-year-old female (141). Treatment approaches are similar to those used for SCC of the vagina, including consideration of combination CRT for patients with gross disease.

CARCINOMA OF THE NEOVAGINA

The neovagina is a surgically constructed vaginal canal, typically described in patients with congenitally deformed or absent genitalia, or patients desiring reconstruction of a functional vagina after surgery for gynecologic malignancy. Various methods have been utilized for neovaginal construction, including split-skin grafts, myocutaneous flaps, and formation of an artificial canal between the rectum and the vagina (142). Given its overall rarity, there are very few reports of in situ or invasive carcinoma arising in the neovagina.

A review of published literature reveals six published reports of carcinoma in situ (143-148). The period of development of carcinoma in situ ranged from 6 months to 20 years after constructive surgery. Invasive carcinoma of the neovagina tends to be poorly differentiated, and most reported cases have been SCC. All reported patients have presented with large tumor masses and evidence of rapid progression, with poor overall outcomes (46,149-152).

Treatment options include radiation, with or without an attempt at radical resection, and, in select cases, lymph node dissection. Of 16 reported cases from a review by Steiner et al (142), 9 received primary radiation alone, 1 received radiation followed by exenteration and intraoperative radiation, and 4 underwent exenteration. Recurrence status was not documented for all patients. Three were found to have rapid disease recurrence within several months. Two patients were free of disease at 10 and 18 months, respectively. One patient had a recurrence-free interval of 3 years, but died a year later from disease.

Although there is no optimal treatment, resection followed by consideration of adjuvant radiation is preferable to definitive radiation alone, as surgery can offer full pathologic diagnosis. The extent of disease, patient characteristics, and treatment goals should guide the choice of treatment.

HISTORY OF PRIOR PELVIC RADIATION

As many as 10% to 50% of patients with VAIN or invasive carcinoma of the vagina have a previous diagnosis of cervical carcinoma (153-161), with an average interval of 14 years between diagnosis of cervical disease to development of vaginal carcinoma (157,162). As a result, a proportion of patients with vaginal cancer have a history of prior pelvic radiation. Reirradiation can be considered in this setting, but there is an increased risk of toxicity, particularly radionecrosis and fistula formation. Xiang et al (163) published a series on 73 patients with a history of RT for cervical carcinoma who received a second diagnosis of vaginal malignancy 5 to 30 years later. All patients received EBRT and brachytherapy for treatment of their initial cancer. Reirradiation for the vaginal malignancy was planned according to site and volume of the vaginal tumor and location and dose of the prior radiation. Patients received brachytherapy, using either radium delivered to the tumor base (30-40 Gy in three to five fractions) or HDR with cobalt-60 to the tumor base (20-35 Gy in three to five fractions), followed by a dose to 0.5 cm below the vaginal mucosa at 20 to 30 Gy in four to six fractions delivered using a vaginal mold. For involvement of the vulva or groin, patients additionally received EBRT to a dose of 30 to 40 Gy. Most patients received RT alone; 11 also received chemotherapy, most typically cisplatin based. The 5-year survival rate was 40.3%, and three patients survived more than 15 years. There were significant side effects with reirradiation: 18 of 73 patients

developed radionecrosis. Other side effects included one (1.4%) vesicovaginal fistula and eight (11%) rectovaginal fistulas, hematuria (12.3%), and moderate to severe rectal sequelae (13.6%).

Beriwal et al (164) reported on the use of HDR interstitial and intracavitary brachytherapy for five patients with recurrent vaginal cancer and a history of prior pelvic RT. Significant grade 3 or higher toxicities were noted in patients who received total EQD2 dose above 140 Gy. Median time from prior RT to recurrence was 4 years (range 6 months to 18 years). The recurrence was within 2 cm of the prior field in two patients and within the previous field for four patients. All patients received EBRT to a median dose of 45 Gy, followed by brachytherapy. For the four patients with prior overlapping fields, the cumulative EQD2 to the vaginal mucosa ranged from 120.7 to 154.54 Gy. Of these patients, one developed a rectovaginal fistula 2 years after treatment and another developed chronic vaginal ulceration with vaginal shortening to 2 cm; the EQD2 values were 142.98 and 154 Gy, respectively.

REFERENCES

1. Herbst AL, Ulfelder H, Poskanzer DC. Adenocarcinoma of the vagina. Association of maternal stilbestrol therapy with tumor appearance in young women. *N Engl J Med*. 1971;284(15):878-881.
2. Herbst AL, Anderson D. Clear cell adenocarcinoma of the vagina and cervix secondary to intrauterine exposure to diethylstilbestrol. *Semin Surg Oncol*. 1990;6:343-346.
3. Herbst AL. Diethylstilbestrol and adenocarcinoma of the vagina. *Am J Obstet Gynecol*. 1999;181(6):1576-1579.
4. Melnick S, Cole P, Anderson D, Herbst A. Rates and risks of diethylstilbestrol-related clear-cell adenocarcinoma of the vagina and cervix. *N Engl J Med*. 1987;316(9):514-516.
5. Robboy SJ, Scully RE, Herbst AL. Pathology of vaginal and cervical abnormalities associated with prenatal exposure to diethylstilbestrol (des). *J Reprod Med*. 1975;15(1):13-18.
6. Robboy SJ, Welch WR, Young RH, Truslow GY, Herbst AL, Scully RE. Topographic relation of cervical ectropion and vaginal adenosis to clear cell adenocarcinoma. *Obstet Gynecol*. 1982;60(5):546-551.
7. Verloop J, Rookus MA, van Leeuwen FE. Prevalence of gynecologic cancer in women exposed to diethylstilbestrol in utero. *N Engl J Med*. 2000;342(24):1838-1839.
8. Hacker NF, Eifel PJ, Van Der Velden J. Cancer of the vagina. *Int J Gynaecol Obstet*. 2015;131:S84-S87.
9. Robboy SJ, Hill EC, Sandberg EC, Czernobilsky B. Vaginal adenosis in women born prior to the diethylstilbestrol era. *Hum Pathol*. 1986;17(5):488-492.
10. Manetta A, Gutrecht EL, Berman ML, DiSaia PJ. Primary invasive carcinoma of the vagina. *Obstet Gynecol*. 1990;76(4):639-642.
11. Herbst AL, Robboy SJ, Scully RE, Poskanzer DC. Clear-cell adenocarcinoma of the vagina and cervix in girls: analysis of 170 registry cases. *Am J Obstet Gynecol*. 1974;119(5):713-724.
12. Jones WB, Koulos JP, Saigo PE, Lewis JL Jr. Clear-cell adenocarcinoma of the lower genital tract: memorial hospital 1974-1984. *Obstet Gynecol*. 1987;70(4):573-577.
13. Senekjian EK, Frey KW, Stone C, Herbst AL. An evaluation of stage II vaginal clear cell adenocarcinoma according to substages. *Gynecol Oncol*. 1988;31(1):56-64.
14. Hanselaar AG, Van Leusen ND, De Wilde PC, Vooijs GP. Clear cell adenocarcinoma of the vagina and cervix. A report of the Central Netherlands Registry with emphasis on early detection and prognosis. *Cancer*. 1991;67(7):1971-1978.
15. Waggoner SE, Anderson SM, Luce MC, Takahashi H, Boyd J. p53 protein expression and gene analysis in clear cell adenocarcinoma of the vagina and cervix. *Gynecol Oncol*. 1996;60(3):339-344.
16. Frank SJ, Deavers MT, Jhingran A, Bodurka DC, Eifel PJ. Primary adenocarcinoma of the vagina not associated with diethylstilbestrol (DES) exposure. *Gynecol Oncol*. 2007;105(2):470-474.
17. Nomura H, Matoda M, Okamoto S, et al. Clinical characteristics of non-squamous cell carcinoma of the vagina. *Int J Gynecol Cancer*. 2015;25(2):320-324.
18. Herbst AL, Norusis MJ, Rosenow PJ, Welch WR, Scully RE. An analysis of 346 cases of clear cell adenocarcinoma of the vagina and cervix with emphasis on recurrence and survival. *Gynecol Oncol*. 1979;7(2):111-122.
19. Senekjian EK, Frey KW, Anderson D, Herbst AL. Local therapy in stage I clear cell adenocarcinoma of the vagina. *Cancer*. 1987;60(6):1319-1324.

20. Senekjian EK, Frey K, Herbst AL. Pelvic exenteration in clear cell adenocarcinoma of the vagina and cervix. *Gynecol Oncol.* 1989;34(3):413-416.

21. Guiou M, Hall WH, Konia T, Scudder S, Leiserowitz G, Ryu JK. Primary clear cell adenocarcinoma of the rectovaginal septum treated with concurrent chemoradiation therapy: a case report. *Int J Gynecol Cancer.* 2008;18(5):1118-1121.

22. Miyamoto DT, Tanaka CK, Viswanathan AN. Concurrent chemoradiation improves survival in patients with vaginal cancer. *Int J Radiat Oncol Biol Phys.* 2010;78(3):S120-S121.

23. Waggoner SE, Mittendorf R, Biney N, Anderson D, Herbst AL. Influence of in utero diethylstilbestrol exposure on the prognosis and biologic behavior of vaginal clear-cell adenocarcinoma. *Gynecol Oncol.* 1994;55(2):238-244.

24. Wharton JT, Tortolero-Luna G, Linares AC, et al. Vaginal intraepithelial neoplasia and vaginal cancer. *Obstet Gynecol Clin North Am.* 1996;23(2):325-345.

25. Herbst AL, Cole P, Norusis MJ, Welch WR, Scully RE. Epidemiologic aspects and factors related to survival in 384 registry cases of clear cell adenocarcinoma of the vagina and cervix. *Am J Obstet Gynecol.* 1979;135(7): 876-886.

26. Fishman DA, Williams S, Small W Jr, et al. Late recurrences of vaginal clear cell adenocarcinoma. *Gynecol Oncol.* 1996;62(1):128-132.

27. Lin LM, Sciubba DM, Gallia GL, Sosnowski J, Weingart JD. Diethylstilbestrol (DES)-induced clear cell adenocarcinoma of the vagina metastasizing to the brain. *Gynecol Oncol.* 2007;105(1):273-276.

28. Tarraza HM Jr, Meltzer SE, DeCain M, Jones MA. Vaginal metastases from renal cell carcinoma: report of four cases and review of the literature. *Eur J Gynaecol Oncol.* 1998;19(1):14-18.

29. Saitoh M, Hayasaka T, Ohmichi M, Kurachi H, Motoyama T. Primary mucinous adenocarcinoma of the vagina: possibility of differentiating from metastatic adenocarcinomas. *Pathol Int.* 2005;55(6):372-375.

30. Nag S, Martínez-Monge R, Copeland LJ, Vacarello L, Lewandowski GS. Perineal template interstitial brachytherapy salvage for recurrent endometrial adenocarcinoma metastatic to the vagina. *Gynecol Oncol.* 1997;66(1):16-19.

31. Staats PN, Clement PB, Young RH. Primary endometrioid adenocarcinoma of the vagina: a clinicopathologic study of 18 cases. *Am J Surg Pathol.* 2007;31(10):1490-1501.

32. Nomoto K, Hori T, Kiya C, et al. Endometrioid adenocarcinoma of the vagina with a microglandular pattern arising from endometriosis after hysterectomy. *Pathol Int.* 2010;60(9):636-641.

33. Haskel S, Chen SS, Spiegel G. Vaginal endometrioid adenocarcinoma arising in vaginal endometriosis: a case report and literature review. *Gynecol Oncol.* 1989;34(2):232-236.

34. Adjetey V, Ganesan R, Downey GP. Primary vaginal endometrioid carcinoma following unopposed estrogen administration. *J Obstet Gynaecol.* 2003;23(3):316-317.

35. Bamford DS. Primary adenocarcinoma of the vagina. *Proc R Soc Med.* 1967;60(10):999-1000.

36. Eckert R, Eckert R. Adenocarcinoma arising in endometriosis. *Am Fam Physician.* 2000;62(4):734-736.

37. Granai CO, Walters MD, Safaii H, Jelen I, Madoc-Jones H, Moukhtar M. Malignant transformation of vaginal endometriosis. *Obstet Gynecol.* 1984;64(4):592-595.

38. Hyman MP. Extraovarian endometrioid carcinoma. Review of the literature and report of two cases with unusual features. *Am J Clin Pathol.* 1977;68(4):522-527.

39. Orr JW Jr, Holimon JL, Sisson PF. Vaginal adenocarcinoma developing in residual pelvic endometriosis: a clinical dilemma. *Gynecol Oncol.* 1989;33(1):96-98.

40. Wirtheimer C. 2 cases of endometrial adenocarcinoma of different origin. *Bull Soc R Belge Gynecol Obstet.* 1964;34:117-129.

41. Tewari DS, McHale MT, Kuo JV, Monk BJ, Burger RA. Primary invasive vaginal cancer in the setting of the Mayer–Rokitansky–Kuster–Hauser syndrome. *Gynecol Oncol.* 2002;85(2):384-387.

42. Ebrahim S, Daponte A, Smith TH, Tiltman A, Guidozzi F. Primary mucinous adenocarcinoma of the vagina. *Gynecol Oncol.* 2001;80(1):89-92.

43. Nasu K, Kai K, Matsumoto H, Mori C, Takai N, Narahara H. Primary mucinous adenocarcinoma of the vagina. *Eur J Gynaecol Oncol.* 2010;31: 679-681.

44. Werner D, Wilkinson EJ, Ripley D, Yachnis A. Primary adenocarcinoma of the vagina with mucinous–enteric differentiation: a report of two cases with associated vaginal adenosis without history of diethylstilbestrol exposure. *J Low Genit Tract Dis.* 2004;8(1):38-42.

45. McCluggage WG, Price JH, Dobbs SP. Primary adenocarcinoma of the vagina arising in endocervicosis. *Int J Gynecol Pathol.* 2001;20(4):399-402.

46. Hiroi H, Yasugi T, Matsumoto K, et al. Mucinous adenocarcinoma arising in a neovagina using the sigmoid colon thirty years after operation: a case report. *J Surg Oncol.* 2001;77(1):61-64.

47. Droegemueller W, Makowski EL, Taylor ES. Vaginal mesonephric adenocarcinoma in two prepubertal children. *Am J Dis Child.* 1970;119(2): 168-170.

48. Shaaban MM. Primary adenocarcinoma of the vagina of mesonephric pattern. Report of a case and review of literature. *Aust N Z J Obstet Gynaecol.* 1970;10(1):55-58.

49. Riva C, Fabbri A, Facco C, Tibiletti MG, Guglielmin P, Capella C. Primary serous papillary adenocarcinoma of the vagina: a case report. *Int J Gynecol Pathol.* 1997;16(3):286-290.

50. Creasman WT, Phillips JL, Menck HR. The national cancer data base report on cancer of the vagina. *Cancer.* 1998;83(5):1033-1040.

51. Frumovitz M, Etchepareborda M, Sun CC, et al. Primary malignant melanoma of the vagina. *Obstet Gynecol.* 2010;116(6):1358-1365.

52. Greggi S, Losito S, Pisano C, Desicato S, Scaffa C. Malignant melanoma of the vagina: report of two cases and review of the literature. *Int Surg.* 2010;95(2):120-125.

53. Ghosh A, Pradhan S, Swami R, Kc SR, Talwar O. Primary malignant melanoma of vagina—a case report with review of literature. *J Nepal Med Assoc.* 2007;46(168):203-205.

54. Weinstock MA. Malignant melanoma of the vulva and vagina in the United States: patterns of incidence and population-based estimates of survival. *Am J Obstet Gynecol.* 1994;171(5):1225-1230.

55. Hu DN, Yu GP, McCormick SA. Population-based incidence of vulvar and vaginal melanoma in various races and ethnic groups with comparisons to other site-specific melanomas. *Melanoma Res.* 2010;20(2):153-158.

56. Gupta JC, Arora MM, Jungalwala BN, Salgia KM. Primary melanoma of the vagina. *BJOG.* 1964;71(5):801-803.

57. Gökaslan H, Sişmanoğlu A, Pekin T, Kaya H, Ceyhan N. Primary malignant melanoma of the vagina: a case report and review of the current treatment options. *Eur J Obstet Gynecol Reprod Biol.* 2005;121(2):243-248.

58. Breslow A. Tumor thickness, level of invasion and node dissection in stage I cutaneous melanoma. *Ann Surg.* 1975;182(5):572-575.

59. Irvin WP Jr, Bliss SA, Rice LW, Taylor PT Jr, Andersen WA. Malignant melanoma of the vagina and locoregional control: radical surgery revisited. *Gynecol Oncol.* 1998;71(3):476-480.

60. Reid GC, Schmidt RW, Roberts JA, Hopkins MP, Barrett RJ, Morley GW. Primary melanoma of the vagina: a clinicopathologic analysis. *Obstet Gynecol.* 1989;74(2):190-199.

61. Shah CA, Goff BA, Lowe K, Peters WA 3rd, Li CI. Factors affecting risk of mortality in women with vaginal cancer. *Obstet Gynecol.* 2009;113(5):1038-1045.

62. Chung AF, Casey MJ, Flannery JT, Woodruff JM, Lewis JL Jr. Malignant melanoma of the vagina—report of 19 cases. *Obstet Gynecol.* 1980;55(6): 720-727.

63. Buchanan DJ, Schlaerth J, Kurosaki T. Primary vaginal melanoma: thirteen-year disease-free survival after wide local excision and review of recent literature. *Am J Obstet Gynecol.* 1998;178(6):1177-1184.

64. Levitan Z, Gordon AN, Kaplan AL, Kaufman RH. Primary malignant melanoma of the vagina: report of four cases and review of the literature. *Gynecol Oncol.* 1989;33(1):85-90.

65. Van Nostrand KM, Lucci JA 3rd, Schell M, Berman ML, Manetta A, DiSaia PJ. Primary vaginal melanoma: improved survival with radical pelvic surgery. *Gynecol Oncol.* 1994;55(2):234-237.

66. Xia L, Han D, Yang W, Li J, Chuang L, Wu X. Primary malignant melanoma of the vagina: a retrospective clinicopathologic study of 44 cases. *Int J Gynecol Cancer.* 2014;24(1):149-155.

67. Jentys W, Sikorowa L, Mokrzanowski A. Primary melanoma of the vagina. *Oncology.* 1975;31(2):83-91.

68. Norris HJ, Taylor HB. Melanomas of the vagina. *Obstet Gynecol Surv.* 1967;22(2):352-355.

69. Geisler JP, Look KY, Moore DA, Sutton GP. Pelvic exenteration for malignant melanomas of the vagina or urethra with over 3 mm of invasion. *Gynecol Oncol.* 1995;59(3):338-341.

70. Stellato G, Iodice F, Casella G, et al. Primary malignant melanoma of the vagina: case report. *Eur J Gynaecol Oncol.* 1998;19(2):186-188.

71. Morrow CP, DiSaia PJ. Malignant melanoma of the female genitalia: a clinical analysis. *Obstet Gynecol Surv.* 1976;31(4):233-271.

72. Miner TJ, Delgado R, Zeisler J, et al. Primary vaginal melanoma: a critical analysis of therapy. *Ann Surg Oncol.* 2004;11(1):34-39.

73. Huang Q, Huang H, Wan T, Deng T, Liu J. Clinical outcome of 31 patients with primary malignant melanoma of the vagina. *J Gynecol Oncol.* 2013;24(4):330-335.

74. DeMatos P, Tyler D, Seigler HF. Mucosal melanoma of the female genitalia: a clinicopathologic study of forty-three cases at Duke University Medical Center. *Surgery*. 1998;124(1):38-48.

75. Cobellis L, Calabrese E, Stefanon B, Raspagliesi F. Malignant melanoma of the vagina. A report of 15 cases. *Eur J Gynaecol Oncol*. 2000;21(3):295-297.

76. Bonner JA, Perez-Tamayo C, Reid GC, Roberts JA, Morley GW. The management of vaginal melanoma. *Cancer*. 1988;62(9):2066-2072.

77. Petru E, Nagele F, Czerwenka K, et al. Primary malignant melanoma of the vagina: long-term remission following radiation therapy. *Gynecol Oncol*. 1998;70(1):23-26.

78. Harwood AR, Cummings BJ. Radiotherapy for mucosal melanomas. *Int J Radiat Oncol Biol Phys*. 1982;8(7):1121-1126.

79. Rogo KO, Andersson R, Edbom G, Stendahl U. Conservative surgery for vulvovaginal melanoma. *Eur J Gynaecol Oncol*. 1991;12(2):113-119.

80. Brand E, Fu YS, Lagasse LD, Berek JS. Vulvovaginal melanoma: report of seven cases and literature review. *Gynecol Oncol*. 1989;33(1):54-60.

81. Ghezelayagh T, Rauh-Hain JA, Growdon WB. Comparing mortality of vaginal sarcoma, squamous cell carcinoma, and adenocarcinoma in the surveillance, epidemiology, and end results database. *Obstet Gynecol*. 2015;125(6):1353-1361.

82. Ahram J, Lemus R, Schiavello HJ. Leiomyosarcoma of the vagina: case report and literature review. *Int J Gynecol Cancer*. 2006;16(2):884-891.

83. Suh MJ, Park DC. Leiomyosarcoma of the vagina: a case report and review from the literature. *J Gynecol Oncol*. 2008;19(4):261-264.

84. Tavassoli FA, Norris HJ. Smooth muscle tumors of the vagina. *Obstet Gynecol*. 1979;53(6):689-693.

85. Ciaravino G, Kapp DS, Vela AM, et al. Primary leiomyosarcoma of the vagina. A case report and literature review. *Int J Gynecol Cancer*. 2000;10(4):340-347.

86. Curtin JP, Saigo P, Slucher B, Venkatraman ES, Mychalczak B, Hoskins WJ. Soft-tissue sarcoma of the vagina and vulva: a clinicopathologic study. *Obstet Gynecol*. 1995;86(2):269-272.

87. Ahuja A, Safaya R, Prakash G, Kumar L, Shukla NK. Primary mixed mullerian tumor of the vagina—a case report with review of the literature. *Pathol Res Pract*. 2011;207(4):253-255.

88. Prempree T, Tang CK, Hatef A, Forster S. Angiosarcoma of the vagina: a clinicopathologic report. A reappraisal of the radiation treatment of angiosarcomas of the female genital tract. *Cancer*. 1983;51(4):618-622.

89. Kounelis S, Jones MW, Papadaki H, Bakker A, Swalsky P, Finkelstein SD. Carcinosarcomas (malignant mixed mullerian tumors) of the female genital tract: comparative molecular analysis of epithelial and mesenchymal components. *Hum Pathol*. 1998;29(1):82-87.

90. Davis PC, Franklin EW 3rd. Cancer of the vagina. *South Med J*. 1975;68(10):1239-1242.

91. Sebenik M, Yan Z, Khalbuss WE, Mittal K. Malignant mixed mullerian tumor of the vagina: case report with review of the literature, immunohistochemical study, and evaluation for human papilloma virus. *Hum Pathol*. 2007;38(8):1282-1288.

92. Sotiropoulou M, Haidopoulos D, Vlachos G, Pilalis A, Rodolakis A, Diakomanolis E. Primary malignant mixed mullerian tumor of the vagina immunohistochemically confirmed. *Arch Gynecol Obstet*. 2005;271(3):264-266.

93. Neesham D, Kerdemelidis P, Scurry J. Primary malignant mixed Müllerian tumor of the vagina. *Gynecol Oncol*. 1998;70(2):303-307.

94. Shibata R, Umezawa A, Takehara K, Aoki D, Nozawa S, Hata J. Primary carcinosarcoma of the vagina. *Pathol Int*. 2003;53(2):106-110.

95. Coronel RG, Palacios RD, Montelongo CA. Vaginal carcinosarcoma (report of a case). *Ginecol Obstet Mex*. 1974;35(209):285-289.

96. McAdam JA, Stewart F, Reid R. Vaginal epithelioid angiosarcoma. *J Clin Pathol*. 1998;51(12):928-930.

97. Tohya T, Katabuchi H, Fukuma K, Fujisaki S, Okamura H. Angiosarcoma of the vagina. A light and electron microscopy study. *Acta Obstet Gynecol Scand*. 1991;70(2):169-172.

98. Hays DM, Shimada H, Raney RB Jr, et al. Sarcomas of the vagina and uterus: the Intergroup Rhabdomyosarcoma Study. *J Pediatr Surg*. 1985;20(6):718-724.

99. Peters WA 3rd, Kumar NB, Andersen WA, Morley GW. Primary sarcoma of the adult vagina: a clinicopathologic study. *Obstet Gynecol*. 1985;65(5):699-704.

100. Suit HD, Mankin HJ, Wood WC, et al. Treatment of the patient with stage M0 soft tissue sarcoma. *J Clin Oncol*. 1988;6(5):854-862.

101. Fein DA, Lee WR, Lanciano RM, et al. Management of extremity soft tissue sarcomas with limb-sparing surgery and postoperative irradiation: do total dose, overall treatment time, and the surgery-radiotherapy interval impact on local control? *Int J Radiat Oncol Biol Phys*. 1995;32(4):969-976.

102. Nielsen OS, Dombernowsky P, Mouridsen H, et al. High-dose epirubicin is not an alternative to standard-dose doxorubicin in the treatment of advanced soft tissue sarcomas. A study of the EORTC soft tissue and bone sarcoma group. *Br J Cancer*. 1998;78(12):1634-1639.

103. Leiser AL, Chi DS, Ishill NM, Tew WP. Carcinosarcoma of the ovary treated with platinum and taxane: the memorial Sloan-Kettering Cancer Center experience. *Gynecol Oncol*. 2007;105(3):657-661.

104. Mok JE, Kim YM, Jung MH, et al. Malignant mixed müllerian tumors of the ovary: experience with cytoreductive surgery and platinum-based combination chemotherapy. *Int J Gynecol Cancer*. 2006;16(1):101-105.

105. Muntz HG, Jones MA, Goff BA, et al. Malignant mixed müllerian tumors of the ovary: experience with surgical cytoreduction and combination chemotherapy. *Cancer*. 1995;76(7):1209-1213.

106. Rutledge TL, Gold MA, McMeekin DS, et al. Carcinosarcoma of the ovary—a case series. *Gynecol Oncol*. 2006;100(1):128-132.

107. Ferry JA, Young RH. Malignant lymphoma, pseudolymphoma, and hematopoietic disorders of the female genital tract. *Pathol Annu*. 1991;26:227-263.

108. Liang R, Chiu E, Loke SL. Non-Hodgkin's lymphomas involving the female genital tract. *Hematol Oncol*. 1990;8(5):295-299.

109. Perren T, Farrant M, McCarthy K, Harper P, Wiltshaw E. Lymphomas of the cervix and upper vagina: a report of five cases and a review of the literature. *Gynecol Oncol*. 1992;44(1):87-95.

110. Mahendran SM. Primary non-Hodgkin's lymphoma of the vagina masquerading as a uterine fibroid in pregnancy. *J Obstet Gynaecol*. 2008;28(4):456-458.

111. Hussein IY, Said MR, Macheta A, Joglekar V. Primary non-Hodgkin's lymphoma of the vagina. *J Obstet Gynaecol*. 2007;27(7):752.

112. Cohn DE, Resnick KE, Eaton LA, deHart J, Zanagnolo V. Non-Hodgkin's lymphoma mimicking gynecological malignancies of the vagina and cervix: a report of four cases. *Int J Gynecol Cancer*. 2007;17(1):274-279.

113. Zafar M, Mehmood A, Abassi MH, Shah SS. Primary non-Hodgkin's lymphoma of vagina associated with pregnancy. *J Coll Physicians Surg Pak*. 2006;16(6):424-425.

114. Garavaglia E, Taccagni G, Montoli S, et al. Primary stage I-IIE non-Hodgkin's lymphoma of uterine cervix and upper vagina: evidence for a conservative approach in a study on three patients. *Gynecol Oncol*. 2005;97(1):214-218.

115. Yoshinaga K, Akahira J, Niikura H, et al. A case of primary mucosa-associated lymphoid tissue lymphoma of the vagina. *Hum Pathol*. 2004;35(9):1164-1166.

116. Engin H, Türker A, Abali H, Uner A, Günalp S. Successful treatment of primary non-Hodgkin's lymphoma of the vagina with chemotherapy. *Arch Gynecol Obstet*. 2004;269(3):208-210.

117. Raspagliesi F, Ditto A, Fontanelli R, Gallino G, Massone PB, De Palo G. Primary non-Hodgkin's lymphoma of the vagina. *Haematologica*. 2000;85(6):666-667.

118. Vang R, Medeiros LJ, Silva EG, Gershenson DM, Deavers M. Non-Hodgkin's lymphoma involving the vagina: a clinicopathologic analysis of 14 patients. *Am J Surg Pathol*. 2000;24(5):719-725.

119. Guarini A, Pavone V, Valentino T, et al. Primary non Hodgkin's lymphoma of the vagina. *Leuk Lymphoma*. 1999;35(5-6):619-622.

120. Skinnider BF, Clement PB, MacPherson N, Gascoyne RD, Viswanatha DS. Primary non-Hodgkin's lymphoma and malakoplakia of the vagina: a case report. *Hum Pathol*. 1999;30(7):871-874.

121. Papadopoulos AJ, Pambakian H, Devaja O, Raju KS. High grade non-Hodgkins stage IEB primary malignant lymphoma of the cervix and upper vagina. A case report. *Eur J Gynaecol Oncol*. 1996;17(6):484-486.

122. Hoffkes HG, Schumann A, Uppenkamp M, et al. Primary non-Hodgkin's lymphoma of the vagina. Case report and review of the literature. *Ann Hematol*. 1995;70(5):273-276.

123. Lonardi F, Ferrari V, Pavanato G, Bonciarelli G, Jirillo A, Balli M. Primary lymphoma of the vagina. A case report. *Haematologica*. 1994;79(2):182-183.

124. Prevot S, Hugol D, Audouin J, et al. Primary non Hodgkin's malignant lymphoma of the vagina. Report of 3 cases with review of the literature. *Pathol Res Pract*. 1992;188(1-2):78-85.

125. Bagella MP, Fadda G, Cherchi PL. Primary non-Hodgkin lymphoma of the vagina: case report. *Clin Exp Obstet Gynecol*. 1989;16(4):100-102.

126. Harris NL, Scully RE. Malignant lymphoma and granulocytic sarcoma of the uterus and vagina. A clinicopathologic analysis of 27 cases. *Cancer*. 1984;53(11):2530-2545.

127. Buchler DA, Kline JC. Primary lymphoma of the vagina. *Obstet Gynecol*. 1972;40(2):235-237.

128. Chorlton I, Karnei RF Jr, King FM, Norris HJ. Primary malignant reticuloendothelial disease involving the vagina, cervix, and corpus uteri. *Obstet Gynecol.* 1974;44(5):735-748.

129. McNicholas MM, Fennelly JJ, MacErlaine DP. Imaging of primary vaginal lymphoma. *Clin Radiol.* 1994;49(2):130-132.

130. Domingo S, Perales A, Torres V, Alcaraz MJ, Pellicer A. Epstein-Barr virus positivity in primary vaginal lymphoma. *Gynecol Oncol.* 2004;95(3):719-721.

131. Pham DC, Guthrie TH, Ndubisi B. HIV-associated primary cervical non-Hodgkin's lymphoma and two other cases of primary pelvic non-Hodgkin's lymphoma. *Gynecol Oncol.* 2003;90(1):204-206.

132. Signorelli M, Maneo A, Cammarota S, et al. Conservative management in primary genital lymphomas: the role of chemotherapy. *Gynecol Oncol.* 2007;104(2):416-421.

133. Gardner GJ, Reidy-Lagunes D, Gehrig PA. Neuroendocrine tumors of the gynecologic tract: a Society of Gynecologic Oncology (SGO) clinical document. *Gynecol Oncol.* 2011;122(1):190-198.

134. Kaminski JM, Anderson PR, Han AC, Mitra RK, Rosenblum NG, Edelson MI. Primary small cell carcinoma of the vagina. *Gynecol Oncol.* 2003;88(3):451-455.

135. Elsaleh H, Bydder S, Cassidy B, Thompson J. Small cell carcinoma of the vagina. *Australas Radiol.* 2000;44(3):336-337.

136. Ulich TR, Liao SY, Layfield L, Romansky S, Cheng L, Lewin KJ. Endocrine and tumor differentiation markers in poorly differentiated small-cell carcinoids of the cervix and vagina. *Arch Pathol Lab Med.* 1986;110(11):1054-1057.

137. Crowder S, Tuller E. Small cell carcinoma of the female genital tract. *Semin Oncol.* 2007;34:57-63.

138. Cai T, Li Y, Jiang Q, Wang D, Huang Y. Paraganglioma of the vagina: a case report and review of the literature. *Onco Targets Ther.* 2014;7:965-968.

139. Hassan A, Bennet A, Bhalla S, Ylagan LR, Mutch D, Dehner LP. Paraganglioma of the vagina: report of a case, including immunohistochemical and ultrastructural findings. *Int J Gynecol Pathol.* 2003;22(4):404-406.

140. Shen JG, Chen YX, Xu DY, Feng YF, Tong ZH. Vaginal paraganglioma presenting as a gynecologic mass: case report. *Eur J Gynaecol Oncol.* 2008;29(2):184-185.

141. Tohya T, Miyazaki K, Katabuchi H, Fujisaki S, Maeyama M. Small cell carcinoma of the endometrium associated with adenosquamous carcinoma: a light and electron microscopic study. *Gynecol Oncol.* 1986;25(3):363-371.

142. Steiner E, Woernle F, Kuhn W, et al. Carcinoma of the neovagina: case report and review of the literature. *Gynecol Oncol.* 2002;84(1):171-175.

143. Lathrop JC, Ree HJ, McDUFF HC Jr. Intraepithelial neoplasia of the neovagina. *Obstet Gynecol.* 1985;65(3 Suppl):91S-94S.

144. Gallup DG, Castle CA, Stock RJ. Recurrent carcinoma in situ of the vagina following split-thickness skin graft vaginoplasty. *Gynecol Oncol.* 1987;26(1):98-102.

145. Imrie JE, Kennedy JH, Holmes JD, McGrouther DA. Intraepithelial neoplasia arising in an artificial vagina. Case report. *Br J Obstet Gynaecol.* 1986;93(8):886-888.

146. Wheelock JB, Schneider V, Goplerud DR. Malignancy arising in the transplanted vagina. *South Med J.* 1986;79(12):1585-1587.

147. Lowe MP, Ault KA, Sood AK. Recurrent carcinoma in situ of a neovagina. *Gynecol Oncol.* 2001;80(3):403-404.

148. Guven S, Guvendag Guven ES, Ayhan A, Gokoz A. Recurrence of high-grade squamous intraepithelial neoplasia in neovagina: case report and review of the literature. *Int J Gynecol Cancer.* 2005;15(6):1179-1182.

149. Munkarah A, Malone JM Jr, Budev HD, Evans TN. Mucinous adenocarcinoma arising in a neovagina. *Gynecol Oncol.* 1994;52(2):272-275.

150. Jackson GW. Primary carcinoma of an artificial vagina. Report of a case. *Obstet Gynecol.* 1959;14(4):534-536.

151. Duckler L. Squamous cell carcinoma developing in an artificial vagina. *Obstet Gynecol.* 1972;40(1):35-38.

152. Rotmensch J, Rosenshein N, Dillon M, Murphy A, Woodruff JD. Carcinoma arising in the neovagina: case report and review of the literature. *Obstet Gynecol.* 1983;61(4):534-536.

153. Lenehan PM, Meffe F, Lickrish GM. Vaginal intraepithelial neoplasia: biologic aspects and management. *Obstet Gynecol.* 1986;68(3):333-337.

154. Chyle V, Zagars GK, Wheeler JA, Wharton JT, Delclos L. Definitive radiotherapy for carcinoma of the vagina: outcome and prognostic factors. *Int J Radiat Oncol Biol Phys.* 1996;35(5):891-905.

155. Andersen ES. Primary carcinoma of the vagina: a study of 29 cases. *Gynecol Oncol.* 1989;33(3):317-320.

156. Ball HG, Berman ML. Management of primary vaginal carcinoma. *Gynecol Oncol.* 1982;14(2):154-163.

157. Gallup DG, Talledo OE, Shah KJ, Hayes C. Invasive squamous cell carcinoma of the vagina: a 14-year study. *Obstet Gynecol.* 1987;69(5):782-785.

158. Kirkbride P, Fyles A, Rawlings GA, et al. Carcinoma of the vagina—experience at the Princess Margaret Hospital (1974-1989). *Gynecol Oncol.* 1995;56(3):435-443.

159. Leung S, Sexton M. Radical radiation therapy for carcinoma of the vagina—impact of treatment modalities on outcome: Peter MacCallum Cancer Institute experience 1970–1990. *Int J Radiat Oncol Biol Phys.* 1993;25(3):413-418.

160. Perez CA, Camel HM, Galakatos AE, et al. Definitive irradiation in carcinoma of the vagina: long-term evaluation of results. *Int J Radiat Oncol Biol Phys.* 1988;15(6):1283-1290.

161. Spirtos NM, Doshi BP, Kapp DS, Teng N. Radiation therapy for primary squamous cell carcinoma of the vagina: Stanford University experience. *Gynecol Oncol.* 1989;35(1):20-26.

162. Davis KP, Stanhope CR, Garton GR, Atkinson EJ, O'Brien PC. Invasive vaginal carcinoma: analysis of early-stage disease. *Gynecol Oncol.* 1991;42(2):131-136.

163. Xiang-E W, Shu-mo C, Ya-qin D, Ke W. Treatment of late recurrent vaginal malignancy after initial radiotherapy for carcinoma of the cervix: an analysis of 73 cases. *Gynecol Oncol.* 1998;69(2):125-129.

164. Beriwal S, Heron DE, Mogus R, Edwards RP, Kelley JL, Sukumvanich P. High-dose rate brachytherapy (HDRB) for primary or recurrent cancer in the vagina. *Radiat Oncol.* 2008;3(1):7.

CHAPTER 3.9

Vaginal Cancer: Follow-Up, Survivorship Issues, and Summary

Diana Miao, Josephine Kang, Amanda Nickles Fader, and Akila N. Viswanathan

Recommendations for posttreatment surveillance are based on Society of Gynecologic Oncology (SGO) guidelines for gynecologic malignancies (1). Patients with early-stage lesions, treated with surgery alone, can be followed every 6 months for 2 years, then annually thereafter. Patients with more advanced lesions are at higher risk of recurrence and are recommended follow-up every 3 months for the first 2 years, then every 6 months for the next 3 years, and annually thereafter.

There is insufficient evidence to support the use of regular cervical or vaginal cytology to detect cancer recurrence. However, the SGO recommends annual cytology as surveillance to detect other gynecologic abnormalities. The routine use of CT or PET as surveillance is not recommended.

OUTCOMES

According to SEER-based data, outcomes for vaginal cancer may be improving. A recent study by Shah et al (2) analyzed records from the SEER database of 2,149 women diagnosed with primary vaginal cancer between 1990 and 2004. The risk of mortality was noted to decrease over time, with a 17% decrease in the risk of death for women diagnosed after 2000 relative to those diagnosed between 1990 and 1994. The authors reported 5-year DSS rates of 84% for stage I, 75% for stage II, and 57% for stages III and IV. An older study by Creasman et al (3) focused on 4,885 women diagnosed with vaginal cancer between 1985 and 1994, and reported 5-year survival rates of 96% for stage 0, 73% for stage I, 58% for stage II, and 36% for stages III and IV, with 85% of invasive cases being SCC.

In general, the rate of locoregional recurrence ranges from 10% to 20% for stage I and 30% to 40% for stage II. Patients with advanced disease often have persistent disease despite treatment. In a series by Dixit et al (4), 68% of failures in patients with stage III disease were due to persistent disease. Most treatment failures occur within 5 years, with a median time to recurrence of 6 to 12 months (5,6), and local recurrence is the most common pattern of treatment failure in most published series. Extravaginal recurrences in the pelvic lymph nodes are less common. The reported rates of distant metastasis vary, ranging from 7% to 33% and usually occur later in the course of disease, with approximately half of all distant metastases presenting at the time of local recurrence (4,7-9).

Patients that have received treatment should be considered for sexual health consultation given the profound impact on desire and function. The use of vaginal dilation is strongly recommended, in conjunction with sexual activity, for women that receive radiation.

SUMMARY

Vaginal cancer is a rare disease, accounting for 1% to 2% of all gynecologic malignancies. Patients presenting with stage I disease should be considered for surgical excision if tumor is small and surgically accessible without undue morbidity. Patients with more advanced disease are managed primarily with RT, often in conjunction with chemotherapy. Surgical resection is typically reserved for treatment failures, given the extensive morbidity of pelvic exenteration.

REFERENCES

1. Fanning J, Manahan KJ, McLean SA. Loop electrosurgical excision procedure for partial upper vaginectomy. *Am J Obstet Gynecol.* 1999;181(6):1382-1385.

2. Shah CA, Goff BA, Lowe K, et al. Factors affecting risk of mortality in women with vaginal cancer. *Obstet Gynecol.* 2009;113(5):1038-1045.

3. Creasman WT, Phillips JL, Menck HR. The national cancer data base report on cancer of the vagina. *Cancer.* 1998;83(5):1033-1040.

4. Dixit S, Singhal S, Baboo HA. Squamous cell carcinoma of the vagina: a review of 70 cases. *Gynecol Oncol.* 1993;48(1):80-87.

5. Frank SJ, Jhingran A, Levenback C, et al. Definitive radiation therapy for squamous cell carcinoma of the vagina. *Int J Radiat Oncol Biol Phys.* 2005;62(1):138-147.

6. Tabata T, Takeshima N, Nishida H, et al. Treatment failure in vaginal cancer. *Gynecol Oncol.* 2002;84(2):309-314.

7. Houghton CR, Iversen T. Squamous cell carcinoma of the vagina: a clinical study of the location of the tumor. *Gynecol Oncol.* 1982;13(3):365-372.

8. Leung S, Sexton M. Radical radiation therapy for carcinoma of the vagina-impact of treatment modalities on outcome: Peter MacCallum cancer institute experience 1970-1990. *Int J Radiat Oncol Biol Phys.* 1993;25(3):413-418.

9. Perez CA, Camel HM, Galakatos AE, et al. Definitive irradiation in carcinoma of the vagina: long-term evaluation of results. *Int J Radiat Oncol Biol Phys.* 1988;15(6):1283-1290.

4

CERVICAL CANCER

Cervix Uteri: Epidemiology, Etiology, Risk Factors, Anatomy, Natural History, and Patterns of Spread

Teresa K. L. Boitano and Charles A. Leath III

EPIDEMIOLOGY

According to the World Health Organization, uterine cervix cancers were the fourth most common malignancy in women, with 604,000 new incident cases reported in 2020 (1,2). An estimated 342,000 women died around the world from uterine cervix cancer in 2020, with approximately 90% of all new cases occurring in low- to middle-income regions (1). In the United States, the American Cancer Society (ACS) projected that over 14,000 new cases of uterine cervix cancer would arise in American women in 2022 and estimated that there would be over 4,200 cervical cancer–related deaths (3). Human papillomavirus (HPV)-related cancer, including uterine cervix cancer, is only one of two cancers (the other, colorectal cancer) that can be effectively screened for as a precancerous lesion. Despite being preventable, the incidence and mortality has remained stable the past several decades instead of decreasing (4). Early detection of uterine cervix cancer is a paramount health care issue, given the overall effectiveness of screening and the implementation of the HPV vaccine.

Currently, around 80% of women in the United States are adherent with cervical cancer screening (CCS) guidelines (5,6). However, despite being a high rate of CCS, anywhere from 20% to 70% of women do not follow up for subsequent evaluation after abnormal screening (7). The lowest adherence rates unfortunately occur in those with lower income and educational rates and racial/ethnic minority individuals (8). Furthermore, Black women have the highest mortality and shortest cancer-specific survival for most cancers of any racial or ethnic group in the United States. Up to 85% of Black women are reportedly being screened, yet they are likely to have higher mortality rates and present with more advanced-stage disease when compared with White women (9).

ETIOLOGY AND RISK FACTORS

The etiology of uterine cervix cancer has been connected to sexual activity, although the exact molecular events implicated in its pathogenesis have not been fully known. Risk factors such as young age of coitarche (10), multiple sexual partners or high-risk sexual partners (11), and a history of sexually transmitted diseases (12), early age at first birth, increasing parity (13), and immunosuppression (ie, HIV infection) correlate with a risk for uterine cervix cancer pathogenesis. Uterine cervix cancer is exceedingly uncommon among females not sexually active (14,15). Low-income (16), low educational status (17), and a history of HPV infection (18) are surrogate risk factors for uterine cervix cancer. Smoking (current smoker or former smoker or never smoker) has been associated with a risk for a malignant uterine cervix cell phenotype (19).

HUMAN PAPILLOMAVIRUS

The HPV is a double-stranded DNA virus that commonly infects humans and inhibits natural tumor suppressor genes. The majority of individuals who are infected with HPV will clear the virus naturally within 12 to 24 months postinfection (20). If the virus is not cleared, then individuals will experience persistent infections that can lead to a preneoplastic lesion. This can eventually lead to cancer. Given the fact that nearly all cervical cancer is caused by these persistent high-risk HPV infections, this has led to major inventions, including (1) screening with high-risk HPV cotesting to identify women with cervical precancer and early cancer for secondary prevention and (2) HPV vaccination to prevent primary HPV infection.

HPV subtypes 16, 18, 31, 33, 35, 45, 52, and 58 (Table 4.1-1) are the most virulent forms associated with cervical intraepithelial neoplasia (CIN) (now coined *high-grade squamous intraepithelial lesion* on biopsy) or cancer (18). HPV infections (single or multiple infections) account for as much as 86% of worldwide incidence of invasive uterine cervix cancer (18). Certainly, immune competence has a role in HPV-related carcinogenesis (21,22)—in as much as a uterine cervix cancer diagnosis might define an AIDS illness event (23). In women of screening age, HPV cotesting (Pap test with HPV genotype testing) is performed and can detect the HPV virus and evaluate for abnormal lesions (24). These lesions are then evaluated and treated per the American Society for Colposcopy and Cervical Pathology (ASCCP) screening guidelines. The goal is to detect and treat the lesions before progression to cervical cancer.

HPVs are nonenveloped viruses utilizing double-stranded closed circular DNA to replicate in the cutaneous and mucosal epithelia of the female and male anogenital tracts (25). HPV DNA encodes six early proteins (E1, E2, E4-E7) and two late proteins (L1, L2) that hijack host cell molecular pathways first to synthesize DNA and then to package it (25). HPV-E6 binds p53, causes its degradation, and thereby removes a G1/S-phase cell cycle restriction checkpoint (26,27). HPV-E6 also disrupts DNA-building block output from the usual rate-limiter ribonucleotide reductase, in that the virus promotes more 2′-deoxyribonucleoside diphosphates (dNDPs) to be supplied freely when demanded (28,29). HPV-E7 degrades hypophosphorylated retinoblastoma protein through a proteosome-dependent pathway (30) that also promotes unchecked activation of a synthesis cell cycle transcription factor (E2F) (31). E2F turns on S-phase proteins critical to DNA replication, like ribonucleotide reductase M2 protein (32). Through an activated telomerase (33), HPV extends host cell life and thus increases HPV-infected cell numbers. Far-reaching outcomes of HPV overriding cell cycle checkpoints include instability of the host cell genome and susceptibility to neoplasia or to an oncogenic phenotype (25). Such observations suggest that throughout its evolution, HPV has targeted at least transcriptional and protein-protein checkpoints in uterine cervix cells to unleash dNDP production by ribonucleotide reductase.

TABLE 4.1-1. Human Papillomavirus (HPV) Genotypes	
Low-Risk Oncogenic HPV	High-Risk Oncogenic HPV
6, 11, 42, 43, 44	16, 18, 31, 33, 35, 39, 45, 51, 52, 56, 58, 59, 68

UTERINE CERVIX ANATOMY

The *cervix uteri* (Latin: neck of the uterus) is a muscular organ in the central pelvis, representing the lower, more narrow, component of the uterus. Macroscopically, the cervix has a conical shape, is truncated at its distal apex, and has its long axis directed backward and downward. It projects posteriorly into the vagina, connecting the vaginal vault to the uterine body hollow (*corpus uteri*) by its endocervical canal (*canalis cervicis uteri*). The supravaginal portion of the cervix (*portio supravaginalis*) extends to the lower uterine segment (isthmus) and has an intimate association with the bladder peritoneum, forming the vesicouterine pouch, an anterior *cul-de-sac* that must be dissected and separated for surgical exposure. The peritoneum covers the supravaginal cervix posteriorly and is reflected upon the rectum, forming the posterior rectouterine cul-de-sac (pouch of Douglas). The vaginal portion of the cervix (*portio vaginalis*) protrudes into the vagina as a round extremity with a circular external aperture between the anterior and posterior vaginal fornices. The vaginal portion of the cervix has two lips, a short anterior and a long posterior. In length, the cervix ranges 2 to 5 cm.

The uterine cervix is fibrous, covered by membranes (*tunica mucosa*) of squamous cells when in contact with the vagina (ectocervix) and by columnar cells when communicating with the uterus (endocervix). A transition from stratified squamous to ciliated columnar cells, coined the *transformation zone*, occurs in the lower one-third of the canal. The length of the transition zone changes throughout life, receding in old age. The preponderance of preneoplastic and neoplastic lesions of the uterine cervix arises from the transformation zone. The ciliated columnar cells secrete viscid alkaline mucus.

The uterine cervix has four cardinal ligaments: one anterior, one posterior, and two transverse (Mackenrodt). The anterior ligament involves the vesicouterine fold of peritoneum, anchoring the supravaginal cervix to the anterior pelvis via the anterior cul-de-sac. The posterior ligament consists of the rectouterine fold of peritoneum, connecting the supravaginal cervix by the rectum to fibrous tissue and nonstriped muscle constituting the uterosacral ligaments. The two transverse ligaments (*ligamentum transversalis coli*) span either side of the uterine cervix and continuously extend into the tissues of the pelvic sidewall surrounding the pelvis iliac blood vessels. The cardinal ligaments anatomically define two surgical spaces, the paravesical space anteriorly and the pararectal space posteriorly. Portions of the cardinal ligament overlie the pelvic ureter (below the uterine artery, above the uterine vein) about 2 cm superior and 2 cm lateral to the external os of the cervix, an anatomic triangle referred to in brachytherapy as *prescription point A*. For completeness, superior to the supravaginal cervix arise the two lateral or broad ligaments (*ligamentum latum uteri*) enveloping the uterine tubes, round ligament of the uterus, the ovary and its ligaments, the epoophoron and paroophoron. The innervation of the uterine cervix derives from sacral (S2-S4) nerve roots.

Blood supply to and from the uterine cervix occurs via the uterine artery and vein, named *terminal tributaries* of the anterior branch of the internal iliac (hypogastric) blood vessels. Collateral arterial anastomoses arise from the ovarian artery (descending aorta), internal pudendal artery (hypogastric artery tributary), and obturator artery (hypogastric artery tributary). A web of venous blood vessels returns blood to the bilateral gonadal and bilateral iliac veins.

The uterine cervix is considered an immunocompetent organ, capable of mounting an immune response to an external pathogen antigen (34,35). In some respects, the bulk of large uterine cervix cancers might represent normal cells, cancer cells, and tumor-infiltrating lymphocytes. Lymphatic drainage appears to be orderly from the uterine cervix to the paracervical and obturator nodes, followed by the internal iliac nodes, external iliac nodes, common iliac nodes, and then ultimately the para-aortic nodes.

First nodal sites of disease commonly include the paracervical and the iliac nodes (36). Left supraclavicular lymph nodes are next echelon extrapelvic distant sites of lymphatic spread. Uterine cervix immunocompetence (37) impacts anticancer proimmune drugs (38) and radiation-induced immune-mediated tumor abscopal response (39).

UTERINE CERVIX DISEASE NATURAL HISTORY

Preinvasive Disease

Uterine cervix cells acquire an oncogenic phenotype through what appears to be a methodical neoplastic process reflected in epithelial cell histology. For uterine cervix squamous cell disease, the histologic terms for preinvasive disease range from atypical cells of undetermined significance (ASC-US), low-grade squamous intraepithelial lesion (LSIL) to high-grade squamous intraepithelial lesion (HSIL). Cervical dysplasia is then classified into three levels based on the depth of invasion ranging from mild to severe: CIN 1, CIN 2, or CIN 3. CIN 1 refers to abnormal cells affecting one-third of the thickness of the epithelium, CIN 2 is between one-third and two-thirds, and CIN 3 is greater than two-thirds. Histologically, HSIL tends to correlate with CIN 3 and most cases of CIN 2 (40).

Most LSIL cases and half of HSIL cases regress to normal cytology within 2 years of first diagnosis by cytology (41). CIN 1 is a low-grade lesion that has a high potential for regression, but CIN 2 and CIN 3 have a higher risk for potential progression to cancer (42). There are some other factors that impact the risk, including HPV status and previous cytology results. The ASCCP guidelines are developed and utilized to inform management plans in patients with abnormal results (24). In general, observation is appropriate for most patients with CIN 1. For patients with CIN 2 who desire future childbearing, consideration can be taken into observation for some patients. However, for CIN 3, treatment is always recommended.

Invasive Disease

The oncogenic potential of uterine cervix cancers follows a more erratic evolution—disease benchmarks are not well chronicled. Uterine cervix cancers follow an International Federation of Gynaecology and Obstetrics (FIGO) clinical staging system (**Table 4.1-2**) (43). Previously, surgical findings or radiographic-guided biopsies of lymph nodes or lung metastasis were not to be used to change or to modify clinical FIGO staging. However, the new 2018 FIGO guidelines call for imaging to be used (if possible) for evaluation of tumor size and spread (44). All uterine cervix cancer histologies are included.

Metastatic Disease

Patterns of spread of uterine cervix cancers are considered predictable and orderly, as pelvic lymph node metastases are low in the absence of deep stromal invasion of the uterine cervix (45,46) and para-aortic lymph node metastases are low when pelvic lymph nodes are uninvolved (47,48).

For instance, the depth of stromal invasion elevates the risk for regional lymph node metastasis. Fifty-one women (1981-1984) who had conization of the cervix for cancer with 3 to 5 mm of invasion (width limited to 7 mm) followed by completion radical hysterectomy plus lymphadenectomy were found to have no lymph node metastases, no recurrences, and no cancer-related deaths over a 5-year observation period (45). Inner third, middle third, and outer third depth of invasion were associated with a frequency of pelvic lymph node metastases of 5% (9/199), 13% (28/210), and 26% (60/227) in a surgicopathologic study (1981-1984) of patients with uterine cervix cancer (49). Invasion into adjoining parametria is associated with a frequency of pelvic lymph node metastases

■ TABLE 4.1-2. Uterine Cervix Clinical Staging

TNM[a]	FIGO[a]	
Primary tumor (T)		
TX		Primary tumor cannot be assessed.
T0		No evidence of primary tumor
Tis	0	Carcinoma in situ (preinvasive carcinoma)
T1	I	Cervical carcinoma confined to uterus (extension to corpus should be disregarded).
T1a	IA	Invasive carcinoma diagnosed only by microscopy. Stromal invasion with a maximum depth of 5 mm measured from the base of the epithelium and a horizontal spread of ≤7 mm. Vascular space involvement, venous or lymphatic, does not affect classification.
T1a1	IA1	Measured stromal invasion ≤3 mm in depth and ≤7 mm in horizontal spread
T1a2	IA2	Measured stromal invasion >3 and ≤5 mm with a horizontal spread ≤7 mm
T1b	IB	Clinically visible lesion confined to the cervix or microscopic lesion >T1a/IA2.
T1b1	IB1	Clinically visible lesion ≤4 cm in greatest dimension
T1b2	IB2	Clinically visible lesion >4 cm in greatest dimension
T2	II	Cervical carcinoma invades beyond uterus, but not pelvic wall or lower third of vagina.
T2a	IIA	Tumor without parametrial invasion
T2a1	IIA1	Clinically visible lesion ≤4 cm in greatest dimension
T2a2	IIA2	Clinically visible lesion >4 cm in greatest dimension
T2b	IIB	Tumor with parametrial invasion
T3	III	Tumor extends to pelvic wall and/or involves lower third of vagina and/or causes hydronephrosis or nonfunctioning kidney.
T3a	IIIA	Tumor involves lower third of vagina, no extension to pelvic wall.
T3b	IIIB	Tumor extends to pelvic wall and/or causes hydronephrosis or nonfunctioning kidney.
T4	IVA	Tumor invades mucosa of bladder or rectum and/or extends beyond true pelvis (bullous edema is not sufficient to classify a tumor as T4).
Regional lymph nodes (N)		
NX		Regional lymph nodes cannot be assessed.
N0		No regional lymph node metastasis
N1	IIIB	Regional lymph node metastasis
Distant metastasis (M)		
M0		No distant metastasis
M1	IVB	Distant metastasis (including peritoneal spread, involvement of supraclavicular, mediastinal, or para-aortic lymph nodes, lung, liver, or bone)

FIGO, International Federation of Gynaecology and Obstetrics; TNM, tumor-node-metastasis.

[a]The American Joint Committee on Cancer definitions of the T categories correspond to clinical stages accepted by the FIGO. Both systems are listed.

Reprinted with permission from Springer; from Edge SB, Byrd DR, Compton CC, et al. *AJCC Cancer Staging Manual*. Springer; 2009; Used with permission of the American College of Surgeons, Chicago, Illinois. The original source for this information is the AJCC Cancer Staging System (2023).

of 43% (19/44) (49). Also in this study, histologic grade 2 or grade 3 disease conferred 14% (52/373) and 22% (39/179) frequencies of pelvic lymph node metastases (49). Lymphovascular invasion (LVSI) was associated with a 25% (70/276) chance of pelvic lymph node metastases (49).

Lymph node metastases are an important clinical consideration and are now taken into account with the 2018 FIGO staging system. For example, an Italian Group study (1986-1991) that investigated 172 patients who had undergone radical abdominal hysterectomy for patients with stage IB or IIA uterine cervix cancer (49), found a 25% (28/114) rate of pelvic node metastases when the cervical diameter measured 4 cm or less, whereas the rate was 31% (17/55) when the cervical diameter measured greater than 4 cm. An American Gynecologic Oncology Group study (1973-1981) found that para-aortic lymph node metastases were associated with initial clinical stage, with rates of 5%, 16%, and 25% for stage IB, II, and III, respectively (48). For 98 patients who had para-aortic lymph node

metastases found at staging laparotomy or at definitive operative management, a 15-month median survival and a 25% probability of 3-year survival were reported (48).

Metastasis to scalene lymph node occurs infrequently, unless uterine cervix cancer involves para-aortic lymph nodes (11% prevalence rate [50]). Distant spread of uterine cervix cancers includes dissemination to the lungs or liver and, less commonly, to the brain and axial or appendicular bones. After intervention, recurrent disease is anticipated within 2 years (47,51).

REFERENCES

1. Ferlay J, Soerjomataram I, Ervik M, et al. *GLOBOCAN 2012 v1.0, Cancer Incidence and Mortality Worldwide. Lyon, France: International Agency for Research on Cancer*. World Health Organization; 2013.

2. World Health Organization. Cervical cancer. 2022. https://www.who.int/news-room/fact-sheets/detail/cervical-cancer

3. Siegel RL, Miller KD, Fuchs HE, Jemal A. Cancer statistics, 2022. *CA Cancer J Clin.* 2022;72(1):7. Epub January 12, 2022.

4. National Cancer Institute. Trends in SEER incidence and U.S. mortality using joinpoint regression program, 1975-2017. 2021. https://seer.cancer.gov/csr/1975_2017/browse_csr.php?sectionSEL=5&pageSEL=sect_05_table.01#d

5. National Cancer Institute. Cervical cancer screening progressreport. cancer.gov: National Institute of Health. 2020. Accessed March 2020. https://progressreport.cancer.gov/detection/cervical_cancer

6. Promotion OoDPaH. Healthy People 2030 online: U.S. Department of Health and Human Services. 2021. https://health.gov/healthypeople/objectives-and-data/browse-objectives/cancer/increase-proportion-females-who-get-screened-cervical-cancer-c-09

7. Katz ML, Young GS, Reiter PL, et al. Barriers reported among patients with breast and cervical abnormalities in the patient navigation research program: impact on timely care. *Womens Health Issues.* 2014;24(1):e155-e162.

8. Miller SM, Tagai EK, Wen KY, et al. Predictors of adherence to follow-up recommendations after an abnormal Pap smear among underserved inner-city women. *Patient Educ Couns.* 2017;100(7):1353-1359.

9. American Cancer Society. Cancer facts & figures for African Americans. American Cancer Society; 2019-2021.

10. Plummer M, Peto J, Franceschi S. Time since first sexual intercourse and the risk of cervical cancer. *Int J Cancer.* 2012;130(11):2638-2644.

11. Lu B, Viscidi RP, Lee JH, et al. Human papillomavirus (HPV) 6, 11, 16, and 18 seroprevalence is associated with sexual practice and age: results from the multinational HPV Infection in Men Study (HIM Study). *Cancer Epidemiol Biomarkers Prev.* 2011;20(5):990-1002.

12. Kjaer SK, Chackerian B, van den Brule AJ, et al. High-risk human papillomavirus is sexually transmitted: evidence from a follow-up study of virgins starting sexual activity (intercourse). *Cancer Epidemiol Biomarkers Prev.* 2001;10(2):101-106.

13. International Collaboration of Epidemiological Studies of Cervical Cancer. Comparison of risk factors for invasive squamous cell carcinoma and adenocarcinoma of the cervix: collaborative reanalysis of individual data on 8,097 women with squamous cell carcinoma and 1,374 women with adenocarcinoma from 12 epidemiological studies. *Int J Cancer.* 2007;120(4):885-891. doi:10.1002/ijc.22357

14. Taylor RS, Carroll BE, Lloyd JW. Mortality among women in 3 Catholic religious orders with special reference to cancer. *Cancer.* 1959;12:1207-1225.

15. Fraumeni JF Jr, Lloyd JW, Smith EM, et al. Cancer mortality among nuns: role of marital status in etiology of neoplastic disease in women. *J Natl Cancer Inst.* 1969;42(3):455-468.

16. McKinnon B, Harper S, Moore S. Decomposing income-related inequality in cervical screening in 67 countries. *Int J Public Health.* 2011;56(2):139-152.

17. Mazor KM, Williams AE, Roblin DW, et al. Health literacy and pap testing in insured women. *J Cancer Educ.* 2014;29(4):698-701.

18. Alemany L, de Sanjose S, Tous S, et al. Time trends of human papillomavirus types in invasive cervical cancer, from 1940 to 2007. *Int J Cancer.* 2014;135(1):88-95.

19. Waggoner SE, Darcy KM, Tian C, et al. Smoking behavior in women with locally advanced cervical carcinoma: a Gynecologic Oncology Group study. *Am J Obstet Gynecol.* 2010;202(3):283.e1-283.e7.

20. Woodman CB, Collins SI, Young LS. The natural history of cervical HPV infection: unresolved issues. *Nat Rev Cancer.* 2007;7(1):11-22.

21. Wang SS, Bratti MC, Rodriguez AC, et al. Common variants in immune and DNA repair genes and risk for human papillomavirus persistence and progression to cervical cancer. *J Infect Dis.* 2009;199(1):20-30.

22. Wang SS, Gonzalez P, Yu K, et al. Common genetic variants and risk for HPV persistence and progression to cervical cancer. *PLoS One.* 2010;5(1):e8667.

23. Maiman M, Fruchter RG, Clark M, et al. Cervical cancer as an AIDS-defining illness. *Obstet Gynecol.* 1997;89(1):76-80.

24. Perkins RB, Guido RS, Castle PE, et al. 2019 ASCCP risk-based management consensus guidelines for abnormal cervical cancer screening tests and cancer precursors. *J Low Genit Tract Dis.* 2020;24(2):102-131. doi:10.1097/LGT.0000000000000525

25. Hebner C, Laimins L. Human papillomaviruses: basic mechanisms of pathogenesis and oncogenicity. *Rev Med Virol.* 2006;16(2):83-97.

26. Cole S, Danos O. Nucleotide sequence and comparative analysis of the human papillomavirus type 18 genome: phylogeny of papillomaviruses and repeated structure of the E6 and E7 gene products. *J Mol Biol.* 1987;193(4):599-608.

27. Werness B, Levine A, Howley P. Association of human papillomavirus type 16 and 18 E6 proteins with p53. *Science.* 1990;248:76-79.

28. Kunos C, Chiu S, Pink J, et al. Modulating radiation resistance by inhibiting ribonucleotide reductase in cancers with virally or mutationally silenced p53 protein. *Radiation Res.* 2009;172(6):666-676.

29. Kunos C, Colussi V, Pink J, et al. Radiosensitization of human cervical cancer cells by inhibiting ribonucleotide reductase: enhanced radiation response at low dose rates. *Int J Radiat Oncol Biol Phys.* 2011;80(4):1198-1204.

30. Gonzalez S, Stremlau M, He X, et al. Degradation of the retinoblastoma tumor suppressor by the human papillomavirus type 16 E7 oncoprotein is important for functional inactivation and is separable from proteosomal degradation of E7. *J Virol.* 2001;75(16):7583-7591.

31. Huang P, Patrick D, Edwards G, et al. Protein domains governing interactions between E2F, the retinoblastoma gene product, and human papillomavirus type 16 E7 protein. *Mol Cell Biol.* 1993;13(2):953-960.

32. Chabes AL, Bjorklund S, Thelander L. S Phase-specific transcription of the mouse ribonucleotide reductase R2 gene requires both a proximal repressive E2F-binding site and an upstream promoter activating region. *J Biol Chem.* 2004;279(11):10796-10807.

33. Klingelhutz A, Foster S, McDougall J. Telomerase activation by the E6 gene product of human papillomavirus type 16. *Nature.* 1996;380(6569):79-82.

34. Hasan UA, Zannetti C, Parroche P, et al. The human papillomavirus type 16 E7 oncoprotein induces a transcriptional repressor complex on the Toll-like receptor 9 promoter. *J Exp Med.* 2013;210(7):1369-1387.

35. de Vos van Steenwijk PJ, Heusinkveld M, Ramwadhdoebe TH, et al. An unexpectedly large polyclonal repertoire of HPV-specific T cells is poised for action in patients with cervical cancer. *Cancer Res.* 2010;70(7):2707-2717.

36. Holman LL, Levenback CF, Frumovitz M. Sentinel lymph node evaluation in women with cervical cancer. *J Minim Invasive Gynecol.* 2014;21(4):540-545.

37. Kobayashi A, Greenblatt RM, Anastos K, et al. Functional attributes of mucosal immunity in cervical intraepithelial neoplasia and effects of HIV infection. *Cancer Res.* 2004;64(18):6766-6774.

38. Kunos C. Novel biological radiochemotherapy approaches in locally advanced-stage cervical cancer management. *Discov Med.* 2014;17(94):179-186.

39. Golden EB, Chhabra A, Chachoua A, et al. Local radiotherapy and granulocyte-macrophage colony-stimulating factor to generate abscopal responses in patients with metastatic solid tumors: a proof-of-principle trial. *Lancet Oncol.* 2015;16(7):795-803.

40. Schiffman M, Solomon D. Clinical practice. Cervical-cancer screening with human papillomavirus and cytologic cotesting. *N Engl J Med.* 2013;369(24):2324-2331.

41. Tainio K, Athanasiou A, Tikkinen KAO, et al. Clinical course of untreated cervical intraepithelial neoplasia grade 2 under active surveillance: systematic review and meta-analysis. *BMJ.* 2018;360:k499. doi:10.1136/bmj.k499

42. Chan JK, Monk BJ, Brewer C, et al. HPV infection and number of lifetime sexual partners are strong predictors for 'natural' regression of CIN 2 and 3. *Br J Cancer.* 2003;89(6):1062-1066. doi:10.1038/sj.bjc.6601196

43. Pecorelli S, Zigliani L, Odicino F. Revised FIGO staging for carcinoma of the cervix. *Int J Gynecol Obstet.* 2009;105(2):107-108.

44. Lee SI, Atri M. 2018 FIGO staging system for uterine cervical cancer: enter cross-sectional imaging. *Radiology.* 2019;292(1):15-24. doi:10.1148/radiol.2019190088

45. Creasman WT, Zaino RJ, Major FJ, et al. Early invasive carcinoma of the cervix (3 to 5 mm invasion): risk factors and prognosis. A Gynecologic Oncology Group study. *Am J Obstet Gynecol.* 1998;178(1 pt 1):62-65.

46. Delgado G, Bundy B, Zaino R, et al. Prospective surgical-pathological study of disease-free interval in patients with stage IB squamous cell carcinoma of the cervix: a Gynecologic Oncology Group study. *Gynecol Oncol.* 1990;38(3):352-357.

47. Landoni F, Maneo A, Colombo A, et al. Randomized study of radical surgery versus radiotherapy for stage Ib-IIa cervical cancer. *Lancet.* 1997;350(9077):535-540.

48. Berman ML, Keys H, Creasman W, et al. Survival and patterns of recurrence in cervical cancer metastatic to periaortic lymph nodes (a Gynecologic Oncology Group study). *Gynecol Oncol.* 1984;19(1):8-16.

49. Delgado G, Bundy B, Fowler WJ, et al. A prospective surgical pathological study of stage I squamous carcinoma of the cervix: a Gynecologic Oncology Group Study. *Gynecol Oncol.* 1989;35(3):314-320.

50. Burke TW, Heller PB, Hoskins WJ, et al. Evaluation of the scalene lymph nodes in primary and recurrent cervical carcinoma. *Gynecol Oncol.* 1987;28(3):312-317.

51. Salani R, Khanna N, Frimer M, Bristow RE, Chen L-M. An update on post-treatment surveillance and diagnosis of recurrence in women with gynecologic malignancies: Society of Gynecologic Oncology (SGO) recommendations. *Gynecol Oncol.* 2017;146:3-10. doi:10.1016/j.ygyno.2017.03.022

CHAPTER **4.2**

Genetics and Molecular Biology of Cervical Cancer

Dmitriy Zamarin

HPV, the causative agent of the majority of cervical cancers, is a nonenveloped virus utilizing double-stranded closed circular DNA to replicate in the cutaneous and mucosal epithelia of the female and male anogenital tracts. Persistent infection with high-risk HPV subtypes with ongoing expression of HPV oncogenes E6 and E7 results in inhibition of the tumor suppressors p53 and Rb, respectively, eventually leading to malignant transformation (1). The E6 and E7 oncoproteins mediate a number or protumorigenic effects, including inhibition of apoptosis, induction of genomic instability, inhibition of telomere shortening, promotion of angiogenesis, and facilitation of invasion and metastasis, among other functions (2-4).

In the process of oncogenic transformation, cervical cancers acquire additional genomic alterations that drive oncogenesis, immune escape, and response to therapy. Several landmark studies have described the genomic landscape of cervical cancer across different populations. Whole-exome sequencing analysis of squamous cell cervical carcinomas revealed frequent alterations in *MAPK1* gene (8%), inactivating mutations in the *HLA-B* gene (9%), and mutations in *EP300* (16%), *FBXW7* (15%), *NFE2L2* (4%), *TP53* (5%), *ERBB2* (6%), *PIK3CA* (14%), *PTEN* (6%), and *STK11* (4%), whereas adenocarcinomas exhibited additional alterations, including *ELF3* (13%) and *CBFB* (8%) (5). These findings were confirmed by subsequent analysis of 228 primary cervical cancers by The Cancer Genome Atlas (TCGA), demonstrating that in addition to the abovementioned alterations, cervical cancers exhibit common mutations in *SHKBP1*, *ERBB3*, *CASP8*, *HLA-A*, and *TGFBR2* (6). The study also identified novel recurrent focal amplification events at 7p11.2 (*EGFR*, 17%), 9p24.1 (*CD274, PDCD1LG2*, 21%), 13q22.1 (*KLF5*, 18%), and 16p13.13 (*BCAR4*, 20%), as well as previously reported amplification events at 3q26.31 (*TERC, MECOM*, 78%), 3q28 (*TP63*, 77%), 8q24.21 (*MYC, PVT1*, 42%), 11q22.1 (*YAP1, BIRC2, BIRC3*, 17%), and 17q12 (*ERBB2*, 17%). Notably, amplifications involving *CD274* (PD-L1) and *PDCD1LG2* (PD-L2) correlated significantly with expression of immune cytolytic effector genes, thus linking genomic alterations to immune response (6).

The majority of the exomes exhibited enrichment for the APOBEC signature, suggesting that APOBEC cytidine deaminase mutagenesis is the predominant source of mutations in cervical cancers. Integrated analysis based on RNA, micro-RNA, protein/phosphoprotein, DNA copy number alterations, and DNA methylation patterns has identified distinct clusters, with significantly shorter overall survival (OS) observed in cervical cancers exhibiting increased expression of Yes-associated protein (YAP) and

features associated with epithelial-to-mesenchymal transition (EMT) and a reactive tumor stroma (6). Finally, analysis of genomic, transcriptomic and epigenomic landscapes of cervical cancers from Ugandan patients identified differences in epigenomes of cervical tumors from individuals infected by different HPV clades (7). Clade A7, encompassing HPV subtypes 18, 45, 59, and 68, appeared to exhibit inferior prognosis, particularly in HIV-infected patients, when compared with the patients infected with HPV clade A9, which encompasses HPV subtypes 16, 52, and 31 (7).

Smaller scale studies have also identified recurrent molecular alterations in rare cervical cancer subtypes. For example, clear cell carcinomas of the cervix have been found to be associated with frequent pathogenic alterations in the Hippo signaling pathway, including recurrent alterations in the *WWTR1* gene (8). Gastric-type cervical adenocarcinomas were found to exhibit frequent mutations in TP53, CDKN2A, KRAS, SKT11, BRCA2, SMAD4, and ERBB2, some of which have clear treatment implications (9,10).

REFERENCES

1. Roden RBS, Stern PL. Opportunities and challenges for human papillomavirus vaccination in cancer. *Nat Rev Cancer*. 2018;18(4):240-254.
2. McLaughlin-Drubin ME, Munger K. The human papillomavirus E7 oncoprotein. *Virology*. 2009;384(2):335-344.
3. Moody CA, Laimins LA. Human papillomavirus oncoproteins: pathways to transformation. *Nat Rev Cancer*. 2010;10(8):550-560.
4. Pal A, Kundu R. Human papillomavirus E6 and E7: the cervical cancer hallmarks and targets for therapy. *Front Microbiol*. 2019;10:3116.
5. Ojesina AI, Lichtenstein L, Freeman SS, et al. Landscape of genomic alterations in cervical carcinomas. *Nature*. 2014;506(7488):371-375.
6. Atlas TCG. Integrated genomic and molecular characterization of cervical cancer. *Nature*. 2017;543(7645):378-384.
7. Gagliardi A, Porter VL, Zong Z, et al. Analysis of Ugandan cervical carcinomas identifies human papillomavirus clade-specific epigenome and transcriptome landscapes. *Nat Genet*. 2020;52(8):800-810.
8. Kim SH, Basili T, Dopeso H, et al. Recurrent WWTR1 S89W mutations and Hippo pathway deregulation in clear cell carcinomas of the cervix. *J Pathol*. 2022;257(5):635-649.
9. Selenica P, Alemar B, Matrai C, et al. Massively parallel sequencing analysis of 68 gastric-type cervical adenocarcinomas reveals mutations in cell cycle-related genes and potentially targetable mutations. *Mod Pathol*. 2021;34(6):1213-1225.
10. Liao X, Xia X, Su W, et al. Association of recurrent APOBEC3B alterations with the prognosis of gastric-type cervical adenocarcinoma. *Gynecol Oncol*. 2022;165(1):105-113.

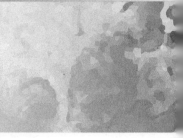

CHAPTER **4.3**

Cervical Cancer: Clinical Presentation and Diagnostic Evaluation

Charles A. Leath III and Teresa K. L. Boitano

PRECLINICAL INVASIVE DISEASE

Screening Cytology

Screening cervical cytology is an effective cancer screening test with high clinical benefit based on its ease of performance, test sensitivity, and ability to detect multiple phases of uterine cervix dysplasia. Nonetheless, a single test may have limited sensitivity for uterine cervix cancer detection (1). Although two primary cellular sampling methods are used, the conventional Pap smear or test and liquid-based cytology, standalone high-risk HPV testing can be used as a standalone screening test or as an adjunct with cytologic assessment.

Screening guidelines and recommendations have been frequently modified over the past decade. In 2013, the U.S. Preventive Services Task Force (USPSTF) recommended cervical cancer screening (CCS) in women aged 21 to 65 years with Pap cytology every 3 years, or for women aged 30 to 65 years who desire a longer screening interval, Pap cytology, and HPV cotesting done every 5 years (2). Moreover, the ACS summarized age-appropriate screening strategies, including the appropriateness of Pap cytology with or without HPV cotesting, follow-up of women after screening, the age at which to exit screening, and screening strategies for women vaccinated against HPV 16 or 18 infections (3). For women aged less than 21 years, no screening is recommended. Women aged 21 to 29 years should consider Pap cytology alone every 3 years. Women aged 30 to 65 years should preferably undergo Pap cytology and HPV cotesting every 5 years. In this category, women with cytology-negative and HPV-positive testing undergo 12-month follow-up with cotesting, or if subsequently found positive for HPV 16 or 18 immediate colposcopy. Women aged 65 years or above may exit screening if prior screening was negative. In women without a personal history or CIN2[+] in the past 20 years as well as the absence of a personal history of cervical cancer, hysterectomy allows discontinuation from further Pap cytology or HPV cotesting, presuming that cervical hysterectomy pathology does not demonstrate either of these conditions. HPV-vaccinated women follow their age-specific recommendations (same as unvaccinated women). The American College of Obstetricians and Gynecologists (ACOG) does not support changing screening intervals (4).

An updated standard terminology via the Bethesda system (2014) was performed to modernize this historically important tool and describes specimen adequacy and dysplastic cytologic abnormalities, and these principles remain in use today. Squamous cell epithelial cell abnormalities include the following: (a) atypical squamous cells of undetermined significance (ASCUS) or atypical squamous cells—cannot rule out high-grade squamous intraepithelial lesion (ASC-H), (b) LSIL, (c) HSIL (encompassing CIN 2 or CIN 3 or carcinoma in situ), and squamous cell carcinoma (5). In addition, glandular epithelial cell abnormalities include the following categories: (a) atypical glandular cells (AGS, specifying endocervix, endometrial, or not otherwise specified origins), (b) AGS favoring neoplastic, (c) endocervical adenocarcinoma in situ (AIS), or (d) adenocarcinoma (5).

Although current screening guidelines are fairly regimented, this has not been the case in clinical practice. Importantly, a large multicenter trial (ASCUS/LSIL Triage Study [ALTS]) of 3,488 women began in 1997 and randomized women to immediate colposcopy versus triage to colposcopy according to Pap cytology and HPV cotesting results (6). Pap cytology reported 86% of cases with an overall CIN 3 or worse diagnosis, whereas HPV cotesting identified 92% (10 pg/mL cutoff) or 96% (1 pg/mL cutoff) of cases with an overall CIN 3 or worse diagnosis. The ALTS study established high-risk HPV testing as the most cost-effective triage test for ASCUS. After this study, the American Society for Colposcopy and Cervical Pathology (ASCCP) and American Society for Clinical Pathology (ASCP) have endorsed HPV cotesting as the preferred method of triage for ASCUS smears detected by liquid-based cytology for women aged 30 years or above (3).

Human Papillomavirus Testing

For women aged 30 years or above undergoing screening in the United States, a recommendation for HPV cotesting as an adjunct to cytology has been made to triage women with ASCUS (7,8). In European nations, HPV tests serve to triage women with ASCUS, to monitor them after CIN treatment, and even to be a standalone primary screening test without cytology (9). Australia (10) and the Netherlands (11) have accepted self-sampling HPV tests as primary screens for their national uterine cervix dysplasia and cancer screening programs. Detection of HPV DNA involves either hybrid capture 2 or polymerase chain reaction technologies. HPV cotesting has become more widespread as a diagnostic aid (6,12-14).

HPV cotesting as either an adjunct to liquid-based cytology or a standalone test was evaluated by a large prospective cohort study (ATHENA, 2008-2009) involving 47,208 American women (8). In that study, the combination of cytology and HPV cotesting was superior to cytology alone for the detection of CIN 3 or worse over a 3-year observation period; however, HPV testing alone identified 64% more CIN 3 or worse lesions (294, 95% confidence interval [CI]: 260-325) than cytology (179, 95% CI, 152-206) and 23% more than cotesting (240, 95% CI, 209-270). ATHENA was the first screening study in American women to support HPV primary screening with triage of HPV-positive women using HPV 16 or 18 genotyping and reflex cytology at age 25 years (8).

Reduced uterine cervix squamous intraepithelial lesion prevalence has arisen out of prophylactic HPV vaccination of adolescent women. A randomized trial reporting 42-month follow-up on 17,622 HPV-naive adolescent women (aged 16-26 years) showed that a prophylactic quadrivalent HPV vaccine (types 6, 11, 16, and 18) administered day 1, month 2, and month 6 sustains immunocompetence against HPV 16 and HPV 18 CIN in those receiving vaccine versus those receiving placebo (15). Long-term high efficacy, immunogenicity, and acceptable safety in adolescent women have been confirmed in a Nordic region extension of the original studies (16). Moreover, Australia instituted in 2007 a nationally funded vaccination program with the quadrivalent HPV vaccine. The initial program launched vaccination as a continuing component of a 12- to 13-year-old schoolgirl health program and funded two catch-up programs targeting 13- to 17-year-old school adolescents and 18- to 26-year-old women in general practice and community well-woman evaluations (17). A 0.38% (95% CI, 0.16-0.61) decrease in a population-wide prevalence of CIN 2 or worse was noticed in the vaccinated cohort between 2007 and 2009, compared with incidence found in the Victorian Cervical Cytology registry (Australia, 2003-2009). In the United Sates, adolescent female vaccination rates are low, and historically, only about 40% of adolescents report receiving the vaccine (18,19). More recent data, however, suggest that HPV vaccination (≤1 dose) among adolescents aged 13 to 17 is now 75.1%, with 58.6% considered UTD including a 61.4% rate in females (20).

Most recently, the ASCCP provided updated guidelines that are more individualized, focusing on risk rather than results, and may recommend either more frequent or less frequent assessments, taking into consideration a patients prior cytology and HPV results (21).

Colposcopy

Colposcopy evaluates the lower genital tract by a colposcope with binocular magnification (5×-30×) via visual assessment in order to perform biopsy(ies) of suspicious precancerous or cancerous lesions. Following an abnormal screening test, colposcopy remains arguably the most important diagnostic tool in uterine cervix cancer prevention (22). Acetic acid or Lugol solution highlights dysplastic change, such as acetowhite plaques or vacuolar abnormalities (including punctations, mosaicism, and abnormal vessel branching), that may signify high-grade lesions. Indications for colposcopy include an abnormal-appearing cervix, persistent postcoital bleeding or discharge, abnormal cytologic results that warrant immediate assessment per guidelines, persistent abnormal cytology, in utero exposure to diethylstilbestrol (DES, a synthetic estrogen), and ASCUS cytology with positive high-risk HPV 16, 18, or 45. Adequate colposcopy examinations involve full visualization of the uterine cervix and its transformation zone. Endocervical curettage (ECC) might be helpful, and yet, its routine practice remains debatable (23). Multiquadrant biopsy improves accuracy of colposcopy, especially when a lesion is not readily visualized (23,24). Most recently, the 2019 ASCCP guidelines suggested that an estimated immediate risk of 4% or greater of diagnosing CIN3+ warrants colposcopy (21).

Conization

Conization of the uterine cervix is a surgical excision of the squamocolumnar junction (transformation zone) and may be either a cold knife conization in the operating room suite or thermal cautery with loop excision in the outpatient office or in the operating room suite. Indications for conization include inadequate colposcopy, positive ECC, persistent CIN 1 (typically >1 year), CIN 2 or CIN 3, carcinoma in situ, *AGC (favor neoplasia) or AIS cytology not explained by colposcopy and biopsy*, and discrepancy among cytology, colposcopy, and pathologic findings. After examination of 447 histopathologic slices from 97 patient conization procedures, small cone height was significantly associated with positive disease margin status: a 20-mm cone height was recommended (25).

Loop Diathermy

Outpatient thermal cautery with loop electrosurgical excision procedure (LEEP or loop diathermy) is an alternative to cold knife conization (26). Studies have demonstrated loop diathermy to be as effective as cold knife conization (27) and laser vaporization (28), with some gynecologists favoring loop diathermy in terms of cost, anesthesia, and ease of use, although thermal artifact may obscure margin status. Return patient visits after loop diathermy might be because to incomplete excision complicated by thermal artifact, secondary hemorrhage, and findings of invasive cancer (26).

CLINICAL INVASIVE DISEASE

Symptoms and Complaints

Uterine cervix cancer presents most often with abnormal vaginal discharge, postcoital bleeding, or nonmenstrual vaginal bleeding, which may, at times, be significant and result in anemia. Well-woman visits might also discover asymptomatic lesions upon pelvic examination or cytologic evaluation. Cancer growth might elicit local pelvic pain or disrupted urination or defecation. Disease spread to regional pelvic or para-aortic lymph nodes may be associated with back pain, or unilateral leg swelling (or even bullous edema) might become evident.

Physical Findings

Gross inspection of the cervix may reveal visible abnormalities to include an abnormal contour of the uterine cervix, which may be the first clue to disease, with necrotic or friable lesions being particularly suspicious. Palpation of the fornices is important to determine the absence or presence of disease extension, and any palpable extension of disease onto the walls of the vagina must be described, if present, and potentially biopsied if pathologic confirmation is needed. Parametrial, sidewall, and uterosacral ligament extension are best felt and described by rectovaginal examination. Nodal disease in the groin, femoral, and scalene lymph node regions should be assessed to guide intervention.

Diagnostic Biopsy

Biopsies should secure sufficient nonnecrotic tissue at depth for the diagnosis of uterine cervix cancers. Multiple biopsies may be necessary for sufficient pathologic assessment, although this may also be associated with a higher risk of bleeding. In general, a marginal biopsy rather than central necrotic tissue biopsy yields superior results.

STAGING

Clinical Staging Procedures

Following initial visual inspection, pelvic examination with rectovaginal palpation provides the basis for clinical cancer staging. An examination under anesthesia, when needed, provides superior visual and manual examination when pain precludes an appropriate and comprehensive pelvic examination. Examination under anesthesia affords opportunities for cystoscopy, proctoscopy, and special instrument biopsy when clinically indicated.

Clinical Laboratory Studies

Anemia and electrolyte abnormalities are commonly noted in women with cervical cancer. Accordingly, a complete peripheral blood count is indicated to assess anemia (<10 g/dL), which may require transfusion of packed red blood cells. Although thrombocytopenia might be found in up to 30% of patients, replacement before therapeutic intervention is uncommon. Serum blood urea nitrogen and creatinine obtained as part of the chemistry panel assess renal insufficiency and dehydration, which might need stabilization and rehydration before cisplatin-based radiochemotherapy. At times, ureteral stents or percutaneous nephrostomy tubes may be necessary to improve renal function if anatomic obstruction related to advanced disease is present. Liver function panels are obtained generally before chemotherapy when indicated. A baseline urinalysis, including pregnancy test, is indicated to exclude pregnancy in potential childbearing patients.

Clinical Serum Tumor Markers

Of historical interest, **Table 4.3-1** lists serum tumor markers for uterine cervix cancer (29,30). Uterine cervix cancers—represented mostly by HPV-competent squamous cell carcinoma or adenocarcinoma—express unique phenotypic fingerprints, which possibly indicative of higher rates of nodal or visceral metastases and poorer disease-specific survival. Prospective trials randomizing go or no-go therapeutic decisions based on serum tumor markers remain elusive. More recently, the potential role of circulating HPV DNA as a possible marker or predictor of response to therapy has been reported (31).

Clinical Radiographic Studies

The FIGO system for cancer staging now incorporates results from both clinical examination and radiographic imaging. Noninvasive chest radiography, intravenous pyelography (IVP), cystoscopy, sigmoidoscopy, and barium enema radiography may aid in clinical evaluation but are not mandatory (32). In resource-limited

areas, physical examination and biopsy are warranted, but limited to no imaging may be available or feasible. Computed tomography (CT), 2-[^{18}F]fluoro-2-deoxy-D-glucose (^{18}F-FDG), positron emission tomography (PET), dual PET/CT, magnetic resonance imaging (MRI), or dual PET/MRI studies can be used when available. In the United States and other countries, these studies are considered important in the care of women with uterine cervix cancer as they improve diagnostic accuracy and inform treatment recommendations.

When compared with operative staging, the previous FIGO clinical staging for uterine cervix cancer understaged 30% of stage IB, 25% of stage IIB, and 40% of stage IIIB patients (33). Abdominopelvic CT or MRI images help sort out cross-sectional anatomy and assist in evaluating prognostic features, such as tumor size and lymph node metastasis. The American College of Radiology Imaging Network (ACRIN) and the Gynecologic Oncology Group (GOG) commenced a intergroup trial (ACRIN 6,651/GOG 183), among 25 sites to prospectively evaluate MRI, CT, clinical examination, and histopathologic analysis for their ability to predict lymph node involvement as verified by lymphadenectomy in 208 women with uterine cervix cancer (34-36). MRI correctly identified 20 (37%) of 54 of cases with surgicopathologic-confirmed lymph node metastases, whereas CT correctly labeled 17 (31%) of 55 cases (36). The investigators concluded that both modalities had an underperforming, low sensitivity for detecting lymph node metastases. However, MRI (area under the curve [AUC] 0.88; $P = .014$) outperformed CT (AUC 0.73) in the ability to measure uterine cervix cancer diameter (35), an important prognostic variable. MRI has, therefore, been associated with a positive predictive value of 61% (95% CI, 48%-73%) among women surgically confirmed for positive pelvic and para-aortic lymph node metastases, a negative predictive value of 66% (95% CI, 55%-75%) among

■ TABLE 4.3-1. Biologic Markers Predicting Lymph Node Metastasis in Uterine Cervix Cancer

Test	Cutoff (ng/mL)	Sensitivity (%)	Specificity (%)	% Node Metastasis	Test Used in Decision for	Reference
Squamous cell carcinoma antigen (SCC-Ag)	>3.5 >3.5	81 71	65 67	35 (34/96) 71 (15/21)	BR PR	(78) (79)
	>3.5	71	67	71 (15/21)	PR	(79)
	>2.0	64	69	64 (23/36)	PR	(80)
	>1.9	66	NR	66 (53/80)	AR	(81)
	>1.5	75	40	75 (215/286)	BR	(82)
	>1.5	NR	NR	30 (35/116)	BR	(83)
Cytokeratin fragment 19 (CYFRA 21.1)	>3.30	36	90	36 (13/36)	PR	(80)
	>3.30	36	90	36 (13/36)	PR	(80)
Cancer antigen 125 (CA 125)	≥30 U/mL	67	84	67 (6/9)	PR	(85)
Human cartilage glycoprotein 39 (YKL-40)	>92.2	21	71	21 (10/47)	ID	(86)
High mobility group box protein 1 (HMGB1)	>28.1	63	40	63 (45/71)	PR	(87)
Uterine cervix circulating tumor cells (CTCs)	E6/E7+	0	78	25 (3/12)	CTC	(88)

AR, adjuvant radiation; BR, biochemical response; CTC, E6+ or E7+ circulating tumor cells; ID, initial detection; NR, not reported; PR, predicting response.

women surgically confirmed for positive pelvic lymph nodes and negative para-aortic lymph nodes and a negative predictive value of 86% (95% CI, 76%-92%) in women with surgically confirmed negative pelvic and para-aortic lymph nodes (37). In cases of parametrial extension, MRI provides superior detail of tumor-related anatomic invasion and affords best contour definition in brachytherapy radiation planning (38).

PET studies have shown that the radiotracer FDG associates with all measures of disease burden, including the prevalence of lymph node metastases, rates of objective (complete or partial) treatment response, and progression-free survival (PFS), in patients with uterine cervix cancer (39-42). FDG proves useful owing to its "look-alike" sugar form, being "trapped" by intracellular hexokinase and being concentrated in overactive cancer cells. A 32-patient surgicopathologic study (1994-1998) of presurgical abdominopelvic PET followed by open surgical lymphadenectomy showed a 75% sensitivity and 92% specificity for uterine cervix cancer metastases in para-aortic lymph nodes (39). A radiographic study of 101 patients (1998-2000) of whole-body PET found that PET-avid para-aortic lymph nodes predicted PFS (40). A retrospective study of 482 patients (1997-2008) investigated imaging-only confirmed sites of lymph node metastases (41). It found 205 (43%) patients with no FDG-avid lymph nodes, 186 (39%) patients with FDG-avid pelvic lymph nodes only, 65 (13%) patients with FDG-avid pelvic and para-aortic lymph nodes, and 26 (5%) patients with FDG-avid pelvic, para-aortic, and supraclavicular lymph nodes. Among 51 patients with uterine cervix cancer (2004-2009) in whom presurgical PET scans were obtained, a 0.33 or less post-therapy: pretherapy standard uptake value maximum ratio of primary cancer metabolic signal was associated in 88% of patients with an at least partial radiochemotherapy treatment response (42). A phase I trial (2006-2008) explored PET-assessed metabolic response to novel radiochemotherapy in patients with uterine cervix cancer (43). Afterward, a prospective phase II clinical trial (2009-2011) in 25 women with advanced-stage uterine cervix or vaginal cancers used a 3-month post-therapy PET-assessed metabolic response as the primary efficacy end point (44,45).

Both ACRIN and GOG worked in concert in a subsequent clinical trial to assess the ability and accuracy of PET imaging to detect nodal metastasis. In ACRIN 6,671/GOG 233, 164 of 169 accrued patients with locally advanced cervical cancer had a pelvic and abdominal lymphadenectomy following the performance of an interpretable preoperative PET with contrast-enhanced CT. Both laparoscopic or extraperitoneal approaches were allowed in order to assess nodes in four bilateral regions, including para-aortic, common iliac, external iliac, and obturator lymph nodes. Of the 164 patients, 109 (66.5%) had interpretable imaging and surgical pathology, clearly limiting definitive conclusions. Nonetheless, PET/CT sensitivity for abdominal lymph node metastasis was 0.50 versus 0.42 for CT alone ($P = .052$), whereas specificity was 0.85 compared with 0.89 ($P = .21$), respectively, suggesting a modest improvement for PET imaging (46).

Pretreatment Para-Aortic Node Operative Staging

Para-aortic lymph node metastases indicate an inferior prognosis and compromised survival (39). It is debatable whether there is a therapeutic advantage to operative removal of para-aortic disease. Historically, either an extraperitoneal approach or transperitoneal approach to para-aortic lymphadenectomy was evaluated in predominantly stage IIB and IIIB cancers and resulted in similar sensitivity and morbidity in a uterine cervix cancer

surgical staging study of 288 patients (1977-1981) (47). Knowledge of para-aortic lymph node disease has been shown to direct care away from surgery toward extended-field radiation therapy (RT) in up to 20% of patients (48). As part of a prospective, multicenter clinical trial (1999-2002), patients with histologically confirmed stage IB2, stage IIA 4 cm or greater, or stage IIB to IVA uterine cervix cancers underwent MRI before pelvic and abdominal lymphadenectomy (37). Lymph nodes less than 1 cm were bisected, whereas those greater than 1 cm were serially sectioned into 5-mm sections for microscopy. Thirty-three patients had 94 metastasis-positive and 659 metastasis-negative lymph nodes removed. Mean size of the long axis of the 60 largest positive and the 209 negative lymph nodes removed did not differ (19 ± 9 mm vs 19 ± 12 mm; $P = .47$). The authors suggested that the negative predictive value of MRI for para-aortic lymph nodes among patients reported to have negative pelvic and para-aortic lymph nodes on MRI is high enough that surgical evaluation and extended-field RT are not necessary. For all others, the positive and negative predictive values of MRI are too low to determine the need for extended-field RT without first performing surgical evaluation. A phase III international trial evaluating lymphadenectomy in locally advanced uterine cervix cancer study (LiLACS) is underway (49).

Sentinel Lymph Node Mapping in Early Uterine Cervix Cancer

The feasibility of sentinel lymph node mapping has been explored in 39 patients with invasive uterine cervix cancer undergoing radical hysterectomy and pelvic lymphadenectomy (50). All patients underwent presurgical lymphoscintigraphy and intraoperative mapping with both a blue dye and a handheld gamma probe. Lymphoscintigraphy revealed at least one sentinel lymph node in 33 (85%) patients, including 21 (55%) patients with bilateral sentinel lymph nodes. All 39 patients had at least one sentinel lymph node identified during surgery. The majority (80%) of sentinel lymph nodes were in the iliac, obturator, and parametrial nodal basins (in descending order of frequency). The remainder were in either the common iliac or the para-aortic nodal basins. A total of 132 nodes were identified clinically as sentinel lymph nodes; 65 (49%) were both blue and hot, 35 (27%) were blue only, and 32 (24%) were hot only. The sensitivity of the sentinel node was 88%, and the negative predictive value was 97%. The German AGO Study Group (1998-2006) identified a 93% sentinel lymph node detection rate, 77% sensitivity, and 94% negative predictive value in 590 women of all uterine cervix cancer stages who underwent lymph node detection after labeling with technetium or patent blue or both (51). Moreover, French investigators reported their experience with sentinel lymph node mapping and dissection in early-stage cervical cancer (stage IA1 with LVSI—IB1 (FIGO 2009)). One hundred thirty-nine patients in their modified IIT population noted that the combination of patent blue and technetium 99 injection had a detection of 97.8% (95% CI 93.8%-99.6%), although the sensitivity was 92.0% (95% CI 74.0%-99.0%) secondary to two false-negative results (52). More recently, these investigators reported 4-year follow-up data for women randomized to sentinel lymph node biopsy alone or followed by pelvic lymphadenectomy and noted similar disease-free rates at 4 years (89.5% vs 93.1%; $P = .53$) (53). Obstacles to widespread adoption include sensitivity of frozen section preparation to detect lymph node metastasis, pathologic expertise, uniformity of surgicopathologic technique, and a determination of whether the clinical impact of presurgical tumor size affects the rate of sentinel lymph node event (54).

REFERENCES

1. Schiffman M, Solomon D. Clinical practice. Cervical-cancer screening with human papillomavirus and cytologic cotesting. *N Engl J Med.* 2013;369(24):2324-2331.

2. Moyer V, LeFevre M, Siu A, et al. Final Recommendation Statement: Cervical Cancer: Screening. United States Preventive Services Task Force; 2013.

3. Saslow D, Solomon D, Lawson HW, et al. American Cancer Society, American Society for Colposcopy and Cervical Pathology, and American Society for Clinical Pathology screening guidelines for the prevention and early detection of cervical cancer. *CA Cancer J Clin.* 2012;62(3):147-172.

4. Committee on Practice Bulletins—Gynecology. ACOG Practice Bulletin Number 131: screening for cervical cancer. *Obstet Gynecol.* 2012;120(5):1222-1238.

5. Nayar R, Wilbur DC. The Pap Test and Bethesda 2014. "The reports of my demise have been greatly exaggerated." (after a quotation from Mark Twain). *Acta Cytol.* 2015;59(2):121-132.

6. Sherman ME, Schiffman M, Cox JT. Effects of age and human papilloma viral load on colposcopy triage: data from the randomized atypical squamous cells of undetermined significance/low-grade squamous intraepithelial lesion triage study (ALTS). *J Natl Cancer Inst.* 2002;94(2):102-107.

7. Monsonego J, Cox JT, Behrens C, et al. Prevalence of high-risk human papilloma virus genotypes and associated risk of cervical precancerous lesions in a large U.S. screening population: data from the ATHENA trial. Gynecol Oncol. 2015;137(1):47-54.

8. Wright TC, Stoler MH, Behrens CM, et al. Primary cervical cancer screening with human papillomavirus: end of study results from the ATHENA study using HPV as the first-line screening test. Gynecol Oncol. 2015;136(2):189-197.

9. Arbyn M, Anttila A, Jordan J, et al. European guidelines for quality assurance in cervical cancer screening. Second edition—summary document. *Ann Oncol.* 2010;21(3):448-458.

10. Sultana F, English DR, Simpson JA, et al. Rationale and design of the iPap trial: a randomized controlled trial of home-based HPV self-sampling for improving participation in cervical screening by never- and under-screened women in Australia. *BMC Cancer.* 2014;14:207.

11. Arbyn M, Castle PE. Offering self-sampling kits for HPV testing to reach women who do not attend in the regular cervical cancer screening program. *Cancer Epidemiol Biomarkers Prev.* 2015;24(5):769-772.

12. Wright TC Jr, Stoler MH, Sharma A, et al. Evaluation of HPV-16 and HPV-18 genotyping for the triage of women with high-risk HPV+ cytology-negative results. Am J Clin Pathol. 2011;136(4):578-586.

13. Sherman ME, Castle PE, Solomon D. Cervical cytology of atypical squamous cells-cannot exclude high-grade squamous intraepithelial lesion (ASC-H): characteristics and histologic outcomes. *Cancer.* 2006;108(5):298-305.

14. Lorenzato M, Clavel C, Masure M, et al. DNA image cytometry and human papillomavirus (HPV) detection help to select smears at high risk of high-grade cervical lesions. *J Pathol.* 2001;194(2):171-176.

15. Dillner J, Kjaer SK, Wheeler CM, et al. Four year efficacy of prophylactic human papillomavirus quadrivalent vaccine against low grade cervical, vulvar, and vaginal intraepithelial neoplasia and anogenital warts: randomised controlled trial. *BMJ.* 2010;341:c3493.

16. Nygard M, Saah A, Munk C, et al. Evaluation of the long-term anti-human papillomavirus 6 (HPV6), 11, 16, and 18 immune responses generated by the quadrivalent HPV vaccine. *Clin Vaccine Immunol.* 2015;22(8):943-948.

17. Brotherton JM, Fridman M, May CL, et al. Early effect of the HPV vaccination programme on cervical abnormalities in Victoria, Australia: an ecological study. *Lancet.* 2011;377(9783):2085-2092.

18. Daley EM, Vamos CA, Buhi ER, et al. Influences on human papillomavirus vaccination status among female college students. *J Women's Health.* 2010;19(10):1885-1891.

19. Liddon NC, Hood JE, Leichliter JS. Intent to receive HPV vaccine and reasons for not vaccinating among unvaccinated adolescent and young women: findings from the 2006-2008 National Survey of Family Growth. *Vaccine.* 2012;30(16):2676-2682.

20. Pingali C, Yankey D, Elam-Evans LD, et al. National, regional, state, and selected local area vaccination coverage among adolescents aged 13-17 years—United States, 2020. *MMWR Morb Mortal Wkly Rep.* 2021;70(35):1183-1190.

21. Perkins RB, Guido RS, Castle PE, et al. 2019 ASCCP risk-based management consensus guidelines for abnormal cervical cancer screening tests and cancer precursors. *J Low Genit Tract Dis.* 2020;24(2):102-131.

22. World Health Organization. *WHO Guidelines for Screening and Treatment of Precancerous Lesions for Cervical Cancer Prevention* (WHO Guidelines Approved by the Guidelines Review Committee). World Health Organization; 2013.

23. Apgar BS, Kaufman AJ, Bettcher C, et al. Gynecologic procedures: colposcopy, treatments for cervical intraepithelial neoplasia and endometrial assessment. *Am Fam Physician.* 2013;87(12):836-843.

24. Davies KR, Cantor SB, Cox DD, et al. An alternative approach for estimating the accuracy of colposcopy in detecting cervical precancer. *PLoS One.* 2015;10(5):e0126573.

25. Kliemann LM, Silva M, Reinheimer M, et al. Minimal cold knife conization height for high-grade cervical squamous intraepithelial lesion treatment. *Eur J Obstet Gynecol Reprod Biol.* 2012;165(2):342-346.

26. Bigrigg MA, Codling BW, Pearson P, et al. Colposcopic diagnosis and treatment of cervical dysplasia at a single clinic visit. Experience of low-voltage diathermy loop in 1000 patients. *Lancet.* 1990;336(8709):229-231.

27. Luesley DM, Cullimore J, Redman CW, et al. Loop diathermy excision of the cervical transformation zone in patients with abnormal cervical smears. *BMJ.* 1990;300(6741):1690-1693.

28. Dey P, Gibbs A, Arnold DF, et al. Loop diathermy excision compared with cervical laser vaporisation for the treatment of intraepithelial neoplasia: a randomised controlled trial. *BJOG.* 2002;109(4):381-385.

29. Li X, Zhou J, Huang K, et al. The predictive value of serum squamous cell carcinoma antigen in patients with cervical cancer who receive neoadjuvant chemotherapy followed by radical surgery: a single-institute study. *PLoS One.* 2015;10(4):e0122361.

30. Weismann P, Weismanova E, Masak L, et al. The detection of circulating tumor cells expressing E6/E7 HR-HPV oncogenes in peripheral blood in cervical cancer patients after radical hysterectomy. *Neoplasma.* 2009;56(3):230-238.

31. Han K, Leung E, Barbera L, et al. Circulating human papillomavirus DNA as a biomarker of response in patients with locally advanced cervical cancer treated with definitive chemoradiation. *JCO Precis Oncol.* 2018;2:1-8.

32. Pecorelli S, Zigliani L, Odicino F. Revised FIGO staging for carcinoma of the cervix. Int J Gynecol Obstet. 2009;105(2):107-108.

33. Lagasse LD, Creasman WT, Shingleton HM, et al. Results and complications of operative staging in cervical cancer: experience of the Gynecologic Oncology Group. *Gynecol Oncol.* 1980;9(1):90-98.

34. Mitchell DG, Snyder B, Coakley F, et al. Early invasive cervical cancer: MRI and CT predictors of lymphatic metastases in the ACRIN 6651/GOG 183 intergroup study. *Gynecol Oncol.* 2009;112(1):95-103.

35. Mitchell DG, Snyder B, Coakley F, et al. Early invasive cervical cancer: tumor delineation by magnetic resonance imaging, computed tomography, and clinical examination, verified by pathologic results, in the ACRIN 6651/GOG 183 Intergroup Study. *J Clin Oncol.* 2006;24(36):5687-5694.

36. Hricak H, Gatsonis C, Chi DS, et al. Role of imaging in pretreatment evaluation of early invasive cervical cancer: results of the intergroup study American College of Radiology Imaging Network 6651-Gynecologic Oncology Group 183. *J Clin Oncol.* 2005;23(36):9329-9337.

37. Gold M, Zhang Z, Marques H, et al. MRI prior to systematic lymphadenectomy in patients with locally advanced cervical cancer. *J Clin Oncol.* 2011;29(suppl 15):5042.

38. Viswanathan AN, Erickson B, Gaffney DK, et al. Comparison and consensus guidelines for delineation of clinical target volume for CT- and MR-based brachytherapy in locally advanced cervical cancer. *Int J Radiat Oncol Biol Phys.* 2014;90(2):320-328.

39. Rose PG, Adler LP, Rodriguez M, et al. Positron emission tomography for evaluating para-aortic nodal metastasis in locally advanced cervical cancer before surgical staging: a surgicopathologic study. *J Clin Oncol.* 1999;17(1):41-45.

40. Grigsby PW, Siegel BA, Dehdashti F. Lymph node staging by positron emission tomography in patients with carcinoma of the cervix. *J Clin Oncol.* 2001;19(17):3745-3749.

41. Kidd E, Siegel B, Dehdashti F, et al. The standardized uptake value for F-18 fluorodeoxyglucose is a sensitive predictive biomarker for cervical cancer treatment response and survival. *Cancer.* 2007;110(8):1738-1744.

42. Kunos C, Radivoyevitch T, Abdul-Karim F, et al. 18F-fluoro-2-deoxy-d-glucose positron emission tomography standard uptake value as an indicator of cervical cancer chemoradiation therapeutic response. *Int J Gynecol Cancer.* 2011;21(6):1117-1123.

43. Kunos C, Waggoner S, Von Gruenigen V, et al. Phase I trial of intravenous 3-aminopyridine-2-carboxaldehyde thiosemicarbazone (3-AP, NSC æ663249) in combination with pelvic radiation therapy and weekly

cisplatin chemotherapy for locally advanced cervical cancer. *Clin Cancer Res.* 2010;16(4):1298-1306.

44. Kunos C, Radivoyevitch T, Waggoner S, et al. Radiochemotherapy plus 3-aminopyridine-2-carboxaldehyde thiosemicarbazone (3-AP, NSC #663249) in advanced-stage cervical and vaginal cancers. *Gynecol Oncol.* 2013;130(1):75-80.

45. Kunos CA, Sherertz TM. Long-term disease control with triapine-based radiochemotherapy for patients with stage IB2-IIIB cervical cancer. *Front Oncol.* 2014;4:184.

46. Atri M, Zhang Z, Dehdashti F, et al. Utility of PET-CT to evaluate retroperitoneal lymph node metastasis in advanced cervical cancer: results of ACRIN6671/GOG0233 trial. *Gynecol Oncol.* 2016;142(3):413-419.

47. Weiser E, Bundy B, Hoskins W, et al. Extraperitoneal versus transperitoneal selective paraaortic lymphadenectomy in the pretreatment surgical staging of advanced cervical carcinoma (a Gynecologic Oncology Group Study). *Gynecol Oncol.* 1989;33(3):283-289.

48. Leblanc E, Narducci F, Frumovitz M, et al. Therapeutic value of pretherapeutic extraperitoneal laparoscopic staging of locally advanced cervical carcinoma. *Gynecol Oncol.* 2007;105(2):304-311.

49. Frumovitz M, Querleu D, Gil-Moreno A, et al. Lymphadenectomy in locally advanced cervical cancer study (LiLACS): phase III clinical trial comparing surgical with radiologic staging in patients with stages IB2-IVA cervical cancer. *J Minim Invasive Gynecol.* 2014;21(1):3-8.

50. Levenback C, Coleman RL, Burke TW, et al. Lymphatic mapping and sentinel node identification in patients with cervix undergoing radical hysterectomy and pelvic lymphadenectomy. *J Clin Oncol.* 2002;20(3):688-693.

51. Altgassen C, Hertel H, Brandstadt A, et al. Multicenter validation study of the sentinel lymph node concept in cervical cancer: AGO Study Group. *J Clin Oncol.* 2008;26(18):2943-2951.

52. Lécuru F, Mathevet P, Querleu D, et al. Bilateral negative sentinel nodes accurately predict absence of lymph node metastasis in early cervical cancer: results of the SENTICOL study. *J Clin Oncol.* 2011;29(13):1686-1691.

53. Favre G, Guani B, Balaya V, Magaud L, Lecuru F, Mathevet P. Sentinel lymph-node biopsy in early-stage cervical cancer: the 4-year follow-up results of the Senticol 2 trial. *Front Oncol.* 2021;10:621518.

54. Holman LL, Levenback CF, Frumovitz M. Sentinel lymph node evaluation in women with cervical cancer. *J Minim Invasive Gynecol.* 2014;21(4):540-545.

CHAPTER 4.4

Surgery for Cervical Cancer

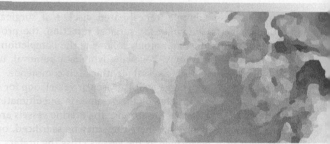

Charles A. Leath III and Teresa K. L. Boitano

Abdominal hysterectomy approaches for the management of cervical cancer including differences among these approaches is well known in clinical practice. Although laparoscopy with or without robotic assistance has been utilized as an alternative surgical approach for the treatment of cervical cancer, recent clinical trial data call into question their safety (1) (see **Table 4.4-1**).

I hysterectomy is satisfactory treatment for high-grade CIN, carcinoma in situ, and clinical stage IA1 invasive cervical cancers. Abdominal, vaginal, laparoscopic, or robot-assisted techniques are described. As noted later, surgeons should consider the appropriateness of a laparoscopic approach for women with stage IA1 cervical cancer with the presence of LVSI.

CLASS I: EXTRAFASCIAL HYSTERECTOMY

The most common type of hysterectomy within gynecologic surgery, for both benign and select malignant conditions, is the class I extrafascial hysterectomy. Specifically, this procedure includes removal of the uterus by detaching it from adnexal structures and round ligaments, separation from the bladder at the vesicouterine fold and past the level of the cervix. The uterine vessels are clamped and ligated at their insertion close to the cervicouterine junction. Surgeons utilize surgical clamps, or electrosurgical devices, in a sequential manner along the lower uterine segment and cervix in order to liberate the uterus and cervix. Ultimately, removal of the uterus occurs by liberating the uterine cervix off from the upper vagina, while consciously avoiding removing excess vaginal tissue in order to ensure adequate vaginal length. The detached specimen includes the pubovesicocervical fascia. Ultimately, the open vaginal cuff is closed with running or interrupted sutures. A class

CLASS II: MODIFIED RADICAL HYSTERECTOMY

The modified radical hysterectomy, or class II hysterectomy, has been increasingly utilized for the surgical management of early-stage operable cervical cancer. As compared with class I hysterectomy, both the class II and class III are technically more challenging and require added surgeon skill for safe performance and completion. Following abdominal entry, the retroperitoneum is opened and the paravesical and pararectal spaces are developed and assessed in order to determine tumor resectability with grossly adequate negative surgical margins. Surgeons may utilize palpation via the index finger of the paravesical space in conjunction with the use of the middle finger in the pararectal space to ensure absent parametrial involvement. Pelvic lymph nodes, to include the common and external iliac as well as the obturator lymph nodes, are palpated for gross involvement. Intraoperative pathologic frozen section may be considered for suspicious nodal

■ TABLE 4.4-1. Surgical Classifications for Hysterectomy

	Intrafascial	Extrafascial (I)	Modified Radical (II)	Radical (III)	Extended (IV)
Uterus	Removed	→	→	→	→
Uterine cervix	Partially removed	Completely removed	→	→	→
Uterine cervix fascia	Partially removed	Completely removed	→	→	→
Upper vagina	None	Small rim removed	Proximal 2 cm removed	Upper 1/3 to 1/2 removed	→
Bladder	Partially mobilized	→	→	Fully mobilized	Partially removed
Rectum	Not mobilized	Rectovaginal septum partially mobilized	→	Rectovaginal septum fully mobilized	→
Ureters	Not mobilized	→	Unroofed in ureteral tunnel	Completely dissected to bladder entry	Partially removed
Cardinal ligaments	Resected medial to ureters	→	Resected at level of ureter	Resected at pelvic sidewall	→
Uterosacral ligaments	Resected at cervix	→	Partially resected	Resected at sacral origin	→

tissue, or suspicious peritoneal-based disease. If surgical evaluation suggests suitability for surgical resection, the procedure moves forward most commonly following the completion of the pelvic lymphadenectomy. Following lymphatic removal, ureteral mobilization and uterine vessel identification commence. The bilateral ureters, often tagged with a vascular vessel loop for ease of manipulation, are dissected off the parametria and ultimately both tunneled to their bladder insertions. The uterine vessels are often identified at their origin, where they may be sacrificed, or alternatively, this is performed as the vessels cross the ureters deeper in the pelvis. The bladder is fully mobilized and dissected off the lower uterine segment past the uterine cervix with exposure of the upper vagina in order to ensure isolation of and ability to include a 2-cm vaginal margin. Finally, the parametrial tissue is extirpated medial to the two ureters, whereas the ureterosacral ligaments are isolated and the proximal portions medial to the ureter are removed. Pelvic lymphadenectomy accompanies the modified radical hysterectomy, although dissection before the class II hysterectomy often improves intraoperative visualization. Traditionally, the class II–modified radical hysterectomy is reserved for small uterine cervical tumors (<2 cm) (FIGO 2018, IB1), taking into account both patient factors and surgical experience and preference.

CLASS III: RADICAL HYSTERECTOMY

As compared with the class II–modified radical hysterectomy, the class III abdominal radical hysterectomy is distinguished by a more extensive parametrial resection. Similar to the class II approach, the paravesical and pararectal spaces are again assessed to ensure resectability. In distinction to the class II hysterectomy, the uterine artery is ligated at its origin from the internal iliac (or hypogastric) artery and mobilized "up and over" the ureter. Both ureters are subsequently tunneled fully to their insertion into the bladder trigone. The uterosacral ligaments are isolated and tissue removed. The bladder is dissected off the anterior uterine cervix, again exposing the upper vagina. The cardinal ligaments are resected to the pelvic sidewall and rectum mobilized to remove elements nearest the sacrum. Traditionally, the upper one third of vagina is removed, although this portion of the procedure may be tailored according to the tumor size and the patient's pelvic anatomy. Pelvic lymphadenectomy and para-aortic node palpation with or without sampling are carried out.

Historically, abdominal, laparoscopic, or robot-assisted techniques were used for completion of class II and class III radical hysterectomy. However, clinical trial results from the LACC trial (NCT00614211), which evaluated both minimally invasive and abdominal approaches, called into question the oncologic safety of laproscopic/robotic technologies in these surgical situations. Six-hundred and thirty-one patients with clinical stage IA1 (LVSI present) to stage IB1 (FIGO 2009) cervical cancer were randomly assigned to abdominal radical hysterectomy and lymph node dissection versus a similar minimally invasive surgery. Disease-free survival for patients undergoing a minimally invasive surgery was 86.0% versus 96.5% (−10.6% difference, 95% CI −16.4 to −4.7) at 4.5 years, which exceeded the prespecified noninferiority margin of 7.2% (1). The rapid dissemination of these trial results translated to a dramatic decline in the utilization of minimally invasive approaches for the surgical management of cervical cancer in the United States (2). Ongoing studies, such as the ROCC (A Trial of Robotic vs Open Hysterectomy Surgery in Cervix Cancer) (NCT 04831580) trial, are looking to confirm or refute the LACC trial results in the context of more stringent quality control, mandated preoperative imaging to confirm tumor size, utilization of an intraperitoneal containment system, as well as avoidance of a uterine manipulator during surgery.

CLASS IV: EXTENDED RADICAL HYSTERECTOMY

Class IV radical hysterectomies are important from a historical standpoint and were targeted for those with distal ureteral or parametrial involvement with tumor, although current indications are limited, considering the availability of modern radiochemotherapy for advanced-stage uterine cervix cancers. Adding to the techniques in a class III radical hysterectomy, the class IV intervention adds complete mobilization and dissection of the ureter off the vesicouterine ligament, ligation and removal of the superior vesicle artery, and removal of the upper three quarters of the vagina. The added radicality of this resection markedly increases the risks for bladder dysfunction and/or for fistula as compared with that seen with class I, II, or III hysterectomy.

CLASS V: EXTENDED RADICAL HYSTERECTOMY OR PELVIC EXENTERATION

The class V–extended radical hysterectomy or pelvic exenteration follows all the steps of the class IV–extended radical hysterectomy, but with the removal of the distal ureter and bladder with the creation of bowel and bladder conduits as needed. An open abdominal or robot-assisted operation is done. Only the bladder is removed in an anterior exenteration, and the rectum and anus are removed in a posterior exenteration. Additional details regarding exenterative surgery are discussed in the subsequent sections.

NEW CLASSIFICATIONS OF RADICAL HYSTERECTOMY

In 2008, new classifications for radical hysterectomy were put forward utilizing terminology based on the lateral extent of surgical extirpation (3). There are four types listed, A through D. More recently, Querleu, Cibula, and Abu-Rustum suggested an update to this alternative surgical classification system (see **Table 4.4-2**). Type A mirrors the class I extrafascial hysterectomy. In this approach, tissues around the uterine cervix are transected medial to the ureters and the uterine vessels are ligated at their cervicouterine union, with a limited vaginal margin removed.

Likewise, type B, which includes subtypes B1 and B2, follows the approach and general techniques of the class II–modified radical hysterectomy and involves surgical incisions through the parametria at the level of the ureter. Subtype B1 does not remove lateral paracervical lymph nodes, whereas subtype B2 includes lateral paracervical lymph nodes removal. The ureter is tunneled under the uterine artery and mobilized laterally. The parametria are then resected to the level of the rolled ureter. A 2-cm vaginal margin is taken.

Type C, including subtypes C1 and C2, varies somewhat from the class III radical hysterectomy. Specifically, for a type C radical hysterectomy, the parametria are removed more laterally next to the hypogastric vessels. Moreover, subtype C1 preserves nearby nerve bundles, whereas subtype C2 does not. The uterosacral

ligaments are removed to the level of the rectum, and the ureters are fully mobilized. Uterine vessels are ligated at their origin. The bladder branches of the hypogastric plexus near the bladder pillars are preserved.

Although uncommon, the type D procedure, including D1 and D2 subtypes, mimics the class IV–extended radical hysterectomy and includes removal of the entire parametrial tissue. Subtype D1 involves parametrial resection with removal of hypogastric vessels, whereas subtype D2 includes the steps in subtype D1 but adds a more extensive removal of fascia and muscular structures. These are rare operations.

ALTERNATIVE OPERATIONS FOR UTERINE CERVIX CANCER

Radical Vaginal Hysterectomy

With the introduction of minimally invasive laparoscopic or robot-assisted lymphadenectomy (4), radical vaginal hysterectomy with concomitant lymphadenectomy gained popularity as an oncologic-surgical procedure, wherein the abdominal incision is omitted, thus improving and shortening postoperative recovery. Importantly, both advanced vaginal surgical skills and minimally invasive surgical knowledge and skills, as neither a pelvic nor para-aortic lymphadenectomy can be performed through the vagina, are required, thus omitting the opportunity of a radical vaginal hysterectomy for most patients with cancer.

A radical vaginal hysterectomy commences with a laparoscopic or robot-assisted lymphadenectomy. Both the paravesical space and the pararectal space may be opened by either traditional or robotic-assisted laparoscopic procedures for exploration of the spaces and determination of surgical ease of uterine cervix tumor removal. The vaginal approach begins with outlining a 2-cm vaginal margin and its ring-like separation of the uterine cervix from the vagina. Vaginal mucosa folds over the uterine cervix and facilitates traction during downward removal of the specimen. Subsequently, the vesicouterine space is opened with bladder pillars identified and ligated. The paravesical space is explored by digital dissection, and the ureters are palpated. Concurrent laparoscopy

■ TABLE 4.4-2. Updated Querleu-Morrow Radical Hysterectomy Anatomic Landmark Classification Sorted by Parametrial Components[a]

Type of Radical Hysterectomy	Lateral Parametrium or Paracervix[b]	Ventral Parametrium[c]	Dorsal Parametrium[d]
A	Medial to identified by nonmobilized ureter	Limited resection	Limited resection
B1	To the ureter at level of mobilization from cervix and lateral parametrium	Partial resection of vesicouterine ligament	Partial resection of rectovaginal-rectouterine ligament and uterosacral peritoneal folds
B2	As earlier in addition to paracervical lymphadenectomy	As earlier	As earlier
C1	To the iliac vessels laterally with caudal portion preserved	Excision of vesicouterine ligament at the bladder	To the rectum with dissection and sparing of hypogastric nerve
C2	To the level of the medial aspect of the iliac vessels	At the bladder with removal of bladder nerves	To the sacrum with hypogastric nerve remove(ed)
D	To the pelvic wall with resection of internal iliac vessels and/or portion of sidewall	At the bladder unless part of an exenteration	At the sacrum unless part of an exenteration

[a]Adapted from Querleu D, Cibula D, Abu-Rustum NR. 2017 update on the Querleu-Morrow classification of radical hysterectomy. *Ann Surg Oncol.* 2017;24: 3406-3412.
[b]Traditional paracolpos tissue.
[c]Vesicouterine ligament both cranial and caudal and lateral to ureter.
[d]Combination of rectouterine and rectovaginal ligaments and the dorsal component of the pelvic autonomic nerves.

may also help augment findings on palpation. Uterine vessels are identified and isolated and ligated at their origin from the hypogastric vessels. The pararectal space is opened, and the uterosacral ligaments are transected midway along their posterior expanse. Then, the ureters are mobilized laterally for parametrial tissue resection. The specimen is retracted downward and removed. The upper vagina is recapitulated and sewn closed in a typical manner with delayed absorbable sutures.

Radical Trachelectomy

For appropriately selected patients with small tumors considering potential fertility preservation, abdominal, vaginal, and minimally invasive procedures have been described for radical trachelectomy (4). A radical trachelectomy begins with a laparoscopic or robot-assisted lymphadenectomy. Following nodal assessment, the vaginal portion replicates the radical vaginal hysterectomy, except that the uterine fundus is retained. Amputating the uterine cervix at the level of the cervicouterine junction achieves the desired procedure, with approximately 1 cm of cervix left behind attached to the uterine fundus, although some gynecologic oncologists prefer that all uterine cervix tissue is removed at surgery. Intraoperative pathologic frozen section analysis confirms margin-free status. A cerclage is performed at the cervicouterine junction, and a probe opens the remaining endocervical canal. The pararectal space is closed, and the upper vagina sewn to the uterine stump by interrupted sutures. As some cervical tissue might remain depending on the tailored surgical procedure done, Pap cytology and pelvic examinations are done per routine screening protocols. Stenosis of the endocervical canal following the procedure has been noted.

Nerve-Sparing Radical Hysterectomy

Secondary to the added surgical dissection, radical hysterectomies may injure the hypogastric nerve plexus, disrupting bladder control and continence at a rate of 5%, in addition to rectal incontinence also secondary to nerve injury. In an attempt to avoid these potential life-altering morbidities, nerve-sparing procedures have been described (5-7). A nerve-sparing radical hysterectomy concentrates on avoiding the hypogastric nerve underneath the ureter lateral to the ureterosacral ligament and bypassing and preserving the inferior hypogastric plexus during removal of the cardinal and vesicouterine ligaments.

Total Pelvic Exenteration

Primary management of cervical cancer via a total pelvic exenteration has been completed in select patients with clinical stage IVA uterine cervix cancer, but its main use remains as a therapeutic option for the management of central pelvic relapses without evidence of extrapelvic disease. Exenterative surgery includes the en bloc removal of the uterine cervix, uterine corpus, bladder, rectum, and vagina. For select anteriorly located recurrences, an anterior pelvic exenteration removes the uterine cervix, uterine corpus, bladder, and vagina, sparing the rectum and need for two ostomies. Alternatively, patients with a more posteriorly located recurrence may undergo a posterior pelvic exenteration that removes the uterine cervix, uterine corpus, rectum, and vagina, thus sparing the bladder and need for a urinary conduit. The procedure, whether tailored or not, is morbid—poor patient health, pelvic sidewall extension, hydronephrosis, and the presence of extrapelvic metastases are relative if not absolute contraindications to the procedure. Perioperative mortality occurs in up to 14% of surgical patients (8). Thorough radiographic imaging such as by PET/CT or PET/MRI is recommended to determine the disease extent before surgery (9,10). Long-term sexual dysfunction and associated psychosocial impact must be considered by the patient and the surgeon before undertaking this procedure (11).

REFERENCES

1. Ramirez PT, Frumovitz M, Pareja R, et al. Minimally invasive versus abdominal radical hysterectomy for cervical cancer. *N Engl J Med.* 2018;379(20):1895-1904. doi:10.1056/NEJMoa1806395
2. Charo LM, Vaida F, Eskander RN, et al. Rapid dissemination of practice-changing information: a longitudinal analysis of real-world rates of minimally invasive radical hysterectomy before and after presentation of the LACC trial. *Gynecol Oncol.* 2020;157(2):494-499. doi:10.1016/j.ygyno.2020.02.018
3. Querleu D, Morrow CP. Classification of radical hysterectomy. *Lancet Oncol.* 2008;9(3):297-303.
4. Debernardo R, Starks D, Barker N, et al. Robotic surgery in gynecologic oncology. *Obstet Gynecol Int.* 2011;2011:139867.
5. Ditto A, Martinelli F, Mattana F, et al. Class III nerve-sparing radical hysterectomy versus standard class III radical hysterectomy: an observational study. *Ann Surg Oncol.* 2011;18(12):3469-3478.
6. Charoenkwan K, Srisomboon J, Suprasert P, et al. Nerve-sparing class III radical hysterectomy: a modified technique to spare the pelvic autonomic nerves without compromising radicality. *Int J Gynecol Cancer.* 2006;16(4):1705-1712.
7. Raspagliesi F, Ditto A, Fontanelli R, et al. Type II versus type III nerve-sparing radical hysterectomy: comparison of lower urinary tract dysfunctions. *Gynecol Oncol.* 2006;102(2):256-262.
8. Petruzziello A, Kondo W, Hatschback SB, et al. Surgical results of pelvic exenteration in the treatment of gynecologic cancer. *World J Surg Oncol.* 2014;12:279.
9. Lakhman Y, Nougaret S, Micco M, et al. Role of MR imaging and FDG PET/CT in selection and follow-up of patients treated with pelvic exenteration for gynecologic malignancies. *Radiographics.* 2015;35(4):1295-1313.
10. Burger IA, Vargas HA, Donati OF, et al. The value of 18F-FDG PET/CT in recurrent gynecologic malignancies prior to pelvic exenteration. *Gynecol Oncol.* 2013;129(3):586-592.
11. Rezk YA, Hurley KE, Carter J, et al. A prospective study of quality of life in patients undergoing pelvic exenteration: interim results. *Gynecol Oncol.* 2013;128(2):191-197.

CHAPTER 4.5

Cervical Cancer: Pathology

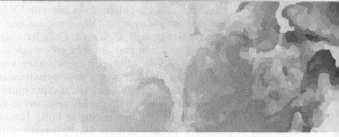

Charles A. Leath III and Teresa K. L. Boitano

SQUAMOUS CELL CARCINOMA

Squamous cell carcinoma remains the most common histologic subtype of cervical cancer and includes microinvasive and, more deeply, invasive squamous cancer cell variants that may differ in biologic behavior, such as verrucous, papillary squamous, transitional, warty, or lymphoepithelioma-like carcinoma.

Preinvasive Disease

HSIL defines full-thickness epithelial neoplasia of the cervix, without penetration of the basement membrane, where the normal maturation steps of a squamous epithelium are absent. Cells often have enlarged oval nuclei, increased nuclear-to-cytoplasm ratios, and mitotic figures (**Figure 4.5-1**). Persistent squamous cell carcinoma in situ became invasive cancer in 22% of New Zealand women over a 5-year period (1).

Microinvasive Disease

Microinvasive squamous cell carcinoma typically arises from squamous intraepithelial neoplasia, originating from surface epithelium and/or from endocervical glands. Microinvasive carcinoma is an irregular, haphazardly arranged minute nest of squamous cells that have penetrated the basement membrane of the surface or glandular epithelium. Cells have abundant eosinophilic cytoplasm, tend to be larger, and are associated with a desmoplastic stromal reaction (**Figure 4.5-2**).

Depth of invasion is critical in assessing if a lesion is a microinvasive squamous cell carcinoma. Specifically, the depth of invasion should be measured from the originating basement membrane.

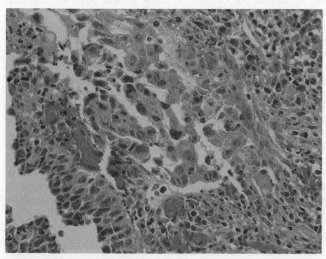

Figure 4.5-2. Microinvasive squamous carcinoma. There is an area of squamous carcinoma in situ (lower left). A nest of invasive carcinoma cells (center) has broken through the basement membrane. The invasive cells are larger, with more abundant cytoplasm and larger, more pleomorphic nuclei. A desmoplastic stroma response is present (right).

When carcinoma arises from the surface epithelium, depth is the distance from the basement membrane of the surface epithelium to the deepest nest of invasive cells. Alternatively, when carcinoma arises from an endocervical gland, the depth is measured from the basement membrane of the gland. When the site of origin, surface epithelium versus endocervical gland, is unclear, the depth should be measured from the basement membrane of the surface epithelium. In addition, any observed nests of superficially invasive squamous cells from small biopsies should be reported along with the dimensions of any invasive tumor. A diagnosis of microinvasive squamous cell carcinoma of the cervix requires a loop diathermy or conization biopsy that encircles the entire lesion with negative margin. A surgicopathologic study of 133 patients with microinvasive cancer of the uterine cervix (1965-1976) noted tumor penetration was less than 1 mm in 38%, 1 to 2 mm in 30%, 2 to 3 mm in 17%, 3 to 4 mm in 12%, and 4 mm or greater in 4% (2). No lymph node metastases were detected at the time of radical hysterectomy in 74 patients. Only two (1.5%) patients developed relapse (2).

Invasive Disease

Invasive squamous cell carcinoma of the uterine cervix arises most often from the progression of untreated or undertreated high-grade dysplasia. This progression may have been detected up to 10 years prior. When considering all preinvasive disease, it has been demonstrated that CIN 2 is 8 times more likely and CIN 3 is 22 times more likely to progress to carcinoma in situ or invasive cancer than CIN 1 (3). HPV is associated with invasive

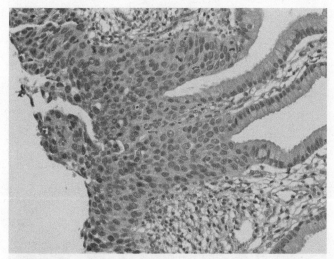

Figure 4.5-1. Squamous carcinoma in situ. The epithelium displays full-thickness atypia. Cells have enlarged, hyperchromatic nuclei, and there is no evidence of maturation.

disease in more than 86% of incident cases (4). Grossly, tumors may be firm indurated masses, polypoid, or ulcerated with or without apparent necrosis. Microscopically, irregular and haphazardly infiltrating nests of cells are noted. Cells have an eosinophilic cytoplasm and nuclei that are enlarged, atypical, and hyperchromatic (**Figure 4.5-3**). Mitoses may be either and or/ both numerous and atypical. Moreover, a desmoplastic stromal reaction occurs around invasive cell nests and is often quite pronounced, perhaps indicating host immune cell response to virally altered uterine cervix cells and manifesting as bulky tumor (5). LVSI may be present, especially in more deeply invasive tumors, and should be noted pathologically.

Although not prognostically significant, squamous cell carcinomas are labeled as keratinizing or nonkeratinizing. Keratinizing squamous cell carcinomas show keratin pearl architecture, whereas nonkeratinizing squamous cell carcinomas lack keratin pearls, with intercellular bridges and display abundant eosinophilic cytoplasm. Small cells lacking neuroendocrine differentiation are classified as nonkeratinizing squamous cell carcinomas.

Tumor grading is also applied to invasive squamous cell carcinomas. Although somewhat rare, grade 1 well-differentiated cancers possess keratin pearls and are composed of predominantly keratinized cells. Although grade 1 cell nuclei demonstrate modest atypia, mitoses are rare. The majority of squamous cell carcinomas are grade 2 moderately differentiated cancers, typically nonkeratinizing, display nuclear pleomorphism and more numerous mitoses, and have an infiltrative pattern. Grade 3 or poorly differentiated cancers may have smaller cells without neuroendocrine differentiation or are pleomorphic with anaplastic nuclei. Grade 3 cancers have a propensity for spindle-shaped cells, which must be distinguished from sarcoma by positive cytokeratin stains.

SQUAMOUS CELL CARCINOMA VARIANTS

Papillary Squamous and Transitional Cell Carcinoma

One variant of cervical carcinoma includes papillary superficial architecture with substantial nuclear atypia. Like other cervical cancers, the most common presenting symptoms include vaginal bleeding and abnormal Pap test results. Examination of the cervix may reveal papillary, polypoid, or granular lesions. Papillary squamous and transitional cell carcinomas may have either thin or thick papillae, with connective tissue cores covered by highly atypical epithelium displaying keratinization. Assessment of the

epithelium occasionally reveals multiple layered cells with oval hyperchromatic nuclei without keratinization and resembles urothelial transitional cell epithelium. At times, nuclear grooves may be present. The majority of these tumors are cytokeratin 7 (CK7) positive and cytokeratin 20 (CK20) negative on immunohistochemical (IHC) analysis; these results are consistent with a squamous cell differentiation. HPV-16 DNA has been detected in addition to shared uroplakin III–negative, p63-positive, and p16^{INK4A}-positive immunophenotype, regardless of light microscopic features (6).

An underlying invasive squamous cell carcinoma may be associated with papillary squamous cell and transitional cell carcinomas. Although this may be an invasive squamous cell carcinoma, other cases of concomitant invasive cancers have been described. Importantly, superficial biopsies displaying only a papillary portion of the neoplasm may be inconclusive. An excisional biopsy of provider choice, appropriate to the patient, should be done to exclude an underlying invasive cancer.

Both local and systemic disease recurrence may occur with these cancer types. Verrucous carcinomas, which display little cell atypia and have a much more indolent clinical course, must be considered and differentiated from papillary squamous cell and transitional cell carcinomas.

Verrucous Carcinoma

Verrucous carcinomas are uncommon cervical cancers that arise in a papillary excrescence of the cervix, resembling condyloma acuminatum (perhaps the "giant condyloma of Buschke and Lowenstein"). Microscopically, pointed "church spire" papillary fronds of squamous epithelium lacking connective tissue cores are noted. Moreover, connective tissue beneath these fronds may display bulbous squamous epithelium nests that invade the stroma with a pushing margin but minor cytologic atypia. Significant nuclear atypia is uncommon and more consistent with another form of uterine cervix carcinoma. It is critically important to delineate verrucous carcinoma versus squamous cell carcinoma as verrucous carcinomas invade local tissues but tend not to metastasize elsewhere. Superficial biopsies are often nondiagnostic as verrucous carcinoma diagnosis necessitates visual inspection of the invasive portion of the tumor.

Warty Carcinoma

Rare papillary neoplasms with condylomatous changes that possess histopathologic features of invasive squamous cell carcinoma at their deep margin are known as *warty* carcinomas (7). HPV-related cellular changes ("koilocytotic atypia") are shown in **Figure 4.5-4**.

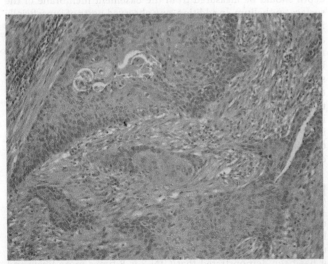

▌ **Figure 4.5-3.** Invasive squamous carcinoma. Small, irregular nests of cells with markedly atypical nuclei are present. They are surrounded by desmoplastic stroma containing inflammatory cells.

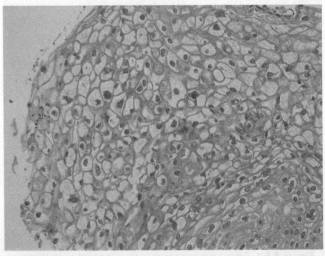

▌ **Figure 4.5-4.** Human papillomavirus changes. This squamous epithelium displays cells with large halos surrounding atypical nuclei ("koilocytotic atypia").

Lymphoepithelioma-Like Carcinoma

Lymphoepithelioma-like carcinoma is another histologic variant of cancer of the uterine cervix that is more commonly seen in the nasopharynx. Presentation may be variable clinically, ranging from a cervical tumor producing modest abnormal vaginal bleeding to a clinically absent tumor detected only by cervical cytology smears. These rare carcinomas present most often in Asian women and have been associated with Epstein-Barr virus infection in those patients (8), although this latter observation remains controversial. Microscopically, nests of cells with large vesicular nuclei with prominent eosinophilic nucleoli in pale eosinophilic cytoplasm are noted. Borders among cells may be indistinct, lending to a syncytial phenotype. A prominent inflammatory infiltrate consisting of lymphocytes, eosinophils, and plasma cells may be prominent. As compared with glassy cell carcinoma (also accompanied by prominent inflammation), lymphoepithelioma-like carcinomas indistinct cell margins and granular eosinophilic cytoplasm are differentiating findings. Moreover, predominantly CD8⁺ suppressor/cytotoxic T cells are present in the lymphocytic infiltrate (9).

ADENOSQUAMOUS CARCINOMA

Adenosquamous carcinomas are tumors consisting of an admixture of both malignant glandular cell and squamous cell elements. Adenosquamous carcinomas have high-risk features, including high-grade tumor cell, the presence of vascular invasion, and an overall aggressive malignant potential. Adenosquamous carcinoma should not be utilized as a surrogate descriptor for poorly differentiated squamous carcinomas, in which mucicarmine stains show only scattered mucin vacuoles. Moreover, this classification is not meant to suggest a true collision tumor, where an adenocarcinoma abuts a squamous cell carcinoma.

ADENOCARCINOMA

Adenocarcinoma of the uterine cervix is the second most common major histologic subtype, although it continues to rise in incidence, accounting for approximately 25% of incident cancer cases (10). In general, AIS is thought to be a precursor lesion for invasive adenocarcinoma (11). High-risk HPV type 18, 33, 35, 45, 51, 58, or 59 confers the risk for adenocarcinoma, although HPV-16 may occur as well (12).

Adenocarcinoma In Situ

Microscopically, AIS generally preserves endocervical gland architecture. Varying degrees of cytologic atypia, including nuclear enlargement and stratification, nuclear hyperchromasia, and mitotic figures, may be present (**Figure 4.5-5**). Most AISs occur near the transformation zone.

Adenocarcinoma

Adenocarcinoma of the uterine cervix demonstrates altered endocervical gland architecture as either solid or cribriform nests of cells, with architectural irregularity or incomplete glands lined by malignant cells, or small buds of highly atypical cells arising from glands involved by AIS. A desmoplastic stromal reaction may be present. Although the FIGO definition of microinvasive carcinoma theoretically applies to all types of cervical cancers, this has not generally been applied to adenocarcinoma of the uterine cervix because an increased incidence of metastatic disease corresponds to incremental increases in the depth of invasive disease.

Mucinous Adenocarcinoma

Endocervical, intestinal, signet-ring cell, minimal deviation, and villoglandular are mucinous adenocarcinoma variants. HPV DNA has been detected in 91% of mucinous adenocarcinomas of the cervix (13).

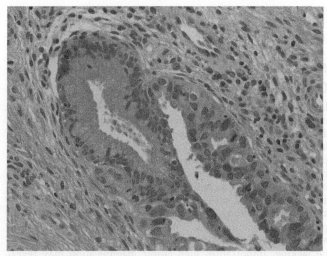

Figure 4.5-5. Adenocarcinoma in situ. Part of this endocervical gland is normal (upper left corner). Stratified cells with atypical, large nuclei and mitotic figures have replaced the remainder of the gland.

Mucinous Adenocarcinoma, Endocervical Variant

The most common type of mucinous adenocarcinoma is the endocervical variant. Microscopically, these lesions are characterized by limited cytoplasmic mucin but irregular, haphazardly arranged tuboloracemose glands are lined by cells resembling those seen in normal endocervical glands. Microscopically, nuclei are stratified, atypical, and basally located (**Figure 4.5-6**). Mitoses are noted. Well-differentiated grade 1 cancers have uniform nuclei with minimal stratification and few mitotic figures. Alternatively, grade 2 moderately differentiated adenocarcinomas have more conspicuous cytologic atypia with more frequent mitoses. In contrast, poorly differentiated grade 3 adenocarcinomas contain prominent pleomorphic nuclei, with solid areas and many more mitoses. Variable desmoplastic stromal response may be noted.

Mucinous Adenocarcinoma, Intestinal Type, Signet-Ring, and Colloid Variants

Rare variants of uterine cervix adenocarcinoma contain goblet cells in endocervical glands; these tumors possess intestinal differentiation. Signet-ring cell and colloid cell carcinomas are exceedingly

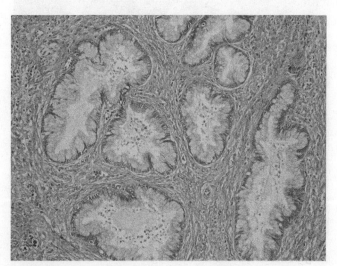

Figure 4.5-6. Well-differentiated glands infiltrate desmoplastic cervical stroma. The glands display a haphazard pattern. Nuclei are basally located but stratified and atypical.

rare in the uterine cervix. Accordingly, it is critical to distinguish these variants of adenocarcinoma from metastatic gastrointestinal (GI) tract cancers.

Mucinous Adenocarcinoma, Minimal Deviation Variant

Less than 1% of uterine cervix adenocarcinomas are the minimal deviation variant of mucinous adenocarcinoma (14) and do not appear to be associated with HPV infection (15). Visual inspection may reveal a normal-appearing cervix, although, pathologically, tumors are firm, tan yellow and may be found in hysterectomy samples. Small biopsies may not result in a definitive diagnosis, and a conization may be necessary. Microscopic assessment reveals disorganized glands infiltrating the cervical stroma, with budding contours or angular peaked outlines. Low-power magnification may note seemingly innocuous benign-appearing glands. For diagnostic purposes, cytologic atypia must be lacking. Importantly, high-power magnification may reveal some nuclear enlargement, stratification, and rare mitotic figures in cells. The infiltrating glands are often lacking a substantial desmoplastic reaction.

Mucinous Adenocarcinoma, Well-Differentiated Villoglandular Variant

Well-differentiated villoglandular adenocarcinomas are generally low-grade adenocarcinomas that appear as either a papillary or polypoid endocervical mass. These lesions may be associated with endocervical AIS. On microscopy, villous, papillary structures are present that assume either long and slender forms or short and broad forms. Moreover, a connective tissue core with inflammatory cells may be present in either. A single stratified layer of cells with endocervical, endometrial, or intestinal differentiation makes up the overlying epithelium. Mild-to-moderate atypia are present in the nuclei, and mitotic figures are infrequent (**Figure 4.5-7**). Invasive adenocarcinoma may exist below papillary areas, often characterized by a desmoplastic stroma among branching glands lined by atypical cells. These tumors lack marked nuclear atypia and epithelial tufting seen in the much more aggressive papillary serous carcinoma of the uterine cervix. Villoglandular uterine cervix cancer may be diagnostically challenging when only small biopsy specimens are available for review; a definitive diagnosis should be made only when

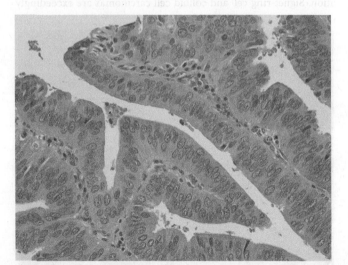

Figure 4.5-7. Well-differentiated villoglandular adenocarcinoma. Long, slender villous processes are covered with epithelium, displaying mild atypia. Nuclei are crowded, but they retain an oval shape and are uniform in size.

viewing conization or hysterectomy surgical specimens. High-grade cytologic findings in villoglandular cancers in addition an underlying obvious invasive adenocarcinoma may include lymphovascular invasion, lymph node metastases, as well as a higher risk of relapse (16).

Adenocarcinoma, Endometrioid Variant

Endometrioid carcinomas are rare and potentially over diagnosed variants of uterine cervical cancers, accounting for 7% of all adenocarcinomas of the uterine cervix. As the name suggests, these tumors have nearly identical pathologic findings to endometrioid cancers of the uterine corpus. Importantly, with these identical appearances, a primary endometrial adenocarcinoma with endocervical extension and/or possible drop metastasis masquerading as a uterine cervix cancer must be excluded, and this can be aided with the use of high-risk HPV in situ hybridization (ISH), IHC, and tumor molecular testing. IHC findings seen in endocervical primary cancers include carcinoembryonic antigen (CEA) positivity, estrogen receptor (ER) negativity, and vimentin negativity, whereas the opposite signature characterizes uterine corpus primary cancers. Adjunctively, HPV markers, such as p16, also favor a uterine endocervix primary cancer.

Adenocarcinoma, Clear Cell Variant

Traditionally, clear cell cancers of the uterine cervix are associated with intrauterine DES exposure; however, clear cell cancers may also occur in the absence of DES exposure. Pathologic assessment reveals a solid pattern with sheets of cells with abundant glycogen-rich clear cytoplasm, atypical nuclei, and numerous mitoses. The tubulocystic pattern includes alternating tubule and cystic spaces lined by oxyphilic, hobnail, or clear cells, whereas the papillary pattern is the least common and consists of mixed solid and tubulocystic areas. Clear cell carcinomas of the cervix are not known to be secondary to HPV infection (15).

Adenocarcinoma, Papillary Serous Variant

Papillary serous uterine cervix cancers are rare tumors not associated with HPV infection (15). Interestingly, there appears to be a bimodal age distribution, occurring in both patients younger than 40 years and patients older than 65 years. Gross pathologic examination is variable and may reveal a nodular mass, an indurated cervix, or no visible abnormality. Microscopically, these cancers appear identical to serous tumors of the endometrium and ovary and primary peritoneal serous carcinomas. Based on their rarity, it is paramount to exclude metastasis or extension of disease from another primary site, especially the endometrium. Fibrous papillae lined by atypical epithelial cells are present pathologically; tufts of malignant-appearing epithelial surface cells or secondary papillae are often present (**Figure 4.5-8**). Cancer cell tufting may cause glandular structures to have misshapen luminal borders. High-grade nuclear atypia with an abundant number of mitoses are observed. Although rare, these are aggressive cancers that often metastasize to pelvic, para-aortic, and groin lymph nodes and hence predict a poor prognosis.

Adenocarcinoma, Mesonephric Variant

Mesonephric duct remnants in the lateral aspects of the uterine cervix may present as lobules of small, round, glandular structures lined by flattened cuboidal epithelium with intraluminal periodic acid–Schiff stain (PAS)-positive material. As compared with cells lining endocervical glans, these cells do not contain intracytoplasmic mucin. Mesonephric-variant adenocarcinomas arise from the lateral mesonephric duct remnants and are extremely rare, with few cases reported. These cancers display ductal, tubular, retiform, solid, and sex cord–like patterns and cells that lack intracytoplasmic mucin.

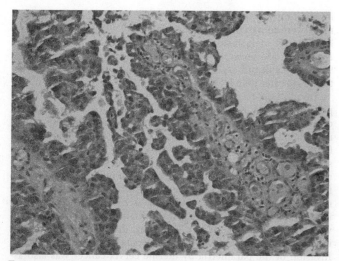

Figure 4.5-8. Serous adenocarcinoma. The papillary structures have a connective tissue core. There is marked tufting and stratification, and the nuclei are markedly atypical.

Adenocarcinoma, Microcystic Endocervical Variant

Microcystic endocervical–variant adenocarcinoma is exceedingly rare, with less than 10 cases described (17). Presentation is similar to other variants with abnormal bleeding and/or cytologic test results. Pathognomonic findings include many low-power microscopic cystic and dilated glands, whereas magnification reveals abundant cytologic atypia and mitoses. Mucinous or intestinal endocervical adenocarcinoma pockets are observed; cells are deeply invasive. Postsurgical recurrences have been recorded.

Glassy Cell Carcinoma

Glassy cell carcinoma is thought to represents an uncommon variant of generally poorly differentiated adenosquamous carcinoma, containing cells with eosinophilic cytoplasm, well-defined margins, and prominent nucleoli in addition to the presence of a plasma cell infiltrate. Relapses of adenosquamous carcinomas or adenocarcinomas following radiation may assume a glassy cell carcinoma appearance (10).

Adenoid Cystic Carcinoma

Adenoid cystic carcinomas of the uterine cervix are aggressive, rare malignancies presenting most often in older patients with bleeding. A cribriform gland pattern, with glands enclosing hyaline or mucinous material, is noted microscopically, whereas nuclei are often large and pleomorphic, both to a greater extent as compared with adenoid basal epithelioma. Both mitoses and necrosis may be present. Cytokeratin effectively stains these cells, although in contrast to the salivary gland variant, this cervical cancer does not exhibit myoepithelial cells, either by IHC for S100 protein or by electron microscopy. Both relapses and metastases may occur.

Adenoid Basal Epithelioma (Carcinoma)

Adenoid basal epitheliomas, originally "adenoid basal carcinoma," are generally indolent, rare neoplasms of the uterine cervix. HPV-16 DNA has been observed in these cancers (15). Some have suggested that these lesions may, in fact, be the precursors for a variety of uterine cervix carcinomas, and as such, subclassification as adenoid basal epitheliomas versus carcinomas should be used. Microscopically, adenoid basal epitheliomas display cell nests with a basaloid appearance and peripheral palisading. Gland lumina are found within nests, although the number of formed glands are

variable. Squamous metaplasia and mitoses are seen infrequently. Adenoid basal epithelioma, in the absence of a coexisting invasive carcinoma, is benign. Importantly, however, this must be distinguished from adenoid cystic carcinoma, given the profound difference in oncologic phenotype. Adenoid basal epitheliomas with carcinomatous components are considered cancers and should be reported accordingly.

NEUROENDOCRINE CANCERS

Standardized diagnostic assessments and labeling of neuroendocrine tumors of the uterine cervix allow epidemiology and natural history chronologies of these cancers (18). IHC chromogranin or synaptophysin stains are utilized to provide needed diagnostic evidence of neuroendocrine differentiation, except in small cell carcinoma of the uterine cervix. Typical carcinoids of the uterine cervix are extremely rare and should be identified with extreme caution as most uterine cervix neuroendocrine tumors are aggressive and too few cases of typical carcinoid have described the histopathology and natural history of this cancer variant. Atypical carcinoids of the uterine cervix are also rare, display organoid cell nests, have a mitotic rate of 5 to 10 foci per high-power microscope field of view, and may have necrosis and display nuclear atypia. Large cell neuroendocrine carcinomas of the uterine cervix (**Figure 4.5-9**) possess numerous mitotic figures (>10 foci per high-power microscope field of view), variable levels of necrosis as well as organoid cell nests with peripheral palisading of nuclei, prominent nucleoli, and eosinophilic cytoplasmic granules. In addition to coexisting AIS or adenocarcinoma of the cervix, LVSI is frequent, thus marking these cancers as highly aggressive neoplasms. As noted, evidence of neuroendocrine differentiation is required with chromogranin or synaptophysin using IHC testing.

Small Cell Carcinoma

The majority of neuroendocrine cancers originating from the uterine cervix are small cell carcinomas. Small cell carcinomas consist of cells having scant cytoplasm, nuclear molding, inconspicuous nuclei with finely stippled chromatin, extensive necrosis, crush artifact, and numerous mitotic figures (**Figure 4.5-10**). Single-cell infiltration of the stroma is commonly noted as is LVSI. Small cell carcinomas, even when a minority is of a mixed tumor, are associated with a poor prognosis and can be difficult to treat with recurrences common.

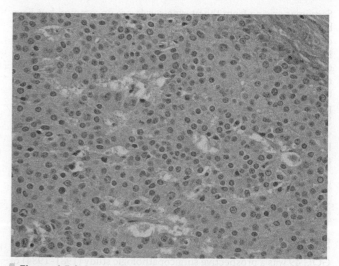

Figure 4.5-9. Large cell neuroendocrine carcinoma. This tumor displays organoid architecture. The tumor cells are much larger than those seen in small cell carcinoma. They have abundant eosinophilic cytoplasm, and there are numerous mitotic figures. Areas of necrosis were present elsewhere in the tumor.

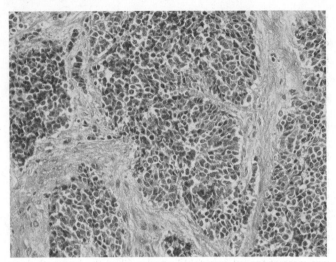

Figure 4.5-10. Small cell neuroendocrine carcinoma. This tumor displays cells that are smaller than those of squamous carcinoma. Nuclei are large and atypical with molding of adjacent nuclei. There is a very high mitotic rate.

MIXED EPITHELIAL AND MESENCHYMAL TUMORS

Various sarcomas have been noted arising from the uterine cervix, including Müllerian adenosarcomas (19). These tumors are polypoid or papillary masses often associated with nonmenstrual bleeding. Cells form benign-appearing glands in a sarcomatous stroma in addition to a periglandular cuff of condensed stroma that may be present. The sarcomatous component demonstrates an inconsistent number of mitotic figures and intermittently may display heterologous elements, such as striated muscle or cartilage. Although Müllerian adenosarcomas are associated with a favorable prognosis, deep invasion and sarcomatous overgrowth are adverse prognostic factors. Malignant mixed Müllerian tumors may involve the cervix and present at a variable stage, with early-stage disease patients generally responding well to therapy (20).

OTHER MALIGNANT TUMORS

Sarcomas arising from the uterine cervix are uncommon but have been seen. A large histopathologic review of 1,583 malignancies of the uterine cervix found only eight (0.5%) sarcomas (21), which included five carcinosarcomas and three unclassified, leiomyosarcomas, or endometrial stromal sarcomas. Other unusual cervical tumors include extranodal lymphomas of typically diffuse B-cell origin (22), primitive neuroectodermal tumors (23), and desmoplastic small round cell tumors (24) which have all been described. Secondary tumors of the uterine cervix may include neoplasms invading from contiguous organs (such as the uterine corpus, urinary bladder, or rectum) or metastases from other organ sites (such as the ovary, uterus, or other visceral organs).

UTERINE CERVIX CANCER PROGNOSTIC FACTORS

Surgicopathologic Factors

GOG 49 was a prospective surgicopathologic study (1981-1984) of untreated stage I uterine cervix cancers, including 732 squamous cell carcinomas, in order to evaluate prognostic factors and cancer outcome (25,26). Per protocol, patients required a radical hysterectomy with pelvic and para-aortic transperitoneal lymphadenectomy

in addition to peritoneal cytology. Grossly visible primary tumors were more commonly associated (85/477, 21%) with pelvic lymph node metastases than occult primary tumors (15/168, 9%; $P = .009$). Moreover, 3-year disease-free survival estimates were 95% for occult tumors, 88% for tumors 3 cm or less, and 68% for tumors greater than 3 cm.

In addition to gross tumor presence or absence, the risk of pelvic lymph node metastases was also associated with the depth of invasion in fractional thirds more so than absolute tumor size in millimeters—5% for inner third (9/199), 13% for middle third (28/210), and 26% (60/227) for outer third ($P = .0001$). This invasive depth was also assessed for 3-year disease-free survival estimates, reporting 94% for inner third, 85% for middle third, and 74% for outer third invasion. LVSI was also associated with an increased risk of pelvic lymph node metastasis, as 25% (70/276) of positive invasion cases had nodal metastases versus 8% (30/366) when invasion was absent ($P = .0001$). Three-year disease-free survival was inferior in positive LVSI cases, 77% versus 89% in negative cases. Invasion of the parametria by uterine cervix cancer was also associated with risk for pelvic lymph node metastases. Forty-three percent (194/44) of cases with parametrial involvement had metastatic pelvic lymph nodes compared with 14% (81/599) of cases when absent ($P = .0001$).

Interestingly, age at diagnosis appeared the least predictive of risk of lymph node metastases (25) and loses more significance when 50 years is used as an arbitrary breakpoint (26). These surgicopathologic data suggest that for a moderately differentiated uterine cervix cancer with middle third invasion and no LVSI or parametrial invasion, the expected probabilities of lymph node metastases in women aged 35, 45, 55, or 65 years are 9%, 8%, 5%, and 3%, respectively (25).

Lymph Node Factors

Metastasis to lymph nodes from uterine cervix cancer has long been acknowledged as a major prognostic factor, with surgical and radiotherapeutic management decisions partially based on the risk for nodal disease. Tumor with 5 mm or less invasion had a pelvic lymph node metastatic rate of 3% (6/177 patients), the lowest risk of nodal disease in a surgicopathologic study (25), although 16 (22%) of 74 patients with uterine extension had pelvic lymph node metastases (25). Grade of tumor also appears to be correlated with nodal involvement as well-, moderately, and poorly differentiated tumors had the risk for pelvic lymph node metastases of 10% (9/93), 14% (52/373), and 22% (39/179), respectively (25); 545 patients with no pelvic node metastases had a 3-year disease-free interval estimate of 86%, whereas 100 patients with positive pelvic node metastases had a 3-year disease-free interval estimate of 74% (26). The 3-year disease-free intervals were 72%, 86%, and 65% for one, two, and three or more positive pelvic nodes, respectively, following surgical resection, suggesting a potentially limited impact on prognosis based on the number of resected positive nodes (26). Despite the well-known and long-standing significant impact of nodal status on prognosis, nodal metastasis was not included in the FIGO staging system until recently, with the updated 2018 FIGO staging (27).

Clinical Stage Factors

Although FIGO staging is important, the unique historical role of clinical stage for cervical cancer has been found to be an inconsistent or even weak-risk factor in an era where radiographic and pathologic information are more powerful prognostic factors. Nonetheless, a multivariate analysis of prognostic variable among 626 women included in therapeutic clinical trials demonstrated a correlation between clinical stage and progression-free interval (28). This secondary analysis of three slightly different trials conducted between 1977 and 1985 included 150 patients who received RT alone, 136 patients who received RT and *Corynebacterium parvum*, 156 patients who received RT plus misonidazole, and 184 patients who received RT and hydroxyurea. Patients underwent para-aortic nodal assessment before therapy, and para-aortic lymph node metastases were associated with 6-fold risk for death and 11-fold risk for short progression-free interval (28). The investigators stated that with increased risk of node positivity, the differential outcomes based on clinical stage decreases. In this summary, and albeit secondary analysis, the investigators concluded that the combination of the most predictive risk factor (node status) with the most commonly used risk factor (clinical stage) presents a clear separation of patients in regard to uterine cervix cancer survival (28).

Histopathology Factors

The role of pathology in clinical outcomes remains controversial and warrants continued assessment. In a study from the U.S. Military Health Care System, 185 women with adenocarcinoma and 88 women with adenosquamous carcinoma were studied for clinical outcomes. Adenosquamous histopathology was associated with a significantly decreased 5-year survival (65% vs 83%; $P < .002$). (29). In a randomized clinical trial of radiation alone versus radiochemotherapy of 243 patients, histopathology lost its prognostic significance when chemotherapy was added (30). To that point, in an analysis of completed GOG chemoradiation clinical trials, although survival for adenocarcinoma or adenosquamous cervical cancer treated by radiation alone was inferior when compared with patients with squamous carcinoma, survival was not lower when cisplatin-based chemotherapy was added for 112 as compared with 842 women with squamous cell cancer ($P = .459$) (31). More recently, Levinson and colleagues suggested that much of the collected knowledge for adjuvant therapy recommendations, including the Sedlis pathologic criteria, for intermediate-risk patients following a radical hysterectomy may not be applicable to patients with adenocarcinoma (32).

Hypoxia and Anemia Factors

Four hundred ninety-four women were treated on two consecutive prospective RT trials, including 278 (56%) with stage II and 216 (44%) with stage III or IV disease (33). Adjusting for patient age, race, performance status, cancer stage, tumor size, cell type, and duration of radiation, mean hemoglobin values during treatment were found to predict disease progression ($P < .0001$). While pretreatment values were not predictive of disease progression, when a 6-week treatment course was divided into 2-week periods (early, middle, and late), hemoglobin values during the late period were the most predictive of disease progression ($P = .0289$). A comprehensive review of translational science confirms the same observations (34).

Anemia is thought to impact patterns of relapse and survival in women with uterine cervix cancer (35), and packed red blood cell infusions are recommended to address this anemia. Recombinant human erythropoietin has been used to stimulate red blood cell production and maintain hemoglobin levels above 12 g/dL. In a GOG trial (36), women with stage IIB-IVA uterine cervix cancer and an initial hemoglobin less than 14 g/dL were randomly assigned to cisplatin radiochemotherapy without or with recombinant human erythropoietin (40,000 units subcutaneously weekly) with a stated objective of maintaining hemoglobin at 12 g/dL or higher. Erythropoietin was to be stopped if hemoglobin was greater than 14 g/dL. Secondary to increased thromboembolic events attributed to erythropoietin, the study closed prematurely with less than 25% of the planned accrual. With a median follow-up of 37 months, 3-year PFS and OS were estimated at 65% and 75% after radiochemotherapy and 58% and 61% after radiochemotherapy plus erythropoietin, respectively. Thromboembolic events occurred in 4 (8%) receiving radiochemotherapy and 11 (19%) receiving radiochemotherapy plus erythropoietin. All thromboembolic events were not treatment related. No deaths occurred from thromboembolic events. With early closure, the role of hemoglobin during chemoradiation greater than 12 g/dL remains unanswered. A second observation deterring the use of erythropoietin is from a surgicopathologic study of 18 patients (1999-2002). Erythropoietin receptor expression was found in 16 (89%) of 18 uterine cervix cancers (37), suggesting the possibility that erythropoietin agents might stimulate the growth of uterine cervix cancer cells. As such, packed red blood cell infusions, not erythropoietin, are recommended to correct anemia, when clinically indicated, in patients with uterine cervix cancer.

Smoking may lead to tissue hypoxia, an important predictor of response to radiation. In GOG trial 165 that randomized 328 women to cisplatin-based radiation or to prolonged venous infusion 5-fluorouracil (5-FU) radiation, 133 (42%) were reported smokers of any kind and 111 (40%) were smokers of nicotine-based products (38). A multivariate analysis revealed a significant increase in the risk of death (but not disease progression) for reported smokers (hazard ratio [HR], 1.51; 95% CI, 1.01-2.27, $P = .04$) and for tobacco-derived smokers (HR, 1.57; 95% CI, 1.03-2.38, $P = .04$). The biologic mechanism of this phenomenon remains under investigation.

Uterine Cervix Cancer Biomarkers and Imaging Correlates

Uterine cervix cancer biomarkers are under investigation (**Table 4.5-1**), including ribonucleotide reductase subunit expression (39).

PET scans have been studied as imaging correlates in uterine cervix cancer trials. In a small prospective trial of 32 patients with stage IIB-IVA cervical cancer, PET has 75% sensitivity and 92% specificity (40). Following chemoradiation, post-treatment FDG-avid uptake (persistent or new) has been negatively associated with metabolic treatment response, development of metastatic disease, and death from uterine cervix cancer (41-43). Consensus recommendations for patients in the National Cancer Institute trials to use of PET as an indicator of therapeutic response have been formulated (44)—a more than 25% increase in FDG standard uptake value (SUV) indicates progressive metabolic disease, a 25% or less increase or a less than 15% decrease in FDG SUV indicates stable metabolic response, a more than 15% reduction in FDG SUV indicates partial metabolic response, and complete absence of FDG SUV indicates complete metabolic response (45). In the modern era of radiotherapy, FDG responses more than 15% are seen with near uniformity and thus makes use of FDG PET imaging to assess uterine cervix cancer response after radiotherapy challenging (46). Kunos and colleagues evaluated a more rigorous "true" metabolic response, defined as a post-therapy/pretherapy uptake ratio of 0.33 or less, and found that this cutoff was more meaningful in assessing treatment response in a small chemoradiation study (46). Additional work by the same investigators in a prospective phase II radiochemotherapy trial found that a post-therapy/pretherapy uptake ratio of 0.33 or less occurred in 96% (23/24 [95% CI, 80%-90%]) of patients treated with radiochemotherapy (47) and none experiencing a local relapse at data lock and publication.

■ TABLE 4.5-1. Gynecologic Oncology Group Protocol 092 Eligibility Criteria		
Lymphovascular Space Involvement	Cervix Stromal Invasion	Tumor Size (cm)
Positive	Deep 1/3	Any
Positive	Middle 1/3	≥2
Positive	Superficial 1/3	≥5
Negative	Deep or middle 1/3	≥4

Alternatively, diffusion-weighted MRI (DWI-MRI), dynamic contrast-enhanced MRI (DCE-MRI), PET-MRI, or traditional MRI may be useful modalities in evaluating response to therapy, recurrence, and OS in cervical cancer. To evaluate serial MRI, scans before, during, and after RT were obtained in 115 women, including 52 also receiving cisplatin (48). Residual MRI tumor volumes of 20% or more detected at 4,000 to 5,000 cGy were independently associated with inferior 5-year local control (53% vs 97%, $P < .001$) and disease-specific survival rates (50% vs 72%, $P = .009$). After completion of radiation delivery, patients having residual MRI tumor volumes of 10% or more had no local control and a 17% disease-specific survival, compared with 91% local control and 72% disease-specific survival when less than 10% of tumor volume remained ($P < .001$).

REFERENCES

1. McIndoe WA, McLean MR, Jones RW, et al. The invasive potential of carcinoma in situ of the cervix. *Obstet Gynecol*. 1984;64(4):451-458.

2. Sedlis A, Sall S, Tsukada Y, et al. Microinvasive carcinoma of the uterine cervix: a clinical-pathologic study. *Am J Obstet Gynecol*. 1979;133(1):64-74.

3. Holowaty P, Miller AB, Rohan T, et al. Natural history of dysplasia of the uterine cervix. *J Natl Cancer Inst*. 1999;91(3):252-258.

4. Alemany L, de Sanjose S, Tous S, et al. Time trends of human papillomavirus types in invasive cervical cancer, from 1940 to 2007. *Int J Cancer*. 2014;135(1):88-95.

5. Sheu BC, Hsu SM, Ho HN, et al. Reversed CD4/CD8 ratios of tumor-infiltrating lymphocytes are correlated with the progression of human cervical carcinoma. *Cancer*. 1999;86(8):1537-1543.

6. Drew PA, Hong B, Massoll NA, et al. Characterization of papillary squamotransitional cell carcinoma of the cervix. *J Low Genit Tract Dis*. 2005;9(3):149-153.

7. Winkler B, Crum CP, Fujii T, et al. Koilocytotic lesions of the cervix. The relationship of mitotic abnormalities to the presence of papillomavirus antigens and nuclear DNA content. *Cancer*. 1984;53(5):1081-1087.

8. Tseng CJ, Pao CC, Tseng LH, et al. Lymphoepithelioma-like carcinoma of the uterine cervix: association with Epstein-Barr virus and human papillomavirus. *Cancer*. 1997;80(1):91-97.

9. Martorell MA, Julian JM, Calabuig C, et al. Lymphoepithelioma-like carcinoma of the uterine cervix. *Arch Pathol Lab Med*. 2002;126(12): 1501-1505.

10. Young RH, Clement PB. Endocervical adenocarcinoma and its variants: their morphology and differential diagnosis. *Histopathology*. 2002;41(3):185-207.

11. Nayar R, Wilbur DC. The Pap Test and Bethesda 2014. "The reports of my demise have been greatly exaggerated." (after a quotation from Mark Twain). *Acta Cytol*. 2015;59(2):121-132.

12. Castellsague X, Diaz M, de Sanjose S, et al. Worldwide human papillomavirus etiology of cervical adenocarcinoma and its cofactors: implications for screening and prevention. *J Natl Cancer Inst*. 2006;98(5):303-315.

13. Pirog EC, Kleter B, Olgac S, et al. Prevalence of human papillomavirus DNA in different histological subtypes of cervical adenocarcinoma. *Am J Pathol*. 2000;157(4):1055-1062.

14. Hart WR. Symposium part II: special types of adenocarcinoma of the uterine cervix. *Int J Gynecol Pathol*. 2002;21(4):327-346.

15. An HJ, Kim KR, Kim IS, et al. Prevalence of human papillomavirus DNA in various histological subtypes of cervical adenocarcinoma: a population-based study. *Mod Pathol*. 2005;18(4):528-534.

16. Kim HJ, Sung JH, Lee E, et al. Prognostic factors influencing decisions about surgical treatment of villoglandular adenocarcinoma of the uterine cervix. *Int J Gynecol Cancer*. 2014;24(7):1299-1305.

17. Tambouret R, Bell DA, Young RH. Microcystic endocervical adenocarcinomas: a report of eight cases. *Am J Surg Pathol*. 2000;24(3):369-374.

18. Albores-Saavedra J, Gersell D, Gilks CB, et al. Terminology of endocrine tumors of the uterine cervix: results of a workshop sponsored by the College of American Pathologists and the National Cancer Institute. *Arch Pathol Lab Med*. 1997;121(1):34-39.

19. McCluggage WG. Mullerian adenosarcoma of the female genital tract. *Adv Anat Pathol*. 2010;17(2):122-129.

20. Sharma NK, Sorosky JI, Bender D, et al. Malignant mixed mullerian tumor (MMMT) of the cervix. *Gynecol Oncol*. 2005;97(2):442-445.

21. Wright JD, Rosenblum K, Huettner PC, et al. Cervical sarcomas: an analysis of incidence and outcome. *Gynecol Oncol*. 2005;99(2):348-351.

22. Muntz HG, Ferry JA, Flynn D, et al. Stage IE primary malignant lymphomas of the uterine cervix. *Cancer*. 1991;68(9):2023-2032.

23. Malpica A, Moran CA. Primitive neuroectodermal tumor of the cervix: a clinicopathologic and immunohistochemical study of two cases. *Ann Diagn Pathol*. 2002;6(5):281-287.

24. Khalbuss WE, Bui M, Loya A. A 19-year-old woman with a cervicovaginal mass and elevated serum CA 125. Desmoplastic small cell tumor. *Arch Pathol Lab Med*. 2006;130(4):e59-e61.

25. Delgado G, Bundy B, Fowler WJ, et al. A prospective surgical pathological study of stage I squamous carcinoma of the cervix: a Gynecologic Oncology Group Study. *Gynecol Oncol*. 1989;35(3):314-320.

26. Delgado G, Bundy B, Zaino R, et al. Prospective surgical-pathological study of disease-free interval in patients with stage IB squamous cell carcinoma of the cervix: a Gynecologic Oncology Group study. *Gynecol Oncol*. 1990;38(3):352-357.

27. Bhatla N, Aoki D, Sharma DN, Sankaranarayanan R. Cancer of the cervix uteri. *Int J Gynaecol Obstet*. 2018;143(suppl 2):22-36. doi:10.1002/ijgo.12611

28. Stehman FB, Bundy BN, DiSaia PJ, et al. Carcinoma of the cervix treated with radiation therapy. I. A multi-variate analysis of prognostic variables in the Gynecologic Oncology Group. *Cancer*. 1991;67(11):2776-2785.

29. Farley JH, Hickey KW, Carlson JW, Rose GS, Kost ER, Harrison TA. Adenosquamous histology predicts a poor outcome for patients with advanced-stage, but not early-stage, cervical carcinoma. *Cancer*. 2003;97(9):2196-2202. doi:10.1002/cncr.11371

30. Monk BJ, Wang J, Im S, et al. Rethinking the use of radiation and chemotherapy after radical hysterectomy: a clinical-pathologic analysis of a Gynecologic Oncology Group/Southwest Oncology Group/Radiation Therapy Oncology Group trial. *Gynecol Oncol*. 2005;96(3):721-728.

31. Rose PG, Java JJ, Whitney CW, et al. Locally advanced adenocarcinoma and adenosquamous carcinomas of the cervix compared to squamous cell carcinomas of the cervix in gynecologic oncology group trials of cisplatin-based chemoradiation. *Gynecol Oncol*. 2014;135(2):208-212.

32. Levinson K, Beavis AL, Purdy C, et al. Beyond Sedlis-A novel histology-specific nomogram for predicting cervical cancer recurrence risk: an NRG/GOG ancillary analysis. *Gynecol Oncol*. 2021;162(3):532-538. doi:10.1016/j.ygyno.2021.06.017

33. Winter WE 3rd, Maxwell GL, Tian C, et al. Association of hemoglobin level with survival in cervical carcinoma patients treated with concurrent cisplatin and radiotherapy: a Gynecologic Oncology Group Study. *Gynecol Oncol*. 2004;94(2):495-501. doi:10.1016/j.ygyno.2004.04.008

34. Fyles AW, Milosevic M, Pintilie M, et al. Anemia, hypoxia and transfusion in patients with cervix cancer: a review. *Radiother Oncol*. 2000;57(1):13-19.

35. Dunst J, Kuhnt T, Strauss HG, et al. Anemia in cervical cancers: impact on survival, patterns of relapse, and association with hypoxia and angiogenesis. *Int J Radiat Oncol Biol Phys*. 2003;56(3):778-787.

36. Thomas G, Ali S, Hoebers FJ, et al. Phase III trial to evaluate the efficacy of maintaining hemoglobin levels above 12.0 g/dL with erythropoietin vs above 10.0 g/dL without erythropoietin in anemic patients receiving concurrent radiation and cisplatin for cervical cancer. *Gynecol Oncol*. 2008;108(2):317-325.

37. Shenouda G, Mehio A, Souhami L, et al. Erythropoietin receptor expression in biopsy specimens from patients with uterine cervix squamous cell carcinoma. *Int J Gynecol Cancer*. 2006;16(2):752-756.

38. Waggoner S, Darcy K, Fuhrman B, et al. Association between cigarette smoking and prognosis in locally advanced cervical carcinoma treated with chemoradiation: a Gynecologic Oncology Group study. *Gynecol Oncol*. 2006;103(3):853-858.

39. Kunos C, Winter K, Dicker A, et al. Ribonucleotide reductase expression in cervical cancer: a radiation therapy oncology group translational science analysis. *Int J Gynecol Cancer*. 2013;23(4):615-621.

40. Rose PG, Adler LP, Rodriguez M, et al. Positron emission tomography for evaluating para-aortic nodal metastasis in locally advanced cervical cancer before surgical staging: a surgicopathologic study. *J Clin Oncol*. 1999;17(1):41-45.

41. Grigsby PW, Siegel BA, Dehdashti F, et al. Posttherapy [18F] fluorodeoxyglucose positron emission tomography in carcinoma of the cervix: response and outcome. *J Clin Oncol*. 2004;22(11):2167-2171.

42. Schwartz J, Siegel B, Dehdashti F, et al. Association of post-therapy positron emission tomography with tumor response and survival in cervical carcinoma. *JAMA*. 2007;298(19):2289-2295.

43. Schwartz J, Grigsby P, Dehdashti F, et al. The role of 18F-FDG PET in assessing therapy response in cancer of the cervix and ovaries. *J Nucl Med*. 2009;50(suppl 5):64S-73S.

44. Shankar L, Hoffman J, Bacharach S, et al. Consensus recommendations for the use of 18F-FDG PET as an indicator of therapeutic response in patients in National Cancer Institute Trials. *J Nucl Med.* 2006;47(6):1059-1066.

45. Young H, Baum R, Cremerius U, et al. Measurement of clinical and subclinical tumor response using 18F-fluorodeoxyglucose and positron emission tomography: review and 1999 EORTC recommendations. *Eur J Cancer.* 1999;35(13):1771-1782.

46. Kunos C, Radivoyevitch T, Abdul-Karim F, et al. 18F-fluoro-2-deoxy-d-glucose positron emission tomography standard uptake value as an indicator of cervical cancer chemoradiation therapeutic response. *Int J Gynecol Cancer.* 2011;21(6):1117-1123.

47. Kunos C, Radivoyevitch T, Waggoner S, et al. Radiochemotherapy plus 3-aminopyridine-2-carboxaldehyde thiosemicarbazone (3-AP, NSC #663249) in advanced-stage cervical and vaginal cancers. *Gynecol Oncol.* 2013;130(1):75-80.

48. Mayr NA, Wang JZ, Lo SS, et al. Translating response during therapy into ultimate treatment outcome: a personalized 4-dimensional MRI tumor volumetric regression approach in cervical cancer. *Int J Radiat Oncol Biol Phys.* 2010;76(3):719-727.

CHAPTER **4.6**

Radiation Therapy, Immunotherapy, and Targeted Therapies in Cervix Cancer

Dmitriy Zamarin, Charles A. Kunos, Casey W. Williamson, Jyoti Mayadev, and Ramez N. Eskander

RADIATION THERAPY

External Beam Radiation Therapy

Conventional Whole Pelvis Radiation

The radiation target has long been both the primary cervix cancer and the pelvic lymph nodes, whether or not known to be involved by metastases (1,2). Two-dimensional (2D) radiation treatment fields or portals for the treatment of uterine cervix cancer were traditionally drawn using bony landmarks of vertebral spine interspaces, pelvic brim dimensions, and, possibly, radiopaque markers for the uterine cervix, vagina, rectum, and bladder. Anteroposterior two-field or anteroposterior and lateral four-field "box" treatment portals irradiate primary disease targets and node-bearing tissue. Intraoperative mapping done in 100 women undergoing radical surgery (3) found common iliac blood vessel bifurcation cephalad to the lumbosacral prominence in 87% of patients. As such, the superior border of traditional anteroposterior portals is placed at the L4-L5 interspace to enclose

the external iliac and internal iliac (hypogastric) lymph nodes or, more commonly, at the L2-L3 interspace to include common iliac lymph nodes. In the same study (3), pelvic width was 12 cm at the obturator fossae and 14 cm at the inguinal ring femoral arteries. Thus, the lateral border of anteroposterior portals is placed 2 cm lateral to the widest pelvic brim to ensure pelvic lymph node inclusion. The inferior border of anteroposterior portals is placed at the lowest extent of the obturator foramen and at least 4 cm below the lowermost extent of uterine cervix disease. Lateral portals use the same superior and inferior border positions as in anteroposterior fields. The posterior border of lateral portals is placed behind the posterior aspect of the sacrum to ensure that the uterosacral and cardinal ligaments are entirely encompassed (3). The anterior border of lateral portals lies in front of the pubic symphysis inferiorly and cuts in superiorly to limit bowel dose but maintains a 3-cm margin on the vertebral bodies so that iliac nodes are dosed appropriately. CT-based RT became standard by the late 1990s (**Figure 4.6-1**), which allows for 3D treatment planning, including quantification of dose to target volumes and organs at risk (OARs).

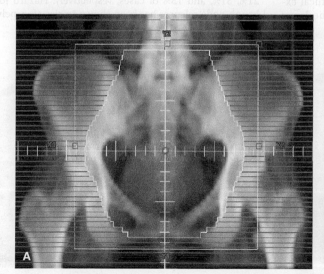
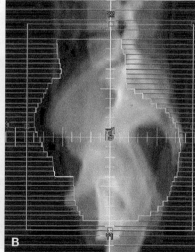

Figure 4.6-1. Standard conventional fields for external beam whole-pelvis radiation therapy. A: Anteroposterior port. B: Lateral port.

Intensity-Modulated Radiation Therapy for Uterine Cervix Cancer

Intensity-modulated radiation therapy (IMRT) uses a multifield radiation beam arrangement with variable beam fluency to generate radiation dose clouds closely conforming to radiation targets. The utilization of IMRT has increased rapidly and, at many institutions, is now standard for both definitive and postoperative RTs for cervical cancer (4). Radiation planning is CT based, with targets and OARs specifically contoured for each patient. MRI and PET image overlays are often used to ensure that targets are not missed, which becomes increasingly important owing to precipitous radiation dose fall-off with the technique and the concomitant drive to reduce toxicity by treating less normal tissue. There are multiple strategies to create planning margins around the targets to account for setup uncertainties and organ motion, including the creation of an internal target volume encompassing the difference in target anatomy between a full and an empty bladder, as well as a validated anisotropic expansion strategy designed to reliably encompass the target structures (5,6). Treatment machines might utilize "step-and-shoot" or "sliding-window" or helical tomotherapy or "volumetric-modulated arc therapy" to deliver the desired radiation dose. Anatomic atlases and contour guidelines have been published and updated (7). An example of the intensity-modulated radiation dose cloud is depicted in **Figure 4.6-2**. Dose-volume histograms plot the proportion of target volume or of an OAR volume planned to receive dose over the course of the radiation prescription. Treating radiation oncologists use this information to balance sufficient delivery of radiation dose with hazard for organ injury. Modern prospective protocols include updated target dose goals and OAR limits to ensure adequate target coverage and prevent excessive dose to critical normal structures. IMRT often results in high target coverage by the prescription dose and low OAR exposure. Grossly involved lymph nodes can be boosted relative to elective nodal doses with either a sequential boost or a simultaneous integrated boost, which appears to be tolerable and efficacious (8). Furthermore, image guidance during treatment, including the use of cone beam CT with the patient on the treatment table immediately before treatment on a weekly or daily basis, allows for near real-time visualization of both target volumes and OARs and can improve treatment accuracy (**Figure 4.6-3**).

There are pitfalls that treating radiation oncologists must be aware of when using IMRT. Target and OAR motions due to respiration, bladder fill, and rectal fill have been documented. With applied radiation dose, central pelvic disease might regress such that intrapelvic target position rests outside the IMRT dose clouds (9). Consensus guidelines have been published (7), and there are online atlases available (eg, www.econtour.org). Early clinical experience suggested that GI and marrow toxicities may be lower with IMRT (10,11). Reports from multiple prospective trials continue to support the use of IMRT. The TIME-C trial included 289 postoperative patients with cervical and endometrial cancer and randomized participants between standard RT and IMRT and showed improvements in bowel and urinary symptoms along with patient-reported diarrhea metrics (12). Similarly, the PARCER trial randomized patients between adjuvant 3D conformal radiation and IMRT and found improvements in toxicity associated with IMRT, including late GI toxicity and several patient-reported measures including diarrhea, appetite, and overall bowel symptoms, with no difference in oncologic outcomes (13). The phase II/III INTERTECC trial enrolled patients with intact cervical cancer and showed a reduction in high-grade neutropenia with image-guided bone marrow–sparing IMRT (14).

Some patients may experience substantial changes in anatomy during the course of treatment, including weight loss, tumor regression, and variation in bowel and/or bladder filling that may not have been fully appreciated at the time of CT simulation. In these cases, adaptive replanning can be considered. Several strategies have been discussed. In one, a "plan-of-the-day" technique involves the generation of a patient-specific library of treatment plans corresponding to different anatomic configurations. Pretreatment cone beam CT scanning can allow for the selection of the library plan most similar to the anatomy that day. Another strategy is simply to repeat the CT simulation either at a scheduled point during the treatment course or as needed upon review of the setup imaging. Interim diagnostic imaging such as MRI can also be helpful. Emerging technologies are also enabling "online" adaptive RT delivery, using the integration of iterative cone beam CT scans for dose calculations and daily replanning (15) or MRI-based online replanning (16).

Extended-Field Radiation Therapy for Uterine Cervix Cancer

Extended-field RT can produce clinical benefit (17). Reluctance to use extended-field radiation portals centers on a perception of excessive radiation dose delivered to the spinal cord, kidneys, and small intestine. Traditional extended-field portals extend the superior border of pelvic radiation portals to include the 12th thoracic vertebral body and involve matching pelvic and para-aortic fields. IMRT can be used to encompass the entire extended field in one plan. A typical extended-field IMRT plan would extend cranially to the L1/L2 interspace or 3-cm cranial to the most superior gross disease (**Figure 4.6-4**).

Clinical stage IB, II, III, or IVA uterine cervix cancers are associated with a risk of para-aortic lymph node metastases in 5%, 21%, 31%, and 13% of cases, respectively. Hazard for para-aortic lymph node relapses has been shown to rise after pelvic field–only

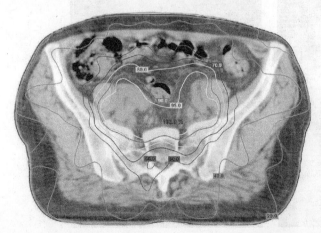
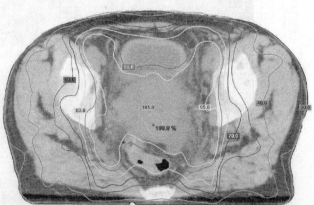

Figure 4.6-2. Typical dose distributions using intensity-modulated radiation therapy to deliver pelvic radiation therapy in uterine cervix cancer.

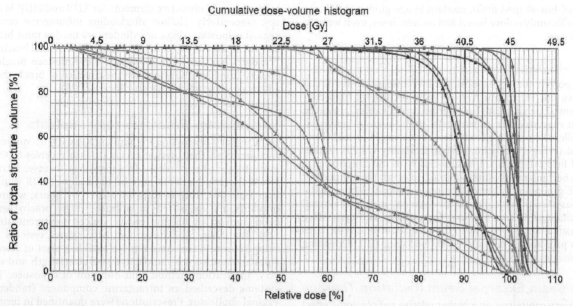

Figure 4.6-3. A dose-volume histogram (DVH) comparing a four-field "box" arrangement (squares) with an intensity-modulated radiation therapy plan (triangles). The DVH plots doses to the planning target volume and the organs at risk.

radiochemotherapy. Given orderly lymphatic dissemination of uterine cervix cancer, adjuvant extended-field RT is a logical treatment strategy that might avoid risks and delays associated with surgical staging of para-aortic lymph nodes. In a randomized trial (17), 10-year relapse rates in the pelvis were 35% for pelvic-only fields and 31% for extended fields. First sites of failure were distant (non–para-aortic metastases) more often in the pelvic-only arm as compared with the extended-field arm (P = .05). The extended-field arm had more grade 4 or above complications, particularly in those patients with prior abdominal surgery (11% vs 2%).

Extended-field radiochemotherapy has been delivered safely in an 86-patient clinical trial. Radiation involved 4,500 cGy to para-aortic lymph nodes in all, 3,960 cGy to the pelvis in clinical stage IB or IIB patients, and 4,860 cGy to the pelvis in clinical stage IIIB or IVA patients. Point A intracavitary brachytherapy prescriptions were 4,000 cGy in IB/IIB patients and 3,000 cGy in IIIB/IVA patients. Point B doses were raised to 6,000 cGy by parametrial boost. Chemotherapy involved cisplatin (50 mg/m²) and 5-FU (4,000 mg/m²)

administered weeks 1 and 5 of RT. Grade 3 or above acute toxicities were mostly GI (19%) or hematologic (15%). Late morbidity risk was 14% at 4 years for mostly rectal complications. Relapses were pelvis only in 21%, distant only in 21%, and pelvis plus distant in 11% of the patients. The RTOG 90-01 randomized patients with locoregionally advanced cervical cancer (with no upfront evidence of para-aortic nodal involvement) to pelvic radiation with concurrent chemotherapy versus para-aortic radiation (without chemotherapy) with an OS benefit in the pelvic chemoradiation group (OS 67% for the pelvic chemoradiation group vs 41% for the para-aortic radiation group, P < .0001). Therefore, the current standard is pelvic chemoradiation, reserving extending field chemoradiation for cases with para-aortic nodal involvement at diagnosis.

Groin Inguinal Lymph Node Radiation

For clinical stage IIIA uterine cervix cancer that involves the distal one third of the vagina, the radiation treatment portal must be widened in the low pelvis to enclose inguinal lymph nodes because of the increased likelihood of metastases. CT cross-sectional anatomy lends itself to measurement of nodal depth and adequate radiation dosing. Two-field radiation portals are commonly used to avoid problems with underdosing and field junctions (18). IMRT techniques have been described (19).

Midline Shield Use Before Brachytherapy

A midline shield has been used to block normal central pelvic tissues during a parametrial boost after a 4,500 cGy dose—a technique using standard two-field anteroposterior fields to boost radiation dose to pelvic sidewall lymph nodes (brachytherapy point B) while blocking midline anatomy (20). A midline shield places brachytherapy prescription point A on the shield edge. Practices introducing a midline shield at 3,000 to 4,000 cGy attempt to protect the bladder and the rectum from excessive delivered radiation dose before brachytherapy, realizing that disease is shielded. Proponents of an early shield argue that intracavitary brachytherapy dose provides sufficient makeup dose to sterilize central pelvic disease. Objectors of an early shield argue that central pelvic disease, once shielded, repairs, redistributes, reoxygenates, and repopulates uterine cervix cancer cells, essentially undoing therapeutic effects of already applied radiation dose. Moreover, relative to

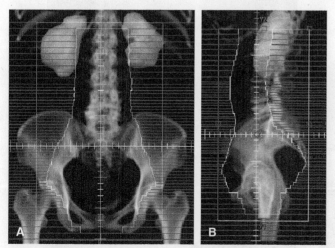

Figure 4.6-4. Portals of extended-field radiation therapy. A: Anteroposterior portal. B: Lateral portal. Yellow shadows indicate kidneys.

conventional box-shaped fields, modern image-guided IMRT can generally sufficiently reduce bowel and rectum doses, even without a midline shield.

Small Field Radiation

Radiation portals for occult postoperative disease or for intact disease have not varied much in 30 years because of high concern for central pelvic relapse of uterine cervix cancer. However, it has been suggested that in surgically staged node-negative patients, smaller-than-standard radiation portals might be useful and meaningful to lower radiation-related morbidity (21,22). Rather than small field RT portals, IMRT, inclusive of the common iliac nodes, has become more commonplace. However, the multicenter EMBRACE group and other institutions do adjust elective nodal coverage based on the risk of nodal involvement, including a "small pelvis" excluding the common iliac for patients with early-stage disease versus a "large pelvis" up to the aortic bifurcations or "large pelvis plus para-aortic" field up to the renal veins (23), depending on the clinical scenario.

Particle Beam External Beam Radiation Therapy

Proton therapy capitalizes on a higher relative radiobiologic effect as compared to photon therapy and a more rapid dose fall-off distal to target depth (the characteristic Bragg peak). This could potentially reduce toxicity, although the reported clinical use of particle beam external beam radiation therapy (EBRT) remains quite limited (24,25). When compared to IMRT plans in a small series, proton plans showed reduced volumes of pelvic bone marrow, bladder, and bowel that received doses in the 10 to 30 Gy range (25). Protons could potentially reduce bowel dose, particularly when large para-aortic fields are needed, and early data also demonstrate feasibility of ovarian sparing (26), but additional prospective studies are needed to clarify the degree to which dosimetric improvements translate to clinical benefits and to what extent routine use might be cost-effective.

Uterine Cervix Brachytherapy

Brachytherapy refers to "short-distance" RT. Uterine corpus and uterine cervix conduit anatomies lend themselves well to the placement of intracavitary applicators for high radiation dose delivery. Treatment can be delivered with a low-dose rate (LDR) or high-dose rate (HDR) system. [137]Cesium and [192]iridium are the most popular radioactive elements for LDR and HDR brachytherapy, respectively. Hollow afterloading intrauterine tandem and vaginal colpostats, rings, or cylinders are used in most brachytherapy practices. For both intracavitary and interstitial brachytherapy, [192]iridium has gained in popularity. The American Brachytherapy Society provides guidelines for the practice of brachytherapy for advanced-stage uterine cervix cancer (27,28).

Intracavitary Brachytherapy Implants

Intracavitary brachytherapy implants usually accompany EBRT treatments so that uterine cervix disease receives 8,000 cGy or more total radiation dose. In early-stage disease, intracavitary brachytherapy implants may be used alone. LDR implants deliver radiation dose in rates measured by hours, whereas HDR implants are measured in minutes. LDR brachytherapy has been applied in uterine cervix cancer treatment since 1913 (29). The Paris, Stockholm, and Manchester systems were developed around the same time to establish a set of standardized rules accounting for radioactive source strength and its geometry, application method, and duration of exposure. The three systems described an intrauterine component (tandem) and a vaginal applicator. Prescriptions were quantified in terms of milligram-hours, that is, the product of the total mass of [226]radium or radium equivalent (eg, [137]cesium) contained in the sources and the duration of the application in hours.

The Manchester system first used units of radiation exposure (Roentgens) rather than milligram-hours in radiation dose prescriptions. The dose in Roentgens was prescribed to specific points, termed point A and point B. Point A was defined as a point 2 cm lateral to the center of the uterine canal and 2 cm from the lateral vaginal fornix mucous membrane in the plane of the uterus. Point A served as a surrogate for average radiation dose delivered to the "paracervical triangle." Point B was defined as 5 cm lateral from the patient's midline at the same level as point A. Point B represented a surrogate for average radiation dose delivered to obturator lymph nodes. A variety of tandem and ovoid applicator loadings aimed for a relatively constant point A dose rate of 50 to 55 cGy/hour. The widely used Fletcher-Suit applicator system, loadings, and reference points A and B in U.S. brachytherapy practices are all derived from the Manchester system.

Computer-assisted isodose curve determinations provide optimal means of point A, point B, bladder, and rectum radiation dose (**Figure 4.6-5**). The International Commission on Radiation

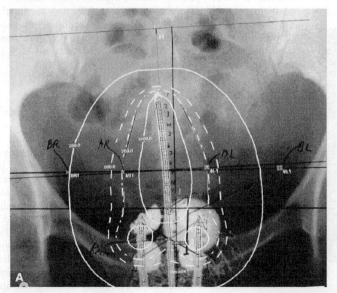
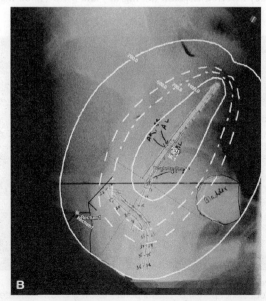

Figure 4.6-5. Axial (A) and (B) sagittal views of tandem and ovoids showing dose distribution superimposed on reconstructed computed tomography images.

Units and Measurements (ICRU) Report No. 38 (ICRU-38) (30) defines radiation dose and volume specifications for the reporting of gynecologic intracavitary brachytherapy. ICRU-38 recommends that reference points, such as point A, not be used, because "such points are located in a region where the dose gradient is high and any inaccuracy in the determination of the distance results in large uncertainties in the absorbed doses evaluated at those points." Instead, ICRU-38 brought forth the concept of a 6,000-cGy reference volume (including the contribution of dose delivered by external beam treatment). A pear-shaped reference volume should be described in terms of its three dimensions according ICRU-38: height (maximum dimension along the intrauterine sources), width (maximum dimension perpendicular to the intrauterine sources), and thickness (maximum dimension perpendicular to the intrauterine sources in the oblique sagittal plane). Opponents of ICRU-38 reporting cite lack of rationale for a 6,000-cGy reference volume, leading to poor acceptance by brachytherapy practitioners (31). ICRU-38 bladder and rectal reference points are used.

Determination of the ICRU-38 bladder reference point involves the use of a Foley catheter placed in the bladder and the Foley balloon filled with 7 cm³ of radiopaque fluid. On a lateral radiograph, the reference point is the posterior balloon surface. Overfill of the Foley balloon will lead to an underestimation of the bladder average dose and an overestimation of the bladder maximum dose. Underfill of the Foley balloon will lead to an overestimation of the bladder average dose and underestimation of the bladder maximum dose.

Determination of the ICRU-38 rectal reference point involves the use of a rectal marker or intravaginal radiopaque mold. On a lateral radiograph, the reference point is the anterior most point along the rectal marker closest to the uterine tandem or lies 5 mm posterior to the posterior aspect of an intravaginal mold or vaginal packing.

The first insertion of an LDR intracavitary implant occurs after 4,000 to 4,500 cGy of EBRT. A prescription dose of 2,000 cGy is common but might be raised for optimal geometry or might be lowered for suboptimal geometry. This is done to decrease lesion size and to improve applicator relationships of the uterine cervix and vagina. Midline shields are employed in some practices, as discussed earlier. A second insertion is performed 1 or 2 weeks later, with a prescription dose of 2,000 cGy or a dose needed to bring the total brachytherapy dose to 4,000 to 4,500 cGy.

However, the use of HDR brachytherapy has substantially increased in recent years, with a survey showing that 85% of respondents in the Unites Stated now employ HDR (32). HDR has several important advantages, including the possibility of outpatient treatment and less exposure to staff. Given the high doses involved, a great deal of care and attention must be placed on the placement of the applicator and the dose delivered to both the target volume and the sensitive OARs.

There are several modern applicator devices available, including tandem and ovoid, tandem and ring, and hybrid applicators, which include supplemental interstitial needles to improve the dose distribution. The choice of applicator depends on tumor size, location, and degree of vaginal and parametrial extent. Smaller tumors with minimal vaginal and/or parametrial involvement can be well covered with an intracavitary device, whereas larger or irregularly shaped tumors with vaginal and/or parametrial involvement may be best treated with a hybrid intracavitary/interstitial approach. Large residual tumors with extensive vaginal or parametrial disease may require a fully interstitial implant. Emerging evidence shows improvements in both target dosing and OAR sparing with a hybrid approach, when indicated (33).

HDR implants are associated with a variety of radiation prescriptions (**Table 4.6-1**). A common practice involves four insertions once or twice weekly and a prescription of 700 cGy per fraction. HDR implants can be scheduled in the fourth or fifth week of daily pelvic external beam radiation or shortly following the completion of EBRT as long as the total treatment package time is less than 8 weeks.

■ **TABLE 4.6-1. Suggested Schedules of HDR-ICBT in the United States**

External Beam Radiation Therapy	HDR-ICBT	EQD2
4,500 cGy in 25 fractions	700 cGy × 4	8,390 cGy
	600 cGy × 5	8,420 cGy
	550 cGy × 5	7,980 cGy
	500 cGy × 6	8,180 cGy
	800 cGy × 3	8,020 cGy

Prescriptions intended for tandem and ovoid, or tandem and ring applicators. EQD2, normalized dose; HDR-ICBT, high-dose rate intracavitary brachytherapy.

Image-Guided Brachytherapy

Although an empiric point A prescription point has proven useful, better understanding of brachytherapy dose distribution using modern imaging techniques enables better radiation dose cloud coverage of tumor and delivery of less radiation dose to normal organs. Guidelines (34,35) for image-based brachytherapy and its reporting have been written (**Table 4.6-2**). Investigators recommend T2-weighted MRI scans as the preferred method for scanning implant geometry. In an image-guided brachytherapy application, gross tumor volume (GTV), clinical tumor volume (CTV), and OARs are contoured, allowing quantitative analysis of implant geometry and doses delivered to both targets and OARs through dose-volume histograms. The radiation dose is then prescribed to the personalized treatment volume that day rather than a fixed geometric point. In a 10-patient case series, MRI was similar to CT when contouring OARs, but CT overestimated uterine cervix tumor widths compared to MRI (36). Tumor width overestimates were adequate for contouring OARs. The investigators suggested that MRI was the preferred imaging modality for image-based brachytherapy because prescription doses were likely to be more accurate anatomically. Limited availability of MRI-compatible applicators and expense has slowed adoption of image-based brachytherapy. Recent studies and a consensus guideline have suggested that primarily CT-based planning can be sufficient for image-guided brachytherapy, although the addition of at least one MRI, with or without instrumentation, is informative in most patients (34,37). The prospective EMBRACE-I study has reported excellent outcomes with modern image-guided brachytherapy, including an actuarial 5-year local control rate of 92% (95% CI 90%-93%), with similar local control across all FIGO stages (38). In addition, the prospective French STIC trial randomized patients between 2D and 3D brachytherapy planning and showed not only that 3D image-guided brachytherapy was feasible, but local control was improved and the incidence of grade 3 to 4 toxicity was reduced by one-half (39).

■ **TABLE 4.6-2. GEC-ESTRO Recommended Parameters for Recording and Reporting MRI-Guided Brachytherapy**

Total Reference Air Kerma (TRAK)
Dose at point A (right, left, mean)
D100 for GTV, HR-CTV, and IR-CTV
D90 for GTV, HR-CTV, and IR-CTV
D0.1cc, D1cc, and D2cc for OAR (eg, rectum, sigmoid, bladder)

GEC-ESTRO, The Groupe Européen de Curiethérapie and the European Society for Therapeutic Radiology and Oncology; GTV, gross tumor volume; HR-CTV, high-risk clinical target volume; IR-CTV, intermediate-risk clinical target volume; MRI, magnetic resonance imaging; OAR, organ at risk.

Brachytherapy Dose Rate Considerations

Radiation dose rate impacts radiobiologic effectiveness (40). Conventional external beam radiation delivered by teletherapy machines delivers radiation dose at a rate ranging from 100 to 300 cGy/minute. Teletherapy radiation doses are fractionated. In contrast, brachytherapy doses can be delivered continuously or in fractions and over a much broader range of dose rates.

ICRU defines LDR brachytherapy as an exposure between 40 and 200 cGy/hour, medium dose rate brachytherapy as between 200 and 1,200 cGy/hour, and HDR brachytherapy as greater than 1,200 cGy/hour. When dose rates are lowered, radiobiologic effects decrease owing to enhanced sublethal DNA damage repair and cancer cell repopulation. Late-responding (slowly proliferating) tissues show enhanced sublethal DNA damage repair, whereas acute-responding (rapidly proliferating) tissues or cancers do not (41). During continuous LDR exposure, late-responding tissues show greater tolerance to radiation exposure. During HDR exposure, late-responding tissues show low tolerance to radiation exposure. Owing to this phenomenon, HDR brachytherapy has a narrower therapeutic window than LDR brachytherapy. Because distance from an HDR source should be maximized to minimize effect on normal tissue, rectal retractors and gauze packing are used in this technique. To allow easier access to the uterine cavity, cervical sleeves may be placed. Pulsed-dose rate brachytherapy provides a workaround of this radiobiologic phenomenon—hourly brief (5 minutes or so) exposures to HDR sources kill cancer cells but preserve late-responding tissues (42). Guidelines for pulsed-dose rate brachytherapy have been written (32). Isoeffective pulsed-dose rate brachytherapy has been reported (43,44). Local disease control rates and technique-related toxicity among LDR, pulsed-dose rate, and HDR brachytherapy techniques appear similar.

Interstitial Implants

Interstitial perineal implants are a treatment option when uterine intracavitary implants are not possible anatomically. Implants are planned and completed using a perineal template, such as the Syed-Neblett Interstitial Template (**Figure 4.6-6**). Fluoroscopy or ultrasound aids in needle positioning during the procedure. Laparoscopy can be used to reduce the risk of bowel perforation by deeply positioned needles. Interstitial brachytherapy may involve CT and MRI fusion preplanning, operative placement of perineal needles using predetermined template maps, postprocedural CT-based planning, and afterloading therapy using [137]cesium and [192]iridium continuous LDR sources or [192]iridium HDR sources. Only experienced radiation oncologists should perform the procedure in centers familiar with the procedure.

Brachytherapy Radiation Doses for Uterine Cervix Cancer

American women with uterine cervix cancer often receive 4,500 cGy in 25 fractions pelvic radiation for therapeutic intent before brachytherapy. LDR brachytherapy typically adds 4,000 cGy to point A over a single or two intracavitary insertions. A range in LDR brachytherapy dose has been accepted, with small less than 1 cm tumors receiving 3,000 cGy prescription doses, whereas larger tumors receive 4,500 to 5,000 cGy prescription doses when normal anatomy permits.

An isoeffective HDR prescription dose may be 25% less than the typical LDR dose. A dose of 2,800 cGy in four equally divided 700 cGy fractions is a common prescription (**Table 4.6-1**). For a median biologic equivalent dose at point A of 101 Gy10 (EQD2 [normalized dose] = 8,400 cGy), a 3-year local control rate as high as 97% has been reported (45). For the same dose, actuarial 3-year grade 3 or above adverse events occurred at a rate of 17%. Another case series found that an EQD2 of 8,500 cGy provided an at least 86% rate of local control and 2-year hazard for grade 3 or above adverse events of 14% (46).

Radiochemotherapy plus image-guided (MRI) adaptive intracavitary brachytherapy (700 cGy × 4 doses) for an EQD2 dose of at least 8,700 cGy as studied in a single-institution 156-patient trial (2001-2008) produced 3-year pelvic disease control rates of 95% in patients with nonbulky stage IB/IIB and 85% in patients with bulky stage IIB/III/IV uterine cervix cancer (47). Late morbidity totaled 188 grade 1 or 2 and 11 grade 3 or 4 late adverse events were documented in 143 assessable patients. Spatial distribution of radiation

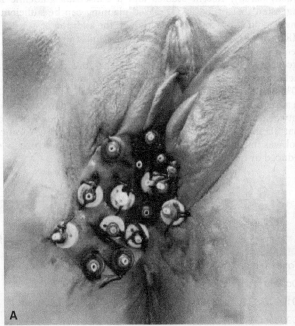
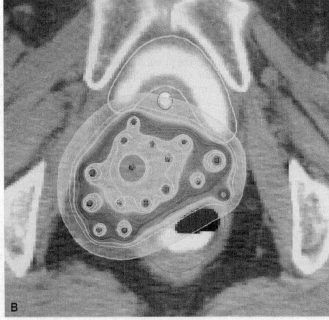

Figure 4.6-6. High-dose rate interstitial brachytherapy for vaginal stump recurrence. A: External view of the application. Vinyl template applicators are used in this case. B: Dose distribution curves superimposed on a relevant computed tomography image. Red line: 100% prescribed isodose line. Orange line: clinical tumor volume. (Special courtesy of Dr. K. Yoshida, Department of Radiology, Osaka National Hospital.)

dose (48), MRI/CT planning techniques (49), and interfraction anatomic variation (50) impact results from radiochemotherapy plus image-guided adaptive intracavitary brachytherapy.

Altered Radiation Fractionation

Conventional pelvic EBRT schedules use a 180- to 200-cGy fraction size delivered once per day, 5 days per week. Pelvic RT plus brachytherapy should be completed by 56 ± 3 days. Nonstandard altered fractionation may employ hypofractionation (larger doses per fraction, lower total dose), hyperfractionation (smaller doses per fraction given more frequently, eg, two or three small 120 cGy fractions per day), accelerated fractionation (standard fraction sizes given twice [BID] or more daily), or concomitant boosts (larger volume irradiation plus additional small fraction irradiation to a reduced volume on the same day). In an accelerated hyperfraction trial (1999-2002), 3,000 cGy pelvic radiation (150 cGy/fraction BID) plus 2,000 cGy pelvic radiation with a midline shield (200 cGy/fraction daily) was delivered. Two to four brachytherapy implants were done. Median treatment time was 35 days. Both a 5-year local control rate of 84% and 5% grade 3 or above adverse rate were reported.

Stereotactic body radiation therapy (SBRT) utilizes hypofractionated RT to precisely deliver high radiation dose with relative sparing of nearby OARs, and its implementation in other disease sites has led to the prospect of an SBRT-based boost. Early dosimetric analysis showed encouraging SBRT plans compared to brachytherapy plans (51), and a small early clinical study showed feasibility for patients who were deemed unable to undergo brachytherapy (52). However, a phase II trial treating patients with an SBRT boost in lieu of brachytherapy was closed prematurely due to lower-than-expected 2-year local control, PFS, and OS, along with higher-than-expected toxicity, including a cumulative 2-year grade 3 or more toxicity of 26.7% (53). Patient selection may have played a role in the development of these discouraging results, but brachytherapy clearly remains the standard of care. Other potential roles for SBRT could be to treat persistent or limited locoregionally recurrent uterine cervix cancer (54) or limited sites of distant disease.

Total Radiation Therapy Treatment Time

Conventional pelvic EBRT plus brachytherapy finishes in 56 ± 3 days. A loss of pelvic disease control of 1% per day is seen when complete RT exceeds this limit (55). In a retrospective review of two prospective randomized clinical trials of 335 patients (56), prolonged radiation (delayed for any cause) was associated with poorer PFS (HR, 1.98; 95% CI, 1.16-3.38, P = .012) and OS (HR, 1.88; 95% CI, 1.08-3.26; P = .024).

Urgent Palliative Radiation for Uterine Cervix Cancer

Urgent palliation of pelvic pain, obstruction, or bleeding may be needed for the patient with uterine cervix cancer. For significant vaginal bleeding, vaginal packing and urgent start of 300 to 400 cGy fraction per day RT may be done. Three or four fractions of radiation allow for conventional CT-based radiation planning. Conventional dose and schedule of EBRT plus brachytherapy typically follows. The use of palliative radiochemotherapy has been explored (57). However, as treatment planning and computational capacity have improved, IMRT plans can often be generated quickly and may often obviate the need to a preliminary 3D conformal plan. Patients with stage IVB or incurable recurrent carcinoma often require palliation of pelvic pain or bleeding, and their general condition may not warrant a prolonged course of external irradiation. A clinical trial of 290 patients (1985-1989) used a radiation dose of 4,440 cGy in 12 fractions (370 cGy BID, known as a "Quad Shot")

with a rest after 1,480 and 2,960 cGy. The rest interval was randomly allocated between 2 and 4 weeks to determine the effects on tumor control. No difference in tumor control was identified (P = .59). A 7% complication rate was noted at 18 months in survivors. This finding represents a significant lower rate of late complications as compared to a 49% rate seen with higher dose per fraction (1,000 cGy in one fraction repeated at 4-week intervals × 3 doses) in a prior trial (58).

IMMUNOTHERAPY AND TARGETED THERAPY APPROACHES IN CERVICAL CANCER

The majority of cervical carcinomas are directly linked to HPV infection, whereby integrated HPV sequences persist in the cancer cells and provide antigenic targets for recognition by the adaptive immune system. To evade the immune response, cervical cancers have evolved a number of immunosuppressive mechanisms. Several therapeutic approaches targeting HPV oncoproteins, cancer surface markers, and mechanisms of immune resistance have been explored with various success in this arena.

Therapeutic Vaccines

Therapeutic vaccines against HPV-associated cancers predominantly target the HPV-16 and HPV-18 E6 and E7 proteins. Therapeutic relevance of vaccination against HPV has been demonstrated in several trials in the setting of preinvasive disease. A study of HLA-restricted peptides HPV16 E7$_{12-20}$ and E7$_{86-93}$ was conducted in patients with high-grade vulvar or cervical lesions, demonstrating an ORR of 50% (59). A Phase II trial of a DNA-based vaccine VGX-3100 targeting HPV-16/18 E6 and E7 demonstrated a similar response of 50% in patients with cervical preinvasive lesions (CIN 2/3) (60).

Unfortunately, in the setting of advanced or recurrent cervical cancer, therapeutic vaccines have been less effective. Axalimogene filolisbac (ADXS11-001) is a live attenuated *Listeria monocytogenes* vaccine that secretes the endogenous Listeriolysin O protein fused with the HPV-16 E7 protein. A phase II trial of ADXS11-001 with or without cisplatin in patients with recurrent/refractory cervical cancer demonstrated a response rate of 14% to 17%, with a median OS of about 8 months (61). A follow-up study (GOG-265) of ADXS11-001 in 50 patients with advanced cervical cancer demonstrated an ORR of 6% and 12-month OS of 38%, which compared favorably with the historical 12-month survival rate of 21% (62). A study of an HPV-16–directed peptide vaccine in 13 patients with advanced cervical cancer demonstrated evidence of an anti-HPV T-cell response in the majority of patients; unfortunately, this did not translate into clinical benefit with no objective clinical responses seen in the study (63). Overall, these findings highlight that although therapeutic anti-HPV vaccines may have a role in the treatment of precancerous lesions, their role in the advanced disease setting remains unknown and may require combinations with other agents.

Adoptive Cell Therapies

Adoptive T-cell therapies are based on collection of T cells from patients followed by their expansion, selection, and manipulation ex vivo before reinfusion into patients, which is typically preceded by myeloablative chemotherapy to facilitate engraftment. Three key adoptive cell therapy approaches include tumor-infiltrating lymphocytes (TILs), T cells modified to express tumor-directed T-cell receptors (TCRs), and T cells modified to express chimeric antigen receptors (CAR T cells).

TIL therapy involves expansion of lymphocytes isolated from a surgically resected specimen. This approach has been explored in several trials in cervical cancer. In a trial of nine patients with metastatic cervical cancer, durable responses were seen in three patients (64). A larger phase II trial of adoptive T-cell therapy in 28 patients with HPV-related cancers (18 cervical) demonstrated response in 28% of patients with cervical cancer (65). C-145-04 is an ongoing phase II trial of TIL therapy in advanced cervical cancers, which demonstrated a response rate of 44% in 27 treated patients in an interim analysis presented at 2019 ASCO (66). Early trials of engineered T cells expressing TCRs directed to HPV-16 E6 or E7 have also demonstrated evidence of activity (67,68).

Antibody-Drug Conjugates

Evolution in antibody engineering strategies has made it possible to use antibodies as delivery vehicles for cytotoxic agents as antibody-drug conjugates (ADCs). Tissue factor (TF) is a cell surface protein that plays a role in the coagulation cascade and in cancer-related signaling pathways (69) and is highly expressed in the majority of cervical cancers (70). Tisotumab vedotin is a monomethyl auristatin E (MMAE)-liked ADC targeting TF. In a phase 2 trial of 102 patients with cervical cancer (innovaTV 204/GOG-3023/ENGOT-cx6), therapy with tisotumab vedotin resulted in ORR of 24%, with a 7% CR rate (71), leading to its accelerated approval by the Food and Drug Administration (FDA) for patients with previously treated cervical cancer. The confirmatory trial of tisotumab vedotin versus single-agent chemotherapy in patients with advanced cervical cancer is ongoing (NCT04697628).

Immune Checkpoint Blockade and Combinations

Activation of antitumor T-cell response is tightly regulated by negative immune regulatory receptors on the surface of T cells, collectively known as *immune checkpoints*. Several immune checkpoints, most commonly CTLA-4, PD-1, and the PD-1 ligand PD-L1, have been explored as therapeutic targets in cervical cancer. KEYNOTE-158 was a basket phase II trial of the PD-1 inhibitor pembrolizumab that included a 98-patient cervical cancer cohort. Twelve patients achieved an objective response, whereby responses were only seen in the patients with tumors expressing PD-L1. Although the ORR was modest, at 14%, those patients who responded to treatment exhibited response durations significantly longer than traditionally seen with chemotherapy. These findings led to the accelerated approval of pembrolizumab by the U.S. FDA for advanced PD-L1–positive, recurrent cervical cancer (72). A separate cohort of the KEYNOTE-158 trial explored tumors exhibiting high tumor mutational burden (TMB), defined as 10 or more mutations per megabase. Findings from the study led to FDA approval of pembrolizumab for patients with TMB 10 or greater, irrespective of cancer type, including cervical cancer (73). A randomized phase III clinical trial EMPOWER-Cervical 1/GOG-3016/ENGOT-cx9 compared cemiplimab, a PD-1 inhibitor, to investigator's choice single-agent chemotherapy in patients with cervical cancer who have progressed on platinum-based chemotherapy (74). In this study of 608 patients, cemiplimab therapy resulted in higher ORR (16.4% vs 6.3%) and OS (12 vs 8.5 months). Objective response of 18% was seen in patients with PD-L1 expression of 1% or greater and 11% in patients with PD-L1 expression of less than 1%. Despite this efficacy signal, lack of alignment regarding postmarketing studies resulted in withdrawal of the U.S. FDA application. Importantly, however, cemiplimab is approved for use in the treatment of recurrent cervical cancer internationally. A phase II trial of the anti–PD-1 inhibitor balstilimab in 161 patients with cervical cancer demonstrated an ORR of 15%, with ORR of 20% in PD-L1–positive tumors and 7.9% in PD-L1–negative tumors (75).

In addition to single-agent PD-1/PD-L1 inhibitors, several studies have focused on combinations of immune checkpoint inhibitors, namely, agents targeting CTLA-4 and PD-1. Combination of ipilimumab, a CTLA-4 inhibitor, and nivolumab, a PD-1 inhibitor, demonstrated a promising ORR of 36% in previously treated and 46% in untreated patients (76). Similarly, a trial of combination of CTLA-4 inhibitor zalifrelimab with balstilimab in 155 patients with previously treated cervical cancer demonstrated an ORR of 25.6%, with response rate of 32.8% observed in the PD-L1–positive cohort (77). A number of additional studies targeting PD-1 and PD-L1 in combination with antibodies targeting other checkpoints such as TIGIT (NCT04300647) or tisotumab vedotin (NCT03786081) are currently ongoing.

Given the potential immunomodulatory role of angiogenesis, several studies have explored antiangiogenic agents in combination with immune checkpoint inhibitors. Addition of bevacizumab to PD-L1 blockade with atezolizumab in bevacizumab-pretreated patients did not appear to increase response rate in an ETCTN-sponsored phase II study, prompting the study discontinuation after accrual of 10 patients to the first stage (78). A combination of a multitargeted tyrosine kinase inhibitor (TKI) apatinib with PD-1 inhibitor camrelizumab in 45 patients with cervical cancer demonstrated an impressive response rate of 55.6%, generating a strong rationale for further evaluation of similar strategies in patients with cervical cancer (79). Trials of other multitargeted TKIs such as lenvatinib and lucitanib in combination with PD-1 inhibitors are currently enrolling patients with different cancer types, including cervical (NCT04042116, NCT04865887).

Combinations of therapeutic vaccines with immune checkpoint inhibitors have also been explored in advanced disease setting. A trial of HPV-16– and HPV-18–directed DNA vaccine GX-188E administered in combination with pembrolizumab in 36 patients with advanced cervical cancer demonstrated an overall response rate (ORR) of 42%, including responses in patients whose tumors were negative for PD-L1 expression (80). These findings compare favorably to single-agent activity of pembrolizumab and generate rationale for further exploration (72).

The activity of PD-1 inhibitors in second-line setting generated strong rationale for their evaluation as part of the upfront regimen in advanced/metastatic disease. In a double-blinded phase 3 trial of platinum-based chemotherapy with bevacizumab per investigator discretion combined with pembrolizumab or placebo, addition of pembrolizumab resulted in improvement of PFS (10.4 vs 8.2 months) in patients with PD-L1 combined positive score of 1 or more. OS at 24 months was 53% in the pembrolizumab group and 41.7% in the placebo group (81). These findings led to FDA approval of pembrolizumab as part of upfront platinum-based regimen for the treatment of metastatic cervical cancer with PD-L1 combined positive score of 1 or more. A similar trial evaluating PD-L1 inhibitor atezolizumab in combination with platinum-based chemotherapy and bevacizumab is ongoing (NCT03556839).

Finally, given the activity of immune checkpoint blockade in the later line setting, several studies are investigating combination of PD-1 or PD-L1 blockade in combination with chemoradiation in the upfront locally advanced setting, including durvalumab, pembrolizumab, and atezolizumab (NCT02635360, NCT03830866, NCT03738228, respectively).

REFERENCES

1. Hreshchyshyn MM, Aron BS, Boronow RC, et al. Hydroxyurea or placebo combined with radiation to treat stages IIIB and IV cervical cancer confined to the pelvis. *Int J Radiat Oncol Biol Phys.* 1979;5(3):317-322.

2. Piver MS, Vongtama V, Emrich LJ. Hydroxyurea plus pelvic radiation versus placebo plus pelvic radiation in surgically staged stage IIIB cervical cancer. *J Surg Oncol.* 1987;35(2):129-134.

3. Greer BE, Koh WJ, Figge DC, et al. Gynecologic radiotherapy fields defined by intraoperative measurements. *Gynecol Oncol.* 1990;38(3):421-424.

4. Gill BS, Lin JF, Krivak TC, et al. National cancer data base analysis of radiation therapy consolidation modality for cervical cancer: the impact of new technological advancements. *Int J Radiat Oncol Biol Phys*. 2014. 90(5):1083-1090. doi:10.1016/j.ijrobp.2014.07.017

5. Khan A, Jensen LG, Sun S, Song WY, Yashar CM, Mundt AJ, Zhang FQ, Jiang SB, Mell LK. Optimized planning target volume for intact cervical cancer. *Int J Radiat Oncol Biol Phys*. 2012;83(5):1500-1505.

6. Williamson CW, Green G, Noticewala SS, et al. Prospective validation of a high dimensional shape model for organ motion in intact cervical cancer. *Int J Radiat Oncol Biol Phys*. 2016;96(4):801-807.

7. Small W Jr, Bosch WR, Harkenrider MM, et al. NRG Oncology/RTOG consensus guidelines for delineation of clinical target volume for intensity modulated pelvic radiation therapy in postoperative treatment of endometrial and cervical cancer: an update. *Int J Radiat Oncol Biol Phys*. 2021;109(2):413-424.

8. Jethwa KR, Jang S, Gonuguntla K, et al. Lymph node-directed simultaneous integrated boost in patients with clinically lymph node-positive cervical cancer treated with definitive chemoradiation: clinical outcomes and toxicity. *Int J Radiat Oncol*. 2018;102(3):E625-E626. doi:10.1016/j.ijrobp.2018.07.1710

9. Beadle BM, Jhingran A, Salehpour M, et al. Cervix regression and motion during the course of external beam chemoradiation for cervical cancer. *Int J Radiat Oncol Biol Phys*. 2009;73(1):235-241.

10. Hasselle MD, Rose BS, Kochanski JD, et al. Clinical outcomes of intensity-modulated pelvic radiation therapy for carcinoma of the cervix. *Int J Radiat Oncol Biol Phys*. 2011;80(5):1436-1445.

11. Chen CC, Lin JC, Jan JS, et al. Definitive intensity-modulated radiation therapy with concurrent chemotherapy for patients with locally advanced cervical cancer. *Gynecol Oncol*. 2011;122(1):9-13.

12. Klopp AH, Yeung AR, Deshmukh S, et al. Patient-reported toxicity during pelvic intensity-modulated radiation therapy: NRG oncology-RTOG 1203. *J Clin Oncol*. 2018;36(24):2538-2544. doi:10.1200/JCO.2017.77.4273

13. Chopra S, Gupta S, Kannan S, et al. Late toxicity after adjuvant conventional radiation versus image-guided intensity-modulated radiotherapy for cervical cancer (PARCER): a randomized controlled trial. *J Clin Oncol*. 2021;39(33):3682-3692.

14. Williamson CW, Sirák I, Xu R, et al. Positron emission tomography-guided bone marrow-sparing radiation therapy for locoregionally advanced cervix cancer: final results from the INTERTECC phase II/III trial. *Int J Radiat Oncol Biol Phys*. 2022;112(1):169-178.

15. Ahunbay EE, Peng C, Holmes S, Godley A, Lawton C, Li XA. Online adaptive replanning method for prostate radiotherapy. *Int J Radiat Oncol Biol Phys*. 2010;77(5):1561-1572. doi:10.1016/j.ijrobp.2009.10.013

16. Visser J, de Boer P, Crama KF, et al. Dosimetric comparison of library of plans and online MRI-guided radiotherapy of cervical cancer in the presence of intrafraction anatomical changes. *Radiat Oncol*. 2019;14:126.

17. Rotman M, Pajak TF, Choi K, et al. Prophylactic extended-field irradiation of para-aortic lymph nodes in stages IIB and bulky IB and IIA cervical carcinomas. Ten-year treatment results of RTOG 79-20. *JAMA*. 1995;274(5):387-393.

18. Dittmer PH, Randall ME. A technique for inguinal node boost using photon fields defined by asymmetric collimator jaws. *Radiother Oncol*. 2001;59(1):61-64.

19. Lim K, Small W Jr, Portelance L, et al. Consensus guidelines for delineation of clinical target volume for intensity-modulated pelvic radiotherapy for the definitive treatment of cervix cancer. *Int J Radiat Oncol Biol Phys*. 2011;79(2):348-355.

20. Fenkell L, Assenholt M, Nielsen SK, et al. Parametrial boost using midline shielding results in an unpredictable dose to tumor and organs at risk in combined external beam radiotherapy and brachytherapy for locally advanced cervical cancer. *Int J Radiat Oncol Biol Phys*. 2011;79(5):1572-1579.

21. Kridelka FJ, Berg DO, Neuman M, et al. Adjuvant small field pelvic radiation for patients with high risk, stage IB lymph node negative cervix carcinoma after radical hysterectomy and pelvic lymph node dissection. A pilot study. *Cancer*. 1999;86(10):2059-2065.

22. Ohara K, Tsunoda H, Nishida M, et al. Use of small pelvic field instead of whole pelvic field in postoperative radiotherapy for node-negative, high-risk stages I and II cervical squamous cell carcinoma. *Int J Gynecol Cancer*. 2003;13(2):170-176.

23. Berger T, Seppenwoolde Y, Pötter R, et al. Importance of technique, target selection, contouring, dose prescription, and dose-planning in external beam radiation therapy for cervical cancer: evolution of practice from EMBRACE-I to II. *Int J Radiat Oncol Biol Phys*. 2019;104(4):885-894.

24. Kagei K, Tokuuye K, Okumura T, et al. Long-term results of proton beam therapy for carcinoma of the uterine cervix. *Int J Radiat Oncol Biol Phys*. 2003;55(5):1265-1271.

25. Lin LL, Kirk M, Scholey J, et al. Initial report of pencil beam scanning proton therapy for posthysterectomy patients with gynecologic cancer. *Int J Radiat Oncol Biol Phys*. 2016;95(1):181-189. doi:10.1016/j.ijrobp.2015.07.2205

26. Vyfhuis MAL, Fellows Z, McGovern N, et al. Preserving endocrine function in premenopausal women undergoing whole pelvis radiation for cervical cancer. *Int J Part Ther*. 2019;6(1):10-17. doi:10.14338/ijpt-d-19-00061.1

27. Viswanathan AN, Thomadsen B. American Brachytherapy Society consensus guidelines for locally advanced carcinoma of the cervix. Part I: general principles. *Brachytherapy*. 2012;11(1):33-46.

28. Lee LJ, Das IJ, Higgins SA, et al. American Brachytherapy Society consensus guidelines for locally advanced carcinoma of the cervix. Part III: low-dose-rate and pulsed-dose-rate brachytherapy. *Brachytherapy*. 2012;11(1):53-57.

29. Heyman J. The combined radium and Rontgen treatment of cancer of the cervix uteri. *Ann Surg*. 1931;93(1):443-450.

30. International Commission on Radiation Units and Measurements. *ICRU Report 38: Dose and Volume Specification for Reporting Intracavitary Therapy in Gynecology*. International Commission on Radiation Units and Measurements; 1985.

31. Potter R, Van Limbergen E, Gerstner N, et al. Survey of the use of the ICRU 38 in recording and reporting cervical cancer brachytherapy. *Radiother Oncol*. 2001;58(1):11-18.

32. Viswanathan AN, Erickson BA. Three-dimensional imaging in gynecologic brachytherapy: a survey of the American Brachytherapy Society. *Int J Radiat Oncol Biol Phys*. 2010;76(1):104-109.

33. Serban M, Kirisits C, de Leeuw A, et al. Ring versus ovoids and intracavitary versus intracavitary-interstitial applicators in cervical cancer brachytherapy: results from the EMBRACE I study. *Int J Radiat Oncol Biol Phys*. 2020;106(5):1052-1062.

34. Viswanathan AN, Erickson B, Gaffney DK, et al. Comparison and consensus guidelines for delineation of clinical target volume for CT- and MR-based brachytherapy in locally advanced cervical cancer. *Int J Radiat Oncol Biol Phys*. 2014;90(2):320-328.

35. Haie-Meder C, Potter R, Van Limbergen E, et al. Recommendations from Gynaecological (GYN) GEC-ESTRO Working Group (I): concepts and terms in 3D image based 3D treatment planning in cervix cancer brachytherapy with emphasis on MRI assessment of GTV and CTV. *Radiother Oncol*. 2005;74(3):235-245.

36. Viswanathan AN, Dimopoulos J, Kirisits C, et al. Computed tomography versus magnetic resonance imaging-based contouring in cervical cancer brachytherapy: results of a prospective trial and preliminary guidelines for standardized contours. *Int J Radiat Oncol Biol Phys*. 2007;68(2):491-498.

37. Eskander RN, Scanderbeg D, Saenz CC, et al. Comparison of computed tomography and magnetic resonance imaging in cervical cancer brachytherapy target and normal tissue contouring. *Int J Gynecol Cancer*. 2010;20(1):47-53.

38. Pötter R, Tanderup K, Schmid MP, et al. MRI-guided adaptive brachytherapy in locally advanced cervical cancer (EMBRACE-I): a multicentre prospective cohort study. *Lancet Oncol*. 2021;22(4):538-547.

39. Charra-Brunaud C, Harter V, Delannes M, et al. Impact of 3D image-based PDR brachytherapy on outcome of patients treated for cervix carcinoma in France: results of the French STIC prospective study. *Radiother Oncol*. 2012;103(3):305-313. doi:10.1016/j.radonc.2012.04.007

40. Hall EJ. *Radiobiology for the Radiologist*. 5th ed. Lippincott Williams & Wilkins; 2000:588.

41. Kunos C, Colussi V, Pink J, et al. Radiosensitization of human cervical cancer cells by inhibiting ribonucleotide reductase: enhanced radiation response at low dose rates. *Int J Radiat Oncol Biol Phys*. 2011;80(4):1198-1204.

42. Fowler J, van Limbergen E. Biological effect of pulsed dose rate brachytherapy with stepping sources if short half-times of repair are present in tissues. *Int J Radiat Oncol Biol Phys*. 1997;37(4):877-883.

43. Swift P, Purser P, Roberts L, et al. Pulsed low dose rate brachytherapy for pelvic malignancies. *Int J Radiat Oncol Biol Phys*. 1997;37(4):811-817.

44. Rogers C, Freel J, Speiser B. Pulsed low dose rate brachytherapy for uterine cervix carcinoma. *Int J Radiat Oncol Biol Phys*. 1999;43(1):95-100.

45. Anker CJ, Cachoeira CV, Boucher KM, et al. Does the entire uterus need to be treated in cancer of the cervix? Role of adaptive brachytherapy. *Int J Radiat Oncol Biol Phys*. 2010;76(3):704-712.

46. Forrest JL, Ackerman I, Barbera L, et al. Patient outcome study of concurrent chemoradiation, external beam radiotherapy, and high-dose rate brachytherapy in locally advanced carcinoma of the cervix. *Int J Gynecol Cancer*. 2010;20(6):1074-1078.

47. Potter R, Georg P, Dimopoulos JC, et al. Clinical outcome of protocol based image (MRI) guided adaptive brachytherapy combined with 3D conformal radiotherapy with or without chemotherapy in patients with locally advanced cervical cancer. *Radiother Oncol*. 2011;100(1):116-123.

48. Schmid MP, Kirisits C, Nesvacil N, et al. Local recurrences in cervical cancer patients in the setting of image-guided brachytherapy: a comparison of spatial dose distribution within a matched-pair analysis. *Radiother Oncol*. 2011;100(3):468-472.

49. Nesvacil N, Potter R, Sturdza A, et al. Adaptive image guided brachytherapy for cervical cancer: a combined MRI-/CT-planning technique with MRI only at first fraction. *Radiother Oncol*. 2013;107(1):75-81.

50. Nesvacil N, Tanderup K, Hellebust TP, et al. A multicentre comparison of the dosimetric impact of inter- and intra-fractional anatomical variations in fractionated cervix cancer brachytherapy. *Radiother Oncol*. 2013;107(1):20-25.

51. Fuller DB, Naitoh J, Lee C, Hardy S, Jin H. Virtual HDRSM CyberKnife treatment for localized prostatic carcinoma: dosimetry comparison with HDR brachytherapy and preliminary clinical observations. *Int J Radiat Oncol Biol Phys*. 2008;70(5):1588-1597. doi:10.1016/j.ijrobp.2007.11.067

52. Haas JA, Witten MR, Clancey O, Episcopia K, Accordino D, Chalas E. CyberKnife boost for patients with cervical cancer unable to undergo brachytherapy. *Front Oncol*. 2012;2:25. doi:10.3389/fonc.2012.00025

53. Albuquerque K, Tumati V, Lea J, Ahn C, Richardson D, Miller D, et al. A phase II trial of stereotactic ablative radiation therapy as a boost for locally advanced cervical cancer. *Int J Radiat Oncol Biol Phys*. 2020;106(3):464-471. doi:10.1016/j.ijrobp.2019.10.042

54. Kunos C, Brindle J, Waggoner S, et al. Phase II clinical trial of robotic stereotactic body radiosurgery for metastatic gynecologic malignancies. *Front Oncol*. 2012;2:181.

55. Petereit D, Sakaria J, Chappell R, et al. The adverse effect of treatment prolongation in cervical carcinoma. *Int J Radiation Oncology Biol Phys*. 1995;32(5):1301-1307.

56. Monk BJ, Tian C, Rose PG, et al. Which clinical/pathologic factors matter in the era of chemoradiation as treatment for locally advanced cervical carcinoma? Analysis of two Gynecologic Oncology Group (GOG) trials. *Gynecol Oncol*. 2007;105(2):427-433.

57. Carrascosa LA, Yashar CM, Paris KJ, et al. Palliation of pelvic and head and neck cancer with paclitaxel and a novel radiotherapy regimen. *J Palliat Med*. 2007;10(4):877-881.

58. Spanos WJ Jr, Wasserman T, Meoz R, et al. Palliation of advanced pelvic malignant disease with large fraction pelvic radiation and misonidazole: final report of RTOG phase I/II study. *Int J Radiat Oncol Biol Phys*. 1987;13(10):1479-1482.

59. Muderspach L, Wilczynski S, Roman L, et al. A phase I trial of a human papillomavirus (HPV) peptide vaccine for women with high-grade cervical and vulvar intraepithelial neoplasia who are HPV 16 positive. *Clin Cancer Res*. 2000;6(9):3406-3416.

60. Trimble CL, Morrow MP, Kraynyak KA, et al. Safety, efficacy, and immunogenicity of VGX-3100, a therapeutic synthetic DNA vaccine targeting human papillomavirus 16 and 18 E6 and E7 proteins for cervical intraepithelial neoplasia 2/3: a randomised, double-blind, placebo-controlled phase 2b trial. *Lancet*. 2015;386(10008):2078-2088.

61. Basu P, Mehta A, Jain M, et al. A randomized phase 2 study of ADXS11-001 listeria monocytogenes-listeriolysin O immunotherapy with or without cisplatin in treatment of advanced cervical cancer. *Int J Gynecol Cancer*. 2018;28(4):764-772.

62. Huh WK, Brady WE, Fracasso PM, et al. Phase II study of axalimogene filolisbac (ADXS-HPV) for platinum-refractory cervical carcinoma: an NRG oncology/gynecologic oncology group study. *Gynecol Oncol*. 2020; 158(3):562-569.

63. van Poelgeest MI, Welters MJ, van Esch EM, et al. HPV16 synthetic long peptide (HPV16-SLP) vaccination therapy of patients with advanced or recurrent HPV16-induced gynecological carcinoma, a phase II trial. *J Transl Med*. 2013;11:88.

64. Stevanovic S, Draper LM, Langhan MM, et al. Complete regression of metastatic cervical cancer after treatment with human papillomavirus-targeted tumor-infiltrating T cells. *J Clin Oncol*. 2015;33(14):1543-1550.

65. Stevanovic S, Helman SR, Wunderlich JR, et al. A phase II study of tumor-infiltrating lymphocyte therapy for human papillomavirus-associated epithelial cancers. *Clin Cancer Res*. 2019;25(5):1486-1493.

66. Jazaeri AA, Zsiros E, Amaria RN, et al. Safety and efficacy of adoptive cell transfer using autologous tumor infiltrating lymphocytes (LN-145) for treatment of recurrent, metastatic, or persistent cervical carcinoma. *J Clin Oncol*. 2019;37(15_suppl):2538.

67. Doran SL, Stevanović S, Adhikary S, et al. T-cell receptor gene therapy for human papillomavirus–associated epithelial cancers: a first-in-human, phase I/II study. *J Clin Oncol*. 2019;37(30):2759-2768.

68. Norberg S, Nagarsheth N, Sinkoe A, et al. Safety and clinical activity of gene-engineered T-cell therapy targeting HPV-16 E7 for epithelial cancers. *J Clin Oncol*. 2020;38(15_suppl):101.

69. Han X, Guo B, Li Y, Zhu B. Tissue factor in tumor microenvironment: a systematic review. *J Hematol Oncol*. 2014;7:54.

70. Zhao X, Cheng C, Gou J, et al. Expression of tissue factor in human cervical carcinoma tissue. *Exp Ther Med*. 2018;16(5):4075-4081.

71. Coleman RL, Lorusso D, Gennigens C, et al. Efficacy and safety of tisotumab vedotin in previously treated recurrent or metastatic cervical cancer (innovaTV 204/GOG-3023/ENGOT-cx6): a multicentre, open-label, single-arm, phase 2 study. *Lancet Oncol*. 2021;22(5):609-619.

72. Chung HC, Ros W, Delord JP, et al. Efficacy and safety of pembrolizumab in previously treated advanced cervical cancer: results from the phase II KEYNOTE-158 study. *J Clin Oncol*. 2019;37(17):1470-1478.

73. Marabelle A, Fakih M, Lopez J, et al. Association of tumour mutational burden with outcomes in patients with advanced solid tumours treated with pembrolizumab: prospective biomarker analysis of the multicohort, open-label, phase 2 KEYNOTE-158 study. *Lancet Oncol*. 2020;21(10):1353-1365.

74. Tewari KS, Monk BJ, Vergote I, et al. Survival with cemiplimab in recurrent cervical cancer. *N Engl J Med*. 2022;386(6):544-555.

75. O'Malley DM, Oaknin A, Monk BJ, et al. Phase II study of the safety and efficacy of the anti-PD-1 antibody balstilimab in patients with recurrent and/or metastatic cervical cancer. *Gynecol Oncol*. 2021;163(2):274-280.

76. Naumann RW, Oaknin A, Meyer T, et al. Efficacy and safety of nivolumab (Nivo) + Ipilimumab (Ipi) in patients (pts) with recurrent/metastatic (R/M) cervical cancer: results from CheckMate 358. *Ann Oncol*. 2019;30:v851-v934.

77. O'Malley DM, Neffa M, Monk BJ, et al. Dual PD-1 and CTLA-4 checkpoint blockade using balstilimab and zalifrelimab combination as second-line treatment for advanced cervical cancer: an open-label phase II study. *J Clin Oncol*. 2022;40(7):762-771.

78. Friedman CF, Snyder Charen A, Zhou Q, et al. Phase II study of atezolizumab in combination with bevacizumab in patients with advanced cervical cancer. *J Immunother Cancer*. 2020;8(2):e001126.

79. Lan C, Shen J, Wang Y, et al. Camrelizumab plus apatinib in patients with advanced cervical cancer (CLAP): a multicenter, open-label, single-arm, phase II trial. *J Clin Oncol*. 2020;38(34):4095-4106.

80. Youn JW, Hur SY, Woo JW, et al. Pembrolizumab plus GX-188E therapeutic DNA vaccine in patients with HPV-16-positive or HPV-18-positive advanced cervical cancer: interim results of a single-arm, phase 2 trial. *Lancet Oncol*. 2020;21(12):1653-1660.

81. Colombo N, Dubot C, Lorusso D, et al. Pembrolizumab for persistent, recurrent, or metastatic cervical cancer. *N Engl J Med*. 2021;385(20):1856-1867.

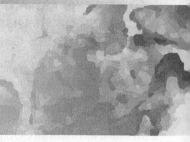

CHAPTER **4.7**

Treatment of Persistent or Recurrent Uterine Cervix Cancer

Charles A. Leath III and Teresa K. L. Boitano

GENERAL CONSIDERATIONS

Death from uterine cervix cancer occurs most often because of uncontrolled, or undertreated, disease in the pelvis. Persistent disease after primary treatment or short-interval relapse of disease in the pelvis may be amenable to salvage surgery or radiation therapy; however, patient desire for treatment and selection of therapeutic intervention are often predicated on disease extent, disease-free interval, impact of prior therapy on pelvic anatomy, patient performance status, and patient comorbidities. The Moore criteria were developed from chemotherapy clinical trials and utilize performance status, race, the presence of pelvic disease, prior cisplatin administration, and disease-free interval (1) and were prospectively validated as part of GOG 240 to help inform both treatment decisions and prognosis for patients with multiple high-risk recurrence factors (2).

If potentially curative salvage treatment is intended, a biopsy of the relapse and restaging radiographic imaging should be acquired. Sciatic pain, leg edema, and hydronephrosis are pathognomonic for pelvic sidewall involvement and as such preclude surgical intervention. PET/CT may be the most accurate restaging test (3). More recently, PET/MRI has also been evaluated in women with primary cervical cancer and may be an imaging consideration, especially if additional information is needed of pelvic soft tissues (4).

RADICAL SURGERY FOR PELVIC DISEASE AFTER PRIOR RADIATION THERAPY

Radical hysterectomy, not planned as part of initial care, has been used as a means of surgical salvage for small (<2 cm) persistent or recurrent uterine cervix cancers (5); however, total pelvic exenteration has more commonly been performed for central pelvic relapses without evidence of extrapelvic disease, with up to one-third of the surgical interventions aborted at some point during the procedure. Exenteration operative time ranges up to 8 hours, average blood loss is 3 L, and postprocedural hospital stay can be up to 23 days (6). Perioperative mortality rates are as high as 14% (7). Complications arise in up to 45% of patients (8), with bowel obstruction (22%), intestinal fistula (15%), and urogenital fistula (8%) as significant adverse events (6). In a retrospective study of 55 patients (1998-2004), tumor-free exenteration surgical margin is associated with a 55% survival estimate, as compared with a 10% survival estimate when margins are positive for tumor (9). Women who are overweight and those with obesity with recurrent disease undergoing exenteration experience

longer operative times and higher wound separation rates than otherwise, but overall postsurgical survival appears equal to normal-weight women (10).

Pelvic anatomy reconstruction may include a combination of urostomy (either continent or incontinent), colostomy, and muscle flap neovagina. Diversion of urine flow by implanting the ureters into an isolated piece of ileum for a separate urostomy with bag reservoir is preferred to a wet colostomy involving implantation of the ureters into a colostomy-diverting fecal flow (11). An ileal urostomy (ileal conduit) is incontinent. Continent internal reservoirs using bowel wall allow for self-catheterization but are associated with a 50% to 65% complication rate from pyelonephritis, ureteral stricture, leak or fistula, renal stone formation, and, even rarely, renal failure (12,13). Muscle flap reconstructions of a neovagina for sexual activity, pelvic tissue fill, and prevention of fistulas have been described (14,15).

RADICAL RADIATION OR RADIOCHEMOTHERAPY FOR PELVIC DISEASE AFTER PRIOR SURGERY

Small (<2 cm) persistent or recurrent disease, or vagina-only relapses, may be amenable to radiation therapy, with durable control exceeding 70% (16,17); 10-year survival estimates in radiotherapy-naive patients are as high as 35% (17). Interstitial brachytherapy (3,000-5,500 cGy) (18,19) and SBRT (2,400 cGy) (20) have been described for disease involving deep pelvic tissues. The use of carboplatin-gemcitabine chemotherapy and SBRT has been explored in a phase I trial (21).

For pelvic or para-aortic lymph node relapses after first-line surgery or radiochemotherapy, conventional radiochemotherapy (>4,500 cGy) (22) or SBRT (800 cGy × 3 doses) (20) has been used. Low toxicity and durable disease control rates exceeding 95% have been documented with either of these two techniques.

Intraoperative electron radiation therapy has been used during radical salvage surgery for persistent or recurrent uterine cervix cancer. The technique is attractive owing to its direct exposure of at-risk tumor-harboring tissue to limited penetration electrons and because of its low radiation dose scatter to normal tissues retracted away or shielded during dose delivery. A single fraction of 1,500 cGy (range 625-2,500 cGy) was used most often in a case series of 86 patients (1983-2010) (23). Adverse events include peripheral neuropathy (19%), ureteral stenosis (5%), and bowel fistula or perforation (5%). Eleven (69%) of 16 women experiencing neuropathy after intraoperative radiation required long-term pain medication.

CHEMOTHERAPY AND BIOLOGIC TARGETED AGENTS FOR PERSISTENT OR RECURRENT UTERINE CERVIX CANCER

Currently, chemotherapy and biologic targeted agents for persistent or recurrent uterine cervix cancer fill a palliative role as metastatic cervical cancer is generally not considered amenable to cure. The standard first-line therapy in these patients includes a platinum agent along with paclitaxel and bevacizumab. This triplet backbone was based on GOG protocol 240 where 452 women were randomly assigned to chemotherapy with or without bevacizumab. The addition of bevacizumab demonstrated a significant improvement in OS when compared with chemotherapy alone (16.8 vs 13.3 months; HR 0.77, 98% CI 0.62-0.95) (24).

More recently, however, and building upon the findings from GOG protocol 240, KEYNOTE-826, a phase III trial evaluated the addition of pembrolizumab to chemotherapy (two-thirds of women also received bevacizumab), which included both combination therapy for up to 6 cycles per a protocol amendment and up to 35 total cycles of pembrolizumab versus placebo. Women in the pembrolizumab group had an improvement in median PFS (10.4 vs 8.2 months; HR 0.65, 95% CI 0.53-0.79). The OS at 24 months in the pembrolizumab group was 50%, compared to only 40% in the placebo group (HR 0.67, 95% CI 0.54-0.84) (25). There is question about the benefit of the use of pembrolizumab in patients with a PD-L1 combined positive score (CPS) of less than 1 (HR 0.94, 95% CI 0.52-1.70).

In an effort to identify alternate treatment options in patients with recurrent or metastatic cervical cancer, the antibody-drug conjugate (ADC) tisotumab vedotin-tftv, which targets TF, was examined. The ORR in a single-arm trial was 24%, with 17% of patients having a partial response and 7% having a complete response (26). An ongoing randomized phase III trial, innovaTV 301, is hoping to confirm the benefit of tisotumab vedotin as compared to standard-of-care chemotherapy options (NCT 04697628).

CONCLUSION

In summary, we have seen significant therapeutic gains in the treatment of metastatic, recurrent uterine cervical carcinoma. GOG protocol 204, which examined various chemotherapy doublet combinations and established carboplatin and paclitaxel as the preferred regimens, showed a median OS of approximately 12 months. As noted earlier, with the addition of the antiangiogenic agent bevacizumab, this median OS was extended to approximately 17 months (24 months in those patients not receiving prior radiation). Most recently, incorporation of pembrolizumab to the GOG 240 regimen resulted in a dramatic improvement in median OS, with median OS not reached in either PD-L1–selected population for pembrolizumab, emphasizing the relevance of continued drug discovery in this space.

REFERENCES

1. Moore DH, Tian C, Monk BJ, Long HJ, Omura GA, Bloss JD. Prognostic factors for response to cisplatin-based chemotherapy in advanced cervical carcinoma: a Gynecologic Oncology Group Study. *Gynecol Oncol.* 2010;116(1):44-49. doi:10.1016/j.ygyno.2009.09.006

2. Tewari KS, Sill MW, Monk BJ, et al. Prospective validation of pooled prognostic factors in women with advanced cervical cancer treated with chemotherapy with/without bevacizumab: NRG oncology/GOG study. *Clin Cancer Res.* 2015;21(24):5480-5487. doi:10.1158/1078-0432.CCR-15-1346

3. Chong A, Ha JM, Jeong SY, et al. Clinical usefulness of (18)F-FDG PET/CT in the detection of early recurrence in treated cervical cancer patients with unexplained elevation of serum tumor markers. *Chonnam Med J.* 2013;49(1):20-26.

4. Esfahani SA, Torrado-Carvajal A, Amorim BJ, et al. PET/MRI and PET/CT radiomics in primary cervical cancer: a pilot study on the correlation of pelvic PET, MRI, and CT derived image features. *Mol Imaging Biol.* 2022;24(1):60-69. doi:10.1007/s11307-021-01658-1

5. Coleman RL, Keeney ED, Freedman RS, et al. Radical hysterectomy for recurrent carcinoma of the uterine cervix after radiotherapy. *Gynecol Oncol.* 1994;55(1):29-35.

6. Berek JS, Howe C, Lagasse LD, et al. Pelvic exenteration for recurrent gynecologic malignancy: survival and morbidity analysis of the 45-year experience at UCLA. *Gynecol Oncol.* 2005;99(1):153-159.

7. Petruzziello A, Kondo W, Hatschback SB, et al. Surgical results of pelvic exenteration in the treatment of gynecologic cancer. *World J Surg Oncol.* 2014;12:279.

8. Westin SN, Rallapalli V, Fellman B, et al. Overall survival after pelvic exenteration for gynecologic malignancy. *Gynecol Oncol.* 2014;134(3):546-551.

9. Marnitz S, Kohler C, Muller M, et al. Indications for primary and secondary exenterations in patients with cervical cancer. *Gynecol Oncol.* 2006;103(3):1023-1030.

10. Iglesias DA, Westin SN, Rallapalli V, et al. The effect of body mass index on surgical outcomes and survival following pelvic exenteration. *Gynecol Oncol.* 2012;125(2):336-342.

11. Bricker EM. Bladder substitution after pelvic evisceration. *Surg Clin North Am.* 1950;30(5):1511-1521.

12. Penalver MA, Angioli R, Mirhashemi R, et al. Management of early and late complications of ileocolonic continent urinary reservoir (Miami pouch). *Gynecol Oncol.* 1998;69(3):185-191.

13. Ungar L, Palfalvi L. Pelvic exenteration without external urinary or fecal diversion in gynecological cancer patients. *Int J Gynecol Cancer.* 2006;16(1):364-368.

14. McCraw JB, Massey FM, Shanklin KD, et al. Vaginal reconstruction with gracilis myocutaneous flaps. *Plast Reconstr Surg.* 1976;58(2):176-183.

15. Sood AK, Cooper BC, Sorosky JI, et al. Novel modification of the vertical rectus abdominis myocutaneous flap for neovagina creation. *Obstet Gynecol.* 2005;105(3):514-518.

16. Ito H, Shigematsu N, Kawada T, et al. Radiotherapy for centrally recurrent cervical cancer of the vaginal stump following hysterectomy. *Gynecol Oncol.* 1997;67(2):154-161.

17. Grigsby PW. Prospective phase I/II study of irradiation and concurrent chemotherapy for recurrent cervical cancer after radical hysterectomy. *Int J Gynecol Cancer.* 2004;14(5):860-864.

18. Randall ME, Evans L, Greven KM, et al. Interstitial reirradiation for recurrent gynecologic malignancies: results and analysis of prognostic factors. *Gynecol Oncol.* 1993;48(1):23-31.

19. Brabham JG, Cardenes HR. Permanent interstitial reirradiation with 198Au as salvage therapy for low volume recurrent gynecologic malignancies: a single institution experience. *Am J Clin Oncol.* 2009;32(4):417-422.

20. Kunos C, Brindle J, Waggoner S, et al. Phase II clinical trial of robotic stereotactic body radiosurgery for metastatic gynecologic malignancies. *Front Oncol.* 2012;2:181.

21. Kunos CA, Sherertz TM, Mislmani M, et al. Phase I trial of carboplatin and gemcitabine chemotherapy and stereotactic ablative radiosurgery for the palliative treatment of persistent or recurrent gynecologic cancer. *Front Oncol.* 2015;5:126.

22. Grigsby PW, Vest ML, Perez CA. Recurrent carcinoma of the cervix exclusively in the paraaortic nodes following radiation therapy. *Int J Radiat Oncol Biol Phys.* 1994;28(2):451-455.

23. Barney BM, Petersen IA, Dowdy SC, et al. Intraoperative electron beam radiotherapy (IOERT) in the management of locally advanced or recurrent cervical cancer. *Radiat Oncol.* 2013;8:80.

24. Tewari KS, Sill MW, Long HJ 3rd, et al. Improved survival with bevacizumab in advanced cervical cancer. *N Engl J Med.* 2014;370(8):734.

25. Colombo N, Dubot C, Lorusso D, et al. Pembrolizumab for persistent, recurrent, or metastatic cervical cancer. *N Engl J Med.* 2021;385(20):1856. Epub September 18, 2021.

26. Coleman RL, Lorusso D, Gennigens C, et al. Efficacy and safety of tisotumab vedotin in previously treated recurrent or metastatic cervical cancer (innovaTV 204/GOG-3023/ENGOT-cx6): a multicentre, open-label, single-arm, phase 2 study. *Lancet Oncol.* 2021;22(5):609. Epub April 9, 2021.

CHAPTER **4.8**

Survivorship Issues Following Treatment for Cervical Cancer

Laura Salama and Don S. Dizon

LONGER TERM COMPLICATIONS FOLLOWING SURGERY-ONLY TREATMENT

Pelvic surgery for cervical cancer is associated with perioperative and late complications. Late sequelae were reported in 3% of patients and include severe actinic cystitis, stress incontinence, and other bladder complications. Severe edema, pelvic lymphocyst, and abdominal hernia occurred in 0%, 8%, and 11% of patients in long term, respectively. Rectal dysfunction (eg, incontinence or constipation) after surgery alone is infrequent (1).

COMPLICATIONS FOLLOWING PREOPERATIVE RADIATION

In a retrospective study on 1,784 patients (2), women having clinical stage IB uterine cervix cancer treated with radiation therapy (RT) had an overall actuarial risk for any long-term complication of 14% at 20 years post-therapy. Significant urinary tract complications occurred in 0.7% per year up to 3 years post-therapy, then tapered to 0.25% per year for the next 22 years. Significant colorectal complications happened at a 1% rate per year in the first 2 years post-therapy and then declined to 0.06% per year for the next 23 years. Radiation-related adverse events are expected to be more common among women undergoing external beam RT plus intracavitary brachytherapy. Prolonged bed rest for intracavitary brachytherapy implants was associated with only a 0.3% risk of life-threatening thromboembolism (11/4,043 patients undergoing 7,662 implants) (3). Overall, RT technique, radiation dose exceeding that prescribed, is associated with radiation-related adverse events.

Improved uterine cervix cancer survival has made long-term hazards from treatment more important, including the risk of developing a second cancer after RT. In the U.S. Surveillance, Epidemiology and End Results (SEER) cancer registries, 8% of all radiotherapy patients surviving longer than 1 year developed a second solid cancer that could be related to prior RT (4).

A contemporary analysis of SEER incidence data identified 9,092 patients diagnosed with cervical cancer between 1993 and 2008 who were treated with RT alone and did not undergo surgery; 0.6% were diagnosed with endometrial cancer, with an average latency to diagnosis of 160 months (range 14-274 months) from the time of diagnosis of cervical cancer. These endometrial tumors were predominantly aggressive histologic types when compared to primary endometrial cancers ($P < .01$). Of these second endometrial cancers, 40% were endometrioid, 42% were clear cell adenocarcinoma, 9% were carcinosarcomas, and 5.5% were leiomyosarcomas compared to 2.3% clear cell adenocarcinomas, 2.3% carcinosarcomas, and 0.5% leiomyosarcomas in the primary endometrial cancer group (5).

LONG-TERM COMPLICATIONS FOLLOWING RADIATION-ONLY TREATMENT

RT predisposes to tissue hardening and fibrosis, especially because the tumor is sterilized and body healing thickens connective tissues. In one clinical trial (6), women randomly allocated to radiation followed by radical hysterectomy had the same incidence of grade 3 or above complications (10%) as compared to women treated by radiation alone (10%). The proportion of women experiencing any toxicity was higher in the radiation and surgery arm (63%) when compared to the radiation-only arm (56%). In another study (7), 35% of women randomized to chemoradiation followed by radical hysterectomy experienced a grade 3 or above toxicity as compared to 13% of women treated with radiation followed by radical hysterectomy. Long-term effects on the skin, GI tract, and genitourinary tract were more common after chemoradiation followed by surgery (4%, five fistulas, one colonic perforation, one intestinal perforation) when compared to treatment with RT alone followed by surgery (2%, five fistulas [three in one patient] and one intestinal obstruction) (8).

LONG-TERM COMPLICATIONS FOLLOWING ADJUVANT RADIATION THERAPY

The administration of adjuvant RT following surgery (typically based on the presence of high-risk factors) can result in a heightened risk of treatment-related toxicity in the long term. In one clinical trial, 29% of patients experienced long-term complications, compared to 24%, and 16% among those treated by surgery only or RT alone, respectively (9). In another clinical trial, women randomized to postsurgical radiochemotherapy had a 17% hazard for grade 4 or above toxicity as compared to 4% after postsurgical radiation alone (10).

COMPLICATIONS FOLLOWING CHEMORADIATION

Most chemoradiation-associated adverse events occur within the first 3 years post-therapy. Chemoradiation has a higher risk of toxicity compared to RT alone. This was shown in a meta-analysis that included 24 randomized trials enrolling 4,921 women treated in the 1980s and 1990s show an increased hazard for adverse event after chemoradiation treatment (11). Long-term complications and risks for second solid cancers attributable to chemoradiation were not well reported. Chemoradiation treatment–related deaths are fortunately rare—six deaths occurred from short-term complications (eg, neutropenic sepsis) and four deaths happened from long-term complications (eg, bowel perforation or fistula). Another retrospective review of 1,243 patients (2001-2002) found grade 3 or above long-term GI or genitourinary complications in 10% of patients receiving chemoradiation versus 8% of patients receiving RT alone (12).

THROMBOEMBOLIC ADVERSE EVENTS

Venous thromboembolic adverse events among women with uterine cervix cancer occur at a rate ranging between 0% and 34% (13-15). Patient risk factors include age, weight, mobility, preexistent hypercoagulable conditions (eg, factor V Leiden or prothrombin gene mutation), and personal history of prior thromboembolic event, venous stasis, or endothelial cell injury. Postsurgical reduced mobility, bed rest during LDR brachytherapy, and radiochemotherapy treatment may exacerbate venous stasis and led to thromboembolic events in 17% of patients (13). Tumor-related factors include pathophysiology, secretion of prothrombotic molecules, and clinical stage (13). Clinical stage is associated with thromboembolic events because direct pelvic sidewall invasion or metastasis resulting in bulky lymph nodes elicits lower extremity venous stasis and thrombus formation. In a clinical trial randomly allocating women with uterine cervix cancer to an erythropoietin-stimulating agent or to no agent, patients in the erythropoietin-stimulating agent arm had a 19% hazard for thromboembolism, whereas those in the no-agent arm had an 8% hazard (16). In the erythropoietin-stimulating agent arm, not all thromboembolic adverse events were linked to the agent (16). Still, erythropoietin-stimulating agents are not recommended for women with uterine cervix cancers. Most thromboembolic adverse events occur within the first 2 years post-therapy.

SEXUAL DYSFUNCTION

Sexual dysfunction is a distressing concern after RT. In one study where sexual health surveys were obtained in 606 women treated between 1991 and 1992 (17), a total of 167 (68%) of 247 women with a history of uterine cervix cancer and 236 (72%) of 330 controls indicated that they engaged in regular vaginal intercourse. Insufficient lubrication (26% of patients with cancer vs 11% control patients), foreshortened vagina (26% vs 3%), and an insufficiently elastic vagina (23% vs 4%) were cited reasons for not engaging in regular vaginal intercourse; 26% of the cancer group reported moderate or much distress due to vaginal changes, as compared to 8% of the control group. Another study conducted in China surveyed 140 women treated for cervical cancer between 2007 and 2010. Results showed 78% of patients experienced sexual dysfunction, scoring a high average score on FACT-Cx (Functional Assessment of Cancer Therapy-Cervix Questionnaire) (18).

The EMBRACE-I, a prospective observational and multicenter trial, used the European Organization for Research and Treatment of Cancer Qualify of Life Questionnaire (EORTC-QLQ-CX24) at baseline and follow-up for analysis of sexual outcomes in 1,045 women with locally advanced cervical cancer treated with chemoradiation and image-guided brachytherapy. The analysis showed that dyspareunia was significantly associated with dryness, vaginal shortening, and tightening (19).

A feasibility study to assess MR-guided brachytherapy consented 27 patients to complete validated sexual adjustment questionnaire (SAQ) at baseline (before brachytherapy) and at follow-ups, along with physician assessment of vaginal toxicity. The study reported no significant changes in sexual adjustment over time ($P = .599$) and worse sexual adjustment ($P = .005$) in patients with FIGO stage IIB or above (20).

INSUFFICIENCY FRACTURES

Insufficiency fracture of the sacroiliac joint is also rare. Patients aged 55 years or above, who weigh more than 55 kg, or received a radiation dose of 5,040 cGy or more with curative intent are more likely to sustain a pelvic insufficiency fracture (21). A 5-year cumulative incidence of pelvic insufficiency fracture was 20%, with 13% requiring narcotic analgesic or hospital admission for the management of pain. In one study, 38 women with cervical cancer who received RT between January 2014 and January 2021 were included in a retrospective comparative analysis examining dynamic changes in ^{18}F-FDG PET at the time of sacral fracture and CT images before RT; analysis revealed that the median time to sacral insufficiency fracture was 13 months (3-42 months), with the main signs on imaging being increased bone density in 92.1%, anterior sacral fracture line in 73.7%, and diffuse or linear uptake parallel to the sacroiliac joint in 97% of patients with average SUV_{max} of 3.1 (22).

REFERENCES

1. Rotman M, Sedlis A, Piedmonte M, et al. A phase III randomized trial of postoperative pelvic irradiation in stage IB cervical carcinoma with poor prognostic features: follow-up of a Gynecologic Oncology Group study. *Int J Radiat Oncol Biol Phys.* 2006;65(1):169-176.

2. Eifel PJ, Levenback C, Wharton JT, et al. Time course and incidence of late complications in patients treated with radiation therapy for FIGO stage IB carcinoma of the uterine cervix. *Int J Radiat Oncol Biol Phys.* 1995;32(5):1289-1300.

3. Jhingran A, Eifel PJ. Perioperative and postoperative complications of intracavitary radiation for FIGO stage I-III carcinoma of the cervix. *Int J Radiat Oncol Biol Phys.* 2000;46(5):1177-1183.

4. Berrington de Gonzalez A, Curtis RE, Kry SF, et al. Proportion of second cancers attributable to radiotherapy treatment in adults: a cohort study in the US SEER cancer registries. *Lancet Oncol.* 2011;12(4):353-360.

5. Papatla K, Houck KL, Hernandez E, Chu C, Rubin S. Second primary uterine malignancies after radiation therapy for cervical cancer. *Arch Gynecol Obstet.* 2019;300(2):389-394. doi:10.1007/s00404-019-05187-9

6. Keys HM, Bundy BN, Stehman FB, et al. Radiation therapy with and without extrafascial hysterectomy for bulky stage IB cervical carcinoma: a randomized trial of the Gynecologic Oncology Group. *Gynecol Oncol.* 2003;89(3):343-353.

7. Keys HM, Bundy BN, Stehman FB, et al. Cisplatin, radiation, and adjuvant hysterectomy compared with radiation and adjuvant hysterectomy for bulky stage IB cervical carcinoma. *N Engl J Med.* 1999;340(15):1154-1161.

8. Stehman F, Ali S, Keys H, et al. Radiation therapy with or without weekly cisplatin for bulky stage 1B cervical carcinoma: follow-up of a Gyneco-logic Oncology Group trial. *Am J Obstet Gynecol.* 2007;197:503.e1-503.e6.

9. Landoni F, Maneo A, Colombo A, et al. Randomized study of radical surgery versus radiotherapy for stage Ib-IIa cervical cancer. *Lancet.* 1997;350(9077):535-540.

10. Peters WI, Liu P, Barrett R, et al. Concurrent chemotherapy and pelvic radiation therapy compared with pelvic radiation therapy alone as adjuvant therapy after radical surgery in high-risk early-stage cancer of the cervix. *J Clin Oncol.* 2000;18(8):1606-1613.

11. Green J, Kirwan J, Tierney J, et al. Concomitant chemotherapy and radiation therapy for cancer of the uterine cervix. *Cochrane Database Syst Rev.* 2005;20(3):CD002225.

12. Vale CL, Tierney JF, Davidson SE, et al. Substantial improvement in UK cervical cancer survival with chemoradiotherapy: results of a Royal College of Radiologists' audit. *Clin Oncol (R Coll Radiol).* 2010;22(7):590-601.

13. Barbera L, Thomas G. Venous thromboembolism in cervical cancer. *Lancet Oncol.* 2008;9(1):54-60.

14. Barbera L, Thomas G. Erythropoiesis stimulating agents, thrombosis and cancer. *Radiother Oncol.* 2010;95(3):269-276.

15. Jacobson G, Lammli J, Zamba G, et al. Thromboembolic events in patients with cervical carcinoma: incidence and effect on survival. *Gynecol Oncol.* 2009;113(2):240-244.

16. Thomas G, Ali S, Hoebers FJ, et al. Phase III trial to evaluate the efficacy of maintaining hemoglobin levels above 12.0 g/dL with erythropoietin vs above 10.0 g/dL without erythropoietin in anemic patients receiving concurrent radiation and cisplatin for cervical cancer. *Gynecol Oncol.* 2008;108(2):317-325.

17. Bergmark K, Avall-Lundqvist E, Dickman PW, et al. Vaginal changes and sexuality in women with a history of cervical cancer. *N Engl J Med.* 1999;340(18):1383-1389.

18. Zhou W, Yang X, Dai Y, Wu Q, He G, Yin G. Survey of cervical cancer survivors regarding quality of life and sexual function. *J Cancer Res Ther.* 2016;12(2):938-944. doi:10.4103/0973-1482.175427

19. Kirchheiner K, Smet S, Jürgenliemk-Schulz IM, et al. Impact of vaginal symptoms and hormonal replacement therapy on sexual outcomes after definitive chemoradiotherapy in patients with locally advanced cervical cancer: results from the EMBRACE-I study. *Int J Radiat Oncol Biol Phys.* 2022;112(2):400-413. doi:10.1016/j.ijrobp.2021.08.036

20. Conway JL, Gerber R, Han K, et al. Patient-reported sexual adjustment after definitive chemoradiation and MR-guided brachytherapy for cervical cancer. *Brachytherapy.* 2019;18(2):133-140. doi:10.1016/j.brachy.2018.09.005

21. Oh D, Huh SJ, Nam H, et al. Pelvic insufficiency fracture after pelvic radiotherapy for cervical cancer: analysis of risk factors. *Int J Radiat Oncol Biol Phys.* 2008;70(4):1183-1188.

22. Ji Y, Shao C, Cui Y, et al. Sacral insufficiency fracture after radiotherapy for cervical cancer: appearance and dynamic changes on 18F-fluorodeoxyglucose positron emission tomography/computed tomography. *Contrast Media Mol Imaging.* 2021;2021:5863530. doi:10.1155/2021/5863530

CHAPTER **4.9**

Cervical Cancer: Future Directions

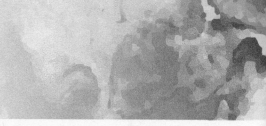

Charles A. Leath III and Teresa K. L. Boitano

Although increased HPV vaccination uptake and appropriate screening and follow-up are vitally important to both prevent and detect preinvasive cervical disease, cervical cancer remains a global challenge for the foreseeable future. Clinical trial results both presented and published over the past several years have dramatically not only impacted current management of women across the cervical cancer spectrum but also resulted in new drug approval and improved clinical outcomes. Nonetheless, several unanswered and important questions remain: (1) the role of less radical surgery in women with early-stage surgically resectable disease; (2) potential of minimally invasive radical hysterectomy for stage IA2-IB2 cervical cancer (≤4 cm); (3) improvement and/or modifications of the chemoradiation backbone for locally advanced cervical cancer; and (4) increasing and improving therapeutic options in the setting of recurrent and metastatic disease.

When considering the role of less radical surgery, both the SHAPE trial (NCT01658930), which is randomly assigning women to either a standard radical hysterectomy with pelvic lymph node dissection versus a simple hysterectomy with lymph node dissection, and GOG 278 (NCT 1649089), whose primary objectives are to assess the impact of either a cold knife conization or simple hysterectomy both in combination with a pelvic lymphadenectomy on quality-of-life (QoL) parameters (lymphedema, bladder, bowel, and sexual function) will inform clinical outcomes and survival. Although findings from the LACC trial resulted in a fairly rapid discontinuation of minimally invasive radical hysterectomy, ongoing studies including ROCC (A Trial of Robotic vs Open Hysterectomy Surgery in Cervix Cancer) (NCT 04831580) with novel surgical modifications including specimen manipulation and tumor containment systems, and mandated preoperative MRI to confirm lesion size, are being performed to determine whether more robust guidelines may inform safe and appropriate minimally invasive candidates.

Although improvement in managing early-stage cervical cancer is important, continued emphasis on determining interventions that may improve outcomes in women with recurrent or metastatic disease at diagnosis is also ongoing. While chemoradiation has been the backbone of treating locally advanced cervical cancer for over two decades, clinical trials have failed to demonstrate significant improvements to the cisplatin-based chemoradiation backbone. Importantly, the renewed emphasis on ensuring adequate and proper brachytherapy delivery and dosing, with an emphasis on avoiding alternative techniques, was recently summarized by both the Society of Gynecologic Oncology (SGO) and the American Brachytherapy Society (ABS) (1). Ongoing clinical trials with novel radiation sensitizers and immune-oncology agents may augment and improve outcomes in locally advanced cervical cancer. In addition, results from clinical trials with cemiplimab (2), tisotumab vedotin (3), and pembrolizumab (4) have demonstrated improved clinical outcomes and resulted in therapeutic drug approval by regulatory agencies. Nonetheless, efforts to improve upon these trial outcomes and in parallel identify potential biomarkers predictive of response are ongoing.

REFERENCES

1. Holschneider CH, Petereit DG, Chu C, et al. Brachytherapy: a critical component of primary radiation therapy for cervical cancer: from the Society of Gynecologic Oncology (SGO) and the American Brachytherapy Society (ABS). *Gynecol Oncol.* 2019;152(3):540-547. doi:10.1016/j.ygyno.2018.10.016

2. Tewari KS, Monk BJ, Vergote I, et al. Survival with cemiplimab in recurrent cervical cancer. *N Engl J Med.* 2022;386(6):544-555. doi:10.1056/NEJMoa2112187

3. Coleman RL, Lorusso D, Gennigens C, et al. Efficacy and safety of tisotumab vedotin in previously treated recurrent or metastatic cervical cancer (innovaTV 204/GOG-3023/ENGOT-cx6): a multicentre, open-label, single-arm, phase 2 study. *Lancet Oncol.* 2021;22(5):609-619. doi:10.1016/S1470-2045(21)00056-5

4. Colombo N, Dubot C, Lorusso D, et al. Pembrolizumab for persistent, recurrent, or metastatic cervical cancer. *N Engl J Med.* 2021;385(20):1856-1867. doi:10.1056/NEJMoa2112435

CORPUS: EPITHELIAL TUMORS

Endometrial Cancer: Introduction, Anatomy, Natural History, and Patterns of Spread

Amy Bregar

INTRODUCTION

Endometrial cancer (EC) accounts for nearly 50% of all new gynecologic cancers diagnosed in the United States. It is the fourth most common malignancy in women and the eighth most common cause of cancer death. The American Cancer Society (ACS) estimated that there were 65,950 new cases of endometrial carcinoma and 12,550 deaths from advanced or recurrent disease in 2022 (1). Worldwide, EC is only second to cervical cancer in frequency. The ACS reported that the incidence has increased by approximately 1% per year since the mid-2000s, with a similar increase in mortality rates of 1% annually from 2015 to 2019, although incidence and mortality rates appear to have stabilized in recent years. Endometrial carcinoma occurs most often in the sixth and seventh decades of life, with an average age at onset of 60 years. It is estimated that 75% to 85% of the cases occur in women aged 50 years and older, and 95% occur in patients over 40 years of age (2,3). Although reported in patients as young as 16 years, EC is rare in women younger than 30 years.

EC is commonly confined to the uterus at diagnosis. Data from the National Cancer Institute's Surveillance, Epidemiology, and End Results (SEER) program demonstrated that stage I disease was found in 73% of patients, and 10% had stage II disease (4). The 26th Annual Report of the International Federation of Gynecology and Obstetrics (FIGO) on 9,386 patients with EC demonstrated that 83% of patients were stage I-II (5). With the favorable disease distribution at presentation, it is not surprising that most patients have a favorable prognosis. Results from FIGO show that 85% to 91% of patients with stage I disease are alive at 5 years, and patients in the SEER database with localized disease have 96% 5-year survival (4,5). As a result, EC has been considered a "good cancer"; that is, most patients present with early-stage, highly curable disease. Despite the favorable characteristics for most patients, those with high-risk factors, including increased age, higher tumor grade, aggressive histology, and advanced stage, face real challenges.

The management of EC continues to evolve. In the past, most patients received some form of pre- or postoperative radiation in combination with a simple hysterectomy. With a better understanding of the relationship between uterine factors and risk of nodal disease and recurrence, selective use of surgical staging was integrated. This was followed by an era during which surgical therapy increasingly included routine use of pelvic and para-aortic lymphadenectomy and more recently the advent and adoption of sentinel lymph node (LN) dissection. Minimally invasive techniques were studied and have been routinely embraced in the surgical management of women with EC. Today, greater emphasis is being placed on the selection of particular patients for whom lymphadenectomy may offer better outcomes and whose avoidance may result in less morbidity. Understanding tumor biology as it relates to predicting recurrence and survival, and how molecular changes can be exploited to direct postoperative therapies represent our current challenges. Over 15 years ago, the National Cancer Institute convened an expert panel to develop a national 5-year plan for research priorities in gynecologic cancers. The resulting report, Priorities of the Gynecologic Cancer Progress Review Group (PRG), specified that an understanding of tumor biology was the central key in controlling gynecologic cancers. For EC, one of the top research priorities defined by the PRG was to identify prognostic and predictive markers for treatment efficacy and toxicity. In a 2006 State of the Science Meeting in Manchester, UK, a series of research questions on prevention, adjuvant treatment, and treatment of advanced or recurrent disease were proposed for setting the stage for a clinical trials agenda over the next 5 years (6). In 2011, the Society of Gynecologic Oncologists (SGO) convened a panel of experts that produced a report, "Pathways to Progress in Women's Cancer." That report detailed areas of research, by disease site, on which the women's cancer community should focus for the next decade. For EC, the recommended road map for the future would include research related to obesity, predicting risk of metastatic disease, targeting therapy based on risk factors and molecular characteristics of disease, and cost-effective care (7). In 2014, given significant advances in the diagnosis and management of EC, the SGO's Clinical Practice Committee reviewed the literature and provided evidence-based practice recommendations (8,9), which were then updated in 2021 (10).

Current clinical controversies center on identifying which patient populations might benefit most from lymphadenectomy, developing alternatives to performing lymphadenectomy, and creating risk models to assist in selection of patients who may benefit most from adjuvant therapies. Although we suspect that an increased use of surgical staging has translated to a better understanding of risk, data also suggest that despite negative nodes, uterine factors play a significant role in risk of recurrence. Current trends also suggest a less frequent use of pelvic radiation therapy (RT) or no use of any radiation (11). There have been important developments in chemotherapy for EC. Combination chemotherapy is increasingly used in the primary management of advanced and recurrent disease and has shown efficacy in an adjuvant setting. How to best integrate RT and which specific techniques to consider are being studied in ongoing clinical trials. Hormonal therapy remains an important option, and our understanding of steroid receptors at a molecular level may help to determine which patients may benefit most (12). Enhanced understanding of biologically relevant targets has fostered the development of new classes of agents that target susceptible pathways in tumor cells, and targeted agents are increasingly integrated into large clinical trials (13-15).

ANATOMY

The uterus is a fibromuscular pelvic organ situated between the bladder and the rectum and enveloped by peritoneal reflections. It is divided into the fundus, isthmus, and cervix. The uterine wall is composed of the outer smooth muscle myometrium and inner cavity lined by glandular endometrial epithelium with supporting stroma (endometrium). Five paired ligaments cover or support the uterus: broad, round, uterosacral, cardinal, and vesicouterine. The uterosacral and cardinal ligaments provide the greatest support within the pelvis and, contrary to cervical cancer, are infrequently involved with tumor spread. Blood is supplied to the uterus by the uterine artery, a branch of the hypogastric artery, which enters the wall of the uterus at the isthmus after it crosses over the ureter. It anastomoses with the ovarian artery in the ovarian ligament.

Malignant transformation of the endometrium is manifest in many fashions, based on the anatomic relationships. Tumor growth may be confined to the endometrium, invade the underlying myometrium, penetrate the uterine serosal surface or adjacent bladder or rectum, or extend into the cervical canal and invade cervical glands or stroma. Peritoneal disease spread may occur via transmigration from the fallopian tubes or through serosal penetration. Hematogenous spread is not uncommon in EC.

The lymphatics of the myometrium drain into the subserosal network of lymphatics, which coalesce into larger channels before leaving the uterus. Lymph flows from the fundus toward the adnexa and infundibulopelvic ligaments. The lymph flow from the lower and middle thirds of the uterus tends to spread in the base of the broad ligaments toward the lateral pelvic sidewall (16). There are four drainage channels from the uterus: from the fundus, in the folds of the broad ligament, along the mesosalpinx and fallopian tubes, and along the round ligaments. The drainage sites are principally reflected in metastatic potential to pelvic and para-aortic LNs and occasionally involve inguinal nodes.

CLASSIFICATION

Our traditional histomorphologic classification of EC was first described by Bokhman in 1983 (17). This simple but somewhat antiquated schema described two clinicopathogenetic types of EC based on metabolic and endocrine influences, pathologic features, and prognosis. Broadly, ECs that are thought to arise in an estrogen-dependent fashion are termed type I, whereas estrogen-independent tumors are classified as type II (Table 5.1-1). Type I tumors are more common (85%), tend to be found in younger women, and develop via a precursor lesion of atypical hyperplasia. These tumors are associated with a predisposing history of hyperestrogenism. They tend to be well differentiated and have minimal myometrial invasion, and as a result typically have

a favorable outcome. *PTEN* loss is common and found in about 83% of these tumors. Type II tumors account for a small percentage of ECs, occur in an older population, and frequently develop in the setting of an atrophic endometrium. About half of all relapses occur in this group. Serous, clear cell, carcinosarcoma, and high-grade endometrioid tumors classically fit into the type II category. Type II tumors are likely to be associated with *TP53* mutations.

Although Bokhman's classification system is helpful in providing a conceptual framework for understanding EC, it does not fit with growing knowledge regarding the molecular underpinnings of EC. In 2013, The Cancer Genome Atlas (TCGA) categorized 370 ECs into four molecular subtypes using genomic, transcriptomic, and proteomic analyses (18). These four molecular subtypes have unique genomic features with distinct prognostic outcomes and clinico-pathologic characteristics. The molecular subtypes first identified by the TCGA (ie, ultramutated, hypermutated, copy number [CN] high, and CN low) have been incorporated into the molecular classification of EC (POLEmut, MMRd, p53 abn, and No Specific Molecular Profile [NSMP]), described in more detail later (19,20). In 2020, the 5th edition of the *World Health Organization (WHO) Classification of Tumours—Female Genital Tumours* was published, which emphasizes the proposed new molecular classification system for ECs (21). Molecular subtypes have been shown to be highly reproducible and, when performed on endometrial sampling, show high concordance with subsequent hysterectomy specimens (19,22-24).

Molecular Subtypes

DNA Polymerase Epsilon Mutated Group (POLEmut)/Ultramutated

These ECs are characterized by a pathogenic mutation in the exonuclease domain of DNA polymerase epsilon (*POLE*), a gene involved in DNA replication and repair (25-28). This mutation results in a remarkably high mutation rate (often >100 mutations per megabase [Mb]), one of the highest mutation frequencies of any solid tumor. The tumors are most often endometrioid histology but can include high-grade and serous tumors. The presence of intratumoral lymphoid infiltrate (or tumor-infiltrating lymphocytes, TILs) is prominent. Women with these tumors tend to be relatively young with a normal body mass index (BMI). Although *POLE*mut tumors can exhibit high-risk pathologic features (such as high-grade and extensive lymphovascular space invasion), they often portend a more favorable prognosis (29-31).

Microsatellite Unstable Group (Mismatch Repair Deficient, MMRd)/Hypermutated

These ECs are notable for a loss of function of one or more of the mismatch repair (MMR) proteins (ie, MLH1, PMS2, MSH2, or MSH6). Epigenetic silencing of *MLH1* via hypermethylation makes up the largest proportion of this subgroup, but the subgroup also encompasses both somatic and germline mutations in other MMR genes. The defect in MMR causes a high mutational burden (>10 mutations/Mb) while exhibiting low levels of somatic CN alterations (deletions or amplifications of genomic material). These ECs occur across a wide age range (younger in patients with Lynch syndrome, a germline mutation in MMR genes) and are not associated with an increased BMI (32,33). Tumors of endometrioid histology make up the bulk of this subgroup, and they are often high grade. Patients who have tumors as a result of Lynch syndrome have a more favorable prognosis compared to those with sporadic MMRd endometrial carcinoma (32).

No Specific Molecular Profile/Copy Number Low Group

These ECs are considered genomically stable, with low levels of somatic CN alterations and moderate mutational burden. By definition, these tumors are MMR-proficient, *POLE* wild type with

■ TABLE 5.1-1. Comparison Between Type I and Type II Endometrial Cancers

	Type I	Type II
Clinical features		
Risk factors	Unopposed estrogen	Age
Race	White > Black	White = Black
Differentiation	Well differentiated	Poorly differentiated
Histology	Endometrioid	Non-endometrioid
Stage	I/II	III/IV
Prognosis	Favorable	Not favorable
Molecular features		
Ploidy	Diploid	Aneuploid
K-ras overexpression	Yes	Yes
HER2/neu overexpression	No	Yes
P53 overexpression	No	Yes
PTEN mutations	Yes	No
MSI	Yes	No

MSI, microsatellite instability.

wild-type pattern p53 immunoreactivity/wild-type p53 on sequencing. This subgroup contains primarily endometrioid tumors that are estrogen and progesterone receptor (ER, PR) positive. These tumors generally have intermediate to favorable outcome, except for tumors with mutations in exon 3 of *CTNNB1* that are associated with a worse prognosis (34).

p53abn/Copy Number High (Serous-Like) Group

The fourth molecular subgroup is characterized by high somatic CN alteration, similar to tubo-ovarian high-grade serous cancer (HGSC). Also similar to HGSC, tumors in this subtype consistently demonstrate abnormal p53 immunostaining/*TP53* mutations. Interestingly, EC molecular pathology does not necessarily correlate with histopathology as it does for HGSC; although a large majority of these tumors are of serous histology, carcinosarcomas, endometrial carcinomas of mixed histology, and a minority of high-grade endometrioid and clear cell carcinomas are also included. HER2 amplification occurs in about 20% of the subtype and some tumors demonstrate homologous recombination deficiency (35,36). Breast cancer susceptibility genes (*BRCA1/2*) mutation carriers have an increased risk for p53abn EC, with *BRCA1* mutation carriers having the highest risk (37). Although this subtype accounts for only 15% of endometrial carcinomas, it accounts for 50% to 70% of endometrial carcinoma–associated mortality (19,38).

It is important to note there can be some apparent molecular overlap. Given that secondary subclonal defects in p53 and MMR can occur in high mutational status tumors, an algorithmic and hierarchical approach to the interpretation of tests is recommended. This would require first assessing for a pathogenic *POLE* mutation, next establishing MMR status, and finally performing p53 immunohistochemistry for classification only in *POLE* and MMR-proficient cases (39).

Clinical Implications

The recognition of the clinical importance of the molecular classification of EC is growing, and data demonstrate that molecular subtype can have important prognostic and treatment implications. Subanalysis of *POLE*mut and *POLE*wild-type EC in the observational arm of the PORTEC-2 trial showed a 10-year recurrence-free survival (RFS) of 100% versus 80.1% (hazard ratio = 0.143; 95% confidence interval = 0.001-0.996; *P* = .049) (40), a finding that has been replicated by multiple studies (29,31,41,42). Further supporting the excellent prognosis of the *POLE*mut subtype, an individual patient meta-analysis of all *POLE*mut ECs found that adjuvant therapy was not associated with improved outcomes, supporting de-escalation of therapy in clinical trials (30). Accordingly, two prospective studies are ongoing, investigating a "less-is-more" approach to *POLE*mut tumors: (1) PORTEC-4a is a multicenter randomized phase III trial in patients with high- to intermediate-risk EC (43,44), and (2) Tailored Adjuvant Therapy in *POLE*-mutated and p53-wild type/no specific molecular profile (NSMP) Early Stage Endometrial Cancer (TAPER) is a prospective cohort study (45).

Although MMRd tumors are generally thought to have an intermediate prognosis, they are particularly susceptible to radiation (46,47). In addition, the U.S. Food and Drug Administration has approved the use of immune checkpoint inhibitors for metastatic or recurrent MMRd ECs with promising response rates even in heavily pretreated disease (48-52), and ongoing trials are investigating immunotherapy in this population in the upfront setting (53,54). Although NSMP encompasses the largest EC subgroup and is considered a relatively heterogeneous molecular group, patients with a mutation in exon 3 of *CTNNB1* have consistently demonstrated significantly worse RFS (34,55,56).

Tumors in the p53abn subgroup are recognized to portend a poor prognosis, accounting for the majority of EC mortality. The PORTEC-3 clinical trial results suggest that patients with p53abn

ECs have superior outcomes when treated with chemotherapy in addition to radiation, as compared to radiotherapy alone (47). Therapies directed at HER2 amplification and poly (ADP-ribose) polymerase (PARP) inhibition have been conducted and are ongoing in this subgroup (35,57,58).

The 2021 SGO evidence-based recommendations state that next-generation sequencing and further molecular classification, including identification of *TP53* mutations, may help guide future treatment decisions (10). The European Society of Gynaecological Oncology (ESGO), European Society for Radiotherapy and Oncology (ESTRO), and European Society of Pathology (ESP) guidelines recommend using these subtypes, when known, to assign risk group and to direct treatment recommendations (59). Notable changes include grouping all early-stage (stage I/II) *POLE*mut ECs as low risk with no adjuvant therapy recommended and classifying stage IA p53abn ECs with any myometrial invasion as high risk and thus recommending chemotherapy (with or without radiation) for these patients.

In summary, the incorporation of molecular subtypes into our understanding of EC may offer more consistent categorization, more useful predictive and prognostic information, and indications for novel treatment paradigms.

REFERENCES

1. Siegel RL, Miller KD, Fuchs HE, Jemal A. Cancer statistics, 2022. *CA Cancer J Clin.* 2022;72:7-33.
2. Gallup DG, Stock RJ. Adenocarcinoma of the endometrium in women 40 years of age or younger. *Obstet Gynecol.* 1984;64:417-420.
3. Norris HJ, Tavassoli FA, Kurman RJ. Endometrial hyperplasia and carcinoma, diagnostic consideration. *Am J Surg Pathol.* 1988;7:839-847.
4. Trimble EL, Harlan LC, Clegg L, Stevens JL. Pre-operative imaging, surgery, and adjuvant therapy for women diagnosed with cancer of the corpus uteri in community practice in the US. *Gynecol Oncol.* 2005;96:741-748.
5. Creasman W, Odicino F, Maisonneuve P, et al. Carcinoma of the corpus uteri. FIGO 26th annual report on the results of treatment in gynecological cancer. *Int J Gynecol Obstet.* 2006;95(suppl 1):S105-S143.
6. Kitchener H, Trimble EL. Endometrial cancer state of the science meeting. *Int J Gynecol Cancer.* 2009;19:134-140.
7. Curtin J, Clarke-Pearson DL. *Pathways to Progress in Women's Cancer. A Research Agenda Proposed by the Society of Gynecologic Oncology.* The Society of Gynecologic Oncology; 2012.
8. SGO Clinical Practice Endometrial Cancer Working Group, Burke WM, Orr J, et al. Endometrial cancer: a review and current management strategies: part I. *Gynecol Oncol.* 2014;134:85-92.
9. SGO Clinical Practice Endometrial Cancer Working Group, Burke WM, Orr J, et al. Endometrial cancer: a review and current management strategies: part II. *Gynecol Oncol.* 2014;134:393-402.
10. Hamilton CA, Pothuri B, Arend RC, et al. Endometrial cancer: a Society of Gynecologic Oncology evidence-based review and recommendations. *Gynecol Oncol.* 2021;160:817-826.
11. Naumann RW, Coleman R. The use of adjuvant radiation therapy in early endometrial cancer by members of the Society of Gynecologic Oncologists in 2005. *Gynecol Oncol.* 2007;105:7-12.
12. Singh M, Zaino R, Filiaci V, Leslie KK. Relationship of estrogen and progesterone receptors to clinical outcome in metastatic endometrial carcinoma: a Gynecologic Oncology Group Study. *Gynecol Oncol.* 2007;106(2):325-333.
13. Engelsen I, Akslen LA, Salverson HB. Biologic markers in endometrial cancer treatment. *APMIS.* 2009;117:693-707.
14. Dedes K, Wetterskog D, Ashworth A, Kaye SB, Reis-Filho JS. Emerging therapeutic targets in endometrial cancer. *Nat Rev Clin Oncol.* 2011;8:261-271.
15. Yen TT, Wang TL, Fader AN, Shih IM, Gaillard S. Molecular classification and emerging targeted therapy in endometrial cancer. *Int J Gynecol Pathol.* 2020;39:26-35.
16. Plentl AA, Friedman EA. *Lymphatic System of the Female Genitalia: The Morphologic Basis of Oncologic Diagnosis and Therapy.* WB Saunders; 1971:116.
17. Bokhman JV. Two pathogenic types of endometrial carcinoma. *Gynecol Oncol.* 1983;10:237-246.
18. Woo HL, Swenerton KD, Hoskins PJ. Taxol is active in platinum-resistant endometrial adenocarcinoma. *Am J Clin Oncol.* 1996;19(3):290-291.

19. Kommoss S, McConechy MK, Kommoss F. Final validation of the ProMisE molecular classifier for endometrial carcinoma in a large population-based case series. *Ann Oncol.* 2018;29:1180-1188.

20. Cosgrove CM, Tritchler DL, Cohn DE. An NRG Oncology/GOG study of molecular classification for risk prediction in endometrioid endometrial cancer. *Gynecol Oncol.* 2018;148:174-180.

21. World Health Organization. *WHO Classification of Tumours: Female Genital Tumours.* 5th ed. International Agency for Research on Cancer; 2020, xii:632.

22. Plotkin A, Kuzeljevic B, De Villa V, et al. Interlaboratory concordance of ProMisE molecular classification of endometrial carcinoma based on endometrial biopsy specimens. *Int J Gynecol Pathol.* 2020;39:537-545.

23. Stelloo E, Nout RA, Naves LC, et al. High concordance of molecular tumor alterations between pre-operative curettage and hysterectomy specimens in patients with endometrial carcinoma. *Gynecol Oncol.* 2014;133:197-204.

24. Abdulfatah E, Wakeling E, Sakr S, et al. Molecular classification of endometrial carcinoma applied to endometrial biopsy specimens: towards early personalized patient management. *Gynecol Oncol.* 2019;154:467-474.

25. Shevelev IV, Hubscher U. The 3′–5′ exonucleases. *Nat Rev Mol Cell Biol.* 2002;3(5):364-376.

26. Rayner E, van Gool IC, Palles C, et al. A panoply of errors: polymerase proofreading domain mutations in cancer. *Nat Rev Cancer.* 2016;16(2):71-81.

27. Church DN, Briggs SE, Palles C, et al. DNA polymerase epsilon and delta exonuclease domain mutations in endometrial cancer. *Hum Mol Genet.* 2013;22(14):2820-2828.

28. Henninger EE, Pursell ZF. DNA polymerase epsilon and its roles in genome stability. *IUBMB Life.* 2014;66(5):339-351.

29. Church DN, Stelloo E, Nout RA, et al. Prognostic significance of POLE proofreading mutations in endometrial cancer. *J Natl Cancer Inst.* 2015;107(1):402.

30. McAlpine JN, Chiu DS, Nout RA, et al. Evaluation of treatment effects in patients with endometrial cancer and POLE mutations: an individual patient data meta-analysis. *Cancer.* 2021;127(14):2409-2422.

31. Meng B, Hoang LN, McIntyre JB, et al. POLE exonuclease domain mutation predicts long progression-free survival in grade 3 endometrioid carcinoma of the endometrium. *Gynecol Oncol.* 2014;134(1):15-19.

32. Post CCB, Stelloo E, Smit VTHBM, et al. Prevalence and prognosis of Lynch syndrome and sporadic mismatch repair deficiency in endometrial cancer. *J Natl Cancer Inst.* 2021;113(9):1212-1220.

33. Vermij L, Smit V, Nout R, Bosse T. Incorporation of molecular characteristics into endometrial cancer management. *Histopathology.* 2020;76(1):52-63.

34. Kurnit KC, Kim GN, Fellman BM, et al. CTNNB1 (beta-catenin) mutation identifies low grade, early stage endometrial cancer patients at increased risk of recurrence. *Mod Pathol.* 2017;30(7):1032-1041.

35. de Jonge MM, Auguste A, van Wijk LM, et al. Frequent homologous recombination deficiency in high-grade endometrial carcinomas. *Clin Cancer Res.* 2019;25(3):1087-1097.

36. Ashley CW, Da Cruz Paula A, Kumar R, et al. Analysis of mutational signatures in primary and metastatic endometrial cancer reveals distinct patterns of DNA repair defects and shifts during tumor progression. *Gynecol Oncol.* 2019;152(1):11-19.

37. de Jonge MM, de Kroon CD, Jenner DJ, et al. Endometrial cancer risk in women with germline BRCA1 or BRCA2 mutations: multicenter cohort study. *J Natl Cancer Inst.* 2021;113(9):1203-1211.

38. Jamieson A, Thompson EF, Huvila J, Gilks CB, McAlpine JN. p53abn Endometrial cancer: understanding the most aggressive endometrial cancers in the era of molecular classification. *Int J Gynecol Cancer.* 2021;31(6):907-913.

39. McCluggage WG, Singh N, Gilks CB. Key changes to the World Health Organization (WHO) classification of female genital tumours introduced in the 5(TH) edition (2020). *Histopathology.* 2022;80(5):762-778.

40. Wortman BG, Creutzberg CL, Putter H, et al. Ten-year results of the PORTEC-2 trial for high-intermediate risk endometrial carcinoma: improving patient selection for adjuvant therapy. *Br J Cancer.* 2018;119(9):1067-1074.

41. McConechy MK, Talhouk A, Leung S, et al. Endometrial carcinomas with POLE exonuclease domain mutations have a favorable prognosis. *Clin Cancer Res.* 2016;22(12):2865-2873.

42. Stasenko M, Tunnage I, Ashley CW, et al. Clinical outcomes of patients with POLE mutated endometrioid endometrial cancer. *Gynecol Oncol.* 2020;156(1):194-202.

43. van den Heerik A, Horeweg N, Nout RA, et al. PORTEC-4a: international randomized trial of molecular profile-based adjuvant treatment for women with high-intermediate risk endometrial cancer. *Int J Gynecol Cancer.* 2020;30(12):2002-2007.

44. ClinicalTrials.gov. PORTEC-4a: molecular profile-based versus standard adjuvant radiotherapy in endometrial cancer (PORTEC-4a). Accessed January 18, 2022. https://clinicaltrials.gov/ct2/show/NCT03469674?cond=PORTEC-4&draw=2&rank=1

45. ClinicalTrials.gov. Tailored adjuvant therapy in POLE-mutated and p53-wildtype early stage endometrial cancer (TAPER). Accessed January 18, 2022. https://clinicaltrials.gov/ct2/show/NCT04705649?term=TAPER+endometrial+cancer&draw=2&rank=1

46. Reijnen C, Küsters-Vandevelde HVN, Prinsen CF, et al. Mismatch repair deficiency as a predictive marker for response to adjuvant radiotherapy in endometrial cancer. *Gynecol Oncol.* 2019;154(1):124-130.

47. Leon-Castillo A, de Boer SM, Powell ME, et al. Molecular classification of the PORTEC-3 trial for high-risk endometrial cancer: impact on prognosis and benefit from adjuvant therapy. *J Clin Oncol.* 2020;38(29):3388-3397.

48. Le DT, Uram JN, Wang H, et al. PD-1 blockade in tumors with mismatch-repair deficiency. *N Engl J Med.* 2015;372(26):2509-2520.

49. U.S. Food & Drug Administration. FDA grants accelerated approval to pembrolizumab for first tissue/site agnostic indication. Accessed January 18, 2022. https://www.fda.gov/drugs/resources-information-approved-drugs/fda-grants-accelerated-approval-pembrolizumab-first-tissuesite-agnostic-indication

50. Marabelle A, Le DT, Ascierto PA, et al. Efficacy of pembrolizumab in patients with noncolorectal high microsatellite instability/mismatch repair-deficient cancer: results from the phase II KEYNOTE-158 study. *J Clin Oncol.* 2020;38(1):1-10.

51. O'Malley DM, Bariani GM, Cassier PA, et al. Pembrolizumab in patients with microsatellite instability-high advanced endometrial cancer: results from the KEYNOTE-158 study. *J Clin Oncol.* 2022;40(7):752-761.

52. Oaknin A, Tinker AV, Gilbert L, et al. Clinical activity and safety of the anti-programmed death 1 monoclonal antibody dostarlimab for patients with recurrent or advanced mismatch repair-deficient endometrial cancer: a nonrandomized phase 1 clinical trial. *JAMA Oncol.* 2020;6(11):1766-1772.

53. ClinicalTrials.gov. Testing the addition of the immunotherapy drug, pembrolizumab, to the usual radiation treatment for newly diagnosed early stage high intermediate risk endometrial cancer. Accessed January 18, 2022. https://clinicaltrials.gov/ct2/show/NCT04214067

54. ClinicalTrials.gov. Testing the addition of the immunotherapy drug pembrolizumab to the usual chemotherapy treatment (paclitaxel and carboplatin) in stage III-IV or recurrent endometrial cancer. Accessed January 18, 2022. https://clinicaltrials.gov/ct2/show/NCT03914612

55. Liu Y, Patel L, Mills GB, et al. Clinical significance of CTNNB1 mutation and Wnt pathway activation in endometrioid endometrial carcinoma. *J Natl Cancer Inst.* 2014;106(9):dju245.

56. Costigan DC, Dong F, Nucci MR, Howitt BE. Clinicopathologic and immunohistochemical correlates of CTNNB1 mutated endometrial endometrioid carcinoma. *Int J Gynecol Pathol.* 2020;39(2):119-127.

57. Fader AN, Roque DM, Siegel E, et al. Randomized phase II trial of carboplatin-paclitaxel compared with carboplatin-paclitaxel-trastuzumab in advanced (stage III-IV) or recurrent uterine serous carcinomas that overexpress Her2/Neu (NCT01367002): updated overall survival analysis. *Clin Cancer Res.* 2020;26(15):3928-3935.

58. Musacchio L, Caruso G, Pisano C, et al. PARP inhibitors in endometrial cancer: current status and perspectives. *Cancer Manag Res.* 2020;12:6123-6135.

59. Concin N, Matias-Guiu X, Vergote I, et al. ESGO/ESTRO/ESP guidelines for the management of patients with endometrial carcinoma. *Int J Gynecol Cancer.* 2021;31(1):12-39.

CHAPTER **5.2**

Endometrial Cancer: Etiology, Epidemiology, Risk Factors, Genetics, and Molecular Biology

Amy Bregar

EPIDEMIOLOGY AND RISK FACTORS

The most important risk factor for the development of EC is age. EC is primarily a disease of postmenopausal women, with median age at diagnosis of 60 years (1). Approximately 85% of cases occur after the age of 50 years; the peak age-specific incidence is from 75 to 79 years, and only 5% of cases are reported in women younger than 40 years (2-4). The ACS has reported that the probability of developing uterine cancer is 1 in 320 from birth until age 49 years, 1 in 157 from age 50 to 59 years, 1 in 94 from age 60 to 69 years, and 1 in 66 from age 70 years and above (5). Not unexpectedly, with an aging U.S. population, the total number of cases of EC has increased yearly, whereas the annual age-adjusted incidence rate peaked in the mid-1970s (33.8 per 100,000) and is most recently reported as 27.4 per 100,000 women from 2014 to 2018 (5).

Race and ethnicity also appear to play a role in the development of EC. The rates of EC are highest in North America and Northern Europe, lower in Eastern Europe and Latin America, and lowest in Asia and Africa (6). Factors accounting for these findings include differences in rates of obesity, use of hormone replacement therapy (HRT), and reproductive factors. In the United States, American Indian and Alaska Native women have the highest age-adjusted incidence of EC at 28.3 (per 100,000 women), compared to non-Hispanic Black (28.1), non-Hispanic White (27.8), Hispanic (24.5), and Asian (20.6) women (5). Non-Hispanic Black women, however, have a much higher mortality rate (9 vs 4.6 per 100,000) and a lower 5-year disease-specific survival (67% vs 86%) compared to non-Hispanic White women (5,7-10). The 2022 ACS annual publication notes that uterine cancer displays one of the highest Black-White survival difference, in absolute terms, among cancer types at 21% (5). Multiple explanations have been suggested to explain the differences in outcomes between racial groups, including differences in frequency of high-risk tumor types, differences in access to care, and differences in medical comorbidities among races. Compared to White women, Black women are more likely to present with higher-grade, advanced-stage cancer with aggressive non-endometrioid histology and mutations in *TP53* associated with poor prognosis (11). However, differences in tumor biology cannot completely account for the disparities in outcomes as Black women have poorer outcomes across nearly all disease stages and histologies (11,12). Growing data report that Black women are less likely to receive guideline-concordant care, which undoubtably contributes, at least in part, to worse outcomes (13-15).

Most cases of EC are thought to be sporadic; however, some cases clearly have a hereditary basis. Lynch syndrome (hereditary nonpolyposis colorectal cancer [HNPCC]) is an autosomal dominant cancer susceptibility syndrome associated with early-onset colon, rectal, ovary, stomach, small bowel, pancreato-biliary, genitourinary, and brain (glioma) cancers and EC. Lynch syndrome–related ECs account for 2% to 5% of all ECs and occur in nearly 10% of women diagnosed with EC who are younger than 50 years (16). The lifetime risk of EC in women with Lynch syndrome is 40% to 60%, a risk similar to that of developing colon cancer. The risk of ovarian cancer is 10% to 12%. In about 50% of cases where patients have both colonic and gynecologic cancers (endometrial or ovarian), the gynecologic cancer precedes the diagnosis of colon cancer (17). The syndrome is most commonly because of germline mutations of one of the DNA mismatch repair genes *MSH2*, *MLH1*, or *MSH6*. In one study, 23% of patients with EC diagnosed at less than 50 years of age, with one relative having a Lynch-type cancer, had a mismatch repair gene mutation (18). Data are growing to suggest that patients with Lynch syndrome–associated EC demonstrated better RFS (19). Prophylactic hysterectomy and bilateral salpingo-oophorectomy (BSO) have been shown to be an effective strategy for preventing ovarian cancer and ECs in these high-risk patients (20). Cowden syndrome, a rare autosomal dominant syndrome resulting from a germline mutation in *PTEN*, is associated with a 13% to 19% lifetime risk of EC, in addition to an increased risk of breast and thyroid cancers (21,22).

Inconsistent data exist regarding the relationship between *BRCA1* and *BRCA2* mutations and the risk of EC (23-27). Germline mutations of *BRCA1* and *BRCA2* account for a large proportion of hereditary breast and ovarian/primary peritoneal cancers. Several studies have suggested that uterine serous cancer is part of the *BRCA1/2* tumor spectrum, but the overall risk is very low. One study of an unselected population of 151 women with uterine papillary serous carcinoma found that 7 women (4.6%) had mutations in *BRCA1*, *TP53*, and *CHEK2* (26). Two percent of subjects had a *BRCA* mutation, which is higher than expected but still quite low. In a large study of 1,083 *BRCA1/2* carriers undergoing risk-reducing BSO without hysterectomy, women with *BRCA1* mutation were noted to have an increased incidence in serous EC compared to what had been historically observed (4 cases observed in 630 women with *BRCA1* mutation followed for a median of 5.1 years; observed-to-expected ratio 22.2, 95% confidence interval [CI] 6.1-56.9) (28). In this study, *BRCA2* mutation did not appear to have an associated increased risk.

Endogenous or exogenous exposure to estrogen is believed to be an important risk factor for the development of endometrial hyperplasia and type I cancers (29). Estrogens not opposed by progestins lead to increased mitotic activity of endometrial cells, resulting in more frequent errors in DNA replication and somatic mutations (30,31). These genetic changes are manifest clinically in endometrial hyperplasia and cancer. Estrogen excess as an etiology for cancers is supported by epidemiologic features of the disease. Patients with excess endogenous sources of estrogen, such as chronic anovulation, nulliparity, early age of menarche, and late menopause, have a higher risk of EC. Occasionally, endometrial hyperplasia or cancer develops in the setting of an estrogen-producing ovarian tumor (granulosa cell tumor) (32).

EC risk is also increased by exogenous sources of unopposed estrogen. The use of unopposed estrogens as part of hormone replacement strategies was first defined as an important risk factor in 1975, when the age-adjusted rate for EC peaked at nearly 33.8 per 100,000 (33). In a meta-analysis of randomized trials of hormone therapy in postmenopausal patients, the increased risk of developing endometrial hyperplasia was statistically significant after 1 year of moderate- or high-dose unopposed estrogen (odds ratio [OR] 8.4 and 10.7, respectively) and after 18 and 24 months of low-dose therapy (OR 2.4) (34). Various case-control and prospective studies have confirmed this finding, with the increased relative risk ranging from 1.5- to 10-fold, depending on duration and dose of use (35-39). Tamoxifen is a selective estrogen receptor modulator (SERM) with both agonist and antagonist properties, depending upon the individual target organ and circulating levels of serum estrogen (40-42). In endometrial tissue, it acts as an estrogen agonist in postmenopausal patients (who have low estrogen levels), whereas it acts as an estrogen antagonist in premenopausal patients (who have high estrogen levels). Accordingly, use of tamoxifen increases the risk of EC in postmenopausal patients in a dose- and duration-dependent fashion. The increased risks of EC are well established for postmenopausal patients and include high-quality data from randomized trials (43-46). In premenopausal patients, the increased risk of EC has not been proven. Tamoxifen does appear to be associated with an increased risk of carcinosarcoma, in addition to sarcomas, although the absolute risk is also low (47-49). The American College of Obstetrics and Gynecology (ACOG) advises that patients taking tamoxifen be advised on the risk of EC and uterine sarcomas (50).

Obesity is an increasingly common problem in the United States and is estimated to account for approximately 57% of ECs (51). Studies have shown that plasma concentrations of androstenedione and estrogens are correlated with body weight in postmenopausal women (52,53). Aromatization of androstenedione to estrone in adipose cells is believed to be the principal mechanism of excess estrogen production (54). Patients with obesity may also have lower circulating sex hormone–binding globulin (leading to increased steroid hormone activity), alterations in concentrations of insulin-like growth factor and its binding proteins, and insulin resistance, all of which may contribute to the increased risk of EC in these patients (55,56). Although much of the data suggest that the relationship is strongest between estrogen exposure and type I cancers, there is evidence that obesity is a risk factor for all ECs (57,58).

Protective Factors

Factors that reduce circulating estrogen levels (weight loss/exercise, cigarette smoking, breastfeeding) appear to be protective against EC. Similarly, progestins antagonize the effects of estrogen on the endometrium and prevent the development of hyperplasia and cancer, when added to estrogens (endogenous or exogenous) (59). Combined estrogen-progestin HRT has been associated with reductions in the risk of EC in most, but not all, studies. Prior use of oral contraceptives is protective against the development of EC (60,61).

NATURAL HISTORY OF DISEASE

A better understanding of the natural history of EC has developed through evaluation of the patterns of spread. In a landmark study, the Gynecologic Oncology Group (GOG) performed a surgical pathologic study (GOG 33) in 621 patients with clinical stage I-occult stage II EC who underwent a standardized surgical procedure including exploration of the abdomen with biopsy of suspicious findings, collection of peritoneal fluid for cytologic evaluation, abdominal hysterectomy and BSO, and pelvic and para-aortic node dissection (62). The results of this study demonstrated important relationships regarding uterine tumor characteristics and spread of disease and should be ingrained into the memory of those caring for patients with ECs.

Overall, 22% of patients with seemingly uterine-confined disease were found to have extrauterine spread. Pelvic and/or para-aortic metastases were found in 11% of patients, 12% had positive peritoneal cytology, 5% had adnexal involvement, and 6% had gross intraperitoneal spread. Nodal metastases were related to tumor grade and depth of myometrial invasion, and patients with positive cytology or adnexal or intraperitoneal spread also had increased frequency of nodal disease.

Patterns of failure in patients with recurrent EC demonstrate, alone or in combination, hematogenous, lymphatic, intraperitoneal, or local/contiguous spread. As attention has increasingly focused on therapies (surgical, radiation, chemotherapy) to reduce particular sites of recurrences, many have argued for defining relationships between initial disease spread and subsequent risk of recurrence (63). In GOG 33, treatment was not specified by protocol, but results showed that outcomes could be predicted by extent of disease found at surgery, thus demonstrating the important relationship between what is learned at surgical staging and recurrence risk (64).

REFERENCES

1. Stelloo E, Bosse T, Nout RA, et al. Refining prognosis and identifying targetable pathways for high-risk endometrial cancer; a TransPORTEC initiative. *Mod Pathol*. 2015;28(6):836-844.
2. Statistics Canada. http://www.statcan.gc.ca
3. Crosbie EJ, Zwahlen M, Kitchener HC, Egger M, Renehan AG. Body mass index, hormone replacement therapy, and endometrial cancer risk: a meta-analysis. *Cancer Epidemiol Biomarkers Prev*. 2010;19(12):3119-3130.
4. Ries LAG, Eisner CL Kosary et al. *SEER Cancer Statistics Review, 1973-1997*. National Cancer Institute; 2000:171-181.
5. Siegel RL, Miller KD, Fuchs HE, Jemal A. Cancer statistics, 2022. *CA Cancer J Clin*. 2022;72:7-33.
6. Parkin DM, Whelan SL, Ferlay J, et al. *Cancer Incidence in Five Continents*. Vol 7: IARC Scientific Publication No 143. IARC; 1997.
7. Cote ML, Ruterbusch JJ, Olson SH, Lu K, Ali-Fehmi R. The growing burden of endometrial cancer: a major racial disparity affecting black women. *Cancer Epidemiol Biomarkers Prev*. 2015;24(9):1407-1415.
8. Rauh-Hain JA, Melamed A, Schaps D, et al. Racial and ethnic disparities over time in the treatment and mortality of women with gynecological malignancies. *Gynecol Oncol*. 2018;149(1):4-11.
9. DeSantis CE, Miller KD, Sauer AG, Jemal A, Siegel RL. Cancer statistics for African Americans, 2019. *CA Cancer J Clin*. 2019;69(3):211-233.
10. Clarke MA, Devesa SS, Havey SV, Wentzensen N. Hysterectomy-corrected uterine corpus cancer incidence trends and differences in relative survival reveal racial disparities and rising rates of nonendometrioid cancers. *J Clin Oncol*. 2019;37(22):1895-1908.
11. Long B, Liu FW, Bristow RE. Disparities in uterine cancer epidemiology, treatment, and survival among African Americans in the United States. *Gynecol Oncol*. 2013;130(3):652-659.
12. Sud S, Holmes J, Eblan M, Chen R, Jones E. Clinical characteristics associated with racial disparities in endometrial cancer outcomes: a surveillance, epidemiology and end results analysis. *Gynecol Oncol*. 2018;148(2):349-356.
13. Doll KM, Khor S, Odem-Davis K, et al. Role of bleeding recognition and evaluation in Black-White disparities in endometrial cancer. *Am J Obstet Gynecol*. 2018;219(6):593.e1-593.e14.
14. Huang AB, Khor S, Odem-Davis K, et al. Impact of quality of care on racial disparities in survival for endometrial cancer. *Am J Obstet Gynecol*. 2020;223(3):396.e1-396.e13.
15. Doll KM, Nguyen A, Alson JG. A conceptual model of vulnerability to care delay among women at risk for endometrial cancer. *Gynecol Oncol*. 2022;164:318-324.
16. Watson P, Lynch H. Extracolonic cancer in hereditary nonpolyposis colorectal cancer. *Cancer*. 1993;71:677-685.
17. Lu K, Dinh M, Kohlman W, et al. Gynecologic cancer as a "sentinel cancer" for women with hereditary nonpolyposis colorectal cancer syndrome. *Obstet Gynecol*. 2005;105:569-574.
18. Berends M, Wu Y, Sijmons R, et al. Toward new strategies to select young endometrial cancer patients for mismatch repair gene mutation analysis. *J Clin Oncol*. 2003;23:4364-4370.
19. Post CCB, Stelloo E, Smit VTHBM, et al. Prevalence and prognosis of lynch syndrome and sporadic mismatch repair deficiency in endometrial cancer. *J Natl Cancer Inst*. 2021;113(9):1212-1220.
20. Schmeler K, Lynch H, Chen L, et al. Prophylactic surgery to reduce the risk of gynecologic cancers in the Lynch syndrome. *N Engl J Med*. 2006;354:261-269.
21. Riegert-Johnson DL, Gleeson FC, Roberts M, et al. Cancer and Lhermitte-Duclos disease are common in Cowden syndrome patients. *Hered Cancer Clin Pract*. 2010;8(1):6.
22. Pilarski R, Stephen JA, Noss R, Fisher JL, Prior TW. Predicting PTEN mutations: an evaluation of Cowden syndrome and Bannayan-Riley-Ruvalcaba syndrome clinical features. *J Med Genet*. 2011;48(8):505-512.

23. Thompson D, Easton DF; Breast Cancer Linkage Consortium. Cancer incidence in BRCA1 mutation carriers. *J Natl Cancer Inst.* 2002;94(18):1358-1365.

24. Moslehi R, Chu W, Karlan B, et al. BRCA1 and BRCA2 mutation analysis of 208 Ashkenazi Jewish women with ovarian cancer. *Am J Hum Genet.* 2000;66(4):1259-1272.

25. Segev Y, Iqbal J, Lubinski J, et al. The incidence of endometrial cancer in women with BRCA1 and BRCA2 mutations: an international prospective cohort study. *Gynecol Oncol.* 2013;130(1):127-131.

26. Pennington KP, Walsh T, Lee M, et al. BRCA1, TP53, and CHEK2 germline mutations in uterine serous carcinoma. *Cancer.* 2013;119(2):332-338.

27. Kitson SJ, Bafligil C, Ryan NAJ, et al. BRCA1 and BRCA2 pathogenic variant carriers and endometrial cancer risk: a cohort study. *Eur J Cancer.* 2020;136:169-175.

28. Shu CA, Pike M, Jotwani A, et al. Uterine cancer after risk-reducing salpingo-oophorectomy without hysterectomy in women with BRCA mutations. *JAMA Oncol.* 2016;2(11):1434-1440.

29. Akhmedkhanov A, Zeleniuch-Jaquotte A, Toniolo P. Role of exogenous and endogenous hormones in endometrial cancer. *Ann N Y Acad Sci.* 2001;943:296-315.

30. Key TJA, Pike MC. The dose effect relationship between unopposed estrogens and endometrial mitotic rate: its central role in explaining and predicting endometrial cancer risk. *Br J Cancer.* 1998;57:205-212.

31. Henderson BE, Feigelson HS. Hormonal carcinogenesis. *Carcinogenesis.* 2000;21:427-433.

32. McDonald TW, Malkasian GD, Gaffey TA. Endometrial cancer associated with feminizing ovarian tumor and polycystic ovarian disease. *Obstet Gynecol.* 1977;49:654-658.

33. Ziel HK, Finkle WD. Increased risk of endometrial carcinoma among users of conjugated estrogens. *N Engl J Med.* 1975;293:1167-1170.

34. Furness S, Roberts H, Marjoribanks J, Lethaby A, Hickey M, Farquhar C. Hormone therapy in postmenopausal women and risk of endometrial hyperplasia. *Cochrane Database Syst Rev.* 2009;(2):CD000402.

35. Henderson BE. The cancer question: an overview of recent epidemiologic and retrospective data. *Am J Obstet Gynecol.* 1989;161(6 Pt 2):1859-1864.

36. Persson I, Adami HO, Bergkvist L, et al. Risk of endometrial cancer after treatment with oestrogens alone or in conjunction with progestogens: results of a prospective study. *BMJ.* 1989;298(6667):147-151.

37. Beral V, Bull D, Reeves G; Million Women Study Collaborators. Endometrial cancer and hormone-replacement therapy in the Million Women Study. *Lancet.* 2005;365(9470):1543-1551.

38. Weiderpass E, Adami HO, Baron JA, et al. Risk of endometrial cancer following estrogen replacement with and without progestins. *J Natl Cancer Inst.* 1999;91(13):1131-1137.

39. Strom BL, Schinnar R, Weber AL, et al. Case-control study of postmenopausal hormone replacement therapy and endometrial cancer. *Am J Epidemiol.* 2006;164(8):775-786.

40. Riggs BL, Hartmann LC. Selective estrogen-receptor modulators—mechanisms of action and application to clinical practice. *N Engl J Med.* 2003;348(7):618-629.

41. Mourits MJ, De Vries EG, Willemse PH, Ten Hoor KA, Hollema H, Van der Zee AG. Tamoxifen treatment and gynecologic side effects: a review. *Obstet Gynecol.* 2001;97(5 Pt 2):855-866.

42. Goldstein SR. The effect of SERMs on the endometrium. *Ann N Y Acad Sci.* 2001;949:237-242.

43. Fisher B, Costantino JP, Wickerham DL, et al. Tamoxifen for the prevention of breast cancer: current status of the National Surgical Adjuvant Breast and Bowel Project P-1 study. *J Natl Cancer Inst.* 2005;97(22):1652-1662.

44. Fisher B, Costantino JP, Wickerham DL, et al. Tamoxifen for prevention of breast cancer: report of the National Surgical Adjuvant Breast and Bowel Project P-1 Study. *J Natl Cancer Inst.* 1998;90(18):1371-1388.

45. Runowicz CD, Costantino JP, Wickerham DL, et al. Gynecologic conditions in participants in the NSABP breast cancer prevention study of tamoxifen and raloxifene (STAR). *Am J Obstet Gynecol.* 2011;205(6):535.e1-535.e5.

46. Davies C, Pan H, Godwin J, et al. Long-term effects of continuing adjuvant tamoxifen to 10 years versus stopping at 5 years after diagnosis of oestrogen receptor-positive breast cancer: ATLAS, a randomised trial. *Lancet.* 2013;381(9869):805-816.

47. Wickerham DL, Fisher B, Wolmark N, et al. Association of tamoxifen and uterine sarcoma. *J Clin Oncol.* 2002;20(11):2758-2760.

48. Bergman L, Beelen ML, Gallee MP, Hollema H, Benraadt J, van Leeuwen FE. Risk and prognosis of endometrial cancer after tamoxifen for breast cancer. Comprehensive Cancer Centres' ALERT Group. Assessment of liver and endometrial cancer risk following tamoxifen. *Lancet.* 2000;356(9233):881-887.

49. Lavie O, Barnett-Griness O, Narod SA, Rennert G. The risk of developing uterine sarcoma after tamoxifen use. *Int J Gynecol Cancer.* 2008;18(2):352-356.

50. Committee Opinion No. 601: tamoxifen and uterine cancer. *Obstet Gynecol.* 2014;123(6):1394-1397.

51. Onstad MA, Schmandt RE, Lu KH. Addressing the role of obesity in endometrial cancer risk, prevention, and treatment. *J Clin Oncol.* 2016;34(35):4225-4230.

52. MacDonald PC, Edman CD, Hemsell DL, et al. Effect of obesity on conversion of plasma androstenedione to estrone in postmenopausal women with and without endometrial cancer. *Am J Obstet Gynecol.* 1978;130:448-455.

53. Judd HL, Lucas WE, Yen SS. Serum 17 beta-estradiol and estrone levels in postmenopausal women with and without endometrial cancer. *J Clin Endocrinol Metab.* 1976;43:272-278.

54. Grodin, JM, Siiteri PK, MacDonald PC. Source of estrogen production in postmenopausal women. *J Clin Endocrinol Metab.* 1973;36:207-214.

55. Potischman N, Swanson CA, Siiteri P, Hoover RN. Reversal of relation between body mass and endogenous estrogen concentrations with menopausal status. *J Natl Cancer Inst.* 1996;88(11):756-758.

56. Amant F, Moerman P, Neven P, Timmerman D, Van Limbergen E, Vergte I. Endometrial cancer. *Lancet.* 2005;366(9484):491-505.

57. McCullough ML, Patel AV, Patel R, et al. Body mass and endometrial cancer risk by hormone replacement therapy and cancer subtype. *Cancer Epidemiol Biomarkers Prev.* 2008;17(1):73-79.

58. Bjorge T, Engeland A, Tretli S, Weiderpass E. Body size in relation to cancer of the uterine corpus in 1 million Norwegian women. *Int J Cancer.* 2007;120(2):378-383.

59. Kaaks R, Lukanova A, Kurzer MS. Obesity, endogenous hormones, and endometrial cancer risk: a synthetic review. *Cancer Epidemiol Biomarkers Prev.* 2002;11(12):1531-1543.

60. Collaborative Group on Epidemiological Studies on Endometrial Cancer. Endometrial cancer and oral contraceptives: an individual participant meta-analysis of 27 276 women with endometrial cancer from 36 epidemiological studies. *Lancet Oncol.* 2015;16(9):1061-1070.

61. Iversen L, Sivasubramaniam S, Lee AJ, Fielding S, Hannaford PC. Lifetime cancer risk and combined oral contraceptives: the Royal College of General Practitioners' Oral Contraception Study. *Am J Obstet Gynecol.* 2017;216(6):580.e1-580.e9.

62. Creasman WT, Morrow CP, Bundy BN, et al. Surgical pathologic spread patterns of endometrial cancer: a Gynecologic Oncology Group study. *Cancer.* 1987;60:2035-2041.

63. Mariani A, Dowdy S, Keeney G, et al. High-risk endometrial cancer subgroups: candidates for target based adjuvant therapy. *Gynecol Oncol.* 2004;95:120-126.

64. Morrow CP, Bundy BN, Kurman RJ, et al. Relationship between surgical-pathological risk factors and outcome in clinical stages I and II carcinoma of the endometrium: a Gynecologic Oncology Group study. *Gynecol Oncol.* 1991;40:55-65.

Endometrial Cancer: Clinical Presentation, Diagnostic Evaluation, and Workup

Amy Bregar

DIAGNOSTIC EVALUATION

Screening

Many ECs develop by way of a precursor lesion. ECs that arise from atypical endometrial hyperplasia/endometrioid intraepithelial neoplasia (AEH/EIN) can be associated with any of the four molecular subtypes described earlier. Serous EC and carcinosarcoma mostly arise from serous endometrial intraepithelial carcinoma (SEIC), but some arise from AEH/EIN. Prompt recognition of precursor lesions, with institution of proper treatment, will prevent cancers and their sequelae. There are no high-quality data to support the efficacy of routine screening (be it imaging, tissue sampling, or cervical cytology) for reducing EC mortality in the general population. The ACOG and the SGO do not recommend routine screening of patients for uterine cancer (1,2). These groups, in addition to the ACS, recommend educating patients about the symptoms of EC and the importance of reporting postmenopausal bleeding to a healthcare provider.

Patients with Lynch syndrome have a markedly increased risk of EC; thus, such patients should be counseled about screening and risk-reducing hysterectomy. The ACS recommends that women with Lynch syndrome be offered yearly endometrial biopsy (EMB) starting at age 35. ACOG suggests an EMB every 1 to 2 years beginning at ages 30 to 35 (3).

In lieu of routine screening, prompt assessment of symptomatic patients and those at high risk should be considered. Because 95% of ECs occur in women aged 40 years and older, and because endometrial hyperplasia tends to occur in premenopausal and perimenopausal women, it is appropriate to evaluate individuals past their fourth decade of life if they experience abnormal bleeding. Similarly, a higher degree of suspicion should be held for younger patients with high-risk characteristics including significant obesity, polycystic ovarian syndrome (PCOS)/chronic anovulation, or tamoxifen exposure.

Prevention

Because of the increased risk of EC associated with unopposed estrogens, women with an intact uterus should rarely, if ever, be prescribed estrogen-only replacement therapy. The addition of progestins to the regimens of patients treated with exogenous estrogen may prevent endometrial hyperplasia and protect against the development of carcinoma (4,5). Continuous or sequential progestin regimens may be used, but the most important factor is administration of a progestin for at least 10 to 14 days each month. In patients with chronic endogenous estrogen exposure, such as obese women with PCOS or chronic anovulation and perimenopausal women with menometrorrhagia, periodic treatment with a progestin to create scheduled withdrawal bleeding and prevent hyperplasia may be considered (6,7). Combined estrogen-progestin oral contraceptives are first-line therapy for women with PCOS. Weight reduction through lifestyle modifications or bariatric surgery should be considered for obese women, and progestin-dominant contraceptives are likely to be protective.

In most cases, patients with AEH/EIN should be treated by hysterectomy to prevent the development of EC (8). Surgery is the definitive therapy as it stops bleeding, prevents cancer, and alleviates the potential for medical failure. Patients with AEH/EIN remain at high risk for recurrence of AEH or cancer during their lifetime, even after successful medical therapy (9). Most importantly, despite a preoperative diagnosis of AEH/EIN, many patients will be found to have a cancer at the time of hysterectomy (9,10). Prospective data from a large surgical pathologic trial conducted by the GOG demonstrated that, of 289 patients with a community diagnosis of AEH, 40% had an EC (10). Neither the type of preoperative EMB (office EMB or dilatation and curettage [D&C]) nor the use of an expert pathology panel was associated with a better ability to predict who had cancer. Patients with significant medical comorbidities, advanced age, or those desiring future fertility may be managed with hormonal therapy (8,11). Although it has been suggested that a D&C should be performed in patients who will be medically managed with progestins for therapeutic effect (surgical curettage of tissue) and to better define the risk of an unrecognized cancer, the data to support these practices are limited. To assess the success of medical therapy, EMBs should be performed at 3- to 4-month intervals, provided cancer is not identified (8,11).

Screening and prevention strategies for women on tamoxifen are more challenging. Women with intact uteri who are taking tamoxifen for either treatment or prevention of breast cancer should be informed of the increased relative risk of developing EC with the use of tamoxifen. This risk is balanced by the reductions in recurrence or development of a contralateral breast cancer. Women on tamoxifen should be encouraged to report abnormal bleeding or vaginal discharge. Screening of asymptomatic women on tamoxifen therapy with ultrasound or EMBs is not recommended (12,13).

CLINICAL PRESENTATION

The classic symptom of endometrial carcinoma is abnormal uterine bleeding, a symptom present in 75% to 90% of cases (2,14). A variety of conditions give rise to abnormal bleeding, but particular suspicion should be held for postmenopausal women and women aged 40 years and over with high-risk factors. Approximately 9% of symptomatic postmenopausal patients are found to have a cancer on biopsy (115). In one series, using age greater than 70 years, diabetes, or nulliparity as risk factors, patients with all three factors had an 87% chance of an AEH/carcinoma diagnosis, whereas only 3% had significant pathology in the absence of all risk factors (116). Additionally, patients with EC may present with vaginal discharge or have a thickened endometrium that is incidentally noted on ultrasound performed for another reason. Pap smear screening is not designed to identify EC, but occasionally patients will have abnormal cervical cytology (atypical glandular cells of undetermined significance, adenocarcinoma in situ). Patients with intraperitoneal disease may present with similar complaints to patients with ovarian cancer, such as abdominal distention, pelvic pressure, and pain.

Historically, when EC was a clinically staged disease (FIGO 1971), fractional D&C was the procedure of choice to evaluate abnormal bleeding. Fractional D&C permitted assessment of uterine size and allowed for endocervical curettage, important steps in the staging process. The standard procedure starts with curettage of the endocervix prior to cervical dilatation. Careful sounding of the uterus is performed followed by dilatation of the cervix, followed by systematic curetting of the entire endometrial cavity. Cervical and endometrial specimens should be kept separate and forwarded for pathologic interpretation.

Pathologic evaluation of the endometrium provides histologic diagnosis and can identify other etiologies of bleeding such as chronic endometritis, atrophy, polyps, cervical cancer, or unusual histologic variants (carcinosarcoma, serous carcinoma, placental nodule), which may alter management. Tissue evaluation by office EMB or D&C offers similar information when adequately performed. Today EMB has largely replaced D&C as the diagnostic procedure of choice. In the GOG hyperplasia study, 63% of the specimens were from EMB (Vabra, Novak, Pipelle) and 37% were from D&C (10). Results of EMBs correlate well with endometrial curetting, and the accuracy in detecting cancer is 91% to 99% (17,18). The accuracy of identifying cancers with EMB is higher in postmenopausal than in premenopausal patients, and a positive study shows cancer is more accurate for identifying disease than it is in excluding it. If office biopsy cannot be obtained (cervical stenosis, patient intolerance of procedure) or results are nondiagnostic, it should be followed by D&C. In cases of abnormal bleeding that persists despite negative biopsy, additional investigation is warranted.

Hysteroscopy has been advocated as an adjuvant to D&C to improve detection of pathology in the evaluation of postmenopausal bleeding based on data demonstrating an improved detection rate (19,20). Hysteroscopy is more accurate in postmenopausal patients and is more accurate in detecting cancer versus other pathologies than it is in identifying cancer or hyperplasia versus other pathologies. One concern is that hysteroscopy may promote transtubal migration of tumor cells, which can be detected as malignant pelvic washings on cytology. In one retrospective study, an OR of 3.88 for positive cytology was seen in hysteroscopic D&Cs compared to D&C alone, and the authors cautioned against hysteroscopy for evaluating EC (21). Similarly, a review of literature suggested that water-based hysteroscopy was associated with increased frequency of positive cytology at the time of hysterectomy (22). Positive peritoneal cytology as the sole extrauterine factor is no longer recognized as a stage-defining characteristic under the FIGO 2009 system, however (23). No prospective studies have been performed to date, and it remains uncertain what effect positive washing produced by hysteroscopy has, if any, on prognosis.

Ultrasound is commonly used as a less invasive tool to evaluate abnormal bleeding. The measurement of endometrial thickness (ET) has been shown to best predict the absence of carcinoma, with a false-negative rate of 4%, using a threshold value of less than 5 mm (24,25). The specific ET used for a cutoff value depends on the menopausal status of the patient population evaluated and on the use of HRT. For example, postmenopausal patients on HRT have a median ET 2 to 3 mm more than those not on HRT (26,27). In a meta-analysis of 85 studies, Smith-Bindman et al (25) reported that a cutoff level of greater than 5 mm would detect 96% of cancers and would have a 39% false-positive rate. Transvaginal ultrasound measuring the lining thickness of the endometrium has excellent negative predictive value (NPV) for ruling out ECs or hyperplasia when the thickness is less than 5 mm, but provides less information when the thickness is more than 5 mm. Given a pretest probability of having EC in a postmenopausal patient with vaginal bleeding of 10%, a normal endometrial stripe is associated with a 1% chance of a cancer. A consensus panel, composed of radiologists, pathologists, and gynecologic oncologists, suggested that when ET is less than 5 mm, the test can be considered negative for EC (28). For patients with ET greater than 5 mm, EMB, D&C with hysteroscopy, or saline infusion sonohysterography should be performed. Saline infusion sonohysterography has been suggested as a more effective way to define findings in the endometrial cavity noted on ultrasound and provide clearer distinction of polyps, fibroids, and

cancers (29). It is more likely to be successful in pre- than postmenopausal patients. The role of vaginal ultrasound in the evaluation of bleeding remains somewhat controversial, because of the importance of histology in defining treatment (for benign and malignant conditions) and the concern about failing to identify cancers. ACOG and the SGO recommend that women with an endometrial stripe greater than 4 mm or a thin strip with persistent endometrial bleeding undergo endometrial sampling (1,30).

DIAGNOSTIC WORKUP

Preoperative Assessment

Following a diagnosis of EC, the surgeon must assess the surgical risks of the patient, evaluate the patient for possible metastatic spread, and determine the most appropriate surgical procedure. Patients with EC are frequently elderly and suffer from obesity, hypertension, diabetes, or cardiac disease. In a series of 595 consecutive patients, Marziale et al (31) found an operability rate of 87%. Preoperative assessment must be performed, occasionally requiring consultation with additional specialists. At a minimum, patients require a thorough examination to evaluate for evidence of cardiac or pulmonary disease and to determine the surgical approach. A chest x-ray and electrocardiogram (ECG), complete blood count, and assessment of electrolytes and renal function are standard in this population. Preoperative counseling includes obtaining permission to remove the uterus, tubes, and ovaries and permission for thorough intra-abdominal exploration with biopsy and tumor resection as indicated, including removal of the pelvic and para-aortic LNs.

Evaluation of Metastatic Spread

A thorough physical examination may discover suspicious supraclavicular, inguinal, and/or occasional pelvic LN as well as suggest the presence of pleural effusions, ascites, or omental caking. The pelvic examination can suggest cervical, vaginal, or adnexal spread. An assessment of uterine size and mobility is important, particularly in patients being considered for vaginal or minimally invasive approaches. A chest radiograph can be considered to evaluate the cardiopulmonary status of the patient and may also demonstrate metastatic disease. For patients without obvious extrauterine disease, surgery is the next step. In cases where intra-abdominal, gross cervical, or distant disease spread is suspected, additional studies such as computed tomography (CT) scans, magnetic resonance imaging (MRI), or cystoscopy and proctoscopy may be needed to assist with surgical planning.

In general, there is very limited need for imaging studies prior to surgery; findings typically do not result in management changes because most patients present with stage I-II disease, and the surgery is essentially the same for patients with stage I-III disease. Imaging studies have significant limitations in detecting nodal disease, which tends to be microscopic in 90% of cases (32,33). In a small series of higher risk patients who underwent preoperative fluorodeoxyglucose (FDG) positron emission tomography (PET)/CT, Signrelli and colleagues showed a 78% sensitivity and 93% NPV (34). GOG 233, a prospective assessment of PET/CT in patients with endometrial and cervical cancer, found that central reader PET/CT interpretation demonstrated a sensitivity, specificity, positive predictive value (PPV) and NPV of 64.6%, 98.6%, 86.1%, and 95.4%, respectively, for EC (35). Imaging after a diagnosis of grade 1 or 2 endometrioid EC to evaluate for metastasis is not necessary; however, given the higher risk of metastasis with high-risk disease (high-grade or high-risk histology), cross-sectional imaging can be considered (1). Cross-sectional imaging can also be obtained if metastatic disease is suspected based on patient history, symptoms, or physical exam findings.

Imaging studies also have utility in selection and counseling of young patients who are considering fertility preservation options. Patients considering fertility-sparing treatment should undergo pelvic imaging to evaluate for myometrial invasion (36). Ultrasound can be used to assess the extent of myometrial invasion; however, in a prospective blinded comparison of the accuracy of preoperative transvaginal ultrasound versus frozen section assessment of myometrial invasion, intraoperative frozen section outperformed transvaginal ultrasound. The sensitivity and specificity of predicting invasion (none, <50%, >50%) of the ultrasound was 75% and 89%, respectively (37). Studies have been inconsistent regarding whether MRI is superior to ultrasound in detecting myometrial invasion (38,39); however, MRI is generally recognized as the preferred imaging modality for EC because it can also assess locoregional disease spread, including cervical extension and deep myometrial invasion (40-45).

Biomarkers that predict the presence of extrauterine disease spread might be useful in triaging patients to referral centers for consideration of surgical staging or to define risk. A variety of biomarkers have been proposed as possible candidates, with CA-125 being the most studied (46-48). Attempts have been made to correlate CA-125 levels with extent of extrauterine disease, as serum levels are frequently elevated in patients with advanced or metastatic EC. Rose et al (49) found serial CA-125 measurements to be most useful in patients with high-risk disease whose initial stage was II, III, or IV or whose tumor was grade 3 or of clear cell or serous histology. Fifteen (94%) of 16 patients with recurrent disease had an elevated CA-125 level. Serial measurements of CA-125 are also used to monitor for recurrence and to assess response to tumor therapy in patients whose levels were initially elevated at diagnosis. In the Laparoscopic Approach to Cancer of the Endometrium (LACE) trial, which compared laparotomy to laparoscopy in the management of early-stage EC, 657 patients had preoperative CA-125 levels that were correlated with extrauterine disease spread. Using a cutoff of 30 U/mL, 15% were noted to have elevated CA-125 levels, and of these 37% had extrauterine disease (50). Accordingly, serum CA-125 can be considered for high-risk disease (high-grade or high-risk histology) or concern for metastatic disease (1).

REFERENCES

1. Hamilton CA, Pothuri B, Arend RC, et al. Endometrial cancer: a Society of Gynecologic Oncology evidence-based review and recommendations. *Gynecol Oncol.* 2021;160:817-826.

2. Practice Bulletin No. 149: endometrial cancer. *Obstet Gynecol.* 2015; 125(4):1006-1026.

3. ACOG Practice Bulletin No. 147: Lynch syndrome. *Obstet Gynecol.* 2014;124(5):1042-1054.

4. The Writing Group for the PEPI Trial. Effects of hormone replacement therapy on endometrial histology in postmenopausal women: the postmenopausal estrogen/progestin interventions (PEPI) trial. *JAMA.* 1996;275:370-375.

5. Maxwell GL, Schildkraut J, Calingaert B, et al. Progestin and estrogen potency of combination oral contraceptives and endometrial cancer risk. *Gynecol Oncol.* 2006;103:535-540.

6. Gambrell RD Jr, Massey FM, Castenada TA, et al. Use of the progestogen challenge test to reduce the risk of endometrial cancer. *Obstet Gynecol.* 1980;55:732-738.

7. Gorodeski IG, Geier A, Lunenfeld B, et al. Progesterone challenge test in postmenopausal women with pathological endometrium. *Cancer Invest.* 1988;6:481-485.

8. The American College of Obstetricians and Gynecologists Committee Opinion No. 631. Endometrial intraepithelial neoplasia. *Obstet Gynecol.* 2015;125(5):1272-1278.

9. Kurman R, Kaminski P, Norris H. The behavior of endometrial hyperplasia. A long-term study of "untreated" hyperplasia in 170 patients. *Cancer.* 1985;56:403-411.

10. Trimble CL, Kauderer J, Zaino R, et al. Concurrent endometrial carcinoma in women with a biopsy diagnosis of atypical endometrial hyperplasia: a Gynecologic Oncology Group study. *Cancer.* 2006;106:812-819.

11. Trimble CL, Method M, Leitao M, et al. Management of endometrial precancers. *Obstet Gynecol.* 2012;120(5):1160-1175.

12. Committee Opinion No. 601: tamoxifen and uterine cancer. *Obstet Gynecol.* 2014;123(6):1394-1397.

13. Runowicz CD. Gynecologic surveillance of women on tamoxifen: first do no harm. *J Clin Oncol.* 2000;18:3457-3458.

14. Seebacher V, Schmid M, Polterauer S, et al. The presence of postmenopausal bleeding as prognostic parameter in patients with endometrial cancer: a retrospective multi-center study. *BMC Cancer.* 2009;9:460.

15. Clarke MA, Long BJ, Del Mar Morillo A, Arbyn M, Bakkum-Gamez JN, Wentzensen N. Association of endometrial cancer risk with postmenopausal bleeding in women: a systematic review and meta-analysis. *JAMA Intern Med.* 2018;178(9):1210-1222.

16. Feldman S, Cook F, Harlow B, et al. Predicting endometrial cancer among women who present with abnormal vaginal bleeding. *Gynecol Oncol.* 1995;56:376-381.

17. Clark TJ, Mann CH, Shah N, et al. Accuracy of outpatient endometrial biopsy in the diagnosis of endometrial cancer: a systematic quantitative review. *Br J Obstet Gynaecol.* 2002;109:313-321.

18. Dijkhuizen FP, Mol B, Brolmann H, et al. The accuracy of endometrial sampling in the diagnosis of patients with endometrial carcinoma and hyperplasia: a meta-analysis. *Cancer.* 2000;89:1765-1772.

19. Leitao MM Jr, Han G, Lee LX, et al. Complex atypical hyperplasia of the uterus: characteristics and prediction of underlying carcinoma risk. *Am J Obstet Gynecol.* 2010;203(4):349.e1-349.e6.

20. Bedner R, Rzepka-Gorska I. Hysteroscopy with directed biopsy versus dilatation and curettage for the diagnosis of endometrial hyperplasia and cancer in perimenopausal women. *Eur J Gynaecol Oncol.* 2007;28(5):400-402.

21. Bradley WH, Boente MP, Brooker D, et al. Hysteroscopy and cytology in endometrial cancer. *Obstet Gynecol.* 2004;104:1030-1033.

22. Revel A, Tsafrir A, Anteby SO, et al. Does hysteroscopy produce intraperitoneal spread of endometrial cancer cells? *Obstet Gynecol Surv.* 2004;59:280-284.

23. Pecorelli S. Revised FIGO staging for carcinoma of the vulva, cervix, and endometrium. *Int J Gynecol Obstet.* 2009;105:109-110.

24. Tabor A, Watt H, Wald N. Endometrial thickness as a test for endometrial cancer in women with post-menopausal vaginal bleeding. *Obstet Gynecol.* 2002;99:663-670.

25. Smith-Bindman R, Kerlikowske K, Feldstein K, et al. Endovaginal ultrasound to exclude endometrial cancer and other endometrial abnormalities. *JAMA.* 1998;280:1510-1517.

26. Conoscenti G, Mier YJ, Fischer-Tamaro L, et al. Endometrial assessment by transvaginal sonography and histological findings after D&C in women with post-menopausal bleeding. *Ultrasound Obstet Gynecol.* 1995;6:108-115.

27. Tongsong T, Pongnarisorn C, Mahanuphap P. Use of vaginosonographic measurements of endometrial thickness in the identification of abnormal endometrium in peri- and postmenopausal bleeding. *J Clin Ultrasound.* 1994;22:479-482.

28. Goldstein R, Bree R, Benson C, et al. Evaluation of the woman with postmenopausal bleeding: Society of Radiologists in Ultrasound-Sponsored Consensus Conference statement. *J Ultrasound Med.* 2001;20:1025-1036.

29. deKroon CD, deBrock GH, Dieben SW, et al. Saline contrast hysterosonography in abnormal uterine bleeding: a systematic review and meta-analysis. *Br J Obstet Gynaecol.* 2003;110:938-947.

30. ACOG Committee Opinion No. 734: the role of transvaginal ultrasonography in evaluating the endometrium of women with postmenopausal bleeding. *Obstet Gynecol.* 2018;131(5):e124-e129.

31. Marziale P, Atlante G, Pozzi M, et al. 426 cases of stage I endometrial carcinoma: a clinicopathological analysis. *Gynecol Oncol.* 1989;32:278-281.

32. Ozalp S, Yalcin OT, Polay S, et al. Diagnostic efficacy of the preoperative lymphoscintigraphy, Ga-67 scintigraphy, and computed tomography for the detection of lymph node metastasis in cases of ovarian or endometrial cancer. *Acta Obstet Gynaecol Scand.* 1999;78:155-159.

33. Zerbe M, Bristow R, Grumbine F, et al. Inability of preoperative computed tomography scans to accurately predict the extent of myometrial invasion and extracorporal spread in endometrial cancer. *Gynecol Oncol.* 2000;78:67-70.

34. Signorelli M, Guerra L, Buda A, et al. Role of the integrated FDG PET/CT in the surgical management of patients with high risk clinical early stage endometrial cancer: detection of pelvic nodal metastases. *Gynecol Oncol.* 2009;115(2):231-235. doi:10.1016/j.ygyno.2009.07.020

35. Gee MS, Atri M, Bandos AI, Mannel RS, Gold MA, Lee SI. Identification of distant metastatic disease in uterine cervical and endometrial cancers with FDG PET/CT: analysis from the ACRIN 6671/GOG 0233 multicenter trial. *Radiology.* 2018;287(1):176-184.

36. SGO Clinical Practice Endometrial Cancer Working Group, Burke WM, Orr J, et al. Endometrial cancer: a review and current management strategies: part II. *Gynecol Oncol.* 2014;134:393-402.

37. Savelli L, Testa A, Mabrouk M, et al. A prospective comparison of the accuracy of transvaginal sonography and frozen section assessment of myometrial invasion in endometrial cancer. *Gynecol Oncol.* 2012;124:549-552.

38. DelMaschio A, Vanzulli A, Sironi S, et al. Estimating the depth of myometrial involvement by endometrial carcinoma: efficacy of transvaginal sonography vs MR imaging. *AJR Am J Roentgenol.* 1993;160(3):533-538.

39. Yamashita Y, Mizutani H, Torashima M, et al. Assessment of myometrial invasion by endometrial carcinoma: transvaginal sonography vs contrast-enhanced MR imaging. *AJR Am J Roentgenol.* 1993;161(3):595-599.

40. Zarbo G, Caruso G, Caruso S, Mangano U, Zarbo R. Endometrial cancer: preoperative evaluation of myometrial infiltration magnetic resonance imaging versus transvaginal ultrasonography. *Eur J Gynaecol Oncol.* 2000;21(1):95-97.

41. Varpula MJ, Klemi PJ. Staging of uterine endometrial carcinoma with ultra-low field (0.02 T) MRI: a comparative study with CT. *J Comput Assist Tomogr.* 1993;17(4):641-647.

42. Sala E, Rockall AG, Freeman SJ, Mitchell DG, Reinhold C. The added role of MR imaging in treatment stratification of patients with gynecologic malignancies: what the radiologist needs to know. *Radiology.* 2013;266(3):717-740.

43. McEvoy SH, Nougaret S, Abu-Rustum NR, et al. Fertility-sparing for young patients with gynecologic cancer: how MRI can guide patient selection prior to conservative management. *Abdom Radiol (NY).* 2017;42(10):2488-2512.

44. Barwick TD, Rockall AG, Barton DP, Sohaib SA. Imaging of endometrial adenocarcinoma. *Clin Radiol.* 2006;61(7):545-555.

45. Kinkel K, Kaji Y, Yu KK, et al. Radiologic staging in patients with endometrial cancer: a meta-analysis. *Radiology.* 1999;212(3):711-718.

46. Todo Y, Okamoto K, Hayashi M, et al. A validation study of a scoring system to estimate the risk of lymph node metastasis for patients with endometrial cancer for tailoring the indication of lymphadenectomy. *Gynecol Oncol.* 2007;104:623-628.

47. Kalogera E, Scholler N, Powless C, et al. Correlation of serum HE4 with tumor size and myometrial invasion in endometrial cancer. *Gynecol Oncol.* 2011;124(2):270-275.

48. Farias-Eisener R, Su F, Robbins T, et al. Validation of serum biomarkers for detection of early- and late-stage endometrial cancer. *Am J Obstet Gynecol.* 2010;202:73.e1-73.e5.

49. Rose PG, Sommers RM, Reale FR, et al. Serial serum CA-125 measurements for evaluation of recurrence in patients with endometrial carcinoma. *Obstet Gynecol.* 1994;84:12-16.

50. Nicklin J, Janda M, Gebski V, et al. The utility of serum CA-125 in predicting extra-uterine disease in apparent early-stage endometrial cancer. *Int J Cancer.* 2012;131(4):885-890. doi:10.1002/ijc.26433

CHAPTER **5.4**

Surgery for Endometrial Cancer

Christine Chin

INTRODUCTION

Staging of Disease

Surgical staging is essential to the treatment and prognostic assessment of patients with EC. Staging is used to inform recommendations on adjuvant therapy. The earliest FIGO staging system was adopted in 1950 and was based solely on the clinical determination of whether tumors were uterine confined (stage I) or had spread beyond the uterus (stage II). These stages were further subdivided into "a" and "b," that is, whether the patient was medically operable or not (1). The FIGO 1971 staging system was updated to consider both grade as well as extent of involvement beyond the corpus into the cervix, bladder, and/or rectum (Table 5.4-1).

In the 1970s a paradigm shift occurred in the management of EC when a series of studies observed that patients with clinically apparent uterine-confined disease had significant risk of occult pelvic and para-aortic LN metastases. Clinical staging was inaccurate and understaged about 15% to 20% of patients (1-3). Although the treatment of EC for decades had consisted of preoperative radium placement followed by hysterectomy and BSO with the pelvic LN often largely ignored, it became clear that the nodal metastatic potential of EC had to be better addressed. Surgical evaluation of LN in EC was reported in the 1960s, but it was not widely embraced (4,5). The GOG undertook the large surgical pathologic study, GOG 33, of clinical stage I EC to better define patterns of spread, with the hope that defining pathologic relationships would lead to a tailored (rather than a universal) approach to the use of radiation and lymphadenectomy (2). Several intrauterine factors including depth of myometrial invasion, disease grade, presence of lymphovascular invasion, and cervical extension were identified as predictors of extrauterine spread. The results of this study subsequently

led to the replacement of clinical staging by surgical staging in the FIGO 1988 staging system. In 2009, FIGO staging was updated such that endocervical glandular involvement no longer upstaged patients (IIA, by FIGO 1988). Furthermore, the status of cytology as a stage-defining criterion (IIIA, by FIGO 1988) was removed, however, with no intent to discontinue the practice of cytologic evaluation as it remains recommended by FIGO. Whereas the

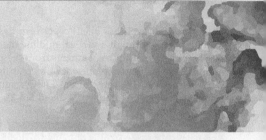

TABLE 5.4-1. Corpus Cancer Clinical Staging, FIGO 1971	
Stage	**Characteristics**
I	Carcinoma is confined to the corpus.
IA	Length of the uterine cavity is 8 cm or less.
IB	Length of the uterine cavity is more than 8 cm.
Histologic subtypes of adenocarcinoma	
G1	Highly differentiated adenomatous carcinoma
G2	Differentiated adenomatous carcinoma with partly solid areas
G3	Predominantly solid or entirely undifferentiated carcinoma
II	Carcinoma involves the corpus and cervix.
III	Carcinoma extends outside the uterus but not outside the true pelvis.
IV	Carcinoma extends outside the true pelvis or involves the bladder or rectum.

FIGO, International Federation of Gynecology and Obstetrics.

From Koskas M, Amant F, Mirza MR, et al. Cancer of the corpus uteri: 2021 update. *Int J Gynecol Obstet.* 2021;155 suppl 1(suppl 1):45-60, John Wiley and Sons.

■ **TABLE 5.4-2. Corpus Cancer Surgical Staging, FIGO 1988**

Stages/Grades	Characteristics
IA G123	Tumor limited to endometrium
IB G123	Invasion to less than half of the myometrium
IC G123	Invasion to less than half of the myometrium
IIA G123	Endocervical glandular involvement only
IIB G123	Cervical stromal invasion
IIIA G123	Tumor invades serosa or adnexa or positive peritoneal cytology.
IIIB G123	Vaginal metastases
IIIC G123	Metastases to pelvic or para-aortic lymph nodes
IVA G123	Tumor invades bladder and/or bowel mucosa.
IVB	Distant metastases including intra-abdominal and/or inguinal LN

FIGO, International Federation of Gynecology and Obstetrics; LN, lymph node.

From Koskas M, Amant F, Mirza MR, et al. Cancer of the corpus uteri: 2021 update. *Int J Gynecol Obstet*. 2021;155 suppl 1(suppl 1):45-60, John Wiley and Sons.

traditional approach has been to perform hysterectomy abdominally (typically through a vertical midline incision) with immediate sampling of peritoneal washings from the pelvis and abdomen, minimally invasive techniques have increasingly been brought to the forefront (6). The most recent FIGO staging system was published in 2018 (6) (see **Tables 5.4-2 and 5.4-3**).

EC staging includes total hysterectomy, BSO, and lymphadenectomy. Although traditionally the operation was performed by open route, most women with early-stage disease undergo minimally invasive surgery, either via conventional laparoscopy or a robotic-assisted platform. Several randomized studies have shown that oncologic outcomes are comparable between open and minimally invasive surgery, with the former approach associated with lower peri- and postoperative complication rates. In the LAP II trial, a total of 1,696 and 920 women with clinical stage I-IIA EC were randomized to laparoscopic and open surgery, respectively (7). Although intraoperative complication rates were similar between the two groups, moderate and severe surgical adverse events were lower in the laparoscopy arm of the study. Five-year survival between the two groups was also similar: 89.8% in both groups (8). In the randomized LACE Janda M trial, a total of 760 women with stage I EC underwent surgical staging by laparoscopy or laparotomy. The study reported similar disease-free survival (DFS) at 4.5 years (81.6% vs 81.3%) as well as overall survival (mortality: 7.4% vs 6.8%) (9). Quality of life was evaluated in a subset of patients participating in the LACE trial and was reported to be better in the women undergoing laparoscopic surgery during the initial postoperative period and up to 6 months after surgery (10). Most of the data on robotic-assisted staging of EC are single- or multi-institutional cohorts (11,12). In a randomized study of 99 women comparing robotic versus laparoscopic staging, the former was associated with shorter operative time and fewer conversions to open surgery and found no differences in number of retrieved LNs, bleeding, or postoperative length of stay (13). Robotic surgery is more costly (11).

Laparotomy is appropriate for women who are not candidates for minimally invasive surgery or who have metastatic disease.

■ **TABLE 5.4-3. Corpus Cancer Surgical Staging, FIGO 2009**

Stages/Grades	Characteristics
IA G123	No or less than half myometrial invasion
IB G123	Invasion equal to or more than half of the myometrium
II G123	Tumor invades the cervical stroma but does not extend beyond the uterus.
IIIA G123	Tumor invades serosa of the corpus uteri and/or adnexa.
IIIB G123	Vaginal and/or parametrial involvement
IIIC1 G123 IIIC2 G123	Metastases to pelvic LN Metastases to para-aortic LN, with or without positive pelvic nodes
IVA G123	Tumor invades bladder and/or bowel mucosa.
IVB	Distant metastases including intra-abdominal and/or inguinal LN
Histopathology, degree of differentiation	
Cases should be grouped by the degree of differentiation of the adenocarcinoma:	
G1	5% or less of a nonsquamous or nonmorular solid growth pattern
G2	6%-50% of a nonsquamous or nonmorular solid growth pattern
G3	More than 50% of a nonsquamous or nonmorular solid growth pattern
Notes on pathologic grading:	
Notable nuclear atypia, inappropriate for the architectural grade, raises the grade of a grade 1 or 2 tumor by 1.	
In serous adenocarcinomas, clear cell adenocarcinomas, and squamous cell carcinomas, nuclear grading takes precedence.	
Adenocarcinomas with squamous differentiation are graded according to the nuclear grade of the glandular component.	
Rules related to staging:	
Because corpus cancer is now surgically staged, procedures previously used for the determination of stages are no longer applicable, such as the finding of fractional D&C to differentiate between stages I and II.	
It is appreciated that there may be a small number of patients with corpus cancer who will be treated primarily with radiation therapy. If that is the case, the clinical staging adopted by FIGO in 1971 would still apply, but designation of that staging system would be noted.	
Ideally, width of the myometrium should be measured, along with the width of tumor invasion.	

D&C, dilatation and curettage; FIGO, International Federation of Gynecology and Obstetrics; LN, lymph node.

From Koskas M, Amant F, Mirza MR, et al. Cancer of the corpus uteri: 2021 update. *Int J Gynecol Obstet*. 2021;155 suppl 1(suppl 1):45-60, John Wiley and Sons.

To complete the surgical staging of EC, the removal of bilateral pelvic and para-aortic LN is also required. The anatomic boundaries of pelvic node dissection are comparable to what is used for a pelvic node dissection with cervical cancer and is outlined by the margins of the circumflex iliac vein distally and the bifurcation of the iliac vessels proximally; the lateral margin is the genitofemoral nerve, and the medial margin is the superior vesical artery. The floor of the dissection is the obturator nerve. Nodal/fatty tissue is skeletonized from these structures. In cases of bulky nodal disease, complete resection/debulking, rather than biopsy to solely demonstrate metastatic disease, is favored where possible. The common iliac nodes can be removed as a separate specimen or divided at a midpoint along the vessels, submitting the inferior half with the pelvic nodes and the superior half with the para-aortic nodes. Particularly on the left side, the common iliac nodes will be quite lateral in location, and sufficient mobilization will be required to visualize these nodes. Removal of para-aortic nodes can be performed through a midline peritoneal incision over the common iliac arteries and aorta, or by mobilizing the right and left colon medially (14,15). In each case, LNs are resected along the upper common iliac vessels on either side and from the lower portion of the aorta and vena cava. At the present time, the inferior mesenteric artery (IMA) is used to demark the superior extent of the para-aortic node dissection, although some prefer to routinely extend the dissection to the level of the renal vessels (15). If suspicious nodes extending to the renal vessels are identified, they should be removed if possible. In cases with gross omental or intraperitoneal disease spread, cytoreductive surgery with total omentectomy, radical peritoneal stripping, and occasionally bowel resection may be required. The goal of reducing the residual disease to no or small volumes, akin to what is performed for ovarian cancer, is increasingly considered (16).

Total vaginal hysterectomy (TVH) with or without postoperative radiation may be another option for managing complicated patients. Patients too medically infirmed to undergo minimally invasive or open surgery or who may only tolerate regional anesthesia may be considered for vaginal hysterectomy. Vaginal hysterectomy has often been cited as the simplest and least morbid approach to hysterectomy and has produced similar treatment outcomes in patients with clinical stage I EC (17-19). It is often used as an alternative to an abdominal approach in obese and poor-surgical-risk patients (20,21). Limitations include the lack of exploration of the intraperitoneal cavity, inability to procure cytologic washings, greater difficulty in performing a salpingo-oophorectomy, and inability to assess LN status. Given that LN metastasis is related to such high-risk features as poor differentiation, unfavorable histologic subtypes, and deep myometrial invasion, the option of TVH for the management of this cancer centers on preoperative uterine pathology and the need for comprehensive surgical staging. TVH is not appropriate for the management of EC in patients with concomitant adnexal pathology.

Management of Lymph Nodes

The most appropriate approach for the evaluation of LNs in women with EC remains controversial, largely because of the fact that data are limited. There are no well-designed studies comparing all available options to one another, and the randomized trials are deemed to be either high-quality studies or of limited interpretation secondary to study design limitations and flaws. In the absence of grossly metastatic disease, the management of retroperitoneal LNs for patients with EC ranges from no dissection to systematic LN dissection (LND) only if the risk of metastasis exceeds a certain threshold, to routine sentinel LN mapping or comprehensive LND in all patients. The value of staging any malignancy relates to the ability to accurately determine the extent of disease at diagnosis and to define comparable patient populations for whom prognosis and recommended therapy are similar. Given the inability to accurately detect disease spread solely based on clinical examination and imaging studies, surgical staging systems that require pathologic evaluation of sampled sites are the current standard (1,6). The principal risks attributable to nodal dissections include increased operative time, potential for blood loss associated with vascular injury, ileus, genitofemoral nerve injury with resulting numbness and paresthesia over medial thighs, lymphocyst formation, and lymphedema. Sentinel LN mapping has been shown to be less morbid compared to comprehensive lymphadenectomy (**Table 5.4-4**) (22-30).

The use of lymphadenectomy in the staging of EC remains a controversial topic, however, its therapeutic benefits independent of the LN status (positive or negative for metastatic disease) remains a controversial topic. The emerging use of sentinel LN mapping in the 2000s, however, has largely transformed the landscape of surgical staging of EC. In fact, the use of less invasive techniques to assess LN status in patients with EC has emerged largely from the lack of evidence that LND carries a therapeutic benefit. Two prospective studies have demonstrated sentinel LN mapping may safely replace comprehensive lymphadenectomy in early-stage EC with less morbidity and high detection rates without a detriment to patient disease outcome (31,32). However, the use of sentinel LN mapping in high-risk patients remains controversial. A recent survey of practice and attitudes of gynecologic oncologists showed frequent utilization for both EC and cervical cancer, with common reasons of non-uptake being uncertainty of data, lack of training, and technology (33).

Nodal Dissection—None

The argument against comprehensive LND centers on the position that most patients are at low risk for nodal disease, treatment decisions can be based on final pathologic information, and despite node dissection the majority of patients who are node-negative do not get benefit (34). Most patients with EC do present with low-risk features. In the entire GOG 33 study population of 621 patients, 75% had grade 1 to 2 tumors, 59% had inner one-third or less myometrial invasion, and only 9% of patients had positive LN (35). The Postoperative Radiation Therapy for Endometrial Cancer (PORTEC) trial evaluated patients with stage IC, grade 1; stage IB-C, grade 2; or stage IB, grade 3 who underwent hysterectomy without LND and compared observation to postoperative pelvic radiation (36). Of note, on the basis of grade and depth of invasion, approximately 60% of patients enrolled in GOG 33 would have had disease characteristics required for eligibility in the PORTEC trial. This patient population managed without nodal dissection had

■ TABLE 5.4-4. Risks Associated With Nodal Dissection: Surgical Complication Rates Associated With Abdominal Hysterectomy + Pelvic and Para-Aortic Lymph Node Dissection

Study	N	Hemorrhage (%)	GU Injury (%)	DVT/PE (%)	Lymphocyst (%)	Other
Morrow et al. 1991 (22)	895	2.2	0.4	2	1.2	–
Homesley et al. 1992 (24)	196	6% transfused	–	4	–	"Serious" 6%
Orr et al. 1997 (23)	396	4.2% transfused	0.6	1.5	1.2	–
Mariani et al. 2006 (25)	96 node(+) patients	–	1	1	3.1	–

DVT/PE, deep vein thrombosis/pulmonary embolism; GU, genitourinary.

favorable outcomes with or without RT (5-year survival rates of 85% observation, 81% with pelvic radiation) in the PORTEC study (36). In a follow-up study including 427 patients with higher risk disease (age >60 years plus grade 1 to 2 and outer 50% invasion, or grade 3 with inner 50% invasion, or stage IIA [1988 FIGO] disease), the PORTEC 2 study compared pelvic RT to vaginal cuff brachytherapy (VCB). None of the patients underwent nodal assessment, and 5-year progression-free survival (PFS) (78%-83%) and survival (80%-85%) suggested that even intermediate-risk patients may be managed without lymphadenectomy, albeit at the cost of requiring adjuvant therapy, with resulting favorable outcomes (37). Trimble et al (38) reported on data from patients with stage I EC collected by SEER from 1988 to 1993 and showed that 5-year relative survival for patients without nodal dissection was 98% compared to 96% in those undergoing nodal dissection and suggested that nodal dissection did not convey a benefit for the overall population. Unfortunately, data on adjuvant therapy use were not available. It is suspected that increased use of radiation in patients who have not undergone LND may produce similar outcomes to patients who have undergone comprehensive staging and who avoid RT. In a nonrandomized trial comparing hysterectomy with or without pelvic lymphadenectomy, followed by RT, 14% of patients ($n = 207$) with negative nodes treated with VCB developed recurrent disease compared to 16% who did not have a lymphadenectomy ($n = 660$) (39). Although the authors noted similar cancer-free survival between the groups, all patients who did not have nodal dissections received both pelvic radiation and VCB to attain these results.

Two randomized trials comparing hysterectomy with or without lymphadenectomy have been reported. A Study in the Treatment of Endometrial Cancer (ASTEC) randomized patients with 1,369 EC to hysterectomy with (LND group) or without (no-LND group) pelvic lymphadenectomy (40). Following surgery, patients with stage I-IIA disease were then randomized again to observation or pelvic RT if they had grade 3, serous, or clear cell histology; greater than 50% myometrial invasion; or endocervical glandular invasion (stage IIA). Nodal status did not alter the use of RT such that node-positive patients could be assigned to observation. Treatment centers were also permitted to use VCB regardless of pelvic radiation assignment based on institutional preference. As a result, a patient with unknown nodal status could receive VCB and not be considered to have received RT. Of the LND group, 54 patients were found to have positive nodes (9%) compared with 9 (1.3%) patients in the no-LND group. The quality of the nodal dissection has been criticized in this study as 8% of patients within the LND group did not get a nodal dissection, 12% had less than 5 nodes removed (median = 12 nodes), and para-aortic node dissection was not performed. There was no difference in PFS (hazard ratio [HR], 1.0) or survival (HR, 1.25; $P = .14$) between the LND groups. Pelvic lymphadenectomy was associated with a longer operative time, and increased frequency of ileus (3% vs 1%), deep venous thrombosis (1% vs 0.1%), lymphocysts (1% vs 0.3%), and wound complications (1% vs 0.3%) compared to the no-LND group. The frequency of transfusions and length of hospitalization were comparable between groups. The authors concluded that the results suggest no evidence of benefit for PFS/overall survival (OS) for pelvic lymphadenectomy and that it "could not be recommended as a routine procedure for *therapeutic* purposes" (40).

A similar study was performed by Italian investigators, Benedetti Panici et al (CONSORT trial). In this trial, 514 patients were assigned to hysterectomy with or without pelvic lymphadenectomy (41). Patients were required to have myometrial invasion, and patients with grade 1 tumors and less than 50% invasion were excluded. In the no-LND group, 22% of patients had nodal dissections because of clinical suspicion, with 14% of these cases, or 3% of the entire no-LND arm, having node-positive disease. In the LND group, the median number of nodes removed was 26. Para-aortic dissection could be performed at the surgeon's discretion and was done in 26% of cases. In the LND group, 13% were found to have positive nodes. Lymphocysts and lymphedema were more

common in the LND group but other early and late complications were similar. Postoperative therapy was not protocol prescribed, but the use of RT was more common in the no-LND group (25% vs 17%). The 5-year DFS was 81% in both groups, and 5-year survival was 90% in the no-LND group versus 86% in the LND group (HR 1.2, $P = .5$). The authors concluded that pelvic lymphadenectomy could not be recommended as a routine procedure for therapeutic purposes (42).

Both the ASTEC (A) and Italian (I) studies have been heavily criticized (43-45). Weaknesses of the studies relate to the absence of treatment in patients identified with positive nodes (A), lack of prescribed adjuvant therapy (I), limited power to show improvements in outcome if one truly existed (A, I), poor quality of the LND (A), absence of para-aortic node dissection (A, I), lack of quality-of-life assessment evaluating the effect of both surgery and downstream use of adjuvant therapy (A, I), and the overrepresentation of low-risk patients (A, I). Despite these limitations, these datasets provide the only level 1 evidence on the role of lymphadenectomy. The studies also suggest that the marginal benefit that lymphadenectomy may provide is likely to be modest for most patients. In addition, the data provide a strong argument that removing negative nodes is unlikely to significantly improve outcomes.

Without nodal information, physicians must rely on intrauterine factors to estimate the probability for pelvic failure to determine the need for postoperative radiation to the pelvis. Risk assessments may be based on nodal positivity estimates from GOG 33 or on uterine factor–derived risk groups treated with or without RT (PORTEC, GOG 2, 36, 37, 46). Nodal positivity is not infrequent in patients with higher risk uterine factors based on GOG 99 or PORTEC models. Nugent and colleagues classified a series of 352 patients with clinical stage 1, endometrioid adenocarcinoma into risk groups based on PORTEC and GOG 99 models. Nodal positivity rates were 20% with PORTEC and 35% with GOG 99 high- to intermediate-risk (HIR) criteria (47). Without specific nodal information, treatments must be based on estimates of risk/probability; this estimation can result in an increase in the use of radiation, particularly if the primary benefit of postoperative radiation is in node-positive patients. Complicating the issue of nodal dissection is that nodal status is only one of several important prognostic factors (47,48). Kwon and colleagues performed a population-based cohort study of 316 patients with EC who underwent lymphadenectomy and reported that pelvic node status was not an independent determinant of survival, whereas prognosis was determined more by uterine factors (48).

The absence of nodal dissection may also lead to poorer outcomes. For example, a subset of 99 patients with stage IC, grade 3 EC, who did not have LND, were not eligible, but were treated with pelvic radiation and followed prospectively within the PORTEC trial (49). Five-year survival for this group of patients was 58%, and 12% had vaginal or pelvic failures despite whole pelvic radiation. It is interesting to note that the outcome of this group is poorer than what has been reported in patients with stage IIIC EC managed by lymphadenectomy followed by radiation (50-52). If patients are not to have nodal dissection, then it would seem reasonable to consider minimally invasive or vaginal approaches to reduce morbidity.

Nodal Dissection—Selective

Surgical staging is the most accurate way to determine the extent of disease spread. Palpation of pelvic LN is not sufficiently accurate, with a sensitivity of 72% in a recent prospective study (10,53). The baseline rate of nodal disease in an "all comer" population of patients with EC is roughly 9% (**Table 5.4-5**). The challenge has been how to identify the smaller portion of patients at high risk from the larger low-risk population. Clearly, subgroups of patients at very high risk (non-endometrioid histology, carcinosarcoma, gross cervical involvement, gross extrauterine disease spread) exist, but these represent a minority of the uterine cancers that are diagnosed every year. Many gynecologic oncologists consider nodal

TABLE 5.4-5. Frequency of Nodal Disease

Study	N	Frequency of Nodal Disease (%)
GOG 33 (54) ASTEC (+LND) (−) LND (40)	621,686,685	991
CONSORT (+ LND) (−) LND (41)	264,250	133
LAP II (55)	2,510	9
PORTEC HIR Criteria (9)	66	20
GOG 99 HIR Criteria (9)	188	35

assessment to be a fundamental step in the evaluation and management of most women with EC, and nodal assessment has been incorporated into the surgical staging of EC since 1988 (6).

Many believe that nodal dissections should be reserved for those with sufficient risk of nodal disease. What risk of nodal disease (3%, 5%, 10%, etc.) warrants LND is debated, that is, at what level one would be comfortable missing unrecognized nodal spread. Equally important in the discussion is the understanding of whether uterine risk factors, independent of nodal status, should drive risk assessment and use of adjuvant therapy and whether adjuvant therapies given to those with node-positive or node status unknown perform similarly.

In 2000, the Mayo group described a model that could classify a group with a low risk of nodal disease spread and high DFS based on frozen section evaluation of the uterus that showed grade 1 to 2 endometrioid tumor, inner 50% invasion, and tumor size less than 2 cm (56). Mariani et al subsequently reported on a prospective experience of 422 patients and reported that 33% of patients with endometrioid-type tumors would qualify as low risk in this model. The authors also showed that 22% patients with risk factors outside of their low-risk model had positive nodal spread at the time of lymphadenectomy (57). Several other investigators have attempted to validate these findings. Convery and colleagues tried to replicate the conditions of Mayo criteria (which are assessed intraoperatively by frozen section) by retrospectively evaluating 602 patients with grade 1 to 2 endometrioid EC and who had intraoperative assessment of tumor (for depth of invasion and/or tumor size) (58). The authors showed that 2/110 (1.8%) patients meeting the Mayo criteria who underwent a lymphadenectomy removing at least eight nodes were found to have metastatic spread to LN. Milam attempted to validate the Mayo criteria using a 971-patient surgical dataset from patients participating in the GOG LAP II trial (randomized trial of laparoscopy vs open hysterectomy with pelvic and para-aortic lymphadenectomy (59)). Of 971 patients with endometrioid adenocarcinoma and complete data, 65 (7%) were identified with positive LN. Patients were classified into a "low-risk" category based on three Mayo criteria: grade 1 to 2 tumor, less than 50% myometrial invasion, and tumor size less than 2 cm. These risk characteristics were assigned based on final pathology report and not frozen section, however, as was used in the Mayo studies. Approximately 40% of patients met the low-risk criteria and of these 3/389 (0.8%) had positive LN. Kang reporting for the Korean GOG retrospectively evaluated 540 patients with endometrioid-type cancers who had undergone preoperative EMB, CA-125 level, and MRI followed by hysterectomy and pelvic lymphadenectomy to create a risk model for predicting nodal disease (60). The model was developed on a 360-patient training set and validated against a 180-patient cohort. Interestingly, the logistic regression model included only data from the MRI and CA-125 level, grade was not an independently significant variable. The authors suggested that based on preoperative information, they could classify 53% of patients as low-risk (<50%) myometrial invasion and absence of enlarged nodes or extrauterine disease by MRI and CA-125 (<35 IU/mL).

Of the low-risk group, only one patient had positive nodal disease (1.7% false-negative rate), suggesting that these patients may avoid an unnecessary lymphadenectomy.

Low-grade tumors appear to represent the most appropriate group for developing criteria to limit lymphadenectomy. Bernardini et al performed a retrospective comparison between two academic institutions' preferences for management of preoperative grade 1 endometrioid EC (61). Of 483 cases with a preoperative grade 1 cancer, final pathology was grade 1 in 357/483 (74%) cases, and 20% were upgraded (grade 2, 18%; grade 3, 2%). In one institution, surgical staging was performed in 50% of cases, and four (3%) patients were identified with nodal disease. At the second institution, LND was performed in only 12% of patients, and three (1.4%) were found to have positive nodal disease. At the second institution, postoperative use of RT was more common (21% vs 7%), although older patient age, capillary space invasion, and cervical involvement were more common at the second site. Despite the differences in surgical practice, the 3-year survival was 96% at both centers. These data indicate that there is little margin to improve outcomes through strategies directed at all patients in this patient population.

Intraoperative assessment of the uterus in patients with low-grade endometrioid adenocarcinoma of the endometrium has been used to guide the surgeon as to when to perform a nodal dissection. Gross inspection of the uterus immediately following its removal can be used to estimate the degree of myometrial invasion. If the uterus is opened by the operating surgeon, care should be taken to avoid distortion of the anatomy. Optimally, the unfixed uterus should be opened by the surgical pathologist, who can grossly estimate the depth of invasion, assess involvement of the cervix, and later sample the tumor for histologic assessment. There is no typical gross appearance of an EC. Most are polypoid or ulcerative. Carcinoma usually differs in texture and color from the surrounding normal endometrium. The normal endometrium is irregular and tan, but a carcinoma is usually shaggy, white to gray-white, and focally hemorrhagic. Areas of myometrial invasion may be visible as gray-white to white, with yellow areas disclosing necrosis (Figures 5.4-1 and 5.4-2). The texture may be soft, friable, or firm depending on the degree of necrosis.

Doering et al (62) reported a 91% accuracy rate for 148 patients for determining the depth of myometrial invasion by gross visual examination of the cut uterine surface. A prospective study indicated that visual inspection of less than or greater than 50% correlated with microscopic assessment in 85% of the cases (63). However, the sensitivity of determining greater than 50% was lower at 72%. Invasion of the myometrium may be more extensive microscopically than is evident visibly because of the characteristic

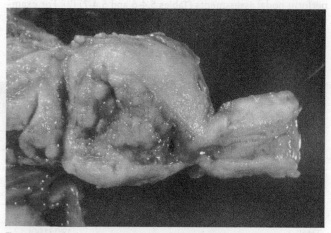

Figure 5.4-1. Endometrioid adenocarcinoma. A polypoid adenocarcinoma of the endometrium that fills much of the lumen and superficially invades the myometrium.

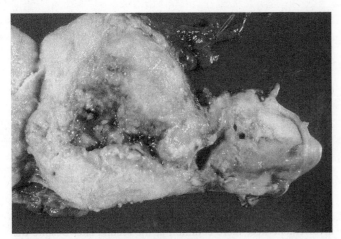

Figure 5.4-2. Endometrial adenocarcinoma. An ulcerating and deeply invasive adenocarcinoma that extends into the uterine cervix.

infiltrative growth pattern of the tumor. In a retrospective study by Goff and Riche, the gross estimation by pathologists of myometrial invasion in grade 2 and 3 tumors was poor (64). With invasion, the uterine cavity usually enlarges and the myometrium thickens, but a small uterus may have myometrial penetration to the serosa.

Selective use of nodal staging highlights the balance between the likelihood of identifying otherwise unrecognized disease against cost, morbidity, and use of adjuvant therapy (with downstream cost, morbidity). The overall surgical complication of lymphadenectomy is approximately 20%. The serious complication rate is 6% or less and is likely to be lower with surgeons who more frequently perform the procedure (65). Downstream utilization of adjuvant therapy, which may occur more frequently in the absence of lymphadenectomy, must also be considered into this balance (66,67). Although the proposed models predicting low-risk disease status appear to be accurate, it is important to understand that the pretest probability of having positive nodes in a large patient population with grade 1 to 2 endometrioid tumors is ~3% to 7%, illustrating the narrow margin in improved outcome (eg, identify 100% of patients with positive nodes and then use adjuvant therapy, which cures 100% of these) that lymphadenectomy may be able to offer in this population of patients. Lymphadenectomy perhaps allows for fine-tuning the management of low-risk patients, but does not appear to be the driver of outcomes.

Historically, data from GOG 33 demonstrated important relationships between tumor grade and depth of invasion and frequency of nodal disease that can be used to decide whether to perform nodal assessments (**Tables 5.4-6 and 5.4-7**) (2). For example, the risk of pelvic nodal disease was 3% for all patients with grade 1 tumors, but was 11% with deeply invasive (outer one-third myometrial invasion) tumors. Patients with grade 3 tumors had a

risk of pelvic nodal metastases of 18%, and 34% with deep invasion. With cervical invasion, the rate of pelvic nodal disease was 16%. Patients with serous or clear cell histology also warrant nodal dissection as ~30% to 50% will have nodal disease, and even in the absence of myometrial invasion, nodal metastases have been reported in up to 36% of patients (68). Some advocate that LN need not be sampled for tumor limited to the endometrium, regardless of grade, because less than 1% of these patients have disease spread to pelvic or para-aortic LN (2,69). A gray zone in deciding about LN sampling is represented by patients whose only risk factor is inner one-half myometrial invasion, particularly if the grade is 2 or 3. This group has 5% or less chance of node positivity. In the most recent survey of SGO members, 35% of respondents reported undergoing lymphadenectomy for grade 1 tumors; however, the use increased to 60% for grade 2 and 90% for grade 3 (15).

Although flawed, the ASTEC and Italian studies (40,41) have suggested that routine nodal dissection may have limited value. If the primary value of lymphadenectomy is to identify patients with positive nodes (as a "diagnostic test"), which define patients who need additional/different postoperative therapy, there is value in defining populations at sufficiently low risk for whom no lymphadenectomy is required.

Nodal Dissection—Routine

Data from 1990 to 2000 provided support for performing uniform comprehensive surgical staging for nearly all patients with EC. The rationale for routine nodal dissection includes the lack of a patient population for whom nodal disease is so low that nodes should be omitted, the inaccuracy of preoperative or intraoperative assessments predicting the risk for nodal disease, the potential for therapeutic benefit in node-positive and node-negative patients, and the lack of significant morbidity associated with the procedure. Postoperative adjuvant decisions are best made with the most complete information. If nodal assessment is the predominant factor by which to categorize patients into risk groups, routine nodal dissection is the best method by which to determine which few patients will require adjuvant therapy.

The factor that constitutes an acceptable rate of nodal disease in EC to warrant the procedure is surgeon dependent. In cervical cancer, routine pelvic lymphadenectomy is advocated for all stage IA2 tumors where nodal positivity rates are 3% to 5% (70). For clinical stage I ovarian cancer, para-aortic dissection is recommended for all, given the 6% risk of para-aortic disease (71). In EC, major complication rates associated with nodal dissection are 2% to 6%, suggesting that this might be an appropriate level of risk to balance against the risk of nodal metastases. Data from GOG 33 show that only patients with tumor limited to the endometrium had a risk of pelvic nodal disease 3% or less, and this group accounted for only 14% of the entire study population.

Frozen section assessment has been the traditional tool to facilitate decisions on selective nodal dissections. Several studies have demonstrated inaccuracies with frozen sections in the

TABLE 5.4-6. Histologic Grade and Depth of Invasion

| Depth | Grade, No. of Patients | | | |
	Grade 1 (%)	Grade 2 (%)	Grade 3 (%)	Total (% of Total)
Endometrium only	44 (24)	31 (11)	11 (7)	86 (14)
Superficial	96 (53)	131 (45)	54 (35)	281 (45)
Middle	22 (12)	69 (24)	24 (16)	115 (19)
Deep	18 (10)	57 (20)	64 (42)	139 (22)
Total	180 (100)	288 (100)	153 (100)	621 (100)

Reprinted from Creasman WT, Morrow CP, Bundy BN, et al. Surgical pathologic spread patterns of endometrial cancer: a Gynecologic Oncology Group study. *Cancer.* 1987;60:2035-2041.

▪ TABLE 5.4-7. Frequency of Nodal Metastasis Among Risk Factors

Risk Factor	No. of Patients	Pelvic No. (%)	Aortic No. (%)
Histology			
Endometrioid adenocarcinoma	599	56 (9)	30 (5)
Others	22	2 (9)	4 (18)
Grade			
1 Well	180	5 (3)	3 (2)
2 Moderate	288	25 (9)	14 (5)
3 Poor	153	28 (18)	17 (11)
Myometrial invasion			
Endometrial	87	1 (1)	1 (1)
Superficial	279	15 (5)	8 (3)
Middle	116	7 (6)	1 (1)
Deep	139	35 (25)	24 (17)
Site of tumor location			
Fundus	524	42 (8)	20 (4)
Isthmus-cervix	97	16 (16)	14 (14)
CLS involvement			
Negative	528	37 (7)	19 (9)
Positive	93	21 (27)	15 (19)
Other extrauterine metastases			
Negative	586	40 (7)	26 (4)
Positive	35	18 (51)	8 (23)
Peritoneal cytology[a]			
Negative	537	38 (7)	20 (4)
Positive	75	19 (25)	14 (19)

CLS, capillary-like space.

[a]Nine patients did not have cytology reported.

Modified with permission from Creasman WT, Morrow CP, Bundy BN, et al. Surgical pathologic spread patterns of endometrial cancer: a Gynecologic Oncology Group study. *Cancer*. 1987;60:2035-2041.

interpretation of grade and depth of myometrial invasion compared to final pathology (72-74). In one prospective evaluation, frozen section determination of depth of invasion correlated with final pathology in 67% of cases but resulted in upstaging in 28% of cases (72). Patients with grade 1 EC or AEH were upstaged in 61% of cases. The clinical significance of these errors has been debated (34), but many believe that such unexpected upstaging justifies routine staging even in seemingly low-risk patients (24,25). Data also suggest that the strategy of routine nodal dissection is more cost-effective than either no staging or selective staging based on frozen section results (72,73).

An assessment of pelvic and para-aortic LN is required to assign stage since the FIGO 2009 staging system and remains in the latest 2018 update (6). The current staging system now separates stage subcategories based on extent of nodal disease (IIIC1, pelvic positive, IIIC2, any para-aortic positive). Two principal nodal basins drain the uterus; the lower and middle portion of the uterus drain laterally to the pelvic LN, the upper corpus and fundus drain to the para-aortic nodes. Nodal assessments should sufficiently examine sites at risk including external iliac, hypogastric, and obturator nodes in the pelvis, common iliac nodes, and para-aortic nodes. LND should be bilateral given the frequency of both left and right para-aortic involvement (75,76). It is interesting to note that GOG 33 only specified right-sided para-aortic removal in the surgical protocol. Likewise, the nodal dissection is more apt to be representative when a larger number of nodes are removed. When LNs are positive, para-aortic nodes are involved ~50% of the time. Isolated para-aortic nodes with negative pelvic nodes are uncommon, particularly with grade 1 to 2 tumors, and are involved in only ~2% of cases (2,77,78). Para-aortic nodal dissection is more difficult to perform than pelvic dissection, by laparotomy or by laparoscopy, and is associated with greater risk. As such, some advocate for pelvic nodal dissections, with performing para-aortic nodal dissections only selectively. In GOG 33, 46% of the positive para-aortic LNs were enlarged, and 98% of the cases with aortic node metastases came from patients with positive pelvic nodes, adnexal or intra-abdominal metastases, or outer one-third myometrial invasion (2). These risk factors affected only 25% of the patients, yet they yielded most of the patients with positive para-aortic node.

The importance of para-aortic nodal spread in node-positive EC cannot be ignored (**Table 5.4-8**). Data from GOG 33 showing that of all patients, isolated para-aortic nodal metastases occurred in 2% are often taken out of context (2). If the goal of nodal dissection is to identify the node-positive patient population and to remove involved nodes, para-aortic disease is seen in 40% to 66%

▪ TABLE 5.4-8. Relationship Between Pelvic and Para-aortic Nodal Involvement in Patients With Node-Positive Endometrial Cancer

Study	N	Surgical Technique	Pelvic (1) Only (%)	Pelvic and Para-aortic (1) (%)	Para-aortic Only (%)	Any Involvement of Para-aortic Nodes (%)
Creasman et al (1987) (2)	70	Routine: sampling	51	31	17	48
Schorge (1996) (81)	35	Selective: lymphadenectomy	74	17	9	26
Hirahatake et al (1997) (82)	42	Routine: systematic lymphadenectomy	57	38	5	42
Onda et al (1997) (50)	30	Routine: systematic lymphadenectomy	33	60	6.6	66
McMeekin et al (2001) (75)	47	Routine: lymphadenectomy	38	41	21	62
Otsuka (2002) (83)	23	Selective: systematic lymphadenectomy	66	33	10	43
Havrilesky (2005) (84)	96	Selective: lymphadenectomy	52	30	18	48

of patients with node-positive/stage IIIC1/2 EC, including isolated positive para-aortic nodes in up to 7% to 21% of cases in certain groups. If only pelvic nodes are removed, when they are positive, para-aortic nodes will be positive in addition in nearly 30% to 40% of cases. It makes less sense to remove only pelvic or only para-aortic nodes given this data. Data would also suggest that when positive, outcomes are improved in patients who have complete surgical resection of para-aortic nodes. Chuang et al (79) reported on their experience with selective pelvic and/or para-aortic dissections and found that failure to systematically remove pelvic and para-aortic nodes resulted in an increased frequency of recurrence in undissected retroperitoneal sites. Similarly, Mariani et al (80) showed that patients at high risk for para-aortic nodal disease (based on invasion >50%, palpable positive pelvic nodes, positive adnexa) who did not have para-aortic dissection or who had biopsy only and who were managed as though para-aortic nodes were positive had 5-year survival of 71% compared to 85% for those patients with positive para-aortic nodes who did undergo complete resection. LN recurrences were detected in 37% of those not having para-aortic dissection compared to none in patients with positive but resected para-aortic nodes, suggesting a possible therapeutic effect of removing involved para-aortic nodes.

A provocative study from Japan (SEPAL study) was published in early 2010 that retrospectively compared the practices of two centers with regard to use of pelvic with or without para-aortic lymphadenectomy (85). At one center, systematic pelvic lymphadenectomy was performed in 325 patients. With a median of 34 pelvic nodes removed, the incidence of stage IIIC disease was 12%. At the second institution, 346 patients underwent pelvic and para-aortic lymphadenectomy. With a median of 59 pelvic and 23 para-aortic nodes resected, stage IIIC disease was identified in 16%. The centers were well matched for stage and tumor grade, but the center where para-aortic lymphadenectomy was performed used adjuvant chemotherapy more commonly (47% vs 27%). Patients were classified into low- versus intermediate- to high-risk groups and outcomes were compared based on lymphadenectomy type. In the intermediate- to high-risk group (but not low-risk group), RFS, disease-specific survival (DSS), and OS were significantly better in those women receiving para-aortic dissections. In a multivariate analysis, age, tumor type, nodal spread, and type of lymphadenectomy were independently associated with improved survival. The authors suggested that if future lymphadenectomy trials were to be conducted, both pelvic and para-aortic lymphadenectomy should be performed (85).

The incidence of isolated para-aortic LN metastasis among patients with negative pelvic LNs confirmed by thorough pelvic LND was investigated in a recent National Cancer Database study examining a total of 14,398 patients diagnosed between 2004 and 2015 with EC. Patients were included if they underwent extensive pelvic LND (defined as at least 10 LNs removed) and underwent para-aortic LN sampling (at least 5 LNs removed). Most patients had endometrioid histology (79.8%) and stage IA disease (68.8%). The overall rate of isolated para-aortic LN metastasis in this low-risk group was 1.6% (86). At the present time, the superior extent of para-aortic dissection should be at least to the level of the IMA. Some suggest that dissections should proceed to the level of the renal vessels given the venous and lymphatic drainage following the infundibulopelvic ligament. In one series, 7 out of 11 patients had positive para-aortic nodes identified above the IMA (82). The Mayo group noted that when para-aortic nodes were positive, 77% of the cases had involvement above the IMA (11). This extended para-aortic dissection is feasible laparoscopically as well (87,88).

The therapeutic value of lymphadenectomy is supported by several reports; however, many are from single institutions, have short follow-up, suffer from selection biases, and do not clearly account for stage migration. Kilgore et al (89) were among the first to report a therapeutic effect of nodal dissections in a series of 649 clinical stage I-occult II patients who were classified based on the extent of nodal dissection. Patients who underwent multiple site pelvic node dissection (defined by nodal dissection of at least four pelvic nodal sites) and had a mean of 11 nodes removed had improved survival over those patients who did not have nodes sampled. The survival advantage for multiple site dissection persisted even when patients were stratified into low-risk (uterine-confined disease) and high-risk (extrauterine disease) groups who received radiation. An explanation for this may be the removal of unrecognized micro metastasis, which goes undetected by standard pathologic processing techniques. Girardi et al (90) performed pelvic lymphadenectomy in 76 patients with EC (mean 37 nodes removed) and reported a 36% nodal positivity rate. Nodal tissue was processed as step serial sections and 37% of positive nodes were less than 2 mm in diameter, suggesting that nodal metastases may be missed in a proportion of node-positive patients processed in a less extensive manner. Others have shown improvement in outcomes following a more complete nodal dissection in node-negative populations. Cragan et al (91) evaluated 509 patients with stage I-IIA who underwent selective pelvic and/or para-aortic lymphadenectomy and found a survival advantage for patients with grade 3 tumors who had greater than 11 pelvic nodes removed, compared to those with 11 or less nodes removed (HR 0.25). For patients with high-risk features (grade 3, >50% myometrial invasion, serous/clear cell tumors), 5-year survival was 82% when greater than 11 nodes were removed versus 64% when 11 or less nodes were removed. Chan et al (92) reported on the effect of a more complete nodal dissection in over 12,000 women with EC tracked in the SEER data system. In patients with high-risk disease (IB/grade 3, IC, II-IV), 5-year survival was proportional to the number of nodes removed, increasing from 75% to 87% when 1 versus greater than 20 nodes were removed. In a multivariate analysis, a more extensive nodal assessment was an independent predictor of survival. Prospective data from the ASTEC and Italian studies suggest that there is no therapeutic benefit to resecting negative LN (40,41). The use of postoperative adjuvant therapy in patients without nodal dissection may obscure the potential benefit of lymphadenectomy, making benefit difficult to measure. Likewise, patients with low-risk uterine factors may be identified with nodal disease.

In patients with positive pelvic and/or para-aortic nodes, complete resection followed by adjuvant therapy results in superior outcomes. Havrilesky et al reported on 91 patients with stage IIIC disease including 39 with microscopic involvement of the LN and 52 with grossly enlarged nodes. Five-year survival was 58% for patients with microscopic LN, 48% for those with grossly positive LN completely resected, and only 22% in cases where the nodes were not resected. The authors felt that this data suggested a therapeutic benefit for lymphadenectomy (84). Bristow evaluated 41 patients with bulky adenopathy who underwent complete resection of involved nodes. Compared with patients who had gross residual disease in LN remaining after surgery, those with resected disease had longer PFS (38 vs 9 months) (93). Mariani et al (25) showed that pelvic sidewall failure at 5 years was 57% for patients who had inadequate nodal dissection and/or no adjuvant radiation compared to 10% when patients had adequate (removal >10 nodes) lymphadenectomy and received radiation. The best outcomes reported for node-positive patients follow complete nodal dissection. For example, in one series of 30 patients with stage IIIC managed with systematic pelvic and para-aortic lymphadenectomy (average number of nodes removed, 66) followed by RT and chemotherapy, 5-year survival was 100% for patients with positive pelvic nodes and 75% for positive para-aortic nodes (50).

The most cogent argument for routine staging is that following thorough nodal assessment, most patients with node-negative disease can accurately be classified as low risk and may avoid pelvic radiation or receive VCB in lieu of pelvic RT. Three randomized trials comparing radiation to observation have failed to demonstrate a survival advantage for adjuvant pelvic RT in patients with stage I-II disease, suggesting that in the absence of nodal disease no therapy is a reasonable option (36,46,94). Indeed, patients with negative nodes and low-risk uterine factors (which account for two-thirds of patients with stage I-II EC) have incredibly low risk of recurrence and death (2% cancer-specific death at 48 months, with or without pelvic radiation) (66). Retrospective studies have shown how the incorporation of a strategy using lymphadenectomy changes the use of postoperative radiation (5,23,66,95,96). In a SEER review of 26,043 women with EC, patients with intermediate-risk disease who underwent nodal assessment were less likely to receive external beam pelvic RT and more likely to receive vaginal brachytherapy compared to women who did not undergo nodal assessment (67). In the absence of nodal disease, recurrence risk is low and OS is high, with no radiation or with the substitution of VCB (37).

Sentinel Lymph Node Mapping

The concept of lymphatic mapping by sentinel LND has been widely accepted into practice in patients with breast cancer and melanoma and is increasingly being used in selected vulvar cancers. It is now supported by randomized evidence to support its use in early-stage EC (31,32). The sentinel LN is the first or first few LNs that receive lymphatic fluid from the organ or regional tissue of interest. The node(s) is thought to be representative of the involvement of the regional drainage area. Theoretically, if the sentinel LN is negative, lymphatic spread to the rest of the drainage area has not occurred yet, thus avoiding the need for complete lymphadenectomy. Sentinel LND not only reduces complications and improves quality of life of patients, but it also provides staging information for evaluating prognosis and guiding adjuvant therapy when used appropriately without a compromise in disease outcomes of EC patients (31). Sentinel LN detection methods may include blue (isosulfan) dye, indocyanine green (ICG), radionuclide tracing method using technetium (TC)-99[m], carbon nanoparticle (CNP), or a combination of these methods. ICG is the most recommended method, especially for patients with minimally invasive surgery and obesity because of its higher overall detection rate bilaterally (97-100). The combined use of methods has been shown to have higher detection rates than using a single method alone, but is often inconvenient and costly (101).

The process of sentinel LN mapping involves injection of a tracer either into the cervix or uterine corpus. Cervical injection is the more common and simpler approach. In recent consensus guidelines, cervical injection is obligatory, whereas hysteroscopic or myometrial injection is not mandatory (100). Superficial injection into the epithelium of the ectocervix penetrates the uterine vessels, isthmus, parametrial, and uterine body, whereas the optional deep injection reaches the para-aortic LNs through the pelvic funnel ligament (100). The detection rate of pelvic LN is higher using cervical injection, with a rate over 80%, however, with the possibility of missing occult para-aortic LN (102). Ditto et al demonstrated that hysteroscopic injection did identify para-aortic LN at a higher rate than cervical injection (29% vs 19.5%, P = .18) as well as isolated para-aortic LN (5.8% vs 0%); however, there was no statistical difference (103). The technique is complicated and may not be suitable for tumors with large size (104). There is also concern regarding potential tubal leakage and tumor dissemination, but this may be mitigated by lowering intrauterine pressure to less than 40 mm Hg when performing hysteroscope (105). In a systematic review of cervical and corpus injections, Cormier et al report that the overall detection rate of cervical injection ranged from 62% to 100% and corpus injection varied from 73% to 95% (102). The detection of para-aortic LN was 39%, 17%, and 2%, respectively, for fundal, deep cervix, and superficial cervix injections. In patients who fail to map, unilateral or bilateral lymphadenectomy of the failed side(s) should follow, and all enlarged or suspicious LNs should be removed.

There are several meta-analyses and systematic reviews as well as two recent prospective trials that evaluate the diagnostic value of sentinel LN mapping; however, we await randomized controlled evidence. In a meta-analysis of 26 series on sentinel node dissection, Kang et al estimated that the detection rate for sentinel

nodes was 78% and the sensitivity was 93%. In a disease where baseline rates of nodal involvement are roughly 10%, this translates to a ~1% false-negative rate (106). Cormier et al conducted a systematic review of 17 studies with patients (n >30) and found the detection rate varied from 60% to 100%, but exceeded 80% in the subgroup of studies with over 100 patients, suggesting the importance of surgeon experience in improving diagnostic accuracy (102). Retrospectively applying a surgical algorithm, they revealed a sensitivity, NPV, and false-negative rate of 95%, 99%, and 5%, respectively. Bodurtha Smith et al reported a meta-analysis of 55 studies including 4,915 patients. The detection rate and bilateral detection rate were 81% and 50%, respectively. The detection rate of para-aortic LN was 17%, the sensitivity and NPV were 96% and 99.7%, respectively (107). Lastly, How et al found in a meta-analysis of 48 studies including 5,348 patients that the detection rate, bilateral detection rate, and para-aortic LN detection rates were 87%, 61%, and 6%, respectively (108). The multicenter Fluorescence Imaging for Robotic Endometrial sentinel lymph node biopsy (FIRES) trial is the largest prospective trial to determine whether sentinel LN biopsy is clinically acceptable compared to standard lymphadenectomy. Compared to previous analyses, 18 surgeons who participated in the trial were instructed and observed in-person to ensure standardization of both their sentinel LN mapping and completion lymphadenectomy technique, some of whom were novices at the inception of the trial. Sentinel LN mapping followed by pelvic LND was completed in 340 patients and para-aortic LND performed in 196 (58%); 86% of patients had successful mapping of at least one sentinel LN, 41 (12%) patients had positive nodes. The sensitivity and NPV were 97.2% and 99.6%, respectively. Sentinel LN biopsy is therefore estimated to not identify metastases in 3% of patients with node-positive disease (31). A second trial by Soliman et al prospectively enrolled 123 patients with high-risk EC (grade 3, serous, clear cell, carcinosarcoma). Preoperative PET/CT and intraoperative sentinel LN biopsy followed by completion lymphadenectomy were performed on all included patients. At least one sentinel LN was identified in 89%, the bilateral detection rate was 58%, 23% of patients had positive LNs. Overall, the sensitivity of sentinel LN was 95% and false NPV was 1.4% (only one patient with negative sentinel LN and positive non-sentinel LNs) (32). Similar success in the use of sentinel LN mapping in high-risk EC has been reported by several other studies (109-114).

There are a number of patient and clinical factors that may affect the successful detection rate of sentinel LN mapping including surgeon experience, tracer type and injection site, and obesity (97-100, 115). The use of pathologic ultrastaging with immunohistochemistry (IHC) staining and serial sectioning may help to improve the detection rate of metastases including low-volume metastatic disease as well as identify disease in previously neglected nodal regions located outside of the routine LND area. The FIRES study reported that 17% of LN-positive patients were found to have sentinel LN in nontraditional sites (presacral, parametrial, and deep iliac) (31). The incidence of low-volume metastatic disease including both micro metastatic disease (<2 mm) and isolated tumor cells (ITCs) discovered by sentinel LN mapping varies from approximately 3.8% up to 19.7%, and the clinical significance of these findings by ultrastaging is still not clear (74). MSKCC reported on a cohort of patients of which 5.2% had low-volume LN disease and 5.6% had macro metastatic disease. The 3-year RFS was significantly higher in the low-volume group (86% vs 71%, P <.001), as many of these patients did receive adjuvant therapy (116). A separate single-center study of 519 patients also found that the 3-year PFS was significantly higher for patients with low-volume disease (95.5% for ITCs and 85.5% for micro metastatic disease) compared to patients with macro metastatic disease in the LN (58.5%) (117). A recently published study by Bogani et al concluded that patients with micro metastatic LN disease should receive adjuvant therapy, whereas the presence of ITCs alone did not necessarily warrant adjuvant therapy and should depend on intrauterine factors (118). In a retrospective review of tissue slides by Goebe et al from sentinel

LN negative patients, patients found to have ITCs (13.5%) on IHC staining did not experience recurrence despite not receiving any adjuvant therapy (119). Overall, ultrastaging may improve the detection of nodal metastasis up to 2 times compared to traditional hematoxylin and eosin (H&E) staining methods; the significance of detected low-volume disease in the LN is an area under investigation, but it appears these patients may perform better than patients who are found to have macro metastatic disease in the LN.

Sentinel LN mapping is gaining widespread utilization in the staging of EC patients. It is now included in national consensus guidelines and supported by FIGO for its use. The use of sentinel LN mapping provides important prognostic information regarding LN involvement and guidance in the selection of adjuvant therapy while decreasing the risk of operative complications.

Minimally Invasive Surgery

After several years of debate and discussion, minimally invasive techniques have been integrated into the management of EC as a standard of care. Techniques utilized in the initial treatment of EC include laparoscopic-assisted vaginal hysterectomy (LAVH), total laparoscopic hysterectomy (TLH), and robotic hysterectomy with concomitant salpingo-oophorectomy and pelvic and para-aortic nodal dissection to stage patients. Minimally invasive staging techniques include transperitoneal and extraperitoneal assessment of nodes and may be done at the time of hysterectomy or at a later time to restage patients following incomplete surgical staging. The decade of the 1990s advanced the use of minimally invasive surgery and introduced the laparoscopic techniques and tools required for comprehensive surgical staging of EC. As the initial debate on LAVH focused on whether laparoscopic techniques could be substituted for abdominal ones, in EC, debate has focused on whether laparoscopic surgical staging could be substituted for open procedures. Initial case reports and small single-institutional series describing technique and demonstrating feasibility were replaced by large series, small randomized trials, and, subsequently, multi-institutional randomized controlled trials (9,10,54,120-136).

Improvements in laparoscopic equipment facilitated the development of LAVH. Building on that experience, and coupled with the introduction of better optics for visualization, laparoscopic resection of LN became possible. Querleu et al (127) were the first to report pelvic lymphadenectomy for cervical cancer in 1991, followed by Nezhat et al (128) who reported in 1992 on the use of laparoscopic pelvic and para-aortic lymphadenectomy with radical hysterectomy in cervical cancer. When first utilized in EC, laparoscopic para-aortic node dissection only evaluated right-sided nodes (78). Techniques have subsequently been developed allowing for dissection to include the left para-aortic nodes and facilitate extraperitoneal approaches (76,77,105-107). Childers et al (54,120) described the initial experience of LAVH in 59 patients with clinical stage I EC. Laparoscopic pelvic and right-sided aortic LN samplings were performed in patients with grade 2 or 3 lesions, or with grade 1 lesions, and greater than 50% myometrial invasion on frozen section. For the group, the mean weight was 69.4 kg, and in two patients, laparoscopic lymphadenectomy was precluded by obesity. Six patients underwent conversion to an open procedure because of intraperitoneal disease, and two patients required laparotomy to manage complications, including a transected ureter and a cystotomy. The mean hospital stay was 2.9 days. Since that time many retrospective series have appeared in the literature describing techniques and presumed advantages (132-136). In general, mean operating times were longer for laparoscopy, but the overall complication rates, length of stay, and hospital charges were lower. With short follow-ups, there was no significant difference in disease recurrence between the two groups.

Prospective data have also emerged. A small prospective, randomized trial comparing laparoscopic-assisted vaginal versus abdominal surgery in patients with EC was reported by Malur et al (124). They randomized 70 patients with EC FIGO stage I-III to laparoscopy-assisted simple or radical vaginal hysterectomy or simple or radical abdominal hysterectomy with or without LN resection. Blood loss and transfusion rates were significantly lower in the laparoscopic group. The number of pelvic and para-aortic LN, duration of surgery, and incidence of postoperative complications were similar for both groups. No significant differences in disease recurrence rate and long-term survival were found between the laparoscopic and laparotomy groups (97.3% vs 93.3% and 83.9% vs 90.9% for stages I, II, and III, respectively). Malzoni and colleagues (136) reported on a 159-patient trial comparing TLH to total abdominal hysterectomy (TAH) with lymphadenectomy. The authors reported less blood loss, shorter hospitalization, and less common ileus with TLH. Operative time was longer (136 vs 123 minutes) with TLH, but there was no difference in number of nodes removed, frequency of stage IIIC disease, ability to do para-aortic dissection, or recurrence. The LACE trial compared TLH ($n = 190$) to TAH ($n = 142$) in 332 patients with stage I EC (with or without lymphadenectomy) (10). The preliminary report designed to specifically assess quality-of-life end points showed that 2.4% of laparoscopic cases required conversion to an open approach, operating time for TLH on average was 30 minutes longer, grade 3 to 4 adverse events were more frequent (23% vs 12%) in the TAH groups, and quality-of-life assessments favored TLH for up to 6 months postsurgery. Concurrent LN assessment was more common with TAH versus TLH (68% vs 41%), and ~20% of patients participating in the study received some form of adjuvant therapy (chemotherapy, RT, or both).

The largest and most comprehensive dataset to date comes from the large prospective, randomized trial conducted by the GOG (LAP II trial) (9). The study was designed to compare laparoscopic hysterectomy with comprehensive surgical staging to the traditional laparotomy technique (using a 2:1 randomization favoring the laparoscopic arm) to determine the complete staging rates, safety, short-term surgical outcomes, and long-term cancer recurrence and survival. The study enrolled 920 patients to the open arm and 1,696 patients to laparoscopy. The rate of conversion from laparoscopy to open procedure was 26% and was most frequently related to poor visibility (15%), extrauterine cancer spread (4%), and bleeding (3%). The conversion rate increased with increasing patient obesity, with the laparoscopic success rate being 90% with a BMI less than 20 kg/m^2, 65% with BMI of 35 kg/m^2, and 34% with BMI of 50 kg/m^2. Median number of removed nodes was similar between each technique as were the frequencies of patients found to have positive LN. Complication rates (combined rates of vascular, urinary, bowel, nerve, or other complications) for those who had an open procedure were 7.6%, compared to 9.5% of patients randomized to laparoscopy. Of the 1,242 patients randomized to laparoscopy who had the procedure successfully completed laparoscopically, the complication rate was 4.9%. Comparing patients who underwent open surgery versus successful completion of laparoscopy, operative time was longer (median 70 minutes), but hospital time was shorter (2 vs 4 days) with laparoscopy. Postoperative arrhythmia, pneumonia, ileus, antibiotic use, and any complications greater than grade 2 were lower in the laparoscopic group. The authors concluded that laparoscopic surgical staging is an acceptable and possibly a better option, particularly when the surgery can be successfully completed laparoscopically.

Results of long-term survival in laparoscopically treated compared to laparotomy-treated EC patients suggest comparable outcomes. Tozzi et al reporting on the first prospective trial ($n = 122$ patients) reported DFS of 91% with LAVH and 94% with laparotomy, with survival of 86% versus 90%, respectively (137). In a subsequent evaluation of recurrence and survival data from the GOG LAP II trial published in 2012, 3-year recurrence rates were 11.4% with laparoscopy versus 10.2% with open surgery, and 5-year survival was 90% in each arm (9). Age and obesity have been suggested as relative contraindications to laparoscopic surgery. In the GOG LAP II trial, the median age was 63 years. Scribner et al (138) evaluated the surgical experience of patients with uterine cancer with age 65 years and above who underwent

LAVH with pelvic and para-aortic lymphadenectomy ($n = 67$) or abdominal hysterectomy with pelvic and para-aortic lymphadenectomy ($n = 45$). Laparoscopic staging could be completed in 78% of patients. In the laparoscopic group, the BMI was 29.5 kg/m^2 (range, 15.9-54.7), and 33% had a history of prior laparotomy. For the 22% of patients who required a conversion to laparotomy, obesity (10%), bleeding (6%), and intraperitoneal disease (5%) were the most frequent reasons. Similar nodal counts (29 laparoscopic, 29 open) were noted, the operative time was longer (236 vs 148 minutes), and hospital stay was shorter (median 3 vs 5.6 days) with laparoscopy. The authors concluded that with the anticipated growth of an aging patient population, laparoscopic management is a viable option.

It has been suggested that obese patients are poor laparoscopic candidates because of difficulties in establishing pneumoperitoneum, poorer visualization, inability to tolerate the steep Trendelenburg positioning needed to facilitate the surgery, and difficulties with ventilation. In the report by Childers et al (54,120), mean patient weight was only 69.4 kg. It is important to recognize that regardless of surgical approach, complete surgical staging is more difficult in an obese patient. Scribner et al (131) compared 55 obese patients (median weight 96.6 kg, median BMI 40 kg/m^2) who underwent LAVH with pelvic and para-aortic lymphadenectomy to 45 patients (median weight 101 kg, median BMI 39 kg/m^2) who had abdominal hysterectomy with pelvic and para-aortic lymphadenectomy. Successful completion of laparoscopy was possible in 64%, with patients with a BMI less than 35 kg/m^2 having an 82% success rate compared to 44% when the BMI was greater than 35 kg/m^2. Eltabbakh (133) evaluated 40 women with BMI between 28 and 60 kg/m^2 who were treated with LAVH and compared them to 40 similar women treated by abdominal approach. Laparoscopic conversion was only required in 8% of patients. Laparoscopic surgery was associated with a longer operative time (195 vs 138 minutes), but more pelvic nodes (mean 11 vs 5), less pain medicine requirement, and shorter hospital stay (2.5 vs 5.6 days) were recorded. TLH has also demonstrated feasibility in heavier patients (139). In the prospective GOG series, there was 80% or more success rate with patients with a BMI of 27 kg/m^2 or less, but even at a BMI of 35 kg/m^2, 65% were able to have successful laparoscopic surgery (102).

Robotic surgery may represent the next step forward in minimally invasive surgery. Since the Food and Drug Administration (FDA) approval for hysterectomy and myomectomy procedures in 2005, there has been an increasing utilization of robotic surgery within gynecologic oncology. To date, greater than 15 series ranging in size from 4 to 405 patients have described robotic experience or compared outcomes to laparoscopy and/or open procedures (**Table 5.4-9**) (140-146). The proposed advantages of robotic surgery include improved visualization with 3-D optics, "wrist-like" motion of instruments allowing greater dexterity, reduction in tremor, easier learning curve for adoption compared

to straight-stick laparoscopy, and more comfortable ergonomics. Published data suggest comparable outcomes with respect to blood loss, nodal counts, and operative time compared to laparoscopy. Mean nodal counts and operative complications are comparable to laparoscopy, with several series suggesting lower postoperative complications compared to open surgery. As with new surgical techniques, there is a learning curve through which additional experience leads to quicker operative times and higher nodal retrieval rates. The Ohio State group has suggested that 20 procedures are required for proficiency (147).

Robotic surgery may offer unique opportunities for obese patients (147,149). Several series suggest that robotics may overcome some of the challenges of laparoscopy and may reduce the morbidity associated with open cases. Seamon and colleagues reported that in a series of 109 obese patients (mean BMI 40 kg/m^2) treated by robotic hysterectomy and staging, the conversion rate was 16% (149). The 92 patients successfully treated by robotic platform were compared to a matched cohort of 162 laparotomy patients. Total nodal counts (~24 nodes in each group) and frequency of adequate lymphadenectomy (defined as at least 10 nodes removed) were similar in both groups, but blood transfusion rate, hospital stay, complications, and wound problems were reduced with robotic surgery.

Arguments have been advanced for and against each of the surgical approaches to EC. Vaginal hysterectomy was once a favored operation, but it did not allow for routine removal of the ovaries in some patients. It also did not permit for surgical resection of LN, inspection of the peritoneal cavity or the retroperitoneum for metastatic disease, or collection of peritoneal fluid for cytology (18). Laparoscopic-assisted or total laparoscopic approaches overcome these limitations, however. Compared to open procedures, LAVH/TLH are thought to lead to reduced incisional complications, wound infections, ileus, hospital stay, cost, and improved rate of recovery and quality of life (8,127,150). Data from prospective studies also showed that short-term (6 weeks to 6 months) patient-assessed quality-of-life assessments favor minimally invasive surgery (151). In patients requiring postoperative radiation, laparoscopic surgical staging followed by RT is suggested to result in fewer bowel adhesions and radiation-induced bowel injuries (132). Criticisms of LAVH/TLH with laparoscopic nodal dissection relate to the learning curve required to master new or unfamiliar procedures, the increased length of operative times, and concerns about the adequacy of the nodal dissection. Studies do suggest that with increased experience, operative times decrease and nodal counts increase (126,133). Laparoscopy also introduced different procedure-related complications (134,135). Rarely, the technique has been associated with port-site recurrences or intraperitoneal dissemination of disease by laparoscopic gas and/or uterine manipulation.

Whether a minimally invasive procedure is comparable to an open approach must be judged by the ability to accurately dissect

■ TABLE 5.4-9. Selected Robotic Surgery Series in EC

Study	N (Robot Cases)	Type of Study	Procedure	OR Time (min) (Mean/Median)	# Nodes (Mean/Median)
Boggess et al (2008) (144)	103	Compare to LSC + Open	Hyst + PPALND	191	33
DeNardis et al (2008) (145)	87	Compare to LSC	Hyst + PPALND	177	19
Veljovich et al (2008) (146)	25	Compare to LSC + Open	Hyst ± LND	283	18
Holloway et al (2009) (147)	100	Case series	Hyst + PPALND	171	19
Seamon et al (2009) (149)	105	Compare to LSC	Hyst + PPALND	242	31
Lowe et al (2009) (150)	405	Case series	Hyst ± LND	172	14
Lim (2011) (148)	122	Compare to LSC	Hyst + PPALND	147	25

EC, endometrial cancer; hyst, hysterectomy; LND, lymph node dissection unspecified; LSC, laparoscopic; Open, laparotomy; OR, odds ratio; PPALND, pelvic, para-aortic lymph node dissection.

appropriate nodal basins, to remove an adequate/representative number of LNs, to identify metastatic disease, and by the rates of recurrence. The technique used to remove the uterus/ovaries is not the source of controversy, although TLH and robotic hysterectomy may facilitate removal of larger uteri or assist in cases with poor descensus compared to LAVH. Comprehensive surgical staging allows for appropriate risk stratification to make appropriate treatment recommendations. Multiple reports demonstrated similar node counts for open, laparoscopic, and robotic techniques in the surgical staging of EC (134,140). In the GOG LAP II trial, median numbers of nodes from pelvic and para-aortic basins, and frequencies of positive nodes were comparable in the surgical arms (9). If laparoscopic nodal dissection cannot be performed, conversion to laparotomy is advised to yield inadequate information for treatment planning.

Minimally invasive surgery must be performed with an acceptable complication rate in order to be considered a viable option. In one series reporting on complication rates with an institution's first 100 pelvic and para-aortic nodal dissections, conversion to manage complications was required in five to control bleeding and one to repair a ureteral injury (18). In another group's experience with 150 patients, seven major vascular injuries were reported, but only 4 patients required laparotomy (127). Querleu et al (150) reported on intraoperative and postoperative complications of laparoscopic node dissection from 1,192 pelvic and para-aortic node dissections. Only 13 open procedures were required to complete the nodal dissections, and a laparotomy was required in seven cases to manage complications. Eleven intraoperative vascular injuries were noted, but none required management by laparotomy. In the GOG LAP II study, intraoperative complications were comparable (7.6% open, 9.5% randomized to laparoscopy, 4.9% successful completion of laparoscopy) (9). Postoperative complications and short-term quality-of-life improvements favored laparoscopy. A meta-analysis of robotic studies for gynecologic conditions noted that for endometrial series, robotic surgery was associated with less blood loss and less frequent conversions to open procedure compared to laparoscopy.

Restaging

One of the more useful roles of minimally invasive surgery is in restaging patients who underwent hysterectomy only. Patients who undergo hysterectomy without nodal dissection and who have pathologic risk factors for potential nodal spread face a difficult dilemma. Patients may elect to receive RT or chemotherapy (presuming nodes are positive), elect observation (presuming nodes are negative), or undergo a second operation. A second laparotomy can be difficult to accept. Laparoscopic staging offers a less invasive option for collecting information. Childers et al (152) reported the initial experience with restaging in 13 patients, finding disease in 3 patients.

Recommendations for Minimally Invasive Surgery

Standard of care today includes minimally invasive surgery in the management of EC. Additional training and experience are required for successful completion of these procedures, just as they are with open procedures. The demonstration of comparable surgical end points (similar numbers of nodes removed, similar frequency of positive nodes, recurrence rates, and survival) along with shortened hospital stays, quicker recovery, and better quality-of-life indicators compared to open procedures suggests that appropriate patients should be counseled regarding this option. Challenges remain on how to increase the minimally invasive training of gynecologic oncologists in practice and fellows in training programs. As with open procedures, defining populations that should be considered for nodal assessment and for postoperative therapies continues to be an important research focus.

Surgical Management of Intraperitoneal Disease

The management of patients with bulky stage III or IV disease depends on the ability to resect disease. In patients with distant metastasis, there may be a limited role for surgery such as to control of vaginal bleeding. In patients with intraperitoneal disease, options include resecting easily removable disease (uterus, adnexa, omentum) versus a more extensive cytoreductive effort. The value of extensive cytoreductive surgery in EC has not been as well studied as it has in ovarian cancer. Historically, limitations in postoperative therapies (lack of enthusiasm for whole abdominal radiation, marginally effective chemotherapy regimens, reliance on hormonal therapy) perhaps reduced interest. Several retrospective reports suggest that survival correlates with volume of residual disease (153-155). Shih et al (156) reported on 58 patients with stage IV endometrioid disease treated from 1977 to 2003, of whom 9 had no gross residual disease, 11 had less than 1 cm residual, and 32 had greater than 1 cm residual. The median survival for the entire population group was 19 months; however, median survival was 42 months for patients with no gross residual disease. In a multivariate analysis of the data, residual disease and the use of postoperative adjuvant chemotherapy were independently associated with survival. Bristow et al (157) demonstrated that optimal cytoreduction (<1 cm) could be obtained in 55% of stage IV patients and required omentectomy (93%), peritoneal stripping (65%), and bowel resection (29%) to do it. In patients with serous histology, similar survival improvements were seen with optimal debulking of intraperitoneal disease (134).

Surgical Recommendations

The contemporary management of EC has significantly changed. We believe that patients must be appropriately counseled with regard to the presumed benefits as well as the potential risks of lymphadenectomy. Data for the ASTEC and Italian lymphadenectomy trials cast doubt as to the benefit of resecting negative nodes, but both studies clearly demonstrate that nodal disease cannot be found unless one searches for it. The clinician is challenged with finding the "needle in the haystack" in a disease where the baseline rate of nodal metastasis is ~9%. The marginal benefit achieved by lymphadenectomy and the downstream costs associated with or without its use in terms of adjuvant therapy, outcomes, and quality of life need to be better defined so that patients and physicians can make choices based on good information. Clinical pathologic models that define low-risk populations for whom lymphadenectomy may be safely omitted appear promising but must be validated prospectively in large series. In the future, biomarker-based testing or sentinel nodal assessment may serve as an alternative to lymphadenectomy but cannot be routinely recommended at this point because the data are immature. Increasing the proportion of patients who undergo minimally invasive surgery to manage EC is an important goal and driven by the data. Patients who a priori are deemed not to be candidates for staging should be considered for vaginal or minimally invasive hysterectomies. Surgical therapy for EC removes the disease and defines populations at risk for recurrence and death. Surgical staging, or the lack of it, defines patient groups as surgically staged node positive or negative, or unstaged. Comprehensive staging most accurately assigns stage and associated prognosis, although the magnitude of the risk assignment is tempered by the frequency of positive nodes, uterine risk factors, and use of adjuvant therapy. Staging also allows for a more tailored approach to the use of adjuvant therapies. For patients with resectable intraperitoneal disease, cytoreductive surgery can result in optimal volumes of residual disease, and perhaps improved outcomes.

REFERENCES

1. Mikuta JJ. International Federation of Gynecology and Obstetrics staging of endometrial cancer 1988. *Cancer*. 1993;71:1460-1463.

2. Creasman WT, Morrow CP, Bundy BN, et al. Surgical pathologic spread patterns of endometrial cancer: a Gynecologic Oncology Group study. *Cancer*. 1987;60:2035-2041.

3. Lewis BU, Stallworthy JA, Cowdell R, et al. Adenocarcinoma of the body of the uterus. *Br J Obstet Gynaecol*. 1970;77:343-348.

4. Dobbie BMW, Taylor C, Waterhouse J. Study of carcinoma of the endometrium. *J Obstet Gynaecol Br Commonw*. 1973;114:106-109.

5. Barakat RR, Lev G, Hummer A, et al. Twelve-year experience in the management of endometrial cancer: a change in surgical and postoperative radiation approaches. *Gynecol Oncol*. 2007;105:150-156.

6. Amant F, Mirza MR, Koskas M, et al. Cancer of the corpus uteri. *Int J Gynecol Obstet*. 2018;143(suppl 2):37-50.

7. Walker JL, Piedmonte MR, Spirtos NM, et al. Laparoscopy compared with laparotomy for comprehensive surgical staging of uterine cancer: Gynecologic Oncology Group Study LAP2. *J Clin Oncol*. 2009;27:5331-5336.

8. Janda M, Gebski V, Davies LC, et al. Effect of total laparoscopic hysterectomy vs total abdominal hysterectomy on disease-free survival among women with stage I endometrial cancer: a randomized clinical trial. *JAMA*. 2017;317:1224-1233.

9. Walker JL, Piedmonte MR, Spirtos NM, et al. Recurrence and survival after random assignment to laparoscopy versus laparotomy for comprehensive surgical staging of uterine cancer: Gynecologic Oncology Group LAP2 study. *J Clin Oncol*. 2012;30:695-700.

10. Janda M, Gebski V, Brand A, et al. Quality of life after total laparoscopic hysterectomy versus total abdominal hysterectomy for stage I endometrial cancer (LACE): a randomised trial. *Lancet Oncol*. 2010;11(8):772-780.

11. Wright JD, Burke WM, Wilde ET, et al. Comparative effectiveness of robotic versus laparoscopic hysterectomy for endometrial cancer. *J Clin Oncol*. 2012;30:783-791.

12. Perrone E, Capasso I, Pasciuto T, et al. Laparoscopic vs. robotic-assisted laparoscopy in endometrial cancer staging: large retrospective single-institution study. *J Gynecol Oncol*. 2021;32(3):e45.

13. Mäenpää MM, Nieminen K, Tomás EI, et al. Robotic-assisted vs traditional laparoscopic surgery for endometrial cancer: a randomized controlled trial. *Am J Obstet Gynecol*. 2016;215:588.e1-588.e7.

14. Morrow CP. Curtin JP. *Surgery for Cervical Neoplasia in Gynecologic Cancer Surgery*. Churchill Livingstone Inc; 1996:451-568.

15. Soliman P, Frumovitz M, Spannuth W, et al. Lymphadenectomy during endometrial cancer staging: practice patterns among gynecologic oncologists. *Gynecol Oncol*. 2010;119:291-294.

16. Morrow CP. Curtin JP. *Surgery for Ovarian Neoplasia in Gynecologic Cancer Surgery*. Churchill Livingstone Inc; 1996:627-716.

17. Candiani GB, Belloni C, Maggi R, et al. Evaluation of different surgical approach in the treatment of endometrial cancer at FIGO stage I. *Gynecol Oncol*. 1990;37:6-8.

18. Massi G, Savino L, Susini T. Vaginal hysterectomy versus abdominal hysterectomy for the treatment of stage I endometrial adenocarcinoma. *Am J Obstet Gynecol*. 1996;174:1320-1326.

19. Scarselli G, Savino L, Ceccherini R, et al. Role of vaginal surgery in the 1st stage endometrial cancer. Experience of the Florence School. *Eur J Gynaecol Oncol*. 1992;13:15-19.

20. Bloss JD, Berman ML, Bloss LP, et al. Use of vaginal hysterectomy for the management of stage I endometrial cancer in the medically compromised patient. *Gynecol Oncol*. 1991;40:74-77.

21. Pitkin RM. Vaginal hysterectomy in obese women. *Obstet Gynecol*. 1977;49:567-569.

22. Morrow CP, Bundy BN, Kumar RJ, et al. Relationship between surgical-pathological risk factors and outcome in clinical stages I and II carcinoma of the endometrium. A Gynecologic Oncology Group study. *Gynecol Oncol*. 1991;40:55-65.

23. Orr JW, Holimon J, Orr P. Stage I corpus cancer: is teletherapy necessary. *Am J Obstet Gynecol*. 1997;176:777-789.

24. Homesley HD, Kadar N, Barrett RJ, et al. Selective pelvic and periaortic lymphadenectomy does not increase morbidity in surgical staging of endometrial carcinoma. *Am J Obstet Gynecol*. 1992;167:1225-1230.

25. Mariani A, Dowdy S, Cliby W, et al. Efficacy of systematic lymphadenectomy and adjuvant radiotherapy in node-positive endometrial cancer patients. *Gynecol Oncol*. 2006;101:200-208.

26. Abu-Rustum N, Alektiar K, Iasonos A, et al. The incidence of symptomatic lower-extremity lymphedema following treatment of uterine corpus malignancies: a 12-year experience at Memorial Sloan-Kettering Cancer Center. *Gynecol Oncol*. 2006;103:714-718.

27. Glaser G, Dinoi G, Multinu F, et al. Reduced lymphedema after sentinel lymph node biopsy versus lymphadenectomy for endometrial cancer. *Int J Gynecol Cancer*. 2021;31(1):85-91.

28. Leitao MM Jr, Zhou QC, Gomez-Hidalgo NR, et al. Patient-reported outcomes after surgery for endometrial carcinoma: prevalence of lower-extremity lymphedema after sentinel lymph node mapping after lymphadenectomy. *Gynecol Oncol*. 2020;156(1):147-153.

29. Casarin J, Multinu F, Tortorella L, et al. Sentinel lymph node biopsy for robotic-assisted endometrial cancer staging: further improvement of perioperative outcomes. *Int J Gynecol Cancer*. 2020;30(1):41-47.

30. Niikura H, Toki A, Nagai T, et al. Prospective evaluation of sentinel node navigation surgery in Japanese patients with low-risk endometrial cancer—safety and occurrence of lymphedema. *Jpn J Clin Oncol*. 2021;51(4):584-589.

31. Rossi EC, Kowalski LD, Scalici J, et al. A comparison of sentinel lymph node biopsy to lymphadenectomy for endometrial cancer staging (FIRES trial): a multicentre, prospective, cohort study. *Lancet Oncol*. 2017;18:384-392.

32. Soliman PT, Westin SN, Dious S, et al. A prospective validation study of sentinel lymph node mapping for high-risk endometrial cancer. *Gynecol Oncol*. 2017;146:234-239.

33. Chambers LM, Vargas R, Michener CM. Sentinel lymph node mapping in endometrial and cervical cancer: a survey of practices and attitudes in gynecologic oncologists. *J Gynecol Oncol*. 2019;30(3):e35.

34. Aalders JG, Thomas G. Endometrial cancer—revisiting the importance of pelvic and para-aortic lymph nodes. *Gynecol Oncol*. 2007;104:222-231.

35. Concin N, Matias-Guiu X, Vergote I, et al. ESGO/ESTRO/ESP guidelines for the management of patients with endometrial carcinoma. *Int J Gynecol Cancer*. 2021;31(1):12-39.

36. Creutzberg CL, van Putten WL, Koper PC, et al. Surgery and postoperative radiotherapy versus surgery alone for patients with stage-1 endometrial carcinoma: multicentre randomised trial. PORTEC Study Group. Post operative radiation therapy in endometrial carcinoma. *Lancet*. 2000;355:1404-1411.

37. Nout RA, Smit VT, Putter H, et al. Vaginal brachytherapy versus pelvic external beam radiotherapy for patients with endometrial cancer of high-intermediate risk (PORTEC-2): an open-label, non-inferiority, randomised trial. *Lancet*. 2010;375:816-823.

38. Trimble E, Kosary C, Park R. Lymph node sampling and survival in endometrial cancer. *Gynecol Oncol*. 1998;71:340-343.

39. COSA-NZ-UK Endometrial Cancer Study Groups. Pelvic lymphadenectomy in high-risk endometrial cancer. *Int J Gynecol Cancer*. 1996;6:102-107.

40. ASTEC Study Group. Efficacy of systematic pelvic lymphadenectomy in endometrial cancer (MRC ASTEC trial): a randomized study. *Lancet*. 2009;373:125-136.

41. Benedetti Panici P, Basile S, Maneschi F, et al. Systematic pelvic lymphadenectomy versus no lymphadenectomy in early-stage endometrial carcinoma: randomized clinical trial. *J Natl Cancer Inst*. 2008;100:1707-1716.

42. Nout RA, Putter H, Jürgenliemk-Schulz, IM, et al. Quality of life after pelvic radiotherapy or vaginal brachytherapy for endometrial cancer: first results of the randomized PORTEC-2 trial. *J Clin Oncol*. 2009;27:3547-3556.

43. Creasman WT, Mutch DE, Herzog TJ. ATEC lymphadenectomy and radiation therapy: are conclusions valid. *Gynecol Oncol*. 2010;116:293-294.

44. Seamon LG, Fowler JM, Cohn DE. Lymphadenectomy for endometrial cancer: the controversy. *Gynecol Oncol*. 2010;117:6-8.

45. Lee TS, Kim JW, Seong S, et al. Benefit of lymphadenectomy in endometrial cancer: can the truth be obtained by randomized controlled trial after ASTEC? *Int J Gynecol Cancer*. 2009;19(8):1467.

46. Keys HM, Roberts JA, Brunetto VL, et al. A phase III trial of surgery with or without adjunctive external pelvic radiation therapy in intermediate risk endometrial adenocarcinoma: a Gynecologic Oncology Group study. *Gynecol Oncol*. 2004;92:744-751.

47. Nugent EK, Bishop EA, Mathews CA, et al. Do uterine risk factors or lymph node metastasis more significantly affect recurrence in patients with endometrioid adenocarcinoma. *Gynecol Oncol*. 2012;125:94-98.

48. Kwon J, Qiu F, Saski R, et al. Are uterine risk factors more important than nodal status in predicting survival. *Obstet Gynecol*. 2009;114:736-743.

49. Creutzberg C, van Putten W, Warlam-Rodenhuis C, et al. Outcome of high-risk stage IC, grade 3 compared with stage I endometrial carcinoma patients: the postoperative radiation therapy in endometrial carcinoma trial. *J Clin Oncol*. 2004;22:1234-1241.

50. Onda T, Yoshikawa H, Mizutani K, et al. Treatment of node positive endometrial cancer with complete node dissection, chemotherapy and radiation therapy. *Br J Cancer*. 1997;75:1836-1841.

51. McMeekin DS, Lashbrook D, Gold M, et al. Analysis of FIGO stage IIIc endometrial cancer patients. *Gynecol Oncol*. 2001;81:273-278.

52. Nelson G, Randall M, Sutton G, et al. FIGO stage IIIC endometrial carcinoma with metastases confined to pelvic lymph nodes: analysis of treatment outcomes, prognostic variables, and failure patterns following adjuvant radiation therapy. *Gynecol Oncol.* 1999;75:211-214.

53. Arango HA, Hoffman MS, Roberts WS, et al. Accuracy of lymph node palpation to determine need for lymphadenectomy in gynecologic malignancies. *Obstet Gynecol.* 2000;95:553-556.

54. Childers JM, Brzechffa P, Hatch K, et al. Laparoscopically assisted surgical staging of endometrial cancer. *Gynecol Oncol.* 1993;51:33-38.

55. Gray LA. Lymph node excision in treatment of gynecologic malignancies. *Am J Surg.* 1964;108:660-663.

56. Mariani A, Webb MJ, Keeney GI, et al. Low risk corpus cancer: is lymphadenectomy or radiotherapy necessary. *Am J Obstet Gynecol.* 2000;182:1506-1519.

57. Mariani A, Dowdy SC, Cliby WA, et al. Prospective assessment of lymphatic dissemination in endometrial cancer: a paradigm shift in surgical staging. *Gynecol Oncol.* 2008;109:11-28.

58. Convery PA, Cantrell LA, DiSanto N, et al. Retrospective review of an intraoperative algorithm to predict lymph node metastasis in low grade endometrial cancer. *Gynecol Oncol.* 2011;123:65-70.

59. Milam M, Java J, Walker JL, et al. Nodal metastasis risk in endometrioid endometrial cancer. *Obstet Gynecol.* 2012;119:286-292.

60. Kang S, Kang WD, Chung HH, et al. Preoperative identification of low-risk group for lymph node metastasis in endometrial cancer: a Korean GOG study. *J Clin Oncol.* 2012;30:1329-1334.

61. Bernardini M, May T, Khalifa M, et al. Evaluation of two management strategies for preoperative grade 1 endometrial cancer. *Obstet Gynecol.* 2009;114:7-15.

62. Doering DL, Barnhill DR, Weiser EB, et al. Intraoperative evaluation of depth of myometrial invasion in stage I endometrial adenocarcinoma. *Obstet Gynecol.* 1989;74:930-933.

63. Franchi M, Ghezzi F, Melpigano M, et al. Clinical value of intraoperative gross examination in endometrial cancer. *Gynecol Oncol.* 2000;76:357-361.

64. Goff BA, Riche LW. Assessment of depth of myometrial invasion in endometrial adenocarcinoma. *Gynecol Oncol.* 1990;38:46-48.

65. Partridge EE, Shingleton H, Menck H. The national cancer data base report on endometrial cancer. *J Surg Oncol.* 1996;61:111-123.

66. Coudge C, Bernhard S, Cloven N, et al. The impact of complete surgical staging on adjuvant treatment decisions in endometrial cancer. *Gynecol Oncol.* 2004;93:536-539.

67. Sharma C, Deeutsch I, Lewin S, et al. Lymphadenectomy influences the utilization of adjuvant radiation treatment for endometrial cancer. *Am J Obstet Gynecol.* 2011;205:562.e1-562.e9.

68. Goff B, Kato D, Schmidt R, et al. Uterine papillary serous carcinoma: patterns of metastatic spread. *Gynecol Oncol.* 1994;54:264-268.

69. Podratz KC, Mariani A, Webb MJ. Staging and therapeutic value of lymphadenectomy in endometrial cancer. *Gynecol Oncol.* 1998;70(2):163-164.

70. Creasman WT, Zaino R, Major FL, et al. Early invasive carcinoma of the cervix (3-5 mm invasion): risk factors and prognosis: a Gynecologic Oncology Group study. *Am J Obstet Gynecol.* 1998;178:62-65.

71. Leblanc E, Querleu D, Narducci F, et al. Surgical staging of early invasive epithelial ovarian tumors. *Semin Surg Oncol.* 2000;19:36-41.

72. Case AS, Rocconi RP, Straughn JM. A prospective blinded evaluation of the accuracy of frozen section for the surgical management of endometrial cancer. *Obstet Gynecol.* 2006;108:1375-1379.

73. Frumovitz M, Slomovitz BM, Singh DK, et al. Frozen section analyses as predictors of lymphatic spread in patients with early-stage uterine cancer. *J Am Coll Surg.* 2004;199:388-393.

74. Frumovitz M, Singh DK, Meyer L, et al. Predictors of final histology in patients with endometrial cancer. *Gynecol Oncol.* 2004;95:463-468.

75. McMeekin DS, Lashbrook D, Gold M, et al. Nodal distribution and its significance in FIGO stage III endometrial cancer. *Gynecol Oncol.* 2001;82:375-379.

76. Flanigan C, Mannel R, Walker J, et al. Incidence and location of para-aortic lymph node metastases in gynecologic malignancies. *J Am Coll Surg.* 1995;181:72-74.

77. Abu-Rustum NR, Gomez J, Alektiar KM, et al. The incidence of isolated para-aortic nodal metastasis in surgically staged endometrial cancer patients with negative pelvic lymph nodes. *Gynecol Oncol.* 2009;115:236-238.

78. Chiang AJ, Yu KJ, Chao KC, et al. The incidence of isolated para-aortic nodal metastasis in completely staged endometrial cancer. *Gynecol Oncol.* 2011;121:122-125.

79. Chuang L, Burke T, Tornos C, et al. Staging laparotomy for endometrial carcinoma: assessment of retroperitoneal lymph nodes. *Gynecol Oncol.* 1995;58:189-193.

80. Mariani A, Webb M, Galli L, et al. Potential therapeutic role of para-aortic lymphadenectomy in node positive endometrial cancer. *Gynecol Oncol.* 2000;76:348-356.

81. Schorge JO, Molpus KL, Goodman A. The effect of postsurgical therapy on stage III endometrial carcinoma. *Gynecol Oncol.* 1996;63(1): 34-39.

82. Hirahatake K, Hareyama H, Sakuragi N, et al. A clinical and pathologic study on para-aortic lymph node metastasis in endometrial carcinoma. *J Surg Oncol.* 1997;65:82-87.

83. Otsuka I, Kubota T, Aso T. Lymphadenectomy and adjuvant therapy in endometrial carcinoma: role of adjuvant chemotherapy. *Br J Cancer.* 2002;87(4):377-380.

84. Havrilesky LJ, Cragun J, Calingaert B, et al. Resection of lymph node metastases influences survival in stage IIIC endometrial cancer. *Gynecol Oncol.* 2005;99(3):689-695.

85. Todo Y, Kato H, Kaneuchi M, et al. Survival effect of para-aortic lymphadenectomy in endometrial cancer (SEPAL study): a retrospective cohort analysis. *Lancet.* 2010;375:1165-1172.

86. Nasioudis D, Holcomb K. Incidence of isolated para-aortic lymph node metastasis in early stage endometrial cancer. *Eur J Obstet Gynecol Reprod Biol.* 2019;242:43-46.

87. Kohler C, Tozzi R, Klemm P, et al. Laparoscopic para-aortic left-sided transperitoneal infrarenal lymphadenectomy in patients with gynecologic malignancies: techniques and results. *Gynecol Oncol.* 2003;91:139-148.

88. Dowdy S, Aletti G, Cliby W. Extra-peritoneal laparoscopic para-aortic lymphadenectomy—a prospective cohort study of 293 patients with endometrial cancer. *Gynecol Oncol.* 2008;111:418-424.

89. Kilgore L, Partridge E, Alvarez R, et al. Adenocarcinoma of the endometrium: survival comparisons of patients with and without pelvic node sampling. *Gynecol Oncol.* 1995;56:29-33.

90. Girardi F, Petru E, Heydarfadai M, et al. Pelvic lymphadenectomy in the surgical treatment of endometrial cancer. *Gynecol Oncol.* 1993;49: 177-180.

91. Cragan J, Havrilesky L, Calingaert B, et al. Retrospective analysis of selective lymphadenectomy in apparent early-stage endometrial cancer. *J Clin Oncol.* 2005;23:3668-3675.

92. Chan J, Cheung M, Huh W, et al. Therapeutic role of lymph node resection in endometrioid corpus cancer: a study of 12,333 patients. *Cancer.* 2006;107:1823-1830.

93. Bristow RE, Zahurak ML, Alexander CJ, et al. FIGO stage IIIC endometrial carcinoma: resection of macroscopic nodal disease and other determinants of survival. *Int J Gynecol Cancer.* 2003;13:664-672.

94. ASTEC/EN.5 Study Group; Blake P, Swart AM, Orton J, et al. Adjuvant external beam radiotherapy in the treatment of endometrial cancer (MRC ASTEC and NCIC CTG EN.5 randomised trials): pooled trial results, systematic review, and meta-analysis. *Lancet.* 2009;373:137-146.

95. Fanning J, Nanavati P, Hilgers R. Surgical staging and high dose rate brachytherapy for endometrial cancer: limiting external radiotherapy to node positive tumors. *Obstet Gynecol.* 1996;87:1041-1044.

96. Mohan D, Samuels M, Selim M, et al. Long term outcomes of therapeutic pelvic lymphadenectomy for stage I endometrial adenocarcinoma. *Gynecol Oncol.* 1998;70:165-171.

97. Ruscito I, Gasparri ML, Braicu EI, et al. Sentinel node mapping in cervical and endometrial cancer: indocyanine green versus other conventional dyes—a meta-analysis. *Ann Surg Oncol.* 2016;23(11):3749-3756.

98. Papadia A, Zapardiel I, Bussi B, et al. Sentinel lymph node mapping in patients with stage I endometrial carcinoma: a focus of bilateral mapping identification by comparing radiotracer Tc99^m with blue dye versus indocyanine green fluorescent dye. *J Cancer Res Clin Oncol.* 2017;143(3):475-480.

99. Eriksson AG, Montovano M, Beavis A, et al. Impact of obesity on sentinel lymph node mapping in patients with newly diagnosed uterine cancer undergoing robotic surgery. *Ann Surg Oncol.* 2016;23(8):2522-2528.

100. Moloney K, Janda M, Frumovitz M, et al. Development of a surgical competency assessment tool for sentinel lymph node dissection by minimally invasive surgery for endometrial cancer. *Int J Gynecol Cancer.* 2021;31(5):647-655.

101. Hou H, Dai Y, Liang S, et al. Sentinel lymph node biopsy is feasible in cervical cancer laparoscopic surgery: a single-center retrospective cohort study. *J Oncol.* 2021;2021:5510623.

102. Cormier B, Rozenholc AT, Gotlieb W, et al; Communities of Practice (CoP) Group of the Society of Gynecologic Oncology of Canada (GOC). Sentinel lymph node procedure in endometrial cancer: a systematic review and proposal for standardization of future research. *Gynecol Oncol.* 2015;138(2):478-485.

103. Ditto A, Casarin J, Pinelli C, et al. Hysteroscopic versus cervical injection for sentinel node detection in endometrial cancer: a multicenter

prospective randomised controlled trial from the Multicenter Italian Trials in Ovarian cancer (MITO) study group. *Eur J Cancer*. 2020;140:1-10.

104. Perrone AM, Casadio P, Formelli G, et al. Cervical and hysteroscopic injection for identification of sentinel lymph node in endometrial cancer. *Gynecol Oncol*. 2008;111(1):62-67.

105. Solima E, Brusati V, Ditto A, et al. Hysteroscopy in endometrial cancer: new methods to evaluate transtubal leakage of saline distension medium. *Am J Obstet Gynecol*. 2008;198(2):214.e1-214.e4.

106. Kang S, Yoo HJ, Hwang JH, et al. Sentinel lymph node biopsy in endometrial cancer: meta-analysis of 26 studies. *Gynecol Oncol*. 2011;123:522-527.

107. Bodurtha Smith AJ, Fader AN, Tanner EJ. Sentinel lymph node assessment in endometrial cancer: a systematic review and meta-analysis. *Am J Obstet Gynecol*. 2017;216(5):459-476.

108. How JA, O'Farrell P, Amajoud Z, et al. Sentinel lymph node mapping in endometrial cancer: a systemic review and meta-analysis. *Minerva Ginecol*. 2018;70(2):194-214.

109. Cusimano MC, Vicus D, Pulman K, et al. Assessment of sentinel lymph node biopsy vs lymphadenectomy for intermediate- and high-grade endometrial cancer staging. *JAMA Surg*. 2021;156(2):157-164.

110. Touhami O, Gregoire J, Renaud M, et al. Performance of sentinel lymph node (SLN) mapping in high-risk endometrial cancer. *Gynecol Oncol*. 2017;147(2):549-553.

111. Basaran D, Brue S, Aviki EM, et al. Sentinel lymph node mapping alone compared to more extensive lymphadenectomy in patients with uterine serous carcinoma. *Gynecol Oncol*. 2020;156(1):70-76.

112. Schlappe BA, Weaver AL, McGree ME, et al. Multicenter study comparing oncologic outcomes after lymph node assessment via a sentinel lymph node algorithm versus comprehensive pelvic and paraaortic lymphadenectomy in patients with serous and clear cell endometrial carcinoma. *Gynecol Oncol*. 2020;156(1):62-69.

113. Nasioudis D, Albright BB, Roy A, et al. Patterns of use and outcomes of sentinel lymph node mapping for patients with high-grade endometrial cancer. *Gynecol Oncol*. 2020;159(3):732-736.

114. Bogani G, Papadia A, Buda A, et al. Sentinel node mapping vs. sentinel node mapping plus back-up lymphadenectomy in high-risk endometrial cancer patients: results from a multi-institutional study. *Gynecol Oncol*. 2021;161(1):122-129.

115. Khoury-Collado F, Glaser GF, Zivanovic O, et al. Improving sentinel lymph node detection rates in endometrial cancer: how many cases are needed? *Gynecol Oncol*. 2009;115(3):453-455.

116. St Clair CM, Eriksson AG, Ducie JA, et al. Low-volume lymph node metastasis discovered during sentinel lymph node mapping for endometrial carcinoma. *Ann Surg Oncol*. 2016;23(5):1653-1659.

117. Plante M, Stanleigh J, Renaud MC, et al. Isolated tumor cells identified by sentinel lymph node mapping in endometrial cancer: does adjuvant treatment matter? *Gynecol Oncol*. 2017;146(2):240-246.

118. Bogani G, Mariani A, Paolini B, et al. Low-volume disease in endometrial cancer: the role of micrometastasis and isolated tumor cells. *Gynecol Oncol*. 2019;153(3):670-675.

119. Goebe EA, St Laurent JD, Nucci MR, et al. Retrospective detection of isolated tumor cells by immunohistochemistry in sentinel lymph node biopsy performed for endometrial carcinoma: is there a clinical significance? *Int J Gynecol Cancer*. 2020;30(3):291-298.

120. Childers JM, Surwit EA. Combined laparoscopic and vaginal surgery for the management of two cases of stage I endometrial cancer. *Gynecol Oncol*. 1992;45:46-51.

121. Boike G, Lurain J, Bruke J. A comparison of laparoscopic management of endometrial cancer with a traditional laparotomy. *Obstet Gynecol*. 1994;52:105.

122. Magrina JF, Mutone NF, Weaver AL, et al. Laparoscopic lymphadenectomy and vaginal or laparoscopic hysterectomy with bilateral salpingo-oophorectomy for endometrial cancer: morbidity and survival. *Am J Obstet Gynecol*. 1999;181:376-381.

123. Homesley HD, Boike G, Spiegel G. Feasibility of laparoscopic management of presumed stage I endometrial carcinoma and assessment of accuracy of myoinvasion estimates by frozen section: a Gynecologic Oncology Group study. *Int J Gynecol Cancer*. 2004;14:341-347.

124. Malur S, Possover M, Michels W, et al. Laparoscopic assisted vaginal hysterectomy versus abdominal surgery in patients with endometrial cancer—a prospective randomized trial. *Gynecol Oncol*. 2001;80:239-244.

125. Gemignani ML, Curtin J, Zelmanovich J, et al. Laparoscopic assisted vaginal hysterectomy for endometrial cancer: clinical outcomes and hospital charges. *Gynecol Oncol*. 1999;73:5-11.

126. Spirtos NM, Schlaerth J, Gross G, et al. Cost and quality of life analyses of surgery for early endometrial cancer: laparotomy versus laparoscopy. *Am J Obstet Gynecol*. 1996;174(6):1795-1799.

127. Querleu D, Leblanc E, Castelain B. Laparoscopic pelvic lymphadenectomy in the staging of early carcinoma of the cervix. *Am J Obstet Gynecol*. 1991;164:579-581.

128. Nezhat CR, Burrell MO, Nezhat FR, et al. Laparoscopic radical hysterectomy with para-aortic and pelvic node dissection. *Am J Obstet Gynecol*. 1992;166:864-865.

129. Spirtos N, Schlaerth J, Spirtos T, et al. Laparoscopic bilateral pelvic and para-aortic lymph node sampling: an evolving technique. *Am J Obstet Gynecol*. 1995;172:105-111.

130. Childers JM, Hatch KD, Tran A, et al. Laparoscopic para-aortic lymphadenectomy in gynecologic malignancies. *Obstet Gynecol*. 1993;82: 741-747.

131. Scribner D, Walker J, Johnson G, et al. Laparoscopic pelvic and para-aortic lymph node dissection: analysis of first 100 cases. *Gynecol Oncol*. 2001;82:498-503.

132. Fowler JM, Carter JR, Carlson JW, et al. Lymph node yield from laparoscopic lymphadenectomy in cervical cancer: a comparative study. *Gynecol Oncol*. 1993;51:187-192.

133. Eltabbakh G, Shamonki M, Moody JM, et al. Laparoscopy as the primary modality for the treatment of women with endometrial cancer. *Cancer*. 2001;91(2):378-387.

134. Harkki-Siren P, Kurki T. A nationwide analysis of laparoscopic complications. *Obstet Gynecol*. 1997;89:108-112.

135. Harkki-Siren P, Sjoberg J. Evaluation and the learning curve of the first one hundred laparoscopic hysterectomies. *Acta Obstet Gynecol Scand*. 1995;74:638-641.

136. Malzoni M, Tinelli R, Cosentino F, et al. Total laparoscopic hysterectomy versus abdominal hysterectomy with lymphadenectomy for early-stage endometrial cancer: a prospective randomized study. *Gynecol Oncol*. 2009;112(1):126-133.

137. Tozzi R, Malur S, Koehler C, et al. Laparoscopy versus laparotomy in endometrial cancer: first analysis of survival of a randomized prospective study. *J Minim Invasive Gynecol*. 2005;12:130-136.

138. Scribner D, Walker J, Johnson G, et al. Surgical management of early stage endometrial cancer in the elderly: is laparoscopy feasible? *Gynecol Oncol*. 2001;83:563-568.

139. Nihura H, Okamoto S, Yoshinaga K, et al. Detection of micrometastases in the sentinel lymph nodes of patients with endometrial cancer. *Gynecol Oncol*. 2007;105:683-686.

140. Boggess JF, Gehrig PA, Cantrell L, et al. A comparative study of 3 surgical methods for hysterectomy with staging for endometrial cancer: robotic assistance, laparoscopy, laparotomy. *Am J Obstet Gynecol*. 2008;199:360-369.

141. DeNardis SA, Holloway RW, Bigsby GE, et al. Robotically assisted laparoscopic hysterectomy versus total abdominal hysterectomy and lymphadenectomy for endometrial cancer. *Gynecol Oncol*. 2008;111:412-417.

142. Veljovich DS, Paley PJ, Drescher CW, et al. Robotic surgery in gynecologic oncology: program initiation and outcomes after the first year with comparison with laparotomy for endometrial cancer staging. *Am J Obstet Gynecol*. 2008;198:679.e1-679.e10.

143. Holloway RW, Ahmad S, DeNardis SA, et al. Robotic-assisted laparoscopic hysterectomy and lymphadenectomy for endometrial cancer: analysis of surgical performance. *Gynecol Oncol*. 2009;115:447-452.

144. Seamon LG, Fowler JM, Richardson DL, et al. A detailed analysis of the learning curve: robotic hysterectomy and pelvic-aortic lymphadenectomy for endometrial cancer. *Gynecol Oncol*. 2009;114:162-167.

145. Lowe MP, Johnson PR, Kamelle SA, et al. A multi-institutional experience with robotic-assisted hysterectomy with staging for endometrial cancer. *Obstet Gynecol*. 2009;114:236-243.

146. Lim PC, Kang E, Park DH. Learning curve and surgical outcome for robotic-assisted hysterectomy with lymphadenectomy: case-matched controlled comparison with laparoscopy and laparotomy for treatment of endometrial cancer. *J Minim Invasive Gynecol*. 2010;17:739-748.

147. Seamon L, Cohn D, Richardson D, et al. Robotic hysterectomy and pelvic-aortic lymphadenectomy for endometrial cancer. *Obstet Gynecol*. 2008;112:1207-1213.

148. Lim P, Kang E, Park DH. A comparative detail analysis of the learning curve and surgical outcome for robotic hysterectomy with lymphadenectomy versus laparoscopic hysterectomy with lymphadenectomy in treatment of endometrial cancer: a case-matched controlled study of the first one hundred and twenty two patients. *Gynecol Oncol*. 2011;120(3):413-418.

149. Seamon LG, Bryant SA, Rheaume PS, et al. Comprehensive surgical staging for endometrial cancer in obese patients-comparing robotics and laparotomy. *Obstet Gynecol*. 2009;114:16-21.

150. Querleu D, Lebanc E, Cartron G, et al. Audit of preoperative and early complications of laparoscopic lymph node dissection in 1000 cancer patients. *Am J Obstet Gynecol*. 2006;195:1287-1292.

151. Kornblith A, Huang H, Walker J, et al. Quality of life of patients with endometrial cancer undergoing laparoscopic FIGO staging compared with laparotomy: a GOG study. *J Clin Oncol.* 2009;27:5337-5342.

152. Childers JM, Spirtos N, Brainard P, et al. Laparoscopic staging of the patient with incompletely staged early adenocarcinoma of the endometrium. *Obstet Gynecol.* 1994;83:597-600.

153. Goff BA, Goodman A, Muntz HG, et al. Surgical stage IV endometrial carcinoma: a study of 47 cases. *Gynecol Oncol.* 1994;52:237-240.

154. Chi DS, Welshinger M, Venkatraman ES, et al. The role of surgical cytoreductive surgery in stage IV endometrial carcinoma. *Gynecol Oncol.* 1997;67(1):56-60.

155. Bristow RE, Zerbe MJ, Rosenshein N, et al. Stage IVB endometrial carcinoma: the role of cytoreductive surgery and determinants of survival. *Gynecol Oncol.* 2000;78:85-91.

156. Shih KK, Gardner G, Barakat R, et al. Surgical cytoreduction in stage IV endometrioid endometrial carcinoma. *Gynecol Oncol.* 2011;122:608-611.

157. Bristow R, Duska L, Montz F. The role of cytoreductive surgery in the management of stage IV uterine papillary serous carcinoma. *Gynecol Oncol.* 2001;81:92-99.

CHAPTER **5.5**

Endometrial Cancer: Pathology and Prognostic Factors

Christine Chin

PATHOLOGIC FACTORS OF PROGNOSTIC SIGNIFICANCE

Pathologic information has been used to estimate the risk of nodal metastasis and to define prognosis (recurrence, survival) in EC. Prognostic factors have been identified within each stage of EC and are probably best served by discussing factors within comparably staged groups, more so than as isolated factors. For example, in GOG 99, which compared observation to pelvic RT in patients with stage I-II EC and pathologically negative LN, a model based on combinations of patient age and tumor grade, depth of invasion, and lymphovascular space invasion (LVI) could predict patients at highest risk for recurrence (1). Similarly, PORTEC identified a combination of two of three factors—age above 60 years, grade 3 tumor, and depth of invasion more than 50%—that defined patients at high risk for local-regional failure when managed by surgery alone (2). Increasingly, risk models are used to counsel patients as to the marginal benefit of postoperative therapies.

Predicting Nodal Disease

On the basis of pathologic information available at the time of surgery, the risk for nodal metastasis may be estimated. Physicians who selectively perform nodal dissections frequently do so based on the presence of uterine risk factors that suggest the potential for nodal disease. In patients who did not undergo a nodal dissection at the time of hysterectomy, decisions to offer RT are commonly based on the estimation of risk for nodal disease based on uterine risk factors. In the surgicopathologic study GOG 33, pelvic and para-aortic nodal disease was more frequent with increasing grade (percentage of pelvic nodal metastases: 3% grade 1, 9% grade 2, 18% grade 3), depth of invasion (1% endometrium only, 5% inner one-third, 6% middle one-third, 25% outer one-third myometrial invasion), and LVI (27% with LVI, 7% without LVI) (3). Pelvic and para-aortic nodal metastases were also more common with cervical involvement, when peritoneal cytology was positive, and when extranodal (adnexal, intraperitoneal sites) disease was found. In a multivariate model, grade, depth of invasion, and intraperitoneal disease were independent predictors of pelvic nodal disease. In a further analysis of patients participating in GOG 33,

47 of 48 patients with para-aortic nodal disease had one or more factors of palpably enlarged para-aortic nodes, grossly positive pelvic nodes, gross adnexal disease, or outer one-third invasion (4). Despite the use of pathology to help predict nodal disease, many believe that LN assessment is superior as it provides actual information on nodal status, as opposed to an estimate, which can then be used to tailor therapy. As previously discussed, patients at very low risk for nodal involvement may also have their risk factors to guide decisions regarding need for adjuvant therapy determined by uterine risk factors, such as tumor size, histology, grade, and depth of invasion (5-9).

Prognostic Factors

International Federation of Gynecology and Obstetrics Stage

Prognostic factors may be used to categorize patients into high- and low-risk groups and to guide the use of adjuvant therapies. Understanding these factors also allows for the development of novel strategies to reduce risk of recurrence or alter patterns of disease failure. Overall, patients at highest risk for recurrence and death have spread of disease outside of the uterus, which is reflected by FIGO stage (4). The prognostic utility of surgicopathologic stage has been confirmed in multiple studies of large numbers of patients, using both univariate and multivariate analyses (3,10-16). FIGO surgical stage is often the single strongest predictor of outcome for women with endometrial adenocarcinoma in studies using multivariate analyses (10). Although the FIGO clinical staging system of 1971 was generally useful, retrospective comparison of the two methods demonstrated the clear superiority of surgicopathologic staging over clinical staging in predicting outcome.

Patients with intraperitoneal or distant metastases (stage IV) have the poorest prognosis, with 5-year survival ranging from 20% to 25% (17). In GOG 122, comparing whole abdominal RT to doxorubicin/cisplatin chemotherapy as primary therapy for patients with EC with less than 2 cm stage III-IV residual disease, stage IV (compared to stage III) disease was an independent predictor of shorter PFS (HR 2.2.9) and survival (HR 1.9) (18). Gross intraperitoneal spread frequently indicates the presence of larger tumor burden as many patients with intraperitoneal disease also have adnexal and nodal disease. In GOG 33, 51% of patients with gross intraperitoneal spread had positive pelvic nodes, whereas only 7% without spread had positive pelvic nodes (3). Prognosis may be modified by the volume of residual disease after cytoreductive surgery (19-22).

Patients with nodal metastases (stage IIIC disease) also have poorer prognosis compared to node-negative populations. FIGO data show 5-year survival to be 57% in patients with stage IIIC disease compared to 74% to 91% when nodes are negative (stage I-II) (17). Patients with positive pelvic but negative para-aortic nodes have a better prognosis compared to those with para-aortic disease (4,23,24). For example, Hoekstra and colleagues reported a series of 85 patients with stage IIIC disease who had a 5-year survival of 61% (24). Patients with positive pelvic nodes had a 5-year survival of 70% compared to 49% when para-aortic disease was present. In 2009, FIGO staging was revised for patients with positive pelvic nodes/negative para-aortic nodes who were reclassified as stage IIIC1, and patients with any positive para-aortic node were classified as stage IIIC2. This change has been validated in two recent reviews (25,26). Two retrospective series have also suggested that patients with nodal disease in addition to positive cytology, adnexa, or serosa have poorer PFS or survival compared to those patients with positive nodes alone (23,27). Lymphadenectomy (28-30), complete surgical resection of bulky nodes (31), and use of chemotherapy (25,28,32,33) have been suggested to improve outcomes in patients and modify the prognostic effect of nodal disease.

Patients with FIGO 1988 stage IIIA disease represent a heterogeneous population having adnexal, peritoneal cytology, and/or serosal involvement, but with negative LN. Positive peritoneal cytology as the sole upstaging factor was dropped in the 2009 FIGO staging revisions as a stage-defining characteristic. In the GOG 33 study, 12% of all patients had positive cytology, and of these, 25% had positive pelvic nodes and 19% had metastases to para-aortic LN (3). Six percent of patients with clinical stage I-II have spread of tumor to the adnexa, and of these, 32% have pelvic node metastases compared with 8% pelvic node positivity if adnexal involvement is not present (3). Twenty percent have positive para-aortic node metastases, which is 4 times greater than if adnexal metastases were not present.

Of patients who are completely staged and found to have no extrauterine disease, 4% to 6% have positive cytology as an isolated finding (3,34,35). Published opinions are mixed about the significance of this finding (36-41). In a review of the literature, Wethington categorized patients into groups based on low-risk uterine features (grade 1-2, <50% depth of invasion, no LVI) with positive peritoneal cytology. In this group, positive cytology occurred in 11% of cases and had a recurrence rate of 4%. Patients with higher risk features plus positive cytology had a 32% risk of recurrence (42). Saga reported that positive peritoneal cytology alone in staged patients ($N = 32$) was associated with a 5-year survival of 87%; however, this was worse than the 97% survival seen in cytology-negative patients (43). In a series of 57 patients with FIGO stage IIIA (1988) disease, cytology appears to carry the same significance as adnexal involvement and was an independent predictor of prognosis (44).

Histologic Cell Types

The histologic classification of endometrial adenocarcinoma is important not only because it facilitates the recognition of lesions as carcinoma but also because the cell type has consistently been recognized as being important in predicting the biologic behavior and probability of survival. Endometrioid adenocarcinoma accounts for the majority of tumors in the uterine corpus and carries a relatively favorable prognosis. Consequently, the virulence of other cell types is usually related to endometrioid adenocarcinoma.

Adenocarcinoma with squamous differentiation is similar to typical endometrioid adenocarcinoma with respect to the distribution by age and frequency of nodal metastasis, and is associated with a slightly increased probability of survival. *Villoglandular carcinoma* has a biologic behavior similar to that of endometrioid adenocarcinoma (45,46). *Serous carcinoma* has been considered an aggressive histologic type, with OS rates varying from 40% to 60% at 5 years (17,47-52). *Clear cell carcinoma* also has a highly aggressive behavior, with 5-year survival rates of 30% to 75% (53-56). One of the problems with using histology as a marker for prognosis is that serous cancers are more likely to have spread at presentation than endometrioid tumors. Patients with serous or clear cell tumors present with stage III-IV disease in 41% and 33%, respectively, compared to 14% with endometrioid type (17). Studies suggest that 40% to 70% of serous tumors will have extrauterine spread at presentation; therefore, complete surgical staging is warranted in this tumor type (57). Given this level of disease spread, it is not surprising that patients with unstaged/clinical stage I serous tumor appear to have similar prognosis to stage III-IV endometrioid types. Once patients with serous or clear cell tumors are appropriately allocated into the correct stage, the importance of histology appears to be less (58-61). For example, Creasman et al evaluated FIGO data and showed that patients with stage I serous tumors had comparable outcomes to those with stage I, grade 3 endometrioid tumors. Five-year survival for stage IB and IC serous tumors was 81% and 55%, respectively, compared to 84% and 66% for grade 3 tumors (61). In patients with advanced and recurrent EC participating in phase III GOG chemotherapy trials, response rate (RR) to chemotherapy was not associated with histologic type, and serous tumor type was not independently associated with PFS (62).

Grade

The degree of histologic differentiation has been considered to be an indicator of tumor spread. The GOG and other studies have confirmed that as grade becomes less differentiated, there is a greater tendency for deep myometrial invasion and, subsequently, higher rates of pelvic and para-aortic LN involvement (3,63-65). Survival has also been consistently related to histologic grade, and in a GOG study of more than 600 women with clinical stage I or occult stage II endometrioid adenocarcinoma, the 5-year relative survival was as follows: grade 1 to 94%; grade 2 to 84%; grade 3 to 72% (4). In patients with early-stage EC participating in the PORTEC trial, the risk of cancer-related death for patients with grade 3 tumors was 4.9 compared to those with grade 1 to 2 tumors (66).

Myometrial Invasion

Deep myometrial invasion is one of the more important factors correlated with a higher probability of extrauterine tumor spread, treatment failure, and recurrence and with diminished probability of survival (**Figure 5.5-1**) (11,67,68). In a GOG study of over 400 women with clinical stage I and occult stage II endometrioid adenocarcinoma, the 5-year relative survival was 94% when the tumor was confined to the endometrium, 91% when the tumor involved the inner third of the myometrium, 84% when the tumor extended into the middle third, and 59% when the tumor invaded into the outer third of the myometrium (4). Even in node-negative patients, deep myometrial invasion retains prognostic information. For example, Mariani et al (69) reported that for stage I (node-negative) patients, deep invasion (>66% myometrial invasion) was an independent predictor for recurrence and distant site of failure.

Lymphovascular Space Invasion

Several studies have suggested that LVI is a strong predictor of recurrence and death, and is independent of depth of myometrial invasion or histologic differentiation (**Figure 5.5-2**) (10,70,71). In a retrospective series of 628 surgically staged patients, the presence of HIR uterine characteristics and LVI were associated with nodal metastases (70). The OR for nodal disease was 4.4 with

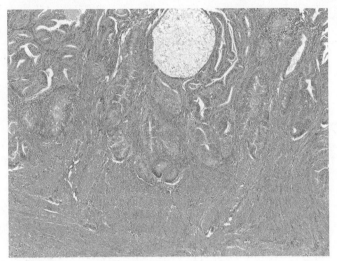

Figure 5.5-1. Myometrial invasion by endometrial adenocarcinoma may be accompanied by a desmoplastic reaction, but often no such reaction is present, as in this case.

HIR factors and 11 for LVI. In this series, the LVI and HIR features were independently associated with PFS and survival. Zaino et al (16) found that LVI was a statistically significant indicator of death from tumor in early clinical stage but not early surgical stage endometrial adenocarcinoma. This suggests that lymphatic invasion helps to identify patients likely to have spread to LN or distant sites, but that its importance is diminished for those in whom thorough sampling of nodes has failed to identify metastasis. Vascular space invasion or capillary-like space (CLS) involvement with tumor exists in approximately 15% of uteri containing adenocarcinoma (3,71,72). Pelvic LN are positive in 27% of cases, which is 4 times more often if malignant cells are found in the CLS than if absent. The risk of para-aortic node metastases when LVI was present was 19%, which is a 6-fold increase over negative CLS involvement (3). Lymphovascular invasion is identified in 35% to 95% of serous carcinomas of the endometrium, where it has generally been associated with an elevated risk of tumor recurrence or death from disease (48,49,51).

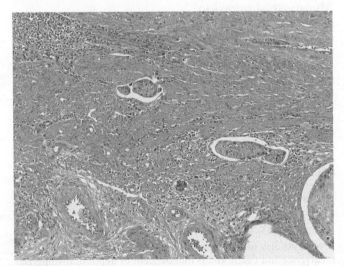

Figure 5.5-2. Lymphatic invasion by endometrial adenocarcinoma. Nests of neoplastic cells occupy the lumen of an endothelial-lined space. Because artifactual retraction of stroma around tumor may simulate lymphatic spaces, true lymphatic invasion is best assessed in the myometrium adjacent to the tumor.

Patterns of Failure

Another way to approach pathologic information is to understand the pathologic relationships that predict particular patterns of failure. For example, in patients with pathologic negative-node, stage I EC, pelvic sidewall recurrences are rare, and failures occur most frequently at the vaginal cuff or at distant sites (67,73,74). Patients with high-risk stage I disease who do not undergo nodal dissections have both pelvic sidewall and distant sites of failure, even with routine use of RT (75). Patients with node-positive disease frequently have recurrences at distant sites, with rare intra-abdominal failures (5,24,27). Patients with stage IV/intraperitoneal disease most commonly fail in the peritoneal cavity. The implications of patterns of failure data are that we may choose our postoperative therapies better by defining patterns of failure for a particular stage distribution or based on the presence of risk factors. The Mayo Clinic group has advocated this approach following a review of patterns of failure data from their group (69,76-79). For example, these investigators suggested that hematogenous, lymphatic, and peritoneal failures could be predicted based on pathologic factors, and that therapy should be directed to reduce failures at these sites depending on pathologic information (80). Whether their finding can be validated in a prospective manner, or if existing therapies effectively control disease at particular sites, needs to be evaluated.

PATHOLOGY

Hyperplasia

The current classification of endometrial hyperplasia accepted by both the International Society of Gynecologic Pathologists (ISGP) and the WHO is based on the schema of Kurman and Norris (81), which divides hyperplasia on the basis of architectural features into simple or complex and on the basis of cytologic features into typical or atypical (**Table 5.5-1**). The resulting classification has four categories as follows: *simple hyperplasia* (SH), *complex hyperplasia* (CH), *simple atypical hyperplasia* (SAH), and *complex atypical hyperplasia* (CAH). SH is defined as an increase in the number of endometrial glands, which may be dilated with little crowding or have an irregular outline and exhibit crowding. CH is characterized by glands with irregular outlines, marked structural complexity, and back-to-back crowding. The designation "atypical hyperplasia" is used to denote a proliferation of glands exhibiting cytologic atypia, recognized as nuclear enlargement, the presence of nucleoli, or a change from an elongated to a more ovoid or round nucleus. The chromatin may be either evenly or irregularly dispersed. The justification for this classification system rests on three retrospective studies that demonstrate a higher rate of progression of CAH to adenocarcinoma (81-84). It is sometimes difficult to apply this system, which requires one to make a distinction between cytologically atypical nuclei and those without atypical nuclei, because a spectrum of nuclear variability actually exists. As noted by Kendall et al (84), the definitions of architectural complexity and nuclear atypia potentially rest on a multitude of criteria, and some but not all criteria may be fully developed in any given case.

■ TABLE 5.5-1. Classification of Endometrial Hyperplasia	
Types of Hyperplasia	**Progressing to Cancer (%)**
Typical	
Simple (cystic without atypia)	1
Complex (adenomatous without atypia)	3
Atypical	
Simple (cystic with atypia)	8
Complex (adenomatous with atypia)	29

Several reports have addressed the reproducibility of diagnoses of hyperplasia (84-86). Intraobserver reproducibility was generally found to be moderate to good, whereas interobserver reproducibility was poor to moderate for various diagnostic categories. These studies probably overestimate the interobserver reproducibility because they used expert gynecologic pathologists and specified the classification to be used. In a prospective study by the GOG, neither community-based nor expert panel diagnosis of atypical hyperplasia was highly accurate (87). The current classification of hyperplasia relies on a combination of multiple architectural and cytologic criteria. It is hardly surprising that interobserver reproducibility is relatively low when multiple criteria are used to classify a lesion, because each pathologist must assign a relative value or weight to each potentially conflicting criterion. Other factors contributing to low reproducibility include (a) the fragmentary nature of curettings, (b) the presence of borderline lesions, (c) uncertainty about the significance of focal hyperplasia, (d) the inadequacy of published descriptions and understanding of terms used to define architectural or cytologic atypia, and (e) the difficulty associated with the translation of verbal descriptions into light microscopic interobserver reproducibility for images.

The gross manifestations of endometrial hyperplasia are highly varied. The endometrium is often of diffusely increased thickness (5-10 mm or greater), vaguely nodular, tan, and soft without hemorrhage or necrosis. However, hyperplasia may be focal or multifocal in a background of polyps or cycling endometrium, or occasionally associated with a diffusely thin endometrial lining. Part of the variability may reflect a reduction in the endometrial thickness (ET) because of prior endometrial sampling. Coexistent adenocarcinoma is present in 1% to 40% of hysterectomies performed to treat hyperplasia, with the latter number reflecting the frequent co-occurrence of carcinoma with atypical CH.

Endometrial Intraepithelial Neoplasia

On the basis of a combination of morphologic, molecular, and morphometric information, Mutter et al have proposed an alternative classification scheme to replace the current WHO hyperplasia terminology (88-91). They have presented data that endometrial EIN is the histopathologic presentation of a monoclonal endometrial preinvasive glandular proliferation that is the immediate pathologic precursor of endometrioid endometrial adenocarcinoma. Monoclonality and forward carryover of EIN mutations into subsequent carcinoma were the original molecular standards used for EIN diagnosis. Computer-assisted morphometric analysis of more than 20 features was carried out initially and the three features seen in molecularly defined precancers enabled an objective delineation of histologic diagnostic criteria (the D-score). The principal components assessed included a reduction in the volume of stroma and an increased variability in nuclear shape gland contour. Several of these features have been translated to characteristics that can be assessed subjectively by the surgical pathologist (**Figure 5.5-3**). These features include the following: (a) the area of the glands exceeds that of stroma; (b) nuclear and cytoplasmic features of the affected glandular cells differ from those of the background glands and may include loss of nuclear polarity or increased nuclear pleomorphism; in the absence of any background glands, a highly abnormal cytology is sufficient; (c) the maximum diameter exceeds 1 mm; (d) benign conditions including disordered proliferation, polyps, and repair are excluded; and (e) the cribriform or maze-like pattern of carcinoma is excluded. There is a high degree of concordance between EIN diagnoses rendered by computer and those made subjectively by pathologists, and either has superior cancer predictive value when compared to the 14-fold increased cancer risk conferred by the presence of atypia compared to lack thereof in the WHO hyperplasia schema. Clinical outcome studies have shown that almost 40% of women with an EIN diagnosis will be diagnosed with EC within 1 year, and for those who do not develop cancer within 12 months, a 45-fold increased risk of

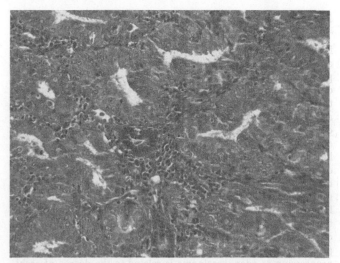

Figure 5.5-3. A lesion that could be classified in two different systems as either endometrial intraepithelial neoplasia or complex atypical hyperplasia based on gland crowding and cytologic atypia. Note the presence of a residual inactive endometrial gland that may be used as a reference for estimating cytologic atypia.

future EC exists. Correspondingly, absence of an EIN lesion in an initial representative biopsy, including those with only benign hyperplasia, confers very high (99%) NPV for concomitant or future adenocarcinoma.

Although EIN shares many features with atypical CH, the two entities are not entirely overlapping. The concept of EIN is appealing because there appears to be a strong biologic basis, with EIN representing a clonal process, whereas disordered proliferation and hyperplasia remain as diffuse endometrial physiologic responses to an abnormal stimulus (unopposed estrogen stimulation).

Simple Hyperplasia

In SH, the endometrium is thicker than usual, with dilated glands that have outpouchings and invaginations, producing an irregular outline to the enlarged glands. The glands are crowded, the stroma is more densely cellular than usual, and some foam cells may exist within the stroma. Follow-up of patients with this condition reveals little or no progression to carcinoma.

Complex Hyperplasia

The endometrium is increased in thickness by back-to-back glands in cases of CH. Most glands have irregular outlines. The two main features differentiating this from SH is the high ratio of glands to stroma, with some back-to-back glands that have very little intervening stroma. Epithelial stratification is a frequent finding, producing an appearance of two to four cell layers. Mitotic activity is highly variable, but may range up to 10 mitotic figures per 10 high-power fields.

Atypical Hyperplasia

Atypical hyperplasia is characterized by cytologic atypia of the glands, which may vary unpredictably according to vagaries of histologic preparation. The architecture may reflect SH or CH, although it is usually complex. The cells lining the glands display nuclear hyperchromatism and nuclear enlargement and have an increased nucleus-to-cytoplasm ratio. Nuclei are irregular in size and shape and have a thickened nuclear membrane, inconspicuous to prominent nucleoli, and a coarse chromatin texture. At times, the nuclei may appear clear with scattered, coarse chromatin clumps.

Progression From Hyperplasia to Cancer

The natural history of endometrial hyperplasia is difficult to define for a variety of reasons, four of which follow: (a) pathologic criteria—criteria and terminology for the various forms of hyperplasia have changed repeatedly; (b) initial sampling—the method of initial diagnosis is often curettage, which removes part or all of the lesion to be studied; (c) coexisting lesions—other lesions such as adenocarcinoma may coexist at the time of diagnosis without our knowledge, because the curettage or biopsy samples only a minority of the endometrium; and (d) subsequent intervention—hormonal or surgical intervention usually interrupts observations of the natural history of the hyperplasia. Nevertheless, there are reasonably good data to support the following assertions: (a) endometrial hyperplasia is commonly a consequence of unopposed prolonged estrogen stimulation; (b) some hyperplasias may regress if the estrogenic stimulus is removed or in response to progestational or antiestrogenic treatment; (c) some hyperplasias coexist with, or progress to, invasive adenocarcinoma; and (d) the probability of progression to adenocarcinoma is related to the degree of architectural or cytologic atypia. Progression from hyperplasia to carcinoma occurs in only 1% of patients with SH and in 3% of patients with CH. Progression from atypical hyperplasia is much higher; 8% of patients with SAH and 29% of those with CAH develop carcinoma (see **Table 5.5-1**) (81). Glandular complexity superimposed on atypia probably places the patient at greater risk than does cytologic atypia alone, but the point is unsettled.

Pathologic Diagnosis

The ISGP and the WHO last revised the classification of uterine tumors in 2003 (92), and the portion pertaining to carcinomas of the endometrium is presented in **Table 5.5-2**. This relatively simple classification scheme accommodates the vast majority of ECs and distinguishes among neoplasms of significantly different prognosis. Mixed carcinomas with two distinctive cell types are relatively common and are defined as those carcinomas in which the secondary component constitutes at least 10% of the neoplasm.

In most endometrial samples, the distinction of adenocarcinoma from hyperplasia is straightforward. However, a small fraction of problematic cases with complex proliferations truly tax the abilities of experts as well as novices to classify them correctly. The diagnosis of a well-differentiated adenocarcinoma is made in the presence of any of the following criteria: (a) irregular infiltration of glands in an altered fibroblastic stroma, (b) a confluent

glandular pattern that results in either a cribriform arrangement or confluent interconnected glands, or (c) extensive papillary growth of epithelium and stroma into glandular lumina (81).

Histologic Grade

The differentiation of a carcinoma is expressed as its grade. Grade 1 lesions are well differentiated and are generally associated with a good prognosis. Grade 2 tumors (**Figure 5.5-4**) are moderately well differentiated and have an intermediate prognosis, and grade 3 reflects poorly differentiated lesions, which frequently have a poor prognosis. Both architectural criteria and nuclear grade are used in the FIGO and ISGP-WHO committee (93) classification of tumors and are applied to endometrioid cell types including variants and mucinous carcinomas (see **Table 5.5-2**). In contrast, serous, clear cell, and undifferentiated carcinomas are considered high grade by definition and are not graded numerically. The architectural grade is determined as follows: grade 1—an adenocarcinoma in which less than 5% of the tumor growth is in solid sheets; grade 2—an adenocarcinoma in which 6% to 50% of the neoplasm is arranged in solid sheets of neoplastic cells; grade 3—an adenocarcinoma in which greater than 50% of the neoplastic cells are in solid masses. Regions of squamous differentiation are excluded from this assessment. The FIGO rules for grading state that notable nuclear atypia, inappropriate for architectural grade, raises the grade of a grade 1 or grade 2 tumor by one. However, FIGO did not define notable nuclear atypia. Justification and clarification for this modification based on extreme nuclear pleomorphism were provided in a recent GOG study. For 715 women with nonserous ECs, three nuclear grades were defined as follows: grade 1—round-to-oval nuclei with even distribution of chromatin and inconspicuous nucleoli; grade 2—irregular, oval nuclei with chromatin clumping and moderate-size nucleoli; and grade 3—large, pleomorphic nuclei with coarse chromatin and large, irregular nucleoli. Patients with tumors of architectural grade 1 or 2, but with a majority of cells having nuclei of grade 3, had a significantly worse behavior, justifying an upgrading by one grade (94).

Taylor et al (95) proposed a two-tiered system for grading endometrial carcinoma based on a study of 85 patients with stage I and II EC. They divided tumors at 10% intervals based on the percentage of solid tumor growth and found that tumor recurrences were confined to the subset with greater than 20% solid tumor. They also found that this binary division yielded a higher degree of interobserver agreement than three architectural grades. Lax et al (96) have presented preliminary data on a binary architectural grading system

TABLE 5.5-2. Classification of Endometrial Carcinoma
Endometrioid adenocarcinoma
Villoglandular
Secretory
Ciliated cell
Adenocarcinoma with squamous differentiation
Mucinous adenocarcinoma
Serous adenocarcinoma
Clear cell adenocarcinoma
Squamous cell carcinoma
Small cell carcinoma
Transitional cell
Undifferentiated (and dedifferentiated) carcinoma
Mixed types
Miscellaneous carcinomas
Metastatic carcinoma

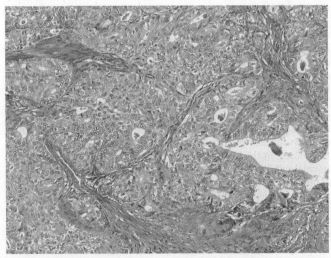

Figure 5.5-4. Endometrioid adenocarcinoma, grade 2. The glandular component is a caricature of proliferative phase glands, with stratification and a shared luminal border to the neoplastic cells. In grade 2 carcinomas, regions of solid neoplastic growth occupy between 5% and 50% of the surface area of the carcinoma.

based on the presence of greater than 50% solid growth, a diffusely infiltrative growth pattern, and tumor cell necrosis. These methods will have to be replicated in a larger patient population before an assessment of their prognostic utility can be made.

Cell Types

Endometrioid Adenocarcinoma

Endometrioid adenocarcinoma is the most common form of carcinoma of the endometrium, comprising 75% to 80% of the cases (3,97). It varies from well differentiated to undifferentiated. Characteristically, the glands of endometrioid adenocarcinoma are formed of tall columnar cells that share a common apical border, resulting in a smoothly delineated, round or oval luminal contour. With decreasing differentiation, there is a preponderance of solid growth rather than gland formation, and the cells lining glandular lumina become more numerous but not necessarily clearly stratified. Stromal invasion manifested by a desmoplastic host response or vascular invasion is often not evident in the biopsy or curettage specimen.

Villoglandular Carcinoma

There has been considerable confusion about the definition and significance of papillary carcinoma of the endometrium. A variety of cell types of endometrial adenocarcinoma with differing biologic behavior, including serous, clear cell, mucinous, and villoglandular carcinoma, may grow in a papillary fashion. Thus, the adjective *papillary* does not represent a cell type but rather an architectural pattern (45,98).

Villoglandular carcinoma is a relatively common subtype of endometrioid adenocarcinoma characterized by neoplastic columnar cells covering delicate fibrovascular cores. The apical cytoplasmic borders are straight, the nuclei are usually low grade, and the tumor cells architecturally resemble those of other endometrioid adenocarcinomas, with which they are often admixed. In the largest study to date, villoglandular carcinomas were better differentiated than ECs, but the age at diagnosis, depth of myometrial invasion, nodal spread, and survival were similar to those of ECs, justifying their classification as a subtype of endometrioid adenocarcinoma (45).

Secretory Carcinoma

Secretory carcinoma is a variant of EC, but it is unusual and represents no more than 2% of the cases (99,100). It is identified by its well-differentiated glandular pattern, consisting of columnar epithelial cells containing intracytoplasmic vacuoles similar to secretory endometrium. It is usually grade 1 architecturally and by nuclear features. There is minimal cellular atypia, stratification, and pleomorphism. The intracellular secretions are not mucin but glycogen. The cellular features of secretory carcinoma differentiate it from clear cell carcinoma, which is more papillary with more pleomorphic nuclei. By its lack of mucin, secretory carcinoma may be differentiated from mucinous carcinoma. Recognition of secretory carcinoma is important because it has a less virulent clinical course (100,101), although the clinical profile of patients is similar to that of patients with adenocarcinoma.

Ciliated Carcinoma

Ciliated carcinoma is rare. Ciliated cells are more commonly identified in endometrial hyperplasia and in benign metaplasia (tubal metaplasia), but they may occur in ECs. Associated with prior exogenous estrogen use, this cell type is reported to have a good prognosis (102).

Adenocarcinoma With Squamous Differentiation

Foci of squamous differentiation are found in about 10% to 25% of endometrial adenocarcinomas (**Figure 5.5-5**). Historically, the tumors were sometimes separated into adenoacanthoma or

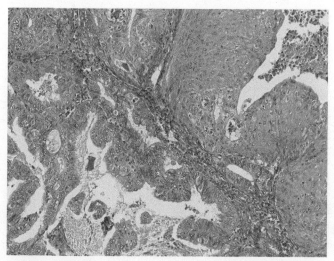

Figure 5.5-5. Endometrioid adenocarcinoma with squamous differentiation. The squamous component may form keratin pearls, but more often simply is characterized by acquisition of more abundant, deeply eosinophilic cytoplasm and distinct cell borders (upper right of figure). The squamous component may appear histologically benign or malignant.

adenosquamous carcinoma based on whether the squamous component appeared histologically benign or malignant (103-107). However, in about 30% of cases, the squamous component is not clearly benign or malignant. In a GOG study of early-stage disease, it was noted that these tumors with squamous regions behave in a fashion similar to ECs without squamous differentiation (108). The squamous areas usually mirror the degree of differentiation, which, coupled with assessment of histologic grade and other conventional prognostic factors, is thus more useful for prognostication and determination of adjuvant therapy than the historic terms *adenoacanthoma* and *adenosquamous carcinoma*, which are confusing and should be abandoned.

Mucinous Adenocarcinoma

Mucinous adenocarcinoma is rare in the endometrium, in contrast to its high frequency in the endocervix. It has been reported to represent between 1% and 9% of endometrial adenocarcinomas (109-111), but the former figure is probably more accurate. If present as the major cellular component of an EC, this tumor resembles mucinous carcinoma seen in the ovary and endocervix. Two patterns occur: In one, the cells are columnar with basally oriented nuclei; in the other, the cells are more pseudostratified, as in an adenocarcinoma of the colon or mucinous carcinoma of the ovary (**Figure 5.5-6**). The characteristic cellular pattern should represent over 50% of the entire tumor. Typically, there are either papillary processes or cystically dilated glands lined by columnar or pseudostratified columnar epithelium. The cytoplasm is positive for carcinoembryonic antigen (CEA), mucicarmine, and periodic acid–Schiff stain, but it is diastase resistant (111). This tumor differs from clear cell carcinoma and secretory endometrium by having more mucin and less glycogen. The glandular architecture is usually well maintained, and most are well differentiated (109). To establish the origin in the endometrium, exclusion of a primary endocervical tumor may be required. If the endocervical sample demonstrates the same neoplasm, the site of origin must be carefully established because this cell type is common in the endocervix (112). Neither the pattern, the type of mucin staining, nor the presence of CEA can reliably distinguish mucinous adenocarcinoma of the endometrium from its more common counterpart in the endocervix (113,114). Mucinous carcinoma of the endometrium has the same prognosis as common EC (110).

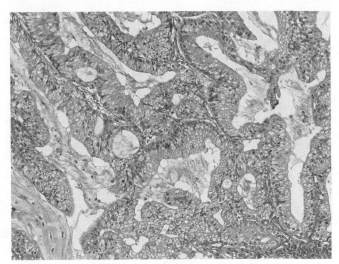

Figure 5.5-6. Mucinous adenocarcinoma. The apical cytoplasm cells as well as the lumina of glands are filled with a pale basophilic mucoid product.

Serous Carcinoma

Serous carcinoma of the endometrium closely resembles serous carcinoma of the ovary and fallopian tube because its papillary growth and cellular features are similar (**Figures 5.5-7 and 5.5-8**). It is usually found in an advanced stage in older women (115). Fibrous papillary fronds are lined by epithelial cells, which are almost devoid of cytoplasm, but which manifest stratification, atypism, pleomorphism, mitotic figures, and bizarre forms. These fronds often detach or demonstrate a terminal growth of tiny papillary excrescences and individual cells, which detach easily (**Figure 5.5-7**). A second pattern of irregular gaping glands lined by cuboidal cells with scalloped, apical borders may be present, particularly in the deeper aspect of the tumor (**Figure 5.5-8**). Lymphatic invasion is commonplace in the myometrium. Distinction from clear cell carcinoma may be difficult but can usually be accomplished on the basis of a greater degree of papillary processes, greater nuclear atypia, and less cytoplasm in papillary serous carcinoma. Psammoma bodies are frequently observed in serous carcinoma, but solid growth is more common in clear cell carcinoma.

Serous carcinoma represents approximately 10% of ECs, which is fortunate because it is an aggressive tumor. The tumors often deeply invade the myometrium, and unlike typical endometrioid

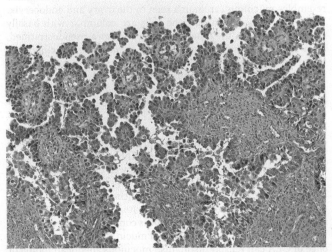

Figure 5.5-7. Serous carcinoma often arises in endometrium of older women, and superficially, portions usually have a highly papillary architecture.

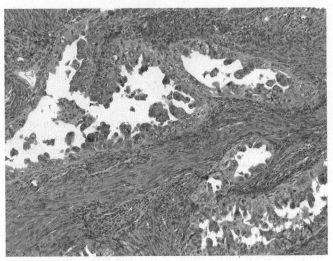

Figure 5.5-8. Serous carcinoma is characterized by high-grade cytologic atypia in cells that do not share a common apical border. The papillary architecture may be replaced by gaping glands at the interface with the myometrium.

adenocarcinoma, there is a propensity for peritoneal spread. Unfortunately, advanced-stage disease or recurrence is common even when serous carcinomas are apparently only minimally invasive or when confined to the endometrium in polyps (47,57,116). Because the metastatic disease is often identified only microscopically, about 60% of patients are upstaged following complete surgical staging (48,57,115). A report by Wheeler et al (117) stressed the prognostic importance of meticulous surgicopathologic staging. They and others found that serous carcinoma truly confined to the uterus had an overall excellent prognosis, whereas patients with extrauterine disease, even if only microscopic in size, almost always suffered recurrence and death from tumor (58,60).

Endometrial intraepithelial carcinoma (EIC) is a histologically distinctive lesion that is specifically associated with serous carcinoma of the endometrium (118-122). Serous carcinomas most often arise from a background of atrophy or polyps rather than hyperplasia (118,119,121), and they are not epidemiologically related to unopposed estrogen stimulation. EIC has been proposed to represent a form of intraepithelial tumor characteristic of serous carcinoma, and it is the precursor to invasive serous carcinoma. Mutations in *p53* that can be detected immunohistochemically as overexpression of the antigen are found in most cases, and the mutation is shared with that found in invasive serous carcinoma (**Figure 5.5-9**). EIC is usually found in the endometrium harboring a serous carcinoma (119), but occasionally occurs in the absence of any invasive carcinoma. In such cases, it may be associated with synchronous serous carcinoma in the peritoneum (120).

Clear Cell Carcinoma

Clear cell adenocarcinoma of the endometrium is generally recognized and defined on the basis of the distinctive clearing of the cytoplasm of neoplastic cells growing in any combination of solid, glandular, tubulocystic, or papillary configurations. About 4% of endometrial adenocarcinomas are of clear cell type (10,123-129). In contrast with the diethylstilbestrol (DES)-related clear cell carcinomas of the vagina and cervix, clear cell carcinoma of the endometrium is almost exclusively a disease of menopausal women. The mean age at diagnosis is about 68 years, which is similar to that of serous adenocarcinoma and about 6 years older than that of typical endometrial adenocarcinoma (10,125,129). It is a biologically aggressive neoplasm, with a 5-year survival rate varying from only about 20% to 65% (10,17,125,127,129).

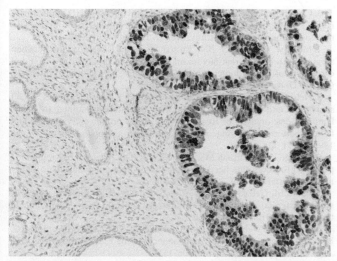

Figure 5.5-9. Endometrial intraepithelial carcinoma (EIC) is the precursor lesion of invasive serous carcinoma. It shares histologic and immunohistochemical features with serous carcinoma, including frequent overexpression of p53. In this case, there is nuclear localization of stain in EIC (right), but no staining of the benign glands or stroma of the polyp in which it has arisen (left).

The hallmark of clear cell carcinoma is the presence of neoplastic cells with optically clear cytoplasm, reflecting an abundance of glycogen. Four basic architectural patterns of clear cell adenocarcinoma exist, including solid, glandular, tubulocystic, and papillary, but most cases display an admixture of patterns. The solid pattern consists of masses of large neoplastic cells of polygonal shape with clear to faintly eosinophilic cytoplasm and distinct cell membranes. The glandular pattern is reminiscent of the tubular glands of endometrioid adenocarcinoma, whereas the tubulocystic pattern is formed of dilated spherical-appearing glands. The papillary pattern is architecturally identical to that of serous carcinoma, with generally short, branching fibrovascular cores, often hyalinized, covered by neoplastic cells. The latter three patterns often have lining cells with a hobnail appearance, resulting from the scalloped apex of individual neoplastic cells that project along the surface (**Figure 5.5-10**).

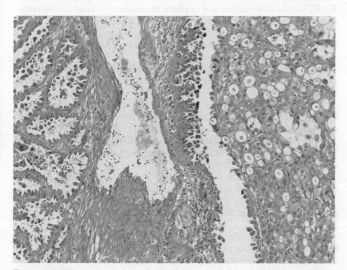

Figure 5.5-10. Clear cell carcinoma. In this tumor, a tubulocystic pattern with a lining of hobnail cells is present on the left, whereas a solid pattern is present on the right. Any mixture of solid, tubulocystic, papillary, or glandular architecture may occur.

Squamous Carcinoma

Although focal squamous differentiation is common in endometrial adenocarcinoma, pure squamous carcinoma of the endometrium is extremely rare, representing less than 1% of EC, and with only about 60 reported cases (130-134). Most patients are postmenopausal, and the average age at diagnosis is about 65 years (130,132). Squamous carcinoma of the endometrium is established as primary in the endometrium after a cervical origin is ruled out. There must be no connection with or spread from benign or malignant cervical squamous epithelium. It is often associated with cervical stenosis, pyometra, and chronic inflammation. About 60% of the cases have been confined to the uterus, and the prognosis for these patients has been relatively good (130). In contrast, less than 15% of women with advanced-stage disease have survived 2 years after diagnosis. Histologic grade does not appear to correlate with the probability of survival.

Undifferentiated Carcinoma

Undifferentiated carcinoma of the endometrium has been described as a distinct tumor type. These neoplasms are composed of a monotonous proliferation of medium-sized, round, or polygonal cells growing in sheets with no specific pattern. Mitotic figures are numerous. No glandular, squamous, or sarcomatous differentiation is detected in routinely stained sections. Keratins and epithelial membrane antigen are detected by immunohistochemistry in fewer than 20% of the cells in most cases, in contrast to diffuse staining in most high-grade endometrioid carcinomas. Selected cases may contain neurosecretory granules in a minority of the cells as demonstrated by immunohistochemical stains. Neurosecretory products are apparently not released into the patient's circulation or are not in an active form because no affected women have manifested symptoms. Most patients present with tumors of advanced stage, and the behavior is usually aggressive. A *glassy cell carcinoma* has also been described, which comprises less than 1% of ECs. It is characterized by cytoplasm that has a ground-glass appearance, as in the cervix. Although few cases have been reported, such as serous and clear cell carcinomas, glassy cell carcinoma appears to be aggressive (135,136).

Carcinosarcomas

Uterine carcinosarcomas (CSs) may not be best classified as sarcomas or mesenchymal tumors any longer, but rather as metaplastic carcinomas of the uterus and are staged per the same FIGO staging system as endometrial adenocarcinomas. Uterine CSs, also known as malignant mixed Müllerian tumors, are lesions containing carcinomatous and sarcomatous elements. Numerous studies have shown that these tumors are clonal malignancies derived from a single stem cell and should be considered metaplastic carcinomas (137). Most CSs are polypoid tumors that fill the endometrial cavity and may protrude through the cervical os. These tumors are soft and fleshy, with areas of necrosis and hemorrhage. Occasionally, they show gross myometrial invasion and may extend into the cervix. The size of the tumor is quite variable, ranging from less than 2 cm to greater than 20 cm in diameter. Microscopically, they demonstrate a typical biphasic pattern with carcinomatous and sarcomatous elements. The carcinoma is usually high grade and reminiscent of serous carcinoma, although some are undifferentiated, endometrioid, clear cell, or even squamous carcinoma. The sarcomatous component is always high grade and may be homologous or heterologous. In homologous tumors, the sarcomatous component is usually high-grade fibrosarcoma, although varieties such as leiomyosarcoma (LMS), malignant fibrous histiocytoma, or undifferentiated sarcoma may be found as well. Heterologous elements are seen in half of the cases. The most common heterologous sarcoma is rhabdomyosarcoma, followed by chondrosarcoma, and, less often, osteosarcoma or liposarcoma (138). Most CSs have myometrial invasion, commonly into less than half of the wall (138). Lymphovascular invasion is present in 60%, and the carcinomatous element is usually the component invading the myometrium and lymphovascular spaces (138,139). Most studies suggest that the behavior of CS is predicted by the carcinomatous component. These tumors typically metastasize through lymphatic channels, similar to endometrial carcinomas. Most metastases and recurrences consist of pure carcinoma (140,141). Histopathologic adverse prognostic factors include heterologous elements (in stage I tumors), a high percentage of sarcomatous components in the main tumor and in the recurrences, and deep myometrial invasion (142,143). Müllerian CS may arise in extrauterine-extraovarian sites. Most have been reported in the peritoneum or retroperitoneum. Some occur at the site of previous RT, and some arise in areas of endometriosis (144-149).

Mixed Cell Type

If an EC manifests two or more different cell types, each representing at least 10% or more of the tumor, the term *mixed cell type* is appropriate.

Metastatic Carcinoma to the Endometrium

Malignancies in other organs may metastasize to the endometrium. The most common extragenital sites are breast, stomach, colon, pancreas, and kidney, although any disseminated tumor could involve the endometrium. The ovaries are the most likely genital sources of metastasis. Metastatic carcinoma presents as abnormal vaginal bleeding, and the initial specimen for evaluation is usually a biopsy or curetting. Although the metastatic disease may appear as a large focus, individual and small groups of malignant cells may subtly intermingle with normal endometrium or myometrium. Lymphatics are usually involved. Special stains for mucin, CEA, or melanin may suggest that the cells are not of endometrial origin. In some instances, unusual cell types, such as signet ring cells, may be present, suggesting a metastasis from the gastrointestinal (GI) tract. It is uncommon but not exceptional for the endometrial sample to be the first indication of an occult primary lesion (150,151).

Simultaneous Tumors

Cancers of an identical cell type may be discovered in the ovary and endometrium simultaneously (152). Usually, the primary site is assigned to the area having the largest tumor mass and most advanced stage. In certain situations, primary malignancies in the endometrium and ovary may coexist. This "field effect" of the "extended Müllerian system" may occur in 15% to 20% of endometrioid carcinomas of the ovary (153,154). In a review of a GOG study of 74 patients with simultaneously detected endometrial and ovarian carcinomas with disease grossly limited to the pelvis, only 16% of women suffered a recurrence of the disease, with a median follow-up of 80 months. This group of patients was atypical, with 86% having endometrioid histology in both sites. Recurrence was statistically related to the presence of microscopic metastases or high histologic grade (155).

Carcinomas of more advanced histologic grade and cell type are more difficult to assign to the field effect because of a higher probability of invasion and metastasis at the time of surgery (101). If the endometrial tumor is less than 5 cm in diameter, the ovarian lesion is unilateral, invasion is less than the middle third, vessels are not involved, and the EC is well differentiated, with metastasis to the ovary unlikely (156).

REFERENCES

1. Goldstein R, Bree R, Benson C, et al. Evaluation of the woman with post-menopausal bleeding. Society of Radiologists in Ultrasound-Sponsored Consensus Conference statement. *J Ultrasound Med*. 2001;20:1025-1036.

2. Scholten A, van Putten WL, Beerman H, et al. Postoperative radiotherapy for stage I endometrial carcinoma: long term outcome of the randomized PORTEC trial with central pathology review. *Int J Radiat Oncol Biol Phys*. 2005;63:834-838.

3. Creasman WT, Morrow CP, Bundy BN, Homesley HD, Graham JE, Heller PB. Surgical pathologic spread patterns of endometrial cancer: a Gynecologic Oncology Group study. *Cancer*. 1987;60:2035-2041.

4. Morrow CP, Bundy BN, Kumar RJ, et al. Relationship between surgical-pathological risk factors and outcome in clinical stages I and II carcinoma of the endometrium. A Gynecologic Oncology Group study. *Gynecol Oncol*. 1991;40:55-65.

5. Nelson G, Randall M, Sutton G, Moore D, Hurteau J, Look K. FIGO stage IIIC endometrial carcinoma with metastases confined to pelvic lymph nodes: analysis of treatment outcomes, prognostic variables, and failure patterns following adjuvant radiation therapy. *Gynecol Oncol*. 1999;75:211-214.

6. Arango HA, Hoffman MS, Roberts WS, et al. Accuracy of lymph node palpation to determine need for lymphadenectomy in gynecologic malignancies. *Obstet Gynecol*. 2000;95:553-556.

7. Janda M, Gebski V, Brand A, et al. Quality of life after total laparoscopic hysterectomy for stage I endometrial cancer (LACE): a randomized trial. *Lancet*. 2010;11(8):772-780.

8. Mariani A, Webb MJ, Keeney GI, Haddock MG, Calori G, Podratz KC. Low risk corpus cancer: is lymphadenectomy or radiotherapy necessary? *Am J Obstet Gynecol*. 2000;182:1506-1519.

9. Mariani A, Dowdy SC, Cliby WA, et al. Prospective assessment of lymphatic dissemination in endometrial cancer: a paradigm shift in surgical staging. *Gynecol Oncol*. 2008;109:11-18.

10. Abeler V, Kjørdstad K, Berle E. Carcinoma of the endometrium in Norway: a histopathological and prognostic survey of a total population. *Int J Gynecol Cancer*. 1992;2:9-22.

11. Boronow R, Morrow C, Creasman W, et al. Surgical staging in endometrial cancer: clinical-pathologic findings of a prospective study. *Obstet Gynecol*. 1984;63:825-832.

12. Gal D, Recio FO, Zamurovic D. The new International Federation of Gynecology and Obstetrics surgical staging and survival rates in early endometrial carcinoma. *Cancer*. 1992;69:200-202.

13. Homesly H, Zaino R. Endometrial cancer: prognostic factors. *Semin Oncol*. 1994;21:71-78.

14. Kosary CL. FIGO stage, histology, histologic grade, age and race as prognostic factors in determining survival for cancers of the female gynecological system: an analysis of 1973-87 SEER cases of cancers of the endometrium, cervix, ovary, vulva, and vagina. *Semin Surg Oncol*. 1994;10:31-46.

15. Wolfson A, Sightler S, Markoe A, et al. The prognostic significance of surgical staging for carcinoma of the endometrium. *Gynecol Oncol*. 1992;45:142-146.

16. Zaino RJ, Kurman RJ, Diana KL, Morrow CP. Pathologic models to predict outcome for women with endometrial adenocarcinoma. *Cancer*. 1996;77:1115-1121.

17. Creasman W, Odicino F, Maisonneuve P, et al. Carcinoma of the corpus uteri: FIGO 26th Annual Report on the Results of Treatment in Gynecological Cancer. *Int J Gynecol Obstet*. 2006;95(suppl 1):S105-S143.

18. Randall M, Filiaci V, Muss H, et al. Randomized phase III trial of WART versus doxorubicin and cisplatin chemotherapy in advanced endometrial carcinoma: a GOG study. *J Clin Oncol*. 2006;24:36-44.

19. Goff BA, Goodman A, Muntz HG, Fuller AF Jr, Nikrui N, Rice LW. Surgical stage IV endometrial carcinoma: a study of 47 cases. *Gynecol Oncol*. 1994;52:237-240.

20. Chi DS, Welshinger M, Venkatraman ES, Barakat RR. The role of surgical cytoreductive surgery in stage IV endometrial carcinoma. *Gynecol Oncol*. 1997;67(1):56-60.

21. Bristow RE, Zerbe MJ, Rosenshein N, Grumbine FC, Montz FJ. Stage IVB endometrial carcinoma: the role of cytoreductive surgery and determinants of survival. *Gynecol Oncol*. 2000;78:85-91.

22. Shih KK, Gardner G, Barakat R, Barakat RR, Chi DS, Leitao MM Jr. Surgical cytoreduction in stage IV endometrioid endometrial carcinoma. *Gynecol Oncol*. 2011;122:608-611.

23. Mariani A, Webb M, Keeney G, et al. Stage IIIC endometrioid corpus cancer includes distinct subgroups. *Gynecol Oncol*. 2002;87:112-117.

24. Hoekstra AV, Kim RJ, Small W, et al. FIGO stage IIIC endometrial carcinoma: prognostic factors and outcomes. *Gynecol Oncol*. 2008;114:273-278.

25. Todo Y, Kato H, Minobe S, et al. A validation study of the new revised FIGO staging system to estimate prognosis for patients with stage IIIC endometrial cancer. *Gynecol Oncol*. 2011;121:126-130.

26. Werner HMJ, Trovik J, Marcickiewicz J, et al. Revision of FIGO surgical staging in 2009 for endometrial cancer validates to improve risk stratification. *Gynecol Oncol*. 2012;125:103-108.

27. McMeekin DS, Lashbrook D, Gold M, Johnson G, Walker JL, Mannel R. Analysis of FIGO stage IIIc endometrial cancer patients. *Gynecol Oncol*. 2001;81:273-278.

28. Mariani A, Dowdy S, Cliby W, et al. Efficacy of systematic lymphadenectomy and adjuvant radiotherapy in node-positive endometrial cancer patients. *Gynecol Oncol*. 2006;101:200-208.

29. Onda T, Yoshikawa H, Mizutani K, et al. Treatment of node positive endometrial cancer with complete node dissection, chemotherapy and radiation therapy. *Br J Cancer*. 1997;75:1836-1841.

30. Chuang L, Burke T, Tornos C, et al. Staging laparotomy for endometrial carcinoma: assessment of retroperitoneal lymph nodes. *Gynecol Oncol*. 1995;58:189-193.

31. Havrilseky LJ, Cragun J, Calingaert B, et al. Resection of lymph node metastases influences survival in stage IIIC endometrial cancer. *Gynecol Oncol*. 2005;99(3):689-695.

32. Takeshima N, Umayahara K, Fujiwara K, Hirai Y, Takizawa K, Hasumi K. Effectiveness of postoperative chemotherapy for para-aortic lymph node metastasis of endometrial cancer. *Gynecol Oncol*. 2006;102:214-217.

33. Todo Y, Kato H, Kaneuchi M, Watari H, Takeda M, Sakuragi N. Survival effect of para-aortic lymphadenectomy in endometrial cancer (SEPAL study): a retrospective cohort analysis. *Lancet*. 2010;375:1165-1172.

34. Homesley HD, Boike G, Spiegel G. Feasibility of laparoscopic management of presumed stage I endometrial carcinoma and assessment of accuracy of myoinvasion estimates by frozen section: a Gynecologic Oncology Group study. *Int J Gynecol Cancer*. 2004;14:341-347.

35. Kennedy A, Peterson G, Becker S, Nunez C, Webster KD. Experience with pelvic washings in stage I and II endometrial carcinoma. *Gynecol Oncol*. 1987;28:50-60.

36. Yazigi R, Piver M, Blumenson I. Malignant peritoneal cytology as an indicator in stage I endometrial cancer. *Obstet Gynecol*. 1983;62:359-362.

37. Grimshaw R, Tupper W, Fraser R, Tompkins MG, Jeffrey JF. Prognostic value of peritoneal cytology in endometrial carcinoma. *Gynecol Oncol*. 1990;36:97-100.

38. Sutton GP. The significance of positive peritoneal cytology in endometrial cancer. *Oncology*. 1990;4:21-26.

39. Konski A, Poulter C, Keys H, Rubin P, Beecham J, Doane K. Absence of prognostic significance, peritoneal dissemination and treatment advantage in endometrial cancer patients with positive peritoneal cytology. *Int J Radiat Oncol Biol Phys*. 1988;14:49-55.

40. Turner D, Gershenson D, Atkinson N, Sneiga N, Wharton AT. The prognostic significance of peritoneal cytology for stage I endometrial cancer. *Obstet Gynecol*. 1989;74:775-780.

41. Kadar N, Homesley H, Malfetano J. Positive peritoneal cytology is an adverse risk factor in endometrial carcinoma only if there is other evidence of extrauterine disease. *Gynecol Oncol*. 1992;46:145-149.

42. Wethington S, Medel NIB, Wright JD, Herzog TJ. Prognostic significance and treatment implications of positive peritoneal cytology in endometrial adenocarcinoma: unraveling a mystery. *Gynecol Oncol*. 2009;115:18-25.

43. Saga Y, Imai M, Joba T, et al. Is peritoneal cytology a prognostic factor of endometrial cancer confined to the uterus. *Gynecol Oncol*. 2006;103:277-280.

44. Havrilesky L, Cragun J, Calingaert B, et al. The prognostic significance of positive peritoneal cytology and adnexal/serosal metastasis in stage IIIa endometrial cancer. *Gynecol Oncol*. 2007;104:401-405.

45. Zaino FJ, Kurman RJ, Brunetto VL, et al. Villoglandular adenocarcinoma of the endometrium: a clinicopathologic study of 61 cases. *Am J Surg Pathol*. 1998;22:1379-1385.

46. Esteller M, Garcia A, Martinez-Palones JM, Xercavins J, Reventos J. Clinicopathologic features and genetic alterations in endometrioid carcinoma of the uterus with villoglandular differentiation. *Am J Clin Pathol*. 1999;111:336-342.

47. Carcangiu ML, Chambers JT. Uterine papillary serous carcinoma: a study on 108 cases with emphasis on the prognostic significance of associated endometrioid carcinoma, absence of invasion, and concomitant ovarian carcinoma. *Gynecol Oncol*. 1992;47:298-305.

48. Chambers JT, Merino M, Kohorn EI, Peschel RE, Schwartz PE. Uterine papillary serous carcinoma. *Obstet Gynecol*. 1987;69:109-113.

49. Abeler VM, Kjørstad KE. Serous papillary carcinoma of the endometrium: a histopathological study of 22 cases. *Gynecol Oncol*. 1990;39:266-271.

50. Chen J, Trost D, Wilkinson E. Endometrial papillary adenocarcinomas: two clinicopathologic types. *Int J Gynecol Pathol*. 1985;4:279-288.

51. Hendrickson M, Ross J, Eifel P, Martinez A, Kempson R. Uterine papillary serous carcinoma: a highly malignant form of endometrial adenocarcinoma. *Am J Surg Pathol*. 1982;6:93-108.

52. Ward BG, Wright RG, Free K. Papillary carcinomas of the endometrium. *Gynecol Oncol*. 1990;39:347-351.

53. Aquino-Parsons C, Lim P, Wong F, Mildenberger M. Papillary serous and clear cell carcinoma limited to endometrial curettings in FIGO stage 1a and 1b endometrial adenocarcinoma: treatment implications. *Gynecol Oncol*. 1998;71:83-86.

54. Carcangiu ML, Chambers JT. Early pathologic stage clear cell carcinoma and uterine papillary serous carcinoma of the endometrium: comparison of clinicopathologic features and survival. *Int J Gynecol Pathol*. 1995;14:30-38.

55. Kanbour-Shakir A, Tobon H. Primary clear cell carcinoma of the endometrium: a clinicopathologic study of 20 cases. *Int J Gynecol Pathol*. 1991;10:67-78.

56. Malpica A, Tornos C, Burke TW, Silva EG. Low-stage clear-cell carcinoma of the endometrium. *Am J Surg Pathol*. 1995;19:769-774.

57. Goff B, Kato D, Schmidt R, et al. Uterine papillary serous carcinoma: patterns of metastatic spread. *Gynecol Oncol*. 1994;54:264-268.

58. Havrilesky L, Alvarez Secord A, Bae-Jump V, et al. Outcomes in surgical stage I uterine papillary serous carcinoma. *Gynecol Oncol*. 2007;105:677-682.

59. Alektiar A, McKee A, Lin O, et al. Is there a difference in outcome between stage I-II endometrial cancer of papillary serous/clear cell and endometrioid FIGO grade 3 cancer? *Int J Radiat Oncol Biol Phys*. 2002;54:79-85.

60. Huh W, Powell M, Leath C, et al. Uterine papillary serous carcinoma: comparisons of outcomes in surgical stage I patients with and without adjuvant therapy. *Gynecol Oncol*. 2003;91:470-475.

61. Creasman WT, Kohler M, Odicino F, Maisonneuve P, Boyle P. Prognosis of papillary serous, clear cell, and grade 3 stage I carcinoma of the uterus. *Gynecol Oncol*. 2004;95:593-596.

62. McMeekin DS, Filiaci V, Thigpen JT, et al. Importance of histology in advanced and recurrent endometrial cancer patients participating in first-line chemotherapy trials: a Gynecologic Oncology Group study. *Gynecol Oncol*. 2007;106:16-22.

63. Chambers SK, Kapp DS, Peschel RE, et al. Prognostic factors and sites of failure in FIGO stage I, grade 3 endometrial carcinoma. *Gynecol Oncol*. 1987;27:180-188.

64. Sutton GP, Geiser HE, Stehman FB, Young PC, Kimes TM, Ehrlich CE. Features associated with survival and disease-free survival in early endometrial cancer. *Am J Obstet Gynecol*. 1989;160:1385-1393.

65. Wharton JT, Mikuta JJ, Mettlin C, et al. Risk factors and current management in carcinoma of the endometrium. *Surg Gynecol Obstet*. 1986;162:515-520.

66. Creutzberg CL, van Putten WL, Koper PC, et al. Surgery and postoperative radiotherapy versus surgery alone for patients with stage-1 endometrial carcinoma: multicentre randomised trial. PORTEC Study Group. Post operative radiation therapy in endometrial carcinoma. *Lancet*. 2000;355:1404-1411.

67. Keys HM, Roberts JA, Brunetto VL, et al. A phase III trial of surgery with or without adjunctive external pelvic radiation therapy in intermediate risk endometrial adenocarcinoma: a Gynecologic Oncology Group study. *Gynecol Oncol*. 2004;92:744-751.

68. Bucy GS, Mendenhall WM, Morgan LS, et al. Clinical stage I and II endometrial carcinoma treated with surgery and/or radiation therapy: analysis of prognostic and treatment-related factors. *Gynecol Oncol*. 1989;33:290-295.

69. Mariani A, Webb M, Keeney G, Lesnick TG, Podratz KC. Surgical stage I endometrial cancer: predictors of distant failure and death. *Gynecol Oncol*. 2002;87:274-280.

70. Guntupalli S, Zigheloim I, Kizer N, et al. Lymphovascular space invasion is an independent risk factor for nodal disease and poor outcomes in endometrioid endometrial cancer. *Gynecol Oncol*. 2012;124:31-35.

71. Sivridis E, Buckley CH, Fox H. The prognostic significance of lymphatic vascular space invasion in endometrial adenocarcinoma. *Br J Obstet Gynaecol*. 1987;94:991-994.

72. Hanson M, van Nagell J, Powell D. The prognostic significance of lymph-vascular space invasion in stage I endometrial cancer. *Cancer*. 1985;55:1753-1757.

73. Straughn JM, Huh W, Kelly J, et al. Conservative management of stage I endometrial carcinoma after surgical staging. *Gynecol Oncol*. 2002;84:194-200.

74. Straughn JM, Huh W, Orr J, et al. Stage IC adenocarcinoma of the endometrium: survival comparisons of surgically staged patients with and without adjuvant therapy. *Gynecol Oncol*. 2003;89:295-300.

75. Creutzberg C, van Putten W, Warlam-Rodenhuis C, et al. Outcome of high-risk stage IC, grade 3 compared with stage I endometrial carcinoma patients: the postoperative radiation therapy in endometrial carcinoma trial. *J Clin Oncol*. 2004;22:1234-1241.

76. Mariani A, Dowdy S, Keeney G, Haddock MG, Lesnick TG, Podratz KC. Predictors of vaginal relapse in stage I endometrial cancer. *Gynecol Oncol*. 2005;97:820-827.

77. Mariani A, Webb M, Kenney G, Aletti G, Podratz KC. Endometrial cancer: predictors of peritoneal failure. *Gynecol Oncol*. 2003;89:236-242.

78. Mariani A, Webb M, Keeney G, Aletti G, Podratz KC. Predictors of lymphatic failure in endometrial cancer. *Gynecol Oncol.* 2002;84:437-442.

79. Mariani A, Webb M, Rao S, Lesnick TG, Podratz KC. Significance of pathologic patterns of pelvic lymph node metastases in endometrial cancer. *Gynecol Oncol.* 2001;80:113-120.

80. Mariani A, Dowdy S, Keeney G, et al. High-risk endometrial cancer subgroups: candidates for target based adjuvant therapy. *Gynecol Oncol.* 2004;95:120-126.

81. Kurman R, Norris H. Evaluation of criteria for distinguishing atypical endometrial hyperplasia from well-differentiated carcinoma. *Cancer.* 1982;49:2547-2559.

82. Huang S, Amparo E, Fu Y. Endometrial hyperplasia: histologic classification and behavior. *Surg Pathol.* 1988;1:215-225.

83. Hunter JE, Tritz DE, Howell MG, et al. The prognostic and therapeutic implications of cytologic atypia in patients with endometrial hyperplasia. *Gynecol Oncol.* 1994;55:66-71.

84. Kendall BS, Ronnett BM, Isacson C, et al. Reproducibility of the diagnosis of endometrial hyperplasia, atypical hyperplasia, and well-differentiated carcinoma. *Am J Surg Pathol.* 1998;22:1012-1019.

85. Bergeron C, Nogales F, Masseroli M, et al. A multicentric European study testing the reproducibility of the WHO classification of endometrial hyperplasia with a proposal of a simplified working classification for biopsy and curettage specimens. *Am J Surg Pathol.* 1999;23:1102-1108.

86. Skov BG, Broholm H, Engel U, et al. Comparison of the reproducibility of the WHO classifications of 1975 and 1994 of endometrial hyperplasia. *Int J Gynecol Pathol.* 1997;16:33-37.

87. Zaino RJ, Kauderer J, Trimble CL, et al. Reproducibility of the diagnosis of atypical endometrial hyperplasia: a Gynecologic Oncology Group study. *Cancer.* 2006;106:804-811.

88. Mutter GL; The Endometrial Collaborative Group. Endometrial intraepithelial neoplasia (EIN): will it bring order to chaos? *Gynecol Oncol.* 2000;76:287-290.

89. Baak JP, Mutter GL. EIN and WHO94. *J Clin Pathol.* 2005;58:1-6.

90. Baak JP, Mutter G, Robboy S, et al. The molecular genetics and morphometry-based endometrial intraepithelial neoplasia classification system predicts disease progression in endometrial hyperplasia more accurately than the 1994 World Health Organization classification system. *Cancer.* 2005;103:2304-2312.

91. Mutter GL, Zaino R, Baak J, Bentley RC, Robboy SJ. Benign endometrial hyperplasia sequence and endometrial intraepithelial neoplasia. *Int J Gynecol Pathol.* 2007;26:103-114.

92. Silverberg S, Kurman R. *Tumors of the Uterine Corpus and Gestational Trophoblastic Disease.* Vol 3. Armed Forces Institute of Pathology; 1992.

93. Zaino RJ, Silverberg SG, Norris HJ, Bundy BN, Morrow CP, Okagaki T. The prognostic value of nuclear versus architectural grading in endometrial adenocarcinoma: a Gynecologic Oncology Group study. *Int J Gynecol Pathol.* 1994;13:29-36.

94. Zaino RJ, Kurman RJ, Diana KL, Morrow CP. The utility of the revised International Federation of Gynecology and Obstetrics histologic grading of endometrial adenocarcinoma using a defined nuclear grading system. *Cancer.* 1995;75:81-86.

95. Taylor R, Zeller J, Lieberman R, O'Connor DM. An analysis of two versus three grades for endometrial carcinoma. *Gynecol Oncol.* 1999;74:3-6.

96. Lax S, Ronntet B, Pizer E, Wu L, Ronnett BM. A binary grading system for uterine endometrioid carcinoma is comparable to FIGO grading for predicting prognosis and has superior interobserver reproducibility. *Mod Pathol.* 1999;12:118A.

97. Fanning J, Evans MC, Peters AJ, Samuel M, Harmon ER, Bates JS. Endometrial adenocarcinoma histologic subtypes: clinical and pathologic profile. *Gynecol Oncol.* 1989;32:288-291.

98. Sutton GP, Brill L, Michael H, Stehman FB, Ehrlich CE. Malignant papillary lesions of the endometrium. *Gynecol Oncol.* 1987;27:294-304.

99. Kusuyama J, Yoshida M, Imai H, Hosomichi T, Mabuchi Y, Yokota H. Secretory carcinoma of the endometrium. *Acta Cytol.* 1989;33:127-130.

100. Toban H, Watkins GJ. Secretory adenocarcinoma of the endometrium. *Int J Gynecol Pathol.* 1985;4:328-335.

101. Christopherson WM, Alberhasky RC, Connelly PF. Carcinoma of the endometrium. I. A clinicopathologic study of clear-cell carcinoma and secretory carcinoma. *Cancer.* 1982;49:1511-1523.

102. Hendrickson MR, Kempson RL. Ciliated carcinoma—a variant of endometrial adenocarcinoma. A report of 10 cases. *Int J Gynecol Pathol.* 1983;2:1-12.

103. Alberhasky RC, Connelly PJ, Christopherson WM. Carcinoma of the endometrium. IV. Mixed adenosquamous carcinoma. A clinical-pathological study of 68 cases with long-term follow-up. *Am J Clin Pathol.* 1982;77:655-664.

104. Julian CG, Daikoku NH, Gillespie A. Adenoepidermoid and adenosquamous carcinoma of the uterus. A clinicopathologic study of 118 cases. *Am J Obstet Gynecol.* 1977;128:106-116.

105. Ng AB, Reagan JW, Storaasli JP, Wentz WB. Mixed adenosquamous carcinoma of the endometrium. *Am J Clin Pathol.* 1973;59:765-781.

106. Salazar OM, DePapp EW, Bonfiglio T, Feldstein ML, Rubin P, Rudolph JH. Adenosquamous carcinoma of the endometrium. An entity with an inherently poor prognosis? *Cancer.* 1977;40:119-130.

107. Silverberg SG, Bolin MG, DeGiorgi LS. Adenoacanthoma and mixed adenosquamous carcinoma of the endometrium. A clinicopathologic study. *Cancer.* 1972;30:1307-1314.

108. Zaino R, Kurman R, Herbold D, et al. The significance of squamous differentiation in endometrial carcinoma. *Cancer.* 1991;68:2293-2302.

109. Melhem MF, Tobon H. Mucinous adenocarcinoma of the endometrium: a clinico-pathological review of 18 cases. *Int J Gynecol Pathol.* 1987;6:347-355.

110. Ross J, Eifel P, Cox R, Kempson RL, Hendrickson MR. Primary mucinous adenocarcinoma of the endometrium. *Am J Surg Pathol.* 1983;7:715-729.

111. Tiltman A. Mucinous carcinoma of the endometrium. *Obstet Gynecol.* 1980;55:244-247.

112. Maier RC, Norris HJ. Coexistence of cervical intraepithelial neoplasia with primary adenocarcinoma of the endocervix. *Obstet Gynecol.* 1980;56:361-364.

113. Maes G, Fleuren GJ, Bara J, Nap M. The distribution of mucins, carcinoembryonic antigen, and mucus-associated antigens in endocervical and endometrial adenocarcinomas. *Int J Gynecol Pathol.* 1988;7:112-122.

114. McCluggage WG, Roberts N, Bharucha H. Enteric differentiation in endometrial adenocarcinomas: a mucin histochemical study. *Int J Gynecol Pathol.* 1995;14:250-254.

115. Wilson TO, Podratz KC, Gaffey TA, Malkasian GD Jr, O'Brien PC, Naessens JM. Evaluation of unfavorable histologic subtypes in endometrial adenocarcinoma. *Am J Obstet Gynecol.* 1990;162:418-423.

116. Chan JK, Loizzi V, Youssef M, et al. Significance of comprehensive surgical staging in noninvasive papillary serous carcinoma of the endometrium. *Gynecol Oncol.* 2003;90:181-185.

117. Wheeler D, Bell K, Kurman R, Sherman ME. Minimal uterine serous carcinoma: diagnostic and clinicopathologic correlation. *Am J Surg Pathol.* 2000;24:797-806.

118. Ambros RA, Sherman ME, Zahn CM, Bitterman P, Kurman RJ. Endometrial intraepithelial carcinoma: a distinctive lesion specifically associated with tumors displaying serous differentiation. *Hum Pathol.* 1995;26:1260-1267.

119. Sherman ME, Bitterman P, Rosenshein NB, et al. Uterine serous carcinoma. A morphologically diverse neoplasm with unifying clinicopathologic features. *Am J Surg Pathol.* 1992;16:600-610.

120. Soslow R, Pirong E, Isacson C. Endometrial intraepithelial carcinoma with associated peritoneal carcinomatosis. *Am J Surg Pathol.* 2000;24:726-732.

121. Spiegel G. Endometrial carcinoma in situ in postmenopausal women. *Am J Surg Pathol.* 1995;19:417-431.

122. Zheng W, Khurana R, Farahmand S, Wang Y, Zhang ZF, Felix JC. p53 immunostaining as a significant adjunct diagnostic method for uterine serous carcinoma. *Am J Surg Pathol.* 1998;22:1463-1473.

123. Abeler VM, Kjørstad KE. Clear cell carcinoma of the endometrium: a histopathological and clinical study of 97 cases. *Gynecol Oncol.* 1991;40:207-217.

124. Abeler VM, Vergote IB, Kjørstad KE, Tropé CG. Clear cell carcinoma of the endometrium. Prognosis and metastatic pattern. *Cancer.* 1996;78:1740-1747.

125. Christopherson W, Alberhasky R, Connelly P. Carcinoma of the endometrium. II. Papillary adenocarcinoma: a clinicopathological study of 46 cases. *Am J Clin Pathol.* 1982;77:534-540.

126. Kurman RJ, Scully RE. Clear cell carcinoma of the endometrium. An analysis of 21 cases. *Cancer.* 1976;37:872-882.

127. Lax SF, Pizer ES, Ronnett BM, Kurman RJ. Clear cell carcinoma of the endometrium is characterized by a distinctive profile of p53, Ki-67, estrogen, and progesterone receptor expression. *Hum Pathol.* 1998;29:551-558.

128. Miller B, Umpierre S, Tornos C, Burke T. Histologic characterization of uterine papillary serous adenocarcinoma. *Gynecol Oncol.* 1995;56:425-429.

129. Webb GA, Lagios MD. Clear cell carcinoma of the endometrium. *Am J Obstet Gynecol.* 1987;156:1486-1491.

130. Goodman A, Zukerberg LR, Rice LW, Fuller AF, Young RH, Scully RE. Squamous cell carcinoma of the endometrium: a report of eight cases and a review of the literature. *Gynecol Oncol.* 1996;61:54-60.

131. Melin JR, Wanner L, Schulz, DM, et al. Primary squamous cell carcinoma of the endometrium. *Obstet Gynecol.* 1979;53:115.

132. Simon A, Kopolovic J, Beyth Y. Primary squamous cell carcinoma of the endometrium. *Gynecol Oncol.* 1988;31:454-461.

133. Tagsjo EB, Rosenberg P, Simonsen E. Primary squamous cell carcinoma of the endometrium. Case report. *Eur J Gynaecol Oncol.* 1993;14:308-310.

134. Yamashina M, Kobara TY. Primary squamous cell carcinoma with its spindle cell variant in the endometrium. A case report and review of literature. *Cancer.* 1986;57:340-345.

135. Christopherson WM, Alberhasky PC, Connelly PJ. Glassy cell carcinoma of the endometrium. *Hum Pathol.* 1982;13:418-421.

136. Hachisuga T, Sugimori H, Kaku T, Matsukuma K, Tsukamoto N, Nakano H. Glassy cell carcinoma of the endometrium. *Gynecol Oncol.* 1990;36:134-138.

137. Hsieh CH, ChangChien CC, Lin H, et al. Can a preoperative CA 125 level be a criterion for full pelvic lymphadenectomy in surgical staging of endometrial cancer? *Gynecol Oncol.* 2002;86:28-33.

138. Nicklin J, Janda M, Gebski V, et al. The utility of serum CA-125 in predicting extra-uterine disease in apparent early-stage endometrial cancer. *Int J Cancer.* 2012;131(4):885-890. doi:10.1002/ijc.26433

139. Tavassoli F, Kraus FT. Endometrial lesions in uteri resected for atypical endometrial hyperplasia. *Am J Clin Pathol.* 1978;70:770-779.

140. Church DN, Stelloo E, Nout RA, et al. Prognostic significance of POLE proofreading mutations in endometrial cancer. *J Natl Cancer Inst.* 2015;107(1):402.

141. McAlpine JN, Chiu DS, Nout RA, et al. Evaluation of treatment effects in patients with endometrial cancer and POLE mutations: an individual patient data meta-analysis. *Cancer.* 2021;127(14):2409-2422.

142. Key TJA, Pike MC. The dose effect relationship between unopposed estrogens and endometrial mitotic rate: its central role in explaining and predicting endometrial cancer risk. *Br J Cancer.* 1998;57:205-212.

143. Cao QJ, Belbin T, Socci N, et al. Distinctive gene expression profiles by cDNA microarrays in endometrioid and serous carcinomas of the endometrium. *Int J Gynecol Pathol.* 2004;23:321-329.

144. Mikuta JJ. International Federation of Gynecology and Obstetrics staging of endometrial cancer 1988. *Cancer.* 1993;71:1460-1463.

145. Heyman J. The so-called Stockholm method and the results of treatment of uterine cancer at the Radiumhemmet. *Acta Radiol.* 1935;16:129-148.

146. Arneson AN, Stanbro WW, Nolan JF. The use of multiple sources of radium within the uterus in the treatment of endometrial cancer. *Am J Obstet Gynecol.* 1948;55:64-78.

147. Asbury RF, Blessing JA, McGuire WP, Hanjani P, Mortel R. Aminothiadiazole (NSC 4728) in patients with advanced carcinoma of the endometrium. A phase II study of the Gynecologic Oncology Group. *Am J Clin Oncol.* 1990;13:39-41.

148. Nolan J, Arneson A. An instrument for inserting multiple capsules of radium within the uterus in the treatment of corpus cancers. *AJR Am J Roentgenol.* 1943;49:504.

149. Lewis GC Jr, Slack NH, Mortel R, et al. Adjuvant progestogen therapy in the primary definitive treatment of endometrial cancer. *Gynecol Oncol.* 1974;2:368-376.

150. Kumar NB, Hart WR. Metastases to the uterine corpus from extravaginal cancers. A clinicopathologic study of 63 cases. *Cancer.* 1982;50:2163-2169.

151. Kumar NB, Schneider V. Metastases to the uterus from extra pelvic primary tumors. *Int J Gynecol Pathol.* 1983;2:134-140.

152. Piura B, Glezerman M. Synchronous carcinomas of endometrium and ovary. *Gynecol Oncol.* 1989;33:261-264.

153. Eifel P, Hendrickson M, Ross J, Ballon S, Martinez A, Kempson R. Simultaneous presentation of carcinoma involving the ovary and uterine corpus. *Cancer.* 1982;50:163-170.

154. Scully RE. *Tumors of the Ovary and Maldeveloped Gonads.* AFIP Pamphlet No. 16. Armed Forces Institute of Pathology; 1982:92.

155. Zaino RJ, Whitney C, Brady MF. Simultaneously detected endometrial and ovarian carcinomas: a clinicopathologic study of 74 cases. *Mod Pathol.* 1998;11:118.

156. Ulbright T, Roth L. Metastatic and independent cancers of the endometrium and ovary. A clinicopathologic study of 34 cases. *Hum Pathol.* 1985;16:28-34.

CHAPTER **5.6**

Therapy for Endometrial Cancer: Radiation, Chemotherapy, Targeted, Immunotherapy, and Other New and Novel Agents

Susana M. Campos and Marcela G. del Carmen

GENERAL MANAGEMENT

Results of Standard Therapy and Their Sequelae

Early uncontrolled trials suggested that progestin therapy after surgery or irradiation was associated with a decreased risk of recurrence in patients with disease confined to the uterus (1). However, large prospective, randomized trials failed to show a survival advantage (2-4). RT has been and remains the standard adjuvant treatment modality for most patients at risk for recurrence. This standard continues

to evolve, however. An older, poorly designed study of adjuvant cytotoxic chemotherapy showed no benefit for patients treated with single-agent doxorubicin and arrested interest in adjuvant chemotherapy for many years (5). By 2006, two prospective trials comparing RT to chemotherapy demonstrated similar outcomes for patients treated with chemotherapy or RT (4,5). Adjuvant chemotherapy improved PFS and survival in patients with advanced-stage disease compared to whole abdominal RT, suggesting an important role for first-line therapy that includes chemotherapy (6). Current research focuses on whether outcomes may be improved by adding chemotherapy either sequentially or concomitantly with radiation.

ADJUVANT RADIATION THERAPY

RT continues to play an important role in the management of EC, although its role is evolving. It is used in the adjuvant setting, as definitive treatment for patients who are medically inoperable, for local recurrence, and for palliation. Historically, patients were treated with preoperative intracavitary brachytherapy with or without external beam RT followed by hysterectomy. This approach has not been completely abandoned but is used infrequently and usually only in patients with gross cervical or parametrial involvement. Today, most patients undergo primary surgery; then, depending on final pathologic review, the need for RT is determined. Radiation can be delivered with external beam irradiation, brachytherapy, or a combination of both. Brachytherapy is most frequently delivered by an intracavitary technique, where an applicator is inserted into an anatomic cavity, such as a tandem positioned in the uterus or cylinder in the vagina. Brachytherapy can also be performed by interstitial application, where needles are placed into the tissues at risk under general anesthesia, most commonly in the setting of vaginal recurrence following hysterectomy. Brachytherapy dose may be delivered with low dose rate (LDR) ^{137}Cs sources, a LDR or pulsed dose rate (PDR) ^{192}Ir source, or a high dose rate (HDR) ^{192}Ir source. With LDR, the patient is admitted to the hospital for the applicator insertion and brachytherapy delivery, and usually requires bed rest for several days. This method exposes other personnel to irradiation, is often costlier, and places the patient at risk for deep venous thrombosis and other medical complications. HDR is typically performed over multiple fractions in the outpatient setting, avoids radiation exposure to personnel, and allows for greater flexibility in the dose distribution by use of a stepping source and remote afterloader. PDR also allows for dose optimization with use of a stepping source and is considered gentler on normal tissues as a low dose of radiation is given every hour over several days. PDR also requires hospital admission but personnel radiation exposure is limited.

Early-Stage Disease

Most of the data on adjuvant radiation in EC pertain to patients with early-stage (I-II) disease, as this is the most common presentation and the focus of several randomized trials. The use of radiation in this group of patients, however, has been undergoing significant changes in practice over the last 10 years. The questions yet to be resolved are clarifying which patients will be best served by adjuvant RT and determining the most appropriate radiation modality, that is, whether pelvic radiation, vaginal brachytherapy, or a combination of both.

Benefit of Adjuvant Radiation

Two prospective, randomized trials compared surgery alone to surgery and postoperative external beam radiation. The first trial was conducted by the GOG (study 99) where 392 patients with stage IB to IIB EC who underwent TAH/BSO and pelvic/para-aortic LN sampling were randomized to observation ($n = 202$) or postoperative pelvic radiation ($n = 190$) to a total dose of 50.4 Gy in 28 fractions (7). The study was designed to allow for an 80% chance of detecting a 58% decrease in the recurrence hazard rate and a 56% decrease in the death hazard rate. Recurrence-free interval (RFI) was the primary end point with all-cause survival as well as RFS as secondary end points. With a median follow-up of 68 months, the 4-year survival rate was 92% in the radiation arm compared with 86% in the observation arm (relative hazard [RH]: 0.86; $P = .557$). The estimated 2-year cumulative incidence of recurrence was 3% versus 12% in favor of the irradiation arm (RH: 0.42; $P = .007$), indicating that radiation decreased the hazard rate of recurrence by the required 58%. Specifically, the rate of vaginal recurrence, the most frequent area of recurrence, was 6.4% (13 out of 202) in the surgery-alone arm compared to 1.05% (2 out of 190) in the

radiation arm. Of interest, the two patients in the surgery arm with tumor recurrence were randomized to radiation but refused adjuvant treatment. In addition, the estimated risk of death from any cause was 14% less in the RT arm, but was not statistically significant. More than half of the deaths were from causes other than treatment or EC, and the paper points out that it was therefore not adequately powered to detect an OS difference, a point often not appreciated by many physicians. This GOG study further identified a subgroup of patients termed HIR, who accounted for two-thirds of the cancer-related deaths and recurrences, and has become a population of interest for further study in currently open trials. The definition of HIR by the GOG is determined by the combination of age and intrauterine risk factors including grades 2 or 3, outer one-third myometrial invasion, and LVI. Patients are considered to fall into the HIR category if they are of age 70 years and above with one risk factor, age 50 years and above with at least two risk factors, or age 18 years and above with all three risk factors. In this HIR patient population, the 4-year cumulative recurrence was 27% without irradiation compared to 13% with irradiation, an absolute benefit of 19%. In contrast, for the low-risk population, there was a 6% versus 2% recurrence rate in unirradiated compared to the irradiated enrollees. The GOG trial 249 was designed to further refine the roles of chemotherapy and RT in the HIR population and randomized women to adjuvant VCB followed by three cycles of carboplatin and paclitaxel versus pelvic irradiation with either 3D conformal therapy or intensity-modulated radiation therapy (IMRT) to 4,500 to 5,040 cGy in 25 to 28 fractions with an optional brachytherapy boost. Publication of GOG 249 is pending; however, there appeared to be no difference in relapse-free or OS between the two adjuvant treatments.

The second trial was the PORTEC study where 714 patients with stage IB grade 2, 3 and IC grade 1, 2 were randomized after TAH/BSO without LN sampling to observation ($n = 360$) or pelvic radiation ($n = 354$) to a total dose of 46 Gy in 23 fractions (8). With a median follow-up of 52 months, the 5-year vaginal/pelvic recurrence rate was 4% in the radiation arm compared to 14% in the observation arm ($P < .001$). The corresponding 5-year survival rates were 81% and 85%, respectively ($P = .37$). In patients with HIR features by the PORTEC definition (where intermediate-risk factors were outer-half invasion, grade 3 or >60 years old, but excluded deeply invasive high-grade tumors; patients were deemed HIR with two of the three factors), the recurrence risk was reduced from 23% to 5% with adjuvant irradiation. It should be noted here that this is different from the GOG HIR definition, and likely a much lower risk population. An update with a median follow-up of 13.3 years has been recently published (9). The actuarial 15-year locoregional recurrence was statistically different at 6% versus 15% for those with adjuvant irradiation compared to observation with no statistical difference in OS or failure-free survival, distant metastases, or secondary cancers. Most recurrences in the observation arm were vaginal (11% of the 15%).

An additional trial, PORTEC 2, was completed as a follow-up study (10). The study population was a HIR population based on the PORTEC definition. As in PORTEC 1, the patients underwent a TAH/BSO without LND and were randomized to 46 Gy in 23 fractions of external beam irradiation or vaginal brachytherapy alone, with either 21 Gy in three fractions of HDR therapy or 30 Gy in one LDR fraction. Four hundred twenty-seven patients were enrolled in this noninferiority trial designed with the primary end point of vaginal recurrence. The research question was whether vaginal brachytherapy was as effective at controlling vaginal recurrence as external beam radiation, with fewer toxic effects and improved quality of life. Secondary end points were locoregional recurrence, distant metastases, OS and DFS, and quality of life. At a median follow-up of 45 months, the estimated 5-year vaginal recurrence rates were 1.8% for brachytherapy alone and 1.6% for external irradiation. The nodal failure rate was significantly different at 3.8% for the brachytherapy-alone arm and 0.5% for external beam irradiation, although this difference was not felt to be clinically meaningful. Distant metastases, DFS, and OS were similar in both arms. Eighty percent of the patients had deeply invasive disease, and over 90% had grade 1 or 2 disease. In fact, with central pathologic review, 48% of the patients that were enrolled with grade 1 disease increased to 78.6% of the study population. Final pathology review revealed that 14% of the patients did not fit pathologic eligibility for the trial, although the outcome was unchanged with these patients excluded on reanalysis. It should not be unexpected that pelvic external beam radiation resulted in a similar vaginal recurrence rate to vaginal brachytherapy. In addition, with this lower risk subgroup compared to the GOG 99 HIR population, it should be noted that the pelvic failure rate was quite low, even in the brachytherapy-only arm. Furthermore, GI toxicity and quality of life were significantly improved in the vaginal brachytherapy arm compared to the external beam arm (11,12). The currently enrolling PORTEC 3 trial randomizes high-risk and advanced-stage patients between external irradiation alone and external irradiation with concurrent and adjuvant chemotherapy. The patients eligible for PORTEC 3 include those with stage IB if the disease is grade 3 and paired with LVI, IC if grade 3, and stages IIIA-C or uterine serous or clear cell carcinoma stages IB-III.

The ASTEC/EN.5 trial was actually two trials with separate randomizations combined as one intergroup trial between the United Kingdom Medical Research Council and the National Cancer Institute of Canada (13). This trial examined women with stage IA grade 3 disease and all grades of IB, and stages I or II uterine serous or clear cell carcinoma. A LND was not required, and positive cytology was not an exclusion criterion. Positive pelvic nodes were allowed in the ASTEC trial. Patients were randomized to external beam radiation or observation, although vaginal brachytherapy was at the institution's choice, even in the observation arm. The primary outcome measure was OS, and 905 women were enrolled from 112 centers and 7 countries. With a median follow-up of 58 months, no statistical survival difference was noted between the two arms, and the site of the first failure was distant in both arms, that is, approximately 7%. The vaginal and pelvic failure rates were 3.7% versus 1.5% and 2.6% versus 1.1% for observation (with 53% receiving VCB) and pelvic irradiation, respectively (13).

Despite the fact that adjuvant radiation consistently and significantly improved locoregional control in these trials, most of the adjuvant treatment debate focuses on the lack of improvement in OS. The end point of OS is the gold standard for any randomized therapeutic trial in cancer, although when considering early-stage EC, the data should be interpreted with caution. First, in GOG 99, the primary end point was not OS but rather PFS, which was significantly better in the radiation arm (7). Second, because of the relatively high incidence of other comorbidities such as hypertension, diabetes mellitus, and obesity as well as other cancers, the chance of dying from an intercurrent illness is as high if not higher than dying from EC. In the RT arm of the PORTEC trial (8), the 8-year mortality rate from EC was 9.6% compared to 14.4% from other causes and 5.3% from other cancers. In the observation arm, the corresponding rates were 7.5%, 10.6%, and 5.3%. Similar data emerged from GOG 99, which reported that approximately half of the deaths were due to causes other than EC or treatment. This led the authors of GOG 99 to state the following: "With this number of intercurrent deaths in both arms, even if RT reduces the risk of EC-related deaths, the size of this trial is not adequate to reliably detect an OS difference." Thus, it is clear that the competing causes of death in this group of patients having a low cancer-related mortality rate make OS a very elusive end point to attain. Third, even in patients who die from EC, the most common cause is distant rather than local relapse. In the PORTEC trial, the 8-year mortality rate from local versus distant relapse was 1.1% and 7.9%, respectively, in the RT group, and 2% and 5.2%, respectively, in the surgery-alone group (8). Furthermore, women in the observation arm who experienced vaginal relapse received salvage RT with 5-year survival rates of 70%. In the PORTEC 2 trial, vaginal control was the primary end point compared to OS in the ASTEC/EN.5

trial (10,13). In the PORTEC 2 study, 62% and 48% died from intercurrent disease in the external beam and brachytherapy arms, respectively, and 38% versus 52% died of EC in the irradiation arm and brachytherapy arm, respectively. In the ASTEC/EN.5 trial, 36% of the deaths were observed to be unrelated to disease or treatment. Therefore, it is unrealistic to expect a local treatment modality such as radiation to alter this pattern of relapse. It is also notable that in the GOG 99 and PORTEC 1 trials, most of the patients did not have poor prognostic features, thus making it difficult to demonstrate any survival advantage to adjuvant radiation. In PORTEC 2, most (80%) of the patients had deeply invasive carcinoma, although those with grade 3 deeply invasive tumors were excluded from the trial. In the ASTEC/EN.5 trial, 75% were deeply invasive but 65% were grades 1 or 2. When the impact of adjuvant radiation in GOG 99 was assessed in the subset of patients with high-risk features (based on age, grade, depth of myometrial invasion, and presence of lymphovascular invasion), the death rate was nonsignificantly lower in the radiation arm (RH: 0.73; 90% CI, 0.43-1.26). The PORTEC 2 study included higher risk patients than PORTEC 1 but was powered as a noninferiority study examining the utility of vaginal brachytherapy to prevent local recurrence. Lee et al in their analysis of the SEER data showed an OS advantage to pelvic radiation for patients with IC grade 1 and grade 3/4 ($P < .001$) EC over those treated with surgery alone in their examination of over 21,000 patients. This survival advantage of adjuvant pelvic radiation was significant even in patients who had surgical LN staging (14). All of these issues need to be considered when assessing the benefit of adjuvant radiation. Such debate is not new in the field of oncology, but it is important to note that other oncologists treating cancers of the breast or rectum, when faced with similar results from prospective, randomized trials, have recognized the importance of a multimodality approach in achieving local-regional control as well as survival.

Type of Radiation

There are two types of radiation (intravaginal brachytherapy and pelvic external beam radiation) that could be used either alone or in combination for early-stage EC. Over the last three decades, the debate about the appropriate radiation modality has undergone a full circle. In the 1970s and mid-1980s, there was a shift from intravaginal brachytherapy alone to pelvic radiation plus intravaginal brachytherapy. Then, in the late 1980s and early 1990s, there was a shift toward pelvic radiation alone. More recently, and with the increase in surgical LN staging, there has been resurgence in the use of intravaginal brachytherapy alone. A recent article by Patel et al (15) documented this by probing the SEER database examining the treatment of FIGO stage I and II EC over the years 1995 to 2005. They examined the treatment of 9,815 patients and found that the proportion of those receiving vaginal brachytherapy alone increased from 12.9% to 32.8% as the use of external beam alone decreased from 56.1% to 45.7% over the same time period. The use of both modalities together also decreased from 31% to 21.4%.

Intravaginal Brachytherapy Alone or Combined With Pelvic Radiation

In a historically important trial, Aalders et al (16) reported on 540 patients with stage IB to IC EC who underwent TAH/BSO without LN sampling and postoperative intravaginal brachytherapy to 60 Gy to the vaginal mucosa. The patients then were randomized to observation ($n = 277$) or to supplemental pelvic radiation to 40 Gy ($n = 263$). A significant reduction in local recurrence rates was seen with the addition of pelvic radiation (1.9% vs 6.9%; $P < .01$). With regard to OS, there was no significant difference between the two arms of the study, but in the subset of patients with grade 3 disease and deep myometrial penetration, there was a survival advantage (cause-specific survival) of 18% versus 7% in favor of the pelvic radiation arm (16).

The data from this trial contributed to the shift in treatment policy from intravaginal brachytherapy alone to external beam pelvic radiation with or without a brachytherapy boost. As outlined earlier, in the ASTEC/EN.5 trial, over 50% of the observation arm received vaginal brachytherapy as well. Because the vagina is the most common site of pelvic failure, this paradigm has become more common. Greven et al (17) reviewed the experience of two institutions to compare the outcome of the two approaches. In that study, there were 270 patients with stage I to II EC: 173 were treated with postoperative pelvic radiation alone, and 97 were treated with a combination of intravaginal and pelvic radiation (17). The corresponding 5-year pelvic control and DFS rates were 96% versus 93% ($P = .32$) and 88% versus 83% ($P = .41$), respectively. This study as well as others called into question whether the addition of vaginal radiation is needed, particularly when vaginal control rates are excellent with pelvic radiation alone in early-stage disease (18,19). Furthermore, some studies have suggested increased toxicity with the combined approach (18). An examination of the SEER database reviewed 3,395 patients with node-negative EC with stages IA, IB, and II disease. Most patients (62.7%) received external beam alone and 37.3% received both external beam and brachytherapy. It was noted that the addition of brachytherapy did not statistically improve survival. A number of other reports (20,21), however, suggest that vaginal vault radiation can be added to pelvic radiation with minimal morbidity and very low rates of recurrence. Some institutions choose to treat to a lower external beam dose of 45 Gy plus a vaginal brachytherapy boost, whereas others prescribe 50.4 Gy to the pelvis without a boost unless higher risk features are present, such as close or positive vaginal margins, extensive LVI, or cervical involvement. As chemotherapy becomes an increasingly common part of the treatment paradigm, the former regimen may spare more bone marrow and bowel. In all randomized studies thus reported (GOG 99, PORTEC 1 and 2, and ASTEC/EN.5), the vaginal recurrence rate following adjuvant pelvic irradiation ranges between 1% and 2%, and therefore, any study to examine whether brachytherapy should be added to external beam RT as a boost would require a very large number of patients and more resources than the question warrants.

Intravaginal Brachytherapy Alone

With the increase in surgical LN staging, the use of postoperative intravaginal brachytherapy alone regained its appeal, the rationale being that full surgical LN staging could potentially eliminate the need for pelvic radiation, whereas vaginal brachytherapy could still address the risk of vaginal cuff recurrence, as demonstrated in PORTEC 2. Several additional reports in the past 10 years also demonstrated a very low rate of recurrence either in the vagina or in the pelvis with such an approach (22-27).

From the above discussion, it is clear that the options available for patients with early-stage endometrioid EC are numerous. Perhaps it is better to consider different options based on the factors identified as risk factors for recurrence—age, grade, depth of invasion, LVI, histology, and whether a nodal dissection was accomplished.

Cancer Limited to the Mucosa (Formerly Stage IA, Grades 1 and 2)

The risk of pelvic LN positivity (28) is 3% or less and the 5-year PFS rate in this group is of the order of 95% to 98%. It is unlikely that postoperative pelvic external beam radiation would add anything to the final outcome (20, 29). The role of intravaginal radiation in these patients is also of questionable benefit because of an almost negligible risk of vaginal recurrence with surgery alone. Straughn et al (30) reported no vaginal recurrence in 103 patients with stage IA grade 1, 2 treated with surgery alone. This is no longer a discreet stage in the 2010 FIGO staging system.

Cancer Limited to the Mucosa, Grade 3

In GOG 33, there were only eight patients with stage IA grade 3 disease, making it difficult to draw any meaningful conclusion (31). There were no relapses in the three patients receiving postoperative radiation as compared with one failure in the five patients who received no postoperative therapy. The risk of LN metastasis in this group of patients is negligible. Straughn et al (30) reported on eight patients with stage IA grade 3 disease treated with surgery alone, with two of the patients developing isolated vaginal recurrence. Again, this subgroup is not formally staged in the new FIGO staging system.

Low-Risk Stage IA, B Grades 1, 2

Straughn et al (30) reported on 296 patients with IB grade 1, 2 and found only 9 (3%) vaginal recurrences and 1 (0.3%) pelvic recurrence. Horowitz et al reported on 62 patients who had surgical LN staging and received adjuvant intravaginal brachytherapy. There was one (1.6%) vaginal recurrence and no pelvic recurrence (24). In comparison, data published by Alektiar et al (32) reported that 233 patients with IB grade 1, 2 showed a vaginal recurrence rate of only 1% and pelvic recurrence of 2% using postoperative intravaginal brachytherapy alone without routine surgical LN staging. In addition, Sorbe et al (33) reported on 110 patients without retroperitoneal LN sampling with IB grade 1, 2 who were part of a prospective, randomized trial evaluating two different intravaginal brachytherapy doses; the rate of vaginal recurrence was 0.9% and pelvic recurrence 1.8%. These patients also often fit the GOG 99, PORTEC 1, and PORTEC 2 trials, with or without lymphadenectomy. Thus, it seems reasonable to suggest that either observation or intravaginal brachytherapy (irrespective of surgical staging) is a reasonable option. But when deciding on whether adjuvant radiation is needed, it is important to address three issues. First, older patients tend to have higher rates of relapse. In the study by Straughn et al (30), 8 of the 10 vaginal/pelvic recurrences were in patients 60 years and above, which was confirmed in the randomized trials. Second, patients with LVI have a higher chance of vaginal recurrence as demonstrated by Mariani et al (34) who reported on 508 patients with stage I EC treated with surgery alone (152 out of 508 were stage IA). The presence of LVI increased the vaginal relapse rate from 3% to 7% ($P = .02$), as was confirmed by the GOG 99 trial among others. Recent publications of patients with HIR and high-risk stage I to III EC suggest LVI to be an independent prognostic factor for relapse and survival (9,35). Third, often the indications for adjuvant radiation are rather arbitrarily based on the amount of myometrial invasion defined in thirds and on whether the tumor is grade 1 versus 2. Yet the amount of myometrial invasion in this group of patients and whether an EC is assigned as grade 1 or 2 do not appear to be significant predictors of outcome (36,37). It is reasonable to observe patients younger than 60 years with stage IA grades 1 and 2 disease without LVI observation, whereas those patients 60 years or more or those with LVI are offered adjuvant brachytherapy. It is worth noting that the most common site of recurrence is the vaginal vault and adjuvant brachytherapy is a low-morbidity treatment. When undecided whether to offer brachytherapy, it should be considered that it is a far less intensive treatment than salvage radiation for recurrent disease.

Intermediate to High-Intermediate Risk Stage IB Grade 3 to IC Grades 1, 2, 3, Stage II

Up until the last 10 years, most data in the literature on this group of patients were based on pelvic radiation either alone or in combination with intravaginal brachytherapy (19,20,38,39). Since 1988 and with the increase in surgical LN staging in the United States, a shift occurred with regard to the role of radiation for stage IB grade 3 and even in stage IC disease. For some time, the treatment decision between whole pelvis RT and VCB alone was primarily based on whether the patient had surgical LN staging. If the decision is made that nodal assessment is necessary, which has been called into question for all early-stage patients, an adequate LN sampling/dissection should, at a minimum, meet the GOG guidelines of sampling the obturator, external iliacs, internal iliacs, common iliacs, and para-aortic LN stations, and the minimum number of nodes sampled should be 10 and above.

Surgically Staged Patients

For patients with IB grade 3 disease, the retrospective data on intravaginal brachytherapy alone after surgical staging were encouraging (**Table 5.6-1**). The average rate of vaginal recurrence and pelvic recurrence was reported as 1.3% for both. This compares favorably with the data from the PORTEC 1 trial where the 5-year rates for vaginal and pelvic recurrence, in the subset of patients with IB grade 3 disease treated with pelvic radiation (n = 35), were 0% and 3%, respectively. A multi-institutional review of 220 patients with stage IC EC by Straughn et al (40) compared adjuvant radiation to no radiation in patients with negative nodes on surgical staging. The investigators concluded that adjuvant radiation is not needed although the 5-year DFS was 74.5% for those treated with surgery alone compared to 92.5% for those treated with adjuvant radiation (P = .0134). It is unlikely that observation alone, even in those patients with full surgical staging, will be the best approach when VCB carries low morbidity and can greatly decrease the 18% statistically significant difference in DFS from a retrospective study in which it is inferred that patients with the worst prognostic features were the ones who received radiation.

Several investigators have shown the feasibility of such an approach with an average vaginal recurrence rate of 1.6% and pelvic control rate of 2.1% (**Table 5.6-2**). Thus, intravaginal brachytherapy alone after surgical staging in patients with IB grade 3 and IC EC seems to provide better local/regional control than surgery alone and in a properly selected patient population with very few pelvic failures (7,24,41-44). As described previously, the GOG 249 trial randomized the HIR population to VCB followed by chemotherapy (carboplatin/paclitaxel for three cycles) or pelvic RT (IMRT or 3D conformal) plus an optional cuff brachytherapy boost for high-risk features, and appeared to show equivalence. Note that LND was optional in this trial. In addition, although LND is not allowed, further information may be gained by the PORTEC 3/EN.7 trial that randomizes patients with (1988 FIGO) stage IB grade 3 with

LVI, stage IC or IIA grade 3, stage IIB, stage IIIA or IIIC, or stages IB to III serous or clear cell EC between pelvic RT alone to 48.6 Gy and the same pelvic RT with two cycles of concurrent cisplatin plus four adjuvant cycles of carboplatin/paclitaxel. In the PORTEC 3 trial, the VCB boost is given in patients with cervical invasion. In the absence of robust evidence, the risk of pelvic failure must be gauged on an individual patient basis to determine whether the risk is sufficient to warrant pelvic radiation versus VCB alone. In the PORTEC trial, 99 patients with stage IC grade 3 tumors were not randomized but were followed prospectively, and all received pelvic irradiation in the absence of LN evaluation. The locoregional recurrence rate in this high-risk group of patients without a node dissection was 12% (5% vaginal), despite adjuvant irradiation. Note that patients with uterine serous and clear cell carcinoma were not identified separately in this trial, so the percentage of these high-risk pathologies is not known, and given the very high distant failure rate, of 31%, this is noted to be a very high-risk subgroup of patients (45).

With the publication of the two randomized trials, ASTEC and CONSORT, questioning the benefit for lymphadenectomy, many gynecologic oncologists in the United States have chosen to evaluate the nodes only in those patients most at risk for metastatic disease—those with deeply invasive tumors, high-grade disease, high-risk histology, older patients, and those with LVI or a combination of factors. Examining the trials where routine lymphadenectomy is performed demonstrates the risk for all stage I patients to be approximately 10% (31,46,47), but selecting the patients at highest risk for disease, although may not change survival, can certainly guide further treatment paradigms.

No Surgical Lymph Node Staging

In those patients with a combination of high-risk features such as grade 3 tumor, high-risk histologies, LVI, advanced age, or deep myometrial invasion, intravaginal brachytherapy may not be adequate treatment. In the Aalders et al (16) randomized trial, the rate of local recurrence in the subset of patients with IB grade 3 to IC was 9.3% (13 of 137) for those treated with brachytherapy alone compared to 1.3% (2 of 146) for those treated with brachytherapy and external radiation. This finding is not unexpected as no LN assessment was performed in that trial. Weiss et al reported on 61 patients with stage IC EC who were treated with postoperative

■ TABLE 5.6-1. Outcome for IB Grade 3 EC After Surgical LN Staging and IVRT Alone

Author	Year	No. of Patients	Median F/U	Vaginal Rec	Pelvic Rec
Fanning	2001	21	52 mo	0%	0%
Horowitz	2002	31	65 mo	0%	0%
Alektiar	2007	21	46 mo	4.8% (1/21)	4.8% (1/21)
Total	–	73	–	1.3% (1/73)	1.3% (1/73)

EC, endometrial cancer; F/U, follow-up; IVRT, intravaginal radiation therapy; LN, lymph node.

■ TABLE 5.6-2. Outcome for IC Endometrial Cancer Grade 1 to 3 After Surgical LN Staging and IVRT Alone

Author	Year	No. of Patients	Median F/U	Vaginal Rec	Pelvic Rec
Horowitz	2002	50	65 mo	2% (1/50)	4% (2/50)
Rittenberg	2003	53	32 mo	0%	1.8% (1/53)
Solheim	2005	40	23 mo	0%	0%
Alektiar	2007	40	46 mo	5% (2/40)	2.5% (1/40)
Total	–	183	–	1.6% (3/183)	2.1% (4/183)

F/U, follow-up; IVRT, intravaginal radiation therapy; LN, lymph node; rec, recurrence.

pelvic radiation alone. With a median follow-up of 69.5 months, there was only one recurrence in the pelvis (1.6%). Their review of the published data from the literature for patients with stage IC disease showed a pelvic recurrence of 1.04% in 240 patients treated with pelvic radiation alone compared to 0.97% in 301 patients treated with pelvic and intravaginal radiation. The authors concluded that pelvic radiation alone is sufficient for local-regional control, and clinical efforts should focus on reducing the risk of distant relapse in this subgroup of patients (48). The results of the PORTEC 3 trial may help further stratify patients who may be appropriate candidates for observation or VCB alone, or those at sufficiently high risk who benefit from intensification of therapy, including a combination of adjuvant irradiation and chemotherapy.

Stage II

It is important to recognize the distinction between gross and occult cervical involvement in EC. Gross cervical involvement increases the risk of parametrial extension as well as spread to pelvic LN in a fashion similar to primary cervical cancer. Patients with gross cervical involvement from EC could undergo radical hysterectomy and pelvic LND or preoperative radiation including pelvic radiation and intracavitary brachytherapy followed by simple hysterectomy. For occult cervical involvement, the treatment often consists of simple hysterectomy with or without LN surgical staging and adjuvant radiation. The type of radiation most often utilized is pelvic radiation and intravaginal brachytherapy. Pitson et al (49) reported on 120 patients treated with such a combination. The 5-year DFS rate was 68% and the rate of pelvic relapse was 5.8% (7 of 120).

There are also emerging data on the role of intravaginal brachytherapy alone in patients with occult cervical involvement who also had surgical LN staging. The rate of pelvic recurrence in four such series ranged from 0% to 6%, but a larger number of patients and longer follow-ups will be necessary in order to confirm this data (24,26,50,51). Stage II EC is now defined by cervical stromal invasion. The new staging system now only encompasses the latter with true cervical stromal invasion into stage II (52). Intravaginal brachytherapy alone could be used for surgically staged patients with mucosal involvement (24,53), whereas those with disease invading into the stroma, with close margins or with a significant amount of cervical disease, should be treated with pelvic radiation with or without intravaginal brachytherapy boost until trial results demonstrate a better option.

Advanced-Stage Disease

Radiation

The outcome of patients with isolated adnexal involvement (stage IIIA) treated with pelvic radiation is fairly good, although the studied patient numbers are small. Connell et al (54) reported on 12 patients treated with postoperative pelvic radiation with a 5-year DFS of 70.9%. The weighted average of 5-year DFS and OS rates from literature review in that study was 78.6% and 67.1%, respectively. Patients with isolated serosal involvement (stage IIIA) have a worse prognosis than those with isolated adnexal involvement. Ashman et al (55) reported on 15 patients with isolated serosal involvement who were treated with pelvic radiation. The 5-year DFS was only 41.5%. If pelvic node involvement (IIIC1) is the only major risk factor, treatment with postoperative pelvic RT can yield a 60% to 72% long-term survival rate (56–58), although distant failure is a problem that new trials evaluating chemotherapy will hopefully change. Patients with stage IIIC2 disease, by virtue of para-aortic node involvement, represent a particularly high-risk group. Following surgery, these patients are generally treated with extended field radiation to encompass the pelvis and the para-aortic regions. With this aggressive approach, several investigators have reported 30% to 40% survival rates in small patient populations (59–61). The

question of whether it is safe to omit radiation even after adequate surgical LN staging in patients with IIIC2 EC was addressed in a study from the Mayo Clinic. Mariani et al reported on 122 patients with node-positive disease; at 5 years, the risk of pelvic recurrence was 57% after inadequate LND and/or no RT compared to 10% with adequate LND (>10 pelvic nodes and ≥5 para-aortic nodes) and radiation. This difference was statistically significant on univariate ($P < .001$) and multivariate analyses ($P = .03$), indicating the need for postoperative radiation even after adequate surgical staging (62). The recognition that a significant number of patients with stage III disease fail in the abdomen (34,57) has prompted a number of investigators to evaluate whole abdominal RT in these patients (63,64), and after a small GOG trial a randomized trial was undertaken (65).

Chemoradiation

In the GOG 122 trial, 396 patients with stage III and optimally debulked stage IV disease were randomized to whole abdomen radiation ($n = 202$) or to doxorubicin-cisplatin chemotherapy ($n = 194$). With a median follow-up of 74 months, there was significant improvement in both PFS (50% vs 38%; $P = .007$) as well as OS (55% vs 42%; $P = .004$), respectively, in favor of chemotherapy (6). To elucidate the right approach for these patients, however, a closer look at this data is warranted. First, the overall absolute rate of relapse was 54% in the radiation arm compared to 50% in the chemotherapy arm, a small difference if any, yet the corresponding 5-year PFS rates were 38% and 50% ($P = .007$), respectively. Why the discrepancy? The answer is that the 5-year PFS rate for the radiation arm was 38%, whereas the chemotherapy arm has two separate 5-year rates. The first one, called unadjusted, was 42%, which is not that significantly different from the 38% rate with radiation, and the second, called "adjusted for stage," was 50%, which was significantly different from the radiation arm. This led us to the second issue: Was the adjustment for stage warranted? The answer is no. Numerically, there were more patients with lymph node involvement in the chemotherapy than the radiation arm, but having positive LN was not an independent predictor of poor outcome in this study. Therefore, the adjustment was not warranted, and if any adjustment was needed it should have gone to the radiation arm because there were more patients with positive cytology in this arm, a factor with an HR of 1.8 (95% CI, 0.89-1.55) in predicting poor outcome. Third, what should be made of the significant difference in OS? There were 15 deaths unrelated to EC or protocol treatment in the radiation arm compared to only 6 in the chemotherapy arm, raising a question about whether the two arms of the study were truly balanced. Finally, the pelvic recurrence rate was lower in the RT arm, which indicates that perhaps both modalities could be used for the advantages they provide—locoregional control for irradiation and distant control for chemotherapy. Another randomized trial comparing adjuvant radiation to chemotherapy (doxorubicin-cisplatin-cyclophosphamide) in patients with stage I to III was recently reported and showed no difference in outcome between the two arms (66). With a median follow-up of 95.5 months, the 5-year DFS was 63% in both arms ($P = .44$), and the 5-year OS rates were 69% in the radiation arm compared to 66% in the chemotherapy arm ($P = .77$). What these two trials show is that chemotherapy at a minimum is equivalent to radiation in this group of patients and ought to be used, not alone, but rather in combination with radiation. Greven et al reported the results of Radiation Therapy Oncology Group (RTOG) 9708 on 44 patients with stage I to III EC who were treated with pelvic radiation and intravaginal brachytherapy given concurrently with cisplatin 50 mg/m^2 on days 1 and 28 of radiation, followed by four cycles of cisplatin (50 mg/m^2) and paclitaxel (Taxol) (175 mg/m^2). The 4-year DFS and OS rates for those with stage III disease (66% of patients) were 72% and 77%, respectively (67).

As the follow-up study to GOG 122, GOG 184 was launched. The combination of irradiation and chemotherapy was used to control disease and was done in a sequential fashion to limit toxicity. Five hundred fifty-two patients with stages III and IV were enrolled (after 66 patients were enrolled, those with upper abdominal disease were excluded) and received tumor volume-directed irradiation (51% received 5,040 cGy pelvis irradiation alone and 49% received 4,320-4,350 cGy of extended field for positive para-aortic disease, or undissected para-aortics) and were then randomized to cisplatin/adriamycin or cisplatin/adriamycin/paclitaxel (68). Growth factors were allowed, and 80% of the patients were able to complete the assigned chemotherapy regimen following full-dose RT. The locoregional recurrence rate (any failure in the pelvis, vagina, or para-aortics as first failure) was 10%, which compares favorably with GOG 122 (isolated failures of 13% in the whole abdominal irradiation [WAI] arm and 18% in the chemotherapy arm); Greven's (69) study of 105 irradiated patients with IIIC disease with a pelvic failure rate of 21%; and Mundt's two series, one describing 30 patients with stage IIIC treated with postoperative pelvic irradiation with an infield failure rate of 23% and the second, a trial of 43 high-risk patients with stage I to IV EC treated with chemotherapy alone who experienced a 21% actuarial rate of pelvic recurrence as their first or only site of recurrence (70,71). The distant failure rate in these trials was unacceptably high ranging from 26% to 55%. The PORTEC 3 trial described earlier and the open GOG 0258 address treatment in this advanced population. In the GOG 0258 trial, stages III or IVA are randomized between volume-directed postoperative irradiation with concurrent cisplatin, followed by four cycles of carboplatin/taxol or six cycles of carboplatin/taxol alone.

SPECIAL SITUATIONS

Positive Cytology Without Adnexal or Serosal Involvement

In this subset of patients, the presence of other adverse features such as aggressive histologies or deep myometrial invasion should be determined first as this is noted but no longer part of the official staging system. The argument to remove it from the staging is that without other factors cytology alone has unclear prognostic value (72). The literature regarding the benefits of treatment in this setting is mixed; even if treatment is beneficial, the appropriate modality still has to be defined. On the basis of the concept that the entire peritoneal cavity is at risk, intraperitoneal radioactive colloidal ^{32}P had been used by some, with results that were better than in historic controls (73) but carried significant toxicity. Eltabbakh et al reported on 27 patients with FIGO grade 1, 2 and <50% myometrial invasion who were treated with intravaginal brachytherapy and megestrol acetate (Megace). None of the patients relapsed or died from their disease. Megace was given for 1 year, and at the end of therapy, 24 patients underwent second-look laparoscopy and peritoneal cytology. In 23 patients, the cytology was negative, and the remaining patients with persistent positive cytology received an additional year of Megace after which cytology was confirmed to be negative (74). Given this, as an isolated risk factor, vaginal brachytherapy with Megace is likely the only adjuvant regimen that may be appropriate in some of these patients.

Definitive Radiation for Inoperable Disease

Patients with medically inoperable stage I to II uterine cancer are usually treated in a fashion similar to those with cervical cancer by using intracavitary applicators with or without pelvic radiation. For patients with clinical stage I grade 1 or 2 and no or minimal evidence of myometrial invasion or LN metastasis on MRI, intracavitary brachytherapy alone may be sufficient, provided the uterus is a size and shape that it can be fully covered with the brachytherapy irradiation. There are several applicator choices with one or two tandems (depending on uterus size) and either a cylinder or ovoids. The American Brachytherapy Society

guidelines have recommended either dosing in the uterus 2 cm from the tandem, and treating the upper several centimeters of vagina, or, in the age of image guidance, dosing to the uterine serosa (75). When pelvic radiation is added to brachytherapy, the dose is usually 45 to 50 Gy supplemented with intracavitary brachytherapy. Rouanet et al (76) treated 250 patients with EC using LDR brachytherapy, which yielded a 5-year DSS of 76.5%. An alternative brachytherapy approach would be to use the Hymen or Simon afterloading system, which consists of multiple Teflon tubes that are inserted into the uterine cavity. With such a treatment approach, Grigsby et al (77) reported that the 5-year PFS rate of patients with clinical stage I disease treated with a combination of external and intracavitary RT was 94% for grade 1 disease, 92% for grade 2 disease, and 78% for grade 3 disease. HDR brachytherapy is increasingly being used and demonstrates equivalent control (78,79). Nguyen (79) and Niazi (80) reported on patients with clinical stage I to II disease treated with HDR alone or with external irradiation and the DSS at 8 years was 76% and at 15 years was 91%. Note that many of these patients, by virtue of being medically inoperable, will die of other causes than their early-stage uterine carcinoma. Intriguingly, Fishman published a study comparing the operable with the inoperable and found that those inoperable patients that did not die of intercurrent disease had a similar median 5-year survival (81). Kucera et al studied a larger population of 228 and using HDR alone found a DSS at 5 years of 85% and 10 years of 75% (82). For several of these studies, image guidance was not available and the expectation is that dosing the radiation in the appropriate area will increase control and DSS. Although uncommonly seen, patients with stage IIIB are definitively treated with irradiation including external beam and intracavitary/interstitial brachytherapy as they are not surgical candidates (83).

RADIATION THERAPY TECHNIQUES

Intravaginal Brachytherapy

Intracavitary vaginal brachytherapy is designed to deliver dose to the vaginal surface and underlying lymphatic channels at risk of harboring residual disease. Choo and colleagues demonstrated that 95% of vaginal lymphatic channels lie within 5 mm of the vaginal mucosa and therefore this modality is well-suited to deliver this dose effectively, and more safely, than with external beam irradiation. Intravaginal brachytherapy can be delivered using LDR to 60 Gy prescribed to the vaginal mucosa or 30 to 35 Gy prescribed to 0.5 cm depth from the vaginal mucosa using either ovoids for the upper several centimeters of vagina or a cylinder, which allows the length treated to be tailored to the clinical situation. Less commonly, the whole length of the vagina needs to be treated and should be considered for those with close or positive margins, extensive LVI, or high-risk histologies. HDR brachytherapy guidelines have been established and published for dose and fractionation, although the most common is 700 cGy for three fractions treated at 5-mm depth according to a survey published by Small et al (84,85). PORTEC 4 is a randomized study that will compare the most common HDR fractionation schemes, including 2,100 versus 1,500 cGy delivered in three fractions.

External Beam Radiation

Pelvic Radiation

Most patients are treated in the postoperative setting. At the time of simulation, the small bowel may be opacified using oral contrast given 60 minutes prior to CT. Vaginal markers are now discouraged as they may displace the vaginal cuff. Patients may be placed in the prone position to displace the small intestines from the radiation field. Prone treatment board allows the abdominal wall and contents to be displaced anteriorly through a hole in the board, to allow displacement of bowel from the pelvis (86). The target volumes are the obturator; external, internal, and lower common iliac nodes; and the proximal two-thirds of the vagina. The presacral and common iliac nodes are encompassed fully in the setting of cervical involvement or pathologic nodal involvement. High-energy linear accelerators (15 MV) are preferred because of their sparing of the skin and subcutaneous tissue when the treatment is a four-field box or when three-dimensional conformal therapy (3DCF) is used, particularly in patients with large tissue separations. The ideal beam arrangement with the conventional four-field pelvic-box technique places the superior border at L5-S1, the inferior border at the bottom of the obturator foramina or at least 3 to 4 cm below the vaginal apex, and the lateral border 1 to 2 cm beyond the widest point of bony pelvis. For the lateral fields, the anterior border is in front of the pubis symphysis to allow external iliac coverage and the posterior border covers S1/S2. The superior and inferior borders are the same for the anterior and posterior fields. All fields are treated daily to a dose of 1.8 Gy. A total dose of 50.4 Gy is given to sterilize microscopic disease, or 45 Gy when combined with intravaginal brachytherapy. 3DCF therapy uses the same beam arrangement, but a planning CT scan is used to outline both tissues at risk and normal tissues. Blocks are placed based on the contours, which allows more accurate targeting and sparing of more normal tissues. Recent evidence suggests decreased acute and late toxicity to the bowel when IMRT is used. Mundt et al demonstrated a significant reduction in acute and chronic GI toxicity when IMRT was compared to historical controls treated with conventional radiation (87-90). IMRT, compared to the four-field box or 3DCF therapy, uses an inverse planning technique to shape the radiation dose to tissues at risk of harboring microscopic disease and to minimize normal tissue dose. Both 3DCF therapy and IMRT use small collimator "leaves" to finely shape the beam. These "leaves" are mobile and block portions of the generated x-rays. If the collimator "leaves" move while the radiation beam is on and vary the beam intensity, areas of tumor and normal tissue can receive a spectrum of doses, hence the term "intensity modulated." Papers have been published on the use of IMRT in postoperative uterine and cervical carcinoma, vulvar carcinoma, whole abdominal RT, vaginal carcinoma, and intact cervical carcinoma. However, because of the daily variation in bladder and rectal filling and the resultant mobility of the upper vagina, the use of IMRT should be undertaken with caution, and experience with contouring, planning, and delivery is essential (91,92). The introduction of new technology such as tomotherapy (a linear accelerator linked to an online CT scanner), cyberknife (a linear accelerator capable of fiducial imaging to target radiation), and cone beam CT (CT scan mounted to the linear accelerator) for image-guided RT assists in daily target and normal tissue localization. Randomized, prospective data comparing this to traditional therapy are lacking, but ongoing trials are evaluating risks, effectiveness, and cost. The NRG TIME-C trial has completed accrual of 1,200 patients and will evaluate patient-reported quality of life, specifically diarrhea at 5 weeks, for patients randomized to 3C versus IMRT.

Extended Field

This technique is mainly used for patients with documented positive para-aortic nodes or patients at risk of disease but without surgical evaluation. Either 3DCF irradiation or IMRT can be utilized (93), although IMRT may significantly reduce the risk of acute and chronic GI toxicity. When para-aortic fields are utilized, attention should be made to the dose delivered to the kidney, especially with increased use of chemotherapy in these patients and when metrics are well known. The lower border is the same as in pelvic radiation, but the upper border is extended in some patients as high as the T12-L1 interspace. The typical dose is 45 Gy at 1.8 Gy per fraction or 1.5 Gy per fraction if patients develop acute GI toxicity.

Whole Abdomen Radiation Therapy

Whole abdominal radiation therapy (WART) is uncommonly used since the publication of GOG 122. The standard approach is anteroposterior (AP)/posteroanterior (PA) open fields with five half-value layer kidney blocks placed over the PA field only (if patient is lying supine) from the start of the treatment. The dose is usually 30.0 Gy at 1.5 Gy per fraction, followed by a 19.8-Gy boost to the pelvis at 1.8 Gy per fraction. The upper border is usually placed 1 cm above the diaphragm, and the lateral borders should extend beyond the peritoneal reflections. The lower border is usually at the bottom of the obturator foramen.

Complications of Radiation

Pelvic Radiation

In GOG 99, the risk of grade 3 or 4 complications was 14% with RT versus 6% without. In the PORTEC 1 randomized trial (7), the overall (grades 1-4) rate of late complications was 26% in the RT group compared to 4% in the observation group ($P < .0001$). Most of the late complications in the RT group, however, were grades 1, 2 (22%), and only 3% were grades 3, 4. It is also important to note that many patients in this trial were treated with AP/PA fields in which the overall rate of complications was 30% compared to 21% for those treated with the four-field box ($P = .06$), and even lower for IMRT. The recent 15-year update notes that second malignancies were diagnosed in 16% of the observation patients and 22% of the irradiation patients, a difference that was insignificant. In PORTEC 2 grades 1 and 2, GI side effects were significantly higher with external beam (delivered using CT planning and with multifield or 3DCF techniques) than with vaginal brachytherapy (53.8% vs 12.6%), but grades 3 and 4 were not reported, which is curious, suggesting it was very low and likely not significantly different between the arms. Late grade 3 GI effects were reported in 2% of those receiving external beam radiotherapy (EBRT) versus <1% of those with vaginal brachytherapy. Alternatively, grade 3 atrophy (marked atrophy with or without narrowing or shortening) was reported in <1% of those with EBRT and 2% with vaginal brachytherapy. There were no grade 4 or 5 toxicities in either arm. In more advanced disease trials, we see a similar pattern. In GOG 122, those with at least one grade 3 and 4 hematologic toxicity between the arms of WART or chemotherapy were 14% versus 88%, respectively. Grade 3 or 4 acute GI toxicity was 13% versus 20% in the WART and chemotherapy arms, respectively. Late grades 3 or 4 GI or genitourinary toxicity between the arms was 13% and <1% for WART and 20% and 3% for chemotherapy, respectively. Many investigators were surprised that the chemotherapy arm had increased acute and late GI effects when compared to WART. Statistical analyses of these results were not reported (6). In GOG 184, where everyone received whole pelvis radiation and 49% pelvis and para-aortic irradiation, the late grade 3 or higher treatment-related GI events were only 5% (68). Acutely pelvic irradiation can cause fatigue, cystitis, diarrhea, skin erythema and breakdown, and vaginitis. Adding a para-aortic field can add nausea and gastritis to the list. VCB is very well tolerated, and complaints during treatment are rare other than discomfort with placement of the device. Late toxicities include intra-abdominal scarring, chronic cystitis or enteritis, bowel obstruction requiring surgery, rectal telangiectasias, and more unusually bone weakening with fracture, fistula formation, kidney or spinal cord damage, second malignancies, menopause if the ovaries are in the field, and WART liver toxicity. With vaginal brachytherapy, vaginal atrophy, narrowing, dryness, and agglutination are possible.

Radiation Therapy for Local Recurrence

RT can be curative in a select group of patients with small vaginal recurrences who have not received prior radiation. The 5-year local control rate ranges from 42% to 65%, and the 5-year OS rate from 31% to 53% (94-96). Creutzberg et al (97) reported on survival after relapse from the PORTEC randomized trial. In patients who were initially randomized to surgery alone ($n = 46$ out of 360), the 5-year survival after vaginal relapse was 65%. But before adopting salvage radiation as a treatment policy for all early-stage EC, a few aspects of this trial need to be addressed. First, the 5-year survival rate from the PORTEC trial is much higher than what is reported in the literature. Most likely, the vaginal recurrences in this trial were detected very early, unlike patients in the community. The extent and size of local recurrence in EC are very significant predictors of outcome (96). Second, this high rate of salvage pertains only to isolated vaginal recurrence. The rate of survival at 3 years for pelvic recurrence in the PORTEC trial was 0%. Third, although the trial does not mention any data on complications, it is not unrealistic to expect a higher complication rate than what is normally seen with adjuvant radiation. With salvage radiation, external beam RT and brachytherapy are often combined and the doses of radiation required are much higher than those used with adjuvant radiation. A study from the M. D. Anderson Cancer Center by Jhingran et al (98) clearly highlights these issues. They reported on 91 patients who were treated with definitive radiation for isolated vaginal recurrence. The 5-year local control and OS rates were 75% and 43%, respectively. The median dose of radiation was 75 Gy, which often included external radiation and brachytherapy. The rate of grade 4 complications (requiring surgery) was 9%. Thus, when talking with a patient about adjuvant radiation versus radiation reserved for salvage, these issues need to be addressed and compared to the excellent local control and low morbidity obtained with adjuvant irradiation. The currently open GOG 0238 trial randomizes patients with recurrence of EC limited to the pelvis and vagina to concurrent cisplatin/irradiation versus standard irradiation alone.

SYSTEMIC THERAPIES

Endometrial Cancer and Cytotoxic Chemotherapy

Early-Stage High-Risk Uterine Cancer

Despite the ability for surgical staging to define a low-risk patient population for most patients with negative pelvic and para-aortic LN, certain subgroups of patients with stage I to II EC have been shown to have a higher risk of recurrence. Defining patients that require adjuvant therapy remains a challenge.

Hogberg et al (99) reported the results of two randomized studies (NSGO-EC-9501/EORTC-55991 and MaNGO-ILIADE-III) examining the role of sequential adjuvant chemotherapy and RT. The two randomized clinical trials included patients with stage I to III EC with no residual tumor and prognostic factors consistent with high-risk disease. These patients were randomly assigned to either adjuvant RT with or without sequential chemotherapy. The authors reported that in the NSGO/EORTC study, the combined modality treatment was associated with a 36% reduction in the risk for relapse or death (HR, 0.064; 95% CI, 0.41-0.99; $P = .04$). A similar HR was reported in the MaNGO study (HR of 0.61), but no significant significance was appreciated. In the combined analysis of these two trials, the estimate of risk for relapse or death was similar with an HR of 0.69 (95% CI, 0.46-1.03; $P = .07$). Careful examination of the two independent studies reveals that the majority of patients in the NSGO-EC-9501/EORTC-55991 trial had stage I disease, whereas patients in the MaNGO-ILIADE-III trial had predominantly stage IIB to IIIC disease. Overall, these results should be interpreted with caution given the heterogeneity of the population studied.

The role of RT alone or in combination with chemotherapy was investigated in GOG 249, a phase III clinical trial that compared the outcomes of pelvic irradiation versus VCB followed by paclitaxel/carboplatin in patients with high-risk early stage. Patients eligible for this clinical trial included stage I endometroid histology with HIR factors, stage II any histology, and stage I/II serous or

clear cell cancer with negative cytology. The majority of patients enrolled in GOG 249 had an endometroid histology (71%). Fifteen percent of patients had uterine serous histology, whereas 5% of the patients had clear cell histology. In the GOG 249 study, there was no difference in RFS or OS when chemotherapy was added to the RT for stage I or II EC (100). It is important to note that these patient populations were heterogeneous.

The results of RTOG 0921, a phase II trial of postoperative IMRT with concurrent cisplatin and bevacizumab followed by four cycles of platinum and taxane, were recently reported. Eligible patients included those who had the following high-risk factors, namely, grade 3 carcinoma with >50% myometrial invasion, grade 2 or 3 disease with any cervical stromal invasion, or known extrauterine extension confined to the pelvis. A total of 30 patients were eligible for treatment. The 2-year OS was 96.7%, whereas the DFS rate was 79.1%. Grade 3 toxicities occurring within the first 90 days included headache, fatigue, syncope, thromboembolic events, hyponatremia, hyperglycemia, vaginal infection, liver function test elevation, febrile neutropenia, and fatigue. The authors noted that no patient developed an infield pelvic failure. The role of bevacizumab in this patient population continues to be explored (101).

As outlined previously, patients enrolled in these earlier studies were heterogeneous. Patients were enrolled on the basis of stage and histology and not based on any molecular characteristics.

One study that is trying to integrate both clinical and molecular characteristics is the PORTEC 4a trial. This an international randomized trial of molecular profile–based adjuvant treatment for women with HIR EC. This trial is centered on defining the role of adjuvant RT in patients with HIR EC. HIR factors are defined as: (a) FIGO stage IA (with invasion) and grade 3; (b) stage IB grade 1 or 2 with age 60 years and above and/or lymphovascular space invasion; (c) stage IB, grade 3 without lymphovascular space invasion; or (d) stage II (microscopic and grade 1). The study employs a molecular-integrated risk model by integrating the molecular subgroups with L1-CAM overexpression, substantial lymphovascular space invasion, and *CTNNB1*-exon 3 mutations. The primary end point is vaginal recurrence. This study does not address the role of chemotherapy in early-stage high-risk uterine cancer (102-104).

At this point in time, we remain uncertain as to which patients with high-risk early-stage uterine cancer should receive chemotherapy, if any. Utilization of the comprehensive genomic analysis of TCGA may help guide future trial design in early-stage uterine cancer that is focused not only on the clinical/pathologic characteristics of the tumor but also on the molecular signature of the tumor (105).

Adjuvant and Advanced Disease

Adjuvant therapy for advanced uterine cancer has been evaluated in multiple clinical trials. Trials have studied different cytotoxic agents either as a single modality or in combination with RT whether administered concurrently or in a sequential manner.

For historical purposes, the initial combinations of cytotoxic therapies in advanced EC explored included the use of cyclophosphamide with doxorubicin (106,107), the addition of cyclophosphamide and doxorubicin to cisplatin (CAP) (108-112), and the addition of doxorubicin to cisplatin (AP) (113-117). Given the lack of additional benefit with a three-drug combination, the AP regimen became the "standard" to which more contemporary approaches were compared.

Chemotherapy Versus Radiation Therapy

GOG 122 compared WART to eight cycles of doxorubicin/cisplatin chemotherapy in patients with *stage III to IV disease who underwent surgical assessment and had a maximum of 2 cm of disease postoperatively* (6). The results demonstrated an improved PFS and OS in patients with chemotherapy, with the reduction in recurrences largely because of reduced abdominal and distant sites of disease. The event rates were high in both arms. The Japanese GOG 2033 trial (118) randomized 385 women with *stages IC to III endometrioid adenocarcinomas* to whole pelvic radiation (WPR) therapy versus chemotherapy using the regimen cisplatin, doxorubicin, and paclitaxel. PFS at 5 years was 83.5% versus 81.8% for whole pelvic RT and chemotherapy, respectively. However, in a subgroup analysis of patients with stage IC over the age of 70 years with grade 3 endometrioid tumors or stage II or IIIA, chemotherapy was associated with improvement over pelvic RT both in terms of PFS (83.8% vs 66.2% respectively, $P = .024$) and OS (89.7% vs 73.6%, respectively, $P = .006$).

Chemotherapy

Given the phase II activity of single-agent taxanes (119-121), the GOG conducted a randomized trial (GOG 163) (122) *for patients with primary stage III and IV or recurrent EC with **measurable disease*** comparing doxorubicin and cisplatin to doxorubicin with 24-hour paclitaxel and granulocyte colony-stimulating factor (G-CSF). There were no significant differences in RR (40% vs 43%), PFS (median 7.2 vs 6 months), or OS (median 12.6 vs 13.6 months) for arms 1 and 2, respectively. The disadvantage of GOG 163 was the lack of platinum in the taxane-containing arm. The addition of a taxane was subsequently studied in GOG 177 (123) (*patients with primary stage III and IV or recurrent EC with **measurable disease***). GOG 177 utilized doxorubicin (60 or 45 mg/m^2 in patients with prior RT) with cisplatin (50 mg/m^2) as the standard arm versus paclitaxel (160 mg/m^2) with doxorubicin (45 mg/m^2) and cisplatin (50 mg/m^2) and G-CSF as the investigational regimen. The primary objective was to determine if the addition of paclitaxel improved RR and PFS and OS. Two hundred seventy-three patients were enrolled, and the study was balanced for history of prior RT (50% vs 46%), serous carcinoma (15% vs 19%), stage, grade, and body surface area. Grade 3 and 4 platelet toxicity was higher in the three-drug arm (21% vs 2%), but other hematologic toxicity was ameliorated with G-CSF: absolute neutrophil count 36% versus 50% and neutropenic fever 3% versus 2%. Nonhematologic grade 3, 4 toxicity was higher in the three-drug arm: GI 59% versus 39% and metabolic 25% versus 13%. RRs were better with the triplet: complete response (CR) 22% versus 7%, partial response (PR) 36% versus 27%, and overall response rate (ORR) 57% versus 34%. Median PFS was 8.3 versus 5.3 months ($P < .0005$), and median OS was 15.3 versus 12.1 months ($P = .0024$). Responses were similar in serous (48%) versus nonserous histology (45%). Overall, paclitaxel, doxorubicin, cisplatin (TAP) chemotherapy increased 12-month survival to 59% compared to 50% with AP with an HR of 0.75 (0.56-0.998). Although the TAP regimen produced an improvement in RR and PFS, survival was minimally increased and was associated with greater toxicity. The combination of paclitaxel and carboplatin as a doublet has also been evaluated in a variety of phase II trials and retrospective studies with RRs in the 43% to 80% range (124,125).

GOG 209, a randomized trial comparing doxorubicin, cisplatin, and paclitaxel (TAP) with carboplatin and paclitaxel (TC) (*stage III, IV or recurrent disease*), was recently reported. TC was not inferior to TAP in terms of PFS (median PFS of TAP vs TP: 13.5 vs 13.3 months: HR, 1.03) and OS (40.3 vs 36.5 months; HR, 1.05) based on interim analysis results. Overall, the toxicity profile favored TC with less sensory neuropathy (sensory neuropathy > grade 1: 26% vs 19%, $P < .01$) (45). Based on the results of GOG 209, the standard backbone of therapy is chemotherapy (126).

Sequence of Therapeutic Modalities

With the current data in mind, the sequence of therapy in patients with advanced surgically resected disease remains in question. Various approaches have been delineated.

GOG 184 (68) randomized 552 women with *stage III disease debulked to a maximum residual of 2 cm or less*, followed by volume-directed RT to doxorubicin and cisplatin (AP) or doxorubicin/cisplatin and paclitaxel (TAP). At 3 years, the proportion of patients alive and free from recurrence was similar (62% AP vs 64% TAP). The overall hazard for recurrence or death of TAP compared to AP was 0.9 (95% CI, 0.69-1.17). In women with gross residual disease at the time of enrollment, TAP was associated with a 50% reduction in the risk of relapse or death (HR, 0.50; 95% CI, 0.26-0.92).

An RTOG phase II study (RTOG 9708) (68) was conducted to assess the feasibility, safety, toxicity, and patterns of recurrence and survival when chemotherapy was combined with adjuvant radiation for patients with high-risk EC. Pathologic requirements included grade 2 or 3 endometrial adenocarcinoma with >50% myometrial invasion, cervical stromal invasion, or pelvic-confined extrauterine disease. Radiation included 45 Gy in 25 fractions to the pelvis along with cisplatin (50 mg/m^2) on days 1 and 28. Vaginal brachytherapy was performed after external beam radiation. Four courses of cisplatin (50 mg/m^2) and paclitaxel (175 mg/m^2) were given at 4-week intervals following completion of RT. Forty-six patients were accrued to the study. Median follow-up was a median of 4.3 years. At 4 years, pelvic, regional, and distant recurrence rates were 2%, 2%, and 19%, respectively. OS and DFS rates at 4 years were 85% and 81%, respectively. Four-year rates for survival and DFS for patients with stage III were 77% and 72%, respectively. There were no recurrences for patients with stage IC, IIA, or IIB. Local-regional control was reported to be excellent following combined modality treatment in all patients, suggesting additive effects of chemotherapy and radiation. Distant metastases continued to occur in more advanced-stage patients.

Secord and colleagues (127) reported a multicenter evaluation of sequential multimodality therapy and clinical outcome for the treatment of advanced EC. A multicenter retrospective analysis of patients with surgical stages III and IV EC from 1993 to 2007 was conducted. Inclusion criteria included a comprehensive staging procedure including hysterectomy, BSO, and/or selective pelvic/aortic lymphadenectomy, and treatment with adjuvant chemotherapy and radiation. One hundred and nine patients with advanced-stage EC were identified who received postoperative adjuvant therapies; 41% ($n = 45$) chemotherapy followed by radiation and then further chemotherapy (CRC), 17% ($n = 18$) radiation followed by chemotherapy (RC), and 42% ($n = 46$) chemotherapy followed by radiation (CR). There was no difference in the frequency of adverse effects because of either chemotherapy ($P = .35$) or RT ($P = .14$), dose modifications ($P = .055$), or delays ($P = .80$) between the various sequencing modalities. There was a significant difference between adjuvant treatment groups for both OS (log-rank $P = .011$) and PFS (log-rank $P = .025$), with those receiving CRC having a superior 3-year OS (88%) and PFS (69%) compared to RC (54% and 47%) or CR (57% and 52%). After adjusting for stage, age, grade, race, histology, and cytoreduction status, the OS HR for therapy was 5.74 (95% CI, 1.96-16.77) for RC and 2.6 (95% CI, 1.01-6.71) for CR, compared to CRC, $P = .003$. When the analysis was restricted to optimally cytoreduced patients, those who were treated with RC were at higher risk for disease progression (HR, 3.53 [95% CI, 1.29-9.71], $P = .024$) and death (HR, 7.24 [95% CI, 2.25-23.37], $P = .001$) than patients who received sequential CRC. The authors reported that sequential CRC was associated with improved survival in women with advanced-stage disease compared to other sequencing modalities with a similar adverse effect profile.

Recently reported were the results of PORTEC 3 (128). This trial studied the role of adjuvant chemoradiotherapy versus radiotherapy for women with high-risk EC. Eligible women had high-risk EC with FIGO 2009 stage I, endometrioid-type grade 3 with deep myometrial invasion or lymphovascular space invasion (or both), endometrioid-type stage II or III, or stage I to III with serous or clear cell histology. Women were randomly assigned (1:1) to receive radiotherapy alone or radiotherapy and chemotherapy (consisting of two cycles of cisplatin 50 mg/m^2 given during radiotherapy, followed by four cycles of carboplatin AUC 5 and paclitaxel 175 mg/m^2). Patients were stratified based on the treatment center, the stage of the disease, the histologic subtype, and whether or not they underwent a lymphadenectomy. Six hundred and sixty patients were included in the final analysis. Median follow-up was 60.2 months. The 5-year OS was 81.8% in the chemoradiation arm versus 76.7% in the radiation arm alone (adjusted HR, 0.76). The 5-year failure-free survival was 75.5% in the chemoradiation arm versus 68.6% in the radiation arm alone ($P = .022$). Grade 3+ adverse events was higher in the chemoradiation arm (60%) when compared to RT alone (12%); $P < .0001$.

When the data were analyzed by stage, patients with stage III EC had the greatest absolute benefit from the combined treatment. Five-year OS for stage III cancer was 78.7% in the chemoradiation group versus 69.8% in the radiation group. Five-year failure-free survival for stage III cancer was 69.3% in the chemoradiation group versus 58.0% in the radiation group (HR, 0.66; 95% CI 0.45-0.97; $P = .031$).

In a post hoc survival analysis of the PORTEC 3 trial, de Boer et al reported a significantly improved OS and failure-free survival with chemoradiotherapy versus radiotherapy alone. At a median follow-up of 72.6 months, the 5-year OS was 81.4% with chemoradiation versus 76.1% with radiation alone (HR, 0.70; $P = .034$), and 5-year failure-free survival was 76.5% versus 69.1% (HR, 0.70 [0.52-0.94]; $P = .016$) (129).

Matei et al (130) recently published the results of GOG 258. This randomized phase III trial compared chemotherapy to chemoradiation therapy in patients with stage III or IVA EC. The primary end point was free survival. The chemoradiotherapy regimen consisted of cisplatin at a dose of 50 mg/m^2 of body surface area given intravenously on days 1 and 29 together with volume-directed external beam RT, followed by carboplatin (AUC 5-6) plus paclitaxel at a dose of 175 mg/m^2 every 21 days for four cycles, with G-CSF support. The sample size was 736 patients. At 60 months, the relapse-free rate was 59% in the chemoradiotherapy group and 58 in the chemotherapy-only group (HR, 0.90; 90% CI, 0.74-1.10). Chemoradiotherapy was associated with a lower incidence of vaginal recurrence, pelvic and para-aortic lymph node recurrence. Distant recurrence was more common in association with chemoradiotherapy. It is important to note that the end point was free survival.

Despite the excellent contributions of all of these trials, the management of advanced EC remains undefined. Many interpretations have been generated on the basis of these studies, but at the present time we remain uncertain as to whether chemotherapy or chemoradiation therapy in advanced uterine cancer offers the best outcome. It is important to note the heterogeneity of the patient population coupled with the specific end points that were measured in each trial. These trials enrolled patients based on clinical/pathologic criteria and not on a molecular basis. It is conceivable that future trials will be more refined and be inconclusive of the molecular signature of the tumor.

Metastatic/Recurrent Disease

Treatment in recurrent or metastatic setting is palliative. Treatment decisions in the management of patients with recurrent or metastatic disease depends on several factors: treatment history (ie, number of prior lines of therapy, residual toxicity, treatment-free interval, platinum-free interval), histologic subtype (endometroid, clear cell, uterine papillary serous, carcinosarcoma), comorbidities, sites of disease, genomic profile, and goals of care.

Endocrine Therapy

Hormonal agents have proven to be valuable, particularly in the patient with recurrent disease, and reviews of their use have been extensively published. RRs to endocrine agents including progestins, antiestrogens, and aromatase inhibitors vary (131-138). The overall response to progestins is approximately 25%. However, some trials demonstrate lower RRs, usually in the range of 15% to 20%. These studies generally used more rigorous response criteria and had multi-institutional participation. A higher dose of

progestin does not appear to increase the RR. In one randomized trial of 200 versus 1,000 mg/d of medroxyprogesterone acetate (MPA), the ORR was actually 25% versus 15% favoring the low-dose arm (139). The time to treatment failure and median OS of the low- versus high-dose regimen, respectively, were 3.2 versus 2.5 months and 11.1 versus 7.0 months, all showing no advantage for an increased dose. Prognostic factors related to response were performance status, grade, and PR level. The RR was only 8% in poorly differentiated tumors. A phase II trial of high-dose megestrol (800 mg orally daily) in 63 patients was associated with an RR of 24% overall, which is similar to lower dose regimens with doses of 40 mg po qid (140). As in the majority of studies with hormonal agents, RRs were statistically higher in patients with grade 1 or 2 lesions (37%) versus grade 3 lesions (8%); $P = .02$. In addition to grade, a long disease-free interval (exceeding 2 or 3 years) and positive ER or PR status have all been associated with an increased frequency of response (131,134,139,140). Age, location of metastatic disease, number of metastatic sites, prior therapy, and weight have also been analyzed by several investigators, but they have not been convincingly linked with response.

Tamoxifen has been investigated in patients with recurrent disease in several studies (137-139,141). Results have varied, but in general, RRs have been modest in untreated patients. A GOG study evaluated 68 patients with advanced or recurrent disease receiving tamoxifen at 20 mg po bid and showed an ORR of 10% (90% CI, 5.7-17.9) (137). The median PFS was short at 1.9 months (90% CI, 1.7-3.2 months) and the OS was 8.8 months (90% CI, 7.0-10.1 months). One small, randomized phase II study comparing megestrol acetate to megestrol acetate with tamoxifen showed no advantage in RR for the combination, with RRs of 20% versus 19%, respectively (142). The lack of synergistic response is supported by observations of EC treated in a nude mouse model. Tumors treated with medroxyprogesterone or tamoxifen plus medroxyprogesterone were devoid of PR during the growth inhibitory and regrowth phase of the tumor resulting from receptor downregulation (143). The possibility of alternating tamoxifen with megestrol acetate to exploit the recruitment of PRs by tamoxifen is an interesting strategy. The GOG performed a phase II study with 56 patients with advanced or recurrent EC who had not previously received chemotherapy or hormonal manipulation (144). Patients were treated with megestrol acetate at 160 mg/d for 3 weeks alternating with tamoxifen 20 mg bid for 3 weeks. An ORR of 27% (90% CI, 17.3-38.4) with a 21.4% CR rate was seen, with the duration of response exceeding 20 months in 8 of 15 responders. The RR was 38% for patients with grade 1 disease and 22% for those with grade 3 disease. In another phase II GOG study, a similar patient population was treated with tamoxifen 40 mg po daily plus alternating weekly cycles of MPA 200 mg po daily (145). Of the 58 evaluable patients, the RR was 33% (6 CR, 13 PR). Although these phase II results are intriguing, a randomized study would be required to determine if alternating hormones are superior to single-hormone approaches. Positive receptor status has been associated with improved DFS and OS rates (146). These data indicate that the receptor status provides important biologic information and that receptor-positive tumors tend to be better differentiated and slower growing than are their receptor-negative counterparts. Chemotherapy had no effect on hormone receptor capacity in a nude mouse model of xenografted EC (147). Other factors, such as changes in vaginal cytology during treatment (148), and results in the subrenal capsule chemosensitivity assay and in the nude mouse model (149) may help predict response to progestins.

Several studies have evaluated gonadotropin-releasing hormone analogs in patients with metastatic EC (150-153). Gallagher et al (151) noted one CR and five PRs to leuprolide or goserelin in 17 patients (35% response; 95% CI, 13%-58%) with metastatic disease. Of note, the duration of remission ranged from 7 to 30 months, and 14 of the 17 patients had been previously treated with progestins. Another report described four responses in seven postmenopausal patients with EC treated with goserelin (153). In vitro studies in human EC cell lines have suggested that such growth inhibition may have been due to apoptosis (154). The GOG studied goserelin at 3.6-mg subcutaneously monthly in 40 patients with advanced or recurrent disease. Seventy-one percent of patients had received prior RT. There were two CRs (5%) and three PRs (7%), with an ORR of 11% (95% CI, 4%-27%). Goserelin is observed to have limited activity in this patient population, and no additional single-agent studies are planned (132).

The aromatase inhibitors have also been studied in patients with uterine cancer. The mechanism of action of aromatase inhibitors works by inhibiting the action of the enzyme aromatase, which converts androgens into estrogens by a process called aromatization. These agents have ER-antagonist activity in breast and uterine tissues and ER-agonist activity in bone. The first reported study to date is from the GOG and evaluated anastrozole at 1-mg po daily orally in 23 unselected patients (ie, 9 patients had grade 2 tumors and 14 patients had grade 3 tumors). A PR rate of 9% was seen (90% CI, 3%-23%) (155).

Another study evaluated the investigational SERM arzoxifene in 37 patients. Twenty-six patients were ER-positive and 22 were PR positive. An RR of 31% (95% CI, 25%-51%) was seen in this selected patient population with a median duration of response of 13.9 months (133).

The role of fulvestrant, a serum estrogen receptor downregulator (SERD), has also been studied in uterine cancer. A phase II study of fulvestrant was conducted in recurrent/metastatic EC by the GOG. Eligible patients with advanced, recurrent, or persistent EC not amenable to curative therapy were treated with fulvestrant at a dose of 250 mg by IM injection every 4 weeks for at least 8 weeks. Sixty-seven patients were enrolled in this study, but 14 patients were excluded. In the 22 ER-negative patients, no patients demonstrated both a CR and PR, and 4 (18%) demonstrated stable disease (as best response). In the 31 ER-positive patients, 1 (3%), 4 (13%), and 9 (29%) patients demonstrated a CR, PR, and stable disease, respectively. The median PFS and OS in the ER-negative patients were 2 and 3 months, respectively, and, in the ER-positive patients 10 and 26 months, respectively (156). Emons and colleagues also reported a phase II study of fulvestrant 250 mg/mo in patients with recurrent or metastatic EC. Thirty-five patients with advanced or recurrent disease were treated. The authors reported 11.4% of patients had a PR and eight patients had stable disease. OS was 13.2 months. The authors highlighted that a loading strategy of fulvestrant as utilized in the breast discipline might improve the efficacy of treatment (157).

Recent studies have explored the combination of targeted therapy with hormonal manipulation. Slomovitz et al (158) reported the results of a phase II study of everolimus and letrozole in patients with recurrent EC. Everolimus was administered orally at 10 mg daily and letrozole was administered orally at 2.5 mg daily. The primary end point was the clinical benefit rate (CBR). Thirty-eight patients were enrolled. Thirty-five patients were evaluable for response. The CBR was 40% (14 of 35 patients). The confirmed objective RR was 32% (11 of 35 patients: nine CRs and two PRs). Patients with endometrioid histology and CTNNB1 mutations responded well to everolimus and letrozole.

The GOG 3007 (159) trial investigated the combination of everolimus and letrozole or hormonal therapy in advanced EC. Patients were randomly assigned to receive everolimus and letrozole in combination (*n* = 37) or hormonal therapy with tamoxifen/medroxyprogesterone acetate (*n* = 36). At a median follow-up of 14 months, median OS could not yet be calculated for the everolimus/letrozole group and was 16.6 months in the hormonal therapy group. Median PFS was 6.3 months for the everolimus/letrozole group and 3.8 months for patients receiving hormonal therapy. Among patients in the everolimus/letrozole study group, those with no prior chemotherapy had a median PFS of 21.6 months, compared with 3.3 months among patients who did have prior chemotherapy. In the hormonal therapy group, those with no prior chemotherapy had a PFS of 6.6 months, compared with 3.2 months among patients who had received prior chemotherapy.

Mirza et al (160) studied the role of palbociclib versus placebo in combination with letrozole for patients with advanced or recurrent EC. Palbociclib is an inhibitor of cyclin-dependent kinases CDK4 and CDK6. Studies in breast cancer have demonstrated the superiority of hormonal therapy plus CDK inhibitors in ER+ HER2-advanced disease. The NSGO ENGOT-EN3/PALEO trial was a multicenter, prospective, double-blind, placebo-controlled, randomized, phase II trial evaluating the efficacy of letrozole when combined with palbociclib against letrozole-placebo combination therapy in women with ER+ advanced or recurrent EC. Eligible patients had stage 4 disease, were ER+, had received no prior endocrine therapy except MPA, and had no prior CDK inhibitors. The primary end point was investigator-assessed PFS. The authors reported an improvement in PFS in patients receiving the combination therapy. Median PFS in the palbociclib and letrozole arm was 8.3 versus 3.0 months in the letrozole arm (*P* = .0376). Disease control rate was also improved in the combination arm (63.6% in the combination arm versus 37.8% in the letrozole arm). Numerous other trials are exploring the role of CDKs in EC (161).

Cytotoxic Chemotherapy

The standard of therapy in patients with metastatic EC is, as previously outlined, based on GOG 209. Despite the tolerability of this combination, PFS is poor. Historically, several trials have explored various agents in the management of metastatic setting. The most commonly studied single agents include cisplatin, carboplatin, doxorubicin, epirubicin, ifosfamide, docetaxel, paclitaxel, and topotecan.

The RR to **cisplatin** dosages of 50 to 60 mg/m^2 given every 3 weeks was similar in patients with prior (25%) (162,163) and no prior chemotherapy (21%) (164-166). **Carboplatin** given in dosages of 300 to 400 mg/m^2 every 4 weeks has been associated with RRs of 29% (167-169), which is similar to cisplatin. **Doxorubicin** in dosages of 55 to 60 mg/m^2 has been associated with an ORR of 26% (106,170,171) and **epirubicin** with an RR of 26% (172). **Liposomal doxorubicin** was reported in a GOG study of 46 patients receiving 50 mg/m^2 every 4 weeks with an ORR of 9.5% (95% CI, 2.7%-26%) (173). It is important to note that 32 patients had received prior doxorubicin therapy. A second study evaluated its efficacy in 19 patients without prior chemotherapy and resulted in a 21% RR (174). Of the antimetabolites, **5-fluorouracil** was given in dosages of 15 mg/kg for 5 consecutive days and then every other day until dose-limiting toxicity occurred. It has displayed a 21% RR in 34 patients, whereas **methotrexate** (175) and **mercaptopurine** (176) have been inactive. **Vincristine** given on a weekly schedule was associated with an RR of 18% in 33 untreated patients (177), but dose-limiting neurotoxicity was substantial. In a phase II trial of **paclitaxel** conducted by the GOG (119), 28 patients with recurrent or advanced EC received a dose of 250 mg/m^2 every 21 days. Patients who had received prior pelvic irradiation were treated at an initial dose of 200 mg/m^2. CRs were noted in four patients (14%) and PRs in six (21%) for an ORR of 36%. A more contemporary GOG study evaluated paclitaxel at 200 mg/m^2 (175 mg/m^2 with prior RT) every 3 weeks in pretreated patients, showing an ORR of 27.3% (95% CI, 15%-42.8%). The median duration of response was 4.2 months, with an OS of 10.3 months (178). A similar study showed an RR of 43% (95% CI, 6%-80%) in patients who had all previously been treated with platinum-based therapy (164). A multicenter trial recently reported showed an RR of 21% with PFS of 12 weeks and OS of 43 weeks in 35 patients receiving weekly **docetaxel** at 35 mg/m^2 (120). **Topotecan** was evaluated in a phase II trial of untreated advanced or recurrent EC administered initially at 1.5 mg/m^2 every day for 5 days every 3 weeks. The trial was suspended for toxicity but reopened and completed at 1 mg/m^2 q day for 5 days (or 0.8 mg/m^2/d for patients with prior RT). An ORR of 20% was seen, with median duration of response of

8 months and OS of 6.5 months (179). A subsequent smaller study by Traina et al using weekly topotecan dosing of 2.5 to 4.0 mg/m² on 2 of 3 weeks' schedule followed by 1 week off showed one PR for 54 weeks with two patients having stable disease for 15 weeks each. Only two patients required dose reduction for toxicity using the weekly schedule (180) **Epothilones**, a novel class of nontaxane microtubule-stabilizing agents, are currently approved for the management of advanced breast cancer. Ixabepilone was reported to have an objective RR of 12%, with a PFS of 2.9 months and a stable disease for at least 8 weeks in 60% of patients (181).

Regardless of the available choices, responses to each successive line of therapy are short-lived. As such, focus has centered on the molecular basis of EC and potential targeted agents.

Targeted Therapy

The molecular background of EC provides a platform that lends itself to targeted therapeutics in patients with advanced recurrent or metastatic disease. The current classification of uterine cancer is now focused into four molecular groups: (1) POLE (ultra-, mutated), (2) microsatellite unstable tumors, (3) CN high tumors with TP53 mutations, and (4) other tumors without these molecular alterations (182).

Biologic agents targeting molecular components are currently under development in numerous clinical trials. Focus has centered on specific histologic subtype- and/or biomarker-driven patient stratification. Evidence suggests that not only are type I and II endometrial tumors distinct entities with diversified genotypic and phenotypic profile (**Table 5.6-3**), but patients within each subtype may also differ molecularly. Hence, efforts have focused on the application of personalized therapies by utilizing biomarkers able to discriminate patients' dominant profile (183,184).

The PI3K/AKT/Mammalian Target of Rapamycin Pathway

The **PI3K/AKT/mammalian target of rapamycin (mTOR) pathway** represents a major signaling pathway downstream of several growth factor receptor kinases (eg, epidermal growth factor receptor (EGFR), platelet-derived growth factor receptor [PDGFR], fibroblast growth factor receptor [FGFR], and insulin growth factor receptor) and is well known to have a pivotal role in cell survival and growth (185,186). The PI3K/AKT/PTEN pathway is the most commonly altered pathway in type I EC (187). Activation of PI3K leads to the phosphorylation of a secondary messenger to form PIP3 (phosphatidylinositol 3, 4, 5-triphosphate). This process is regulated by PTEN, which dephosphorylates PIP3 to PIP2. Activation of PI3K, resulting in PIP3, subsequently leads to AKT activation. AKT promotes cell growth, proliferation, reduces apoptosis, and increases angiogenesis. Two important regulators of the process include the mammalian target of rapamycin complexes mTORC 1 and 2.

The most common mechanisms of PI3K activation are loss of the phosphatase and tensin homolog (PTEN) tumor suppressor protein function and activating mutations in catalytic PI3K subunit, p110α, which is encoded by the *PIK3CA* gene. Cells that are deficient in PTEN may have a resulting activation of the PI3K pathway. The function of the tumor suppressor gene *PTEN* includes inhibition of cell migration, spreading, and adhesion (188-192). The *PTEN* gene is located on chromosome 10q23, and about 40% of ECs display loss of heterozygosity of chromosome 10q23, which suggests the involvement of *PTEN* in this disease (188-193). *PTEN* mutations in 30% to 50% of EC tumors make this the most frequent genetic alteration known in

TABLE 5.6-3. Molecular Aberrations of EC by Type

Molecular Aberration	Type I (Endometrioid) EC (%)	Type II (Non-endometrioid) EC (%)	Aberrant Pathway
PTEN loss	80-83	5	PI3K/AKT/mTOR pathway
PIK3CA Mutation amplification	24-40 2-14	2,046	PI3K/AKT/mTOR pathway
PIK3R1 mutation	43	12	PI3K/AKT/mTOR pathway
AKT mutation	3	0	PI3K/AKT/mTOR pathway
K-RAS mutation	10-30	0-10	Ras-Raf-Mek-Erk pathway
MSI	15-45	0-5	—
a-catenin (CTNNB1) mutation	14-50	0	Wnt/β-catenin/LEF-1 pathway
E-cadherin loss	5-50	60-90	Wnt/β-catenin/LEF-1 pathway
TP53 mutation	10-20	90	Tumor suppression
p16 loss	8	45	Cyclin D/CDK4-CDK6/RB
HER2 Overexpression Amplification	3-10 1	32-43 17-29	Cell surface receptor
FGFR-2 mutation	12-16	1	Cell surface receptor
EGFR overexpression mutation	46 unknown	340	Cell surface receptor
IGFIR overexpression	70	Unknown	Cell surface receptor
Chromosomal instability STK15, BUB1, CCNB2 LOH at multiple loci			—
EphA2 overexpression	48	Unknown	Transmembrane protein
EpCAM overexpression	Unknown	96	Transmembrane protein
HIF1a overexpression	25%	80%	Gene transcription nuclear protein
ARID1A mutation	29-40	18-26	Transcription-regulating process

EC, endometrial cancer.

this disease (192-194). Genes for the catalytic subunit of PI3K (PI3KCA) are frequently amplified (2%-14% type I ECs, 46% type II) or mutated (30% type I-II) in EC, leading to constitutive activation (183).

mTOR is a conserved serine/threonine kinase that lies downstream of the phosphatidylinositol 3 kinase/PTEN/AKT pathway and is composed of two subunits, mTORC1 and mTORC2. Activated AKT phosphorylates mTOR directly or indirectly by phosphorylating TSC2 (tuberous sclerosis complex 2), which in turn stimulates mTORC1. Subsequently, mTORC1 phosphorylates several transcription factors, namely, S6K-1 (ribosomal S6 kinase-1) and 4E-BP1 eukaryote translation initiation factor (4E-binding protein-1 [4EBP1]), thereby leading to the synthesis of proteins involved in proliferation and survival. The second subunit mTORC2 is well less defined but may mediate activation of AKT in response to mTORC1 inhibitors (186,195,196).

Genomic aberrations in the PI3K pathway in EC has made this an attractive target for biologic agents (197-199). Representative trials targeting this pathway are listed next.

A phase II trial (200) of **temsirolimus** in recurrent or metastatic EC (chemotherapy naïve, with up to one prior line of hormonal therapy) demonstrated encouraging results with five confirmed PRs (26%) out of 19 evaluable patients. Three of the PRs were in patients with papillary serous tumors. Evaluation of a second cohort, women who must have had treatment with one prior regimen of cytotoxic chemotherapy, revealed an RR of 7% (2/27). Overall, temsirolimus activity was seen in all histologic subgroups and grades, regardless of PTEN loss. The most frequent drug-related toxicities were fatigue, mucocutaneous irritation (acne-like maculopapular rashes, mucositis, stomatitis, and diarrhea), and pneumonitis. Grade 3 toxic effects were rare and included lymphopenia, neutropenia, thrombocytopenia, hyperglycemia, and hyperlipidemia. Temsirolimus has also been studied in combination with paclitaxel/carboplatin and has demonstrated good tolerability in a phase I trial (201), prompting the initiation of a phase II study. A reported GOG study combining temsirolimus with alternating hormones, megestrol acetate, and tamoxifen, was closed secondary to high levels of venous thrombosis and insufficient additional activity to warrant further study (202). Alvarez et al (203) reported a trial of the combination of bevacizumab and temsirolimus in the treatment of recurrent or persistent EC. Eligible patients had persistent or recurrent endometrial cancer (EMC) after receiving one to two prior cytotoxic regimens. Patients had to have measurable disease. Treatment consisted of bevacizumab 10 mg/kg every other week and temsirolimus 25 mg IV weekly until disease progression or prohibitory toxicity. Primary end points were PFS at 6 months and ORR. Forty-nine patients were evaluable. Adverse events included two GI-vaginal fistulas, epistaxis, two intestinal perforations, and thrombosis/embolism. The authors reported that three patient deaths were possibly treatment related. Twelve patients (24.5%) experienced clinical responses (one CR and 11 PRs), and 23 patients (46.9%) survived progression free for at least 6 months. Median PFS and OS were 5.6 and 16.9 months, respectively. The authors concluded that the combination of temsirolimus and bevacizumab was active; however, it was associated with significant toxicity in this pretreated group.

Previously outlined were the results of the phase II utilizing everolimus and letrozole (158,159). Recently reported were the results of a randomized phase II trial. Patients with chemotherapy-naïve stage III/IVA (with measurable disease) and stage IVB or recurrent (with or without measurable disease) EC were randomly assigned to treatment with PC plus bevacizumab (arm 1), PC plus temsirolimus (arm 2), or ixabepilone and carboplatin (IC) plus bevacizumab (arm 3). The primary end point was PFS. GOG 209 was used as a historical control. PFS duration was not significantly increased in any experimental arm compared with historical controls (204).

ANGIOGENESIS

Vascular Endothelial Growth Factor Receptor Ligand

Angiogenesis mediates the growth of several solid tumors including that of EC. Overexpression of vascular endothelial growth factor (VEGF) has been associated with poor prognostic factors in EC such as deep myometrial invasion and LN metastasis (205-207). VEGF expression seems highly variable depending on histologic subtype and disease stage, with early-stage well-differentiated lesions expressing the highest levels (208). To date, treatment of recurrent EC with antiangiogenic agents has revealed mixed results.

The most significant developments in this class of agents have centered on suppressing the vascular endothelial growth factor receptor (VEGFR) ligand. **Bevacizumab** (Avastin, Roche) (15 mg IV every 3 weeks) was investigated in GOG 229E, a study in patients with recurrent or persistent measurable EC after receiving one or two prior cytotoxic regimens (209). Of 52 evaluable patients, 13.5% had objective response (one CR and six PRs), whereas 40.4% of patients survived progression free for at least 6 months. Median PFS and OS were 4.2 and 10.5 months, respectively. Although no GI perforations or fistulas occurred, two episodes of grades 3 to 4 hemorrhage and thromboembolism were reported.

Two randomized phase II trials evaluating the addition of bevacizumab to carboplatin and paclitaxel in advanced or recurrent EC have been reported. Previously described was the GOG 86P, which was a three-arm trial that evaluated the addition of bevacizumab, temsirolimus, or ixabepilone to carboplatin and paclitaxel in 349 patients. There was no difference in PFS when compared to carboplatin and paclitaxel (204). In contrast, there was an improvement in median OS in the carboplatin/paclitaxel/bevacizumab arm when compared to the historical control, namely, GOG 209 (34 vs 22.7 months, $P < .039$).

The MITO END-2 trial (210) was a randomized phase II trial of 108 patients with advanced or recurrent EC. Patients were randomized to carboplatin and paclitaxel and/or bevacizumab. Bevacizumab was continued as maintenance therapy. The authors reported PFS of 10.5 versus 13.7 months (HR, 0.84; $P = .43$), an ORR of 53.1% versus 74.4% and OS of 29.7 vs 40.0 months (HR, 0.71; $P = .24$). The PFS increase became significant when an exploratory analysis was performed. However, patients treated with bevacizumab experienced a significant increase in 6-month disease control rate (70.4% vs 90.7%).

Vascular Endothelial Growth Factor Receptor Inhibitors

Tyrosine kinase receptor inhibitors are among the various targeted therapeutics that were studied. Despite multiple studies, the role of these agents did not provide a signal that they would be instrumental in the management of patients with EC. Several VEGFR inhibitors are currently utilized in combination with other agents such as pembrolizumab and olaparib. It is important to distinguish these combinatorial agents with the data that are listed for historical purposes.

For historical purposes, sunitinib malate (211), sorafenib (Nexavar, Bayer) (212) and thalidomide (Thalomid, Celgene) (213) did not lead to significant objective responses in the corresponding phase II clinical trials and were deemed to no further investigation. Additional agents studied included brivanib, cediranib, BIBF-1120, and the VEGF-Trap aflibercept (GOG 229-F). Powell and colleagues (214) reported a phase II trial of brivanib in recurrent or persistent EC. Eligible patients received up to two prior cytotoxic agents, had measurable disease, and had a performance status of <2. Treatment consisted of brivanib 800 mg daily. Primary end points included PFS at 6 months and objective tumor response.

Forty-three patients were eligible. Eight patients (18.6%) had responses (one CR and seven PRs) and 13 patients (30.2%) had a PFS at 6 months. The median PFS and OS were 3.3 and 10.7 months, respectively. Bender and colleagues (215) evaluated a phase II trial of cediranib in the treatment of persistent EC. Cediranib was administered at 30 mg daily. Forty-eight patients were evaluable for efficacy and toxicity. A PR was observed in 12.5% of patients. Fourteen patients (29%) had a 6-month event-free survival. Median PFS was 3.65 months and median OS was 12.5 months. Vascular disorders accounted for the majority of grade 3 toxicities that included hypertension and pulmonary embolus. Diarrhea and fatigue were also reported. One patient sustained a colonic perforation. BIBF-1120 (216) (nintedanib), a potent small-molecule triple-receptor tyrosine kinase inhibitor of PDGFR-α and -β, FGFR, and VEGFR, was also recently reported. Patients were treated with single-agent nintedanib at 200 mg daily. This agent failed to show sufficient activity. Coleman et al (217) evaluated aflibercept in a similar patient population. Aflibercept, which targets VEGF and placental growth factor, was administered at 4 mg/kg IV q 14 days (q 28-day cycle). The PFS at 6 months was 41%; median PFS and OS were 2.9 and 14.6 months, respectively. The agent was associated with significant grade 3 to 4 toxicities including cardiovascular, constitutional, hemorrhage, and metabolic toxicities. Current VEGFR inhibitors in combination are listed in the following sections.

Mismatch Repair

MSI is found in 20% to 45% of type I tumors (0%-5% type II tumors) and is caused by inactivation of DNA repair genes such as MLH1, MSH2, MSH6, and PMS2 (218-220). Tumors with MSI have instability (insertions and deletions) in the simple repeated sequences found in coding and noncoding elements of many genes. Resulting frame-shift mutations may inactivate some genes including *PTEN*. MSI was first described in HNPCC. One of the most common extracolonic tumors associated with this disease is EC, and MSI has been demonstrated in both hereditary and sporadic tumors (221). MSI in EC has been reported to be between 9% and 43% (222-226). In 71% to 92% of sporadic EC, MSI has been found to be associated with hypermethylation of the *hMLH1* promoter region, whereas it seems to be less common in the promoter region of *hMSH2* (1,227). It is likely that methylation of the promoter region is an important mechanism of *hMLH1* gene inactivation in EC (228-232) and a precursor to MSI.

Universal MMR testing is now the standard of care for all uterine cancer diagnosis either by IHC that tests for the loss of expression of MMR proteins or by a polymerase chain reaction (PCR) assay that assesses MSI.

Role of Immunotherapy in the Management of Patients With Endometrial Cancer

Immunotherapy has advanced the management of patients with EC. POLE-mutated and MSI-H/MMRd ECs are associated with tumor-infiltrating lymphocytes, making them responsive checkpoint inhibitors.

Numerous trials have explored the role of immunotherapy in EC. The KEYNOTE 28 study was designed to evaluate the safety and efficacy of pembrolizumab, an anti–programmed death 1 monoclonal antibody, in patients with programmed death ligand 1 (PD-L1)-positive advanced solid tumors. Ott et al (233) reported the results in patients with advanced, locally advanced, or metastatic PD-L1-positive EC who had experienced progression after standard therapy. Patients received pembrolizumab 10 mg/kg every 2 weeks for up to 24 months or until progression or unacceptable toxicity. Primary efficacy end point was objective RR. Secondary end points included safety, duration of response, PFS, and OS. Twenty-four patients were enrolled. Three patients (13.0%) achieved confirmed PR. Three additional patients (13.0%) achieved

stable disease, with a median duration of 24.6 weeks. One patient who achieved PR had a polymerase E mutation.

The FDA granted accelerated approval of pembrolizumab for patients with MSI-H or deficient MMR (dMMR) that progressed following prior treatment.

Oaknin et al (234) reported the clinical activity of dostarlimab, an anti-PD-1 antibody that binds with high affinity to the PD-1 receptor, in patients with recurrent or advanced dMMR EC. The primary end point was objective RR and duration of response. The authors reported a confirmed response in 30 patients with an objective RR of 42.3%. The FDA approved dostarlimab for adult patients with dMMR recurrent or advanced solid tumors that have progressed on or following prior treatment and who have no satisfactory alternative treatment options.

As outlined by the The Cancer Genome Atlas (TCGA) data, POLE-mutated endometrial tumors are characterized by an extremely high mutational rate. The FDA approved pembrolizumab for the treatment of patients with unresectable or metastatic tumor mutational burden–high (TMB-H; ≥10 mutations/megabase [mut/Mb]) solid tumors, as determined by an FDA-approved test, that have progressed following prior treatment and who have no satisfactory alternative treatment option (235). This has expanded the role of immunotherapy to include both MSI tumors and those that have an ultramutated profile like the POLE-mutated ECs.

Although the role of immunotherapy is immensely advantageous in MSI-H/POLE-mutated EC, it is important to note that the majority of endometrial tumors are microsatellite stable (MSS). Recent advances have been made in this population of patients as well. Makker et al have published several studies highlighting the benefit of pembrolizumab and lenvatinib in the management of patients with MSS endometrial tumors. KEYNOTE 146 (236) is a phase II single-arm study of pembrolizumab and lenvatinib for MSS EC. In this study, patients with pathologically confirmed and metastatic EC, with less than or equal to two prior lines of systemic therapy, were treated with lenvatinib (20 mg/d) and pembrolizumab 200 mg q 3 weeks. The primary end point was ORR at week 24. The authors of this study reported an ORR of 38.3% in patients that were not MSI-H or deficient MMR. The results of this trial led to the randomized trial of lenvatinib and pembrolizumab versus chemotherapy with either doxorubicin or paclitaxel called KEYNOTE 775 (237). The primary end points were PRS and OS. A total of 827 patients (697 with proficient MMR [pMMR] disease and 130 with dMMR disease) were randomly assigned to receive lenvatinib plus pembrolizumab or chemotherapy. The median PFS was longer with lenvatinib plus pembrolizumab than with chemotherapy (pMMR population: 6.6 vs 3.8 months). The median OS was longer with lenvatinib plus pembrolizumab than with chemotherapy (pMMR population: 17.4 vs 12.0 months). Adverse events (grade 3+) occurred in 88.9% of the patients who received lenvatinib plus pembrolizumab and in 72.7% of those who received chemotherapy.

Given the results of this trial, an upfront trial called the ENGOT-en9LEAP-001 trial is being conducted, which is a phase III study of first-line pembrolizumab plus lenvatinib versus chemotherapy in advanced or recurrent EC.

Several trials in EC are currently being explored utilizing the combination of checkpoint inhibitors and chemotherapy in the upfront setting. These trials include the NRG-018 trial (NCT03914612) that adds pembrolizumab to the backbone of carboplatin and paclitaxel and the RUBY trial (ENGOT-EN-6; GOG3031; NCT03981796), which is a combination of dostarlimab and chemotherapy.

HER2/neu

HER2/neu is a proto-oncogene, the product of which is a transmembrane growth factor receptor, p185erb-2, which shares some homology with EGFR. It is normally expressed at low levels in the cycling endometrium. HER2/neu is frequently overexpressed or amplified in 10% to 30% of type I and 40% to 80% of type II ECs (238) and has been associated with advanced stage (239), decreased differentiation, aggressive cell types, particularly including the clear cell type (240) and deep myometrial invasion. The significance of HER2/neu amplification or overexpression as a predictor of survival is somewhat unclear, with no apparent association of overexpression to outcome being identified in several studies (241), (242-250), but a statistically significant relationship exists in most others even after adjusting for other known risk factors. In addition to its potential utility as an indicator of poor prognosis, systemic therapy using antibodies directed against the HER2/neu protein has been investigated for patients with tumors that express the protein at high levels. **Trastuzumab** monotherapy failed to demonstrate significant activity in the recent GOG 181-B study (251). No responses were achieved, although 12 of 34 women experienced stabilization. Given the higher rates of HER2 overexpression seen in type II tumors, Fader et al (252) conducted a randomized phase II trial of carboplatin-paclitaxel with and without trastuzumab in patients with advanced or recurrent uterine serous carcinoma who overexpress HER2/neu. Eligible patients had primary stage III or IV or recurrent HER2/neu-positive disease. Patients were randomly assigned to receive carboplatin-paclitaxel (control arm) for six cycles with or without intravenous trastuzumab (experimental arm) until progression or unacceptable toxicity. The primary end point was PFS. The authors reported a median PFS of 8.0 (control) versus 12.6 months (experimental; $P = .005$; HR, 0.44). The median PFS was 9.3 (control) versus 17.9 (experimental) months among 41 patients with stage III or IV disease undergoing primary treatment ($P = .013$; HR, 0.40) and 6.0 (control) versus 9.2 months (experimental), respectively, among 17 patients with recurrent disease ($P = .003$; HR, 0.14; 90% CI, 0.04-0.53).

Recently, Fader et al (253) and colleagues reported an updated OS analysis. After a median follow-up of 25.9 months, the median PFS favored the triple-agent arm. The median PFS was 8.0 versus 12.9 months (HR, 0.46) in the control and trastuzumab arms, respectively. The median PFS was 9.3 versus 17.7 months among 41 patients with stage III to IV disease undergoing primary treatment (HR, 0.44). OS was higher in the trastuzumab arm compared with the control arm, with medians of 29.6 versus 24.4 months (HR, 0.58; $P = .046$). The benefit was most pronounced in those with stage III to IV disease, with survival median not reached in the trastuzumab arm versus 24.4 months in the control arm (HR, 0.49; $P = .041$).

WEE1 Inhibitors

WEE1 kinase is a key regulator of the G2/M- and S-phase cell-cycle checkpoints. WEE-1 inhibition has two major effects, namely the dysregulation of the G2/M checkpoint and an increase in replication stress. Cells with TP53 mutation/loss have lost their G1/S checkpoint, which leads to early entry into S-phase, an increase in replication stress, and an increased dependency on the G2/M checkpoint. Liu et al (254) recently reported a phase II study of the WEE1 inhibitor adavosertib in recurrent uterine serous carcinoma. This was a single-arm two-stage phase II study with two end points: namely objective RR and rate of PFS at 6 months (PFS6). The authors reported an objective RR of 29.4% (95% CI, 15.1-47.5). Sixteen patients were progression free at 6 months, for a PFS6 rate of 47.1% (95% CI, 29.8-64.9). Median PFS was 6.1 months, and median duration of response was 9.0 months. Frequent treatment-related adverse events included diarrhea (76.5%), fatigue (64.7%), nausea (61.8%), and hematologic adverse events.

The Poly (Adenosine Diphosphate Ribose) Polymerase

Poly (adenosine diphosphate ribose) polymerase (PARP) is a family of nuclear, multifunctional enzymes that mediates the recruitment of the DNA repair machinery through the base-excision repair pathway (255). The antineoplastic effect of PARP inhibitors stems from their ability to enhance the genomic instability of tumor cells by simultaneously targeting DNA repair pathways and exploiting their intrinsic deficiencies in the homologous recombination pathway through the phenomenon of synthetic lethality (255). PTEN loss is considered a component of BRCA-ness phenotype. It impedes repair of DNA double-strand breaks via homologous recombination, thereby creating cellular susceptibility to PARP inhibition (256). Preclinical data have shown a correlation between in vitro sensitivity to PARP inhibition and mutated PTEN status in EC cell lines (257), providing a strong rationale for testing PARP inhibitors in EC, especially type I, which harbors PTEN functional loss in 80% of cases.

Recently reported were the results a randomized, phase II study comparing single-agent olaparib, single-agent cediranib, and the combination of cediranib/olaparib in women with recurrent, persistent, or metastatic EC (Trial NRG GY012) (258). Eligible patients had to have received at least one prior platinum-containing chemotherapy but two or less prior lines of chemotherapy for recurrent EC. Cediranib was administered 30 mg po daily and olaparib 300 mg po bd. The combination was dosed as such: cediranib 20 mg po qd/olaparib 300 mg po bid. The primary end point was PFS. Patients were stratified by histology (serous vs endometrioid). The median PFS was 3.8 months for cediranib, 2.0 months for olaparib, and 5.5 months for the combination of cediranib and olaparib. The efficacy of the combination of cediranib and olaparib was not significantly different when compared to single-agent cediranib. Single-agent olaparib demonstrated poor efficacy. This study continues to explore other combinations with, for example, olaparib and capivasertib, olaparib and durvalumab, and cediranib and durvalumab.

REFERENCES

1. Kauppila A, Kujansuu E, Vihko R. Cytosol estrogen and progestin receptors in endometrial carcinoma of patients treated with surgery, radiotherapy, and progestin. Clinical correlates. Cancer. 1982;50(10):2157-2162.

2. Macdonald RR, Thorogood J, Mason MK. A randomized trial of progestogens in the primary treatment of endometrial carcinoma. Br J Obstet Gynaecol. 1988;95:166-174.

3. Vergote I, Kjorstad K, Abeler V, et al. A randomized trial of adjuvant progestogen in early endometrial cancer. Cancer. 1989;64:1011.

4. von Minckwitz G, Loibl S, Brunnert K, et al. Adjuvant endocrine treatment with medroxyprogesterone acetate or tamoxifen in stage I and II endometrial cancer—a multicentre, open, controlled, prospectively randomised trial. Eur J Cancer. 2002;38:2265-2271.

5. Morrow C, Bundy B, Homesley H, et al. Doxorubicin as an adjuvant following surgery and radiation therapy in patients with high-risk endometrial carcinoma, stage I and occult stage II: a Gynecologic Oncology Group study. Gynecol Oncol. 1990;36:166-171.

6. Randall M, Filiaci V, Muss H, et al. Randomized phase III trial of WART versus doxorubicin and cisplatin chemotherapy in advanced endometrial carcinoma: a GOG study. J Clin Oncol. 2006;24:36-44.

7. Keys HM, Roberts JA, Brunetto VL, et al. A phase III trial of surgery with or without adjunctive external pelvic radiation therapy in intermediate risk endometrial adenocarcinoma: a Gynecologic Oncology Group study. Gynecol Oncol. 2004;92:744-751.

8. Creutzberg CL, van Putten WL, Koper PC, et al. Surgery and postoperative radiotherapy versus surgery alone for patients with stage-1 endometrial carcinoma: multicentre randomised trial. PORTEC Study Group. Post Operative Radiation Therapy in Endometrial Carcinoma. Lancet. 2000;355:1404-1411.

9. Guntupalli S, Zighelboim I, Kizer N, et al. Lymphovascular space invasion is an independent risk factor for nodal disease and poor outcomes in endometrioid endometrial cancer. Gynecol Oncol. 2012;124:31-35.

10. Nout RA, Smit VT, Putter H, et al. Vaginal brachytherapy versus pelvic external radiotherapy for patients with endometrial cancer of high-intermediate risk (PORTEC 2): an open lable, non inferiority, randomized trial. Lancet. 2010;375:816-823.

11. Nout RA, Putter H, Jürgenliemk-Schulz IM, et al. Quality of life after pelvic radiotherapy or vaginal brachytherapy for endometrial cancer: first results of the randomized PORTEC-2 trial. J Clin Oncol. 2009;27:3547-3556.

12. Nout RA, Putter H, Jürgenliemk-Schulz IM, et al. Five year quality of life of endometrial cancer patients treated in the randomized PORTEC 2 trial and comparison with norm data. Eur J Cancer. 2012;48(11):1638-1648.

13. ASTEC/EN.5 Study Group, Blake P, Swart AM, et al. Adjuvant external beam radiotherapy in the treatment of endometrial cancer (MRC ASTEC and NCIC CTG EN.5 randomized trials): pooled trial results, systematic review, and meta-analysis. *Lancet.* 2009;373:137-146.

14. Lee CM, Szabo A, Shrieve DC, et al. Frequency and effect of adjuvant radiation therapy among women with stage I endometrial adenocarcinoma. *JAMA.* 2006;295(4):389-397.

15. Patel MK, Cote ML, Ali-Fehmi R, et al. Trends in the utilization of adjuvant vaginal cuff brachytherapy and/or external beam radiation treatment in stage I and II endometrial cancer: a surveillance, epidemiology, and end-results study. *Int J Radiat Oncol Biol Phys.* 2012;83(1):178-184.

16. Aalders J, Abeler V, Kolstad P, et al. Postoperative external irradiation and prognostic parameters in stage I endometrial carcinoma: clinical and histopathologic study of 540 patients. *Obstet Gynecol.* 1980;56:419-427.

17. Greven KM, D'Agostino RB Jr, Lanciano RM, et al. Is there a role for a brachytherapy vaginal cuff boost in the adjuvant management of patients with uterine-confined endometrial cancer? *Int J Radiat Oncol Biol Phys.* 1998;42:101-104.

18. Randall ME, Wilder J, Greven K, et al. Role of intracavitary cuff boost after adjuvant external irradiation in early endometrial carcinoma. *Int J Radiat Oncol Biol Phys.* 1990;19:49-54.

19. Rush S, Gal D, Potters L, et al. Pelvic control following external beam radiation for surgical stage I endometrial adenocarcinoma. *Int J Radiat Oncol Biol Phys.* 1995;33:851-854.

20. Kucera H, Vaura N, Weghoupt K. Benefit of external irradiation in pathologic stage I endometrial carcinoma: a prospective clinical trial of 605 patients who received postoperative vaginal irradiation and additional pelvic irradiation in the presence of unfavorable prognostic factors. *Gynecol Oncol.* 1990;38:99-104.

21. Nori D, Merimsky O, Batata M, et al. Postoperative high dose-rate intravaginal brachytherapy combined with external irradiation for early stage endometrial cancer: a long-term follow-up. *Int J Radiat Oncol Biol Phys.* 1994;30:831-837.

22. Orr JW, Holimon J, Orr P. Stage I corpus cancer: is teletherapy necessary. *Am J Obstet Gynecol.* 1997;176:777-789.

23. Mohan D, Samuels M, Selim M, et al. Long term outcomes of therapeutic pelvic lymphadenectomy for stage I endometrial adenocarcinoma. *Gynecol Oncol.* 1998;70:165-171.

24. Horowitz NS, Peters WA III, Smith MR, et al. Adjuvant high dose rate vaginal brachytherapy as treatment of stage I and II endometrial carcinoma. *Obstet Gynecol.* 2002;99:235-240.

25. Anderson JM, Stea B, Hallum AV, et al. High-dose-rate postoperative vaginal cuff irradiation alone for stage IB and IC endometrial cancer. *Int J Radiat Oncol Biol Phys.* 2000;46:417-425.

26. MacLeod C, Fowler A, Duval P, et al. High-dose-rate brachytherapy alone post-hysterectomy for endometrial cancer. *Int J Radiat Oncol Biol Phys.* 1998;42:1033-1039.

27. Petereit DG, Tannehill SP, Grosen EA, et al. Outpatient vaginal cuff brachytherapy for endometrial cancer. *Int J Gynecol Cancer.* 1999;9:456-462.

28. Maxwell GL, Schildkraut J, Calingaert B, et al. Progestin and estrogen potency of combination oral contraceptives and endometrial cancer risk. *Gynecol Oncol.* 2006;103:535-540.

29. Elliot P, Green D. The efficacy of postoperative vaginal irradiation in preventing vaginal recurrence in endometrial cancer. *Int J Gynecol Cancer.* 1994;4:84.

30. Straughn JM, Huh W, Kelly J, et al. Conservative management of stage I endometrial carcinoma after surgical staging. *Gynecol Oncol.* 2002;84:194-200.

31. Creasman WT, Morrow CP, Bundy BN, et al. Surgical pathologic spread patterns of endometrial cancer: a Gynecologic Oncology Group study. *Cancer.* 1987;60:2035-2041.

32. Alektiar KM, McKee A, Venkatraman E, et al. Intravaginal high-dose-rate brachytherapy for stage IB (FIGO grade 1, 2) endometrial cancer. *Int J Radiat Oncol Biol Phys.* 2002;53:707-713.

33. Sorbe B, Staumits A, Karlsson L. Intravaginal high-dose-rate brachytherapy for stage I endometrial cancer: a randomized study of two dose-per-fraction levels. *Int J Radiat Oncol Biol Phys.* 2005;62(5):1385-1389.

34. Mariani A, Webb M, Kenney G, et al. Endometrial cancer: predictors of peritoneal failure. *Gynecol Oncol.* 2003;89:236-242.

35. Narayan K, Khaw P, Bernshaw D, et al. Prognostic significance of lymphovascular space invasion and nodal involvement in intermediate- and high-risk endometrial cancer patients treated with curative intent using surgery and adjuvant radiotherapy. *Int J Gynecol Cancer.* 2012;22:260-266.

36. Alektiar KM, McKee A, Lin O, et al. The significance of the amount of myometrial invasion in patients with stage IB endometrial carcinoma. *Cancer.* 2002;95:316-321.

37. Scholten AN, Creutzberg CL, Noordijk EM, et al. Long-term outcome in endometrial carcinoma favors a two—instead of a three—tiered grading system. *Int J Radiat Oncol Biol Phys.* 2002;52:1067-1074.

38. Irwin C, Levin W, Fyles A, et al. The role of adjuvant radiotherapy in carcinoma of the endometrium—results in 550 patients with pathologic stage I disease. *Gynecol Oncol.* 1998;70:247-254.

39. Piver M, Hempling R. A prospective trial of post-operative vaginal radium/cesium for grade 1–2 less than 50% myometrial invasion and pelvic radiation therapy for grade 3 or deep myometrial invasion in surgical stage I endometrial adenocarcinoma. *Cancer.* 1990;66:133.

40. Straughn JM, Huh W, Orr J, et al. Stage IC adenocarcinoma of the endometrium: survival comparisons of surgically staged patients with and without adjuvant therapy. *Gynecol Oncol.* 2003;89:295-300.

41. Chadha M, Nanavati PJ, Liu P, et al. Patterns of failure in endometrial carcinoma stage IB grade 3 and IC patients treated with postoperative vaginal vault brachytherapy. *Gynecol Oncol.* 1999;75:103-107.

42. Alektiar KM, Chi D, Barakat RR. Risk stratification of death from endometrial cancer in patients with early stage disease. *Int J Radiat Oncol Biol Phys.* 2007;69(3):S387-S388.

43. Solhjem MC, Petersen IA, Haddock MG. Vaginal brachytherapy alone is sufficient adjuvant treatment of surgical stage I endometrial cancer. *Int J Radiat Oncol Biol Phys.* 2005;62(5):1379-1384.

44. Rittenberg PVC, Lotocki RJ, Heywood MS, et al. High-risk surgical stage 1 endometrial cancer: outcomes with vault brachytherapy alone. *Gynecol Oncol.* 2003;89(2):288-294.

45. Creutzberg C, van Putten W, Warlam-Rodenhuis C, et al. Outcome of high-risk stage IC, grade 3 compared with stage I endometrial carcinoma patients: the postoperative radiation therapy in endometrial carcinoma trial. *J Clin Oncol.* 2004;22:1234-1241.

46. ASTEC Study Group. Efficacy of systematic pelvic lymphadenectomy in endometrial cancer (MRC ASTEC trial): a randomized study. *Lancet.* 2009;373:125-136.

47. Benedetti Panici P, Basile S, Maneschi F, et al. Systematic pelvic lymphadenectomy versus no lymphadenectomy in early-stage endometrial carcinoma: Randomized clinical trial. *J Natl Cancer Inst.* 2008;100:1707-1716.

48. Weiss MF, Connell PP, Waggoner S, et al. External pelvic radiation therapy in stage IC endometrial carcinoma. *Obstet Gynecol.* 1999;93:599-602.

49. Pitson G, Colgan T, Levin W, et al. Stage II endometrial carcinoma: prognostic factors and risk classification in 170 patients. *Int J Radiat Oncol Biol Phys.* 2002;53:862-867.

50. Fanning J. Long-term survival of intermediate risk endometrial cancer (stage IG3, IC, II) treated with full lymphadenectomy and brachytherapy without teletherapy. *Gynecol Oncol.* 2001;82:371-374.

51. Ng TY, Nicklin JL, Perrin LC, et al. Postoperative vaginal vault brachytherapy for node-negative stage II (occult) endometrial carcinoma. *Gynecol Oncol.* 2001;81:193-195.

52. Pecorelli S. Revised FIGO staging for carcinoma of the vulva, cervix, and endometrium. *Int J Gynecol Obstet.* 2009;105:109-110.

53. Rittenberg PVC, Lotocki RJ, Heywood MS, et al. Stage II endometrial carcinoma: limiting post-operative radiotherapy to the vaginal vault in node-negative tumors. *Gynecol Oncol.* 2005;98(3):434-438.

54. Connell PP, Rotmensch J, Waggoner S, et al. The significance of adnexal involvement in endometrial carcinoma. *Gynecol Oncol.* 1999;74:74-79.

55. Ashman JB, Connell PP, Yamada D, et al. Outcome of endometrial carcinoma patients with involvement of the uterine serosa. *Gynecol Oncol.* 2001;82:338-343.

56. Nelson G, Randall M, Sutton G, et al. FIGO stage IIIC endometrial carcinoma with metastases confined to pelvic lymph nodes: analysis of treatment outcomes, prognostic variables, and failure patterns following adjuvant radiation therapy. *Gynecol Oncol.* 1999;75:211-214.

57. Greven K, Corn B, Lanciano RM. Pathologic stage III endometrial carcinoma. *Cancer.* 1993;71:3697.

58. Mariani A, Webb MJ, Keeney GL, et al. Stage IIIC endometrioid corpus cancer includes distinct subgroups. *Gynecol Oncol.* 2002;87:12-17.

59. Corn BW, Lanciano RM, Greven KM, et al. Endometrial carcinoma with para-aortic lymphadenopathy: patterns of failure and opportunity for cure. *Int J Radiat Oncol Biol Phys.* 1992;24:223.

60. Hicks ML, Piver S, Jeffrey LP, et al. Survival in patients with para-aortic lymph node metastases from endometrial adenocarcinoma clinically limited to the uterus. *Int J Radiat Oncol Biol Phys.* 1993;26:607.

61. Rose PG, Cha SD, Tak WK, et al. Radiation therapy for surgically proven para-aortic node metastasis in endometrial carcinoma. *Int J Radiat Oncol Biol Phys.* 1992;24:229-233.

62. Mariani A, Dowdy S, Cliby W, et al. Efficacy of systematic lymphadenectomy and adjuvant radiotherapy in node-positive endometrial cancer patients. *Gynecol Oncol.* 2006;101:200-208.

63. Gibbons S, Martinez A, Schary M, et al. Adjuvant whole abdominopelvic irradiation for high-risk endometrial carcinoma. *Int J Radiat Oncol Biol Phys.* 1991;21:1019-1025.

64. Martinez A, Podratz K. Results of whole abdomino-pelvic radiation with nodal boost for patients with endometrial cancer at high risk of failure in the peritoneal cavity. *Hematol Oncol Clin North Am.* 1988;2:431.

65. Sutton G, Axelrod J, Bundy B, et al. Whole abdominal radiotherapy in the adjuvant treatment of patients with stage III and IV endometrial cancer: a Gynecologic Oncology Group study. *Gynecol Oncol.* 2005;97(3):755-763.

66. Maggi R, Lissoni A, Spina F, et al. Adjuvant chemotherapy vs. radiotherapy in high-risk endometrial carcinoma: results of a randomised trial. *Br J Cancer.* 2006;95(3):266-271.

67. Greven K, Winter K, Underhill K, et al. Final analysis of RTOG 9708: adjuvant postoperative irradiation combined with cisplatin/paclitaxel chemotherapy following surgery for patients with high-risk endometrial cancer. *Gynecol Oncol.* 2006;103(1):155-159.

68. Homesley HD, Filiaci V, Gibbons SK, et al. A randomized phase III trial in advanced endometrial carcinoma of surgery and volume directed radiation followed by cisplatin and doxorubicin with or without paclitaxel: a Gynecologic Oncology Group study. *Gynecol Oncol.* 2009;112:543-552.

69. Janda M, Gebski V, Brand A, et al. Quality of life after total laparoscopic hysterectomy versus total abdominal hysterectomy for stage I endometrial cancer (LACE): a randomised trial. *Lancet Oncol.* 2010;11:772-781.

70. Mundt AJ, Murphy KT, Rotmensch J, et al. Surgery and postoperative radiation therapy in FIFO stage IIIC endometrial carcinoma. *Int J Radiat Oncol Biol Phys.* 2001;50:1154-1160.

71. Mundt AJ, McBride R, Rotmensch J, et al. Significant pelvic recurrence in high risk pathologic stage I-IV endometrial carcinoma patients after chemotherapy alone: implications for adjuvant radiation therapy. *Int J Radiat Oncol Biol Phys.* 2001;50:1145-1153.

72. Milosevic MF, Dembo AJ, Thomas GM. The clinical significance of malignant peritoneal cytology in stage I endometrial carcinoma. *Int J Gynecol Cancer.* 1992;2:225-235.

73. Soper JT, Creasman WT, Clarke-Pearson DL, et al. Intraperitoneal chromic phosphate 32P suspension therapy of malignant peritoneal cytology in endometrial carcinoma. *Am J Obstet Gynecol.* 1985;153:191-196.

74. Eltabbakh GH, Piver MS, Hempling RE, et al. Excellent long-term survival and absence of vaginal recurrences in 332 patients with low-risk stage I endometrial adenocarcinoma treated with hysterectomy and vaginal brachytherapy without formal staging lymph node sampling: report of a prospective trial. *Int J Radiat Oncol Biol Phys.* 1997;38:373-380.

75. Nag S, Erickson B, Parikh S, et al. The American Brachytherapy Society recommendations for high-dose-rate brachytherapy for carcinoma of the endometrium. *Int J Radiat Oncol Biol Phys.* 2000;48:779-790.

76. Rouanet P, Dubois JB, Gely S, et al. Exclusive radiation therapy in endometrial carcinoma. *Int J Radiat Oncol Biol Phys.* 1993;26:223-228.

77. Grigsby P, Kuske R, Perez CA, et al. Medically inoperable stage I adenocarcinoma of the endometrium treated with radiotherapy alone. *Int J Radiat Oncol Biol Phys.* 1986;13:483.

78. Knocke TH, Kucera H, Weidinger B, et al. Primary treatment of endometrial carcinoma with high-dose-rate brachytherapy: results of 12 years of experience with 280 patients. *Int J Radiat Oncol Biol Phys.* 1997;37:359-365.

79. Nguyen TV, Petereit DG. High-dose-rate brachytherapy for medically inoperable stage I endometrial cancer. *Gynecol Oncol.* 1995;59:370-375.

80. Niazi TM, Souhami L, Portelance L, et al. Long term results of high dose rate brachytherapy in the primary treatment of medically inoperable stage I-II endometrial carcinoma. *Int J Radiat Oncol Biol Phys.* 2005;63:1108-1113.

81. Fishman DA, Roberts KB, Chambers JT, et al. Radiation therapy as exclusive treatment for medically inoperable patients with stage I and II endometrioid carcinoma with endometrium. *Gynecol Oncol.* 1996;61(2):189-196.

82. Kucera H, Knocke TH, Kucera E, et al. Treatment of endometrial carcinoma with high-dose-rate brachytherapy alone in medically inoperable stage I patients. *Acta Obstet Gynecol Scand.* 1998;77:1008-1012.

83. Nicklin JL, Petersen RW. Stage 3B adenocarcinoma of the endometrium: a clinicopathologic study. *Gynecol Oncol.* 2000;78:203-207.

84. Small W Jr, Beriwal S, Demanes DJ, et al. American Brachytherapy Society consensus guidelines for adjuvant vaginal cuff brachytherapy after hysterectomy. *Brachytherapy.* 2012;1:58-67.

85. Small W Jr, Erickson B, Kwakwa F. American Brachytherapy Society survey regarding practice patterns of postoperative irradiation for endometrial cancer: current status of vaginal brachytherapy. *Int J Radiat Oncol Biol Phys.* 2005;63:1502-1507.

86. Ghosh K, Padilla LA, Murray KP, et al. Using a belly board device to reduce the small bowel volume within pelvic radiation fields in women with postoperatively treated cervical carcinoma. *Gynecol Oncol.* 2001;83:271-275.

87. Mundt AJ, Lujan AE, Rotmensch J, et al. Intensity-modulated whole pelvic radiotherapy in women with gynecologic malignancies. *Int J Radiat Oncol Biol Phys.* 2002;52(5):1330-1337.

88. Mundt AJ, Mell LK, Roeske JC. Preliminary analysis of chronic gastrointestinal toxicity in gynecology patients treated with intensity-modulated whole pelvic radiation therapy. *Int J Radiat Oncol Biol Phys.* 2003;56(5):1354-1360.

89. Roeske JC, Lujan A, Rotmensch J, et al. Intensity-modulated whole pelvic radiation therapy in patients with gynecologic malignancies. *Int J Radiat Oncol Biol Phys.* 2000;48:1613-1621.

90. Lujan AE, Mundt AJ, Roeske JC, et al. Intensity-modulated radiotherapy as a means of reducing dose to bone marrow in gynecologic patients receiving whole pelvic radiotherapy. *Int J Radiat Oncol Biol Phys.* 2003;57:516-521.

91. Buchali A, Koswig S, Dinges S, et al. Impact of the filling status of the bladder and rectum on their integral dose distribution and the movement of the uterus in the treatment planning of gynaecological cancer. *Radiother Oncol.* 1999;52:29-34.

92. Huh, SJ, Park W, Han Y. Interfractional variation in position of the uterus during radical radiotherapy for cervical cancer. *Radiother Oncol.* 2004;71:73-79.

93. Salama JK, Mundt AJ, Roeske J, et al. Preliminary outcome and toxicity report of extended-field, intensity-modulated radiation therapy for gynecologic malignancies. *Int J Radiat Oncol Biol Phys.* 2006;65:1170-1176.

94. Curran WJ, Whittington R, Peters AJ, et al. Vaginal recurrences of endometrial carcinoma: the prognostic value of staging by a primary vaginal carcinoma system. *Int J Radiat Oncol Biol Phys.* 1988;15:803-808.

95. Sears J, Greven K. Prognostic factors and treatment outcome for patients with locally recurrent endometrial cancer. *Cancer.* 1994;74:1303-1308.

96. Wylie J, Irwin C, Pintilie M, et al. Results of radical radiotherapy for recurrent endometrial cancer. *Gynecol Oncol.* 2000;77:66-72.

97. Creutzberg CL, van Putten WL, Koper PC, et al. Survival after relapse in patients with endometrial cancer: results from a randomized trial. *Gynecol Oncol.* 2003;89:201-209.

98. Jhingran A, Burke TW, Eifel PJ, et al. Definitive radiotherapy for patients with isolated vaginal recurrence of endometrial carcinoma after hysterectomy. *Int J Radiat Oncol Biol Phys.* 2003;56:1366-1372.

99. Hogberg T, Signorelli M, de Oliveira CF, et al. Sequential adjuvant chemotherapy and radiotherapy in endometrial cancer-results from two randomised studies. *Eur J Cancer.* 2010;46(13):2422-2431.

100. McMeekin DS, Filiaci VL, Aghajanian C, et al. A randomized phase III trial of pelvic radiation therapy (PXRT) versus vaginal cuff brachytherapy followed by paclitaxel/carboplatin chemotherapy (VCB/C) in patients with high risk (HR), early-stage endometrial cancer (EC): a Gynecologic Oncology Group trial. *Gynecol Oncol.* 2014;134(2):438.

101. Viswanathan AN, Moughan J, Miller BE, et al. NRG Oncology/RTOG 0921: a phase 2 study of postoperative intensity modulated radiotherapy with concurrent cisplatin and bevacizumab followed by carboplatin and paclitaxel for patients with endometrial cancer. *Cancer.* 2015;121:2156-2163.

102. van den Heerik ASVM, Horeweg N, Nout RA, et al. PORTEC-4a: international randomized trial of molecular profile-based adjuvant treatment for women with high-intermediate risk endometrial cancer. *Int J Gynecol Cancer.* 2020;12:2002-2007.

103. Talhouk A, McConechy MK, Leung S, et al. A clinically applicable molecular-based classification for endometrial cancers. *Br J Cancer.* 2015;113:299-310.

104. Stelloo E, Nout RA, Osse EM, et al. Improved risk assessment by integrating molecular and clinicopathological factors in early-stage endometrial cancer-combined analysis of the PORTEC cohorts. *Clin Cancer Res.* 2016;22:4215-4224.

105. Kommoss FK, Karnezis AN, Kommoss F, et al. L1Cam further stratifies endometrial carcinoma patients with no specific molecular risk profile. *Br J Cancer.* 2018;119:480-486.

106. Campora E, Vidali A, Mammoliti S, et al. Treatment of advanced or recurrent adenocarcinoma of the endometrium with doxorubicin and cyclophosphamide. *Eur J Gynaecol Oncol.* 1990;11(3):181-183.

107. Muggia FM, Chia G, Reed LJ, et al. Doxorubicin-cyclophosphamide: effective chemotherapy for advanced endometrial adenocarcinoma. *Am J Obstet Gynecol.* 1977;128(3):314-319.

108. Seski JC, Edwards CL, Gershenson DM, et al. Doxorubicin and cyclophosphamide chemotherapy for disseminated endometrial cancer. *Obstet Gynecol.* 1981;58(1):88-91.

109. Edmonson JH, Krook JE, Hilton JF, et al. Randomized phase II studies of cisplatin and a combination of cyclophosphamide-doxorubicin-cisplatin (CAP) in patients with progestin-refractory advanced endometrial carcinoma. *Gynecol Oncol.* 1987;28(1):20-24.

110. Burke TW, Stringer CA, Morris M, et al. Prospective treatment of advanced or recurrent endometrial carcinoma with cisplatin, doxorubicin, and cyclophosphamide. *Gynecol Oncol.* 1991;40(3):264-267.

111. Dunton CJ, Pfeifer SM, Braitman LE, et al. Treatment of advanced and recurrent endometrial cancer with cisplatin, doxorubicin, and cyclophosphamide. *Gynecol Oncol.* 1991;41(2):113-116.

112. Hancock KC, Freedman RS, Edwards CL, et al. Use of cisplatin, doxorubicin, and cyclophosphamide to treat advanced and recurrent adenocarcinoma of the endometrium. *Cancer Treat Rep.* 1986;70(6):789-791.

113. Barrett RJ, Blessing JA, Homesley HD, et al., Circadian-timed combination doxorubicin-cisplatin chemotherapy for advanced endometrial carcinoma. A phase II study of the Gynecologic Oncology Group. *Am J Clin Oncol.* 1993;16(6):494-496.

114. Pasmantier MW, Coleman M, Silver RT, et al. Treatment of advanced endometrial carcinoma with doxorubicin and cisplatin: effects on both untreated and previously treated patients. *Cancer Treat Rep.* 1985;69(5):539-542.

115. Seltzer V, Vogl SE, Kaplan BH. Adriamycin and cis-diamminedichloroplatinum in the treatment of metastatic endometrial adenocarcinoma. *Gynecol Oncol.* 1984;19(3):308-313.

116. Thigpen JT, Brady MF, Homesley HD, et al. Phase III trial of doxorubicin with or without cisplatin in advanced endometrial carcinoma: a Gynecologic Oncology Group study. *J Clin Oncol.* 2004;22(19):3902-3908.

117. Trope C, Johnsson JE, Simonsen E, et al. Treatment of recurrent endometrial adenocarcinoma with a combination of doxorubicin and cisplatin. *Am J Obstet Gynecol.* 1984;149(4):379-381.

118. Susumu N, Sagae S, Udagawa Y, et al. Randomized phase III trial of pelvic radiotherapy vs cisplatin-based combined chemotherapy in patients with intermediate and high-risk endometrial cancer: a JGOG study. *Gynecol Oncol.* 2008;108:236-233.

119. Ball HG, Blessing JA, Lentz SS, et al. A phase II trial of paclitaxel in patients with advanced or recurrent adenocarcinoma of the endometrium: a Gynecologic Oncology Group study. *Gynecol Oncol.* 1996;62(2):278-281.

120. Gunthert AR, Ackermann S, Beckmann MW, et al. Phase II study of weekly docetaxel in patients with recurrent or metastatic endometrial cancer: AGO Uterus-4. *Gynecol Oncol.* 2007;104(1):86-90.

121. Lincoln S, Blessing JA, Lee RB, et al. Activity of paclitaxel as second-line chemotherapy in endometrial carcinoma: a Gynecologic Oncology Group study. *Gynecol Oncol.* 2003;88(3):277-281.

122. Fleming GF, Filiaci VL, Bentley RC, et al. Phase III randomized trial of doxorubicin + cisplatin versus doxorubicin + 24-h paclitaxel + filgrastim in endometrial carcinoma: a Gynecologic Oncology Group study. *Ann Oncol.* 2004;15(8):1173-1178.

123. Fleming GF, Brunetto VL, Cella D, et al. Phase III trial of doxorubicin plus cisplatin with or without paclitaxel plus filgrastim in advanced endometrial carcinoma: a Gynecologic Oncology Group study. *J Clin Oncol.* 2004;22(11):2159-2166.

124. Hoskins PJ, Swenerton KD, Pike JA, et al. Paclitaxel and carboplatin, alone or with irradiation, in advanced or recurrent endometrial cancer: a phase II study. *J Clin Oncol.* 2001;19(20):4048-4053.

125. Sovak MA, Dupont J, Hensley ML, et al. Paclitaxel and carboplatin in the treatment of advanced or recurrent endometrial cancer: a large retrospective study. *Int J Gynecol Cancer.* 2007;17(1):197-203.

126. Miller D, Filiaci V, Fleming G, et al. Randomized phase III noninferiority trial of first line chemotherapy for metastatic recurrent endometrial carcinoma: a Gynecologic Oncology Group study. 2012 Annual Meeting on Women's Cancer (SGO): late breaking abstract 1. *Gynecol Oncol.* 2012;125:771-773.

127. Secord AA, Havrilesky LJ, O'Malley DM, et al. A multicenter evaluation of sequential multimodality therapy and clinical outcome for the treatment of advanced endometrial cancer. *Gynecol Oncol.* 2009;114(3):442-447.

128. de Boer SM, Powell M, Mileshkin, et al. Adjuvant chemoradiotherapy versus radiotherapy alone for women with high-risk endometrial cancer (PORTEC-3): results of an international, open-label, multicentre, randomised, phase 3 trial. *Lancet Oncol.* 2018;19(3):295-309.

129. de Boer SM, Powell M, Mileshkin, et al. Adjuvant chemoradiotherapy versus radiotherapy in women with high-risk endometrial cancer (PORTEC3): patterns of recurrence and post hoc survival analysis of a randomized phase 3 trial. *Lancet Oncol.* 2019;20(9);1273-1285.

130. Matei D, Filiaci V, Randall M, et al. Adjuvant chemotherapy plus radiation therapy for locally advanced endometrial cancer. *NEJM.* 2019;380:2317-2326.

131. Podratz KC, O'Brien PC, Malkasian GD Jr, et al. Effects of progestational agents in treatment of endometrial carcinoma. *Obstet Gynecol.* 1985;66:106-110.

132. Asbury RF, Brunetto VL, Lee RB, et al. Goserelin acetate as treatment for recurrent endometrial carcinoma: a Gynecologic Oncology Group study. *Am J Clin Oncol.* 2002;25:557-560.

133. McMeekin DS, Gordon A, Fowler J, et al. A phase II trial of arzoxifene, a selective estrogen response modulator, in patients with recurrent or advanced endometrial cancer. *Gynecol Oncol.* 2003;90:64-69.

134. Piver MS, Barlow JJ, Lurain JR, et al. Medroxyprogesterone acetate (Depo-Provera) vs. hydroxyprogesterone caproate (Delalutin) in women with metastatic endometrial adenocarcinoma. *Cancer.* 1980;45:268-272.

135. Quinn MA, Cauchi M, Fortune D. Endometrial carcinoma: steroid receptors and response to medroxyprogesterone acetate. *Gynecol Oncol.* 1985;21:314-319.

136. Slavik M, Petty WM, Blessing JA, et al. Phase II clinical study of tamoxifen in advanced endometrial adenocarcinoma: a Gynecologic Oncology Group study. *Cancer Treat Rep.* 1984;68:809-811.

137. Thigpen T, Brady MF, Homesley HD, et al. Tamoxifen in the treatment of advanced or recurrent endometrial carcinoma: a Gynecologic Oncology Group study. *J Clin Oncol.* 2001;19:364-367.

138. Thigpen JT, Brady MF, Alvarez RD, et al. Oral medroxyprogesterone acetate in the treatment of advanced or recurrent endometrial carcinoma: a dose-response study by the Gynecologic Oncology Group. *J Clin Oncol.* 1999;17:1736-1744.

139. Lentz SS, Brady MF, Major FJ, et al. High-dose megestrol acetate in advanced or recurrent endometrial carcinoma: a Gynecologic Oncology Group study. *J Clin Oncol.* 1996;14:357-361.

140. Quinn MA, Campbell JJ, Murray R, et al. Tamoxifen and aminoglutethimide in the management of patients with advanced endometrial carcinoma not responsive to medroxyprogesterone. *Aust N Z J Obstet Gynaecol.* 1981;21:226-229.

141. Pandya KJ, Yeap BY, Weiner LM, et al. Megestrol and tamoxifen in patients with advanced endometrial cancer: an Eastern Cooperative Oncology Group study (E4882). *Am J Clin Oncol.* 2001;24:43-46.

142. Satyaswaroop PG, Clarke CL, Zaino RJ, et al. Apparent resistance in human endometrial carcinoma during combination treatment with tamoxifen and progestin may result from desensitization following downregulation of tumor progesterone receptor. *Cancer Lett.* 1992;62:107-114.

143. Fiorica JV, Brunetto VL, Hanjani P, et al. Phase II trial of alternating courses of megestrol acetate and tamoxifen in advanced endometrial carcinoma: a Gynecologic Oncology Group study. *Gynecol Oncol.* 2004;92:10-14.

144. Whitney C, Brunetto V, Zaino R, et al. Phase II study of medroxyprogesterone acetate plus tamoxifen in advanced endometrial carcinoma: a Gynecologic Oncology Group study. *Gynecol Oncol.* 2004;92:4-9.

145. Geisinger K, Homesely H, Morgan T, et al. Endometrial adenocarcinoma. A multiparameter clinicopathologic analysis including the DNA profile and the sex steroid hormone receptors. *Cancer.* 1986;58:1518-1525.

146. Kauppila A. Oestrogen and progestin receptors as prognostic indicators in endometrial cancer. A review of the literature. *Acta Oncol.* 1989;28:561-566.

147. Vering A, Michel RT, Mitze M, et al. Influence of chemotherapy on hormone receptor concentration in a xenotransplanted endometrial cancer. *Eur J Obstet Gynecol Reprod Biol.* 1992;45:131-138.

148. Bonte J, Decoster JM, Ide P. Vaginal cytologic evaluation as a practical link between hormone blood levels and tumor hormone dependency in exclusive medroxyprogesterone treatment of recurrent or metastatic endometrial adenocarcinoma. *Acta Cytol.* 1977;21:218-224.

149. Stratton JA, Mannel RS, Rettenmaier MA, et al. Treatment of advanced and recurrent endometrial carcinoma: correlation of patient response to hormonal and cytotoxic chemotherapy and the response predicted by the subrenal capsule chemo sensitivity assay. *Gynecol Oncol.* 1989;32:55-59.

150. Zaino RJ, Satyaswaroop PG, Mortel R. Hormonal therapy of human endometrial adenocarcinoma in a nude mouse model. *Cancer Res.* 1985;45:539-541.

151. Gallagher CJ, Oliver RT, Oram DH, et al. A new treatment for endometrial cancer with gonadotrophin releasing-hormone analogue. *Br J Obstet Gynaecol.* 1991;98:1037.

152. De Vriese G, Bonte J. Possible role of goserelin, an LH-RH agonist, in the treatment of gynaecological cancers. *Eur J Gynaecol Oncol.* 1993;14:187-191.

153. Kleinman D, Douvdevani A, Schally AV, et al. Direct growth inhibition of human endometrial cancer cells by the gonadotropin-releasing hormone antagonist SB-75: role of apoptosis. *Am J Obstet Gynecol.* 1994;170:96-102.

154. Chan S. A review of selective estrogen receptor modulators in the treatment of breast and endometrial cancer. *Semin Oncol.* 2002;29(3 suppl 11):129-133.

155. Rose PG, Brunetto VL, VanLe L, et al. A phase II trial of anastrozole in advanced recurrent or persistent endometrial carcinoma: a Gynecologic Oncology Group study. *Gynecol Oncol.* 2000;78(2):212-216.

156. Covens AL, Filiaci V, Gersell D, et al. Phase II study of fulvestrant in recurrent/metastatic endometrial carcinoma: a Gynecologic Oncology Group study. *Gynceol Oncol.* 2011;120(2):185-188.

157. Emons Gunther A, Thiel F, et al. Phase II study of fulvestrant 250 mg/month in patients with recurrent or metastatic endometrial cancer: a study of the Arbeitsgemeinschaft Gynäkologische Onkologie. *Gynceol Oncol.* 2013;129:495-499.

158. Slomovitz BM, Jiang Y, Yates MS, et al. Phase II study of everolimus and letrozole in patients with recurrent endometrial carcinoma. *J Clin Oncol.* 2015;33(8):930-936.

159. Slomovitz BM, Filiaci V, Coleman R., et al. GOG 3007, a randomized phase II (RP2) trial of everolimus and letrozole (EL) or hormonal therapy (medroxyprogesterone acetate/tamoxifen, PT) in women with advanced, persistent or recurrent endometrial carcinoma (EC): a GOG Foundation study. *Gynecol Oncol.* 2018;149(1):2.

160. Mirza MR, Salutari V, Mendiola C, et al. Palbociclib versus placebo in combination with letrozole for patients with advanced or recurrent endometrial cancer: the NSGO ENGOT-EN3/PALEO trial. *J Clin Oncol.* 2017;35:15(suppl, TPS5612-TPS5612).

161. Giannone G, Tuninetti V, Ghisoni E, et al. Role of cyclin-dependent kinase inhibitors in endometrial cancer. *Int J Mol Sci.* 2019;20(9):2353.

162. Nagamani M, Stuart CA. Specific binding and growth-promoting activity of insulin in endometrial cancer cells in culture. *Am J Obstet Gynecol.* 1998;179:6-12.

163. Thigpen JT, Blessing JA, Lagasse LD, et al. Phase II trial of cisplatin as second-line chemotherapy in patients with advanced or recurrent endometrial carcinoma. A Gynecologic Oncology Group study. *Am J Clin Oncol.* 1984;7(3):253-256.

164. Deppe G, Cohen CJ, Bruckner HW. Treatment of advanced endometrial adenocarcinoma with cis-dichlorodiammine platinum (II) after intensive prior therapy. *Gynecol Oncol.* 1980;10(1):51-54.

165. Seski JC, Edwards CL, Herson J, et al. Cisplatin chemotherapy for disseminated endometrial cancer. *Obstet Gynecol.* 1982;59(2):225-228.

166. Thigpen JT, Blessing JA, Homesley H, et al. Phase II trial of cisplatin as first-line chemotherapy in patients with advanced or recurrent endometrial carcinoma: a Gynecologic Oncology Group study. *Gynecol Oncol.* 1989;33(1):68-70.

167. Burke TW, Munkarah A, Kavanagh JJ, et al. Treatment of advanced or recurrent endometrial carcinoma with single-agent carboplatin. *Gynecol Oncol.* 1993;51(3):397-400.

168. Green JB III, Green S, Alberts DS, et al. Carboplatin therapy in advanced endometrial cancer. *Obstet Gynecol.* 1990;75(4):696-700.

169. Long HJ, Pfeifle DM, Wieand HS, et al. Phase II evaluation of carboplatin in advanced endometrial carcinoma. *J Natl Cancer Inst.* 1988;80(4):276-278.

170. Horton J, Begg CB, Arseneault J, et al. Comparison of adriamycin with cyclophosphamide in patients with advanced endometrial cancer. *Cancer Treat Rep.* 1978;62(1):159-161.

171. Thigpen JT, Buchsbaum HJ, Mangan C, et al. Phase II trial of adriamycin in the treatment of advanced or recurrent endometrial carcinoma: a Gynecologic Oncology Group study. *Cancer Treat Rep.* 1979;63(1):21-27.

172. Calero F, Asins-Codoñer E, Jimeno J, et al. Epirubicin in advanced endometrial adenocarcinoma: a phase II study of the Grupo Ginecologico Espanol para el Tratamiento Oncologico (GGETO). *Eur J Cancer.* 1991;27(7):864-866.

173. Muggia FM, Blessing JA, Sorosky J, et al. Phase II trial of the pegylated liposomal doxorubicin in previously treated metastatic endometrial cancer: a Gynecologic Oncology Group study. *J Clin Oncol.* 2002;20(9):2360-2364.

174. Escobar PF, Markman M, Zanotti K, et al. Phase 2 trial of pegylated liposomal doxorubicin in advanced endometrial cancer. *J Cancer Res Clin Oncol.* 2003;129(11):651-665.

175. Muss HB, Blessing JA, Hatch KD, et al. Methotrexate in advanced endometrial carcinoma. A phase II trial of the Gynecologic Oncology Group. *Am J Clin Oncol.* 1990;13(1):61-63.

176. Dvorak O. Cytembena treatment of advanced gynaecological carcinomas. *Neoplasma.* 1971;18(5):461-464.

177. Broun GO, Blessing JA, Eddy GL, et al. A phase II trial of vincristine in advanced or recurrent endometrial carcinoma. A Gynecologic Oncology Group study. *Am J Clin Oncol.* 1993;16(1):18-21.

178. Woo HL, Swenerton KD, Hoskins PJ. Taxol is active in platinum-resistant endometrial adenocarcinoma. *Am J Clin Oncol.* 1996;19(3):290-291.

179. Wadler S, Levy DE, Lincoln ST, et al. Topotecan is an active agent in the first-line treatment of metastatic or recurrent endometrial carcinoma: Eastern Cooperative Oncology Group Study E3E93. *J Clin Oncol.* 2003;21(11):2110-2114.

180. Traina TA, Sabbatini P, Aghajanian C, et al. Weekly topotecan for recurrent endometrial cancer: a case series and review of the literature. *Gynecol Oncol.* 2004;95(1):235-241.

181. Dizon DS, Blessing JA, McMeekin DS, et al. Phase II trial of ixabepilone as second-line treatment in advanced endometrial cancer: Gynecologic Oncology Group Trial 129-P. *J Clin Oncol.* 2009;27(19):3104-3108.

182. The Cancer Genome Atlas Research Network. Integrated genomic characterization of endometrial cancer. *Nature.* 2013;497:67-72.

183. Dedes K, Wetterskog D, Ashworth A, et al. Emerging therapeutic targets in endometrial cancer. *Nat Rev Clin Oncol.* 2011;8:261-271.

184. Westin SN, Broaddus RR. Personalized therapy in endometrial cancer: challenges and opportunities. *Cancer Biol Ther.* 2012;13(1):1-13.

185. Yeramian A, Moreno-Bueno G, Dolcet X, et al. Endometrial carcinoma: molecular alterations involved in tumor development and progression. *Oncogene.* 2013;32(4):403-413.

186. Hennessy BT, Smith DL, Ram PT, et al. Exploiting the PI3K/AKT pathway for cancer drug discovery. *Nat Rev Drug Discov.* 2005;4(12):988-1004.

187. Naumann RW. The role of the phosphatidylinositol 3-kinase (PI3K) pathway in the development and treatment of uterine cancer. *Gynecol Oncol.* 2011;123(2):411-420.

188. Sansal I, Sellers W. The biology and clinical relevance of the PTEN tumor suppressor pathway. *J Clin Oncol.* 2004;22:2954-2963.

189. Lee JO, Yang H, Georgescu MM, et al. Crystal structure of the PTEN tumor suppressor: implications for its phosphoinositide phosphatase activity and membrane association. *Cell.* 1999;99:323-334.

190. Li J, Yen C, Liaw D, et al. PTEN, a putative protein tyrosine phosphatase gene mutated in human brain, breast, and prostate cancer. *Science.* 1997;275:1943-1947.

191. Maxwell GL, Risinger JI, Gumbs C, et al. Mutation of the PTEN tumor suppressor gene in endometrial hyperplasias. *Cancer Res.* 1998;58(12):2500-2503.

192. Tamura M, Gu J, Matsumoto K, et al. Inhibition of cell migration, spreading, and focal adhesions by tumour suppressor PTEN. *Science.* 1998;280:1614-1617.

193. Peiffer SL, Herzog TJ, Tribune DJ, et al. Allelic loss of sequences from the long arm of chromosome 10 and replication errors in endometrial cancers. *Cancer Res.* 1995;55:1922-1926.

194. Kong D, Suzuki A, Zou TT, et al. PTEN1 is frequently mutated in primary endometrial carcinomas. *Nat Genet.* 1997;17:143-144.

195. Meric-Bernstam F, Gonzalez-Angulo AM. Targeting the mTOR signaling network for cancer therapy. *J Clin Oncol.* 2009;27(13):2278-2287.

196. Cantley LC. The phosphoinositide 3-kinase pathway. *Science.* 2002;296(5573):1655-1657.

197. Slomovitz BM, Wu W, Broaddus RR, et al. mTor inhibition is a rational target for the treatment of endometrial cancer. *J Clin Oncol.* 2004;22(14):5076.

198. Engelman JA. Targeting PI3K signaling in cancer: opportunities, challenges and limitations. *Nat Rev Cancer.* 2009;9(8):550-562.

199. Dancey JE. Clinical development of mammalian target of rapamycin inhibitors. *Hematol Oncol Clin North Am.* 2002;16(5):1101-1114.

200. Oza AM, Elit L, Tsao MS, et al. Phase II study of temsirolimus in women with recurrent or metastatic endometrial cancer: a trial of the NCIC Clinical Trials Group. *J Clin Oncol.* 2011;29(24):3278-3285.

201. Kollmannsberger C, Hirte H, Siu LL, et al. Temsirolimus in combination with carboplatin and paclitaxel in patients with advanced solid tumors: a NCIC-CTG, phase I, open-label dose-escalation study (IND 179). *Ann Oncol.* 2012;23(1):238-244.

202. Fleming GF, Filiaci VL, Hanjani P, et al. Hormone therapy plus temsirolimus for endometrial carcinoma (EC): Gynecologic Oncology Group Trial #248. *J Clin Oncol.* 2011;29(5 suppl):5014.

203. Alvarez EA, Brady WE, Walker JL, et al. Phase II trial of combination bevacizumab and temsirolimus in the treatment of recurrent or persistent endometrial carcinoma: a Gynecologic Oncology Group study. *Gynecol Oncol.* 2013;129(1):22-27.

204. Aghajanian C, Filiaci V, Dizon DS, et al. A phase II study of frontline paclitaxel/carboplatin/bevacizumab, paclitaxel/carboplatin/temsirolimus, or ixabepilone/carboplatin/bevacizumab in advanced/recurrent endometrial cancer. *Gynecol Oncol.* 2018;150(2):274-281.

205. Stefansson IM, Salvesen HB, Akslen LA. Vascular proliferation is important for clinical progress of endometrial cancer. *Cancer Res.* 2006;66(6):3303-3309.

206. Salvesen HB, Iversen OE, Akslen LA. Prognostic significance of angiogenesis and Ki-67, p53, and p21 expression: a population-based endometrial carcinoma study. *J Clin Oncol.* 1999;17(5):1382-1390.

207. Kamat AA, Merritt WM, Coffey D, et al. Clinical and biological significance of vascular endothelial growth factor in endometrial cancer. *Clin Cancer Res.* 2007;13(24):7487-7495.

208. Gehrig PA, Bae-Jump VL. Promising novel therapies for the treatment of endometrial cancer. *Gynecol Oncol.* 2010;116(2):187-194.

209. Aghajanian C, Sill MW, Darcy KM, et al. Phase II trial of bevacizumab in recurrent or persistent endometrial cancer: a Gynecologic Oncology Group study. *J Clin Oncol.* 2011;29(16):2259-2265.

210. Lorusso D, Ferrandina G, Colombo N, et al. Carboplatin-paclitaxel compared to Carboplatin-Paclitaxel-Bevacizumab in advanced or recurrent endometrial cancer: MITO END-2–a randomized phase II trial. *Gynecol Oncol.* 2019;155(3):406-412.

211. Correa R, Mackay H, Hirte HW, et al. A phase II study of sunitinib in recurrent or metastatic endometrial carcinoma: a trial of the Princess Margaret Hospital, the University of Chicago, and California Cancer Phase II Consortia. *J Clin Oncol.* 2010;28(15 suppl):5038.

212. Nimeiri HS, Oza AM, Morgan RJ, et al. A phase II study of sorafenib in advanced uterine carcinoma/carcinosarcoma: a trial of the Chicago, PMH, and California Phase II Consortia. *Gynecol Oncol.* 2010;117(1):37-40.

213. McMeekin DS, Sill MW, Benbrook D, et al. A phase II trial of thalidomide in patients with refractory endometrial cancer and correlation with angiogenesis biomarkers: a Gynecologic Oncology Group study. *Gynecol Oncol.* 2007;105(2):508-516.

214. Powell MA, Sill MW, Goodfellow PJ, et al. A phase II trial of brivanib in recurrent or persistent endometrial cancer: an NRG Oncology/Gynecologic Oncology Group study. *Gynecol Oncol.* 2014;135(1):38-43.

215. Bender D, Sill MW, Lankes HA, et al. A phase II evaluation of cediranib in the treatment of recurrent or persistent endometrial cancer: an NRG Oncology/Gynecologic Oncology Group study. *Gynecol Oncol.* 2015;138(3):507-512.

216. Dizon DS, Sill MW, Schilder JM, et al. A phase II evaluation of nintedanib (BIBF-1120) in the treatment of recurrent or persistent endometrial cancer: an NRG Oncology/Gynecologic Oncology Group study. *Gynecol Oncol.* 2014;135(3):441-445.

217. Coleman RL, Sill MW, Lankes HA, et al. A phase II evaluation of aflibercept in the treatment of recurrent or persistent endometrial cancer: a Gynecologic Oncology Group study. *Gynecol Oncol.* 2012;127(3):538-543.

218. Jiricny J. The multifaceted mismatch-repair system. *Nat Rev Mol Cell Biol.* 2006;7(5):335-346.

219. MacDonald ND, Salvesen HB, Ryan A, Iversen OE, Akslen LA, Jacobs IJ. Frequency and prognostic impact of microsatellite instability in a large population-based study of endometrial carcinomas. *Cancer Res.* 2000;60(6):1750-1752.

220. Basil JB, Goodfellow PJ, Rader JS, Mutch DG, Herzog TJ. Clinical significance of microsatellite instability in endometrial carcinoma. *Cancer.* 2000;89(8):1758-1764.

221. Dunlop MG, Farrington SM, Carothers AD, et al. Cancer risk associated with germline DNA mismatch repair gene mutations. *Hum Mol Genet.* 1997;6(1):105-110.

222. Black D, Soslow RA, Levine DA, et al. Clinicopathologic significance of defective DNA mismatch repair in endometrial carcinoma. *J Clin Oncol.* 2006;24(11):1745-1753.

223. Caduff RF, Johnston CM, Svoboda-Newman SM, Poy EL, Merajver SD, Frank TS. Clinical and pathological significance of microsatellite instability in sporadic endometrial carcinoma. *Am J Pathol.* 1996;148(5):1671-1678.

224. Duggan BD, Felix JC, Muderspach LI, Tourgeman D, Zheng J, Shibata D. Microsatellite instability in sporadic endometrial carcinoma. *J Natl Cancer Inst.* 1994;86(16):1216-1221.

225. Helland A, Børresen-Dale AL, Peltomäki P, et al. Microsatellite instability in cervical and endometrial carcinomas. *Int J Cancer.* 1997;70(5):499-501.

226. Risinger JI, Berchuck A, Kohler MF, Watson P, Lynch HT, Boyd J. Genetic instability of microsatellites in endometrial carcinoma. *Cancer Res.* 1993;53(21):5100-5103.

227. Esteller M, Levine R, Baylin SB, Ellenson LH, Herman JG. MLH1 promoter hypermethylation is associated with the microsatellite instability phenotype in sporadic endometrial carcinomas. *Oncogene.* 1998;17(18):2413-2417.

228. Lax SF, Kendall B, Tashiro H, Slebos RJ, Hedrick L. The frequency of p53, K-ras mutations, and microsatellite instability differs in uterine endometrioid and serous carcinoma: evidence of distinct molecular genetic pathways. *Cancer.* 2000;88(4):814-824.

229. Lalloo F, Evans G. Molecular genetics and endometrial cancer. *Best Pract Res Clin Obstet Gynaecol.* 2001;15(3):355-363.

230. De Luca A, Carotenuto A, Rachiglio A, et al. The role of the EGFR signaling in tumor microenvironment. *J Cell Physiol.* 2008;214(3):559-567.

231. Bilbao C, Lara PC, Ramirez R, et al. Microsatellite instability predicts clinical outcome in radiation-treated endometrioid endometrial cancer. *Int J Radiat Oncol Biol Phys.* 2010;76(1):9-13.

232. Resnick KE, Frankel WL, Morrison CD, et al. Mismatch repair status and outcomes after adjuvant therapy in patients with surgically staged endometrial cancer. *Gynecol Oncol.* 2010;117(2):234-238.

233. Ott PA, Bang YJ, Berton-Rigaud D, et al. Safety and antitumor activity of pembrolizumab in advanced programmed death ligand 1-positive endometrial cancer: results From the KEYNOTE-028 study. *J Clin Oncol.* 2017;35(22):2535-2541.

234. Oaknin A, Tinker AV, Gilbert L, et al. Clinical activity and safety of the anti-programmed death 1 monoclonal antibody dostarlimab for patients with recurrent or advanced mismatch repair-deficient endometrial cancer: a nonrandomized phase 1 clinical trial. *JAMA Oncol.* 2020;6(11):1766-1772.

235. Marcus L, Fashoyin-Aje LA, Donoghue M, et al. FDA approval summary: pembrolizumab for the treatment of tumor mutational burden-high solid tumors. *Clin Cancer Res.* 2021;27:4685-4689.

236. Makker V, Taylor MH, Aghajanian C, et al. Lenvatinib plus pembrolizumab in patients with advanced endometrial cancer. *J Clin Oncol.* 2020;38(26):2981-2992.

237. Makker, V, Colombo N, Herraez AC, et al. Lenvatinib plus pembrolizumab for advanced endometrial cancer. *N Engl J Med.* 2022;386(5):437-448.

238. Samarnthai N, Hall K, Yeh IT. Molecular profiling of endometrial malignancies. *Obstet Gynecol Int.* 2010;2010:162363.

239. Berchuck A, Rodriguez G, Kinney RB, et al. Overexpression of HER-2/neu in endometrial cancer is associated with advanced stage disease. *Am J Obstet Gynecol.* 1991;164:15-21.

240. Reinartz JJ, George E, Lindgren BR, Niehans GA. Expression of p53, transforming growth factor alpha, epidermal growth factor receptor, and c-erbB-2 in endometrial carcinoma and correlation with survival and known predictors of survival. *Hum Pathol.* 1994;25:1075-1083.

241. Rolitsky CD, Theil KS, McGaughy VR, Copeland LJ, Niemann TH. HER-2/neu amplification and overexpression in endometrial carcinoma. *Int J Gynecol Pathol.* 1999;18:138-143.

242. Santin AD, Bellone S, Van Stedum S, et al. Determination of HER2/neu status in uterine serous papillary carcinoma: comparative analysis of immunohistochemistry and fluorescence in situ hybridization. *Gynecol Oncol.* 2005;98:24-30.

243. Slomovitz BM, Broaddus RR, Burke TW, et al. Her-2/neu overexpression and amplification in uterine papillary serous carcinoma. *J Clin Oncol.* 2004;22:3126-3132.

244. Kohler MF, Carney P, Dodge R, et al. p53 overexpression in advanced-stage endometrial adenocarcinoma. *Am J Obstet Gynecol.* 1996;175:1246-1252.

245. Backe J, Gassel AM, Krebs S, Müller T, Caffier H. Immunohistochemically detected HER-2/neu-expression and prognosis in endometrial carcinoma. *Arch Gynecol Obstet.* 1997;259:189-195.

246. Pisani AL, Barbuto DA, Chen D, Ramos L, Lagasse LD, Karlan BY. HER-2/neu, p53, and DNA analyses as prognosticators for survival in endometrial carcinoma. *Obstet Gynecol.* 1995;85:729-734.

247. Hetzel DJ, Wilson TO, Keeney GL, Roche PC, Cha SS, Podratz KC. HER-2/neu expression: a major prognostic factor in endometrial cancer. *Gynecol Oncol.* 1992;47:179-185.

248. Nazeer T, Ballouk F, Malfetano JH, Figge H, Ambros RA. Multivariate survival analysis of clinicopathologic features in surgical stage I endometrioid carcinoma including analysis of HER-2/neu expression. *Am J Obstet Gynecol.* 1995;173:1829-1834.

249. Saffari B, Jones LA, el-Naggar A, Felix JC, George J, Press MF. Amplification and overexpression of HER-2/neu (c-erbB2) in endometrial cancers: correlation with overall survival. *Cancer Res.* 1995;55:5693-5698.

250. Morrison C, Fanagolo V, Ramirez N, et al. HER-2 is an independent prognostic factor in endometrial cancer: association with outcome in a large cohort of surgically staged patients. *J Clin Oncol.* 2006;24:2376-2385.

251. Fleming GF, Sill MW, Darcy KM, et al. Phase II trial of trastuzumab in women with advanced or recurrent, HER2-positive endometrial carcinoma: a Gynecologic Oncology Group study. *Gynecol Oncol.* 2010;116(1):15-20.

252. Fader AN, Roque DM, Siegel E, et al. Randomized phase II trial of carboplatin-paclitaxel versus carboplatin-paclitaxel-trastuzumab in uterine serous carcinomas that overexpress human epidermal growth factor receptor 2/neu. *J Clin Oncol.* 2018;36(20):2044-2051.

253. Fader AN, Roque DM, Siegel E, et al. Randomized phase II trial of carboplatin-paclitaxel compared with carboplatin-paclitaxel-trastuzumab in advanced (stage III-IV) or recurrent uterine serous carcinomas that overexpress Her2/Neu (NCT01367002): updated overall survival analysis. *Clin Cancer Res.* 2020;26(15):3928-3935.

254. Liu JF, Xiong N, Campos SM, et al. Phase II study of the wee1 inhibitor adavosertib in recurrent uterine serous carcinoma. *J Clin Oncol.* 2021;39(14):1531-1539.

255. Forster MD, Dedes KJ, Sandhu S, et al. Treatment with olaparib in a patient with PTEN-deficient endometrioid endometrial cancer. *Nat Rev Clin Oncol.* 2011;8(5):302-306.

256. Javle M, Curtin NJ. The role of PARP in DNA repair and its therapeutic exploitation. *Br J Cancer.* 2011;105(8):1114-1122.

257. Mendes-Pereira AM, Martin SA, Brough R, et al. Synthetic lethal targeting of PTEN mutant cells with PARP inhibitors. *EMBO Mol Med.* 2009;1(6-7):315-322.

258. Rimel BJ. A randomized, phase II study comparing single-agent olaparib, single agent cediranib, and the combination of cediranib/olaparib in women with recurrent, persistent or metastatic endometrial cancer. *Gynecol Oncol.* 2021;162:S43-S44.

CHAPTER **5.7**

Treatment of Persistent and Recurrent Endometrial Cancer

Susana M. Campos

MANAGEMENT OF PATIENTS WITH SEROUS, CLEAR CELL HISTOLOGY

Serous cancer and, to a lesser extent, clear cell ECs tend to spread in a fashion similar to ovarian cancer with a high propensity for upper abdominal relapse. Chemotherapy is used to treat this high-risk histology.

On the basis of the RRs of paclitaxel and carboplatin in other tumors of serous histology, trials investigating paclitaxel and carboplatin in uterine papillary serous carcinomas (UPSCs) have reported RRs of 60% to 70% (1,2). A single-institution phase II trial for advanced-stage uterine papillary serous histology administered paclitaxel and platinum-based chemotherapy for three cycles followed by volume-directed RT. Patients then received an additional three cycles of chemotherapy. The most common toxicity was hematologic and occurred during chemotherapy following RT. The PFS for the nine women treated is 46.4 months (3). A similar study administered four cycles of platinum with paclitaxel or epirubicin followed by whole pelvic and vaginal brachytherapy. The 5-year OS for this group was 58.9% (4). As outlined earlier (5,6) trastuzumab has improved PFS in patients with advanced or recurrent disease.

With regard to stage I disease, the available data for designing a treatment plan are retrospective. A study of 74 stage I patients with UPSC between 1987 and 2004 who underwent complete staging at Yale University was reported (7). Patients were divided into those who had no residual cancer in the hysterectomy specimen versus those who did. Stage IA patients who had residual cancer in the hysterectomy specimen and who were treated with platinum-based chemotherapy had no recurrences (*n* = 7) versus 6 of 14 (43%) who did not receive treatment. Of 15 patients with stage IB disease, there were no recurrences in the treated group but 10 of 13 nontreated patients (77%) recurred. Platinum-based chemotherapy was associated with improved PFS (*P* < .01) and OS (*P* < .05). Furthermore, no patient who received radiation to the

vaginal cuff recurred at the cuff versus 6 of 31 (19%) of those who did not receive vaginal cuff irradiation. Recognizing the limits of retrospective studies, these data support the potential benefit of a regimen of platinum-based chemotherapy with cuff irradiation in patients with UPSC. Randomized, prospective data are needed to accurately define the best approach in these patients.

The rarity of these tumor types has made histology-based clinical trials difficult to perform. It is hoped that as we incorporate molecular biology in clinical trials, the treatment for rare histologic subtypes of uterine cancer may evolve.

REFERENCES

1. Zanotti KM, Belinson JL, Kennedy AW, et al. The use of paclitaxel and platinum-based chemotherapy in uterine papillary serous carcinoma. *Gynecol Oncol.* 1999;74:272-277.

2. Ramondetta L, Burke TW, Levenback C, et al. Treatment of uterine papillary serous carcinoma with paclitaxel. *Gynecol Oncol.* 2001;82:156-161.

3. Gehrig PA. Uterine papillary serous carcinoma: a review. *Expert Opin Pharmacother.* 2007;8:809-816.

4. Low JS, Wong EH, Tan HS, et al. Adjuvant sequential chemotherapy and radiotherapy in uterine papillary serous carcinoma. *Gynecol Oncol.* 2005;97:171-177.

5. Fader AN, Roque DM, Siegel E, et al. Randomized phase II trial of carboplatin-paclitaxel versus carboplatin-paclitaxel-trastuzumab in uterine serous carcinomas that overexpress human epidermal growth factor receptor 2/neu. *J Clin Oncol.* 2018;36(20):2044-2051.

6. Fader AN, Roque DM, Siegel E, et al. Randomized phase II trial of carboplatin–paclitaxel compared with carboplatin–paclitaxel–trastuzumab in advanced (stage III–IV) or recurrent uterine serous carcinomas that overexpress Her2/Neu (NCT01367002): updated overall survival analysis. *Clin Cancer Res.* 2020;26(15):3928-3935.

7. Kelly MG, O'Malley DM, Hui P, et al. Improved survival in surgical stage I patients with uterine papillary serous carcinoma (UPSC) treated with adjuvant platinum-based chemotherapy. *Gynecol Oncol.* 2005;98(3):353-359.

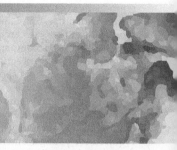

CHAPTER **5.8**

Endometrial Cancer: Special Conditions

Allison Gockley

FERTILITY-SPARING TREATMENT

Approximately 5% of women with EC are diagnosed under the age of 40 years (1). The main risk factors leading to EC in young women include increased BMI, nulliparity, anovulation, as well as Lynch syndrome (2). Although hysterectomy and surgical staging are considered the standard of care, for some younger women, hysterectomy is unacceptable because of a desire to maintain fertility. EC in younger women may be associated with early-stage, low-grade disease, making medical management an attractive option to some (3-7). However, not all young women with EC are candidates for fertility-sparing treatment. In one registry study, only 18% of patients with EC aged 45 years and younger were diagnosed with stage IA, grade 1 tumors (8). Following a diagnosis of EC by either D&C (preferred to confirm grade) or biopsy, an MRI of the pelvis should be obtained to evaluate for myometrial invasion, lymphadenopathy, and adnexal pathology (2). MRI has been shown to be superior to transvaginal ultrasound in detecting deep myometrial invasion, and advanced MRI techniques can aid in this process (9,10). Patients with grade 1 tumors without myometrial invasion or evidence of extrauterine spread are thought to be the best candidates. Fertility-sparing treatment should be undertaken using shared decision-making with the patient and in conjunction with an infertility specialist.

Medical Management

Current evidence establishes administration of medroxyprogesterone acetate (MPA) at a dose of 400 to 600 mg/d or megestrol acetate (MA) at a dose of 160 to 320 mg/d for at least 6 months and recommends performing a follow-up assessment of treatment response using D&C and imaging (11). Progestin therapy has been successful in reversing malignant changes in up to 76% to 81% of cases (5,6). Increasingly, there has been a consideration for progestin-based intrauterine devices (IUDs), although the data are limited. In a 2012 systematic review of the literature, 74% of AEH and 72% of patients with grade 1 EC achieved a pathologic CR for 6 months or longer with oral progestins (12). The range of CRs for AEH was 50% to 95%, and for grade 1 cancer was 50% to 100%. The mean time required to achieve the CR was 6 months. Of 22 patients with EC with grade 1 tumors treated with IUD, 68% achieved a CR. In a study by Park et al, in women aged 40 years and less with grade 1 endometrioid EC treated with daily oral MPA or MA, complete RRs of 77.7% were achieved after a median follow-up of 66 months. In this study, MPA correlated with a lower risk of recurrence (13).

Because response may be temporary or incomplete, periodic sampling of the endometrium is advised. Penner and colleagues suggested that lack of response to progestin therapy is more common when the first-response assessment shows lack of response, despite adjacent stromal decidualization (14).

Although several papers do not report significant toxicity among patients treated with high-dose oral progestins, adverse events such as thrombophlebitis, pulmonary emboli, weight gain, hypertension, and headaches may lead to low patient compliance (15,16). The levonorgestrel (LNG)-IUD is a reasonable option for patient with EC desiring fertility-sparing treatment, because it avoids any compliance issues associated with oral progestins and minimizes systemic side effects.

Other studies advocate for dual-modality progesterone therapy. The Korean Gynecologic Oncologic Group has reported that the 6-month RR of LNG-IUD associated with oral MPA at 500 mg/d in fertility-sparing patients was 37% and PR was attained in 25.7% of patients. The authors note that a higher RR may be seen with extended durations of treatment (17). In a prospective observational study of 16 patients with EC aged 40 years or younger, the overall complete remission rate with LNG-IUD and 500 mg/d oral MPA was 87.5%, and the time to remission was 9.8 months. There were no cases of progressive disease reported and three women achieved pregnancies (18). Other studies advocate for a hysteroscopic resection followed by progesterone therapy and report complete RRs in excess of 90% (19,20).

Current national guidelines support MA, MPA, or LNG-IUD as options for fertility-sparing treatment for eligible young women with EC. Fertility-sparing treatment is generally continued for 6 to 12 months with repeat sampling or D&C in 3 to 6 months (21). Women with persistence of disease should be referred for surgery and then advised to undergo hysterectomy.

Emerging data suggest that assessing tumor progesterone status may lead to improved identification of patients with EC who are likely to respond to progesterone-based treatment. Although data are limited, RR of 72% for progesterone-positive tumors have been reported in contrast to 12% for progesterone-negative tumors (22). Factors that may influence response to progesterone treatment include insulin resistance status (23) and tumor molecular classification. In a study of 57 patients with EC younger than 40 years, tumors were categorized by the Proactive Molecular Risk Classifier. This study noted that patients with dMMR had a significantly lower CR or PR to progesterone therapy as compared to those with wild-type p53 tumors (44.4% vs 82.2%, $P = .18$) (24). Future work in this area is likely to improve risk stratification for women seeking fertility-sparing EC treatment (21,25). The risk of recurrence following fertility-sparing treatment ranges from 25% to 40% (13,26). Hysterectomy with staging should be recommended once childbearing is complete (27).

Pregnancy Outcomes

There are several studies that describe successful pregnancies following fertility-sparing treatment for EC. Park et al reported the experience of 141 women with stage IA G1 EC. A total of 70 (49.6%) of the 141 patients tried to conceive, with 44 (62.9%) receiving fertility treatments. The authors reported that fertility treatments were not associated with a higher incidence of cancer recurrence. A total of 44 patients (8.3%) achieved more than one viable pregnancy (13). Similarly, in a systematic review of reproductive outcomes for patients with grade 1 adenocarcinoma treated with progestins, Gunderson et al showed that nearly 35% of those with a history of carcinoma became pregnant (26).

A case series accompanied by a systematic review reported 77 live births, with pregnancies resulting from assisted reproductive treatments and spontaneous conceptions. One maternal death was seen because of recurrent disease (28). Women with a history of EC may require assisted reproduction treatments in up to 60% of cases (6). Pregnancy outcomes reported in the literature are encouraging; however, given the complexity of care required for young women with EC, consultation with a reproductive endocrinologist and maternal-fetal medicine specialist is recommended (21,29).

Ovarian Preservation

Although the standard of care includes removal of the bilateral fallopian tubes and ovaries during surgical staging of EC, ovarian preservation may be considered in premenopausal women meeting criteria for fertility-sparing treatment. In a single-institution review, among patients with EC with pelvic-confined disease, the risk of microscopic ovarian involvement was exceeding low at 0.8% (30). A Korean Gynecologic Oncology Group Study demonstrated that among women with stage I to II EC who underwent ovarian preservation, there was no impact on RFS and there were no recurrences in patients with stage IA disease (31). Retrospective data also suggest that for women with stage I to II disease, ovarian preservation is not associated with an adverse effect on recurrence of OS (32). If the ovaries are retained, the bilateral fallopian tubes should be removed (2).

REFERENCES

1. Trimble EL, Harlan LC, Clegg LX, et al. Pre-operative imaging, surgery and adjuvant therapy for women diagnosed with cancer of the corpus uteri in community practice in the United States. *Gynecol Oncol.* 2005; 96:741-748.

2. Hamilton CA, Pothuri B, Arend RC, et al. Endometrial cancer: a society of gynecologic oncology evidence-based review and recommendations, part II. *Gynecol Oncol.* 2021;160(3):827-834.

3. Ushijima K, Yahata H, Yoshikawa H, et al. Multicenter phase II study of fertility-sparing treatment with medroxyprogesterone acetate for endometrial carcinoma and atypical hyperplasia in young women. *J Clin Oncol.* 2007;25:2798-2803.

4. Leitao MM, Chi DS. Fertility-sparing options for patients with gynecologic malignancies. *Oncologist.* 2005;10:613-622.

5. Jadoul P, Donnez J. Conservative treatment may be beneficial for young women with atypical endometrial hyperplasia or endometrial adenocarcinoma. *Fertil Steril.* 2003;80:1315-1324.

6. Ramirez PT, Frumovitz M, Bodurka DC, Sun CC, Levenback C. Hormonal therapy for the management of grade 1 endometrial adenocarcinoma: a literature review. *Gynecol Oncol.* 2004;95(1):133-138.

7. Soliman PT, Oh JC, Schmeler KM, et al. Risk factors for young premenopausal women with endometrial cancer. *Obstet Gynecol.* 2005;105: 575-580.

8. Navarria I, Usel M, Rapiti E, et al. Young patients with endometrial cancer: how many could be eligible for fertility-sparing treatment? *Gynecol Oncol.* 2009;114(3):448-451.

9. Alcázar JL, Gastón B, Navarro B, Salas R, Aranda J, Guerriero S. Transvaginal ultrasound versus magnetic resonance imaging for preoperative assessment of myometrial infiltration in patients with endometrial cancer: a systematic review and meta-analysis. *J Gynecol Oncol.* 2017;28(6):e86.

10. Himoto Y, Lakhman Y, Fujii S, et al. Multiparametric magnetic resonance imaging facilitates the selection of patients prior to fertility-sparing management of endometrial cancer. *Abdom Radiol (NY).* 2021;46(9): 4410-4419.

11. Rodolakis A, Biliatis I, Morice P, et al. European society of gynecological oncology task force for fertility preservation: clinical recommendations

12. Baker J, Obermair A, Gebski V, et al. Efficacy of oral or intrauterine device-delivered progestin in patients with complex endometrial hyperplasia with atypia or early endometrial adenocarcinoma: a meta-analysis and systematic review of the literature. *Gynecol Oncol.* 2012;125:263-270.

13. Park JY, Kim DY, Kim JH, et al. Long-term oncologic outcomes after fertility-sparing management using oral progestin for young women with endometrial cancer (KGOG 2002). *Eur J Cancer.* 2013;49(4):868-874.

14. Penner KR, Dorigo O, Aoyama C, et al. Predictors of resolution of complex atypical hyperplasia or grade 1 endometrial adenocarcinoma in premenopausal women treated with progestin therapy. *Gynecol Oncol.* 2012;124:542-548.

15. VAN Heertum K, Liu J. Differential effects of progestogens used for menopausal hormone therapy. *Clin Obstet Gynecol.* 2018;61(3):454-462.

16. Thigpen JT, Brady MF, Alvarez RD, et al. Oral medroxyprogesterone acetate in the treatment of advanced or recurrent endometrial carcinoma: a dose-response study by the Gynecologic Oncology Group. *J Clin Oncol.* 1999;17(6):1736-1744.

17. Kim MK, Seong SJ, Kang SB, et al. Six months response rate of combined oral medroxyprogesterone/levonorgestrel-intrauterine system for early-stage endometrial cancer in young women: a Korean Gynecologic-Oncology Group Study. *J Gynecol Oncol.* 2019;30(2):e47.

18. Kim MK, Seong SJ, Kim YS, et al. Combined medroxyprogesterone acetate/levonorgestrel-intrauterine system treatment in young women with early-stage endometrial cancer. *Am J Obstet Gynecol.* 2013;209(4):358. e1-358.e3584.

19. Gallo A, Catena U, Saccone G, Di Spiezio Sardo A. Conservative surgery in endometrial cancer. *J Clin Med.* 2021;11(1):183.

20. Giampaolino P, Di Spiezio Sardo A, Mollo A, et al. Hysteroscopic endometrial focal resection followed by levonorgestrel intrauterine device insertion as a fertility-sparing treatment of atypical endometrial hyperplasia and early endometrial cancer: a retrospective study. *J Minim Invasive Gynecol.* 2019;26(4):648-656.

21. Cavaliere AF, Perelli F, Zaami S, et al. Fertility sparing treatments in endometrial cancer patients: the potential role of the new molecular classification. *Int J Mol Sci.* 2021;22(22):12248.

22. Ehrlich CE, Young PC, Stehman FB, Sutton GP, Alford WM. Steroid receptors and clinical outcome in patients with adenocarcinoma of the endometrium. *Am J Obstet Gynecol.* 1988;158(4):796-807.

23. Wang Y, Zhou R, Zhang X, Liu H, Shen D, Wang J. Significance of serum and pathological biomarkers in fertility-sparing treatment for endometrial cancer or atypical hyperplasia: a retrospective cohort study. *BMC Womens Health.* 2021;21(1):252.

24. Chung YS, Woo HY, Lee JY, et al. Mismatch repair status influences response to fertility-sparing treatment of endometrial cancer. *Am J Obstet Gynecol.* 2021;224(4):370.e1-370.e13.

25. Puechl AM, Spinosa D, Berchuck A, et al. Molecular classification to prognosticate response in medically managed endometrial cancers and endometrial intraepithelial neoplasia. *Cancers (Basel).* 2021;13(11):2847.

26. Gunderson CC, Fader AN, Carson KA, Bristow RE. Oncologic and reproductive outcomes with progestin therapy in women with endometrial hyperplasia and grade 1 adenocarcinoma: a systematic review. *Gynecol Oncol.* 2012;125(2):477-482.

27. Frumovitz M, Gershenson DM. Fertility-sparing therapy for young women with endometrial cancer. *Expert Rev Anticancer Ther.* 2006;6(1):27-32.

28. Chao AS, Chao A, Wang CJ, Lai CH, Wang HS. Obstetric outcomes of pregnancy after conservative treatment of endometrial cancer: case series and literature review. *Taiwan J Obstet Gynecol.* 2011;50(1):62-66.

29. Park JY, Seong SJ, Kim TJ, et al. Pregnancy outcomes after fertility-sparing management in young women with early endometrial cancer. *Obstet Gynecol.* 2013;121(1):136-142.

30. Lin KY, Miller DS, Bailey AA, et al. Ovarian involvement in endometrioid adenocarcinoma of uterus. *Gynecol Oncol.* 2015;138(3):532-535.

31. Lee TS, Kim JW, Kim TJ, et al. Ovarian preservation during the surgical treatment of early stage endometrial cancer: a nation-wide study conducted by the Korean Gynecologic Oncology Group. *Gynecol Oncol.* 2009;115(1):26-31.

32. Lee TS, Lee JY, Kim JW, et al. Outcomes of ovarian preservation in a cohort of premenopausal women with early-stage endometrial cancer: a Korean Gynecologic Oncology Group study. *Gynecol Oncol.* 2013;131(2):289-293.

CHAPTER **5.9**

Endometrial Cancer: Follow-Up and Survivorship Issues

Allison Gockley

SURVEILLANCE

Posttreatment follow-up and surveillance is a significant component of caring for women with EC. Both SGO and other national guidelines recommend clinical follow-up every 3 to 6 month for the first 2 years following diagnosis and then every 6 to 12 months thereafter (1). These visits should include a review of symptoms to elicit any symptoms concerning for recurrence (pelvic pain, vaginal bleeding, etc.) and pelvic exam including speculum exam. There is no evidence that routine cytology (Pap smears) or imaging studies are beneficial in the surveillance of women with EC. In 2011, SGO guidelines supporting these recommendations were presented and adherence to these guidelines has shown to decrease surveillance costs without affecting patient outcomes (2). However, if there is concern on physical exam or review of symptoms for recurrence, imaging with CT or PET/CT is recommended. For patients who previously had stage III or IV disease, CT of the chest, abdomen, and pelvis every 6 months is an option (1). Serum CA-125 may be used in surveillance of patients who had elevated CA-125 prior to treatment or in those with advanced disease or serous EC (3). Patients with advanced-stage or high-risk EC should be followed by an oncologist for at least 5 years; however, it is reasonable for patients with low-risk EC to follow with a gynecologist after 2 years have elapsed since their treatment (751).

SURVIVORSHIP ISSUES

Obesity is one of the predominant risk factors for EC and should be a focus of posttreatment survivorship. Although obesity has not been shown to impact EC recurrence (4), it has been shown to be inversely correlated with quality of life in obese EC survivors (5). Morbidly obese EC women with a BMI of more than 40 had significantly shorter OS and were almost 25% more likely to die from causes other than EC compared with women with a BMI of less than 40. In fact, at three and half years from diagnosis, cardiovascular disease–related death exceeds cancer-related risk of death (6). Therefore, cardiac risk reduction and weight loss as appropriate are important cornerstones of treatment and cannot be overstated with patients with EC. Interventions include lifestyle changes (weight loss, increasing physical activity, heart-healthy diet, etc.) and bariatric surgery (7). The Survivors of Uterine CanCer Empowered by Exercise and Healthy Diet (SUCCEED) trial randomized 75 obese and overweight EC survivors to 6 months of nutrition, exercise, and behavioral modification counseling or routine care. At 6 and 12 months, the intervention group demonstrated sustained weight loss, increased physical activity, and increased fruit/vegetable intake (8). Although obesity may be difficult to discuss and address, it is of paramount importance to EC survivors, and surveillance visits should incorporate these discussions and referrals to supporting services as feasible.

Sexual Health

Sexual health following EC treatment is an important aspect of survivorship for many women. Treatment for EC often includes surgery, chemotherapy, radiation, or a combination of these modalities, which can lead to anatomic and hormonal changes in the vulvovaginal tract as well as psychosocial changes (9). In one study of 72 women with early-stage EC, 89% of women reported sexual dysfunction (10). Sexual dysfunction among EC survivors is common even without adjuvant treatment. In one study comparing sexual function of women following benign hysterectomy to women following hysterectomy for EC, women with EC were noted to have more entry dyspareunia at 1 year as well as decreased arousal, desire, and entry dyspareunia at 2 years (11). For women who receive adjuvant radiation, sexual function may not be significantly different between vaginal brachytherapy and external beam radiation. The PORTEC 2 trial demonstrated no differences in sexual function between the vaginal brachytherapy and external beam radiation arms at quality-of-life assessments at 5 years posttreatment (12). However, women in this trial undergoing radiation (either vaginal or pelvic) reported worse sexual function as compared to age-matched healthy population.

There are several validated tools available for screening: Vaginal Assessment Scale (VAS), Vulvar Assessment Scale (VuAS), Female Sexual Function Index (FSFI), Female Sexual Medicine Clinical Assessment Form (FSMCAF), Sexual Activity Questionnaire (SAF), PROMIS sexual function items (PROMIS-SxF), Menopausal Symptom Checklist (MSCL), Brief Sexual Symptom Checklist for Women (BSSC-W), etc. If sexual dysfunction is identified, women may benefit from referral to a multidisciplinary women's sexual health clinic (13). Pelvic floor physical therapy can also be helpful. In one multicenter prospective interventional study of 31 patients with EC and cervical cancer, a 12-week course of pelvic floor physical therapy resulted in 90% of women feeling "much" or "very much" improved (14). Additionally, sex therapists can address the multifactorial nature of sexual dysfunction. Certified sex therapists can be found on the website of the American Association of Sexuality Educators, Counselors, and Therapists (AASECT.org).

For women suffering from vulvovaginal estrogen-deprivation symptoms, the recommended first-line treatment includes nonhormonal interventions. Vaginal moisturizers and lubricants are recommended. A single-arm trial of hyaluronic acid–based vaginal moisturizer reported improvement in vulvovaginal symptoms and increased sexual activity among EC survivors (15). For women with refractory symptoms, it is reasonable to consider local vaginal hormone treatments using shared decision-making with EC survivors. Historical nonrandomized data suggest that HRT may be safe in EC survivors. A matched control study suggested that women with EC who received estrogen replacement therapy actually experienced a significantly longer RFS as compared to patients with EC who did not undergo estrogen replacement therapy (P = .006) (16). A GOG trial investigating estrogen versus placebo following surgery for patients with early-stage EC closed because of poor accrual. Among the over 1,000 women randomized, EC recurrence rates were not significantly different between groups: 2.3% in the estrogen group and 1.9% in the placebo group (17). Because of the early closure of this trial, it is not possible to make definitive conclusions based on this data; however, other data support the safety of this intervention. A meta-analysis of nearly 900 hormonal users versus over 1,000 patients not using hormonal therapy reported no increased risk of recurrence among women using hormonal therapy (18), and several other nonrandomized studies support this conclusion (19,20). A meta-analysis of over 1,800 patients with EC treated with hormone therapy reported a DFS HR of 0.90 with no significant difference between women treated with hormone therapy and those that were not (21). A short course of low-dose estrogen therapy may be discussed with patients with early-stage and low-grade disease; however, further research is needed in this area.

For women undergoing RT, coordination with radiation oncology providers to encourage use of vaginal dilators is appropriate. Dilator therapy can play a critical role in the vaginal patency and reducing dyspareunia (15,22). Although dilators have not been shown to prevent vaginal stenosis, some studies report improved sexual function, although compliance remains challenging. Research efforts continue to focus on using multimodal treatments aimed at reducing radiation-related vaginal stenosis (23,24).

Although many sexual health concerns for patients with EC may be related to physical/anatomic alterations, the psychological impact of cancer diagnosis, treatment, and survivorship can be significant and may affect multiple domains of health, including sexual health. Multidisciplinary care with social workers, mental health providers, support groups, and psychoeducational interventions can improve sexual health and should be considered (25,26).

Survivorship Considerations for Young Women

Although most women diagnosed with EC are postmenopausal, up to 25% are premenopausal and 4% are women under 40 years (27). The number of young women diagnosed with EC is expected to increase because of increasing prevalence of obesity coupled with nulliparity and anovulation. Lynch syndrome also predisposes women to EC and accounts for 9% of EC among women under age 50 (28). Fertility-sparing treatment of young women with EC was already discussed. Following EC treatment, young survivors may face early menopause if ovaries were removed or radiated during treatment. The North American Menopause Society (NAMS) defines induced menopause as cessation of menstruation following bilateral oophorectomy or iatrogenic ablation of ovarian function resulting from delivery of chemotherapy or pelvic radiation (29). Induced menopause can be more abrupt and severe in symptomatology as compared to natural menopause. Symptoms following oophorectomy manifest within days and within 12 weeks following pelvic radiotherapy (30). Women who experience abrupt surgical menopause may benefit from multidisciplinary care with menopause specialists in order to support bone and cardiovascular health as well as support for sexual health and other menopausal symptoms. Vasomotor symptoms can be addressed with hormonal or nonhormonal medications as well as behavioral interventions (31).

REFERENCES

1. Hamilton CA, Pothuri B, Arend RC, et al. Endometrial cancer: a society of gynecologic oncology evidence-based review and recommendations. *Gynecol Oncol.* 2021;160(3):817-826.

2. Schwartz ZP, Frey MK, Philips S, Curtin JP. Endometrial cancer surveillance adherence reduces utilization and subsequent costs. *Gynecol Oncol.* 2017;146(3):514-518.

3. Salani R, Backes FJ, Fung MF, et al. Posttreatment surveillance and diagnosis of recurrence in women with gynecologic malignancies: Society of Gynecologic Oncologists recommendations. *Am J Obstet Gynecol.* 2011; 204(6):466-478.

4. Martra F, Kunos C, Gibbons H, et al. Adjuvant treatment and survival in obese women with endometrial cancer: an international collaborative study. *Am J Obstet Gynecol.* 2008;198(1):89.e1-89.e898.

5. Smits A, Lopes A, Bekkers R, Galaal K. Body mass index and the quality of life of endometrial cancer survivors—a systematic review and meta-analysis. *Gynecol Oncol.* 2015;137(1):180-187.

6. Ward KK, Shah NR, Saenz CC, McHale MT, Alvarez EA, Plaxe SC. Cardiovascular disease is the leading cause of death among endometrial cancer patients. *Gynecol Oncol.* 2012;126(2):176-179.

7. Laskey RA, McCarroll ML, von Gruenigen VE. Obesity-related endometrial cancer: an update on survivorship approaches to reducing cardiovascular death. *BJOG.* 2016;123(2):293-298.

8. von Gruenigen V, Frasure H, Kavanagh MB, et al. Survivors of uterine cancer empowered by exercise and healthy diet (SUCCEED): a randomized controlled trial. *Gynecol Oncol.* 2012;125(3):699-704.

9. Rizzuto I, Oehler MK, Lalondrelle S, Sexual and psychosexual consequences of treatment for gynaecological cancers. *Clin Oncol (R Coll Radiol).* 2021;33(9):602-607.

10. Onujiogu N, Johnson T, Seo S, et al. Survivors of endometrial cancer: who is at risk for sexual dysfunction? *Gynecol Oncol.* 2011;123(2):356-359.

11. Aerts L, Enzlin P, Verhaeghe J, Poppe W, Vergote I, Amant F. Sexual functioning in women after surgical treatment for endometrial cancer: a prospective controlled study. *J Sex Med.* 2015;12(1):198-209.

12. Nout RA, Putter H, Jürgenliemk-Schulz IM, et al. Five-year quality of life of endometrial cancer patients treated in the randomised post operative radiation therapy in endometrial cancer (PORTEC-2) trial and comparison with norm data. *Eur J Cancer.* 2012;48(11):1638-1648.

13. Li JY, D'Addario J, Tymon-Rosario J, et al. Benefits of a multidisciplinary women's sexual health clinic in the management of sexual and menopausal symptoms after pelvic radiotherapy. *Am J Clin Oncol.* 2021;44(4):143-149.

14. Cyr MP, Dumoulin C, Bessette P, et al. Feasibility, acceptability and effects of multimodal pelvic floor physical therapy for gynecological cancer survivors suffering from painful sexual intercourse: a multicenter prospective interventional study. *Gynecol Oncol.* 2020;159(3):778-784.

15. Carter J, Stabile C, Seidel B, Baser RE, Goldfarb S, Goldfrank DJ. Vaginal and sexual health treatment strategies within a female sexual medicine program for cancer patients and survivors. *J Cancer Surviv.* 2017;11(2):274-283.

16. Suriano KA, McHale M, McLaren CE, Li KT, Re A, DiSaia PJ. Estrogen replacement therapy in endometrial cancer patients: a matched control study. *Obstet Gynecol.* 2001;97(4):555-560.

17. Barakat RR, Bundy BN, Spirtos NM, Bell J, Mannel RS, Gynecologic Oncology Group Study. Randomized double-blind trial of estrogen replacement therapy versus placebo in stage I or II endometrial cancer: a gynecologic oncology group study. *J Clin Oncol.* 2006;24(4):587-592.

18. Shim SH, Lee SJ, Kim SN. Effects of hormone replacement therapy on the rate of recurrence in endometrial cancer survivors: a meta-analysis. *Eur J Cancer.* 2014;50(9):1628-1637.

19. 767. Chapman JA, DiSaia PJ, Osann K, Roth PD, Gillotte DL, Berman ML. Estrogen replacement in surgical stage I and II endometrial cancer survivors. *Am J Obstet Gynecol.* 1996;175(5):1195-1200.

20. Creasman WT, Henderson D, Hinshaw W, Clarke-Pearson DL. Estrogen replacement therapy in the patient treated for endometrial cancer. *Obstet Gynecol.* 1986;67(3):326-330.

21. Londero AP, Parisi N, Tassi A, Bertozzi S, Cagnacci A. Hormone replacement therapy in endometrial cancer survivors: a meta-analysis. *J Clin Med.* 2021;10(14):3165.

22. Crean-Tate KK, Faubion SS, Pederson HJ, Vencill JA, Batur P. Management of genitourinary syndrome of menopause in female cancer patients: a focus on vaginal hormonal therapy. *Am J Obstet Gynecol.* 2020;222(2):103-113.

23. Stahl JM, Qian JM, Tien CJ, et al. Extended duration of dilator use beyond 1 year may reduce vaginal stenosis after intravaginal high-dose-rate brachytherapy. *Support Care Cancer.* 2019;27(4):1425-1433.

24. Miles T, Johnson N. Vaginal dilator therapy for women receiving pelvic radiotherapy. *Cochrane Database Syst Rev.* 2014;2014(9):Cd007291.

25. Brotto LA, Heiman JR, Goff B, et al. A psychoeducational intervention for sexual dysfunction in women with gynecologic cancer. *Arch Sex Behav.* 2008;37(2):317-329.

26. Huffman LB, Hartenbach EM, Carter J, Rash JK, Kushner DM. Maintaining sexual health throughout gynecologic cancer survivorship: a comprehensive review and clinical guide. *Gynecol Oncol.* 2016;140(2):359-368.

27. Ibeanu O, Modesitt SC, Ducie J, von Gruenigen V, Agueh M, Fader AN. Hormone replacement therapy in gynecologic cancer survivors: why not? *Gynecol Oncol.* 2011;122(2):447-454.

28. Lu KH, Schorge JO, Rodabaugh KJ, et al. Prospective determination of prevalence of lynch syndrome in young women with endometrial cancer. *J Clin Oncol*. 2007;25(33):5158-5164.

29. Shifren JL, Gass ML, NAMS Recommendations for Clinical Care of Midlife Women Working Group. The North American menopause society recommendations for clinical care of midlife women. *Menopause*. 2014;21(10):1038-1062.

30. Hinds L, Price J. Menopause, hormone replacement and gynaecological cancers. *Menopause Int*. 2010;16(2):89-93.

31. Del Carmen MG, Rice LW. Management of menopausal symptoms in women with gynecologic cancers. *Gynecol Oncol*. 2017;146(2):427-435.

CHAPTER **5.10**

Endometrial Cancer: Future Directions

Allison Gockley

Over a decade ago, the National Cancer Institute convened an expert panel to develop research priorities in gynecologic cancers. The resulting report, Gynecologic Cancer Strategic Priorities, specified that understanding tumor biology was the central key toward controlling gynecologic cancers. Updated in 2021, this report now focuses on the identification of EC subtypes with optimization of treatments aimed toward molecular and genetic features of each patient's tumor. The hope for a better understanding of EC at a genetic and molecular level is being realized. The GOG 210 study, a prospective surgical pathologic study that created an annotated tissue repository from over 6,000 patients with more than 36,000 specimens, serves as a resource for discovery and validation of predictive and prognostic biomarkers. This collaborative research endeavor has led to numerous publications, further elucidating pathologic treatment and prognostic factors for women with EC and will continue to serve as a foundational tool in the future (1-4). In addition, TCGA Research Network has reported an analysis of over 300 ECs with array-based analyses and second-generation sequencing that will provide information on genome CN, gene expression profiles, methylation status, whole-exome sequencing and has deepened the understanding for molecular classification of ECs (5). It is expected that the knowledge from these datasets will drive clinical research and patient care. Increasingly, we can expect that therapies offered to our patients will be based on a more complete understanding of molecular pathways and that therapies may be matched to address specific genetic changes. Additionally, investigations into racial/ethnic differences in presentation, pathology, and clinical course among women with EC continue to shed light on opportunities to improve care and reduce disparities (6,7).

SUMMARY

EC is the most common gynecologic malignancy, and an understanding of presentation, surgical management, and treatment options is required for gynecologic oncologists. Surgical therapy is a mainstay of EC with lymphadenectomy and laparoscopy increasingly integrated. A thorough knowledge of the relationships between uterine factors and extrauterine disease spread is essential. Surgical staging defines extent of disease and largely defines risk of recurrence. Pelvic radiation is associated with better local control, but no improvement in survival for patients with stage I to II EC in randomized trials. Chemotherapy is increasingly integrated into upfront management of advanced-stage EC and may have a role in early-stage disease. Combination RT and chemotherapy is under evaluation. Targeted agents hold promise; however, a better understanding of molecular and genetic changes is required to improve efficacy.

REFERENCES

1. Brooks RA, Tritchler DS, Darcy KM, et al. GOG 8020/210: risk stratification of lymph node metastasis, disease progression and survival using single nucleotide polymorphisms in endometrial cancer: an NRG oncology/gynecologic oncology group study. *Gynecol Oncol*. 2019;153(2):335-342.

2. Felix AS, Brasky TM, Cohn DE, et al. Endometrial carcinoma recurrence according to race and ethnicity: an NRG oncology/gynecologic oncology group 210 study. *Int J Cancer*. 2018;142(6):1102-1115.

3. Devor EJ, Miecznikowski J, Schickling BM, et al. Dysregulation of miR-181c expression influences recurrence of endometrial endometrioid adenocarcinoma by modulating NOTCH2 expression: an NRG oncology/gynecologic oncology group study. *Gynecol Oncol*. 2017;147(3):648-653.

4. Creasman WT, Ali S, Mutch DG, et al. Surgical-pathological findings in type 1 and 2 endometrial cancer: an NRG oncology/gynecologic oncology group study on GOG-210 protocol. *Gynecol Oncol*. 2017;145(3):519-525.

5. Cancer Genome Atlas Research Network, Kandoth C, Schultz N, et al. Integrated genomic characterization of endometrial carcinoma. *Nature*. 2013;497(7447):67-73.

6. Alson JG, Nguyen A, Hempstead B, et al. "We are a powerful movement": evaluation of an endometrial cancer education program for black women. *Prog Community Health Partnersh*. 2021;15(4):439-452.

7. Reid HW, Broadwater G, Montes de Oca MK, et al. Distress screening in endometrial cancer leads to disparity in referral to support services. *Gynecol Oncol*. 2022;164:622-627.

6

CORPUS: MESENCHYMAL TUMORS

Mesenchymal Tumors: Introduction, Anatomy, Natural History, and Patterns of Spread

Tiffany Y. Sia and Mario M. Leitao Jr

INTRODUCTION

Mesenchymal tumors of the uterine corpus are rare, accounting for between 3% and 7% of all uterine cancers (1,2). The outcomes of many of these tumors seem to be less favorable than in many of the more common uterine carcinomas. However, outcomes do vary significantly based on specific histology. These tumors are believed to arise from the mesenchymatous portion of the uterine corpus involving the myometrium or the connective tissue elements of the endometrium and are often considered to be uterine "sarcomas." The World Health Organization (WHO) classification of mesenchymal uterine corpus tumors is summarized in **Table 6.1-1** (3). Although uterine carcinosarcomas (CS) used to be considered uterine sarcomas, they are now considered metaplastic carcinomas of the uterus (1). Nevertheless, this group of malignancies is described as "uterine CS," which is addressed in this chapter. A key concept is that uterine sarcomas are a heterogeneous mixture of tumor histologies with vastly different clinical presentations, responses to therapy, and outcomes. Until recently, much of the available literature has been extremely limited, as most studies had previously combined all uterine sarcomas into a single cohort. However, the development of molecular profiling techniques has allowed for further subclassification of uterine sarcoma subtypes through identification of specific gene rearrangements and mutations. Although uterine sarcomas remain extremely rare, this additional subclassification allows for more specific treatment and prognostic information to be made available, especially through collaboration via rare tumor registries.

ANATOMY

Mesenchymal cells, also known as *stromal cells*, are a cell type found throughout the body that gives rise to connective tissue and are capable of forming bone, cartilage, fat, and muscle. They tend to be more or less organized within the extracellular matrix adjacent to epithelial cells (4). Epithelial cells, in contrast, line organs, vessels, and cavities and remain separated from the adjacent tissues by a basal lamina (**Figure 6.1-1**). Abnormal proliferation of uterine mesenchymal cells gives rise to a variety of mesenchymal tumors. General tumor subtypes include smooth muscle tumors and endometrial stromal tumors; however, other mixed epithelial and mesenchymal tumors, as well as miscellaneous mesenchymal tumors, may arise (**Table 6.1-1**). Despite the heterogeneity of uterine sarcomas, the majority of tumors originate in the connective tissue of the uterus and grow in size, sometimes spreading into the endometrium and, in aggressive cases, metastasizing distantly via hematogenous or lymphatic spread.

NATURAL HISTORY

Uterine sarcomas comprise a heterogeneous group of tumors, and tumor biology depends heavily on histology. The most aggressive histologies, such as leiomyosarcoma (LMS) and CS, tend to grow rapidly and present with distant metastases. As such, survival rates are lower than for other sarcomas. Studies of uterine LMS have estimated 5-year overall survival (OS) rates to be between 54% and 55%, 29% and 33%, 25% and 36%, and 13% and 22% for stages I, II, III, and IV disease, respectively (5,6). Uterine CS tend to occur in older postmenopausal women, and at the time of diagnosis, over one-third of cases have already spread beyond the uterus (7). Even after resection and treatment, the recurrence rate of CS is 64%, and 5-year OS is estimated at 30%.

On the other end of the spectrum, uterine sarcomas such as low-grade endometrial stromal sarcomas (ESS) and adenosarcomas (AS) have a slow-growing, indolent course. In an analysis of The National Cancer Institute's Surveillance, Epidemiology, and End Results (SEER) database, Chan et al analyzed 831 women with

---

TABLE 6.1-1. WHO Categorization of Mesenchymal Tumors of the Uterine Corpus

Smooth muscle tumors

- Leiomyoma
- Intravenous leiomyomatosis
- Smooth muscle tumor of uncertain/low malignant potential (STUMP)
- Metastasizing leiomyoma
- Leiomyosarcoma
- Conventional (spindle cell) variant
- Myxoid variant
- Epithelioid variant

Endometrial stromal and related tumors

- Endometrial stromal nodule
- Low-grade endometrial stromal sarcoma
- High-grade endometrial stromal sarcoma
- Undifferentiated uterine sarcoma

Miscellaneous mesenchymal tumors

- Uterine tumor resembling ovarian sex cord tumor (UTROSCT)
- Perivascular epithelioid cell tumor
- Inflammatory myofibroblastic tumor (IMT)
- Other mesenchymal tumors

Mixed epithelial and mesenchymal tumors

- Adenomyoma
- Atypical polypoid adenomyoma
- Adenosarcoma

WHO, World Health Organization.

Based on uptodate which references WHO Classification of Tumours Editorial Board. *Female Genital Tumours* [Internet]. International Agency for Research on Cancer; 2020. Accessed July 16, 2020. (WHO classification of tumours series, 5th ed.; vol. 4). https://tumourclassification.iarc.who.int/

https://www.uptodate.com/contents/staging-treatment-and-prognosis-of-endometrial-stromal-sarcoma-and-related-tumors-and-uterine-adenosarcoma?search=uterine%20sarcoma&topicRef=3211&source=see_link#H1374342169

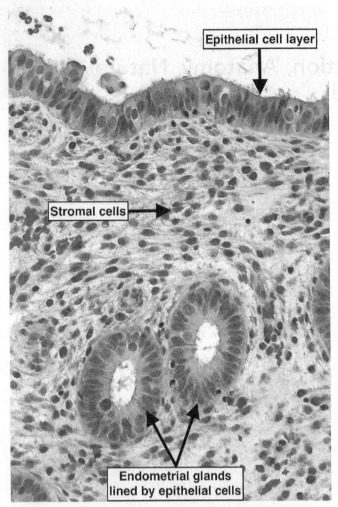

Epithelial cell layer

Stromal cells

Endometrial glands
lined by epithelial cells

Figure 6.1-1. Endometrium in proliferative phase. The endometrium is composed of a layer of epithelial cells resting on stromal cells. Endometrial glands lined by epithelial cells also tunnel from the surface of the endometrium through the base of the stroma, which may be found in cross section.

all grades of ESS and found the median age at diagnosis to be 52 years, with 60% of patients presenting with stage I disease. A 5-year disease-specific survival rate was 91%, 95%, and 42% for grades 1, 2, and 3 disease, respectively. Younger age at diagnosis was associated with improved OS (8).

In another analysis of SEER data, Arend et al contrasted the natural history of CS with AS and reported that 45.6% of patients with CS presented with stage III or IV tumors compared to only 10.5% of patients with AS. A 5-year survival for stage IA AS was 84% compared to 62% for stage IA CS; similarly, 5-year survival for stage III tumors was 48% in AS as opposed to 24% for CS (9). Older age at diagnosis is also associated with decreased survival. AS with sarcomatous overgrowth, in which the sarcomatous component comprises more than 25% of the tumor, are associated with worse prognosis, with recurrence rates of 44% compared to 14% for AS without sarcomatous overgrowth (10). In a case series of 17 patients with AS with sarcomatous overgrowth, 31% of patients died of their disease compared to 7% of women without sarcomatous overgrowth (10).

PATTERNS OF SPREAD

Uterine LMS has a propensity for hematogenous spread, resulting in distant metastases, high local failure rates, and low OS. The most frequent affected metastatic sites are the lung, followed by the cranium, skin and soft tissues, and bone. LMS has also been reported to metastasize to the thyroid and salivary glands, heart,

liver, pancreas, adrenal gland, and breast. Metastases tend to be histologically identical to the primary tumors, and a wide range of time intervals to the development of first metastases have been reported, requiring long-term follow-up (11). Uterine CS have a propensity for extrauterine spread and, during staging surgery, are most often found to also affect the cervix, ovary, and peritoneum (12). The tumors frequently invade the myometrium and lymphatic spaces, and lymph node positivity has been reported to be around 28% (12,13). Recurrences can be classified into locoregional recurrences, affecting the central pelvis, pelvic wall, para-aortic lymph nodes, or distal vagina, or distant recurrences, which include the upper abdomen and inguinal region.

For low- and high-grade ESS, lymph node involvement has been reported to be 10%, though the utility of nodal dissection and effect on oncologic outcome remain to be determined (8). In a retrospective cohort study of 56 patients with low-grade ESS, despite an indolent and slow-growing course, 41% of patients had metastases beyond the pelvis or had recurrences characterized by abdominal pain, mass, vaginal bleeding, or backache (14). Recurrences of ESS in the lung have also been reported (15). Similarly, AS have been associated with a low rate of nodal metastases, with rates ranging between 3% and 7% (9). Recurrences of AS are almost always confined to the vagina, pelvis, or abdomen, suggesting metastatic spread through direct extension rather than hematogenous spread (16).

REFERENCES

1. D'Angelo E, Prat J. Uterine sarcomas: a review. *Gynecol Oncol.* 2010;116 (1):131-139.

2. Felix A, Cook L, Gaudet M, et al. The etiology of uterine sarcomas: a pooled analysis of the epidemiology of endometrial cancer consortium. *Br J Cancer.* 2013;108:727-734. doi:10.1038/bjc.2013.2

3. WHO Classification of Tumours Editorial Board. *Female Genital Tumours* [Internet]. International Agency for Research on Cancer; 2020.

4. Thiery JP, Acloque H, Huang RY, Nieto MA. Epithelial-mesenchymal transitions in development and disease. *Cell.* 2009;139(5):871-890.

5. Zivanovic O, Jacks LM, Iasonos A, et al. A nomogram to predict post-resection 5-year overall survival for patients with uterine leiomyosarcoma. *Cancer.* 2012;118(3):660-669. doi:10.1002/cncr.26333

6. Seagle BL, Sobecki-Rausch J, Strohl AE, Shilpi A, Grace A, Shahabi -S. Prognosis and treatment of uterine leiomyosarcoma: a national cancer database study. *Gynecol Oncol.* 2017;145(1):61-70.

7. Cherniack AD, Shen H, Walter V, et al. Integrated molecular characterization of uterine carcinosarcoma. *Cancer Cell.* 2017;31(3):411-423. doi:10.1016/j.ccell.2017.02.010

8. Chan JK, Kawar NM, Shin JY, et al. Endometrial stromal sarcoma: a population-based analysis. *Br J Cancer.* 2008;99:1210-1215. doi:10.1038/sj.bjc.6604527

9. Arend R, Bagaria M, Lewin SN, et al. Long-term outcome and natural history of uterine adenosarcomas. *Gynecol Oncol.* 2010;119(2):305-308. doi:10.1016/j.ygyno.2010.07.001

10. Kaku T, Silverberg SG, Major FJ, Miller A, Fetter B, Brady MF. Adenosarcoma of the uterus: a gynecologic oncology group clinicopathologic study of 31 cases. *Int J Gynecol Pathol.* 1992;11(2):75-88. PMID: 1316323.

11. Bartosch C, Afonso M, Pires-Luís AS, et al. Distant metastases in uterine leiomyosarcomas: the wide variety of body sites and time intervals to metastatic relapse. *Int J Gynecol Pathol.* 2017;36(1):31-41. doi:10.1097/PGP.0000000000000284

12. Callister M, Ramondetta LM, Jhingran A, Burke TW, Eifel PJ. Malignant mixed Müllerian tumors of the uterus: analysis of patterns of failure, prognostic factors, and treatment outcome. *Int J Radiat Oncol Biol Phys.* 2004;58(3):786-796. doi:10.1016/S0360-3016(03)01561-X

13. Norris HJ, Taylor HB. Mesenchymal tumors of the uterus. 3. A clinical and pathologic study of 31 carcinosarcomas. *Cancer.* 1966;19(10):1459-1465. doi:10.1002/1097-0142(196610)19:10<1459::aid-cncr2820191019>3.0.co;2-a

14. Dai Q, Xu B, Wu H, You Y, Wu M, Li L. The prognosis of recurrent low-grade endometrial stromal sarcoma: a retrospective cohort study. *Orphanet J Rare Dis.* 2021;16(1):160. doi:10.1186/s13023-021-01802-8

15. Garavaglia E, Pella F, Montoli S, Voci C, Taccagni G, Mangili G. Treatment of recurrent or metastatic low-grade endometrial stromal sarcoma: three case reports. *Int J Gynecol Cancer.* 2010;20(7):1197-1200. doi:10.1111/igc.0b013e3181ef6d87

16. Clement PB, Scully RE. Mullerian adenosarcoma of the uterus: a clinicopathologic analysis of 100 cases with a review of the literature. *Hum Pathol.* 1990;21:363-381.

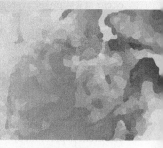

CHAPTER **6.2**

Mesenchymal Tumors: Etiology, Epidemiology, and Risk Factors

Tiffany Y. Sia, Mario M. Leitao Jr, and Lora Hedrick Ellenson

HISTOLOGIC DISTRIBUTION

The histopathologic criteria for uterine sarcomas have evolved significantly over the past few years and are frequently shifting. Generally, pure mesenchymal uterine sarcomas contain homologous elements, which are normally found in uterine tissues such as smooth muscle, endometrial stroma, or vascular tissue. More uncommonly, uterine sarcomas such as rhabdomyosarcomas or primitive neuroectodermal tumors may also contain heterologous elements, such as skeletal muscle, bone, or fat. Uterine sarcomas may also contain mixed epithelial and mesenchymal tumors, such as AS or adenomyomas. CS, which contain both carcinoma and sarcoma tissue types, had previously been considered part of the uterine sarcoma subgroup, but in 2009, the International Federation of Gynaecology and Obstetrics (FIGO) reclassified them as metaplastic uterine carcinomas.

Given the rarity of uterine sarcomas, many series do not include or specify sarcoma subtypes, and many of these studies report on very small patient cohorts. By combining series with at least 100 cases, we see that the most common uterine sarcomas are LMS, which account for over two-thirds of uterine sarcomas, followed by ESS that account for approximately 25% of uterine sarcomas (1-6) **(Figure 6.2-1A,B)**. All other subtypes are exceedingly rare, comprising less than 10% (1-7) **(Figure 6.2-1B)**. Although LMS has become the most common subtype of uterine sarcoma, it comprises only 1% to 2% of all uterine malignancies.

In 2009, Abeler and colleagues (7) reported on a large series of uterine sarcomas (*n* = 419) from the Norwegian Cancer Registry (which describes histologic subtype distribution). This series excluded CS altogether. Of the 419 included sarcomas, 62% were LMS, 20% were ESS, and 18% were various other subtypes, including undifferentiated sarcomas (6%), AS (5.5%), sarcoma not otherwise specified (NOS) (4.5%), rhabdomyosarcoma (<1%), giant cell sarcoma (<1%), and perivascular epithelioid cell tumors (PEComa; <1%) (7).

Age Distribution

Patients with CS and AS tend to be older at the time of diagnosis compared to those with LMS and ESS. The mean/median ages

reported in the published series range from 42 to 51 years for ESS (1,2,6-13), 48 to 57 years for LMS (1,2,6,7,14-16), 57 to 67 years for CS (1,2,6,17,18), 58 to 66 years for AS (7, 19), and 46 years for undifferentiated sarcomas (9). Thus, many patients with CS and AS are postmenopausal at the time of diagnosis, whereas patients with LMS, ESS, or undifferentiated sarcomas may be premenopausal or perimenopausal at diagnosis. The mean age for patients diagnosed with smooth muscle tumors of uncertain malignant potential (STUMP) is 43 years, and many of these patients are likely to be premenopausal (20). This has potential implications in terms of patient fertility. The other tumor subtypes are so rare that it is difficult to discern a particular pattern of age distribution among them.

Racial Distribution

In general, Black patients have a higher incidence of developing both uterine sarcomas and CS than White women. Brooks et al (21) reported that the age-adjusted incidence of uterine sarcomas in African American women was twice that of White women or women of other races (1.5 vs 0.9 per 100,000). Similarly, Sherman et al (22) reported an incidence of uterine sarcomas of 1.2 and 0.8 per 100,000 women for Black and non-Hispanic White women, respectively. Felix and colleagues (23) noted that African American race was more prevalent among 82 (20.7%) LMS cases compared to 98 (6.1%) EMS cases.

Incidence of CS tumors followed a similar pattern. Zelmanowicz et al (24) noted that women with CS are more likely to be of African American descent (among 453 patients and controls, 28% vs 4% other, *P* = .001) than those with endometrial adenocarcinomas. Incidence rates for CS ranged between 1 to 4 and 0.6 to 1.7 per 100,000 women of Black and non-Hispanic White heritage, respectively (21,22).

RISK FACTORS

Prior Radiation Exposure

Prior exposure to pelvic radiotherapy (RT) is thought to increase the risk of developing a subsequent uterine sarcoma, primarily CS and undifferentiated sarcoma. However, prior pelvic RT is not thought to increase the risk for uterine LMS or STUMP. In a large series from the Mayo Clinic, only 1 (0.6%) of 208 patients with LMS had received prior pelvic RT (25). In a study from MD Anderson Cancer Center, none of 41 patients with STUMP had a history of pelvic RT (20). In a study by Christopherson et al (26), only 2 of 33 patients with uterine LMS had a history of RT.

In the series of CS reported by Norris et al in 1966 (27), 9 (29%) of 31 patients had received pelvic RT 7 to 26 years before diagnosis. In a 1986 report by Meredith et al (28) on 1,208 uterine malignancies, only 30 (2.4%) patients had received prior pelvic RT. Interestingly, only eight patients had received RT for a gynecologic malignancy; others had pelvic RT for a benign diagnosis. Of irradiated patients, 5 (17%) developed CS, with a crude association of 11%. The risk of endometrial adenocarcinoma after radiation was much less than 2%. It has been suggested that postirradiation CS

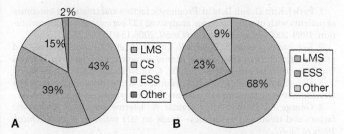

Figure 6.2-1. Histologic distribution of uterine sarcomas in series with at least 100 cases, (A) including CS and (B) excluding CS. AS, adenosarcoma; CS, carcinosarcoma; ESS, endometrial stromal sarcoma; LMS, leiomyosarcoma.

occur at a younger average age than those arising de novo (29). Pothuri et al (30) compared the clinicopathologic characteristics of 23 cases of uterine cancers occurring in patients with prior history of cervical cancer treated with pelvic RT, to 527 cases of uterine cancers in patients with no history of pelvic RT. CS and undifferentiated sarcomas accounted for 9 (39%) of the 23 radiation-associated malignancies, compared to 33 (8%) of the sporadic cases (30). It appears that radiation-associated malignancies tend to have a worse outcome, possibly due to the lack of early symptomatology. In the setting of other, very rare uterine sarcoma subtypes, definitive assessment is precluded.

Hormone Exposure and Obesity

It has been suggested that exposure to hormonal medications, including tamoxifen, may increase the risk of uterine sarcomas. The association of estradiol-progestin therapy was assessed by Jaakkola et al (31) using data from the Finnish Cancer Registry (which captures nearly 100% of all cancers in Finland) and the Reimbursement Registry of the Social Insurance Institution of Finland. Uterine sarcomas occurred in 76 of the 243,857 (0.03%) women identified as having used estradiol-progestin therapy for more than 6 months. CS were not included in this analysis. The use of estradiol-progestin therapy was associated with a 60% elevation in risk for any uterine sarcoma (standardized incidence ratio [SIR], 1.6; 95% confidence interval [CI], 1.2-1.9). It was mostly associated with LMS (SIR, 1.8; 95% CI, 1.3-2.4); no statistically significant association with ESS was identified (SIR, 1.4; 95% CI, 0.9-2.1). In addition, the elevated risk was noted only in women who had used estradiol-progestin therapy for 5 years or more.

The Epidemiology of Endometrial Cancer Consortium (E2C2) recently published a pooled analysis of 15 cohort and case-control observational studies (23). This is the largest series to date assessing risk factors for uterine sarcoma ($n = 229$) and CS ($n = 244$) versus endometrioid endometrial carcinomas ($n = 7,623$) and normal controls ($n = 28,829$). Uterine sarcomas included all sarcomas of the uterus, with 98 ESS and 82 LMS. Oral contraceptive use, postmenopausal estrogen (ER)-alone use, and postmenopausal ER-progesterone (PR) use were not associated with uterine sarcoma or CS. No association was found when LMS and ESS were analyzed separately. Thus, it seems that the association of hormonal use with the risk of uterine sarcoma or CS is not strong. As the risk is exceedingly low, these data should not dissuade the use of hormones in appropriate cases.

Interestingly, the E2C2 analyses (23) suggested an association of obesity (body mass index [BMI] ≥30 kg/m^2) with uterine sarcoma (odds ratio [OR] = 1.73 [95% CI, 1.22-2.46]) and CS (OR = 2.25 [95% CI, 1.60-3.15]). Obesity was also associated with ESS (OR = 1.74 [95% CI, 1.03-2.93]), but not with LMS (OR = 1.56 [95% CI, 0.88-2.77]). As ESS is known to be ER driven, the association with obesity is understandable. However, the association of obesity with CS in this analysis requires further study and validation.

Tamoxifen Use

Tamoxifen use among patients with breast cancer may also increase the risk of uterine malignancies, including sarcomas. The proposed mechanism behind this increased risk is estrogenic agonist activity on the uterus, and the effect appears to be dose related. Using data from the National Israeli Cancer Registry, Lavie and colleagues (32) reported on 1,507 cases of women with breast cancer diagnosed from 1987 to 1988. They noted that uterine cancers developed in 17 (1.9%) of 886 women treated with tamoxifen, compared to only 4 (0.6%) of 621 women who did not receive tamoxifen (OR, 3.1; 95% CI, 1-9.1). The risk of uterine cancer was associated with increased duration of tamoxifen use. A significant association was seen with more than 4 years of tamoxifen use (OR, 6.6; 95% CI, 2.0-21.1), whereas the use of tamoxifen for 2 years or less was not associated with an increased risk (OR, 2.1; 95% CI, 0.4-11.6). Uterine sarcomas developed in only four patients in the entire cohort: two CS and two rhabdomyosarcomas. All four occurred in patients who received tamoxifen, suggesting a possible association of tamoxifen use and risk of uterine sarcoma. Hoogendoorn and colleagues (33) reported that among patients diagnosed with uterine cancer, CS accounted for a much larger proportion of cases in those who had received prior tamoxifen therapy compared to those who had not (15% vs 4%). Furthermore, a secondary analysis of National Surgical Adjuvant Breast and Bowel Project (NSABP) trials included more than 17,000 women who were randomized to take tamoxifen or placebo and found that the incidence of both endometrial adenocarcinoma and uterine sarcoma was increased with tamoxifen, with sarcomas making up 10% of uterine malignancies in the cohort (34). The same group performed a review of adverse events reported for Nolvadex (tamoxifen citrate) through AstraZeneca's global drug safety database and found that for 12 million patient-years, 942 uterine malignancies were reported. Sarcomas made up 15% of the cohort, and 73% of all reported sarcomas were CS. Women taking tamoxifen therapy should undergo annual gynecologic examinations and seek evaluation for any gynecologic symptoms such as pelvic pressure or abnormal uterine bleeding.

Hereditary Predisposition

Hereditary predisposition to certain uterine sarcomas has also been suggested, but this remains to be elucidated. Using the Danish Hereditary Nonpolyposis Colorectal Cancer (HNPCC) Registry, Nilbert et al (35) identified 164 HNPCC families with predisposing mutations; sarcomas of various sites represented only 1% ($n = 14$) of 1,570 malignant diagnoses. Three sarcomas were uterine: one was a CS in a 44-year-old with loss of MSH2 and MSH6 expression; another CS was seen in a 55-year-old with loss of MSH6 expression; and another was an LMS in a 44-year-old with loss of MSH2 and MSH6 expression. Recently, it has been suggested that the prevalence of uterine LMS is increased in women with hereditary retinoblastoma (36) and that women with a germline mutation in the *SMARCA4* gene are at increased risk for small cell carcinoma of the ovary, hypercalcemic type, as well as undifferentiated uterine sarcomas (37,38). Because of the high risk of endometrial sarcoma, prophylactic hysterectomy is strongly recommended in women from HNPCC kindreds after childbearing is complete. No such recommendation exists for women with hereditary retinoblastoma or for women with germline *SMARCA4* pathogenic or likely pathogenic variants, given the rarity of the tumors and the limited data. However, we believe that it is reasonable to consider prophylactic total hysterectomy, with retention of ovaries, in women with a history of retinoblastoma who have completed childbearing. For women with a germline *SMARCA4* pathogenic or likely pathogenic variant who have completed childbearing, it may be reasonable to pursue prophylactic bilateral salpingo-oophorectomy with or without hysterectomy or careful endometrial surveillance after discussion with the patient.

REFERENCES

1. Park J, Kim D, Suh D, et al. Prognostic factors and treatment outcomes of patients with uterine sarcoma: analysis of 127 patients at a single institution, 1989-2007. *J Cancer Res Clin Oncol.* 2008;134:1277-1287.

2. Koivisto-Korander R, Butzow R, Koivisto A, et al. Clinical outcome and prognostic factors in 100 cases of uterine sarcoma: experience in Helsinki University Central Hospital 1990-2001. *Gynecol Oncol.* 2008;111:74-81.

3. Kahanpaa K, Wahlstrom T, Grohn P, et al. Sarcomas of the uterus: a clinicopathologic study of 119 patients. *Obstet Gynecol.* 1986;67:417-424.

4. George M, Pejovic MH, Kramar A. Uterine sarcomas: prognostic factors and treatment modalities—study on 209 patients. *Gynecol Oncol.* 1986;24:58-67.

5. Olah KS, Gee H, Blunt S, et al. Retrospective analysis of 318 cases of uterine sarcoma. *Eur J Cancer.* 1991;27:1095-1099.

6. Pautier P, Genestie C, Rey A, et al. Analysis of clinicopathologic prognostic factors for 157 uterine sarcomas and evaluation of grading score validated for soft tissue sarcoma. *Cancer.* 2000;88:1425-1431.

7. Abeler VM, Royne O, Thoresen S, et al. Uterine sarcomas in Norway. A histopathological and prognostic survey of a total population from 1970 to 2000 including 419 patients. *Histopathology*. 2009;54:355-364.

8. Lee CH, Mariño-Enriquez A, Ou W, et al. The clinicopathologic features of YWHAE-FAM22 endometrial stromal sarcomas: a histologically high-grade and clinically aggressive tumor. *Am J Surg Pathol*. 2012;36:641-653.

9. Jin Y, Pan L, Wang X, et al. Clinical characteristics of endometrial stromal sarcoma from and academic medical hospital in China. *Int J Gynecol Cancer*. 2010;20:1535-1539.

10. Vera AA, Guadarrama MB. Endometrial stromal sarcoma: clinicopathological and immunophenotype study of 18 cases. *Ann Diag Pathol*. 2011;15:312-317.

11. Cheng X, Yang G, Schmeler KM, et al. Recurrence patterns and prognosis of endometrial stromal sarcoma and the potential of tyrosine kinase-inhibiting therapy. *Gynecol Oncol*. 2011;121:323-327.

12. Shah LP, Bryant CS, Kumar S, et al. Lymphadenectomy and ovarian preservation in low-grade endometrial stromal sarcoma. *Obstet Gynecol*. 2008;112:1102-1108.

13. dos Santos LA, Garg K, Diaz JP, et al. Incidence of lymph node and adnexal metastasis in endometrial stromal sarcoma. *Gynecol Oncol*. 2011;121:319-322.

14. Garg G, Shah JP, Liu R, et al. Validation of tumor size as staging variable in the revised International Federation of Gynecology and Obstetrics stage I leiomyosarcoma: a population-based study. *Int J Gynecol Cancer*. 2010;20:1201-1206.

15. Loizzi V, Cormio G, Nestola D, et al. Prognostic factors and outcomes in 28 cases of uterine leiomyosarcoma. *Oncology*. 2011;81:91-97.

16. Zivanovic O, Leitao MM, Iasonos A, et al. Stage-specific outcomes of patients with uterine leiomyosarcoma: a comparison of the international federation of gynecology and obstetrics and american joint committee on cancer staging systems. *J Clin Oncol*. 2009;27:2066-2072.

17. Park J, Kim D, Kim J, et al. The role of pelvic and/or para-aortic lymphadenectomy in surgical management of apparently early carcinosarcoma of uterus. *Ann Surg Oncol*. 2010;17:861-868.

18. Pradhan TA, Stevens EE, Ablavsky M, et al. FIGO staging for carcinosarcoma: can the revised staging system predict overall survival. *Gynecol Oncol*. 2011;123:221-224.

19. Clement PB, Scully RE. Mullerian adenosarcoma of the uterus: a clinicopathologic analysis of 100 cases with a review of the literature. *Hum Pathol*. 1990;21:363-381.

20. Guntupalli SR, Ramirez PT, Anderson ML, et al. Uterine smooth muscle tumor of uncertain malignant potential: a retrospective analysis. *Gynecol Oncol*. 2009;113:324-326.

21. Brooks SE, Zhan M, Cote T, et al. Survival epidemiology and end results analysis of 267 cases of uterine sarcomas, 1989–1999. *Gynecol Oncol*. 2004;93:204-208.

22. Sherman ME, Devesa SS. Analysis of racial differences in incidence, survival, and mortality for malignant tumors of the uterine corpus. *Cancer*. 2003;98(1):176-186. doi:10.1002/cncr.11484

23. Felix A, Cook L, Gaudet M, et al. The etiology of uterine sarcomas: a pooled analysis of the epidemiology of endometrial cancer consortium. *Br J Cancer*. 2013;108:727-734. doi:10.1038/bjc.2013.2

24. Zelmanowicz A, Hildesheim A, Sherman MA, et al. Evidence for a common etiology for endometrial carcinomas and malignant mixed müllerian tumors. *Gynecol Oncol*. 1998;69:253-257.

25. Giuntoli RL, Metzinger DS, DiMarco CS, et al. Retrospective review of 208 patients with leiomyosarcoma of the uterus: prognostic indicators, surgical management, and adjuvant therapy. *Gynecol Oncol*. 2003;89:460-469.

26. Christopherson WM, Williamson EO, Gray LA. Leiomyosarcoma of the uterus. *Cancer*. 1972;29:1512-1517.

27. Norris HJ, Roth E, Taylor HB. Mesenchymal tumors of the uterus. *Obstet Gynecol*. 1966;28:57-63.

28. Meredith RJ, Eisert DR, Kaka Z, et al. An excess of uterine sarcomas after pelvic irradiation. *Cancer*. 1986;58:2003-2007.

29. Varala-Duran J, Nochomovitz LE, Prem KA, et al. Post irradiation mixed Müllerian tumors of the uterus. *Cancer*. 1980;45:1625-1631.

30. Pothuri B, Ramondetta L, Eifel P, et al. Radiation-associated endometrial cancers are prognostically unfavorable tumors: a clinicopathologic comparison with 527 sporadic endometrial cancers. *Gynecol Oncol*. 2006;103:948-951.

31. Jaakkola S, Lyytinen HK, Pukkala E, et al. Use of estradiol-progestin therapy associates with increased risk for uterine sarcomas. *Gynecol Oncol*. 2011;122:260-263.

32. Lavie O, Barnett-Griness O, Narod SA, et al. The risk of developing uterine sarcoma after tamoxifen use. *Int J Gynecol Cancer*. 2008;18:352-356.

33. Hoogendoorn WE, Hollema H, van Boven HH, et al. Prognosis of uterine corpus cancer after tamoxifen treatment for breast cancer. *Breast Cancer Res Treat*. 2008;112:99-108.

34. Wickerham DL, Fisher B, Wolmark N, et al. Association of tamoxifen and uterine cancer. *J Clin Oncol*. 2002;20(11):2758-2760. doi:10.1200/JCO.2002.20.11.2758

35. Nilbert M, Therkildsen C, Nissen A, et al. Sarcomas associated with hereditary nonpolyposis colorectal cancer: broad anatomical and morphological spectrum. *Fam Cancer*. 2009;8:209-213.

36. Francis JH, Kleinerman RA, Seddon J, et al. Increased risk of secondary uterine leiomyosarcoma in hereditary retinoblastoma. *Gynecol Oncol*. 2012;124:254-259.

37. Connor YD, Miao D, Lin DI, et al. Germline mutations of SMARCA4 in small cell carcinoma of the ovary, hypercalcemic type and in SMARCA4-deficient undifferentiated uterine sarcoma: clinical features of a single family and comparison of large cohorts. *Gynecol Oncol*. 2020;157(1):106-114. doi:10.1016/j.ygyno.2019.10.031

38. Lin DI, Allen JM, Hecht JL, et al. *SMARCA4* inactivation defines a subset of undifferentiated uterine sarcomas with rhabdoid and small cell features and germline mutation association. *Mod Pathol*. 2019;32:1675-1687. doi:10.1038/s41379-019-0303-z

CHAPTER **6.3**

Mesenchymal Tumors: Clinical Presentation and Diagnostic Evaluation and Workup

Tiffany Y. Sia and Mario M. Leitao Jr

CLINICAL PRESENTATION

Presenting Symptoms and Signs

The most common presenting symptom of uterine sarcoma is abnormal vaginal bleeding (1-6) (**Table 6.3-1**). Patients also often present with an abdominopelvic mass, or a mass that is palpable on physical examination (1,5). Rarely, a mass can be found protruding through the cervix. Because presenting symptoms are the same as those in patients with benign uterine myomas, LMS and ESS are often incidentally diagnosed after surgery for presumed uterine fibroids. For example, ESS was an incidental finding in 42% of cases reported by Memorial Sloan Kettering Cancer Center (7). Therefore, it is quite likely that the vast majority of patients ultimately diagnosed with LMS or ESS would have some abnormal enlargement of the uterus, discovered after presentation with abnormal vaginal

■ **TABLE 6.3-1. Common Presenting Symptoms in Patients With Uterine Sarcomas (Percentage of Cases Describing the Symptoms)**

Symptom	ESS (%) (4,12,14)	CS (%) (4)	LMS (%) (4,27)	AS (%) (22,38)
Asymptomatic	14	7	11	12
Abnormal vaginal bleeding	68	68	53	61
Abdominopelvic mass	14	16	48	—
Abdominopelvic pain	18	9	23	20
Uterine enlargement	64	—	—	—
Uterine cavity lesion	21	—	—	—
Vaginal discharge	4	—	—	—
Abdominal distention	—	—	—	2

AS, adenosarcoma; CS, carcinosarcoma; ESS, endometrial stromal sarcoma; LMS, leiomyosarcoma.

Santos P, Cunha TM. Uterine sarcomas: clinical presentation and MRI features. *Diagn Interv Radiol.* 2015;21(1):4-9. doi:10.5152/dir.2014.14053. https://www.ncbi.nlm.nih.gov/pmc/articles/PMC4463355/

bleeding. Vaginal bleeding in a postmenopausal female should be evaluated appropriately, with endometrial sampling and, possibly, a pelvic ultrasound (US). Any enlarging pelvic mass in a postmenopausal female is suspicious for a malignant process. Proper assessment of symptoms and signs in premenopausal patients is a challenge, and diagnosis of malignancy is often delayed because multiple benign conditions are likely to cause such symptoms.

DIAGNOSTIC EVALUATION/WORKUP

Physical Examination and Preoperative Imaging

Uterine sarcomas typically present with physical examination findings of an enlarged abdominopelvic mass, although the uterus may sometime be normal in size. These physical examination findings are similar to those of benign uterine myomas. In addition, preoperative pelvic imaging is of limited accuracy in differentiating benign from malignant uterine lesions, especially in the absence of obvious extrauterine disease; nevertheless, it is often utilized as part of the initial evaluation of these patients.

On magnetic resonance imaging (MRI), LMS typically present as a large infiltrating myometrial mass with heterogeneous T1 signal hypointensity, T2 intermediate-to-high signal intensity, and with central hyperintensity indicative of necrosis (**Table 6.3-2**) (8). Compared to benign leiomyomas, LMS are generally larger and demonstrate more rapid growth and more necrosis. However, even leiomyomas may at times demonstrate regular growth and areas of increased signal intensity on T2-weighted images. Namimoto et al (9) reported 100% sensitivity and specificity using a combination of

■ **TABLE 6.3-2. MRI Features of Uterine Sarcomas, Leiomyoma, and Endometrial Carcinoma**

	LMS	ESS	UES	AS	Leiomyoma	Endometrial Carcinoma
Localization	Myometrium	Generally endometrium; can be located in myometrium	Generally endometrium; can be located in myometrium	Endometrium	Myometrium	Endometrium
Margins	Irregular and ill-defined	Irregular and nodular	Markedly irregular and nodular	Regular and well demarcated	Regular	Regular or irregular
T1 signal	Hypointense and heterogeneous (hemorrhage, calcifications)	Hypointense	Heterogeneous	Predominantly hypointense, heterogeneous	Low-to-intermediate signal; high signal foci—hemorrhagic degeneration	Hypo-to-isointense signal to normal endometrium
T2 signal	Intermediate-to-high signal	Hyperintense and heterogeneous; bands of low signal corresponding to preserved myometrium	Heterogeneous (extensive hemorrhage and necrosis)	Multiseptated cystic appearance; can show multiple small hyperintense foci	Low signal (nondegenerated); high signal—cystic, myxoid degeneration	Hyperintense and heterogeneous relative to normal endometrium
Contrast enhancement	Early and heterogeneous	Moderate (more intense than endometrial carcinoma) and heterogeneous	Marked (generally more intense than normal myometrium) and heterogeneous	Marked (generally isointense compared to normal myometrium) and heterogeneous	Variable	Hypointense compared to normal myometrium
DWI	Generally more restriction (lower ADC values) than leiomyomas	High signal and low ADC	High signal and low ADC	Low signal (low grade nature)	Variable; generally higher ADC values than LMS	High signal and low ADC

ADC, apparent diffusion coefficient; AS, adenosarcoma; DWI, diffusion-weighted imaging; ESS, endometrial stromal sarcoma; LMS, leiomyosarcoma; UES, undifferentiated endometrial sarcoma. Table 3 from Santos P, Cunha TM. Uterine sarcomas: clinical presentation and MRI features. *Diagn Interv Radiol.* 2015;21(1):4-9. https://www.ncbi.nlm.nih.gov/pmc/articles/PMC4463355/

diffusion-weighted imaging (DWI) and T2-weighted MRI in distinguishing uterine sarcomas from benign lesions, compared to DWI alone. This seems promising, but it is unlikely to be utilized in clinical practice, and its accuracy may not be reliably reproducible. For example, Cornfeld and colleagues (10), using various objective MRI criteria, reported that MRI showed very poor accuracy in distinguishing leiomyomas with atypical imaging features from malignant uterine mesenchymal tumors. Using various MRI-specific criteria, the sensitivity of this imaging modality in identifying uterine sarcoma ranged from only 17% to 56%; however, specificity was 80% to 100% (10). A retrospective review by Lakhman and colleagues noted high accuracy when three of four of the following features were identified on MRI: nodular borders, hemorrhage, "T2 dark" area(s), and central unenhanced area(s) (11) (**Figure 6.3-1**). The sensitivity and specificity were reported as 100% and 95%, respectively. The positive and negative predictive values were reported as 95% and 100%, respectively. However, this retrospective series was enriched for LMS ($N = 19$) and compared to only 22 atypical leiomyomata.

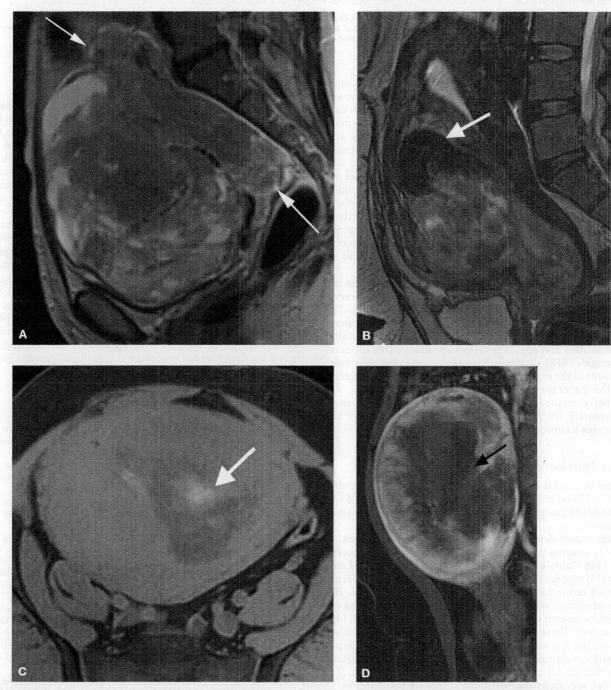

Figure 6.3-1. Illustrations of the four qualitative magnetic resonance features that demonstrated the strongest statistical associations with leiomyosarcoma at histopathology. **A:** Sagittal T2-weighted image shows a large uterine mass with nodular superior and posterior borders (white arrows). **B:** Sagittal T2-weighted image demonstrates "T2 dark" area in the myometrial mass (white arrow). **C:** Noncontrast T1-weighted fat-saturated image illustrates the presence of intralesional hemorrhage (white arrow). **D:** Sagittal contrast-enhanced T1-weighted fat saturated image shows the presence of central unenhanced areas (black arrow). Reprinted by permission from Springer: From Lakhman Y, Veeraraghavan H, Chaim J, et al. Differentiation of uterine leiomyosarcoma from atypical leiomyoma: diagnostic accuracy of qualitative MR imaging features and feasibility of texture analysis. *Eur Radiol.* 2017;27(7):2903-2915. doi:10.1007/s00330-016-4623-9

■ **TABLE 6.3-3. Test Characteristics Using Dynamic MRI and Serum LDH in Predicting Uterine LMS From Degenerating Leiomyomas**

Test	Sensitivity (%)	Specificity (%)	Accuracy (%)	PPV (%)	NPV (%)
Total serum LDH	100	87.7	86.6	38.5	100
MRI	100	96.9	97.1	71.4	100
Dynamic MRI	100	87.5	90.5	71.4	100
LDH & MRI	100	99.2	99.3	90.9	100

LDH, lactate dehydrogenase; LMS, leiomyosarcoma; MRI, magnetic resonance imaging; NPV, negative predictive value; PPV, positive predictive value.

Used with permission of BMJ Publishing Group, from Goto A, Takeuchi S, Sugimura K, et al. Usefulness of Gd-DTPA contrast-enhanced dynamic MRi and serum determination of LDH and its isozymes in the differential diagnosis of leiomyosarcoma from degenerated leiomyoma of the uterus. *Int J Gynecol Cancer*. 2002;12:354-361; permission conveyed through Copyright Clearance Center, Inc

ESS tends to appear as an endometrial polypoid mass with low signal on T1-weighted images and heterogeneous increased T2 signal (**Table 6.3-2**) (8). Compared to endometrial carcinomas, ESS tumors tend to be larger, have a more irregular margin, showcase nodular extension into the myometrium, and extend along vessels and lymphatic systems. ESS may sometimes present as a myometrial mass but also demonstrate rapid and invasive growth, lymphatic and vascular invasion, and higher incidence of necrosis compared to intramural leiomyomas. Undifferentiated endometrial sarcoma (UES) often presents similarly but may also manifest with intramyometrial worm-like extension bands of low signal intensity within areas of myometrial involvement on T2-weighted images owing to marked vascular and lymphatic invasion (8). Multiple nodular masses may also be seen with UES.

AS tumors typically present as a polypoid mass within the endometrial cavity and may sometimes protrude through the cervical os. The uterus may be enlarged with a thin myometrium. The polypoid mass may appear to have multiseptated cystic areas along with heterogeneous solid components that fill the uterine cavity. Areas of necrosis may appear as hyperintense foci within the mass on T2-weighted MRI, and after administration of gadolinium, solid components of the mass may show enhancement on T2-weighted images like that of the myometrium (**Table 6.3-2**).

Neither computed tomography (CT) nor positron emission tomography/CT (PET/CT) can reliably detect the difference between benign leiomyomas and uterine sarcomas (12).

Tumor Markers

There are no reliable serum tumor markers for uterine sarcoma. Serum CA-125 is elevated in 17% to 33% of LMS, ESS, and CS (1). It should not be routinely used in the evaluation and diagnosis of these tumors.

Serum lactate dehydrogenase (LDH) may be an interesting additive to imaging in the evaluation of uterine lesions concerning for LMS (**Table 6.3-3**). In a prospective trial, Goto and colleagues (13) reported an accuracy of 99.3% in predicting uterine LMS when serum LDH was combined with dynamic MRI. The positive predictive value (PPV) was 91% using the combined assessment, compared to 39% for LDH alone and 71% for MRI (dynamic or not). These results are impressive and require further validation, but it is simple enough to obtain a serum LDH in patients with concerning lesions of the uterus. Another important point is that the series by Goto et al, as well as other series, report a high specificity and nearly 100% negative predictive value (NPV) for MRI, with or without LDH. This may be useful for patients who do not wish to undergo surgery, especially those desiring fertility. It may also help in deciding upon the surgical approach for patients with presumed benign leiomyomas as well as suspicious lesions.

Endometrial Sampling

Preoperative endometrial assessment with office pipelle or dilation and curettage (D&C) under anesthesia is of limited accuracy and has yielded a preoperative diagnosis in only 33% to 68% of patients with sarcomas (2,14). However, endometrial assessments should be performed in all women who present with abnormal vaginal bleeding.

CS often presents with vaginal bleeding in a postmenopausal female and can often be diagnosed with endometrial assessment, as it is a lesion arising in the endometrium. However, true uterine sarcomas often lack an endometrial component or endometrial involvement and can be missed by endometrial sampling. Bansal et al (15) reported that invasive tumor was diagnosed in 86% of uterine sarcoma cases through preoperative endometrial sampling. The correct histology was noted in only 64% of the cases ultimately diagnosed as uterine sarcoma (15). However, a majority of sarcomas in this series (32/46; 70%) were correctly diagnosed as CS on final pathology, as well as four LMS, two ESS, and eight other sarcomas (15). Minimally invasive needle biopsy has been proposed to diagnose uterine sarcomas; however, given the heterogeneous nature of the tumor, multiple sampling sites are often needed, and there is concern that the procedure may spill malignant cells into the peritoneal cavity.

References

1. Park J, Kim D, Suh D, et al. Prognostic factors and treatment outcomes of patients with uterine sarcoma: analysis of 127 patients at a single institution, 1989-2007. *J Cancer Res Clin Oncol*. 2008;134:1277-1287.

2. Jin Y, Pan L, Wang X, et al. Clinical characteristics of endometrial stromal sarcoma from an academic medical hospital in China. *Int J Gynecol Cancer*. 2010;20(9):1535-1539. PMID: 21370596.

3. Cheng X, Yang G, Schmeler KM, et al. Recurrence patterns and prognosis of endometrial stromal sarcoma and the potential of tyrosine kinase-inhibiting therapy. *Gynecol Oncol*. 2011;121:323-327.

4. Clement PB, Scully RE. Mullerian adenosarcoma of the uterus: a clinicopathologic analysis of 100 cases with a review of the literature. *Hum Pathol*. 1990;21:363-381.

5. Brooks SE, Zhan M, Cote T, et al. Survival epidemiology and end results analysis of 267 cases of uterine sarcomas, 1989–1999. *Gynecol Oncol*. 2004;93:204-208.

6. Francis JH, Kleinerman RA, Seddon J, et al. Increased risk of secondary uterine leiomyosarcoma in hereditary retinoblastoma. *Gynecol Oncol*. 2012;124:254-259.

7. dos Santos LA, Garg K, Diaz JP, et al. Incidence of lymph node and adnexal metastasis in endometrial stromal sarcoma. *Gynecol Oncol*. 2011;121:319-322.

8. Santos P, Cunha TM. Uterine sarcomas: clinical presentation and MRI features. *Diagn Interv Radiol*. 2015;21(1):4-9. doi:10.5152/dir.2014.14053

9. Namimoto T, Yamashita Y, Awai K, et al. Combined use of T2-weighted and diffusion-weighted 3-T MR imaging for differentiating uterine sarcomas from benign leiomyomas. *Eur Radiol*. 2009;19:2756-2764.

10. Cornfeld D, Israel G, Martel M, et al. MRI appearance of mesenchymal tumors of the uterus. *Eur J Radiol*. 2010;74:241-249.

11. Lakhman Y, Veeraraghavan H, Chaim J, et al. Differentiation of uterine leiomyosarcoma form atypical leiomyoma: diagnostic accuracy of qualitative MR imaging features and feasibility of texture analysis. *Eur Radiol* 2017;27:2903-2915.

12. Kitajima K, Murakami K, Kaji Y, Sugimura K. Spectrum of FDG PET/CT findings of uterine tumors. *AJR Am J Roentgenol*. 2010;195(3):737-743. doi:10.2214/AJR.09.4074

13. Goto A, Takeuchi S, Sugimura K, et al. Usefulness of Gd-DTPA contrast-enhanced dynamic MRI and serum determination of LDH and its isozymes in the differential diagnosis of leiomyosarcoma from degenerated leiomyoma of the uterus. *Int J Gynecol Cancer*. 2002;12:354-361.

14. Sagae S, Yamashita K, Ishioka S, et al. Preoperative diagnosis and treatment results in 106 patients with uterine sarcoma in Hokkaido, Japan. *Oncology*. 2004;67(1):33-39. doi:10.1159/000080283

15. Bansal N, Herzog TJ, Burke W, et al. The utility of preoperative endometrial sampling for the detection of uterine sarcomas. *Gynecol Oncol*. 2008;110:43-48.

CHAPTER **6.4**

Surgery for Newly Diagnosed Uterine Corpus Mesenchymal Tumors

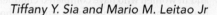

Tiffany Y. Sia and Mario M. Leitao Jr

SURGERY FOR NEWLY DIAGNOSED PATIENTS

Surgery is a cornerstone in the treatment of most soft-tissue sarcomas, including uterine sarcomas. Many women with uterine sarcomas are premenopausal at the time of initial diagnosis; therefore, concerns about fertility and premature menopause should be considered. Furthermore, given the lack of definitive tumor markers or imaging findings that are predictive of uterine sarcoma, diagnosis is frequently achieved on review of final pathology. In cases where the diagnosis is known preoperatively or where a high suspicion for neoplasm exists, surgery to remove the primary tumor—most often hysterectomy—and inspection of the peritoneal cavity are central to the initial management of these patients. In this section, we discuss preoperative workup, the approach to patients with resectable disease, fertility-sparing surgery, the necessity of performing nodal evaluation, and the role of oophorectomy. The role of cytoreductive procedures for extra-uterine disease at the time of diagnosis are also discussed, as also the scenario of patients diagnosed postoperatively after myomectomy or hysterectomy. Finally, uterine morcellation for surgical specimen removal is addressed.

PREOPERATIVE OR INTRAOPERATIVE DIAGNOSIS

Preoperative Workup

For patients who are diagnosed with uterine sarcomas on preoperative biopsy, imaging of the chest, abdomen, and pelvis is recommended to evaluate for distant metastases. For women who are found to have widespread unresectable metastases, surgery is not recommended as first-line treatment as the healing process can impede administration of systemic therapy. Imaging to determine the extent of disease may also help with surgical planning, as resection of all visible disease is important for patient outcomes. In a study of 106 patients with uterine sarcoma diagnosed preoperatively, patients with CS and LMS who underwent complete gross resection of all visible disease had 5-year survival rates of 78.8% and 73%, respectively, which was significantly higher than 5-year survival in patients who had residual disease (1).

Resectable Disease

In patients with either uterine-confined disease or disease that can be completely excised, we recommend proceeding with primary surgery consisting of hysterectomy with bilateral salpingectomy and resection of all intra-abdominal and retroperitoneal disease. The role of concurrent oophorectomy or lymphadenectomy is discussed in subsequent sections. In LMS, HG-ESS, UES, and CS, optimal surgical cytoreduction to less than 2 cm of residual disease or less has been associated with longer OS (2,3). If the disease is deemed unresectable, the patient should be offered systemic therapy rather than surgery.

Uterine Preservation

Myomectomy, or tumor resection with preservation of the uterus, is an option in younger women diagnosed with STUMP or other atypical leiomyomata of the uterus who wish to preserve fertility. Unfortunately, a total hysterectomy (never supracervical) must be performed in a majority of malignant mesenchymal tumors of the uterus. There is no clear option for preserving the uterus in patients diagnosed with LMS, undifferentiated (or high-grade) ESS, or CS. Uterine preservation has been described in eight women diagnosed with "LMS," and successful pregnancies were reported (4). However, it is unclear from this report whether these were all truly high-grade LMS, or whether some, or all, were STUMPs or other tumors of less malignant histologies (4). In a systemic review of fertility-sparing treatment in uterine sarcomas, OS was poorer in the fertility-sparing treatment group for LMS (43% compared to 73% in published literature), suggesting a possible aggravation of tumor during the original surgery (5). Until further conclusive investigation is conducted and reported, total abdominal hysterectomy (TAH) must still be recommended.

The management of endometrial stromal tumors is somewhat challenging. A confirmed endometrial stromal nodule does not require complete hysterectomy, as it is a benign lesion. However, it may be difficult to confirm whether such a tumor is an endometrial stromal nodule or an ESS without a significant amount of normal myometrium around it, and to state with confidence that there are no infiltrating margins with or without angioinvasion (6). Therefore, a TAH should be recommended in postmenopausal women

■ TABLE 6.4-1. Lymph Node and Ovarian Metastases in Uterine LMS

| Series | Lymph Node Metastasis | | Ovarian Metastasis | |
	All Cases	Occult Metastasis[a]	All Cases	Occult Metastasis[a]
Ayhan (15)	3/34 (8.8%)	1/27 (3.7%)	—	—
Major (16)	—	2/57 (3.5%)	—	2/59 (3.4%)
Leitao (17)	3/37 (8%)	1/27 (3.7%)	—	—
Goff (18)	—	0/9 (0%)	—	—
Gadducci (19)	—	0/4 (0%)	—	—
Giuntoli (13)	4/36 (11%)	—	—	—
Park (11)	0/11 (0%)	—	—	—
Koivisto (12)	0/15 (0%)	—	—	—
Kapp (14)	23/357 (6.4%)	—	—	—
Total	33/490 (6.7%)	3/124 (2.4%)	4/108 (3.7%)	4/130 (3.1%)

[a]Occult metastasis means nodal metastasis in clinically normal lymph nodes and disease clinically confined to the uterine corpus and/or cervix.

and in women who have completed childbearing. Sometimes, TAH may also be necessary even in women who wish to have children. Uterine preservation in the setting of ESS has been reported in a very young (16-year-old) girl (7) and in a 25-year-old who went on to carry a successful pregnancy (8). However, a systematic review of fertility-sparing treatments in LG-ESS demonstrated a recurrence rate of 54% that was higher than the rate of recurrence in standard treatment, although an increased risk of death was not appreciated (2%) (5).

Similarly, uterine preservation in well-selected patients with uterine AS has been reported in the literature, but its practice is rare and outside the standard of care. As tumors usually present as a polypoid mass within the endometrial cavity, uterine-preserving surgery has previously involved hysteroscopic resection or D&C with polypectomy. In a case series detailing 10 cases of fertility-preserving surgery in AS, two women received adjuvant chemotherapy, and two women had persistent disease confined to the uterus on imaging that was retreated with D&C (9). Three women suffered a recurrence, and time between initial resection and recurrence ranged from 10 months (in a patient with sarcomatous overgrowth) to up to 8 years. Nevertheless, in women who choose to undergo uterine preservation, intensive monitoring and close surveillance are required, and a plan for definitive hysterectomy is recommended.

Role of Nodal Evaluation or Lymphadenectomy

Two important questions to ask when deciding whether to perform a procedure—in particular, nodal dissections of nonenlarged lymph nodes and removal of ovaries in premenopausal women—are as follows: (1) What is the risk of microscopic disease in those organs? (2) Is there a benefit to removing those organs? Lymph node metastasis in adult soft-tissue sarcomas is less than 3%, with some variation among histologic subtypes (10). Routine regional lymphadenectomy is not recommended for patients with adult soft-tissue sarcomas, but resection of bulky isolated metastases can be considered (10).

The risk of lymph metastasis in LMS overall is approximately 7% (11-19) (Table 6.4-1). However, the rate of occult lymph node metastasis is less than 3% (15-17). There is no clear benefit to routine lymphadenectomy in patients who present with uterine LMS confined to the uterus and/or clinically normal lymph nodes (11,13-15,20).

The rate of overall and occult lymph node metastasis in ESS is 16% and 6%, respectively (11,12,19,21-25) (Table 6.4-2). Deep myometrial invasion and extensive lymph-vascular space invasion (LVSI) further increase the risk of occult metastasis (23). These features are often not obvious at the time of hysterectomy. Though

■ TABLE 6.4-2. Lymph Node and Ovarian Metastases in ESS (Low Grade)

| Series | Lymph Node Metastasis | | Ovarian Metastasis | |
	All Cases	Occult Metastasis[a]	All Cases	Occult Metastasis[a]
Park (11)	2/17 (12%)	—	—	—
Koivisto (12)	1/13 (8%)	—	—	—
Dos Santos (23)	7/36 (19%)	2/20 (10%)	11/87 (13%)	0/62 (0%)
Goff (18)	—	0/7 (0%)	—	—
Gadducci (19)	—	0/2 (0%)	—	—
Riopel (24)	3/8 (38%)	1/6 (17%)	—	—
Cheng (21)	4/18 (22%)	—	—	—
Shah (22)	7/100 (7%)	—	—	—
Signorelli (25)	3/19 (16%)	1/16 (6.3%)	—	—
Total	27/211 (12.8%)	4/51 (7.8%)	11/87 (13%)	0/62 (0%)

[a]Occult metastasis means nodal metastasis in clinically normal lymph nodes and disease clinically confined to the uterine corpus and/or cervix.

lymph node assessment may provide prognostic information regarding stage, there is no clear known survival advantage to routine lymphadenectomy in these patients (22,26). Nevertheless, it may be reasonable to consider lymphadenectomy at the time of hysterectomy, recognizing that the therapeutic or predictive value of this in ESS is unknown. In cases where ESS is diagnosed postoperatively, reoperation to complete a lymphadenectomy is not likely to be of any benefit in ESS that does not exhibit deep stromal invasion or extensive LVSI.

The rate of lymph node metastasis in AS is approximately 3% (27). Lymphadenectomy during primary surgery for AS has not been shown to offer OS nor progression free survival (PFS) benefit (28). UES are believed to behave similarly, but clear data are lacking. The role of lymphadenectomy beyond debulking of enlarged lymph nodes is still to be determined.

CS have a higher rate of overall (27%) and occult (20%) lymph node metastasis compared to LMS and ESS (11,12,16,27,29,30) (Table 6.4-3). Lymphadenectomy has been associated with improved survival, which may be attributed to removal of micrometastatic foci and reduction of recurrence risk in node-negative patients, or upstaging of node-positive patients who then will go on to receive adjuvant RT to the nodal beds (31,32). The current standard is that all patients, regardless of stage, receive postoperative systemic chemotherapy. Therefore, it is quite possible that the therapeutic benefit of lymphadenectomy, if any, in patients with CS may be tempered by this. However, nodal dissection in this setting is recommended given the high rates of nodal positivity and remains standard treatment. As full lymphadenectomy presents with increased risks of lymphedema, a single-institution study comparing outcomes of patients with uterine CS undergoing sentinel lymph node mapping and patients who underwent routine lymphadenectomy demonstrated high mapping rates and similar PFS (33). Recently, a cohort study of 156 patients with high-grade endometrial cancer subtypes including 17 (11%) patients with CS demonstrated that sentinel lymph node biopsy had as much accuracy and prognostic ability as full lymphadenectomy (34).

Role of Oophorectomy

The risk of ovarian metastasis is very low in LMS (16,17) (Table 6.4-1). Routine oophorectomy, especially in premenopausal patients with uterine-confined disease, provides no benefit. In a retrospective cohort study of 225 women with stage I LMS using the National Cancer Database, ovarian conservation did not have an impact on 5-year survival (35). Similarly, an analysis of SEER database found no difference in mortality between women with stage I LMS who underwent ovarian preservation and women who underwent oophorectomy even after controlling for age and FIGO substage and excluding patients who underwent RT (36). These data support retention of the ovaries in premenopausal women with LMS who want to retain ovarian function.

Occult ovarian metastasis in ESS is rare (23) (Table 6.4-3). Ovarian preservation appears to be associated with a higher risk of recurrence; however, this has no impact on OS, and these patients do very well in general (15,37-39). BSO is recommended to reduce the risk of recurrence, but this should be carefully discussed with young premenopausal women. The risk of ovarian metastasis and therapeutic benefit is difficult to discern, because of a lack of large series addressing it in this and other rare uterine sarcomas. However, it is important to note that in the majority of recurrences, secondary cytoreductive surgery (CRS) may be used as a salvage treatment option.

In uterine AS, incidence of tumor spread to the adnexa ranges from 0% to 17%, with an occult ovarian metastasis rate of up to 8% (40,41). The rarity of the tumor, the wide range of reported adnexal metastases, and high rates of estrogen receptor/progesterone receptor (ER/PR) positivity make consensus regarding ovarian preservation in premenopausal patients with uterine-confined disease difficult to reach. Hence, hysterectomy with concurrent oophorectomy is recommended at the time of primary surgery, especially in patients whose histology demonstrates sarcomatous overgrowth (28). Performance of oophorectomy in premenopausal patients will also allow for adjuvant hormonal therapy as a treatment option for metastatic or recurrent disease, although uncertainties remain regarding their efficacy (28,40,41).

For patients with CS, occult ovarian metastasis can be seen in approximately 12% of women (16) (Table 6.4-3). BSO should be recommended for these patients; fortunately, many are postmenopausal.

Cytoreductive Surgery for Patients With Extrauterine Disease at Initial Diagnosis

CRS in patients presenting with uterine sarcoma has not been well described. In a single-institution study of 96 patients who presented with metastatic uterine LMS, the median PFS in patients undergoing a complete gross resection was 14.2 months, compared to 6.8 months for those who had surgery and visible residual disease (P = .002) (42). OS was 31.9 months compared to 20.2 months, respectively (P = .04) (42). On multivariable analysis, complete CRS maintained an independent association with PFS, but not with OS. The lack of independent statistical association with OS in this study may be explained by the relatively small number of cases studied.

Leath et al studied the impact of surgical cytoreduction in ESS and found that optimal cytoreduction with residual disease less than 2 cm was associated with increased median OS for patients with HG-ESS (52 vs 2 months, P = .007) (2). However, this survival difference was not seen in patients with LG-ESS. At the time of their 2007 study, the classification of HG-ESS would have included the current HG-ESS and UES groups.

Given the aggressiveness of uterine CS, metastatic disease outside the uterus is often found at the time of diagnosis. For advanced

TABLE 6.4-3. Lymph Node and Ovarian Metastases in Uterine Carcinosarcoma

| Series | Lymph Node Metastasis | | Ovarian Metastasis | |
	All Cases	Occult Metastasis[a]	All Cases	Occult Metastasis[a]
Major (16)	—	51/287 (18%)	—	36/300 (12%)
Park (11)	—	13/41 (32%)	—	—
Park (29)	8/37 (22%)	—	—	—
Koivisto (12)	6/24 (25%)	—	—	—
Arend (27)	726/2709 (14%)	—	—	—
Galaal (30)	19/34 (56%)	—	—	—
Total	759/2804 (27.1%)	64/328 (19.5%)	—	36/300 (12%)

[a]Occult metastasis means nodal metastasis in clinically normal lymph nodes and disease clinically confined to the uterine corpus and/or cervix.

uterine CS, complete gross resection of all visible disease has been associated with a significant survival benefit compared to patients with residual disease (median 52 vs 9 months) (43). Furthermore, in patients with stage IV CS undergoing neoadjuvant chemotherapy, patients who underwent interval CRS with complete reduction followed by postoperative chemotherapy had significantly PFS compared to patients who had residual disease after cytoreduction and did not undergo postoperative chemotherapy (11.5 vs 1.5 months, $P < .001$). Similar findings were seen when assessing for cause-specific survival (23.8 vs 2.2 months) (44).

Therefore, CRS may be a reasonable consideration in highly select cases, in which complete resection of tumor is believed to be feasible without the need for extensive procedures such as exenteration. The potential benefit of surgery should be weighed against the potential risks, and these cases must be individually managed.

POSTOPERATIVE DIAGNOSIS

In patients who are diagnosed with uterine sarcomas including LMS and ESS incidentally after myomectomy or supracervical hysterectomy, imaging with a CT of the chest, abdomen, and pelvis or combination of MRI and CT scan should be performed to evaluate for metastatic disease. If the patient is a surgical candidate, then operation to remove the uterus, fallopian tubes, and cervix as well as staging should be performed (45). Removal of the ovaries and lymph node evaluation should be considered and have been discussed in earlier sections of this chapter. Removal of the uterus, tubes, and cervix allows for the potential removal of residual disease left behind at the original surgery, and additional surgical staging allows for the option to tailor postoperative therapies should the patient require them. Initial uterus-preserving surgery does not appear to be associated with poorer survival in patients who are ultimately diagnosed with unexpected uterine sarcoma as long as surgical reexploration is performed immediately (46). In patients who are diagnosed with a uterine sarcoma after total hysterectomy with no residual disease noted on postoperative imaging, a second procedure solely for the purposes of surgical staging is not recommended.

In patients diagnosed with CS after hysterectomy who are surgical candidates for cytoreduction with no evidence of extra-abdominal metastatic disease, a second surgery for cytoreduction and lymphadenectomy is recommended. In patients with widely metastatic disease or who are deemed not surgical candidates, the role of systemic therapy should be addressed.

Uterine Morcellation

Laparoscopy has become the standard, preferred approach in the management of women with benign and malignant gynecologic conditions. Morcellation of the uterus, either for removal of the specimen during minimally invasive procedures, for myomectomy for fertility preservation, or for supracervical hysterectomy, has been commonplace for many years. Although diagnosis of CS is rare after uterine morcellation procedures as patients are generally older and postmenopausal, it is not unusual that an LMS or ESS is incidentally diagnosed after some form of morcellation, or less-than-total hysterectomy. Morcellation of a uterine LMS is associated with worse outcome. Perri et al (47) reported a significantly higher rate of recurrence and lower OS in women who had undergone something less than a TAH and were subsequently diagnosed with uterine LMS. The hazard ratios (HR) for recurrence and survival in TAH compared to other types of resection (myomectomy, morcellation, or supracervical hysterectomy) was 0.39 and 0.36, respectively. Park et al (48) reported a series in which the 5-year disease-free survival (DFS) was 40% in women who underwent tumor morcellation and were subsequently diagnosed with LMS, compared to 65% in patients with LMS who did not undergo morcellation ($P = .04$). Similarly, the 5-year OS was 46% after morcellation, compared to 73% in

patients who were not morcellated ($P = .04$) (48). Morcellation also appears to have a negative impact on the risk of recurrence in ESS, but no adverse impact on OS (49).

The true impact of morcellation of uterine LMS is difficult to fully understand because of the very small cohorts and overall poor quality of published reports. Bogani and colleagues (50) reported the results of an extensive meta-analysis on the impact of morcellation and outcomes in patients with unsuspected uterine LMS. Following an exhaustive review of the available medical literature databases, they identified 60 potential studies. After applying rigorous inclusion material, only four studies remained in the meta-analysis. These included 202 patients (75 morcellated, 127 nonmorcellated); all were analyzed retrospectively. The 75 morcellated cases included patients who had undergone open, vaginal, laparoscopic, or hysteroscopic morcellation. Significantly higher rates of overall recurrence, intra-abdominal recurrence, and death were noted in the morcellated cohort. The combined death rate for morcellated versus nonmorcellated was 48% and 29% (OR = 2.42 [95% CI, 1.19-4.92]; $P = .01$). The rate of extra-abdominal recurrence was not significantly different (50). The authors clearly noted a high risk of bias in all four studies. In a study comparing outcomes of women who underwent power morcellation at the time of laparoscopic hysterectomy or myomectomy compared to TAH and were found to have occult uterine sarcoma, morcellation was associated with higher disease-specific mortality, with a 20% increased risk of mortality within 5 years (51).

The higher risk of recurrence and death may be a consequence of disseminated, unrecognized sarcoma during morcellation. The difference in intra-abdominal recurrence rates noted by Bogani and colleagues is very similar to that reported by Oduyebo et al (52) in a small (but the largest available) series of cases of disseminated disease identified at the time of reexploration, immediately after morcellation, from an unrecognized LMS. Disseminated sarcomatosis was noted in two out of seven patients (28.6%) with uterine LMS who underwent immediate reexploration before noted recurrence. All seven were presumed to be stage I at the time of initial surgery. Both patients recurred and one died; the other had only 8 months of follow-up. In the five cases without disease at reexploration, four (80%) have not recurred and are alive without evidence of disease at a median follow-up of 23.4 months (range, 3.5-48.2 months) (52). The true value of reexploration cannot be definitively stated based on such a small series. In addition, one cannot comment on whether immediate reexploration and possible debulking would alter the outcomes. However, immediate reexploration and possible debulking are reasonable considerations. Reexploration may provide information to help guide decisions regarding additional therapies. At a minimum, it provides prognostic information and a clearer understanding of the patient's current disease state.

Despite the potential adverse impact of morcellation on outcomes in patients ultimately diagnosed with LMS and ESS, we cannot definitively conclude that morcellation or myomectomy is entirely inappropriate in the management of patients with presumed benign leiomyomas. The risk of LMS and ESS in patients undergoing surgery for presumed benign leiomyoma is quite low. In a combined series of four studies with a total of 4,981 patients, the risk of LMS and ESS after surgery for presumed benign leiomyoma was only 0.24% and 0.06%, respectively (53-56). This risk is no greater in those undergoing surgery for an indication of rapidly enlarging leiomyoma (54). The risk of unexpected malignancy is associated with age. In two large public database analyses, the risk of any uterine cancer was exceedingly low in women less than 40 years of age, but increased significantly with increasing patient age (57,58). Neither study specifically assessed the prevalence or risk of uterine sarcoma.

In April 2014, the U.S. Food and Drug Administration (FDA) issued a safety communication regarding uterine power morcellation (59). This communication was not an outright ban. It encouraged thoughtful decision-making when considering morcellation, but strongly discouraged it. The FDA communication also specified a need for careful patient counseling regarding the risks of power morcellation before consenting patients for surgery. While the FDA communication comments only on power morcellation, similar concerns remain with respect to myomectomy and supracervical (subtotal) hysterectomy that, as stated previously, are not morcellated. In addition, little has been mentioned regarding uterine artery embolization of presumed uterine fibroids. In response to the FDA communication, many institutions decided to ban the use of power morcellation altogether. Patient safety is always the prime consideration in surgery. However, when morcellation is completely abandoned, there are many other consequences that must be taken into account. Barron and colleagues (60) reported a decrease in minimally invasive hysterectomies and myomectomies following the FDA announcement. Similarly, Harris et al (61) reported a decrease in minimally invasive hysterectomy. An increase in surgical complications and readmissions was also noted. It is reasonable to obtain preoperative pelvic MRI when a less-than-total hysterectomy for presumed benign leiomyoma is planned. Appropriate imaging will help localize the tumors, and provides an excellent NPV. Serum LDH may also be useful in determining when morcellation may be less than optimal. Morcellation should be avoided in patients with highly suspicious MRI findings and elevated serum LDH and in postmenopausal patients with enlarging uterine masses, new uterine masses, or newly symptomatic uterine masses. Proper and thoughtful patient selection is likely much more important in surgical decision-making than is the complete abandonment of a particular surgical tool. In December 2013, the Society of Gynecologic Oncology issued a position statement on morcellation, recommending that patients be counseled regarding the risk of occult malignancy before undergoing this procedure. They asserted that morcellation is generally contraindicated in the presence of known or suspected malignancy and may be inadvisable in the treatment of premalignant conditions or risk-reducing surgeries (62).

More recently, in 2020, the FDA released an updated safety communication, recommending that laparoscopic power morcellation of myomectomy or hysterectomy be performed only within a tissue containment system with specifically designated laparoscopic power morcellators (63). The safety communication also stated that laparoscopic power morcellators should not be used in postmenopausal women or women older than 50 years, or women whose specimens are able to be removed vaginally or through a mini-laparotomy incision.

REFERENCES

1. Sagae S, Yamashita K, Ishioka S, et al. Preoperative diagnosis and treatment results in 106 patients with uterine sarcoma in Hokkaido, Japan. *Oncology.* 2004;67(1):33-39. doi:10.1159/000080283

2. Leath CA 3rd, Huh WK, Hyde J Jr, et al. A multi-institutional review of outcomes of endometrial stromal sarcoma. *Gynecol Oncol.* 2007;105(3):630-634. doi:10.1016/j.ygyno.2007.01.031

3. Tanner EJ, Garg K, Leitao MM Jr, Soslow RA, Hensley ML. High grade undifferentiated uterine sarcoma: surgery, treatment, and survival outcomes. *Gynecol Oncol.* 2012;127(1):27-31. doi:10.1016/j.ygyno.2012.06.030

4. Lissoni A, Cormio G, Bonazzi C, et al. Fertility-sparing surgery in uterine leiomyosarcoma. *Gynecol Oncol.* 1998;70:348-350.

5. Dondi G, Porcu E, De Palma A, et al. Uterine preservation treatments in sarcomas: oncological problems and reproductive results: a systematic review. *Cancers (Basel).* 2021;13(22):5808. doi:10.3390/cancers13225808

6. Dionigi A, Oliva E, Clement PB, et al. Endometrial stromal nodules and endometrial stromal tumors with limited infiltration: a clinicopathologic study of 50 cases. *Am J Surg Pathol.* 2002;26:567-581.

7. Stadsvold JL, Molpus KL, Baker JJ, et al. Conservative management of a myxoid endometrial stromal sarcoma in a 16-year-old nulliparous woman. *Gynecol Oncol.* 2005;99:243-245.

8. Yan L, Tian Y, Fu Y, et al. Successful pregnancy after fertility-preserving surgery for endometrial stromal sarcoma. *Fertil Steril.* 2010;93:269.e1-269.e3.

9. L'Heveder A, Jones BP, Saso S, et al. Conservative management of uterine adenosarcoma: lessons learned from 20 years of follow-up. *Arch Gynecol Obstet.* 2019;300(5):1383-1389.

10. Fong Y, Coit DG, Woodruff JM, et al. Lymph node metastasis from soft tissue sarcoma in adults: analysis of data from a prospective database of 1772 sarcoma patients. *Ann Surg.* 1993;217:72-77.

11. Park J, Kim D, Suh D, et al. Prognostic factors and treatment outcomes of patients with uterine sarcoma: analysis of 127 patients at a single institution, 1989-2007. *J Cancer Res Clin Oncol.* 2008;134:1277-1287.

12. Koivisto-Korander R, Butzow R, Koivisto A, et al. Clinical outcome and prognostic factors in 100 cases of uterine sarcoma: experience in Helsinki University Central Hospital 1990-2001. *Gynecol Oncol.* 2008;111:74-81.

13. Giuntoli RL, Metzinger DS, DiMarco CS, et al. Retrospective review of 208 patients with leiomyosarcoma of the uterus: prognostic indicators, surgical management, and adjuvant therapy. *Gynecol Oncol.* 2003;89:460-469.

14. Kapp DS, Shin JY, Chan JK. Prognostic factors and survival in 1396 patients with uterine leiomyosarcomas: emphasis on impact of lymphadenectomy and oophorectomy. *Cancer.* 2008;112:820-830.

15. Ayhan A, Aksan G, Gultekin M, et al. Prognosticators and the role of lymphadenectomy in uterine leiomyosarcomas. *Arch Gynecol Obstet.* 2009;280:79-85.

16. Major FJ, Blessing JA, Silverberg SG, et al. Prognostic factors in early-stage uterine sarcoma: a gynecologic oncology group study. *Cancer.* 1993;71:1702-1709.

17. Leitao MM, Sonoda Y, Brennan MF, et al. Incidence of lymph node and ovarian metestases in leiomyosarcoma of the uterus. *Gynecol Oncol.* 2003;91:209-212.

18. Goff BA, Rice LW, Fleischhacker D, et al. Uterine leiomyosarcoma and endometrial stromal sarcoma: lymph node metastases and sites of recurrence. *Gynecol Oncol.* 1993;50:105-109.

19. Gadducci A, Landoni F, Sartori E, et al. Uterine leiomyosarcoma: analysis of treatment failures and survival. *Gynecol Oncol.* 1996;62:25-32.

20. Garg G, Shah JP, Liu R, et al. Validation of tumor size as staging variable in the revised international federation of gynecology and obstetrics stage I leiomyosarcoma: a population-based study. *Int J Gynecol Cancer.* 2010;20:1201-1206.

21. Cheng X, Yang G, Schmeler KM, et al. Recurrence patterns and prognosis of endometrial stromal sarcoma and the potential of tyrosine kinase-inhibiting therapy. *Gynecol Oncol.* 2011;121:323-327.

22. Shah LP, Bryant CS, Kumar S, et al. Lymphadenectomy and ovarian preservation in low-grade endometrial stromal sarcoma. *Obstet Gynecol.* 2008;112:1102-1108.

23. dos Santos LA, Garg K, Diaz JP, et al. Incidence of lymph node and adnexal metastasis in endometrial stromal sarcoma. *Gynecol Oncol.* 2011;121:319-322.

24. Riopel J, Plante M, Renaud MC, et al. Lymph node metastases in low-grade endometrial stromal sarcoma. *Gynecol Oncol.* 2005;96:402-406.

25. Signorelli M, Fruscio R, Dell'Anna T, et al. Lymphadenectomy in uterine low-grade endometrial stromal sarcoma: an analysis of 19 cases and a literature review. *Int J Gynecol Cancer.* 2010;20:1363-1366.

26. Chan JK, Kawar NM, Shin JY, et al. Endometrial stromal sarcoma: a population-based analysis. *Br J Cancer.* 2008;99:1210-1215.

27. Arend R, Bagaria M, Lewin SN, et al. Long−term outcome and natural history of uterine adenosarcomas. *Gynecol Oncol.* 2010;119:305-308.

28. Nathenson MJ, Ravi V, Fleming N, et al. Uterine adenosarcoma: a review. *Curr Oncol Rep.* 2016;18:68. doi:10.1007/s11912-016-0552-7

29. Park J, Kim D, Kim J, et al. The role of pelvic and/or para-aortic lymphadenectomy in surgical management of apparently early carcinosarcoma of uterus. *Ann Surg Oncol.* 2010;17:861-868.

30. Galaal K, Kew FM, Tam KF, et al. Evaluation of prognostic factors and treatment outcomes in uterine carcinosarcoma. *Eur J Obstet Gynecol Reprod Biol.* 2009;143:88-92.

31. Nemani D, Mitra N, Guo M, et al. Assessing the effects of lymphadenectomy and radiation therapy in patients with uterine carcinosarcoma: a SEER analysis. *Gynecol Oncol.* 2008;111:82-88.

32. Vorgias G, Fotiou S. The role of lymphadenectomy in uterine carcinosarcomas (malignant mixed mullerian tumours): a critical literature review. *Arch Gynecol Obstet.* 2010;282(6):659-664. doi:10.1007/s00404-010-1649-0

33. Schiavone MB, Zivanovic O, Zhou Q, et al. Survival of patients with uterine carcinosarcoma undergoing sentinel lymph node mapping. *Ann Surg Oncol.* 2016;23:196-202. doi:10.1245/s10434-015-4612-2

34. Cusimano MC, Vicus D, Pulman K, et al. Assessment of sentinel lymph node biopsy vs lymphadenectomy for intermediate-and high-grade endometrial cancer staging. *JAMA Surg.* 2021;156(2):157-164. doi:10.1001/jamasurg.2020.5060

35. Sia TY, Huang Y, Gockley A, et al. Trends in ovarian conservation and association with survival in premenopausal patients with stage I leiomyosarcoma. *Gynecol Oncol.* 2021;161(3):734-740. doi:10.1016/j.ygyno.2021.03.027

36. Nasioudis D, Chapman-Davis E, Frey M, Holcomb K. Safety of ovarian preservation in premenopausal women with stage I uterine sarcoma. *J Gynecol Oncol.* 2017;28(4):e46. doi:10.3802/jgo.2017.28.e46

37. Jin Y, Pan L, Wang X, et al. Clinical characteristics of endometrial stromal sarcoma from and academic medical hospital in China. *Int J Gynecol Cancer.* 2010;20:1535-1539.

38. Li N, Wu L, Zhang H, et al. Treatment options in stage I endometrial stromal sarcoma: a retrospective analysis of 53 cases. *Gynecol Oncol.* 2008;108:306-311.

39. Yoon A, Park JY, Park JY, et al. Prognostic factors and outcomes in endometrial stromal sarcoma with the 2009 FIGO staging system: a multicenter review of 114 cases. *Gynecol Oncol.* 2014;132(1):70-75. doi:10.1016/j.ygyno.2013.10.029

40. Carroll A, Ramirez PT, Westin SN, et al. Uterine adenosarcoma: an analysis on management, outcomes, and risk factors for recurrence. *Gynecol Oncol.* 2014;135:455-461.

41. Tanner EJ, Toussaint T, Leitao MM, et al. Management of uterine adenosarcomas with and without sarcomatous overgrowth. *Gynecol Oncol.* 2013;129(1):140-144.

42. Leitao MM Jr, Zivanovic O, Chi DS, et al. Surgical cytoreduction in patients with metastatic uterine leiomyosarcoma at the time of initial diagnosis. *Gynecol Oncol.* 2012;125:409-413.

43. Tanner EJ, Leitao MM Jr, Garg K, et al. The role of cytoreductive surgery for newly diagnosed advanced-stage uterine carcinosarcoma. *Gynecol Oncol.* 2011;123(3):548-552.

44. Matsuo K, Johnson MS, Im DD, et al. Survival outcome of women with stage IV uterine carcinosarcoma who received neoadjuvant chemotherapy followed by surgery. *J Surg Oncol.* 2018;117(3):488-496.

45. Einstein MH, Barakat RR, Chi DS, et al. Management of uterine malignancy found incidentally after supracervical hysterectomy or uterine morcellation for presumed benign disease. *Int J Gynecol Cancer.* 2008;18(5):1065-1070. doi:10.1111/j.1525-1438.2007.01126.x

46. Lee JY, Kim HS, Nam EJ, Kim SW, Kim S, Kim YT. Outcomes of uterine sarcoma found incidentally after uterus-preserving surgery for presumed benign disease. *BMC Cancer.* 2016;16(1):675. doi:10.1186/s12885-016-2727-x

47. Perri T, Korach J, Sadetzki S, et al. Uterine leiomyosarcoma: does the primary surgical procedure matter? *Int J Gynecol Cancer.* 2009;19:257-260.

48. Park J, Park S, Kim D, et al. The impact of tumor morcellation during surgery on the prognosis of patients with apparently early uterine leiomyosarcoma. *Gynecol Oncol.* 2011;122:255-259.

49. Park J, Kim D, Kim J, et al. The impact of tumor morcellation during surgery on the outcomes of patients with apparently early low-grade endometrial stromal sarcoma of the uterus. *Ann Surg Oncol.* 2011;18:3453-3461.

50. Bogani G, Cliby WA, Aletti GD. Impact of morcellation on survival outcomes of patients with unexpected uterine leiomyosarcoma: a systematic review and meta-analysis. *Gynecol Oncol.* 2015;137:167-172.

51. Xu X, Lin H, Wright JD, et al. Association between power morcellation and mortality in women with unexpected uterine cancer undergoing hysterectomy or myomectomy. *J Clin Oncol.* 2019;37(35):3412-3424. doi:10.1200/JCO.19.00562

52. Oduyebo T, Rauh-Hain AJ, Meserve EE, et al. The value of re-exploration in patients with inadvertently morcellated uterine sarcoma. *Gynecol Oncol.* 2014;132:360-365.

53. Leibsohn S, D'Ablaing G, Mishell DR Jr, et al. Leiomyosarcoma in a series of hysterectomies performed for presumed uterine leiomyomas. *Am J Obstet Gynecol.* 1990;162:968-976.

54. Parker WH, Fu YS, Berek JS. Uterine sarcoma in patients operated on for presumed leiomyoma and rapidly growing leiomyoma. *Obstet Gynecol.* 1994;83:414-418.

55. Takamizawa S, Minakami H, Usui R, et al. Risk of complications and uterine malignancies in women undergoing hysterectomy for presumed benign leiomyomas. *Gynecol Obstet Invest.* 1999;48:193-196.

56. Leung F, Terzibachian JJ, Gay C, et al. Hysterectomies performed for presumed leiomyomas: should the fear of leiomyosarcoma make us apprehend non laparotomic surgical routes? *Gynecol Obstet Fertil.* 2009;37:109-114.

57. Wright JD, Tergas AI, Cui R, et al. Use of electric power morcellation and prevalence of underlying cancer in women who undergo myomectomy. *JAMA Oncol.* 2015;1:69-77.

58. Perkins RB, Handal-Orefice R, Hanchate AD, et al. Risk of undetected cancer at the time of laparoscopic supracervical hysterectomy and laparoscopic myomectomy: implications for the use of power morcellation. *Womens Health Issues.* 2016;26(1):21-26.

59. U.S. Food & Drug Administration. FDA discourages use of laparoscopic power morcellation for removal of uterus or uterine fibroids. Accessed July 19, 2023. https://wayback.archive-it.org/7993/20170722215731/https://www.fda.gov/MedicalDevices/Safety/AlertsandNotices/ucm393576.htm

60. Barron KI, Richard T, Robinson PS, et al. Association of the U.S. Food and Drug Administration morcellation warning with rates of minimally invasive hysterectomy and myomectomy. *Obstet Gynecol.* 2015;126:1174-1180.

61. Harris JA, Swenson CW, Uppal S, et al. Practice patterns and postoperative complications before and after US Food and Drug Administration safety communication on power morcellation. *Am J Obstet Gynecol.* 2016;214:98.e1-98.e13.

62. Society of Gynecologic Oncology. Morcellation updates. Accessed July 19, 2023. https://www.sgo.org/news/statement-of-the-society-of-gynecologic-oncology-to-the-food-and-drug-administrations-obstetrics-and-gynecology-medical-devices-advisory-committee-concerning-safety-of-laparoscopic-power-morc/

63. U.S. Food & Drug Administration. UPDATE: The FDA recommends performing contained morcellation in women when laparoscopic power morcellation is appropriate. Date Issued: February 25, 2020. Accessed May 24, 2022. https://www.fda.gov/medical-devices/safety-communications/update-perform-only-contained-morcellation-when-laparoscopic-power-morcellation-appropriate-fda

CHAPTER **6.5**

Pathology of Uterine Mesenchymal Tumors

Amir Momeni-Boroujeni and Lora Hedrick Ellenson

INTRODUCTION

This chapter focuses on the pathology of uterine sarcomas and highlights the most salient molecular features with diagnostic implications in each category. As mentioned in other chapters, uterine sarcomas are uncommon tumors that arise from the mesenchymal components of the uterine corpus. The 2020 WHO classification of mesenchymal uterine corpus tumors is summarized in **Table 6.5-1** (1).

Malignant mesenchymal tumors can be classified as either pure mesenchymal tumors or tumors with mixed epithelial and mesenchymal components. In the first group, the most common is

■ **TABLE 6.5-1. Mesenchymal Tumors Specific to the Uterus**

Leiomyoma NOS
  Lipoleiomyoma
  Leiomyoma, apoplectic
  Leiomyoma, hydropic
  Dissecting leiomyoma
  Cellular leiomyoma
  Myxoid leiomyoma
  Epithelioid leiomyoma
  Symplastic leiomyoma
  Leiomyomatosis NOS
Intravenous leiomyoma
Smooth muscle tumor of uncertain malignant potential
  Epithelioid smooth muscle tumor of uncertain malignant potential
  Myxoid smooth muscle tumor of uncertain malignant potential
  Spindle smooth muscle tumor of uncertain malignant potential
Metastasizing leiomyoma
Leiomyosarcoma NOS
  Spindle leiomyosarcoma
  Epithelioid leiomyosarcoma
  Myxoid leiomyosarcoma
Endometrial stromal nodule
Endometrial stromal sarcoma, low grade
Endometrial stromal sarcoma, high grade
Undifferentiated sarcoma
Uterine tumor resembling ovarian sex cord tumor
Perivascular epithelioid tumor, benign
Perivascular epithelioid tumor, malignant
Inflammatory myofibroblastic tumor
  Epithelioid myofibroblastic tumor
Mixed epithelial and mesenchymal tumors
  Adenomyoma NOS
  Atypical polypoid adenomyoma
  Adenosarcoma

NOS, not otherwise specific.

leiomyosarcoma (LMS), followed by endometrial stromal sarcoma (ESS) and (rarely) other tumors that are not specific to the uterus, including rhabdomyosarcoma, liposarcoma, angiosarcoma, chondrosarcoma, osteosarcoma, and alveolar soft-part sarcoma. Adenosarcoma is a malignant mixed epithelial and mesenchymal tumor in which the mesenchymal component is malignant and the epithelial component is benign. In addition, there are three rare mesenchymal tumors that occur in the uterus: uterine tumors resembling ovarian sex cord tumors (UTROSCTs), perivascular epithelioid cell tumors (PEComas), and inflammatory myofibroblastic tumor (IMT). These entities are usually benign; however, they can be malignant and, more problematically, can be confused with sarcomas of the uterus.

OVERVIEW OF MOLECULAR LANDSCAPE OF UTERINE MESENCHYMAL TUMORS

Uterine mesenchymal sarcomas just like their extrauterine counterparts are mainly driven by two molecular pathogenetic mechanisms; on the one hand, a subset of the tumors, including the majority of uterine LMS, are driven by chromosomal instability often caused by deleterious alterations of the p53 signaling pathway (2), whereas ESS are mainly driven by epigenetic instability brought about by fusions involving the polycomb repressive complex (PRC) proteins (3).

The most common genomic alteration in uterine LMS are mutations or deletions of the *TP53* gene (4); one of the roles of the P53 protein is to inhibit the structural chromosome instability in postmitotic cells (5). As a result, most uterine LMS show considerable chromosomal instability as manifested by genome fragmentation and frequent copy number losses and gains (6). Other common alterations involve cell cycle regulators such as *RB1* and *CDKN2A*,

genes encoding for proteins involved in alternative lengthening of telomeres such as *ATRX* and *DAXX* as well as PI3K pathway alterations such as *PTEN* (2).

ESS are generally categorized into two groups: low grade and high grade. Low-grade ESS often have fusions involving the PRC2 complex, including JAZF1::SUZ12 and JAZF1::PHF1 (7), whereas high-grade ESS often harbor fusions or alterations of *BCOR* gene (a member of the PRC1 complex) or *YWHAE* gene (8). All of these proteins are involved in epigenetic regulation, and these fusions are believed to cause epigenetic instability, leading to tumor growth and proliferation (3). In addition, low-grade ESS are often ER dependent and can be treated with hormonal blockade. However, some of these tumors acquire ESR1 resistance mutations in response to hormonal blockade, leading to a more aggressive form of the disease (9).

Some, less common, uterine mesenchymal neoplasms harbor fusions involving kinase proteins. For example, IMTs harbor anaplastic lymphoma kinase (*ALK*) fusions, or the fibrosarcoma-like sarcomas harbor *NTRK1*, *NTRK2*, or *NTRK3* fusions (8). These fusions make the tumors sensitive to targeted therapies, which have been shown to be effective against these fusions in pan-cancer studies.

Overall, as our understanding of the molecular basis of uterine mesenchymal tumors increases, it will provide improved diagnostic and prognostic tools and may allow for the development of targeted therapies for these tumors.

Leiomyosarcomas and Other Smooth Muscle Tumors

LMS are malignant smooth muscle tumors that usually arise de novo. Recent studies have shown that some of these tumors have areas of benign morphology, suggesting progression from leiomyoma to LMS (10,11); however, clonality studies support this progression in only a small percentage of cellular or symplastic leiomyomas (11,12). LMS is usually a solitary, poorly circumscribed mass with a soft and fleshy consistency. The cut surface is variegated, with gray areas intermixed with yellow areas of necrosis, and sometimes hemorrhagic areas. The epicenter of the tumor is the myometrium. Most LMS tumors are intramural. Occasionally, they extend into the cervix or beyond the uterus through the serosa (**Figure 6.5-1**).

LMS most commonly exhibit spindle morphology, but some have epithelioid or myxoid morphology. The criterion for malignancy is dependent on the morphology (see later). Microscopically, most LMS are overtly malignant with hypercellularity, coagulative tumor cell necrosis (TCN), abundant mitoses, atypical mitoses, marked cytologic atypia, and infiltrative borders (**Figure 6.5-2**). Some lack one or more of these features, and occasionally, the differential diagnosis between a benign and a malignant lesion is controversial. The three most important criteria are coagulative TCN, high mitotic rate, and significant cytologic atypia. In conventional LMS (spindle cell type), the diagnosis of malignancy is rendered when any two of the following three criteria are present: TCN, diffuse moderate-to-severe cytologic atypia, and 10 or more mitoses per 10 high-power fields (HPF) (13). TCN is characterized by an abrupt transition from viable to necrotic tissue (**Figure 6.5-3**). In contrast, hyaline necrosis, which is seen in some leiomyomas, has an area of hyalinized tissue between the necrotic and viable tumor.

Five studies in the literature have addressed the diagnosis and clinical behavior of borderline smooth muscle tumors classified as atypical leiomyomas, tumors with low malignant potential, and tumors of uncertain malignant potential (14-18). The overall recurrence rate, based on these studies, is 8.6%. Most tumors recurred as STUMP, although one recurred as LMS (14). Most patients were alive and free of disease when these studies were published; one study reported three disease-specific deaths, all occurring more than 6 years after initial diagnosis (15). There are tumors that lack one of the three major diagnostic criteria (mitoses, atypia, necrosis) but show other worrisome features, such as infiltrative borders,

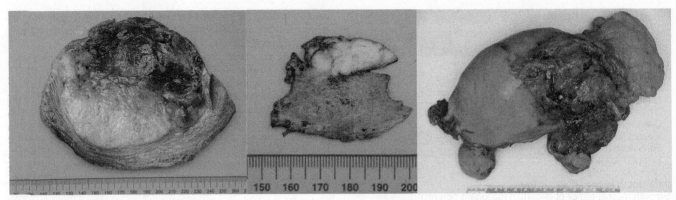

Figure 6.5-1. Leiomyosarcoma, gross.

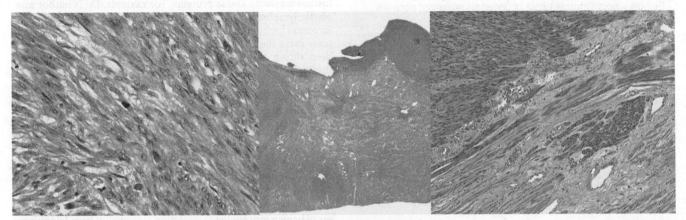

Figure 6.5-2. Leiomyosarcoma, microscopic with cytologic atypia, mitotic figures, and myoinvasion.

lymphovascular invasion, atypical mitoses, or bizarre nuclei. Classification of these tumors is often problematic. It is recommended that any unusual cases be reviewed by a gynecologic pathologist.

Leiomyomas with bizarre nuclei often have atypical cells including multinucleated cells, which often exhibit smudgy chromatin and abundant eosinophilic cytoplasm and may have prominent nucleoli. These tumors may pose a diagnostic challenge for pathologists due to occasional marked nuclear atypia; however, they are distinguished from LMS by a lack of mitotic activity and coagulative TCN. Fumarate hydratase (FH)-deficient leiomyoma

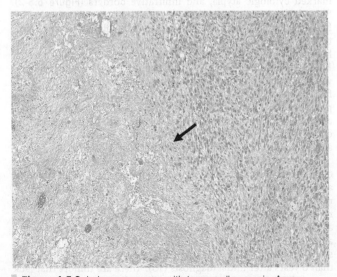

Figure 6.5-3. Leiomyosarcoma with tumor cell necrosis. Arrow shows abrupt transition between necrosis and viable tumor.

constitutes a portion of uterine leiomyomas with bizarre nuclei. These tumors are caused by a deficiency in an enzyme called fumarate hydratase, which is responsible for converting fumarate to malate in the citric acid cycle. This deficiency leads to an accumulation of fumarate and succinate in cells, which can lead to the development of leiomyomas. These lesions have distinct histopathologic features, including staghorn vessels, and large orangeophilic nucleoli surrounded by perinucleolar halo. Identification of these tumors, especially in young patients, should prompt an investigation for germline *FH* gene alterations that give rise to the hereditary leiomyomatosis and renal cell carcinoma syndrome (19).

Infarct-type necrosis of benign leiomyomas is sometimes seen during pregnancy, after uterine artery embolization, thermal balloon endometrial ablation, therapy with tranexamic acid, or therapy with high-dose progestins. In addition, pedunculated submucosal leiomyomas may undergo spontaneous torsion and infarction, even protruding through the cervix. Infarcted leiomyomas should not be confused with LMS. As noted before, infarct-type necrosis is not TCN. In addition, infarcted leiomyomas are not associated with significant cytologic atypia, high mitotic index, atypical mitoses, or invasive borders. An accurate clinical history may be useful in many of these cases.

The classification criteria of smooth muscle tumors with either myxoid or epithelioid features differ from the criteria used for spindle cell tumors. Epithelioid tumors have cells that are round rather than spindle shaped, mimicking epithelial cells (hence the term "epithelioid") (**Figure 6.5-4**). Tumors with epithelioid morphology are considered malignant if they have one or more of the following: moderate-to-severe cytologic atypia, four or more mitoses per 10 HPF, or TCN. A previous study suggests that epithelioid tumors may behave more aggressively than spindle cell tumors, with a higher tendency to metastasize (20). Myxoid LMS is rare and may be histologically deceiving. They are characterized by one or

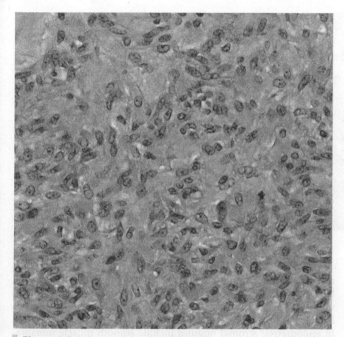

Figure 6.5-4. Leiomyosarcoma, epithelioid.

more of the following: moderate-to-severe cytologic atypia, TCN, greater than one mitoses per 10 HPF, or infiltrative borders (21) (**Figure 6.5-5**). Given that they may be relatively bland, the presence of the infiltrative borders is often one of the most easily recognized criteria. Myxoid LMS portends a long-term survival similar to that of other LMS tumors, but at least one study reported better 5-year survival (73%) compared to ordinary LMS (49%) (22).

Some smooth muscle tumors demonstrate histologic features that are not worrisome enough to render an unequivocal diagnosis of sarcoma. These lesions can be classified as atypical leiomyomas, smooth muscle tumors with low malignant potential (low probability of an unfavorable outcome), or STUMP, depending on the histologic features. **Table 6.5** summarizes the classification of uterine smooth muscle tumors based on histologic characteristics. This classification is largely based upon a large retrospective study

from Stanford University, published in 1994 (13)—the largest to date. Tumors that clinically and pathologically appear to be leiomyomas, but have up to 15 mitoses per 10 HPF, behave in a benign manner and are classified as mitotically active leiomyomas (13,23). Leiomyomas are more likely to have a high mitotic count if they are excised during the secretory phase of the menstrual cycle, during pregnancy, or while patients are receiving exogenous PR therapy.

The histologic parameters of LMS that have been associated with poor prognosis include mitotic index (24,25), lymphovascular invasion (24), size (25), diffuse high-grade cytologic atypia (26), and lack ER and PR expression by immunohistochemistry (IHC) (27). However, many of these characteristics have not been associated with outcome; therefore, they are not entirely validated.

Benign Metastasizing Leiomyoma

Benign metastasizing leiomyoma (BML) is characterized by the presence of a uterine leiomyoma associated with one or more extrauterine smooth muscle tumors that are histologically benign. The most common site of metastasis is the lung, although metastases have also been described in the retroperitoneum, mediastinal lymph nodes, soft tissue, and bone. Before rendering a diagnosis of BML, the pathologist should sample tissue extensively to rule out any aggressive components. The pathogenesis of these tumors is unclear. Some animal experiments suggest that BML may be secondary to lymphatic and hematologic spread, coelomic metaplasia, and intraperitoneal seeding (a pathogenesis similar to that of endometriosis) (28).

ENDOMETRIAL STROMAL NEOPLASMS

In the most recent (2020) WHO publication, endometrial stromal tumors are classified as endometrial stromal nodules, low-grade ESS, and high-grade ESS (29). Both endometrial stromal nodules and low-grade ESS are composed of cells identical to those found in the stroma of proliferative endometrium, whereas high-grade ESS are composed of cells with cytologic atypia. The differential diagnosis between an endometrial stromal nodule and an ESS is important, because nodules are benign. Differential diagnosis is based upon the presence of infiltrating margins with or without angioinvasion in ESS. These two features are not seen in stromal nodules,

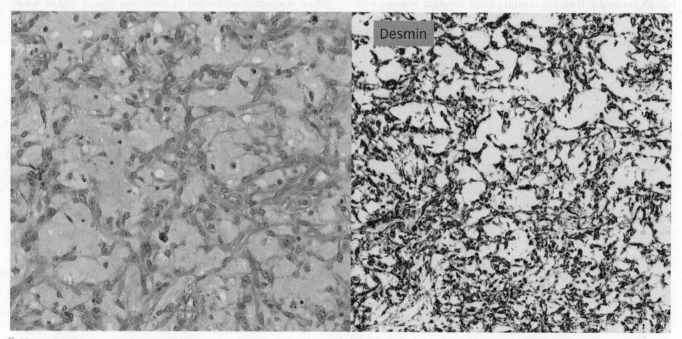

Figure 6.5-5. Leiomyosarcoma, myxoid.

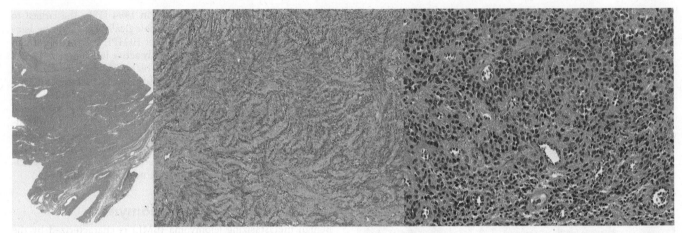

Figure 6.5-6. Endometrial stromal nodule, microscopic.

which are always well circumscribed, with pushing (well-defined) margins (30). Thus this distinction cannot be made on endometrial sampling specimens and requires evaluation of a hysterectomy specimen.

STROMAL NODULE

Stromal nodules are the least common of the pure endometrial stromal neoplasms. They are usually solitary masses, with diameters ranging from 1.2 to 22 cm, with an average of 7.1 cm (31). On cut section, endometrial stromal nodules are fleshy and often tan yellow in color. Microscopically, they are composed of uniformly bland, small cells resembling normal endometrial stromal cells, with fusiform nuclei and scant cytoplasm. Abundant arterioles, reminiscent of the spiral arterioles of the normal endometrium, are also present. The mitotic index is low, with most tumors having fewer than five mitoses per 10 HPF. Most endometrial stromal nodules are cellular; some have variable amounts of intercellular collagen, which occasionally forms dense collagen bands or nodules (**Figure 6.5-6**). Another common finding is the presence of clusters of foamy histiocytes within the tumor. The borders between the tumor and the adjacent myometrium are microscopically pushing. Occasionally, they demonstrate more irregular borders with

minimal areas of tumor extending into the adjacent myometrium, but should have three or fewer finger-like projections less than 3 mm from the tumor margin (30). Endometrial stromal nodules lack any associated lymphovascular invasion. Other changes seen in endometrial stromal nodules include smooth muscle metaplasia, cystic degeneration, sex cord–like areas, and necrosis.

Endometrial stromal nodules are sometimes confused with cellular leiomyomas. As both tumors are benign, the misdiagnosis of one for the other is probably of no clinical consequence in a hysterectomy specimen. In a curettage specimen, however, the differential diagnosis is more important. Some histologic features favor a leiomyoma: blood vessels with thick muscular walls, cleft-like spaces, and merging with adjacent myometrium. A battery of IHC stains may be useful. CD10 is usually present in endometrial stromal cells, and smooth muscle tumors stain positively for desmin and H-caldesmon; however there is considerable overlap so caution is warranted.

Low-Grade Endometrial Stromal Sarcoma

Low-grade ESS is characterized by uniformly bland cells resembling endometrial stromal cells. On gross examination, some comprise a single visible mass, whereas others have multiple masses or diffuse myometrial infiltration by worm-like masses (**Figure 6.5-7**).

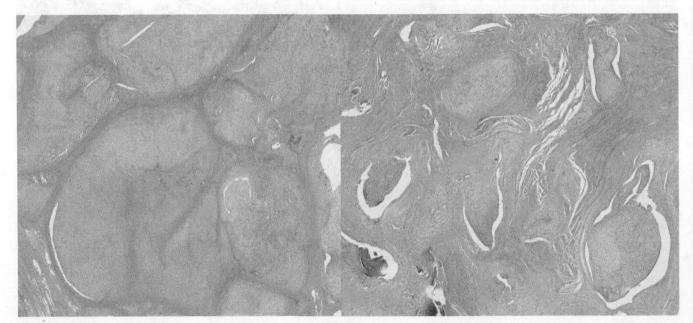

Figure 6.5-7. Endometrial stromal sarcoma, low grade.

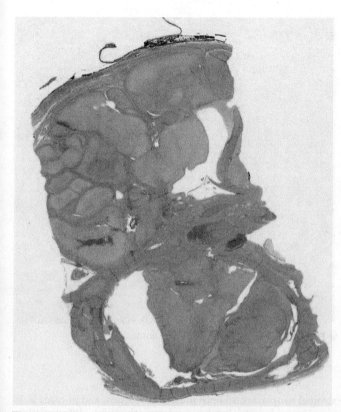

Figure 6.5-8. Endometrial stromal sarcoma, low grade.

Typically, these tumors permeate the myometrial wall, in some cases, up to the serosa (**Figure 6.5-8**). Most have fewer than 10 mitoses per 10 HPF. Some ESS tumors have unusual histologic features that may confound the diagnosis, including myxoid changes, fibroblastic and/or smooth muscle differentiation, epithelioid changes, and extensive endometrioid glandular differentiation (32-35).

Low-grade ESS is usually positive for ER, PR, and CD10, and approximately 65% have genetic fusions involving polycomb family genes. The most characteristic translocation of these tumors generates a fusion of the *JAZF1-SUZ12* genes, with JAZF1-PHF1, EPC1-PHF1 and MEAF6-PHF1 also occurring in a significant number of reported tumors (8,36,37). The presence of the specific gene fusion may be useful in diagnosing difficult cases or recurrent tumors (38).

Low-grade ESS may occur in extrauterine sites, including the ovary, fallopian tube, cervix, vagina, vulva, pelvis, abdomen, retroperitoneum, placenta, sciatic nerve, or round ligament (39-43). Some are associated with endometriosis. Histologically, they are similar to uterine ESS, and a uterine tumor must be excluded before defining the lesion as a primary extrauterine ESS.

Low-grade ESS is an indolent tumor, and patients often have a protracted clinical course, even after a recurrence. The most important prognostic factor is stage. Patients with stage I/II disease have a greater than 90% 5-year survival, which drops to 50% for stage III/IV disease.

High-Grade Endometrial Stromal Sarcoma

High-grade ESS is an infiltrative tumor showing confluent destructive growth, often invading deeply into the myometrial wall. These tumors have areas of high-grade cytology with a brisk mitotic count of greater than 10 mitoses per 10 HPF, necrosis, and often lymphovascular invasion (**Figure 6.5-9**). Approximately 50% have an admixed low-grade component, which is usually fibroblastic. These tumors may demonstrate the same histologic variants seen in other endometrial stromal tumors, including rosettes, glandular, and sex cord–like patterns. The morphology and immunophenotype vary with the underlying genetic abnormality. The three most common abnormalities are YWHAE-NUTM2A/B and ZC3H7B-BCOR fusions and BCOR internal tandem repeats (BCOR ITD) (8). All three demonstrate diffuse expression of cyclin D1, but tumors with YWHAE-NUTM2A/B fusion and BCOR ITD usually have diffuse expression of BCOR, whereas it can be more focal or negative in ZC3H7B-BCOR-driven tumors (44). In addition, the ZC3H7B-BCOR tumors usually express CD10 with variable expression of ER and PR, whereas these are negative in YWHAE-NUTM2A/B fusion tumors (45).

In comparison with low-grade ESS, patients with high-grade ESS have more recurrences and are more likely to die of disease (46).

Undifferentiated Uterine Sarcomas

Undifferentiated uterine sarcomas are rare and account for only 6% of all uterine sarcomas (22). They demonstrate cytologic atypia to the extent that they cannot be recognized as arising from endometrial stroma or smooth muscle. Morphologically, these high-grade lesions resemble undifferentiated mesenchymal tumors and behave as high-grade sarcomas (22,47,48). It is important to exclude YWHAE, JAZF1, and NTRK rearrangements as tumors with these alterations should not be included in this category.

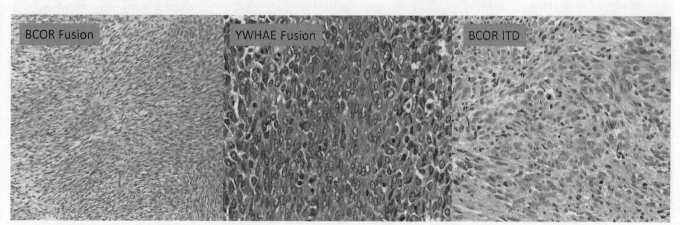

Figure 6.5-9. Endometrial stromal sarcoma, high grade.

Müllerian Adenosarcoma

Müllerian AS are mixed Müllerian tumors composed of malignant stroma and benign epithelium. Most AS arise in the endometrium and, rarely, in the endocervix, lower uterine segment, and myometrium (49). Grossly, the majority are solitary polypoid masses with a spongy appearance, secondary to the presence of small cysts. Occasionally, these tumors appear as multiple polyps or masses and may be multicentric. Their size varies from 1 to 17 cm (mean, 5 cm).

Microscopically, Müllerian AS have a benign epithelial component, usually covering the surface of the polyps and in the form of benign glands uniformly distributed throughout the tumor. The mesenchymal component is usually a low-grade sarcoma that resembles endometrial stroma. The presence of hypercellular stroma around the glands is common, and some tumors have a leaflike papillary growth pattern (**Figure 6.5-10**). It may be difficult to arrive at a diagnosis of AS because of the very low-grade nature of this tumor. A minority of cases have sarcomatous overgrowth, in which more than 25% of the tumor is composed of pure sarcoma. In these cases, the sarcoma is typically high grade, and the lesions are aggressive (50,51) (**Figure 6.5-11**). The histologic parameters associated with increased risk of recurrence include sarcomatous overgrowth, lymphovascular invasion, and myometrial invasion (52,53).

Most AS without sarcomatous overgrowth express ER and PR in the sarcomatous component, which may be used for therapeutic purposes. However, hormonal receptors are negative in AS with sarcomatous overgrowth (50,54). Besides sarcomatous overgrowth, the only other histopathologic features associated with decreased survival are myometrial invasion (49,50,55,56) and the presence of lymphovascular invasion (PMID: 25449308) (53). Müllerian AS have been described in extrauterine sites, including the ovary, and in areas of endometriosis in the vagina, rectovaginal septum, gastrointestinal tract, urinary bladder, pouch of Douglas, peritoneum, and liver (57-64).

Uterine Tumor Resembling Ovarian Sex Cord Tumor

In 1976, Clement and Scully (65) coined the term "uterine tumors resembling ovarian sex cord tumor" (UTROSCT) to describe a series of uterine neoplasms with sex cord–like pattern. Since then, sex cord–like patterns have been demonstrated in endometrial

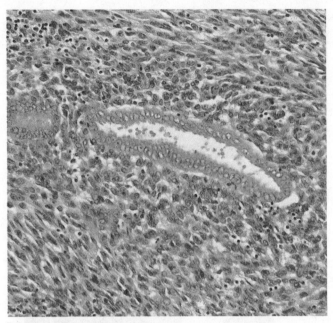

Figure 6.5-11. Adenosarcoma, high grade.

stromal neoplasms, smooth muscle neoplasms, and in cases lacking clear endometrial stroma and smooth muscle differentiation. The term *UTROSCT* should be reserved for this last category. UTROSCTs are tumors of uncertain histogenesis/lineage. Immunohistochemically, these tumors coexpress epithelial, myoid, and sex cord markers (66,67). This immunoprofile can also be seen in ESS with sex cord–like areas. However, UTROSCT lacks the typical *JAZF1-SUZ12* translocation frequently seen in endometrial stromal tumors (68). Recent studies have found rearrangements involving the *ESR1* or *GREB1* genes with a large number of partners including NCOA1, NCOA2, NCOA3, and CTNNB1 as well as others (69,70). UTROSCTs are rare, usually submucosal, and well circumscribed, with a yellow cut surface. Histologically, they are composed of sertoliform tubules with low mitotic activity and little nuclear atypia (65-67) (**Figure 6.5-12**). Most behave in a benign manner, but since they can recur, they are best considered of low malignant potential.

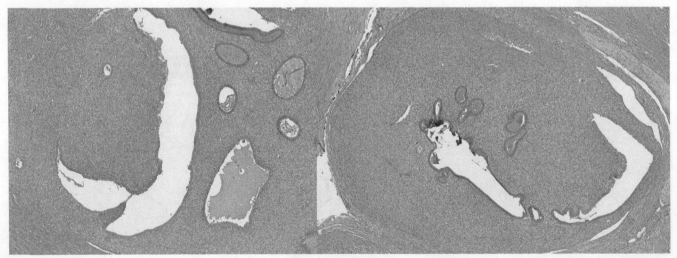

Figure 6.5-10. Adenosarcoma, low grade.

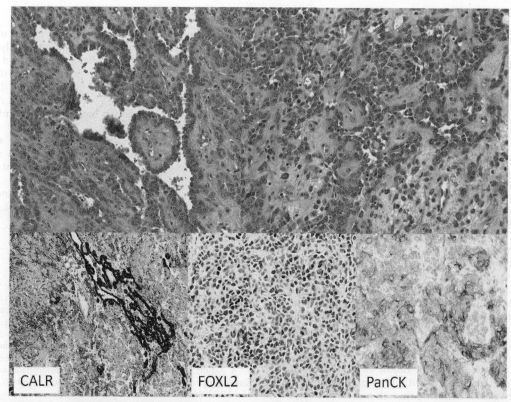

Figure 6.5-12. Uterine tumor resembling ovarian sex cord tumor, hematoxylin and eosin and immunohistochemistry.

PERIVASCULAR EPITHELIOID CELL TUMORS

PEComas are rare neoplasms presumably derived from perivascular epithelioid cells that coexpress melanocytic and smooth muscle markers. Other tumors belonging to the same family include angiomyolipoma, clear cell/sugar tumor of the lung, lymphangioleiomyomatosis, and myomelanocytic tumor of the ligamentum teres/falciform ligament. PEComas have been described in a variety of locations, including visceral organs, soft tissues, skin, oral mucosa, orbit, and base of skull (71). The uterus and gastrointestinal tract are the most common locations for visceral PEComas. About 8% of PEComas occur in patients with the tuberous sclerosis complex. Most of these tumors coexpress melanocytic (HMB45, Melan-A, microphthalmia transcription factor, S-100 protein) and smooth muscle markers (desmin, SMA, H-caldesmon). Most uterine PEComas are histologically and clinically benign. They can appear as either grossly well-circumscribed or focally infiltrative masses (72). Histologically, they are composed of epithelioid cells with abundant clear or eosinophilic cytoplasm, sometimes associated with spindle cells, and a prominent vasculature (71,73) **(Figure 6.5-13)**.

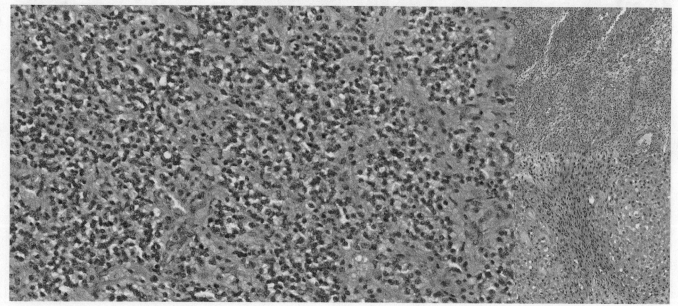

Figure 6.5-13. Perivascular epithelioid cell tumor.

Approximately 25% of reported cases develop metastases and/or recurrences. Most malignant tumors have more than one of these histologic features: size greater than 5 cm, high-grade nuclear features, infiltration of surrounding tissue, necrosis, mitoses greater than 1 per 50 HPF, and lymphovascular invasion. However, there is not a single reliable prognostic indicator other than the presence of lymphovascular invasion (71,73-75).

A distinct subset including some uterine PEComas harbor *TFE3* gene fusions and show immunoreactivity for TFE3 protein (76,77). These tumors tend to have distinctive nested/alveolar morphology. In the past, *TFE3* gene fusions were described only in alveolar soft-part sarcomas and in some renal cell carcinomas. PEComas with *TFE3* gene fusions seem to occur in younger people without tuberous sclerosis.

INFLAMMATORY MYOFIBROBLASTIC TUMOR

IMTs are rare mesenchymal lesions considered to be of intermediate biologic potential. The most common sites for these tumors include the lung, mesentery, omentum, and retroperitoneum. A few cases have been reported in the uterus (78,79), where they present as polypoid masses in the lower uterine segment, or bulky myometrial masses. IMTs range in size from 1 to 12 cm. They are composed of spindle and epithelioid myofibroblastic cells admixed with lymphoplasmacytic infiltrate in variably myxoid background (**Figure 6.5-14**). Expression of ALK protein by IHC is characteristic of almost all IMTs and can be used in the differential diagnosis with other uterine spindle cell tumors that are negative (including smooth muscle tumors, ESS, and CS) (78), whereas a small subset can harbor alterations of *ROS1* and *NTRK3* genes (80,81). Most IMTs behave indolently. However, a recent series reported three cases with aggressive behavior, including local recurrence, extrauterine spread, or distant metastases. The aggressive tumors were reportedly larger and characterized by a higher percentage of myxoid stroma, higher mitotic count, and necrosis, compared to indolent tumors (82). Given the positive ALK expression, patients with IMT may benefit from targeted therapy.

Other Rare Uterine Sarcomas

Rarely, other sarcomas may be found in the uterine corpus. Rhabdomyosarcomas, although more commonly arising in the cervix of children, have also been encountered in the corpus in adults. These tumors may be of embryonal or pleomorphic histology. They are aggressive, with a 5-year disease-specific survival of only 29%. Patients with pleomorphic rhabdomyosarcoma have a worse prognosis than those with embryonal histology (22,83,84).

Uterine liposarcomas are rare tumors. Some arise in uterine lipoleiomyomas (85), others are associated with smooth muscle tumors and may represent LMS with divergent differentiation (84,86).

Other rare sarcomas described in the uterus include angiosarcoma, Ewing sarcoma, alveolar soft-part sarcoma, osteosarcoma, chondrosarcoma, and fibrosarcoma (84).

REFERENCES

1. Moch H. *WHO Classification of Tumours*. Volume 4: Female Genital Tumours. International Agency for Research on Cancer; 2020:6.

2. Hensley ML, Chavan SS, Solit DB, Genomic landscape of uterine sarcomas defined through prospective clinical sequencing. *Clin Cancer Res.* 2020;26(14):3881-3888. doi:10.1158/1078-0432.CCR-19-3959

3. Nacev BA, Jones KB, Intlekofer AM, et al. The epigenomics of sarcoma. *Nat Rev Cancer.* 2020;20(10):608-623. doi:10.1038/s41568-020-0288-4

4. Astolfi A, Nannini M, Indio V, et al. Genomic database analysis of uterine leiomyosarcoma mutational profile. *Cancers (Basel).* 2020;12(8):2126. doi:10.3390/cancers12082126

5. Dalton WB, Yu B, Yang VW. p53 suppresses structural chromosome instability after mitotic arrest in human cells. *Oncogene.* 2010;29(13):1929-1940. doi:10.1038/onc.2009.477

6. de Almeida BC, Dos Anjos LG, Dobroff AS, et al. Epigenetic features in uterine leiomyosarcoma and endometrial stromal sarcomas: an overview of the literature. *Biomedicines.* 2022;10(10):2567. doi:10.3390/biomedicines10102567

7. Tavares M, Khandelwal G, Muter J, et al. JAZF1-SUZ12 dysregulates PRC2 function and gene expression during cell differentiation. *Cell Rep.* 2022;39(9):110889. doi:10.1016/j.celrep.2022.110889

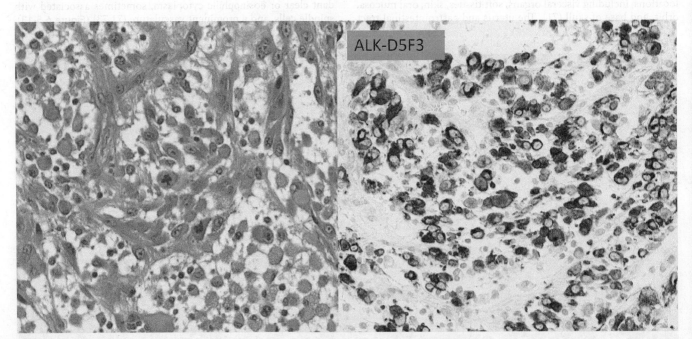

Figure 6.5-14. Inflammatory myofibroblastic cell tumor, hematoxylin and eosin and immunohistochemistry.

8. Momeni-Boroujeni A, Chiang S. Uterine mesenchymal tumours: recent advances. *Histopathology*. 2020;76(1):64-75. doi:10.1111/his.14008

9. Dessources K, Miller KM, Kertowidjojo E, et al. ESR1 hotspot mutations in endometrial stromal sarcoma with high-grade transformation and endocrine treatment. *Mod Pathol*. 2022;35(7):972-978. doi:10.1038/s41379-021-01003-5

10. Mittal K, Joutovsky A. Areas with benign morphologic and immunohistochemical features are associated with some uterine leiomyosarcomas. *Gynecol Oncol*. 2007;104(2):362-365. doi:10.1016/j.ygyno.2006.08.034

11. Mittal KR, Chen F, Wei JJ, et al. Molecular and immunohistochemical evidence for the origin of uterine leiomyosarcomas from associated leiomyoma and symplastic leiomyoma-like areas. *Mod Pathol*. 2009;22(10):1303-1311. doi:10.1038/modpathol.2009.96

12. Zhang P, Zhang C, Hao J, et al. Use of X-chromosome inactivation pattern to determine the clonal origins of uterine leiomyoma and leiomyosarcoma. *Hum Pathol*. 2006;37(10):1350-1356. doi:10.1016/j.humpath.2006.05.005

13. Bell SW, Kempson RL, Hendrickson MR. Problematic uterine smooth muscle neoplasms. A clinicopathologic study of 213 cases. *Am J Surg Pathol*. 1994;18(6):535-558.

14. Guntupalli SR, Ramirez PT, Anderson ML, Milam MR, Bodurka DC, Malpica A. Uterine smooth muscle tumor of uncertain malignant potential: a retrospective analysis. *Gynecol Oncol*. 2009;113(3):324-326. doi:10.1016/j.ygyno.2009.02.020

15. Giuntoli RL 2nd, Gostout BS, DiMarco CS, Metzinger DS, Keeney GL. Diagnostic criteria for uterine smooth muscle tumors: leiomyoma variants associated with malignant behavior. *J Reprod Med*. 2007;52(11):1001-1010.

16. Ip PP, Cheung AN, Clement PB. Uterine smooth muscle tumors of uncertain malignant potential (STUMP): a clinicopathologic analysis of 16 cases. *Am J Surg Pathol*. 2009;33(7):992-1005. doi:10.1097/PAS.0b013e3181a02d1c

17. Ng JS, Han A, Chew SH, Low J. A clinicopathologic study of uterine smooth muscle tumours of uncertain malignant potential (STUMP). *Ann Acad Med Singap*. 2010;39(8):625-628.

18. Veras E, Zivanovic O, Jacks L, Chiappetta D, Hensley M, Soslow R. "Low-grade leiomyosarcoma" and late-recurring smooth muscle tumors of the uterus: a heterogenous collection of frequently misdiagnosed tumors associated with an overall favorable prognosis relative to conventional uterine leiomyosarcomas. *Am J Surg Pathol*. 2011;35(11):1626-1637. doi:10.1097/PAS.0b013e31822b44d2

19. Chan E, Rabban JT, Mak J, Zaloudek C, Garg K. Detailed morphologic and immunohistochemical characterization of myomectomy and hysterectomy specimens from women with hereditary leiomyomatosis and renal cell carcinoma syndrome (HLRCC). *Am J Surg Pathol*. 2019;43(9):1170-1179. doi:10.1097/PAS.0000000000001293

20. Jones MW, Norris HJ. Clinicopathologic study of 28 uterine leiomyosarcomas with metastasis. *Int J Gynecol Pathol*. 1995;14(3):243-249. doi:10.1097/00004347-199507000-00008

21. Botsis D, Koliopoulos C, Kondi-Pafitis A, Creatsas G. Myxoid leiomyosarcoma of the uterus in a patient receiving tamoxifen therapy: a case report. *Int J Gynecol Pathol*. 2006;25(2):173-175. doi:10.1097/01.pgp.0000185407.93308.ce

22. Abeler VM, Røyne O, Thoresen S, Danielsen HE, Nesland JM, Kristensen GB. Uterine sarcomas in Norway. A histopathological and prognostic survey of a total population from 1970 to 2000 including 419 patients. *Histopathology*. 2009;54(3):355-364. doi:10.1111/j.1365-2559.2009.03231.x

23. Perrone T, Dehner LP. Prognostically favorable "mitotically active" smooth-muscle tumors of the uterus. A clinicopathologic study of ten cases. *Am J Surg Pathol*. 1988;12(1):1-8. doi:10.1097/00000478-198801000-00001

24. Pelmus M, Penault-Llorca F, Guillou L, et al. Prognostic factors in early-stage leiomyosarcoma of the uterus. *Int J Gynecol Cancer*. 2009;19(3):385-390. doi:10.1111/IGC.0b013e3181a1bfbc

25. D'Angelo E, Espinosa I, Ali R, et al. Uterine leiomyosarcomas: tumor size, mitotic index, and biomarkers Ki67, and Bcl-2 identify two groups with different prognosis. *Gynecol Oncol*. 2011;121(2):328-333. doi:10.1016/j.ygyno.2011.01.022

26. Wang WL, Soslow R, Hensley M, et al. Histopathologic prognostic factors in stage I leiomyosarcoma of the uterus: a detailed analysis of 27 cases. *Am J Surg Pathol*. 2011;35(4):522-529. doi:10.1097/PAS.0b013e31820ca624

27. Iasonos A, Keung EZ, Zivanovic O, et al. External validation of a prognostic nomogram for overall survival in women with uterine leiomyosarcoma. *Cancer*. 2013;119(10):1816-1822. doi:10.1002/cncr.27971

28. Awonuga AO, Shavell VI, Imudia AN, Rotas M, Diamond MP, Puscheck EE. Pathogenesis of benign metastasizing leiomyoma: a review. *Obstet Gynecol Surv*. 2010;65(3):189-195. doi:10.1097/OGX.0b013e3181d60f93

29. Dionigi A, Oliva E, Clement PB, Young RH. Endometrial stromal nodules and endometrial stromal tumors with limited infiltration: a clinicopathologic study of 50 cases. *Am J Surg Pathol*. 2002;26(5):567-581. doi:10.1097/00000478-200205000-00003

30. Conklin CM, Longacre TA. Endometrial stromal tumors: the new WHO classification. *Adv Anat Pathol*. 2014;21(6):383-393. doi:10.1097/PAP.0000000000000046

31. Chang KL, Crabtree GS, Lim-Tan SK, Kempson RL, Hendrickson MR. Primary uterine endometrial stromal neoplasms. A clinicopathologic study of 117 cases. *Am J Surg Pathol*. 1990;14(5):415-438. doi:10.1097/00000478-199005000-00002

32. Oliva E, Young RH, Clement PB, Scully RE. Myxoid and fibrous endometrial stromal tumors of the uterus: a report of 10 cases. *Int J Gynecol Pathol*. 1999;18(4):310-319. doi:10.1097/00004347-199910000-00004

33. Yilmaz A, Rush DS, Soslow RA. Endometrial stromal sarcomas with unusual histologic features: a report of 24 primary and metastatic tumors emphasizing fibroblastic and smooth muscle differentiation. *Am J Surg Pathol*. 2002;26(9):1142-1150. doi:10.1097/00000478-200209000-00004

34. Oliva E, Clement PB, Young RH. Epithelioid endometrial and endometrioid stromal tumors: a report of four cases emphasizing their distinction from epithelioid smooth muscle tumors and other oxyphilic uterine and extrauterine tumors. *Int J Gynecol Pathol*. 2002;21(1):48-55. doi:10.1097/00004347-200201000-00009

35. Clement PB, Scully RE. Endometrial stromal sarcomas of the uterus with extensive endometrioid glandular differentiation: a report of three cases that caused problems in differential diagnosis. *Int J Gynecol Pathol*. 1992;11(3):163-173.

36. Micci F, Gorunova L, Gatius S, et al. MEAF6/PHF1 is a recurrent gene fusion in endometrial stromal sarcoma. *Cancer Lett*. 2014;347(1):75-78. doi:10.1016/j.canlet.2014.01.030

37. Dickson BC, Lum A, Swanson D, et al. Novel EPC1 gene fusions in endometrial stromal sarcoma. *Genes Chromosomes Cancer*. 2018;57(11):598-603. doi:10.1002/gcc.22649

38. Nucci MR, Harburger D, Koontz J, Dal Cin P, Sklar J. Molecular analysis of the JAZF1-JJAZ1 gene fusion by RT-PCR and fluorescence in situ hybridization in endometrial stromal neoplasms. *Am J Surg Pathol*. 2007;31(1):65-70. doi:10.1097/01.pas.0000213327.86992.d1

39. Chang KL, Crabtree GS, Lim-Tan SK, Kempson RL, Hendrickson MR. Primary extrauterine endometrial stromal neoplasms: a clinicopathologic study of 20 cases and a review of the literature. *Int J Gynecol Pathol*. 1993;12(4):282-296.

40. Irvin W, Pelkey T, Rice L, Andersen W. Endometrial stromal sarcoma of the vulva arising in extraovarian endometriosis: a case report and literature review. *Gynecol Oncol*. 1998;71(2):313-316. doi:10.1006/gyno.1998.5142

41. Kondi-Paphitis A, Smyrniotis B, Liapis A, Kontoyanni A, Deligeorgi H. Stromal sarcoma arising on endometriosis. A clinicopathological and immunohistochemical study of 4 cases. *Eur J Gynaecol Oncol*. 1998;19(6):588-590.

42. Lacroix-Triki M, Beyris L, Martel P, Marques B. Low-grade endometrial stromal sarcoma arising from sciatic nerve endometriosis. *Obstet Gynecol*. 2004;104(5 pt 2):1147-1149. doi:10.1097/01.AOG.0000128114.97877.33

43. Sato K, Ueda Y, Sugaya J, Ozaki M, Hisaoka M, Katsuda S. Extrauterine endometrial stromal sarcoma with JAZF1/JJAZ1 fusion confirmed by RT-PCR and interphase FISH presenting as an inguinal tumor. *Virchows Arch*. 2007;450(3):349-353. doi:10.1007/s00428-006-0345-8

44. Chiang S, Lee CH, Stewart CJR, et al. BCOR is a robust diagnostic immunohistochemical marker of genetically diverse high-grade endometrial stromal sarcoma, including tumors exhibiting variant morphology. *Mod Pathol*. 2017;30(9):1251-1261. doi:10.1038/modpathol.2017.42

45. Momeni-Boroujeni A, Mohammad N, Wolber R, et al. Targeted RNA expression profiling identifies high-grade endometrial stromal sarcoma as a clinically relevant molecular subtype of uterine sarcoma. *Mod Pathol*. 2021;34(5):1008-1016. doi:10.1038/s41379-020-00705-6

46. Lee CH, Mariño-Enriquez A, Ou W, et al. The clinicopathologic features of YWHAE-FAM22 endometrial stromal sarcomas: a histologically high-grade and clinically aggressive tumor. *Am J Surg Pathol*. 2012;36(5):641-653. doi:10.1097/PAS.0b013e31824a7b1a

47. D'Angelo E, Spagnoli LG, Prat J. Comparative clinicopathologic and immunohistochemical analysis of uterine sarcomas diagnosed using the World Health Organization classification system. *Hum Pathol*. 2009;40(11):1571-1585. doi:10.1016/j.humpath.2009.03.018

48. Evans HL. Endometrial stromal sarcoma and poorly differentiated endometrial sarcoma. *Cancer*. 1982;50(10):2170-2182. doi:10.1002/1097-0142(19821115)50:103.0.co;2-k

49. Clement PB, Scully RE. Mullerian adenosarcoma of the uterus: a clinicopathologic analysis of 100 cases with a review of the literature. *Hum Pathol.* 1990;21(4):363-381. doi:10.1016/0046-8177(90)90198-e

50. Clement PB. Müllerian adenosarcomas of the uterus with sarcomatous overgrowth. A clinicopathological analysis of 10 cases. *Am J Surg Pathol.* 1989;13(1):28-38. doi:10.1097/00000478-198901000-00004

51. Momeni Boroujeni A, Kertowidjojo E, Wu X, et al. Mullerian adenosarcoma: clinicopathologic and molecular characterization highlighting recurrent BAP1 loss and distinctive features of high-grade tumors. *Mod Pathol.* 2022;35(11):1684-1694. doi:10.1038/s41379-022-01160-1

52. Bernard B, Clarke BA, Malowany JI, et al. Uterine adenosarcomas: a dual-institution update on staging, prognosis and survival. *Gynecol Oncol.* 2013;131(3):634-639. doi:10.1016/j.ygyno.2013.09.011

53. Carroll A, Ramirez PT, Westin SN, et al. Uterine adenosarcoma: an analysis on management, outcomes, and risk factors for recurrence. *Gynecol Oncol.* 2014;135(3):455-461. doi:10.1016/j.ygyno.2014.10.022

54. Soslow RA, Ali A, Oliva E. Mullerian adenosarcomas: an immunophenotypic analysis of 35 cases. *Am J Surg Pathol.* 2008;32(7):1013-1021. doi:10.1097/PAS.0b013e318161d1be

55. Arend R, Bagaria M, Lewin SN, et al. Long-term outcome and natural history of uterine adenosarcomas. *Gynecol Oncol.* 2010;119(2):305-308. doi:10.1016/j.ygyno.2010.07.001

56. Gallardo A, Prat J. Mullerian adenosarcoma: a clinicopathologic and immunohistochemical study of 55 cases challenging the existence of adenofibroma. *Am J Surg Pathol.* 2009;33(2):278-288. doi:10.1097/PAS.0b013e318181a80d

57. Anderson J, Behbakht K, De Geest K, Bitterman P. Adenosarcoma in a patient with vaginal endometriosis. *Obstet Gynecol.* 2001;98(5 pt 2):964-966. doi:10.1016/s0029-7844(01)01545-9

58. Liu L, Davidson S, Singh M. Müllerian adenosarcoma of vagina arising in persistent endometriosis: report of a case and review of the literature. *Gynecol Oncol.* 2003;90(2):486-490. doi:10.1016/s0090-8258(03)00266-x

59. Raffaelli R, Piazzola E, Zanconato G, Fedele L. A rare case of extrauterine adenosarcoma arising in endometriosis of the rectovaginal septum. *Fertil Steril.* 2004;81(4):1142-1144. doi:10.1016/j.fertnstert.2003.09.053

60. Yantiss RK, Clement PB, Young RH. Neoplastic and pre-neoplastic changes in gastrointestinal endometriosis: a study of 17 cases. *Am J Surg Pathol.* 2000;24(4):513-524. doi:10.1097/00000478-200004000-00005

61. Vara AR, Ruzics EP, Moussabeck O, Martin DC. Endometrioid adenosarcoma of the bladder arising from endometriosis. *J Urol.* 1990;143(4):813-815. doi:10.1016/s0022-5347(17)40105-4

62. Murugasu A, Miller J, Proietto A, Millar E. Extragenital mullerian adenosarcoma with sarcomatous overgrowth arising in an endometriotic cyst in the pouch of Douglas. *Int J Gynecol Cancer.* 2003;13(3):371-375. doi:10.1046/j.1525-1438.2003.13187.x

63. Dincer AD, Timmins P, Pietrocola D, Fisher H, Ambros RA. Primary peritoneal mullerian adenosarcoma with sarcomatous overgrowth associated with endometriosis: a case report. *Int J Gynecol Pathol.* 2002;21(1):65-68. doi:10.1097/00004347-200201000-00012

64. N'Senda P, Wendum D, Balladur P, Dahan H, Tubiana JM, Arrivé L. Adenosarcoma arising in hepatic endometriosis. *Eur Radiol.* 2000;10(8):1287-1289. doi:10.1007/s003300000322

65. Clement PB, Scully RE. Uterine tumors resembling ovarian sex-cord tumors. A clinicopathologic analysis of fourteen cases. *Am J Clin Pathol.* 1976;66(3):512-525. doi:10.1093/ajcp/66.3.512

66. Hurrell DP, McCluggage WG. Uterine tumour resembling ovarian sex cord tumour is an immunohistochemically polyphenotypic neoplasm which exhibits coexpression of epithelial, myoid and sex cord markers. *J Clin Pathol.* 2007;60(10):1148-1154. doi:10.1136/jcp.2006.044842

67. de Leval L, Lim GS, Waltregny D, Oliva E. Diverse phenotypic profile of uterine tumors resembling ovarian sex cord tumors: an immunohistochemical study of 12 cases. *Am J Surg Pathol.* 2010;34(12):1749-1761. doi:10.1097/PAS.0b013e3181f8120c

68. Staats PN, Garcia JJ, Dias-Santagata DC, et al. Uterine tumors resembling ovarian sex cord tumors (UTROSCT) lack the JAZF1-JJAZ1

translocation frequently seen in endometrial stromal tumors. *Am J Surg Pathol.* 2009;33(8):1206-1212. doi:10.1097/PAS.0b013e3181a7b9cf

69. Chang B, Bai Q, Liang L, Ge H, Yao Q. Recurrent uterine tumors resembling ovarian sex-cord tumors with the growth regulation by estrogen in breast cancer 1-nuclear receptor coactivator 2 fusion gene: a case report and literature review. *Diagn Pathol.* 2020;15(1):110.

70. Kao YC, Lee JC. An update of molecular findings in uterine tumor resembling ovarian sex cord tumor and GREB1-rearranged uterine sarcoma with variable sex-cord differentiation. *Genes Chromosomes Cancer.* 2021;60(3):180-189.

71. Folpe AL, Mentzel T, Lehr HA, Fisher C, Balzer BL, Weiss SW. Perivascular epithelioid cell neoplasms of soft tissue and gynecologic origin: a clinicopathologic study of 26 cases and review of the literature. *Am J Surg Pathol.* 2005;29(12):1558-1575. doi:10.1097/01.pas.0000173232.22117.37

72. Bennett JA, Ordulu Z, Pinto A, et al. Uterine PEComas: correlation between melanocytic marker expression and TSC alterations/TFE3 fusions. *Mod Pathol.* 2022;35(4):515-523. doi:10.1038/s41379-021-00855-1

73. Vang R, Kempson RL. Perivascular epithelioid cell tumor ('PEComa') of the uterus: a subset of HMB-45-positive epithelioid mesenchymal neoplasms with an uncertain relationship to pure leiomyoma to pure smooth muscle tumors. *Am J Surg Pathol.* 2002;26(1):1-13. doi:10.1097/00000478-200201000-00001

74. Fadare O. Perivascular epithelioid cell tumor (PEComa) of the uterus: an outcome-based clinicopathologic analysis of 41 reported cases. *Adv Anat Pathol.* 2008;15(2):63-75. doi:10.1097/PAP.0b013e31816613b0

75. Schoolmeester JK, Howitt BE, Hirsch MS, Dal Cin P, Quade BJ, Nucci MR. Perivascular epithelioid cell neoplasm (PEComa) of the gynecologic tract: clinicopathologic and immunohistochemical characterization of 16 cases. *Am J Surg Pathol.* 2014;38(2):176-188. doi:10.1097/PAS.0000000000000133

76. Argani P, Aulmann S, Illei PB, et al. A distinctive subset of PEComas harbors TFE3 gene fusions. *Am J Surg Pathol.* 2010;34(10):1395-1406. doi:10.1097/PAS.0b013e3181f17ac0

77. Agaram NP, Sung YS, Zhang L, et al. Dichotomy of genetic abnormalities in PEComas with therapeutic implications. *Am J Surg Pathol.* 2015;39(6):813-825. doi:10.1097/PAS.0000000000000389

78. Rabban JT, Zaloudek CJ, Shekitka KM, Tavassoli FA. Inflammatory myofibroblastic tumor of the uterus: a clinicopathologic study of 6 cases emphasizing distinction from aggressive mesenchymal tumors. *Am J Surg Pathol.* 2005;29(10):1348-1355. doi:10.1097/01.pas.0000172189.02424.91

79. Gupta N, Mittal S, Misra R. Inflammatory pseudotumor of uterus: an unusual pelvic mass. *Eur J Obstet Gynecol Reprod Biol.* 2011;156(1):118-119. doi:10.1016/j.ejogrb.2011.01.002

80. Bennett JA, Wang P, Wanjari P, Diaz L, Oliva E. Uterine inflammatory myofibroblastic tumor: first report of a ROS1 fusion. Genes Chromosomes Cancer. 2021;60(12):822-826. doi:10.1002/gcc.22986

81. Alassiri AH, Ali RH, Shen Y, et al. ETV6-NTRK3 Is Expressed in a Subset of ALK-Negative Inflammatory Myofibroblastic Tumors. *Am J Surg Pathol.* 2016;40(8):1051-1061. doi:10.1097/PAS.0000000000000677

82. Parra-Herran C, Quick CM, Howitt BE, Dal Cin P, Quade BJ, Nucci MR. Inflammatory myofibroblastic tumor of the uterus: clinical and pathologic review of 10 cases including a subset with aggressive clinical course. *Am J Surg Pathol.* 2015;39(2):157-168. doi:10.1097/PAS.0000000000000330

83. Ferguson SE, Gerald W, Barakat RR, Chi DS, Soslow RA. Clinicopathologic features of rhabdomyosarcoma of gynecologic origin in adults. *Am J Surg Pathol.* 2007;31(3):382-389. doi:10.1097/01.pas.0000213352.87885.75

84. Fadare O. Heterologous and rare homologous sarcomas of the uterine corpus: a clinicopathologic review. *Adv Anat Pathol.* 2011;18(1):60-74. doi:10.1097/PAP.0b013e3182026be7

85. McDonald AG, Dal Cin P, Ganguly A, et al. Liposarcoma arising in uterine lipoleiomyoma: a report of 3 cases and review of the literature. *Am J Surg Pathol.* 2011;35(2):221-227. doi:10.1097/PAS.0b013e31820414f7

86. Fadare O, Khabele D. Pleomorphic liposarcoma of the uterine corpus with focal smooth muscle differentiation. *Int J Gynecol Pathol.* 2011;30(3):282-287. doi:10.1097/PGP.0b013e31820086a4

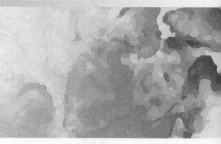

CHAPTER **6.6**

Radiation Therapy for Uterine Corpus Mesenchymal Tumors

Matthew M. Harkenrider

UTERINE SARCOMAS

Much of the published literature on uterine sarcomas is retrospective in design, with limited numbers, and often spanning many years. Furthermore, these studies often have significant heterogeneity with sarcomas of different cell types. In addition, there may not be routine central pathology review of the original hysterectomy permanent slides to verify cell type. These retrospective studies have not achieved statistical power to reach definite conclusions, especially regarding the impact of postoperative radiation therapy (PORT) on outcomes for patients with uterine sarcomas (1-31).

There is only one published phase III randomized trial comparing observation versus PORT in surgically staged patients with FIGO 1988 stages I and II uterine sarcomas. The European Organisation for Research and Treatment of Cancer (EORTC) Gynecological Cancer Group (GCG) 55874 trial accrued patients from 1988 to 2001. Eligible patients underwent an initial surgical resection that involved mandatory TAH-BSO and recommended lymph node sampling (~25% underwent lymph node sampling). Because of the time period of this trial's inception, there were no recommendations regarding either collection of peritoneal washings or omentectomy. The study enrolled 224 patients for randomization from 36 institutions. Patient histologies included the following: 99 LMS, 92 CS, 30 ESS, 1 myxoid LMS, and 2 unclassified cell types.

The inclusion of CS in this study makes the inclusion population heterogeneous as CS is a histology arising from the uterine epithelium with biphasic development creating its mixed histology. In this study, CS tumors were those with mixed epithelial and sarcomatoid components without elements of LMS or stromal components. It must be noted that there was a central pathology review of tumor samples; however, no distinction was made regarding low-grade ESS and high-grade undifferentiated uterine sarcomas (UUS). Eligible study patients were randomized to undergo either observation or PORT, consisting two-dimensional or three-dimensional treatment planning to a dose of 50.4 Gy in 28 fractions (32).

The primary objective of this EORTC-GCG trial was to determine whether patients receiving PORT had reduced rates of pelvic recurrence and to assess if decreased pelvic recurrences translated into a reduction in distant metastases. At a median follow-up of 6.8 years, there was a significant reduction in locoregional recurrence from 21% with PORT compared to 40% with observation (*P* = .004). The improvement in locoregional control with PORT did not translate to a decrease in distant metastases though. Distant metastases occurred as a component of failure in 46% of patients in the PORT arm versus 32% in the observation arm. The primary cause of death was malignant disease in 81% (39/48) of PORT patients and 93% (43/46) of observation patients. There was no significant difference in PFS or OS (32) (**Figures 6.6-1 and 6.6-2**).

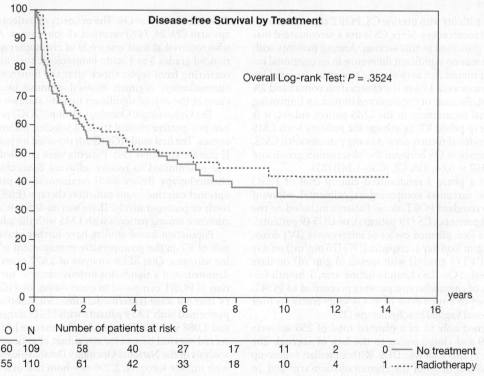

▪ **Figure 6.6-1.** Disease-free survival from EORTC-GCG 55874 comparing postoperative radiation therapy versus observation in patients with uterine sarcoma.

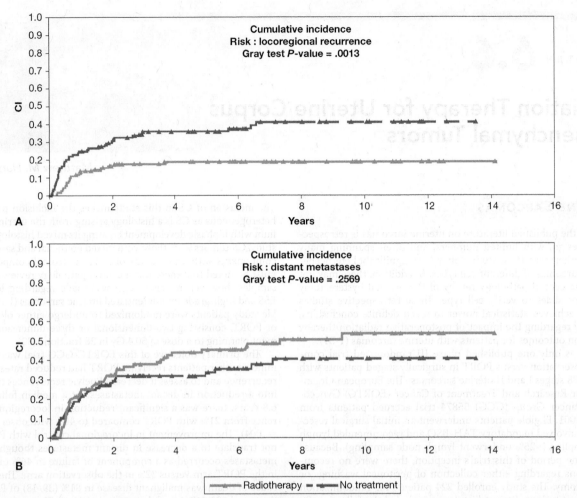

Figure 6.6-2. Cumulative incidence of (A) locoregional recurrence and (B) distant metastases of postoperative adjuvant radiation therapy versus observation in patients with uterine sarcoma.

With respect to patients with uterine CS, PORT significantly reduced locoregional recurrences. Since CS is not a sarcomatoid histology, CS are not discussed in this section. Among patients with uterine LMS, there was no significant difference in locoregional recurrence or distant metastases between the two arms. Isolated locoregional recurrences were 14% in the observation cohort and 2% in the PORT cohort. Because of the observed impact on improving isolated locoregional recurrences in the LMS patient subset, it is reasonable to reserve pelvic RT as salvage for patients with LMS with isolated locoregional recurrences. Among patients with LMS, there was no difference in OS between the observation group and the PORT group (HR = 0.64; 95% CI, [0.36-1.14]) (32).

SARCGYN was a phase 3 randomized clinical trial of FIGO stages I-III uterine sarcomas comparing experimental adjuvant chemoradiation to standard PORT alone. Patients included on the study had LMS (53 patients), CS (19 patients), or UUS (9 patients). Chemotherapy was four planned cycles of intravenous (IV) doxorubicin ["A"] (50 mg/m^2) on day 1, cisplatin ["P"] (75 mg/m^2) on day 3, and ifosfamide ["I"] (3 g/m^2/d) with mesna (3 g/m^2/d) on days 1 and 2 every 3 weeks. On the chemoradiation arm, 1 month following completion of chemotherapy, patients proceeded to PORT. PORT was delivered to a total dose of 45 Gy in 25 fractions over 5 weeks, with optional vaginal brachytherapy (33).

This study accrued only 81 of a planned total of 256 subjects from 2001 to 2009 and closed owing to the lack of accrual. The primary end point of this trial was DFS. With a median follow-up of 4.3 years, 15 (38.5%) of 39 in the chemoradiation arm and 26 (61.9%) of 42 in the PORT arm relapsed. The 3-year DFS was significantly improved with the addition of chemotherapy at 55% versus 41% for PORT alone (P = .048). There was no significant

difference in 3-year OS. The majority of patients in the chemotherapy arm (29/39, 74%) received all four cycles. Among the patients who received at least one cycle of chemotherapy, a majority experienced grades 3 to 4 acute hematologic toxicities, with two deaths occurring from septic shock after the fourth cycle. Although this chemotherapy regimen showed promise by improving DFS, it came at the cost of significant toxicity and two deaths (33).

The Gynecologic Oncology Group (GOG) previously conducted two prospective clinical trials of selected patients with uterine sarcomas. The first study (GOG 20) reported on patients with stage I or II uterine sarcomas (34). Patients were enrolled from 1973 to 1982 and randomized to receive adjuvant doxorubicin or no adjuvant chemotherapy. Before study randomization, patients could receive optional external beam radiation therapy (EBRT) either preoperatively or postoperatively. There was no difference in locoregional recurrence among patients with LMS with the addition of EBRT (35).

Population-based studies have further attempted to clarify the role of RT in the postoperative management of patients with uterine sarcoma. One SEER analysis of 2,677 cases of uterine sarcoma demonstrated a significant improvement in survival with the addition of PORT compared to observation for FIGO stages II, III, and IV (but not stage I) uterine sarcoma (36). Another SEER analysis was performed with 1,819 patients with FIGO stages I and II uterine CS and 1,088 with FIGO stages I and II uterine LMS. There was no observed survival benefit for any subset of patients with LMS (37). An analysis of the National Oncology Database identified 3,650 patients with uterine sarcoma, 2,206 of whom had definitive surgery (1,128 CS, 529 LMS, and 361 ESS). There was no significant difference on survival for patients receiving PORT compared to those receiving no adjuvant therapy. However, there was significant improvement in locoregional relapse-free survival from 85% with observation to 93% with PORT ($P < .001$) (38). An analysis of the National Cancer Database did not show any difference in survival among patients with LMS treated with PORT or chemoradiation (39). A study of 38 premenopausal patients with LMS from the Alberta Cancer Registry found improved survival among patients undergoing PORT on univariate analysis, but this improvement in survival was not maintained on multivariate analysis (40). Another analysis of the National Cancer Database investigated the role of adjuvant therapy for patients with ESS. They found that the use of adjuvant RT improved survival among patients with high-grade ESS (41).

There are mixed data regarding the role of RT in the postoperative management of patients with uterine sarcoma. Interpretation of these data remains challenging as studies are routinely limited in patient numbers, slow to accrue prospectively, and heterogeneous regarding histologic subtypes. These studies are often confounded with the inclusion of patients of CS. Available data demonstrate mixed outcomes regarding the role of PORT for patients with uterine LMS. While PORT may decrease risk of locoregional recurrence, routine use of PORT in the adjuvant management of patients with uterine sarcoma is not likely to improve development of extrapelvic recurrences nor survival. The use of PORT in uterine sarcomas remains reasonable among patients who have high-risk features of close or positive surgical margins, locoregionally recurrent disease, or in palliation of symptoms in recurrent or metastatic patients.

REFERENCES

1. Zhang YY, Li Y, Qin M, Cai Y, Jin Y, Pan LY. High-grade endometrial stromal sarcoma: a retrospective study of factors influencing prognosis. *Cancer Manag Res.* 2019;11:831-837. doi:10.2147/CMAR.S187849

2. Hou HL, Meng MB, Chen XL, et al. The prognosis factor of adjuvant radiation therapy after surgery in uterine sarcomas. *Onco Targets Ther.* 2015;8:2339-2344. doi:10.2147/OTT.S88186

3. Vongtama V, Karlen JR, Piver SM, et al. Treatment, results and prognostic factors in stage I and II sarcomas of the corpus uteri. *Am J Obstet Gynecol.* 1976;126:139-147.

4. Salazar OM, Bonfiglio TA, Patten SF, et al. Uterine sarcomas: natural history, treatment and prognosis. *Cancer.* 1978;42:1152-1160.

5. Perez CA, Askin F, Baglan RJ, et al. Effects of irradiation on mixed Müllerian tumors of the uterine sarcomas. *Cancer.* 1979;43:1274-1284.

6. Hoffmann W, Schmandt S, Koradiotherapymann RD, et al. Radiotherapy in the treatment of uterine sarcomas: a retrospective analysis of 54 cases. *Gynecol Obstet Invest.* 1996;42:49-57.

7. Knocke TH, Kucera H, Dorfler D, et al. Results of postoperative radiotherapy in the treatment of sarcomas of the corpus uteri. *Cancer.* 1998;83:1972-1979.

8. Ferrer F, Sabater S, Farruterine B, et al. Impact of radiotherapy on local control and survival in uterine sarcomas: a retrospective study from the GRUP oncologic catala-occita. *Int J Radiat Oncol Biol Phys.* 1999;44:47-52.

9. Chauveinc L, Deniaud E, Plancher C, et al. Uterine sarcomas: the curie institute experience. Prognostic factors and adjuvant treatments. *Gynecol Oncol.* 1999;72:232-237.

10. Soumarova R, Horova H, Seneklova Z, et al. Treatment of uterine sarcoma: a survey of 49 patients. *Arch Gynecol Obstet.* 2002;266:92-95.

11. Livi L, Paiar F, Shah N, et al. Uterine sarcoma: twenty-seven years of experience. *Int J Radiat Oncol Biol Phys.* 2003;57:1366-1373.

12. Dusenbery KE, Potish RA, Agenta PA, et al. On the apparent failure of adjuvant pelvic radiotherapy to improve survival for women with uterine sarcomas confined to the uterus. *Am J Clin Oncol.* 2005;28:295-300.

13. Dusenberry KE, Potish RA, Judson P. Limitations of adjuvant radiotherapy for uterine sarcomas spread beyond the uterus. *Gynecol Oncol.* 2004;94:191-196.

14. Sorbe B, Johansson B. Prophylactic pelvic irradiation as part of primary therapy in uterine sarcomas. *Int J Oncol.* 2008;32:1111-1117.

15. Sahinler I, Atalar B, Tecer GM, et al. Postoperative radiotherapy in the treatment of uterine sarcomas: long-term results and analysis of prognostic factors. *J BUON.* 2010;15:480-488.

16. Rovirosa A, Ascaso C, Ordi J, et al. How to deal with prognostic factors and radiotherapy results in uterine neoplasms with a sarcomatous component. *Clin Transl Oncol.* 2009;11:681-687.

17. Magnuson WJ, Petereit DG, Anderson BM, et al. Impact of adjuvant pelvic radiotherapy in stage I uterine sarcoma. *Anticancer Res.* 2015;35:365-370.

18. Hou HL, Meng MB, Chen XL, et al. The prognosis of adjuvant radiation therapy after surgery in uterine sarcomas. *Onco Targets Ther.* 2015;8:2339-2344.

19. Pautier P, Rey A, Haie-Meder C, et al. Adjuvant chemotherapy with cisplatin, ifosfamide, and doxorubicin followed by radiotherapy in localized uterine sarcomas: results of a case-control study with radiotherapy alone. *Int J Gynecol Cancer.* 2004;14:1112-1117.

20. Denschlag D, Masoud G, Gilbert L. Prognostic factors and outcome in women with uterine sarcoma. *Eur J Surg Oncol.* 2006;33:91-95.

21. Yoney A, Eren B, Eskici S, et al. Retrospective analysis of 105 cases with uterine sarcoma. *Bull Cancer.* 2008;95:E10-E17.

22. Gadducci A, Sartori E, Landoni F, et al. Endometrial stromal sarcoma: analysis of treatment failure and survival. *Gynecol Oncol.* 1996;63:247-253.

23. Bodner K, Bodner-Adler B, Obermair A, et al. Prognostic parameters in endometrial stromal sarcoma: a clinicopathologic study in 31 patients. *Gynecol Oncol.* 2001;81(2):160-165.

24. Tanz R, Mahfound T, Bazine A, et al. Endometrial stromal sarcoma: prognostic factors and impact of adjuvant therapy in early stages. *Hematol Oncol Stem Cell Ther.* 2012;5:31-35.

25. Malouf GG, Duclos J, Rey A, et al. Impact of adjuvant treatment modalities on the management of patients with stage I-II endometrial sarcoma. *Ann Oncol.* 2010;21:2102-2106.

26. Geller MA, Argenta P, Bradley W, et al. Treatment and recurrence patterns in endometrial stromal sarcomas and the relation to c-kit. *Gynecol Oncol.* 2004;95:632-636.

27. Valduvieco I, Rovirosa A, Colomo L, et al. Endometrial stromal sarcoma. Is there a place for radiotherapy. *Clin Transl Oncol.* 2010;12:226-230.

28. Rios I, Rovirosa A, Morales J, et al. Undifferentiated uterine sarcoma: a rare, not well known aggressive disease: report of 13 cases. *Arch Gynecol Obstet.* 2014;290:993-997.

29. Weitmann HD, Knocke TH, Kucera H, et al. Radiation therapy in the treatment of endometrial stromal sarcoma. *Int J Radiat Oncol Biol Phys.* 2001;49:739-748.

30. Barney B, Tward JD, Skidmore T, et al. Does radiotherapy or lymphadenectomy improve survival in endometrial stromal sarcoma? *Int J Gynecol Cancer.* 2009;19:1232-1238.

31. Leath CA, Huh WK, Hyde J Jr, et al. A multi-institutional review of outcomes of endometrial stromal sarcoma. *Gynecol Oncol.* 2007;105:630-634.

32. Reed NS, Mangioni C, Malmstrom H, et al. Phase III randomized study to evaluate the role of adjuvant pelvic radiotherapy in the treatment of uterine sarcomas stages I and II: an European Organisation for Research and Treatment of Cancer Gynaecological Cancer Group Study (protocol 55874). *Eur J Cancer.* 2008;44:808-818.

33. Pautier P, Floquet A, Gladieff L, et al. A randomized clinical trial of adjuvant chemotherapy with doxorubicin, ifosfamide, and cisplatin followed by radiotherapy versus radiotherapy alone in patients with localized uterine sarcomas (SARCGYN study). A study of the French Sarcoma Group. *Ann Oncol.* 2013;24:1099-1104.

34. Omura GA, Blessing JA, Major F, et al. A randomized clinical trial of adjuvant adriamycin in uterine sarcomas: a gynecologic oncology group study. *J Clin Oncol.* 1985;3:1240-1245.

35. Hornback NB, Omura G, Major FJ. Observations on the uterine sarcomas of adjuvant radiation therapy in patients with stage I and II uterine sarcoma. *Int J Radiat Oncol Biol Phys.* 1986;12:2127-2130.

36. Brooks SE, Zhan M, Cote T, et al. Survival epidemiology and end results analysis of 2677 cases of uterine sarcomas, 1989–1999. *Gynecol Oncol.* 2004;93:204-208

37. Wright JD, Venkatraman ES, Shah M, et al. The role of radiation in improving survival for early-stage carcinosarcoma and leiomyosarcoma. *Am J Obstet Gynecol.* 2008;199:536.e1-536.e8.

38. Sampath S, Schultheiss TE, Ryu JK, et al. The role of adjuvant radiation in uterine sarcomas. *Int J Radiat Oncol Biol Phys.* 2010;76:728-734.

39. Costales AB, Radeva M, Ricci S. Characterizing the efficacy and trends of adjuvant therapy versus observation in women with early stage (uterine confined) leiomyosarcoma: a National Cancer Database Study. *J Gynecol Oncol.* 2020;31(3):e21. doi:10.3802/jgo.2020.31.e21

40. Singh N, Al-Ruwaisan M, Batra A, Itani D, Ghatage P. Factors affecting overall survival in premenopausal women with uterine leiomyosarcoma: a retrospective analysis with long-term follow-up. *J Obstet Gynaecol Can.* 2020;42(12):1483-1488. doi:10.1016/j.jogc.2020.05.016

41. Seagle BL, Shilpi A, Buchanan S, Goodman C, Shahabi S. Low-grade and high-grade endometrial stromal sarcoma: a national cancer database study. *Gynecol Oncol.* 2017;146(2):254-262. doi:10.1016/j.ygyno.2017.05.036

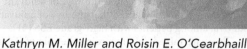

CHAPTER **6.7**

Chemotherapy for Uterine-Limited and Advanced Uterine Sarcomas

Kathryn M. Miller and Roisin E. O'Cearbhaill

INTRODUCTION

Uterine sarcomas, although far less common than endometrial carcinomas, exhibit two features that suggest a need for systemic therapy: a recurrence rate of at least 50%, even in early-stage disease (1,2); and a high propensity for distant failure. The comparatively low incidence of uterine sarcomas has made randomized controlled trials difficult. Despite this, cooperative group studies have provided data from phase 2 and 3 trials supporting the rational selection of systemic antineoplastic treatment.

Uterine sarcomas are heterogeneous. Historically, uterine CS (malignant mixed Müllerian tumors) and LMS constituted 90% of cases entered into clinical trials as they were the only subtypes of uterine sarcomas presenting in sufficient numbers to allow meaningful phase 3 studies. However, as understanding has evolved in regard to molecular differences and chemotherapy response, they are now studied separately, with uterine CS treated similarly to endometrial cancers (see Chapter 5.5).

LIMITED OR COMPLETELY RESECTED DISEASE

Uterine sarcoma is associated with a high rate of distant metastasis, even in the absence of intraperitoneal or lymph node involvement, due to hematogenous and lymphatic dissemination (3). Therefore, the role of adjuvant systemic antineoplastic therapy has been investigated in patients with apparently limited disease that has been fully resected. A meta-analysis of almost 2,000 patients with localized, resectable soft-tissue sarcomas (STS) (including uterine sarcomas) in small randomized trials of adjuvant anthracycline-based chemotherapy showed improved outcomes with chemotherapy compared to local treatment alone. Absolute risk reduction of 12% in recurrence and 11% in death were associated with doxorubicin-based regimens combined with ifosfamide (4). Application of these data to uterine sarcoma is somewhat stymied, however, by the range of tumor sites and the heterogeneity of sarcoma subtypes included in this meta-analysis.

The largest randomized trial to date (a phase 3 GOG trial of 156 evaluable patients) concluded that there was no significant difference between adjuvant chemotherapy versus no further therapy in patients with stage I or II uterine sarcoma. The recurrence rate and median survival of patients treated with doxorubicin compared to no therapy were 41% versus 53% and 73 versus 55 months, respectively. However, this trial did not segregate different histologic subtypes and included 48 patients with uterine CS (5). Adjuvant pelvic RT was optional and was not balanced between the arms. The fact that there was no protocol-specified schedule of imaging for recurrence may also have affected the results. Previous studies reported that a chemotherapy regimen consisting of a combination of cyclophosphamide, vincristine, doxorubicin, and dacarbazine yielded a 68% to 89% 5-year survival in stage I uterine sarcomas (6-8).

Uterine Leiomyosarcoma

Two factors continue to limit the study of adjuvant therapy in uterine LMS: the relatively low frequency of the disease, which makes it difficult to complete randomized trials in a reasonable period of time; and the lack of highly active therapeutic agents.

The demonstrated activity of gemcitabine plus docetaxel in metastatic uterine LMS led to the investigation of this combination in the adjuvant setting (9,10). A phase 2, single-institution trial of four cycles of fixed-dose-rate gemcitabine and docetaxel following complete resection of stage I to IV disease in 23 patients with high-grade LMS has been reported (11). Among the 18 patients with early-stage disease, 59% remained disease free at 2 years, with a median PFS of 39 months. Among the entire cohort, the median follow-up time was 49 months, with a 2-year PFS rate of 45% and median PFS of 13 months. Although these numbers appeared superior to a historical 2-year PFS rate of 30%, the clinical application of these findings is challenged by the absence of a control arm and the small number of patients enrolled in the trial.

The Sarcoma Alliance for Research through Collaboration (SARC) subsequently conducted a phase 2, multicenter study of four cycles of adjuvant fixed-dose-rate gemcitabine plus docetaxel followed by four cycles of doxorubicin in 47 patients with uterus-limited LMS (12). Although 78% of the patients remained progression free at 2 years, the percentage dropped to 50% at 3-year follow-up (13). Of note, age, menopausal status, hormone receptor status, grade, mitotic rate, or FIGO stage was not significantly associated with PFS.

A phase 3 multicenter, randomized superiority trial (GOG 277) compared four cycles of gemcitabine plus docetaxel followed by four cycles of doxorubicin to the current standard of observation alone, to determine whether adjuvant chemotherapy improved outcomes for patients with uterus-limited high-grade LMS (NCT01533207). The study was closed because of poor accrual after 38 patients from a target accrual of 216 were enrolled over a 4-year period. Despite the small numbers in each arm, there was no difference observed in the number of recurrences or PFS. OS was slightly worse in the adjuvant chemotherapy arm. These data support the rationale for observation as standard of care.

Low-Grade Endometrial Stromal Sarcoma

There are no data to support the use of adjuvant chemotherapy in patients who have had complete resection of low-grade ESS confined to the uterus. The standard approach for these patients is observation alone. The role of adjuvant hormonal therapy for these patients has not been evaluated prospectively. Given the hormone-sensitive nature of these tumors, it is believed that ER replacement therapy may be detrimental in patients with low-grade ESS (14).

Adenosarcoma

Because of the rarity of these tumors, there are no prospective data on the role of adjuvant systemic therapy for patients with completely resected AS. Patients without sarcomatous overgrowth are often treated similarly to patients with ESS. The presence of sarcomatous overgrowth is associated with an increased propensity for disease spread and recurrence (15,16). In a retrospective single-institution review of uterine AS, only one (20%) of five patients with sarcomatous overgrowth was progression free at 2 years, whereas 14 patients without sarcomatous overgrowth remained progression free at 2 years (17). Management of patients with sarcomatous overgrowth is often extrapolated from data regarding high-grade STS. Patients with STS should be encouraged to participate in clinical trials.

Rhabdomyosarcomas

Rhabdomyosarcoma (RMS) is exceedingly rare in adults, with a tendency for early metastatic spread and aggressive behavior. Adjuvant treatment recommendations vary by subtype. Pleomorphic RMS typically affects adults, is extremely rare, and usually excluded from RMS clinical trials. The best systemic therapy has not been defined for this histologic subtype, but treatment following STS guidelines is reasonable (4,18,19). For nonpleomorphic RMS and the more commonly affected pediatric population, the Intergroup Rhabdomyosarcoma Study Group (IRSG) has defined treatment protocols that have dramatically improved outcomes (20-23). The use of a multimodal approach, including surgery, systemic therapy, and radiation in the treatment of local disease, has corresponded to increased survival rates of up to 80% in childhood RMS (23). Therefore, adjuvant therapy in adults has been extrapolated from pediatric RMS treatment paradigms. With varying doses and schedules, the most widely used regimen includes vincristine and dactinomycin, with or without cyclophosphamide (VA, VAC), or vincristine, dactinomycin, and ifosfamide (VAI-Europe) (22,23). However, a modified every-3-week schedule consisting of vincristine and dactinomycin and cyclophosphamide has been proposed, as weekly vincristine causes significant neurotoxicity in adults.

Despite the use of similar multidrug regimens, published series have reported inferior outcomes in adult patients as compared with children, with 5-year OS as low as 31% to 47% (24-27). Both the rarity of adult RMS and range of systemic therapy options have made it challenging to determine the most effective treatment for these patients. Even so, it appears that outcomes for fully resected disease are most favorable when managed with multimodal strategies like those used for childhood RMS, and collaboration with pediatric sarcoma specialists should be considered. Enrollment in clinical trials should additionally be encouraged for adults, particularly as most RMS trials allow enrollment up to age 50 (28).

NEOADJUVANT CHEMOTHERAPY

To date, there have been no published prospective studies evaluating the role of neoadjuvant chemotherapy in the treatment of uterine sarcoma. The theoretical appeal of neoadjuvant therapy is that it might potentially facilitate improved surgical outcomes through tumor shrinkage and permit in vivo assessment of chemosensitivity to first-line drug therapy. The role of PET as an intermediate end point biomarker to assess early treatment response in patients with STS undergoing neoadjuvant chemotherapy is under investigation (29).

CHEMOTHERAPY FOR METASTATIC DISEASE

Single-Agent Therapies

Leiomyosarcoma

Numerous single agents have been and continue to be tested in patients with LMS (**Table 6.7-1**). Unfortunately, the results have been unimpressive (30-52). Doxorubicin and ifosfamide as primary single-agent chemotherapy are the most active in recurrent and advanced uterine LMS. In 1983, the GOG demonstrated seven responses among 28 (25%) patients treated every 3 weeks with single-agent doxorubicin (36). Because of these results, doxorubicin is considered the most active single agent. The GOG subsequently reported that treatment with liposomal doxorubicin yielded one complete (3.2%) and four partial (13%) responses but conferred no advantage compared to historical results using doxorubicin alone (30). However, given the lower risk of cardiotoxicity, liposomal doxorubicin may be considered for certain patients in whom doxorubicin therapy is precluded. The GOG demonstrated that ifosfamide had moderate activity, with six partial responses among 35 (17%) patients (33).

As in other types of STS, gemcitabine has demonstrated activity, with one (2.3%) complete response and eight (18%) partial responses observed in a GOG phase 2 trial of persistent or recurrent uterine LMS (39). The median duration of response (DOR) was only 4.8 months. A similar response rate (19%, based on five partial responses) was found by Pautier et al, who reported a median PFS of 5.5 months. In a small phase II study of temozolomide, an oral alkylating prodrug with the same active metabolite as dacarbazine, in advanced STS, a partial response was seen in two (18%) of 11 patients with LMS (51). Single-agent paclitaxel demonstrated limited activity, with a 9% overall response in 33 patients (32). IV single-agent etoposide demonstrated an overall response of 11% in 28 patients (46), whereas prolonged oral etoposide yielded an overall response of 6.9% in 29 patients (45). However, no complete or partial responses were observed in another GOG phase 2 study of single-agent IV etoposide (100 mg/m^2 daily for 3 days every 3 weeks) (34). Topotecan was tested in 36 patients, with complete response in 1 (3%), partial response in 3 (8%), stable disease in 12 (33%), and tumor progression in 20 (56%) patients (31).

A phase 2 study of the marine-derived drug trabectedin, with a 24-hour infusion schedule in 20 chemotherapy-naïve patients who had advanced or recurrent uterine LMS, demonstrated a partial response rate of 10%, and 50% of the patients remained progression free for at least 6 months (53). A phase 3 study of trabectedin versus dacarbazine led to the FDA approval of trabectedin for patients with LMS and liposarcoma, who previously received anthracycline-based therapy. A total of 212 of the 518 patients on this study had uterine LMS. Patients were randomized 2:1 to trabectedin 1.5 mg/m^2 with a 24-hour IV infusion, or to dacarbazine. The response rate was 9.9% with a median PFS of 4 months in the trabectedin arm versus 6.9% and 1.5-month PFS in the dacarbazine arm (54). Gadducci et al subsequently performed a multicenter, randomized phase 2 study of trabectedin in patients with persistent, recurrent, or metastatic uterine LMS who previously received at least one prior line of chemotherapy including doxorubicin with or without ifosfamide or gemcitabine with or without docetaxel. Out of 108 evaluable patients treated with single-agent trabectedin, the 6-month PFS was 35.2%. An ORR of 23.5% (27/115) was observed in the per protocol population (55). Moreover, trabectedin was well tolerated and appeared to maintain its activity, independent of prior lines of systemic therapy.

A small phase 2 trial of vinorelbine in patients who had failed before doxorubicin-based chemotherapy demonstrated a partial response in one (6%) of 16 patients with LMS (50). Single-agent cisplatin also yielded a poor overall response in phase 2 trials: 3% to 5% (35,49). In a small study published in 2002, the antifolate compound trimetrexate was associated with an overall response of 4.3% in 28 patients who had received prior treatment (44). Mitoxantrone (48), diaziquone (38), amonafide (47), aminothiadiazole (37), piperazinedione (56), and ixabepilone (57) were inactive as single agents. A phase 2 trial comparing doxorubicin and docetaxel for advanced STS demonstrated no objective responses in the docetaxel group (58). In a phase 2 study of LMS, eribulin, a fully synthetic analog of the marine sponge product halichondrin B, showed some promise (59). However, in the phase 3 study that led to FDA approval of eribulin for the treatment of liposarcoma, no apparent advantage was conferred by eribulin, compared to the significantly less expensive dacarbazine, in the uterine LMS subgroup (60).

■ **TABLE 6.7-1. Chemotherapy in Leiomyosarcoma of the Uterus**

Drug	n	Prior Therapy	Schedule	Overall Response (%)	Reference
Single-agent chemotherapy					
Primary chemotherapy					
Liposomal doxorubicin	32	11 RT	50 mg/m² q 4 wk	16	Sutton et al (30)
Topotecan	36	8 RT	1.5 mg/m² × 5 d q 3 wk	11	Miller et al (31)
Paclitaxel	33	8 RT	175 mg/m² q 3 wk	9	Sutton et al (32)
Ifosfamide	35	15 RT	1.5 g/m² × 5 d q 4 wk (1.2 g/m² if prior RT)	17	Sutton et al (33)
Etoposide	28	7 RT	100 mg/m² × 3 d q 3 wk	0	Thigpen et al. (34)
Cisplatin	33	8 RT	50 mg/m² q 3 wk	3	Thigpen et al (35)
Doxorubicin	28	NA	60 mg/m² q 3 wk	25	Omura et al (36)
Piperazinedione	19	NA	9 mg/m² q 3 wk	5[a]	Thigpen et al (56)
Aminothiadiazole	20	NA	125 mg/m² q 1 wk	0	Asbury et al (37)
Diaziquone	24	NA	22.5 mg/m² q 3 wk	0	Slayton et al (38)
Trabectedin	20	7 RT	1.5 mg/m² over 24 hr q 3 wk	10	Monk et al (53)
Nonprimary chemotherapy					
Gemcitabine	44	11 RT, 35 CT	1,000 mg/m² weekly × 3 q 4 wk	21	Look et al (39)
	31	20 RT, 31 CT	1,250 mg/m² weekly × 2 q 3 wk	3.2[b]	Svancarova et al (153)
	29	15 RT, 19 CT	1,250 mg/m² weekly × 3 q 4 wk	3[b]	Okuno et al (40)
	56	NA	1,000 mg/m² weekly × 3 q 4 wk	18[b]	Patel et al. (41)
	22	16 RT, 21 CT	1,000 mg/m² weekly × 3 q 4 wk (fixed-dose rate)	19	Pautier et al (52)
Paclitaxel	48	15 RT, 33 CT	175 mg/m² q 3 wk (135 mg/m² if prior RT)	8.4	Gallup et al (42)
Trabectedin	54	54 CT	1.5 mg/m² over 24 hr q 3 wk	4[b]	Yovine et al (91)
	49	49 CT	1-1.8 mg/m² over 1-3 hr q 3 wk	4.1[b]	Twelves et al (154)
	35	21 RT, 4 CT	1.5 mg/m² over 24 hr q 3 wk	17[b]	Garcia-Carbonero et al (43)
	115	115 CT	1.3 mg/m² over 24 hr q 3 wk	23.5	Gadducci et al (55)
Trimetrexate	23	7 RT, 10 CT	5 mg/m² orally × 5 d q 2 wk	4.3	Smith et al (44)
Etoposide	29	6 RT, 27 CT	50 mg/m² orally × 21 d q 4 wk	6.9	Rose et al (45)
	28	7 RT, 27 CT	100 mg/m² days 1, 3, 5 q 4 wk	11	Slayton et al (46)
Amonafide	26	8 RT, 25 CT	300 mg/m² × 5 d q 3 wk	4	Asbury et al (47)
Mitoxantrone	12	12 CT	12 mg/m² q 3 wk	0	Muss et al (48)
Cisplatin	19	19 CT	50 mg/m² q 3 wk	5	Thigpen et al (155)
Temozolomide	11	NA	180 mg/m² orally × 5 d q 4 wk	18[c]	Talbot et al (51)
Vinorelbine	16	16 CT	30 mg/m² weekly × 8	6[c]	Fidias et al (50)
Combination chemotherapy					
Doxorubicin *plus*	20	NA	60 mg/m² q 3 wk	30	Omura et al (36)
Dacarbazine			250 mg/m² × 5 d q 3 wk		
Dacarbazine *plus*	18	7 RT	750 mg/m² q 4 wk	28	Long et al (62)
Mitomycin			6 mg/m² q 4 wk		
Doxorubicin			40 mg/m² q 4 wk		
Cisplatin			60 mg/m² q 4 wk		
Dacarbazine *plus*	10	10 No CT	750 mg/m² q 4 wk	80	Edmonson et al (156)
Mitomycin			6 mg/m² q 4 wk		
Doxorubicin			40 mg/m² q 4 wk		
Cisplatin			60 mg/m² q 4 wk		
Mitomycin *plus*	35	8 RT	8 mg/m² q 3 wk	23	Edmonson et al (63)

■ TABLE 6.7-1. Chemotherapy in Leiomyosarcoma of the Uterus (*continued*)

Drug	n	Prior Therapy	Schedule	Overall Response (%)	Reference
Doxorubicin			40 mg/m^2 q 3 wk		
Cisplatin			60 mg/m^2 q 3 wk		
Hydroxyurea *plus*	38	11 RT	2 g orally × 1 d q 4 wk	18	Currie et al (64)
Dacarbazine			700 mg/m^2 q 4 wk		
Etoposide			300 mg/m^2 × 2 d q 4 wk		
Ifosfamide *plus*	33	9 RT, 33 No CT	5 mg/m^2 q 3 wk	30	Sutton et al (65)
Doxorubicin			50 mg/m^2 q 3 wk		
Gemcitabine *plus*	34	14 RT, 16 CT	900 mg/m^2 days 1, 8 q 3 wk (675 mg/m^2 if prior RT)	53[c]	Hensley et al (66)
Docetaxel			100 mg/m^2 day 8 q 3 wk (75 mg/m^2 if prior RT)		
Gemcitabine *plus*	42	42 No CT	900 mg/m^2 days 1, 8	36	Hensley et al (10)
Docetaxel			100 mg/m^2 day 8 q 3 wk		
Gemcitabine *plus*	48	17 RT, 48 CT	900 mg/m^2 days 1, 8 (675 mg/m^2 if prior RT)	27	Hensley et al (9)
Docetaxel			100 mg/m^2 day 8 q 3 wk (75 mg/m^2 if prior RT)		
Gemcitabine *plus*	24	12 RT, 18 CT	900 mg/m^2 days 1, 8 (675 mg/m^2 if prior RT)	24	Pautier et al (52)
Docetaxel	—	—	100 mg/m^2 day 8 q 3 wk (75 mg/m^2 if prior RT)		
Gemcitabine *plus*	8	No RT, 4 CT	900 mg/m^2 days 1, 8	38	Takano et al (57)
Docetaxel	—	—	70 mg/m^2 day 8 q 3 wk		
Gemcitabine *plus*	54	11 RT, No CT	900 mg/m^2 days 1, 8 (675 mg/m^2 if prior RT)	32	Hensley et al (120)
Docetaxel			75 mg/m^2 day 8 q 3 wk (60 mg/m^2 if prior RT)		
Doxorubicin *plus*	38	38 No CT	60 mg/m^2 q 3 wk	19[a]	Muss et al (67)
Cyclophosphamide			500 mg/m^2 q 3 wk		
Gemcitabine *plus*	9	NA	800 mg/m^2 days 1, 8	22	Dileo et al (68)
Vinorelbine			25 mg/m^2 days 1, 8 q 3 wk		
Temozolomide *plus*	11	10 CT	150 mg/m^2 orally days 1-7 q 2 wk	9.1	Boyar et al (70)
Thalidomide			200 mg orally daily		
Doxorubicin *plus*	47	17 RT, No CT	60 mg/m^2 q 3 wk	60	Pautier et al (71)
Trabectedin			1.1 mg/m^2 3-hr q 3 wk		

All chemotherapy agents were given intravenously unless specified.

CT, chemotherapy; NA, not available; RT, radiation therapy.

[a]Uterine sarcoma.
[b]Adult soft-tissue sarcoma.
[c]Adult leiomyosarcoma.
[d]Female genital tract leiomyosarcoma.

Combination Therapy

Leiomyosarcoma

Combination chemotherapy yields greater response rates (**Table 6.7-2**) (9,10,36,61-69) than single-agent strategies. In 1983, the GOG demonstrated that the combination of doxorubicin and dacarbazine resulted in an overall response rate of 30%. Two years later, the same group demonstrated a 19% response rate using the combination of doxorubicin and cyclophosphamide (67). Both of the phase 3 trials were too small to draw any definite conclusions. However, as noted earlier, these trials did enable researchers to observe that LMS had a different chemotherapeutic response profile compared to uterine CS. This resulted in the separation of the two different histologic entities in subsequent trials.

In 1996, the GOG demonstrated an 18% overall response in patients treated with a combination of dacarbazine, etoposide, and hydroxyurea (64). In the same year, using a combination of ifosfamide and doxorubicin, the GOG demonstrated an overall response rate of 30% in patients with advanced LMS and no history of prior treatment (65). A later GOG study showed that treatment with mitomycin, doxorubicin, and cisplatin produced an overall response rate of 23% in 35 patients. Pulmonary toxicity was appreciable,

■ TABLE 6.7-2. Grade 3 to 4 Adverse Effects of Chemotherapy in Leiomyosarcoma (Overall Response Rate >5%).

Drug	n	Prior Therapy	Schedule	Overall Response (%)	Leukopenia (%)	Neutropenia (%)	Thrombocytopenia (%)	Anemia (%)	GI (%)	Others	Reference
Liposomal doxorubicin	32	11 RT	50 mg/m² q 4 wk	16	13	16	NA	23	19	Dermatotoxicity 6.5%	Sutton et al (30)
Topotecan	36	8 RT	1.5 mg/m² × 5 d q 3 wk	11	33	90	13	16	17		Miller et al (31)
Paclitaxel	33	8 RT	175 mg/m² q 3 wk	9	9.1	33	3	3	0	No neurotoxicity	Sutton et al (32)
	48	15 RT, 33 CT	175 mg/m² q 3 wk	8.4	6.3	17	0	17	42		Gallup et al (42)
Ifosfamide	35	15 RT	1.5 g/m² × 5 d q 4 wk	17	34	NA	0	0	3	Neurotoxicity 3%, granulocytopenia 11%, dermatotoxicity 14%	Sutton et al (33)
Doxorubicin	28	NA	60 mg/m² q 3 wk	25	16	NA	4	NA	2		Omura et al (36)
Oral etoposide	29	6 RT, 27 CT	50 mg/m² orally × 21 d q 4 wk	6.9	24	35	18	12	6	Neurotoxicity 6%	Rose et al (45)
Gemcitabine	44	11 RT, 35 CT	1,000 mg/m² weekly × 3 q 4 wk	21	27	34	11.4	6.8	14		Look et al (39)
	22	16 RT, 21 CT	1,000 mg/m² weekly × 3 q 4 wk	19	37	32	11	1	0		Pautier et al (52)
Trabectedin	20	7RT	1.5 mg/m² over 24 hr q 3 wk	10	55	80	15	5	0	Hepatotoxicity 10%	Monk et al (53)
	134	134CT	1.5 mg/m² over 24 hr q 3 wk	10	NA	37	17	14	15	Hepatotoxicity 26% Rhabdomyolysis 1%	Demetri et al (54)
	115	115 CT	1.3 m/m² over 24 hr q 3 wk	23.5%	12	22	4	5	7	Hepatotoxicity 3%	Gadducci et al (55)
Trabectedin plus doxorubicin	47	17 RT, No CT	1.1 mg/m² over 3 hr q 3 wk	60	76	78	37	27	19	Hepatotoxicity 39%	Pautier et al (71)
Dacarbazine	78	78 CT	1 g/m² q 3 wk	7	NA	21	18	12	4		Demetri et al (54)
Temozolomide	11	NA	180 mg/m² orally × 5 d q 4 wk	18	0	0	0	4	4	Fatigue 4%	Talbot et al (51)
Vinorelbine	16	16 CT	30 mg/m² weekly × 8	6	NA	NA	NA	NA	NA	Grade 3 toxicity 67%	Fidias et al (50)
Doxorubicin plus Dacarbazine	20	NA	60 mg/m² q 3 wk / 250 mg/m² × 5 d q 3 wk	30	35	NA	13	NA	9		Omura et al (36)
Dacarbazine plus mitomycin plus doxorubicin plus cisplatin	18	7 RT	750 mg/m² q 4 wk / 6 mg/m² q 4 wk / 40 mg/m² q 4 wk / 60 mg/m² q 4 wk	28	67	78	94	61	44		Long et al (62)

Regimen	Reference	No. of patients	Prior RT/CT	Dose							Toxicity
Mitomycin *plus* doxorubicin *plus* cisplatin	Edmonson et al (63)	35	8 RT	8 mg/m² q 3 wk 40 mg/m² q 3 wk 60 mg/m² q 3 wk	23	NA	NA	NA	NA	NA	Pulmonary toxicity 8%
Hydroxyurea *plus* dacarbazine *plus* etoposide	Currie et al (64)	38	11 RT	2 g orally × 1 d q 4 wk 700 mg/m² q 4 wk 300 mg/m² × 2 d q 4 wk	18	NA	29	3	NA	NA	NA
Ifosfamide *plus* doxorubicin	Sutton et al (65)	33	9 RT	5 g/m²/24 hr q 3 wk 50 mg/m² q 3 wk	30	NA	49	0	0	0	Cardiac toxicity 3%
Gemcitabine *plus* docetaxel	Hensley et al (66)	34	14 RT, 16 CT	900 mg/m² days 1, 8 q 3 wk 100 mg/m² day 8 q 3 wk	53	NA	21	29	15	12	Dyspnea 21%, fatigue 21%
	Hensley et al (9)	42	42 No CT	As above	36	17	14	14	24	14	NA
	Hensley et al (10)	48	17 RT, 48 CT	As above	27	23	21	40	25	6.3	Fluid retention syndrome 19%
	Pautier et al (52)	24	12 RT, 18 CT	As above 75 mg/m² day 8 q 3 wk	24	11	14	26	8	0	NA
	Hensley et al (120)	54	11 RT, No CT	900 mg/m² days 1, 8 q 3 wk	32	NA	23	28	33	25	NA
Gemcitabine *plus* vinorelbine	Dileo et al (68)	9	NA	800 mg/m² days 1, 8 25 mg/m² days 1,8 q3 wk	22	28	40	10	5	10	NA
Temozolomide *plus* thalidomide	Boyar et al (70)	11	10 CT	150 mg/m² orally × 7 q 2 wk 200 mg orally daily	9.1	4	4	4	8	8	Neurotoxicity 12%
Sunitinib	Hensley et al (125)	23	23 CT	50 mg orally daily × 4 of 6 wk	8.7	13	17	13	17	30	NA
Bevacizumab *plus* doxorubicin	D'Adamo et al (119)	7	NA	15 mg/kg q 3 wk 75 mg/m²	28	NA	NA	18	6	NA	Alopecia 100% Cardiotoxicity gr ≥2 35%

All chemotherapy agents were given intravenously unless specified.

CT, chemotherapy; GI, gastrointestinal system; NA, not available; RT, radiation therapy.

however (63). On the basis of this study, the GOG conducted a phase 2 trial of dacarbazine, doxorubicin, mitomycin, and cisplatin (DAMP), which produced a 28% response rate. However, the complexity and toxicity of this regimen precluded further investigation, and the study was closed after the first stage of accrual (62).

Fixed-dose-rate gemcitabine plus docetaxel has proved highly active and tolerable (40% overall response rate) in both treated and untreated patients with unresectable uterine LMS (69). As initial therapy for metastatic uterine LMS, this combination chemotherapy yielded a 36% response rate (2 complete and 13 partial responses) among 42 patients. The response rate for the doublet was 27% in the second-line setting, with a median PFS of greater than 5.6 months. In a more recent French study, the response rate for the doublet as second-line therapy for uterine LMS was 24% (5 partial responses among 22 patients, with a median PFS of 4.7 months). In the Gadducci et al's study, gemcitabine with or without docetaxel naïve patients were randomized to either single-agent trabectedin or gemcitabine 900 and docetaxel 75 mg/m^2. Results were in line with previously published data, with a median PFS of 6.9 months in doublet arm as compared to 4.1 months in the trabectedin-only arm (55).

A phase 2 trial of gemcitabine plus dacarbazine reported a 19% response rate for the doublet, compared to 13% for dacarbazine alone, in 32 previously treated patients with LMS. A phase 2 trial of fixed-dose-rate gemcitabine and vinorelbine in patients with advanced STS yielded a response rate of 22% in nine patients with uterine LMS but conferred no advantage over the historical results achieved with single-agent gemcitabine (68). A combination of temozolomide and thalidomide in advanced LMS yielded a partial response in two (10%) cases, with no complete response (70).

Pautier et al reported an impressive response rate of 60% (28 complete responses) and a median PFS of 8.2 months among 47 patients with uterine LMS enrolled in a nonrandomized phase 2 trial of doxorubicin plus 3-hour trabectedin as first-line treatment for advanced LMS (71). An additional 28% (13 patients) had stable disease. Conversely, another randomized phase 2 study of 3-hour trabectedin plus doxorubicin versus doxorubicin alone as first-line therapy for STS was stopped early owing to futility, with a reported 13% response rate for the combination regimen and 20% rate for doxorubicin alone. The caveat to this cross-trial comparison is that the sequence of chemotherapy administration was different in the two trials; in addition, the latter trial was conducted in a population of patients with heterogeneous STS. Given the significant toxicity associated with the combination regimen, including elevated transaminases, myelosuppression, and febrile neutropenia, further validation is required before this combination could be recommended.

The effort in LMS treatment continues to focus on identifying active drugs and combination regimens in phase 2 trials. A pooled analysis of phase 2 studies (undertaken in 2005) compared the response rates of single-agent versus combination therapy. It showed that patients who received first- or second-line chemotherapy for the treatment of metastatic LMS had a higher response rate with combination chemotherapy than with single-agent chemotherapy (72). The European GeDDiS trial, a phase 3 comparison of single-agent doxorubicin versus gemcitabine plus docetaxel as first-line treatment in 257 patients with locally advanced or metastatic STS, failed to show any difference in OS between the two regimens. In fact, the HR favored the superiority of doxorubicin (HR, 1.28, P = .07). This also held true in the subgroup analysis of 72 patients with uterine LMS. Although a higher incidence of oral mucositis and febrile neutropenia was associated with doxorubicin, in general, it was better tolerated. Only one (2%) patient in the doxorubicin arm withdrew from treatment early because of unacceptable toxicity, whereas 13 (16%) patients in combined gemcitabine and docetaxel arm experienced significant grade 3 or 4 fatigue and diarrhea. Nevertheless, the higher objective response rates associated with combination therapy may be crucial for select patients with imminent life-threatening organ compromise.

Ongoing clinical trials include investigation of locoregional delivery and combination chemotherapy for recurrent or metastatic LMS. NCT04727242 is a phase 2 trial of locally recurrent uterine LMS, which aims to evaluate the efficacy of hyperthermic intraperitoneal chemotherapy (HIPEC) with gemcitabine followed by postoperative dacarbazine. The combination of trabectedin, gemcitabine, and dacarbazine in advanced LMS is being examined in a phase 2 trial, which is currently enrolling patients (NCT0453271). Efforts are also underway to explore cytotoxic agents known to be active in other cancer types. An example of such a trial is the not-yet recruiting phase 1b/2 trial investigating lurbinectedin, an alkylating agent approved in small cell lung cancer, with doxorubicin versus doxorubicin monotherapy in advanced LMS (NCT05099666). The advent of immunotherapy and other targeted agents has resulted in many combinatorial chemotherapy trials, which are discussed in a later section.

Endometrial Stromal Sarcoma

In metastatic ESS, reports support hormonal therapy for patients in the low-grade subgroup, and chemotherapy for patients with high-grade tumors (73). In a retrospective review of 74 patients with low-grade stromal sarcoma, none of the 10 patients who received chemotherapy responded to treatment, compared to 27% of patients treated with hormonal therapy (74). The use of hormonal therapy in this setting is discussed in a later section. Randomized phase 3 trials of stromal sarcomas are limited because of the rarity of this disease. Two randomized trials compared single agent and combination chemotherapy in advanced uterine sarcoma but did not report the response rate of stromal sarcomas separately. The GOG reported a phase 2 study of ifosfamide treatment in 21 cases of recurrent or metastatic ESS. Three patients attained complete responses and four had partial responses, for an overall response rate of 33.3% (65). Another noncontrolled study showed a 50% response rate to doxorubicin therapy in 10 patients with recurrent ESS (75). Much of the other literature consists of case reports and retrospective studies involving a small number of cases. Published chemotherapy regimens include carboplatin plus paclitaxel (76); doxorubicin, cisplatin, and ifosfamide (77); doxorubicin plus ifosfamide (78); doxorubicin, vincristine, and cyclophosphamide (79); and prolonged oral etoposide (80).

Adenosarcoma

In a small retrospective series of AS, three of the five patients treated with doxorubicin- and/or ifosfamide-containing salvage chemotherapy showed a brief partial response (17). Similar response rates were reported in another retrospective series of patients with recurrent disease treated with doxorubicin plus ifosfamide (81). More recently, in a retrospective analysis of 78 patients with recurrent AS, the response rate was 31.2% for doxorubicin-based regimens and 14.3% for gemcitabine plus docetaxel. The median PFS was superior for doxorubicin plus ifosfamide (15.4 months) compared to gemcitabine plus docetaxel (5.0 months), platinum-based regimens (5.7 months), or other doxorubicin-based regimens (6.5 months), although there was no significant difference in OS (82).

High-Grade Undifferentiated Endometrial Sarcoma

There are no prospective trials of chemotherapy specifically for high-grade UES. Case reports of response to ifosfamide- and doxorubicin-based regimens have been documented in the literature (77,83). Gemcitabine plus docetaxel may also have activity in high-grade UES, as evidenced by a small retrospective case series reporting a 75% response rate among six patients treated with that combination. In that series, the response rate of five patients treated with doxorubicin was 40%. All responses were of short duration.

The response rate to second-line chemotherapy was only 19%, and no patient responded to retreatment with a regimen that they had previously responded to. A phase 2 trial of first-line chemotherapy for recurrent or metastatic ESS reported a 33% response rate but did not segregate high- versus low-grade tumors (84). Owing to the paucity of data available to guide systemic treatment, patients with these tumors should be encouraged to participate in clinical trials.

PEComa

There are no prospective data on cytotoxic therapy for PEComa. A case report of a 9-year-old girl with uterine PEComa reported radiographic response following two cycles of neoadjuvant vincristine, ifosfamide, and doxorubicin, but analysis of the surgical specimen did not show any tumor response. Case reports of tamoxifen- or anthracycline-based chemotherapy following surgical resection of gynecologic PEComa do not suggest any benefit from adjuvant therapy (85). For metastatic or recurrent disease, chemotherapy similarly does not appear to be effective (86). Certain targeted and biologic agents, in particular mammalian target of rapamycin (mTOR) inhibitors, have demonstrated efficacy in this rare tumor, which is discussed in the biologic and targeted therapy section later in this chapter. Generally, patients with uterine PEComa should be encouraged to participate in clinical trials.

Rhabdomyosarcoma

Because of the rarity of uterine RMS, there are no prospective data to guide optimal therapy. In a case series of pediatric patients with RMS of the genital tract, complete responses have been reported with the administration of neoadjuvant ifosfamide, vincristine, and dactinomycin combination chemotherapy (28). Generally, first-line regimens of VAC and VAI-Europe as discussed previously in the adjuvant therapy section are used in the metastatic setting. Other recommended regimens include vincristine, doxorubicin, and cyclophosphamide alternating with ifosfamide and etoposide based on pediatric data (87). Referral to experienced tertiary cancer centers and collaboration with pediatric sarcoma specialists for multimodality treatment planning and risk stratification are recommended for patients with nonpleomorphic uterine RMS (including the alveolar and embryonal subtypes). Enrollment in clinical trials should be encouraged.

Liposarcoma

Uterine liposarcoma is another rare tumor. In contemplating treatment, we must extrapolate from the management of nonuterine liposarcomas, for which agents such as doxorubicin, ifosfamide, trabectedin, and dacarbazine are reportedly active. Eribulin, a synthetic analog of halichondrin B, is an FDA-approved treatment for unresectable or metastatic liposarcoma previously treated with anthracycline-based therapy (88).

TOXICITY OF SYSTEMIC THERAPIES

The most common toxicities of chemotherapy are hematologic and gastrointestinal toxicities. The grade 3 to 4 adverse effects of chemotherapy with overall response rate higher than 5% in LMS are listed in **Table 6.7-2**. Combination chemotherapy is associated with a much higher incidence of grade 3 to 4 toxicities compared with the single-agent regimens. In the GOG study, the overall response rate of combination ifosfamide plus cisplatin was 54%; however, the rate of grades 3 to 4 of leukopenia was 97%, and six deaths occurred before the first dose reduction of ifosfamide (89). The more recent GOG phase 3 trial with ifosfamide plus paclitaxel reported a 45% overall response rate, with tolerable toxicities (90); this seems to be a relatively effective and safe regimen. Ifosfamide should be used with caution in older patients, however, because of the risk of encephalopathy. Consideration of reduced-dose regimens may still be reasonable in older patients with good performance status.

Among other phase 2 trials of different chemotherapy regimens, liposomal doxorubicin plus paclitaxel, doxorubicin, cisplatin, and etoposide plus cisplatin plus doxorubicin were reported to have less toxicity, with moderate effect. Despite the routine use of growth factor support with gemcitabine and docetaxel, myelosuppression—particularly in previously treated patients—is still the predominant toxicity encountered with this combination (9,10). Lower limb edema is also more common in the second-line setting. Trabectedin requires central venous access and is associated with fatigue, myelosuppression, transaminitis, and vomiting (91). Steroid premedication is required to reduce hepatotoxicity.

Newer agents may have a more tolerable toxicity profile compared to standard chemotherapy drugs, but more prospective data are needed. PICASSO III, a phase 3 trial, investigated palifosfamide-tris as an alternative agent to ifosfamide in combination with doxorubicin in patients with STS. Unfortunately, there was no significant difference in PFS, and a higher incidence of serious adverse events was observed in the experimental arm (92).

SYSTEMIC THERAPY: SUMMARY

The current role of chemotherapy in the management of uterine sarcomas involves palliative-intent therapy for patients with advanced disease. Unfortunately, the use of adjuvant chemotherapy in the setting of limited or completely resected has not demonstrated survival benefit. In LMS, the active drugs are doxorubicin, ifosfamide, gemcitabine, and docetaxel. Hormonal, targeted, and novel therapies have shown promise in the treatment of these rare tumors and are discussed in the next section.

HORMONAL, TARGETED, IMMUNOTHERAPY, AND OTHER, NEW, AND NOVEL

Hormonal Therapy

Although the role of hormonal therapy is clear in breast and endometrial cancers, it has not been extensively evaluated in mesenchymal uterine tumors. Few uterine sarcomas contain sufficient ER or PR protein to influence therapy, exceptions being low-grade ESS or stromal nodules. ER and PR have been identified in 55.5% and 55.8%, respectively, of samples from patients with various types of uterine sarcomas, but the median concentrations are substantially lower than those observed in breast or endometrial cancers. ESS tumors reportedly have higher receptor levels (93). Uniquely, low-grade ESS is hormonally responsive in roughly two-thirds of cases, and long-term maintenance therapy should be beneficial.

Endometrial Stromal Sarcoma

Adjuvant Therapy

The role of adjuvant hormonal therapy in completely resected low-grade ESS remains unclear. In one retrospective study of 22 patients with resected low-grade ESS, 31% (N = 4 of 13 patients) treated with adjuvant megestrol acetate recurred versus 67% (N = 6 of 9 patients) who did not receive hormonal treatment (14).

In a second retrospective report of 31 women with low-grade ESS, those treated with postoperative medroxyprogesterone had a lower recurrence rate compared with those who were not (14% vs 29%), although this did not translate to differences in 5-year OS rates (86% vs 83%) (94).

Metastatic/Recurrent Endometrial Stromal Sarcoma

Progestins, gonadotropin-releasing hormone (GnRH) analogs (95), or aromatase inhibitors (AIs) (73,96) have been used in the treatment of patients with advanced or recurrent ESS, and several case reports are associated with gain in long-term stability. A retrospective study of patients with low-grade ESS reported a response rate of 27% (five complete responses and three partial responses), stable disease in 53% (16 patients), and a median time to progression of 24 months in a subgroup of patients receiving hormonal therapy (74). A significant majority received megestrol acetate. In a retrospective report of 13 patients with metastatic low-grade ESS, initial treatment with hormonal therapy resulted in an ORR of 46.2% (6 partial responses) and clinical benefit of 92%. Median PFS in those who received hormonal therapy was 3 years (97).

Lantta et al reported two cases of patients with extensive intraperitoneal low-grade ESS, associated with high levels of PR, who achieved complete response on hormonal therapy (98). Three cases with high levels of PR were reported by Baker et al, all of which achieved partial responses or stabilization of disease on oral megestrol acetate (99). In a collaborative survey of endolymphatic stromal myosis, Piver et al recorded complete or partial responses to hormonal therapy in six (46%) of 13 patients treated with progestational agents (100). Scribner and Walker reported on one patient with extensive ESS of the uterus whose tumor was reduced to resectable size by administration of leuprolide acetate and megestrol acetate (101). Low-grade ESS has also been reported to express srp27, an ER-induced 24-DK protein suggesting hormone responsiveness (102).

Medroxyprogesterone acetate has induced major responses in ESS pulmonary metastatic lesions (103,104). GnRH analogs reportedly controlled tumor progression in one case of recurrent low-grade ESS with moderate ER and PR positivity (95). Medroxyprogesterone acetate and AIs, such as letrozole, were reportedly highly effective and conferred sustained progression control in six of 10 cases of low-grade stromal sarcomas (105). Spano et al presented two cases of ESS with lung metastases treated with aminoglutethimide; both patients achieved complete responses and remained disease free for 14 and 7 years, respectively (73). In a phase 2 trial of mifepristone, a selective PR modulator, in recurrent uterine cancer, no responses (0%) were seen in two patients with low-grade ESS (106).

In a phase 2 trial performed by Ramondetta et al, mifepristone (RU-486) was administered daily to patients with PR-positive advanced/recurrent endometrioid adenocarcinoma or LG-ESS (106). Three of 12 patients achieved stable disease, one of which had LG-ESS, and no objective responses were observed. Given the poor response rate, the authors concluded against the efficacy of single-agent mifepristone in this population.

The FUCHsia Study (NCT03926936) is an international, multicenter phase 2 study currently enrolling patients with recurrent/metastatic ER-positive low-grade gynecologic malignancies to evaluate the efficacy of intramuscular fulvestrant. Included tumor types are LG-ESS, low-grade endometrial carcinoma, sex cord stromal tumors, and low-grade serous ovarian cancer. The primary objective is ORR with goal enrollment is 200 participants.

A phase 2 trial comparing the PFS between AIs interruption and AIs maintenance strategies in patients with a locally advanced or metastatic LG-ESS is ongoing (NCT03624244).

Other Uterine Sarcomas

Adenosarcomas and Leiomyosarcoma

There are anecdotal reports of responses to hormonal therapy in AS and low-grade LMS (107). A retrospective study of an AI in selected patients with advanced, predominantly low-volume, LMS reported partial responses in three (9%) patients. Patients whose tumors did not express ER or PR derived no benefit (108). No objective responses were seen in a phase 2 study of letrozole in 27 previously treated patients with advanced ER- or PR-positive uterine LMS (109). The best response was stable disease in 14 (54%) patients. All three patients who received letrozole for more than

24 weeks had tumors expressing ER and PR in more than 90% of tumor cells. A phase 2 prospective study comparing letrozole to observation alone for newly diagnosed uterine LMS was unfortunately terminated due to low accrual with only nine patients enrolled. Of the four patients treated with letrozole, one progressed on study. Of the five who underwent observation only, two progressed (NCT00414076).

PEComa

In metastatic PEComa with progression on mTOR inhibition, the efficacy of antiestrogen therapy (exemestane with or without luteinizing hormone-releasing hormone [LHRH] analog) in combination with sirolimus was reported in a small retrospective case series (110). With a median follow-up of 13 months, three (43%) patients had partial response and three (43%) experienced stable disease, resulting in a remarkable disease control rate of 86% and a median response duration of 11 months. The authors conclude that the addition of an antiestrogen treatment may help overcome resistance to sirolimus in advanced PEComa, although more data are needed.

BIOLOGIC AND TARGETED THERAPY

In light of the high rates of recurrence and poor response to RT and chemotherapy, biologic and targeted therapy may hold more promise in the treatment of uterine sarcoma and other types of STS. Recent advances in understanding the biology of uterine sarcoma, with respect to probable treatment targets, have concentrated on vascular endothelial growth factor (VEGF), tyrosine kinase receptors, the phosphatidyl 3-kinase (PI3K)/Akt pathway, and actionable genetic alterations. **Table 6.7-3** highlights the current FDA approvals compendia listed of various targeted/biologic therapies in sarcoma.

Angiogenesis Inhibitors

Pazopanib, an oral antiangiogenic multitarget kinase inhibitor, has been investigated in many uterine sarcoma subtypes. In a phase 2 study of STS, only one partial response (2.4%) was reported among 41 patients receiving single-agent pazopanib in the LMS cohort (111). LMS03, a phase 2 trial of second-line therapy pazopanib and gemcitabine, followed by pazopanib alone, failed to show benefit for patients with advanced LMS (112). In the phase 3 PALETTE trial of pazopanib versus placebo as second-line therapy for metastatic STS (46% LMS), the response rate in the pazopanib group was 6%. There was a 3-month increase in PFS. Although this did not translate into significant improvement in OS, pazopanib is now FDA approved for patients with advanced STS who previously received chemotherapy (113). Its use as monotherapy versus combination with gemcitabine is currently being examined in an ongoing international phase 2 trial (NCT02203760).

Although no prospective studies exist for the use of pazopanib in malignant PEComa, case reports have reported response to single-agent therapy, particularly after progression on mTOR inhibitors (114).

Emoto et al demonstrated inhibition of a VEGF-expressing malignant mixed tumor cell line by TNP-470, an angiogenesis inhibitor (115). Another angiogenesis inhibitor, thalidomide, failed to demonstrate any activity in recurrent or persistent uterine LMS (116). A phase 2 study of sorafenib, a small molecule B-Raf and VEGF receptor inhibitor, was also negative, and only one (3%) partial was seen among 37 patients with adult LMS (117). No responses were observed in a phase 2 trial of aflibercept in recurrent or metastatic gynecologic CS or uterine LMS (118).

A phase 2 study of doxorubicin with bevacizumab in 17 chemotherapy-naïve patients with STS reported a lower-than-anticipated response rate of 12%, with significant cardiotoxicity

■ **TABLE 6.7-3. Current FDA Approvals/Biologic Therapies in Sarcomas**

Cancer Type	Cancer Subtype/ Biomarker	Drug/Drug Combination	Line	Overall Response or Outcome	FDA Approval	Reference
Soft-tissue sarcoma	Excluding adipocytic subtypes and GIST	Pazopanib	2+ (post anthracycline)	6%	Yes	van der Graaf et al (PALETTE) (113)
Soft-tissue sarcoma	Liposarcoma	Eribulin	2+	OS 13.5 mo in eribulin arm vs 11.5 mo in dacarbazine arm	Yes	Schoffski et al (58)
Uterine sarcoma	UPS only	Pembrolizumab	2+	23%	No	Tawbi et al (SARC-028)(150)
Soft-tissue sarcoma	*NTRK* gene fusion	Larotrectinib	1+	75%	Yes	Drilon et al (141)
Soft-tissue sarcoma	*NTRK* gene fusion	Entrectinib	2+	57%	Yes	Doebele et al (STARTRK-1, STARTRK-2, and ALKA-372-001) (157)
Soft-tissue sarcoma	Malignant PEComa	*nab*-sirolimus	1+	39%	Yes	Wagner et al (AMPECT) (141)
Inflammatory myofibroblastic tumor	ALK translocation	Crizotinib Ceritinib Brigatinib	1+ 1+ 1+		Yes No No	Butrynski et al (146) Shaw et al (158) Gettinger et al (149)

FDA, Food and Drug Administration; GIST, gastrointestinal stromal tumor; OS, overall survival; UPS, undifferentiated pleomorphic sarcoma.

Demetri GD, von Mehren M, Jones RL, et al. Efficacy and safety of trabectedin or dacarbazine for metastatic liposarcoma or leiomyosarcoma after failure of conventional chemotherapy: results of a phase iii randomized multicenter clinical trial. *J Clin Oncol*. 2016;34(8):786-793. doi:10.1200/jco.2015.62.4734; Duska LR, Blessing JA, Rotmensch J, et al. A phase II evaluation of ixabepilone (IND #59699, NSC #710428) in the treatment of recurrent or persistent leiomyosarcoma of the uterus: an NRG Oncology/Gynecologic Oncology Group Study. *Gynecol Oncol*. 2014;135(1):44-48. doi:10.1016/j.ygyno.2014.07.101; Pautier P, Floquet A, Chevreau C, et al. Trabectedin in combination with doxorubicin for first-line treatment of advanced uterine or soft-tissue leiomyosarcoma (LMS-02): a non-randomised, multicentre, phase 2 trial. *Lancet Oncol*. 2015;16(4):457-464. doi:10.1016/s1470-2045(15)70070-7; Hensley ML, Miller A, O'Malley DM, et al. Randomized phase III trial of gemcitabine plus docetaxel plus bevacizumab or placebo as first-line treatment for metastatic uterine leiomyosarcoma: an NRG Oncology/Gynecologic Oncology Group study. *J Clin Oncol*. 2015;33(10):1180-1185. doi:10.1200/jco.2014.58.3781; Takano T, Niikura H, Ito K, et al. Feasibility study of gemcitabine plus docetaxel in advanced or recurrent uterine leiomyosarcoma and undifferentiated endometrial sarcoma in Japan. *Int J Clin Oncol*. 2014;19(5):897-905. doi:10.1007/s10147-013-0627-5; Pautier P, Floquet A, Penel N, et al. Randomized multicenter and stratified phase II study of gemcitabine alone versus gemcitabine and docetaxel in patients with metastatic or relapsed leiomyosarcomas: a Federation Nationale des Centres de Lutte Contre le Cancer (FNCLCC) French Sarcoma Group Study (TAXOGEM study). *Oncologist*. 2012;17(9):1213-1220. doi:10.1634/theoncologist.2011-0467

(≥grade 2 in 35% of patients) (119). Among the seven patients with uterine LMS, there were two (28%) partial responses. The addition of bevacizumab to fixed-dose-rate gemcitabine plus docetaxel failed to improve overall response rate, PFS, or OS in a GOG phase 3 trial. A total of 107 chemotherapy-naïve patients with advanced or recurrent uterine LMS were accrued to the placebo-controlled trial of gemcitabine plus docetaxel, with or without bevacizumab. The trial was closed early after the planned interim analysis failed to show superiority in the experimental arm. In fact, median PFS was observed to be shorter in the bevacizumab-containing arm versus the control arm: 4.2 and 6.2 months, respectively (120).

Tyrosine Kinase Inhibitors

Since the discovery that high proto-oncogene *c-kit* expression in gastrointestinal stromal tumors (GIST) may be amenable to control with **tyrosine kinase inhibitors** such as imatinib mesylate and sunitinib, there has been some interest in this treatment for uterine sarcomas (121). However, the expression of *c-kit* in uterine sarcomas varies considerably in different studies (122-124). The GOG investigated sunitinib maleate as a second- or third-line therapy for LMS of the uterus. The trial was reported as negative, with only two partial responses (9%) noted among 23 patients (125).

Regorafenib, a multitargeted tyrosine kinase inhibitor, has been investigated in STS. REGOSARC, a placebo-controlled phase 2 trial, examined the use of regorafenib in advanced STS previously treated with anthracycline treatment (126). In the LMS cohort, PFS was 3.7 versus 1.8 months with placebo

($P < .005$), and activity was seen in other nonadipocytic sarcomas. In another phase 2 trial of regorafenib in advanced STS, of 21 evaluable patients in the intention to treat population, one experienced partial response (4.8%) and five had stable disease (57.1%) per RECIST; 62% of patients were progression free at 8 weeks ($N = 13$ of 21) (127).

Many trials are examining the use of tyrosine kinase inhibitors such as cabozantinib, anlotinib, vimseltinib, and sunitinib, either alone or in combination with other agents (NCT04200443, NCT03016819, NCT04242238, NCT03277924). Pazopanib, the oral antiangiogenic tyrosine kinase inhibitor, is discussed earlier.

PI3K/AKT/mTOR Pathway

Leiomyosarcoma

Loss of PTEN function results in upregulation of the PI3K/Akt signaling pathway and has been associated with high-grade and recurrent LMS (128). mTOR is a central regulator of this pathway. Ridaforolimus (formerly deforolimus), an mTOR inhibitor, demonstrated no response in a study of 56 patients with LMS, but 36% had disease stabilization at 16 weeks (129). A phase 3 study of ridaforolimus as maintenance strategy in patients with metastatic sarcoma who derived benefit from chemotherapy reported a disappointing 3-week increase in PFS (130). In hopes of greater activity with combination therapy, everolimus is currently being assessed in conjunction with ribociclib, a selective CDK4/6 inhibitor, in advanced LMS (NCT03114527).

PEComa

The use of mTOR inhibitors in malignant PEComas has increased in recent years with greater understanding of molecular pathology in these rare tumors. Somatic inactivating mutations of *TSC1* or *TSC2* have been observed in sporadic PEComas, loss of which is associated with increased mTOR activity and sensitivity to rapalogs (131-133). A retrospective study of 15 patients with unresectable or metastatic PEComa treated with sirolimus after prior chemotherapy ($N = 4$) or as upfront therapy ($N = 11$) demonstrated remarkable efficacy, regardless of treatment line (134). The OR was 73% ($N = 11/15$), and all patients achieved a period of disease control. Of the three patients with a gynecologic PEComa, one achieved complete response with a DOR of 62.1 months, one achieved partial response with DOR of 16 months, and one stable disease with DOR 9.2 months. Another retrospective review of eight patients with uterine PEComa treated with mTOR inhibitors showed a less robust response with one partial response (12.5%) and three (37.5%) stable disease (135). Case reports have reported durable response with the use of alternate mTOR inhibitor following progression on first-line mTOR inhibitor, representing another possible treatment strategy in the care of these tumors with limited available options (136).

In November 2021, the FDA granted approval to *nab*-sirolimus, a nanoparticle albumin-bound mTOR inhibitor, for the treatment of locally advanced unresectable or metastatic malignant PEComas based on the results of AMPECT, a phase 2 trial by Wagner et al (137). In this single-arm trial of 31 patients, patients with malignant PEComa were treated weekly for 2 weeks with IV nab-sirolimus in 3-week cycles. The overall response rate was 39% ($N = 12$ of 31), with 1 complete and 11 partial responses. Sixteen (52%) patients had stable disease. Moreover, responses were durable with median DOR not reached, with a median follow-up of 2.5 years.

Histone Deacetylase Inhibitors

Aberrant activity of epigenetic enzymes, such as histone deacetylases (HDACs), has been linked to tumorigenesis. HDAC inhibitors appear to exert greater apoptotic effects in tumor cells compared to normal, healthy cells. It is hypothesized that the enhanced sensitivity of tumor cells to HDAC inhibitors is due to the altered expression of apoptotic genes, as a result of alterations in the cancer epigenome (138). The activity of the HDAC inhibitor mocetinostat in combination with gemcitabine in the treatment of metastatic LMS resistant to prior gemcitabine-containing therapy was investigated in a phase 2 clinical trial. Out of 18 evaluable patients, best responses included 1 partial response (seen in a patient with uterine LMS) and 12 stable disease (five of which had uterine LMS). Unfortunately, given that median PFS was only 2 months in conjunction with the underwhelming response rate, the study was halted after completion of the first stage (139).

Targeted Therapy for Tumor Genomic Alterations

Tumor genomic profiling may help identify novel therapies for uterine sarcomas. Hensley et al performed prospective molecular characterization of 107 advanced metastatic uterine sarcomas. Sequenced tumors included LMS ($N = 80$), high-grade non-LMS ($N = 22$), low-grade ESS ($N = 4$), and STUMP ($N = 2$) (Hensley 2020, CCR) (140). Potentially actionable mutations were identified in 45% of patients ($N = 48$), 17% ($N = 8$) of whom received matched therapy with two achieving clinical responses. Interestingly, *BRCA2* alterations were identified in seven patients. Five additional patients with *BRCA2* alterations (four somatic and one germline mutation) were subsequently identified. These patients received PARP inhibitor–containing therapy as part of either a clinical trial or as off-label use for a germline *BRCA* mutation. All five had radiologic response to treatment, including one with a complete response to PARP inhibition.

PARP Inhibition

The utility of PARP inhibition in uterine sarcomas is not currently well described, but efforts are ongoing to evaluate its efficacy. Two phase 2 trials are examining the combination of Olaparib with trabectedin plus ipilimumab in LMS (NCT04076579 and NCT03138161), and a phase 2 trial of niraparib monotherapy in advanced LMS is not yet open to accrual (NCT05174455).

NTRK Gene Fusions

NTRK gene fusions are oncogenic driver mutations observed in a variety of solid tumors, including STS. Larotrectinib, a TRK inhibitor, was approved by the FDA in 2018 for *NTRK* fusion–positive tumors with no satisfactory alternative treatment options. The approval was initially based on the results of three single-arm clinical trials that included 55 patients with unresectable or metastatic solid tumors harboring an *NTRK* gene fusion (141). The ORR was 75%, including 13% ($N = 7$) complete responses and 62% ($N = 34$) partial responses. Eleven patients with STS were included, although the overall frequency of TRK alterations in sarcoma is reported to be low (142). Follow-up studies have continued to demonstrate durable and robust response in this population, supporting the rationale for routine *NTRK* gene fusion testing regarding of tumor type (143,144).

Entrectinib (RXDX-101) is an oral inhibitor of *NTRK* and c-ros oncogene 1 (*ROS1*), which is approved for the treatment of patients with advanced *NTRK* fusion–positive solid tumors and for *ROS1*-positive non–small cell lung cancers (NSCLCs). Currently, its use is being investigated in a phase 2 basket study of patients with solid tumors harboring *NTRK*, *ROS1*, or *ALK* rearrangements (NCT02568267).

Despite these advancements in tumor genomics, our ability to translate results of genetic sequencing into effective therapeutic strategies is still in its infancy. An example of this is a negative clinical trial of alisertib, a highly selective small molecule inhibitor of Aurora A kinase (145). Genome-wide transcriptional profiling of uterine LMS demonstrated frequent overexpression of gene products of the mitotic spindle apparatus, including Aurora A kinase; preclinical models in uterine LMS have shown activity for alisertib; disappointingly, however, no clinically meaningful activity was seen in the phase 2 study.

ALK Rearrangements
Inflammatory Myofibroblastic Tumors

In regard to *ALK*-positive tumors, molecular profiling efforts have demonstrated frequency of *ALK* rearrangements in up to 50% of IMTs. IMTs are intermediate- or low-grade malignant myofibroblastic neoplasms, which typically arise in the lung, abdomen, or retroperitoneum. Small case reports have shown remarkable efficacy of ALK inhibitors, such as crizotinib, alectinib, ceritinib, and brigatinib, and are now considered standard of care for IMTs with *ALK* translocations (146-149).

IMMUNOTHERAPY

Immunotherapy has been catapulted to the forefront of cancer care for many types of solid and hematologic malignancies. Although immune checkpoint blockade (ICB), a cornerstone of immunotherapy strategy, has demonstrated promising results in other gynecologic cancers, results have been modest in sarcoma. The inherent tumor heterogeneity and lack of well-established antigen targets in sarcomas represent challenges to immunotherapy use in this population.

Soft-Tissue Sarcoma

SARC028 was one of the first phase 2 trials evaluating the use of ICB in sarcoma (150). A total of 80 patients were treated with pembrolizumab (monoclonal antibody to programmed cell death-1 protein [PD-1]), 40 of which had STS. There were only seven responses, with greatest response observed in undifferentiated pleomorphic sarcoma (UPS) and dedifferentiated liposarcoma (DDLPS). Trials investigating combination ICB therapy in advanced/metastatic sarcoma have also been disappointing. The Alliance A091401 study examined the use of nivolumab (anti–PD-1) with or without ipilimumab (anticytotoxic T-lymphocyte–associated protein 4 [CTLA-4]) with 38 patients in each arm (151). There were two responses in the nivolumab-only arm and six responses in the combination arm; again, the greatest benefit was seen in UPS and DDLPS histologies.

Leiomyosarcoma

Although ICB monotherapy in LMS is still being studied (NCT03241745), the strategy of combined ICB continues to be of greater interest. NCT04239443, a phase 2 trial, is accruing patients with advanced NSCLC, STS, and uterine cancers (including sarcoma) for combination therapy with a PD-1 monoclonal antibody and apatinib, a tyrosine kinase inhibitor that inhibits VEGF-2. NCT02428192 is a currently enrolling phase 2 trial, investigating the use of nivolumab with or without ipilimumab in advanced uterine LMS.

Additional combinatorial strategies of immunotherapy and cytotoxic or other targeted therapies are being explored in various sarcoma subtypes. TTI-621 is a novel immune checkpoint inhibitor that blocks CD47, thereby delivering a prophagocytic signal to macrophages and natural killer cells (152). The combination of TTI-621 plus doxorubicin is currently being investigated in the use of metastatic high-grade LMS in a phase 1/2 trial (NCT04996004). The EAGLES trial (NCT03536780) is enrolling patients with advanced LMS to investigate avelumab, a PD-L1 inhibitor, plus gemcitabine in the second-line setting. Similarly, the use of retifanlimab, a PD-1 inhibitor, is being examined in combination with gemcitabine and docetaxel for advanced STS, including LMS (NCT04577014). A phase 2 trial of nivolumab, a PD-1 inhibitor, in combination with rucaparib, a PARP inhibitor, in refractory LMS is underway (NCT04624178). The combination of pembrolizumab, a PD-L1 inhibitor, and lenvatinib, an oral multiple receptor kinase inhibitor, an FDA-approved combination for advanced endometrial cancer, is currently being studied in advanced LMS (NCT04784247).

NOVEL AGENTS

New innovations continue to provide promising advances for the future of antineoplastic therapies. ATX-101, a small molecule peptide composed of a novel human proliferating cell nuclear antigen (PCNA), has been shown to potentiate other cytotoxic and targeted agents in preclinical studies. A phase 2 trial evaluating its use in advanced DDLPS and LMS has not yet opened to accrual. APX005M, a novel CD40 monoclonal antibody that has demonstrated activity in pancreatic carcinoma, is being studied in combination with doxorubicin in advanced sarcoma (NCT03719430). INBRX-109 is a death receptor 5 agonistic antibody being studied in phase 1 studies of advanced solid tumors including sarcoma (NCT03715933). A phase 1/2 study with BA3011, a novel antibody-drug conjugate, is evaluating its safety and efficacy with or without and a PD-1 inhibitor in advanced solid tumors (phase 1) and advanced sarcoma (phase 2) (NCT03425279). Finally, the use of PTC596, an oral small molecule tubulin-binding agent, is under investigation in a phase 1b study in combination with dacarbazine for advanced LMS (NCT03761095).

HORMONAL, TARGETED, IMMUNOTHERAPY, AND OTHER, NEW, AND NOVEL THERAPY: SUMMARY

Hormonal therapy, including progestational agents, GnRH analogs, and AIs, has a role in the treatment of advanced or recurrent low-grade ESS. The efficacy of immunotherapy, biologic, and targeted therapies remains unclear in these rare tumors, but numerous clinical trials are attempting to elucidate best monotherapy or combination strategies. Further advances in our understanding of the biology of uterine sarcomas are needed to provide more treatment targets and make long-term disease control possible. Efforts to identify additional active agents continue.

REFERENCES

1. Dinh TA, Oliva EA, Fuller AF Jr, Lee H, Goodman A. The treatment of uterine leiomyosarcoma. Results from a 10-year experience (1990-1999) at the massachusetts general hospital. *Gynecol Oncol.* 2004;92(2):648-652. doi:10.1016/j.ygyno.2003.10.044

2. Zivanovic O, Leitao MM, Iasonos A, et al. Stage-specific outcomes of patients with uterine leiomyosarcoma: a comparison of the international federation of gynecology and obstetrics and american joint committee on cancer staging systems. *J Clin Oncol.* 2009;27(12):2066-2072. doi:10.1200/JCO.2008.19.8366

3. Rose PG, Piver MS, Tsukada Y, Lau T. Patterns of metastasis in uterine sarcoma. An autopsy study. *Cancer.* 1989;63(5):935-938. doi:10.1002/1097-0142(19890301)63:5<935::aid-cncr2820630525>3.0.co;2-9

4. Pervaiz N, Colterjohn N, Farrokhyar F, Tozer R, Figueredo A, Ghert M. A systematic meta-analysis of randomized controlled trials of adjuvant chemotherapy for localized resectable soft-tissue sarcoma. *Cancer.* 2008;113(3):573-581. doi:10.1002/cncr.23592

5. Omura G, Blessing J, Major F, et al. A randomized clinical trial of adjuvant adriamycin in uterine sarcomas: a gynecologic oncology group study. *J Clin Oncol.* 1985;3(9):1240-1245.

6. Odunsi K, Moneke V, Tammela J, et al. Efficacy of adjuvant CYVADIC chemotherapy in early-stage uterine sarcomas: results of long-term follow-up. *Int J Gynecol Cancer.* 2004;14(4):659-664. doi:10.1111/j.1048-891X.2004.14420.x

7. Hempling RE, Piver MS, Baker TR. Impact on progression-free survival of adjuvant cyclophosphamide, vincristine, doxorubicin (adriamycin), and dacarbazine (CYVADIC) chemotherapy for stage I uterine sarcoma. A prospective trial. *Am J Clin Oncol.* 1995;18(4):282-286.

8. Piver MS, Lele SB, Marchetti DL, Emrich LJ. Effect of adjuvant chemotherapy on time to recurrence and survival of stage I uterine sarcomas. *J Surg Oncol.* 1988;38(4):233-239. doi:10.1002/jso.2930380406

9. Hensley ML, Blessing JA, Degeest K, Abulafia O, Rose PG, Homesley HD. Fixed-dose rate gemcitabine plus docetaxel as second-line therapy for metastatic uterine leiomyosarcoma: a gynecologic oncology group phase II study. *Gynecol Oncol.* 2008;109(3):323-328. doi:10.1016/j.ygyno.2008.02.024

10. Hensley ML, Blessing JA, Mannel R, Rose PG. Fixed-dose rate gemcitabine plus docetaxel as first-line therapy for metastatic uterine leiomyosarcoma: a gynecologic oncology group phase II trial. *Gynecol Oncol.* 2008;109(3):329-334. doi:10.1016/j.ygyno.2008.03.010

11. Hensley ML, Ishill N, Soslow R, et al. Adjuvant gemcitabine plus docetaxel for completely resected stages I-IV high grade uterine leiomyosarcoma: results of a prospective study. *Gynecol Oncol.* 2009;112(3):563-567.

12. Hensley ML, Wathen K, Maki RG, et al. Adjuvant treatment of high-risk primary uterine leiomyosarcoma with gemcitabine/docetaxel (GT), followed by doxorubicin (D): results of phase II multicenter trial SARC005. *J Clin Oncol.* 2010;28(15 suppl):10021.

13. Hensley ML, Wathen JK, Maki RG, et al. Adjuvant therapy for high-grade, uterus-limited leiomyosarcoma: results of a phase 2 trial (SARC 005). *Cancer.* 2013;119(8):1555-1561. doi:10.1002/cncr.2/942

14. Chu MC, Mor G, Lim C, Zheng W, Parkash V, Schwartz PE. Low-grade endometrial stromal sarcoma: hormonal aspects. *Gynecol Oncol.* 2003;90(1):170-176. doi:10.1016/s0090-8258(03)00258-0

15. Fadare O. Heterologous and rare homologous sarcomas of the uterine corpus: a clinicopathologic review. *Adv Anat Pathol.* 2011;18(1):60-74. doi:10.1097/PAP.0b013e3182026be7

16. Shi Y, Liu Z, Peng Z, Liu H, Yang K, Yao X. The diagnosis and treatment of Mullerian adenosarcoma of the uterus. *Aust N Z J Obstet Gynaecol.* 2008;48(6):596-600. doi:10.1111/j.1479-828X.2008.00914.x

17. Tanner EJ, Toussaint T, Leitao MM Jr, et al. Management of uterine adenosarcomas with and without sarcomatous overgrowth. *Gynecol Oncol.* 2013;129(1):140-144. doi:10.1016/j.ygyno.2012.12.036

18. Edmonson JH, Ryan LM, Blum RH, et al. Randomized comparison of doxorubicin alone versus ifosfamide plus doxorubicin or mitomycin, doxorubicin, and cisplatin against advanced soft tissue sarcomas. *J Clin Oncol.* 1993;11(7):1269-1275. doi:10.1200/jco.1993.11.7.1269

19. Adjuvant chemotherapy for localised resectable soft-tissue sarcoma of adults: meta-analysis of individual data. Sarcoma meta-analysis collaboration. *Lancet.* 1997;350(9092):1647-1654.

20. Maurer HM, Beltangady M, Gehan EA, et al. The Intergroup Rhabdomyosarcoma Study-I. A final report. *Cancer.* 1988;61(2):209-220. doi:10.1002/1097-0142(19880115)61:2<209::aid-cncr2820610202>3.0.co;2-l

21. Maurer HM, Gehan EA, Beltangady M, et al. The intergroup rhabdomyosarcoma study-II. *Cancer.* 1993;71(5):1904-1922. doi:10.1002/1097-0142(19930301)71:5<1904::aid-cncr2820710530>3.0.co;2-x

22. Crist W, Gehan EA, Ragab AH, et al. The third intergroup rhabdomyosarcoma study. *J Clin Oncol.* 1995;13(3):610-630. doi:10.1200/jco.1995.13.3.610

23. Crist WM, Anderson JR, Meza JL, et al. Intergroup rhabdomyosarcoma study-IV: results for patients with nonmetastatic disease. *J Clin Oncol.* 2001;19(12):3091-3102. doi:10.1200/jco.2001.19.12.3091

24. Little DJ, Ballo MT, Zagars GK, et al. Adult rhabdomyosarcoma: outcome following multimodality treatment. *Cancer.* 2002;95(2):377-388. doi:10.1002/cncr.10669

25. Ferrari A, Dileo P, Casanova M, et al. Rhabdomyosarcoma in adults. A retrospective analysis of 171 patients treated at a single institution. *Cancer.* 2003;98(3):571-580. doi:10.1002/cncr.11550

26. Sultan I, Qaddoumi I, Yaser S, Rodriguez-Galindo C, Ferrari A. Comparing adult and pediatric rhabdomyosarcoma in the surveillance, epidemiology and end results program, 1973 to 2005: an analysis of 2,600 patients. *J Clin Oncol.* 2009;27(20):3391-3397. doi:10.1200/jco.2008.19.7483

27. Ogilvie CM, Crawford EA, Slotcavage RL, et al. Treatment of adult rhabdomyosarcoma. *Am J Clin Oncol.* 2010;33(2):128-131. doi:10.1097/COC.0b013e3181979222

28. Gerber NK, Wexler LH, Singer S, et al. Adult rhabdomyosarcoma survival improved with treatment on multimodality protocols. *Int J Radiat Oncol Biol Phys.* 2013;86(1):58-63. doi:10.1016/j.ijrobp.2012.12.016

29. Herrmann K. 18F-FDG-PET/CT imaging as an early survival predictor in patients with primary high-grade soft tissue sarcomas undergoing neoadjuvant therapy. *Clin Cancer Res.* 2012;18(7):2024-2031. doi:10.1158/1078-0432.ccr-11-2139

30. Sutton G, Blessing J, Hanjani P, Kramer P. Phase II evaluation of liposomal doxorubicin (Doxil) in recurrent or advanced leiomyosarcoma of the uterus: a gynecologic oncology group study. *Gynecol Oncol.* 2005;96(3):749-752. doi:10.1016/j.ygyno.2004.11.036

31. Miller DS, Blessing JA, Kilgore LC, Mannel R, Van Le L. Phase II trial of topotecan in patients with advanced, persistent, or recurrent uterine leiomyosarcomas: a gynecologic oncology group study. *Am J Clin Oncol.* 2000;23(4):355-357.

32. Sutton G, Blessing JA, Ball H. Phase II trial of paclitaxel in leiomyosarcoma of the uterus: a gynecologic oncology group study. *Gynecol Oncol.* 1999;74(3):346-349. doi:10.1006/gyno.1999.5463

33. Sutton GP, Blessing JA, Barrett RJ, McGehee R. Phase II trial of ifosfamide and mesna in leiomyosarcoma of the uterus: a gynecologic oncology group study. *Am J Obstet Gynecol.* 1992;166(2):556-559. doi:0002-9378(92)91671-V

34. Thigpen T, Blessing JA, Yordan E, Valea F, Vaccarello L. Phase II trial of etoposide in leiomyosarcoma of the uterus: a gynecologic oncology group study. *Gynecol Oncol.* 1996;63(1):120-122. doi:10.1006/gyno.1996.0289

35. Thigpen JT, Blessing JA, Beecham J, Homesley H, Yordan E. Phase II trial of cisplatin as first-line chemotherapy in patients with advanced or recurrent uterine sarcomas: a gynecologic oncology group study. *J Clin Oncol.* 1991;9(11):1962-1966.

36. Omura GA, Major FJ, Blessing JA, et al. A randomized study of adriamycin with and without dimethyl triazenoimidazole carboxamide in advanced uterine sarcomas. *Cancer.* 1983;52(4):626-632.

37. Asbury R, Blessing JA, Smith DM, Carson LF. Aminothiadiazole in the treatment of advanced leiomyosarcoma of the uterine corpus. A gynecologic oncology group study. *Am J Clin Oncol.* 1995;18(5):397-399.

38. Slayton RE, Blessing JA, Look K, Anderson B. A phase II clinical trial of diaziquone (AZQ) in the treatment of patients with recurrent leiomyosarcoma of the uterus. A gynecologic oncology group study. *Invest New Drugs.* 1991;9(2):207-208.

39. Look KY, Sandler A, Blessing JA, Lucci JA 3rd, Rose PG. Phase II trial of gemcitabine as second-line chemotherapy of uterine leiomyosarcoma: a gynecologic oncology group (GOG) Study. *Gynecol Oncol.* 2004;92(2):644-647. doi:10.1016/j.ygyno.2003.11.023

40. Okuno S, Edmonson J, Mahoney M, Buckner JC, Frytak S, Galanis E. Phase II trial of gemcitabine in advanced sarcomas. *Cancer.* 2002;94(12):3225-3229. doi:10.1002/cncr.10602

41. Patel SR, Gandhi V, Jenkins J, et al. Phase II clinical investigation of gemcitabine in advanced soft tissue sarcomas and window evaluation of dose rate on gemcitabine triphosphate accumulation. *J Clin Oncol.* 2001;19(15):3483-3489.

42. Gallup DG, Blessing JA, Andersen W, Morgan MA. Evaluation of paclitaxel in previously treated leiomyosarcoma of the uterus: a gynecologic oncology group study. *Gynecol Oncol.* 2003;89(1):48-51. doi:10.1016/s0090-8258(02)00136-1

43. Garcia-Carbonero R, Supko JG, Maki RG, et al. Ecteinascidin-743 (ET-743) for chemotherapy-naive patients with advanced soft tissue sarcomas: multicenter phase II and pharmacokinetic study. *J Clin Oncol.* 2005;23(24):5484-5492. doi:10.1200/JCO.2005.05.028

44. Smith HO, Blessing JA, Vaccarello L. Trimetrexate in the treatment of recurrent or advanced leiomyosarcoma of the uterus: a phase II study of the gynecologic oncology group. *Gynecol Oncol.* 2002;84(1):140-144. doi:10.1006/gyno.2001.6482

45. Rose PG, Blessing JA, Soper JT, Barter JF. Prolonged oral etoposide in recurrent or advanced leiomyosarcoma of the uterus: a gynecologic oncology group study. *Gynecol Oncol.* 1998;70(2):267-271. doi:10.1006/gyno.1998.5080

46. Slayton RE, Blessing JA, Angel C, Berman M. Phase II trial of etoposide in the management of advanced and recurrent leiomyosarcoma of the uterus: a gynecologic oncology group study. *Cancer Treat Rep.* 1987;71(12):1303-1304.

47. Asbury R, Blessing JA, Buller R, Malfetano JH, Walker J, Sevin BU. Amonafide in patients with leiomyosarcoma of the uterus: a phase II gynecologic oncology group study. *Am J Clin Oncol.* 1998;21(2):145-146.

48. Muss HB, Bundy BN, Adcock L, Beecham J. Mitoxantrone in the treatment of advanced uterine sarcoma. A phase II trial of the gynecologic oncology group. *Am J Clin Oncol.* 1990;13(1):32-34.

49. Thigpen JT, Blessing JA, Orr JW Jr, DiSaia PJ. Phase II trial of cisplatin in the treatment of patients with advanced or recurrent mixed mesodermal sarcomas of the uterus: a gynecologic oncology group study. *Cancer Treat Rep.* 1986;70(2):271-274.

50. Fidias P, Demetri G, Harmon D. Navelbine shows activity in previously treated sarcoma patients: phase II results from MGH/Dana Farber/Partner's cancer care study. *Proc Am Soc Clin Oncol.* 1998;17:1977.

51. Talbot SM, Keohan ML, Hesdorffer M, et al. A phase II trial of temozolomide in patients with unresectable or metastatic soft tissue sarcoma. *Cancer.* 2003;98(9):1942-1946. doi:10.1002/cncr.11730

52. Pautier P, Floquet A, Penel N, et al. Randomized multicenter and stratified phase II study of gemcitabine alone versus gemcitabine and docetaxel in patients with metastatic or relapsed leiomyosarcomas: a Federation Nationale des Centres de Lutte Contre le Cancer (FNCLCC) French Sarcoma Group Study (TAXOGEM study). *Oncologist.* 2012;17(9):1213-1220. doi:10.1634/theoncologist.2011-0467

53. Monk BJ, Blessing JA, Street DG, Muller CY, Burke JJ, Hensley ML. A phase II evaluation of trabectedin in the treatment of advanced, persistent, or recurrent uterine leiomyosarcoma: a gynecologic oncology group study. *Gynecol Oncol.* 2012;124:48-52. http://www.ncbi.nlm.nih.gov/pubmed/21996263

54. Demetri GD, von Mehren M, Jones RL, et al. Efficacy and safety of trabectedin or dacarbazine for metastatic liposarcoma or leiomyosarcoma after failure of conventional chemotherapy: results of a phase III randomized multicenter clinical trial. *J Clin Oncol.* 2016;34(8):786-793. doi:10.1200/jco.2015.62.4734

55. Gadducci A, Grosso F, Scambia G, et al. A phase II randomised (calibrated design) study on the activity of the single-agent trabectedin in metastatic or locally relapsed uterine leiomyosarcoma. *Br J Cancer.* 2018;119(5):565-571. doi:10.1038/s41416-018-0190-y

56. Thigpen JT, Blessing JA, Homesley HD, Hacker N, Curry SL. Phase II trial of piperazinedione in patients with advanced or recurrent uterine sarcoma. A gynecologic oncology group study. *Am J Clin Oncol.* 1985;8(5):350-352. doi:10.1097/00000421-198510000-00002

57. Takano T, Niikura H, Ito K, et al. Feasibility study of gemcitabine plus docetaxel in advanced or recurrent uterine leiomyosarcoma and undifferentiated endometrial sarcoma in Japan. *Int J Clin Oncol.* 2014;19(5):897-905. doi:10.1007/s10147-013-0627-5

58. Verweij J, Lee SM, Ruka W, et al. Randomized phase II study of docetaxel versus doxorubicin in first-and second-line chemotherapy for locally advanced or metastatic soft tissue sarcomas in adults: a study of the

european organization for research and treatment of cancer soft tissue and bone sarcoma group. *J Clin Oncol.* 2000;18(10):2081-2086.

59. Schoffski P, Ray-Coquard IL, Cioffi A, et al. Activity of eribulin mesylate in patients with soft-tissue sarcoma: a phase 2 study in four independent histological subtypes. Clinical trial, phase II multicenter study research support, Non-U.S. Gov't. *Lancet Oncol.* 2011;12(11):1045-1052. doi:10.1016/S1470-2045(11)70230-3

60. Blay JY, Schoffski P, Bauer S, et al. Eribulin versus dacarbazine in patients with leiomyosarcoma: subgroup analysis from a phase 3, open-label, randomised study. *Br J Cancer.* 2019;120(11):1026-1032. doi:10.1038/s41416-019-0462-1

61. Shah JP, Bryant CS, Kumar S, Ali-Fehmi R, Malone JM Jr, Morris RT. Lymphadenectomy and ovarian preservation in low-grade endometrial stromal sarcoma. *Obstet Gynecol.* 2008;112(5):1102-1108. doi:10.1097/AOG.0b013e31818aa89a

62. Long HJ 3rd, Blessing JA, Sorosky J. Phase II trial of dacarbazine, mitomycin, doxorubicin, and cisplatin with sargramostim in uterine leiomyosarcoma: a gynecologic oncology group study. *Gynecol Oncol.* 2005;99(2):339-342. doi:10.1016/j.ygyno.2005.06.002

63. Edmonson JH, Blessing JA, Cosin JA, Miller DS, Cohn DE, Rotmensch J. Phase II study of mitomycin, doxorubicin, and cisplatin in the treatment of advanced uterine leiomyosarcoma: a gynecologic oncology group study. *Gynecol Oncol.* 2002;85(3):507-510. doi:10.1006/gyno.2002.6661

64. Currie J, Blessing JA, Muss HB, Fowler J, Berman M, Burke TW. Combination chemotherapy with hydroxyurea, dacarbazine (DTIC), and etoposide in the treatment of uterine leiomyosarcoma: a gynecologic oncology group study. *Gynecol Oncol.* 1996;61(1):27-30. doi:10.1006/gyno.1996.0091

65. Sutton G, Blessing JA, Malfetano JH. Ifosfamide and doxorubicin in the treatment of advanced leiomyosarcomas of the uterus: a gynecologic oncology group study. Clinical trial clinical trial, phase II multicenter study research support, U.S. Gov't, P.H.S. *Gynecol Oncol.* 1996;62(2):226-229. doi:10.1006/gyno.1996.0220

66. Hensley ML, Maki R, Venkatraman E, et al. Gemcitabine and docetaxel in patients with unresectable leiomyosarcoma: results of a phase II trial. *J Clin Oncol.* 2002;20(12):2824-2831. doi:10.1200/JCO.2002.11.050

67. Muss HB, Bundy B, DiSaia PJ, et al. Treatment of recurrent or advanced uterine sarcoma. A randomized trial of doxorubicin versus doxorubicin and cyclophosphamide (a phase III trial of the gynecologic oncology group). *Cancer.* 1985;55(8):1648-1653.

68. Dileo P, Morgan J, Zahrieh D, et al. Gemcitabine and vinorelbine combination chemotherapy for patients with advanced soft tissue sarcomas: results of a phase II trial. *Cancer.* 2007;109(9):1863-1869.

69. Hensley ML, Anderson S, Soslow R, et al. Activity of gemcitabine plus docetaxel in leiomyosarcoma (LMS) and other histologies: report of an expanded phase II trial. *J Clin Oncol.* 2004;22(14 suppl):9010.

70. Boyar MS, Hesdorffer M, Keohan ML, Jin Z, Taub RN. Phase II study of temozolomide and thalidomide in patients with unresectable or metastatic leiomyosarcoma. *Sarcoma.* 2008;2008:412503. doi:10.1155/2008/412503

71. Pautier P, Floquet A, Chevreau C, et al. Trabectedin in combination with doxorubicin for first-line treatment of advanced uterine or soft-tissue leiomyosarcoma (LMS-02): a non-randomised, multicentre, phase 2 trial. *Lancet Oncol.* 2015;16(4):457-464. doi:10.1016/s1470-2045(15)70070-7

72. Kanjeekal S, Chambers A, Fung MF, Verma S. Systemic therapy for advanced uterine sarcoma: a systematic review of the literature. *Gynecol Oncol.* 2005;97(2):624-637. doi:10.1016/j.ygyno.2005.01.041

73. Spano JP, Soria JC, Kambouchner M, et al. Long-term survival of patients given hormonal therapy for metastatic endometrial stromal sarcoma. *Med Oncol.* 2003;20(1):87-93. doi:10.1385/MO:20:1:87

74. Cheng X, Yang G, Schmeler KM, et al. Recurrence patterns and prognosis of endometrial stromal sarcoma and the potential of tyrosine kinase-inhibiting therapy. *Gynecol Oncol.* 2011;121(2):323-327. doi:10.1016/j.ygyno.2010.12.360

75. Berchuck A, Rubin SC, Hoskins WJ, Saigo PE, Pierce VK, Lewis JL Jr. Treatment of endometrial stromal tumors. *Gynecol Oncol.* 1990;36(1):60-65. doi:10.1016/0090-8258(90)90109-x

76. Szlosarek PW, Lofts FJ, Pettengell R, Carter P, Young M, Harmer C. Effective treatment of a patient with a high-grade endometrial stromal sarcoma with an accelerated regimen of carboplatin and paclitaxel. *Anticancer Drugs.* 2000;11(4):275-278. doi:10.1097/00001813-200004000-00008

77. Yamawaki T, Shimizu Y, Hasumi K. Treatment of stage IV "high-grade" endometrial stromal sarcoma with ifosfamide, adriamycin, and cisplatin. Case reports. *Gynecol Oncol.* 1997;64(2):265-269. doi:10.1006/gyno.1996.4537

78. Ihnen M, Mahner S, Janicke F, Schwarz J. Current treatment options in uterine endometrial stromal sarcoma: report of a case and review of the literature. *Int J Gynecol Cancer.* 2007;17(5):957-963. doi:10.1111/j.1525-1438.2007.00889.x

79. Lehrner LM, Miles PA, Enck RE. Complete remission of widely metastatic endometrial stromal sarcoma following combination chemotherapy. *Cancer.* 1979;43(4):1189-1194. doi:10.1002/1097-0142(197904)43:4<1189::aid-cncr2820430405>3.0.co;2-e

80. Lin YC, Kudelka AP, Tresukosol D, et al. Prolonged stabilization of progressive endometrial stromal sarcoma with prolonged oral etoposide therapy. *Gynecol Oncol.* 1995;58(2):262-265. doi:10.1006/gyno.1995.1223

81. Carroll A, Ramirez PT, Westin SN, et al. Uterine adenosarcoma: an analysis on management, outcomes, and risk factors for recurrence. *Gynecol Oncol.* 2014;135(3):455-461. doi:10.1016/j.ygyno.2014.10.022

82. Nathenson MJ, Conley AP, Lin H, Fleming N, Ravi V. Treatment of recurrent or metastatic uterine adenosarcoma. *Sarcoma.* 2017;2017:4680273. doi:10.1155/2017/4680273

83. Thomas MB, Keeney GL, Podratz KC, Dowdy SC. Endometrial stromal sarcoma: treatment and patterns of recurrence. *Int J Gynecol Cancer.* 2009;19(2):253-256. doi:10.1111/IGC.0b013e3181999c5f

84. Sutton G, Blessing JA, Park R, DiSaia PJ, Rosenshein N. Ifosfamide treatment of recurrent or metastatic endometrial stromal sarcomas previously unexposed to chemotherapy: a study of the gynecologic oncology group. Clinical trial clinical trial, phase II multicenter study research support, U.S. Gov't, P.H.S. *Obstet Gynecol.* 1996;87(5 Pt 1):747-750.

85. Dusenbery KE, Potish RA, Argenta PA, Judson PL. On the apparent failure of adjuvant pelvic radiotherapy to improve survival for women with uterine sarcomas confined to the uterus. *Am J Clin Oncol.* 2005;28(3):295-300. doi:10.1097/01.coc.0000156919.04133.98

86. Bleeker JS, Quevedo JF, Folpe AL. "Malignant" perivascular epithelioid cell neoplasm: risk stratification and treatment strategies. *Sarcoma.* 2012;2012:541626. doi:10.1155/2012/541626

87. Sandler E, Lyden E, Ruymann F, et al. Efficacy of ifosfamide and doxorubicin given as a phase II "window" in children with newly diagnosed metastatic rhabdomyosarcoma: a report from the intergroup rhabdomyosarcoma study group. *Med Pediatr Oncol.* 2001;37(5):442-448. doi:10.1002/mpo.1227

88. Schoffski P, Maki RG, Italiano A. Randomized, open-label multicenter, phase III study of eribulin versus dacarbazine in patients (pts) with leiomyosarcoma (LMS) and adipocytic sarcoma (ADI). *J Clin Oncol.* 2015;33(18 suppl).

89. Sutton G, Brunetto VL, Kilgore L, et al. A phase III trial of ifosfamide with or without cisplatin in carcinosarcoma of the uterus: a gynecologic oncology group study. *Gynecol Oncol.* 2000;79(2):147-153. doi:10.1006/gyno.2000.6001

90. Homesley HD, Filiaci V, Markman M, et al. Phase III trial of ifosfamide with or without paclitaxel in advanced uterine carcinosarcoma: a gynecologic oncology group study. *J Clin Oncol.* 2007;25(5):526-531. doi:10.1200/JCO.2006.06.4907

91. Yovine A, Riofrio M, Blay JY, et al. Phase II study of ecteinascidin-743 in advanced pretreated soft tissue sarcoma patients. *J Clin Oncol.* 2004;22(5):890-899. doi:10.1200/JCO.2004.05.210

92. Ryan CW, Merimsky O, Agulnik M, et al. PICASSO III: a phase III, placebo-controlled study of doxorubicin with or without palifosfamide in patients with metastatic soft tissue sarcoma. *J Clin Oncol.* 2016;34(32):3898-3905. doi:10.1200/JCO.2016.67.6684

93. Sutton GP, Stehman FB, Michael H, Young PC, Ehrlich CE. Estrogen and progesterone receptors in uterine sarcomas. *Obstet Gynecol.* 1986;68(5):709-714.

94. Amant F, De Knijf A, Van Calster B, et al. Clinical study investigating the role of lymphadenectomy, surgical castration and adjuvant hormonal treatment in endometrial stromal sarcoma. *Br J Cancer.* 2007;97(9):1194-1199. doi:10.1038/sj.bjc.6603986

95. Burke C, Hickey K. Treatment of endometrial stromal sarcoma with a gonadotropin-releasing hormone analogue. *Obstet Gynecol.* 2004;104(5 pt 2):1182-1184. doi:10.1097/01.AOG.0000133533.05148.aa

96. Maluf FC, Sabbatini P, Schwartz L, Xia J, Aghajanian C. Endometrial stromal sarcoma: objective response to letrozole. *Gynecol Oncol.* 2001;82(2):384-388. doi:10.1006/gyno.2001.6238

97. Thanopoulou E, Aleksic A, Thway K, Khabra K, Judson I. Hormonal treatments in metastatic endometrial stromal sarcomas: the 10-year experience of the sarcoma unit of royal marsden hospital. *Clin Sarcoma Res.* 2015;5:8. doi:10.1186/s13569-015-0024-0

98. Lantta M, Kahanpaa K, Karkkainen J, Lehtovirta P, Wahlstrom T, Widholm O. Estradiol and progesterone receptors in two cases of endometrial stromal sarcoma. *Gynecol Oncol.* 1984;18(2):233-239. doi:10.1016/0090-8258(84)90031-3

99. Baker TR, Piver MS, Lele SB, Tsukada Y. Stage I uterine adenosarcoma: a report of six cases. *J Surg Oncol*. 1988;37(2):128-132. doi:10.1002/jso.2930370213

100. Piver MS, Rutledge FN, Copeland L, Webster K, Blumenson L, Suh O. Uterine endolymphatic stromal myosis: a collaborative study. *Obstet Gynecol*. 1984;64(2):173-178.

101. Scribner DR Jr, Walker JL. Low-grade endometrial stromal sarcoma preoperative treatment with Depo-Lupron and Megace. *Gynecol Oncol*. 1998;71(3):458-460. doi:10.1006/gyno.1998.5174

102. Navarro D, Cabrera JJ, Leon L, et al. Endometrial stromal sarcoma expression of estrogen receptors, progesterone receptors and estrogen-induced srp27 (24K) suggests hormone responsiveness. *J Steroid Biochem Mol Biol*. 1992;41(3-8):589-596. doi:10.1016/0960-0760(92)90389-z

103. Mansi JL, Ramachandra S, Wiltshaw E, Fisher C. Endometrial stromal sarcomas. *Gynecol Oncol*. 1990;36(1):113-118. doi:10.1016/0090-8258(90)90120-a

104. O'Brien AA, O'Briain DS, Daly PA. Aggressive endometrial stromal sarcoma responding to medroxyprogesterone following failure of tamoxifen and combination chemotherapy. Case report. *Br J Obstet Gynaecol*. 1985;92(8):862-866. doi:10.1111/j.1471-0528.1985.tb03062.x

105. Pink D, Lindner T, Mrozek A, et al. Harm or benefit of hormonal treatment in metastatic low-grade endometrial stromal sarcoma: single center experience with 10 cases and review of the literature. *Gynecol Oncol*. 2006;101(3):464-469. doi:10.1016/j.ygyno.2005.11.010

106. Ramondetta LM, Johnson AJ, Sun CC, et al. Phase 2 trial of mifepristone (RU-486) in advanced or recurrent endometrioid adenocarcinoma or low-grade endometrial stromal sarcoma. Clinical trial, phase II research support, N.I.H., extramural. *Cancer*. 2009;115(9):1867-1874. doi:10.1002/cncr.24197

107. Krumholz BA, Lobovsky FY, Halitsky V. Endolymphatic stromal myosis with pulmonary metastases. Remission with progestin therapy: report of a case. *J Reprod Med*. 1973;10(2):85-89.

108. O'Cearbhaill R, Zhou Q, Iasonos A, et al. Treatment of advanced uterine leiomyosarcoma with aromatase inhibitors. *Gynecol Oncol*. 2010;116(3):424-429. doi:10.1016/j.ygyno.2009.10.064

109. George S, Feng Y, Manola J, et al. Phase 2 trial of aromatase inhibition with letrozole in patients with uterine leiomyosarcomas expressing estrogen and/or progesterone receptors. *Cancer*. 2014;120(5):738-743. doi:10.1002/cncr.28476

110. Sanfilippo R, Fabbroni C, Fucà G, et al. Addition of antiestrogen treatment in patients with malignant PEComa progressing to mTOR inhibitors. *Clin Cancer Res*. 2020;26(20):5534-5538. doi:10.1158/1078-0432.Ccr-20-1191

111. Sleijfer S, Ray-Coquard I, Papai Z, et al. Pazopanib, a multikinase angiogenesis inhibitor, in patients with relapsed or refractory advanced soft tissue sarcoma: a phase II study from the european organisation for research and treatment of cancer-soft tissue and bone sarcoma group (EORTC study 62043). *J Clin Oncol*. 2009;27(19):3126-3132. doi:10.1200/JCO.2008.21.3223

112. Pautier P, Penel N, Ray-Coquard I, et al. A phase II of gemcitabine combined with pazopanib followed by pazopanib maintenance, as second-line treatment in patients with advanced leiomyosarcomas: a unicancer french sarcoma group study (LMS03 study). *Eur J Cancer*. 2020;125:31-37. doi:10.1016/j.ejca.2019.10.028

113. van der Graaf WT, Blay JY, Chawla SP, et al. Pazopanib for metastatic soft-tissue sarcoma (PALETTE): a randomised, double-blind, placebo-controlled phase 3 trial. Research support, Non-U.S. Gov't. *Lancet*. 2012;379(9829):1879-1886. doi:10.1016/S0140-6736(12)60651-5

114. Liapi A, Mathevet P, Herrera FG, Hastir D, Sarivalasis A. VEGFR inhibitors for uterine metastatic perivascular epithelioid tumors (PEComa) resistant to mTOR inhibitors. A case report and review of literature. Mini review. *Front Oncol*. 2021;11:641376. doi:10.3389/fonc.2021.641376

115. Emoto M, Ishiguro M, Iwasaki H, Kikuchi M, Kawarabayashi T. Effect of angiogenesis inhibitor TNP-470 on the growth, blood flow, and microvessel density in xenografts of human uterine carcinosarcoma in nude mice. *Gynecol Oncol*. 2003;89(1):88-94. doi:10.1016/s0090-8258(02)00155-5

116. McMeekin DS, Sill MW, Benbrook D, et al. A phase II trial of thalidomide in patients with refractory endometrial cancer and correlation with angiogenesis biomarkers: a gynecologic oncology group study. *Gynecol Oncol*. 2007;105(2):508-516. doi:10.1016/j.ygyno.2007.01.019

117. Maki RG, D'Adamo DR, Keohan ML, et al. Phase II study of sorafenib in patients with metastatic or recurrent sarcomas. *J Clin Oncol*. 2009;27(19):3133-3140. doi:10.1200/jco.2008.20.4495

118. Mackay HJ, Buckanovich RJ, Hirte H, et al. A phase II study single agent of aflibercept (VEGF Trap) in patients with recurrent or metastatic gynecologic carcinosarcomas and uterine leiomyosarcomas. A trial of the princess margaret hospital, Chicago and California cancer phase II consortia. *Gynecol Oncol*. 2012;125(1):136-140. doi:10.1016/j.ygyno.2011.11.042

119. D'Adamo DR, Anderson SE, Albritton K, et al. Phase II study of doxorubicin and bevacizumab for patients with metastatic soft-tissue sarcomas. *J Clin Oncol*. 2005;23(28):7135-7142. doi:10.1200/JCO.2005.16.139

120. Hensley ML, Miller A, O'Malley DM, et al. Randomized phase III trial of gemcitabine plus docetaxel plus bevacizumab or placebo as first-line treatment for metastatic uterine leiomyosarcoma: an NRG oncology/gynecologic oncology group study. *J Clin Oncol*. 2015;33(10):1180-1185. doi:10.1200/jco.2014.58.3781

121. Maki RG. Recent advances in therapy for gastrointestinal stromal tumors. *Curr Oncol Rep*. 2007;9(3):165-169. doi:10.1007/s11912-007-0017-0

122. Rushing RS, Shajahan S, Chendil D, et al. Uterine sarcomas express KIT protein but lack mutation(s) in exon 11 or 17 of c-KIT. *Gynecol Oncol*. 2003;91(1):9-14. doi:10.1016/s0090-8258(03)00442-6

123. Winter WE 3rd, Seidman JD, Krivak TC, et al. Clinicopathological analysis of c-kit expression in carcinosarcomas and leiomyosarcomas of the uterine corpus. *Gynecol Oncol*. 2003;91(1):3-8. doi:10.1016/j.ygyno.2003.06.001

124. Huh WK, Sill MW, Darcy KM, et al. Efficacy and safety of imatinib mesylate (Gleevec) and immunohistochemical expression of c-Kit and PDGFR-beta in a gynecologic oncology group phase II trial in women with recurrent or persistent carcinosarcomas of the uterus. Clinical trial, phase IIMulticenter studyresearch support, N.I.H., extramural research support, N.I.H., intramural research support, Non-U.S. Gov't. *Gynecol Oncol*. 2010;117(2):248-254. doi:10.1016/j.ygyno.2010.01.002

125. Hensley ML, Sill MW, Scribner DR Jr, et al. Sunitinib malate in the treatment of recurrent or persistent uterine leiomyosarcoma: a gynecologic oncology group phase II study. Clinical trial, phase II multicenter study research support, N.I.H., extramural. *Gynecol Oncol*. 2009;115(3):460-465. doi:10.1016/j.ygyno.2009.09.011

126. Mir O, Brodowicz T, Italiano A, et al. Safety and efficacy of regorafenib in patients with advanced soft tissue sarcoma (REGOSARC): a randomised, double-blind, placebo-controlled, phase 2 trial. *Lancet Oncol*. 2016;17(12):1732-1742. doi:10.1016/s1470-2045(16)30507-1

127. Marrari A, Bertuzzi A, Bozzarelli S, et al. Activity of regorafenib in advanced pretreated soft tissue sarcoma: results of a single-center phase II study. *Medicine (Baltimore)*. 2020;99(26):e20719. doi:10.1097/md.0000000000020719

128. Hu J, Khanna V, Jones M, Surti U. Genomic alterations in uterine leiomyosarcomas: potential markers for clinical diagnosis and prognosis. Comparative Study Research Support, Non-U.S. Gov't. *Genes Chromosomes Cancer*. 2001;31(2):117-124. doi:10.1002/gcc.1125

129. Chawla SP, Staddon AP, Baker LH, et al. Phase II study of the mammalian target of rapamycin inhibitor ridaforolimus in patients with advanced bone and soft tissue sarcomas. Clinical trial, phase II multicenter study research support, Non-U.S. Gov't. *J Clin Oncol*. 2012;30(1):78-84. doi:10.1200/JCO.2011.35.6329

130. Blay JY, Chawla SP, Ray-Coquard I, et al. Phase III, placebo-controlled trial (SUCCEED) evaluating ridaforolimus as maintenance therapy in advanced sarcoma patients following clinical benefit from prior standard cytotoxic chemotherapy: long-term (≥24 months) overall survival results. *J Clin Oncol*. 2012;30(15 suppl):10010.

131. Agaram NP, Sung YS, Zhang L, et al. Dichotomy of genetic abnormalities in PEComas with therapeutic implications. *Am J Surg Pathol*. 2015;39(6):813-825. doi:10.1097/pas.0000000000000389

132. Flechter E, Zohar Y, Guralnik L, Passhak M, Sela GB. Long-lasting stable disease with mTOR inhibitor treatment in a patient with a perivascular epithelioid cell tumor: a case report and literature review. *Oncol Lett*. 2016;12(6):4739-4743. doi:10.3892/ol.2016.5231

133. Kwiatkowski DJ, Choueiri TK, Fay AP, et al. Mutations in TSC1, TSC2, and MTOR are associated with response to rapalogs in patients with metastatic renal cell carcinoma. *Clin Cancer Res*. 2016;22(10):2445-2452. doi:10.1158/1078-0432.Ccr-15-2631

134. Świtaj T, Sobiborowicz A, Teterycz P, et al. Efficacy of sirolimus treatment in PEComa-10 years of practice perspective. *J Clin Med*. 2021;10(16):3705. doi:10.3390/jcm10163705

135. Sanfilippo R, Jones RL, Blay JY, et al. Role of chemotherapy, VEGFR inhibitors, and mTOR inhibitors in advanced perivascular epithelioid cell tumors (PEComas). *Clin Cancer Res*. 2019;25(17):5295-5300. doi:10.1158/1078-0432.Ccr-19-0288

136. Kopparthy P, Murphy M. Rapid and durable response with nab-sirolimus after everolimus failure in a patient with perivascular epithelioid cell tumors (PEComas) of the uterus. *Cureus*. 2021;13(5):e14951. doi:10.7759/cureus.14951

137. Wagner AJ, Ravi V, Riedel RF, et al. nab-Sirolimus for patients with malignant perivascular epithelioid cell tumors. *J Clin Oncol*. 2021;39(33):3660-3670. doi:10.1200/JCO.21.01728

138. Bolden JE, Shi W, Jankowski K, et al. HDAC inhibitors induce tumor-cell-selective pro-apoptotic transcriptional responses. *Cell Death Dis*. 2013;4:e519. doi:10.1038/cddis.2013.9

139. Choy E, Ballman K, Chen J, et al. SARC018_SPORE02: phase II study of mocetinostat administered with gemcitabine for patients with metastatic leiomyosarcoma with progression or relapse following prior treatment with gemcitabine-containing therapy. *Sarcoma*. 2018;2018:2068517. doi:10.1155/2018/2068517

140. Hensley ML, Chavan SS, Solit DB, et al. Genomic landscape of uterine sarcomas defined through prospective clinical sequencing. *Clin Cancer Res*. 2020;26(14):3881-3888. doi:10.1158/1078-0432.Ccr-19-3959

141. Drilon A, Laetsch TW, Kummar S, et al. Efficacy of larotrectinib in TRK fusion–positive cancers in adults and children. *N Engl J Med*. 2018;378(8):731-739. doi:10.1056/NEJMoa1714448

142. Stransky N, Cerami E, Schalm S, Kim JL, Lengauer C. The landscape of kinase fusions in cancer. *Nat Commun*. 2014;5:4846. doi:10.1038/ncomms5846

143. Bazhenova L, Lokker A, Snider J, et al. TRK fusion cancer: patient characteristics and survival analysis in the real-world setting. *Target Oncol*. 2021;16(3):389-399. doi:10.1007/s11523-021-00815-4

144. Hong DS, DuBois SG, Kummar S, et al. Larotrectinib in patients with TRK fusion-positive solid tumours: a pooled analysis of three phase 1/2 clinical trials. *Lancet Oncol*. 2020;21(4):531-540. doi:10.1016/s1470-2045(19)30856-3

145. Hyman DM, Sill MW, Lankes HA, et al. A phase 2 study of alisertib (MLN8237) in recurrent or persistent uterine leiomyosarcoma: an NRG oncology/gynecologic oncology group study 0231D. *Gynecol Oncol*. 2017;144(1):96-100. doi:10.1016/j.ygyno.2016.10.036

146. Butrynski JE, D'Adamo DR, Hornick JL, et al. Crizotinib in ALK-rearranged inflammatory myofibroblastic tumor. *N Engl J Med*. 2010;363(18):1727-1733. doi:10.1056/NEJMoa1007056

147. Xavier CB, Canedo FSNA, Lima FAS, et al. Complete response to alectinib following crizotinib in an ALK-positive inflammatory myofibroblastic tumor with CNS involvement. *Curr Probl Cancer Case Rep*. 2021;4:100117. doi:10.1016/j.cpccr.2021.100117

148. Ono A, Murakami H, Serizawa M, et al. Drastic initial response and subsequent response to two ALK inhibitors in a patient with a highly aggressive ALK-rearranged inflammatory myofibroblastic tumor arising in the pleural cavity. *Lung Cancer*. 2016;99:151-154. doi:10.1016/j.lungcan.2016.07.002

149. Gettinger SN, Bazhenova LA, Langer CJ, et al. Activity and safety of brigatinib in ALK-rearranged non-small-cell lung cancer and other malignancies: a single-arm, open-label, phase 1/2 trial. *Lancet Oncol*. 2016;17(12):1683-1696. doi:10.1016/s1470-2045(16)30392-8

150. Tawbi HA, Burgess M, Bolejack V, et al. Pembrolizumab in advanced soft-tissue sarcoma and bone sarcoma (SARC028): a multicentre, two-cohort, single-arm, open-label, phase 2 trial. *Lancet Oncol*. 2017;18(11):1493-1501. doi:10.1016/S1470-2045(17)30624-1

151. D'Angelo E, Ali RH, Espinosa I, et al. Endometrial stromal sarcomas with sex cord differentiation are associated with PHF1 rearrangement. *Am J Surg Pathol*. 2013;37(4):514-521. doi:10.1097/PAS.0b013e318272c612

152. Ansell SM, Maris MB, Lesokhin AM, et al. Phase I study of the CD47 blocker TTI-621 in patients with relapsed or refractory hematologic malignancies. *Clin Cancer Res*. 2021;27(8):2190-2199. doi:10.1158/1078-0432.Ccr-20-3706

153. Svancarova L, Blay JY, Judson IR, et al. Gemcitabine in advanced adult soft-tissue sarcomas. A phase II study of the EORTC Soft Tissue and Bone Sarcoma Group. *Eur J Cancer*. 2002;38:556-559.

154. Twelves C, Hoekman K, Bowman A, et al. Phase I and pharmacokinetic study of YondelisTM (Ecteinascidin-743; ET-743) administered as an infusion over 1 h or 3 h every 21 days in patients with solid tumours. *Eur J Cancer*. 2003;339:1842-1851.

155. Thigpen JT, Blessing JA, Wilbanks GD. Cisplatin as second-line chemotherapy in the treatment of advanced or recurrent leiomyosarcoma of the uterus. A phase II trial of the Gynecologic Oncology Group. *Am J Clin Oncol*. 1986;9:18-20.

156. Edmonson JH, Marks RS, Buckner JC, et al. Contrast of response to dacarbazine, mitomycin, doxorubicin, and cisplatin (DMAP) plus GM-CSF between patients with advanced malignant gastrointestinal stromal tumors and patients with other advanced leiomyosarcomas. *Cancer Invest*. 2002;20:605-612.

157. Doebele RC, Drilon A, Paz-Ares L, et al. Entrectinib in patients with advanced or metastatic NTRK fusion-positive solid tumours: integrated analysis of three phase 1-2 trials. *Lancet Oncol*. 2020;21(2):271-282. doi:10.1016/S1470-2045(19)30691-6

158. Shaw AT, Kim TM, Crinò L, et al. Ceritinib versus chemotherapy in patients with ALK-rearranged non-small-cell lung cancer previously given chemotherapy and crizotinib (ASCEND-5): a randomised, controlled, open-label, phase 3 trial. *Lancet Oncol*. 2017;18(7):874-886. doi:10.1016/S1470-2045(17)30339-X

CHAPTER **6.8**

Surgery for Persistent and Recurrent Uterine Sarcomas

Tiffany Y. Sia and Mario M. Leitao Jr

SURGERY FOR RECURRENT DISEASE

Data are limited with respect to CRS of recurrent uterine sarcomas. However, CRS may be considered in many of these cases, especially if the patient has had a relatively long disease-free interval and the sites of recurrence appear amenable to a complete surgical resection. Surgery is often considered for recurrent ESS because of the relative indolence of these tumors, long disease-free intervals, and lack of other effective treatments. Currently, the approach to CS is often extrapolated from data for endometrial carcinomas.

Resection of recurrent LMS has been described. Surgery for other sarcomas is often considered, but there are no data regarding these very rare uterine sarcomas.

Surgical cytoreduction of recurrent uterine LMS, with or without pulmonary involvement, has been reported to provide a possible survival benefit. Leitao and colleagues (1) reported a survival benefit with optimal resection (defined as largest residual tumor mass ≤1 cm in diameter) of pulmonary and extrapulmonary first recurrences of uterine LMS among 41 patients who underwent resection. Median survival was 3.9 years after an optimal resection compared to only 0.7 years after suboptimal resection ($P = .002$). The only other prognostic factor was time to first recurrence. Median survival was 5.1 years in cases with a time to first recurrence of greater than 12 months, compared to 1.5 years in cases with a time to recurrence of 12 months or less ($P = .005$). Tumor grade, thoracic versus nonthoracic procedures, sites of first recurrence, and use of adjuvant therapy after resection were not associated with survival. In a larger series by Giuntoli et al (2), secondary cytoreduction in patients with recurrent uterine LMS was also associated with a survival benefit. Secondary cytoreduction to no gross residual was independently associated with survival after adjusting for site of recurrence, use of chemotherapy, RT, combined surgery and chemotherapy, and recurrence time (2). Similar to the findings of Leitao et al, a longer time to recurrence was also prognostic of outcome but with 6 months used for the cutoff. Cybulska and colleagues updated the earlier experience reported by Leitao et al within a cohort of 62 patients (3). A complete gross resection was obtained in 93% of these cases. The median OS was 54 months after a complete gross resection compared to 38.7 months after traditional "optimal" resection and only 1.7 months if suboptimal (>1 cm residual) ($P < .001$). Secondary surgical cytoreduction in patients with recurrent LMS is a worthwhile consideration if a complete gross resection is feasible.

Khoury-Collado et al (4) described an updated series of 21 patients (from 1997 to 2011) with uterine cancers who developed recurrence in the pelvis after prior RT and underwent pelvic exenteration. The cases included uterine sarcomas ($n = 6$), CS ($n = 2$), AS ($n = 2$), LMS ($n = 1$), and ESS ($n = 1$). In the two CS cases, there was a short time between prior therapy and exenteration, and the median survival after exenteration was only 6 months. The median survival after exenteration for the four other sarcomas was not reached, and the 5-year OS was 66%. Pelvic exenteration may also be a reasonable consideration for patients with isolated pelvic recurrences after prior RT. However, it must be recognized that these operations are quite morbid, and the reported outcomes are based on very small numbers of highly selected patients with uterine sarcomas.

As uterine sarcomas, particularly LMS, frequently metastasize to the lungs, the role of pulmonary metastasectomy has been investigated. In a single-institution retrospective cohort study of pulmonary resections performed for LMS compared to other sarcomas, the LMS cohort presented with fewer pulmonary lesions and fewer involved lobes and had a median OS of 70 months compared to 24 months for other histologies (5). Other factors associated with survival in the LMS cohort were longer disease-free interval from time of primary tumor resection to development of pulmonary metastases and disease-free interval between pulmonary resection to second pulmonary recurrence (5,6). Generally, in recurrent uterine sarcomas without other extrathoracic disease, resection of pulmonary metastases is associated with a survival benefit. Levenback and colleagues (7) reported a 5-year survival rate of 43% after resection of pulmonary metastases in a group of 45 uterine sarcomas including 38 LMS, 4 ESS, and 3 CS. Unilateral pulmonary recurrence was associated with better survival after metastasectomy than bilateral recurrence (mean survival 39 vs 27 months; $P = .02$).

REFERENCES

1. Leitao MM, Brennan MF, Hensley M, et al. Surgical resection of pulmonary and extrapulmonary recurrences of uterine leiomyosarcoma. *Gynecol Oncol.* 2002;87:287-294.
2. Giuntoli RL 2nd, Garrett-Mayer E, Bristow RE, et al. Secondary cytoreduction in the management of recurrent uterine leiomyosarcoma. *Gynecol Oncol.* 2007;106:82-88.
3. Cybulska P, Sioulas V, Orfanelli T, et al. Secondary surgical resection for patients with recurrent uterine leiomyosarcoma. *Gynecol Oncol.* 2019;154:333-337.
4. Khoury-Collado F, Einstein MH, Bochner BH, et al. Pelvic exenteration with curative intent for uterine malignancies. *Gynecol Oncol.* 2012;124:42-47.
5. Burt BM, Ocejo S, Mery CM, et al. Repeated and aggressive pulmonary resections for leiomyosarcoma metastases extends survival. *Ann Thorac Surg.* 2011;92:1202-1207.
6. Anraku M, Yokoi K, Nakagawa K, et al. Pulmonary metastases from uterine malignancies: results of surgical resection in 133 patients. *J Thorac Cardiovasc Surg.* 2004;127(4):1107-1112.
7. Levenback C, Rubin SC, McCormack PM, et al. Resection of pulmonary metastases from uterine sarcomas. *Gynecol Oncol.* 1992;45:202-205.

CHAPTER **6.9**

Uterine Sarcomas: Follow-Up, Survivorship Issues, and Future Directions

Tiffany Y. Sia and Mario M. Leitao Jr

SURVEILLANCE RECOMMENDATIONS

Given the wide range in tumor biology and rarity of uterine sarcomas, post-treatment surveillance varies widely by histology and provider. Generally, symptom assessment and physical examinations (consisting of a thorough speculum examination with visualization of the vaginal mucosa and vaginal cuff, bimanual pelvic examination, and digital rectovaginal examination) are recommended every 3 to 4 months for the first 2 to 3 years after diagnosis and then every 6 to 12 months for the next 2 years. Patient should receive information regarding symptoms of recurrence, which may include vaginal, bladder, or rectal bleeding; pelvic pressure; changes in bowel or bladder habits; decreased appetite; weight loss; pain in the abdomen, pelvis, or back; cough; dyspnea; or swelling in the abdomen and extremities.

Given the high propensity for uterine LMS and ESS to recur with distant metastases, CT imaging of the chest, abdomen, and pelvis is recommended every 3 to 6 months for the first 3 years and then every 6 to 12 months for the next 2 years. MRI of the abdomen and pelvis combined with chest CT may also be considered, reserving PET/CT scans if clinically concerned for metastases or to clarify imaging findings. Annual to biannual imaging may be considered for an additional 5 years, though practice patterns on long-term surveillance vary.

Surveillance for uterine CS follows surveillance recommendations for other high-risk endometrial carcinomas and consists of symptom assessment and physical examination every 3 months for 2 years, then every 6 months for up to year 5, then annually. Vaginal cytology as a screening tool is no longer recommended as its utility has been limited, and recurrences are usually able to be detected by physical examination or symptoms alone (1,2).

Menopause Symptom Management

Women experiencing symptoms of premature menopause and estrogen deprivation following BSO are at higher risk of osteopenia and osteoporosis, coronary heart disease, and cognitive impairment, not to mention vasomotor symptoms, sleep disturbance, and joint pain (3). Sexual health is also frequently negatively impacted by gynecologic cancer and its treatment, which includes not only pelvic surgery but also pelvic radiation and chemotherapy.

However, menopausal hormone replacement therapy for uterine sarcomas cannot be recommended at this time as nearly 50% of uterine LMS express ERs and PRs and ER and PR are expressed in 70% and 90% of LG-ESS cases, respectively. Furthermore, given the high hormone receptor positivity rates, antiestrogen therapies such as AIs have shown efficacy in treating metastatic or recurrent ESS and small case series have demonstrated modest effect of AIs in LMS, with clinical stability rates of up to 32% and median PFS of 2.9 months (4).

As such, for women experiencing vasomotor symptoms after BSO for uterine sarcomas, we recommend treatment with non-hormonal therapies, which include paced breathing techniques; avoidance of caffeine, alcohol, and tobacco; and drugs such as selective norepinephrine reuptake inhibitors and selective serotonin reuptake inhibitors. For women under the age of 45, a dual energy x-ray absorptiometry scan (DEXA) is recommended to assess bone mineral density of the spine and hip, and all women should be counseled regarding adequate calcium (1,200 mg elemental calcium daily) and vitamin D (800-1,000 IU/d) intake. Sexual dysfunction may be managed by a multidisciplinary approach, which may involve water or silicone-based lubricants, pelvic floor physical therapy, and a psychologist or sex therapist (3).

FUTURE DIRECTIONS

Traditionally, identification and classification of uterine sarcomas has relied on histologic morphology, immunohistochemical staining, and fluorescence in situ hybridization (FISH) technology. More recently, the adoption of next-generation sequencing for molecular profiling has allowed for discovery of new ways of classifying this diverse group of mesenchymal neoplasms and has led to the discovery of novel fusions and prognostic biomarkers.

For example, the identification of frequent translocations leading to novel gene fusions within low-grade ESS (*JAZF1-SUZ12*) has led to the adoption of fusion testing as part of the workup for uterine sarcomas (5,6). Within the HG-ESS category, fusion testing has allowed for the detection of three HG-ESS subtypes: tumors harboring the *YWHAE-NUTM2* fusion (which are associated with a low-grade fibrous spindle cell component with low mitotic index), tumors with fusions involving exons 6 and 7 of *BCOR* and exons 6, 11, and 10 of *ZC3H7B* (which are composed of high-grade spindle cells within myxoid matrix), and tumors with *BCOR* exon 15 internal tandem duplications (which contain round and spindle cell components with high mitotic index and frequently present with lymphovascular invasion) (5,6).

Neurotrophic tyrosine kinase receptor (*NTRK*) gene rearrangements have been found in more than 60% of uterine

sarcomas, and treatment with a TRK inhibitor such as larotrectinib or entrectinib may be considered in patients with tumors containing the rearrangement (7). Finally, the category of USS, which comprises a morphologically heterogeneous cohort of tumors and is a diagnosis of exclusion, has been reexamined through the lens of molecular profiling. In one study of 10 tumors originally diagnosed as USS, application of gene fusion testing, immunohistochemistry, and FISH reclassified 70% of the samples as HG-ESS after testing revealed characteristic gene rearrangements (8). The discovery of the SMARCA4-deficient UUS subtype has led to refinement of a previously heterogeneous cohort of patients and has allowed patients with this rare subtype of tumor to enroll in clinical trials using targeted therapies such as EZH2 inhibitors.

Recently, there has been interest in examining the role of hyperthermic intraperitoneal chemotherapy (HIPEC) in patients with disseminated recurrent peritoneal malignancies, including uterine LMS. A meta-analysis of 11 studies including 75 patients found that though the overall mortality of cytoreductive surgery combined with HIPEC (CRS-HIPEC) was relatively high at 4.0%, CRS-HIPEC was a potential treatment options for disseminated peritoneal uLMS, with 3-year OS of 47% to 73.4% (9). One systematic review comparing the effectiveness of CRS-HIPEC ($N = 4$) with CRS alone ($N = 9$) found 3-year PFS rates of 71.4% versus 0%, though the difference was not significant, likely due to small cohort size (10). Despite limited interpretation of data given small sample sizes, additional studies are justified in determining the treatment effectiveness of CRS-HIPEC in this patient population.

Similarly, given the poor response rate of recurrent uterine LMS to chemotherapy, trials of new systemic therapies and targeted treatments such as anti-VEGF therapies, dacarbazine, trabectedin, and tyrosine kinase inhibitors such as pazopanib are underway, though thus far responses have been modest in small cohorts. Though treatment with single agent nivolumab, a PD-L1 inhibitor, has shown no benefit in uLMS in a phase II study (11), several clinical trials are underway studying immunotherapeutic agents in combination with either RT or chemotherapy, as roughly 75% of LMS are PD-L1 positive and have high T-cell infiltration compared to other uterine smooth muscle tumors (12).

Finally, identification of uterine sarcoma subtypes using molecular profiling techniques has potential implications for biomarker-directed therapies and allows for further characterization and understanding of the biology of these tumors. Given the rarity of these tumors, collaboration between centers through clinical trials enrollment and data sharing, as well as confirmation of pathology is required to generate meaningful information regarding natural history, treatment responses, and patterns of recurrence.

REFERENCES

1. Bristow RE, Purinton SC, Santillan A, Diaz-Montes TP, Gardner GJ, Giuntoli RL II. Cost-effectiveness of routine vaginal cytology for endometrial cancer surveillance. *Gynecol Oncol.* 2006;103(2):709-713.

2. Salani R, Khanna N, Frimer M, Bristow RE, Chen LM. An update on post-treatment surveillance and diagnosis of recurrence in women with gynecologic malignancies: Society of Gynecologic Oncology (SGO) recommendations. *Gynecol Oncol.* 2017;146(1):3-10.

3. Faubion SS, MacLaughlin KL, Long ME, Pruthi S, Casey PM. Surveillance and care of the gynecologic cancer survivor. *J Womens Health (Larchmt).* 2015;24(11):899-906. doi:10.1089/jwh.2014.5127

4. O'Cearbhaill R, Zhou Q, Iasonos A, et al. Treatment of advanced uterine leiomyosarcoma with aromatase inhibitors. *Gynecol Oncol.* 2010;116:424-429.

5. Chiang S, Ali R, Melnyk N, et al. Frequency of known gene rearrangements in endometrial stromal tumors. *Am J Surg Pathol.* 2011;35(9):1364-1372. doi:10.1097/PAS.0b013e3182262743

6. Parra-Herran C, Howitt BE. Uterine mesenchymal tumors: update on classification, staging, and molecular features. *Surg Pathol Clin.* 2019;12(2):363-396.

7. Cocco E, Scaltriti M, Drilon A. NTRK fusion-positive cancers and TRK inhibitor therapy. *Nat Rev Clin Oncol.* 2018;15(12):731-747. doi:10.1038/s41571-018-0113-0

8. Cotzia P, Benayed R, Mullaney K, et al. Undifferentiated uterine sarcomas represent under-recognized high-grade endometrial stromal sarcomas. *Am J Surg Pathol.* 2019;43(5):662-669.

9. Matsuzaki S, Matsuzaki S, Chang EJ, Yasukawa M, Roman LD, Matsuo K. Surgical and oncologic outcomes of hyperthermic intraperitoneal chemotherapy for uterine leiomyosarcoma: a systematic review of literature. *Gynecol Oncol.* 2021;161(1):70-77.

10. Díaz-Montes TP, El-Sharkawy F, Lynam S, et al. Efficacy of hyperthermic intraperitoneal chemotherapy and cytoreductive surgery in the treatment of recurrent uterine sarcoma. *Int J Gynecol Cancer.* 2018;28(6):1130-1137.

11. Ben-Ami E, Barysauskas CM, Solomon S, et al. Immunotherapy with single agent nivolumab for advanced leiomyosarcoma of the uterus: results of a phase 2 study. *Cancer.* 2017;123(17):3285-3290. doi:10.1002/cncr.30738

12. Shanes ED, Friedman LA, Mills AM. PD-L1 expression and tumor-infiltrating lymphocytes in uterine smooth muscle tumors: implications for immunotherapy. *Am J Surg Pathol.* 2019;43(6):792-801. doi:10.1097/PAS.0000000000001254

GESTATIONAL TROPHOBLASTIC DISEASE: MOLAR PREGNANCY AND GESTATIONAL TROPHOBLASTIC NEOPLASIA

Epidemiology, Genetics, and Pathology in Gestational Trophoblastic Disease

Sue Yazaki Sun, Gabriela Paiva, and Antonio Braga

INTRODUCTION

Gestational trophoblastic disease (GTD) comprises a heterogeneous group of rare conditions characterized by abnormal proliferation of placental trophoblast, with benign and malignant clinical forms (1). It includes the premalignant partial hydatidiform mole (PHM) and complete hydatidiform mole (CHM), and malignant forms, collectively called gestational trophoblastic neoplasia (GTN) (2). Most cases of GTN result from persistence of molar pregnancies after primary treatment and are diagnosed by elevation or stabilization of human chorionic gonadotropin (hCG) hormone values, measured weekly after uterine evacuation, and does not require histologic confirmation. GTN can also originate from any pregnancy event (term pregnancy, abortion, ectopic pregnancy), and its diagnosis will be suspected due to abnormal uterine bleeding or the presence of metastases without a defined primary site. The histopathologic forms of GTN are invasive mole (IM), choriocarcinoma (CCA), placental site trophoblastic tumor (PSTT), and epithelioid trophoblastic tumor (ETT) (3,4).

There are other benign entities of GTD, rare, less known, and studied, such as exaggerated placental site reaction and placental site nodule (3,5). They are usually incidental findings after abortion, childbirth, or hydatidiform mole, without the need for follow-up. However, when a placental site nodule has cellular atypia, it requires follow-up, as 10% to 15% may coexist with or develop into PSTT/ETT (6,7).

All forms (benign or malignant) of GTD have serum hCG levels as a reliable biochemical marker of disease progression to GTN, response to treatment, as well as post-treatment surveillance. This ensures early recognition of malignant progression of CHM and PHM through a plateaued or rising hCG level, which occurs in 15% to 20% and 0.5% to 5% of cases, respectively (6,8,9).

Earlier detection of molar pregnancy with ultrasonography, the use of hCG as a biomarker, advances in uterine evacuation, and the development of highly effective chemotherapy have transformed survival outcomes for these patients such that cure rates are now nearly 100%, especially when treated in reference centers (9,10).

EPIDEMIOLOGY

Epidemiologic differences related to the incidence of GTD may cover not only genetic, immunologic, environmental, and nutritional aspects but also the methodologic variability among published studies (2). It is difficult to establish the true incidence of hydatidiform mole, as well as defining the risk factors that contribute to the development of GTD. Interpretation and comparison between studies are limited owing to inconsistencies and uncertainties in the population at risk, no centralized databases, and the rarity of the disease (11).

Wide regional variations are described, worldwide incidence of GTD is around 0.57 to 2 per 1,000 pregnancies, with higher rates reported from Asia, Latin America, the Middle East, and Africa (12). The incidence of hydatidiform mole in Japan and the Republic of Korea used to be 2- to 3-fold higher than Europe or North America; however, contemporary studies reported that the incidence has fallen to what is reported in the rest of the world (13,14). Of note, the reported incidence of CCA ranges from 1 in 40,000 pregnancies in North America and Europe to 9.2 and 3.3 per 40,000 pregnancies in Southeast Asia and Japan, respectively (2).

The two main risk factors for GTD are extremes of maternal age (15) and a previous history of GTD (16). In one report, adolescence and advanced maternal age were specifically associated with increased incidence of CHM, but not of PHM (17). The risk of developing CHM in a population of women of childbearing age is nearly 2-fold higher for women younger than 21 years and above than 35 years and 7.5 times higher for women over 40 years, suggesting an increased risk of abnormal gametogenesis and fertilization of the ovum produced at reproductive age extremes (18-21).

Reproductive immaturity or senescence predisposes women to ovulation of an empty ovum to a greater degree than it permits abnormal fertilization by two sperm, which could explain the increased incidence of complete as opposed to partial moles at the extremes of age (17).

Patients under age 16 and above than age 45 had the highest relative risks of CHM (15,19). While adolescents with CHM are not at a higher risk of developing GTN (20), studies have shown that women older than 40 years with complete molar pregnancy are more likely to develop GTN and require additional treatment (22,23).

Reproductive history is of interest as a risk factor for trophoblastic disease. American and British studies have reported that women with a history of molar pregnancy (CHM, PHM, or GTN) have a 1% to 2% chance of molar recurrence in subsequent pregnancies, compared to an incidence of 0.1% in the general population. The recurrence rate is much higher after two molar pregnancies (16%-28%) (8). After two molar gestations, the risk of a third mole is 15% to 20% (24-26), and the risk is not decreased by change of partner (27). In addition, these patients are more likely to develop persistent gestational trophoblastic tumor in their later episodes of molar pregnancy (28,29). Rarely, CHM has a biparental chromosomal pattern and is associated with a mutation in the gene *NLRP7* or *KHDC3L* (30-32). This has been reported in familial recurrent molar pregnancy. A history of abortion increases the risk of both complete and partial moles 2-to 3-fold compared with women without a history of miscarriage (33,34). No difference in risk was reported for spontaneous or induced abortions (35).

Race/ethnicity is a risk factor for both complete and partial molar pregnancy. Most significantly, Asian women are more than twice as likely as Whites to develop CHM, and far less likely to develop PHM (2,36). Black women showed a lower risk of developing PHM, when compared to Whites (36,37). Hispanic women presented significantly lower risk of CHM and PHM, compared to Whites. However, regional variation in genetic, behavioral, socioeconomic, and cultural factors among self-identified Hispanics may explain the discrepancy between study findings concerning the risk for PHM in this population (38,39). A similar pattern of risk for CHM and PHM was noted for Black women as Hispanics (36).

Diet has also been suggested to have a role in the risk of developing molar pregnancy, in view of the high frequency of GTD in some regions where malnutrition is common and could help explain global differences in the incidence of CHM. Regions with a higher incidence of vitamin A deficiency also have a higher incidence of molar pregnancy. Case-control studies have been performed to identify risk factors for molar pregnancy. Studies from both the United States and Italy have indicated that the risk for complete molar pregnancy increases progressively with decreasing intake of animal fat and dietary carotene, a vitamin A precursor. They also showed an inverse relationship between dietary animal fat and animal protein and the risk for CHM (40,41). On the other hand, another study from the United States found no significant relationship between the dietary intake of carotene, fat, or protein and risk for PHM (34).

GENETICS

In most cases, CHMs are diploid and entirely derived from the paternal genome (42). It usually arises when an ovum without maternal chromosomes is fertilized by one sperm that then duplicates its DNA, resulting in a 46,XX homozygous androgenetic karyotype and the exclusion of the maternal chromosomal complement (43-45). Some complete moles (15%-25%) can arise after dispermic fertilization of an "empty" ovum and are either 46,XY or 46,XX. In either case, maternal chromosomes are lost before, or shortly after, fertilization. However, while nuclear DNA is entirely paternal in CHM, mitochondrial DNA remains maternal in origin (46,47) (**Figure 7.1-1**) (8).

PHM is triploid with maternal and paternal genetic origin with two sets of paternal haploid chromosomes and one set of maternal haploid chromosomes (**Figure 7.1-1**) (48,49). They usually result from fertilization of an ovum by two sperms or, very occasionally, a diploid sperm and may be 69,XXX, 69,XXY, or, less frequently, 69,XYY (50,51). Occasionally, molar pregnancies represent tetraploid or mosaic conceptions. In PHM, there is usually evidence of a fetus or fetal red blood cells.

Microsatellite short tandem repeat (STR) genotyping enables precise diagnosis of CHM and PHM by identifying the absence of maternal genetic contribution and diandric triploidy, respectively (6).

Although molar pregnancies are sporadic for the most part, a history of prior GTD increases the risk of a subsequent molar pregnancy to about 1% to 2% after one mole and to approximately 16% to 28% after two or more hydatidiform moles (28,29,52).

In patients who have had at least two episodes of molar pregnancy, assisted reproductive technology may help achieve normal fertilization of oocytes. However, standard in vitro fertilization (IVF) techniques and selection of oocytes and embryos presumed to be normal may still result in hydatidiform mole. In addition, the use of a donor ovum may also be employed to reduce the risk of molar disease (27).

A small number of patients with recurrent CHMs have an inherited predisposition to molar pregnancies and diploid biparental CHM rather than the typical androgenetic origin (**Figure 7.1-1**). In these cases, the molar phenotype is due to an autosomal recessive condition, the familial recurrent hydatidiform mole (FRHM) that predisposes women to recurrent pregnancy loss, usually CHM (53,54). Mutations in two maternal effect genes have been associated with this condition: *NLRP7* (75%-80% of cases) (31) and, more rarely, *KHDC3L* (32), which results in global imprinting alteration, leading to preferential expression of paternally imprinted genes in villous trophoblast (55,56). Women with FRHM are unlikely to achieve a normal pregnancy, except through ovum donation from an unaffected individual (8). A smaller number of women with recurrent molar pregnancies have recurrent androgenetic CHMs (53). Nevertheless, these women may also have normal pregnancies, do not have other affected family members, and have no effect

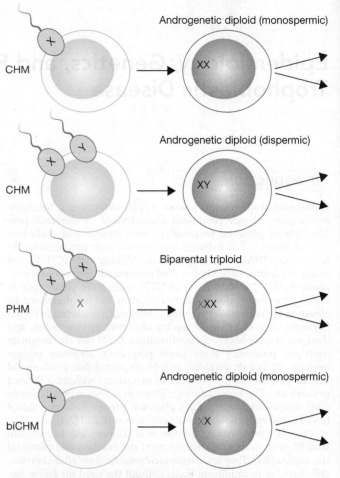

Figure 7.1-1. Cytogenetics of the complete (CHM) and partial hydatidiform mole (PHM). In CHM, we can observe a phenomenon of diandric diploidy arising by cytogenetic mechanisms of parthenogenesis, whereas in PHM, there is dignic triploidy, for the most part, by dyspermia. We also show the cytogenetic origin of the rare cases of biparental repetitive CHM. Reprinted from Seckl MJ, Sebire NJ, Berkowitz RS. Gestational trophoblastic disease. *Lancet.* 2010;376:717-729 with permission from Lancet.

gene mutations (46). For these patients, IVF with preimplantation genetic diagnosis can achieve a normal pregnancy (54).

Genetic analysis can also be helpful for GTN, when tissue is available, identifying the genotype of the causative pregnancy, when having both maternal and paternal chromosomes if the tumor originated in a term pregnancy, hydropic abortion, or PHM but only paternal genes if the causative pregnancy was a CHM (29,46). Because the interval from the causative pregnancy to the time of GTN diagnosis carries prognostic information, genotyping can be helpful, particularly in patients with multiple pregnancies (1,2). Genetics can also be important in the differential diagnosis between gestational and nongestational tumors, such as lung and gastric cancers, that can occasionally present as gestational CCA, but will have a genotype reflecting that of the patient (48,55).

PATHOLOGY

Molar pregnancies and GTN originate from the placental trophoblast, which is derived from the outermost layer of the blastocyst, called the trophectoderm (56). The trophoblast is composed of cytotrophoblast, syncytiotrophoblast, and intermediate trophoblast.

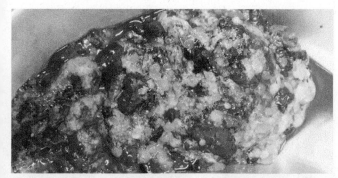

Figure 7.1-2. Macroscopy of complete hydatidiform mole with early gestational age (8 weeks of gestation).

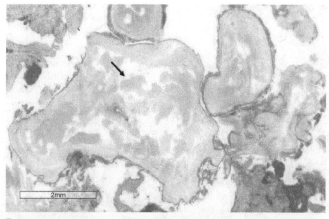

Figure 7.1-4. Complete hydatidiform mole microscopy. Note the presence of a voluminous central cistern (black arrow) and vesselless stroma and moderate trophoblast hyperplasia (blue arrow).

Syncytiotrophoblast invades the endometrial stroma upon implantation of the blastocyst and secretes hCG and other proteins to regulate the implantation site microenvironment. Cytotrophoblast fuses with syncytiotrophoblast to form the chorionic villi that cover the chorionic sac. Nonvillous cytotrophoblast differentiates into intermediate trophoblast, categorized as either implantation site or chorion type. Implantation site intermediate trophoblast loses the ability to proliferate but invades the maternal decidua and myometrium in a highly controlled manner, migrating to the maternal spiral arteries to facilitate oxygen and waste transfer between the fetus and the mother.

When regulatory mechanisms are impaired, invasive and vascular tumors arise. For example, TGF-β and a proteoglycan, decorin, have an inhibitory effect on nonvillous trophoblast cell growth, migration, and invasion, and this negative regulation is lost in trophoblast lesions (57,58).

All molar pregnancies are derived from the placenta and have in common the presence of enlarged, edematous, and vesicular villi showing variable amounts of abnormally proliferative trophoblast (59).

In CHM, both hydropic villi and trophoblastic proliferation are diffuse and cytologic atypia and mitosis are frequently observed in the trophoblast component (60,61).

Macroscopically, CHM presents with vesicles throughout the placenta and absence of fetal tissue and ovular membranes (**Figure 7.1-2**). In the second trimester, the vesicles present as large, swollen hydropic villi interspersed with blood clots similar to a "bunch of grapes" (**Figure 7.1-3**). The vesicles are translucent, filled with clear fluid, with a diameter of 1 to 1.5 mm in the first trimester

and 1.5 to 2.0 cm in the second trimester, weighing up to 2,000 g and occupying up to 3 L. Each vesicle is the chorionic villi that has become macroscopic by the accumulation of fluid in the villous stroma, leading to edematous degeneration. Microscopically, classic CHMs show enlarged, hydropic villi, generally moderate to marked, circumferential trophoblastic hyperplasia, often with cytologic atypia and prominent central cistern formation (**Figure 7.1-4**). Early CHMs, however, may be difficult to distinguish from nonmolar miscarriages on macroscopic examination. Fetal parts are absent (62). CHM is now more commonly diagnosed in the first trimester, and the degree of villous chorionic swelling and trophoblastic hyperplasia is more limited (59).

The *p57* gene is a gene with a paternal imprint but expressed by the mother. In CHM where there is no maternal genome, p57 is not expressed in chorionic villi (**Figure 7.1-5**). In contrast, PHM and nonmolar pregnancies have a maternal genome and express the *p57* gene. Therefore, immunohistochemical staining of p57 shows the absence of nuclear positivity in the villous cytotrophoblast and stromal nuclei (negative staining) with retained expression in intermediate trophoblastic cells and maternal decidua (secondary to epigenetic relaxation) (62). It cannot differentiate partial mole from hydropic spontaneous abortions, but it may be useful to distinguish partial from complete mole, especially in the first trimester of pregnancy, when morphologic features are not well characterized. So, the main applicability of p57 is in the differential diagnosis between CHM, in which it will be negative, and PHM, in which it will be positive (63).

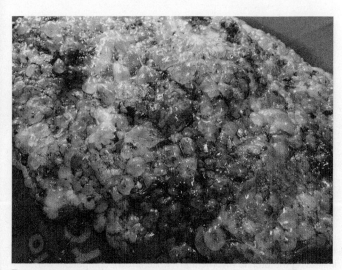

Figure 7.1-3. Macroscopy of complete hydatidiform mole in the second trimester (14 weeks of gestation).

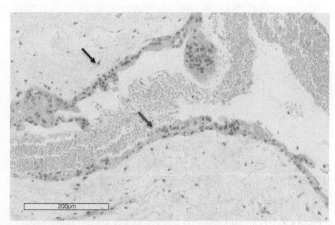

Figure 7.1-5. Immunoreactivity negative for p57 protein in the villous stroma (black arrow) and the cytotrophoblast (red arrow), indicative of the diagnosis of complete mole.

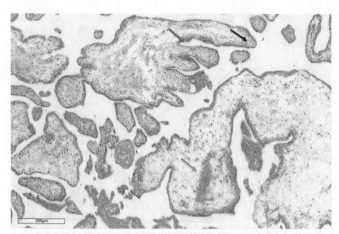

Figure 7.1-6. Partial hydatidiform mole microscopy. Note the double population of hydopic villi alongside smaller villi. There are also digitiform processes (black arrow) with inclusions (red arrow) and trophoblast invaginations (blue arrow).

In PHM, hydropic villi and trophoblastic proliferation are focal (**Figure 7.1-6**). There is expression of p57 (**Figure 7.1-7**). The villi are smaller than in CHM, and cell atypia is mild (60). There may be areas of normal-appearing placenta (**Figure 7.1-8**). If fetal tissue is well developed, the tissues will show malformations consistent with triploidy, such as syndactyly (1) (**Figure 7.1-9**).

Macroscopically, PHM is usually not as voluminous as in CHM with limited villous hydrops.

It is characterized by the focal presence of vesicles in the placenta, sometimes associated with the presence of conceptus and/or ovular membranes. The vesicles are smaller (1-5 mm in the first trimester and up to 2 cm in the second trimester) and intertwine areas of normal villi. The fetus is small and has multiple congenital anomalies.

Microscopically, PHMs have two distinct populations of villi. There are large, edematous villi, which at least focally have central cisterns, much like in CHM, although less prominent. There is a second population of small villi that usually show some degree of stromal fibrosis. As in CHM, there is abnormal trophoblastic proliferation around villi, but this finding is usually focal and can be hard to identify. Trophoblastic pseudoinclusions are frequently present and, although not pathognomonic of PHM, are highly suggestive (61,62).

IM is diagnosed histologically by identifying direct myometrial invasion by hydropic villi with trophoblastic proliferation in the myometrium (**Figure 7.1-10**). Hydropic villi invade the

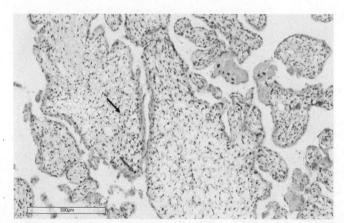

Figure 7.1-7. Immunoreactivity positive for p57 protein in the villous stroma (black arrow) and in the cytotrophoblast (red arrow) confirming the diagnosis of partial hydatidiform mole.

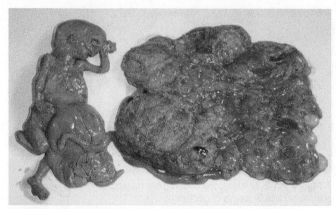

Figure 7.1-8. Macroscopy of a partial hydatidiform mole. We can see a malformed fetus with adnexa (umbilical cord and ovular membrane), placenta with a normal area, interspersed with vesicles, generally smaller in diameter than those of the complete hydatidiform mole.

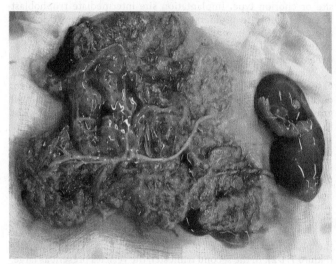

Figure 7.1-9. Case of partial hydatidiform mole with fetal presence and evident malformation (phocomelia), present in triploidy.

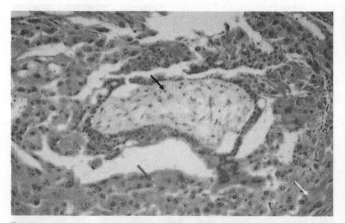

Figure 7.1-10. Chorionic villus (black arrow) and neoplastic trophoblast (red arrow) with marked atypia and hyperplasia infiltrating the uterine myometrium (white arrow), compatible with invasive mole.

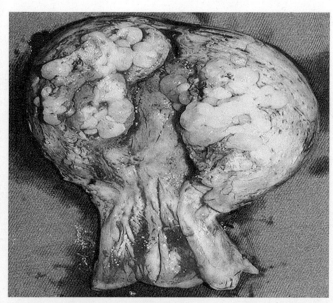

Figure 7.1-11. Invasive mole. Note the invasive nature of this entity in myometrial intimacy, clearly showing the presence of chorionic villi in the myometrium.

myometrium or blood vessels, and the lesion may be hemorrhagic, erosive, and extending from the cavity to the myometrium (**Figure 7.1-11**) (45,60,61). Histologically, the IM differs from the CCA by the presence of villi, which are absent in the CCA (64,65).

CCA is a highly malignant trophoblastic cell tumor developing in relation to a gestational event, comprising neoplastic trophoblasts in intermediate trophoblasts, cytotrophoblasts, and syncytiotrophoblasts. Cytologic atypia is very common, and most cases have high mitotic counts. The trophoblast presents cellular atypia with large, pleomorphic nuclei and abnormal mitotic figures (**Figure 7.1-12**). Aneuploidy is often identified. Central necrosis and hemorrhage are frequently seen in CCA tumor nodules. There are no chorionic villi. Deep myometrial invasion is common and can lead to uterine perforation (**Figure 7.1-13**) (60-62,65).

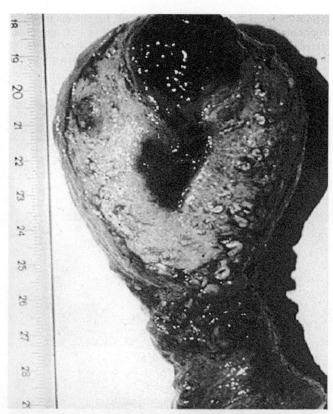

Figure 7.1-13. Macroscopy of choriocarcinoma. Note the darkened myometrial lesion, due to its hypervascular nature, in close contact with the uterine serosa, signaling the risk of uterine perforation. Note the absence of villous structures.

Macroscopically, CCA is characterized by a tumor that invades adjacent tissues and blood vessels, with central necrosis. Microscopically, it is characterized by proliferation of syncytium and cytotrophoblast interspersed with necrosis and hemorrhage; the intermediate trophoblast presents multinucleated giant cells with large nuclei and abnormal mitotic figures (8,64,65).

Apart from the uterus, it can be found in tubes, ovaries, vagina, lung, liver, spleen, kidneys, bowel, or brain (**Figures 7.1-14 to 7.1-19**) (8).

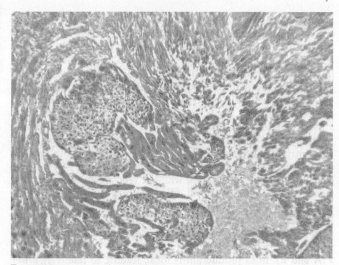

Figure 7.1-12. Choriocarcinoma microscopy. Proliferation of malignant epithelioid cells infiltrating the myometrium, with a biphasic pattern consisting of mononucleated sheets of cytotrophoblast/intermediate trophoblast enveloped by multinucleated syncytiotrophoblast.

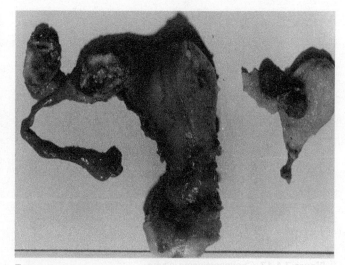

Figure 7.1-14. Choriocarcinoma in fallopian tube.

No single marker is sensitive or specific for the diagnosis of trophoblastic tumors, and therefore, a panel of immunomarkers is used. Tumors stain strongly for hCG and inhibin α in the cytotrophoblast and syncytiotrophoblast, human placental

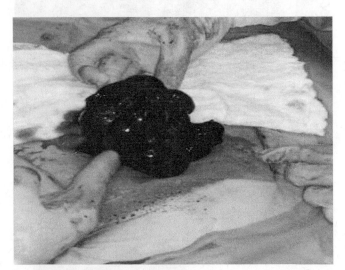

Figure 7.1-15. Choriocarcinoma in ovary.

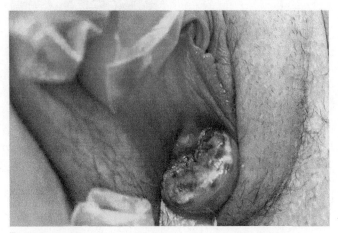

Figure 7.1-16. Choriocarcinoma in vagina.

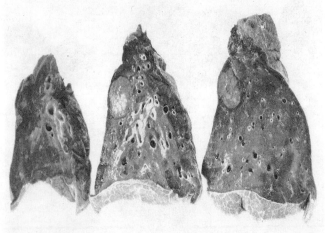

Figure 7.1-17. Choriocarcinoma in lung.

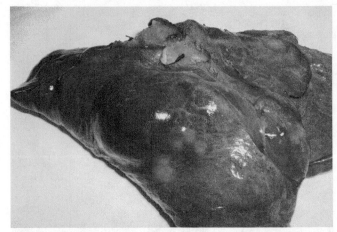

Figure 7.1-18. Choriocarcinoma in liver.

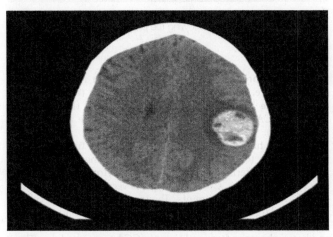

Figure 7.1-19. Choriocarcinoma in brain.

lactogen (hPL), and inhibin α in the intermediate trophoblast, and cytokeratin in all trophoblast cells and Ki-67 is diffusely expressed in approximately half of the cells. GATA-3 is a recent addition with approximately 80% of CCA that shows nuclear positivity of variable intensity (62,66). Genotyping analysis can identify unique paternal alleles and distinguish the gestational CCA of germ cell origin and somatic carcinoma with trophoblast differentiation (6).

PSTT lesions are uncommon and are usually diploid and monomorphic, characterized by the absence of villi, proliferation of cytotrophoblastic cells of the intermediate type, without syncytiotrophoblastic cells and with low mitotic counts. Macroscopically, it has fleshy consistency, white or yellow color and polypoid appearance (**Figure 7.1-20**). It grows from the uterine cavity outward, invading the endometrium, myometrium, and perimetrium, in this sequence, causing hemorrhage and necrosis (67). Compared with CCA, there is less hemorrhage, necrosis, and vascular invasion, but there is a higher risk of lymphatic metastasis (**Figure 7.1-21A and B**). hCG production is focal, leading to relatively lower serum levels. Microscopically, PSTT is formed by sheets or nests of round or polygonal monomorphic cells, with eosinophilic cytoplasm and a hyperchromatic and irregular nucleus (**Figure 7.1-21 C**) (67,68).

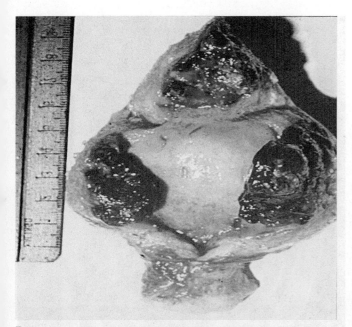

Figure 7.1-20. Macroscopy of the intrauterine placental site trophoblastic tumor. Multiple uterine lesions are observed with a hypervascular mass in the endometrium and myometrium.

Typically, the immunohistochemical profile of PSTT is strongly positive for hPL (**Figure 7.1-21D**) (67,69). Other tumor-associated biomarkers include cytokeratins (diffusely positive), epidermal growth factor receptor (strongly positive), and endothelial growth factor (strongly positive) (68-70).

ETT is rare and also derived from intermediate cytotrophoblastic cells. They often arise in the cervix or lower uterine segment, invading deeply into the surrounding tissues. Its diameter can vary from 0.5 to 15 cm. Macroscopically, a necrotic and hemorrhagic lesion is identified (**Figure 7.1-22**). Microscopically, this tumor comprises relatively small intermediate trophoblast cell nests with frequent eosinophilic cytoplasm and strong p63 expression. Intermediate trophoblast cells are uniform and monomorphic growing in rounded nests, leaves, and, occasionally, cords (**Figure 7.1-23**). It has a hyaline-like matrix and extensive necrosis surrounding blood vessels in a map-like distribution called geographic necrosis. The immunohistochemical profile of ETT is positive for cytokeratins, inhibin α, epithelial membrane antigen, hCG, and hPL, among others. The Ki-67 index in ETT is significantly lower than that in CCA (**Figure 7.1-24**). Cyclin E staining is higher in ETT than in placental site nodule and can help in differentiating between the two. p63 is reliably positive in ETT and is a useful marker in the differential diagnosis with other malignant trophoblastic tumors (**Figure 7.1-25**) (60,65,67,71).

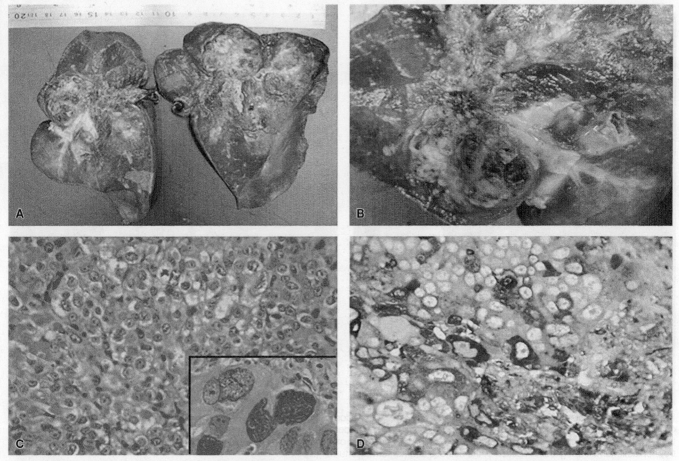

Figure 7.1-21. Pulmonary lobe with necrohemorrhagic areas (A and B), which on histopathology shows proliferation of the intermediate trophoblast (C), and which, by immunohistochemistry, was proved to be a metastatic pulmonary placental site trophoblast tumor with high immunoreactivity for human placental lactogen (D).

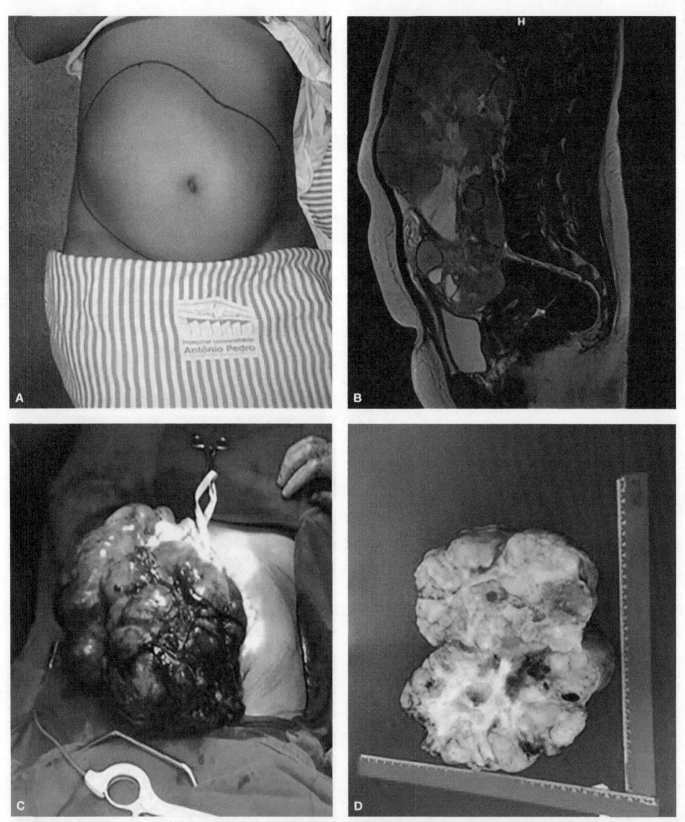

Figure 7.1-22. Patient presents to the emergency department with abdominal pain; physical examination identified a voluminous rigid mass occupying the entire abdomen (A). Magnetic resonance imaging of the abdomen and pelvis showed a close relationship between the mass and the uterus (B). Laparotomy found a mass with a macroscopic appearance of an epithelioid trophoblastic tumor (C). Macroscopy of epithelioid trophoblastic tumor. Longitudinal section of the necrotic and hemorrhagic tumor (D).

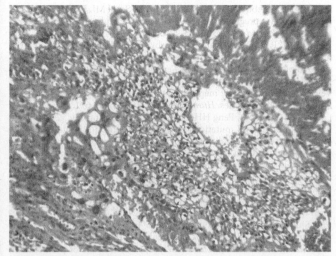

Figure 7.1-23. Epithelioid trophoblastic tumor microscopy. Proliferation of monomorphic epithelioid cells with clear cytoplasm and mild to focally moderate atypia.

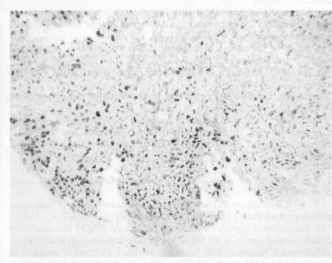

Figure 7.1-24. Epithelioid trophoblastic tumor microscopy. Ki-67 proliferative index exceeding 20%.

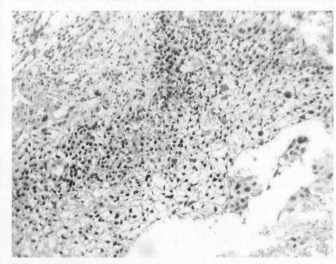

Figure 7.1-25. Epithelioid trophoblastic tumor microscopy. Diffuse immunopositivity for p63.

REFERENCES

1. Berkowitz RS, Goldstein DP. Current advances in the management of gestational trophoblastic disease. *Gynecol Oncol.* 2013;128(1):3-5.

2. Lurain JR. Gestational trophoblastic disease. I. Epidemiology, pathology, clinical presentation and diagnosis of gestational trophoblastic disease, and management of hydatidiform mole. *Am J Obstet Gynecol.* 2010;203:531-539.

3. Horn LC, Einenkel J, Hoehn AK. Classification and morphology of gestational trophoblastic disease. *Curr Obstet Gynecol Rep.* 2014;3(1):44-54.

4. Braga A, Mora P, de Melo AC, et al. Challenges in the diagnosis and treatment of gestational trophoblastic neoplasia worldwide. *World J Clin Oncol.* 2019;10(2):28-37.

5. Genest DR, Berkowitz RS, Fisher RA, Newlands ES, Fehr M. Gestational trophoblastic disease. In: Tavassoli FA, Devilee P, eds. *World Health Organization Classification of Tumors.* Tumors of the breast and female genital tract. IARC Press; 2003:250-254.

6. Ngan HYS, Seckl MJ, Berkowitz RS, et al. Diagnosis and management of gestational trophoblastic disease: 2021 update. *Int J Gynaecol Obstet.* 2021;155(1):86-93.

7. Kaur B, Short D, Fisher RA, Savage PM, Seckl MJ, Sebire NJ. Atypical placental site nodule (APSN) and association with malignant gestational trophoblastic disease; a clinicopathologic study of 21 cases. *Int J Gynecol Pathol.* 2015;34:152-158.

8. Seckl MJ, Sebire NJ, Berkowitz RS. Gestational trophoblastic disease. *Lancet.* 2010;376:717-729.

9. Clark JJ, Slater S, Seckl MJ. Treatment of gestational trophoblastic disease in the 2020s. *Curr Opin Obstet Gynecol.* 2021;33(1):7-12.

10. Braga A, Uberti EM, Fajardo Mdo C, et al. Epidemiological report on the treatment of patients with gestational trophoblastic disease in 10 Brazilian referral centers: results after 12 years since international FIGO 2000 consensus. *J Reprod Med.* 2014;59(5-6):241-247.

11. Bracken MB. Incidence and aetiology of hydatidiform mole: an epidemiological review. *Br J Obstet Gynaecol.* 1987;94:1123-1135.

12. Strohl AE, Lurain JR. Clinical epidemiology of gestational trophoblastic disease. *Curr Obstet Gynecol Rep.* 2013;3(1):40-43.

13. Yuk JS, Baek JC, Park JE, Jo HC, Park JK, Cho IA. Incidence of gestational trophoblastic disease in South Korea: a longitudinal, population-based study. *PeerJ.* 2019;20(7):e6490.

14. Matsui H, Kihara M, Yamazawa K, Mitsuhashi A, Seki K, Sekiya S. Recent changes of the incidence of complete and partial mole in Chiba prefecture. *Gynecol Obstet Invest.* 2007;63:7-10.

15. Savage PM, Sita-Lumsden A, Dickson S, et al. The relationship of maternal age to molar pregnancy incidence, risks for chemotherapy and subsequent pregnancy outcome. *J Obstet Gynaecol.* 2013;33(4):406-411.

16. Parazzini F, Mangili G, La Vecchia C, et al. Risk factors for gestational trophoblastic disease: a separate analysis of complete and partial hydatidiform moles. *Obstet Gynecol.* 1991;78(6):1039-1045.

17. Gockley AA, Melamed A, Joseph NT, et al. The effect of adolescence and advanced maternal age on the incidence of complete and partial molar pregnancy. *Gynecol Oncol.* 2016;140(3):470-473.

18. Parazzini F, La Vecchia C, Pampallona S. Parental age and risk of complete and partial hydatidiform mole. *Br J Obstet Gynaecol.* 1986;93(6):582-585.

19. Sebire NJ, Foskett M, Fisher RA, et al. Risk of partial and complete hydatidiform molar pregnancy in relation to maternal age. *BJOG.* 2002;109(1):99-102.

20. Braga A, Growdon WB, Bernstein M, et al. Molar pregnancy in adolescents. *J Reprod Med.* 2012;57(5-6):225-230.

21. Rauh-Hain JA, Growdon WB, Braga A, Goldstein DP, Berkowitz RS. Gestational trophoblastic neoplasia in adolescents. *J Reprod Med.* 2012;57(5-6):237-242.

22. Elias KM, Shoni M, Bernstein M, Goldstein DP, Berkowitz RS. Complete hydatidiform mole in women aged 40 to 49 years. *J Reprod Med.* 2012;57(5-6):254-258.

23. Elias KM, Goldstein DP, Berkowitz RS. Complete hydatidiform mole in women older than age 50. *J Reprod Med.* 2010;55(5-6):208-212.

24. Bagshawe KD, Dent J, Webb J. Hydatidiform mole in England and Wales 1973-83. *Lancet.* 1986;328:673-677.

25. Garrett LA, Garner EI, Feltmate CM, Goldstein DP, Berkowitz RS. Subsequent pregnancy outcomes in patients with molar pregnancy and persistent gestational trophoblastic neoplasia. *J Reprod Med.* 2008;53:481-486.

26. Sebire NJ, Fisher RA, Foskett M, Rees H, Seckl MJ, Newlands ES. Risk of recurrent hydatidiform mole and subsequent pregnancy outcome following complete or partial hydatidiform molar pregnancy. *BJOG.* 2003;110:22-26.

27. Tuncer ZS, Bernstein MR, Wang J, Goldstein DP, Berkowitz RS. Repetitive hydatidiform mole with different male partners. *Gynecol Oncol.* 1999;75(2):224-226.

28. Sand PK, Lurain JR, Brewer JL. Repeat gestational trophoblastic disease. *Obstet Gynecol.* 1984;63:140-144.

29. Berkowitz RS, Im SS, Bernstein MR, Goldstein DP. Gestational trophoblastic disease: subsequent pregnancy outcome, including repeat molar pregnancy. *J Reprod Med.* 1998;43:81-86.

30. Wang CM, Dixon PH, Decordova S, et al. Identification of 13 novel NLRP7 mutations in 20 families with recurrent hydatidiform mole; missense mutations cluster in the leucine-rich region. *J Med Genet.* 2009;46:569-575.

31. Murdoch S, Djuric U, Mazhar B, et al. Mutations in NALP7 cause recurrent hydatidiform moles and reproductive wastage in humans. *Nat Genet.* 2006;38:300-302.

32. Parry DA, Logan CV, Hayward BE, et al. Mutations causing familial biparental hydatidiform mole implicate c6orf221 as a possible regulator of genomic imprinting in the human oocyte. *Am J Hum Genet.* 2011;89:451-458.

33. Parazzini F, Mangili G, La Vecchia C, Negri E, Bocciolone L, Fasoli M. Risk factors for gestational trophoblastic disease: a separate analysis of complete and partial hydatidiform moles. *Obstet Gynecol.* 1991;78:1039-1045.

34. Berkowitz RS, Bernstein MR, Harlow BL, et al. Case-control study of risk factors for partial molar pregnancy. *Am J Obstet Gynecol.* 1995;173(3 pt 1):788-794.

35. Acaia B, Parazzini F, La Vecchia C, Ricciardiello O, Fedele L, Battista Candiani G. Increased frequency of complete hydatidiform mole in women with repeated abortion. *Gynecol Oncol.* 1988;31(2):310-314.

36. Melamed A, Gockley AA, Joseph NT, et al. Effect of race/ethnicity on risk of complete and partial molar pregnancy after adjustment for age. *Gynecol Oncol.* 2016;143(1):73-76.

37. Hayashi K, Bracken MB, Freeman DH Jr, Hellenbrand K. Hydatidiform mole in the United States (1970-1977): a statistical and theoretical analysis. *Am J Epidemiol.* 1982;115(1):67-77.

38. Smith HO, Hilgers RD, Bedrick EJ, et al. Ethnic differences at risk for gestational trophoblastic disease in New Mexico: a 25-year population-based study. *Am J Obstet Gynecol.* 2003;188(2):357-366.

39. Drake RD, Rao GG, McIntire DD, Miller DS, Schorge JO. Gestational trophoblastic disease among hispanic women: a 21-year hospital-based study. *Gynecol Oncol.* 2006;103(1):81-86.

40. Parazzini F, La Vecchia C, Mangili G, et al. Dietary factors and risk of trophoblastic disease. *Am J Obstet Gynecol.* 1988;158(1):93-99.

41. Berkowitz RS, Cramer DW, Bernstein MR, Cassells S, Driscoll SG, Goldstein DP. Risk factors for complete molar pregnancy from a case-control study. *Am J Obstet Gynecol.* 1985;152(8):1016-1020.

42. Kajii T, Ohama K. Androgenetic origin of hydatidiform mole. *Nature.* 1977;268:633-634.

43. Yamashita K, Ishikawa M, Shimizu T, Kuroda M. HLA antigens in husband-wife pairs with trophoblastic tumour. *Gynaecol Oncol.* 1981;12:68-74.

44. Fisher RA, Newlands ES. Gestational trophoblastic disease: molecular and genetic studies. *J Reprod Med.* 1998;43:81-97.

45. Seckl MJ, Sebire NJ, Fisher RA, Golfier F, Massuger L, Sessa C. ESMO guidelines working group. Gestational trophoblastic disease: ESMO clinical practice guidelines for diagnosis, treatment and follow-up. *Ann Oncol.* 2013;24(6):39-50.

46. Fisher RA, Maher GJ. Genetics of gestational trophoblastic disease. *Best Pract Res Clin Obstet Gynecol.* 2021;74:29-41.

47. Kajii T, Ohama K. Androgenetic origin of hydatidiform mole. *Nature.* 1977; 268(5621): 633-4.

48. Lawler SD, Fisher RA, Pickthall VJ, Povey S, Evans MW. Genetic studies on hydatidiform moles. I. The origin of partial moles. *Cancer Genet Cytogenet.* 1982;5:309-320.

49. Jacobs PA, Szulman AE, Funkhouser J, Matsuura JS, Wilson CC. Human triploidy: relationship between parental origin of the additional haploid complement and development of partial hydatidiform mole. *Ann Hum Genet.* 1982;46:223-231.

50. Eagles N, Sebire NJ, Short D, Savage PM, Seckl MJ, Fisher RA. Risk of recurrent molar pregnancies following complete and partial hydatidiform moles. *Hum Reprod.* 2015;30:2055-2063.

51. Savage P, Sebire N, Dalton T, Carby A, Seckl MJ, Fisher RA. Partial molar pregnancy after intracytoplasmic sperm injection occurring as a result of diploid sperm usage. *J Assist Reprod Genet.* 2013;30:761-764.

52. Moglabey YB, Kircheisen R, Seoud M, El Mogharbel N, Van den Veyver I, Slim R. Genetic mapping of a maternal locus responsible for familial hydatidiform moles. *Hum Mol Genet.* 1999;8:667-671.

53. Kou YC, Shao L, Peng HH, et al. A recurrent intragenic genomic duplication, other novel mutations in NLRP7 and imprinting defects in recurrent biparental hydatidiform moles. *Mol Hum Reprod.* 2008;14:33-40.

54. Deveault C, Qian JH, Chebaro W, et al. NLRP7 mutations in women with diploid androgenetic and triploid moles: a proposed mechanism for mole formation. *Hum Mol Genet.* 2009;18:888-897.

55. Ogilvie CM, Renwick PJ, Khalaf Y, Braude PR. First use of preimplantation genotyping in prevention of recurrent diandric complete hydatidiform mole. *Reprod Biomed Online.* 2009;19:224-227.

56. Shih IM, Kurman RJ. The pathology of intermediate trophoblastic tumors and tumor-like lesions. *Int J Gynecol Pathol.* 2001;20(1):31-47.

57. Xu G, Guimond MJ, Chakraborty C, et al. Control of proliferation, migration, and invasiveness of human extravillous trophoblast by decorin, a decidual product. *Biol Reprod.* 2002;67(2):681-689.

58. Xu G, Chakraborty C, Lala PK. Expression of TGF-beta signaling genes in the normal, premalignant, and malignant human trophoblast: loss of smad3 in choriocarcinoma cells. *Biochem Biophys Res Commun.* 2001;287(1):47-55.

59. Mosher R, Goldstein DP, Berkowitz R, Bernstein M, Genest DR. Complete hydatidiform mole. Comparison of clinicopathologic features, current and past. *J Reprod Med.* 1998;43(1):21-27.

60. Soper JT. Gestational trophoblastic disease: current evaluation and management. *Obstet Gynecol.* 2021;137(2): 355-370.

61. Bentley RC. Pathology of gestational trophoblastic disease. *Clin Obstet Gynecol.* 2003;46(3):513-522.

62. Kaur B. Pathology of gestational trophoblastic disease (GTD). *Best Pract Res Clin Obstet Gynaecol.* 2021;74:3-28.

63. Mondal SK, Mandal S, Bhattacharya S, Panda UK, Ray A, Alsi SM. Expression of P57 immunomarker in the classification and differential diagnosis of partial and complete hydatidiform moles. *J Lab Physicians.* 2019;11:270-274.

64. Altieri A, Franceschi S, Ferlay J, Smith J, La Vecchia C. Epidemiology and etiology of gestational trophoblastic diseases. *Lancet Oncol.* 2003;4:670-678.

65. Hui P. Gestational trophoblastic tumors: a timely review of diagnostic pathology. *Arch Pathol Lab Med.* 2019;143:65-74.

66. International Agency for Research on Cancer. *WHO Classification of Female Genital Tumours.* 5th ed. World Health Organization; 2020:309e22.

67. Brown J, Naumann RW, Seckl MJ, Schink J. 15 Years of progress in gestational trophoblastic disease: scoring, standardization, and salvage. *Gynecol Oncol.* 2016;144(1):200-207.

68. Gadducci A, Carinelli S, Guerrieri ME, Aletti GD. Placental site trophoblastic tumor and epithelioid trophoblastic tumor: clinical and pathological features, prognostic variables and treatment strategy. *Gynecol Oncol.* 2019;153(7):684-693.

69. Rey Valzacchi GM, Odetto D, Chacon CB, Wernicke A, Xiang Y. Placental site trophoblastic disease. *Int J Gynecol Cancer.* 2020;30(1):144-149.

70. De Nola R, Schönauer LM, Fiore MG, Loverro M, Carriero C, Di Naro E. Management of placental site trophoblastic tumor: two case reports. *Medicine (Baltimore).* 2018;97(48):134-139.

71. Ronnett BM. Hydatidiform moles: differential diagnosis, diagnostic reproducibility, genetics and ancillary techniques to refine diagnosis. *Diagn Histopath.* 2019;25(2):35-52.

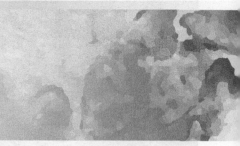

CHAPTER 7.2

Management of Molar Pregnancy

Kevin M. Elias, Neil S. Horowitz, and Ross S. Berkowitz

INTRODUCTION

The management of molar pregnancy can be divided into two phases. The first consideration is making the diagnosis, which relies on clinical suspicion, ultrasonographic findings, and an elevated hCG level. Attendant medical complications need to be managed, followed by surgical evacuation of the pregnancy. The second phase is postmolar surveillance, where the primary focus is on monitoring for progression from benign molar pregnancy to GTN. The likelihood of requiring chemotherapy depends on whether the pathology reveals complete or partial mole and maternal age, but timely diagnosis of progression reduces the risk of medical complications from high disease burden and the likelihood that multiagent chemotherapy will be required to achieve remission. Here, we review the initial assessment of the patient with suspected molar pregnancy and principles of postmolar care.

Patient Assessment

Molar pregnancy should be in the differential diagnosis for any woman presenting with abnormal uterine bleeding, an elevated hCG level, and an intrauterine mass. Other considerations include early pregnancy, spontaneous abortion, and other forms of GTN. Nonmolar hydropic abortion and placental mesenchymal dysplasia are frequently mistaken for molar pregnancies because both present with villous edema and dilated cystic spaces on ultrasound (1). As noted earlier, in cases of histologic uncertainty, molecular genotyping can distinguish between nonmolar and molar gestations.

Classically, CHM was associated with a uterine size greater than expected for gestational age, markedly elevated serum hCG levels, vaginal bleeding, and theca lutein cysts. Early-onset hyperemesis gravidarum and preeclampsia were also relatively common (2,3). However, most molar pregnancies are now diagnosed in the first trimester due to routine hCG testing and access to transvaginal ultrasound (4-5). This has changed the clinical presentation of CHM

(Table 7.2-1) (6,7). At the New England Trophoblastic Disease Center, whereas the median gestation at the time of uterine evacuation used to be 16 weeks, in more recent years, it has fallen to 9 weeks. Although vaginal bleeding in early pregnancy remains the most common symptom, patients may be asymptomatic and diagnosed with a missed abortion on routine ultrasound (8). Nearly identical trends have been reported in Brazil, Italy, and China (9-11). Because of early gestational ages, around one-third of CHM and two-thirds of PHM are misdiagnosed on ultrasound as cases of missed abortion, and the molar histology is only recognized after uterine evacuation (12). This highlights the importance of routine histologic assessment of products of conception (13).

The evaluation of a patient with a suspected molar pregnancy should include a transvaginal ultrasound, a quantitative serum hCG measurement, and a physical examination, including a pelvic examination (14). A transvaginal pelvic ultrasound is the only required imaging study. The characteristic vesicular or "snowstorm" pattern imparted by the generalized swelling of the chorionic villi normally appears by 8 weeks of gestation (Figure 7.2-1) (15). At earlier gestational ages, only an intrauterine mass may be evident. Partial moles are frequently misdiagnosed as missed abortions, but cystic spaces in the placenta and a ratio of transverse to anteroposterior dimension of the gestational sac greater than 1.5 may raise concern for PHM (Figure 7.2-2) (16,17). A speculum examination is essential to exclude cervical or vaginal metastases and to evaluate for vaginal bleeding. A thorough lung examination should evaluate for pulmonary edema or effusions, a basic neurologic exam should exclude focal neurologic deficits, and an abdominal examination may note an enlarged uterus or adnexal masses.

Rarely, molar pregnancy can occur in twin gestations along with a normal fetus. In these cases, partial mole must also be excluded. Twin molar gestations are high-risk pregnancies and are associated with preeclampsia and vaginal hemorrhage (18). In a review of 72 cases of multiple gestations with complete mole and coexisting fetus among five centers in the United States and Brazil, the overall

TABLE 7.2-1. Change in Presentation of Complete Mole Over Time at the New England Trophoblastic Disease Center			
	1965-1975 (N = 306)	1988-1993 (N = 74)	1994-2013 (N = 180)
Median gestational age at evacuation, weeks	16	12	9
Vaginal bleeding, N (%)	297 (97%)	62 (84%)	80 (46%)
Hyperemesis, N (%)	80 (26%)	6 (8%)	25 (14%)
Uterine size greater than dates, N (%)	156 (51%)	21 (28%)	34 (24%)
Preeclampsia, N (%)	83 (27%)	1 (1%)	2 (1%)
Respiratory insufficiency, N (%)	6 (2%)	0 (0%)	2 (1%)
Progression to GTN, N (%)[a]	57 (18.6%)	15/64 (23%)	33/172 (19%)

GTN, gestational trophoblastic neoplasia.

[a]Numbers reflect patients completing hCG surveillance.

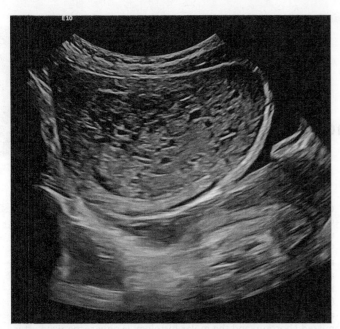

Figure 7.2-1. Sonogram at 11 weeks of gestational age showing a thickened endometrium with innumerable cystic spaces consistent with complete molar pregnancy.

rate of GTN was 46%. Elective termination of pregnancy was not associated with a reduction in GTN risk, and 60% of 60 continued pregnancies resulted in viable live birth (19). Similar findings were reported from Charing Cross Hospital in the United Kingdom, where 20 of 28 continued pregnancies resulted in live births (20).

Serum hCG is the key laboratory measure for assessing molar pregnancies. Of note, hCG assays vary in their capacity to measure different hCG isoforms, such as total hCG, hyperglycosylated hCG (hCG-H), nicked hCG, hCG missing the β-subunit C-terminal peptide, free α-subunit, free β-subunit, nicked free b-subunit, and the urine β-core fragment (21). Molar pregnancies and other forms for GTD often produce a larger proportion of hCG fragments compared to normal pregnancies (22). Providers should always order a "tumor-specific" hCG test, not a pregnancy hCG test, whenever possible. If the clinical presentation is highly suspicious for a molar pregnancy, but the hCG test is negative, a serial dilution of the sample should be requested. A false-negative hCG may occur when hCG values are extremely high. Known as the "hook effect," this occurs in sandwich assays when an overabundance of hCG saturates

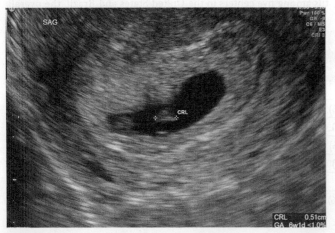

Figure 7.2-2. Sonogram at 6 weeks of gestational age from a missed abortion, subsequently diagnosed as a partial molar pregnancy, with the crown rump length (CRL) of the fetus indicated.

the capture antibody and prevents formation of the capture and detect antibody complex (23). False-positive hCG results may occur with low-level hCG, either from pituitary hCG or from heterophile antibodies (such as anti-mouse antibodies) (14). Placing a patient on high-dose oral contraceptives or gonadotropin hormone-releasing hormone (GnRH) agonists can suppress pituitary hCG. Comparing urine hCG values to serum hCG values can help distinguish heterophile antibodies as these do not cross the glomerulus.

Initial Management

Surgery is the cornerstone of initial therapy for molar pregnancies. Most patients undergo surgical uterine evacuation via dilation and curettage (24). The technique is quick, effective, and preserves fertility. Ultrasound guidance is associated with lower rates of complications from pregnancy termination and is advisable to ensure complete evacuation of uterine contents (25). Electric and manual vacuum aspiration are similarly safe and efficacious (26,27). In select patients who do not desire future fertility, particularly those older than 40 years with complete mole, hysterectomy is a reasonable alternative to evacuation. By eliminating any locally invasive disease, total hysterectomy substantially reduces the chances of GTN and the likelihood that a patient will require chemotherapy (28,29). In a meta-analysis focused on patients older than 40 years with molar pregnancies, primary hysterectomy reduced the chances of postmolar GTN by 80% compared to uterine evacuation (30). Medical methods of pregnancy termination should not be used for molar pregnancies due to a higher rate of incomplete uterine evacuation (31).

The technique for uterine evacuation is analogous to pregnancy termination for other indications. Patients should have an active type and screen. Patients who are RhD-negative should receive anti-D immune globulin at the time of treatment (32). Blood products should be available. Mechanical dilation of the cervix is performed with serial graduated Hegar or Hanks dilators. A simple guideline is to dilate to a diameter to accommodate a cannula diameter equal to or 1 mm smaller than the number of weeks of gestation of a similarly sized normal intrauterine pregnancy. Disruption of the pregnancy may induce brisk bleeding, and the rate of bleeding is substantially more than that encountered during normal pregnancy termination. At the time of anesthesia induction, an oxytocin infusion may promote myometrial contraction and decreases blood loss. As noted earlier, sonographic guidance can ensure a complete evacuation and shorten the procedure time. In cases of severe bleeding, uterine tamponade may be achieved with a Bakri balloon or a 30-mL Foley catheter. Uterine artery embolization may be required to control hemorrhage, but emergent hysterectomy is rare.

Following uterine evacuation, prophylactic chemotherapy is not usually required. In select cases where follow-up is unavailable or unreliable and the risk of GTN is high (age >40 years, preevacuation hCG levels >100,000, or very large theca lutein cysts), a single dose of pulsed actinomycin-D (Act-D) postoperatively may be considered (33,34). However, this should be balanced against potentially unnecessary chemotoxicity and the risk of induction of resistance to subsequent therapy.

Postmolar Surveillance

Following uterine evacuation, weekly hCG levels are followed until undetectable (35). A rising hCG, defined as a level that progressively increases more than 10% across three values during at least a 2-week period (eg, on days 1, 7, and 14), or a plateaued hCG level, defined as four measurements that remain within ±10% over at least a 3-week period (eg, days 1, 7, 14, and 21) meet criteria for GTN (36). Chemotherapy should be promptly initiated. Persistence of an elevated hCG level more than 6 months following evacuation or an hCG level greater than 20,000 IU/L at 4 weeks postevacuation suggest a higher risk of GTN but are no longer considered sufficient indications to begin chemotherapy (5,37).

Historically, all patients were advised to continue weekly surveillance until levels were below the lower limit of normal on a local assay for 3 weeks and then monthly for 6 months. However, the overall likelihood of experiencing a reelevation of the hCG level once a single normal value is reached is less than 1% (38-40). For partial moles, the risk approaches 0% (41). In the largest series from the Charing Cross Hospital, comprising more than 20,144 consecutive cases of molar pregnancy, only 29 (0.14%) cases had a reelevation in hCG after achieving one normal level (42). For CHM, the risk of GTN after hCG normalization was 1:406, whereas for PHM, the risk of GTN after hCG normalization was 1:3,195. Thus, surveillance guidelines have been modified to stop surveillance after a single normal value for partial moles and 3 months for complete moles (43,44).

Maternal age is the most important risk factor for predicting postmolar GTN. While adolescents have a higher risk of developing CHM, they have similar risks of progression to postmolar GTN (45,46). However, women older than 40 will develop GTN in more than 50% of cases, and women older than 50 will develop GTN in 60% of cases (28,29,47). The higher likelihood of requiring chemotherapy for older women with CHM is an important factor when counseling patients about the risks of primary hysterectomy versus uterine evacuation. However, rates of GTN following PHM are low, regardless of maternal age (48).

The rate of hCG decline following uterine evacuation is prognostic for the risk of progression to GTN. If the hCG takes more than 56 days to normalize, the risk of GTN increases by 3.8-fold (42). In a series from the Netherlands, a single hCG value at 4 weeks postevacuation had 97.5% specificity for predicting GTN (49). Other models have considered the slope of the hCG regression curve (50). Importantly, all these models require correlation with a locally derived nomogram related to local hCG testing patterns and patient population; thus, the external validity of these regression curves has not been established (51-53). However, the hCG regression curve after molar evacuation is not clinically significantly influenced by the patient's age, race, ethnicity, the presence of obesity, or the use of hormonal contraception (54).

Ideally, the risk of postmolar GTN would be estimated from biomarkers present in molar tissue at the time of uterine evacuation (55). Ki-67, a proliferation marker used commonly in many malignancies, has been examined by several groups, but the results have been inconsistent across studies, with some reports suggesting a strong correlation with progression to GTN and others observing no association (56-59). Markers of apoptosis, that is, programmed cell death, have also attracted interest because altered apoptotic responses are a common feature of many placental diseases (60). Expression of the proapoptotic enzyme caspase-3 is associated with a lower risk of GTN; in a study of 780 cases of CHM, a caspase-3 apoptotic index 4% or more had a 97% negative predictive value for GTN (61). Conversely BCL2, a key upstream regulator of apoptosis, is lower in the villi of CHM destined to progress to GTN compared to those which spontaneously regress, and expression of the microRNAs miR-181b-5p and miR-181d-5p, which negatively regulate BCL2, is higher (62). In fact, a continuum of BCL2 expression has been described from normal placentas to molar pregnancies to choriocarcinoma, with expression essentially absent among choriocarcinoma (63,64). Progression of CHM to GTN is also associated with reduced expression of miRNAs in the 14q32 cluster and lower expression of the protein DIO3 (65,66).

Contraception During Human Chorionic Gonadotropin Surveillance

Interval pregnancy should always be considered with a new rise in hCG. As the likelihood of developing GTN after a single normal hCG value is less than 1% and the risk of a repeat molar pregnancy if another gestation occurs is also 1% to 2%, distinguishing true "relapse" from the development of a second molar pregnancy is difficult. Thus, reliable contraception is essential during gonadotropin surveillance.

Oral contraceptives are generally preferred because in addition to providing contraception, estrogen-containing preparations suppress pituitary hCG. Historically, there were concerns that oral contraceptives might hormonally stimulate trophoblastic tumors and increase the risk for chemotherapy (67). However, this finding was noted to be confounded by maternal age (68). Subsequent studies from both the United Kingdom and Brazil have decidedly shown that use of hormonal contraception is not associated with the development of postmolar GTN or delayed time to hCG remission (69,70). We strongly recommend oral contraception use during postmolar hCG monitoring.

REFERENCES

1. Marinho M, Nogueira R, Soares C, Melo M, Godinho C, Brito C. Placental spectrum features between mesenchymal dysplasia and partial hydatidiform mole coexisting with a live fetus. *J Clin Ultrasound.* 2021;49:841-846.

2. Curry SL, Hammond CB, Tyrey L, Creasman WT, Parker RT. Hydatidiform mole: diagnosis, management, and long-term followup of 347 patients. *Obstet Gynecol.* 1975;45:1-8.

3. Kohorn EI. Molar pregnancy: presentation and diagnosis. *Clin Obstet Gynecol.* 1984;27:181-191.

4. Sun SY, Melamed A, Joseph NT, et al. Clinical presentation of complete hydatidiform mole and partial hydatidiform mole at a regional trophoblastic disease center in the United States over the past 2 decades. *Int J Gynecol Cancer.* 2016;26:367-370.

5. Braga A, Torres B, Burla M, et al. Is chemotherapy necessary for patients with molar pregnancy and human chorionic gonadotropin serum levels raised but falling at 6months after uterine evacuation? *Gynecol Oncol.* 2016;143:558-564.

6. Soto-Wright V, Bernstein M, Goldstein DP, Berkowitz RS. The changing clinical presentation of complete molar pregnancy. *Obstet Gynecol.* 1995;86:775-779.

7. Sun SY, Melamed A, Goldstein DP, et al. Changing presentation of complete hydatidiform mole at the New England trophoblastic disease center over the past three decades: does early diagnosis alter risk for gestational trophoblastic neoplasia? *Gynecol Oncol.* 2015;138:46-49.

8. Sebire NJ, Rees H, Paradinas F, Seckl M, Newlands E. The diagnostic implications of routine ultrasound examination in histologically confirmed early molar pregnancies. *Ultrasound Obstet Gynecol.* 2001;18:662-665.

9. Braga A, Moraes V, Maesta I, et al. Changing trends in the clinical presentation and management of complete hydatidiform mole among Brazilian women. *Int J Gynecol Cancer.* 2016;26:984-990.

10. Mangili G, Garavaglia E, Cavoretto P, Gentile C, Scarfone G, Rabaiotti E. Clinical presentation of hydatidiform mole in northern Italy: has it changed in the last 20 years? *Am J Obstet Gynecol.* 2008;198:302.e1-302.e4.

11. Hou JL, Wan XR, Xiang Y, Qi QW, Yang XY. Changes of clinical features in hydatidiform mole: analysis of 113 cases. *J Reprod Med.* 2008;53:629-633.

12. Memtsa M, Johns J, Jurkovic D, Ross JA, Sebire NJ, Jauniaux E. Diagnosis and outcome of hydatidiform moles in missed-miscarriage: a cohort-study, systematic review and meta-analysis. *Eur J Obstet Gynecol Reprod Biol.* 2020;253:206-212.

13. Tasci Y, Dilbaz S, Secilmis O, Dilbaz B, Ozfuttu A, Haberal A. Routine histopathologic analysis of product of conception following first-trimester spontaneous miscarriages. *J Obstet Gynaecol Res.* 2005;31:579-582.

14. Berkowitz RS, Goldstein DP. Current management of gestational trophoblastic diseases. *Gynecol Oncol.* 2009;112:654-662.

15. Benson CB, Genest DR, Bernstein MR, Soto-Wright V, Goldstein DP, Berkowitz RS. Sonographic appearance of first trimester complete hydatidiform moles. *Ultrasound Obstet Gynecol.* 2000;16:188-191.

16. Fine C, Bundy AL, Berkowitz RS, Boswell SB, Berezin AF, Doubilet PM. Sonographic diagnosis of partial hydatidiform mole. *Obstet Gynecol.* 1989;73:414-418.

17. Savage JL, Maturen KE, Mowers EL, et al. Sonographic diagnosis of partial versus complete molar pregnancy: a reappraisal. *J Clin Ultrasound.* 2017;45:72-78.

18. Irani RA, Holliman K, Debbink M, et al. Complete molar pregnancies with a coexisting fetus: pregnancy outcomes and review of literature. *AJP Rep.* 2022;12:e96-e107.

19. Lin LH, Maesta I, Braga A, et al. Multiple pregnancies with complete mole and coexisting normal fetus in North and South America: a retrospective multicenter cohort and literature review. *Gynecol Oncol.* 2017;145:88-95.

20. Sebire NJ, Foskett M, Paradinas FJ, et al. Outcome of twin pregnancies with complete hydatidiform mole and healthy co-twin. *Lancet.* 2002;359:2165-2166.

21. Cole LA, Butler S. Detection of hCG in trophoblastic disease. The USA hCG reference service experience. *J Reprod Med.* 2002;47:433-444.

22. Stenman UH, Alfthan H, Hotakainen K. Human chorionic gonadotropin in cancer. *Clin Biochem.* 2004;37:549-561.

23. Herskovits AZ, Chen Y, Latifi N, Ta RM, Kriegel G. False-negative urine human chorionic gonadotropin testing in the clinical laboratory. *Lab Med.* 2020;51:86-93.

24. Berkowitz RS, Horowitz NS, Elias KM. Hydatidiform mole: treatment and follow-up. In: Goff B, ed. *UpToDate.* Wolters Kluwer; 2021. https://www.uptodate.com/contents/hydatidiform-mole-treatment-and-follow-up

25. Acharya G, Morgan H, Paramanantham L, Fernando R. A randomized controlled trial comparing surgical termination of pregnancy with and without continuous ultrasound guidance. *Eur J Obstet Gynecol Reprod Biol.* 2004;114:69-74.

26. Padron L, Rezende Filho J, Amim Junior J, et al. Manual compared with electric vacuum aspiration for treatment of molar pregnancy. *Obstet Gynecol.* 2018;131:652-659.

27. Braga A, Padron L, Rezende-Filho J, Elias K, Horowitz N, Berkowitz R. Treatment of hydatidiform mole using manual vacuum aspiration: technical and tactical aspects. *Int J Gynecol Cancer.* 2021;31:1299-1300.

28. Elias KM, Shoni M, Bernstein M, Goldstein DP, Berkowitz RS. Complete hydatidiform mole in women aged 40 to 49 years. *J Reprod Med.* 2012;57:254-258.

29. Elias KM, Goldstein DP, Berkowitz RS. Complete hydatidiform mole in women older than age 50. *J Reprod Med.* 2010;55:208-212.

30. Zhao P, Lu Y, Huang W, Tong B, Lu W. Total hysterectomy versus uterine evacuation for preventing post-molar gestational trophoblastic neoplasia in patients who are at least 40 years old: a systematic review and meta-analysis. *BMC Cancer.* 2019;19:13.

31. Tidy JA, Gillespie AM, Bright N, Radstone CR, Coleman RE, Hancock BW. Gestational trophoblastic disease: a study of mode of evacuation and subsequent need for treatment with chemotherapy. *Gynecol Oncol.* 2000;78:309-312.

32. van't Veer MB, Overbeeke MA, Geertzen HG, van der Lans SM. The expression of Rh-D factor in human trophoblast. *Am J Obstet Gynecol.* 1984;150:1008-1010.

33. Uberti EM, Diestel MC, Guimaraes FE, De Napoli G, Schmid H. Single-dose actinomycin D: efficacy in the prophylaxis of postmolar gestational trophoblastic neoplasia in adolescents with high-risk hydatidiform mole. *Gynecol Oncol.* 2006;102:325-332.

34. Wang Q, Fu J, Hu L, et al. Prophylactic chemotherapy for hydatidiform mole to prevent gestational trophoblastic neoplasia. *Cochrane Database Syst Rev.* 2017;9:CD007289.

35. Ngan HYS, Seckl MJ, Berkowitz RS, et al. Diagnosis and management of gestational trophoblastic disease: 2021 update. *Int J Gynaecol Obstet.* 2021;155(suppl 1):86-93.

36. Mangili G, Lorusso D, Brown J, et al. Trophoblastic disease review for diagnosis and management: a joint report from the international society for the study of trophoblastic disease, european organisation for the treatment of trophoblastic disease, and the gynecologic cancer intergroup. *Int J Gynecol Cancer.* 2014;24:S109-S116.

37. Braga A, Biscaro A, do Amaral Giordani JM, et al. Does a human chorionic gonadotropin level of over 20,000 IU/L four weeks after uterine evacuation for complete hydatidiform mole constitute an indication for chemotherapy for gestational trophoblastic neoplasia? *Eur J Obstet Gynecol Reprod Biol.* 2018;223:50-55.

38. Wolfberg AJ, Growdon WB, Feltmate CM, et al. Low risk of relapse after achieving undetectable HCG levels in women with partial molar pregnancy. *Obstet Gynecol.* 2006;108:393-396.

39. Wolfberg AJ, Berkowitz RS, Goldstein DP, Feltmate C, Lieberman E. Postevacuation hCG levels and risk of gestational trophoblastic neoplasia in women with complete molar pregnancy. *Obstet Gynecol.* 2005;106:548-552.

40. Braga A, Maesta I, Matos M, Elias KM, Rizzo J, Viggiano MG. Gestational trophoblastic neoplasia after spontaneous human chorionic gonadotropin normalization following molar pregnancy evacuation. *Gynecol Oncol.* 2015;139:283-287.

41. Descargues P, Hajri T, Massardier J, et al. Gestational trophoblastic neoplasia after human chorionic gonadotropin normalization in a retrospective cohort of 7761 patients in France. *Am J Obstet Gynecol.* 2021;225:401.e1-401.e9.

42. Coyle C, Short D, Jackson L, et al. What is the optimal duration of human chorionic gonadotrophin surveillance following evacuation of a molar pregnancy? A retrospective analysis on over 20,000 consecutive patients. *Gynecol Oncol.* 2018;148:254-257.

43. Horowitz NS, Berkowitz RS, Elias KM. Considering changes in the recommended human chorionic gonadotropin monitoring after molar evacuation. *Obstet Gynecol.* 2020;135:9-11.

44. Albright BB, Shorter JM, Mastroyannis SA, Ko EM, Schreiber CA, Sonalkar S. Gestational trophoblastic neoplasia after human chorionic gonadotropin normalization following molar pregnancy: a systematic review and meta-analysis. *Obstet Gynecol.* 2020;135:12-23.

45. Soares RR, Maesta I, Colon J, et al. Complete molar pregnancy in adolescents from North and South America: clinical presentation and risk of gestational trophoblastic neoplasia. *Gynecol Oncol.* 2016;142:496-500.

46. Braga A, Growdon WB, Bernstein M, et al. Molar pregnancy in adolescents. *J Reprod Med.* 2012;57:225-230.

47. Palmer JE, Hancock BW, Tidy JA. Influence of age as a factor in the outcome of gestational trophoblastic neoplasia. *J Reprod Med.* 2008;53:565-574.

48. Savage PM, Sita-Lumsden A, Dickson S, et al. The relationship of maternal age to molar pregnancy incidence, risks for chemotherapy and subsequent pregnancy outcome. *J Obstet Gynaecol.* 2013;33:406-411.

49. Hoeijmakers YM, Eysbouts YK, Massuger L, et al. Early prediction of post-molar gestational trophoblastic neoplasia and resistance to methotrexate, based on a single serum human chorionic gonadotropin measurement. *Gynecol Oncol.* 2021;163:531-537.

50. Zhao P, Wang S, Zhang X, Lu W. A novel prediction model for post-molar gestational trophoblastic neoplasia and comparison with existing models. *Int J Gynecol Cancer.* 2017;27:1028-1034.

51. Eysbouts Y, Brouwer R, Ottevanger P, et al. Serum human chorionic gonadotropin normogram for the detection of gestational trophoblastic neoplasia. *Int J Gynecol Cancer.* 2017;27:1035-1041.

52. Kim BW, Cho H, Kim H, et al. Human chorionic gonadotrophin regression rate as a predictive factor of postmolar gestational trophoblastic neoplasm in high-risk hydatidiform mole: a case-control study. *Eur J Obstet Gynecol Reprod Biol.* 2012;160:100-105.

53. Kang WD, Choi HS, Kim SM. Prediction of persistent gestational trophobalstic neoplasia: the role of hCG level and ratio in 2 weeks after evacuation of complete mole. *Gynecol Oncol.* 2012;124:250-253.

54. Gockley AA, Lin LH, Davis M, et al. Impact of clinical characteristics on human chorionic gonadotropin regression after molar pregnancy. *Clinics (Sao Paulo).* 2021;76:e2830.

55. Sebire NJ, Seckl MJ. Immunohistochemical staining for diagnosis and prognostic assessment of hydatidiform moles: current evidence and future directions. *J Reprod Med.* 2010;55:236-246.

56. Cheung AN, Ngan HY, Collins RJ, Wong YL. Assessment of cell proliferation in hydatidiform mole using monoclonal antibody MIB1 to Ki-67 antigen. *J Clin Pathol.* 1994;47:601-604.

57. Hasanzadeh M, Sharifi N, Esmaieli H, Daloee MS, Tabari A. Immunohistochemical expression of the proliferative marker Ki67 in hydatidiform moles and its diagnostic value in the progression to gestational trophoblastic neoplasia. *J Obstet Gynaecol Res.* 2013;39:572-577.

58. Jeffers MD, Richmond JA, Smith R. Trophoblast proliferation rate does not predict progression to persistent gestational trophoblastic disease in complete hydatidiform mole. *Int J Gynecol Pathol.* 1996;15:34-38.

59. Nagib RM, M A Zaki M, Wageh A, Abdelrazik M. Can Ki67 and caspase predict molar progression? *Fetal Pediatr Pathol.* 2019;38:444-448.

60. Sharp AN, Heazell AE, Crocker IP, Mor G. Placental apoptosis in health and disease. *Am J Reprod Immunol.* 2010;64:159-169.

61. Braga A, Maesta I, Rocha Soares R, et al. Apoptotic index for prediction of postmolar gestational trophoblastic neoplasia. *Am J Obstet Gynecol.* 2016;215:336.e1-336.e12.

62. Lin LH, Maesta I, St Laurent JD, et al. Distinct microRNA profiles for complete hydatidiform moles at risk of malignant progression. *Am J Obstet Gynecol.* 2021;224:372.e1-372.e30.

63. Sakuragi N, Matsuo H, Coukos G, et al. Differentiation-dependent expression of the BCL-2 proto-oncogene in the human trophoblast lineage. *J Soc Gynecol Investig.* 1994;1:164-172.

64. Candelier JJ, Frappart L, Yadaden T, et al. Altered p16 and Bcl-2 expression reflects pathologic development in hydatidiform moles and choriocarcinoma. *Pathol Oncol Res.* 2013;19:217-227.

65. Laban M, El-Swaify ST, Refaat MA, Ibrahim EA, Abdelrahman RM. Prediction of neoplastic transformation of hydatidiform mole: current evidence. *Reprod Sci.* 2021;28:3010-3012.

66. St Laurent JD, Lin LH, Owen DM, et al. Loss of selenoprotein iodothyronine deiodinase 3 expression correlates with progression of complete

hydatidiform mole to gestational trophoblastic neoplasia. *Reprod Sci.* 2021;28:3200-3211.

67. Stone M, Dent J, Kardana A, Bagshawe KD. Relationship of oral contraception to development of trophoblastic tumour after evacuation of a hydatidiform mole. *Br J Obstet Gynaecol.* 1976;83:913-916.

68. Berkowitz RS, Marean AR, Goldstein DP, Bernstein MR. Oral contraceptives and post-molar trophoblastic tumours. *Lancet.* 1980;2:752.

69. Braga A, Maesta I, Short D, Savage P, Harvey R, Seckl MJ. Hormonal contraceptive use before hCG remission does not increase the risk of gestational trophoblastic neoplasia following complete hydatidiform mole: a historical database review. *BJOG.* 2016;123:1330-1335.

70. Dantas PRS, Maesta I, Filho JR, et al. Does hormonal contraception during molar pregnancy follow-up influence the risk and clinical aggressiveness of gestational trophoblastic neoplasia after controlling for risk factors? *Gynecol Oncol.* 2017;147:364-370.

CHAPTER **7.3**

Management of Low-Risk Gestational Trophoblastic Neoplasia

Neil S. Horowitz, Ross S. Berkowitz, and Kevin M. Elias

GESTATIONAL TROPHOBLASTIC NEOPLASIA

GTN, unlike any other malignancy, is diagnosed based mainly on hCG criteria. Although occurring after any pregnancy event, GTN most commonly is diagnosed after a molar pregnancy and more rarely after a term, abortion, or ectopic pregnancy. There are four distinct histologic types of GTN: IM, CCA, PSTT, and ETT (1-4). Management of the first two histologies is similar and based on International Federation of Gynaecology and Obstetrics (FIGO) staging and World Health Organization (WHO) risk score, whereas management of PSTT and ETT is predominately surgical with adjuvant therapy administered for those with advanced stage or long interval (>48 months) since the antecedent pregnancy (1-5) (**Table 7.3-1**). This chapter focuses on the management of low-risk GTN.

Diagnosis of Gestational Trophoblastic Neoplasia

After a molar pregnancy has been evacuated, hCG assessment is undertaken on a weekly basis until the levels are undetectable or until FIGO criteria for GTN are met (2,5). Updated in 2021, the FIGO/WHO criteria are as follows (2-4,6):

- hCG increases more than 10% across three values during at least a 2-week period (ie, days 1, 7, 14).
- hCG plateaus ± 10% across four measurements during at least a 3-week period (ie, days 1, 7, 14, 21).
- Histologic diagnosis of CCA

Historically, a slowly falling but persistently elevated hCG greater than 6 months after molar evacuation was considered diagnostic for GTN. However, two large cohort studies (7,8) found that 80% or more of these patients with a falling hCG at 6 months after evacuation that were managed expectantly, spontaneously achieved undetectable levels. For those in whom the hCG did not normalize, subsequent treatment was successful and survival was not compromised (7,8).

Human Chorionic Gonadotropin

hCG is part of the heterodimer glycoprotein hormone family consisting of an α-subunit identical to luteinizing hormone (LH), follicle-stimulating hormone (FSH), and thyroid-stimulating hormone (TSH) and a unique β-subunit (9,10). There are multiple isoforms of hCG that can be present in the circulation. The two most common, regular hCG and hyper glycosolated hCG (hCG-H), are produced almost exclusively by cytotrophoblast and syncytiotrophoblast of the placenta, GTN, germ cell, and other somatic tumors, such as bladder or lung, with trophoblastic elements. hCG-H contains more sugar residues and is thought to promote trophoblastic growth and invasion (11). Not surprising, the ratio of hCG-H to total hCG increases with the invasiveness of tumors such that hCG-H comprises approximately 5% of total hCG in complete moles, 30% of total hCG in IMs, and 60% of total hCG in CCA (12). Enzymatic degradation and dissociation of α and β subunits give rise to all the other variants of the hCG, including free subunits (α, β, and hCG-H), nicked forms (nicked hCG, nicked hCG-H, nicked hCG-H free subunit, nicked hCG-β, nicked free β-subunit), and hCG β-subunit core fragment (13). This last fragment results from the urine degradation of hCG free β-subunit and is only detectable in urine (9,13).

All common commercially available hCG assays are sandwich-type immunoassays that measure the β-subunit, the intact hCG, and

■ TABLE 7.3-1. FIGO Staging

Stage I	Disease confined to uterine corpus
Stage II	GTN extends outside uterus but is limited to the genital structures (adnexa, vagina, broad ligament)
Stage III	GTN extends to the lungs, with or without known genital tract involvement
Stage IV	All other metastatic sites

FIGO, International Federation of Gynaecology and Obstetrics; GTN, gestational trophoblastic disease.

From Horowitz NS, Eskander RN, Adelman MR, Burke W. Epidemiology, diagnosis, and treatment of gestational trophoblastic disease: a society of gynecologic oncology evidenced-based review and recommendations. *Gynecol Oncol.* 2021;163:605.

From Berkowitz RS, Horowitz NS, Elias KM. Gestational trophoblastic neoplasia: Epidemiology, clinical features, diagnosis, staging and risk stratification. In: Goff B, Dizon Ds, eds. *UpToDate.* Wolters Kluwer; 2022.

almost all the major variants described earlier (9,10). These sandwich assays are highly sensitive and can detect serum hCG levels as low as 1 to 2 mIU/mL, while urine assays can only detect hCG levels 20 mIU/mL or greater (10). Fortunately, hCG is an exquisitely sensitive tumor marker, thus allowing for easy diagnosis, monitoring response to treatment, and identifying recurrence of GTN. This is most successful if the same assay is used consistently throughout the course of care as there can be great variation between assays.

False-negative and false-positive results for hCG can occur at the extremes of value. Markedly elevated hCG, usually when hCG greater than 1,000,000 IU/L, can produce a phenomenon known as the "hook effect," in which the fixed, solid-phase antibodies and the labeled, soluble antibodies are saturated preventing sandwich formation and a negative result. In the setting of presumed GTD/GTN if hook effect is suspected, the true hCG value can be obtained with serial dilutions of the sample before analysis (9,14,15). In addition, false-negative results can occur if the tumor secretes a form of hCG not detected or underdetected by a particular assay. When there is a persistently low but positive hCG level, defined as an hCG less than 1,000 IU/L with no more than a 2-fold variation over at least a 3-month period and in the absence of tumor on imaging, one must consider false-positive results like phantom hCG, quiescent GTD, or other sources of hCG such as the pituitary (9,10,16,17). Phantom hCG results from heterophile antibodies that interfere with the immunoassay. This can be confirmed if hCG elevation is noted only in serum and not in urine, by using two separate commercial assays in which the results vary greatly or are negative in repeat assay, or by persistent elevated hCG despite serial dilution of the serum (10,16). In quiescent GTD, the hCG is usually less than 200 mIU/mL. This occurs when there are residual slow-growing or inactive trophoblastic cells. This is most common after molar pregnancies but can be seen after CCA. Active disease can occur in approximately 20% of cases and is diagnosed by two doublings of the total hCG or a rise in hCG-H to greater than 20% (16-19). The pituitary gland produces a small amount of hCG, which becomes more pronounced around menopause, before ovulation, or in women in whom multiagent, high-dose chemotherapy has temporarily stopped ovarian function. These are all times with high LH levels. Pituitary hCG is typically less than 10 mIU/mL but can range between 20 and 40 mIU/mL. Pituitary hCG can be distinguished from real trophoblastic hCG by placing the patient on higher dose oral contraceptive or GnRH agonist which will suppress pituitary hCG production (9,10,16,19).

PSTT and ETT are often associated with low level of hCG. As these tumors originate from intermediate trophoblast rather than synchiotrophoblast, hCG production is low and typically consists of more free β-subunit (9,10).

Staging of Gestational Trophoblastic Neoplasia

Once criteria for GTN have been met, women need to undergo staging. Staging has two components. The FIGO stage to determine the anatomic extent and spread of disease and the WHO risk score to determine the likelihood of disease progression and/or resistance to single-agent chemotherapy (4,5). The most common sites of metastases include the lung (70%) and vagina (20%), and as such, physical/pelvic examination in addition to laboratory evaluations (complete blood count, chemistry, hepatic, thyroid, and hCG test) is critical (20). A pelvic ultrasound is useful to assess uterine and intrauterine tumor size, which are components of the WHO risk score calculation. A chest x-ray rather than a computed tomography (CT) scan is explicitly recommended by FIGO for staging as approximately 40% of patients with a negative chest x-ray will have micrometastases on chest CT scan (21-25). These micrometastases have been associated with chemotherapy resistance but have not been shown to worsen overall survival. Using chest CT can increase the WHO risk score, potentially leading to inappropriate use of more toxic multiagent chemotherapy, without improving outcome. If the plain chest x-ray shows metastases, then CT scan of the chest, abdomen, and pelvis and a brain magnetic resonance imaging (MRI) are warranted to check for other sites of disease (26). Using the information garnered from these assessments, WHO risk score is calculated (3-4,6). Women with stage I or stage II/III with WHO prognostic score less than 7 are considered to have low-risk disease (Table 7.3.2).

■ TABLE 7.3-2. WHO Risk Score

	Scores			
	0	1	2	4
Age (yr)	<40	≥40	—	
Antecedent pregnancy	Mole	Abortion	Term	
Interval months from index pregnancy	<4	4 to <7	7 to <13	≥13
Pretreatment serum hCG (IU/L)	$<10^3$	10^3 to $<10^4$	10^4 to $<10^5$	$>10^5$
Largest tumor size (including uterus)	3 to <5 cm	≥5 cm		
Site of metastases	Lung	Kidney/spleen	Gastrointestinal/liver	Brain
Number of metastases	—	1-4	5-8	>8
Previous failed chemotherapy	—	—	Single drug	2 or more drugs

Format for reporting to FIGO Annual Report: In order to stage and allot a risk factor score, a patient's diagnosis is allocated to a stage as represented by a Roman numeral I, II, III, and IV. This is then separated by a colon from the sum of all the actual risk factor scores expressed in Arabic numerals for example, stage II:4, stage IV:9. This stage and score will be allotted for each patient. Lung involvement is based on chest x-ray and not computed tomography scan.

Definition of Risk Categories:

Low risk—Stage I or stage II/III with a WHO prognostic score <7.

High risk—Stage IV disease or any stage and WHO score ≥7.

Ultra-high risk—Any stage with WHO score >12.

FIFO, International Federation of Gynecology and Obstetrics; hCG, human chorionic gonadotropin; WHO, World Health Organization.

From Horowitz NS, Eskander RN, Adelman MR, Burke W. Epidemiology, diagnosis, and treatment of gestational trophoblastic disease: a society of gynecologic oncology evidenced-based review and recommendations. *Gynecol Oncol.* 2021;163:605.

From Berkowitz RS, Horowitz NS, Elias KM. Gestational trophoblastic neoplasia: epidemiology, clinical features, diagnosis, staging and risk stratification. In: Goff B, Dizon Ds, eds. *UpToDate.* Wolters Kluwer; 2022.

Treatment for Low-Risk Gestational Trophoblastic Neoplasia

Single-agent chemotherapy utilizing either methotrexate (MTX) or Act-D is the mainstay of treatment of low-risk GTN (2-4,26-28) (**Table 7.3.3**). Alternatively, for women who have completed childbearing, hysterectomy, usually with a single dose of adjunctive chemotherapy, also provides excellent cure rates (29-32), or for those who desire to avoid chemotherapy, a second curettage offers an alternative (33-36).

Methotrexate

MTX is an antimetabolite that is highly effective at treating low-risk GTN. Given its effectiveness, low toxicity profile, and cost-effectiveness, it is our treatment of choice at the New England Trophoblastic Disease Center (NETDC) (37-39). There are a variety of schedules and doses of MTX utilized, but in our experience, 8-day MTX with folinic acid (FA) is very effective and well tolerated (38-46). In a recent review by Maesta et al (38), 325 women with low-risk GTN were treated between 1974 and 2014 with 8-day MTX-FA or 1-day MTX infusion with FA. Compared to the 1-day infusion, 8-day MTX was noted to have a higher sustained remission (84% vs 62%, $P < .001$) and lower rate of MTX resistance (7.3% vs 34.5% $P < .001$). Although there was a higher rate of need to change to second-line therapy due to treatment-related adverse events (5.3% vs 0% $P = .001$), the overall incidence was low and predominately consisted of gastrointestinal toxicities, hematologic abnormalities, fatigue, and eye disorders that were self-limited and resolved with no long-term sequelae. Although we use a dose of 1 mg/kg/d of MTX in our 8-day regimen at NETDC, a recent retrospective, multicenter study by Mangili and colleagues compared that dose to a fixed dose of 50 mg/d (45). These authors showed no difference in the number of cycles required to obtain remission, rates of resistance, or relapse, and no difference in toxicity. One difficulty with the 8-day MTX regimen is need for a weekend administration, which is not necessarily available at all institutions. Importantly, a modified 8-day regimen (with MTX treatment on the eighth day rather than the seventh day) has been employed, thus avoiding weekend administration without compromise to

oncologic outcomes (46). For most multiday regimens, FA is an important component to abrogate toxicity. Traditionally, dosing for FA is weight based using 0.1 mg/kg. However, Poli et al (47) recently showed that when compared to weigh-based dosing, a fixed dose of FA at 15 mg was associated with a similar primary remission rate (76.8% vs 81.5% $P = .33$) with less delay in treatment due to toxicity (6.8% vs 2.8% $P < .01$), thus providing a highly practical, equally effective, and preferable FA dose. This is now our standard practice at NETDC.

Alternative dosing and treatment schedules of MTX have been used with equivalent success as the 8-day regimen. The 5-day MTX regimen (0.3-0.5 mg/kg, intramuscular [IM] or intravenous [IV], for 5 consecutive days every 2 weeks) is the treatment of choice at the Brewer Trophoblastic Disease Center and has shown primary remission rates of 80% to 90% and toxicity of approximately 5% (43,44). High-dose MTX, with 100 mg/m^2 IV push followed by 12-hour infusion of MTX 200 mg/m^2, has a lower complete remission rate (69%-90%) but avoids multiple visits for treatment and, therefore, may be more convenient (38). Finally, weekly IM MTX at 30 to 50 mg/m^2 is widely used, given its ease of schedule, low toxicity, and familiarity for many physicians (40,41). Although it can achieve remission rates of 49% to 74%, the time to remission and duration of therapy tend to be prolonged to 15 to 20 weeks in some cases, which may be unacceptable to some patients.

Actinomycin-D

Act-D is the preferred first-line therapy for some centers and can be administered 10 to 12 µg/kg for 5 days every 2 weeks or more commonly as a "pulsed" administration every 14-day infusion with dose of 1.25 mg/m^2 (48-53). Total dose is often capped at 2,000 mg to limit toxicities. Efficacy with Act-D is similar for both the 5-day and pulse regimens and ranges from 70% to 90% (49). Toxicities with Act-D seem to be greater than MTX and primarily consist of hematologic, hyperemesis, alopecia, and local tissue injury with extravasation. Because of the higher toxicity, Act-D is often used as second-line therapy (54,55).

Regardless of which single agent one starts with, the survival for women with low-risk disease approaches 100% but may require sequential use of single agents, combination chemotherapy, and/or surgery to achieve remission (28). Given this excellent outcome, the choice of initial chemotherapy is often left to clinician or institutional preference; however, there have been several trials and a Cochrane review comparing MTX to Act-D (56-61). The Cochrane review included seven randomized controlled trials encompassing 667 patients and concluded that Act-D was associated with higher cure rates (relative risk 0.65, 95% CI 0.57-0.95) and higher adverse events. The meta-analysis was limited by significant heterogeneity in dosing and treatment schedule of MTX or Act-D (61).

One of the largest studies included in the meta-analysis was a randomized controlled trial from the Gynecologic Oncology Group (#174) that compared weekly MTX 30 mg/m^2 IM to pulsed Act-D (56). This trial showed complete response rates were 58% and 73%, respectively, with time to remission being 8 weeks for both but requiring fewer courses of Act-D. As highlighted in this study, the response rate to single-agent chemotherapy for women with FIGO/WHO score 5 or 6 was 9% and 40% for MTX and Act-D, respectively. Although some elect to use multiagent chemotherapy for these patients with FIGO/WHO score 5 or 6, there are some women who will respond to single-agent chemotherapy and, therefore, able to avoid the unnecessary exposure to more toxic multiagent regimens. A recent international multicenter retrospective study evaluated patients with WHO score of 5 or 6 to better understand which patients can receive single-agent chemotherapy and those who should be treated primarily with multiagent chemotherapy (62). Of 431 patients with GTN and WHO score of 5 or 6, 60% achieved remission with first- or second-line single-agent chemotherapy. In this study, first-line chemotherapy was 8-day MTX-FA, and the second-line single-agent therapy was Act-D. Primary multiagent chemotherapy was recommended for

TABLE 7.3-3. Single-Agent Regimens for Low-Risk Gestational Trophoblastic Neoplasia	
Actinomycin-D Regimens (Max Dose 2,000 µg)	**Primary Remission Rates (%)**
Daily 10-12 µg IV × 5 d every 2 wk	77-94
Pulse 1.25 mg/m^2 IV every 2 wk	69-90
Methotrexate Regimens	
Multiday (every 2 wk)	
5-d 0.3-0.5 mg/kg IV or IM × 5 d	87-93
No FA	74-90
8-d 1 mg/kg IV or IM days 1, 3, 5, 7	70-80
FA 15 mg PO days 2, 4, 6, 8	69-90
8-d 50 mg IM days 1, 3, 5, 7	
FA 7.5 mg PO days 2, 4, 6, 8	49-74
Weekly	
30-50 mg/m^2 IM	69-90
High dose	
100 mg/m^2 IV over 30 min	
200 mg/m^2 IV over 12 hr	
FA 15 mg PO every 12 hr × 6 doses	
starting 24 hr after MTX	

FA, folinic acid/leucovorin; IM, intramuscular; IV, intravenous; PO, by mouth.

Adapted from Berkowitz RS, Horowitz NS, Elias KM. Gestational trophoblastic neoplasia: epidemiology, clinical features, diagnosis, staging and risk stratification. In: Goff B, Dizon Ds eds. *UpToDate*. Wolters Kluwer; 2022.

women with metastatic CCA, no CCA, and no metastatic disease but with hCG greater than 411,000 mIU/mL, or CCA or metastatic disease with hCG greater than 149,000 mIU/mL (62).

Alternative Single Agents

The majority of trophoblastic centers use either MTX or Act-D as their first-line chemotherapy for low-risk GTN. With that said, other single-agent regimens have been used with equally good results. Etoposide at a dose of 100 mg/m^2 IV daily × 5 days or as an oral agent has been shown to be a highly active agent, however, given its significant toxicity and risk of secondary malignancies limit its use in low-risk disease (63,64). The preferred single-agent treatment in China is fluorouracil (5-FU) at a dose of 30 mg/kg daily for 10 days. This regimen produced remission rates of 85% to 93% in low-risk patients with mild toxicity (65,66).

Consolidation

After hCG normalization is achieved, patients should receive consolidation with the last effective agent to help prevent relapse. Lybol et al showed that three rather than two cycles of consolidation therapy decreased the rate of relapse from 8% to 4% (67).

Resistance/Relapse

Despite excellent initial response rates to single-agent chemotherapy, approximately 30% of patients with low-risk GTN will develop resistance to single-agent chemotherapy and approximately 2% to 8% who achieve initial remission will relapse (1-4,68). Resistance is typically defined as a rising hCG after two cycles of treatment or hCG plateau (<10% change) over three cycles or the development of new metastases (1-4), whereas relapse is noted as a rising hCG after hCG remission and after excluding other possible sources, like a new pregnancy. The median time to relapse is 6 months. Less commonly (≤5%) patients need to change to second-line therapy due to toxicity (38,68). hCG levels and regression curves, uterine artery pulsatility index with or without serum BMP-9 levels, and clinical factors such as antecedent pregnancy or number of cycles of chemotherapy have all been investigated to try and predict patients who are destined to develop MTX-resistant disease or relapse; however, none are widely used in clinical practice (69-73).

At the time of resistance/relapse, the choice of second-line therapy (alternative single-agent vs multiagent chemotherapy regimen) can be determined by restaging and recalculating the WHO score, or as has been done at Charing Cross, using the hCG at the time of resistance (74,75). Over time, the hCG cutoff whereby patients developing resistance to first-line single-agent therapy could be treated with the alternative single agent (MTX followed by Act-D or vice versa) has slowly risen. Historically, at the Charing Cross, a cutoff of 300 mIU/mL (74) was used to determine second-line therapy; however, in a recent review from this center of 609 patients with low-risk GTN treated with 8-day MTX-FA, 57% (348/609) achieved complete remission and 25% (153/609) developed resistance with a hCG less than or equal to 1,000 mIU/mL. When these patients were switched to Act-D, 92.8% of patients achieved complete remission. The remaining patients were all cured with EMA-CO. Although using a higher hCG cutoff significantly decreased the likelihood of remission with the alternative single agent, a number of women were spared the toxicity of EMA-CO, and those who did experience sequential single-agent therapy failure were all ultimately cured, thus justifying the higher cutoff (75). Other trophoblastic centers that use MTX as first-line therapy argue that Act-D should be used, regardless of hCG value at the time of resistance given the reported response rates of 70% to 75% (54,55). It appears that the response rate of Act-D as a second-line agent is similar whether administered as a 5-day regimen or pulsed. Compared to pulsed Act-D, the 5-day regimen had a faster time to hCG remission and required fewer cycles to achieve remission; however, it was associated with higher rates of thrombocytopenia, mucositis, and alopecia (54).

In an effort to avoid the toxicity of multiagent chemotherapy for those who develop MTX-resistant low-risk disease, alternative single agents have been used. Carboplatin as a single agent showed promise as a second-line therapy with excellent tolerability and approximate 80% response rate when used at the Sheffield Trophoblastic Center (76); however, similar results were not reproducible in Brazil where the remission rate was 48% and 70% of patients had delays in their treatment secondary to toxicity (77). A recent study from France evaluated the immunotherapy avelumab as second-line therapy for MTX-resistant disease (78). They showed an approximately 55% remission rate with acceptable toxicity and a subsequent normal pregnancy after treatment. Importantly, for women with low-risk disease who experience second-line single-agent chemotherapy failure, the cure rate remains 100% with the use of multiagent chemotherapy and/or surgery.

Surgery

Second curettage is commonly employed to treat/minimize hemorrhage in patients with postmolar GTN (33,34), but also it has been proposed as primary treatment of nonmetastatic low-risk GTN in lieu of single-agent chemotherapy (35,36). Retrospective studies show remission rates for curettage ranging from less than 20% to approximately 70% and uterine perforation rate of between 4.8% and 8% (33-36). However, in the only prospective study by Osborne and colleagues (35), approximately 40% of women with low-risk GTN treated with second curettage were cured and avoided chemotherapy altogether. The authors reported only 1 (1.5%) uterine perforation. Although the trial did not identify any clinical features predictive of success with this approach, those at extremes of reproductive age (>39 or <19 years old) were less likely to respond to second curettage and there were no responses for those with WHO scores of 5 or 6 or hCG greater than 100,000 mIU/mL.

Hysterectomy also plays a role in the management of low-risk GTN. This is particularly true for those women who have completed their families and have chemotherapy-resistant disease in the uterus (30-32). Bolze et al (30) reported an 82% remission rate for first-line hysterectomy in management of low-risk disease. FIGO score of 5 to 6 (OR-8.9, 95% CI, 1.60-64.9) and CCA (OR-14.2, 95% CI, 1.78-138.1) were associated with the need for salvage chemotherapy (29). At the NETDC between 1965 and 2018, 40 women with stage I GTN underwent primary hysterectomy and one course of adjuvant chemotherapy and all achieved remission (28). More common for women with low-risk disease is the use of hysterectomy as an adjunct to chemotherapy. Eysbouts reported on 109 patients who underwent hysterectomy as part of their management of both low- and high-risk GTN (31). After hysterectomy, complete remission was achieved in 66% of those with localized disease, but only 15% in those with metastatic disease. Importantly in those with localized disease, after hysterectomy, the number of cycles and duration of treatment to remission were shorter as compared to age-matched controls. Even with apparent localized disease, some advocate a single dose of chemotherapy, typically Act-D, at the time of hysterectomy to address potential occult metastatic disease (32). As there is a risk of recurrence even after hysterectomy, these women still require hCG surveillance once they have reached remission. Though limited, newer data suggest that a laparoscopic hysterectomy and its inherent benefits can be performed without compromising oncologic outcome (29).

Given the relative chemotherapy resistance of PSTT and ETT, hysterectomy is the standard of management for these histologies with lymphadenectomy reserved for those with enlarged nodes (5,79,80). Although there have been small series of cases of patients with PSTT and ETT undergoing local uterine resection, the role of fertility-preserving surgery is not well defined in these patients (81). Chemotherapy is reserved for those patients with factors such as advanced stage or more than 48 month interval from antecedent pregnancy.

A more in-depth review of hysterectomy or other surgeries such as thoracotomy, for the management of relapsed or resistant disease, is covered in the high-risk GTN section of this chapter.

Surveillance

For women with low-risk GTN, once chemotherapy is completed and they remain asymptomatic, they should undergo surveillance with monthly hCG × 12 months (1-4). During that year or in subsequent years, if they become symptomatic (ie, abnormal bleeding), hCG should be obtained to exclude recurrence. In a population-based cohort study from the United Kingdom, approximately 75% of recurrences happened within the first year after completion of treatment and with risk of recurrence thereafter being incredibly low at less than 1% per year (82). During the year of surveillance, ideally, women would be on hormonal contraception to minimize risk of subsequent pregnancy and to suppress pituitary hCG, thus reducing difficulties interpreting hCG. Oral contraceptive with estrogen-progestins offers excellent protection against pregnancy without increasing the risk of GTN or recurrence rates (83).

REFERENCES

1. Ngan HYS, Seckl MJ, Berkowitz RS, et al. Diagnosis and management of gestational trophoblastic disease: 2021 update. *Int J Gynaecol Obstet.* 2021;155(suppl 1):86-93.

2. Horowitz NS, Eskander RN, Adelman MR, Burke W. Epidemiology, diagnosis, and treatment of gestational trophoblastic disease: a Society of Gynecologic Oncology evidenced-based review and recommendations. *Gynecol Oncol.* 2021;163:605-613.

3. Lok C, van Trommel N, Massuger L, Golfier F, Seckl M. Practical clinical guidelines of EOTTD for the treatment and referral of gestational trophoblastic disease. *Eur J Cancer.* 2020;130:228-240.

4. Seckl MJ, Sebire NJ, Berkowitz RS. Gestational trophoblastic disease. *Lancet.* 2010;376:717-729.

5. Frijstein MM, Lok CAR, van Trommel NE, et al. Management and prognostic factors of epithelioid trophoblastic tumors: results from the international society for the study of trophoblastic diseases database. *Gynecol Oncol.* 2019;152(2):361-367.

6. Berkowitz RS, Horowitz NS, Elias KM. Gestational trophoblastic neoplasia: epidemiology, clinical features, diagnosis, staging and risk stratification. In: Goff B, Dizon DS, eds. *UpToDate.* Wolters Kluwer; 2022.

7. Braga A, Torres B, Burla M, et al. Is chemotherapy necessary for patients with molar pregnancy and human chorionic gonadotropin serum levels raised but falling at 6 months after uterine evacuation? *Gynecol Oncol.* 2016;143(3):558-564.

8. Agarwal R, Teoh S, Short D, Harvey R, Salvage PM, Seckl MJ. Chemotherapy and human chorionic gonadotropin concentrations 6 months after uterine evacuation of molar pregnancy: a retrospective cohort study. *Lancet.* 2012;379:130-135.

9. Goff, B. Human chorionic gonadotropin: testing in pregnancy and gestational trophoblastic disease and causes of low persistent levels. In: Goff B, Barss VA, eds. *UpToDate.* Wolters Kluwer; 2019.

10. Richard H. Human chorionic gonadotropin: biochemistry and measurement in pregnancy and disease. In: Goff B, Barss VA, eds. *UpToDate.* Wolters Kluwer; 2019.

11. Cole LA. Hyerglycosolated hCG. *Placenta.* 2010;31(8):653-664.

12. Cole LA, Dai D, Butler SA, et al. Gestational trophoblastic diseases: 1. Pathophysiology of hyperglycosylated hCG. *Gynecol Oncol.* 2006;102(2):145-150.

13. Stenman UH, Tiitinen A, Alfthan H, Valmu L. The classification, functions and clinical use of different isoforms of hCG. *Hum Reprod Update.* 2006;12(6):769-784.

14. Al-Mahdili HA, Jones GR. High-dose hook effect in six automated human chorionic gonadotropin assays. *Ann Clin Biochem.* 2010;47(pt 4):383-385.

15. Winder AD, Mora AS, Berry E, Lurain JR. The "hook effect" causing a negative pregnancy test in a patient with an advanced molar pregnancy. *Gynecol Oncol Rep.* 2017;21:34-36.

16. Cole LA, Khanlian SA, Giddings A, et al. Gestational trophoblastic diseases: 4. Presentation with persistent low positive human chorionic gonadotropin test results. *Gynecol Oncol.* 2006;102(2):165-172.

17. Muller CY, Cole LA. The quagmire of hCG and hCG testing in gynecologic oncology. *Gynecol Oncol.* 2009;112:663-672.

18. Kelly LS, Birken S, Puett D. Determination of hyperglycosylated human chorionic gonadotropin produced by malignant gestational trophoblastic neoplasia and male germ cell tumors using a lectin-based immunoassay and surface plasmon resonance. *Mol Cell Endocrinol.* 2007;260-262:33-39.

19. Khanlian SA, Smith HO, Cole LA. Persistent low levels of human chorionic gonadotropin: a premalignant gestational trophoblastic disease. *Am J Obstet Gynecol.* 2003;188(5):1254-1259.

20. Berkowitz RS, Goldstein DP. Chorionic tumors. *N Engl J Med.* 1996;335(23):1740-1748.

21. Frijstein MM, Lok CAR, van Trommel NE, ten Kate-Booij MJ, Massuger LFAG. Lung metastases in low-risk gestational trophoblastic neoplasia: a retrospective cohort study. *BJOG.* 2020;127(3):389-395.

22. Gamer EI, Garrett A, Goldstein DP, Berkowitz RS. Significance of chest computed tomography findings in the evaluation and treatment of persistent gestational trophoblastic neoplasia. *J Reprod Med.* 2004;49:411-414.

23. Ngan HY, Chan FL, Au VW, et al. Clinical outcome of micrometastases in the lung in stage IA persistent gestational trophoblastic disease. *Gynecol Oncol.* 1998;70:192-194.

24. Price JM, Lo C, Abdi S, et al. The role of computed tomography scanning of the thorax in the Initial assessment of gestational trophoblastic neoplasia. *Int J Gynecol Cancer.* 2015;25:1731-1736.

25. Parker VL, Winter MC, Whitby E, et al. Computed tomography chest imaging offers no advantage over chest X-ray in the initial assessment of gestational trophoblastic neoplasia. *Br J Cancer.* 2021;124(6):1066-1071.

26. Tidy J, Seck M, Hancock BW; on behalf of the Royal College of Obstetricians and Gynaecologists. Management of gestational trophoblastic disease. *BJOG.* 2021;128:e1-e27.

27. Lawrie TA, Alazzam M, Tidy J, Hancock BW, Osborne R. First-line chemotherapy in low-risk gestational trophoblastic neoplasia. *Cochrane Database Syst Rev.* 2016;2016(6):CD007102.

28. Berkowitz RS, Horowitz NS, Elias KM. Initial management of low-risk gestational trophoblastic neoplasia. In: Goff B, Dizon DS eds. *UpToDate.* Wolter Kluwer; 2021.

29. Sugrue R, Foley O, Elias KM, et al. Outcomes of minimally invasive versus open abdominal hysterectomy in patients with gestational trophoblastic disease. *Gynecol Oncol.* 2021;160(2):445-449.

30. Bolze PA, Mathe M, Hajri T, et al. First-line hysterectomy for women with low-risk non-metastatic gestational trophoblastic neoplasia no longer wishing to conceive. *Gynecol Oncol.* 2018;150:282-287.

31. Eysbouts YK, Massuger LFAG, IntHout J, Lok CAR, Sweep FCGJ, Ottewanger FB. The added value of hysterectomy in management of gestational trophoblastic neoplasia. *Gynecol Oncol.* 2017;145(3):536-542.

32. Clark RM, Nevadunsky NS, Ghosh S, et al. The evolving role of hysterectomy in gestational trophoblastic neoplasia at the New England Trophoblastic Disease Center. *J Reprod Med.* 2010;55(5-6):194-198.

33. Goldstein DP, Garner EL, Feltmate CM, Berkowitz RS. The role of repeat uterine evacuation in the management of persistent gestational trophoblastic disease. *Gynecol Oncol.* 2004;95:421-422.

34. Pezeshki M, Hancock BW, Silcocks P, et al. The role of repeat uterine evacuation in the management of persistent gestational trophoblastic disease. *Gynecol Oncol.* 2004;95:423-429.

35. Osborne RJ, Filiaci VL, Schink JC, et al. Second curettage for low-risk nonmetastatic gestational trophoblastic neoplasia. *Obstet Gynecol.* 2016;128(3):535-542.

36. van Trommel NE, Massuger LF, Verheijen RH, et al. The curative effect of a second curettage in persistent trophoblastic disease: a retrospective cohort survey. *Gynecol Oncol.* 2005;99:6-13.

37. Shah NT, Barroilhet L, Berkowitz RS, et al. A cost analysis of first-line chemotherapy for low-risk gestational trophoblastic neoplasia. *J Reprod Med.* 2012;57:211-218.

38. Maesta I, Nitecki R, Horowitz NS, et al. Effectiveness and toxicity of first-line methotrexate chemotherapy in low-risk postmolar gestational trophoblastic neoplasia: the New England trophoblastic disease center experience. *Gynecol Oncol.* 2018;148(1):161-167.

39. Berkowitz RS, Goldstein DP, Bernstein MR. Ten years experience with methotrexate and folinic acid as primary therapy for gestational trophoblastic disease. *Gynecol Oncol.* 1986;23(1):111-118.

40. Homesley HD, Blessing JA, Schlaerth J, et al. Rapid escalation of weekly intramuscular methotrexate for nonmetastatic gestational trophoblastic disease: a gynecologic oncology group study. *Gynecol Oncol.* 1990;39:305-308.

41. Homesley HD, Blessing JA, Rettenmaier M, et al. Weekly intramuscular methotrexate for nonmetastatic gestational trophoblastic disease. *Obstet Gynecol.* 1988;72:413-418.

42. Wong LC, Ngan HY, Cheng DK, Ng TY. Methotrexate infusion in low-risk gestational trophoblastic disease. *Am J Obstet Gynecol.* 2000;183:1579-1582.

43. Lurain JR, Elfstrand EP. Single-agent methotrexate chemotherapy for the treatment of nonmetastatic gestational trophoblastic tumors. *Am J Obstet Gynecol.* 1995;172(pt1):574-579.

44. Chapman-Davis E, Hoekstra AV, Rademaker AW, et al. Treatment of nonmetastatic and metastatic low-risk gestational trophoblastic neoplasia: factors associated with resistance to single-agent methotrexate chemotherapy. *Gynecol Oncol.* 2012;125:572-575.

45. Mangili G, Cioffi R, Danese S, et al. Does Methotrexate (MTX) dosing in a 8-day MTX/FA regimen for the treatment of low-risk gestational trophoblastic neoplasia affect outcome? The MITO-9 study. *Gynecol Oncol.* 2018;151(3):449-452.

46. Braga A, Araujo C, Mora P, et al. Comparison of treatment for low-risk GTN with standard 8-day MTX/FA regimen versus modified MTX/FA regimen without chemotherapy on the weekend. *Gynecol Oncol.* 2020;15(3):598-605.

47. Poli JG, Paiva G, Feitas F, et al. Folinic acid rescue during methotrexate treatment for low-risk gestational trophoblastic neoplasia—how much is just right? *Gynecol Oncol.* 2021;162(3):638-644.

48. Li L, Wan X, Feng F, et al. Pulse actinomycin D as first-line treatment of low-risk post molar non-choriocarcinoma gestational trophoblastic neoplasia. *BMC Cancer.* 2018;18(1):585.

49. Mu X, Song L, Li Q, Yin R, Zhao X, Wang D. Comparison of pulsed actinomycin D and 5-day actinomycin D as first-line chemotherapy for low-risk gestational trophoblastic neoplasia. *Int J Gynaecol Obstet.* 2018;143(2):225-231.

50. Osathanondh R, Goldstein DP, Pastorfide GB. Actinomycin D as the primary agent for gestational trophoblastic disease. *Cancer.* 1975;36:863-866.

51. Twiggs LB. Pulse actinomycin D scheduling in nonmetastatic gestational trophoblastic neoplasia: cost-effective chemotherapy. *Gynecol Oncol.* 1983;16:190-195.

52. Petrilli ES, Twiggs LB, Blessing JA, et al. Single-dose actinomycin-D treatment for nonmetastatic gestational trophoblastic disease. A prospective phase II trial of the Gynecologic oncology group. *Cancer.* 1987;60:2173-2176.

53. Schlaerth JB, Morrow CP, Nalick RH, Gaddis O Jr. Single-dose actinomycin D in the treatment of postmolar trophoblastic disease. *Gynecol Oncol.* 1984;19:53-56.

54. Maesta I, Nitecki R, Desmarais CCF, et al. Effectiveness and toxicity of second-line actinomycin D in patients with methotrexate-resistant postmolar low-risk gestational trophoblastic neoplasia. *Gynecol Oncol.* 2020;157(2):372-378.

55. Prouvot C, Golfier F, Massardier J, et al. Efficacy and safety of second-line 5-day dactinomycin in cases of methotrexate failure for gestational trophoblastic neoplasia. *Int J Gynecol Cancer.* 2018;5:1038-1044.

56. Osborne RJ, Filiaci V, Schink JC, et al. Phase III trial of weekly methotrexate or pulsed dactinomycin for low-risk gestational trophoblastic neoplasia: a gynecologic oncology group study. *J Clin Oncol.* 2011;29(7):825-831.

57. Schink JC, Filiaci V, Huang HQ, et al. An international randomized phase III trial of pulse actinomycin-D versus multi-day methotrexate for the treatment of low risk gestational trophoblastic neoplasia; NRG/GOG275. *Gynecol Oncol.* 2020;158(2):354-360.

58. Lertkhachonsuk AA, Israngura N, Wilailak S, Tangtrakul S. Actinomycin D versus methotrexate-folinic acid as the treatment of stage I, low-risk gestational trophoblastic neoplasia: a randomized controlled trial. *Int J Gynecol Cancer.* 2009;19:985-988.

59. Yarandi F, Mousavi A, Abbaslu F, et al. Five-day intravascular methotrexate versus biweekly actinomycin-D in the treatment of low-risk gestational trophoblastic neoplasia: a clinical randomized trial. *Int J Gynecol Cancer.* 2016;26:971-976.

60. Matsui H, Iitsuka Y, Seki K, Sekiya S. Comparison of chemotherapies with methotrexate, VP-16 and actinomycin-D in low-risk gestational trophoblastic disease. Remission rates and drug toxicities. *Gynecol Obstet Invest.* 1998;46:5-8.

61. Alazzam M, Tidy J, Osborne R, et al. First-line chemotherapy in low-risk gestational trophoblastic neoplasia. *Cochrane Database Syst Rev.* 2012;12:CD008891.

62. Braga A, Paiva G, Ghorani E, et al. Predictors for single-agent resistance in FIGO score 5 or 6 gestational trophoblastic neoplasia: a multicenter retrospective cohort study. *Lancet Oncol.* 2021;22:1188-1198.

63. Wong LC, Choo YC, Ma HK. Use of oral VP16-213 as primary chemotherapeutic agent in treatment of gestational trophoblastic disease. *Am J Obstet Gyencol.* 1984;150(8):924-927.

64. Hitchins RN, Holden L, Newlands ES, et al. Single agent etoposide in gestational trophoblastic tumours. Experience at Charing Cross Hospital 1978-1987. *Eur J Cancer Clin Oncol.* 1988;24:1041-1046.

65. Sung HC, Wu PC, Yang HY. Reevaluation of 5-fluorouracil as a single therapeutic agent for gestational trophoblastic neoplasms. *Am J Obstet Gynecol.* 1984;150:69-75.

66. Song HZ, Yang XY, Xiang Y. Forty-five year's experience of the treatment of choriocarcinoma and invasive mole. *Int J Gynaecol Obstet.* 1998;60(suppl 1):S77-S83.

67. Lybol C, Sweep FC, Harvey R, et al. Relapse rates after two versus three consolidation courses of methotrexate in the treatment of low-risk gestational trophoblastic neoplasia. *Gynecol Oncol.* 2012;125(3):576-579.

68. Jareemit N, Horowitz NS, Goldstein DP, Berkowitz RS, Elias KM. Outcomes for relapsed versus resistant low risk gestational trophoblastic neoplasia following single-agent chemotherapy. *Gynecol Oncol.* 2020;159(3):751-757.

69. Coulder F, Massardier J, You B, et al. Predictive factors of relapse in low-risk gestational trophoblastic neoplasia patients successfully treated with methotrexate alone. *Am J Obstet Gynecol.* 2016;215(1):80.e1-80.e7.

70. Harvey R, Elias KM, Lim A, et al. Uterine artery pulsatility index and serum BMP-9 predict resistance to methotrexate therapy in gestational trophoblastic neoplasia: a cohort study. *Curr Probl Cancer.* 2021;45(1):100622.

71. You B, Harvey R, Henin E, et al. Early prediction of treatment resistance in low-risk gestational trophoblastic neoplasia using population kinetic modelling of hCG measurements. *Br J Cancer.* 2013;108:1810-1816.

72. Growdon WB, Wolfberg AJ, Goldstein DP, et al. Evaluating methotrexate treatment in patients with low-risk postmolar gestational trophoblastic neoplasia. *Gynecol Oncol.* 2009;112:353-357.

73. van Trommel NE, Massuger LF, Schijf CP, et al. Early identification of resistance to first-line single-agent methotrexate in patients with persistent trophoblastic disease. *J Clin Oncol.* 2006;24:52-58.

74. Sita-Lumsden A, Short D, Lindsay I, et al. Treatment outcomes for 618 women with gestational trophoblastic tumours following a molar pregnancy at Charing Cross Hospital, 2000-2009. *BR J Cancer.* 2012;107(11):1810-1814.

75. Cortes-Charry R, Hennah L, Froeling FEM, et al. Increasing the human chorionic gonadotrophin cut-off to ≤1000 IU/l for starting actinomycin D in post-molar gestational trophoblastic neoplasia developing resistance to methotrexate spares more women multi-agent chemotherapy. *ESMO Open.* 2021;6(3):100110.

76. Winter MC, Tidy JA, Hilts A, et al. Risk adapted single-agent dactinomycin or carboplatin for second-line treatment of methotrexate resistant low-risk gestational trophoblastic neoplasia. *Gynecol Oncol.* 2016;143(3):565-570.

77. Mora PAR, Sun SY, Velarde GC, et al. Can carboplatin or etoposide replace actinomycin-D for second-line treatment of methotrexate resistant low-risk gestational trophoblastic neoplasia? *Gynecol Oncol.* 2019;153(2):277-285.

78. You B, Bolze PA, Lotz JP, et al. Avelumab in patients with gestational trophoblastic tumors with resistance to single-agent chemotherapy: cohort a of the TROPHIMMUN phase II trial. *J Clin Oncol.* 2020;38(27):3129-3137.

79. Horowitz NS, Goldstein DP, Berkowitz RS. Placental site trophoblastic tumors and epithelioid trophoblastic tumors: biology, natural history, and treatment modalities. *Gynecol Oncol.* 2017;144(1):208-214.

80. Lan C, Li Y, He J, Liu J. Placental site trophoblastic tumor: lymphatic spread and possible target markers. *Gynecol Oncol.* 2010;116(3):430-437.

81. Shen X, Xiang Y, Guo L, et al. Fertility preserving treatment in young patients with placental site trophoblastic tumors. *Int J Gynecol Cancer.* 2012;22:869-874.

82. Balachandran K, Salawu A, Ghorani E, et al. When to stop human chorionic gonadotrophin (hCG) surveillance after treatment with chemotherapy for gestational trophoblastic neoplasia (GTN): a national analysis on over 4,000 patients. *Gynecol Oncol.* 2019;155(1):8-12.

83. Dantas PRS, Maesta I, Filho JR, et al. Does hormonal contraception during molar pregnancy follow-up influence the risk and clinical aggressiveness of gestational trophoblastic neoplasia after controlling for risk-factors? *Gynecol Oncol.* 2017;147:364-370.

Management of High-Risk Gestational Trophoblastic Neoplasia

Antonio Braga, Fernanda Freitas Oliveira Cardoso, and Izildinha Maestá

HIGH-RISK GESTATIONAL TROPHOBLASTIC NEOPLASIA

GTN is uniquely sensitive to chemotherapy, which is the major treatment modality for patients with high-risk disease. The exception to this is PSTT and/or ETT, which are relatively resistant to chemotherapy as compared with IM or CCA. The cure rate for high-risk GTN, most commonly CCA, is greater than 80%, and for low-risk disease, it approaches 100% (1), primarily because of the inherent sensitivity of trophoblastic neoplasms to chemotherapy, the effective use of hCG as a marker of early disease, the identification of predictive factors of treatment response that has permitted individualization of therapy, and the use of combined treatment strategies. Given the rarity of these tumors, we recommend all patients undergo treatment at specialized centers wherever possible.

High-risk GTN is defined as stage IV disease or stages I, II, and III disease with a risk factor score greater than 6. These patients have an increased risk of developing chemoresistance to single-agent chemotherapy and are treated more aggressively with multiagent chemotherapy, reaching cure rates of approximately 80% to 90% (2). Evidence of the greater likelihood of resistance to single-agent chemotherapy comes from early work at the National Cancer Institute where only 36% of patients with high-risk GTN achieved remission with single-agent treatment (3).

The primary treatment should be a multiagent etoposide-based regimen. The preferred regimen for these patients is etoposide, high-dose MTX with FA, and Act-D alternating with cyclophosphamide and vincristine (EMA-CO) (**Table 7.4-1**) because it improves both primary remission and survival rates in patients with high-risk GTN, reporting complete response rates of 71% to 78% and long-term survival rates of 85% to 94% (4-6). The survival rates exceed the complete primary response rates because GTN is a unique malignancy where secondary therapies often result in cure.

However, a 2012 Cochrane review found that regimens that incorporate etoposide and cisplatin are also effective options, though the lack of randomized trials prevented an analysis to define the optimal regimen (7). Nevertheless, EMA-CO has emerged as the regimen of choice for initial treatment of high-risk GTN worldwide. This is predominantly based on retrospective data that consistently show it is active in high-risk GTN and is associated with a low toxicity profile (7,8). These data support the use of EMA-CO as a primary treatment for high-risk GTN, as it appears to be as effective (if not more so), compared to other combination regimens, and better tolerated. The Charing Cross Group has reported the use of induction low-dose etoposide (100 mg/m^2) and cisplatin (20 mg/m^2) on days 1 and 2 every 7 days with good results and no treatment-related toxicities, but its use is suggested only in selected patients with high tumor burden; they also report a 94% remission rate with EMA-CO by carefully excluding nongestational tumors using genetic analysis (9).

Treatment with EMA should alternate with CO every 2 to 3 weeks. Although a treatment delay or dose reduction may be required due to side effects, these should be avoided as both have been associated with less than optimal outcomes. Treatment delay or dose reduction because of side effects increases the likelihood of tumor resistance and treatment failure (10-12). Employment of growth factor support helps minimize hematologic toxicity and avoid delays (13).

Floxuridine (FUDR)-based multiagent chemotherapy (floxuridine, actinomycin-D, etoposide, and vincristine, FAEV regimen) has been used in China for several decades to treat high-risk GTN instead of EMA-CO with favorable outcomes. The Peking GTD group reported that FAEV regimen achieved a complete remission rate of 63.6% among patients with GTN who were referred to Peking Union Medical College Hospital because of progression on prior chemotherapy (14). Another study reported that 60.4% of patients with relapsed or chemoresistant GTN achieved

■ TABLE 7.4-1. EMA-CO Chemotherapy Regimen for High-Risk Gestational Trophoblastic Neoplasia

Day	Order	Drug	Dose	Route	Diluent and Rate
1	1	Actinomycin-D	0.5 mg	IV bolus	n/a
1	2	Etoposide	100 mg/m^2	IV	1,000 mL 0.9% NaCl over 1 hr[a]
1	3	Methotrexate	100 mg/m^2	IV bolus	n/a
1	4	Methotrexate	200 mg/m^2	IV	1,000 mL 0.9% NaCl over 12 hr
2	1	Actinomycin-D	0.5 mg	IV bolus	n/a
2	2	Etoposide	100 mg/m^2	IV	1,000 mL 0.9% NaCl over 1 hr
2	3	Folinic acid rescue	15 mg	PO	Every 12 hr for 4 doses (initiating 24 hr after start of methotrexate)
8	1	Vincristine	1 mg/m^2 (maximum 2 mg)	IV	50 mL 0.9% NaCl over 15 min
8	2	Cyclophosphamide	600 mg/m^2	IV	100 mL 0.9% NaCl over 30 min

EMA-CO, etoposide, methotrexate, actinomycin-D, cyclophosphamide, and vincristine; IV, intravenous.

[a]Hypotension following rapid IV administration has been reported. Longer infusion times may be required based on the patient's tolerance.

complete remission by FAEV chemotherapy (15). The major toxicity associated with the FAEV regimen is neutropenia; however, it was shown to be managed with administration of granulocyte colony-stimulating factor (G-CSF) (16). Treatment for high-risk GTN should be continued until the hCG level becomes undetectable and remains so for 3 consecutive weeks. Once achieved, consolidation treatment of at least three courses of EMA-CO is often administered to reduce the risk of relapse. Though aggressive multiagent therapy is associated with higher levels of toxicity than single-agent therapy, single-agent therapy is not appropriate for high-risk GTN, because the success rate of secondary chemotherapy after failure of single-agent therapy ranges between 20% and 50% (17).

Of note, while some patients meet the definition of having low-risk GTN (ie, prognostic score 5 and 6), those who present with hCG concentrations of 410,000 IU/L or higher with no metastatic disease and no CCA, those with metastatic disease or histopathologic evidence of CCA and pretreatment hCG concentrations of 150,000 IU/L or higher, and those with metastatic disease and CCA appear to be at significant risk for chemoresistance to single-agent chemotherapy (6). In these patients, we suggest first-line multiagent chemotherapy.

For patients in whom combination chemotherapy is indicated, treatment may result in ovarian insufficiency. Therefore, the use of oral contraceptives is suggested to suppress the pituitary gland's production of LH, which aims to protect the ovaries from the toxicity of chemotherapy and also suppress the pituitary production of hCG, which could falsely suggest the presence of active disease if not suppressed (18,19). In addition, strict hormonal contraception allows for the reliable use of the biologic marker of this disease, hCG, by ensuring the absence of pregnancy and thereby allowing assessment of response to treatment and monitoring for relapse. Importantly, after controlling for risk factors, hormonal contraception does not influence the risk or clinical aggressiveness of GTN (20).

Ultrahigh-Risk Gestational Trophoblastic Neoplasia

Patients with widely metastatic disease as evidenced by a very high WHO/FIGO score (≥13) are at significant risk for pulmonary, intraperitoneal, or intracranial hemorrhage, and this risk may be mitigated by starting treatment with low-dose induction chemotherapy. The use of induction low-dose etoposide 100 mg/m^2 and cisplatin 20 mg/m^2 (EP), days 1 and 2, every 7 days, has been used at the Charing Cross since 1995 to reduce early deaths before commencing EMA-CO or EMA-EP (21,22). EP induction was given to 23.1% of 140 high-risk patients (33/140 patients) with a large disease burden for one to four cycles, and the early death rate was reduced to only 0.7%, compared with 7.2% in a cohort treated before 1995 (9).

The prevalence of ultrahigh-risk GTN was 8.1% in the Chinese GTN cohort (16) and 21% in the French cases (23). While Bolze et al showed that the 5-year death rate approached 38.4% for patients with FIGO score 13 or higher treated with EMA-CO with or without low-dose EP, those 143 patients with ultrahigh-risk GTN 94 (65.7%) patients had achieved complete remission after treatment with FAEV, 15.9% (15/94) relapse rate, and a 5-year overall survival rate of 67.9%. Even so, it is not possible to compare the efficacy between the EMA-CO and the FAEV regimen on ultrahigh-risk patients, owing to scarcity of studies focusing on these patients.

Ultrahigh-risk GTN is associated with a higher frequency of resistance to standard first-line MTX- and etoposide-based regimens. The results of the multivariate analysis of a Chinese study revealed that nonmolar antecedent pregnancy (relative risk [RR] 4.689, 95% CI, 1.448-15.189, P = .010), brain metastases (RR 2.280, 95% CI, 1.248-4.163, P = .007), previous multiagent chemotherapy failure (RR 5.345, 95% CI, 2.222-12.857, P = .000), and surgery (RR 0.336, 95% CI, 0.177-0.641, P = .001) all had influence on the prognosis of patient with ultrahigh-risk GTN (16). However, the use of platinum-containing regimens for the treatment of ultrahigh-risk GTN (ie, both EMA-EP and paclitaxel-cisplatin/paclitaxel-etoposide [TP/TE]) is recommended, especially the case in patients with liver metastases, multiple brain metastases, and those with a prolonged time from the antecedent pregnancy (**Tables 7.4-2 and 7.4-3**).

Patients With Brain Metastases

For patients with brain metastases, a neurosurgical consult should be obtained before treatment. These patients are at risk for complications directly related to their brain metastases or as a result of treatment, which may require urgent or emergent intervention (eg, craniotomy for intracerebral bleeding).

For these patients, a modification of systemic EMA-CO that uses a higher MTX dose (1,000 mg/m^2 over 24 hours) than what is routinely administered could be used (24). The higher dose of parenteral MTX allows for adequate levels of MTX within the cerebrospinal fluid (CSF) (25). In addition, these patients should receive dexamethasone to decrease cerebral edema; however, prophylactic antiepileptic drugs are generally not recommended in most patients, provided there is no history of an antecedent seizure.

■ TABLE 7.4-2. EMA-EP Chemotherapy Regimen for High-Risk Gestational Trophoblastic Neoplasia

Day	Order	Drug	Dose	Route	Diluent and Rate
1	1	Actinomycin-D	0.5 mg	IV bolus	100 mL 0.9% NaCl over 15 min
1	2	Etoposide	100 mg/m^2	IV	250 mL 0.9% NaCl over 1 hr[a]
1	4	Methotrexate	300 mg/m^2	IV bolus	1,000 mL 0.9% NaCl over 12 hr
2	3	Folinic acid rescue	15 mg	PO	Every 12 hr for 4 doses (initiating 24 hr after start of methotrexate)
8	1	Etoposide	150 mg/m^2	IV	**250 mL 0.9% NaCl over 1 hr**[a]
8	2	Cisplatin	75 mg/m^2	IV	1,000 mL 0.9% NaCl over 3 hr[b]
9-14	1	Filgrastim	300 µg	SC	n/a

EMA-EP, etoposide, methotrexate, actinomycin-D, etoposide and cisplatin; IV, intravenous.

[a]Hypotension following rapid IV administration has been reported. Check blood pressure every 15 minutes during the etoposide infusion. Longer infusion times may be required based on the patient's tolerance.

[b]Pre- and posthydration therapy required for cisplatin: 1. Administer 10 mmol magnesium sulfate (MgSO$_4$) (±KCl 20 mmol/L if indicated) in 1,000 mL sodium chloride 0.9% over 1 hour. Administer cisplatin as described earlier. Posthydration: Administer 1,000 mL 0.9% NaCl over 1 hour. Mannitol 10% may be used to as per local policy to induce diuresis, although there is no conclusive evidence that this is required. The routine use of furosemide to increase urine flow is not recommended unless there is evidence of fluid overload.

■ TABLE 7.4-3. TP/TE Salvage Chemotherapy Regimen for High-Risk Gestational Trophoblastic Neoplasia

Day	Order	Drug	Dose	Route	Diluent and Rate
1	1	Premedications[a]			
1	2	Paclitaxel	135 mg/m^2	IV	250 mL 0.9% NaCl over 3 hr
1	3	Mannitol	10%	IV	500 mL over 1 hr
1	4	Cisplatin	60 mg/m^2	IV	1,000 mL 0.9% NaCl over 3 hr
1	5	Posthydration	1,000 mL	IV	0.9 NaCl + KCl 20 mmol + 1 g MgSO$_4$ over 2 hr
15	1	Premedications[a]			
15	2	Paclitaxel	135 mg/m^2	IV	2,50 mL 0.9% NaCl over 3 hr
15	3	Etoposide	150 mg/m^2	IV	1,000 mL 0.9% NaCl over 1 hr

IV, intravenous; PO, orally; TP/TE, paclitaxel-cisplatin/paclitaxel-etoposide.

[a]The choice of premedications may vary among institutions: 1. Dexamethasone 20 mg PO 12 hour before paclitaxel; 2. Dexamethasone 20 mg PO 6 hour before paclitaxel; 3. Ondansetron 8 mg PO 8/8 hour during the treatment; 4. Ranitidine 50 mg IV 100 mL 0.9% over 30 minutes; 5. Chlorpheniramine 10 mg IV bolus.

A typical regimen is as follows:

Etoposide: 100 mg/m^2 IV over 60 minutes on days 1 and 2
MTX: 1,000 mg/m^2 IV over 24 hours on day 1
Act-D: 0.5 mg IV bolus on days 1 and 2
Leucovorin calcium: 30 mg IM or orally every 12 hours for 3 days, starting 32 hours after treatment with MTX
Cyclophosphamide: 600 mg/m^2 IV on day 8
Vincristine: 1.0 mg/m^2 IV on day 8

At these high doses of MTX, significant renal toxicity can occur, typically from crystallization of the MTX in the renal tubules. Renal dysfunction can lead to decreased MTX clearance, which leads to more significant nonrenal toxicities (eg, myelosuppression, mucositis). Adequate hydration and alkalinization of the urine with sodium bicarbonate can help prevent these problems (26).

Finally, these patients should be closely followed during treatment, which can be done using serial imaging and hCG monitoring. **Figure 7.4-1** presents a case report of GTN treatment of patient with brain metastasis.

Role for Intrathecal Therapy

The need for intrathecal (IT) therapy in these patients is controversial (25,27), and its use alongside high-dose EMA-CO is based on institutional preferences. If administered, MTX is given as a 12.5-mg dose IT on day 8, followed by leucovorin calcium 15 mg at 24 and 36 hours. However, one study that included 15 patients treated with EMA-CO plus IT MTX reported that 87% (13 patients) achieved a sustained remission without the use of whole-brain irradiation (27). An update of this study reported that 23 (85%) of 27 patients with brain metastases achieved complete remission with EMA-CO or EMA-EP (etoposide and cisplatin on day 8) plus IT MTX (28).

Radiation

As with the role of IT MTX, the role of cranial radiation therapy is also controversial. For patients who present with brain metastases, whole-brain radiation (3,000 cGy in 200 cGy fractions) or, in selected patients, surgical excision with stereotactic radiation is indicated and is usually performed at the start of chemotherapy to lower the risk of hemorrhage (29,30). In these patients, the EMA-CO regimen is modified such that MTX is increased to 1 g/m^2 with 30 mg of FA every 12 hours for 3 days starting 32 hours after the start of infusion (27). At some centers, such as the NETDC, cranial radiotherapy (20-30 Gy in 2 Gy daily fractions) or stereotactic radiotherapy is given concurrently with high-dose

MTX chemotherapy. In addition to shrinking the brain metastases, concomitant cranial irradiation increases the MTX concentration within the central nervous system (CNS) (30) and reduces the risk of cerebral hemorrhage before eradication of tumor and may improve survival (31,32). However, the use of concurrent MTX and cranial irradiation also increases the likelihood of treatment-related toxicity, especially leukoencephalopathy. IT and high-dose MTX may also be used. Patients are also treated with dexamethasone to decrease edema and phenytoin sodium to prevent seizure. During therapy, patients undergo serial CT scans or MRIs to monitor the lesions. Once a complete response has been achieved, hCG levels in the CSF should be measured, ideally by radioimmunoassay to detect low levels of protein. The plasma-to-CSF ratio of hCG should be less than 60 (31). Patients with brain metastases have a cure rate of 50% to 85% depending on symptoms and the number, size, and location of brain lesions.

Alternatives Regimens

In many centers, a modified EMA-CO regimen that incorporates cisplatin is preferentially administered to patients with a WHO risk score 12 or greater. The most commonly used combination replaces vincristine and cyclophosphamide (used in EMA-CO) with etoposide and cisplatin on day 8 (EMA-EP). EMA-EP, either alone or in combination with surgery, induced complete remission in 16 (76%) of 21 patients with EMA-CO resistance (33). Among patients with ultrahigh-risk GTN (FIGO score ≥13), only 97 (67.9%) of 143 and 23 (63.9%) of 36 achieved complete remission (16,22).

While no randomized trials have compared EMA-CO with cisplatin-containing regimens, a retrospective study evaluated outcomes among 83 patients treated with cisplatin-containing treatment and 103 patients treated with EMA-CO (34). Compared with EMA-CO, incorporation of cisplatin was associated with a slightly lower remission rate (85% vs 92%), a lower number of cycles to achieve a normal hCG level (three vs five courses), and more toxicity, including fever, nephropathy, nausea, and diarrhea. As EMA-EP is very toxic, great attention to renal and bone marrow function is required (35).

In China, the preferred regimen as primary therapy in ultrahigh-risk GTN is FAEV. Among 30 patients with stage IV GTN, primary treatment with FAEV was administered, and 24 (80%) patients achieved complete and sustained remission with tolerable toxicity (36). Among six patients with resistance, two died from progressive disease and four achieved remission with other regimens. The major adverse event of FAEV regimen was hematologic toxicity.

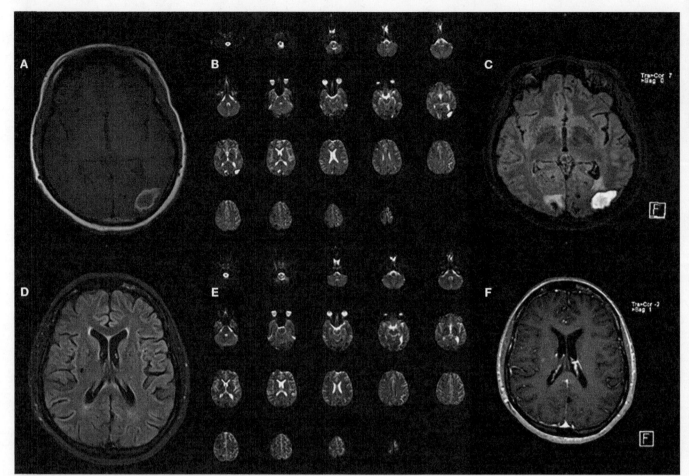

Figure 7.4-1. A case of a Brazilian 26-year-old primigravida, presenting with amenorrhea, nausea and vomiting, and right inferotemporal visual field loss 9 months postpartum. **Her condition remained undiagnosed from** December 2013 to July 2014, when she was referred to a Gestational Trophoblastic Disease Reference Center (São Paulo State University, Botucatu Medical School). Magnetic resonance of the brain revealed a 3.5-cm tumor in the left occipital lobe (A-C). Chest tomography showed two lung nodules, and **three-phase computed tomography revealed two liver nodules**. Serum hCG was 1,722,560 IU/L, FIGO stage IV: WHO/FIGO score 17. Initial inpatient care consisting of radiotherapy (2,400 cGy) and chemotherapy (induction low-dose etoposide-cisplatin) was followed by a modified EMA-EP regimen. After 4 EMA-EP cycles, the patient received no chemotherapy for 21 days due to grade 4 myelosuppression with febrile neutropenia. Subsequently, three EMA-EP cycles were given at a reduced dose (80%). Nonetheless, there was hCG elevation (4.6-6.1 IU/L). The patient was then switched to paclitaxel-carboplatin/paclitaxel-etoposide achieving complete remission after one cycle of this regimen. Only one consolidation cycle was used due to bone marrow toxicity. The patient is now healthy, with a normal visual field and normal (D, E, F) hCG for the past 5 years. EMA-EP, etoposide, methotrexate, actinomycin-D, etoposide and cisplatin; FIGO, International Federation of Gynaecology and Obstetrics; hCG, human chorionic gonadotropin; WHO, World Health Organization.

Surgery

Approximately 50% of patients with high-risk, metastatic GTN will require adjuvant surgical procedures, usually hysterectomy and pulmonary resection, for chemotherapy-resistant disease or to control hemorrhage and sepsis (37). Selected patients with focal disease may be the candidates for partial lung, liver, or brain resection. For women with excessive vaginal bleeding, selective arterial embolization may be beneficial (38) (**Figure 7.4-2**) (39).

In general, hysterectomy is not required and can be avoided, particularly in women who desire future fertility. However, it may be indicated after chemotherapy, especially for heavy bleeding, large bulky intrauterine disease, or in the presence of sepsis (40). Hysterectomy may also be performed to manage chemotherapy resistance and to reduce tumor burden (41, 42). For patients undergoing a hysterectomy, it is important to note that the removal of the ovaries is usually not indicated, even when they are enlarged, often due to theca lutein cysts, because metastatic disease involving the ovary is rare. Symptomatic ovarian theca lutein cysts can be aspirated if indicated, but otherwise will regress spontaneously after

treatment. Furthermore, the preferred approach to hysterectomy, laparoscopic versus laparotomy, has not been well defined and usually is left to the discretion of the surgeon. However, it appears that laparoscopic hysterectomy maintains the same high effectiveness with less toxicity (43).

Intra-abdominal metastases may require resection, as they are often less responsive to chemotherapy (44). In addition, these metastases may cause complications, particularly hemorrhage (45). Some studies suggest that clinical parameters may predict the outcome following surgical resection.

In one series of 33 patients who underwent various surgical procedures for resistant or recurrent GTN, successful outcome was achieved mostly in patients with the following characteristics: a single preoperative disease site, underwent salvage surgery within 1 year of initial diagnosis, non-CCA histology, and/or a total WHO score of less than 8 (46). In another report of 61 patients with chemoresistant GTN undergoing surgical salvage, the clinical factors that predicted treatment failure were age over 35, hCG greater than 10,000 IU/L, antecedent nonmolar pregnancy, and metastases outside the lungs (47).

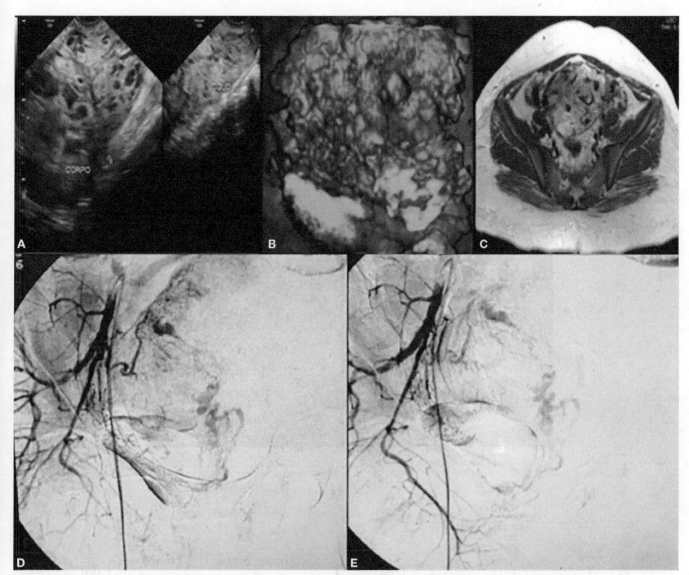

Figure 7.4-2. A case of a Brazilian 23-year-old primigravida, with complete hydatidiform mole without surveillance of hCG after uterine evacuation. Two months later, the patient presented to the emergency with heavy vaginal bleeding and was referred to a Gestational Trophoblastic Disease Reference Center (Universidade Federal de São Paulo, Escola Paulista de Medicina). She was diagnosed with high-risk GTN stage/score III:7. The sonographic examination revealed enlarged uterus with a heterogeneous mass constituted of multiple large vessels invading and causing disarrangement of the myometrium. Uterine images before chemotherapy (June 9, 2016) demonstrating loss of myometrium stratification due to heterogeneous image, mainly vascular, invading the whole uterus and cervix (A). Pelvic transvaginal ultrasonography B-mode (B). Transvaginal three-dimensional high-definition flow multiplanar view scan (C). The patient developed progressive worsening of vaginal bleeding after chemotherapy with etoposide, methotrexate, actinomycin D, cyclophosphamide, and vincristine (EMA-CO) regimen. She underwent blood transfusion and embolization of uterine arteries due to severe vaginal hemorrhage episodes with complete control of bleeding. Pelvic angiogram: ongoing embolization (D) and completed embolization (E) (July 6, 2016). The hCG reached a negative value after the third cycle, and there was a complete regression of the anomalous vascularization of the uterus as well as full recovery of the uterine anatomy. GTN, gestational trophoblastic neoplasia; hCG, human chorionic gonadotropin. (From Silva ACBD, Passos JP, Signorini Filho RC, Braga A, Mattar R, Sun SY. Uterine rescue in high-risk gestational trophoblastic neoplasia treated with EMA-CO by uterine arteries embolization due to arteriovenous malformations. Resgate uterino em neoplasia trofoblástica gestacional de alto risco tratada com EMA-CO por embolização de artérias uterinas devido a malformações arteriovenosas. *Rev Bras Ginecol Obstet.* 2021;43(4):323-328.)

Management of persistent liver metastases (**Figure 7.4-3**) (48) can be a particularly difficult and challenging problem. Selective embolization or hepatic resection may be used in cases to control bleeding or excise resistant tumor (49). Because of their hypervascular nature, biopsy should not be performed because of the potential for life-threatening hemorrhage.

Resection of chemoresistant pulmonary disease can be curative. Favorable prognostic indicators include normalization of hCG within to 2 weeks after resection of a pulmonary metastasis (50), and a separate series reported that successful outcomes

were possible even after multiple resections (51). When evaluating patients for thoracotomy, it is important to remember that fibrotic lung nodules may mimic areas of active disease. Criteria that predict favorable outcome include the absence of other systemic metastases, presence of a unilateral solitary nodule, no uterine involvement, and serum hCG less than 1,500 IU/L.

Craniotomy can play a vital role in the management of GTN cerebral metastases. It is indicated for the resection of peripheral, solitary, drug-resistant lesions and can be lifesaving, especially with a neurologic emergency due to intracranial hemorrhage or

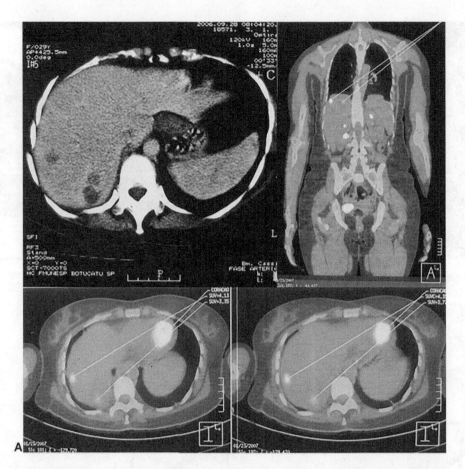

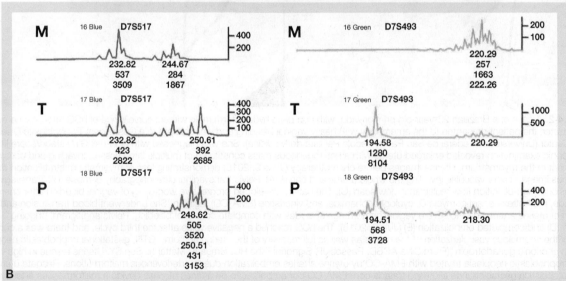

Figure 7.4-3. A: A 28-year-old patient with a history of hydatidiform mole and term pregnancy was diagnosed with gestational primary pulmonary choriocarcinoma. After EMA-CO/EP-EMA treatment, she was referred to our center. Upon admission, she had a 3.5-cm isolate mass in the right lung. FIGO staging and WHO/FIGO score were III:13. Following lower right lobectomy, hCG dropped from 1,202.6 to 5.2 mUI/mL. Because consolidation treatment with paclitaxel-ifosfamide resulted in hCG elevation, bleomycin-etoposide-cisplatin was used. During therapy, hepatic metastasis was detected and high-dose EP-EMA (methotrexate 1.0 g/m²) was administered. Following initial positive response, the EP portion of the regimen was omitted due to nephrotoxicity. Subsequently, hepatic metastasis and hCG increased (1,519.0 mUI/mL). Positron emission tomography scan revealed that only the right lobe of the liver was affected. Systemic infection prevented the scheduling of right hepatectomy. hCG increased 2-fold weekly (31,434.0 mUI/mL), and due to the rupture of an hepatic metastatic lesion, emergency hepatectomy was performed. Postoperatively, hCG dropped but resumed increasing. The treatment using 5-fluoracyl/actinomycin-D failed and tumor infiltration led to liver insufficiency, which caused death. Choriocarcinoma samples matched with peripheral blood samples from the patient and her partner were used to confirm the gestational origin of the tumor using polymorphic microsatellite markers. EMA-CO, etoposide, methotrexate, actinomycin D, cyclophosphamide, and vincristine; EMA-EP, etoposide, methotrexate, actinomycin D, etoposide and cisplatin; FIGO, International Federation of Gynaecology and Obstetrics; hCG, human chorionic gonadotropin; WHO, World Health Organization.

increased intracranial pressure (24,28). Resection of intracranial disease can also result in remission. Among seven patients who underwent craniotomy for drug-resistant disease, five (71%) achieved complete remission (52).

Chemoresistance or Relapsed Disease

GTN is resistant to chemotherapy when hCG levels plateau or increase, in two consecutive hCG values over a 2-week interval, regardless of whether new metastases develop, while the patient is undergoing treatment. In contrast, a diagnosis of relapse is made when there are two elevations of hCG concentrations in the absence of pregnancy after remission is attained. Both conditions are challenging in the treatment of GTN.

Despite the success of primary therapy with EMA-CO, roughly 30% to 40% of women with high-risk GTN will have an incomplete response to first-line therapy or will relapse from remission and will need additional multiagent chemotherapy with or without other treatment modalities (53-57). Risk factors for resistant or relapse disease in most studies appear to be related to a large initial tumor burden, inadequate primary therapy, and in patients who defaulted on potential treatments or noncompliant follow-up (58).

Common reasons for treatment failure for GTN are the use of single-agent chemotherapy for patients with high-risk disease and inappropriate use of weekly IM MTX chemotherapy for treatment of patients with metastatic disease, FIGO scores 7 or greater, and/or nonpostmolar CCA. It is recommended that clinicians request advice from or referral for treatment to centers with expertise in management of GTN for patients who have single-agent therapy failure for low-risk disease and for any patient with high-risk disease.

All patients who develop chemoresistant or relapse disease require reassessment of extent of disease. In addition, this evaluation should be repeated each time a new treatment is indicated.

Patients who recur or develop resistance often have multiorgan involvement, particularly if they were previously treated for high-risk GTN. Therefore, reimaging with chest, abdominal, and pelvic CT scans and brain MRI should be performed to help guide treatment options. For patients in whom the diagnosis is questionable, positron emission tomography (PET) scanning may aid in the differential characterization of active disease (which should be PET positive) from fibrotic tumor nodules.

Second-Line Combination Therapy

Although there are no universally accepted evidence-based guidelines for second-line treatment for patients who develop resistant or recurrent disease on first-line EMA-CO, our approach is as follows.

For patients previously treated with EMA-CO, we administer the multiagent chemotherapy combination consisting of EMA-EP. Neutropenia may become an issue for patients receiving EMA-CO followed by EMA-EP, and in our clinical experience, prolonged neutropenia develops by the second or third cycle. Therefore, growth factor support (ie, filgrastim) is usually required. In addition to chemotherapy, these patients may benefit from surgical excision of localized, persistent tumor (59). In one report of 21 patients who had previously received EMA-CO, EMA-EP (either alone or in combination with surgery) induced remission in 16 (76%) (60). In a separate report that included 49 patients, the complete remission rate was 82% (37).

Patients who were not treated with EMA-CO in the first-line setting should undergo treatment with this combination in the second-line setting.

For patients with resistant or relapsed disease despite two prior combination regimens, a number of alternative regimens can be administered. However, none of these regimens have been used in a sufficient number of patients to identify one as being the optimal choice. It is important to restage patients before the initiation of a new regimen so that the extent of disease may be appropriately characterized and to evaluate for a potential role for surgical treatment.

Multiagent Therapy

Paclitaxel and etoposide alternating biweekly with paclitaxel and cisplatin (TE-TP) has had encouraging results in heavily pretreated patients. It appears to have tolerable toxicity, though the experience remains quite limited.

In one report of two patients, both had a complete remission with TE-TP (61). In a separate series of 16 patients (including six previously treated with cisplatin), 19% and 31% had a complete and partial remission, respectively (62). Despite the lack of randomized clinical trials, it should be noted that the TE-TP regimen has good clinical tolerability, less toxicity, and can be an alternative second-line therapy for high-risk GTN, with the advantage of introducing two new drugs (taxol and platinum) rather than continued exposure to EMA and addition of only one new drug, platinum.

The combination of bleomycin, etoposide, and cisplatin (BEP) is widely used to treat germ cell tumors of the ovary and testicle. In one report of 16 patients with EMA-CO–resistant disease, 11 (69%) patients had a complete response and nine (56%) survived (57).

The combination of ifosfamide, etoposide, and cisplatin (ICE) is often administered to men with recurrent or chemorefractory testicular cancer. Its use in women with recurrent or resistant GTN is limited. In one experience that included six patients, four had a complete remission and three ultimately survived (57).

High-dose FU in conjunction with Act-D is commonly used in Asia, though the experience with this regimen is limited. For example, one series of 11 patients reported a complete remission rate of 82% (63).

Very limited data suggest that single-agent treatment may provide benefit in patients with previously treated recurrent, advanced, or metastatic GTN. These include paclitaxel, capecitabine, and pegylated liposomal doxorubicin.

New Treatments

Standard treatments for GTN rely on chemotherapy: single agents for low-risk disease and polychemotherapy for high-risk disease or disease resistant to single agents. However, 0.5% to 5.0% of women die as a result of multidrug resistance, necessitating novel approaches. Risk factors for poor survival include drug-refractory disease, liver or brain metastases, and PSTT and ETT that develop more than4 years after the antecedent pregnancy (64). We have few options for unresectable multidrug-resistant GTN, and immunotherapy may be a lifesaving treatment. Anticancer T-cell activity is regulated by multiple suppressive mechanisms, including tumor-expressed proteins that regulate cell death. Monoclonal antibodies that block the activity of these tumor-expressed proteins have important effects on different cancers. The rationale for immunotherapy in this disease is histologic evidence that trophoblasts, including all forms of GTN, strongly express programmed cell death ligand 1 (PD-L1) (65).

Pembrolizumab, a humanized monoclonal antibody to the PD-L1 receptor, has shown to be effective in treating chemoresistant high-risk GTN (64). These authors reported four GTN cases with metastatic disease and chemoresistance to multiple combination chemotherapy regimens reporting remission in three of four patients. With these results, the authors presented evidence in favor of pembrolizumab as an important advance in the management of drug-resistant GTN and suggested that tumor-infiltrating lymphocytes and HLA-G expression are predictors of good response. However, in MTX-resistant GTN, avelumab, another monoclonal antibody PD-L1 inhibitor, cured only approximately 50% of patients; therefore, it may not be considered a therapeutic option in GTN resistant to polychemotherapy (66,67).

These provocative data point to the potential role of immune checkpoint inhibitors like pembrolizumab for resistant GTN and warrant further evaluation (65).

Placental Site Trophoblastic Tumor and Epithelioid Trophoblastic Tumor

PSTT and ETT are rare types of GTN, with an incidence of 1 in 100,000 pregnancies and representing 1% to 2% of GTN cases (68,69), that arise from intermediate trophoblast. PSTT and ETT are important forms of GTN with unique pathology, natural history, and treatment paradigms. Both PSTT and ETT are relatively newly recognized disease entities, with the first description of PSTT as a "trophoblastic pseudotumor of the uterus" being from 1976 (70) and ETT from 1988 (71).

PSTT and ETT both exhibit slow growth rates and remain confined to the uterus (stage I, nonmetastatic) for extended periods of time. As a result, there is often a paucity of symptoms other than vaginal bleeding or amenorrhea (72-75). Other symptoms are contingent upon sites of metastases, which ultimately occur in 30% to 50% of women with PSTT and ETT (76,77). Similar to other types of GTN, common sites of metastasis include the lung, vagina, and CNS, with the lung being the most common site. However, there is thought to be a higher propensity for retroperitoneal node involvement. Assessment of metastatic disease in patients with PSTT/ETT is, therefore, crucial in prognosis. The potential role of PET, in the evaluation of metastatic GTN, has not yet been well studied (78). The available information indicates that the PET does not add to GTN staging when compared to conventional imaging workup that is less expensive and more widely available. PET may help evaluate metastases in unusual sites or to differentiate active metastatic nodules from necrotic and/or hemorrhagic tissue following chemotherapy and in cases of chemoresistance or relapse, notably in patients with PSTT or ETT, as well as for guiding surgical intervention (78,79). Both false-positive and false-negative results can occur with FDG-PET imaging so careful co-evaluation with other imaging modalities is desirable (80).

FIGO staging and prognostic scoring for GTN do not correlate well with outcome in PSTT and ETT. A few risk factors generally appear to be associated with favorable or unfavorable outcomes. Advanced age (>34 years old), deep myometrial invasion (>50%), and tumor size (>1 cm^3) have been associated with worse outcome for women with PSTT. A high mitotic rate has also correlated with a higher risk of recurrence, and advanced-stage disease, defined as stages II to IV, has been associated with relapse and worse survival (81). The most important factors for increased risk of death from PSTT are metastasis and interval from antecedent pregnancy greater than 4 years.

Risk factors for ETT are even less well established. Given the clinical similarities between PSTT and ETT, it is assumed that many of the same risk factors for PSTT would apply to ETT (82,83). The world's largest case series of patients with ETT is from the International Society for the Study of Trophoblastic Diseases database (84). These authors presented data on 54 patients diagnosed with ETT or mixed PSTT/ETT. Eleven of them did not survive. Interval since antecedent pregnancy more than 48 months and advanced-stage disease were prognostic factors of overall survival. (84).

Localized Disease

Treatment decisions for PSTT and ETT are made predominantly upon stage of disease with some consideration of high-risk factors. Given the relative chemotherapy resistance of PSTT and ETT, hysterectomy, without removal of the ovaries in premenopausal women, is the treatment of choice for localized disease confined to the uterus in women who no longer desire fertility preservation (81). Patients with uterine-confined disease may be cured with primary hysterectomy alone without adjuvant chemotherapy (83,85).

The role of lymphadenectomy in the surgical management of PSTT is controversial and may be performed in patients with presumed stage I PSTT, when deep myometrial invasion or bulky lymph nodes are present (81).

Although there is no conclusive evidence currently available to support adjuvant chemotherapy in stage I PSTT, it is reasonable to discuss the role of adjuvant chemotherapy in patients with a long time interval from the antecedent pregnancy (ie, >4 years). While some may administer adjuvant chemotherapy in stage I disease due to deep myometrial invasion or serosal involvement, there are currently no data to support this recommendation.

For young women in whom fertility preservation is important, there are several case series of local uterine resection with varying degrees of success. Given the discrepant results, the role of fertility-preserving therapy is still controversial and requires extensive counseling (81).

Metastatic Disease

Unlike IM or CCA, PSTT and ETT are relatively chemotherapy resistant. As such, treatment of advanced-stage, metastatic, or locally advanced disease with chemotherapy alone is not recommended. Patients with metastatic disease should be treated with intensive combination chemotherapy and surgery. In the United Kingdom experience with PSTT, 60% of patients treated with chemotherapy alone had no or an incomplete response to chemotherapy. Long-term disease control was only achieved with either surgery alone or surgery and chemotherapy combined (72). Multimodality therapy for PSTT and ETT with complete surgical resection appears to be more critical for ETT than PSTT (72-75,82,83,85). Depending upon sites and extent of metastases, surgical resection needs to be individualized and may necessitate thoracic procedures, hepatic resection or other upper abdominal procedures, bowel resection, and/or craniotomy. The role of surgery after normalization of serum hCG in patients with PSTT is uncertain. Because PSTT and ETT are less sensitive to chemotherapy and hCG is a less sensitive tumor marker, some experts, having found viable tumor in resected residual lesions, recommend resection of residual masses after completion of chemotherapy (72). For other forms of GTN, surgical resection of residual masses after normalization of hCG has shown no benefit (86).

Given the rarity of these diseases and the lack of controlled trials, the optimal chemotherapy regimen to treat PSTT and ETT is not known. Despite the lack of any conclusive differences between regimens such as EMA-CO, EMA-EP, or other platinum- and non–platinum-based regimens, the preferential first-line therapy is EMA-EP (81). Based predominately on the experience at the Charing Cross, this regimen achieved a 100% remission in those patients who had less than 2-year interval from antecedent pregnancy, a 20% remission in those with interval greater than 2 years, and an overall survival of 50% for patients with metastatic PSTT (59). Because this regimen is associated with significant hematologic toxicity, alternative active and less toxic regimens, such as TP/TE, are gaining favor (62).

Regimens for recurrent or resistant PSTT and ETT are needed. Available regimens include gemcitabine, high-dose chemotherapy with stem cell rescue, combination BEP, and other platinum- and FU-based regimens (57,87). However, new therapeutic strategies for these diseases are needed, and targeted biologic agents should be further evaluated.

Survival

Long-term survival for patients with stage I PSTT after hysterectomy, with or without lymphadenectomy, is approaching 90% at 10 years. For patients with stages II to IV disease, overall survival at 10 years is approximately 50% after surgical resection and chemotherapy. Long-term remission after recurrence is approximately 30% with greater than 5-year follow-up (72). Schmid et al (72) in an updated series of 62 patients with PSTT indicated that the only independent predictor of survival was time from antecedent pregnancy at less than 4 years or at 4 years or more. For patients with ETT, there are limited data concerning survival. The world's largest case series of patients with ETT is from the International Society for the Study of Trophoblastic Diseases database (84). Among 45 patients with ETT and 9 mixed PSTT/ETT, 39 patients survived, including 22 patients with complete sustained hCG remission for at least 1 year. Patients treated with surgery as first-line treatment had early-stage disease and all survived. Most patients treated with multiple lines of chemotherapy with or without surgery had FIGO stages II to IV disease (55%). Eleven of them did not survive. Interval since antecedent pregnancy greater than 48 months and advanced-stage disease were prognostic factors of overall survival. Concerning treatment, surgery seems adequate for early-stage disease with a shorter interval, whereas advanced-stage disease requires a combination of treatment modalities (84).

Surveillance After Treatment

After remission is achieved, serum hCG should be measured monthly until there have been undetectable hCG levels for 12 months (65). In a population-based cohort study from the United Kingdom, 86% of recurrences in patients with high-risk GTN occurred within 1 year of treatment cessation and 95% occurred within 2 years (88). These data support discontinuing routine monitoring after 1 year. Until then, hormonal contraception should be encouraged. Pregnancy can be allowed after 12 months with normal hCG levels.

If a patient develops a rising hCG after remission, it is important to consider alternative sources for this elevation. These would include a new conception, which could be new molar pregnancy or a new intrauterine pregnancy, or pituitary hCG, which is more common if the ovaries experience significant damage following intensive combination chemotherapy (89).

REFERENCES

1. Freitas F, Braga A, Viggiano M, et al. Gestational trophoblastic neoplasia lethality among Brazilian women: a retrospective national cohort study. *Gynecol Oncol.* 2020;158(2):452-459.

2. Braga A, Mora P, de Melo AC, et al. Challenges in the diagnosis and treatment of gestational trophoblastic neoplasia worldwide. *World J Clin Oncol.* 2019;10:28-37.

3. Ross GT, Goldstein DP, Hertz R, Lipsett MB, Odell WD. Sequential use of methotrexate and actinomycin D in the treatment of metastatic choriocarcinoma and related trophoblastic diseases in women. *Am J Obstet Gynecol.* 1965;93(2):223-229.

4. Newlands ES, Bagshawe KD, Begent RH, et al. Results with the EMA/CO (etoposide, methotrexate, actinomycin D, cyclophosphamide, vincristine) regimen in high risk gestational trophoblastic tumours, 1979 to 1989. *Br J Obstet Gynaecol.* 1991;98(6):550-557.

5. Escobar PF, Lurain JR, Singh DK, et al. Treatment of high-risk gestational trophoblastic neoplasia with etoposide, methotrexate, actinomycin D, cyclophosphamide, and vincristine chemotherapy. *Gynecol Oncol.* 2003;91(3):552-557.

6. Braga A, Paiva G, Ghorani E, et al. Predictors for single-agent resistance in FIGO score 5 or 6 gestational trophoblastic neoplasia: a multicentre, retrospective, cohort study. *Lancet Oncol.* 2021;22(8):1188-1198.

7. Deng L, Zhang J, Wu T, Lawrie TA. Combination chemotherapy for primary treatment of high-risk gestational trophoblastic tumour. *Cochrane Database Syst Rev.* 2013;1:CD005196.

8. Kim SJ, Bae SN, Kim JH, et al. Effects of multiagent chemotherapy and independent risk factors in the treatment of high-risk GTT-25 years experiences of KRI-TRD. *Int J Gynaecol Obstet.* 1998;60(suppl 1):S85-S96.

9. Alifrangis C, Agarwal R, Short D, et al. EMA/CO for high-risk gestational trophoblastic neoplasia: good outcomes with induction low-dose etoposide-cisplatin and genetic analysis. *J Clin Oncol.* 2013;31(2):280-286.

10. Berkowitz RS, Goldstein DP. Current management of gestational trophoblastic diseases. *Gynecol Oncol.* 2009;112:654-662.

11. Seckl MJ, Sebire NJ, Berkowitz RS. Gestational trophoblastic disease. *Lancet.* 2010;376:717-729.

12. Lurain JR. Gestational trophoblastic disease. II. Classification and management of gestational trophoblastic neoplasia. *Am J Obstet Gynecol.* 2011;204:11-18.

13. Kanis MJ, Greendyk R, Sobecki-Rausch J, Dayno M, Lurain JR. Use of granulocyte colony stimulating factors (G-CSFs) with multiagent chemotherapy for gestational trophoblastic neoplasia (GTN). *Gynecol Oncol.* 2017;145(suppl 1):218.

14. Wan X, Xiang Y, Yang X, et al. Efficacy of the FAEV regimen in the treatment of high-risk, drug-resistant gestational trophoblastic tumor. *J Reprod Med.* 2007;52:941-944.

15. Feng F, Xiang Y, Wan X, Geng S, Wang T. Salvage combination chemotherapy with floxuridine, dactinomycin, etoposide, and vincristine (FAEV) for patients with relapsed/chemoresistant gestational trophoblastic neoplasia. *Ann Oncol.* 2011;22:1588-1594.

16. Kong Y, Yang J, Jiang F, et al. Clinical characteristics and prognosis of ultra high-risk gestational trophoblastic neoplasia patients: a retrospective cohort study. *Gynecol Oncol.* 2017;146(1):81-86.

17. Ngan HYS, Seckl MJ, Berkowitz RS, et al. Update on the diagnosis and management of gestational trophoblastic disease. *Int J Gynaecol Obstet.* 2018;143(suppl 2):79-85.

18. Berkowitz RS, Horowitz NS, Elias KM. Initial management of high-risk gestational trophoblastic neoplasia. In: Goff B, Dizon DS, eds. *UpToDate.* Wolters Kluwer; 2021. Accessed February 19, 2022. https://www.uptodate.com/contents/initial-management-of-high-risk-gestational-trophoblastic-neoplasia#

19. Cole LA, Sasaki Y, Muller CY. Normal production of human chorionic gonadotropin in menopause. *N Engl J Med.* 2007;356(9):1184-1186.

20. Dantas PRS, Maestá I, Rezende-Filho J, et al. Does hormonal contraception during molar pregnancy follow-up influence the risk and clinical aggressiveness of gestational trophoblastic neoplasia after controlling for risk factors? *Gynecol Oncol.* 2017;147(2):364-370.

21. Ngan HYS, Seckl MJ, Berkowitz RS, et al. Diagnosis and management of gestational trophoblastic disease: 2021 update. *Int J Gynaecol Obstet.* 2021;155(suppl 1):86-93.

22. Maestá I, Moreira MFS, Rezende-Filho K, et al. Outcomes in the management of high risk gestational trophoblastic neoplasia in trophoblastic disease centers in South America. *Int J Gynecol Cancer.* 2020;30(9):1366-1371.

23. Bolze PA, Riedl C, Massardier J, et al. Mortality rate of gestational trophoblastic neoplasia with a FIGO score of ≥13. *Am J Obstet Gynecol.* 2016;214(3):390.e1-390.e8.

24. Newlands ES, Holden L, Seckl MJ, McNeish I, Strickland S, Rustin GJ. Management of brain metastases in patients with high-risk gestational trophoblastic tumors. *J Reprod Med.* 2002;47(6):465-471.

25. Newlands ES. The management of recurrent and drug-resistant gestational trophoblastic neoplasia (GTN). *Best Pract Res Clin Obstet Gynaecol.* 2003;17(6):905-923.

26. Howard SC, McCormick J, Pui CH, Buddington RK, Harvey RD. Preventing and managing toxicities of high-dose methotrexate. *Oncologist.* 2016;21(12):1471-1482.

27. Rustin GJ, Newlands ES, Begent RH, et al. Weekly alternating etoposide, methotrexate, and actinomycin/vincristine and cyclophosphamide chemotherapy for the treatment of CNS metastases of choriocarcinoma. *J Clin Oncol.* 1989;7(7):900-903.

28. Savage P, Kelpanide I, Tuthill M, Short D, Seckl MJ. Brain metastases in gestational trophoblast neoplasia: an update on incidence, management and outcome. *Gynecol Oncol.* 2015;137(1):73-76.

29. Barber EL, Schink JC, Lurain JR. Hepatic metastasis in gestational trophoblastic neoplasia: patient characteristics, prognostic factors, and outcomes. *J Reprod Med.* 2014;59(5-6):199-203.

30. Herrington S. Enhancing cure and palliation: radiation therapy in the treatment of metastatic gestational trophoblastic neoplasia. *Semin Oncol.* 1995;22(2):185-192.

31. Athanassiou A, Begent RH, Newlands ES, et al. Central nervous system metastases of choriocarcinoma: 23 years' experience at Charing Cross Hospital. *Cancer.* 1983;52(9):1728-1735.

32. Yordan EL Jr, Schlaerth J, Gaddis O, Morrow CP. Radiation therapy in the management of gestational choriocarcinoma metastatic to the central nervous system. *Obstet Gynecol.* 1987;69(4):627-630.

33. Altintas A, Vardar MA. Central nervous system involvement in gestational trophoblastic neoplasia. *Eur J Gynaecol Oncol.* 2001;22(2):154-156.

34. Lybol C, Thomas CMG, Blanken EA, et al. Comparing cisplatin-based combination chemotherapy with EMA/CO chemotherapy for the treatment of high risk gestational trophoblastic neoplasia. *Eur J Cancer.* 2013;49(4):860-867.

35. Patel SM, Arora R, Tiwari R, et al. Management of "ultra-high risk" gestational trophoblastic neoplasia at a tertiary center in India. *Indian J Med Paediatr Oncol.* 2020;41:345-350.

36. Yang J, Xiang Y, Wan X, Feng F, Ren T. Primary treatment of stage IV gestational trophoblastic neoplasia with floxuridine, dactinomycin, etoposide and vincristine (FAEV): a report based on our 10-year clinical experiences. *Gynecol Oncol*. 2016;143(1):68-72.

37. Lurain JR, Singh DK, Schink JC. Role of surgery in the management of high-risk gestational trophoblastic neoplasia. *J Reprod Med*. 2006;51(10):773-776.

38. Lim AK, Agarwal R, Seckl MJ, et al. Embolization of bleeding residual uterine vascular malformations in patients with treated gestational trophoblastic tumors. *Radiology*. 2002;222(3):640-644.

39. Silva ACBD, Passos JP, Signorini Filho RC, Braga A, Mattar R, Sun SY. Uterine rescue in high-risk gestational trophoblastic neoplasia treated with EMA-CO by uterine arteries embolization due to arteriovenous malformations [Resgate uterino em neoplasia trofoblástica gestacional de alto risco tratada com EMA-CO por embolização de artérias uterinas devido a malformações arteriovenosas]. *Rev Bras Ginecol Obstet*. 2021;43(4):323-328.

40. Cagayan MS. High-risk metastatic gestational trophoblastic neoplasia. Primary management with EMA-CO (etoposide, methotrexate, actinomycin D, cyclophosphamide and vincristine) chemotherapy. *J Reprod Med*. 2012;57(5-6):231-236.

41. Eysbouts YK, Massuger LFAG, IntHout J, Lok CAR, Sweep FCGJ, Ottevanger PB. The added value of hysterectomy in the management of gestational trophoblastic neoplasia. *Gynecol Oncol*. 2017;145(3):536-542.

42. Clark RM, Nevadunsky NS, Ghosh S, Goldstein DP, Berkowitz RS. The evolving role of hysterectomy in gestational trophoblastic neoplasia at the New England Trophoblastic Disease Center. *J Reprod Med*. 2010;55(5-6):194-198.

43. Sugrue R, Foley O, Elias KM, et al. Outcomes of minimally invasive versus open abdominal hysterectomy in patients with gestational trophoblastic disease. *Gynecol Oncol*. 2021;160(2):445-449.

44. Soper JT. Surgical therapy for gestational trophoblastic disease. *J Reprod Med*. 1994;39(3):168-174.

45. Soper JT. Role of surgery and radiation therapy in the management of gestational trophoblastic disease. *Best Pract Res Clin Obstet Gynaecol*. 2003;17(6):943-957.

46. Lehman E, Gershenson DM, Burke TW, Levenback C, Silva EG, Morris M. Salvage surgery for chemorefractory gestational trophoblastic disease. *J Clin Oncol*. 1994;12(12):2737-2742.

47. Soper JT. Identification and management of high-risk gestational trophoblastic disease. *Semin Oncol*. 1995;22(2):172-184.

48. Maestá I, Leite FV, Michelin OC, Rogatto SR. Primary pulmonary choriocarcinoma after human chorionic gonadotropin normalization following hydatidiform mole: a report of two cases. *J Reprod Med*. 2010;55(7-8):311-316.

49. Lok CAR, Reekers JA, Westermann AM, der Velden JV. Embolization for hemorrhage of liver metastases from choriocarcinoma. *Gynecol Oncol*. 2005;98(3):506-509.

50. Fleming EL, Garret L, Growdon WB, et al. The changing role of thoracotomy in gestational trophoblastic neoplasia at the New England Trophoblastic Disease Center. *J Reprod Med*. 2008;53(7):493-498.

51. Alifrangis C, Wilkinson MJ, Stefanou DC, Virk JS, Anderson J, Seckl MJ. Role of thoracotomy and metastatectomy in gestational trophoblastic neoplasia: a single center experience. *J Reprod Med*. 2012;57(7-8):350-358.

52. Evans AC, Soper JT, Clarke-Pearson DL, Berchuck A, Rodriguez GC, Hammond CB. Gestational trophoblastic disease metastatic to the central nervous system. *Gynecol Oncol*. 1995;59(2):226-230.

53. Lurain JR, Nejad B. Secondary chemotherapy for high-risk gestational trophoblastic neoplasia. *Gynecol Oncol*. 2005;97(2):618-623.

54. Yang J, Xiang Y, Wan X, et al. Recurrent gestational trophoblastic tumor: management and risk factors for recurrence. *Gynecol Oncol*. 2006;103(2):587-590.

55. Ngan HYS, Tam KF, Lam KW, et al. Relapsed gestational trophoblastic neoplasia: a 20-year experience. *J Reprod Med*. 2006;51(10):829-834.

56. Powles T, Savage PM, Stebbing J, et al. A comparison of patients with relapsed and chemo-refractory gestational trophoblastic neoplasia. *Br J Cancer*. 2007;96(5):732-737.

57. Lurain JR, Schink JC. Importance of salvage therapy in the management of high-risk gestational trophoblastic neoplasia. *J. Reprod Med*. 2012;57:219-224.

58. Berkowitz RS, Horowitz NS, Elias KM. Management of resistant or recurrent gestational trophoblastic neoplasia. In: Goff B, Dizon DS, eds. *UpToDate*. Wolters Kluwer; 2021.

59. Newlands ES, Mulholland PJ, Holden L, Seckl MJ, Rustin GJ. Etoposide and cisplatin/etoposide, methotrexate, and actinomycin D (EMA) chemotherapy for patients with high-risk gestational trophoblastic tumors refractory to EMA/cyclophosphamide and vincristine chemotherapy and patients presenting with metastatic placental site trophoblastic tumors. *J. Clin Oncol*. 2000;18:854-859.

60. Bower M, Newlands ES, Holden L, et al. EMA/CO for high-risk gestational trophoblastic tumors: results from a cohort of 272 patients. *J Clin Oncol*. 1997;15(7):2636-2643.

61. Osborne R, Covens A, Mirchandani D, Gerulath A. Successful salvage of relapsed high-risk gestational trophoblastic neoplasia patients using a novel paclitaxel-containing doublet. *J Reprod Med*. 2004;49(8):655-661.

62. Wang J, Short D, Sebire NJ, et al. Salvage chemotherapy of relapsed or high—risk gestational trophoblastic neoplasia (GTN) with paclitaxel/cisplatin alternating with paclitaxel/etoposide (TP/TE). *Ann Oncol*. 2008;19(9):1578-1583.

63. Matsui H, Suzuka K, Iitsuka Y, et al. Salvage combination chemotherapy with 5-fluorouracil and actinomycin D for patients with refractory, high-risk gestational trophoblastic tumors. *Cancer*. 2002;95(5):1051-1054.

64. Ghorani E, Kaur B, Fisher RA, et al. Pembrolizumab is effective for drug-resistant gestational trophoblastic neoplasia. *Lancet*. 2017;390(10110):2343-2345.

65. Braga A, Elias KM, Horowitz NS, Berkowitz RS. Treatment of high-risk gestational trophoblastic neoplasia and chemoresistance/relapsed disease. *Best Pract Res Clin Obstet Gynaecol*. 2021;74:81-96.

66. You B, Bolze PA, Lotz JP, et al. Avelumab in patients with gestational trophoblastic tumors with resistance to single-agent chemotherapy: cohort A of the TROPHIMMUN phase II trial. *J Clin Oncol*. 2020;38(27):3129-3137.

67. You B, Bolze P, Lotz J, et al. 273 Avelumab in patients with gestational trophoblastic tumorsresistant to polychemotherapy: efficacy outcomes of cohort B of TROPHIMMUN phase II trial. *Int J Gynecol Cancer*. 2021;31:A344.

68. Lybol C, Thomas CM, Bulten J, van Dijck JA, Sweep FC, Massuger LF. Increase in the incidence of gestational trophoblastic disease in the Netherlands. *Gynecol Oncol*. 2011;121:334-338.

69. Li J, Shi Y, Wan X, Qian H, Zhou C, Chen X. Epithelioid trophoblastic tumor: a clinico-pathological and immunohistochemical study of seven cases. *Med Oncol*. 2011;28(1):294-299.

70. Kurman RJ, Scully RE, Norris HJ. Trophoblastic pseudotumor of the uterus: an exaggerated form of syncytial endometritis simulating a malignant tumor. *Cancer*. 1976;38:1214-1226.

71. Shih IM, Kurman RJ. Epithelioid trophoblastic tumor: a neoplasm distinct from choriocarcinoma and placental site trophoblastic tumor simulating carcinoma. *Am J Surg Pathol*. 1998;22:1393-1403.

72. Schmid P, Nagai Y, Agarwal R, et al. Prognostic markers and long-term outcome of placental-site trophoblastic tumors: a retrospective observational study. *Lancet*. 2009;374:48-55.

73. Zhao J, Lu WG, Feng FZ, et al. Placental site trophoblastic tumor: a review of 108 cases and their implications for prognosis and treatment. *Gynecol Oncol*. 2016;142:102-108.

74. Feltmate CM, Genest DR, Wise L, Bernstein MR, Goldstein DP, Berkowitz RS. Placental site trophoblastic tumor: a 17-year experience at the New England Trophoblastic Disease Center. *Gynecol Oncol*. 2001;82:415-419.

75. Papadopoulos AJ, Foskett M, Seckl M, et al. Twenty-five years' clinical experience with placental site trophoblastic tumor. *J Reprod Med*. 2002;47:460-464.

76. Lan C, Li Y, He J, Liu J. Placental site trophoblastic tumor: lymphatic spread and possible target markers. *Gynecol Oncol*. 2010;116(3):430-437.

77. Zhou Y, Lu H, Yu C, Tian Q, Lu W. Sonographic characteristics of placental site trophoblastic tumor. *Ultrasound Obstet Gynecol*. 2013;41(6):679-684.

78. Lima LL, Parente RC, Maestá I, et al. Clinical and radiological correlations in patients with gestational trophoblastic disease. *Radiol Bras*. 2016;49(4):241-250.

79. Mapelli P, Mangili G, Picchio M, et al. Role of 18F-FDG PET in the management of gestational trophoblastic neoplasia. *Eur J Nucl Med Mol Imaging*. 2013;40(4):505-513.

80. Dhillon T, Palmieri C, Sebire NJ, et al. Value of whole body 18FDG-PET to identify the active site of gestational trophoblastic neoplasia. *J Reprod Med*. 2006;51(11):879-887.

81. Horowitz NS, Goldstein DP, Berkowitz RS. Placental site trophoblastic tumors and epithelioid trophoblastic tumors: biology, natural history, and treatment modalities. *Gynecol Oncol*. 2017;144(1):208-214.

82. Zang X, Lu W, Lu B. Epithelioid trophoblastic tumor: an outcome based literature review of 78 reported cases. *Int J Gynecol Cancer*. 2013;23(7):1334-1338.

83. Davis MR, Howitt BE, Quade BJ, et al. Epithelioid trophoblastic tumor: a single institution case series at the New England Trophoblastic Disease Center. *Gynecol Oncol*. 2015;137:456-461.

84. Frijstein MM, Lok CAR, van Trommel NE, et al. Management and prognostic factors of epithelioid trophoblastic tumors: results from the International Society for the Study of Trophoblastic Diseases database. *Gynecol Oncol.* 2019;152(2):361-367.

85. Goldstein DP, Berkowitz RS. Current management of gestational trophoblastic neoplasia. *Hematol Oncol Clin North Am.* 2012;26(1):111-131.

86. Bouchard-Fortier G, Ghorani E, Short D, et al. Following chemotherapy for gestational trophoblastic neoplasia, do residual lung lesions increase the risk of relapse? *Gynecol Oncol.* 2020;158(3):698-701.

87. Agarwal R, Alifrangis C, Everard J, et al. Management and survival of patients with FIGO high risk gestational trophoblastic neoplasia: the UK experience, 1995-2010. *J Reprod Med.* 2014;59:7-12.

88. Balachandran K, Salawu A, Ghorani E, et al. When to stop human chorionic gonadotrophin (hCG) surveillance after treatment with chemotherapy for gestational trophoblastic neoplasia (GTN): a national analysis on over 4,000 patients. *Gynecol Oncol.* 2019;155(1):8-12.

89. Elias KM, Berkowitz RS, Horowitz NS. Continued hCG surveillance following chemotherapy for gestational trophoblastic neoplasia: when is enough enough? *Gynecol Oncol.* 2019;155(1):1-2.

CHAPTER **7.5**

Gestational Trophoblastic Disease: Postdiagnosis and Treatment, Long-Term Sequelae, and Quality-of-Life Issues

Neil S. Horowitz, Kevin M. Elias, and Ross S. Berkowitz

INTRODUCTION

GTD comprises a spectrum of interrelated diseases ranging from benign conditions such as complete and partial molar pregnancies to rare and aggressive malignancies that can present with widely metastatic disease. These malignancies are referred to as gestational trophoblastic neoplasia (GTN). With the use of single- or multiagent chemotherapies and adjuvant surgery when necessary, these conditions are highly curable and have excellent prognosis (1-3). As these diseases affect young women in their reproductive years, it is important to understand the impact of this diagnosis and treatment on future fertility, general health, and psychosocial well-being.

FUTURE FERTILITY

The impact of chemotherapy on fertility is related to the gonadotoxicity of the agents used, the number of cycles received, and age of the patient at the time of treatment (4). Anti-Müllerian hormone (AMH) is produced by the granulosa cells of small, growing follicles and is often used as a marker of ovarian reserve (5,6). An abnormal AMH may predict diminished fertility or poor response to in vitro protocols. Chemotherapy is known to have adverse effects on ovarian function and increase the risk of primary ovarian insufficiency. Studies, mostly in patients with breast cancer, have shown that AMH levels decline rapidly, to nearly undetectable levels, after initiation of treatment with variable rates and degrees of recovery (7-10). In a prospective study on 34 patients with GTN treated with chemotherapy, AMH levels were evaluated before, during, and after chemotherapy. Similar to what was seen in patients with breast cancer, the authors showed that after three cycles of chemotherapy, AMH levels decreased. This was more pronounced after multiagent chemotherapy, especially those that contained etoposide, than after single-agent Act-D (11). Post-treatment, the AMH levels continued to decline, but 3 months following chemotherapy, AMH levels began to increase. The impact of low AMH levels is unclear as some authors have shown that despite low serum AMH levels, spontaneous pregnancies can occur (12).

The chemotherapies used to treat GTN have varying risk of inducing permanent ovarian dysfunction and amenorrhea (4). The

American Society of Clinical Oncology (ASCO) has reported on fertility preservation for patients with cancer and in which they evaluate the risk of inducing permanent amenorrhea for various chemotherapy agents (13). The two most common agents in treating low-risk disease, MTX and Act-D, have very low risk (<20%) of inducing ovarian failure and amenorrhea, whereas cisplatin has an intermediate risk (20%-80%) (13). Cyclophosphamide was defined as both a high-risk agent (>80%) if given for more than six cycles, in combination with other agents and/or to women age greater than 40 years and an intermediate-risk agent in those aged 30 to 39 years (13). The other major chemotherapy commonly used to treat GTN, etoposide was not evaluated in the ASCO review. The impact of this cessation of ovarian function was confirmed in a large review by Savage et al. In a survey of 1,903 patients treated for GTN between 1958 and 2000, the authors assembled data on incident rates of subsequent malignancies and age of menopause after a variety of chemotherapy regimens (14). For those who provided data on their menopausal status, they noted the risk of menopause by age of 40 in the overall cohort was 5% and was 15% by the age of 45. The risk varied depending upon chemotherapy exposure. The incidence of premature menopause (<40 years) was 1%, and early menopause (age <45) after MTX was 7%, which was comparable to the general population incidence of less than 1% and 5%, respectively. Treatment with EMA-CO, on the other hand, carried significantly higher rates of premature menopause and early menopause, 13% and 36%, respectively (14). These rates of menopause are consistent with the rate reported after MTX by Wong et al and Coiffi et al (15,16).

Multiple reviews of fertility and reproductive outcomes after molar pregnancies and treatment of GTN have been performed (17-26). The impact of single-agent versus multiagent chemotherapy on these outcomes is hard to determine as most studies are not large enough to do this type of subgroup analysis. Overall, the fertility rate after chemotherapy for GTN has been reported to be as high as 87% among those wishing to conceive (26). Some studies suggest that fertility/conception rates are lower for those treated with multiagent chemotherapy (26), whereas others show no difference (16,22). Uniformally, studies have shown that the rates of live births, miscarriage, malformations, and obstetrical complications are no different between those with a diagnosis of GTD or GTN requiring chemotherapy and the general population

(16-21). In one of the largest reviews from the NETDC, the rate of live births was 67%, spontaneous abortions was 18%, preterm deliveries 6.6%, congenital malformations 1.5%, and stillbirths was 1.5% (17). Although there does not seem to be a difference in perinatal outcomes between those with GTD/GTN and the general population, the one exception is the risk of a new molar pregnancy, which increases with successive molar pregnancies. In a study of 16,000 women, Eagles et al (27) reported that after a complete molar pregnancy, the risk of a second molar pregnancy increased from approximately 1 in 1,000 to 1 in 100 and the risk for a third molar pregnancy increased to 25% after two consecutive moles (27,28). An elevated risk of subsequent molar pregnancy after a partial molar pregnancy was also present but much smaller.

After completing treatment for GTN, women are monitored for recurrence with serial hCG for at least 12 months and are advised to avoid pregnancy during this surveillance as a new conception during this time would complicate management (1-3). The use of estrogen-progestin contraceptive is recommended as it has a low failure rate and has not been shown to increase the risk of developing GTN when used after a molar pregnancy nor worsen the course of GTN (29,30). Despite these recommendations, women often get pregnant before the end of the surveillance. The impact of these "early" conceptions on perinatal outcome was recently evaluated in a large meta-analysis. Madi et al (18) examined perinatal outcomes of first pregnancies following remission of GTN and the impact of time between the end of chemotherapy and subsequent pregnancy. The authors reported that pregnancies occurring before completion of surveillance did not have unfavorable perinatal outcomes (malformation, stillbirths, or prematurity) but were associated with a higher rate of abortions/miscarriages. Women who followed recommendations and became pregnant 12 months or more after completion of chemotherapy, the abortion rate was 8.92% (95% CI, 4.99-15.45). This is sharply contrasted by those pregnancies that occurred 6 months or less after chemotherapy completion, in which case the rate of abortion was 53.86% (95% CI, 27.21-78.47), and for those who became pregnant between 6 and 12 months where the rate was 16.47% (95% CI, 10.0-25.91%) (18). Similar higher rates of miscarriage in pregnancies that are conceived early after completion of chemotherapy is supported by other authors (21,24).

The impact of immunotherapy on future fertility is not well established. Pembrolizumab has been used increasingly for salvage treatment for women with heavily pretreated chemotherapy-resistant GTN (31). In addition, in the TROPHIMMUNE study, avelumab was used to treat women with low-risk disease that was resistant to MTX (32). Given the mechanisms of action of these agents, there has been concern about the loss of immunotolerance during future pregnancies and thus significant impact on a woman's ability to conceive or carry a pregnancy. Although there are no described pregnancies after pembrolizumab, Bolze et al reported on a patient treated on the TROPHIMMUN trial who conceived and delivered a healthy newborn at 39 weeks of gestation (33).

For patients with a prior history of GTD/GTN, who ultimately go on to have a future pregnancy, we recommend an early trimester ultrasound to ensure a normally developing pregnancy and for all patients to have an hCG level measured 6 to 8 weeks at the end of the pregnancy event whether term or preterm delivery, miscarriage, or ectopic, to ensure complete remission and exclude occult GTN. The placenta does not need to be sent to pathology routinely, but if upon inspection there are any abnormalities, pathologic evaluation is warranted (2,34).

Secondary Malignancies

Fortunately for all women with low-risk GTN and for many with high-risk or ultrahigh-risk disease, cure is the expected outcome (1-3). As these women are young and have long life expectancies after treatment for their GTN, the impact of chemotherapy on long-term quality-of-life (QoL) and health issues is critical to consider. This is especially true regarding the risk of secondary malignancies as many of the chemotherapy regimens for GTN contain alkylating agents, which have been shown to double the risk of future malignancies when used for other curable cancers. To assess the risk of secondary malignancies in patients treated for GTN, Savage et al (14) conducted a large survey of patients treated at the Charing Cross. Analyzing data from approximately 1,900 patients treated with both single- and multiagent chemotherapy, and with a mean follow-up of approximately 17 years, they noted 86 patients developed a future malignancy, compared to an expected rate of 79 (standardized incident ratio [SIR], 1.1; 95% CI, 0.9-1.3). The overall risk was low after MTX-FA, but EMA-CO or other multiagent chemotherapy regimens were associated with increase rates of oral cancer, melanoma, meningioma, and leukemia. The risk of secondary cancers was directly related to the number of cycles of chemotherapy and inversely related to the age of the patient at the time of treatment. This was particularly significant for those who received 13 or more cycles of chemotherapy (SIR = 2.5) or were under 20 years old (SIR = 2.3, 95% CI, 1.0-5.2) at the time of treatment (14).

Psychosocial Consequences

As cure is generally anticipated for patients with GTN, it is critically important to understand both the short- and long-term psychosocial consequences of the diagnosis and treatment of this disease. From the moment of diagnosis, couples are jolted from the excitement and joyful anticipation of a new pregnancy to a state of worry and distress associated with the loss of a pregnancy and potentially life-threatening cancer. Not surprising, this is associated with psychological, social, and relationship adaptations that are necessary to deal with this new reality. Although the research into the psychosocial consequences of GTD has been limited, three important areas have emerged: identity/reproduction, psychological health, and relationship/sexual dysfunction (35).

Identity/Childbearing

Historically, reproductive capacity has been closely linked to femininity and gender identity. Because motherhood carries many social expectations and feelings, a woman's self-esteem can be affected by the knowledge that her pregnancy is imperfect (36). There is a natural extension of this sense of imperfection to worries about future fertility. In a study of 110 women diagnosed with GTN at the NETDC, 40% felt loss of control over their reproductive futures, 35% were not content with their current family size, 17% expressed anger in regard to the threat to their fertility, and 31% mourned the loss of the pregnancy associated with GTN (37). The fact that these feelings persisted 5 to 10 years after their diagnosis speaks to the impact that reproductive concerns have on the psychosocial well-being of patients with GTN. Furthermore, several studies have shown that reproductive concerns and stress related to fertility are higher for women with more severe disease, younger age, and nulliparity, whereas those with less social support and less spiritual well-being also have worse psychosocial outcomes (37-42).

Psychological Adaptation

Although the prognosis for GTD/GTN is excellent, it is clear that women experience emotional and psychological stress during the acute phase of their illness/treatment and that this persists into surveillance and long-term follow-up (41,42). Much of this distress is expressed as anxiety and depression. A recent study by Blok et al (41) reported a rated of anxiety of 47% and depression of 27%. The source of the anxiety and depression stemmed from feelings of defectiveness, loss of pregnancy, and fear of future infertility. As mentioned earlier, levels of distress were greater and persisted for longer periods of time for women who needed chemotherapy or presented with metastatic disease, whereas patients with children or who had experienced previous pregnancy loss had lower levels of distress.

In a cross-sectional study of patients from the NETDC and the United Kingdom diagnosed with GTN 5 to 10 years before the study, Wenzel et al (37) described the QoL and long-term psychosocial impact of the diagnosis of molar pregnancy, nonmetastatic, and metastatic GTN. Although the overall QoL of the cohort was quite good, 51% of respondents expressed that they would likely participate in a counseling program years after their diagnosis to discuss psychosocial issues raised by having GTN and 74% stated that they would have attended a support group program during the initial treatment if it had been offered. In addition, women noted that during or shortly after treatment, the frequency of functional QoL problems (20%) and emotional problems (19%) was equivalent to that of treatment side effects (22%). As patients transitioned into survivorship, emotional distress persisted but with the added fears of recurrence and future reproductive difficulties. Approximately one-third of patients expressed that more support and more medical information/communication would be helpful in addressing these fears and distress. Not surprisingly, women with metastatic disease compared to those without metastases had clinically significant range of distress and reported that they needed more than a year from completing treatment before life felt back to normal. The long-term psychological morbidity of GTN was also highlighted by Stafford et al (43). In their analysis of 176 women diagnosed with GTN a mean 4.7 years earlier, 22% had elevated levels of depression and 26% had elevated levels of anxiety. Up to 50% of women were troubled by some GTD-specific traumatic stress expressed as intrusive thoughts or attempts to avoid GTD-related stimuli. These poor psychological outcomes were more common and more severe in socially disadvantaged women (less educated, unmarried, unemployed, poor) and in those who failed to conceive after their GTD diagnosis. Multiple studies suggest that spiritual well-being and social support were desired by patients and were protective for QoL (37,40,42-44). As shown by Victoria Diniz et al, some of this support can come through Facebook or other social media platforms (45).

Relationship Issues/Sexual Function

Despite a growing appreciation of psychosocial impact of GTD/GTN on patients, there is little research on impact of this disease on partners and sexual function. In one of the few studies focusing on male partners of women with the diagnosis of GTN, 32% met criteria for clinical anxiety, whereas 12% had depression (46). This rate of anxiety was twice the expected rate in the community. Much of this anxiety was related to frustration with the diagnosis, loss of control over fertility and inability to have more children, and their partner's health. Similar to women with GTN, having other children was associated with less anxiety and depression and overall improved QoL. Despite these levels of anxiety in both women and men, studies suggest that the diagnosis of GTD does not affect overall marital satisfaction, with most females and males describing their relationships as supportive and satisfactory and perhaps even better after the GTN diagnosis (43,47,48). However, failure to conceive in the future introduces significant stress, erodes the relationship, and leads to more dissatisfaction. Despite these strong relationships, 20% to 50% of women with molar pregnancy or GTN report some level of both short- and long- term sexual dysfunction (40,43). This primarily is reported as a loss of sexual desire both during the active phase of their disease and as a long-term sequelae. Often, this sexual dysfunction is attributed by women and their partners to the diagnosis of GTD/GTN rather than physical change or stress (35). This is interesting in the context of a study by Cagayan (49) in which 40% of women treated for GTN experienced dyspareunia and reported lubrication issues, both of which can contribute to sexual dysfunction and could be related to the treatment toxicities rather than the disease itself.

Survivorship issues are becoming more important for all women with cancer. Given the young age of women diagnosed with GTD/GTN and the impact this can have on future health, psychological

well-being, and relationships, it is critical that more work be done in understanding the psychosocial impact of this disease over time and that clinicians be empowered to address these concerns in their patients.

REFERENCES

1. Ngan HYS, Seckl MJ, Berkowitz RS, et al. Diagnosis and management of gestational trophoblastic disease: 2021 update. *Int J Gynaecol Obstet.* 2021;155(suppl 1):86-93.

2. Horowitz NS, Eskander RN, Adelman MR, Burke W. Epidemiology, diagnosis, and treatment of gestational trophoblastic disease: a Society of Gynecologic Oncology evidenced-based review and recommendations. *Gynecol Oncol.* 2021;163:605-613.

3. Lok C, van Trommel N, Massugar L, Golfier F, Seckl M. Practical clinical guidelines of EOTTD for the treatment and referral of gestational trophoblastic disease. *Eur J Cancer.* 2020;130:228-240.

4. Joneborg U, Coopmans L, van Trommel N, Seckl M, Lok CAR. Fertility and pregnancy outcome in gestational trophoblastic disease. *Int J Gynecol Cancer.* 2021;31(3):399-411.

5. Lee MM, Donahue PK, Hasegawa T, et al. Mullerian inhibiting substance in humans: normal levels from infancy to adulthood. *J Clin Endocrinol Metab.* 1996;81:571-576.

6. deVet A, Laven JS, de Jong FH, et al. Antimullerian hormone serum levels: a putative marker for ovarian aging. *Fertil Steril.* 2002;77:357-362.

7. Ruddy KJ, Schaid DJ, Batzler A, et al. Antimullerian hormone as a serum biomarker for risk of chemotherapy-induced amenorrhea. *J Natl Cancer Inst.* 2021;113(8):1105-1108.

8. Partridge AH, Ruddy KJ, Gelber S, et al. Ovarian reserve in women who remain premenopausal after chemotherapy for early stage breast cancer. *Fertil Steril.* 2010;94(2):638-644.

9. Gracia CR, Sammel MD, Freeman E, et al. Impact of cancer therapies on ovarian reserve. *Fertil Steril.* 2012;97(1):134-140.

10. Iwase A, Sugita A, Hirokawa W, et al. Anti-Müllerian hormone as a marker of ovarian reserve following chemotherapy in patients with gestational trophoblastic neoplasia. *Eur J Obstet Gynecol Reprod Biol.* 2013;167(2):194-198.

11. Bi X, Zhang J, Cao D, et al. Anti-Müllerian hormone levels in patients with gestational trophoblastic neoplasia treated with different chemotherapy regimens: a prospective cohort study. *Oncotarget.* 2017;8(69):113920-113927.

12. Ghorani E, Ramaswami R, Smith RJ, Savage PM, Seckl MJ. Anti-Müllerian hormone in patients treated with chemotherapy for gestational trophoblastic neoplasia does not predict short-term fertility. *J Reprod Med.* 2016;61(5-6):205-209.

13. Loren AW, Mangu PB, Beck LN, et al. Fertility preservation for patients with cancer: American Society of Clinical Oncology clinical practice guidelines. *J Clin Oncol.* 2013;31:2500-2510.

14. Savage P, Cooke R, O'Nions J, et al. Effects of single-agent and combination chemotherapy for gestational trophoblastic tumors on risks of second malignancy and early menopause. *J Clin Oncol.* 2015;33(5):472-478.

15. Wong JMK, Liu D, Lurain JR. Reproductive outcomes after multiagent chemotherapy for high-risk gestational trophoblastic neoplasia. *J Reprod Med.* 2014;59:204-208.

16. Cioffi R, Bergamini A, Gadducci A, et al. Reproductive outcomes after gestational trophoblastic neoplasia. A comparison between single-agent and multiagent chemotherapy: retrospective analysis from the MITO-9 group. *Int J Gynecol Cancer.* 2018;28:332-337.

17. Vargas R, Barroilhet LM, Esselen K, et al. Subsequent pregnancy outcomes after complete and partial molar pregnancy, recurrent molar pregnancy, and gestational trophoblastic neoplasia: an update from the New England Trophoblastic Disease Center. *J Reprod Med.* 2014;59(5-6): 188-194.

18. Madi JM, Paganella MP, Litvin IE, et al. Perinatal outcomes of first pregnancy after chemotherapy for gestational trophoblastic neoplasia: a systematic review of observational studies and meta-analysis. *Am J Obstet Gynecol.* 2022;226:633-645.e8. doi:10.1016/j.ajog.2021.10.004

19. Ayahn A, Ergeneli MH, Yuce K, et al. Pregnancy after chemotherapy for gestational trophoblastic disease. *J Reprod Med.* 1990;35(5):522-524.

20. Amr MF. Return of fertility after successful chemotherapy treatment of gestational trophoblastic tumors. *Int J Fertil Womens Med.* 1999;44(3):146-149.

21. Braga A, Maestá I, Michelin OC, et al. Maternal and perinatal outcomes of first pregnancy after chemotherapy for gestational trophoblastic neoplasia in Brazilian women. *Gynecol Oncol.* 2009;112(3):568-571.

22. Woolas RP, Bower M, Newlands ES, Seckl M, Short D, Holden L. Influence of chemotherapy for gestational trophoblastic disease on subsequent pregnancy outcome. *Br J Obstet Gynaecol*. 1998;105(9):1032-1035.

23. Lok CA, van der Houwen C, ten Kate-Booij MJ, van Eijkeren MA, Ansink AC. Pregnancy after EMA/CO for gestational trophoblastic disease: a report from the Netherlands. *BJOG*. 2003;110(6):560-566.

24. Matsui H, Iitsuka Y, Suzuka K, et al. Early pregnancy outcomes after chemotherapy for gestational trophoblastic tumor. *J Reprod Med*. 2004;49(7):531-534.

25. Tranoulis A, Georgiou D, Sayasneh A, et al. Gestational trophoblastic neoplasia: a meta-analysis evaluating reproductive and obstetrical outcomes after administration of chemotherapy. *Int J Gynecol Cancer*. 2019;29:1021-1031.

26. Kim JH, Park DC, Bae SN, Namkoong SE, Kim SJ. Subsequent reproductive experience after treatment for gestational trophoblastic disease. *Gynecol Oncol*. 1998;71(1):108-112.

27. Eagles N, Sebire NJ, Short D, Savage PM, Seckl MJ, Fisher RA. Risk of recurrent molar pregnancies following complete and partial hydatidiform moles. *Hum Reprod*. 2015;30(9):2055-2063.

28. Sebire NJ, Fisher RA, Foskett M, Rees H, Seckl MJ, Newlands ES. Risk of recurrent hydatidiform mole and subsequent pregnancy outcome following complete or partial hydatidiform molar pregnancy. *BJOG*. 2003;110(1):22-26.

29. Dantas PRS, Maesta I, Filho JR, et al. Does hormonal contraception during molar pregnancy follow-up influence the risk and clinical aggressiveness of gestational trophoblastic neoplasia after controlling for risk-factors? *Gynecol Oncol*. 2017;147:364-370.

30. Braga A, Maestá I, Short D, Savage P, Harvey R, Seckl MJ. Hormonal contraceptive use before hCG remission does not increase the risk of gestational trophoblastic neoplasia following complete hydatidiform mole: a historical database review. *BJOG*. 2016;123(8):1330-1335.

31. Ghorani E, Kaur B, Fisher RA, et al. Pembrolizumab is effective for drug-resistant gestational trophoblastic neoplasia. *Lancet*. 2017;390(10110):2343-2345.

32. You B, Bolze PA, Lotz JP, et al. Avelumab in patients with gestational trophoblastic tumors with resistance to single-agent chemotherapy: cohort A of the TROPHIMMUN phase II trial. *J Clin Oncol*. 2020;38(27):3129-3137.

33. Bolze PA, You B, Lotz JP, et al. Successful pregnancy in a cancer patient previously cured of a gestational trophoblastic tumor by immunotherapy. *Ann Oncol*. 2020;31:823-825.

34. Berkowitz RS, Horowitz NS, Elias KM. Initial management of low-risk gestational trophoblastic neoplasia. In: Goff B, Dizon DS, eds. *UpToDate*. Wolters Kluwer; 2021.

35. Horowitz NS, Wenzel LB. Psychosocial consequences of gestational trophoblastic disease. In Hancock BW, Seckl M, Berkowitz RS

eds. Chapter 22. *Gestational Trophoblastic Disease*. 5th Ed. International Society for the Study of Trophoblastic Disease, 2022.

36. Bibring G, Dwyer T, Huntington D, et al. A study of the psychological processes in pregnancy and the earliest mother—child relationship. *Psychoanal Study Child*. 1961;16:9-72.

37. Wenzel L, Berkowitz R, Newlands ES, et al. Quality of life after gestational trophoblastic disease. *J Reprod Med*. 2002;47:387-394.

38. Di Mattei VE, Carnelli L, Bernardi M, et al. An investigative study into psychological and fertility sequelae of gestational trophoblastic disease: the impact on patients' perceived fertility, anxiety and depression. *PLoS One*. 2015;10(6):e0128354.

39. Lok CA, Donken M, Calff MM, et al. Psychologic impact of follow up after low risk gestational trophoblastic disease. *J Reprod Med*. 2011;56:47-52.

40. Wenzel LB, Berkowitz RS, Robinson SE, et al. The psychological, social, and sexual consequences of gestational trophoblastic disease. *Gynecol Oncol*. 1992;46:74-81.

41. Blok LJ, Frijstein MM, Eysbouts YK, et al. The psychological impact of gestational trophoblastic disease: a prospective observational multicentre cohort study. *BJOG*. 2022;129(3):444-449.

42. Ireson J, Jones G, Winter MC, Radley SC, Hancock BW, Tidy JA. Systematic review of health-related quality of life and patient-reported outcome measures in gestational trophoblastic disease: a parallel synthesis approach. *Lancet Oncol*. 2018;19(1):e56-e64.

43. Stafford L, McNally OM, Gibson P, Judd F. Long-term psychological morbidity, sexual functioning, and relationship outcomes in women with gestational trophoblastic disease. *Int J Gynecol Cancer*. 2011;21(7):1256-1263.

44. Cagayan MS, Llarena RT. Quality of life of gestational trophoblastic neoplasia survivors: a study of patients at the Philippine general hospital trophoblastic disease section. *J Reprod Med*. 2010;55(7-8):321-326.

45. Victoria Diniz M, Sun SY, Barsottini C, et al. Experience with the use of an online community on Facebook for Brazilian patients with gestational trophoblastic disease: netnography study. *J Med Internet Res*. 2018;20(9):e10897.

46. Quinlivan JA, Ung KA, Petersen RW. The impact of molar pregnancy on the male partner. *Psychooncology*. 2012;21:970-976.

47. Wenzel LB, Berkowitz RS, Robinson SE, et al. Psychological, social and sexual effects of gestational trophoblastic disease on patients and their partners. *J Reprod Med*. 1994;39(3):163-167.

48. Ngan HY, Tang GW. Psychosocial aspects of gestational trophoblastic disease in Chinese residents of Hong Kong. *J Reprod Med*. 1986;31:173-178.

49. Cagayan MS. Sexual dysfunction as a complication of treatment of gestational trophoblastic neoplasia. *J Reprod Med*. 2008;53(8):595-599.

EPITHELIAL OVARIAN CANCER

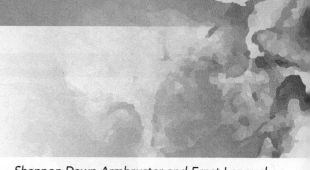

CHAPTER 8.1

Epidemiology and Risk Factors

Shannon Dawn Armbruster and Ernst Lengyel

In this section, "ovarian cancer" (OC) generally refers to a Müllerian cancer arising in the peritoneum, fallopian tube, or the ovary; we use the term "ovarian cancer" as it is highly recognized by the medical community. This section covers risk factors for developing OC. Prognostic factors after OC are discussed in this section.

Established genetic risk factors for OC include genetic factors, such as a known genetic predisposition (eg, BRCA1/2 and HNPCC) and a strong family history for breast cancer and OC. Hormonal and reproductive factors include parity, breastfeeding, early menarche, late menopause, menopausal hormonal treatment, oral contraceptive (OCP) use, and endometriosis. The relative risks (RR) associated with endocrinologic factors and obesity are small, although important, because they are potentially subject to modulation. The most important risk factor, after having a first-degree relative with the disease, is age. Women younger than 40 years without a positive family history are rarely diagnosed with epithelial ovarian cancer (EOC). Fifty percent of all cases of OC in the United States occur in women over the age of 65 years. A large meta-analysis including more than 1.3 million women showed that most risk factors show heterogeneity across OC histologic subtypes. For example, reproductive and hormonal risk factors are more strongly associated with clear cell and endometrioid OCs, whereas smoking is associated with mucinous tumors (1). This suggests that there is no unifying etiology for "ovarian cancer" and that the different histologic subtypes must be considered separately to understand the specific risk profile, biology, and clinical behavior.

EPIDEMIOLOGY

EOC is second only to breast cancer as a cause of death from gynecologic cancer in the United States and Europe. The Surveillance, Epidemiology, and End Results (SEER) data project approximately 20,000 new cases of OC and almost 13,000 deaths from OC in the United States each year (2). It is estimated that in the United States, 1 individual in 70 will develop OC (lifetime incidence) and 1 individual in 100 will die of the disease. Incidence rates are higher in the United Kingdom impacting 1:50 individuals and range from 0.9% to 2.2% cumulative risk across Europe. Mortality rates in Europe range from 0.9% to 1.7%. Reports for the global OC burden, which includes low malignant potential (LMP) cancers (the U.S. and European numbers exclude them), are that 313,959 patients developed EOC and over 207,000 succumbed to the disease in 2020 (3).

OC rates vary between different countries and appear to be linked to socioeconomic status and reproductive patterns. North America and most of the industrialized countries of Europe have high incidence rates, whereas the disease is rare in Asia and Africa. The lowest rates of OC are in Middle Africa (**Figure 8.1-1**). Although the reasons for this difference are not well understood, countries with a high incidence rate are generally characterized by smaller family sizes, high-fat diets, higher socioeconomic status,

older age, and a predominantly Caucasian population. Once a woman moves from a country with a low incidence of OC to one with a high incidence, her risk for the disease tends to approach that of her adopted country rather than her country of origin. There are significant geographical and racial differences in the proportions of newly diagnosed OCs: Out of all EOC, the incidence of clear cell carcinoma is high in Korea (10%) and Taiwan (19%), whereas it is 1% to 5% in Europe and North America (4).

Diagnosis usually occurs at advanced stages. The fatality rate of OC is high (70%), and 80% of deaths occur within 5 years of diagnosis. Reports from Europe predict a 17% decrease in the incidence of OC in the United Kingdom and 7% in the European Union (EU) between 2017 and 2022 (5). In line with this trend, the age-adjusted mortality in the United States declined by 38% from 9.8 in 100,000 to 6.0 in 100,000 per year from 1975 to 2019 (6). The incidence of OC decreased in both Black women (10.3→8.6/100,000) and White women (15.3→10.5/100,000). Although there is disparity in mortality rates between U.S. Whites and Blacks (6.7 vs 5.7 per 100,000 women per year), the incidence rates by race are more disparate (11.3 per 100,000 women per year among Whites vs 9.0 among Blacks) (6).

It has been hypothesized that this decline in mortality resulted from advances in treatment and a decline in OC incidence, due to risk-reducing surgery and because of the known protective effect of OCPs, which were introduced in the 1960s. Today, 80% to 85% of U.S. women have taken OCP at some point in their life. Paralleling the reduction in mortality, the age-adjusted OC incidence fell by 26% from 16.3 in 100,000 to 9.6 in 100,000 women from 1975 to 2018. The decline in incidence was then followed by a decline in mortality, supporting the hypothesis that OCP contributed to this effect. Still, despite the widespread use of OCP, it is estimated that, because of the expanding and aging U.S. population, the annual number of OC cases will increase from 21,000 to 28,591 in the years from 2010 to 2030 (7).

Weight/Body Mass Index

Strong evidence exists to support the relationship of weight and height to the risk of developing OC. The International Agency for Research on Cancer established a working group in 2016 that identified OC as one of 13 cancers linked to excess adiposity (8). This causal relationship is supported by several studies including a cohort study of 2.7 million Korean women noting a statistically significant association between the incidence of OC and increasing body mass index (BMI) ($P < .0001$) (3). In this prospective cohort study that followed 495,477 women for 6 years, BMI and OC mortality were also significantly associated. For women with a BMI of 35 to 39, the RR of developing OC was 1.5 (95% confidence interval [CI] 1.1-2). Confounding variables may moderate this association as was seen in a 2012 meta-analysis, which reported that the RR for OC per 5 kg/m^2 increase in BMI was 1.1 among those who did _not_ take hormone replacement therapy (HRT) but only 0.95 in women on HRT (9).

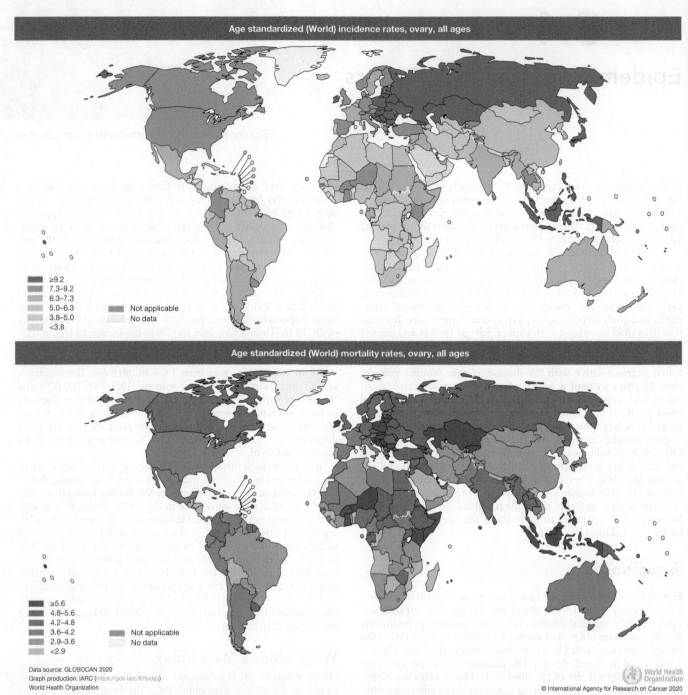

Figure 8.1-1. Age-standardized (World) incidence and mortality rates, ovary, all ages. (From World Health Organization. Globocan. 2020. https://gco.iarc.fr/today/data/factsheets/cancers/25-Ovary-fact-sheet.pdf)

The association between increasing BMI and OC subtype has also been studied (10). Higher BMI is associated with increased risk for borderline serous (recent BMI, odds ratio [OR] 1.24 per 5 kg/m², CI 1.18-1.3), invasive endometrioid (OR 1.17, CI 1.11-1.23), and invasive mucinous (OR 1.19, CI 1.06-1.32) tumors. Low-grade serous invasive tumors (RR 1.13, CI 1.03-1.25) and high-grade serous invasive cancers in premenopausal women (RR 1.11, CI 1.04-1.18) were also associated with an increased BMI, but high-grade serous postmenopausal cancers were not.

For those diagnosed with OC, obesity appears to have an impact on survival. A large meta-analysis demonstrated worse survival with higher BMI (per 5-unit increase: RR = 1.06, 95% CI:

1.02-1.11) (11). Bariatric surgical intervention is associated with decreased rates of developing OC (OR 0.38), supporting a contributing role of obesity to OC initiation and progression (12).

Height has also been reported as a risk factor. In 2012, a meta-analysis that summarized 47 studies involving 25,157 women with OC and 81,311 women without the disease found a small but significant increase in RR (1.07) of OC per 5-cm increase in height (9). Pooled data from the Ovarian Cancer Association Consortium (OCAC) studies support the association of height (pooled-OR [pOR] = 1.06) and OC risk, including invasive cancer (pOR = 1.06) and borderline (pOR = 1.15) tumors (13).

Reproductive Factors: Menstrual Cycles, Pregnancy, Breastfeeding, and Infertility

Several epidemiologic studies have indicated that early menarche and late menopause increase the risk of OC, whereas increased parity, breastfeeding, and the use of OCPs reduce that risk. Early menarche has been associated with increased OC risk in a meta-analysis including Chinese and European individuals (14). Adding to this evidence are several case-control studies, showing that pregnancy lowers OC risk and that the risk reduction is greater with each additional pregnancy. Gravidity is consistently associated with decreased OC risk. Compared with nulligravid women, women with a single pregnancy have an RR of 0.6 to 0.8. Each additional pregnancy decreases the risk by another 10% to 15% (15). The unifying feature of these reproductive factors is an increase or decrease in the number of ovulations that a woman experiences throughout her lifetime. However, a pregnancy after age 35 is more protective against OC than a pregnancy in a woman 25 years or below, regardless of the number of times she has given birth, suggesting that pregnancy at older ages involves mechanisms of risk reduction other than cessation of ovulation (16). Results of a more recent meta-analysis also support this relationship. Specifically, when controlled for parity, older age at last birth is associated with a lower risk of OC (RR: 0.76; 95% CI 0.63-0.93). Data regarding the impact of pregnancy and number of ovulatory cycles on survival are contradictory (17). A cohort study including 1,421 OC survivors reported a 29% reduction in mortality risk for parous women when compared to nulliparous women. However, women with higher cumulative number of ovulatory cycles had a decreased risk of OC-specific death (hazard ratio [HR] = 0.63; 95% CI 0.43-0.94). Mucinous tumors are not associated with any ovulation-related factors, except parity, suggesting a different tumor biology (1).

The relationship between infertility and the risk of OC has been studied, yielding mixed results. A meta-analysis that included over 10,000 patients with OC and 6.2 million participants supported this association (OR = 1.5; 95% CI 1.35-1.69) (18). Another meta-analysis reported the incidence of OC increased by 30% for women undergoing in vitro fertilization (IVF) and 40% in women receiving clomiphene citrate compared to women not undergoing fertility treatment (19). In this analysis, the incidence of borderline tumors was higher in the fertility-treatment group (OR 1.69, CI 1.27-2.25), but overall, when including all histologic subtypes, fertility treatment was not associated with a significant increase in OC incidence (OR 1.19; CI 0.98-1.46). The precise mechanism of this increased risk is unknown, and these findings are limited by a lack of knowledge of individuals hereditary cancer risk or other risk factors, making them more likely to undergo fertility treatment (such as obesity) that could also increase their risk. These mixed data suggest, but do not prove, an association between infertility and OC risk.

A number of studies have found a reduced risk of OC associated with breastfeeding, that is long-lasting and not related to parity (15). Breastfeeding provides 20% to 30% reduction in OC risk and has its strongest effect on high-grade serous ovarian cancer (HGSOC) (20). A pooled analysis including 13 case-control studies from the OCAC including over 20,000 women reported the value of breastfeeding for 1 to 3 months (18% risk reduction) as well as for 12 months or greater (34% reduction). In addition, this reduction in risk (OR, 0.56; 95% CI, 0.47-0.66) not only lasted for 10 years but also persisted (OR, 0.83, 95% CI, 0.77-0.90) for 30 years (20). Given the risk reduction seen with breastfeeding and increasing parity, the combination benefit was explored using data pooled from 32 studies (15). The combined benefit of two births and less than 6 months of breastfeeding resulted in a 0.5-fold reduction in EOC risk. Suppression of ovulation and decreased gonadotropin levels have been proposed as explanatory of the reduced risk, but further studies are needed to confirm this hypothesis and to clarify relations by histologic subtype.

Contraceptives and Ovarian Cancer Risk Reduction

To date, OCPs use has been consistently shown to be protective against OC. OCPs were first introduced in the United States in the 1960s. Most formulations include estrogen, progesterone, or a combination of the two. In addition to suppressing ovulation, OCPs also reduce pituitary secretion of gonadotropins and protect against chronic inflammation associated with pelvic inflammatory disease (PID). The use of OCP appears to decrease a woman's risk for OC by 30% to 60%. Specifically, women who use OCP for at least 5 years reduce their risk of OC by an average of 50%, with a concomitant decrease in mortality (21-23) (**Figure 8.1-2**). The largest pooled analysis, a meta-analysis reanalyzing data from 45 epidemiologic studies, which included 23,257 women with OC and 87,303 controls, showed that the use of OCP in high-income countries reduced OC incidence from 1.2 to 0.8 and mortality from 0.7 to 0.5 per 100 users (23). The data also showed a solid duration-response relationship between OC incidence and OCP use because the level of protection conferred clearly increased with duration of use (22) (**Figure 8.1-3**). In addition, the data confirmed that the protective effect continues for decades after OCPs are discontinued and suggested that the earlier a woman begins using OCP, the greater the reduction in her risk for developing OC (22). An analysis stratifying the effects of OCP by histologic subtypes showed that a 5-year increase in OCP duration reduced the risk of serous cancer, endometrioid cancer, and clear cell cancer by 14% to 15% (1). However, it is unclear which is more important for a protective effect—the age at which women begin taking OCP or the duration of use. Interestingly, OCP had little effect on risk for mucinous OCs, which is consistent with the distinct biology of these tumors (1,24).

The mechanisms underlying the profound and long-lasting protection against OC provided by OCP use are not well understood. The protective effects may be mediated by suppression of ovulation, reduction of gonadotropin levels, and/or induction of apoptosis (21). Moreover, OCPs suppress the levels of follicle-stimulating hormone (FSH), luteinizing hormone (LH), and estradiol, which all can promote tumor cell proliferation. In view of the protective effects of parity and breastfeeding, however, a primary mechanism of protection may well involve suppression of ovulation, which reduces the number of lifetime ovulatory cycles and the associated injury to the epithelial cells on the surface of the ovary. According to an older hypothesis (the "incessant ovulation" hypothesis) (25), OC develops from an aberration in the repair process of the surface epithelium, which is ruptured and repaired during each ovulatory cycle. In support of this theory, it is well known that domestic egg-laying hens, which are forced to ovulate incessantly, have a high incidence of lesions believed to be ovarian-derived tumors with peritoneal carcinomatosis (26). Alternative hypotheses center on the ability of OCP to treat endometriosis and reduce the risk of acquiring PID, two conditions known to be associated with OC (see later in this chapter). However, these hypotheses are at odds with the origin of OC in the fallopian tube, further elucidated in Chapter 7.1.

A case-control study has shown that progestin-only contraceptive users have a reduced risk (0.39) for developing OC (27). Moreover, the increase in progestin levels seen during pregnancy suggests that the protective effect of pregnancy may involve progestins as well as the reduction in the number of lifetime ovulations (22). Studies in primates indicate that the progestin component of OCP has a chemopreventive effect by inducing apoptosis of ovarian surface cells that have undergone genetic damage (28). The levonorgestrel-releasing Intrauterine device (IUD) is associated with a significant risk reduction of OC and endometrial cancer. In a Norwegian cohort study including 104,318 women (NOWAC study), the incidence rate of OC among ever users of a levonorgestrel-releasing IUD was 16.7 per 100,000 person-years

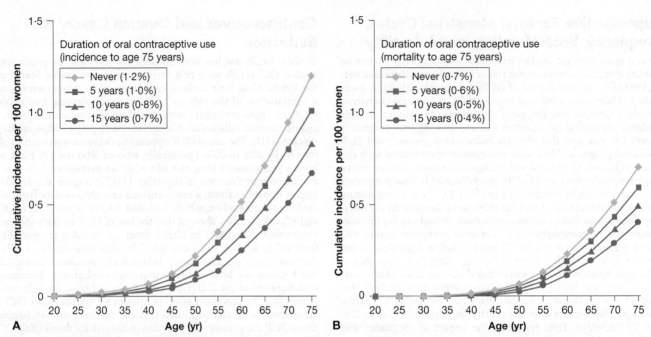

Figure 8.1-2. Absolute risk of ovarian cancer (OC) for women in high-income countries, by duration of use of oral contraceptives. A: Cumulative incidence of OC per 100 women. B: Cumulative mortality from OC per 100 women. (From Beral V, Doll R, Hermon C, et al. Ovarian cancer and oral contraceptives: collaborative reanalysis of data from 45 epidemiological studies including 23,257 women with ovarian cancer and 87,303 controls. *Lancet.* 2008;371:303-314.)

compared to 38.1 among never users (29). Depot medroxyprogesterone acetate (DMPA) is an injectable progestin-only contraceptive. Ever use of DMPA was associated in a pooled analysis of seven studies with a 35% decreased risk of OC (OR 0.65; 95% CI 0.5-0.85) (30). It is accepted that progestin/progesterone play a protective role against the development of OC.

Chemoprevention

The majority of theoretical models of OC chemoprevention have been based on the assumption that the origin of OC is the ovarian surface epithelium (OSE). As the paradigm has shifted to identifying the epithelial surface of the fallopian tube as the site of

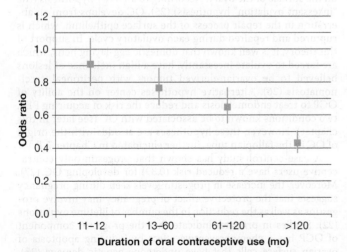

Figure 8.1-3. Relationship between duration of oral contraceptive pill use and ovarian cancer incidence. There is no evidence of heterogeneity. The estimated value of sigma (σ) is 0.15. (From Beral V, Doll R, Hermon C, et al. Ovarian cancer and oral contraceptives: collaborative reanalysis of data from 45 epidemiological studies including 23,257 women with ovarian cancer and 87,303 controls. *Lancet.* 2008;371:303-314.)

origin, it is not clear how to interpret the previous theories (31). Receptors for most members of the steroid hormone superfamily, including receptors for progestins, retinoids, androgens, and vitamin D, are present in the ovary and fallopian tube (32). Progestins, retinoids, and vitamin D have been shown to exert a broad range of common biologic effects in epithelial cells, including induction of apoptosis, upregulation of transforming growth factor-β (TGF-β), cellular differentiation, and inhibition of proliferation. It is yet to be demonstrated that these agents are active in the fallopian tube epithelium.

Retinoids are natural and synthetic derivatives of vitamin A. They have potential for cancer prevention owing to a broad range of biologic effects on epithelial cells through their ability to induce differentiation. Epidemiologic and laboratory evidence suggests a potential role for retinoids as preventive agents for OC, but it has not entered clinical practice because of the paucity of data. The most significant evidence supporting a rationale for retinoids as chemopreventive agents for OC is that of a chemoprevention study in Italy, which suggested an OC preventive effect from the retinoid 4-HPR. Among women randomized to receive either 4-HPR or placebo in a trial designed to evaluate 4-HPR as a chemopreventive for breast carcinoma, significantly fewer OC cases were noted in the 4-HPR group as compared to controls (33). Subsequently, a meta-analysis including 10 case-control and 5 cohort studies show a reduced risk of OC with vitamin A intake, especially in North American populations (33).

Vitamin D is a fat-soluble vitamin that is essential as a positive regulator of calcium homeostasis. The vitamin D receptor and the retinoic acid receptors share strong homology and readily dimerize, making it likely that vitamin D and retinoids have common signaling pathways in the cell. Vitamin D has been shown to have diverse biologic effects in epithelial cells relevant to cancer prevention, including retardation of growth, induction of cellular differentiation, induction of apoptosis, and upregulation of TGF-β. However, a meta-analysis also failed to show a protective effect of vitamin D on OC risk (RR 1.02, CI 0.62-1.03) (34).

Epidemiologic studies have suggested that the use of nonsteroidal anti-inflammatory drugs (NSAIDs) may lower OC risk. Several biologic mechanisms have been proposed to account for the chemopreventive effects of NSAIDs, including inhibition of ovulation, inhibition of COX, downregulation of prostaglandins, enhancement of the immune response, and induction of apoptosis. A meta-analysis including 8 cohort and 15 case-control studies showed an inverse relationship between aspirin use and OC risk (RR = 0.89, 95% CI, 0.83-0.96) (35). Subsequently, a cohort study including over 204,000 women investigated the association of analgesics and OC risk (36). An inverse association was observed with low-dose (≤100 mg) aspirin (HR = 0.77; 95% CI 0.61, 0.96), but not with standard dose (325 mg) aspirin or acetaminophen. Non-aspirin NSAID was associated with increased cancer risk when comparing the use with nonuse (HR, 1.19; 95% CI, 1.00-1.41), as well as based on the duration of use (P = .02 for trend) and cumulative average tablets per week (P = .03 for trend). Analysis of the Prostate, Lung, Colorectal, and Ovarian (PLCO) trial showed that in women younger than 70 years, there was inverse association for daily use of aspirin, suggesting a modest effect of daily, low-dose aspirin in reducing OC risk (37). In a report summarizing 17 studies, frequent aspirin was associated with a 13% reduction of OC risk in all OC histologic subtypes, including a 14% reduction for high-grade serous cancers (HGSCs). The risk reduction was independent of most other OC risk factors (obesity, family history of breast cancer/OC, parity, OCP use) (38).

The role of β-blockers has been examined in patients with OC to decrease adrenergic activation and thus decrease OC growth and metastasis and has been associated with a significant improvement in overall survival (OS) (39). However, a recent meta-analysis did not support this finding, indicating no relationship between postdiagnosis use of β-blockers and improved survival (40). The role of β-blockers for chemoprevention of OC has yet to be defined.

In summary, despite a growing body of preclinical data indicating chemopreventive effects of several agents, clinical research exploring their efficacy to reduce rates of OC is hindered by the relatively low incidence of the disease, insufficient understanding of the preclinical course of OC, the lack of validated preclinical biomarkers, and inadequate screening strategies.

Hormone Replacement Therapy

Currently, the primary indications for the prescription of HRT are severe postmenopausal symptoms and not the prevention of chronic disease. Several prospective cohort studies examined the relationship of postmenopausal estrogen or estrogen/progestin HRT to the risk of developing OC. In the prospective, double-blind Women's Health Initiative (WHI) randomized trial, over 8,000 women who had not had a hysterectomy were randomized to either placebo or 0.625-mg conjugated equine estrogen with 2.5-mg medroxyprogesterone acetate (41). After an average of 5.6 years of follow-up, 20 women in the estrogen/progestin group were diagnosed with an invasive OC versus 12 in the placebo group, which was not a significant difference (HR: 1.64; 0.78-3.45). The observational "Million Women study" showed an increased risk with estrogen-only HRT (RR 1.49; CI 1.2-1.81) and, like the Breast Cancer Detection Demonstration Project, showed a lower risk with estrogen/progestin combination therapy (RR 1.15; CI 1-1.33) (42). This study also reviewed the cumulative incidence of gynecologic cancers, including ovarian, endometrial, and breast cancer in women taking HRT. The gynecologic cancer incidence per 1,000 women over 5 years increased from 19 per 1,000 in "never users" to 26 per 1,000 in current users of estrogen-only HRT and to 35 per 1,000 in current users of estrogen/progestin combinations (**Figure 8.1-4**). The strength of this study, which followed nearly 1 million women, was that the results were adjusted for age at menopause, OCP use, BMI, smoking, and physical activity. HRT was found to be unrelated to the risk of mucinous OC. Other data indicate that regular use of vaginal and transdermal estrogen may carry a slightly increased risk of OC (42,43).

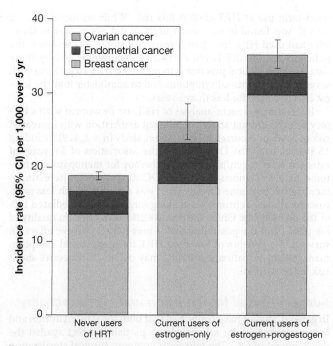

Figure 8.1-4. Standardized incidence rate (95% CI) for ovarian, endometrial, and breast cancer per 100 women in the study cohort over a 5-year period, for current users of various types of HRT and for never users. Incidence rates are standardized by age, region of residence, socioeconomic status, time since menopause, parity, use of oral contraceptives, body mass index, and alcohol consumption. Rates apply to women with a uterus and ovaries. CI, confidence interval; HRT, hormone replacement therapy. (Fig. 3 from Havrilesky LJ, Moorman PG, Lowery WJ, et al. Oral contraceptive pills as primary prevention for ovarian cancer: a systematic review and meta-analysis. *Obstet Gynecol.* 2013;122:139.)

In 2015, a meta-analysis of 52 epidemiologic studies (17 prospective) was published. It included a total of 21,488 postmenopausal women with OC and found the RR of OC to be increased by 1.14 (CI 1.10-1.19, P < .0001) in patients taking HRT (44). The risk was related to the recency of use. The greatest risk was in current HRT users (RR 1.41, CI 1.32-1.5), and risk decreased with the length of time since last use of HRT. In both current and recent users, the OC risk was significantly increased with the use of both estrogen-only (RR 1.32, CI 1.23-1.41) and estrogen-progesterone (RR 1.25, 95% CI: 1.16-1.34) combinations. Interestingly, the RR did not differ between nonepithelial and epithelial tumors and was increased for the two most common tumor histologic subtypes: serous (RR 1.53, 95% CI 1.40-1.66, P <.0001) and endometrioid (RR 1.42, CI 1.2-1.67; P < .0001), but not for the less common mucinous and clear cell (RR 0.75, CI 0.57-0.98, P = .04) subtypes. The RR of developing OC when taking HRT was independent of age at initiation of HRT. The authors concluded that "5 years of HRT use, starting at age 50, would result in one additional OC per 1,000 users."

A more recent meta-analysis of 34 studies (n = 3.3 million participants) was published in 2019 (45). The pooled RR of OC was 1.29 (95% CI 1.19-1.4) for menopausal HRT. Subgroup analyses supported this relationship for North America (1.41, 95% CI: 1.23-1.61), Europe (1.22, 95% CI: 1.12-1.34), and Asia (1.76, 95% CI: 1.09-2.85), but not for Australia (0.96, 95% CI: 0.57-1.61). Similar to previous studies, the risk was increased for only serous and endometrioid tumors. However, this meta-analysis did not evaluate dosage, and only included patients who were on standard or high doses of HRT. It also did not offer information on whether lower doses confer a lower risk, which is particularly relevant now, since most of the women taking HRT in the United States are currently on low-dose regimens. The study did indicate, however, that short-term use of HRT confers less risk. While an increased risk for OC was found in all current users, it did not persist in those who had used HRT less than 5 years and stopped. Therefore, the judicious use of HRT is not necessarily contraindicated by these data. Current clinical practice is to prescribe HRT to patients with severe postmenopausal symptoms and to administer it at the lowest effective dose for less than 5 years.

Interestingly, a meta-analysis of HRT use by women with a history of EOC did not show a significant association with increased risk of death or recurrence (46). A large study ($n = 6,419$) including 15 studies from the OCAC noted the association of 5+ years of estrogen or estrogen/progesterone therapy for menopausal symptoms, before diagnosis, and better OC survival (47). Interestingly, menopausal hormone therapy (HT) was associated with less macroscopic disease at primary debulking surgery, which mediated 17% of the relationship. Given the positive effects of HRT on quality of life (QoL) and the possibility that it may have a positive effect on survival, the benefits of low-dose HRT for menopausal symptom management in patients with OC may outweigh concerns about risk for recurrence.

Surgery: Tubal Interruption and Hysterectomy

In general, studies have confirmed that both tubal interruption and hysterectomy without salpingectomy partially protect against the development of OC. The four most common surgical sterilization methods, tubal ligation, thermal injury, rings, and clips are probably equally effective in reducing risk. A large prospective cohort study, the Nurses' Health Study (48), confirmed the findings of smaller case-control studies, showing an RR of 0.33 (CI 0.16-0.64) of developing OC in women who had a tubal ligation. Tubal ligation was shown to almost halve the risk of clear cell cancers and endometrioid tumors (RR 0.54; CI 0.43-0.69) and reduce the risk of grade III (RR 0.77, CI 0.67-0.89), but not grade I, serous papillary tumors. It had no impact on the development of mucinous OC (1,49). The same study also reported a weak inverse relationship between hysterectomy and OC (RR 0.67; CI 0.45-1) and found that the effect of hysterectomy was greater when the surgery was performed at an earlier age (48), a finding that was not confirmed in a cohort study of 1.1 million U.K. women (49). In analysis by the Ovarian Cancer Cohort Consortium, tubal ligation was associated with reduced risk of endometrioid (RR 0.6, CI 0.41-0.88) and clear cell (RR 0.35, CI 0.18-0.69) cancers, but not with a reduced risk of serous tumors, and hysterectomy was associated with a reduced risk only for clear cell cancers (1). A meta-analysis including 40,609 OC cases and 368,452 controls showed no association of hysterectomy and subsequent OC risk, tubal ligation with a decreased risk of EOC (OR 0.7, CI 1.28-1.57), and endometriosis associated with increased risk (OR 1.42, CI 1.28-1.57) (50). However, another meta-analysis reports a 30% reduced risk of endometrioid and clear cell cancer following a simple hysterectomy for benign gynecologic disease. No risk reduction was seen for serous or mucinous histologic subtypes (51).

A retrospective case-control study evaluated the effect of tubal ligation in patients with *BRCA1* mutations (52). Like women unselected for genetic risk, *BRCA1* mutation carriers who had undergone a tubal ligation had a considerably reduced risk of developing OC (OR 0.39; CI 0.22-0.7). Those who both had a tubal ligation and had used OCP in the past had an even lower OR of developing OC (OR 0.28; CI 0.15-0.52). Possible explanations for the protective effect of tubal interruption against OC include (a) an impaired blood supply to the ovaries/distal fallopian tube through the superior branch of the uterine artery, which causes most women to enter menopause earlier and experience fewer lifetime ovulations; (b) an occlusion of the tube that blocks the upward flow of carcinogens and endometrial tissue from the uterus and reduces pelvic infection rates; and (c) the reduced presence and decreased proliferation of progenitor cells in the fimbriated end of the fallopian tube (53).

Opportunistic salpingectomy is recommended to decrease OC incidence. Molecular data suggest that many of the serous, clear cell, and endometroid carcinomas originate at the distal end of the fallopian tube that have undergone metaplastic changes (31). Given these findings, investigations into the clinical relevance of salpingectomies have been undertaken. A recent meta-analysis demonstrated a 50% reduction in the risk of OC for patients undergoing bilateral salpingectomy compared to controls (54). A second population-based study of 60,153 women included 25,889 individuals who underwent opportunistic salphingectomy and 32080 individuals who underwent hysterectomy alone or tubal ligation between 2008 and 2017 (55). At the point of data analysis in 2021, no cases of serous carcinoma were diagnosed, although the age-expected rate was 5.27 cancer diagnoses. There were less than five EOC diagnoses in the salpingectomy arm, compared to the expected rate of 8.68. In comparison, the tubal ligation arm had 15 serous carcinomas and 21 epithelial carcinomas (**Figure 8.1-5**). Based on prediction models, the authors estimated that opportunistic salpingectomy reduces the risk of epithelial serous OC by about 80%. Thus, organizations such as The Society of Gynecologic Oncology and the American College of Obstetricians and Gynecologists recommend salpingectomy for women already undergoing pelvic surgery to reduce this risk of OC.

Inflammation: Pelvic Inflammatory Disease and Endometriosis

Chronic inflammation, with its attendant increase in cell proliferation and potential for DNA disruption, has been proposed as a precursor for many cancers, including OC. Endometriosis and PID, both of which induce chronic inflammatory states, are associated with OC.

PID is a generalized infection of the female genital tract. Several small case-control studies have suggested that PID is associated with OC. However, this association only gained wide acceptance with the publication of a large study comparing the OC incidence of 68,000 women who had experienced PID versus 136,000 who had not (56). In this well-designed study, the HR for OC in patients with a history of PID (adjusted appropriately for confounding factors) was twice as high (HR 1.92) as that of controls and was even higher (HR 2.46) in women who had at least five episodes of PID. Another meta-analysis supported the association of PID with OC risk (RR: 1.24, 95% CI 1.06-1.44), but this relationship was strongest for Asian women (RR = 1.69, 95% CI 1.22-2.34), but not significant among White women (RR 1.18, 95% CI 1.00-1.39) (57). These findings were challenged by a recent pooled analysis of 13 case-control trials from the OCAC that included 9,162 women with OC, 2,454 women with borderline tumors, and 14,736 control participants, supporting an association of borderline tumors with one episode of PID (OR = 1.10) and two or more PID episodes (OR 2.14), but no association between PID and OC (58). It is evident that PID does impact the ovaries, increasing the risk of pathology; however, the extent of risk for developing borderline versus invasive cancer remains unknown.

Endometriosis, characterized by the ectopic growth of endometrial glands in the ovary and the abdominal cavity, affects 10% of women of reproductive age. In smaller case-control studies and one large meta-analysis (1), a history of endometriosis has been consistently shown to be associated with clear cell and endometrioid ovarian carcinoma, with an OR of approximately 2. In many endometrioid and clear cell OCs, endometriosis is detected histologically adjacent to the carcinoma. Combining data from 13 OC case-control studies (7,900 patients with OC), the OCAC published a definitive report that self-reported endometriosis increased the risk of clear cell (OR 3.05; CI 2.4-3.8) and endometrioid OC (OR 2.04; CI 1.7-2.5) (59). In this report, endometriosis was also associated, for the first time, with low-grade serous cancers (LGSCs) (OR 2.11; CI 1.4-3.2), suggesting that these cancers, which are generally believed to arise from serous borderline tumors (SBTs), can

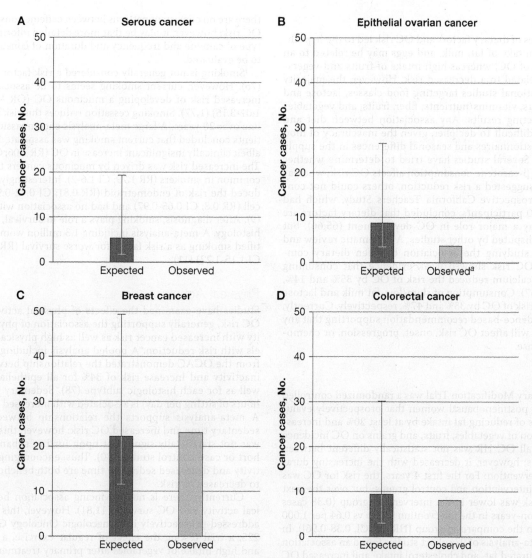

Figure 8.1-5. Expected versus observed cancers in the opportunistic salphingectomy group. There were no serous cancers in the OS group by the end of follow-up. Given the age-adjusted rate at which serous ovarian cancers occurred in the control group and the follow-up time in the OS group, 5.27 (95% CI, 1.78-19.29) serous cancers were expected (Figure 8.1-5A). The same is true for all epithelial ovarian cancers (EOCs). The expected number of EOCs in the OS group was 8.68 (95% CI, 3.36-26.58) cancers, and the actual number was ≤5 (exact number not presented to protect patient privacy) (Figure 8.1-5B). In contrast, there were 15 serous cancers in the control group and 21 EOCs (including 6 nonserous cancers). No differences existed between expected and observed numbers of breast or colorectal cancers (Figures 8.1-5C and D). CI, confidence interval; OS, overall survival. (From Hanley GE, Pearce CL, Talhouk A, et al. Outcomes from opportunistic salpingectomy for ovarian cancer prevention. *JAMA Netw Open.* 2022;5(2):e2147343. doi:10.1001/jamanetworkopen.2021.47343)

also arise from endometriotic implants. Adjusted for histology and International Federation of Gynaecology and Obstetrics (FIGO) stage, women with endometriosis-associated OC have similar survival to women with non–endometriosis-associated OC (60). There are two pathologic subtypes of endometriosis: displaced benign ectopic endometrial glands and atypical endometriosis. Endometriosis with cytological atypia and complex hyperplasia ("atypical endometriosis"), present in 2% to 3% of all patients who undergo surgery for endometriosis, is most likely a direct precursor for type I/low-grade OCs (61). This hypothesis was supported by a study in which *ARID1A* gene mutations were detected in 30% of endometrioid and 46% of clear cell cancers, as well as in areas of atypical endometriosis that were adjacent to the cancers (62). Many genes expressed in endometriosis are also detected in endometrioid OC but do not overlap with genes expressed in HGSCs (63). Surprisingly, cancer-associated somatic mutations (*ARID1A, PIK3CA, KRAS, PPP2R1A*) are often found in the epithelial compartment of endometriotic glands without any evidence of transformation. This

suggests that the presence of "driver mutations" alone is not sufficient nor indicative of likely progression to cancer (64). In summary, endometriosis is associated with three histologic subtypes of OC: endometrioid, clear cell, and low-grade serous (60). The risk of LGSC is 3.77 times higher (CI 1.24-11.48) in patients with endometriosis, but the risk of HGSC is not increased (1). In the general population, the risk of developing OC is one woman in 76 (1/31%), the lifetime risk of women with endometriosis is just slightly higher (1.8%) (6) and does not justify an oophorectomy solely for the purpose to reduce endometriosis-associated cancer risk.

Other Risk Factors: Diet, Smoking, and Exercise

Dietary, lifestyle, and social factors have been suggested to play a role in OC risk. These relationships have been primarily investigated via observational studies.

Dietary Factors

Ecologic studies of dietary factors and OC risk led to the hypothesis that high intake of fat, milk, and eggs may be related to an increased risk of OC, whereas high intake of fruits and vegetables may be related to a decreased risk. However, the majority of the observational studies targeting food classes, lactose and dairy foods, fats, vitamins/nutrients, fiber, fruits, and vegetables provide conflicting results. Any association between diet and cancer risk is difficult to decipher, given the inaccuracy of food frequency questionnaires and seasonal differences in the supply of fresh food. Several studies have tried to determine whether vitamin A and β-carotene consumption affects OC risk, whereas some studies suggested a risk reduction, others could not confirm it. The prospective California Teachers Study, which had almost 100,000 participants, concluded that dietary factors are unlikely to play a major role in OC development (65,66), but this has been disputed by other studies. A systematic review and meta-analysis studying the association between dietary components and OC risk showed weak evidence that consuming black tea and calcium reduced the risk of OC by 35% and 14%, respectively (67). Consumption of skim/low-fat milk and lactose increased the risk of OC by 35% and 47%, respectively. Currently, there is no evidence-based recommendation supporting that any change in diet will affect OC risk, onset, progression, or chemotherapy response.

Fat Intake

The WHI Dietary Modification Trial was a randomized controlled trial in 48,835 postmenopausal women that prospectively evaluated the effects of reducing fat intake by at least 20% and increasing consumption of vegetables, fruits, and grains on OC incidence (68). The overall OC HR was not statistically different between the two groups; however, it decreased with the increasing duration of the intervention: For the first 4 years, the risk for OC was similar in the intervention and control groups; but over the next 4 years, the risk was lower in the intervention group (0.38 cases per 1,000 person-years in the intervention group vs 0.64 per 1,000 person-years in the comparison group [HR 0.6; CI, 0.38-0.96]). In addition, a meta-analysis of 97 cohort studies found an association of total fat, saturated fat, and cholesterol intake and increased OC risk (69). However, not all analyses support these findings, including two meta-analyses reporting no association of trans-fatty acid intake and OC risk (67,70).

Fruits and Vegetables and Micronutrient Intake

Although a number of studies have suggested that OC risk might be reduced by higher consumption of fruits and vegetables or fiber, others, including a pooling project of 12 cohort studies, fail to support such relationships (71). However, a more recent meta-analysis including 97 cohort studies reports an association of the intake of green leafy vegetables, allium vegetables, fiber, and flavonoids with risk reduction (69). Some studies have shown inverse associations with particular nutrients, such as vitamins A, C, and E; β-carotene; or methionine, but results have been inconsistent across studies. Meta-analyses evaluating folate, vitamin D, or the major carotenoids and OC risk report no substantial relationships (72).

Alcohol, Caffeine, and Cigarette Smoking

Several studies have examined OC risk in relation to alcohol consumption. Most investigations, including a meta-analysis (73), have not found any convincing relationships. A recent dose-response meta-analysis found no association between the consumption of coffee and OC risk (RR: 1.08; 95% CI, 0.089-1.33) (74). Further support comes from another meta-analysis reporting no relationship between OC incidence and caffeine or coffee intake (75). Overall,

there are no consistent patterns between caffeine consumption and OC risk; however, it may be that more detailed information on the type of caffeine and frequency and duration of consumption need to be evaluated.

Smoking is not generally considered a risk factor for all EOCs (76). However, current smoking seems to be associated with an increased risk of developing a mucinous OC (OR = 1.78; CI = 1.01-3.15) (1,77). Smoking cessation reduces this risk back to baseline over 20 years. A large meta-analysis encompassing 28,114 patients concluded that current smoking was associated with a small albeit clinically insignificant increase in OC (RR 1.06; CI 1.01-1.11). The increased risk was driven by mucinous cancers that are more common in smokers (RR 1.79; CI 1.6-2). Interestingly, smoking reduced the risk of endometrioid (RR 0.81; CI 0.72-0.92) and clear cell (RR 0.8; CI 0.65-0.97) and had no association with serous OC (9). After diagnosis, smoking plays a role in survival, regardless of histology. A meta-analysis including 1.3 million women also identified smoking as a risk factor for worse survival (RR = 1.17; 95% CI 1.15-1.22) (11).

Physical Activity

Studies have examined the effects of physical activity levels on OC risk, generally supporting the association of physical inactivity with increased cancer risk as well as high physical activity levels with risk reduction. A pooled analysis including nine studies from the OCAC demonstrated the relationship between chronic inactivity and increase risk of 34% for all epithelial cancers, as well as for each histologic subtype (78). Sedentary behavior (6+ hours of sitting per day) is associated with increased OC risk (79). A meta-analysis supports the relationship between increased sedentary time and increased OC risk; however, this relationship was not statistically significant upon further subanalyses of cohort or case-control studies (80). Thus, encouraging physical activity and decreased sedentary time are both beneficial strategies to decrease OC risk.

Currently, there is no convincing association between physical activity and OC survival (11,81). However, this issue will be addressed prospectively in Gynecologic Oncology Group (GOG) 225, a trial testing the effect of regular exercise, a low-fat diet, and high intake of vegetables after primary treatment for OC on progression-free survival (PFS). All participants have been accrued, and the results are pending data maturation.

Given that individuals can be exposed to several risks, a pooled analysis was undertaken (n = 7,022 OC survivors) that demonstrated an increased mortality rate when participants were current smokers, overweight/obese, and physically inactive compared to nonsmoking, normal weight, active women (82). Furthermore, the association for joint exposures exceeded that of a single exposure. No associations between these factors and PFS were seen.

In summary, although some data are incongruent, there is no reason not to encourage patients to make healthy dietary choice, avoid tobacco products, and be physically active for their overall health. These activities and choices may have protective effect against OC. In addition, the factors that decrease the number of lifetime ovulations reduce the risk of developing OC, whereas hereditary factors increase the risk. From a practical, clinical standpoint, only a positive family history will raise the suspicion of a predisposition to OC in an asymptomatic woman.

CONCLUSIONS

Much of the clinical and epidemiologic evidence concerning risk factors for OC implicates ovulatory activity. Conditions associated with reduced ovulation (eg, pregnancy and OCP use) consistently reduce risk. Combining these and other menstrual factors into single "ovulatory age" or "lifetime ovulatory cycles" indexes has generally produced the expected associations with OC risk; that is, older ovulatory ages or higher cycle counts increase risk. However, the misclassification inherent in these indexes is sufficient to generate different risk estimates, and the magnitude of risk reduction for short-term OCP use or a single pregnancy or breastfeeding exceeds the proportional decrease in ovulatory cycles that would be expected to be associated with these exposures.

A popular unifying hypothesis is that OC is the result of accumulated exposure to circulating pituitary gonadotropins. Although this is consistent with the parity, menopause, and OCP associations, there is no support for high gonadotropin levels being related to increased risk. This theory also fails to account for the risks associated with clinical infertility, and it predicts that menopausal HT use would decrease risk, because both exposures are associated with reduced gonadotropin levels.

A second explanation points to a biologic effect of ovulation on OSE. Ovulation prompts a cascade of epithelial events, including minor trauma, increased local concentrations of estrogen-rich follicular fluid, and increased epithelial proliferation, followed by local inflammation and wound repair. Such

proliferation, particularly near the point of ovulation, can recruit inclusions into the ovarian parenchyma. Some or all of these "incessant ovulation" events may lie on the causal path to OC. This is consistent with most of the endocrine-related risk factors, except for the risks associated with clinical infertility, but then increasing evidence indicates that a large subset of HGSOCs arise from high-grade intraepithelial serous carcinomas in the fallopian tube and spread to the ovary (31).

No single theory adequately incorporates the available data. A unifying hypothesis may lie in a combination of ovulation, hormones, and local effects on the fallopian tube and ovary. Additional factors, such as predisposing genetic alterations; androgens, progestins, and other hormones; inflammation; and endometriosis, also appear to be important.

OC epidemiology presents both simple and complex patterns, varying with histologic subtypes (**Figure 8.1-6**). Rates have largely remained unchanged over the past 40 years. A clear picture has emerged for some protective factors, such as OCPs and parity, but risk associated with other important public health issues, such as smoking, obesity, and physical activity, remains uncertain. Although it is tempting to attribute the differences to

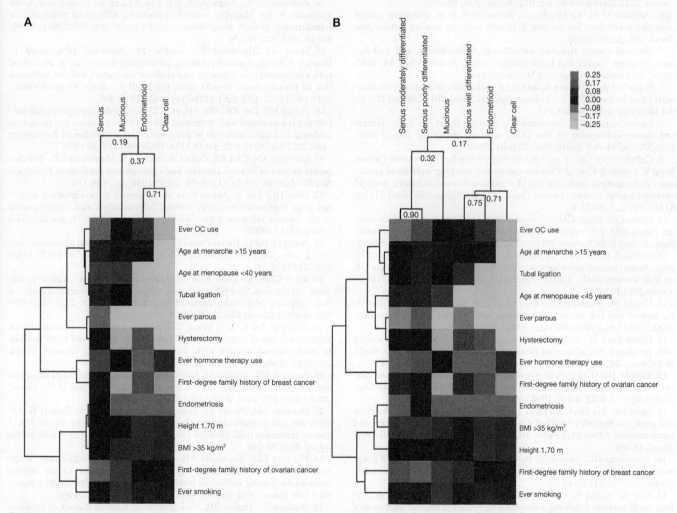

Figure 8.1-6. Unsupervised hierarchical clustering of ovarian cancer histologic subtypes by their associations with risk factors. Unsupervised hierarchical clustering of the (A) four subtypes and (B) that includes the serous subtype divided into well-, moderately, and poorly differentiated carcinomas by using β-estimates, complete linkage, and an uncentered correlation similarity metric. The categories used in the cluster analysis were ever versus never parous, ever versus never oral contraceptive (OC) use, ever versus never tubal ligation, ever versus never endometriosis, age at menarche >15 versus ≤11 years, age at menopause <40 versus 50 to 55 years, ever versus never menopausal hormone therapy use, ever versus never hysterectomy, family history of breast cancer (yes vs no), family history of ovarian cancer (yes vs no), body mass index (BMI) >35 versus 20 to 25 kg/m², height (per 5-cm increase), and ever versus never smoking. The color scale shows the range of β-values for each exposure. (From Wentzensen N, Poole EM, Trabert B, et al. Ovarian cancer risk factors by histologic subtype: an analysis from the ovarian cancer cohort consortium. *J Clin Oncol.* 2016;34(24):2888-2898. doi:10.1200/JCO.2016.66.8178)

histology-specific associations, such hypotheses will require substantially more epidemiologic, clinical, and genetic data before their acceptance is certain. Consistent risk factors for high-grade serous tumors, the most fatal subtype, also remain elusive. Continued attempts to account for the differences between studies should help delineate spurious associations from the etiologically relevant risk factors.

REFERENCES

1. Wentzensen N, Poole EM, Trabert B, et al. Ovarian cancer risk factors by histologic subtype: an analysis from the ovarian cancer cohort consortium. *J Clin Oncol*. 2016;34(24):2888-2898. doi:10.1200/JCO.2016.66.8178

2. Siegel RL, Miller KD, Fuchs HE, Jemal A. Cancer statistics, 2022. *CA Cancer J Clin*. 2022;72(1):7-33. doi:10.3322/caac.21708

3. Sung H, Ferlay J, Siegel RL, et al. Global cancer statistics 2020: GLOBOCAN estimates of incidence and mortality worldwide for 36 cancers in 185 countries. *CA Cancer J Clin*. 2021;71(3):209-249. doi:10.3322/caac.21660

4. Iida Y, Okamoto A, Hollis RL, Gourley C, Herrington CS. Clear cell carcinoma of the ovary: a clinical and molecular perspective. *Int J Gynecol Cancer*. 2021;31(4):605-616. doi:10.1136/ijgc-2020-001656

5. Dalmartello M, La Vecchia C., Bertuccio P, et al. European cancer mortality predictions for the year 2022 with focus on ovarian cancer. *Ann Oncol*. 2022;33(3):330-339.

6. National Cancer Institute Surveillance, Epidemiology, and End Results Program. Cancer stat facts: ovarian cancer. Accessed July 14, 2022. https://seer.cancer.gov/statfacts/html/ovary.html

7. Sopik V, Iqbal J, Rosen B, Narod SA. Why have ovarian cancer mortality rates declined? Part I. Incidence. *Gynecol Oncol*. 2015;138(3):741-749. doi:10.1016/j.ygyno.2015.06.017

8. Lauby-Secretan B, Scoccianti C, Loomis D, et al. Body fatness and cancer—viewpoint of the IARC working group. *N Engl J Med*. 2016;375(8):794-798. doi:10.1056/NEJMsr1606602

9. Collaborative Group on Epidemiological Studies of Ovarian Cancer, Beral V, Gaitskell K, et al. Ovarian cancer and smoking: individual participant meta-analysis including 28,114 women with ovarian cancer from 51 epidemiological studies. *Lancet Oncol*. 2012;13(9):946-956. doi:10.1016/S1470-2045(12)70322-4

10. Olsen CM, Nagle CM, Whiteman DC, et al. Obesity and risk of ovarian cancer subtypes: evidence from the ovarian cancer association consortium. *Endocr Relat Cancer*. 2013;20(2):251-262. doi:10.1530/ERC-12-0395

11. Gaitskell K, Hermon C, Barnes I, et al. Ovarian cancer survival by stage, histotype, and pre-diagnostic lifestyle factors, in the prospective UK million women study. *Cancer Epidemiol*. 2022;76:102074. doi:10.1016/j.canep.2021.102074

12. Khalid SI, Maasarani S, Wiegmann J, et al. Association of bariatric surgery and risk of cancer in patients with morbid obesity. *Ann Surg*. 2022;275(1):1-6. doi:10.1097/SLA.0000000000005035

13. Dixon-Suen SC, Nagle CM, Thrift AP, et al. Adult height is associated with increased risk of ovarian cancer: a Mendelian randomisation study. *Br J Cancer*. 2018;118(8):1123-1129. doi:10.1038/s41416-018-0011-3

14. Yang H, Dai H, Li L, et al. Age at menarche and epithelial ovarian cancer risk: a meta-analysis and Mendelian randomization study. *Cancer Med*. 2019;8(8):4012-4022. doi:10.1002/cam4.2315

15. Sung HK, Ma SH, Choi JY, et al. The effect of breastfeeding duration and parity on the risk of epithelial ovarian cancer: a systematic review and meta-analysis. *J Prev Med Public Health*. 2016;49(6):349-366. doi:10.3961/jpmph.16.066

16. Whiteman DC, Siskind V, Purdie DM, Green AC. Timing of pregnancy and the risk of epithelial ovarian cancer. *Cancer Epidemiol Biomarkers Prev*. 2003;12(1):42-46.

17. Kim SJ, Rosen B, Fan I, et al. Epidemiologic factors that predict long-term survival following a diagnosis of epithelial ovarian cancer. *Br J Cancer*. 2017;116(7):964-971. doi:10.1038/bjc.2017.35

18. Jiang YT, Gong TT, Zhang JY, et al. Infertility and ovarian cancer risk: evidence from nine prospective cohort studies. *Int J Cancer*. 2020;147(8):2121-2130. doi:10.1002/ijc.33012

19. Barcroft JF, Galazis N, Jones BP, et al. Fertility treatment and cancers-the eternal conundrum: a systematic review and meta-analysis. *Hum Reprod*. 2021;36(4):1093-1107. doi:10.1093/humrep/deaa293

20. Babic A, Sasamoto N, Rosner BA, et al. Association between breastfeeding and ovarian cancer risk. *JAMA Oncol*. 2020;6(6):e200421. doi:10.1001/jamaoncol.2020.0421

21. Schildkraut JM, Calingaert B, Marchbanks PA, Moorman PG, Rodriguez GC. Impact of progestin and estrogen potency in oral contraceptives on ovarian cancer risk. *J Natl Cancer Inst*. 2002;94(1):32-38. doi:10.1093/jnci/94.1.32

22. Havrilesky LJ, Moorman PG, Lowery WJ, et al. Oral contraceptive pills as primary prevention for ovarian cancer: a systematic review and meta-analysis. *Obstet Gynecol*. 2013;122(1):139-147. doi:10.1097/AOG.0b013e318291c235

23. Collaborative Group on Epidemiological Studies of Ovarian Cancer, Beral V, Doll R, Hermon C, Peto R, Reeves G. Ovarian cancer and oral contraceptives: collaborative reanalysis of data from 45 epidemiological studies including 23,257 women with ovarian cancer and 87,303 controls. *Lancet Lond Engl*. 2008;371(9609):303-314. doi:10.1016/S0140-6736(08)60167-1

24. Lengyel E. Ovarian cancer development and metastasis. *Am J Pathol*. 2010;177(3):1053-1064. doi:10.2353/ajpath.2010.100105

25. Casagrande JT, Louie EW, Pike MC, Roy S, Ross RK, Henderson BE. "Incessant ovulation" and ovarian cancer. *Lancet Lond Engl*. 1979;2(8135):170-173. doi:10.1016/s0140-6736(79)91435-1

26. Treviño LS, Buckles EL, Johnson PA. Oral contraceptives decrease the prevalence of ovarian cancer in the hen. *Cancer Prev Res*. 2012;5(2):343-349. doi:10.1158/1940-6207.CAPR-11-0344

27. Risch HA. Hormonal etiology of epithelial ovarian cancer, with a hypothesis concerning the role of androgens and progesterone. *J Natl Cancer Inst*. 1998;90(23):1774-1786. doi:10.1093/jnci/90.23.1774

28. Rodriguez GC, Nagarsheth NP, Lee KL, et al. Progestin-induced apoptosis in the Macaque ovarian epithelium: differential regulation of transforming growth factor-beta. *J Natl Cancer Inst*. 2002;94(1):50-60. doi:10.1093/jnci/94.1.50

29. Jareid M, Thalabard JC, Aarflot M, Bøvelstad HM, Lund E, Braaten T. Levonorgestrel-releasing intrauterine system use is associated with a decreased risk of ovarian and endometrial cancer, without increased risk of breast cancer. Results from the NOWAC study. *Gynecol Oncol*. 2018;149(1):127-132. doi:10.1016/j.ygyno.2018.02.006

30. Phung MT, Lee AW, Wu AH, et al. Depot-Medroxyprogesterone acetate use is associated with decreased risk of ovarian cancer: the mounting evidence of a protective role of progestins. *Cancer Epidemiol Biomarkers Prev*. 2021;30(5):927-935. doi:10.1158/1055-9965.EPI-20-1355

31. Karnezis AN, Cho KR, Gilks CB, Pearce CL, Huntsman DG. The disparate origins of ovarian cancers: pathogenesis and prevention strategies. *Nat Rev Cancer*. 2017;17(1):65-74. doi:10.1038/nrc.2016.113

32. Dinh HQ, Lin X, Abbasi F, et al. Single-cell transcriptomics identifies gene expression networks driving differentiation and tumorigenesis in the human fallopian tube. *Cell Rep*. 2021;35(2):108978. doi:10.1016/j.celrep.2021.108978

33. Wang Q, He C. Dietary vitamin A intake and the risk of ovarian cancer: a meta-analysis. *Biosci Rep*. 2020;40(4):BSR20193979. doi:10.1042/BSR20193979

34. Xu J, Chen K, Zhao F, et al. Association between vitamin D/calcium intake and 25-hydroxyvitamin D and risk of ovarian cancer: a dose-response relationship meta-analysis. *Eur J Clin Nutr*. 2021;75(3):417-429. doi:10.1038/s41430-020-00724-1

35. Zhang D, Bai B, Xi Y, Wang T, Zhao Y. Is aspirin use associated with a decreased risk of ovarian cancer? A systematic review and meta-analysis of observational studies with dose-response analysis. *Gynecol Oncol*. 2016;142(2):368-377. doi:10.1016/j.ygyno.2016.04.543

36. Barnard ME, Poole EM, Curhan GC, et al. Association of analgesic use with risk of ovarian cancer in the nurses' health studies. *JAMA Oncol*. 2018;4(12):1675-1682. doi:10.1001/jamaoncol.2018.4149

37. Hurwitz LM, Pinsky PF, Huang WY, Freedman ND, Trabert B. Aspirin use and ovarian cancer risk using extended follow-up of the PLCO cancer screening trial. *Gynecol Oncol*. 2020;159(2):522-526. doi:10.1016/j.ygyno.2020.08.038

38. Hurwitz LM, Townsend MK, Jordan SJ, et al. Modification of the association between frequent aspirin use and ovarian cancer risk: a meta-analysis using individual-level data from two ovarian cancer consortia. *J Clin Oncol*. 2022;40:4207-4217. doi:10.1200/JCO.21.01900

39. Watkins JL, Thaker PH, Nick AM, et al. Clinical impact of selective and nonselective beta-blockers on survival in patients with ovarian cancer. *Cancer*. 2015;121(19):3444-3451. doi:10.1002/cncr.29392

40. Wen ZY, Gao S, Gong TT, et al. Post-Diagnostic beta blocker use and prognosis of ovarian cancer: a systematic review and meta-analysis of 11 cohort studies with 20,274 patients. *Front Oncol*. 2021;11:665617. doi:10.3389/fonc.2021.665617

41. Anderson GL, Judd HL, Kaunitz AM, et al. Effects of estrogen plus progestin on gynecologic cancers and associated diagnostic procedures: the women's health initiative randomized trial. *JAMA*. 2003;290(13):1739-1748. doi:10.1001/jama.290.13.1739

42. Beral V, Million Women Study Collaborators, Bull D, Green J, Reeves G. Ovarian cancer and hormone replacement therapy in the million women study. *Lancet Lond Engl.* 2007;369(9574):1703-1710. doi:10.1016/S0140-6736(07)60534-0

43. Mørch LS, Løkkegaard E, Andreasen AH, Krüger-Kjaer S, Lidegaard O. Hormone therapy and ovarian cancer. *JAMA.* 2009;302(3):298-305. doi:10.1001/jama.2009.1052

44. Collaborative Group On Epidemiological Studies of Ovarian Cancer, Beral V, Gaitskell K, et al. Menopausal hormone use and ovarian cancer risk: individual participant meta-analysis of 52 epidemiological studies. *Lancet Lond Engl.* 2015;385(9980):1835-1842. doi:10.1016/S0140-6736(14)61687-1

45. Liu Y, Ma L, Yang X, et al. Menopausal hormone replacement therapy and the risk of ovarian cancer: a meta-analysis. *Front Endocrinol.* 2019;10:801. doi:10.3389/fendo.2019.00801

46. Li D, Ding CY, Qiu LH. Postoperative hormone replacement therapy for epithelial ovarian cancer patients: a systematic review and meta-analysis. *Gynecol Oncol.* 2015;139(2):355-362. doi:10.1016/j.ygyno.2015.07.109

47. Brieger KK, Peterson S, Lee AW, et al. Menopausal hormone therapy prior to the diagnosis of ovarian cancer is associated with improved survival. *Gynecol Oncol.* 2020;158(3):702-709. doi:10.1016/j.ygyno.2020.06.481

48. Hankinson SE, Hunter DJ, Colditz GA, et al. Tubal ligation, hysterectomy, and risk of ovarian cancer. A prospective study. *JAMA.* 1993;270(23):2813-2818.

49. Gaitskell K, Green J, Pirie K, Reeves G, Beral V, Million Women Study Collaborators. Tubal ligation and ovarian cancer risk in a large cohort: substantial variation by histological type. *Int J Cancer.* 2016;138(5):1076-1084. doi:10.1002/ijc.29856

50. Wang C, Liang Z, Liu X, Zhang Q, Li S. The Association between endometriosis, tubal ligation, hysterectomy and epithelial ovarian cancer: meta-analyses. *Int J Environ Res Public Health.* 2016;13(11):1138. doi:10.3390/ijerph13111138

51. Huo X, Yao L, Han X, et al. Hysterectomy and risk of ovarian cancer: a systematic review and meta-analysis. *Arch Gynecol Obstet.* 2019;299(3):599-607. doi:10.1007/s00404-018-5020-1

52. Narod SA, Sun P, Ghadirian P, et al. Tubal ligation and risk of ovarian cancer in carriers of BRCA1 or BRCA2 mutations: a case-control study. *Lancet Lond Engl.* 2001;357(9267):1467-1470. doi:10.1016/s0140-6736(00)04642-0

53. Tiourin E, Velasco VS, Rosales MA, Sullivan PS, Janzen DM, Memarzadeh S. Tubal ligation induces quiescence in the epithelia of the fallopian tube fimbria. *Reprod Sci.* 2015;22(10):1262-1271. doi:10.1177/1933719115574345

54. Yoon SH, Kim SN, Shim SH, Kang SB, Lee SJ. Bilateral salpingectomy can reduce the risk of ovarian cancer in the general population: a meta-analysis. *Eur J Cancer.* 2016;55:38-46. doi:10.1016/j.ejca.2015.12.003

55. Hanley GE, Pearce CL, Talhouk A, et al. Outcomes from opportunistic salpingectomy for ovarian cancer prevention. *JAMA Netw Open.* 2022;5(2):e2147343. doi:10.1001/jamanetworkopen.2021.47343

56. Lin HW, Tu YY, Lin SY, et al. Risk of ovarian cancer in women with pelvic inflammatory disease: a population-based study. *Lancet Oncol.* 2011;12(9):900-904. doi:10.1016/S1470-2045(11)70165-6

57. Zhou Z, Zeng F, Yuan J, et al. Pelvic inflammatory disease and the risk of ovarian cancer: a meta-analysis. *Cancer Causes Control.* 2017;28(5):415-428. doi:10.1007/s10552-017-0873-3

58. Rasmussen CB, Kjaer SK, Albieri V, et al. Pelvic inflammatory disease and the risk of ovarian cancer and borderline ovarian tumors: a pooled analysis of 13 case-control studies. *Am J Epidemiol.* 2017;185(1):8-20. doi:10.1093/aje/kww161

59. Pearce CL, Templeman C, Rossing MA, et al. Association between endometriosis and risk of histological subtypes of ovarian cancer: a pooled analysis of case-control studies. *Lancet Oncol.* 2012;13(4):385-394. doi:10.1016/S1470-2045(11)70404-1

60. Kim HS, Kim TH, Chung HH, Song YS. Risk and prognosis of ovarian cancer in women with endometriosis: a meta-analysis. *Br J Cancer.* 2014;110(7):1878-1890. doi:10.1038/bjc.2014.29

61. Vercellini P, Somigliana E, Buggio L, Bolis G, Fedele L. Endometriosis and ovarian cancer. *Lancet Oncol.* 2012;13(5):e188-e189. doi:10.1016/S1470-2045(12)70198-5

62. Wiegand KC, Shah SP, Al-Agha OM, et al. ARID1A mutations in endometriosis-associated ovarian carcinomas. *N Engl J Med.* 2010;363(16):1532-1543. doi:10.1056/NEJMoa1008433

63. Banz C, Ungethuem U, Kuban RJ, Diedrich K, Lengyel E, Hornung D. The molecular signature of endometriosis-associated endometrioid ovarian cancer differs significantly from endometriosis-independent endometrioid ovarian cancer. *Fertil Steril.* 2010;94(4):1212-1217. doi:10.1016/j.fertnstert.2009.06.039

64. Anglesio MS, Papadopoulos N, Ayhan A, et al. Cancer-associated mutations in endometriosis without cancer. *N Engl J Med.* 2017;376(19):1835-1848. doi:10.1056/NEJMoa1614814

65. Chang ET, Lee VS, Canchola AJ, et al. Dietary patterns and risk of ovarian cancer in the California teachers study cohort. *Nutr Cancer.* 2008;60(3):285-291. doi:10.1080/01635580701733091

66. Chang ET, Lee VS, Canchola AJ, et al. Diet and risk of ovarian cancer in the California teachers study cohort. *Am J Epidemiol.* 2007;165(7):802-813. doi:10.1093/aje/kwk065

67. Sun H, Gong TT, Xia Y, et al. Diet and ovarian cancer risk: an umbrella review of systematic reviews and meta-analyses of cohort studies. *Clin Nutr Edinb Scotl.* 2021;40(4):1682-1690. doi:10.1016/j.clnu.2020.11.032

68. Prentice RL, Thomson CA, Caan B, et al. Low-fat dietary pattern and cancer incidence in the women's health initiative dietary modification randomized controlled trial. *J Natl Cancer Inst.* 2007;99(20):1534-1543. doi:10.1093/jnci/djm159

69. Khodavandi A, Alizadeh F, Razis AFA. Association between dietary intake and risk of ovarian cancer: a systematic review and meta-analysis. *Eur J Nutr.* 2021;60(4):1707-1736. doi:10.1007/s00394-020-02332-y

70. Michels N, Specht IO, Heitmann BL, Chajès V, Huybrechts I. Dietary trans-fatty acid intake in relation to cancer risk: a systematic review and meta-analysis. *Nutr Rev.* 2021;79(7):758-776. doi:10.1093/nutrit/nuaa061

71. Koushik A, Hunter DJ, Spiegelman D, et al. Fruits and vegetables and ovarian cancer risk in a pooled analysis of 12 cohort studies. *Cancer Epidemiol Biomarkers Prev.* 2005;14(9):2160-2167. doi:10.1158/1055-9965.EPI-05-0218

72. Wang K, Zhang Q, Yang J. The effect of folate intake on ovarian cancer risk: a meta-analysis of observational studies. *Medicine (Baltimore).* 2021;100(3):e22605. doi:10.1097/MD.0000000000022605

73. Caprio GG, Picascia D, Dallio M, et al. Light alcohol drinking and the risk of cancer development: a controversial relationship. *Rev Recent Clin Trials.* 2020;15(3):164-177. doi:10.2174/1574887115666200628143015

74. Salari-Moghaddam A, Milajerdi A, Surkan PJ, Larijani B, Esmaillzadeh A. Caffeine, type of coffee, and risk of ovarian cancer: a dose-response meta-analysis of prospective studies. *J Clin Endocrinol Metab.* 2019;104(11):5349-5359. doi:10.1210/jc.2019-00637

75. Shafiei F, Salari-Moghaddam A, Milajerdi A, Larijani B, Esmaillzadeh A. Coffee and caffeine intake and risk of ovarian cancer: a systematic review and meta-analysis. *Int J Gynecol Cancer.* 2019;29(3):579-584. doi:10.1136/ijgc-2018-000102

76. Tworoger SS, Gertig DM, Gates MA, Hecht JL, Hankinson SE. Caffeine, alcohol, smoking, and the risk of incident epithelial ovarian cancer. *Cancer.* 2008;112(5):1169-1177. doi:10.1002/cncr.23275

77. Soegaard M, Jensen A, Høgdall E, et al. Different risk factor profiles for mucinous and nonmucinous ovarian cancer: results from the Danish MALOVA study. *Cancer Epidemiol Biomarkers Prev.* 2007;16(6):1160-1166. doi:10.1158/1055-9965.EPI-07-0089

78. Cannioto RA, LaMonte MJ, Kelemen LE, et al. Recreational physical inactivity and mortality in women with invasive epithelial ovarian cancer: evidence from the ovarian cancer association consortium. *Br J Cancer.* 2016;115(1):95-101. doi:10.1038/bjc.2016.153

79. Hildebrand JS, Gapstur SM, Gaudet MM, Campbell PT, Patel AV. Moderate-to-vigorous physical activity and leisure-time sitting in relation to ovarian cancer risk in a large prospective US cohort. *Cancer Causes Control.* 2015;26(11):1691-1697. doi:10.1007/s10552-015-0656-7

80. Biller VS, Leitzmann MF, Sedlmeier AM, Berger FF, Ortmann O, Jochem C. Sedentary behaviour in relation to ovarian cancer risk: a systematic review and meta-analysis. *Eur J Epidemiol.* 2021;36(8):769-780. doi:10.1007/s10654-020-00712-6

81. Moorman PG, Jones LW, Akushevich L, Schildkraut JM. Recreational physical activity and ovarian cancer risk and survival. *Ann Epidemiol.* 2011;21(3):178-187. doi:10.1016/j.annepidem.2010.10.014

82. Minlikeeva AN, Cannioto R, Jensen A, et al. Joint exposure to smoking, excessive weight, and physical inactivity and survival of ovarian cancer patients, evidence from the ovarian cancer association consortium. *Cancer Causes Control.* 2019;30(5):537-547. doi:10.1007/s10552-019-01157-3

CHAPTER **8.2**

Hereditary Ovarian Cancer: BRCA and HNPCC—Panel Testing

Shannon Dawn Armbruster and Ernst Lengyel

The study of familial breast cancer and OC began in 1866 when the French physician and pathologist Paul Broca noted a much larger-than-expected incidence of cancer in his wife's family. Over four generations, 10 out of the 24 women in her family died from breast cancer, whereas several more individuals of both sexes developed other malignancies. He concluded that this excess of cancers could not reasonably be attributed to chance (1). We now estimate that approximately 18% of invasive EOCs are the result of autosomal dominant genetic factors with high disease penetrance, predominantly germline mutations in the *BRCA1* or *BRCA2* genes (65%-85%), in mismatch repair (*MMR*) genes (10%-15%) (2,3) or in genes linked to Lynch syndrome (*MLH1, MSH2, MSH6, PMS2*) (4). As of this writing (July 2022), at least 12 suspected hereditary OC genes have been identified (**Table 8.2-1**). These hereditary mutations are the strongest known risk factors for the development of OC. They may also provide targets for therapy, as is the case with *BRCA1/2* mutations and PARP inhibitors (PARPi) or mismatch repair deficiencies (MMRd) and immunotherapy.

BIOLOGY OF BRCA-ASSOCIATED OVARIAN CANCER

The *BRCA* genes are inherited in an autosomal dominant manner, which means that every first-degree relative of a mutation carrier has a 50% chance of carrying a mutation (**Figure 8.2-1**). The *BRCA* genes function as classic tumor suppressors, with loss of function of both alleles required for cancer formation. Those impacted are initially heterozygous for the *BRCA* gene mutation(s) in all cells and then the sporadic loss of wild-type allele in epithelial breast or fallopian/ovarian cells results in a predisposition to cancer.

The two BRCA proteins regulate cell cycle checkpoints and gene expression. Their most important function is participation in a specific DNA repair pathway, homologous recombination, which is used for the high-fidelity repair of double-strand DNA breaks. Because cells with *BRCA1/2* mutations lack the ability to repair double-strand breaks, they have increased genomic instability and a predisposition to malignant transformation. The ability of cells with *BRCA* mutations to repair DNA cross-links induced by platinum salts is impaired, which is hypothesized to explain the increased platinum sensitivity of patients with *BRCA* mutations (see later in this chapter). Another pathway important in the biology of OC is the Fanconi anemia pathway. The *PALB2* gene, which is part of this pathway, binds *BRCA1/2* at sites of DNA damage.

The prevalence of *BRCA1* or *BRCA2* mutations (over 1,000 have been identified) in the general population is about 1:300 to 1:800. However, specific ethnic populations founded by small ancestral groups, such as French Canadians, Icelanders, Hispanics, and Ashkenazi Jews, have a higher mutation rate arising from spontaneous "founder mutations." For example, 2% to 3% of all Jewish women of Eastern European descent have one of three founder mutations (two in *BRCA1* 187delAG and 5382insC; one in *BRCA2* 6174 delT). The cumulative lifetime risk of developing OC for women with a pathogenic variant *BRCA1* mutation has been estimated at 39% to 46% and for women with a *BRCA2* mutation at 10% to 27%. The largest study reviewing the care of women with BRCA mutations found that the OC cumulative risk to age 80 years was 44% for BRCA1 (95% CI, 36%-53%) and 17% for BRCA2 (95% CI, 11%-25%) carriers. In the same study, the cumulative risk of developing breast cancer by age 80 was 72% for BRCA1 mutation carriers and 69% for BRCA2 mutation carriers (5).

▪ TABLE 8.2-1. Multiplex Testing of Hereditary Ovarian Cancer

	Gene Name	Penetrance	Relative Risk
Mismatch repair/Lynch-HNPCC	*MLH1, MSH2* *MSH6* *PMS2* *EPCAM*		High Low No elevated risk
Tumor suppressor	*TP53, PTEN*		
Double-strand DNA break repair genes	*BRCA1, BRCA2* *ATM, CHEK2, NBN*	High Low	>4 <1.5
Fanconi anemia pathway	*BRIP1* *RAD51C* *RAD51D* *PALB2* *BARD1* *MRE11A, RAD50,* *FANCP*	Moderate Moderate Moderate Low	2.6-11 <3.4-14.6 4.8-12
	STK11/LKB1		

Currently, there are 12 genes (*italicized*) associated with hereditary breast/ovarian cancer syndromes. The role of risk-reducing surgery in individuals with mutations in moderate-penetrance genes is less clear. The risk of ovarian cancer may be higher in patients with a family history of ovarian cancer.

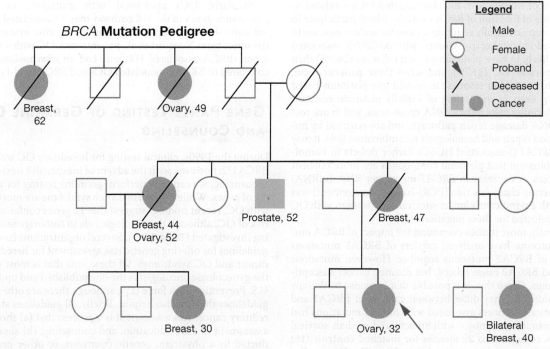

Figure 8.2-1. Family pedigree illustrating BRCA mutation.

In comparison, the lifetime risk for OC for women in the general population is 1.3% (5,6). Some mutations may be more specifically related to OC risk than others. OC cluster regions have been identified within the *BRCA1* gene from c.1380 to c.4062 (within exon 11) and within the *BRCA2* gene from c.3249 to c.5681 (near c.5946 dekT) and from c.6645 to c.7471, which carry a higher risk of OC than breast cancer. The wide variation in penetrance observed may also reflect the interaction of the genetic mutation with other genetic and/or environmental factors and suggests that these genes may function as "gatekeepers" and, when lost, allow other genetic alterations to accumulate. Of note, borderline tumors are not associated with *BRCA1/2* mutations. The age of a *BRCA1/2* mutation carrier, however, is very relevant to the absolute risk of OC or breast cancer. The older an individual becomes without developing either cancer, the lower the risk (7). There are several online tools for calculating the probability of a *BRCA1/2* mutation and cancer risk, regardless of gene status. One is the Breast and Ovarian Analysis of Disease Incidence and Carrier Estimation Algorithm (BOADICEA [CanRisk]: https://www.canrisk.org/), which is used to calculate the risk of breast cancer and OC (8). It takes into consideration family history of breast cancer, OC and other cancers, a history of oophorectomy, weight, and mammographic breast density. The pretest counseling of women interested in germline testing should include a pedigree evaluation, use of one of the mathematical models, a summary of genetic testing recommendations, a discussion of the implications of genetic testing including outcomes and how it could affect relatives, and, finally, financial considerations of genetic testing. The general studies have shown that genetic testing does not lead to psychological dysfunction, but a few patients respond to severe anxiety when offered multigene panel testing.

CLINICAL FEATURES OF *BRCA*-ASSOCIATED OVARIAN CANCER

In general, people with *BRCA* mutation who develop OC do so at a younger age are more likely to have cancers of high-grade serous histology originating in the fallopian tube, are less likely to have borderline or mucinous tumors, and have, in the short term, a better prognosis than matched controls with sporadic OC (2,9). A breast cancer precedes the OC diagnosis in 37% of *BRCA1*-associated cases and 37% of *BRCA2*-associated cases (10).

While most series have found that *BRCA*-associated cancers are usually of high-grade serous histology, one review suggested that *BRCA1*- and *BRCA2*-associated tumors are similar in histology and grade to sporadic cancers. In one study of 1,119 *BRCA1/2*-associated OCs (10), the subtypes associated with these mutations included 67% serous, 12% endometrioid, 2% clear cell, and 1% mucinous cancers. Similarly, Norquist et al found BRCA mutations in 240 (16.0%) of 1,498 HGSCs, 7 (10.9%) of 64 high-grade endometrioid cancers, 4 (6.9%) of 58 clear cell cancers, and 4 (5.7%) of 70 LGSCs; no BRCA mutations were identified in those with low-grade endometrioid cancers or mucinous tumors (3). In another series of *BRCA*-associated OCs with centralized pathology review, cancers in *BRCA* carriers were compared to those in noncarriers (11). Mutation-associated tumors were of significantly higher grade and stage and less often mucinous than non–mutation-associated tumors. No mucinous and no borderline tumors were found in the mutation-associated group. Primary peritoneal carcinoma occurred rarely in both groups. In a large cohort of patients with serous cancer, 44% of all the mutations identified occurred in the absence of a family history (2). Another study that included 1,342 patients diagnosed with EOC from the province of Ontario reported a *BRCA1/2* mutation frequency of 13.4% (12). This study used multiplex ligation-dependent probe amplification and, therefore, detected the large deletions that normally elude general sequencing. In this study, women with OC in their fourth life decade had the highest mutation rate (24%), as did women of Italian (43%), Jewish (30%), or Indo-Pakistani (29%) origin. Importantly, 8% of the mutation carriers detected by the screening had no first-degree relative with OC or breast cancer. Among Ashkenazi Jewish women with OC, there is an estimated 29% to 40% chance that the disease is related to a *BRCA1* or *BRCA2* mutation (13). Therefore, genetic testing solely based on family history alone can no longer be recommended.

OC in a *BRCA1/2* mutation carrier has specific clinical characteristics when compared to sporadic OC. Interestingly, in this series, tumors associated with mutations in BRCA1 or BRCA2 also had improved outcomes compared to patients with silencing of BRCA1 due to methylation of the BRCA1 promoter, suggesting that the mechanism of loss of BRCA function may be relevant to the biology and clinical behavior of these tumors. It is probable that the improved

5-year survival of women with *BRCA*-associated OCs is related to the fact that loss of function of *BRCA* proteins, which participate in DNA damage repair, initially results in a more favorable response to platinum-based chemotherapy. Women with *BRCA1/2*-associated OCs are less likely to have platinum-resistant disease (14.9%) than those with sporadic OC (31.7%), and when these patients recur, they tend to have a higher response to second-line platinum-based chemotherapy, even in the setting of initially platinum-resistant disease (2). Platinum salts induce DNA cross-links, which are recognized by DNA damage repair pathways, and are repaired by nucleotide excision repair and homologous recombination (14). It may be because *BRCA1/2*-associated HGSCs harbor defects in homologous recombination that platinum compounds are more efficient in these cancers. A decrease in *BRCA1* messenger RNA (mRNA) levels (polymerase chain reaction [PCR]-based measurement) was associated with a significantly longer survival in 57 women with OC who were unselected for these mutations (15).

Until recently, most studies examining the impact of BRCA mutations on outcome have analyzed carriers of BRCA1 mutations and carriers of BRCA2 mutations together. However, mutations in BRCA1 and BRCA2 cause related, but distinct, cancer susceptibility syndromes. Given this, it is possible that response to therapy and clinical outcome may differ between carriers of BRCA1 and BRCA2 mutations. Cancers associated with *BRCA1* mutations had a relatively favorable prognosis, with an actuarial median survival of 77 months compared to 29 months for matched controls (16) (**Figure 8.2-2**). Yang et al reexamined data from The Cancer Genome Atlas (TCGA) ovarian project. In this report, patients with BRCA2-associated OC had markedly better outcome than those with BRCA wild-type tumors (HR = 0.33; 95% CI, 0.16-0.69) (17). BRCA1-associated tumors also appeared to have a somewhat better outcome than BRCA wild-type tumors (HR = 0.76; 95% CI, 0.43-1.35), but this result did not reach statistical significance. Bolton et al reported on a pooled series of 3,879 invasive EOCs genotyped for BRCA mutations and found that in a model adjusted for age at diagnosis, stage, grade, and histology, both BRCA2 (HR = 0.49; 95% CI, 0.39-0.61) and BRCA1 (HR = 0.73; 95% CI, 0.64-0.84) had improved outcome compared to BRCA wild-type tumors (18). Tests of heterogeneity also demonstrated that HR for BRCA2 mutation carriers was significantly different from that for BRCA1 mutation carriers. However, larger studies have shown that although *BRCA1*-related cancers have a better initial prognosis, this advantage decreases over time and eventually reverses at 8 years (3,16). The 5- and 10-year survival rate is 42/30% for noncarriers, 45/25% for *BRCA1* mutation carriers, and 54/35% for *BRCA2* carriers. These data may evolve as OS data become available for PARPi.

Similarly, OCs associated with mutations in moderate-penetrance genes in the HR pathway may be associated with different natural history depending upon the specific mutated gene. In the series from Norquist et al., patients with OC with a mutation in a non–BRCA-associated HR gene had an intermediate prognosis compared to BRCA2-associated OCs and BRCA wild-type OCs (3).

GENE PANEL TESTING OF GERMLINE DNA AND COUNSELING

During the 1990s, clinical testing for hereditary OC was limited to BRCA1/2; however, with the advent of inexpensive next-generation sequencing, we can now perform germline testing for a wide variety of genes. While BRCA and Lynch syndrome are most associated with OC, recent findings suggest that 12 genes confer an increased risk of OC, although their biologic role in tumorigenesis is still being investigated (**Table 8.2-1**). Several organizations have proposed guidelines for offering genetic risk assessment for hereditary breast cancer and OC syndromes. Of these, one that is most relevant for the gynecologic oncologist is the one published and updated by the U.S. Preventive Task force (19), although there are other consensus guidelines that are also helpful. Briefly, all guidelines state that hereditary cancer risk assessment is a process that (a) should include assessment of risk, education, and counseling; (b) should be conducted by a physician, genetic counselor, or other provider with experience in cancer genetics; and (c) may include genetic testing after appropriate counseling and consent is obtained.

Specifically, the American College of Obstetrics and Gynecology (ACOG) states that it is reasonable to offer genetic risk assessment to any woman who has greater than a 5% to 10% chance of having a BRCA1 or BRCA2 mutation. Specific constellations of personal and family history that meet this threshold are outlined in **Table 8.2-2**. Given that 16% to 18% of HGSOCs and fallopian tube cancers (including 8%-10% of patients with no significant family history) and a significant proportion of other high-grade EOC and fallopian tube cancers segregate a BRCA1 or BRCA2 mutation, the Society of Gynecologic Oncology (SGO) and other consensus guidelines recommend genetic risk assessment and testing for BRCA1 and BRCA2 mutations in all women with high-grade EOC, irrespective of age of diagnosis or family history. There are also several brief risk prediction models, such as BRCAPRO, BOADICEA, and IBIS, that can assist in predicting the likelihood of a patient having a mutation in BRCA1 or BRCA2 (19). Each of these models, however, has unique advantages and limitations, and selecting the appropriate model is generally best done with the assistance of a genetics professional.

Based on three pivotal studies, most laboratories perform multiplex testing (3,4,20). While the specific panels used may vary slightly, most commercial and academic panels include whole-exome sequencing for gene variation detection and whole transcriptome sequencing for RNA characterization. In a cohort of 1,915 patients with OC identified from GOG clinical study protocols 218 & 262 and the Washington University gynecologic tissue bank (3), 18% were found to have a pathogenic germline mutation. Approximately 15% had mutations in *BRCA1* (9.5%) or *BRCA2* (5.1%), whereas 3% had mutations in the Fanconi anemia pathway. *BRIP1*, a Fanconi anemia pathway gene, is the third most frequent germline mutation in patients with OC (0.9%-1.6%), conferring an RR of OC of about 3.4 (lifetime risk 5.8%). While *PALB2* increases breast cancer risk, its contribution to OC risk is limited, with a RR ratio of 2.9; the cumulative risk ratio is 4.8%, which was modulated by a significant family history of OC (21). Of note, for patients with a *CHEK2* mutation, there is no established OC risk, and its detection does not justify a risk-reducing salpingo-oophorectomy (RRSO). DNA *MMR* genes indicating Lynch syndrome were altered in 0.4% of cases (3). Current consensus guideline recommendations include an RRSO for all BRCA1/2, BRIP1, RAD51C/D, MLH1, and MSH2 germline mutation carriers. Every mutation predisposes to cancer development at a different age. Given the detrimental effect of an RRSO on well-being, reproduction, and

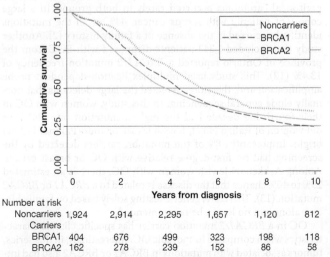

Figure 8.2-2. Kaplan-Meier estimates of cumulative survival according to BRCA1/2 mutation status. Reprinted from Candido-dos-Reis FJ, Song H, Goode EL, et al. Germline mutation in BRCA1 or BRCA2 and ten-year survival for women diagnosed with epithelial ovarian cancer. *Clin Cancer Res.* 2015;21:652-657, with permission from AACR

Number at risk					
Noncarriers	1,924	2,914	2,295	1,657	1,120	812
Carriers						
BRCA1	404	676	499	323	198	118
BRCA2	162	278	239	152	86	58

Patients with one or more of the following have an increased chance of having an inherited predisposition to breast, ovarian, tubal, or peritoneal cancer, and genetic counseling and testing may be offered:

- Epithelial ovarian, tubal, or peritoneal cancer
- Breast cancer at age 45 or younger
- Breast cancer AND close relative[a] with breast cancer at age 50 or younger
- Breast cancer AND close relative[a] with ovarian, tubal, or peritoneal cancer
- Breast cancer at age 50 or younger with limited family history
- Breast cancer AND 2 or more close relatives[a] with breast cancer (any age)
- Breast cancer AND 2 or more close relatives[a] with pancreatic or aggressive prostate cancer
- Two breast cancer primaries, one diagnosed before age 50
- Triple-negative breast cancer diagnosed at age 60 or younger
- Breast cancer and Ashkenazi Jewish ancestry
- Pancreatic cancer and two or more close relatives[a] with breast, ovarian, tubal, peritoneal, pancreatic, or aggressive prostate cancer

Patients without cancer, but with one or more of the following, have an increased chance of having an inherited predisposition to breast, ovarian, tubal, or peritoneal cancer, and genetic counseling and testing may be offered:

- First-degree or several close relatives[a] that meet the above criteria
- Close relative[a] with known BRCA1 or BRCA2 mutation, or other actionable mutations associated with hereditary breast and ovarian cancer syndrome
- Close relative[a] with male breast cancer

ACOG, American College of Obstetricians and Gynecologists.

[a]Close relative is first, second, or third degree.

Adapted from ACOG Practice Bulletin No 182: Hereditary Breast and Ovarian Cancer Syndrome. *Obstet Gynecol.* 2017.

health, recommendations have been developed for each specific gene (**Figure 8.2-3**—threshold) (22). In view of the rapid pace of changes in our understanding of the cancer risks associated with these genes, it is recommended that patients with germline mutations associated with breast cancer/OC have an ongoing discussion with experienced provider, to determine if changes in management are warranted (**Figure 8.2-4**).

If patients are selected based solely on clinical criteria (young age, family history, and serous tumor type) for germline testing, a

significant proportion of patients with mutations would have been missed. It is estimated that about one-third of patients found to have a non-*BRCA1/2* mutation will experience a change in clinical management (eg, RRSO, colorectal screening, additional family testing) (4). However, some controversy over the use of panel testing remains. It should be realized that we do not understand the significance of germline variants, including copy number variations or mosaicism, for most of the genes in **Table 2.8-1**, and at this point, the presence of variants not clearly associated with increased risk should not guide medical decision-making, especially not such an invasive procedure as an RRSO.

All patients with a diagnosis of invasive EOC should be offered genetic counseling and germline testing. The identification of a *BRCA* mutation or defect in the homologous recombination pathway can impact their treatment, because it could indicate an increased sensitivity to PARPi as well as to platinum compounds both in the first- and second-line settings (2). While the upfront treatment (carboplatin/paclitaxel) for *BRCA* mutation–associated OCs is currently the same as treatment for sporadic OCs, the use of PARPi following first-line platinum-based not only shows a durable PFS benefit for patients with BRCA mutations (23) but also has benefit for patients with HRD when combined with bevacizumab (24). Thus, if germline testing does not identify a mutation, somatic testing should be completed as these results can impact treatment options. Women diagnosed with clear cell, endometrioid, or mucinous OC should be offered somatic tumor testing for *MMR* genes. Somatic testing of the tumor can identify other targets beyond BRCA1/2 targets that are useful for subsequent lines of therapy, such as immunotherapy for MMRd, microsatellite instability-high (MSI-high), or patients with high tumor mutational burden. In a population-based study in Georgia and California, including 6,001 patients with OC, somatic testing of the tumor tissue yielded pathogenic variants in BRCA1 (8.7%), BRCA2 (5.8%), BRIP1 (0.92%), MSH2 (0.8%), and RAD51C (0.58%) (25).

Aside from the treatment implication, germline genetic testing can impact a patient's family members. The unaffected first-degree female relatives of *BRCA* mutation carriers have a 50% probability of carrying the same mutation and can be specifically tested for it. Those first-degree relatives who are found to be *BRCA* negative can be informed that they are not at a significantly greater risk of developing OC than the general population, whereas those who carry the mutation can be counseled on risk-reducing strategies. Given that an RRSO reduces the risk of developing OC and fallopian tube cancer by about 80%, it is clinically meaningful to be aware that a woman carries a *BRCA* mutation. Negative findings in multigene testing may reassure relatives that they are not at increased risk for OC despite a family history and thereby provide useful clinical information that will assist with her care and inform screening recommendations.

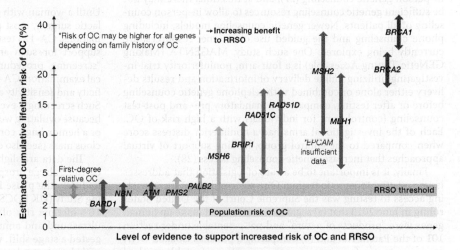

Figure 8.2-3. Clinical guide for RRSO for ovarian cancer (OC) by cancer susceptibility genes. RRSO, risk-reducing salpingo-oophorectomy. (From Liu YL, Breen K, Catchings A, et al. Risk-reducing bilateral salpingo-oophorectomy for ovarian cancer: a review and clinical guide for hereditary predisposition genes. *JCO Oncol Pract.* 2022;18(3):201-209.)

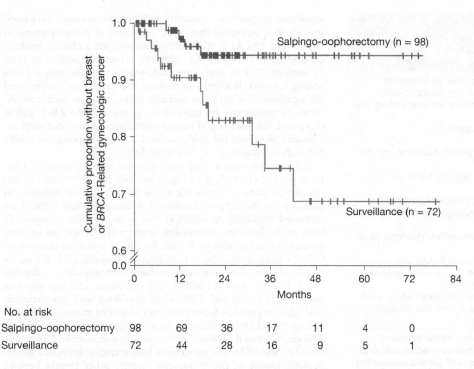

Figure 8.2-4. Kaplan-Meier estimates of the time to breast cancer or BRCA-related gynecologic cancer among women electing risk-reducing salpingo-oophorectomy and women electing surveillance for ovarian cancer. $P = .006$ by the log-rank test for the comparison between the actuarial mean times to cancer. A Cox proportional hazards model for multiple end points, which took into account the different proportions of women in the two groups who had breast tissue at risk, yielded a hazard ratio for subsequent breast cancer or BRCA-related gynecologic cancer after risk-reducing salpingo-oophorectomy of 0.25 (95% confidence interval, 0.08-0.74).

We believe genetic testing should, therefore, be routinely offered to all women with high-grade EOC, regardless of family history, which is in alignment with guidelines from the American Society of Clinical Oncology (ASCO) and other consensus guidelines (26). It is important that clinical decisions are not made based on variants of uncertain significance (VUS). The ClinVar database has up-to-date information on the pathogenicity of mutations (https://www.ncbi.nlm.nih.gov/clinvar/). An alternative reliable database is the Clinical Genome Resource: https://www.clinicalgenome.org/. Progressively, circulating tumor DNA (ctDNA) assays are used with may identify both somatic and germline mutations.

Considerable expertise and time are needed to counsel women at risk for hereditary cancer. A genetic counselor or physician with expertise in treating hereditary cancers in women can provide the patient not only appropriate medical information but also skilled consideration for her concerns and emotional support. BRCA- and Lynch syndrome–directed genetic counseling is important for the effective assessment of risk for the patient and her family and for decision-making regarding preventive strategies and therapies. However, most women who undergo genetic testing do not receive in-person genetic counseling (27), and at this time, there may not be sufficient genetic counseling resources to allow in-person counseling of all patients. Newer genetic counseling models, including phone counseling and the guided use of internet resources, are currently being explored. One such study, MAGENTA (Making GENetic Testing Accessible) is a four-arm, noninferiority trial investigating utilizing online delivery of information and results delivery either alone or combined with telephone genetic counseling before or after testing, compared to mandatory pre- and post-test counseling (control arm) for individuals with a high risk of OC. Each of the investigational arms had a noninferior distress score when compared to the control group, lending support of virtual approaches that increase genetic counseling access (28).

Finally, it is important to be aware of legislation that addresses issues relating to genetic testing. One piece of legislation impacting access to testing was the Supreme Court of the United States ruling in June 2013 that (a) segments of DNA that make up human genes were "products of nature" and not patentable under section 101 of the Patent Act and (b) comparing a patient's isolated DNA sequence to a reference sequence was not a patentable method (29). Currently, there is little standardization with respect to how individual labs ensure analytic and clinical validity of sequencing

results. This creates difficulties for providers in choosing labs and interpreting results. In addition, the prospect of increasingly comprehensive genetic information on each patient has the potential to create discrimination and privacy issues. The 2008 Genetic Information Nondiscrimination Act (GINA) prohibits health insurers and employers from discriminating based on genetic information (30). Rules governing patient privacy and confidentiality prevent a physician from disclosing genetic test results to a relative without permission from the patient. The ASCO guidelines suggest that the ethical duty to warn a relative of genetic risk is satisfied if the doctor explains to the patient that a hereditary cancer syndrome has implications for other family members, advises the patient to share information with them, and offers genetic counseling for those family members who are interested and at risk.

FOLLOW-UP OF BRCA1/2-POSITIVE PATIENTS WHO DO NOT WANT TO UNDERGO RISK-REDUCING SALPINGO-OOPHORECTOMY

Until a woman with a BRCA1/2 mutation chooses to have prophylactic surgery, most practitioners will follow her with pelvic examinations, CA-125 testing, and pelvic ultrasound, albeit the scientific support for such an approach is weak. The current often-used "screening" procedures of the general population for OC using clinical examination, CA-125, and pelvic ultrasound have very low specificity and sensitivity and cannot detect OC at a curable stage (31,32). Such screening is even less efficient in young premenopausal women because ovulating women may have functional cysts, endometriosis, or a hemorrhagic corpus luteum, which can be mistaken for a suspicious mass (see also differential diagnosis of adnexal mass).

The data are slightly more encouraging for BRCA1/2 mutation carrier. A large prospective trial targeting women at familial/inherited risk, the phase I of the U.K. Familial Ovarian Cancer Screening Study (UK FOCSS), including 3,563 women with a greater than 10% lifetime risk of OC, were followed with annual transvaginal ultrasound and annual CA-125 blood tests (33). The results suggested a stage shift, with only 6 (26%) of 23 cancers not associated with Lynch syndrome in women screened according to protocol diagnosed at stage IIIc or higher. This contrasted with six (86%) of seven cancers being of advanced stage in women with delayed screening. This research group has now completed phase II of the study, in which participants ($n = 4,348$) were followed with annual transvaginal ultrasound and every 4-month CA-125 determinations, interpreted by the risk of ovarian cancer algorithm (ROCA) algorithm (33). Within 1-year screening, 19 patients were diagnosed with OC or fallopian tube cancer, 13 of which were screen detected and six were symptomatic. Five (38.5%) of the 13 screening-detected cancers were stages I to II (CI, 13.9%-68.4%), compared to five (83.3%) of the six occult cancers that were stages I to II (CI, 35.9%-99.6%). The model sensitivity was 94.7% (95% CI: 74%, 99.9%), positive predictive value (PPV) was 10.8% (95% CI: 6.5%, 16.5%), and negative predictive value was 100% (95% CI: 100%, 100%). Cancers diagnosed less than 1 year from screening were more likely to be stages I to II, compared to those diagnosed more than a year after screening (36.8% vs 94.4%). Given the shift in stage at diagnosis, ROCA-based screening is an option for individuals who defer or decline RRSO, but compliance with an every 3 months ultrasound and biomarker follow-up model is low and the survival implications of this strategy remain unknown (34).

Patients should have regular breast examinations as well as annual breast magnetic resonance imaging (MRI). Prophylactic bilateral mastectomy should also be discussed with BRCA mutation carriers, and patients should be informed of the techniques available for removing and reconstructing the breast and of the expected psychosocial and sexual effects.

Most studies have shown that the reproductive and hormonal factors that affect OC risk in the general population also affect risk for women who carry BRCA1 and BRCA2 mutations. The use of OCPs reduced the risk of OC in women with BRCA1 (OR, 0.56) and BRCA2 mutations (OR, 0.39). The six studies that addressed this question were analyzed together in a meta-analysis (35), showing that the OR for developing OC was 0.65 (CI, 0.47-0.66) in BRCA1 mutation carriers using OCPs, 0.65 (CI 0.34-1.24) for BRCA2 mutation carriers, and 0.58 (0.46-0.73) for the combined BRCA1/2 group. In summary, OCP use is inversely associated with OC risk, whereas a modest but not statistically significant increased risk was observed for breast cancer. The International BRCA1/2 Carrier Cohort Study confirmed an inverse relationship between OCP use and OC risk (36). The duration of use was the most important protective factor, and the reduction with a longer duration of use was present more than 15 years after stopping OCPs. There is a significantly reduced risk of OC associated with the use of levonorgestrel-releasing IUD and contraceptive injections (DMPA), which is comparable in magnitude to OCP use (37).

Breastfeeding is associated with a reduction in OC risk in both women without (38) and with a BRCA1/2 mutation (40) by 24% and 23%, respectively. The benefit increases with the duration of breastfeeding and a history of OCP use. In BRCA1/2 mutation carriers, parity and tubal ligation were not significant protective factors (39).

PROPHYLACTIC RISK-REDUCING SALPINGO-OOPHORECTOMY FOR PREVENTION OF *BRCA*-ASSOCIATED OVARIAN CANCER

Indications for Surgery for BRCA1/2 Mutations

Counseling about RRSO should balance the risks and symptoms associated with surgical menopause with the morbidity and high mortality of advanced serous OC and the low sensitivity and specificity of current screening methods for OC in carriers of cancer susceptibility genes like *BRCA1/2*. In contrast, the evidence does strongly support the efficacy of RRSO for prevention in unaffected women (**Table 8.2-3**). In 2002, two large prospective series clearly demonstrated that RRSO reduced the risk of developing Müllerian carcinoma (OC, fallopian tube, and peritoneal cancer) in patients with *BRCA1/2* mutations (40,41). In addition, three large prospective studies showed that the RRSO group had significantly fewer *BRCA*-related gynecologic and breast cancers than the surveillance group (7,40,42).

Another larger prospective study reported the effects of RRSO in *BRCA1* and *BRCA2* germline mutation carriers separately (12). Among 1,079 patients, RRSO reduced OC risk in women with *BRCA1* mutations by 85% and reduced breast cancer risk in women with *BRCA2* mutations by 72%. There was also a 39% reduction in breast cancer risk in women with *BRCA1* mutations and a reduction in OCs in women with *BRCA2* mutations, but these were not statistically significant. The absence of a significant reduction in OC in *BRCA2* mutation carriers may have been partially attributable to the fact that most women with *BRCA2*-associated OC are over 60 years old, whereas the median age of the women in the study was 46 years. In another large study coordinated by the Toronto group, 1,828 known carriers of a *BRCA1* or *BRCA2* mutation were identified from an international registry of 32 centers (43). The overall reduction in risk of Müllerian cancers with RRSO was 80%; the estimated cumulative incidence of peritoneal cancer at 20 years after RRSO was 4.3%, with most cases occurring less than 5 years after RRSO.

Given the strong evidence that RRSO reduces all-cause, breast cancer–specific, and OC–specific mortality, ACOG, SGO, and other consensus guidelines have all recommended prophylactic salpingo-oophorectomy in women with OC syndromes. Because the median age of diagnosis of OC among women with a hereditary risk is 50 years for BRCA1 carriers and 60 years for BRCA2 carriers, the recommended age for prophylactic surgery is at the completion of childbearing, or between age 35 and 40 years for BRCA1 carriers and 40 and 45 years for BRCA2 carriers. Although the incidence of premenopausal OC is higher in BRCA1 carriers than BRCA2

TABLE 8.2-3. Prospective Observational Studies of Risk-Reducing Salpingo-Oophorectomy in Patients With BRCA1/2 Mutations

Author, Journal, Year	Study Period	RRSO	Surveillance	Mean Follow-up (yrs)	Ovarian Cancer RRSO vs No RRSO	Hazard Ratio	Comment	Reference
Kauff, *NEJM*, 2002	1995-2001	98	72	2.1	1 vs 5	0.15 (0.02-1.31)		Kauff et al (40)
Domcheck, *JAMA*, 2010	1974-2008	465	1,092	3.7	10 vs 98	0.28 (0.12-0.69)	No breast cancer in 247 women with RRM	Domchek et al (42)
Finch, *JCO*, 2014	1995-2011	3513	2,270	5.6	32 vs 108	0.2 (0.13-0.3)	46 women had an occult cancer at RRSO	Finch et al (7)

RRM, risk-reducing mastectomy; RRSO, risk-reducing salpingo-oophorectomy.

carriers, removal of the ovaries before menopause is recommended for both groups. Women with *BRCA2* mutations have a 26% to 34% risk of developing breast cancer by the age of 50, and the evidence suggests that the breast cancer risk reduction conferred by RRSO is greater when the ovaries are removed before natural menopause (3,44). In addition, because there is an approximate 15% risk of OC after age 60 years among BRCA carriers, bilateral salpingo-oophorectomy (BSO) is also justified at older ages for women who still have intact ovaries. RRSO *after* a primary diagnosis of breast cancer significantly reduces breast cancer–specific mortality in *BRCA1* mutation carriers (HR 0.38; CI 0.19-0.77), but not in *BRCA2* carriers, and mostly benefits patients with estrogen receptor (ER)-negative breast cancer (45). The data also suggest that oophorectomy is most beneficial during the first year of treatment.

Surgery: Risk-Reducing Salpingo-Oophorectomy

Because RRSO substantially decreases OC risk by as much as 80%, the benefits of prophylactic surgery clearly outweigh the associated risks (7,42). Prospective follow-up of a large international cohort of 2,482 BRCA carriers found not only a lower risk of OC but also a significantly lower all-cause mortality (HR 0.40; 95% CI, 0.26-0.61) and OC-specific mortality (HR 0.21; 95% CI, 0.06-0.76) (42). The incidence of primary peritoneal cancer following BSO is reported to be approximately 2% to 5% (43). The origin of peritoneal cancers after RRSO is not entirely clear. Some of these may represent recurrence of occult ovarian or tubal malignancies that were not recognized on initial pathologic evaluation, highlighting the need for careful pathologic evaluation of the entire ovary and fallopian tube at the time of RRSO. It has also been speculated that peritoneal cancer can arise from exfoliated tubal cells (endosalpingiosis) that implant on the peritoneum and undergo malignant transformation in that location. Lastly, some have suggested that peritoneal malignancies can arise exclusively in the peritoneum through Müllerian metaplasia. Irrespective of the origin, it is important that patients undergoing RRSO be informed of the small possibility of primary peritoneal cancer occurring after the procedure. It is unclear if an RRSO reduces breast cancer risk. Some studies suggest a reduction by 48% (42,43), whereas a more recent prospective study did not find a statistical difference in breast cancer incidence between BRCA1/2 carriers undergoing surgery or observation (46).

The informed consent discussion for RRSO surgery should include not only information about the general risks of surgery but also information about the likely side effects of surgical menopause. Permission to perform a full staging or debulking procedure if cancer is found should also be obtained. The rate of occult cancer detected with RRSO (which requires an additional surgical procedure) in a population-based study of BRCA1/2 mutation carriers (5,782 patients) undergoing RRSO was 4.2% (7).

While RRSO is now part of standard management for women with BRCA1 and BRCA2 mutations, the role of concomitant hysterectomy is controversial, as it is not clear if women with BRCA mutations are at increased risk of uterine cancer. Shu et al reported the results of a multicenter prospective study in which 1,083 women with deleterious BRCA1 or BRCA2 mutation were followed for a median of 5.1 years after RRSO (47). Eight incident uterine cancers were observed (4.3 expected; O/E = 1.9, P = .09). Stratifying by subtype, the authors found no increased risk of endometrioid endometrial carcinoma or sarcoma. Five serous/serous-like endometrial carcinomas were observed (four BRCA1+; one BRCA2+) 7.2 to 12.9 years after RRSO (BRCA1: 0.18 expected; O/E = 22.2, P < .001; BRCA2: 0.16 expected; O/E = 6.4, P = .15). Using these data, the authors estimated that a BRCA1 mutation carrier undergoing RRSO at age 45 had a 2.6% to 4.7% risk of serous uterine cancer through age 70. More recent observational data have indicated BRCA mutation carriers have an increased risk of endometrial cancer compared to the general population, with the absolute risk by 75 years of age being 3% for endometrial cancer and 1.1% for serous carcinomas (48). Other additional situations merit

consideration of completing a hysterectomy. First, hysterectomies can reduce endometrial cancer risk for patients with Lynch syndrome, as discussed later in this section. Other rationale for a hysterectomy includes uterine pathology (eg, fibroids, incontinence, menorrhagia), to simplify HRT (use of estrogen only), or tamoxifen use as an estrogen antagonist for breast cancer chemoprophylaxis, which increases the risk of endometrial cancer as a uterine estrogen agonist. Less than 10% of patient's undergoing RRSO required a hysterectomy for standard indications (ie, prolapse or fibroids). Therefore, hysterectomy solely to avoid future surgery is not supported.

It is usually possible to perform RRSO laparoscopically as an outpatient procedure. Occasionally, a laparotomy will be necessary due to extensive intra-abdominal/pelvic adhesions. After a thorough surveillance of the entire abdominal cavity, including the upper abdomen, peritoneal washings are performed and abnormal areas biopsied. Washing should be performed at the time of peritoneal entry in all women undergoing RRSO as malignant cells leading to upstaging of disease have been found in peritoneal cytology specimens (49). The ureter is visualized, and the infundibulopelvic vessels are transected about 2 cm superior to the ovary to ensure that the entire ovary has been removed. The tube and the superior branch of the uterine artery are transected very close to the uterine cornea. A frozen section is only prepared if there is a gross abnormality of the ovary or any other suspicious tumor. Random biopsies of the omentum and peritoneum have not been found to lead to improved detection of occult cancers (50). Some patients presenting for RRSO will have had a previous reconstruction of their breast using some variation of a rectus abdominis myocutaneous flap. Because these procedures can lead to umbilical translocation in relation to the aortic bifurcation, higher camera port placement or a single site approach may be required (51). In general, RRSO is associated with a very low risk of operative complications. In a Memorial Sloan-Kettering study, 4 out of 80 RRSOs performed laparoscopically had complications caused by adhesions and trocar injuries, which are known complications associated with operative laparoscopy (40). With improved optical equipment and direct visualization trocars, the current rate may be lower.

Because many experts believe that HGSOC arises in the fallopian tube (52), the option of removing the fallopian tube and leaving the ovary in situ is being debated. Bilateral salpingectomy with ovarian retention (BSOR) and radical fimbriectomy have been proposed as a temporary solution, which will prolong the production of ovarian hormone for BRCA1/2 carriers, thus postponing the onset of premature menopause (53). A population-based, retrospective cohort study of all women in British Columbia involving 25,889 women who underwent opportunistic salpingectomy had significantly fewer serous and epithelial OC (54). Current recommendations support salpingectomy alone for patients with a lifetime risk of OC that is less than 5% (40). A trial studying BSOR with delayed oophorectomy (NCT01907789) is currently underway, but results are not yet available. Thus, given the paucity of evidence, this approach is not standard of care for individuals with a genetic predisposition for OC.

Postoperative Results

Women who have chosen to undergo RRSO generally report a good overall QoL. The operation is often accompanied by a significant decrease in perceived risk and, therefore, a decrease in anxiety (55). Acute surgical menopause, however, can have a significant negative effect on QoL. Menopause affects bone health and can cause a decrease in sexual desire along with vaginal atrophy and dyspareunia, which affect sexual functioning, leading to a further decrease in sexual desire, discomfort, and avoidance of intimacy (56). In addition, patients having an RRSO are at a higher risk for cardiovascular disease (adjusted HR [aHR] 1.82; 95% CI: 1.18-2.79) compared to patients who underwent hysterectomy or salpingectomy, without oophorectomy (57). Many patients also suffer from vasomotor symptoms, such as hot flashes and night sweats, which lead to sleep disturbances. These symptoms can be alleviated, but not eliminated, by HRT (56). It has been reported that *BRAC1/2* mutation carriers who received short-term HRT (~3 years duration) after RRSO preserved the reduction in breast cancer risk offered by the surgery (HR 0.38 vs 0.37) (44). This was confirmed by Eisen et al, who showed that HRT after RRSO is not associated with an increase in breast cancer risk in *BRCA* mutation carriers (58). Still, decision-making regarding menopausal therapies in women with *BRCA* mutations who are at increased risk of breast cancer is challenging because of the theoretical risk that HRT will promote the growth of occult breast tumors. In addition, results from the WHI have influenced women and physicians to avoid the use of cyclic estrogen/progestin HRT. Alternative treatments for vasomotor symptoms, such as venlafaxine and gabapentin, which are less effective than HRT, should be discussed in counseling. None of the "natural" treatments for hot flashes have been shown to be more effective than placebo.

Pathology and Prognosis after Risk-Reducing Salpingo-Oophorectomy Specimens

A family history of OC and/or *BRCA* mutation status should be shared with the pathologist because only one slide form of the isthmus, ampulla, and fimbriae of the fallopian tube and one cross section of the ovary of patients with benign gynecologic disease are normally reviewed (50). In the setting of a known history of genetic predisposition to breast cancer and OC, most pathologists will submit the entirety of the fallopian tubes and ovaries for microscopic examination. The SEE-FIM (Sectioning and Extensively Examining the FIMbriated ends) protocol is now widely used for RRSO specimens, which is further discussed in "Pathology" section. When this method is utilized, serous tubal intraepithelial carcinoma (STIC), a putative precursor to invasive serous carcinoma, is identified in as many as 5% to 8% of specimens obtained at the time of RRSO in women with mutations in BRCA1 or BRCA2 (50). Patients in whom small high-grade invasive serous cancers are found incidentally at RRSO generally receive adjuvant chemotherapy. The role of adjuvant therapy in the management of STIC is less clear. Wethington et al evaluated the clinical outcome of patients found to have STIC at RRSO (59). Of 593 patients in this study, isolated STIC was diagnosed in 12 (2%) patients. Seven patients subsequently underwent hysterectomy and omentectomy, six patients had pelvic node dissections, and five patients had para-aortic node dissections. Apart from positive peritoneal washings in one patient, no invasive or metastatic disease was identified. None of the patients received adjuvant chemotherapy. At a median follow-up of 28 months (range, 16-44 months), no recurrences were identified. The authors concluded that the yield of surgical staging is low in patients with STICs, and short-term clinical outcomes are favorable. A more recent systematic review identified 78 patients with STIC lesions, reporting a rate of primary peritoneal carcinoma of 4.5% (60). A meta-analysis summarized 17 studies including 3,121 women undergoing an RRSO, of whom 115 had an STIC (49). If an STIC is present at the time of RRSO for a pathologic variant of BRCA1/2 mutation, the 5- and 10-year risks of peritoneal carcinomatosis was 10.5% and 27.5%, respectively. For women without an STIC, it was 0.3% and 0.9%, respectively. However, individuals diagnosed with STIC lesions should undergo genetic testing if not completed presurgery, given the 10% chance of BRCA mutation associated with the finding. Given that there is a risk of peritoneal carcinomatosis in patients with STIC, the European Society of Gynaecological Oncology (ESGO) guidelines advise to consider staging surgery in cases of an STIC (61). The role of systemic chemotherapy remains undefined but is not recommended.

Microscopic occult carcinomas have been identified in RRSO specimens in about 2% to 9% of *BRCA* mutation carriers, generally involving the tubal fimbriae. In one prospective series, seven OCs and three tubal carcinomas (and one case in which washings showed malignant cells but no primary cancer was identified) were found among 490 women who underwent RRSO (43). Powell and colleagues report that of 111 consecutive BRCA-positive patients treated at a single institution, 9% had occult neoplasia (50). Suspicious epithelial cells, clearly distinct from mesothelial cells, are occasionally identified in cytology specimens. Colgan et al found malignant cells in 3 of 35 pelvic washings. One microscopic ovarian surface carcinoma and one in situ tubal carcinoma were found; no carcinoma could be identified in the third patient (62). Twenty-two percent of specimens showed endosalpingiosis. Positive cytology specimens only rarely lead to the discovery of early-stage tubal carcinomas, although sometimes, as mentioned, malignant cells are present in washings at RRSO and there is no identifiable carcinoma by histology (43).

BIOLOGY AND CLINICAL FEATURES OF LYNCH SYNDROME–ASSOCIATED OVARIAN CANCERS

EOC is also a component of hereditary nonpolyposis colorectal cancer syndrome (HNPCC), which refers to patients who fulfill the Amsterdam criteria (Table 8.2-4) for Lynch syndrome II. The Amsterdam II criteria are age and family history–based prediction tools that enrich for patients who are likely to have a hereditary origin of their cancer and have a specificity of about 61%. Newer prediction tools such as MMRpredict (63), MMRpro (64), and PREMM5 (65) utilize clinical and germline data to determine the probability of having a germline Lynch–associated gene mutation with population-based specificity of 64%, 85%, and 73%, respectively. Dr Henry Lynch, who gave his name to the syndrome, characterized it as autosomal dominant cancer susceptibility syndrome (66). Most will have Lynch syndrome on germline molecular testing with a germline mutation in one of the *MMR* genes (*MLH1, MSH2, MSH6, PMS2*). Identifying patient with MMRd is important as they could be amenable to targeted therapy with checkpoint inhibitors. In the general population, Lynch syndrome occurs in about 1 in 300 individuals (67), making it the most common inherited cancer predisposition syndrome. Unfortunately, most people are not aware of their risk. In addition to a predisposition to develop colorectal and endometrial cancer, woman with this syndrome have a 10% to 13% lifetime risk for developing OC (27%-71% risk of developing endometrial cancer) (68,69). The mean age of diagnosis for OC in women with Lynch syndrome is 42 to 48 years (70-72), which is substantially lower than the mean age of diagnosis of OC in the general population. In addition, cancers present at an earlier stage, being confined to the pelvis (68). They also have a higher percentage of low-grade tumors than the general population. A series of Lynch-related OC reported a stage breakdown, with endometrioid, clear cell, and mucinous histologies seen in 35%, 28%, and 5% of patients, respectively (71). One study reported that 12% of MMRd OCs are serous (72). In a cohort of women with HNPCC and at least two primary cancers, more than half were initially diagnosed with a gynecologic cancer, which preceded the development of a colorectal cancer. Fourteen percent of these women had synchronous cancers, where a colorectal and a gynecologic cancer were found simultaneously (69). Other cancers associated with Lynch syndrome include cancers of the stomach, small bowel, renal pelvis and ureter, and brain.

■ TABLE 8.2-4. Lynch Syndrome: Amsterdam II Criteria

At least three relatives with a Lynch syndrome–associated cancer (colorectal, endometrial, small bowel, ureter, renal cancer)
One relative should be a first-degree relative
Two successive generations
One should be diagnosed <age 50
Familial adenomatous polyposis should be excluded in colon cancer cases
Pathologic verification of tumors

Lynch syndrome describes patients and families with a germline mutation in *MLH1*, *MSH6*, *PMS2*, or loss of expression of *MSH2* due to deletion of the *EPCAM* gene, all involved in the highly conserved DNA MMR pathway. These group of genes correct base substitutions and insertion/deletion mismatches of base pairings occurring during DNA replication. If the MMR system is dysfunctional, the uncorrected mutation rate accompanying DNA synthesis increases 1,000-fold, leading to widespread genomic instability. Lynch syndrome–related tumors exhibit a lengthening or shortening of DNA repeat sequences, which leads to MSI, caused by an inability to repair DNA replication errors and a marker of hypermutation. Patients with Lynch syndrome have a germline mutation in one allele of an *MMR* gene and then the second allele is inactivated somatically by a random mutation, loss of heterozygosity (LOH), or epigenetic silencing by promoter hypermethylation (*MLH1*), leading of failure repairing the DNA mismatches occurring during normal DNA synthesis. MMRd cancers are highly immunogenic because of the production of numerous neoantigens due to their hypermutated genomes, possibly explaining why they respond to immunotherapies. *MSH2* and *MLH1* account for about 90% of the mutations detected in families with Lynch syndrome. *MSH2* is particularly associated with an excess of endometrial and ovarian carcinomas. Other genes in the MMR family, including *MSH6*, *PMS1*, and *PMS2*, account for 10% of HNPCC-related cancers (68).

To identify patients with a diagnosis of endometrial cancer at risk for HNPCC, two approaches are used for patients who have endometrial cancer to identify any somatic, tumor mutations: For MSI analysis, DNA is extracted from macro-dissected endometrial tumors using paraffin sections, and short tandem repeats (2-5 nucleotides) are amplified in specific, predefined gene regions. The ovarian or endometrial tumors are characterized as MSI-stable, MSI-low (<30%), or MSI-high if more than 30% of markers are unstable based on the number of allelic shifts. MSI-high tumors suggest that the patient has Lynch syndrome. Immunohistochemical (IHC) stains on the tumor are performed for *MSH2*, *MSH6*, *MLH1*, and *PMS2*. If an MMR protein is absent, despite appropriate controls, confirmatory sequencing may be performed or, in the case of MLH1, methylation testing using a methylation-specific PCR for the MLH1 proximal promoter region, which suggests a somatic methylation events and, therefore, sporadic cancer. MSI can be due to epigenetic changes as well as to Lynch syndrome. MSI or IHC leads to a similar rate of MMRd tumors, but IHC allows to identify which specific protein is lost. Of note, tumor tissue–based testing does not identify patients with Lynch syndrome, it stratifies their risk for the condition triaging patients for germline genetic testing. Despite having loss of MMR protein expression, 10% to 15% of tumors with loss of either the MLH1 or PMS2 protein and 35% to 40% of tumors with loss of the MSH2 or MSH6 protein remain unexplained after comprehensive genetic evaluation, leading to counseling and management challenges. Recent data have suggested a fraction of these may be caused by biallelic somatic mutations, but clinical testing for this possibility is not widely available.

A French multicenter study reviewed the cancer incidence in 537 families with Lynch syndrome (73). For women in the study, the cumulative risk for Lynch syndrome–associated cancers was 19% by age 50 and 54% by age 70. The age-specific cumulative risk for OC by age 70 was 20% for *MLH1* mutation carriers, 24% for *MSH2* mutation carriers, and 1% for those with *MSH6* mutations. The authors found that by age 70, *MSH6* mutation carriers have a much lower risk of endometrial and ovarian cancer (16% and 1%, respectively) compared to *MLH1* (54% and 20%, respectively) or *MSH2* (21% and 24%, respectively) mutation carriers. These findings raise the question of whether women with a *MSH6* mutation need prophylactic surgery, especially if no other family member has been affected by cancer and none of the Amsterdam II criteria are met. However, a smaller cohort study did not confirm this low OC risk in women affected by *MSH6* mutations (71). This study from the combined Swedish/Danish cancer registry found that the distribution of OC histologic subtypes in patients with Lynch syndrome differed considerably from the sporadic OC population. They reported that

35% of the OCs associated with Lynch syndrome were endometrioid and 17% were clear cell, both much higher percentages than are seen in sporadic cases. *PMS2* mutations are associated with only a small increased risk of OC and have only a 3% lifetime risk of OC and present at a later age (51-59 years) (67). These patients could have risk-reducing surgery later. A cancer risk algorithm enables interactive calculation of remaining lifetime risks for cancer in patients with Lynch syndrome (www.plsd.eu) (67). The survival of OC in patients with any of the four Lynch syndrome mutations appears to be more favorable than for sporadic cancers.

PROPHYLACTIC SURGERY FOR PREVENTION OF LYNCH SYNDROME–ASSOCIATED CANCERS

As with *BRCA1/2* patients, RRSO is a very effective method for the prevention of OC in patients with a Lynch syndrome mutation (Table 8.2-5). Because of the possibility of synchronous tumors at the time of diagnosis, the preoperative workup should include a vaginal ultrasound to detect any ovarian masses and a thickened endometrial stripe, an endometrial biopsy to exclude an occult endometrial cancer, and a colonoscopy to search for polyps and colon cancer. Results of these studies will affect the extent of the surgery and the surgical approach (minimally invasive vs open surgery) as will a previous history of a radiation or surgery for colon cancer. In a large study combining all patients with Lynch syndrome followed at MD Anderson, UCSF, and Creighton University, none of 61 patients who underwent RRSO and a hysterectomy developed OC or uterine cancer (70). However, 12 (5.5%) of the 223 patients who chose surveillance developed OC and 33% developed endometrial cancer. Consistent with the French study (73), half of the patients who developed OC had an *MLH1* mutation and the other half an *MSH2* mutation, whereas none had an *MSH6* mutation. It is also important to note that occult endometrial cancers have been found in asymptomatic women at the time of risk-reducing hysterectomy and RRSO (74). Regardless, RRSO and hysterectomy are highly effective in preventing gynecologic cancers in women affected by HNPCC. Women with Lynch syndrome and OC have a better prognosis, with a 5-year survival of 88%.

Women with Lynch syndrome should be seen starting around age 25 by a knowledgeable gynecologist to learn about symptoms associated with cancers with Lynch syndrome that predispose them

---

■ TABLE 8.2-5. Risk-Reducing Recommendations for Carriers of BRCA1 and BRCA2 Mutations

Breast
- Clinical breast examination every 6-12 mo, age 25+ yr
- Annual breast MRI with contrast, age 25-29 yr
- Annual mammogram, age 30-75 yr
- RRSO to reduce breast cancer risk when childbearing is complete or between age 35-40 yr (BRCA1 mutation) or between 40 and 45 yr (BRCA2 mutation)
- Consider chemoprevention with tamoxifen, raloxifene, or aromatase inhibitors if the 5-yr Gail model is at least 3%
- Consider RRM

Ovary/fallopian tube
- RRSO to reduce ovary/fallopian tube cancer risk when childbearing is complete and between age 35 and 40 yr (BRCA1 mutation) or between 40 and 45 yr (BRCA2 mutation)
- Consider chemoprevention with oral contraceptives
- Consider transvaginal ultrasound and CA-125 if RRSO is not undertaken

Uterine
- Consider hysterectomy at the time of RRSO if BRCA1 mutation

MRI, magnetic resonance imaging; RRM, risk-reducing mastectomy; RRSO, risk-reducing salpingo-oophorectomy;

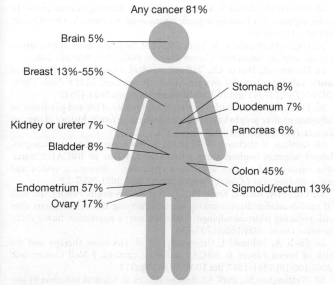

Figure 8.2-5. Risk of developing various cancers with Lynch syndrome. (From Ryan NAJ, McMahon RFT, Ramchander NC, Seif MW, Evans DG, Crosbie EJ. Lynch syndrome for the gynaecologist. *Obstet Gynaecol.* 2021;23:9-20. doi:10.1111/tog.12706)

(Figure 8.2-5). The discussion should include family planning given the 50% chance of passing a defective *MMR* gene to the next generation (autosomal dominant) and the (expensive) option of IVF combined with preimplantation genetic testing. Several risk-reducing strategies are available, such as OCPs (36), a levonorgestrel-coated IUD (37), and aspirin (75). A critical question for patients with Lynch syndrome is at what age a hysterectomy/BSO should be performed. Two studies reported that the median age for endometrial and OC in these patients is 46 to 48 and 42 to 48 years, respectively, much younger than for sporadic OC (70,71). The mean age of diagnosis for OC in women with Lynch syndrome is 45 years, and the average age of women with MMRd OC is 48 years (72). Moreover, a significant number of the women in one study (21%-42%) developed OC before age 40. However, the French study found that the risk of developing OC for all Lynch syndrome mutation carriers by age 40 does not exceed 2% to 3% (43). Still, a prudent approach is to perform the hysterectomy and RRSO after the age of 35, or once childbearing is completed. Obviously, such an early intervention requires extensive counseling, balancing the consequences of surgical menopause treated with HRT with the benefits of avoiding OC and endometrial cancer. There is no clear contraindication to estrogen replacement therapy after risk-reducing surgery.

For patients undergoing colonic resection for a Lynch-associated colorectal cancer, it may be reasonable to discuss concomitant hysterectomy with BSO. However, for premenopausal patients who are diagnosed with Lynch syndrome at the same time as their colorectal cancer, substantial fertility and psychosocial issues will be associated with this approach.

For patients with Lynch syndrome who prefer not to undergo prophylactic surgery, there is no scientifically proven screening option for OC, whereas every other year, colonoscopies reduce death from Lynch syndrome. According to most experts, transvaginal ultrasound and CA-125 are acceptable examinations in patients with mutations, if the patient is fully aware that these interventions will not necessarily diagnose OC early and might even be harmful, due to possible complications of surgical follow-up for a false-positive result (31). However, given that 66% to 81% of HNPCC-associated OCs are diagnosed during stages I and II because of their endometrioid and clear cell histology (70-72), a vaginal ultrasound is a reasonable choice for surveillance in a woman who is hesitant to undergo prophylactic surgery. Although it has not been thoroughly studied, chemoprevention with OCP together with screening for OC and endometrial cancer is currently used in women who want to delay surgery.

REFERENCES

1. Broca P, Satrústegui ASM, Ribera J, Sans AFC, Asselin P. *Traité des Tumeurs.* P. Asselin; 1866.
2. Alsop K, Fereday S, Meldrum C, et al. BRCA mutation frequency and patterns of treatment response in BRCA mutation-positive women with ovarian cancer: a report from the Australian ovarian cancer study group. *J Clin Oncol.* 2012;30:2654-2663.
3. Norquist BM, Harrell MI, Brady MF, et al. Inherited mutations in women with ovarian carcinoma. *JAMA Oncol.* 2016;2(4):482-490.
4. Desmond A, Kurian AW, Gabree M, et al. Clinical actionability of multigene panel testing for hereditary breast and ovarian cancer risk assessment. *JAMA Oncol.* 2015;1(7):943-951.
5. Kuchenbaecker KB, Hopper JL, Barnes DR, et al. Risks of breast, ovarian, and contralateral breast cancer for BRCA1 and BRCA2 mutation carriers. *JAMA.* 2017;317(23):2402-2416.
6. Torre LA, Trabert B, DeSantis CE, et al. Ovarian cancer statistics, 2018. *CA Cancer J Clin.* 2018;68(4):284-296.
7. Finch APM, Lubinski J, Møller P, et al. Impact of oophorectomy on cancer incidence and mortality in women with a BRCA1 or BRCA2 mutation. *J Clin Oncol.* 2014;32(15):1547-1553. doi:10.1200/JCO.2013 .53.2820
8. Centre for Cancer Genetic Epidemiology. BOADICEA. 2016. http:// ccge.medschl.cam.ac.uk/boadicea/
9. Rubin SC, Benjamin I, Behbakht K, et al. Clinical and pathological features of ovarian cancer in women with germ-line mutations of BRCA1. *N Engl J Med.* 1996;335:1413-1416.
10. Mavaddat N, Barrowdale D, Andrulis IL, et al. Pathology of breast and ovarian cancers among BRCA1 and BRCA2 mutation carriers: results from the consortium of investigators of modifiers of BRCA1/2 (CIMBA). *Cancer Epidemiol Biomarkers Prev.* 2012;21(1):134-147.
11. Werness BA, Ramus SJ, DiCioccio R. Histopathology, FIGO stage, and BRCA mutation status of ovarian cancers from the gilda radner familial ovarian cancer registry. *Int J Gynecol Pathol.* 2004;23:29-34.
12. Zhang Z, Royer R, Li S, et al. Frequencies of BRCA1 and BRCA2 mutations among 1342 patients with invasive ovarian cancer. *Gynecol Oncol.* 2011;121:353-357.
13. Modan B, Hartge P, Hirsch-Yechezel G. Oral contraceptives and the risk of ovarian cancer among carriers and noncarriers of a BRCA1 and BRCA2 mutation. *N Engl J Med.* 2001;345:235-240.
14. Lord CJ, Ashworth A. The DNA damage response and cancer therapy. *Nature.* 2012;481:287-292.
15. Quinn GP, Bell BA, Bell MY, et al. The guinea pig syndrome: improving clinical trial participation among thoracic patients. *J Thorac Oncol.* 2007;2(3):191-196. doi:10.1097/JTO.0b013e318031cdb6
16. Candido-dos-Reis FJ, Song H, Goode EL, et al. Germline mutation in BRCA1 or BRCA2 and ten-year survival for women diagnosed with epithelial ovarian cancer. *Clin Cancer Res.* 2015;21(3):652-657.
17. Yang D, Khan S, Sun Y, et al. Association of BRCA1 and BRCA2 mutations with survival, chemotherapy sensitivity, and gene mutator phenotype in patients with ovarian cancer. *JAMA.* 2011;306(14):1557-1565.
18. Bolton KL, Chenevix-Trench G, Goh C, et al. Association between BRCA1 and BRCA 2 mutations and survival in women with invasive epithelial ovarian cancer. *J Am Med Assoc.* 2012;307(4):382-390.
19. US Preventive Services Task Force, Owens DK, Davidson KW, et al. Risk assessment, genetic counseling, and genetic testing for BRCA-related cancer: US preventive services task force recommendation statement. *JAMA.* 2019;322(7):652-665.
20. Walsh T, Casadei S, Lee MK, et al. Mutations in 12 genes for inherited ovarian, fallopian tube and peritoneal carcinoma identified by massively parallel sequencing. *Proc Natl Acad Sci U S A.* 2011;108(44):18032-18037.
21. Yang X, Leslie G, Doroszuk A, et al. Cancer risks associated with germline PALB2 pathogenic variants: an international study of 524 families. *J Clin Oncol.* 2020;38(7):674-685.
22. Liu YL, Breen K, Catchings A, et al. Risk-reducing bilateral salpingo-oophorectomy for ovarian cancer: a review and clinical guide for hereditary predisposition genes. *JCO Oncol Pract.* 2022;18(3):201-209.
23. Banerjee S, Moore KN, Colombo N, et al. Maintenance olaparib for patients with newly diagnosed advanced ovarian cancer and a BRCA mutation (SOLO1/GOG 3004): 5-year follow-up of a randomised, double-blind, placebo-controlled, phase 3 trial. *Lancet Oncol.* 2021;22:1721-1731.
24. Ray-Coquard I, Pautier P, Pignata S, et al. Olaparib plus bevacizumab as first-line maintenance in ovarian cancer. *N Engl J Med.* 2019;381(25):2416-2428.
25. Kurian AW, Ward KC, Howlader N, et al. Genetic testing and results in a population-based cohort of breast cancer patients and ovarian cancer patients. *J Clin Oncol.* 2019;37(15):1305-1315.

26. Konstantinopoulos PA, Norquist B, Lacchetti C, et al. Germline and somatic tumor testing in epithelial ovarian cancer: ASCO guideline. *J Clin Oncol.* 2020;38(11):1222-1245.

27. Armstrong J, Toscano M, Kotchko N, et al. Utilization and outcomes of BRCA genetic testing and counseling in a national commercially insured population: the about study. *JAMA Oncol.* 2015;1:1251-1260.

28. Rayes N, Bowen DJ, Coffin T, et al. MAGENTA (making genetic testing accessible): a prospective randomized controlled trial comparing online genetic education and telephone genetic counseling for hereditary cancer genetic testing. *BMC Cancer.* 2019;19(1):648.

29. Kesselheim AS, Cook-Deegan RM, Winickoff DE, Mello MM. Gene patenting—the supreme court finally speaks. *N Engl J Med.* 2013;369(9):869-875.

30. Leib JR, Hoodfar E, Haidle JL, Nagy R. The new genetic privacy law. *Community Oncol.* 2008;5(6):351-354.

31. Buys S, Partridge E, Black A, et al. Effect of screening on ovarian cancer mortality. *J Am Med Assoc.* 2011;305(27):2295-2303.

32. Menon U, Gentry-Maharaj A, Burnell M, et al. Ovarian cancer population screening and mortality after long-term follow-up in the UK collaborative trial of ovarian cancer screening (UKCTOCS): a randomised controlled trial. *Lancet.* 2021;397(10290):2182-2193.

33. Rosenthal AN, Fraser LSM, Philpott S, et al. United Kingdom familial ovarian cancer screening study. *J Clin Oncol.* 2017;35(13):1411-1420.

34. Nanez A, Stram DA, Garcia C, Powell CB. Ovarian cancer surveillance in the clinical follow up of women with known BRCA1 or BRCA2 pathogenic variants in a large health care system. *Gynecol Oncol.* 2021;163(1):134-141.

35. Moorman PG, Havrilesky LJ, Gierisch JM, et al. Oral contraceptives and risk of ovarian cancer and breast cancer among high-risk women: a systematic review and meta-analysis. *J Clin Oncol.* 2013;31(33):4188-4198.

36. Schrijver LH, Antoniou AC, Olsson H, et al. Oral contraceptive use and ovarian cancer risk for BRCA1/2 mutation carriers: an international cohort study. *Am J Obstet Gynecol.* 2021;225(1):51.e1-51.e17.

37. Xia YY, Gronwald J, Karlan B, et al. Hereditary ovarian cancer clinical study. *Gynecol Oncol.* 2022;164(3):514-521.

38. Babic A, Sasamoto N, Rosner BA, et al. Association between breastfeeding and ovarian cancer risk. *JAMA Oncol.* 2020;6(6):e200421. doi:10.1001/jamaoncol.2020.0421

39. Kotsopoulos J, Gronwald J, McCuaig JM, et al. Hereditary ovarian cancer clinical study. *Gynecol Oncol.* 2020;159(3):820-826.

40. Kauff ND, Stagopan JM, Robson ME, et al. Risk-reducing salping-oophorectomy in women with a BRCA1 or BRCA2 mutation. *N Engl J Med.* 2002;346(21):1609-1615.

41. Rebbeck TR, Lynch HT, Neuhausen SL, et al. Prophylactic oophorectomy in carriers of BRCA1 or BRCA2 mutations. *N Engl J Med.* 2002;346(21):1616-1622.

42. Domchek SM, Friebel TM, Singer CF, et al. Association of risk-reducing surgery in BRCA1 or BRCA2 mutation carriers with cancer risk and mortality. *JAMA.* 2010;304(9):967-975.

43. Finch A, Beiner M, Lubinski J, et al. Salpingo-oophorectomy and the risk of ovarian, fallopian tube, and peritoneal cancers in women with a BRCA1 or BRCA2 mutation. *J Am Med Assoc.* 2006;296(2):185-192.

44. Eisen A, Lubinski J, Kljin J, et al. Breast cancer risk following bilateral oophorectomy in BRCA 1 and BRCA 2 mutation carriers: an international case-control study. *J Clin Oncol.* 2005;23(30):7491-7496.

45. Metcalfe K, Lynch HT, Foulkes WD, et al. Effect of oophorectomy on survival after breast cancer in BRCA1 and BRCA2 mutation carriers. *JAMA Oncol.* 2015;1(3):306-313.

46. Heemskerk-Gerritsen BA, Seynaeve C, Asperen CJ, et al. Breast cancer risk after salpingo-oophorectomy in healthy BRCA1/2 mutation carriers: revisiting the evidence for risk reduction. *J Natl Cancer Inst.* 2015;107(5):djv033.

47. Shu CA, Pike MC, Jotwani AR, et al. Uterine cancer after risk-reducing salpingo-oophorectomy without hysterectomy in women with BRCA mutations. *JAMA Oncol.* 2016;2:1434-1440. doi:10.1001/jamaoncol.2016.1820

48. Jonge MM, Kroon CD, Jenner DJ, et al. Endometrial cancer risk in women with germline BRCA1 or BRCA2 mutations: multicenter cohort study. *J Natl Cancer Inst.* 2021;113(9):1203-1211.

49. Steenbeek MP, Bommel MHD, Bulten J, et al. Risk of peritoneal carcinomatosis after risk-reducing salpingo-oophorectomy: a systematic review and individual patient data meta-analysis. *J Clin Oncol.* 2022;40(17):1879-1891.

50. Powell BC, Chen LM, McLennan J, et al. Risk-reducing salpingo-oophorectomy (RRSO) in BRCA mutation carriers. *Int J Gynecol Cancer.* 2011;21(5):846-851.

51. Muller CY, Coleman R, Adams WP. Laparoscopy in patients following transverse rectus abdominis myocutaneous flap reconstruction. *Obstet Gynecol.* 2000;96:132-135.

52. Bowtell DD, Bohm S, Ahmed AA, et al. Rethinking ovarian cancer II: reducing mortality from high-grade serous ovarian cancer. *Nat Rev Cancer.* 2015;15(11):668-679.

53. Daly MB, Dresher CW, Yates MS, et al. Salpingectomy as a means to reduce ovarian cancer risk. *Cancer Prev Res Phila.* 2015;8(5):342-348.

54. Hanley GE, Pearce CL, Talhouk A, et al. Outcomes from opportunistic salpingectomy for ovarian cancer prevention. *JAMA Netw Open.* 2022;5(2):e2147343. doi:10.1001/jamanetworkopen.2021.47343

55. Elit L, Esplen MJ, Butler K, Narod SA. Quality of life and psychosocial adjustment after prophylactic oophorectomy for a family history of ovarian cancer. *Fam Cancer.* 2001;1(3-4):149-156.

56. Kershaw V, Hickey I, Wyld L, Jha S. The impact of risk reducing bilateral salpingo-oophorectomy on sexual function in BRCA1/2 mutation carriers and women with lynch syndrome: a systematic review and meta-analysis. *Eur J Obstet Gynecol Reprod Biol.* 2021;265:7-17.

57. Valle HA, Kaur P, Kwon JS, Cheifetz R, Dawson L, Hanley GE. Risk of cardiovascular disease among women carrying BRCA mutations after risk-reducing bilateral salpingo-oophorectomy: a population-based study. *Gynecol Oncol.* 2021;162(3):707-714.

58. Eisen A, Lubinski J, Gronwald J, et al. Hormone therapy and the risk of breast cancer in BRCA1 mutation carriers. *J Natl Cancer Inst.* 2008;100(19):1361-1367. doi:10.1093/jnci/djn313

59. Wethington SL, Park KJ, Soslow RA, et al. Clinical outcome of isolated serous tubal intraepithelial carcinomas (STIC). *Int J Gynecol Cancer.* 2013;23(9):1603-1611.

60. Patrono MG, Iniesta MD, Malpica A, et al. Clinical outcomes in patients with isolated serous tubal intraepithelial carcinoma (STIC): a comprehensive review. *Gynecol Oncol.* 2015;139(3):568-572.

61. Colombo N, Sessa C, Bois AD, et al. ESMO-ESGO consensus conference recommendations on ovarian cancer: pathology and molecular biology, early and advanced stages, borderline tumours and recurrent disease. *Int J Gynecol Cancer.* 2019;29(4):728-760.

62. Colgan TJ, Murphy J, Cole D, Narod SA, Rosen B. Occult carcinoma in prophylactic oophorectomy specimens: prevalence and association with BRCA germline mutation status. *Am J Surg Pathol.* 2001;25:1283-1289.

63. Barnetson RA, Tenesa A, Farrington SM, et al. Identification and survival of carriers of mutations in DNA mismatch-repair genes in colon cancer. *N Engl J Med.* 2006;354(26):2751-2763.

64. Chen S, Wang W, Lee S, et al. Prediction of germline mutations and cancer risk in the lynch syndrome. *JAMA.* 2006;296(12):1479-1487.

65. Kastrinos F, Uno H, Ukaegbu C, et al. Development and validation of the PREMM5 model for comprehensive risk assessment of lynch syndrome. *J Clin Oncol.* 2017;35(19):2165-2172.

66. Lynch HT, Shaw MW, Magnuson CW, Larsen AL, Krush AJ. Hereditary factors in cancer. Study of two large midwestern kindreds. *Arch Intern Med.* 1966;117(2):206-212.

67. Dominguez-Valentin M, Sampson JR, Seppala TT, et al. Cancer risks by gene, age, and gender in 6350 carriers of pathogenic mismatch repair variants: findings from the prospective lynch syndrome database. *Genet Med.* 2020;22(1):15-25.

68. Lynch HT, Chapelle A. Hereditary colorectal cancer. *N Engl J Med.* 2003;348:919-932.

69. Lu KH, Dinh M, Kohlmann W, et al. Gynecologic cancer as a "sentinel cancer" for women with hereditary nonpolyposis colorectal cancer syndrome. *Obstet Gynecol.* 2005;105(3):569-574.

70. Schmeler KM, Lynch HT, Chen LM, et al. Prophylactic surgery to reduce the risk of gynecologic cancers in the lynch syndrome. *N Engl J Med.* 2006;354:261-269.

71. Ketabi Z, Bartuma K, Bernstein I, et al. Ovarian cancer linked to lynch syndrome typically presents as early-onset, non-serous epithelial tumors. *Gynecol Oncol.* 2011;121:462-465.

72. Atwal A, Snowsill T, Dandy MC, et al. The prevalence of mismatch repair deficiency in ovarian cancer: a systematic review and meta-analysis. *Int J Cancer.* 2022;151:1626-1639.

73. Bonadona V, Bonaïti B, Olschwang S, et al. Cancer risk associated with germline mutations in MLH1, MSH2, and MSH6 genes in lynch syndrome. *J Am Med Assoc.* 2011;305(22):2304-2310.

74. Pistorius S, Kruger S, Hohl R, et al. Occult endometrial cancer and decision making for prophylactic hysterectomy in hereditary nonpolyposis colorectal cancer patients. *Gynecol Oncol.* 2006;102(2):189-194.

75. Hurwitz LM, Townsend MK, Jordan SJ, et al. Modification of the association between frequent aspirin use and ovarian cancer risk: a meta-analysis using individual-level data from two ovarian cancer consortia. *J Clin Oncol.* 2022;40:4207-4217. doi:10.1200/JCO.21.01900

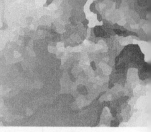

CHAPTER **8.3**

Natural History of the Disease: Patterns of Spread

Kathryn A. Mills and Ernst Lengyel

MUCINOUS, CLEAR CELL, AND ENDOMETRIOID OVARIAN CANCER

Mucinous neoplasms are frequently the largest of all ovarian tumors. They can reach diameters of 30 to 40 cm, often compressing adjacent organs (**Figure 8.3-1**). Intact removal of these tumors may be challenging owing to their weight, the large veins that drain from them, and difficulties visualizing the ureter during the procedure. However, mucinous tumors, especially the largest, tend to be benign. Indeed, 80% of these tumors are benign mucinous cystadenomas, and when malignant, most mucinous tumors are either borderline or low-grade invasive mucinous tumors. While high-grade invasive mucinous cancers are very aggressive and resistant to chemotherapy, they are rare. Only 0.5% to 1.5% of advanced OCs have a mucinous histology. One large study found that 71% of invasive mucinous tumors found in the ovary were metastases from the gastrointestinal (GI) tract (colon, pancreas, and appendix), and only 29% were truly primary mucinous OCs (1,2). These primary invasive mucinous tumors are often confined to the ovary without surface involvement and are unilateral (metastases are more often bilateral) and of a significant size (≥13 cm) (2). Often, patients with mucinous tumors have an elevated level of one of two tumor markers, CEA or CA19-9, that are also often associated with GI malignancies. In addition, they are frequently found in younger patients, with recent data confirming 26% of patient diagnosed with mucinous OC were under age 44 (3). If a tumor is confined to the ovary, FIGO (2014) 1A, and removed as part of a salpingo-oophorectomy (no cystectomy), the risk of residual tumor or upstaging is very low, especially in expansile mucinous OC. Mucinous OCs rarely metastasize to regional lymph nodes; therefore, lymph node dissection is not necessary, unless the intraoperative frozen section diagnosis is equivocal on histologic subtype.

Pseudomyxoma peritonei is a condition caused by the production of mucin by glandular cells in the peritoneal cavity. These cells have a benign glandular histology, but their behavior is biologically malignant because the mucin-producing cells implant diffusely on the abdominal and pelvic peritoneum. The cells then produce thick mucin that encases the bowel and pelvic organs, frequently leading to tumor cachexia and bowel obstruction. The most common origins of pseudomyxoma peritonei are currently thought to be appendiceal neoplasms or ruptured benign mucoceles of the appendix with secondary involvement of the ovary. Patients with pseudomyxoma peritonei can progress for months or years without symptoms. Although their disease often has an indolent course, it is rarely fully eliminated (10-year survival is 50%-60%) (4,5). Currently, it is generally recommended that patients receive aggressive cytoreductive surgery with complete peritonectomy and hyperthermic intraperitoneal chemotherapy (HIPEC) in a specialized center, although there are no randomized data to support this strategy (5).

Endometrioid cancer and clear cell cancers of the ovary are the most common malignancies that arise from endometriosis. Invasive endometrioid OC accounts for about 10% of all ovarian carcinomas and occurs most often in perimenopausal patients. Up to 7% of patients of reproductive age (29 and 47 years) with an endometrioid endometrial cancer have a synchronous early-stage endometrioid OC (6) (**Figure 8.3-2**). These cancers are often associated with endometriosis (7). Molecularly, these tumors are often clonally related, representing metastatic disease from either the uterus or the ovary.

Clear cell OC, which makes up 5% to 10% of all ovarian carcinomas, is also associated with some unique presenting symptoms at the time of diagnosis, which include a higher frequency of thromboembolic events, hypercalcemia, and paraneoplastic syndromes (8); a higher propensity for hematologic and lymphatic spread; and a higher rate of bony metastasis than high-grade serous carcinomas (HGSCs). Recurrences of clear cell cancers are often multifocal, pelvic, extrapelvic, and intrathoracic, and sometimes, women present with a brain metastasis.

Because of the large size of the primary tumor and the biology driving these tumors, nonserous histologies are more likely to be discovered at an early stage (FIGO I/II) (8). They typically do not have the pattern of transcoelomic spread along peritoneal surfaces seen with serous cancers, and unlike HGSOC, they often do not respect anatomic intraperitoneal (IP) planes. Locally, they are characterized by thick adhesions to the pelvis and can invade adjacent pelvic organs, including the muscularis of the colon, the small bowel mesentery, and the pelvic sidewall. Advanced endometrioid and mucinous tumors (FIGO III/IV) implant into the abdominal wall and metastasize to the parenchyma of intra-abdominal organs, such as the liver and spleen (2).

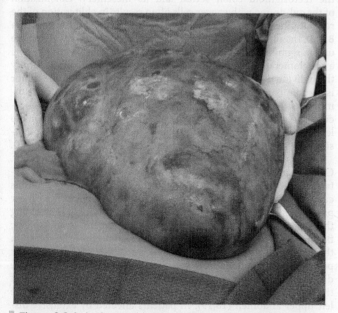

■ **Figure 8.3-1.** A 42-year-old patient with a multicystic adnexal mass originating from the left ovary. The specimen was 20 cm × 15 cm and weighed 5 pounds. The frozen section returned as a mucinous borderline tumor.

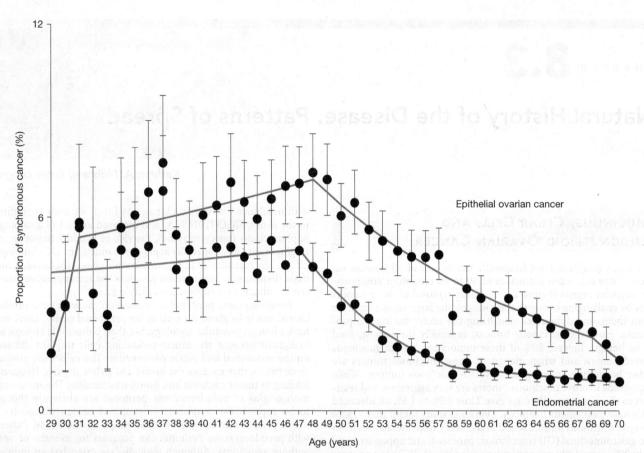

Figure 8.3-2. Proportion of synchronous endometrial and ovarian cancer by age. Blue line depicts a trend of proportion of women with endometrial cancer who had synchronous ovarian cancer. Red line depicts a trend of proportion of women with epithelial ovarian cancer who had synchronous endometrial cancer. Dots represent percent proportion, and error bars represent 95% confidence interval. (From Matsuo K, Machida H, Blake EA, et al. Trends and outcomes of women with synchronous endometrial and ovarian cancer. *Oncotarget.* 2018;9(47):28757-28771.)

SEROUS PAPILLARY OVARIAN CANCER

Serous carcinomas originating from Müllerian epithelium, which includes ovarian, peritoneal, and fallopian tube cancers, are characterized by transcoelomic spread (9). Since 1999, there have been new insights into the origin of serous "ovarian" cancer, and a putative precursor lesion in the fallopian tube, STIC, has been identified (10,11). It is now believed that most serous "ovarian" cancer originates in the fallopian tube as STIC (12). A small tumor can be more easily assigned to a particular anatomic site, but if the tumor is widely disseminated, it is not possible to clearly identify where a serous tumor originated. In the absence of an STIC lesion, serous cancers are generally categorized as ovarian primaries. However, this is not crucial from a clinical standpoint, because the dissemination patterns of serous papillary ovarian, fallopian tube, and peritoneal cancer are clinically indistinguishable by virtue of their propensity to exfoliate malignant cells into the peritoneal cavity, patient survival is very similar, and management is the same, regardless of primary site. A study (13) as well as clinical experience suggest that all three tumor subtypes grow quickly and disseminate on mesothelial cell–covered body cavities, including the peritoneal cavity or pleural space. Once the cancer cells detach from the ovarian or fallopian tube tumor, they float in the ascites as single cells or as multicellular spheroids. The cells follow the normal clockwise circulation of peritoneal fluid up the right paracolic gutter and to the undersurface of the right hemidiaphragm, where they may implant and grow as surface nodules. All IP mesothelium-covered surfaces are at risk, with frequent involvement of the peritoneum, diaphragm, omentum, to a lesser degree the hepatic flexure and splenic hilum, bowel and bowel mesentery, and appendix (14).

The most common sites involved in locoregional metastasis are the contralateral ovary, the peritoneum of the cul-de-sac, and the rectosigmoid colon serosa and its mesentery. Colonization of the cul-de-sac with cancer cells often results in obliteration of the rectouterine space. In patients with extensive pelvic disease (**Figure 8.3-3**), the uterus, bladder dome, sidewall peritoneum overlying the ureter, sigmoid colon, ovarian tumor masses, and appendix become a conglomerate pelvic tumor, and it can be very difficult to identify the individual organs or any anatomic borders (15,16). If the tumor is predominantly on the patient's right side, a large conglomerate tumor mass is found in the right lower quadrant involving the ileocecum, appendix, and right ovary. If the tumor is predominantly on the left side, the conglomerate tumor includes the left ovary, the rectosigmoid and its mesentery, and the left side of the uterus (**Figure 6.3**).

The most frequent site of distant metastasis is the omentum. Other than metastases to the contralateral ovary, an omental metastasis is often the largest tumor in the abdominal cavity. Serous cancers initially infiltrate the infracolic omentum, but as the cancer progresses, the entire omentum is replaced by tumor (17), reaching the lower stomach and extending from the hepatic to the splenic flexure (**Figure 8.3-4**). Because the omentum reaches the spleen in the left upper quadrant, there is often a solid tumor at the lower pole of the spleen and at the splenic hilum directly adjacent to the distal pancreas, which sometimes requires an en bloc resection of the distal pancreas and the spleen in order to completely clear the left upper abdomen (18,19). In patients affected by extensive disease, the lesser omentum, which is attached to the lesser curvature of the stomach, is also involved. Despite extensive involvement of the omentum by serous carcinoma, there is almost never invasion of the gastric or transverse colon muscularis because the tumor is

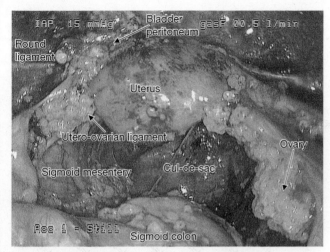

Figure 8.3-3. Laparoscopic intraoperative image of the pelvis of a patient with disseminated high-volume disease suggestive of ovarian cancer on computed tomography scan. Tumor implants on the sigmoid colon, sigmoid mesentery, pelvic sidewall, ovary, utero-ovarian ligament, and bladder peritoneum.

typically on the serosal surface. It is almost always possible to develop a plane between the tumor and the muscularis and remove the tumor nodules and plaques without a colon or gastric resection. However, if the integrity of transverse colon is in question after resection, a partial colectomy may be required. Another important observation is tumor almost never extends in to the retroperitoneal space or deep to the lesser sac, because serous tumors metastasize on the mesothelial cell–covered surfaces. Extensive surface involvement of the abdominal or pleural cavity will cause ascites and a pleural effusion, respectively. Patients with extensive intra-abdominal tumor involvement sometimes have extensive involvement of the small bowel mesentery. A condition described due to its appearance as "rose budding" will occur when tumor constricts the blood supply to the bowel and limits bowel mobility because of the short mesenteric root. Often, these tumors are deemed unresectable because they compromise all blood supply to the small bowel from the

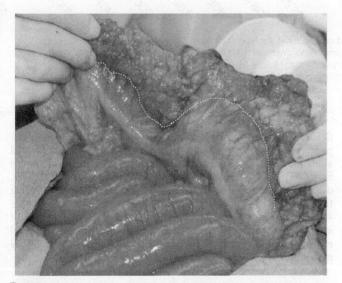

Figure 8.3-4. Patient with FIGO stage IIIC ovarian cancer with an omental cake. The omentum is completely transformed by tumor nodules. The omentum is lifted superiorly, toward the patient's head. The omental tumor can almost always be dissected off the transverse colon along an avascular plane (white dotted line), allowing entry into the lesser sac. FIGO, International Federation of Gynaecology and Obstetrics.

superior mesenteric artery and impair venous return through the superior mesenteric vein. In very advanced disease, serous cancers tend to agglutinate the loops of small bowel and cause a high-grade bowel obstruction at many levels (jejunum, ileum). If such findings are noted on preoperative imaging, strong consideration should be given to neoadjuvant chemotherapy.

Women with advanced serous OC, who have disseminated miliary disease covering the entire peritoneal surface, including the diaphragms, often have large-volume ascites (20). The ascitic fluid generally contains mesothelial, inflammatory, and tumor cells (14). Rarely, serous tumors will metastasize to the mesothelial cell–covered pericardium, causing a pericardial effusion (21).

Because FIGO stage IV serous OC is defined by several anatomic locations in the upper abdomen and/or a malignant pleural effusion, it represents a very heterogeneous group. Peritoneal-pleural lymphatic communication through the diaphragm allows transdiaphragmatic spread of tumor into the mesothelium-covered pleural space, leading to malignant pleural effusion. Because serous cancers have a preference for implantation on the right diaphragm, most patients with stage IV disease have a right-sided malignant pleural effusion (37%-48%). Other metastasis patterns that define FIGO stage IVB disease include parenchymal liver metastases, supraclavicular/axillary lymphadenopathy, parenchymal lung metastases, mediastinal adenopathy, and distal vaginal or perineal metastases (22,23). While serous OC disseminates extensively within the abdominal cavity, intrapulmonary metastasis, or other intraparenchymal involvement, for example, intrahepatic, spleen, or kidney tumors are rare. If these are found, the differential diagnosis should be expanded to include a different OC histotype (clear cell, mucinous, or carcinosarcoma) or a different tumor origin (GI, pancreatic, breast cancer).

Advanced invasive LGSCs, which represent about 9% of all EOCs, have a tumor distribution pattern that is very similar to that of HGSCs, with metastasis to the omentum (83%), fallopian tube (63%), pelvic peritoneum (49%), and uterine serosa (46%) (24), although rarely metastasize to lymph nodes.

LYMPH NODE METASTASIS

Exfoliation followed by implantation is one of two primary modes of OC dissemination. The other is via the retroperitoneal lymphatics draining the ovary. This path follows the superior ovarian blood supply in the infundibulopelvic ligament, which contains the ovarian artery and vein as well as extensive lymphatics that terminate in lymph nodes near the aorta and vena cava up to the level of the renal vessels. The next lymph node stations are at the celiac trunk, from which tumor cells may continue up to the mediastinal and supraclavicular lymph nodes. Lymph channels also pass laterally through the broad ligament and parametrial channels to terminate in the pelvic sidewall lymphatics, including the external iliac, obturator, and hypogastric chains (25). Spread may also occur along the course of the round ligament, resulting in the involvement of the inguinal lymphatics. The principal lymphatic drainage of the ovary and fallopian tube appears to be via the para-aortic lymph nodes. Lymph node metastases are often correlated with the stage and extent of intra-abdominal disease involvement, but involvement may be present without obvious disseminated spread, so lymph node exploration should still be performed in the absence of visible peritoneal disease (26). Retroperitoneal node involvement has been found in 23% of suspected stage I disease, 31% of stage 2, 72% of stage 3, and 87% of stage 4 HGSOC. Other histologic subtypes have a lower incidence of lymph node metastasis (27) (**Figure 8.3-5**).

The initial spread of OC, by both the IP and lymphatic routes, is clinically occult. As many as 20% of women with the appearance of FIGO stage I/II OC have microscopic metastatic disease, most frequently to the omentum or lymph nodes (28). Histologic type (serous), grade (III), stage (II), and CA-125 (high) at diagnosis are risk factors for lymph node metastasis (27). The true extent of disease in early-stage OC can be detected only by histologic examination of visually normal tissues sampled during surgical staging (29).

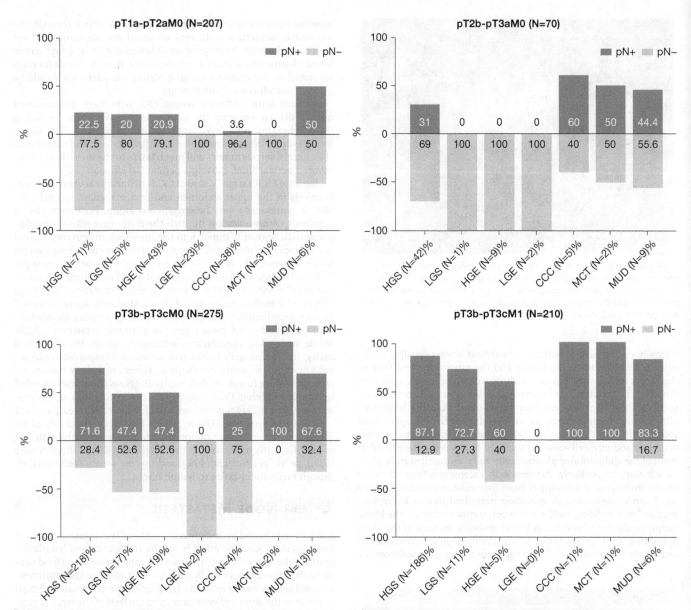

Figure 8.3-5. Frequency (%) of patients with affected lymph nodes based on histologic subtype in all patients based on pT stage; high-grade serous (HGS), low-grade serous (LGS), low-grade endometrioid LGE), high-grade endometrioid (HGE), clear cell tumors (CCC), mucinous tumors (MCT), and mixed/undifferentiated (MUD). (Reprinted by permission from Springer: From Heitz F, Harter P, du Bois A. Stage- and histologic subtype-dependent frequency of lymph node metastases in patients with epithelial ovarian cancer undergoing systematic pelvic and paraaortic lymphadenectomy. *Ann Surg Oncol.* 2018;25(7):2053-2059.)

Approximately 7% of patients with cancer that appears to be confined to the ovaries will have metastases only to the para-aortic nodes, skipping the pelvic lymph nodes (27). Many patients with apparently localized disease will also have occult disease found in peritoneal washings or in biopsies of the diaphragm and omentum.

RECURRENT OVARIAN CANCER

The majority (80%) of patients with advanced OC who undergo a combination of platinum- and taxane-based chemotherapy will have a recurrence, despite an initial complete response to primary treatment. Of all patients with OC, 75% will have an intra-abdominal recurrence; the remainder have extraperitoneal/intrahepatic or distant metastasis with or without intra-abdominal recurrence (30). Twenty-two percent of recurrences occur outside the peritoneal cavity. The locations of intra-abdominal recurrences include the remnants of the omentum, especially at the splenic

flexure; the small and large bowel mesentery; and the epiploic appendices, which are peritoneal pouches filled with fat and located along the colon and IP rectum. The majority of deaths occur in the first 2 years (53%), and while only 48% of patients survive 5 years, overall survival has actually been slowly improving (31). Following the increased use of IP chemotherapy with the publication of GOG #182 (32), several retrospective studies reported a higher rate of extra-abdominal recurrences, including brain metastasis, pleural effusions, and mediastinal disease. More pleural and parenchymal metastases are observed after bevacizumab treatment (33).

REFERENCES

1. Bookman MA, Brady MF, McGuire WP, et al. Evaluation of new platinum-based treatment regimens in advanced-stage ovarian cancer: a phase III trial of the gynecologic cancer intergroup. *J Clin Oncol.* 2009;27(9):1419-1425.

2. Zaino R, Brady MF, Lele S, Michael H, Greer BE, Bookman MA. Advanced stage mucinous adenocarcinoma of the ovary is both rare and highly lethal. *Cancer.* 2011;117:554-562.

3. Peres LC, Cushing-Haugen KL, Kobel M, et al. Invasive epithelial ovarian cancer survival by histotype and disease stage. *J Natl Cancer Inst.* 2019;111:60-68.

4. Sugerbaker PH. New standard of care for appendiceal epithelial neoplasms and pseudomyxoma peritonei. *Lancet Oncol.* 2006;7:69-76.

5. Passot G, Vaudoyer D, Villeneuve L, et al. What made hyperthermic intraperitoneal chemotherapy an effective curative treatment for peritoneal surface malignancy: a 25-year experience with 1,125 procedures. *J Surg Oncol.* 2016;113(7):796-803.

6. Matsuo K, Machida H, Blake EA, et al. Trends and outcomes of women with synchronous endometrial and ovarian cancer. *Oncotarget.* 2018;9(47):28757-28771.

7. Bennett JA, Pesci A, Morales-Oyarvide V, Silva A, Nardi V, Oliva E. Incidence of mismatch repair protein deficiency and associated clinico-pathologic features in a cohort of 104 ovarian endometrioid carcinomas. *Am J Surg Pathol.* 2019;43(2):235-243.

8. Gadducci A, Multinu F, Cosio S, Carinelli S, Ghioni M, Aletti GD. Clear cell carcinoma of the ovary: epidemiology, pathological and biological features, treatment options and clinical outcomes. *Gynecol Oncol.* 2021;162(3):741-750.

9. Tan D, Agarwal R, Kaye SB. Mechanisms of transcoelomic metastasis in ovarian cancer. *Lancet.* 2006;7:925-934.

10. Dubeau L. The cell of origin of ovarian epithelial tumors and the ovarian surface epithelium dogma: does the emperor have no clothes? *Gynecol Oncol.* 1999;72(3):437-442.

11. Piek JM, Diest PJ, Zweemer RP, et al. Dysplastic changes in prophylactically removed fallopian tubes of women predisposed to developing ovarian cancer. *J Pathol.* 2001;195(4):451-456.

12. Kuhn E, Kurman RJ, Vang R, et al. TP53 mutations in serous tubal intraepithelial carcinoma and concurrent pelvic high-grade serous carcinoma-evidence supporting the clonal relationship of the two lesions. *J Pathol.* 2012;226:421-426.

13. Brown PO, Palmer C. The preclinical natural history of serous ovarian cancer: defining the target for early detection. *PLoS Med.* 2009; 6(7):1-11.

14. Lengyel E. Ovarian cancer development and metastasis. *Am J Pathol.* 2010;177(3):1053-1064. doi:10.2353/ajpath.2010.100105

15. Bristow RE, Carmen M, Kaufman H, Montz FJ. Radical oophorectomy with primary stapled colorectal anastomosis for resection of locally advanced epithelial ovarian cancer. *J Am Coll Surg.* 2003;197:565-574.

16. Aletti GD, Podratz KC, Jones MB, Cliby WA. Role of rectosigmoidectomy and stripping of pelvic peritoneum in outcomes of patients with advanced ovarian cancer. *J Am Coll Surg.* 2006;203(4):521-526.

17. Sehouli J, Senyuva F, Fotopoulou C, et al. Intra-abdominal tumor dissemination pattern and surgical outcome in 214 patients with primary ovarian cancer. *J Surg Oncol.* 2009;99:424-427.

18. Kehoe SM, Eisenhauer EL, Chi DS. Upper abdominal surgical procedures: liver mobilization and diaphragm peritonectomy/resection, splenectomy, and distal pancreatectomy. *Gynecol Oncol.* 2008; 111:51-55.

19. Chi DS, Eisenhauer EL, Zivanovic O, et al. Improved progression-free and overall survival in advanced ovarian cancer as a result of a change in surgical paradigm. *Gynecol Oncol.* 2009;114(1):26-31. doi:10.1016/j.ygyno.2009.03.018

20. Ayantunde A, Parsons S. Pattern and prognostic factors in patients with malignant ascites: a retrospective study. *Ann Oncol.* 2007; 18:945-949.

21. Kooy J, Findley R, Nelson G, Chu P. Cytology positive pericardial effusion causing tamponade in patients with high grade serous carcinoma of the ovary. *Gynecol Oncol Rep.* 2020;33:100621.

22. Winter WE, Maxwell GL, Tian C, et al. Tumor residual after surgical cytoreduction in prediction of clinical outcome in stage IV epithelial ovarian cancer: a gynecological oncology group study. *J Clin Oncol.* 2008;26(1):83-89.

23. Wimberger P, Wehling M, Lehmann N, et al. Influence of residual tumor on outcome in ovarian cancer patients with FIGO stage IV disease. *Ann Surg Oncol.* 2010;17:1642-1648.

24. Gershenson D, Sun CC, Lu K, et al. Clinical behavior of stage II-IV low-grade serous carcinoma of the ovary. *Obstet Gynecol.* 2006; 108(2):361-368.

25. Mangan CE, Rubin SC, Rabin DS, Mikuta JJ. Lymph node nomenclature in gynecologic oncology. *Gynecol Oncol.* 1986;23:222-226.

26. Morice P, Joulie F, Camatte S, et al. Lymph node involvement in epithelial ovarian cancer: analysis of 276 pelvic and paraaortic lymphadenectomies and surgical implications. *J Am Coll Surg.* 2003;197:198-205.

27. Heitz F, Harter P, Ataseven B, et al. Stage- and histologic subtype-dependent frequency of lymph node metastases in patients with epithelial ovarian cancer undergoing systematic pelvic and paraaortic lymphadenectomy. *Ann Surg Oncol.* 2018;25(7):2053-2059.

28. Timmers PJ, Zwinderman AH, Coens C, Vergote I, Trimbos JB. Understanding the problem of inadequately staging early ovarian cancer. *Eur J Cancer.* 2010;46(5):880-884.

29. Maggioni A, Panici PB, Dell'Anna T, et al. Randomised study of systematic lymphadenectomy in patients with epithelial ovarian cancer macroscopically confined to the pelvis. *Br J Cancer.* 2006;95:699-704.

30. Cormio G, Rossi C, Cazzolla A, et al. Distant metastases in ovarian carcinoma. *Int J Gynecol Cancer.* 2003;13:125-129.

31. Surveillance E, Program ER. Cancer stats facts: ovarian cancer. 2022. https://seer.cancer.gov/statfacts/html/ovary.html

32. Armstrong DK, Bundy B, Wenzel L, et al. Intraperitoneal cisplatin and paclitaxel in ovarian cancer. *N Engl J Med.* 2006;354(1):34-43. doi:10.1056/NEJMoa052985

33. Petrillo M, Amadio G, Salutari V, et al. Impact of bevacizumab containing first line chemotherapy on recurrent disease in epithelial ovarian cancer: a case-control study. *Gynecol Oncol.* 2016;142(2):231-236.

CHAPTER 8.4

Ovarian Cancer: Etiology, Genetics, and Molecular Biology

Charles N. Landen Jr and Ernst Lengyel

Historically, the origin of EOC was believed to be from the invagination of OSE into the ovarian stroma forming inclusion cysts, which had the potential to undergo malignant transformation (1). However, as more careful examination of pathologic specimens from prophylactic BSO in patients with a BRCA mutation and subsequently tumor debulking specimens has demonstrated, it is now believed that most OCs, at least serous subtypes, originate in the fallopian tubes. Almost all incidental cancers from prophylactic BSO specimens have been found in the fallopian tube, and up to 15% of women with *BRCA1/2* mutations who undergo prophylactic BSO harbor premalignant STIC lesions (2). STIC lesions are often accompanied by p53 mutations, also at the fimbriated end of the fallopian tube suggesting that STIC is the precursor lesion for invasive ovarian carcinoma. Although these changes were originally thought to be present only in women with *BRCA1* or *BRCA2* mutations, there is growing evidence pointing to the existence of these precursor lesions among women who develop sporadic serous OC (3). Careful examination of the fallopian tubes obtained at the time of prophylactic debulking surgery has also identified a high prevalence of STIC lesions in the fimbriated end of the fallopian tube. The distal fallopian tube, therefore, is increasingly being seen as the origin of tubal cancer, OC, and peritoneal serous OC.

In 2006, the TCGA began with studies in glioblastoma and HGSOC (4). The National Institutes of Health committed major resources to TCGA to have since collected and characterized the genomic landscape of more than 20,000 primary cancers across 33 cancer types. A national network of research and technology teams pooled the results of their efforts to create an economy of scale and develop an infrastructure for making the data publicly accessible (5). Each cancer underwent comprehensive genomic characterization and analysis. The data generated by TCGA are available and widely used by the cancer research community through the CBIO Data Portal (6,7). The analyses included sequencing of the entire coding regions (exomes) of each cancer. The levels of gene expression, including mRNA and microRNA, were measured either through microarray-based platforms or using second-generation sequencing techniques to sequence the RNA transcriptome. Copy number alterations and methylation events were also assessed through microarray platforms. Some tumors were also hybridized to reverse-phase protein arrays when sufficient biomaterial was available. For some subtypes, clinical information is also available, allowing assessment of outcomes associated with molecular abnormalities. A more thorough description of the findings of the TCGA and other profiling studies is found in this chapter.

OVARIAN CANCER ETIOLOGY

Classically, there were many theories as to how and why OCs develop. These were mainly based on epidemiologic and clinical features that placed patients at increased risk, including incessant ovulation, hormonal stimulation by FSH and LH, and inflammation.

Incessant ovulation was first postulated based on the observation that patients with a greater number of ovulatory cycles were at increased risk by Fathalla in 1971 (8). Those with multiple pregnancies, increased time of lactation, and OCP use were at reduced risk. However, patients who undergo tubal ligation (thus not interfering with ovulation), and those on progesterone-only contraception (which does not inhibit ovulation), are also at reduced risk. Patients with polycystic ovary syndrome (PCOS) with fewer ovulatory cycles are at somewhat increased risk, weakening the importance of ovulation alone as a primary factor.

The median age of OC development is 61, about 10 years after the onset of menopause, raising the question of whether increased FSH and LH associated with menopause initiate a cascade of changes, ultimately leading to malignant transformation. Indeed, FSH and LH receptors are expressed by more than 60% of EOCs, and exogenous FSH and LH can activate multiple oncogenes, such as MAP kinase (MAPK), EGFR, HER2, C-MYC, β-catenin, cyclin G2, IGF-1, and β-1 integrin. In preclinical mouse models, exposure to excess FSH and LH increases tumor growth, metastasis, and invasion. However, no study has convincingly demonstrated that FSH or LH can lead to malignant transformation. Collectively, studies suggest that FSH and LH may promote OC growth, but not initiation.

Cytokines are also implicated in OC growth, so a role in inflammation has been postulated. Patients are at reduced risk if they are chronic users of aspirin, NSAIDs, and acetaminophen. Patients could be at increased risk if exposed to high doses of inflammation-inducing substances, such as talc and asbestos, but the data on the cancer-inducing effect of talc are ambiguous. There might be a dose effect as some data suggest that talc could be carcinogenic when used for a long time in high quantities on the perineum. Downstream effectors of inflammation do contribute to

cancer growth, such as STAT3, nitric oxide synthase, vascular endothelial growth factor (VEGF), and NF-κB. However, again, there is no convincing evidence that these agents actually cause malignant transformation.

Genetic and molecular profiling, as well as clinical and pathologic observations of BRCA patients and their associated fallopian tubes, have led to the current belief that most "ovarian" cancers, especially those of serous histology, originate in the fallopian tube with a mutation in TP53. Loss or dysfunction of P53 leads to numerous chromosomal abnormalities, allowing an accumulation of insults that ultimately result in malignant transformation. However, especially for the additional subtypes, the abovementioned physiologic conditions may still play an important etiologic role.

EOCs are heterogeneous with respect to behavior (borderline vs invasive), grade, and histologic type. It has become increasingly clear that there are striking differences in the molecular pathogenesis of various disease subsets. The family of OCs has often been divided in two types, reflective of their rate of growth, origin, and genetic abnormalities, with type I encompassing high-grade lesions and type II being low-grade serous ovarian cancer (LGSOC) (9) (**Figure 8.4-1**). Type I tumors are more often confined to an ovarian mass at diagnosis owing to their slower growth rate. They include low-grade serous, mucinous, and most endometrioid and clear cell carcinomas. They are more genetically stable and are characterized by mutations in a number of genes, including KRAS, BRAF, PTEN, CTNNB1, ARID1A, and PPP2R1A. Low-grade cancers develop mostly through an intermediary premalignant borderline histologic type. Because the etiology of mucinous OCs is poorly understood, they are often included in type I because of the nature of their slower growth rate. Type II cancers have a higher growth rate and typically present at an advanced stage. These include and are predominantly high-grade serous lesions but also include high-grade endometrioid, clear cell, carcinosarcoma, and undifferentiated cancers. This group of tumors has a high level of genetic instability, with frequent chromosomal gains and losses and mutation of TP53.

Endometrioid and clear cell cancers are thought to develop in deposits of endometriosis on the ovary or other pelvic structures (10-12). The origin of mucinous OCs is less clear, and some may arise from preexisting dermoid cysts (teratomas). Historically, the majority of mucinous ovarian tumors represented unrecognized metastatic GI cancers. Molecular analysis by copy number variation, variant analysis, and sequencing have demonstrated that most mucinous OCs share features and likely evolve from benign mucinous and borderline tumors of the ovary (13). They retain high copy number variation and frequent p53 mutations seen in other high-grade OCs. It has also been postulated that some mucinous and Brenner tumors arise from embryonic rests near the ovary.

As our understanding of the molecular pathogenesis of OC continues to mature, it is likely that the various OC subsets will increasingly be thought of as distinct entities with respect to diagnosis, treatment, and prevention. In view of this, each of the subtypes is discussed separately in the subsequent section.

OVARIAN CANCER GENETICS AND GENOMICS

HGSC is characterized by the nearly ubiquitous presence of TP53 mutations (4,14-16). Missense or nonsense mutations of TP53 are considered the earliest molecular event in high-grade serous carcinogenesis. A schematic of the common alterations in HGSOC is shown in **Figure 8.4-2**.

BRCA1 is an essential factor in the repair of DNA double-strand breaks. Double-strand breaks are the most cytotoxic DNA lesions because they cause full disruption of a chromosome, possibly leading to deletions, insertions, duplications, and translocations of chromosomes (17). It has been long recognized that approximately

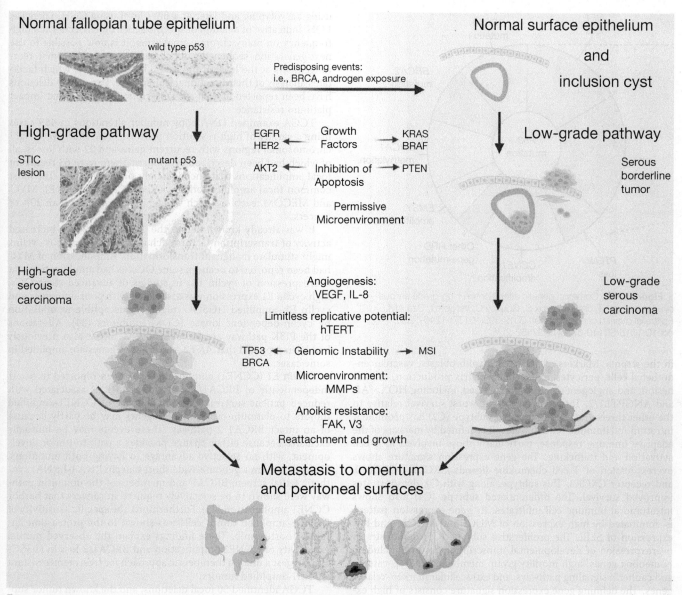

Figure 8.4-1. Molecular changes leading to low- and high-grade ovarian cancer. Schematic. STIC, serous tubal intraepithelial carcinoma.

12% to 15% of HGSCs occur in patients with germline mutations in *BRCA1* and *BRCA2* genes. Recent studies showed that up to 50% of HGSCs are related to inactivation of *BRCA1/2* genes by either germline or somatic mutation, or through epigenetic mechanisms. The term *BRCAness* is applied to these tumors that share deficient homologous recombination DNA repair pathways, leading to marked genomic instability. The cases with high levels of genomic aberrations have been shown to have improved survival, at least in the short term (18). The impaired HR is thought to be responsible for superior sensitivity to platinum-based chemotherapy. Interesting, some of this advantage may be lost over time, when 10-year survival is examined. One study demonstrated a lower 10-year survival (25%) than noncarriers (30%), with a long-term advantage to BRCA2 carriers (35%) (19).

A majority of alterations of *BRCA1/2* genes are truncating mutations; however, a small proportion of missense mutations have been described in cases with somatic mutations (20). The data regarding a favorable outcome in BRCA-deficient patients are somewhat conflicting as some studies have shown that BRCA2, but not BRCA1, deficiency is associated with improved survival and chemotherapy response (21). Some studies also suggest that the

survival benefits seen early are no longer seen 10 to 15 years after diagnosis (19).

The primary molecular insult attributable to OC is global chromosomal instability. Point mutations in oncogenes and tumor suppressor genes other than *TP53*, *BRCA1*, and *BRCA2* are relatively uncommon in HGSC (4). However, structural variations (gains and losses due to increased or decreased copy number) are frequent, resulting in a chromosomally unstable or C-class malignancy (dominated by copy number changes) (22). A large study of the gene expression patterns in a cohort of ovarian that included HGSCs, endometrioid carcinoma, as well as a group of borderline tumors described six groups (C1-C6) with distinct expression profiles (23). All borderline tumors clustered into the C3 subtype. Group C6 was composed almost exclusively of endometrioid carcinomas of low and intermediate grades. HGSCs, along with some high- and intermediate-grade endometrioid carcinoma, were distributed over four groups (C1, C2, C4, and C5). TCGA initiative validated these findings and termed the expression profile-based subtypes of HGSC as *Immunoreactive, Differentiated, Proliferative, and Mesenchymal* (4). The mesenchymal subtype (C1) is characterized by extensive stromal desmoplasia and immune cell infiltration

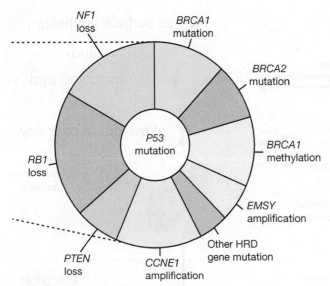

Figure 8.4-2. Common genetic alterations in high-grade serous ovarian cancer. (From Lheureux S, Gourley C, Vergote I, Oza AM. Epithelial ovarian cancer. *Lancet*. 2019;393(10177):1240-1253. doi:10.1016/S0140-6736(18)32552-2)

in the stroma. Markers of activated myofibroblasts, vascular endothelial cells, pericytes, extracellular matrix production, cell adhesion, and angiogenesis are overexpressed, including HOX, FAP, and ANGPTL1/2. This subtype has the worst survival relative to the other three. The immunoreactive subtype (C2) has prominent intratumoral immune cell infiltrates. It is defined by markers of the adaptive immune response, particularly those involved in T-cell activation and trafficking. The gene expression signature shows overexpression of T-cell chemokine ligands CXCL11, CXCL10, and receptor CXCR3. This subtype, along with C4, demonstrates improved survival. The differentiated subtype (C4) also shows intratumoral immune cell infiltrates. Its gene expression pattern is dominated by high expression of MUC1 and MUC16 and low expression of SLPI. The proliferative subtype (C5) demonstrates overexpression of developmental transcription factors, including homeobox genes, high motility group members, WNT/β-catenin and cadherin signaling pathways, and extracellular marker–related genes. The defining gene expression signature consists of high expression of HMGA2, SOX11, MCM2, and PCN and low expression of MUC1 and MUC16.

In addition to describing four subtypes of OC based on expression profiles, TCGA integrated analysis, including mutations, expression profiling, and amplification/deletions identified the most frequent pathways perturbed in some way. The most important of these was the observation that up to 50% of patients with OC have some abnormity in homologous recombination (**Figure 8.4-2**), which has become increasing important as the use of PARPi is much more effective in patients with this abnormality, whether acquired through inherited defects or somatically derived.

HIGH-GRADE SEROUS OVARIAN CANCER

HGSOC was the second cancer analyzed in the TCGA project (4). This comprehensive genomic analysis confirmed prior findings; most notably, these cancers are characterized by a high degree of genomic instability with many copy number alterations and inactivation of TP53 and BRCA1/2 and other genes in the HR DNA repair pathway. Some previously unreported alterations also were discovered. This section puts the TCGA data in perspective with prior studies.

Most HGSOCs have extensive genetic instability. Initially, gains and losses of various segments of the genome were demonstrated

using karyotyping and later at a finer level using CGH. Likewise, LOH, indicative of deletion of specific genetic loci, occurs at a high frequency on many chromosomal arms. It is now possible to use next-generation sequencing to characterize chromosomal rearrangements at the level of the actual base sequence, which facilitates analysis of their functional significance. Large gene deletions have been reported as well as transcriptional fusions that impact platinum resistance.

TCGA examined DNA copy number alterations in 489 cases using a variety of high-resolution platforms (4). There were eight chromosomal regions with recurrent gains and 22 with losses, all of which had been described previously. There were 63 recurrent focal amplifications that encoded eight or fewer genes. The most common focal amplifications included CCNE1 (cyclin E), MYC, and MECOM, each of which was amplified in more than 20% of cancers.

It was already known before the TCGA study that increased activity of transcription factors such as MYC and various cyclins might stimulate malignant transformation. Amplification of MYC had been reported to occur in some OCs, as had amplification and overexpression of cyclin E1. In studies of advanced-stage OCs, high cyclin E1 expression was associated with poor outcomes and cyclin E1–amplified HGSOC might be susceptible to inhibition by cyclin-dependent kinase (CDK) inhibitors (24). Alterations of the PI3K pathway are frequent in OC, and it also previously had been reported that AKT2 and PIK3CA genes are amplified in some cases.

Cyclin E1 (CCNE1) amplification has been reported to occur independently of BRCA1/2 mutation, and it is associated with reduced patient survival. The insensitivity of CCNE1-amplified tumors to platinum cross-linking agents may be partly because of an intact BRCA1/2 pathway. These events may be mutually exclusive because either change provides a path to tumor development, with no selective advantage to having both mutations. Using data from a genome-wide short hairpin RNA (shRNA) synthetic lethal screen, BRCA1 and members of the ubiquitin pathway were shown to be selectively required in cancers that harbor CCNE1 amplification (25). Furthermore, the specific sensitivity of CCNE1-amplified tumor cells was shown to the proteasome inhibitor bortezomib. These findings explain the observed mutual exclusivity of CCNE1 amplification and BRCA1/2 loss in HGSCs and suggest a unique therapeutic approach for treatment-resistant CCNE1-amplified tumors.

TCGA identified 50 focal deletions, and the known tumor suppressor genes PTEN, RB, and NF1 were deleted, albeit only in a small fraction of cases. The latter two genes also were targeted by mutations, consistent with the two-hit paradigm of tumor suppressor gene inactivation. Although mutations in the RB1 tumor suppressor gene are not a common feature of OCs, evidence suggests that the inactivation of RB1 greatly enhances tumor formation in the presence of TP53 mutations (26). HGSOC exhibits RB1 and NF1 loss due to gene breakage (~15%). Many other candidate genes are in regions that are recurrently amplified or deleted in HGSOCs, most notably amplified regions of *1p23.2, 3q29, 8q24.3, 12q.13.11,* and *19q13.2,* and deleted regions of *1q36.11, 4q34.3, 5q13.1, 6q27, 15q15.1, 18q23,* and *22q13.33.* Considerable effort will be required to elucidate which of these represent driver events in some cancers, as opposed to alterations of no consequence for tumorigenesis or progression.

Cancer is characterized by the rapid, uncontrolled proliferation of cells usurping the cell cycle machinery responsible for controlled cell division, which is tightly regulated by proliferative and antiproliferative signals. In principle, the cell cycle is regulated through the interaction of serine/threonine CDKs and cyclins. The cell cycle is initiated by cyclin D1-D3, which forms a complex with and activates CDK4/6. This leads to the phosphorylation of RB1, removing the inhibitory control of the E2F transcription factor on E-type cyclins that drives the G_1- to S-phase transition. The negative regulation of CDK4/6 activity is mediated by the INK4 family of cell cycle inhibitors (INK4B: p16 encoded by *CDKN2A* gene). CDK inhibitors like p16 inhibit cyclinD-CDK4/6 function through binding to CDK4/6, thereby preventing premature entry into S phase. The cdk inhibitors act as tumor suppressors by virtue of their inhibition of cell cycle progression from G1 to S phase. The expression of several cdk inhibitors appears to be decreased in some OCs. CDKN2A (p16) undergoes homozygous deletions, and CDKN2A and CDKN2B (p15) may be inactivated via transcriptional silencing due to promoter methylation rather than mutation and/or deletion. Likewise, decreased expression of the p21/WAF1 cdk inhibitor has been noted in a significant fraction of OCs despite the absence of inactivating mutations. Loss of p27 (CDKN1B) also may occur and correlates with poor survival in some studies (27). It has been suggested that aberrant expression of p27 in the cytoplasm may be most associated with poor outcome (28). Treatment of preclinical OC models with ribociclib, a CDK4/6 inhibitor, inhibited the proliferation of several OC cell lines and worked synergistically with cisplatin (29), and a phase I study showed some surprising responses using the CDK4/6 inhibitor ribociclib with carboplatin and paclitaxel (30).

The TCGA performed sequencing of the coding regions and splice sites of approximately 18,500 genes in DNA isolated initially from 316 HGSOCs. The extent of this sequencing effort in OC was unprecedented and would not have been possible without the recent development of massively parallel next-generation sequencing technologies. Although several genes are mutated at low frequencies, *TP53* and *BRCA1/2* were confirmed to be the most frequently mutated genes in high-grade OCs (**Figure 8.4-3**).

Studies validated the prior finding that mutation of the *TP53* tumor suppressor gene is the most frequent genetic event in HGSOCs (4,14,15). About two-thirds of HGSOCs have TP53 missense mutations in the DNA-binding regions of exons 5 through 8 that result in p53 protein overexpression due to increased protein stability. Codons 175, 248, and 273 are mutational hot spots. Owing to their nonfunctional transcriptional activity, these missense mutants act as dominant negative transforming genes. Loss of the other copy of the *TP53* gene is not required. Interestingly, in subsequent ultra-sensitive sequencing studies, *TP53* mutations can even be found in normal tissue and in fluids, even from newborns, and increase in frequency with age (31). It may be that, like with BRCA, the fallopian tube is particularly susceptible to malignant transformation when P53 is mutated, more so than other tissues. This also carries implications for attempts to use P53 as a biomarker for early detection in low-invasive fluids.

Although genetic alterations are at the heart of carcinogenesis, the most important aspect of tumor behavior is at the protein level. An integrative analysis of sequence, mRNA, and proteomic expression identified multiple pathways critical to carcinogenesis: DNA replication, cell-cell communications, cytokine signaling, erythrocytes/platelets, extracellular matrix, the complement cascade, and metabolism (14). Survival outcomes could also be predicted by specific proteomic signatures, and elements of these signatures could be used in the future as a biomarker.

TP53 mutations are early events that are found in the earliest premailgnant lesions in the fallopian tube. In pioneering work, P53 protein overexpression (as a result of a cell increasing P53 production because the protein product is functionally ineffective) was noted in both invasive cells and premalignant STIC lesions. More importantly, through laser microdissection of the STIC and invasive portions in the same patient, the exact same P53 mutations were identified in the distinct tissues (**Figure 8.4-4**) (32,33).

Most HGSOCs that do not overexpress p53 protein have *TP53* null mutations that result in truncated protein products (34). These are usually accompanied by loss of the other copy of the gene, consistent with the classic two-hit model of tumor suppressor gene inactivation. The TCGA study reported *TP53* mutations in more than 95% of samples, suggesting that this is essentially a requisite event in the development of these cancers. Subsequent pathology

review of the few cases lacking mutations found that these were probably not HGSCs (4).

miRNAs play an important role in the initiation and progression of HGSOC. The Let-7 family induces the DNA-binding factor HMGA2, which regulates chromatin conformation, thereby regulating many genes. Indeed, overexpression of HMGA2 correlates with survival and is associated with poorly associated tumors (35).

BRCA1 and BRCA2. BRCA1 and BRCA2 germline mutations were found in 9% and 8% of high-grade serous cases, respectively, in the TCGA study, and somatic mutations in each gene occurred in an additional 3% (4). Silencing of BRCA1 due to promoter methylation was observed in 11% of cases. Defective HR repair of double-stranded DNA damage due to loss of BRCA1/2 was predicted in 31% of HGSOCs. Other genes in the HR pathway are inactivated in some cancers, and the HR pathway may be compromised in approximately half of all cases. A subsequent analysis of germline and somatic alterations in TCGA ovarian carcinoma cases suggests that truncation variants and large deletions exist across Fanconi pathway genes in 20% of cases (36).

Patients with HGSC associated with BRCA1 or BRCA2 mutations have increased sensitivity to platinum chemotherapy and favorable survival relative to sporadic cases. More recently, studies have suggested that the initial favorable outcome seen in BRCA1/2 carriers does not persist with longer follow-up (37). The emergence of platinum resistance in these cancers may occur due to "revertant mutations" in which the normal BRCA1 or BRCA2 sequence is restored (38).

Cancers with defects in the double-stranded DNA HR repair pathway can be targeted effectively by inducing a second hit in the form of inhibition of the single-stranded DNA repair pathway. This concept of synthetic lethality—the combination of two genetic alterations, which on their own are nonlethal, but together result in a lethal phenotype—led to an interest in inhibitors of enzymes such as PARP that are involved in single-stranded base excision repair. Inhibition of PARP leads to the persistence of DNA lesions normally repaired by HR and makes HR-deficient cells particularly sensitive to chemotherapy-induced DNA injury. PARPi are selective for cells with defects in the repair of double-strand DNA breaks by HR, particularly in the context of BRCA1 or BRCA2 mutation. While normal cells can repair the damage and survive, the BRCA-deficient cells cannot activate the HR system and, therefore, die (17).

While only about 20% of HGSOCs have germline BRCA1 or BRCA2 mutations, sporadic OCs can harbor acquired genetic and epigenetic defects in BRCA1/2 and in other HR genes and proteins, such as *RAD51C/D*, *PALB2*, and *BRIP1*, that may contribute to a "BRCAness profile". Given the shared role that *BRCA1* and *BRCA2* have with other DNA repair genes, defects in these genes lead to severe chromosomal instability, which influences recurrence rates and may increase sensitivity to platinum drugs and PARPi. Of concern is that with more frequent use of PARPi, resistance has become a significant clinical problem. Several cancer cell defense mechanisms contribute to resistance, including (a) the ability to get into the cancer cell, (b) the activity and abundance of PAR chains, (c) reactivation of homologous recombination, and (d) protection of the replication fork (**Figure 8.4-5**) (17).

Investigators with the Australian Ovarian Cancer Study performed whole-genome sequencing of tumor and germline DNA from 92 patients with primary refractory, resistant, sensitive, and matched acquired resistant disease (39). It was shown that gene breakage commonly inactivates the tumor suppressors *RB1*, *NF1*, *RAD51B*, and *PTEN* and contributes to acquired chemotherapy resistance. CCNE1 amplification was common in primary resistant and refractory diseases. Several molecular events were associated with acquired resistance, including multiple independent reversions of germline BRCA1 or BRCA2 mutations in individual patients, loss of BRCA1 promoter methylation, an alteration in molecular subtype, and recurrent promoter fusion associated with overexpression of the drug efflux pump MDR1. Clonal evolution

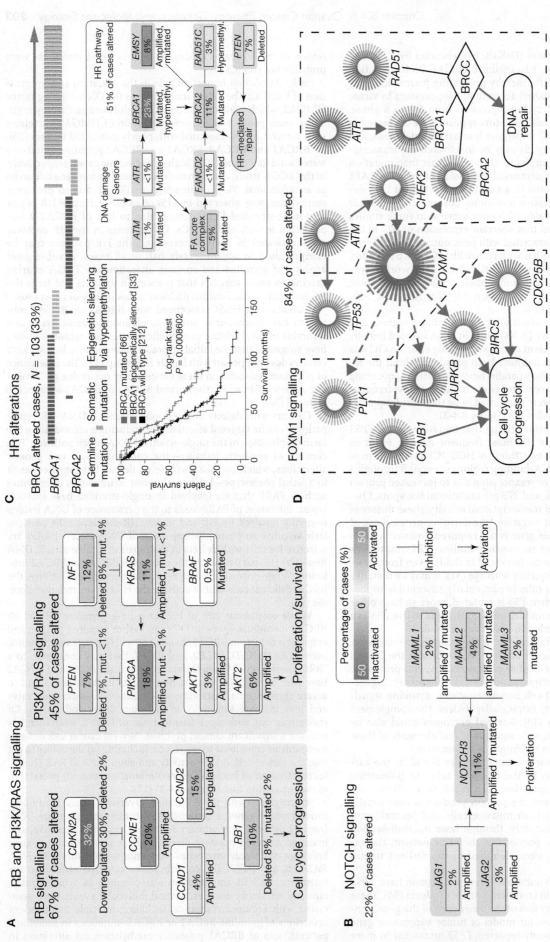

Figure 8.4-3. Altered pathways in HGS-OvCa, identified by curated analysis, and (B) NOTCH pathway, identified by HotNet analysis, are commonly altered. Alterations are defined by somatic mutations, DNA copy number changes, or, in some cases, by significant upregulation or downregulation compared to expression in diploid tumors. Alteration frequencies are in percentage of all cases; activated genes are in red, inactivated genes are in blue. (C) Genes in the HR pathway are altered in up to 49% of cases. Survival analysis of BRCA status shows divergent outcome for BRCA mutated cases (exhibiting better overall survival) than BRCA wild type, and BRCA1 epigenetically silenced cases exhibiting worse survival. (D) The FOXM1 transcription factor network is activated in 87% of cases. Each gene is depicted as a multiring circle in which its copy number (outer ring) and gene expression (inner ring) are plotted such that each "spoke" in the ring represents a single patient sample, with samples sorted in increasing order of FOXM1 expression. Excitatory (red arrows) and inhibitory interactions (blue lines) were taken from the NCI Pathway Interaction Database. Dashed lines indicate transcriptional regulation. (Reprinted by permission from Springer: Cancer Genome Atlas Research Network. Integrated genomic analyses of ovarian carcinoma [published correction appears in Nature. 2012;490(7419):298]. *Nature.* 2011;474(7353):609–615. doi:10.1038/nature10166)

304

INV
p53
Fimbria
A
B
T
T
T
OVARY
TIC
INV
TIC
C
D
E

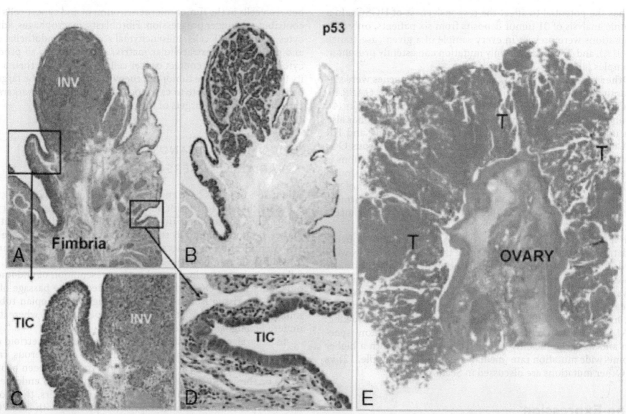

■ **Figure 8.4-4.** Coexisting serous carcinomas on the tubal fimbria (A-D) and ovarian surface (E). A microscopic focus of intraepithelial (TIC) and invasive fallopian tube carcinoma involving the fimbria (A, INV) exhibits strong p53 immunostaining (B). The invasive portion (INV) is flanked by TIC (C and D). One of the ovaries (E) is shown, exhibiting the largest tumor mass on the surface (T). (From Kindelberger DW, Lee Y, Miron A, et al. Intraepithelial carcinoma of the fimbria and pelvic serous carcinoma: evidence for a causal relationship. *Am J Surg Pathol*. 2007;31(2):161-169. doi:10.1097/01.pas.0000213335.40358.47)

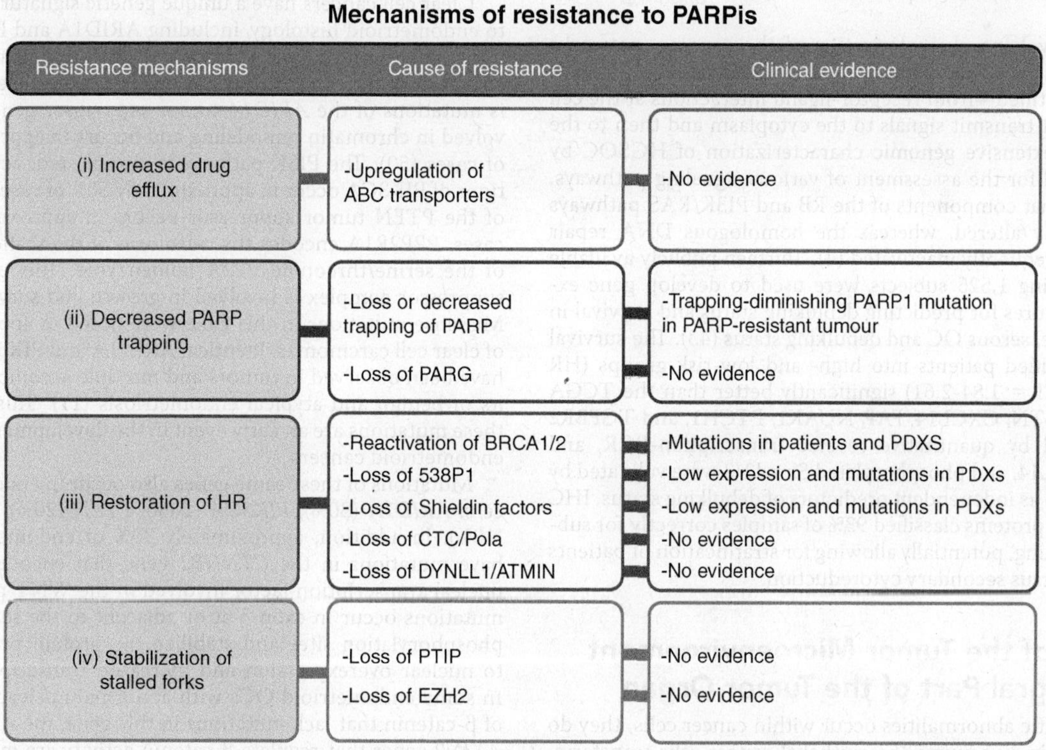

Mechanisms of resistance to PARPis
Resistance mechanisms
Cause of resistance
Clinical evidence
(i) Increased drug efflux
-Upregulation of ABC transporters
-No evidence
(ii) Decreased PARP trapping
-Loss or decreased trapping of PARP
-Trapping-diminishing PARP1 mutation in PARP-resistant tumour
-Loss of PARG
-No evidence
(iii) Restoration of HR
-Reactivation of BRCA1/2
-Mutations in patients and PDXS
-Loss of 538P1
-Low expression and mutations in PDXs
-Loss of Shieldin factors
-Low expression and mutations in PDXs
-Loss of CTC/Pola
-No evidence
-Loss of DYNLL1/ATMIN
-No evidence
(iv) Stabilization of stalled forks
-Loss of PTIP
-No evidence
-Loss of EZH2
-No evidence
Trends in Cell Biology
Sylvie M. Noordermeer, Haico van Aikum. Trends in Cell Biology, 2019, 29(10), 820-834.

■ **Figure 8.4-5.** Mechanisms of PARP inhibitor resistance. (From Noordermeer, S. M. and H. van Attikum (2019). "PARP Inhibitor Resistance: A Tug-of-War in BRCA-Mutated Cells." *Trends Cell Biol* 29(10): 820-834.)

also has the potential to affect the responsiveness of HGSCs. In a genomic analysis of 31 tumor deposits from six patients, only 52% of mutations were present in every sample of a given case (range 10%-91%), and *TP53* was the only mutation consistently present in all samples (40).

Other mutations. In the TCGA study, six other genes were significantly mutated, including *RB1, NF1, FAT3, CSMD3, GABRA6,* and *CDK12*, but none was mutated in more than 6% of cancers (4). *RB1* and *NF1* are tumor suppressor genes, whereas *CDK12* has also been implicated in both the regulation of RNA splicing and HR DNA repair. *FAT3* and *GABRA6* are not expressed in serous OCs or in the fallopian tube, and the significance of these mutations is unclear. A number of other known oncogenic mutations were found in KRAS, NRAS, PIK3CA, and BRAF, but at low frequencies of less than 1%. These mutations have been shown to have transforming activity and probably represent important drivers of some cancers but may highlight cases misdiagnosed as high-grade serous.

In a subsequent analysis of the TCGA whole-exome sequencing data, mutations of eight members of the ADAMTS family were noted in 10.4% of cases and were associated with a significantly higher chemotherapy sensitivity and better overall survival (OS) (58 vs 41.3 months) (41). ADAMTS family members are metalloproteases that play roles in cell adhesion, migration, blood clotting, inflammation, angiogenesis, and connective tissue modeling. ADAMTS-mutated cases exhibited a distinct mutation spectrum and were significantly associated with tumors with a higher genome-wide mutation rate (median mutations per sample, 121 vs 69). Other mutations are discussed in Section 2 (42).

Gene Expression

Microarray chips that contain sequences complementary to thousands of genes have been created that allow global assessment of the level of expression of each gene. More recently, RNA sequencing has become technically feasible at a reasonable cost, provides a more accurate and direct representation of gene expression, and is replacing microarrays as the preferred method for gene expression quantification.

With the evolving characterization of the genome, networks of molecular signals that regulate cellular proliferation and death have been identified—from receptor-ligand interactions at the cell membrane that transmit signals to the cytoplasm and then to the nucleus. The extensive genomic characterization of HGSOC by TCGA allowed for the assessment of various signaling pathways. It was found that components of the RB and PI3K/RAS pathways were frequently altered, whereas the homologous DNA repair pathway was frequently inactivated (4). Thirteen publicly available data sets totaling 1,525 subjects were used to develop gene expression signatures for predicting debulking status and survival in advanced-stage, serous OC and debulking status (43). The survival signature stratified patients into high- and low-risk groups (HR = 2.19; 95% CI = 1.84-2.61) significantly better than the TCGA signature. POSTN, CXCL14, FAP, NUAK1, PTCH1, and TGFBR2 were validated by quantitative reverse transcription-PCR, and POSTN, CXCL14, and phosphorylated Smad2/3 were validated by IHC ($P < .001$) as independent predictors of debulking status. IHC for these three proteins classified 93% of samples correctly for suboptimal debulking, potentially allowing for stratification of patients for primary versus secondary cytoreduction.

The Role of the Tumor Microenvironment as an Integral Part of the Tumor Organ

Although genetic abnormalities occur within cancer cells, they do not live alone in a vacuum. The epithelial cancer cells transform, grow, and metastasize within the surrounding microenvironment, and there is a crosstalk between them. Although it is difficult to discern whether the microenvironment plays an initiating or permissive role in carcinogenesis, there is most definitively crosstalk between cells in the tumor microenvironment and cancer cells that contribute to cancer progression. Fibroblasts, macrophages, adipocytes, regulatory T cells, mesenchymal stem cells, endothelial cells and pericytes, the extracellular matrix, and exosomes all produce cytokines or directly contact cancer cells and modulate their activity (44,45). Cells in the tumor microenvironment could be targeted because they contribute to carcinogenesis, serve as biomarkers for early detection, and targets of therapy.

ENDOMETRIOID AND CLEAR CELL OVARIAN CANCERS

About 20% of EOCs have endometrioid or clear cell histology, and these are thought to arise in pelvic endometriosis, on the ovary, or in the pelvic peritoneum. This presumption is based on the pattern of spread (more commonly stage I or II primarily involving the pelvis), identification of adjacent endometriosis tissue, and common molecular alterations between cancer and endometriosis (46). The fallopian tube is also implicated in the presentation of endometrioid and clear cell OCs, which are attributed to the passage of endometriosis tissue from the uterus through the fallopian tube to implant on the surface of the ovary or the peritoneum, where it can undergo malignant transformation.

In general, clear cell cancers and low-grade endometrioid cancers have less genetic instability than high-grade serous cases. Ovarian endometrioid and clear cell subtypes have been profiled based on the TCGA-identified subtypes identified for endometrial cancers of the uterus. Similar to endometrial cancers, these ovarian subtypes follow a similar expression pattern, with rare POLE mutations, some MSI-high tumors, and more frequent P53 mutations, but most with no specific molecular profile. The clinical prognosis for these subtypes also follows what is seen in uterine endometrial cancers in that those with POLE mutations have an excellent prognosis and those with *TP53* mutations having a poor prognosis (47).

Clear cell cancers have a unique genetic signature as compared to endometrioid histology, including ARID1A and PIK3CA mutations, and even an increased rate of expression of histone-modifying enzymes (48,49). The most common alteration in clear cell cancers is mutations of the *ARID1A* tumor suppressor gene, which is involved in chromatin remodeling and occurs in approximately 50% of cases (50). The PI3K pathway is also altered; activating mutations of PIK3CA occur in approximately 50% of cases, and deletion of the PTEN tumor suppressor occurs in approximately 20% of cases. PPP2R1A encodes the α-isoform of the scaffolding subunit of the serine/threonine PP2A holoenzyme. This putative tumor suppressor complex is involved in growth and survival pathways. Missense mutations in this gene were noted in approximately 5% of clear cell carcinomas. Identical ARID1A and PIK3CA mutations have been observed in tumors and multiple accompanying deposits of benign and atypical endometriosis (11). This suggests that these mutations are an early event in the development of clear cell/endometrioid cancers.

Mutations of these same genes also occur in endometrioid cancers: *ARID1A* (30%), *PIK3CA* (20%), *PTEN* (20%), and *PPP2R1A* (10%). In addition, approximately 30% of endometrioid cancers have mutations in the *CTNNB1* gene that encodes β-catenin, a nuclear transcription factor involved in the WNT pathway. These mutations occur in exon 3 at or adjacent to the serine/threonine phosphorylation sites and stabilize the protein product, leading to nuclear overexpression and increased transcriptional activity. In some endometrioid OCs with abnormal nuclear accumulation of β-catenin that lack mutations in this gene, the *APC, AXIN1*, or *AXIN2* genes that regulate β-catenin activity are mutated (51). In general, endometrioid OCs have specific molecular signatures that overlap with endometrioid uterine cancer. This suggests that in addition to the mutations that are also present in clear cell cancers, endometrioid cancers frequently have alterations in the WNT signaling pathway. Mouse models in which the WNT and the PI3K/ PTEN pathways are inactivated lead to the development of endometriosis and endometrioid cancers (52). Although endometrioid OCs are believed to arise from ectopic endometrium, and there is considerable overlap in pathogenic mutations, the frequency of mutations differs between endometrioid OCs and endometrioid endometrial cancers.

In one comparative study, PTEN mutations were more frequent in low-grade endometrial endometrioid carcinomas (67%) compared with low-grade ovarian endometrioid carcinomas (17%) (53). In contrast, CTNNB1 mutations were significantly more common in low-grade ovarian endometrioid carcinomas (53%) compared with low-grade endometrial endometrioid carcinomas (28%). High-grade endometrioid OCs typically have molecular features similar to HGSOCs, including genetic instability and TP53 mutations. These tumor types may be difficult to classify by pathologists based on light microscopy.

An integrated molecular profile of endometrioid cancers was reported in 2020 (51). In addition to previously reported upregulation of characteristic oncogenes, they found that a subset of tumors harbors p53 mutations, homologous recombination deficiency (HRD), and widespread copy number variation. This subtype may carry the most heterogeneity of origin of any of the OC subtypes, highlighting the importance of profiling patients for emerging therapeutics.

Proteomic analysis of ovarian clear cell carcinomas demonstrates distinct active pathways compared to other high-grade OCs, with alterations in lipid and purine metabolism and the complement system (54). Distinctive pathways between clear cell and endometrioid subtypes were identified as well—although this is not definitive for a difference in etiology, it does suggest a variance in their evolution to cancer and may be responsible for the increased chemoresistance seen in clear cell cancers. Four distinct subgroups could be identified among clear cell tumors, with associated differences in clinical outcome.

In another transcriptomic analysis of a cohort of Chinese patients, clear cell cancers could be separated into immune (22%) and nonimmune (78%) (55). The immune group was enriched in PD-1 expression, which may have implications for the efficacy of checkpoint inhibitors, as well as angiogenesis and PI3K-AKT-mTOR signaling. The nonimmune clear cell cancer group was characterized predominantly by upregulation of metabolic pathways.

The molecular profiling of endometrioid and clear cell subtypes has been exploited in drug development, with small molecule inhibitors generated against the WNT pathway and ARID1A, with clinical trials ongoing.

SYNCHRONOUS ENDOMETRIOID OVARIAN AND ENDOMETRIAL CANCERS

Synchronous endometrioid cancers of the ovary and uterus are sometimes encountered in the endometrium and ovary and are indistinguishable microscopically. Based on pathology review, these tumors are diagnosed as synchronous cancers. However, molecular data strongly suggest that most endometrioid OCs are likely metastases from endometrial primaries and are clonally related: Both the ovarian and endometrioid tumors had similar repertoires of somatic mutations and gene copy number alterations, indicating that they are clonally related and likely constitute metastasis from one side to the other (56,57). The sporadic nonsynonymous mutations (which change protein sequences) found in both the ovarian and endometrial tumors included PTEN, PIK3CA, K-ras, ARID1A, and CTNNB1 (β-catenin). In general, the molecular profiles of synchronous endometrioid ovarian/uterine cancer are very similar to endometrioid endometrial cancer as defined by the TCGA (58,59). This implies that the endometrium could be the origin of most synchronous cases rather than the ovary. One exception is ovarian tumors with a TP53 mutation, which is rare in endometrioid endometrial cancer.

BORDERLINE AND INVASIVE LOW-GRADE SEROUS OVARIAN CANCERS

Similar to HGSCs, it is thought that borderline cancer and LGSC likely arise from fallopian tube epithelium. However, LGSCs have a distinct biology and clinical behavior. They are characterized by younger average age, indolent clinical course, and long-term survival but relative chemotherapy resistance. The underlying genetic alterations in borderline and low-grade tumors are different from those of high-grade cancers. Almost all LGSCs express the ER, whereas progesterone receptor (PR) expression is more variable (25%-50%) (60). LGSCs have a low somatic mutation burden and always a low HRD score, suggesting that they are distinct entities rather than a single disease with varying degrees of differentiation (61). Moreover, LGSC rarely expresses PD-L1 and are MSI-stable (60). It is, therefore, unlikely that immune checkpoint inhibitors are effective in LGSOC.

LGSCs have frequent copy number loss on chromosome 1p and homozygous deletion of the CDKN2A/2b genetic locus, a cell cycle inhibitor discussed earlier (60,62). An additional frequent gene mutation is USP9X, a ubiquitin specific protease playing a role in tissue hemostasis, mTOR regulation, which acts as a tumor suppressor gene in the context of LGSC. Mutations in USP9X are also not seen in HGSOC. Mutations in USP9X and EIF1AX are associated with the mTOR pathway found in LGSC and may represent drivers of progression from SBT to LGSC. Compared to SBTs, LGSC copy number alterations include loss of 9p, homozygous deletion of the CDKN2A/2B locus, and hemizygous deletion of 1p36 (62,63). These copy number changes have been suggested as another potential mechanism of progression.

The MAPK pathway, which regulates cell proliferation and migration through a sequence of phosphorylated proteins, is one of the characteristic features of LGSC. Activating mutations in codons 12 and 13 of the KRAS oncogene are common in SBTs, occurring in about 25% to 50% of cases but also in some LGSOCs (64). In addition, the activating mutation V600E in the BRAF gene, which is a downstream effector of KRAS, occurs in about 20% of SBT (65). Mutations in KRAS and BRAF have also been noted in benign epithelial cysts adjacent to SBTs, suggesting that this is an early event in their development. Mutations in these MAPK genes are mutually exclusive and result in constitutive activation of the MAPK pathway in 47% of LGSCs (27% K-RAS, 13% B-RAF, 9% N-RAS) (61). Patients with MAPK mutations have a significantly longer PFS (32 vs 24 months) and OS (48 vs 90 months) compared to those without an MAPK mutation (60). In contrast, HGSC very rarely has mutations in the MAPK pathway. Inhibition of MEK, which is part of the MAPK cascade with trametinib, has shown clinical activity, with a recent trial in patients with recurrent disease demonstrating a meaningful increase in PFS compared to standard of care (median PFS 13.0 vs 7.2 months) (66). Interestingly, PFS did not correlate with mutations status (about 30% mutation rate in both groups), although overall response rate (ORR) was higher in patients with KRAS, BRAF, or NRAS mutations (50% vs 9%, $P = .11$). The independence of response to an MEK inhibitor from MAPK mutation status was confirmed in a parallel study (60).

The gene expression pattern of low-grade endometrioid tumors clustered into a distinct C6 subtype and is characterized by low expression of proliferation markers (KI67, TOP2A, CCNB1, CDC2, and KIF11) and overexpression of transcriptional targets of the β-catenin complex correlating with the presence of β-catenin mutations and reflecting deregulation of the WNT signaling pathway (23).

MUCINOUS OVARIAN CANCER

Historically, mucinous OCs were often misdiagnosed as metastases from the GI tract. However, some mucinous carcinomas clearly arise from the ovary, perhaps from mucinous cystadenomas, mucinous borderline tumors (MBTs), or teratomas (dermoid cysts).

The data on molecular genetic profiles of mucinous carcinomas are relatively limited. Some studies have demonstrated KRAS mutations in more than half of MBTs and mucinous carcinomas and are missense changes in the hotspot codons (67). Identical KRAS mutations have been found in mucinous carcinomas and adjacent mucinous cystadenomas and borderline tumors, suggesting that the latter lesions represent premalignant precursors. Exhaustive exome sequencing analysis of these tumors revealed mutations in known drivers, such as KRAS, BRAF, and CDKN2A (13). In addition, a high percentage of mucinous ovarian carcinomas had TP53 mutations (52%), and recurrent mutations were found in RNF43, ELF3, GNAS, ERBB3, and KLF5. Another targeted sequencing study in mucinous tumors found similar results with mutations in KRAS, TP53, CDKN2A, PIK3CA, PTEN, BRAF, FGFR2, STK11, CTNNB1, SRC, SMAD4, GNA11, and ERBB2 (68). Proven and potential RAS pathway–activating changes were observed in all but one case, suggesting the potential of targeting this pathway.

Molecular analyses of mucinous cystadenomas, mucinous borderline, and mucinous OCs support an evolution from benign to borderline to malignant transformation at the mutation and chromosomal aberration level (13). Early events appear to be KRAS or CDKN2A mutations, as they are noted even in benign specimens, with increasing chromosomal instability and copy number alterations as tumors transition to a malignant phenotype.

Anglesio et al demonstrated HER2/neu (ERBB2) amplification in 18% of mucinous carcinomas and a smaller proportion (6%) of MBTs. Anecdotal responses to trastuzumab have been reported in patients with HER2/neu-amplified tumors (69).

FUTURE DIRECTIONS

The availability of new molecular profiling platforms of multiple targets (DNA, RNA, protein, epigenetic) has exponentially increased our understanding of the genetic and epigenetic perturbations, leading to OC carcinogenesis. Developing technologies such as single-cell sequencing may shed additional light on the genetic chaos and evolution of heterogeneous tumors. Evaluation of not just the cancer cells themselves, but the surrounding nonmalignant cells, such as inflammatory and vascular components, should be undertaken to understand the complexity of the entire tumor microenvironment. The next frontier in understanding OC is to obtain a compartmental resolved characterization of gene and protein expression. Novel methods like spatial transcriptomics and proteomics as well as spatial epigenetic information that gives cues to chromatin accessibility by transcription factors will allow to identify the specific gene/protein expression for every single cell in the tumor organ (70,71). Single-cell sequencing studies in OC have demonstrated not only heterogeneity among cancer specimens but even among benign fallopian tube epithelium, potentially allowing for biomarker discovery of risk and a better understanding of the immune landscape of serous OC (72,73).

The identification of the fallopian tube as the primary site of origin of the ovarian family of cancers, at least of the serous subtype, has led to new opportunities for prevention and early detection. Removal of the fallopian tubes during concomitant gynecologic cancers will likely reduce the incidence in the coming years, given the encouraging data from Canada (74). In addition, ubiquitous germline genetic screening and genomic somatic characterization of every OC will identify high-risk patients and allow tailoring treatment.

An understanding of the differences between OC subtypes requires that these entities be studied separately rather than grouped together as a single disease. Although the fallopian tube is the likely origin of serous cancer, there are many cases in which there is an alternate pathway to carcinogenesis. Profiling studies often do not have corresponding clinical information, which is required to understand which molecular changes are clinically important as biomarkers relevant to prognosis, treatments, and outcomes. This includes the oncologic outcome and preexisting risk factors such as concurrent diseases and medication use (ie, aspirin) that may confer risk or differential response to treatment. Prospective collection of both clinical information and molecular profiling is necessary to fully understand the spectrum of this disease. Translational end points should be incorporated into all clinical trials so that biomarkers of response can be identified to individualize treatment. Again, collaborative efforts to pool similar samples, especially of the rare subtypes, are urgently needed (75).

REFERENCES

1. Auersperg N. The origin of ovarian cancers-hypotheses and controversies. *Front Biosci.* 2013;5:709-719.
2. Rebbeck TR, Kauff ND, Domchek SM. Meta-analysis of risk reduction estimates associated with risk-reducing salpingo-oophorectomy in BRCA1 or BRCA2 mutation carriers. *J Natl Cancer Inst.* 2009;101(2):80-87.
3. Bogaerts JMA, Steenbeek MP, Bommel MHD, et al. Recommendations for diagnosing STIC: a systematic review and meta-analysis. *Virchows Arch.* 2022;480(4):725-737.
4. Cancer Genome Atlas Research Network. Integrated genomic analyses of ovarian carcinoma. *Nature.* 2011;474:609-615.
5. National Cancer Institute. The cancer genome atlas program. Accessed December 4, 2022. https://www.cancer.gov/about-nci/organization/ccg/research/structural-genomics/tcga
6. Cerami E, Gao J, Dogrusoz U, et al. The cBio cancer genomics portal: an open platform for exploring multidimensional cancer genomics data. *Cancer Discov.* 2012;2(5):401-404. doi:10.1158/2159-8290.CD-12-0095
7. Gao J, Aksoy BA, Dogrusoz U, et al. Integrative analysis of complex cancer genomics and clinical profiles using the cBioPortal. *Sci Signal.* 2013;6(269):pl1. doi:10.1126/scisignal.2004088
8. Fathalla M. Factors in the causation and incidence of ovarian cancer. *Obstet Gynecol Surv.* 1972;27:751-768.
9. Landen CN, Birrer MJ, Sood AK. Early events in the pathogenesis of epithelial ovarian cancer. *J Clin Oncol.* 2008;26(6):995-1005.
10. Kim HS, Kim TH, Chung HH, Song YS. Risk and prognosis of ovarian cancer in women with endometriosis: a meta-analysis. *Br J Cancer.* 2014;110(7):1878-1890. doi:10.1038/bjc.2014.29
11. Anglesio MS, Yong PJ. Endometriosis-associated ovarian cancers. *Clin Obstet Gynecol.* 2017;60(4):711-727.
12. Similä-Maarala J, Soovares P, Pasanen A, et al. TCGA molecular classification in endometriosis-associated ovarian carcinomas: novel data on clear cell carcinoma. *Gynecol Oncol.* 2022;165(3):577-584.
13. Cheasley D, Wakefield MJ, Ryland GL, et al. The molecular origin and taxonomy of mucinous ovarian carcinoma. *Nat Commun.* 2019;10(1):3935.
14. Zhang H, Liu T, Zhang Z, et al. Integrated proteogenomic characterization of human high-grade serous ovarian cancer. *Cell.* 2016;166(3):755-765.
15. Thorsson V, Gibbs DL, Brown SD, et al. The immune landscape of cancer. *Immunity.* 2018;48(4):812-830.e14.
16. Reddy J, Fonseca MAS, Corona RI, et al. Predicting master transcription factors from pan-cancer expression data. *Sci Adv.* 2021;7(48):eabf6123.
17. Noordermeer SM, Attikum H. PARP inhibitor resistance: a tug-of-war in BRCA-mutated cells. *Trends Cell Biol.* 2019;29(10):820-834.
18. Baumbusch LO, Helland A, Wang Y, et al. High levels of genomic aberrations in serous ovarian cancers are associated with better survival. *PLoS One.* 2013;8(1):e54356.
19. Candido-dos-Reis FJ, Song H, Goode EL, et al. Germline mutation in BRCA1 or BRCA2 and ten-year survival for women diagnosed with epithelial ovarian cancer. *Clin Cancer Res.* 2015;21(3):652-657.
20. Birkbak NJ, Kochupurakkal B, Izarzugaza JMG, et al. Tumor mutation burden forecasts outcome in ovarian cancer with BRCA1 or BRCA2 mutations. *PLoS One.* 2013;8(11):e80023. doi:10.1371/journal.pone.0080023
21. Yang D, Khan S, Sun Y, et al. Association of BRCA1 and BRCA2 mutations with survival, chemotherapy sensitivity, and gene mutator phenotype in patients with ovarian cancer. *JAMA.* 2011;306(14):1557-1565.
22. Ciriello G, Miller ML, Aksoy BA, Senbabaoglu Y, Schultz N, Sander C. Emerging landscape of oncogenic signatures across human cancers. *Nat Genet.* 2013;45(10):1127-1133.
23. Tothill RW, Tinker AV, George J, et al. Novel molecular subtypes of serous and endometrioid ovarian cancer linked to clinical outcome. *Clin Cancer Res.* 2008;14(16):5198-5208.
24. Au-Yeung G, Lang F, Azar WJ, et al. Selective targeting of cyclin E1-amplified high-grade serous ovarian cancer by cyclin-dependent kinase 2 and AKT inhibition. *Clin Cancer Res.* 2017;23(7):1862-1874.
25. Etemadmoghadam D, Weir BA, Au-Yeung G, et al. Synthetic lethality between CCNE1 amplification and loss of BRCA1. *Proc Natl Acad Sci U S A.* 2013;110(48):19489-19494.

26. Flesken-Nikitin A, Choi KC, Eng JP, Shmidt EN, Nikitin A. Induction of carcinogenesis by concurrent inactivation of p53 and Rb1 in the mouse ovarian surface epithelium. *Cancer Res.* 2003;63:3459-3463.

27. Korkolopoulou P, Vassilopoulos I, Konstantinidou AE, et al. The combined evaluation of p27Kip1 and Ki-67 expression provides independent information on overall survival of ovarian carcinoma patients. *Gynecol Oncol.* 2002;85(3):404-414.

28. Rosen DG, Yang G, Cai KQ, et al. Subcellular localization of p27kip1 expression predicts poor prognosis in human ovarian cancer. *Clin Cancer Res.* 2005;11(2 Pt 1):632-637.

29. Iyengar M, O'Hayer P, Cole A, et al. CDK4/6 inhibition as maintenance and combination therapy for high grade serous ovarian cancer. *Oncotarget.* 2018;9(21):15658-15672.

30. Coffman LG, Orellana TJ, Liu T, et al. Phase I trial of ribociclib with platinum chemotherapy in ovarian cancer. *JCI Insight.* 2022;7:e160573.

31. Salk JJ, Loubet-Senear K, Maritschnegg E, et al. Ultra-sensitive TP53 sequencing for cancer detection reveals progressive clonal selection in normal tissue over a century of human lifespan. *Cell Rep.* 2019;28(1):132-144.e3.

32. Kindelberger DW, Lee Y, Miron A, et al. Intraepithelial carcinoma of the fimbria and pelvic serous carcinoma: evidence for a causal relationship. *Am J Surg Pathol.* 2007;31(2):161-169.

33. Bergsten TM, Burdette JE, Dean M. Fallopian tube initiation of high grade serous ovarian cancer and ovarian metastasis: mechanisms and therapeutic implications. *Cancer Lett.* 2020;476:152-160.

34. Eckert MA, Pan S, Hernandez KM, et al. Genomics of ovarian cancer progression reveals diverse metastatic trajectories including intraepithelial metastasis to the fallopian tube. *Cancer Discov.* 2016;6(12):1342-1351.

35. Shell S, Park SM, Radjabi AR, et al. Let-7 expression defines two differentiation stages of cancer. *Proc Natl Acad Sci U S A.* 2007;104(27):11400-11405.

36. Berger AC, Korkut A, Kanchi RS, et al. A comprehensive pan-cancer molecular study of gynecologic and breast cancers. *Cancer Cell.* 2018;33(4):690-705.e9.

37. Heemskerk-Gerritsen BAM, Hollestelle A, Asperen CJ, et al. Progression-free survival and overall survival after BRCA1/2-associated epithelial ovarian cancer: a matched cohort study. *PLoS One.* 2022;17(9):e0275015.

38. Sakai W, Swisher EM, Karlan BY, et al. Secondary mutations as a mechanism of cisplatin resistance in BRCA2-mutated cancers. *Nature.* 2008;451(7182):1116-1120.

39. Patch AM, Christie EL, Etemadmoghadam D, et al. Whole-genome characterization of chemoresistant ovarian cancer. *Nature.* 2015;521(7553):489-494.

40. Bashashati A, Ha G, Tone A, et al. Distinct evolutionary trajectories of primary high-grade serous ovarian cancers revealed through spatial mutational profiling. *J Pathol.* 2013;231(1):21-34.

41. Liu Y, Yasukawa M, Chen K, et al. Association of somatic mutations of ADAMTS genes with chemotherapy sensitivity and survival in high-grade serous ovarian carcinoma. *JAMA Oncol.* 2015;1(4):486-494.

42. Norquist BM, Harrell MI, Brady MF, et al. Inherited mutations in women with ovarian carcinoma. *JAMA Oncol.* 2016;2(4):482-490.

43. Riester M, Wei W, Waldron L, et al. Risk prediction for late-stage ovarian cancer by meta-analysis of 1525 patient samples. *J Natl Cancer Inst.* 2014;106(5):dju048.

44. Curtis M, Mukherjee A, Lengyel E. The tumor microenvironment takes center stage in ovarian cancer metastasis. *Trends Cancer.* 2018;4(8):517-519.

45. Vickman RE, Faget DV, Beachy P, et al. Deconstructing tumor heterogeneity: the stromal perspective. *Oncotarget.* 2020;11(40):3621-3632.

46. Prat J, D'Angelo E, Espinosa I. Ovarian carcinomas: at least five different diseases with distinct histological features and molecular genetics. *Hum Pathol.* 2018;80:11-27.

47. D'Alessandris N, Travaglino A, Santoro A, et al. TCGA molecular subgroups of endometrial carcinoma in ovarian endometrioid carcinoma: a quantitative systematic review. *Gynecol Oncol.* 2021;163(2):427-432.

48. Gadducci A, Multinu F, Cosio S, Carinelli S, Ghioni M, Aletti GD. Clear cell carcinoma of the ovary: epidemiology, pathological and biological features, treatment options and clinical outcomes. *Gynecol Oncol.* 2021;162(3):741-750.

49. Gaitskell K, Hermon C, Barnes I, et al. Ovarian cancer survival by stage, histotype, and pre-diagnostic lifestyle factors, in the prospective UK million women study. *Cancer Epidemiol.* 2022;76:102074. doi:10.1016/j.canep.2021.102074

50. Cybulska P, Paula ADC, Tseng J, et al. Molecular profiling and molecular classification of endometrioid ovarian carcinomas. *Gynecol Oncol.* 2019;154(3):516-523.

51. Pierson WE, Peters PN, Chang MT, et al. An integrated molecular profile of endometrioid ovarian cancer. *Gynecol Oncol.* 2020;157(1):55-61.

52. Dinulescu DM, Ince TA, Quade BJ, Shafer SA, Crowley D, Jacks T. Role of K-ras and Pten in the development of mouse models of endometriosis and endometrioid ovarian cancer. *Nat Med.* 2005;11(1):63-70.

53. McConechy MK, Ding J, Senz J, et al. Ovarian and endometrial endometrioid carcinomas have distinct CTNNB1 and PTEN mutation profiles. *Mod Pathol.* 2014;27(1):128-134.

54. Ji JX, Cochrane D, Negri GL, et al. The proteome of clear cell ovarian carcinoma. *J Pathol.* 2022;258(4):325-338.

55. Ye S, Li Q, Wu Y, et al. Integrative genomic and transcriptomic analysis reveals immune subtypes and prognostic markers in ovarian clear cell carcinoma. *Br J Cancer.* 2022;126(8):1215-1223.

56. Anglesio MS, Wang YK, Maassen M, et al. Synchronous endometrial and ovarian carcinomas: evidence of clonality. *J Natl Cancer Inst.* 2016;108(6):djv428.

57. Schultheis AM, Ng CK, Filippo MR, et al. Massively parallel sequencing-based clonality analysis of synchronous endometrioid endometrial and ovarian carcinomas. *J Natl Cancer Inst.* 2016;108(6):djv427.

58. Reijnen C, Kusters-Vandevelde HVN, Ligtenberg MJL, et al. Molecular profiling identifies synchronous endometrial and ovarian cancers as metastatic endometrial cancer with favorable clinical outcome. *Int J Cancer.* 2020;147(2):478-489.

59. Ortiz M, Wabel E, Mitchell K, Horibata S. Mechanisms of chemotherapy resistance in ovarian cancer. *Cancer Drug Resist.* 2022;5(2):304-316.

60. Gershenson DM, Sun CC, Westin SN, et al. The genomic landscape of low-grade serous ovarian/peritoneal carcinoma and its impact on clinical outcomes. *Gynecol Oncol.* 2022;165(3):560-567.

61. Cheasley D, Nigam A, Zethoven M, et al. Genomic analysis of low-grade serous ovarian carcinoma to identify key drivers and therapeutic vulnerabilities. *J Pathol.* 2021;253(1):41-54.

62. Hunter SM, Anglesio MS, Ryland GL, et al. Molecular profiling of low grade serous ovarian tumours identifies novel candidate driver genes. *Oncotarget.* 2015;6(35):37663-37677.

63. Kuo KT, Guan B, Feng Y, et al. Analysis of DNA copy number alterations in ovarian serous tumors identified new molecular genetic changes in low-grade and high-grade carcnomas. *Cancer Res.* 2009;69(9):4036-4042.

64. Mok SC, Bell DA, Knapp RC, et al. Mutation of K-ras protooncogene in human ovarian epithelial tumors of borderline malignancy. *Cancer Res.* 1993;53(7):1489-1492.

65. Singer G, Oldt R, Cohen Y, et al. Mutations in B-raf and K-ras characterize the development of low-grade ovarion serous carcinoma. *J Natl Cancer Inst.* 2003;95(6):484-486.

66. Gershenson DM, Miller A, Brady WE, et al. Trametinib versus standard of care in patients with recurrent low-grade serous ovarian cancer (GOG 281/LOGS): an international, randomised, open-label, multicentre, phase 2/3 trial. *Lancet.* 2022;399(10324):541-553.

67. Vereczkey I, Serester O, Dobos J, et al. Molecular characterization of 103 ovarian serous and mucinous tumors. *Pathol Oncol Res.* 2011;17(3):551-559.

68. Mackenzie R, Kommoss S, Winterhoff BJ, et al. Targeted deep sequencing of mucinous ovarian tumors reveals multiple overlapping RAS-pathway activating mutations in borderline and cancerous neoplasms. *BMC Cancer.* 2015;15:415. doi:10.1186/s12885-015-1421-8

69. Anglesio MS, Kommoss S, Tolcher MC, et al. Molecular characterization of mucinous ovarian tumours supports a stratified treatment approach with HER2 targeting in 19% of carcinomas. *J Pathol.* 2013;229(1):111-120.

70. Deng Y, Bartosovic M, Ma S, et al. Spatial profiling of chromatin accessibility in mouse and human tissues. *Nature.* 2022;609:375-383.

71. Mund A, Coscia F, Kriston A, et al. Deep visual proteomics defines single-cell identity and heterogeneity. *Nat Biotechnol.* 2022;40(8):1231-1240.

72. Hu Z, Artibani M, Alsaadi A, et al. The repertoire of serous ovarian cancer non-genetic heterogeneity revealed by single-cell sequencing of normal fallopian tube epithelial cells. *Cancer Cell.* 2020;37(2):226-242.e7.

73. Regner MJ, Wisniewska K, Garcia-Recio S, et al. A multi-omic single-cell landscape of human gynecologic malignancies. *Mol Cell.* 2021;81(23):4924-4941.

74. Hanley GE, Pearce CL, Talhouk A, et al. Outcomes from opportunistic salpingectomy for ovarian cancer prevention. *JAMA Netw Open.* 2022;5(2):e2147343. doi:10.1001/jamanetworkopen.2021.47343

75. Virani S, Baiocchi G, Bowtell D, et al. Joint IARC/NCI international cancer seminar series report: expert consensus on future directions for ovarian carcinoma research. *Carcinogenesis.* 2021;42(6):785-793.

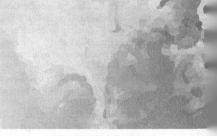

CHAPTER **8.5**

Ovarian Cancer: Clinical Presentation and Diagnostic Workup

Ernst Lengyel and Kathryn A. Mills

CLINICAL PRESENTATION OF PATIENTS WITH A BENIGN ADNEXAL MASS OR EARLY-STAGE OVARIAN CANCER

The diagnosis and treatment of patients with ovarian masses is difficult because of the diversity of clinical presentation, the plethora of differential diagnoses, and the wide range of therapeutic options (**Table 8.5-1**). Historically, almost all patients with small adnexal tumors were considered asymptomatic; the mass is usually discovered incidentally using imaging during a workup for other conditions (**Figure 8.5-1**). However, in a recent retrospective review of the patients enrolled in GOG 157, over 70% of patients had one or more symptoms; the problem is that these symptoms are typically nonspecific and commonly include vague complaints of pain or fullness (1). With increasing size, adnexal masses cause pelvic pressure and pain by compressing surrounding structures. In the same review, nearly half of patients with masses over 15 cm complained of multiple symptoms (1). A larger pelvic tumor can cause genitourinary symptoms, including urinary urgency, urinary frequency, and dyspareunia, because the tumor pushes on the bladder. Posteriorly, a fixed pelvic tumor can compress the sigmoid colon, causing severe constipation, pain, or even a bowel obstruction. Compression of the ureter by a mass densely adherent to the pelvic sidewall may cause ureteral dilatation and hydronephrosis. It is the local compression of organs in the pelvis that defines the symptoms patients present with. These symptoms can occur in both benign disease and early/late OC, depending on what organ the mass impinges. It is impossible to differentiate a benign from a malignant ovarian mass by clinical examination alone. Borderline ovarian tumors, nonserous malignant EOC (endometrioid, clear cell, mucinous), and nonepithelial (germ cell, stromal cell) malignant tumors frequently present as large adnexal masses at an early stage without any further abdominal dissemination. In one study, 67% to 75% of all endometrioid, mucinous, and clear cell cancer all presented as FIGO stage I/II disease (2), whereas in another report, 80% of high-grade serous tumors were FIGO stage III/IV (**Figure 8.5-2**) (3).

An ovarian mass becomes a surgical emergency if a patient has a sudden onset of abdominal pain. The differential diagnosis in this situation includes rupture, torsion, and possible infarction of the ovarian mass. In addition, severe abdominal pain can also be caused by a hemorrhage inside a cyst, which distends it, or by the rupture of a blood-filled cyst, causing hemoperitoneum. Sudden abdominal pain associated with an adnexal mass is often accompanied by malaise, nausea and vomiting, low-grade fever, an elevated white blood cell count, and elevated C-reactive protein levels, which are all caused by peritoneal irritation as well as, rarely, hypotension from hemorrhage. In the presence of acute pain, peritoneal signs, rigidity, and rebound tenderness, urgent expert surgical evaluation should be considered. Evaluation is most often performed laparoscopically. Delaying surgery can result in infarction, ongoing hemorrhage, peritonitis, and sepsis. Vaginal bleeding in a patient with an adnexal mass could be an indication of synchronous endometrial cancer and OC (4) or an estrogen-producing granulosa cell

tumor. Sertoli-Leydig cell tumors, which can cause bleeding, can also lead to virilization.

CLINICAL PRESENTATION OF PATIENTS WITH ADVANCED OVARIAN CANCER

The clinical presentation of advanced OC is varied. Treating physicians are often surprised by how unspecific symptoms women with advanced OC may experience, despite extensive disease burden. Nonspecific symptoms associated with advanced OC include anorexia, fatigue, early satiety, and loss of appetite. While significant weight loss is unusual in OC because of diffuse ascites production, tumor cachexia can be a presenting sign in patients with high-volume disease and long-standing partial bowel obstruction.

Often, patients have nonspecific pelvic and abdominal symptoms, including bloating and diffuse, dull, constant abdominal pain caused by the infiltration of the peritoneum and the bowel mesentery, or by extensive ascites. Involvement of the small bowel can cause changes in the frequency of bowel movements, with alternating constipation and diarrhea. If the tumor has metastasized to the omentum, there may be upper abdominal discomfort with nausea, belching, early satiety, and fullness. The abdominal cavity may also be distended by several liters of ascites, which can cause a significant increase in abdominal circumference, leading to marked discomfort. Extensive ascites can cause significant fatigue, anorexia, pain, nausea/vomiting, and incontinence from pressure on the bladder. In addition, ascites can cause dyspnea, because the lower lung lobes are compressed by the abdominal distension. Signs of bowel obstruction, urinary symptoms (frequency, pressure), intense pelvic pain, and ascites are likely to indicate miliary dissemination on the peritoneal surfaces and large-volume advanced disease. Moreover, patients with advanced OC sometimes present with deep venous thrombosis (DVT) from large tumors pressing on pelvic veins or as part of the hypercoagulopathy associated with advanced-stage cancer, especially in HGSOC and clear cell cancer (5).

Because overt symptoms often develop late, when the cancer is already advanced, OC has been called the "silent killer" or "the cancer that whispers." Given that the survival of patients with early (FIGO stages I and II disease) is about 80% and patients with advanced disease (stages III and IV) have a 20% to 30% survival rate, it is critical to diagnose the disease early. In general, there are no specific symptoms that assist in diagnosing OC early and that screening for OC has not been effective (6,7). A retrospective chart review of women enrolled in the UKTOCS OC screening trial did not demonstrate reduction in deaths due to disease, even though some stage shift to earlier diagnosis was noted (7).

Whether clinically symptomatic disease can be picked up earlier is not clear. In one study, the authors noted that many ultimately diagnosed with OC have abdominal symptoms, urinary frequency, and pain for 3 months or longer before diagnosis (8). The study suggested that patients with OC tend to have a combination of symptoms (eg, increased abdominal size/bloating, early satiety, pelvic/abdominal pain, urinary urge, incontinence), which

TABLE 8.5-1. Differential Diagnosis of an Adnexal Mass

Definition	Description	Mean Age	Clinical Presentation	Imaging	Therapy	Comments
Ectopic pregnancy	Tubal pregnancy, most common in the fimbriated end	Reproductive-aged women	Positive pregnancy test. History of PID, tubal surgery, fertility treatment, or previous ectopic pregnancies. Pelvic pain, anemia	Pelvic ultrasound	Methotrexate or laparoscopy with salpingectomy or salpingostomy, laparotomy if hemodynamically unstable	Clinical emergency. 10%–15% recurrence risk
Physiologic, functional cysts	Follicular cyst—preovulatory cyst Corpus luteum cyst—postovulatory cyst caused by hemorrhage or cyst formation. Theca lutein cysts are caused by hCG stimulation of the ovary. "Other": paratubal cysts	Reproductive-aged women	Depending on size, lower abdominal pain, dyspareunia, and signs of latent torsion. On examination freely mobile and unilateral. May present as an acute abdomen when ruptured, torsed, or infarcted: unilateral intermittent, acutely worsening pelvic pain	Pelvic ultrasound. Often >7 cm	Persists for weeks. Oral contraceptives might cause involution/resolution and help with the diagnosis. If a cyst does not resolve within 8 weeks, laparoscopy should be considered	Most frequent benign masses in reproductive-aged women. A bleeding corpus luteum can cause an acute abdomen, anemia, and hemoperitoneum
Hydrosalpinx	Fluid-filled fallopian that leads to cystic dilatation. When the fluid is pus, it is considered salpingitis with or without PID	Reproductive-aged women	Asymptomatic, infertility, or torsion	Tortuous shapes of the distended tube	Diagnosed by ultrasound and HSG	Hydrosalpinx is caused by PID, ectopic pregnancy, endometriosis, or fallopian tube cancer
Polycystic ovaries	Endocrine disorder. Multiple follicle cysts enlarging the ovaries to 2–5 their normal size	Reproductive-aged woman	Irregular menstrual cycles, anovulation, amenorrhea, acne, hirsutism, subfertility, metabolic syndrome	Pelvic ultrasound, hormonal tests (DHEA-S, androstenedione, testosterone, FSH). Glucose-tolerance test	Oral contraceptives, metformin, glitazones, weight loss, clomiphene, spironolactone	Often associated with peripheral insulin resistance. Higher risk of endometrial hyperplasia and endometrial cancer
Serous and mucinous cystadenomas	Serous—Cystic: thin-walled, unilocular. Mucinous—cystic thicker wall but may be multicystic	Reproductive-aged women	Serous 5–20 cm, mucinous up to 40 cm	Pelvic/abdominal ultrasound shows clear fluid or mucinous more echogenic	Laparoscopic drainage and removal or laparoscopic cystectomy	May present with torsion or rupture
Adenofibroma	Type of stromal tumor	Reproductive-aged women	Depends on size: intermittent torsion, frequency	Pelvic/abdominal ultrasound shows a unilocular or multilocular solid or a plain solid tumor	Observation, laparoscopic removal if tumor growth or causes symptoms	Because appearance is solid on ultrasound, often read as malignant. CA-125 often normal. MRI will show solid components with a density of fibrous stroma
Germ cell tumors	Benign: teratoma (dermoid) Malignant: immature teratoma/dysgerminoma	Young reproductive-aged patients	Bilateral in 20%. Elevated β-hCG, AFP, LDH, (CA-125)	Ultrasound, might show calcifications on x-ray or CT. Solid, partially cystic	Laparoscopic cystectomy removing the entire capsule. If malignant salpingo-oophorectomy, staging	Malignancy found < 1% of occurrences

(continued)

TABLE 8.5-1. Differential Diagnosis of an Adnexal Mass (continued)

Definition	Description	Mean Age	Clinical Presentation	Imaging	Therapy	Comments
Sex cord stromal cell tumors	Benign: fibromas, thecomas, Brenner cell tumors Malignant: granulosa cell tumor, Sertoli-Leydig cell tumor	30–menopause, but also postmenopausal patients	Solid, firm tumors resembling fibroids. May produce hormones: estradiol, and inhibin. May cause irregular bleeding, uterine hyperplasia	Ultrasound/CT. Solid homogeneous tumors. Granulosa cell tumors are heterogeneous and often cause rupture	Laparoscopic or laparotomy for ovarian cystectomy or oophorectomy depending on size	In postmenopausal patients, benign stromal cell tumors are often preoperatively interpreted as being malignant. The CA-125 is normal or only slightly elevated
Peritoneal inclusion cysts	Cystic	Any age	History of multiple pelvic/abdominal surgeries or recurrent pelvic infections or peritoneal dialysis	Ultrasound: multiple thin-walled cysts, CT, MRI can often help to establish a diagnosis	Differential hydrosalpinx. Observation vs ultrasound or CT-guided aspiration with cytology. Surgical intervention for severe symptoms or hydronephrosis. Higher risk for perioperative morbidity (bowel, ureter injury)	
Fibroids	Benign. Broad ligament or pedunculated fibroids misdiagnosed as cancer	30–55 yr	Often asymptomatic. Degeneration or infarction can occur and cause acute pain	Ultrasound, rarely CT or MRI. If degenerated will have heterogeneous appearance	Observation versus surgical intervention with myomectomy or hysterectomy. Growing fibroid postmenopausal DD sarcoma	Common in African American women. Pedunculated fibroids may be mistaken for an adnexal mass
Endometriosis	1–10 cm endometriotic cysts filled with blood, adherent to surrounding organs. Often bilateral. Endometriotic implants occur in the pelvic peritoneum including the cul-de-sac and bladder peritoneum. Nodularity of the uterosacral ligaments	30–45 yr	Pelvic pain. Dyspareunia. May have cyclical pain with menses, infertility, and dyspareunia. May present with acute pain from rupture, rarely torsion. Hydronephrosis. CA-125 100–300 U/mL	Pelvic/abdominal ultrasound. Diagnostic laparoscopy	Conservative treatment. Anti-inflammatory drugs, OCP, GnRH analogs. Laparoscopy with removal of endometriomas and coagulation of endometriotic nodules. The extent of surgery depends on symptoms and desire for future fertility	Common in White nulliparous women. Ovarian endometrioma is also called a "chocolate cyst"
PID/Salpingitis	Tubo-ovarian abscess complicate PID in 15% of all woman	Young, sexually active patients	History of PID. Pelvic pain, malaise, vaginal discharge (GO, chlamydia), cervical motion tenderness. Fever, chills, leukocytosis, CRP ↑, Platelets ↑. CA-125: 100–500 U/mL. Lactate ↑ Coagulopathy if septic	Ultrasound showing one or more masses that are homogeneous, cystic, possibly with air-fluid levels and septations	Combination antibiotic treatment, CT-guided abscess drainage. Laparoscopy or laparotomy if an abscess cannot be drained or if the patient has signs and symptoms of sepsis, hemodynamically unstable	High recurrence risk. Complications: infertility, chronic pelvic pain
Appendicitis and appendiceal abscess	Appendicitis right-sided tenderness, rebound	Younger patients	Fever, guarding, rebound tenderness. Malaise, Migrating pain from umbilicus to RLQ, nausea, vomiting, absence of vaginal discharge. Leukocytosis, CRP ↑, platelets ↑, CA-125 ~100–200 U/mL	Ultrasound and CT imaging with contrast. No distinct mass (25% appendicolith). CT with IV contrast shows dilated inflamed appendix. Concerning features: abscess: enhancement, irregular borders, perforation	Localized appendicitis (80%): Nonoperative treatment with antibiotics and analgesia. Laparoscopic appendectomy for peritonitis, patients with sepsis, perforation, nonresponder, and recurrence	A difficult differential in children and young women. Consider PID and pregnancy

Diverticulitis and diverticular abscess	Diverticulitis mostly in the sigmoid colon causing left-sided pain	Older patients. Obesity, smoking	Fever, guarding, rebound tenderness. Malaise, tachycardia, LLQ pain, nausea, vomiting. Pain leukocytosis, CRP ↑, platelets ↑, CA-125 ~100-200 U/mL	Ultrasound and CT imaging with contrast. Features consistent with abscess: enhancement, irregular borders. Possible microperforation. Thickening sigmoid wall. Air bubbles	Combination parenteral antibiotic treatment. Percutaneous abscess drainage. Bowel rest, pain control. Surgery if patient has sepsis and for definitive treatment. Laparoscopic sigmoid resection with colostomy for perforated diverticulitis	Presentation in very old patients might be subtle. High recurrence risk
Colon cancer	Gastrointestinal malignancy with possible metastasis to ovaries	After age 40 unless HNPCC	Anemia, irregular stools. Induration and irregularity. Family history. ↑ CEA	Sigmoidoscopy/colonoscopy. CT scan	If localized surgery, colon resection	60%-70% occur on the left side but cecal cancer can present as right adnexal mass
Early invasive epithelial ovarian cancer	Early serous ovarian cancer, endometrioid, mucinous, or clear cell ovarian cancer	Over age 50 is most common unless high-risk mutation carrier (BRCA1 or BRCA2, Lynch, etc) in premenopausal women 35-50	CA-125 ↑ only in 50%. Normal in mucinous and clear cell cancer	Papillary surface excrescences, areas of necrosis, internal solid elements. Hydronephrosis	Surgical intervention: consider starting with a laparoscopy to establish a diagnosis. Avoid spillage if possible. Referral to gynecologic oncologist for full staging	Differential of ovarian malignancy: invasive serous cancer, endometrioid, clear cell cancer. Borderline tumors
Advanced invasive epithelial ovarian cancer	Serous carcinoma with ascites and metastasis to upper abdomen	Postmenopausal women	Persistent bloating, general abdominal pain, early satiety. Vaginal bleeding. CA-125 ↑ in 80%, HE4 ↑, platelets ↑	Suspicious adnexal mass and ascites, upper abdominal disease	Exploratory laparotomy, staging, tumor debulking. Referral to gynecologic oncologist for debulking	Differentiate between high- and low-volume disease. High-volume disease often requires upper abdominal procedures and bowel surgery
Metastasis	Gastric (Krukenberg), colon, breast, and uterine cancer	All patients with advanced or recurrent disease are at risk	CA-125 can be elevated. Other tumor markers might be helpful (CEA, CA19-9, CA15-3)	Bilateral solid complex masses in patients with prior cancer history	Excision can be considered for symptomatic relief or if it is the only site of metastatic disease	Poor prognosis compared to ovarian cancer
Rare differential diagnoses	• Pelvic kidney • Disseminated abdominal tuberculosis: Young woman unlikely to have ovarian cancer. Women from endemic areas, populations at risk (prison, facilities, immigrants), ascites, CA-125 ↑, absence of a dominant adnexal mass.					

AFP, α-fetoprotein; CRP, C-reactive protein; CT, computed tomography; DD, dedifferentiated; DHEA-S, dehydroepiandrosterone sulfate; GnRH, gonadotropin-releasing hormone; FSH, follicle-stimulating hormone; hCG, human chorionic gonadotrophin; HNPCC, hereditary nonpolyposis colorectal carcinoma; HSG, hysterosalpingogram; IV, intravenous; LDH, lactate dehydrogenase; LLQ, left lower quadrant; MRI, magnetic resonance imaging; OCP, oral contraceptive; PID, pelvic inflammatory disease; RLQ, right lower quadrant.

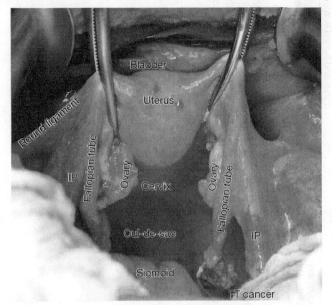

Figure 8.5-1. Patient with left fallopian tube cancer hanging off the left tubal fimbriae fallopian tube (FT) and infundibulopelvic (ip) artery and vein.

The ACOG and SGO consensus guidelines recommend referral to a gynecologic oncologist for postmenopausal women with elevated CA-125, ascites, a nodular/fixed pelvic mass, or evidence of abdominal/distant metastasis (11). In premenopausal women, a very elevated CA-125, ascites, or evidence of abdominal or distant metastasis should also trigger a referral. These guidelines have a PPV of 39.6% for premenopausal women and 64.6% for postmenopausal women. A benign condition that can closely mimic the constellation of symptoms described in the consensus guidelines is Meigs syndrome (12). This syndrome is characterized by a cytologically benign pleural effusion and ascites, which resolve upon removal of a concomitant ovarian tumor, usually an ovarian fibroma or thecoma.

DIAGNOSIS OF OVARIAN CANCER

The correct clinical diagnosis of an ovarian mass is difficult and requires considerable experience and clinical judgment (**Table 8.5-1**). Age is a very important factor in assessing an adnexal mass because many ovarian tumors have a predilection for a particular age group. In premenarchal girls, an adnexal mass is often germ cell in origin, whereas young women in their reproductive years are most likely to have benign findings. In postmenopausal patients, a complex adnexal mass is particularly concerning for an epithelial cancer, because a normal postmenopausal ovary is atrophic and small (1.5 cm × 1 cm × 0.5 cm) (**Table 8.5-1**). On average, the volume of a normal ovary is 10 cm^3 in postmenopausal and 20 cm^3 in premenopausal women.

An adnexal mass in a woman of reproductive age is a significant diagnostic challenge, because most are benign and maintaining fertility remains an important consideration. However, it is also critical that malignant tumors are not missed. The differential diagnosis of an adnexal mass/cyst is described in detail in **Table 8.5-1**. There are several categories of benign masses, including functional cysts,

are more severe, more frequent, and of more recent onset than those symptoms reported by patients without cancer who present to a primary care clinic. However, these symptoms are nonspecific and overlap with several common disorder like irritable bowel syndrome, dyspepsia, and menopause. In addition, several studies have concluded that the appraisal of symptoms alone is not likely to lead to an earlier diagnosis (9,10).

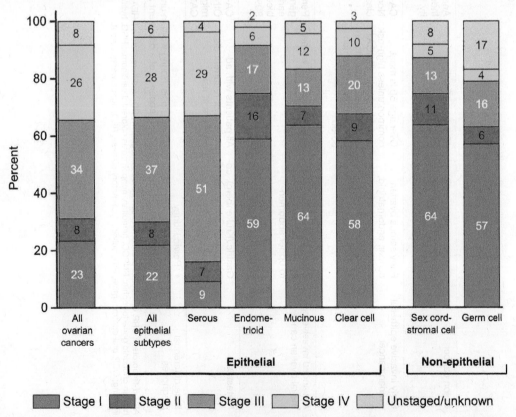

Figure 8.5-2. Stage distribution for ovarian cancer by histologic subtype. (From Torre LA, Trabert B, DeSantis CE, et al. Ovarian cancer statistics, 2018. *CA Cancer J Clin*. 2018;68(4):284-296.)

adenomas, nonmalignant germ cell tumors (mature teratomas/dermoids), nonmalignant sex cord stromal tumors (fibromas), and endometriosis. The most common benign solid ovarian tumors are ovarian fibromas (fibroma/fibrothecoma/cystadenofibroma). Another common solid tumor is a pedunculated fibroid, which may be interpreted on imaging as an adnexal mass. Infectious conditions that may present with similar signs and symptoms include PID/tubo-ovarian abscess (13), appendicitis (14), and diverticulitis (15). For women in their reproductive years, the decision to pursue surgery or to observe will depend on the degree of clinical suspicion based on the factors detailed earlier and her desire for future fertility.

In some patients, there is no distinct adnexal mass but a conglomerate tumor in the lower abdomen. The differential diagnosis for this includes multiple confluent pelvic abscesses, an advanced OC, an advanced endometrial cancer/sarcoma, colon or appendiceal cancer, and retroperitoneal tumors. A metastatic breast, colon, or lung cancer tumor should be considered in the presence of an atypical pattern of metastasis, or abnormal mammogram or chest x-ray (16,17). It should be remembered, however, that although OC is much more prevalent in postmenopausal women than premenopausal women, the most common cause of an adnexal mass in a postmenopausal patient is still a benign tumor. This is either caused by hormonal imbalances that can exist during perimenopause or developed when one is postmenopausal, driven by hormones secreted by the postmenopausal ovary. In postmenopausal women, simple unilocular cysts can be monitored, but women with solid or complex masses should be offered surgery or followed at very close intervals. Surgery may begin with a minimally invasive approach that can be converted to an open procedure if the frozen section suggests a borderline tumor or malignancy that necessitates exploratory laparotomy for full surgical evaluation.

When formulating a diagnosis of an adnexal mass, the most important factors to consider are the patient's age, menopausal status, family history of cancer, clinical examination, and the results of serum testing (such as WBC, platelets, CA-125, CEA, and HE-4) and imaging studies (ultrasound/CT/MRI) (**Tables 8.5-1 and 8.5-2**). Owing to the lethality of OC, it is considered advisable to "err on the side of caution." The fear of not detecting a malignancy, which could delay diagnosis or lead to inadequate surgery, has shaped the clinical response to adnexal masses for decades. The current treatment paradigm is that every postmenopausal woman with a solid adnexal mass should have a surgical exploration to determine histology. Given that early-stage OC has a much better prognosis than advanced-stage disease, many operations are performed with the goal of "catching" a cancer early. Because only histology can exclude the presence of an OC, about 5% to 10% of all women will, at some point, undergo surgery to rule out an OC, despite the fact that most adnexal masses are benign (18).

CLINICAL EXAMINATION

A focused clinical examination should begin with an assessment of supraclavicular and axillary lymph nodes, a breast examination, and percussion of the lungs to detect a pleural effusion. The abdomen should also be evaluated for the presence of an umbilical hernia or tumor. The involvement of the umbilicus by an OC is colloquially called *Sister Mary Joseph nodule*, named after an assistant to Dr William Mayo, who identified the lesion as a sign of advanced malignancy. The abdomen should also be inspected for surgical scars and visible veins (*caput medusae*) caused by impaired central venous return from extensive intra-abdominal disease. The size and mobility of the adnexal mass should be assessed, and the abdomen examined for the presence of ascites, costovertebral angle tenderness from hydronephrosis, and enlarged inguinal lymph nodes. In a patient with extensive ascites, the bowel floats on top of the ascites, leading to central tympany on examination, whereas in patients with a large tumor, the tympany is lateral.

On gynecologic examination, a prominent cystocele can be indicative of ascites. The bimanual and rectovaginal examination should attempt to evaluate and characterize the adnexal mass in respect to size, borders (smooth/irregular), mobility (fixed/mobile), and location. Invasive OCs often have irregular borders and can be fixed to the pelvic sidewall and fill the cul-the-sac. Pelvic examination findings may also include involvement of the parametrium by tumor, or nodularity of the rectovaginal septum, and pain. It may not be possible to differentiate the uterus from the tumor, and the cervix is sometimes dislocated anteriorly behind the pubic symphysis. Some ovarian tumors are behind the uterus and can be best palpated with a rectovaginal examination after the bladder is emptied. While a fixed mass is more suggestive of a malignant neoplasm than a mobile mass, this is not pathognomonic, because a malignant neoplasm that is localized may be mobile and an ovarian tumor associated with endometriosis or pelvic infection may be fixed. Unfortunately, there are no examination findings that can accurately distinguish a benign from a malignant adnexal mass. Still, despite best efforts and experience, the pelvic examination is less accurate than ultrasound and/or CT in detecting and characterizing an adnexal mass, especially if the patient is obese or if the uterus is significantly enlarged.

■ TABLE 8.5-2. Differential Diagnosis of an Adnexal Mass by Age		
History	**Age**	**Differential Diagnosis**
Age Pregnancy Menopausal status Family history	Premenarchal	Germ cell tumors, mature teratomas, rhabdomyosarcomas
	Young reproductive age (15-25 yr)	Functional cysts, ectopic pregnancy, pelvic inflammatory disease (PID)/salpingitis/tubo-ovarian abscess (TOA), mature teratomas (dermoid), appendicitis/appendiceal abscess, polycystic ovaries, juvenile granulosa cell tumor, dysgerminoma, endodermal sinus tumor, tuberculosis
	Middle reproductive age (25-35 yr)	Endometriosis, functional cysts, polycystic ovaries, serous/mucinous cystadenomas, PID/salpingitis/TOA, mature teratomas (dermoid), Sertoli-Leydig cell tumor
	Advanced reproductive age (35-45 yr)	Stromal cell tumors (fibroma/fibrothecoma/cystadenofibroma), pedunculated fibroids, peritoneal cysts, adult granulosa cell tumor, synchronous ovarian/endometrial cancer
	Perimenopausal (46-52 yr)	Functional cysts, fibroids, ovarian cancer, synchronous ovarian/endometrial cancer, breast cancer metastasis, clear cell and endometrioid ovarian cancer
	Postmenopausal (<52 yr)	Serous/mucinous cystadenomas, ovarian cancer, colon cancer and metastasis from other cancer, benign stromal cell tumors, diverticulitis/diverticular abscess

LABORATORY TESTS

The laboratory workup for patients with suspected OC generally includes a complete blood count and chemistry panel. Patients with OC are often hemoconcentrated, whereas patients with GI malignancies are frequently anemic. Patients with OC often have thrombocytosis (a poor prognostic marker) (5) and may have low albumin level, which is indicative of prolonged low oral intake leading to tumor cachexia and malnutrition and is associated with higher perioperative and postoperative morbidity. A pregnancy test should be part of the workup for all premenopausal women because uterine/adnexal enlargement can be due to pregnancy.

Tumor markers can be potentially used for screening for OC in the general or in high-risk populations (eg, BRCA1/2 carrier), risk stratification deciding about surgery or who should perform surgery (generalist, minimally invasive surgeon, or gynecologic oncologist), differential diagnosis (Table 8.5-1), prognosis, predicting and monitoring response to therapy, and detecting cancer recurrence. The performance of a tumor marker depends on its sensitivity (percentage of patients with cancer correctly identified as a result of a positive test), specificity (percentage of the population without cancer correctly identified as a result of a negative test), and PPV (percentage of patients with positive test that who the cancer, true positives). An ideal OC tumor marker should have a 100% sensitivity, specificity, and PPV. However, in practice, such a marker does not exist. As all tumor marker in clinical for OC are tumor associated rather than tumor specific and are elevated in multiple cancers, benign and physiologic conditions, they lack specificity. In addition, if sensitivity is low, a normal result may not exclude malignancy. Tumor markers discovered thus far contribute to differential diagnosis but are not themselves diagnostic. This restricts their use, with few exceptions, to contributing to the initial clinical diagnosis of an adnexal mass (Table 8.5-1) and monitoring therapeutic response and follow-up.

The CA-125 Tumor Marker

The CA-125 tumor marker (normal <35 U/mL), initially described by Dr Robert Bast, is the most thoroughly investigated serum marker used to diagnose OC (19). It is expressed on both Müllerian (tubal, endometrial, endocervical) and coelemic (pericardium, pleura, peritoneum, ovarian surface) epithelium.

A number of gynecologic conditions can falsely elevate CA-125 levels. In premenopausal women, the differential of an elevated CA-125 includes many diseases associated with acute or chronic inflammation, to the extent that CA-125 can be regarded as an acute-phase reactant. CA-125 can be elevated in patients with PID, peritoneal tuberculosis, endometriosis, fibroids, pregnancy, liver cirrhosis, systemic lupus erythematosus, and inflammatory bowel disease. Moreover, CA-125 is not specific to OC because it is increased, albeit modestly, in most metastatic solid tumors, including GI, breast, and endometrial cancer. Patients with mucinous OC often have elevated CEA values, but this tumor marker is also nonspecific and is increased in patients with GI malignancies, especially colon and gastric cancer, but also in smokers. A ratio of CA-125/CEA greater than 25 is used clinically to exclude a GI malignancy and has been employed in randomized trials (20). Whether a raised CA-125 in asymptomatic postmenopausal women is a predictor of nongynecologic cancer is not clear. Data from a Norwegian trial of 5,500 women showed that breast and lung cancers were overrepresented among women with elevated CA-125 (21). In addition, an elevated CA-125 was a risk factor for death from malignant disease. These data indicate that steps should be taken to rule out other malignancies such as breast, lung, and pancreas in asymptomatic postmenopausal women with rising CA-125 levels and no evidence of gynecologic malignancy. In general, the CA-125, as a serum biomarker, underperforms in premenopausal women, early-stage malignancies, and several histologic subtypes.

CA-125 for Screening

CA-125 is not useful for screening. An acceptable screening method for detecting early-stage OC requires a sensitivity of greater than 75% and a specificity of at least 96.6% to achieve a PPV of at least 10%. Two large randomized controlled trials showed no difference in reduction of OC death between the screening and no screening arms (22,23). Therefore, the U.S. Preventive Task Force recommends against screening of unaffected, asymptomatic, individuals (6).

The UKTOCS study with over 200,000 study participants has used multimodal strategies, including repeated CA-125 measurements (7,23). Two screening strategies were tested: primary ultrasound screening versus multimodality screening (CA-125 followed by ultrasound). They then annually measured CA-125 and used the ROCA for an interpretation of rises in CA-125 over time. The ROCA establishes a CA-125 baseline for each woman and evaluates for changes in slope, monitoring for significant increases in CA-125 levels, when patients are evaluated by transvaginal ultrasound. Unfortunately, the results of the UKTOCS study were negative as screening with CA-125 and ultrasound did not affect OS (7). The only positive finding was a subtle stage shift with FIGO (2014) stages I and IV cancer incidence 47% higher and 25% lower, respectively compared to the unscreened group.

The PLCO Cancer Screening Trial (1993-2001) randomized 78,216 postmenopausal women either to annual screening with a fixed cutoff value for CA-125 (<35 U/mL) and ultrasound or to usual medical care (22). Ultrasounds were done yearly for 3 consecutive years and CA-125 yearly for 5 years. Borderline tumors were considered false positive and were not considered malignant neoplasms. The results showed that screening does not improve mortality from OC. False-positive screening results were returned in 3,285 patients; 1,080 (32.9%) underwent surgery, and of these, 15% (163 women) experienced 222 major complications (20.6 complication rate/100 surgeries). The number of patients diagnosed in late-stage OC was similar in the screening and observation group, suggesting that screening does not detect OC at an earlier stage. In addition, it reported the PPV for CA-125 alone was only 3.7%.

The inability to detect early OC using a yearly screening approach is probably due to the very fast growth rate of HGSC once it is fully transformed, which reduces the time during which screening can detect preinvasive or early invasive OC (24). Another reason that screening tends to be ineffective may be the extent of OC disease heterogeneity. In summary, pelvic examinations, CA-125, and ultrasound have not been conclusively shown to significantly decrease mortality from OC in either low- or high-risk populations. If a woman wants to reduce her risk, tubal ligation, OCPs, or a prophylactic salpingo-oophorectomy may currently be the best strategy for primary prevention.

Primary Diagnosis

Only 50% of stage I disease is associated with an elevated serum CA-125, which is one reason that CA-125 is not a good screening method for early-stage OC (25). Even in advanced-stage cancers, the marker has a 20% to 25% false-negative rate. However, 80% of patients with OC of any stage who are over 50 years have an elevated CA-125 (26). In addition, serum levels of CA-125 generally reflect disease burden in women with initially elevated levels and in patients with ascites.

A meta-analysis by Myers et al studied the performance of CA-125 as a serum marker to distinguish between benign and malignant adnexal masses (27). In premenopausal women with an adnexal mass, an increased CA-125 predicts a malignancy with the following statistical performance: sensitivity: 50% to 74%, specificity 26% to 92%, and PPV 5% to 67%. For postmenopausal women the performance is much better: sensitivity 69% to 87%, specificity 81% to 100%, and a PPV 73% to 100%. The CA-125 is highest in serous and lowest in mucinous OC. Although it can be elevated, clear cell cancer and endometrioid OC often have lower CA-125 values than with HGSCs, hovering around 200 U/mL or else, remaining within normal range (26,28).

In summary, CA-125 is most useful in distinguishing between a benign and malignant mass when used in conjunction with clinical history (age, menopausal status, family history) and imaging, but the specificity is low (29). Accompanied by other factors, it may help triage women with an adnexal mass for surgery or observation and to surgery with a gynecologic oncologist or a general obstetrician-gynecologist.

Monitoring Response to Treatment

CA-125 is also helpful in the evaluation of response to therapy in patients with an established diagnosis of OC and can assist in the diagnosis of recurrence after completion of adjuvant therapy. It is now established that serum CA-125 levels reflect progression or regression of disease in over 90% of patients with OC with elevated preoperative levels (**Figure 8.5-3**). Despite the widespread use of serum CA-125 levels to monitor the clinical course of OC and its response to chemotherapy, CA-125 should not be used as the sole criterion to determine clinical response. Studies involving second-look laparotomy have confirmed that CA-125 values of less than 35 U/mL do not exclude active disease (30). Serial measurements and following the trend of CA-125 are more informative than a cutoff. Most clinicians use a 50% or higher decrease in CA-125 or a 75% response from pretreatment levels to define response. A multicenter French study showed that prechemotherapy CA-125, its half-life, nadir concentration, and time to nadir have a univariate prognostic value for disease-free survival (DSF) and OS (31). Following first-line therapy, a fast doubling time of CA-125 is of concern for recurrence and platinum-resistant disease.

Detecting Recurrence

Among patients with elevated CA-125 levels at diagnosis, serial monitoring following initial chemotherapy can lead to the early detection of recurrent disease. A risk of recurrence is increased in those with either a relative increase in CA-125 of 100% (OR = 23.7; 95% CI, 2.9-192.5) or an absolute increase of 5 kU/L (OR = 8.4; 95%

CI, 2.2-32.6) or 10 kU/L (OR = 71.2; 95% CI, 4.8 to >999.9), thus suggesting that progressive low-level increase in serum CA-125 levels is strongly predictive of disease recurrence (29). Whether to use CA-125 in follow-up or wait for a symptomatic presentation of disease has been a subject of much debate. The MRC OVO5/EORTC55955 trial showed no benefit in CA-125 monitoring in the follow-up of patients with OC, as those randomized to immediate (based on CA-125 levels) or delayed chemotherapy (the latter when signs and symptoms of recurrence were present) did not demonstrate a difference in survival (early arm: median 25.7 months, 95% CI, 23.0-27.9; delayed arm: median 27.1, 95% CI, 22.8-30.9; HR 0.98, 95% CI, 0.80-1.20; $P = .85$) (32).

The usual pattern of CA-125 throughout a clinical course of the disease is presented in **Figure 8.5-3**. CA-125 remains the best-performing biomarker for OC when tumors of mucinous origin are excluded.

The HE4 Tumor Marker

Human epididymis (HE)4 is a secreted glycoprotein expressed on human OC cells (33). There is no evidence that HE4 performs better than CA-125 as a first- or second-line test in screening. A case-control set (using preclinical samples collected 6 months before diagnosis) nested within PLCO showed that CA-125 remained the single best biomarker for OC (sensitivity of 86%) followed closely by HE4 (73%) (34). In terms of outcome, however, there is no clear advantage in diagnosing HE4-associated rather than TVS-associated tumors. A 2020 study nested within the UK-TOCS screening trial sought to evaluate CA-125, transvaginal ultrasound, and HE4 in the differential diagnosis of an incidentally identified adnexal mass in those who being screened (35). There was no improvement in the sensitivity by incorporating HE4 levels into the model.

A meta-analysis by Olsen showed that HE4 assays had a pooled sensitivity of 80% (CI 74%-84%) and a mean specificity of 84% (CI 80%-88%) in correctly identifying adnexal masses (36). At a 15% prevalence of OC, the negative predictive value would be 96% (CI 94%-97%) in the differentiation of benign and malignant adnexal masses.

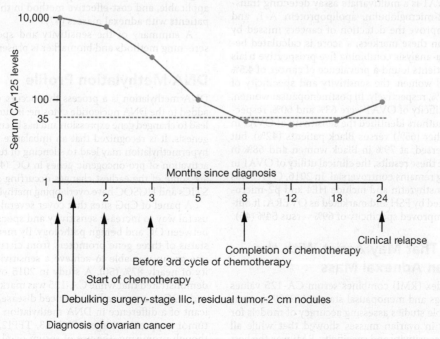

Figure 8.5-3. Correlation between serum CA-125 and clinical course in ovarian cancer.

A combination of HE4 and CA-125 enhances both sensitivity (90% CI 0.87-0.92) and specificity (85% CI 0.82-0.87) compared to either test used alone (37). In mucinous tumors, HE4 performs better than CA-125, and its serum level is less affected by endometriosis and benign disease than CA-125, resulting in increased specificity, while maintaining sensitivity. The added value of HE4 is that it is expressed in about half of all patients who do not express CA-125. HE4 can also be elevated in other cancers, such as mesothelioma, lung, endometrial, breast, GI, renal, and transitional cell carcinomas (38).

The performance of HE4 can, however, be improved by being incorporated into an algorithm that includes CA-125 and menopausal status (Risk of Malignancy, ROMA index) (39). The ROMA gives a risk of OC with a value more than 13.1% in predicting a high risk of EOC in premenopausal women and a value more than 27.7% when used in the postmenopausal population. Another multicenter trial evaluated 472 women undergoing surgery for an adnexal mass (40). When taking premenopausal and postmenopausal women together, ROMA had a sensitivity of 93.8%, a specificity of 74.9%, and a negative predictive value of 99.0%. Based on these data, the ROMA algorithm was Food and Drug Administration (FDA) approved for distinguishing benign from malignant masses. It is most widely used in practice to clarify when to triage patients with adnexal masses to gynecologic oncology for initial management. Emerging data suggest it may also be more cost-effective to utilize ROMA for referral decisions (41). Lastly, including age, rather than menopausal status, along with CA-125 and HE4, is called the Copenhagen Index (CPH-I), and this has also been evaluated in a similar setting. A recent evaluation in 2016 compared the ROMA against the CPH-I. While the best results were noted in determining cancer from benign lesions, with the CPH-I slightly outperforming ROMA (both approached 89% sensitivity and 85% specificity), neither performed well in the evaluation of nonepithelial and borderline tumors (42). In the United States, HE4 is FDA approved for use in monitoring for recurrent or progressive disease. In a study from 2012, the combination of HE4 plusCA-125 in the detection of recurrent disease had a sensitivity of 76% and a specificity of 100% (43).

OVA1

OVA1 was the first panel of multiple protein serum markers that was approved by the FDA for further assessment of malignancy in an adnexal mass. OVA1 is a multivariate assay detecting transferrin, prealbumin, β2-microglobulin, apolipoprotein A-1, and CA-125, which may improve the detection of cancers missed by CA-125 alone. Based on these markers, a score is calculated between 0 and 10. A meta-analysis combining five prospective trials with a total of 2,305 patients found a prevalence of cancer of 4.5% (44). In premenopausal women, the sensitivity and specificity of OVA1 were 51% and 77%, respectively. In postmenopausal women, the sensitivity and specificity of OVA1 were 63% and 60%, respectively. In addition, the authors identified the sensitivity of OVA1 in White women was higher (65%) versus Black patients (42%), but the specificity was reversed, at 79% in Black women and 68% in White patients. Despite these results, the clinical utility of OVA1 in the preoperative setting remains controversial. In 2016, OVA1 was changed to remove transthyretin and include HE4 and β2-microglobulin and was replaced by FSH and marketed as OVERA. It outperforms OVA1 with improved specificity of 69% versus 54% (45).

Other Markers That May Assist With the Differential of an Adnexal Mass

Risk of malignancy index (RMI) combines serum CA-125 values with ultrasound findings and menopausal status. A 2009 systematic review of 109 eligible studies assessing accuracy of models for predicting malignancy in ovarian masses showed that while all models had acceptable sensitivity and specificity, RMI was the best predictor at that time (46). Using a value of 200 as the cutoff, the

■ TABLE 8.5-3. Sensitivity and Specificity of All Different Screening Methods and Biomarker

Screening Methods and Biomarkers	True positive Sensitivity	True negative Specificity
Ultrasound	84.9%	77.6%
CA125	>35 U/mL: 78%	78%
CA125 and HE4	88.7%	74.7%
CA125 and SMRP	44.1%-86.5%	95% - 98%
RMI (CA125, Pelvic sonography, Menopausal status)	>50: 95.1%* >200: 87.4%+	76.5%* 56.8%+
ROMA (CA125, HE4, menopausal status)	93.8%	74.9%
OVA1 (CA125, transferrin, transthyretin, apolipoprotein A-1, β-2- macroglobulin)	92.4%	53.5%
OVERA (CA125, HE4, apolipoprotein A-1, FSH and transferrin)	87.2%-91.3%	66.1%-69.1%

For symptomatic patients!

pooled estimate for sensitivity for preoperative assessment of an adnexal mass was 78%, with a specificity of 87%. There were many modifications of the RMI since 1990 (by varying the cutoff levels, incorporating CA19-9), the performance between RMI I-IV is comparable. Despite the lower accuracy of the RMI in borderline, stage I invasive, and nonepithelial OC, the RMI is a simple, easily applicable, and cost-effective method in the primary evaluation of patients with adnexal masses (47).

A summary of the sensitivity and specificity of all different screening methods and biomarker is presented in **Table 8.5-3**.

DNA Methylation Profile

DNA methylation is a process that occurs when methyl groups are added to the DNA nucleotide cytosine; in turn, when altered, this can lead to changed gene expression and has been correlated with carcinogenesis. It is recognized that an imbalance of hypomethylation and hypermethylation may lead to silencing of tumor suppressors and/or activation of pro-oncogenic genes in OC (48). Methylation changes are some of the earliest changes occurring at the pre-STIC stage as STICs and HGSOC have overlapping methylation profiles (49).

A panel of CpG sites that cover several genes may be the most useful way to increase sensitivity and specificity for differentiating between OC and benign pathology. By measuring the methylation status of three gene promoters from circulating DNA in plasma, one group was able to achieve a sensitivity of 90% and specificity of nearly 87% (50). A study in 2015 of 114 patients with OC demonstrated that while CA-125 was markedly lower in those with early OC as compared to advanced disease, there was not as significant of a difference in DNA methylation findings when studying tumor suppressor targets RUNX3, TFPI2, and OPCML (51). Although promising, the use of serum or plasma DNA methylation as a means for early OC detection has not yet become widespread.

Carcinoembryonic Antigen

CEA was first identified in 1965 in the serum of rabbits immunized with colon carcinoma (52). It is an oncofetal glycoprotein that belongs to the immunoglobulin family and is found in small amounts in the adult colon. Elevated levels are associated with colon, lung, and pancreatic cancers, but CEA levels may also be raised in benign diseases of the liver, GI tract, and lung and in smokers. It is mostly used in follow-up of patients with colon cancer.

In patients with OC, elevated levels of CEA can be found in the majority of patients with mucinous histology (53). Similarly, some data report that even up to 50% of those with other histologies will have at least a mild elevation (54). In ovarian borderline tumors, however, the reported rates of elevated CEA vary widely from 3% to 60%, and in some cases, CEA was not significantly different between patients with adnexal masses of benign and borderline etiologies (55-57).

It may be more helpful to consider utilizing CEA in combination with CA-125 to help differentiate ovarian malignancy from metastatic implants from another primary (colorectal, eg) to the ovary, but CEA is also elevated in breast, pancreatic, lung, and thyroid cancer, as well in mucinous adenocarcinomas of the cervix. In patients with a CA-125/CEA ratio of greater than 25, OC, rather than a metastatic implant, was noted in 82% of cases (58). This may guide preoperative counseling as well as additional imaging or evaluations needed before a planned operation.

IMAGING OF ADNEXAL MASSES AND EARLY OVARIAN CANCER: ULTRASOUND AND MAGNETIC RESONANCE IMAGING

In patients with adnexal masses, a pelvic ultrasound, as well as a complete history, physical examination, and a CA-125, is generally needed to provide the information necessary to determine whether surgery is required. Because the patient history and the clinical examination alone cannot reliably differentiate between benign and malignant masses, imaging is commonly performed to help establish a diagnosis and treatment plan.

Ultrasound can detect and characterize ovarian size and morphology. While vaginal ultrasound provides high-resolution imaging of the ovary, for large ovarian masses, an abdominal ultrasound will complement the vaginal scan. Defined ultrasound criteria help diagnose functional cysts, cystadenomas, dermoids, and endometriomas.

with a high degree of certainty, allowing the choice of conservative, nonoperative treatment. Benign tumors often appear on ultrasound as unilateral with smooth walls, a few smooth cysts, no solid elements or papillary projections, and an absence of ascites. Functional cysts have thin walls and are fluid filled. In general, most benign tumors are cystic and mobile. The risk of malignancy in unilocular cystic tumors (even if they are >10 cm) and septated cystic ovarian tumors is extremely low. In the absence of solid areas or papillary projections, these cysts are never malignant, and 38% to 80% resolve within 1 year (18). Dermoids are often cystic with hyperechoic areas (teeth, hair). Endometriomas have low-level, layered echoes (blood) and thick walls. In contrast, malignant tumors are partially solid and cystic, often bilateral, irregular, fixed, and often accompanied by ascites. Patients with tumors that display these features require surgical exploration. Homogeneous solid tumors often require surgical exploration because on ultrasound, it is very difficult to differentiate them from a malignancy, but the most common finding is an ovarian fibroma or a pedunculated fibroid (**Table 8.5-1**).

Several sonography-based predictive models have been developed to differentiate between benign and malignant tumors to introduce objectivity and simplicity in reading scans by ultrasonographers with various levels of experience. Ueland published a morphology index based on ovarian volume and morphologic complexity (**Figure 8.5-4**) (26,59). The risk of malignancy was related to structural complexity, tumor volume, and a total morphology index score. There was only one malignancy found in 315 tumors with a morphology index less than 5, indicating that the score is very useful in identifying low-risk tumors. Among 127 patients with a morphology index 5 or higher, there were 52 invasive or borderline tumors. A group of investigators from Kentucky expanded this finding by adding serial examinations to determine whether a change in the morphology index over time could aid in deciding if a patient with an adnexal mass needed surgery (60). Adnexal masses that were found to be malignant showed an increase of 1.6 points per month in the morphology index, whereas the scores of benign ovarian tumors only increased 0.3 per month.

The International Ovarian Tumor Analysis (IOTA) group has two main models (61). The IOTA simple rule considers five benign and five malignant ultrasound features: If one or more malignant features ("M-features") apply in the absence of benign features ("B-features"), the mass is considered malignant (**Table 8.5-4**). If a mass has one or more benign features in the absence of malignant ("M-features"), the mass is considered benign. If a mass has both benign and malignant features, the mass cannot be classified using

Size	>4-6 cm
Ovarian volume	Length x width x height x 0.523. Premenopausal > 20 cm³. Postmenopausal > 10 cm³.
Morphology	Thick septations > 3 mm (differentiate from a papillary projection) Complex solid and cystic (multilocular) Solid enhancing nodules Papillary projections
Vascularization	Pulsatility index (PI) > 1. Resistive Index (RI) >0.4. Central intramural blood flow
Other findings	Ascites (≥60) Uterine invasion Peritoneal thickening, carcinomatosis

A

MORPHOLOGY INDEX

	TUMOR VOLUME	TUMOR STRUCTURE	
0	<10 cm³		
1	10-50 cm³		
2	>50-100 cm³		
3	>100-200 cm³		
4	>200-500 cm³		
5	>500 cm³		

B

Figure 8.5-4. Imaging characteristics of a malignant adnexal mass. A: Criteria for malignancy. B: Morphology index with sonographic examples. (A: Adapted from van Nagell JR Jr, Miller RW. Evaluation and management of ultrasonographically detected ovarian tumors in asymptomatic women. *Obstet Gynecol.* 2016;127:848-858; Forstner R, Meissnitzer M, Cunha TM. Update on imaging of ovarian cancer. *Curr Radiol Rep.* 2016;4:31. Miller RW, Ueland FR. Risk of malignancy in sonographically confirmed ovarian tumors. *Clin Obstet Gynecol.* 2012;55:52-64. B: From Elder JW, Pavlik EJ, Long A, et al. Serial ultrasonographic evaluation of ovarian abnormalities with a morphology index. *Gynecol Oncol.* 2014;135:8-12.)

■ TABLE 8.5-4. Malignant (M) and Benign (B) Features of the IOTA Simple Rules

	Benign Features		Malignant Features
B1	Unilocular cyst	M1	Irregular solid tumor
B2	Presence of solid components with the largest <7 mm	M2	Presence of ascites
B3	Presence of acoustic shadows	M3	At least four papillary structures
B4	Smooth, multilocular tumor with the largest diameter <100 mm	M4	Irregular, multilocular solid tumor ≥100 mm
B5	No blood flow (color score 1)	M5	Very strong blood flow (color score 4)

IOTA, International Ovarian Tumor Analysis.

the simple rules and needs additional evaluation. This classification works well to classify 77% of adnexal masses with a sensitivity of 92% and a specificity of 96% (62).

A more sophisticated model expanded this approach using an Assessment of Different NEoplasias in the adneXa (ADNEX) model to differentiate between five types of ovarian tumors: benign, borderline, stage I, stage II-IV OC, and metastatic cancer (63). It is available online and as an App. An online calculator is available for free or can be downloaded as an App.

A large prospective study of 5,909 patients evaluated in 24 primarily European centers established the parameter for the ADNEX model (63). The final model had four clinical variables (age, family history, referral center) and six ultrasound variables (lesion diameter, proportion of solid tissue, <10 cysts, # of papillary projections, acoustic shadow, ascites) (Table 8.5-5). In contrast to the simple rule, Doppler is not part of the model. The sensitivity of the model is 97% and the specificity 71% at a 10% risk cutoff. The area under the receiver operating curve (AUC), differentiating between benign and malignant masses, was 0.94, indicating that the model discriminated very well between the two. The model was also designed to be used by nonexperts, which may help those with less experience evaluating pelvic ultrasound to more accurately characterize ovarian masses. However, when establishing the model, all patients in the study underwent surgery, biasing the model toward more severe pathology that did not warrant expectant management.

An additional model, the O-RADS (Ovarian-Adnexal Reporting and Data System) ultrasound, was published in 2020 by the American College of Radiology to assist those who perform and interpret pelvic ultrasound for malignancy (Figure 8.5-5) (64). This system, similar to the mammography categorization, uses a range from 1, being normal-appearing ovary, to 5, being high risk (>50% risk) of malignancy. By these criteria, patients with masses categorized with a 1 or 2 do not require follow-up imaging or other

■ TABLE 8.5-5. IOTA ADNEX Model (Online Calculator)

Clinical Features	Sonographic Features
Age of the patient at examination	Maximum diameter of lesion (mm) (log-transformed)
Serum CA-125 (U/mL)	Maximal diameter of the largest solid part (mm)
Oncology center (referral center for GYN-ONC)	Number of papillary projections
	>10 cyst locules
	Acoustic shadow present
	Ascites (fluid outside the pelvis present)

GYN-ONC, gynecologic oncologist; IOTA, International Ovarian Tumor Analysis.

intervention. The O-RADS system classifies six classic benign lesions as O-RADS category 2, where the risk of malignancy is under 1% (Figure 8.5-5A). Adnexal masses with O-RADS category 4 or 5 should have surgery (Figure 8.5-5B). Those with a score of 3 should have additional imaging, such as with an MRI or repeat ultrasound with an adnexal ultrasound specialist. One study with 30% cancer prevalence showed that the system is extremely accurate at categorizing malignant masses with a score of 4 or 5, with a more than 98% sensitivity, and that it can be accurately used by radiologists of all experience levels (65). The O-RADS performed with lower sensitivity (91%) and specificity (82%) in a different multicenter study where the prevalence of cancer was lower (8%) (66). Although not yet studied in the community setting, it is expected that the specificity of the O-RADS reporting system will drop even further because the incidence of malignancy is much lower (1%-2%).

Sometimes, color-flow Doppler is used to aid in distinguishing benign from malignant tumors. The neovascularization of malignant tumors is characterized by an absence of tunica media in tumor blood vessels, leading to reduced flow resistance, which can be detected by Doppler. Resistance to blood flow is measured by calculating the pulsatility index (PI) and resistive index (RI). However, these indices, as independent variables, are unreliable for predicting OC because the location of tumor vessels is variable (18).

A study evaluating ultrasound findings in 111 patients with pathologically confirmed early FIGO (2014) stages I and II OC revealed that early-stage HGSOCs rarely presented as a mass less than 5 cm size without a solid component. The average size of an even early-stage malignant mass was 9.6 cm. Not one case of cancer was identified in a purely cystic mass (67). The risk of adverse events (malignancy, torsion, rupture) during follow-up of adnexal masses with benign ultrasound morphology by use of ultrasound is very low, and 20% of all adnexal tumors, even in postmenopausal patients, resolved spontaneously (68). Along the same lines, a retrospective study of 878 lesions categorized simplified "classic" (simple cysts, hemorrhagic cysts, endometriomas, and dermoids) versus "nonclassic" (anything else) adnexal masses based on ultrasound appearance. The malignancy rate for "classic," clearly as benign identified lesions was less than 1%, whereas the finding of blood flow in a 60-year-old with a "nonclassic" lesion carried a 50% rate of malignancy. The overall sensitivity for malignancy was 93% (69). These two studies utilized ultrasound in a simple, binary model to differentiate benign from malignant adnexal masses, where frequently occurring adnexal masses (cystadenoma, endometriosis, teratoma) are instantly diagnosed based on "classic" features.

Overall, these findings suggested that small, cystic appearing lesions, and "classic" adnexal tumors can, and should, be observed to avoid surgical morbidity.

Often, ovarian masses are indeterminate on grayscale ultrasound and, although they provide an insufficient rationale to proceed to surgery, are sufficiently concerning that a second imaging test is ordered for further characterization. Contrast-enhanced MRI is the preferred advanced modality for an ultrasound-indeterminate adnexal lesion because of its high specificity. When combined with conventional MRI, diffusion-weighted imaging (DWI) further improves the tissue contrast of conventional MRI and allows a better characterization of an adnexal mass. The ability to exclude malignancy is one of the greatest strengths of referring sonographically indeterminate adnexal lesions to MRI. An MRI study can differentiate between simple fluid, atypical fluid (mucinous), fresh blood, old hematoma, solid tissue, stromal tissue, and fat (70,71). As with ultrasound, several criteria have been established to differentiate a benign from a malignant mass, including the presence of septations, solid elements and papillary projections, and solid tissue intensity on T2-weighted MRI. Injection of gadolinium-contrast agents adds further information, because solid malignant components within a mass take up the contrast. This also allows a better differentiation of cystic from solid lesions, especially endometriomas, stromal cell tumors, and teratomas. In 2020, an O-RADS MRI risk score was established to provide a stratification system for assigning the probability of malignancy to adnexal lesions based on MRI features (72). Like the O-RADS ultrasound, it has five levels. A total of 203 (18.0%) patients had at least one malignant adnexal or nonadnexal pelvic mass. No invasive cancer was assigned a score of 2, and high inter-rater agreement with a kappa of 0.78. In a premenopausal woman with an indeterminate ultrasound and a negative contrast-enhanced MRI, the risk of malignancy is 2%, whereas a positive MRI increases the risk of malignancy in the same patient to 80%. An MRI of an adnexal mass that is assigned a score of 4 has a 50% PPV for malignancy and score 5 has a 90% risk of malignancy (73).

American College of Radiology™

O-RADS™ US v2022 — Assessment Categories

Release Date: November 2022

O-RADS Score	Risk Category [IOTA Model]	Lexicon Descriptors		Management Pre-menopausal	Management Post-Menopausal
0	Incomplete Evaluation [N/A]	Lesion features relevant for risk stratification cannot be accurately characterized due to technical factors		Repeat US study or MRI	
1	Normal Ovary [N/A]	No ovarian lesion		None	
		Physiologic cyst: follicle (≤3 cm) or corpus luteum (typically ≤3 cm)			
2	Almost Certainly Benign [<1%]	Simple cyst	≤3 cm	N/A (see follicle)	None
			>3 cm to 5 cm	None	Follow-up US in 12 months*
			>5 cm but <10 cm	Follow-up US in 12 months*	Follow-up US in 12 months*
		Unilocular, smooth, non-simple cyst (internal echoes and/or incomplete septations) - - - - - - - - - - - Bilocular, smooth cyst	≤3 cm	None	Follow-up US in 12 months*
			>3 cm but <10 cm	Follow-up US in 6 months*	
		Typical benign ovarian lesion (see "Classic Benign Lesions" table)	<10 cm	See "Classic Benign Lesions" table for descriptors and management	
		Typical benign extraovarian lesion (see "Classic Benign Lesions" table)	Any size		
3	Low Risk [1 – <10%]	Typical benign ovarian lesion (see "Classic Benign Lesions" table), ≥10 cm		Imaging: • If not surgically excised, consider follow-up US within 6 months** • If solid, may consider US specialist (if available) or MRI (with O-RADS MRI score)† Clinical: Gynecologist	
		Uni- or bilocular cyst, smooth, ≥10 cm			
		Unilocular cyst, irregular, any size			
		Multilocular cyst, smooth, <10 cm, CS <4			
		Solid lesion, ± shadowing, smooth, any size, CS = 1			
		Solid lesion, shadowing, smooth, any size, CS 2–3			
4	Intermediate Risk [10 – <50%]	Bilocular cyst without solid component(s)	Irregular, any size, any CS	Imaging: Options include: • US specialist (if available) or • MRI (with O-RADS MRI score)† or • Per gyn–oncologist protocol Clinical: Gynecologist with gyn–oncologist consultation or solely by gyn–oncologist	
		Multilocular cyst without solid component(s)	Smooth, ≥10 cm, CS <4		
			Smooth, any size, CS 4		
			Irregular, any size, any CS		
		Unilocular cyst with solid component(s)	<4 pps or solid component(s) not considered a pp; any size, any CS		
		Bi- or multilocular cyst with solid component(s)	Any size, CS 1–2		
		Solid lesion, non-shadowing	Smooth, any size, CS 2–3		
5	High Risk [≥50%]	Unilocular cyst, ≥4 pps, any size, any CS		Imaging: Per gyn-oncologist protocol Clinical: Gyn-oncologist	
		Bi- or multilocular cyst with solid component(s), any size, CS 3–4			
		Solid lesion, ± shadowing, smooth, any size, CS 4			
		Solid lesion, irregular, any size, any CS			
		Ascites and/or peritoneal nodules††			

GLOSSARY

Smooth and irregular: refer to inner walls/septation(s) for cystic lesions, and outer contour for solid lesions; irregular inner wall for cysts = <3 mm in height	Solid: excludes blood products and dermoid contents; solid lesion = ≥80% solid; solid component = protrudes ≥3 mm (height) into cyst lumen off wall or septation
Shadowing: must be diffuse or broad to qualify; excludes refractive artifact	pp = papillary projection; subtype of solid component surrounded by fluid on 3 sides
CS = color score; degree of intralesional vascularity; 1 = none, 2 = minimal flow, 3 = moderate flow, 4 = very strong flow	Bilocular = 2 locules; multilocular = ≥3 locules; bilocular smooth cysts have a lower risk of malignancy, regardless of size or CS
Postmenopausal = ≥1 year amenorrhea (early = <5 yrs; late = ≥5 yrs); if uncertain or uterus surgically absent, use age >50 years (early = >50 yrs but <55 yrs, late = ≥55 yrs)	

*Shorter imaging follow-up may be considered in some scenarios (eg, clinical factors). If smaller (≥10–15% decrease in average linear dimension), no further surveillance. If stable, follow-up US at 24 months from initial exam. If enlarging (≥10–15% increase in average linear dimension), consider follow-up US at 12 and 24 months from initial exam, then management per gynecology. For changing morphology, reassess using lexicon descriptors. Clinical management with gynecology as needed.

**There is a paucity of evidence for defining the optimal duration or interval for imaging surveillance. Shorter follow-up may be considered in some scenarios (eg, clinical factors). If stable, follow-up at 12 and 24 months from initial exam, then as clinically indicated. For changing morphology, reassess using lexicon descriptors.

† MRI with contrast has higher specificity for solid lesions, and cystic lesions with solid component(s).

†† Not due to other malignant or non-malignant etiologies; specifically, must consider other etiologies of ascites in categories 1–2.

A

Figure 8.5-5. American College of Radiology ovarian adnexal reporting and system (O-RADS) ultrasound risk stratification table. A: O-RADS ultrasound risk stratification and management system. Classic benign lesions categorized as O-RADS 2. B: O-RADS categories 1-5 correlation with the IOTA system and suggested management. (From Andreotti RF, Timmerman D, Strachowski LM, et al. O-RADS US risk stratification and management system: a consensus guideline from the ACR ovarian-adnexal reporting and data system committee. *Radiology.* 2020;294:168-185. Figures 2 and 3)

O-RADS™ US v2022 — Classic Benign Lesions

Release Date: November 2022

Lesion	Descriptors and Definitions For any atypical features on initial or follow-up exam, use other lexicon descriptors (eg, unilocular, multilocular, solid, etc.)	Management If sonographic features are only suggestive, and overall assessment is uncertain, consider follow-up US within 3 months

Typical Hemorrhagic Cyst	Unilocular cyst, **no internal vascularity***, <u>and at least one</u> of the following:
	• Reticular pattern (fine, thin intersecting lines representing fibrin strands)
	• Retractile clot (intracystic component with straight, concave, or angular margins)
		Imaging:
		○ Premenopausal:
		  • ≤5 cm: None
		  • >5 cm but <10 cm: Follow-up US in 2–3 months
		○ Early postmenopausal (<5 years):
		  • <10 cm, options to confirm include:
		    ▪ Follow–up US in 2–3 months _or_
		    ▪ US specialist (if available) _or_
		    ▪ MRI (with O–RADS MRI score)
		○ Late postmenopausal (≥5 years):
		  • Should not occur; recategorize using other lexicon descriptors.
		
		Clinical: Gynecologist**

Typical Dermoid Cyst	Cystic lesion with ≤3 locules, **no internal vascularity***, <u>and at least one</u> of the following: • Hyperechoic component(s) (diffuse or regional) with shadowing • Hyperechoic lines and dots • Floating echogenic spherical structures	Imaging: ○ ≤3 cm: May consider follow-up US in 12 months† ○ >3 cm but <10 cm: If not surgically excised, follow-up US in 12 months† Clinical: Gynecologist**

Typical Endometrioma	Cystic lesion with ≤3 locules, **no internal vascularity***, homogeneous low–level/ground glass echoes, and smooth inner walls/septation(s)
	• ± Peripheral punctate echogenic foci in wall
		Imaging:
		○ Premenopausal:
		  • <10 cm: If not surgically excised, follow-up US in 12 months†
		○ Postmenopausal:
		  • <10 cm <u>and initial exam</u>, options to confirm include
		    ▪ Follow–up US in 2–3 months _or_
		    ▪ US specialist (if available) _or_
		    ▪ MRI (with O-RADS MRI score)
		
		  Then, if not surgically excised, recommend follow-up US in 12 months†
		
		Clinical: Gynecologist**

Typical Paraovarian Cyst	Simple cyst separate from the ovary	Imaging: None Clinical: Gynecologist**
Typical Peritoneal Inclusion Cyst	Fluid collection with ovary at margin or suspended within that conforms to adjacent pelvic organs • ± Septations (representing adhesions)	Imaging: None Clinical: Gynecologist**
Typical Hydrosalpinx	Anechoic, fluid–filled tubular structure • ± Incomplete septation(s) (representing folds) • ± Endosalpingeal folds (short, round projections around inner walls)	

*Excludes vascularity in walls or intervening septation(s)

**As needed for management of clinical issues

† There is a paucity of evidence for defining the need, optimal duration or interval of timing for surveillance. If stable, consider US follow-up at 24 months from initial exam, then as clinically indicated. Specifically, evidence does support **an increased risk of malignancy in endometriomas following menopause and those present greater than 10 years.**

B

Figure 8.5-5. (continued)

Given the high sensitivity and specificity, MRI is a very good (though often more expensive) test for predicting whether a mass is benign or malignant. However, it is not able to clearly differentiate between borderline and invasive tumors. A meta-analysis found that the average sensitivity and specificity of MRI in distinguishing a borderline or malignant tumor from a benign tumor were 92% (95% CI, 89%-94%) and 85% (95% CI, 82%-87%), respectively. While this sensitivity is similar to that reported by ultrasound, the specificity of MRI is superior. A comparison of color Doppler, CT scans, and MRI showed that of all three modalities, contrast-enhanced MRI is most helpful in further characterizing an adnexal mass that is indeterminate on ultrasound (70).

CT allows the detection and characterization of an adnexal mass but performs less well than MRI as a secondary imaging modality following grayscale ultrasound. Even when intravenous (IV) contrast is given, CT offers lower soft-tissue contrast than MRI (70). CT has a sensitivity of 87% but a low specificity of 16% in differentiating a benign from a malignant ovarian mass (74). In general, CT plays a much more critical role in the evaluation of advanced OC, but not in the differential of a benign versus borderline versus a malignant adnexal mass.

Given the high a priori probability that a mass in a premenopausal patient is benign, a reasonable approach is to further characterize an ultrasound-indeterminate adnexal lesion by MRI. If the MRI is reassuring, the patient can be followed with a combination of clinical examination, serial ultrasounds, and CA-125 every 3 to 6 months to capture a malignant adnexal tumor not detected during the initial workup (71,75). If the mass is stable, the follow-up interval can be extended.

Although the imaging approaches described earlier are very useful in the evaluation of an adnexal mass, other factors will affect the final decision to perform surgery. It is important to stress to the patient that while imaging and clinical judgment can be used to characterize many ovarian masses, only histologic examination can confirm the diagnosis. If the size of a mass changes over time or the sonographic morphology or vascularity/Doppler changes, surgery should be considered. Clinical aspects that factor into the decision to perform surgery include the patient's age, clinical symptoms, fertility preferences, family history of breast cancer and/or OC, medical comorbidities, and the number and extent of previous surgeries. Increased biomarker (CA-125, HE4) in a patient with a sonographic benign–looking mass may also persuade the gynecologist to perform surgery. Pain, and not a concern for malignancy, is often the reason to perform surgery, be it chronic pain, acute-onset pain, suspected torsion, or a cyst rupture with or without hemorrhage. Urinary symptoms (frequency, urinary tract infection [UTI]) from a large adnexal mass can become a clinically significant problem when even a benign unilocular mass that otherwise would be observed requires surgical removal. Sometimes, adnexal surgery is performed as part of a different procedure or an adnexal mass is removed because it is discovered intraoperatively.

IMAGING OF ADVANCED OVARIAN CANCER: COMPUTED TOMOGRAPHY, POSITRON EMISSION TOMOGRAPHY SCAN, AND MAGNETIC RESONANCE IMAGING

Because of its reasonable cost and wide availability, CT scanning with oral and IV contrast is currently the preoperative imaging modality most often used in patients with a high clinical suspicion for OC. Frequently, patients are found to have an adnexal mass or advanced disease after a CT scan of the abdomen and pelvis ordered for nonspecific clinical symptoms. A CT scan of the pelvis is able to characterize the adnexal mass and discern any involvement of the surrounding organs (bladder, sigmoid, ureter, and pelvic sidewall). In the upper abdomen, retroperitoneal adenopathy, omental and mesenteric involvement, and intrahepatic liver involvement can be detected reliably by CT scans with IV contrast. Often, the CT scan of the abdomen and pelvis is extended to the chest, which allows detection of intrapulmonary metastasis, pleural effusion, and pleural disease. These findings predict a lower chance of optimal cytoreduction (76).

Preoperative CT scans can identify the presence of disease in anatomic regions of the abdominal cavity that are difficult or technically impossible to resect (eg, stomach, lesser sac, liver, small bowel mesentery, and adenopathy above the renal vessels). The sensitivity to detect disease is limited: omental dissemination (90%-98%), diaphragmatic implants (43%-93%), and bowel involvement (38%-55%). In respect to lymph nodes, the sensitivity is 43% and the specificity 95% (77). Peritoneal dissemination is often associated with ascites and appears as a thick peritoneum with irregular surface indicating small-volume peritoneal disease.

Bristow and colleagues identified 13 diagnostic features and devised a score to predict the chances of optimal cytoreduction in patients with advanced OC (78). The 13 factors included in the score were peritoneal thickening; peritoneal implants greater than 2 cm; small and large bowel mesenteric disease greater than 2 cm; omental extension to stomach, spleen, or lesser sac; extension of the tumor to the pelvic sidewall/parametria/hydroureter; large-volume ascites; suprarenal and infrarenal lymphadenopathy; diaphragm involvement; inguinal canal disease; liver lesions greater than 2 cm; and porta hepatis/gallbladder disease. Using this model, the authors were able to predict surgical outcomes at their own institution with 93% accuracy. However, a multi-institutional validation study showed an accuracy of only 34% to 46% (79). This validation study identified disease on the diaphragm and large bowel mesentery implants as the only statistically significant predictors of suboptimal cytoreduction, and even when the score was limited to these two factors, there was a 33% false-positive rate.

In a joint prospective study at Memorial Sloan-Kettering and MD Anderson Cancer Center involving 350 patients, Suidan and colleagues sought to determine whether a CT of the abdomen and pelvis could predict the likelihood of suboptimal debulking (80). Three clinical (age ≥60 years, CA-125 ≥500 U/mL, American Society of Anesthesiology [ASA] 3/4) and six radiologic criteria were significantly associated with suboptimal debulking to more than 1 cm residual tumor size. The radiologic criteria included (1) suprarenal retroperitoneal lymph nodes greater than 1 cm, (2) diffuse small bowel adhesions/thickening, (3) tumors greater than 1 cm in the small bowel mesentery, (4) root of the superior mesenteric artery, (5) perisplenic area, and (6) lesser sac. Forty-eight patients receiving neoadjuvant chemotherapy during the study period were excluded. This prognostic model was found to have a predictive accuracy of 0.758. It does seem that surgical outcome depends on so many factors other than preoperative anatomical disease distribution (comorbidities, surgeon philosophy, advanced surgical techniques, perioperative resources) that overall preoperative CT scanning poorly predicts surgical resectability. Therefore, for most patients, surgical evaluation of the peritoneal cavity, which often includes a diagnostic laparoscopy, is required to evaluate the resectability of disease (81,82). Still, a patient whose CT scan clearly indicates high-volume ovarian disease and/or with poor performance status should be evaluated carefully before a decision is made to proceed with primary debulking and serious consideration should be given to neoadjuvant chemotherapy.

PET has been integrated with CT scan for the diagnosis of OC and the evaluation of disease recurrence (83,84). CT/PET combines the high anatomic resolution afforded by CT scan with a functional study of tumor fluoro-deoxy glucose (FDG) uptake. While PET scans have very high sensitivity, they have low specificity because of increased FDG uptake in benign metabolically active tissues and inflammatory changes. In a single-institution prospective study of 101 patients, the combined CT/PET scan had a sensitivity of 100% and specificity of 92% in the correct diagnosis of tumors that were suspicious on ultrasound (85). CT/PET scans seem to be especially useful in further characterizing a suspected recurrence. In a retrospective study, PET/CT showed a sensitivity of 82% and a specificity of 87% in correctly identifying recurrent disease, which was superior to CA-125 or CT/MRI scans used alone (84). CT/PET scans were also found to be particularly effective in the diagnosis of retroperitoneal lymph nodes (86). Unfortunately, PET scan–based imaging has not been shown effective at discrimination of resectability (87) or in differentiation of benign and borderline tumors, either.

While CT provides good spatial resolution, MRI is a nonradioactive imaging modality that provides excellent soft-tissue contrast resolution. In addition to its utility in the diagnosis of an indeterminate ovarian mass as described earlier, MRI is also an excellent modality for the characterization of nonadnexal pelvic pathology (eg, diverticulitis) and for the further characterization of the extent of OC in the upper abdomen and peritoneal implants. The T1-weighted MRI images, after administration of contrast (gadolinium), allow for the detection of peritoneal metastases and bowel implants. They also can determine whether the bowel mesentery or diaphragm is involved by cancer and whether a liver tumor is benign or malignant, or is on the surface of the liver or intrahepatic. MRI is better than CT or ultrasound in the diagnosis of small peritoneal metastases (87% DWI MRI vs 35% CT) (88), but CT imaging is superior in identifying involvement of the omentum by OC. One more recent study evaluated advanced MRI technology for prediction of OC resectability in 50 preoperative patients with suspected disseminated disease using the peritoneal cancer index (PCI), which is usually used in GI-related malignancy. Interobserver rate was only fair between participating radiologists ($\kappa = 0.42$), and the population was enriched with low-volume disease patients, making wider patient applicability questionable (89).

In recurrent cancer, MRI is especially useful for differentiating postsurgical changes from a recurrence on the vaginal cuff, small bowel mesentery, splenic hilum, liver surface, or diaphragm. The reported sensitivity of MRI for recurrent OC ranges from 62% to 91% and the specificity from 40% to 100%, depending primarily on tumor size (83).

DIFFERENTIAL DIAGNOSIS OF OVARIAN CANCER

The most common cause of malignant ascites in women is OC, but patients with metastatic breast, pancreatic, and gastric cancer, which usually has concomitant intrahepatic metastasis, can also present with ascites (**Table 8.5-1**). Therefore, other cancers should be considered in patients with extensive ascites and CA-125 values around 200 U/mL. Reviewing patients with ascites who presented to an oncology clinic, Ayantunde found diagnoses to be OC (37%), pancreatico-biliary cancer (21%), gastric cancer (18%), colon cancer (4%), and breast cancer (3%) (90). Nonmalignant causes of ascites include pancreatitis, tuberculosis, hepatitis, systemic lupus erythematosus, cirrhosis, ovarian torsion, and Meigs syndrome. Tuberculotic granulomas on the peritoneum combined with ascites are clinically indistinguishable from serous OC. A paracentesis will both establish a diagnosis of malignancy and improve the dyspnea, pain, nausea, and vomiting that the patient may be experiencing as a result of large-volume ascites.

While serous OC disseminates extensively within the abdominal cavity or to retroperitoneal lymph nodes, it will only rarely have metastasized elsewhere at the time of initial presentation. Imaging studies that suggest intrapulmonary metastasis or intraparenchymal metastases in the liver, spleen, or kidney, especially in the absence of significant IP disease or the absence of a significant ovarian tumor, should broaden the differential diagnosis to include a less common OC histotype (clear cell, mucinous, or carcinosarcoma) or a different tumor origin (GI: colon/gastric/appendiceal or breast cancer). Younger age and bilateral ovarian tumors may also be a sign that the ovarian tumors are of metastatic origin.

Gastric cancers tend to cause drop metastases to the ovary, referred to as a Krukenberg tumors, after Friedrich Krukenberg, a German gynecologist and pathologist. Because GI malignancies are apt to metastasize to the ovary owing to its extensive blood supply, these cancers are important differential diagnoses for women presenting with disseminated intra-abdominal disease on imaging. Indeed, 9% of all patients with colon cancers have metastases to the ovary, and the ovarian tumor is often bigger than the primary colonic tumor. One to 3% of all patients operated on for a presumed OC metastasis are found to have an extragenital cancer (16). Patients who present with predominantly GI symptoms, anemia, a high CEA, low CA-125, and a positive hemoccult test should undergo an esophagogastroduodenoscopy and a colonoscopy with biopsies. A CA-125/CEA serum ratio greater than 25 has high discriminative power to differentiate between OC and colon cancer, but might not be able to exclude a mucinous tumor (58).

The median survival for patients who present with peritoneal and ovarian metastasis from colon cancer is only 10 months.

Breast cancer can also metastasize to the ovary, and it is the most frequent (84%) primary cause of ovarian metastasis of non-GI origin. Metastasis of breast cancer to the ovary was found at autopsy in 23% to 39% patients who died of breast cancer. The median survival after diagnosis of breast cancer metastasized to the ovary is 26 to 54 months (17). To determine if an ovarian mass is a breast cancer metastasis or a new OC in patient with a history of breast cancer, the stage and histology and other prognostic factors (ER/PR, HER2/neu, proliferation) of the previous breast disease should be considered. Patients with stage IV breast disease are much more likely to have distant metastasis than patients with early-stage tumors, and lobular breast cancer metastasizes more often to the ovary than invasive ductal cancer (91). Most patients with ovarian metastasis from breast cancer are premenopausal (77%) and present with abdominal distension in the absence of ascites. Often, these patients have bilateral ovarian involvement (64%), a high CA15-3, and a low CA-125. However, patients with breast cancer and abdominal carcinomatosis can have a high CA-125, which makes the differentiation from OC challenging. On pelvic ultrasound, breast cancer metastases to the ovary tend to be more solid appearing than a primary OC, which is often multicystic. The benefit of surgery in the treatment of breast cancer metastatic to the ovaries has not been proven and may be limited to the palliation of symptoms by removing a single mass. Retrospective studies have suggested a possible survival benefit for surgery in patients with no residual disease after the operation but found no benefit in the setting of widely metastatic disease (17). The 5-year survival for women with ovarian metastasis from breast cancer is 26%, which is much higher than that for those with ovarian metastasis from colorectal and gastric cancer (8% and 1%, respectively), but lower than the median survival for primary OC (16). OC is the most common nonbreast secondary malignancy after treatment for breast cancer. Indeed, a history of breast cancer is associated with a 2- to 4-fold increase in the risk of developing OC, and this rate is higher in patients with hereditary breast cancer and OC syndrome.

REFERENCES

1. Chan JK, Tian C, Kesterson JP, et al. Symptoms of women with high-risk early-stage ovarian cancer. *Obstet Gynecol.* 2022;139(2):157-162.

2. Gadducci A, Multinu F, Cosio S, Carinelli S, Ghioni M, Aletti GD. Clear cell carcinoma of the ovary: epidemiology, pathological and biological features, treatment options and clinical outcomes. *Gynecol Oncol.* 2021;162(3):741-750.

3. Torre LA, Trabert B, DeSantis CE, et al. Ovarian cancer statistics, 2018. *CA Cancer J Clin.* 2018;68(4):284-296.

4. Matsuo K, Machida H, Blake EA, et al. Trends and outcomes of women with synchronous endometrial and ovarian cancer. *Oncotarget.* 2018;9(47):28757-28771.

5. Stone RL, Nick AM, McNeish IA, et al. Paraneoplastic thrombocytosis in ovarian cancer. *N Engl J Med.* 2012;366(7):610-618.

6. Henderson JT, Webber EM, Sawaya GF. Screening for ovarian cancer: updated evidence report and systematic review for the US preventive services task force. *JAMA.* 2018;319(6):595-606.

7. Menon U, Gentry-Maharaj A, Burnell M, et al. Ovarian cancer population screening and mortality after long-term follow-up in the UK Collaborative Trial of Ovarian Cancer Screening (UKCTOCS): a randomised controlled trial. *Lancet.* 2021;397(10290):2182-2193.

8. Goff BA, Mandel LS, Melancon CH, Muntz HG. Frequency of symptoms of ovarian cancer in women presenting to primary care clinics. *JAMA.* 2004;291(22):2705-2712.

9. Rossing MA, Wicklund KG, Cushing-Haugen KL, Weiss NS. Predictive value of symptoms for early detection of ovarian cancer. *J Natl Cancer Inst.* 2010;102:222-229.

10. Lim AWW, Mesher D, Gentry-Maharaj A, et al. Predictive value of symptoms for ovarian cancer: comparison of symptoms reported by questionnaire, interview, and general practitioner notes. *J Natl Cancer Inst.* 2012;104:114-124.

11. Gynecologic Practice SGO. Committee opinion No. 716: the role of the obstetrician-gynecologist in the early detection of epithelial ovarian cancer in women at average risk. *Obstet Gynecol.* 2017;130(3):e146-e149.

12. Ray A, Masch WR, Saukkonen K, Harrison BT. Case records of the Massachusetts general hospital: case 18-2016. A 52-year-old woman with a pleural effusion. *N Engl J Med.* 2016;374(24):2378-2387.

13. Taira T, Broussard N, Bugg C. Pelvic inflammatory disease: diagnosis and treatment in the emergency department. *Emerg Med Pract.* 2022;24(12):1-24.

14. Talan DA, Saverio S. Treatment of acute uncomplicated appendicitis. *N Engl J Med.* 2021;385(12):1116-1123.

15. Young-Fadok TM. Diverticulitis. *N Engl J Med.* 2018;379(17): 1635-1642.

16. Skirnisdottir I, Garmo H, Holmberg L. Non-genital tract metastases to the ovaries presented as ovarian tumors in Sweden 1990-2003: occurrence, origin and survival compared to ovarian cancer. *Gynecol Oncol.* 2007;105(1):166-171.

17. Ayhan A, Guvenal T, Salman MC, Ozyuncu O, Sakinci M, Basaran M. The role of cytoreductive surgery in nongenital cancers metastatic to the ovaries. *Gynecol Oncol.* 2005;98:235-241.

18. Nagell JR Jr, Miller RW. Evaluation and management of ultrasonographically detected ovarian tumors in asymptomatic women. *Obstet Gynecol.* 2016;127(5):848-858.

19. Bast RC, Feeney M, Lazarus H, Nadler LM, Colvin RB, Knapp RC. Reactivity of a monoclonal antibody with human ovarian carcinoma. *J Clin Invest.* 1981;68:1331-1337.

20. Vergote I, Tropé CG, Amant F, et al. Neoadjuvant chemotherapy or primary surgery in stage IIIC or IV ovarian cancer. *N Engl J Med.* 2010;363(10):943-953. doi:10.1056/NEJMoa0908806

21. Sjovall K, Nilsson B, Einhorn N. The significance of serum CA 125 elevation in malignant and nonmalignant diseases. *Gynecol Oncol.* 2002;85(1):175-178.

22. Buys S, Partridge E, Black A, et al. Effect of screening on ovarian cancer mortality. *JAMA.* 2011;305(27):2295-2303.

23. Jacobs IJ, Menon U, Ryan A, et al. Ovarian cancer screening and mortality in the UK Collaborative Trial of Ovarian Cancer Screening (UKCTOCS): a randomised controlled trial. *Lancet.* 2016;387(10022):945-956.

24. Brown PO, Palmer C. The preclinical natural history of serous ovarian cancer: defining the target for early detection. *PLoS Med.* 2009;6(7):1-11.

25. Mann W, Patsner B, Coher H, Loesch M. Preoperative serum CA-125 levels in patients with surgical stage I invasive ovarian adenocarcinoma. *J Natl Cancer Inst.* 1998;80:208-213.

26. Miller RW, Ueland FR. Risk of malignancy in sonographically confirmed ovarian tumors. *Clin Obstet Gynecol.* 2012;55(1):52-64.

27. Myers ER, Bastian LA, Havrilesky LJ, et al. Management of adnexal mass. *Evid Rep Technol Assess (Full Rep).* 2006;(130):1-145.

28. Nagell JR Jr, Miller RW, DeSimone CP, et al. Long-term survival of women with epithelial ovarian cancer detected by ultrasonographic screening. *Obstet Gynecol.* 2011;118(6):1212-1221.

29. Santillan A, Garg R, Zahurak ML, et al. Risk of epithelial ovarian cancer recurrence in patients with rising serum CA-125 levels within the normal range. *J Clin Oncol.* 2005;23(36):9338-9343.

30. Gallion HH, Hunter JE, Nagell JR, et al. The prognostic implications of low serum CA 125 levels prior to the second-look operation for stage III and IV epithelial ovarian cancer. *Gynecol Oncol.* 1992;46(1):29-32.

31. Riedinger JM, Wafflart J, Ricolleau G, et al. CA 125 half-life and CA 125 nadir during induction chemotherapy are independent predictors of epithelial ovarian cancer outcome: results of a French multicentric study. *Ann Oncol.* 2006;17(8):1234-1238.

32. Rustin GJ, Burg ME, Griffin CL, Guthrie D, Lamont A, Jayson GC. Early versus delayed treatment of relapsed ovarian cancer (MRC OVO5/EORTC 55955): a randomised trial. *Lancet.* 2010;376(9747):1155-1163.

33. Rauh-Hain JA, Melamed A, Buskwofie A, Schorge JO. Adnexal mass in the postmenopausal patient. *Clin Obstet Gynecol.* 2015;58(1):53-65.

34. Cramer DW, Bast RC Jr, Diamandis EP, et al. Ovarian cancer biomarker performance in prostate, lung, colorectal, and ovarian cancer screening trial specimens. *Cancer Prev Res (Phila).* 2011;4(3):365-374.

35. Gentry-Maharaj A, Blyuss O, Ryan A, et al. Multi-marker longitudinal algorithms incorporating HE4 and CA125 in ovarian cancer screening of postmenopausal women. *Cancers (Basel).* 2020;12:1931.

36. Olsen M, Lof P, Stiekema A, et al. The diagnostic accuracy of human epididymis protein 4 (HE4) for discriminating between benign and malignant pelvic masses: a systematic review and meta-analysis. *Acta Obstet Gynecol Scand.* 2021;100(10):1788-1799.

37. Zhen S, Bian LH, Chang LL, Gao X. Comparison of serum human epididymis protein 4 and carbohydrate antigen 125 as markers in ovarian cancer: a meta-analysis. *Mol Clin Oncol.* 2014;2(4):559-566.

38. Galgano MT, Hampton GM, Frierson HF Jr. Comprehensive analysis of HE4 expression in normal and malignant human tissues. *Mod Pathol.* 2006;19(6):847-853.

39. Moore RG, McMeekin DS, Brown AK, et al. A novel multiple marker bioassay utilizing HE4 and CA125 for the prediction of ovarian cancer in patients with a pelvic mass. *Gynecol Oncol.* 2009;112(1):40-46.

40. Moore RG, Miller MC, Disilvestro P, et al. Evaluation of the diagnostic accuracy of the risk of ovarian malignancy algorithm in women with a pelvic mass. *Obstet Gynecol.* 2011;118(2 Pt 1):280-288.

41. Underkofler K, Morell A, Esquivel R, Simone F, Miller M, Moore R. Cost-analysis comparison of initial clinical risk assessment and ROMA score for the triage of women with pelvic masses. *Gynecol Oncol.* 2021;162:120-121.

42. Yoshida A, Derchain SF, Pitta DR, Andrade LA, Sarian LO. Comparing the Copenhagen index (CPH-I) and Risk of Ovarian Malignancy Algorithm (ROMA): two equivalent ways to differentiate malignant from benign ovarian tumors before surgery? *Gynecol Oncol.* 2016;140(3):481-485.

43. Plotti F, Capriglione S, Terranova C, et al. Does HE4 have a role as biomarker in the recurrence of ovarian cancer? *Tumor Biol.* 2012;33(6):2117-2123.

44. Dunton CJ, Hutchcraft ML, Bullock RG, Northrop LE, Ueland FR. Salvaging detection of early-stage ovarian malignancies when CA125 is not informative. *Diagnostics (Basel).* 2021;11(8):1440.

45. Ghose A, Gullapalli SVN, Chohan N, et al. Applications of proteomics in ovarian cancer: dawn of a new era. *Proteomes.* 2022;10(2):16.

46. Geomini P, Kruitwagen R, Bremer GL, Cnossen J, Mol BWJ. The accuracy of risk scores in predicting ovarian malignancy. *Obstet Gynecol.* 2009;113(2):384-394.

47. Huwidi A, Abobrege A, Assidi M, Buhmeida A, Ermiah E. Diagnostic value of risk of malignancy index in the clinical evaluation of ovarian mass. *Mol Clin Oncol.* 2022;17(1):118.

48. Hentze JL, Hogdall CK, Hogdall EV. Methylation and ovarian cancer: can DNA methylation be of diagnostic use? *Mol Clin Oncol.* 2019;10(3):323-330.

49. Pisanic TR, Wang Y, Sun H, et al. Methylomic landscapes of ovarian cancer precursor lesions. *Clin Cancer Res.* 2020;26(23):6310-6320. doi:10.1158/1078-0432.CCR-20-0270

50. Liggett TE, Melnikov A, Yi Q, et al. Distinctive DNA methylation patterns of cell-free plasma DNA in women with malignant ovarian tumors. *Gynecol Oncol.* 2011;120(1):113-120.

51. Wang B, Yu L, Yang GZ, Luo X, Huang L. Application of multiplex nested methylated specific PCR in early diagnosis of epithelial ovarian cancer. *Asian Pac J Cancer Prev.* 2015;16(7):3003-3007.

52. Gold P, Freedman SO. Demonstration of tumor-specific antigens in human colonic carcinomata by immunological tolerance and absorption techniques. *J Exp Med.* 1965;121(3):439-462.

53. Tholander B, Taube A, Lindgren A, et al. Pretreatment serum levels of CA-125, carcinoembryonic antigen, tissue polypeptide antigen, and placental alkaline phosphatase, in patients with ovarian carcinoma, borderline tumors, or benign adnexal masses: relevance for differential diagnosis. *Gynecol Oncol.* 1990;39(1):16-25.

54. Anger H, Gleissenberger U. Carcino-embryogenic antigen (CEA) in patients with genital tumors (author's transl). *Geburtshilfe Frauenheilkd.* 1977;37(7):604-608.

55. Engelen MJ, Bruijn HW, Hollema H, et al. Serum CA 125, carcinoembryonic antigen, and CA 19-9 as tumor markers in borderline ovarian tumors. *Gynecol Oncol.* 2000;78(1):16-20.

56. Nomelini RS, Silva TM, Murta BMT, Murta EF. Parameters of blood count and tumor markers in patients with borderline ovarian tumors: a retrospective analysis and relation to staging. *ISRN Oncol.* 2012;2012:947831.

57. Messalli EM, Grauso F, Balbi G, Napolitano A, Seguino E, Torella M. Borderline ovarian tumors: features and controversial aspects. *Eur J Obstet Gynecol Reprod Biol.* 2013;167(1):86-89.

58. Sørensen SS, Mosgaard BJ. Combination of cancer antigen 125 and carcinoembryonic antigen can improve ovarian cancer diagnosis. *Dan Med Bull.* 2011;58(11):A4331.

59. Ueland FR, DePriest PD, Pavlik EJ, Kryscio RJ, Nagell J. Preoperative differentiation of malignant from benign ovarian tumors: the efficacy of morphology indexing and doppler flow sonography. *Gynecol Oncol.* 2003;91(1):46-50.

60. Elder JW, Pavlik EJ, Long A, et al. Serial ultrasonographic evaluation of ovarian abnormalities with a morphology index. *Gynecol Oncol.* 2014;135(1):8-12.

61. Manegold-Brauer G, Timmerman D, Hoopmann M. Evaluation of adnexal masses: the IOTA concept. *Ultraschall Med.* 2022;43:550-569.

62. Timmerman D, Ameye L, Fischerova D, et al. Simple ultrasound rules to distinguish between benign and malignant adnexal masses before surgery: prospective validation by IOTA group. *BMJ.* 2010;341:c6839.

63. Calster B, Hoorde K, Valentin L, et al. Evaluating the risk of ovarian cancer before surgery using the ADNEX model to differentiate between benign, borderline, early and advanced stage invasive, and secondary

metastatic tumours: prospective multicentre diagnostic study. *BMJ.* 2014;349:g5920.

64. Strachowski L. M., Jha P., Phillips C. H., Blanchette Porter M. M., Froyman W., Glanc P. et al. O-RADS US v2022: An Update from the American College of Radiology's Ovarian-Adnexal Reporting and Data System US Committee. *Radiology,* 2023:308:e23068.

65. Cao L, Wei M, Liu Y, et al. Validation of American College of Radiology Ovarian-adnexal Reporting and Data System Ultrasound (O-RADS US): analysis on 1054 adnexal masses. *Gynecol Oncol.* 2021;162(1):107-112.

66. Jha P, Gupta A, Baran TM, et al. Diagnostic performance of the ovarian-adnexal reporting and data system (O-RADS) ultrasound risk score in women in the United States. *JAMA Netw Open.* 2022;5(6):2216370.

67. Suh-Burgmann E, Brasic N, Jha P, Hung YY, Goldstein RB. Ultrasound characteristics of early-stage high-grade serous ovarian cancer. *Am J Obstet Gynecol.* 2021;225(4):401-409.

68. Froyman W, Landolfo C, Cock B, et al. Risk of complications in patients with conservatively managed ovarian tumours (IOTA5): a 2-year interim analysis of a multicentre, prospective, cohort study. *Lancet Oncol.* 2019;20(3):448-458.

69. Gupta A, Jha P, Baran TM, et al. Ovarian cancer detection in average-risk women: classic-versus nonclassic-appearing adnexal lesions at US. *Radiology.* 2022;303:603-610.

70. Kinkel K, Lu Y, Mehdizade A, Pelte M, Hricak H. Indeterminate ovarian mass at US: incremental value of second imaging test for characterization—meta-analysis and bayesian analysis. *Radiology.* 2005;236(1):85-94.

71. Anthoulakis C, Nikoloudis N. Pelvic MRI as the "gold standard" in the subsequent evaluation of ultrasound-indeterminate adnexal lesions: a systematic review. *Gynecol Oncol.* 2014;132(3):661-668.

72. Thomassin-Naggara I, Poncelet E, Jalaguier-Coudray A, et al. Ovarian-adnexal reporting data system magnetic resonance imaging (O-RADS MRI) score for risk stratification of sonographically indeterminate adnexal masses. *JAMA Netw Open.* 2020;3(1):1919896.

73. Sadowski EA, Thomassin-Naggara I, Rockall A, et al. O-RADS MRI risk stratification system: guide for assessing adnexal lesions from the ACR O-RADS committee. *Radiology.* 2022;303(1):35-47.

74. Balan P. Ultrasonography, computed tomography and magnetic resonance imaging in the assessment of pelvic pathology. *Eur J Radiol.* 2006;58:147-155.

75. Liu J, Xu Y, Wang J. Ultrasonography, computed tomography and magnetic resonance imaging for diagnosis of ovarian carcinoma. *Eur J Radiol.* 2007;62(3):328-334.

76. Borley J, Wilhelm-Benartzi C, Yazbek J, et al. Radiological predictors of cytoreductive outcomes in patients with advanced ovarian cancer. *BJOG.* 2015;122(6):843-849.

77. Onda T, Tanaka YO, Kitai S, Hung YY, et al. Stage III disease of ovarian, tubal and peritoneal cancers can be accurately diagnosed with pre-operative CT. Japan clinical oncology group study JCOG0602. *Jpn J Clin Oncol.* 2021;51(2):205-212.

78. Bristow RE, Duska L, Lambrou N, et al. A model for predicting surgical outcome in patients with advanced ovarian carcinoma using computed tomography. *Cancer.* 2000;89:1532-1540.

79. Axtell A, Lee MH, Bristow RE, et al. Multi-Institutional reciprocal validation study of computed tomography predictors of suboptimal primary cytoreduction in patients with advanced ovarian cancer. *J Clin Oncol.* 2007;25(4):384-389.

80. Suidan RS, Ramirez PT, Sarasohn DM, et al. A multicenter prospective trial evaluating the ability of preoperative computed tomography scan and serum CA-125 to predict suboptimal cytoreduction at primary debulking surgery for advanced ovarian, fallopian tube, and peritoneal cancer. *Gynecol Oncol.* 2014;134(3):455-461.

81. Nick AM, Coleman RL, Ramirez PT, Sood AK. A framework for a personalized surgical approach to ovarian cancer. *Nat Rev Clin Oncol.* 2015;12(4):239-245.

82. Petrillo M, Vizzielli G, Fanfani F, et al. Definition of a dynamic laparoscopic model for the prediction of incomplete cytoreduction in advanced epithelial ovarian cancer: proof of a concept. *Gynecol Oncol.* 2015; 139(1):5-9.

83. Gadducci A, Cosio S. Surveillance of patients after initial treatment of ovarian cancer. *Crit Rev Oncol Hematol.* 2009;71:43-52.

84. Antunovic L, Cimitan M, Borsatti E, et al. Revisiting the clinical value of 18 F-FDG PET/CT in detection of recurrent epithelial ovarian carcinomas. *Clin Nucl Med.* 2012;37(8):184-188.

85. Risum S, Hogdall C, Loft A, et al. The diagnostic value of PET/CT for ovarian cancer—a prospective study. *Gynecol Oncol.* 2007;105: 145-149.

86. Dauwen H, Calster B, Deroose CM, et al. PET/CT in the staging of patients with a pelvic mass suspicious for ovarian cancer. *Gynecol Oncol.* 2013;131(3):694-700.

87. Michielsen K, Vergote I, Beeck KO, et al. Whole-body MRI with diffusion-weighted sequence for staging of patients with suspected ovarian cancer: a clinical feasibility study in comparison to CT and FDG-PET/CT. *Eur Radiol.* 2014;24(4):889-901.

88. Michielsen K, Dresen R, Vanslembrouck R, et al. Diagnostic value of whole body diffusion-weighted MRI compared to computed tomography for pre-operative assessment of patients suspected for ovarian cancer. *Eur J Cancer.* 2017;83:88-98.

89. Garcia Prado J, Hernando CG, Delgado DV, et al. Diffusion-weighted magnetic resonance imaging in peritoneal carcinomatosis from suspected ovarian cancer: diagnostic performance in correlation with surgical findings. *Eur J Radiol.* 2019;121:108696.

90. Ayantunde A, Parsons S. Pattern and prognostic factors in patients with malignant ascites: a retrospective study. *Ann Oncol.* 2007;18: 945-949.

91. Mathew A, Rajagopal PS, Villgran V, et al. Distinct pattern of metastases in patients with invasive lobular carcinoma of the breast. *Geburtshilfe Frauenheilkd.* 2017;77(6):660-666.

CHAPTER **8.6**

Surgery for Ovarian Cancer

Oliver Zivanovic and Ernst Lengyel

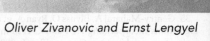

INTRODUCTION AND DEFINITIONS

Surgery plays an important role at every phase of OC treatment, and patients with OC should be seen by gynecologic oncologist whenever a major treatment decision is made to consider if surgery is a treatment option. Patients newly diagnosed with OC usually undergo surgery for the purpose of pathologic diagnosis,

cytoreduction, symptom relief, and tumor staging. Indeed, both the old 1988 and new 2014 FIGO staging systems (**Table 8.6-1**) require that surgery be performed to confirm the histologic diagnosis and to determine the true extent of the disease. The staging does not change when the patient has a recurrence. In the recurrent disease setting, a surgical biopsy can confirm a diagnosis and may provide therapeutic benefit, because the removal of an isolated mass may

■ **TABLE 8.6-1. 1988 and 2013 FIGO Ovarian Cancer Staging**

Surgical FIGO—Ovarian Cancer Staging Rio de Janeiro—1988		Surgical FIGO—Ovarian Cancer Staging Rome—2013		
I	Tumors limited to one or both ovaries	I	Tumor confined to ovaries or *fallopian tubes*	
IA	Tumor limited to one ovary; capsule intact; no tumor on ovarian surface; no malignant cells in ascites/peritoneal washings	IA	Tumor limited to one ovary, capsule intact or *fallopian tube*, no tumor on ovarian or fallopian tube surface, no malignant cells in ascites or peritoneal washings	
IB	Tumor limited to both ovaries; capsule intact; no tumor on ovarian surface; no malignant cells in ascites/peritoneal washings	IB	Tumor involves both ovaries; capsule intact or *fallopian tubes*, no malignant cells in ascites or peritoneal washings	
IC	Tumor limited to ovaries with any of the following: capsule ruptured, tumor on ovarian surface, positive washings/ascites	IC1-3	Tumor limited to one or both ovaries/fallopian tubes	
			IC1	Surgical spill intraoperatively
			IC2	Capsule rupture before surgery or tumor on ovarian or fallopian tube surface
			IC3	Malignant cells in the ascites or peritoneal washings
II	Tumor involves one or both ovaries with pelvic extension or implants	II	Tumor involves one or both ovaries or *fallopian tube* with pelvic extension (below the pelvic brim) or *primary peritoneal cancer*	
IIA	Extension and/or implants on uterus or fallopian tube; negative washings/ascites	IIA	Extension and/or implants on uterus and/or fallopian tubes	
IIB	Extension or implants onto other pelvic structures; negative washings/ascites	IIB	Extension to other pelvic intraperitoneal tissues	
IIC	Pelvic extension (IIA or IIB) or implants with positive peritoneal washings/ascites			
III	Microscopic peritoneal implants outside the pelvis; or limited to the pelvis with extension to the small bowel or omentum	III	Tumor involves one or both ovaries or fallopian tubes, or primary peritoneal cancer, with cytologically or histologically confirmed spread to the peritoneum outside the pelvis and/or metastasis to the *retroperitoneal* lymph nodes	
IIIA	Microscopic peritoneal metastases beyond pelvis	IIIA	IIIA1	Positive retroperitoneal lymph nodes only IIIA1(i) Metastasis ≤10 mm IIIA1(ii) Metastasis >10 mm
			IIIA2	Microscopic, extrapelvic (above the pelvic brim), peritoneal involvement and/or positive retroperitoneal lymph nodes
IIIB	Macroscopic peritoneal metastases beyond pelvis <2 cm in size	IIIB	Macroscopic, extrapelvic, peritoneal metastasis ≤2 cm and/or positive retroperitoneal lymph nodes. Includes extension to capsule of liver/spleen	
IIIC	Macroscopic peritoneal metastases beyond pelvis >2 cm and/or positive retroperitoneal or inguinal lymph nodes (pT3B N1 or pT3C)	IIIC	Macroscopic, extrapelvic, peritoneal metastasis >2 cm and/or positive retroperitoneal lymph nodes. Includes extension to capsule of liver/spleen (no parenchymal involvement)	
IV	Distant metastasis including pleural effusion with positive cytology. Distant metastases outside the peritoneal cavity. Parenchymal liver/splenic metastasis	IV	Distant metastasis excluding peritoneal metastasis	
		IVA	Pleural effusion with positive cytology/biopsy	
		IVB	Hepatic and/or splenic parenchymal metastasis, metastasis to extra-abdominal organs (including inguinal lymph nodes and lymph nodes outside the abdominal cavity) Bowel infiltration—transmural with mucosal involvement and umbilical deposit	

Comments on FIGO 2013 (Prat and Oncology 2014): There is no stage I primary peritoneal cancer. Dense adhesions of pelvic tumors containing tumor cells justify upgrading apparent stage I tumors to stage II. Rectum invasion is stage IIB. Positive para-aortic lymph node metastases are considered regional lymph nodes (2013 FIGO IIIA1(ii). Involvement of retroperitoneal lymph nodes must be proven cytologically or histologically. Examples of metastatic sites that upstage tumors to 2013 FIGO IVB: mesenteric lymph nodes, for example, colon or small bowel mesentery, transmural bowel infiltration, subcutaneous/umbilicus/abdominal wall, extra-abdominal lymph nodes (inguinal, axillary) and umbilical metastasis. Changes between 1988 FIGO and 2013 FIGO are italicized.

From Berek JS, Renz M, Kehoe S, et al. Cancer of the ovary, fallopian tube, and peritoneum: 2021 update. *Int J Gynecol Obstet*. 2021;155 suppl 1(suppl 1):61-85, John Wiley and Sons.

render a patient macroscopically tumor free and provide tissue for molecular testing and possible targeted treatment. In patients with recurrent disease involving extensive tumor dissemination, removal of tumor masses ("debulking" or "cytoreduction") accomplishes significant symptom relief, and, in select patients, limited surgery may result in the palliation of bowel obstruction. Clinically, there is a distinction between "low-volume advanced-stage disease" and "high-volume advanced-stage disease" because the lower the volume at presentation, the greater the possibility that surgery will result in an absence of residual disease and better survival (1).

The most important prognostic factors predicting long-term survival from OC are the FIGO stage and the amount of disease remaining after cytoreductive surgery. Patients with OC will benefit from treatment by a gynecologic oncologist or physicians familiar with the disease and skilled in its surgical management.

The widely used 1988 FIGO staging system for OC was replaced in 2013 by a new staging system approved by FIGO in 2013 (**Table 8.6-1**) (2). Of note, both para-aortic and inguinal lymph nodes are included in FIGO stage IIIC disease, whereas mesenteric lymph nodes (eg, nodes in the mesentery of the colon) are considered FIGO stage IV disease.

The terms for common surgical procedures, as they are used in this chapter, are defined in **Table 8.6-2**.

▪ **TABLE 8.6-2. Terms for Common Surgical Procedures**

Procedure	Definition
Paracentesis Thoracentesis	Drainage of presumed malignant fluid/ascites in a patient with intra-abdominal (paracentesis) tumor masses or a pleural effusion (thoracentesis) to establish a diagnosis with cytology before initiation of chemotherapy, to confirm a recurrence, or to provide symptomatic relief.
Biopsy	Biopsy of disseminated disease or an adnexal mass to establish a pathologic diagnosis before initiation of chemotherapy. Most commonly CT and sometimes ultrasound guided.
Staging surgery	Surgery to evaluate extent of disease guiding treatment decisions (chemotherapy: yes/no) for early-stage disease.
Interval cytoreduction or interval debulking	Cytoreductive surgery after a biopsy only or a primary suboptimal debulking or a limited surgery (eg, hysterectomy/BSO) followed by induction chemotherapy, most commonly carboplatin/paclitaxel.
Second-look surgery	Surgery performed at the completion of primary chemotherapy in patients who do not have evidence of disease by CT scan or CA-125 to determine whether there is residual disease in order to plan for additional chemotherapy. Currently rarely performed.
Secondary cytoreductive surgery	Surgery in a patient with recurrent disease who has completed primary treatment, including primary debulking and/or chemotherapy, and had been without evidence of disease for at least 6 mo. The procedure is most commonly performed for platinum-sensitive patients with oligometastatic disease. Also called "secondary debulking" by some physicians.
Palliative surgery	Surgery performed to relieve symptoms, most commonly performed for a malignant bowel obstruction with the goal to remove the obstruction or perform a diversion. Rarely performed for pain relief. Not primarily intended to remove tumors.
Staging surgery	Surgery to evaluate extent of disease guiding treatment decisions (chemotherapy: yes/no) for early-stage disease.
Posterior pelvic exenteration	*En bloc* resection of bladder serosa, uterus, sigmoid colon, and proximal rectum, as well as ovarian/fallopian tube masses, cul-de-sac tumors with complete parietal pelvic peritonectomy to encompass all pan-pelvic disease (25).
Surgery: Complete debulking Result: No macroscopic disease	Complete resection (99): Cytoreduction of all tumors independent of preoperative tumor load to microscopic residual disease at the completion of surgery—no gross residual tumors left. R0 resection.
Surgery: Optimal debulking Result: Macroscopic disease up to 1 cm	Minimal residual (99): Macroscopic disease up to 1 cm in diameter after primary surgery. Also called by some physicians "optimal cytoreduction." R1 resection.
Surgery: Suboptimal debulking Result: Macroscopic disease >1 cm	Gross residual (99): Primary cytoreduction resulting in macroscopic disease >1 cm in size at the end of surgery. R2 resection.

BSO, bilateral salpingo-oophorectomy; CT, computed tomography.

EARLY-STAGE OVARIAN CANCER

Optimal staging in early OC includes careful inspection and/or palpation, biopsies of peritoneal surfaces (diaphragm, paracolic gutters, bladder, and cul-de-sac peritoneum), pelvic and diaphragmatic washings, removal of the affected ovary, an infracolic or infragastric omentectomy, and a systematic pelvic and para-aortic lymph node dissection (3). An appendectomy can, though rarely, change the final staging. However, sometimes, there is microscopic disease on the tip of the appendix, especially if it is attached to the right ovary. Preserving the contralateral ovary and the uterus in young patients desiring fertility is considered acceptable in appropriately selected cases of early-stage epithelial invasive and borderline OC. Every effort should be made to remove an ovarian mass intact, although it is not clear whether intraoperative rupture affects prognosis. Rupture of an ovarian mass is often associated with thick/dense adhesions, especially in endometrioid and clear cell cancers. If these adhesions contain tumor cells, tumors that otherwise appear to be FIGO stage I should be upstaged to FIGO stage II (**Table 8.6-1**).

Thorough surgical staging of early OC is important for establishing the correct FIGO stage in order to determine prognosis and choice of therapy (chemotherapy vs observation) and/or the role of maintenance therapy. In a study of 86 patients with OC grossly confined to the ovary, approximately 30% of the patients who underwent completion surgery were upstaged. Sixty percent of these patients were upstaged because of microscopic disease in biopsy specimens from adhesions or the omentum, whereas the others had either uterine or fallopian tube metastases or positive lymph nodes. Occult metastases were associated with increasing tumor grade and the presence of ascites (4). Other predictors that residual disease will be present after primary surgery include a high preoperative CA-125 level and positive cytology from pelvic or diaphragmatic washings (5).

For women presenting with early-stage disease, complete staging may obviate the need for cytotoxic chemotherapy. A retrospective subset analysis of patients with FIGO stage I-IIA disease enrolled in the Adjuvant ChemoTherapy In Ovarian Neoplasm (ACTION) trial found that complete surgical staging was statistically significantly associated with better outcomes, presumably because the unstaged group included patients with occult FIGO stage III disease (6,7). In this trial, patients were randomly assigned to adjuvant chemotherapy or observation after they had undergone either complete or incomplete staging surgery. Although the trial was not designed to compare different surgical staging procedures (and extent of surgical staging was not randomized), a subgroup analysis of patients with a poorly differentiated tumor found that the optimally surgically staged group (*n* = 78) had a significantly longer (*P* < .009) 10-year cancer-specific survival of 85% compared to 56% in patients who were not completely staged (*n* = 78). This improved outcome was independent of age, presumed stage, histology, and whether or not chemotherapy was given. Moreover, the benefit of adjuvant chemotherapy was seen only in patients with incomplete surgical staging. Incompletely staged patients with a poorly differentiated, grade III tumor were found to derive the greatest benefit from adjuvant chemotherapy. However, the role of chemotherapy in relation to staging remains uncertain. The separate International Collaborative Ovarian Neoplasm 1 (ICON1) trial suggested that both incompletely and completely staged patients with early-stage disease may benefit from adjuvant chemotherapy (8,9). The role of adjuvant chemotherapy in early-stage OC is particularly questionable in patients with clear cell or endometrioid carcinoma of the ovary, often diagnosed at a younger age and lower stage than the more common high-grade serous epithelial carcinoma of the ovary. Here, adjuvant chemotherapy in patients with FIGO stages IA and IB disease has not been shown to have an impact on survival, probably because clear cell and endometrioid OC are less responsive to standard chemotherapy than HGSCs (10). Therefore, accurate staging is of great importance in patients with presumably early-stage EOC and can help determine the need for adjuvant chemotherapy.

The surgical approach to the staging of presumed early-stage OC will depend on patient comorbidities and the number of previous abdominal operations, as well as on how skilled the surgeon is at minimally invasive surgery. Retrospective studies suggest that both a minimally invasive approach and an open laparotomy allow for comprehensive surgical staging. Concerns regarding the minimally invasive approaches include limited visibility of both diaphragms, the inability to palpate tissue, and the longer operating time. Lymph node counts and the size of the omental specimen obtained are similar for both procedures. Given that bulky disease is only rarely detected in patients with early-stage OC, a minimally invasive surgical approach is preferable, because it involves less blood loss, a shorter hospital stay, and faster recovery with less pain and allows patients to start chemotherapy earlier. However, specialized surgical training and experience is necessary (11). Another concern with the laparoscopic approach is the possibility of port site metastasis, although this risk seems to be small (1.18%) and such metastases are often a sign of disseminated intra-abdominal disease (12). In early OC, restaging involves multiple biopsies of the diaphragmatic, abdominal, and pelvic/bladder peritoneum, as well as, at the least, a unilateral salpingo-oophorectomy, omentectomy, pelvic and para-aortic lymph node dissection, and peritoneal washings for cytology. Patients who do not want to preserve fertility will also have a hysterectomy and removal of the contralateral ovary and tubes.

In most cases, patients with presumed early-stage invasive OC (eg, found incidentally) should be offered staging, even if this means a second surgical procedure, particularly if this can be done

minimally invasive. Exceptions here are mucinous and low-grade endometrioid OC because the risk of lymph node metastases is extremely low (13). If surgical staging is not feasible, decisions with regard to adjuvant treatment should be weight carefully against observation, taking into consideration the detailed histology, imaging results, and patient comorbidities. Often, such patients will be treated with adjuvant chemotherapy to account for possible high-risk disease.

The Role of Lymph Node Dissection in Early and Advanced Ovarian Cancer

When treating both early and advanced OC, a surgeon should make two decisions: (a) whether to perform a lymph node sampling and (b) whether to remove only enlarged or palpably suspicious lymph nodes or to perform a systematic lymph node dissection, removing all visible pelvic and para-aortic lymph nodes within defined anatomic borders. Dye studies have shown that the lymphatic drainage of the ovaries originates under the ovarian surface. Lymph fluid predominantly drains superiorly, along both ovarian vascular pedicles (14). On the left side, the lymphatics follow the infundibulopelvic vein until it drains into the left renal vein. The high left infrarenal, para-aortic lymph nodes often harbor lymph node metastasis and are a known site of (isolated) recurrence. The right infundibulopelvic vein and its accompanying lymphatics reach the inferior vena cava (IVC) about 1 to 3 cm below the right renal vein. Cancer cells are then able to continue traveling along a net of lymphatic vessels covering the IVC and the interaortocaval space to lymph nodes at the base of the celiac axis and then through the caval opening in the diaphragm into the chest, reaching thoracic, mediastinal, or prescalene lymph nodes. Secondary lymph drainage routes are along lymphatics draining inferiorly through the utero-ovarian ligament to lymph nodes in the broad ligament and along the external iliac artery to the round ligament and then to inguinal lymph nodes. This spread pattern explains why inguinal lymph node metastasis is sometimes detected in patients with OC. There is also minor lymph drainage to lymphatics along the internal iliac artery or lymph nodes in the obturator fossa (15). Ovarian lymph drainage does not reach the uterus, explaining why intrauterine or cervical metastases are rare in serous OC.

It is recommended that both the pelvic and high, infrarenal para-aortic lymph nodes should be removed when a systematic lymph node dissection is performed in patients with early OC (8,9) (Figure 8.6-1). However, given the lymphatic drainage of the

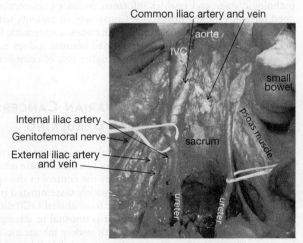
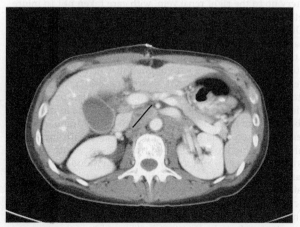

Figure 8.6-1. Pelvic and high para-aortic lymph node dissection in a patient with FIGO stage IIIC serous ovarian cancer and bulky para-aortic (computed tomography scan, upper panel) and pelvic lymph node (lower panel) metastasis that were surgically removed. Before the lymph node dissection, a posterior exenteration was performed—the next step was to perform an end-to-end anastomosis, the descending colon with the rectum (not shown). She was optimally debulked (microscopic disease). FIGO, International Federation of Gynaecology and Obstetrics; IVC, inferior vena cava.

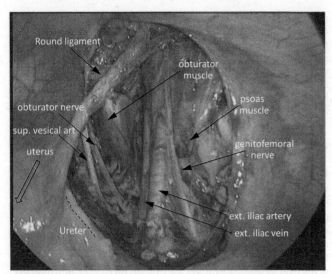

Figure 8.6-2. Right pelvic space anatomy showing the anatomic structures identified during a complete pelvic lymph node (LN) dissection. The borders of a pelvic LN dissection are as follows: lateral—the genitofemoral nerve, medial—the superior vesical artery, and posterior—the obturator nerve. In this specific patient, 13 pelvic LNs were removed.

ovaries, the removal of high para-aortic lymph nodes is the most important procedure (16). The anatomic borders of a pelvic lymph node dissection are laterally, the external iliac artery and the genitofemoral nerve that travels on the psoas muscle; superiorly, the bifurcation of the external and internal iliac artery to the inguinal ligament; and medially, the anterior division of the hypogastric artery and the ureter (**Figure 8.6-2**). By slightly elevating and lateralizing the external iliac vein, the surgeon exposes the obturator fossa and the obturator nerve and then clears the lymph nodes superior to the nerve, which should be observed at all times during the deep pelvic lymph node dissection. To enable right para-aortic lymph node dissection, the descending colon and terminal ileum are mobilized by incising the peritoneum around the cecum to expose the IVC and interaortocaval space. The cecum is reflected medially by incising the peritoneum on the right side along Toldt line on the right and the cecum mesentery, which allows reflection of the entire cecum and part of the right hemicolon to the left. The dissection is begun on the right common iliac artery. The precaval fatty tissue containing lymph nodes is then removed from the common iliac artery up to the right renal vein, with care taken not to injure the ureter, renal vessels, or the third/horizontal part of the duodenum. Of note, the superior mesenteric artery/vein is anterior to the third part of the duodenum. To remove the left para-aortic lymph nodes, the fat/lymph node containing tissue lateral to the aorta between the bifurcation of the left common iliac artery and the left renal vein is removed. Although it is rarely necessary, the inferior mesenteric artery can be ligated to accomplish a high para-aortic dissection. Because the lymph nodes rest on top of the lumbar vertebral bodies, care must be taken not to injure the lumbar veins. A systematic lymph node dissection is associated with increased operating time, blood loss, and blood transfusions. Acute complications of the surgery include, rarely, bowel injury (duodenum), venous vascular injuries (IVC, external iliac, hypogastric vein), nerve (obturator, genitofemoral nerves), and ureteral injuries. Long-term complications include lower extremity lymphedema, adhesive disease, and formation of lymphoceles, which can become chronic and sometimes infected, requiring drainage, obliteration, or surgery (17). The rate of positive lymph nodes is very low in mucinous OC and in patients with low-grade endometrioid OC. Lymph node dissection probably can be omitted in for patients with these histologic subtypes of OC (13,17-19).

Several retrospective studies have indicated that the rate of positive lymph nodes in patients of all FIGO stages who undergo a systematic pelvic and para-aortic lymph node dissection is 25% to 53%, with most of the positive lymph nodes found in the high para-aortic and interaortocaval regions (16,18,20). Because imaging and intraoperative palpation of lymph node beds have a low sensitivity and specificity for the detection of lymph node metastasis, several studies have investigated the role of a systematic pelvic and para-aortic lymph node dissection. In a prospective trial, Maggioni and colleagues randomized 310 patients diagnosed with early FIGO 1988 stages I and II OC, who had undergone optimal surgical debulking, to receive either a systematic lymph node dissection or lymph node sampling (21). Patients with all major histologic subtypes were represented in the study: serous (39%), endometrioid (21%), mucinous (13%), and clear cell tumors (13%). Positive lymph nodes (which upstage a patient to FIGO 1988 stage IIIC or FIGO 2013 stage IIIA1) were found in 9% of patients in the sampling group and in 22% of the systematic lymph node dissection group ($P < .05$), suggesting that 13% were upstaged because of the lymph node dissection. Of those with negative lymph nodes, 66% of the patients in the control arm and 51% in the systematic lymphadenectomy arm received chemotherapy ($P < .03$), suggesting that, in an unstaged patient, physicians tend to err on the side of overtreatment. The patients in the systematic lymph node dissection arm spent an average of 90 minutes longer in surgery, lost 300 mL more blood, and significantly more patients received blood transfusions (22% vs 36%, $P < .05$). Both groups had similar rates of postoperative complications. There was no difference in PFS or OS between the two groups, but the study was underpowered for the detection of a small benefit.

The 1988 FIGO staging categorized patients with lymph node metastasis or IP metastasis as FIGO IIIC. Patients with an OC limited to the pelvis with positive retroperitoneal lymph nodes have a significantly longer 5-year PFS and OS than patients with a pelvic tumor and IP disease. Therefore, the new 2014 FIGO (**Table 8.6-1**) staging subclassified patients with "only" retroperitoneal lymph node metastasis as stage IIIA1. A review of the large GOG #182 trial (22) analyzed patients who underwent cytoreduction to microscopic residual disease. The median PFS was 21 months for patients with positive lymph nodes and IP disease greater than 2 cm before surgery, 29 months with negative lymph nodes and disease greater than 2 cm, and 48 months for patients who had positive lymph nodes but preoperative IP disease less than 2 cm (23).

In summary, systematic lymph node dissection provides important prognostic and staging information for patients with suspected early-stage OC, which assists with assigning the correct pathologic stage and enables informed decisions concerning the need for adjuvant chemotherapy. Conversely, in patients with advanced OC and clinically normal lymph nodes, a systematic lymph node dissection should not be performed because it does not improve survival but is associated with higher risk of complications and mortality.

ADVANCED EPITHELIAL OVARIAN CANCER: RATIONALE FOR SURGICAL DEBULKING

Surgical debulking is central to the initial management of advanced FIGO stage III/IV OC, and the extent of residual disease after surgery is the only prognostic factor under the control of the operating surgeon. The concept of removing widely disseminated tumors within the abdominal cavity is specific to epithelial OC/fallopian/peritoneal, and appendiceal cancers. It is unusual to attempt primary tumor debulking in patients with widely metastatic colon, breast, or gastric cancer. One reason surgical debulking of OC is technically feasible is that serous OC is usually confined within the peritoneal borders of the abdominal cavity. It spreads along the peritoneal, diaphragmatic surfaces without deep invasion (24) into abdominal organs, and this allows dissection along a surgical plane between an organ and the attached tumor. For example, while the omental tumor is often large and densely attached to the transverse colon, it is often not necessary to perform a transverse colon resection and it is frequently possible to sharply dissect the tumor off without injuring the colon muscularis. In patients with deep infiltration of the colon with impending large bowel obstruction, sometimes, an en bloc resection with a portion of transverse colon is necessary to achieve a complete gross resection. The omental tumor often reaches the splenic hilum and distal pancreas but rarely invades the parenchyma of these organs, and most of the times, it is possible to dissect the diseased omentum from the pancreas and spleen. In cases when tumor is invading the splenic hilum or the tail of the pancreas, en bloc resection with spleen and distal pancreas is necessary to achieve a complete gross resection. While ovarian tumors can occlude the pelvis completely and transform the pelvic peritoneum into thick tumor plaques, the pelvis can usually be completely cleared of tumors with a modified posterior exenteration (25). Serous OC tumors never extend via direct invasion beyond the lining of the peritoneal surfaces, and a retroperitoneal dissection allows the entire tumor-covered peritoneal reflection to be removed (**Figure 8.6-3A,B**) (25). In contrast, uterine and ovarian sarcomas and carcinosarcomas, and colon and breast cancers often grow retroperitoneally, making a complete resection more challenging.

Several theories have been put forward to explain the strong association of surgical debulking to a state of no visible residual disease with patient survival ("microscopic disease"). One factor could be that the ability to surgically remove all disease correlates with other biologic factors that predispose to better outcomes. However, large bulky tumors may contain necrotic or hypoxic areas that have a low growth fraction and are resistant to chemotherapy. Optimal debulking could then, theoretically, drive remaining microscopic tumor cells into the cell cycle, rendering them more susceptible to cytotoxic chemotherapy.

In advanced "high tumor volume" OC, staging traditionally takes place as part of the initial debulking surgery, with the goal of removing all visible disease and, possibly, implanting a port for IP chemotherapy (26) or HIPEC. In patients with extensive tumor dissemination combined with a chronic bowel obstruction, the cancer leads to tumor-associated cachexia with a catabolic metabolic status, limiting the patient's ability to maintain reasonable nutritional status. Removal of tumor masses ("debulking") produces significant symptom relief from tumors externally pressing on organs in the pelvis or the upper abdomen. Surgical tumor debulking can also reduce ascites production and improve the nutritional and functional status of the patient, resulting in a higher QoL.

Overall, there is no uniform surgical approach to the treatment of advanced OC. Patient (age, nutritional status, comorbidities) and intraoperative factors (disease location, adhesions from previous surgeries, intraoperative stability/anesthesia, blood loss) and the surgical skills of the physician as well as the available infrastructure will determine the extent of surgical resection in the individual patient. It requires significant surgical training and experience to successfully remove pelvic and upper abdominal disease with an acceptable complication rate. In Europe, a gynecologist generally collaborates closely with a general surgeon, who usually performs the bowel resections and upper abdominal debulking (eg, diaphragm stripping, splenectomy). In North America, the majority of debulking, including gastrointestinal (GI) procedures, is performed by a gynecologic oncologist with the consultation of a hepatobiliary surgeon should extensive mobilization of the liver or a liver resection be necessary. Although the comparative efficacy of these two approaches has never been studied, studies on both sides of the Atlantic have shown that high-volume centers have a higher rate of optimal surgical debulking in advanced OC. The resectability of extensive disease with acceptable morbidity is likely to reflect a combination of surgical experience, technique, anesthesia care, critical and postoperative care, and nursing. Optimal debulking rates of up to 70% to 80% have been reported in various centers

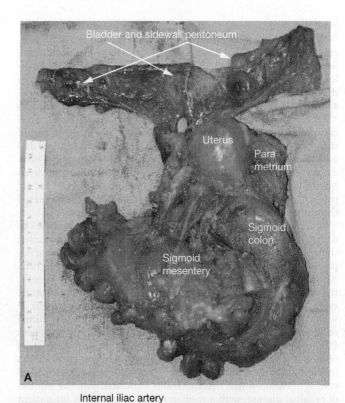

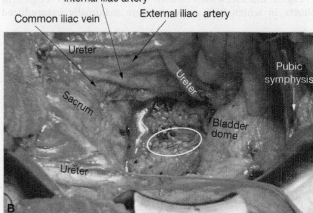

Figure 8.6-3. Posterior pelvic exenteration. (A) En bloc resection of sigmoid colon and its mesentery, uterus, cervix, parametrium, and tumor-studded pelvic peritoneum (cul-de-sac, pelvic sidewall, bladder). (B) Pelvis after a posterior pelvic exenteration. The pelvis is tumor free and deperitonealized. The white circle indicates the stapled rectal stump. The next surgical step is reanastomosing the descending colon with the rectum.

(27,28), but 50% is an accepted quality measure (3). Several centers have shown that a dedicated surgical team and a multidisciplinary effort can improve complete and optimal cytoreduction rates over time (29). Size and tumor distribution at the beginning and end of surgery should be carefully documented in the operative report in order to define the two most important prognostic factors (stage and residual disease).

The characterization of surgical outcome based on the amount of residual disease at the end of surgery is an accepted measure of surgical success, with the caveat that tumor measurements have a high degree of interobserver variability. Although many surgeons had previously recommended a maximal debulking effort for patients with advanced OC (eg, Joe V. Meigs; Surgeon at MGH), it was not until a retrospective study by the American gynecologic oncologist C. Tom Griffiths in 1975 that an inverse relationship between residual tumor size and survival was established (30). Since that time, a number of retrospective studies and meta-analyses have reported the prognostic value of residual disease for both PFS and OS (22,23,27,31-33). In 1992, Hoskins and colleagues reviewed survival and surgical results in two GOG studies that enrolled patients with FIGO stages III and IV disease (GOG #52, #97) (34,35). Defining three different groups (microscopic vs <2 cm vs >2 cm residual disease), the authors found that survival is inversely related to the volume of residual disease at the end of surgery. Notably, they also found that, in patients with residual disease greater than 2 cm, increments in the size of residual disease did not appreciably affect survival. Later, Chi and colleagues from Memorial Sloan-Kettering showed that the introduction of radical pelvic dissection and upper abdominal debulking surgery increased the number of patients who could be optimally debulked (28).

In the largest (4,312 women) phase III OC trial performed to date (GOG #182), the Gynecological Cancer InterGroup studied the addition of a third chemotherapy group to the standard carboplatin and paclitaxel regimen in women with stage III/IV OC (22). Although the addition of a third drug did not show any benefit, the extent of cytoreductive surgery was shown to be significantly correlated with PFS and OS. Patients with FIGO stages III and IV who had no macroscopic disease at the end of surgery, minimal residual disease (<1 cm), or gross residual disease had a median PFS of 29, 16, and 13 months, respectively, and a median OS of 68, 44, and 30 months, respectively. Breakdown by stage is shown in **Figure 8.6-4**. A meta-analysis of 81 studies by Bristow and colleagues also showed that survival is associated with the amount of residual disease, with a median OS of 22.7 months for patient cohorts in which 25% or fewer were maximally cytoreduced

(≤3 cm residual tumor) and a median OS of 33.9 months for patient cohorts with 75% or greater rates of maximal cytoreduction (27). Each 10% increase in the proportion of patients who were maximally cytoreduced was associated with a 5.5% increase in median cohort survival time.

Improved survival with complete tumor resection is also seen in patients with FIGO stage IV disease. Winter et al, reviewing the experience of GOG #111, #132, #152, and #162, showed that patients with residual disease greater than 5 cm, multiple stage IV defining sites of metastasis (parenchymal liver disease, pleural effusion), and clear cell cancer/mucinous OC had a significantly worse survival (31). The median PFS and OS for stage IV patients whose tumor was reduced to microscopic disease were better than those for patients with any amount of visible residual cancer. Patients with residual disease where the single largest lesion is 0.1 to 1.0 cm and 1.1 to 5.0 cm had comparable survival, and patients with residual tumor bigger than 5 cm had the worst prognosis. These data have been interpreted to suggest that, even in patients with FIGO stage IV disease, cytoreduction to microscopic disease should be the primary goal at initial surgery. A positive association of stage IV disease optimally debulked to microscopic residual disease with longer survival was also confirmed by review of three prospective phase III German AGO trials (AGO-OVAR #3, #5, #7) (36).

Presurgical large metastatic tumor load plays an important role in prognosis (34). An important question is whether every patient benefits from surgical debulking, independent of the extent of disease at the beginning of surgery. In GOG #52, patients with large-volume disease at the beginning of surgery, who were optimally debulked using an aggressive upper abdominal procedure, still had shorter survival than patients who initially had low-volume

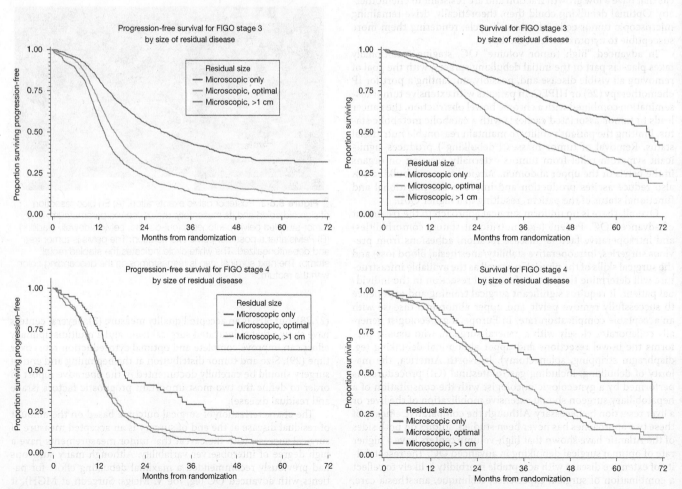

Figure 8.6-4. Outcomes by residual disease in GOG #182. FIGO, International Federation of Gynaecology and Obstetrics; GOG, Gynecologic Oncology Group. (Courtesy of Drs. Bookman, Brady, and Lengyel of the Gynecologic Oncology Group.)

disease, even if the surgical outcome was similar (34). Du Bois and colleagues, summarizing the AGO experience from three prospective phase III trials (3,126 patients from AGO-OVAR #3, #5, #7) with identical inclusion criteria, concluded that complete surgical debulking is associated with improved prognosis in any FIGO substage but cannot completely overcome the prognostic impact of preoperative disease load (32). Resection to microscopic disease was associated with a longer median OS (microscopic disease: 99.1 months CI 83.5 not reached; residual <1 cm: 29.6 months CI 27.4-32.2; residual >1 cm: 29.6 months CI 27.4-32). Similarly, Zivanovic and colleagues evaluated the impact of upper abdominal disease on surgical outcome and survival (37). In their study, 526 patients with FIGO stage IIIC ovarian carcinoma who underwent primary cytoreduction followed by platinum-based chemotherapy were evaluated. Optimal versus suboptimal cytoreduction was significantly associated with improved median PFS and OS in patients with no, minimal (≤1 cm), and bulky (>1 cm) upper abdominal disease. On multivariate analysis, patients with bulky upper abdominal disease who underwent optimal cytoreduction had a 28% decreased risk of relapse (HR, 0.72; 95% CI: 0.53-0.99; $P = .04$) and a 33% decreased risk of death (HR, 0.67; 95% CI: 0.47-0.96; $P = .03$) compared to patients who underwent suboptimal cytoreduction. In this study, the presence of large-volume disease found during surgical exploration did not preclude the benefit of optimal cytoreduction. Extending these studies, Horowitz et al analyzed the impact of preoperative disease burden on survival by studying the impact of aggressive surgery on patients with high- and low-volume disease from GOG #182 (1). Of 1,636 patients with large-volume disease preoperatively (upper abdominal disease-diaphragm/spleen/liver/pancreas), 199 (12%) were reduced to microscopic disease, but these patients still had a worse PFS and OS compared to patients with preoperative low-volume

disease (**Figure 8.6-5**). Therefore, both the preoperative tumor burden, including the extent of upper abdominal disease and the extent of surgical resection (postoperative tumor burden), influence the PFS and OS of patients with advanced OC.

For metastatic LGSOC, it is also important to attempt maximal surgical debulking as microscopic residual disease results in better survival (97 vs 35 months), when compared to women with residual disease greater than 1 cm (38). However, the success rate of complete cytoreduction of patients with LGSCs is lower than in HGSOC (52%), which might be explained by deeper invasion of low-grade tumors into healthy tissue, which makes it more difficult to dissect them off the tissue. Because the average age of patients with LGSOC is much younger (~47 years), it is also important to take fertility aspects into consideration.

In summary, surgical cytoreduction plays a very important role in the management of advanced OC. However, patients with very extensive carcinomatosis and extensive upper abdominal disease and/or mesenteric involvement have little to no benefit from primary debulking procedures, when suboptimally debulked (1). Surgery alone is never curative in advanced disease and, therefore, should only be attempted as part of a combined treatment plan, including postoperative chemotherapy. As discussed later, it is not possible to predict with accuracy which patients can undergo optimal cytoreduction, because CA-125, CT, and PET imaging lack sufficient specificity (39-41). Laparoscopy has been used to determine resectability, though it is not clear if it impacts prognosis (33,42). Still, direct visualization of tumor distribution by laparoscopy can provide useful information and may help decide if an upfront debulking should be performed. The overall goal of cytoreductive surgery for patients with advanced-stage FIGO III/IV OC should be, whenever feasible, the complete cytoreduction of all visible disease. The reports of improved outcomes with radical

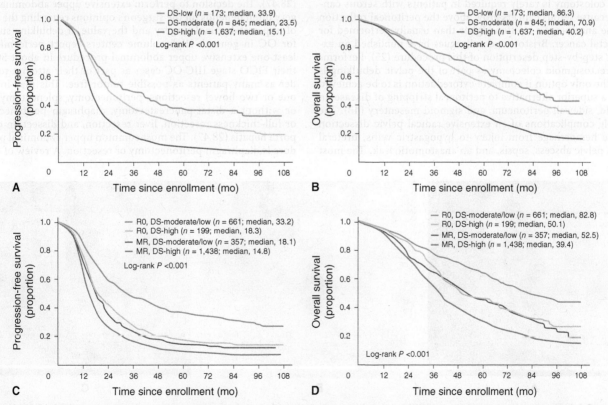

▌ **Figure 8.6-5.** (A) Progression-free and (B) overall survival (C) stratified by preoperative disease burden and (D) further characterized by residual disease for those with high, moderate, and low disease scores. DS, preoperative disease status; MR, minimal residual <1 cm of residual disease; R0, complete surgical resection. (From Horowitz NS, Miller A, Rungruang B, et al. Does aggressive surgery improve outcomes? Interaction between preoperative disease burden and complex surgery in patients with advanced-stage ovarian cancer: an analysis of GOG 182. *J Clin Oncol.* 2015;33(8):937-943.)

debulking suggest that patients should be counseled about this option. However, it is important to remember that, although we justify surgical cytoreduction because it provides symptom relief and it has been shown, in numerous retrospective reviews, to be associated with improved survival, the clinical benefits of radical surgery in OC have never been studied in a prospective random-ized trial. In general, complex surgical pelvic and upper abdominal procedures should be judiciously used in patients with resectable disease, when there is a high chance that removal of all visible tu-mors can be achieved.

SURGICAL DEBULKING—PELVIC AND UPPER ABDOMINAL PROCEDURES

Surgery for patients with advanced OC should start with a vertical midline incision extending from the pubic symphysis to above the umbilicus. This allows visualization of the entire abdominal cavity, including the diaphragms, and permits the safe evaluation and re-section of upper abdominal disease. With a careful exploration of the abdominal cavity, the surgeon will be able to evaluate the extent of the disease and plan the surgical approach. Particular attention should be paid to the upper abdomen because the disease distri-bution in that region will often determine whether a patient can undergo optimal cytoreduction.

Patients with advanced OC and high-volume disease usually have extensive tumor burden in the pelvis with encasement of the reproductive organs and sigmoid colon (**Figure 8.3-1**). However, it is almost always possible to completely remove pelvic disease. This requires a modified posterior exenteration, an en bloc resec-tion of the tumor-studded bladder, peritoneum, uterus, sigmoid colon, and proximal rectum, as well as ovarian/fallopian tube masses, cul-de-sac tumors, and, possibly, the appendix removed (**Figure 8.6-3**). A low colorectal anastomosis (25,43) should fol-low; a colostomy is rarely required in patients with serous can-cers because serous cancers grow above the peritoneal reflection and the anastomosis is often higher than usually performed for colorectal cancer. Bristow and colleagues have published an ex-cellent step-by-step description of this procedure (25). Perform-ing a rectosigmoid colectomy as part of the pelvic debulking is often the only option if complete cytoreduction is to be achieved and is a superior alternative to peritoneal stripping of disease on sigmoid, sidewall peritoneum, and sigmoid mesentery (43). The possible complications of an extensive radical pelvic dissection include hemorrhage from injury to hypogastric veins, ureteral injury, pelvic abscess, sepsis, and an anastomotic leak. The most

important feature of the anastomosis is that it be tension free, which can require mobilization of the splenic flexure and liga-tion of the inferior mesenteric artery and vein. Anastomotic leaks are dangerous complications often associated with emergency surgery, prolonged hospital stay, intensive care unit (ICU) ad-mission, and mortality. Traditionally, leak rates from colorectal surgery have been reported to be as high as 20% to 35%, but after the adoption of the air leak test and the EEA stapler, these rates have improved to 5% to 15% and have remained there since. More specifically in the gynecologic literature, anastomotic leaks have been reported to occur at a rate of 2% to 7% in patients having undergone debulking surgery for OC requiring bowel resection and are associated with a mortality rate of up to 21%, mostly sec-ondary to sepsis (44). Poor oxygenation due to diminished blood supply is believed to play an important role, resulting in leakage and failed anastomosis, as does a preexisting abnormal microbi-ome (45). Therefore, continuous efforts have been made in the search for accurate methods to assess intestinal viability and per-fusion before or during surgical procedures. More recently, the use of near-infrared (NIR) imaging to assess vascular perfusion of the anastomosis has been used. Moukarzel and colleagues have evaluated 410 patients who underwent a rectosigmoid resection and anastomosis for gynecologic malignancies (46). The majority of patients underwent surgery for advanced OC. Of those, NIR imaging was used in 133 patients to assess the perfusion of the anastomosis. NIR assessment of the anastomosis was associated with a decrease in postoperative complications and a decrease in the use of diverting ileostomies (**Figure 8.6-6**). A randomized trial is ongoing to prospectively evaluate the intraoperative use of NIR imaging for patients undergoing rectosigmoid resection for advanced OC (ARIA 2 trial).

Patients with serous OC who require a modified posterior exenteration often need one or more upper abdominal proce-dures as well if complete surgical debulking is to be accomplished (28,47). The decision to perform extensive upper abdominal sur-gery often depends on the surgeon's opinions regarding the value of upper abdominal surgery and the value of debulking surgery for OC in general. High-volume centers report performing at least one extensive upper abdominal procedure in about 50% of their FIGO stage IIIC OC cases as part of their attempt to ren-der as many patients as possible tumor free. This may include one or two bowel resections, peritonectomy, splenectomy with or without a distal pancreatectomy, diaphragm peritonectomy or full-thickness resection, liver resection, and dissection of the porta hepatis (28,47). The most common upper abdominal proce-dure is diaphragm peritonectomy or resection. A review of GOG

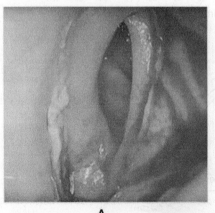
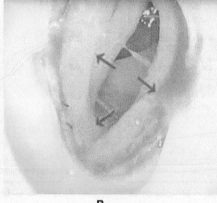
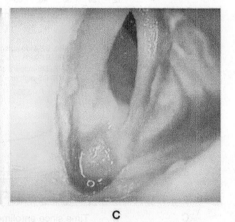

A	**B**	**C**

Figure 8.6-6. The use of indocyanine green (ICG) in assessing anastomotic perfusion of a rectosigmoid resection anastomosis. A: View of rectosigmoid anastomosis via proctoscopy. B: Use of near-infrared with ICG demonstrating an area concerning for inadequate perfusion in the proximal portion (red arrows). C: After anastomotic revision, bowel perfusion appreciable along the entire anastomosis. (Courtesy of Allie Straubhar and Dennis Chi © MSKCC 2019.)

#182, limited to patients with FIGO stage III or IV disease who were optimally debulked (<1 cm), showed that 18% (482/2,655 patients) had undergone upper abdominal procedures (23). The most common procedure was diaphragm surgery (13%), followed by splenectomy and liver surgery (4% each), pancreatectomy (0.5%), and porta hepatis surgery (0.2%). An excellent description of en bloc resection of extensive left upper quadrant disease has been published by Hoffman et al (48). By using upper abdominal procedures, the authors were able to achieve complete cytoreduction in a high percentage of patients, and OS of patients with upper abdominal disease who were completely cytoreduced was superior to OS of patients with upper abdominal disease who were not completely cytoreduced. However, the preoperative tumor load continues to largely define PFS and OS. Even when aggressive upper abdominal surgery is used to reduce the tumor to microscopic disease, the survival of patients who present with high-volume disease worsen than that of patients who present with low-volume disease (1). As a word of caution, extensive involvement of the upper abdomen with disease may preclude an optimal debulking; complex upper abdominal surgery should be performed only when the entire disease can be removed with acceptable morbidity. Laparoscopy is often not able to accurately evaluate the extent of upper abdominal disease, specifically retrohepatic spaces and small bowel mesentery.

Magtibay and colleagues reported on 112 patients at the Mayo Clinic who underwent a splenectomy as part of OC debulking (49). The most common indications were metastatic parenchymal involvement (46%), perisplenic involvement from an omental tumor that reached the splenic hilum (42%), and intraoperative trauma (13%). Complications included wound infections (6%), postoperative pneumonitis (4.5%), thromboembolic events (8%), and sepsis (4.5%). The overall perioperative mortality was 5%. A similar complication rate was reported in a 2015 study (50). Out of 121 patients, 38% had a complication, but severe complications were observed only in 19%. Postoperative hematologic changes such as a second peak in leukocytosis and a longer duration of thrombocytosis are associated with an increased risk of infections or thromboembolic events (51). Complications were most often observed when ovarian debulking surgery was paired with pancreatectomy or biliary surgery, causing abscess formation, pancreatic fistulas, and/or leakage. The 90-day postoperative mortality rate in this retrospective study was 0.9%.

Common complications after splenectomy and distal pancreatectomy are pancreatic leaks, which can result in prolonged hospital stay and readmissions and may require drainage but, if managed appropriately, do not result in delay of chemotherapy (52). Patients often present with fever, left upper quadrant pain, and shortness of breath due to concomitant left pleural effusion. A diagnosis of a pancreatic leak is often established with CT imaging. A rim-enhancing left upper quadrant fluid collection is accompanied with elevated white blood count. Interventional radiology drainage of fluid collection is the treatment of choice. Alternatively, transgastral drainage of left upper quadrant fluid collection is often possible. Amylase levels of the fluids collection are often high. Typically, pancreatic leaks are self-limiting after adequate drainage. The use of octreotide may decrease the duration of a pancreatic leak. Perioperative treatment with pasireotide decreased the rate of clinically significant postoperative pancreatic fistula, leak, or abscess in a randomized, double-blind trial of perioperative subcutaneous pasireotide in patients undergoing either pancreaticoduodenectomy or distal pancreatectomy (53).

Long abdominal surgery also increases the risk of hernia formation, as does obesity, wound infection, and diabetes. Patients undergoing elective splenectomy should be vaccinated 2 weeks before or after surgery to reduce the risk of overwhelming postsplenectomy infection due to organisms like *Streptococcus pneumoniae*, *Haemophilus influenzae* type B, and *Neisseria meningitidis*. Polyvalent pneumococcal, *H. influenzae* b, and meningococcal vaccinations

are recommended. Surgical site infection bundles have been used to reduce the risk of postoperative infections (54). Including patients undergoing surgery for OC in an enhanced recovery program reduces postoperative complications, reduces hospital stay, and allows patients to begin chemotherapy earlier than would otherwise be deemed safe (55). Postoperative thrombosis prophylaxis with extended prophylactic use of low-molecular-weight heparin has been shown to reduce the risk of postoperative thromboembolic disease.

ROLE OF LYMPH NODE DISSECTION IN SURGERY FOR ADVANCED OVARIAN CANCER

A prospective randomized Italian trial of 427 patients with advanced OC (stages IIIB-IV) compared extensive systematic lymph node dissection with resection of only enlarged ("bulky") lymph nodes and concluded that, although positive lymph nodes are a negative prognostic marker, systematic lymph node dissection did not contribute to the benefit of optimal tumor debulking (16). Systematic lymph node dissection improved PFS (median PFS, 22 vs 29 months), but not OS (median OS, 59 vs 56 months). The addition of systematic lymph node dissection resulted in greater blood loss, more transfusions, and added operative time. The perioperative and late morbidity of a systematic lymph node dissection was 28%, whereas morbidity for the resection of only enlarged lymph nodes was 18%. Most of this excess morbidity was caused by lymphocyst formation and lymphedema. Therefore, even in experienced hands, a systematic lymph node dissection carries significant morbidity, which should be factored into decision-making. The study took over 12 years to recruit patients from 13 centers. However, it is worth noting that 63% of the patients in this study had residual tumor after debulking surgery, which might obviate any benefit of lymph node dissection. The German AGO retrospectively reviewed data from three large phase III trials (AGO-OVAR #3, #5, #7) of chemotherapy in advanced EOC. They found that in the subgroup of patients with no residual disease and no enlarged lymph nodes, a systematic lymph node dissection was associated with a small statistically significant survival benefit (median OS, 108 vs 83 months) (20).

In 2019, Harter and colleagues have published the randomized Lymphadenectomy In Ovarian Neoplasms (LION) trial in patients with advanced ovarian neoplasms (17). Patients with newly diagnosed advanced FIGO IIB-IV OC who had undergone macroscopically complete resection and had normal lymph nodes both before and during surgery were intraoperatively randomized to either undergo or not undergo lymphadenectomy. The primary end point was OS. A total of 647 patients underwent randomization. Among patients who underwent lymphadenectomy, the median number of removed nodes was 57 (35 pelvic and 22 para-aortic nodes). The median OS was 69.2 months in the no-lymphadenectomy group and 65.5 months in the lymphadenectomy group (HR for death in the lymphadenectomy group, 1.06; 95% CI, 0.83-1.34; $P = .65$). Systematic pelvic and para-aortic lymphadenectomy in patients with advanced OC who had undergone intra-abdominal macroscopically complete resection and had normal lymph nodes both before and during surgery was not associated with longer OS or PFS than no lymphadenectomy and was associated with a higher risk of postoperative complications and mortality. The lymph node dissection was associated with a higher risk of postoperative complications (blood loss, infections, ICU admissions, lymphocele) and mortality, but there was no meaningful difference in QoL. In summary, the current practice in advanced OC is to remove enlarged/suspicious lymph nodes as part of tumor debulking, but does not support the use of systemic lymph node dissection at the time of advanced OC surgery.

NEOADJUVANT CHEMOTHERAPY

Because of the potential morbidity of cytoreductive surgery and the chemosensitivity of OC, multiple studies have evaluated the role of neoadjuvant chemotherapy with the goal to reduce the tumor burden preoperatively and decrease operative time, and complexity of surgery and complications. The EORTC-GCG and NCIC performed a phase III trial (EORTC #55971) randomizing 718 patients with 1988 FIGO stage IIIC or IV OC to either neoadjuvant platinum-containing chemotherapy followed by interval debulking or primary debulking surgery followed by platinum-based chemotherapy (56). The largest residual tumor after surgery was less than 1 cm in 80% of patients treated with the neoadjuvant approach, whereas this was only accomplished in 42% of all patients who underwent upfront debulking. There was a trend toward less blood loss, fewer postoperative infections, and fewer thromboembolic complications in the neoadjuvant treatment group, as well as a shorter operative time. Most importantly, there was no significant difference in PFS (12 months in both groups) or OS (29/30 months) between the two groups, and this was independent of the rate of optimal debulking accomplished in a specific center. The study was criticized for its low PFS and OS results; however, most patients had adverse prognostic factors at the time of randomization: 74% had tumors larger greater than 5 cm (61% >10 cm) in size at baseline, indicating that study participants had very advanced disease. Another related criticism of the study was the low rate of optimal debulking. In the primary debulking group, 19.4% of all patients were reduced to microscopic disease, whereas the rate was 51.2% for the neoadjuvant group. The phase III CHORUS trial randomly assigned 552 women to either primary surgery or neoadjuvant chemotherapy (three cycles preoperatively and three cycles postoperatively) also found no significant difference in OS between the two groups (PFS: 10.7 vs 12 months; OS 22.6 vs 24.1 months) (57). There were fewer complications in the neoadjuvant group, and more patients in the neoadjuvant group had an improvement in global QoL. Fourteen (6%) patients died in the primary surgery group, which is a much higher mortality rate than has been previously reported in phase III trials of advanced OC, and may be related to the advanced stage or poor performance status of the patients entered on the study. The median operative time in both groups was short, at 120 minutes, and debulking to microscopic disease was accomplished in only 17% of the women who had primary surgery compared to 39% of those who had primary chemotherapy ($P = .0001$). In the primary surgery group, 27% did not have a BSO, 24% did not have a hysterectomy, and only 20% had upper abdominal surgery. The findings from these two trials are not generalizable to large-volume centers reporting complete gross resection rates of over 50% and significantly longer PFS and OS.

Results of these studies started a heated discussion on the role of neoadjuvant chemotherapy and the best timing of cytoreductive surgery in the frontline treatment of OC. This discussion is still ongoing. There are no preoperative factors or imaging studies that can be used to predict the success of interval cytoreduction surgery (39). For patients with 1988/2013 FIGO stage I-IIIB disease, primary surgery is currently the standard treatment. An exploratory analysis of the EORTC #55971 study showed that women with less extensive metastatic disease did better with primary surgery, whereas patients with metastatic tumors that are larger than 4.5 cm and patients with 1988 FIGO stage IV did better with neoadjuvant chemotherapy (58). Physicians who feel a primary surgical approach is preferable even in women with large tumor volume note results such as those from a retrospective analysis of patients treated at Memorial Sloan-Kettering Cancer Center during the time of EORTC trial who underwent very complex surgery (including upper abdominal surgery), with high rates of optimal debulking, and reported that these patients experienced results that appear superior to those seen in the CHORUS and EORTC trials,

with a PFS and OS of 17 and 50 months, respectively (59). Results from the Trial of Radical Upfront Surgical Therapy (TRUST) in advanced OC have completed recruitment and are awaited (60). Finally, one retrospective study from the Mayo Clinic objectively identified cohorts of patients at high risk for postoperative complications and appeared to have limited benefit from primary cytoreductive surgery (PCS) (61). In patients who were 75 years or above with an ASA 3 or higher or serum albumin levels 3 or lower and in patients who had stage IV disease, the risk of major complications was over 60%, and there was no survival benefit in favor of optimal cytoreduction. Therefore, such patients who meet these criteria should be offered neoadjuvant chemotherapy.

Given the randomized data, in patients with extensive tumor burden, ascites, poor performance status, low albumin level and several comorbidities, obesity, and older age, neoadjuvant chemotherapy is an acceptable treatment strategy. The current standard, especially for a healthier, younger patient with disease that is deemed to be surgically resectable, is primary surgery with the goal of accomplishing a complete tumor debulking with no visible residual disease. For patients who are medically fit to undergo cytoreductive surgery, CT imaging, thoracoscopy, and laparoscopy can be used to determine which patients are likely to undergo complete gross resection (33,40).

HYPERTHERMIC INTRAPERITONEAL CHEMOTHERAPY

The use of intraoperative HIPEC in patients undergoing cytoreductive surgery for advanced OC has been the subject of debate in recent years. Some experts recommend HIPEC for all patients undergoing cytoreductive surgery (62), whereas others judge it to be investigational at this time (63). The rationale for HIPEC in patients with OC is the pharmacologic advantage of IP chemotherapy with high dose-density in the peritoneum while only resulting in low systemic exposure (64). The use of sequential normothermic postoperative platinum-based IP chemotherapy has been associated with improved PFS and OS but remains underused owing to increased toxicity (26,65). In addition, the results of GOG 252 failed to show an OS benefit with incorporation of IP compared to IV chemotherapy when maintenance bevacizumab was also administered (66).

HIPEC differs from the postoperative IP treatment in that chemotherapy is administered intraoperatively using the opportune time window when the patient is undergoing a cytoreductive surgery. In 2018, van Driel et al reported the first randomized trial evaluating the use of cisplatin as HIPEC in patients undergoing interval cytoreductive surgery after three cycles of neoadjuvant platinum- and taxane-based chemotherapy (67). In this trial, 250 patients were randomized to either surgery alone or surgery with 90 minutes of HIPEC with cisplatin at a dose of 100 mg/m^2. Postoperatively, the patients completed three cycles of IV standard chemotherapy. The median recurrence-free survival was 10.7 months in the surgery group and 14.2 months in the surgery-plus-HIPEC group (HR for disease recurrence or death, 0.66; 95% CI, 0.50-0.87; $P = .003$). At a median follow-up of 4.7 years, 76 (62%) patients in the surgery group and 61 (50%) patients in the surgery-plus-HIPEC group had died (HR, 0.67; 95% CI, 0.48-0.94; $P = .02$). The median OS was 33.9 months in the surgery group and 45.7 months in the surgery-plus-HIPEC group. The percentage of patients who had adverse events of grade 3 or 4 was similar in the two groups (25% in the surgery group and 27% in the surgery-plus-HIPEC group, $P = .76$). In another randomized clinical trial by Lim et al, a total of 184 patients with stage III or IV OC with residual tumor size less than 1 cm were randomized (1:1) to an HIPEC (41.5°C, 75 mg/m^2 of cisplatin, 90 minutes) or control group (68). The primary end point was PFS. OS and adverse events were key secondary end points. Although the primary analysis did not show a benefit of HIPEC for the entire cohort in an unplanned subgroup analysis, patients who underwent interval cytoreductive surgery after neoadjuvant chemotherapy derived a benefit from HIPEC, confirming the results of van Driel et al. In this subgroup, the median PFS was 15.4 months (interquartile range [IQR], 10.6-21.1 months) in the control group and 17.4 months (IQR, 13.8-31.5 months) in the HIPEC group (HR for disease progression or death, 0.60; 95% CI, 0.37-0.99; $P = .04$), and the median OS was 48.2 months (IQR, 33.8-61.3 months) in the control group and 61.8 months (IQR, 46.7 months to not reported) in the HIPEC group (HR, 0.53; 95% CI, 0.29-0.96; $P = .04$). An ongoing randomized trial is exploring the use of HIPEC with cisplatin (100 mg/m^2) in the primary cytoreductive setting (69).

Lei et al reported a retrospective study including patients with EOC undergoing PCS with or without the addition of HIPEC (70). Within the cohort of 584 patients, 425 underwent PCS plus HIPEC and 159 underwent PCS alone. At a median follow-up of 42.2 months, the addition of HIPEC led to a nearly 16-month increase in survival for the PCS-HIPEC group (median, 49.8 months; 95% CI, 45.2-60.2 months) compared with the PCS group (median, 34.0 months; 95% CI, 28.9-42.3 months). The 3-year OS was also increased by nearly 11 percentage points for the PCS-HIPEC group (60.5%; 95% CI, 55.5%-65.2%) versus the PCS group (49.6%; 95% CI, 41.2%-57.5%). Remarkably, the improvement in survival was found in patients who underwent both optimal (<1 cm) and suboptimal cytoreduction, although the improvement in median survival time did not reach significance in the suboptimal cohort.

In the recurrent setting, in a randomized phase 2 trial, Zivanovic et al failed to show that HIPEC with carboplatin (800 mg/m^2) improved PFS and OS in patients undergoing secondary cytoreductive surgery for platinum-sensitive recurrent OC (71). These results confirm the results of Spiliotis et al who saw a benefit of HIPEC in patients with platinum-resistant disease, but not in those with platinum-sensitive recurrent disease (72).

In summary, HIPEC is safe for patients treated in centers with expertise. HIPEC with cisplatin at 100 mg/m^2 improves PFS and OS at the time of interval cytoreductive surgery in patients with stage III OC and can be considered in this patient population. But, this needs to be confirmed in a more contemporary treatment setting (PARPi, bevacizumab, immune therapy). There are no robust data supporting the role of HIPEC in the primary cytoreductive setting. Prospective trials are ongoing. HIPEC with carboplatin at 800 mg/m^2 in the recurrent setting did not result in improved PFS or OS. There is no high-level evidence to support HIPEC in the recurrent OC setting.

SUMMARY OF PRIMARY DEBULKING SURGERY FOR OVARIAN CANCER

Many factors contribute to how long a patient with advanced OC survives. Inherent genetic characteristics of the tumor may play a more important role in OS than stage or cytoreductive surgical debulking. However, the study of genetic factors in relation to surgical treatment is in its infancy. At present, the degree of surgical debulking is the only prognostic factor that can be influenced by the surgeon. We know that among patients with advanced-stage III/V OC, those who undergo a complete debulking have the most favorable prognosis. Whether a complete resection is performed is, at least in part, determined by the surgeon's skill and willingness to engage in a maximal surgical effort. Once the decision has been made to proceed, the goal of every operation in patients with advanced-stage III/IV OC should be a complete resection of all visible tumors to microscopic disease (73).

However, ultraradical surgery, involving the addition of upper abdominal procedures to pelvic tumor debulking, will increase morbidity, and not every patient is a good candidate for such an aggressive approach (74). Large-volume involvement of the upper abdomen, extended small and large bowel surface and

mesentery involvement or multiple liver metastases, will preclude an optimal debulking. Wright and colleagues, reviewing a large administrative database with over 28,000 patients, showed that the complication rate of extensive OC debulking (eg, surgical site, medical, infectious complications) increases with age. Women younger than 50 years, 70 to 80 years, and those older than 80 years have a 17.1%, 29.7%, and 31.5% complication rates, respectively (74).

Two groups of factors should contribute to the decision whether to take a patient to surgery and perform a radical debulking procedure (61): (a) a careful preoperative evaluation of patient-related risk factors: Patients with significant comorbidities and low performance status (ASA preoperative score 3 or 4, poor nutritional status, low albumin <3 g/dL) have a low likelihood of optimal debulking to microscopic disease and are at risk of significant perioperative and postoperative morbidity; (b) a critical evaluation of the extent of disease with particular attention to upper abdominal tumor burden, ascites, and upper abdominal tumor distribution. Patients with one or more of these risk factors often have a prolonged postoperative recovery, because they have limited ability to withstand a long operation. Furthermore, once a complication occurs, the patient may not receive chemotherapy and is more likely to succumb to disease within 3 months. For these patients, neoadjuvant chemotherapy is a well-studied alternative to a debulking surgery and has been shown to produce similar outcomes and less morbidity.

Sometimes, it is not possible to preoperatively decide if radical debulking surgery is feasible because of the limited ability of CT scans to predict success (39). Several scoring systems have been developed to select patients who can be completely cytoreduced. All agree that mesenteric retraction and miliary dissemination of tumor nodules on the serosa of the small bowel predict unresectability to microscopic disease. Staging laparoscopy offers an opportunity to evaluate disease extent with a minimal complication rate using a laparoscopy-based scoring system (Fagotti score or Predictive Index [PI]) (75). The Fagotti score includes the evaluation of peritoneal and diaphragmatic carcinomatosis, omental caking, need for a large/small bowel resection (excluding sigmoid resection), involvement of the stomach, lesser sac or spleen, and liver surface lesions, assigning a score of 2 for each feature present (42). A score greater than 10 predicts that it will be impossible to completely cytoreduce a tumor to microscopic disease. At MD Anderson, the Fagotti score is used to standardize care. Patients with scores less than 8 receive initial cytoreductive surgery, whereas those with scores greater than 8 receive neoadjuvant chemotherapy (73). A group from Memorial Sloan-Kettering Cancer Center identified CT imaging criteria, CA-125, and ASA score criteria to help identify which patients are likely to undergo optimal versus suboptimal cytoreduction (76). A refined model to predict residual disease after PCS was validated and can help with clinical decision-making (77).

Second-look laparotomy was often performed in the 1980s after primary surgery and adjuvant cisplatin-based therapy for prognostic information and to determine the need for further treatment. Chemotherapy was generally continued for those found to have residual small-volume disease. Second-look surgery is no longer generally performed, because no therapy instituted as a result of disease found during these procedures altered prognosis. Reoperation following chemotherapy also introduces unnecessary morbidity. About one-third of patients with advanced OC were found to be free of disease at a second-look laparotomy, yet over half of these patients eventually experienced a recurrence.

In summary, the extent of primary surgical cytoreduction in patients with advanced OC and multiple comorbidities should be determined for every patient individually. If there is doubt, until more data become available, it is reasonable to treat these patients with neoadjuvant chemotherapy followed by debulking surgery.

INTERVAL DEBULKING FOR SUBOPTIMALLY DEBULKED PATIENTS

The term *interval debulking surgery* refers to a surgical procedure in a patient with the persistent abdominal disease after an initial surgical debulking effort and neoadjuvant chemotherapy (typically 3-4 cycles) (**Table 8.6-2**). There is conflicting evidence from two large prospective, randomized trials regarding whether interval debulking surgery can improve survival in patients for whom an initial surgical effort did not achieve optimal results (78,79). In a multicenter EORTC trial, patients with suboptimal (>1 cm) disease remaining after primary cytoreduction were treated with three cycles of cyclophosphamide and cisplatin (78). Those without progression were randomized to interval debulking surgery and additional chemotherapy versus additional chemotherapy alone. With approximately 140 patients randomized to each arm, patients undergoing interval debulking showed a statistically significant improvement in both progression-free interval and median survival. The survival of patients with residual lesions of more than 1 cm after the interval debulking surgery was similar to that of patients who did not undergo the surgery. None of the patients in the interval debulking group died, and morbidity was minimal. The long-term results from this study showed that after 5 years, PFS and OS were still significantly better for the patients in the interval debulking group and that being randomized to interval debulking remained an independent prognostic factor for improved survival (80). However, this trial used a chemotherapy regimen cyclophosphamide/cisplatin, which is not used anymore for upfront treatment. GOG 152 was a randomized trial also evaluated interval secondary cytoreduction in patients with advanced FIGO stage III/IV OC with suboptimal (>1 cm) residual disease but reached different conclusions (79). Five hundred fifty patients were enrolled within 6 weeks of initial surgery. After three cycles of paclitaxel and cisplatin, patients without evidence of tumor progression were randomized to receive either secondary cytoreduction and three additional cycles of chemotherapy or chemotherapy alone. At the time of the 2004 report2004, median PFS and OS (**Figure 8.6-7**) for the interval cytoreduction group were 10.5 and 33.9 months, respectively, compared to 10.7 and 33.7 months for the chemotherapy-alone group.

A consistent lack of effect was seen in all patients, regardless of the residual tumor size at the end of the interval debulking surgery.

Several theories have been advanced to explain the difference in outcomes between the GOG and European studies. One point raised is that there were differences in the extent of the initial cytoreduction surgery. In the GOG trial, both the initial and interval cytoreductive operations were clearly defined and were performed almost exclusively by trained gynecologic oncologists, whereas in the EORTC trial, the extent of the initial surgery was not clearly defined and, as a result, surgery was most often performed by general gynecologists. As a result, residual disease following primary surgery measured less than 5 cm in about two-thirds of the GOG patients, compared to one-third of the patients in the EORTC trial. Following chemotherapy, residual disease greater than 1 cm was found in 56% of the GOG patients versus 65% of the European patients. In addition, the chemotherapeutic regimens used in the GOG trial, paclitaxel and platinum, may have been more effective than the platinum and cyclophosphamide combination used by the EORTC. Less effective chemotherapy would increase the benefit of interval cytoreduction in the EORTC trial, which found conversion from suboptimal to optimal residual tumor in 45% of patients as compared to 36% in the GOG trial. Differences in outcomes may also be related to different post-treatment surveillance and the availability of more effective second-line therapies, because the EORTC trial completed accrual in May 1993 before paclitaxel was introduced into clinical care. It is of interest to note that the similar median and OS in both arms of the GOG trial were substantially longer than those reported in the best (interval cytoreduction) arm of the EORTC trial. We can conclude that patients who had an initial maximal effort at cytoreduction resulting in suboptimal debulking are unlikely to benefit from interval cytoreduction. However, patients with advanced OC who previously only had a biopsy, removal of the ovary, or just a simple hysterectomy with bilateral removal of the ovaries/fallopian tube, partial removal of ovarian tumors, or, in general, a limited surgical attempt may benefit from a second surgery that involves maximal debulking.

SECONDARY CYTOREDUCTIVE SURGERY FOR RECURRENT DISEASE

Despite modest improvements in adjuvant chemotherapy for OC and aggressive primary debulking surgery (including upper abdominal procedures), the majority (70%) of patients with advanced EOC will have a recurrence (22). Because there is currently no chemotherapy that can cure recurrent OC, surgical resection of recurrent disease is an option for a select group of patients.

In 1992, a retrospective study of secondary cytoreduction for recurrent disease showed an OS of 29 months for patients cytoreduced to microscopic residual disease, whereas patients with any visible disease after surgery had a median survival of only 9 months (81). The Descriptive Evaluation of preoperative Selection KriTeria for Operability in recurrent OVARian cancer (DESKTOP OVAR I) trial enrolled 267 patients with recurrent OC who had secondary cytoreductive surgery and found that patients with carcinomatosis had 19.9 months median survival versus 45.3 months for patients without disseminated disease ($P < .0001$) (82). In this trial, a score (the "AGO score") was developed to predict optimal operability in this recurrent patient group, using criteria for a positive score that included good performance status (European Cooperative Oncology Group [ECOG] ≤1), complete debulking at first surgery, and less than 500 cc of ascites The score was then tested in the DESKTOP II prospectively: 76% of the patients who fulfilled all three criteria had an optimal debulking to no residual disease (83). One-third of the patients who had surgery suffered at least one minor or major complication. However, the AGO score was found to have no independent prognostic value.

A retrospective study from the Mayo Clinic that applied the AGO score to 192 women who had secondary cytoreductive

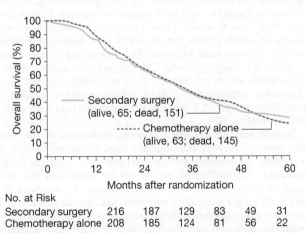

P = 0.92 for the comparison between the groups by the log-rank test

Figure 8.6-7. Overall survival of patients with advanced ovarian cancer who underwent interval debulking surgery compared with treatment with chemotherapy-only Gynecologic Oncology Group trial. (From Rose PG, Nerenstone S, Brady MF, et al. Secondary surgical cytoreduction for advanced ovarian carcinoma. *N Engl J Med.* 2004;351(24):2489-2497. Copyright © 2004 Massachusetts Medical Society. Reprinted with permission from Massachusetts Medical Society)

surgery between 1998 and 2013 found that a positive AGO score predicted an R0 resection in 84.3% of cases (84). Thus, a positive AGO score does indicate that secondary debulking surgery for recurrent OC is likely to be successful. However, 64.4% of patients with a negative score also achieved an R0 resection. The median disease-free interval for the entire group was 1.9 years. OS was longer for patients with complete (5.4 years), optimal (2.4 years), or suboptimal cytoreduction (1.3 years).

A small subset of patients (4%-5%) will present with isolated recurrences in retroperitoneal lymph nodes. Several small retrospective studies found that complete resection of lymph nodes limited to one anatomic region (60% are high para-aortic) is associated with significantly improved survival (85). This finding is consistent with the better prognosis of patients who present with localized disease in the pelvis and retroperitoneal lymph node metastasis. If this is the only site of disease, postoperative radiation of the lymph node bed might also reduce the risk of recurrence.

Four prospective randomized phase III trials evaluated the impact of secondary cytoreductive surgery on survival: the DESKTOP III trial (86), the GOG #213 trial (87), the SOC-1 trial (88), and the SOCceR trial (unpublished). All randomized patients with potentially resectable platinum-sensitive disease to secondary cytoreduction or no surgery. GOG 213 and DESKTOP 3/SOC-1 were published with contradictory results (86,87). In GOG #213, 485 patients with recurrent platinum-sensitive OC who had received one previous therapy, had an interval during which no platinum-based chemotherapy was used (platinum-free interval) of 6 months or more, and had investigator-determined resectable disease (to no macroscopic residual disease) were randomly assigned to undergo secondary surgical cytoreduction and then receive platinum-based chemotherapy or to receive platinum-based chemotherapy alone (87). Adjuvant chemotherapy (paclitaxel-carboplatin or gemcitabine-carboplatin) and use of bevacizumab were at the discretion of the investigator. The primary end point was OS. Complete gross resection was achieved in 67% of the patients assigned to surgery who underwent the procedure. Platinum-based chemotherapy with bevacizumab followed by bevacizumab maintenance was administered to 84% of the patients overall. In this trial involving patients with platinum-sensitive, recurrent OC, secondary surgical cytoreduction followed by chemotherapy did not result in longer OS than chemotherapy alone. The HR for death (surgery vs no surgery) was 1.29 (95% CI, 0.97-1.72; $P = .08$), which corresponded to a median OS of 50.6 and 64.7 months, respectively. The DESKTOP 3 trial randomly assigned 407 patients to recurrent platinum-sensitive OC to undergo secondary cytoreductive surgery and then receive platinum-based chemotherapy or receive platinum-based chemotherapy alone (86). The primary end point of DESKTOP 3 was time from randomization to death. Unlike in the GOG 213 trial, patients were eligible if they presented with a positive AGO score, defined as an ECOG performance status score of 0 (on a 5-point scale, with higher scores indicating greater disability), ascites of less than 500 mL, and complete resection at initial surgery. The primary end point was OS. Complete resection was achieved in 75.5% of the patients in the surgery group who underwent the procedure. The median OS was 53.7 months in the surgery group and 46.0 months in the no-surgery group (HR for death, 0.75; 95% CI, 0.59-0.96; $P = .02$). Patients with a complete resection had the most favorable outcome, with a median OS of 61.9 months. No perioperative mortality within 30 days after surgery was observed, and it took an average of 35 days before a woman began chemotherapy. It is important to note that older patients did benefit from secondary cytoreduction. Finally, the SOC-1 trial from China enrolled 357 women with platinum-free interval of at least 6 months who were predicted to have resectable disease based on the iMODEL to chemotherapy alone or secondary cytoreduction (88). The iMODEL score includes six criteria: FIGO stage, residual disease at primary debulking, length of platinum-free interval, ECOG performance status, CA-125 level at recurrence, presence of ascites, and a

PET-CT. Median PFS was 17.4 months in the surgery group and 11.9 months in the no-surgery group (HR 0.58; 95% CI 0.45-0.74; $P < .0001$), favoring the surgery group. OS results were immature. A meta-analysis reviewing published studies between 1983 and 2021 concluded that maximal cytoreductive surgery at relapse resulting in maximal tumor debulking improves significantly the OS platinum-sensitive patients with OC (89).

Based on the available literature, the following selection criteria for secondary debulking seem reasonable: patients with (a) a disease-free interval longer than 12 months, (b) platinum-sensitive disease with additional chemotherapy options, (c) oligometastatic or localized IP or retroperitoneal disease with the absence of ascites and carcinomatosis, and (d) a good performance status (90). For all other patients, the potential morbidity and limited benefit associated with suboptimal secondary cytoreduction should be carefully weighed against the possible benefit of surgery. In cases where radiologic studies do not provide a clear preoperative picture of disease extent, a diagnostic laparoscopy to assess resectability may assist with the decision. In appropriately selected patients, secondary cytoreduction is associated with an improved patient outcome, with the largest benefit in patients from whom all visible disease is removed. Very rarely is surgery indicated in platinum-resistant recurrences and, in our opinion, should be performed only if a PET/CT shows only one or two lesions and the absence of ascites.

PALLIATIVE SURGERY INCLUDING SURGERY FOR MALIGNANT BOWEL OBSTRUCTION

The primary goal of palliative surgery is to relieve symptoms and improve the QoL, rather than prolong survival. Bowel obstruction is one of the main causes of both distress and death from OC. Others are extensive ascites, intractable pleural effusions, sepsis from a bowel perforation, and tumor cachexia (91,92). A malignant bowel obstruction is the most common reason for a hospital admission for patients with OC during the last year of life. The median survival of patients admitted with a bowel obstruction is around 3 months. The tumor, although it does not deeply invade the bowel, connects and then kinks bowel loops and/or encases the bowel mesentery, limiting bowel mobility and blood supply and causing a combination of mechanic bowel obstruction and adynamic ileus. Other etiologies can be extrinsic compression of the bowel lumen by intra-abdominal tumors or retroperitoneal lymph nodes pushing on the pyloric antrum or the duodenum. In patients without a recurrence, who underwent an extensive debulking procedure or received previous IP chemotherapy, adhesions, an old hematoma or a new incisional hernia may also be the cause of a bowel obstruction.

Patients with advanced disease tend to present to the emergency department with one or more of the following signs and symptoms: tachypnea/dyspnea because of cranial displacement of the diaphragm/atelectasis of lower lung lobes or a malignant pleural effusion, tachycardia from dehydration and pain, or a low-grade fever from the dehydration and chronic inflammation associated with a long-standing obstruction. Symptoms of a bowel obstruction include nausea and vomiting, the absence of gas or bowel movements, periumbilical cramping and a combination of dull and sharp abdominal pain, and abdominal distension. If the obstruction is high in the jejunum or duodenum, the distension might be subtle. Sometimes, patients complain of colicky pain from peristaltic waves of bowel against a focal, narrow point of obstruction. Changing bowel habits and loose stools are typical of a partial obstruction. Often, patients also have a DVT because of active, advanced disease affecting coagulation and prolonged immobility.

Instant nausea and vomiting after oral intake or projectile vomiting is an indication of a very proximal obstruction of the stomach or duodenum that cannot be relieved by surgery. If the patient has an adynamic ileus from peritoneal carcinomatosis, auscultation will show an absence of bowel sounds, but if there is a complete bowel obstruction, bowel sounds will be high pitched. Proximal bowel obstruction may be caused by either an extensive upper abdominal tumor load or enlarged high para-aortic lymph nodes causing extrinsic compression of the duodenum or jejunum. The abdomen of patients with a proximal bowel obstruction is often not distended, which can give the mistaken impression that the problem is limited, although the patients suffer from severe nausea and bilious emesis. Laboratory analysis often shows hemoconcentration, thrombocytosis, low albumin, and hypokalemic, hypochloremic metabolic alkalosis, which is a sign of repeated vomiting and/or long-standing nasogastric tube drainage. Patients with a volvulus or chronic bowel ischemia may have metabolic acidosis, leukocytosis, and an increase in lactate. While a bowel obstruction is a clinical diagnosis, a supine and upright abdominal x-ray ("GI obstruction series") will show air-fluid levels. A chest x-ray may reveal free air. A CT scan of the abdomen and pelvis with oral and IV contrast or a small bowel follow-through will permit the evaluation of the small/large bowel over its entire length and will help determine whether there is partial or complete bowel obstruction and if there are multiple sites of obstruction or a single transition point. The bowel is often dilated proximal to the transition point and collapsed distally.

Treatment options at this point include palliative care with symptom control, a percutaneous endoscopic gastrostomy (PEG) tube placed surgically of by interventional radiology, parenteral nutrition, palliative chemotherapy, stents for gastric outlet obstruction or single site colonic obstruction, and, as last, resort palliative surgery. Initial treatment for a malignant bowel obstruction should be conservative and may include bowel rest and hydration to correct metabolic abnormalities, which are signs of a long-standing obstruction. Additional supportive measures include treatment with octreotide to reduce secretions, antiemetics, corticosteroids to reduce inflammation and act as antiemetics, and narcotics for adequate pain management. In selected patients, it is possible to accomplish a temporary surgical correction and relieve the blockage by either removing the tumors obstructing the bowel or performing a diversion that may involve a colostomy, ileostomy, or a limited bowel resection with intestinal bypass. Preoperative contraindications to an attempted surgical correction of a malignant bowel obstruction include an adynamic ileus caused by carcinomatosis or extensive ascites, diffusely metastatic cancer with bowel obstructions on multiple levels, and involvement of the proximal ileum, duodenum, or stomach. Relative contraindications to palliative surgery for a malignant bowel obstruction are a long-standing obstruction, significant deconditioning and tumor cachexia (low serum albumin), multiple previous abdominal surgeries, and rapidly progressing chemotherapy-resistant disease (93). A very proximal obstruction of the stomach or duodenum cannot usually be relieved by surgery. Before surgery, consideration should be given to a large bowel stent if the obstruction is distal.

Because the purpose of palliative surgery is to improve the QoL, the procedure must be short and limited, with the lowest possible complication rate. A review of patients with OC at a single institution who underwent palliative surgery for bowel obstruction found that, in experienced hands and with appropriately selected patients, a surgical correction was possible in 84% of all patients and successful palliation, defined as the ability to tolerate oral intake for at least 60 days after surgery, was achieved in 71% of patients (94). In 16% of patients, a gastrostomy tube was placed, and most of the other patients received an ileostomy or a colostomy, or the obstructed area was bypassed. The rate of major surgical complications was 22% and included enterocutaneous fistula formation, abscess formation, bacterial peritonitis, thromboembolic events, and death. The median survival for patients who were able to receive chemotherapy (70%) was 9.7 months, whereas it was 2.4 months for those not treated with chemotherapy. A low preoperative albumin (<2.5 mg/dL), ascites (<2 L), and carcinomatosis were found to be relative contraindications to surgery in another study (93).

Palliative surgery for bowel obstruction in patients with OC is associated with significant mortality (15%-25%), whether it is an elective or an emergency procedure. Successful palliation (adequate oral intake >60 days) is achieved in 53% to 71% of patients, and the inoperability rate is around 20% (93-95). These results highlight the importance of discussing possible outcomes with patients, fostering realistic expectations, and learning how the patient defines successful palliation.

Excessive ascites production is also often encountered in patients with progressive disease. Ultrasound-guided IP catheter placement is safe and can be performed intermittently as an outpatient procedure. Visceral injury followed by peritonitis is very rare with this procedure, but with repeated paracentesis, the ascites may become loculated and drainage incomplete. Often, repeated paracenteses are necessary, and in this case, a permanent indwelling abdominal catheter can be placed, and the patient or her family instructed on how to drain the ascites. Potassium-sparing diuretics (triamterene, spironolactone) or antiangiogenic therapy may also reduce ascites production.

Fluorescence-Guided Surgery

Novel intraoperative visualization techniques, such as NIR fluorescence imaging, are being explored in the field of surgical oncology. NIR fluorescence imaging is a real-time imaging technique that combines an NIR fluorescent agent with a specialized imaging system that can detect fluorescence after excitation with NIR light (650-900 nm). The number of tumor-targeted fluorescent agents has substantially increased in the past two decades. Vascular endothelial growth factor α (EGF-α), indocyanine green (ICG), methylene blue (MB), CEA, and folate receptor α have been used as fluorescent agents (96). A phase 2 open-label study evaluated the use of pafolacianine injection (OTL38) for intraoperative imaging of folate receptor positive in patients undergoing surgery for OC (97). In this study, 44 patients were evaluated. OTL38 was safe and detected additional implants in over 50%. No survival outcomes were reported. This leads to a phase 3 confirmatory study for real-time detection of folate receptor–positive OC in patients undergoing surgery (98). The objectives were to confirm safety and efficacy of pafolacianine (0.025 mg/kg IV), given 1 hour or more before intraoperative NIR imaging to detect macroscopic lesions, which are often small IP lesions, not detected by palpation and normal white light. In 33.0% of patients (95% CI, 24.3-42.7; $P < .001$), pafolacianine with NIR imaging identified additional cancer on tissue not planned for resection and not detected by white light assessment and palpation, exceeding the prespecified threshold of 10%. The drug was well tolerated. Again, no survival outcomes were reported. The authors concluded that pafolacianine may offer an important real-time adjunct to current surgical approaches for OC.

REFERENCES

1. Horowitz NS, Miller A, Rungruang B, et al. Does aggressive surgery improve outcomes? Interaction between preoperative disease burden and complex surgery in patients with advanced-stage ovarian cancer: an analysis of GOG 182. *J Clin Oncol*. 2015;33(8):937-943.

2. Prat JG, Oncology FC. Staging classification for cancer of the ovary, fallopian tube, and peritoneum. *Int J Gynaecol Obstet*. 2014;124(1):1-5.

3. Verleye L, Ottevanger PB, Graaf W, Reed NS, Vergote I. EORTC-GCG process quality indicators for ovarian cancer surgery. *Eur J Cancer*. 2009;45:517-526.

4. Garcia-Soto AE, Boren T, Wingo SN, Heffernen T, Miller DS. Is comprehensive surgical staging needed for thorough evaluation of early-stage ovarian carcinoma? *Am J Obstet Gynecol*. 2012;206(3):242.e1-242.e2425.

5. Ayhan A, Gultekin M, Celik NY, et al. Occult metastasis in early ovarian cancers: risk factors and associated prognosis. *Am J Obstet Gynecol*. 2007;196:81.e1-81.e816.

6. Trimbos JB, Vergote I, Bolis G, et al. Impact of adjuvant chemotherapy and surgical staging in early-stage ovarian carcinoma: European organisation for research and treatment of cancer—adjuvant chemotherapy in ovarian neoplasm trial. *J Natl Cancer Inst*. 2003;95(2):113-125.

7. Timmers PJ, Zwinderman AH, Coens C, Vergote I, Trimbos JB. Understanding the problem of inadequately staging early ovarian cancer. *Eur J Cancer*. 2010;46(5):880-884.

8. Colombo N, Guthrie D, Chiari S, et al. International collaborative ovarian neoplasm trial 1: a randomized trial of adjuvant chemotherapy in women with early-stage ovarian cancer. *J Natl Cancer Inst*. 2003;95(2):125-132.

9. Collinson F, Qian W, Fossati R, et al. Optimal treatment of early-stage ovarian cancer. *Ann Oncol*. 2014;25(6):1165-1171.

10. Oseledchyk A, Leitao MM Jr, O'Cearbhaill RE, et al. Adjuvant chemotherapy in patients with stage I endometrioid or clear cell ovarian cancer in the platinum era: a surveillance, epidemiology, and end results cohort study, 2000-2013. *Ann Oncol*. 2017;28(12):2985-2993.

11. Chi DS, Abu-Rustum NR, Sonoda Y, et al. The safety and efficacy of laparoscopic surgical staging of apparent stage I ovarian and fallopian tube cancers. *Am J Obstet Gynecol*. 2005;192:1614-1619.

12. Zivanovic O, Sonoda Y, Diaz JP, et al. The rate of port-site metastases after 2251 laparoscopic procedures in women with underlying malignant disease. *Gynecol Oncol*. 2008;111:431-437.

13. Heitz F, Harter P, Ataseven B, et al. Stage- and histologic subtype-dependent frequency of lymph node metastases in patients with epithelial ovarian cancer undergoing systematic pelvic and paraaortic lymphadenectomy. *Ann Surg Oncol*. 2018;25(7):2053-2059.

14. DiRe F, Fontanelli R, Raspagliesi F, DiRe E. Pelvic and para-aortic lymphadenetomy in cancer of the ovary. *Bailliere Clin Obstet Gynaecol*. 1989;3:131-138.

15. Eichner E, Bove ER. In vivo studies on the lymphatic drainage of the human ovary. *Obstet Gynecol*. 1954;3(3):287-297.

16. Benedetti P, Maggioni A, Hacker NF, et al. Systematic aortic and pelvic lymphadenectomy versus resection of bulky nodes only in optimally debulked advanced ovarian cancer: a randomized clinical trial. *J Natl Cancer Inst*. 2005;97(8):560-566.

17. Harter P, Sehouli J, Lorusso D, et al. A randomized trial of lymphadenectomy in patients with advanced ovarian neoplasms. *N Engl J Med*. 2019;380(9):822-832.

18. Morice P, Joulie F, Camatte S, et al. Lymph node involvement in epithelial ovarian cancer: analysis of 276 pelvic and paraaortic lymphadenectomies and surgical implications. *J Am Coll Surg*. 2003;197:198-205.

19. Schmeler KM, Frumovitz M, Deavers M, et al. Prevalence of lymph node metastasis in primary mucinous carcinoma of the ovary. *Obstet Gynecol*. 2010;116(2):269-273.

20. Bois A, Reuss A, Harter P, Pujade-Lauraine E, Ray-Coquard I, Pfisterer J. Potential role of lymphadenectomy in advanced ovarian cancer: a combined exploratory analysis of three prospectively randomized phase III multicenter trials. *J Clin Oncol*. 2010;28(10):1733-1739.

21. Maggioni A, Panici PB, Dell'Anna T, et al. Randomised study of systematic lymphadenectomy in patients with epithelial ovarian cancer macroscopically confined to the pelvis. *Br J Cancer*. 2006;95:699-704.

22. Bookman MA, Brady MF, McGuire WP, et al. Evaluation of new platinum-based treatment regimens in advanced-stage ovarian cancer: a phase III trial of the gynecologic cancer intergroup. *J Clin Oncol*. 2009;27(9):1419-1425.

23. Rodriguez N, Miller A, Richard SD, et al. Upper abdominal procedures in advanced stage ovarian or primary peritoneal carcinoma patients with minimal or no gross residual disease: an analysis of gynecologic oncology group (GOG) 182. *Gynecol Oncol*. 2013;130(3):487-492.

24. Lengyel E. Ovarian cancer development and metastasis. *Am J Pathol*. 2010;177(3):1053-1064. doi:10.2353/ajpath.2010.100105

25. Bristow RE, Carmen M, Kaufman H, Montz FJ. Radical oophorectomy with primary stapled colorectal anastomosis for resection of locally advanced epithelial ovarian cancer. *J Am Coll Surg*. 2003;197:565-574.

26. Armstrong DK, Bundy B, Wenzel L, et al. Intraperitoneal cisplatin and paclitaxel in ovarian cancer. *N Engl J Med*. 2006;354(1):34-43. doi:10.1056/NEJMoa052985

27. Bristow RE, Tomacruz RS, Armstrong DK, Trimble EL, Montz FJ. Survival effect of maximal cytoreductive surgery for advanced ovarian carcinoma during the platinum era: a meta-analysis. *J Clin Oncol*. 2002;20(5):1248-1259.

28. Chi DS, Eisenhauer EL, Zivanovic O, et al. Improved progression-free and overall survival in advanced ovarian cancer as a result of a change in surgical paradigm. *Gynecol Oncol*. 2009;114(1):26-31. doi:10.1016/j.ygyno.2009.03.018

29. Tseng JH, Cowan RA, Zhou Q, et al. Continuous improvement in primary debulking surgery for advanced ovarian cancer: do increased complete gross resection rates independently lead to increased progression-free and overall survival? *Gynecol Oncol*. 2018;151(1):24-31.

30. Griffiths CT. Surgical resection of tumor bulk in the primary treatment of ovarian carcinoma. *Natl Cancer Inst Monogr*. 1975;42:101-104.

31. Winter WE, Maxwell GL, Tian C, et al. Tumor residual after surgical cytoreduction in prediction of clinical outcome in stage IV epithelial ovarian cancer: a gynecological oncology group study. *J Clin Oncol*. 2008;26(1):83-89.

32. Bois A, Reuss A, Pujade-Lauraine E, Harter P, Ray-Coquard I, Pfisterer J. Role of surgical outcome as prognostic factor in advanced epithelial ovarian cancer: a combined exploratory analysis of prospectively randomized phase 3 multicenter trials. *Cancer*. 2009;115(6):1234-1244.

33. Fagotti A, Vizzielli G, Iaco P, et al. A multicentric trial (Olympia-MITO 13) on the accuracy of laparoscopy to assess peritoneal spread in ovarian cancer. *Am J Obstet Gynecol*. 2013;209(5):462.e1-462.e11.

34. Hoskins WJ, Bundy BN, Thigpen JT, Omura GA. The influence of cytoreductive surgery on recurrence-free interval and survival in small-volume stage III epithelial ovarian cancer: a gynecologic oncology group study. *Gynecol Oncol*. 1992;47:159-166.

35. Hoskins WJ, McGuire WP, Brady MF, et al. The effect of diameter of largest residual disease on survival after primary cytoreductive surgery in patients with suboptimal residual epithelial ovarian carcinoma. *Am J Obstet Gynecol*. 1994;170(4):974-979.

36. Wimberger P, Wehling M, Lehmann N, et al. Influence of residual tumor on outcome in ovarian cancer patients with FIGO stage IV disease. *Ann Surg Oncol*. 2010;17:1642-1648.

37. Zivanovic O, Sima CS, Iasonos A, et al. The effect of primary cytoreduction on outcomes of patients with FIGO stage IIIC ovarian cancer stratified by the initial tumor burden in the upper abdomen cephalad to the greater omentum. *Gynecol Oncol*. 2010;116(3):351-357.

38. Grabowski JP, Harter P, Heitz F, et al. Operability and chemotherapy responsiveness in advanced low-grade serous ovarian cancer. An analysis of the AGO Study Group metadatabase. *Gynecol Oncol*. 2016;140(3):457-462.

39. Axtell A, Lee MH, Bristow RE, et al. Multi-institutional reciprocal validation study of computed tomography predictors of suboptimal primary cytoreduction in patients with advanced ovarian cancer. *J Clin Oncol*. 2007;25(4):384-389.

40. Suidan RS, Ramirez PT, Sarasohn DM, et al. A multicenter prospective trial evaluating the ability of preoperative computed tomography scan and serum CA-125 to predict suboptimal cytoreduction at primary debulking surgery for advanced ovarian, fallopian tube, and peritoneal cancer. *Gynecol Oncol*. 2014;134(3):455-461.

41. Boj SF, Hwang CI, Baker LA, et al. Organoid models of human and mouse ductal pancreatic cancer. *Cell*. 2015;160(1-2):324-338.

42. Fagotti A, Ferrandina G, Fanfani F, et al. A laparoscopy-based score to predict surgical outcome in patients with advanced ovarian carcinoma: a pilot study. *Ann Surg Oncol*. 2006;13(8):1156-1161.

43. Aletti GD, Podratz KC, Jones MB, Cliby WA. Role of rectosigmoidectomy and stripping of pelvic peritoneum in outcomes of patients with advanced ovarian cancer. *J Am Coll Surg*. 2006;203(4):521-526.

44. Grimm C, Harter P, Alesina PF, et al. The impact of type and number of bowel resections on anastomotic leakage risk in advanced ovarian cancer surgery. *Gynecol Oncol*. 2017;146(3):498-503.

45. Williamson AJ, Alverdy JC. Influence of the microbiome on anastomotic leak. *Clin Colon Rectal Surg*. 2021;34(6):439-446.

46. Moukarzel LA, Byrne ME, Leiva S, et al. The impact of near-infrared angiography and proctoscopy after rectosigmoid resection and anastomosis performed during surgeries for gynecologic malignancies. *Gynecol Oncol*. 2020;158(2):397-401.

47. Kehoe SM, Eisenhauer EL, Chi DS. Upper abdominal surgical procedures: liver mobilization and diaphragm peritonectomy/resection, splenectomy, and distal pancreatectomy. *Gynecol Oncol*. 2008;111:51-55.

48. Hoffman MS, Tebes SJ, Sayer RA, Lockhart J. Extended cytoreduction of intraabdominal metastatic ovarian cancer in the left upper quadrant utilizing en bloc resection. *Am J Obstet Gynecol*. 2007;197(2):209.e1-209.e4, 209.e4-209.e5.

49. Magtibay PM, Adams PB, Silverman MB, Cha SS, Podratz KC. Splenectomy as part of cytoreductive surgery in ovarian cancer. *Gynecol Oncol*. 2006;102:369-374.

50. Benedetti Panici P, Donato V, Fischetti M, et al. Predictors of postoperative morbidity after cytoreduction for advanced ovarian cancer: analysis and management of complications in upper abdominal surgery. *Gynecol Oncol*. 2015;137(3):406-411.

51. Filippova OT, Kim SW, Cowan RA, et al. Hematologic changes after splenectomy for ovarian cancer debulking surgery, and association with infection and venous thromboembolism. *Int J Gynecol Cancer*. 2020;30(8):1183-1188.

52. Kehoe SM, Eisenhauer EL, Abu-Rustum NR, et al. Incidence and management of pancreatic leaks after splenectomy with distal pancreatectomy

performed during primary cytoreductive surgery for advanced ovarian, peritoneal and fallopian tube cancer. *Gynecol Oncol.* 2009;112(3): 496-500.

53. Allen PJ, Gonen M, Brennan MF, et al. Pasireotide for postoperative pancreatic fistula. *N Engl J Med.* 2014;370(21):2014-2022.

54. Schiavone MB, Moukarzel L, Leong K, et al. Surgical site infection reduction bundle in patients with gynecologic cancer undergoing colon surgery. *Gynecol Oncol.* 2017;147(1):115-119.

55. Sanchez-Iglesias JL, Gomez-Hidalgo NR, Perez-Benavente A, et al. Importance of enhanced recovery after surgery (ERAS) protocol compliance for length of stay in ovarian cancer surgery. *Ann Surg Oncol.* 2021;28(13):8979-8986.

56. Vergote I, Tropé CG, Amant F, et al. Neoadjuvant chemotherapy or primary surgery in stage IIIC or IV ovarian cancer. *N Engl J Med.* 2010;363(10):943-953. doi:10.1056/NEJMoa0908806

57. Kehoe S, Hook J, Nankivell M, et al. Primary chemotherapy versus primary surgery for newly diagnosed advanced ovarian cancer (CHORUS): an open-label, randomised, controlled, non-inferiority trial. *Lancet.* 2015;386(9990):249-257. doi:10.1016/S0140-6736(14)62223-6

58. van Meurs HS, Tajik P, Hof MHP, et al. Which patients benefit most from primary surgery or neoadjuvant chemotherapy in stage IIIC or IV ovarian cancer? An exploratory analysis of the European organisation for research and treatment of cancer 55971 randomised trial. *Eur J Cancer.* 2013;49(15):3191-3201. doi:10.1016/j.ejca.2013.06.013

59. Chi DS, Musa F, Dao F, et al. An analysis of patients with bulky advanced stage ovarian, tubal, and peritoneal carcinoma treated with primary debulking surgery (PDS) during an identical time period as the randomized EORTC-NCIC trial of PDS vs neoadjuvant chemotherapy (NACT). *Gynecol Oncol.* 2012;124:10-14.

60. Reuss A, Bois A, Harter P, et al. TRUST: trial of radical upfront surgical therapy in advanced ovarian cancer (ENGOT ov33/AGO-OVAR OP7). *Int J Gynecol Cancer.* 2019;29(8):1327-1331.

61. Aletti GD, Eisenhauer E, Santillan A, et al. Identification of patient groups at highest risk from traditional approach to ovarian cancer treatment. *Gynecol Oncol.* 2011;120:23-28.

62. Steffen T, Haller L, Bijelic L, et al. Decision-making analysis for hyperthermic intraperitoneal chemotherapy in ovarian cancer: a survey by the executive committee of the peritoneal surface oncology group international (PSOGI). *Oncology.* 2021;99(1):41-48.

63. Schwameis R, Chiva L, Harter P. There is no role for hyperthermic intraperitoneal chemotherapy (HIPEC) in ovarian cancer. *Int J Gynecol Cancer.* 2022;32(4):578.

64. Zivanovic O, Abramian A, Kullmann M, et al. HIPEC ROC I: a phase I study of cisplatin administered as hyperthermic intraoperative intraperitoneal chemoperfusion followed by postoperative intravenous platinum-based chemotherapy in patients with platinum-sensitive recurrent epithelial ovarian cancer. *Int J Cancer.* 2015;136(3):699-708.

65. Wright AA, Cronin A, Milne DE, et al. Use and effectiveness of intraperitoneal chemotherapy for treatment of ovarian cancer. *J Clin Oncol.* 2015;33:2841-2847. doi:10.1200/JCO.2015.61.4776

66. Walker JL, Brady MF, Wenzel L, et al. Randomized trial of intravenous versus intraperitoneal chemotherapy plus bevacizumab in advanced ovarian carcinoma: an NRG oncology/gynecologic oncology group study. *J Clin Oncol.* 2019;37(16):1380-1390. doi:10.1200/JCO.18.01568

67. van Driel WJ, Koole SN, Sikorska K, et al. Hyperthermic intraperitoneal chemotherapy in ovarian cancer. *N Engl J Med.* 2018;378(3):230-240. doi:10.1056/NEJMoa1708618

68. Lim MC, Chang SJ, Park B, et al. Survival after hyperthermic intraperitoneal chemotherapy and primary or interval cytoreductive surgery in ovarian cancer: a randomized clinical trial. *JAMA Surg.* 2022; 157(5):374-383.

69. Koole S, Stein R, Sikorska K, et al. Primary cytoreductive surgery with or without hyperthermic intraperitoneal chemotherapy (HIPEC) for FIGO stage III epithelial ovarian cancer: OVHIPEC-2, a phase III randomized clinical trial. *Int J Gynecol Cancer.* 2020;30(6):888-892.

70. Lei Z, Wang Y, Wang J, et al. Evaluation of cytoreductive surgery with or without hyperthermic intraperitoneal chemotherapy for stage III epithelial ovarian cancer. *JAMA Netw Open.* 2020;3(8):e2013940.

71. Zivanovic O, Chi DS, Zhou Q, et al. Secondary cytoreduction and carboplatin hyperthermic intraperitoneal chemotherapy for platinum-sensitive recurrent ovarian cancer: an MSK team ovary phase II study. *J Clin Oncol.* 2021;39(23):2594-2604.

72. Spiliotis J, Halkia E, Lianos E, et al. Cytoreductive surgery and HIPEC in recurrent epithelial ovarian cancer: a prospective randomized phase III study. *Ann Surg Oncol.* 2015;22(5):1570-1575.

73. Nick AM, Coleman RL, Ramirez PT, Sood AK. A framework for a personalized surgical approach to ovarian cancer. *Nat Rev Clin Oncol.* 2015;12(4):239-245.

74. Wright J, Lewin SN, Deutsch I, et al. Defining the limits of radical cytoreductive surgery for ovarian cancer. *Gynecol Oncol.* 2011;123:467-473.

75. Petrillo M, Vizzielli G, Fanfani F, et al. Definition of a dynamic laparoscopic model for the prediction of incomplete cytoreduction in advanced epithelial ovarian cancer: proof of a concept. *Gynecol Oncol.* 2015;139(1):5-9.

76. Suidan RS, Ramirez PT, Sarasohn DM, et al. A multicenter assessment of the ability of preoperative computed tomography scan and CA-125 to predict gross residual disease at primary debulking for advanced epithelial ovarian cancer. *Gynecol Oncol.* 2017;145(1):27-31.

77. Coll AP, Chen M, Taskar P, et al. GDF15 mediates the effects of metformin on body weight and energy balance. *Nature.* 2020;578(7795): 444-448.

78. Burg MEL, Lent M, Buyse M, et al. The effect of debulking surgery after induction chemotherapy on the prognosis in advanced epithelial ovarian cancer. *N Engl J Med.* 1995;332(10):629-634.

79. Rose PG, Nerenstone S, Brady MF, et al. Secondary surgical cytoreduction for advanced ovarian carcinoma. *N Engl J Med.* 2004;351(24):2489-2497.

80. van der Burg ME. Advanced ovarian cancer. *Curr Treat Options Oncol.* 2001;2:109-118.

81. Jänicke F, Hölscher M, Kuhn W, et al. Radical surgical procedure improves survival time in patients with recurrent ovarian cancer. *Cancer.* 1992;70:2129-2136.

82. Harter P, Hahmann M, Lueck HJ, et al. Surgery for recurrent ovarian cancer: role of peritoneal carcinomatosis. Exploratory analysis of the DESKTOP I trial about risk factors, surgical implications, and prognostic value of peritoneal carcinomatosis. *Ann Surg Oncol.* 2009;13(12):1702-1710.

83. Harter P, Sehouli J, Reuss A, et al. Prospective validation study of a predictive score for operability of recurrent ovarian cancer. *Int J Gynecol Cancer.* 2011;21(2):289-295.

84. Janco JM, Kumar A, Weaver AL, McGree ME, Cliby WA. Performance of AGO score for secondary cytoreduction in a high-volume U.S. center. *Gynecol Oncol.* 2016;141(1):140-147.

85. Rungruang B, Miller A, Richard SD, et al. Should stage IIIC ovarian cancer be further stratified by intraperitoneal vs. retroperitoneal only disease?: a gynecologic oncology group study. *Gynecol Oncol.* 2012; 124:53-58.

86. Harter P, Sehouli J, Vergote I, et al. Randomized trial of cytoreductive surgery for relapsed ovarian cancer. *N Engl J Med.* 2021;385(23): 2123-2131.

87. Coleman RL, Spirtos NM, Enserro D, et al. Secondary surgical cytoreduction for recurrent ovarian cancer. *N Engl J Med.* 2019;381(20): 1929-1939.

88. Shi T, Zhu J, Feng Y, et al. Secondary cytoreduction followed by chemotherapy versus chemotherapy alone in platinum-sensitive relapsed ovarian cancer (SOC-1): a multicentre, open-label, randomised, phase 3 trial. *Lancet Oncol.* 2021;22(4):439-449.

89. Baek MH, Park EY, Ha HI, et al. Secondary cytoreductive surgery in platinum-sensitive recurrent ovarian cancer: a meta-analysis. *J Clin Oncol.* 2022;40(15):1659-1670.

90. Díaz-Montes TP, Bristow RE. Secondary cytoreduction for patients with recurrent ovarian cancer. *Curr Oncol Rep.* 2012;7:451-458.

91. Radwany SM, Gruenigen VE. Palliative and end-of-life care for patients with ovarian cancer. *Clin Obstet Gynecol.* 2012;55(1):173-184.

92. Hope JM, Pothuri B. The role of palliative surgery in gynecologic cancer cases. *Oncologist.* 2013;18(1):73-79.

93. Perri T, Korach J, Ben-Baruch G, et al. Bowel obstruction in recurrent gynecologic malignancies: defining who will benefit from surgical intervention. *Eur J Surg Oncol.* 2014;40(7):899-904.

94. Pothuri B, Vaidya A, Aghajanian C, Venkatraman ES, Barakat RR, Chi DS. Palliative surgery for bowel obstruction in recurrent ovarian cancer: an updated series. *Gynecol Oncol.* 2003;89:306-313.

95. Kolomainen DF, Daponte A, Barton DP, et al. Outcomes of surgical management of bowel obstruction in relapsed epithelial ovarian cancer (EOC). *Gynecol Oncol.* 2012;125(1):31-36.

96. Galema HA, Meijer RPJ, Lauwerends LJ, et al. Fluorescence-guided surgery in colorectal cancer; a review on clinical results and future perspectives. *Eur J Surg Oncol.* 2022;48(4):810-821.

97. Randall LM, Wenham RM, Low PS, Dowdy SC, Tanyi JL. A phase II, multicenter, open-label trial of OTL38 injection for the intra-operative imaging of folate receptor-alpha positive ovarian cancer. *Gynecol Oncol.* 2019;155(1):63-68. doi:10.1016/j.ygyno.2019.07.010

98. Tanyi JL, Randall LM, Chambers SK, et al. A phase III study of pafolacianine injection (OTL38) for intraoperative imaging of folate receptor-positive ovarian cancer (Study 006). *J Clin Oncol.* 2023;41: 276-284.

99. Zapardiel I, Morrow CP. New terminology for cytoreduction in advanced ovarian cancer. *Lancet Oncol.* 2011;12:214.

CHAPTER **8.7**

Ovarian Cancer: Pathology

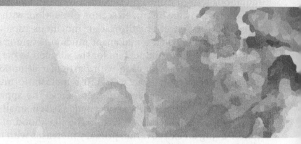

Agnes Julia Bilecz and Ricardo R. Lastra

CLASSIFICATION

Epithelial tumors comprise about half of all ovarian tumors and account for 40% of benign and over 95% of malignant tumors. The 2020 WHO classification of ovarian epithelial tumors is summarized in **Table 8.7-1** (1).

The apparent histotype distribution of OC has changed significantly in the past decades, largely due to changes in the pathologic criteria applied when diagnosing ovarian neoplasms. These changes reflect our improved understanding of the pathophysiologic

TABLE 8.7-1. 2020 WHO Classification of Ovarian Epithelial Tumors

Serous tumors	Serous cystadenoma
	Serous adenofibroma
	Surface papilloma
	Serous borderline tumor
	Low-grade serous carcinoma
	High-grade serous carcinoma
Mucinous tumors	Mucinous cystadenoma
	Mucinous adenofibroma
	Mucinous borderline tumor
	Mucinous carcinoma
Endometrioid tumors	Endometrioid cystadenoma
	Endometrioid adenofibroma
	Endometrioid borderline tumor
	Endometrioid carcinoma
Clear cell tumors	Clear cell cystadenoma
	Clear cell adenofibroma
	Clear cell borderline tumor
	Clear cell carcinoma
Seromucinous tumors	Seromucinous cystadenoma
	Seromucinous adenofibroma
	Seromucinous borderline tumor
Brenner tumors	Brenner tumor
	Borderline Brenner tumor
	Malignant Brenner tumor
Other carcinomas	Mesonephric-like adenocarcinoma
	Undifferentiated and dedifferentiated carcinomas
	Carcinosarcoma
	Mixed carcinoma

World Health Organization (WHO). Female Genital Tumors. Vol 4. 5th ed. WHO International Agency for Research on Cancer; 2020.
From IARC 2020

mechanisms. A study comparing interobserver reproducibility for diagnoses rendered based on the 2003 and 2014 WHO classification of tumors of the gynecologic tract demonstrated that, when using the 2003 criteria, the interobserver agreement was only 54% compared to 98% when utilizing the 2014 criteria (2). For instance, the recent description of a subset of HGSCs, especially those associated with HRD demonstrating variant morphology, has led to the reclassification of many cases of ovarian endometrioid carcinomas, transitional cell carcinomas, and mixed epithelial carcinomas as HGSC. The distinction between primary and metastatic mucinous carcinomas has also evolved significantly, with primary ovarian mucinous carcinomas now being regarded as rather rare entities. Carcinosarcoma, previously thought to be a very rare primary ovarian tumor, now appears to comprise 5% of ovarian carcinomas in the United States, likely due to more thorough sampling with the identification of small sarcomatous components in otherwise typical HGSCs (**Table 8.7-2**). The incidence of different histotypes varies among geographic regions (3). For example, clear cell carcinomas are more common in Japan as compared to North America. The extent to which these differences may reflect variation in diagnostic criteria or other aspects of pathology practice remains to be determined.

INTRAOPERATIVE CONSULTATION (FROZEN SECTION)

Maximizing the yield of frozen section evaluation of ovarian lesions relies on three fundamental pieces of information: clinical history including abnormal tumor markers (CEA, CA-125), macroscopic evaluation, and microscopic interpretation. The value of clinical information and the operative findings to the pathologist should not be underestimated, and two-way intraoperative communication between the pathologist and the surgeon is essential. The ideal scenario would include obtaining the patient's pertinent history and imaging results before the anticipated frozen section (4). In addition, frozen section should only be requested when necessary to guide surgical management, as unnecessary and "curiosity" frozen sections waste valuable resources and increase the likelihood of diagnostic errors (5).

The main purpose of intraoperative pathology consultation of an ovarian mass is to determine whether the lesion is borderline or malignant, indicating that surgical staging is necessary. This distinction is relatively straight forward in most cases, with the estimated sensitivity being over 95% (6,7). However, a simple diagnosis of "malignant" is not always sufficient because the extent of surgical staging will depend on other factors, such as the tumor histotype, patient age, and the desire to retain fertility. Moreover, metastatic neoplasms to the ovary represent approximately 5% to 15% of malignant ovarian masses, and surgical staging is generally not indicated in these cases. This may be the case even in the absence of a known history of malignancy, as instances in which the ovarian lesion may indeed represent the sentinel finding of an occult primary do occur. In this context, it is important to mention that the distinction of a primary ovarian lesion (particularly a mucinous lesion) from a metastatic tumor can be challenging and not always possible on frozen section evaluation, with discrepancy rates for frozen sections of ovarian mucinous tumors exceeding 30% (8). Hence, when a malignant mucinous tumor is diagnosed intraoperatively, it is important for the surgeon to perform a complete abdominal exploration with particular attention to the GI and pancreatobiliary tracts, as most metastatic mucinous carcinomas to the ovaries arise in these sites. The appendix should be removed even if it appears normal, as even small appendiceal neoplasms can disseminate (9,10). The likelihood of a mucinous tumor being an extraovarian primary increases with the degree of cytologic atypia, gross and microscopic complexity, and the presence of extraovarian disease. Simple unilocular mucinous cysts are nearly always benign primary ovarian tumors, although ovarian metastases of pancreatic adenocarcinomas and low-grade appendiceal mucinous neoplasms (LAMNs) can both present as cystic tumors lined by deceptively bland mucinous epithelium (11,12). Once any degree of atypia is present, an extraovarian primary should be considered in addition to a primary ovarian MBT. If unequivocal evidence of mucinous carcinoma is identified within the ovary, the likelihood of this representing metastatic disease to the ovary is approximately 80%. If peritoneal disease in the form of pseudomyxoma peritonei (PMP) (see "Mucinous Tumors Associated with Pseudomyxoma Peritonei" section) or metastatic adenocarcinoma is present, the likelihood of an extraovarian primary much higher, as most true primary ovarian mucinous carcinomas are diagnosed as an early stage I (**Table 8.7-2**). Features that may aid the pathologist in more definitively determining whether the lesion is primary versus metastatic include unilateral versus bilateral ovarian involvement, tumor size, and ovarian surface involvement, with most primary ovarian mucinous lesions being large and unilateral (13).

If frozen section demonstrates a lesion with endometrioid morphology, the possibility of colorectal metastasis needs to be considered, particularly in patients over the age of 40. The average size of primary ovarian endometrioid carcinomas is 15 cm, with bilaterality only observed in approximately 17% of patients and squamous differentiation being often present. In contrast, metastatic diseases from colorectal primaries tend to be smaller than 12 cm, are often bilateral, and lack squamous differentiation. Focal mucinous differentiation can be observed in endometrioid lesions, but the presence of an extensive mucinous component, goblet cells, or signet-ring cell is characteristic of metastases from GI primaries (4).

It is somewhat less important to distinguish borderline tumors from carcinoma intraoperatively, as full staging is indicated for both, although a more through staging is performed when there is a high index of suspicion for malignancy based on frozen section and intraoperative findings (see earlier). In this sense, low-grade serous neoplasms present a unique intraoperative challenge. These lesions can be extremely heterogeneous, with LGSCs nearly always containing benign-appearing areas resembling a cystadenoma or SBT, and because the amount of tissue that can be examined

intraoperatively is limited, errors due to sampling do occur. Approximately 20% to 30% of tumors diagnosed as SBTs on frozen examination prove to be LGSCs on further sampling (7,14). The likelihood of a tumor interpreted as SBT during frozen section, which later is proven to be an LGSC on permanent evaluation, increases with tumor size. In one study, tumors measuring more than 8 cm diagnosed as SBT on frozen section were found to have invasive carcinoma in 22.4% of cases, compared to 3.2% in cases of tumors of smaller size (15). In challenging cases, a frozen section diagnosis of "at least borderline tumor" is considered pathologically appropriate but not really helpful for the surgeon, as more accurate tumor classification requires extensive sampling that is not feasible during intraoperative assessment (4). Whether a complete staging with its attendant possible morbidity should be undertaken depends on the findings at exploration, the level of suspicion for carcinoma on the part of both the pathologist and the surgeon, and the patient's preferences.

COLLEGE OF AMERICAN PATHOLOGISTS, 2020 WORLD HEALTH ORGANIZATION, AND INTERNATIONAL COLLABORATION ON CANCER REPORTING GUIDELINES

The College of American Pathologists (CAP) has issued guidelines for the reporting of OC, which are regularly updated, and recommends using the WHO classification and nomenclature for histologic types (1).

Recommendations for Reporting

Site assignment, including laterality, is now a core data element for complete reporting. Criteria for site assignment are also based on the 2020 WHO classification. Possible primary sites include ovaries, fallopian tubes, tubo-ovarian, and primary peritoneal localizations. Site assignment as "undesignated" should be avoided, whereas "tubo-ovarian" primaries should be reserved for select cases (ie, small biopsies, HGSC developing in patients with prior surgical treatment but incomplete tubal examination, and a subset of post-treatment resection specimens).

Assessment of ovarian surface involvement and tumor rupture is required. Communication between the pathologist and the surgeon, or review of the operative report, is, therefore, important to record this information. For advanced-stage disease, documenting the size of the largest extrapelvic peritoneal nodule is required, and although this is often evident from the gross pathologic examination, input from the surgeon may be necessary in cases of an incomplete tumor resection.

Other required elements of the checklist include specimen type, procedure, specimen integrity, tumor size, histologic type, number of sampled regional lymph nodes, number of metastatic lymph

■ **TABLE 8.7-2. Incidence of Malignant Epithelial Tumors of the Ovary**

Patient Characteristics	High-Grade Serous, n (%)	Low-Grade Serous, n (%)	Endometrioid, n (%)	Clear Cell, n (%)	Mucinous, n (%)	Carcinosarcoma, n (%)	Malignant Brenner, n (%)
Total	17,837 (63.4)	708 (2.5)	2,782 (9.9)	2,695 (9.6)	2,641 (9.4)	1,381 (4.9)	74 (0.3)
Disease stage							
Localized	882 (5.0)	144 (20.3)	1,275 (45.8)	929 (34.5)	1,274 (48.2)	75 (5.4)	42 (56.8)
Regional	3,057 (17.1)	186 (26.3)	1,177 (42.3)	1,021 (37.9)	661 (25.0)	267 (19.3)	19 (25.7)
Distant	13,898 (78.9)	378 (53.4)	330 (11.9)	745 (27.6)	706 (26.7)	1,039 (75.2)	13 (17.6)

Based on Peres LC, Cushing-Haugen KL, Kobel M, et al. Invasive epithelial ovarian cancer survival by histotype and disease stage. *J Natl Cancer Inst.* 2018;111(1):60-68.

nodes and size of largest nodal metastasis, extent of involvement of other organs, status of peritoneal and pleural fluid specimens (see "Cytopathology" section), and pTNM stage with adequate TNM descriptors (based on the current AJCC Staging Manual). Grade is required only for malignant tumors, whereas borderline tumors are not graded. For mucinous and endometrioid carcinomas, the use of the three-tier FIGO system is recommended. HGSCs and LGSCs have to be distinguished. Clear cell carcinomas and carcinosarcomas are not graded, as these are high grade by definition. Assessment of response to neoadjuvant chemotherapy using the highly reproducible three-tier chemotherapy response score (CRS) is now a required element to report in post-therapy cases (see "High-Grade Serous Carcinoma of Ovarian, Tubal, and Peritoneal Origin" section) (16). The FIGO stage should be included in report. The International Collaboration on Cancer Reporting (ICCR) data set for reporting are generally in line with the CAP and WHO recommendations and also include primary site assignment for HGSC as a core data element (17).

Recommendations Regarding Gross Examination

Sectioning and extensive evaluation of the fimbriae (SEE-FIM protocol) is recommended for RRSO specimens and in select HGSC cases where careful macroscopic examination fails to identify tubal involvement (18). The SEE-FIM protocol requires the entire ovaries and fallopian tubes to be submitted for histologic evaluation. This involves serially sectioning the tube transversely at 2 mm intervals, stopping before the fimbriae. The fimbria is amputated and sectioned longitudinally, thereby maximizing exposure (19). Optimal sampling of macroscopically normal-appearing omentum requires at least 10 blocks to be submitted for histologic evaluation to reach 95% sensitivity in pathologic detection of microscopic omental metastases (20).

Recent Changes in Classification and Terminology

The 2020 WHO classification of female genital tumors contains several minor changes from the 2014 edition. The 2020 fifth edition further emphasizes that HGSCs and LGSCs are two distinctly different tumor types with fundamental differences in morphology, pathogenesis, molecular genetics, and patient outcomes. The fimbriated end of the fallopian tube is now considered to represent the primary site of the majority of HGSCs.

The term "invasive peritoneal implant"—previously used in the context of SBTs—is no longer recommended. These invasive proliferations are now designated LGSCs of the peritoneum in the absence of macroscopic or microscopic ovarian involvement. When ovarian involvement is present—with or without detectable ovarian invasion—the invasive lesions are considered metastases, and the ovarian tumor is diagnosed as LGSC. The use of terms such as "atypical proliferative tumor," "noninvasive LGSC," and "tumor of low malignant potential" is no longer recommended. The micropapillary variant of SBT is no longer equated with noninvasive LGSC (see "Serous Borderline Tumor" section).

The current recommended terminology for lesions previously termed mixed Müllerian cystadenomas/adenofibromas or endocervical-type/Müllerian MBTs is seromucinous cystadenoma/adenofibroma or seromucinous borderline tumor (SMBT). Seromucinous carcinomas are no longer a distinct entity but are now regarded as a subtype of endometrioid carcinomas demonstrating mucinous differentiation.

The category of mixed carcinoma has been reintroduced in the WHO fifth edition, specifying that these lesions are exceedingly rare, and the diagnosis should only be rendered when the components are unequivocally different and preferably exhibit different immunophenotypes.

Mesonephric-like adenocarcinoma (MLAC) and dedifferentiated carcinoma are newly added variants of ovarian epithelial tumors, both morphologically resembling their endometrial counterparts. Ovarian carcinosarcoma is currently regarded as a variant of an epithelial malignancy that is dedifferentiated and not a genuine mixed mesenchymal-epithelial tumor.

CYTOPATHOLOGY

Often, fluid cytology specimens are used in evaluation of ovarian epithelial neoplasms. These include peritoneal fluids obtained by aspiration of pleural or ascitic fluid and peritoneal washings. Fine-needle aspirates (FNA) of primary ovarian lesions should be avoided to minimize the risk of peritoneal seeding and upstaging the patient in case this is a localized lesion.

The cytologic evaluation of ascitic fluids plays a significant role in the primary diagnosis of a subset ovarian neoplasms, particularly those associated to ascites (**Figure 8.7-1**). A retrospective study involving 313 women with chemonaïve invasive OC reported positive ascites cytology in only 67.1% of the cases, and there was no significant correlation between positive cytology and stage, grade, or histology (21). Importantly, the distinction between SBT and LGSC cells cannot be reliably made on cytology specimens, and the ICCR recommends the cytology results to be correlated with the histopathologic findings in such cases (17).

Cytologic samples of peritoneal fluid—either through aspiration of ascitic fluid upon entering the peritoneal cavity or through washings before surgical manipulation of the tumor—are routinely obtained as part of the staging procedures of ovarian neoplasms, and the findings are relevant to the substaging of FIGO stage I disease. As such, the presence of tumor cells in peritoneal washings warrants tumor staging as stage FIGO IC. In a retrospective study including cases of various histotypes, 24% of peritoneal washings were positive for tumor cells and 83% of the tumors were upstaged when the cytology result was positive. Positive cytology was detected in about 22% to 30% of SBTs, serous, endometrioid, mucinous, and clear cell ovarian carcinomas, whereas only in 10% of MBT cases (22).

Peritoneal washing is often performed at the time of RRSO in high-risk women, and occult carcinoma is rarely identified in these cytology specimens. A prospective study involving 644 women undergoing RRSO between 1999 and 2017 identified occult STICs in nine cases and HGSCs in eight cases on final histology (23). Two of the nine STIC cases and four of the eight HGSC cases had positive

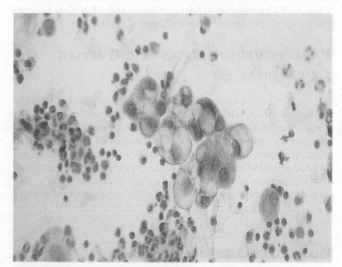

Figure 8.7-1. Three-dimensional clusters and single cells of high-grade serous carcinoma in ascites fluid specimen. Tumor cells exhibit significant nuclear pleomorphism and prominent nucleoli.

peritoneal cytology. The study reports one case where the primary tumor was only found after examination of multiple recuts, which was triggered by the positive cytology result. In summary, malignant cells reported in washings at RRSO rarely lead to the discovery of early-stage HGSC, but cytology samples are required for appropriate staging.

Endometriosis and endosalpingiosis involving peritoneal surfaces may shed epithelial fragments into peritoneal washings or ascites. In addition, benign fallopian tube epithelium (particularly if salpingitis is present) and benign eutopic endometrial tissue may also be shed into the fluid via retrograde menstruation through the fallopian tubes. If the cells in the fluid are not obviously malignant, comparison of the cytologic features of the epithelium in the fluid with those of the neoplastic tissue sections is critical. The presence of cilia within epithelial cells is generally considered to represent a finding that confirms the benign nature of these cells. Conversely, cytologic abnormalities mimicking malignancy may be caused by chemotherapy as well as radiation; accordingly, review of the patient's clinical history is important in the interpretation of cytologic findings.

Evaluation of pleural effusions and/or FNA of potential metastatic disease may be useful in patients who appear to have inoperable disease. Although cell blocks can be used for IHC staining, it is generally preferred to obtain tissue cores of solid masses for better characterization. The cores or FNAs are often performed under ultrasound or CT guidance.

BORDERLINE TUMORS

A distinct subset of low-grade ovarian epithelial tumors not displaying invasion occasionally exhibit malignant behavior. These tumors have been designated borderline tumors since the early 1970s. Even though originally intended as a provisional term, the borderline category has become entrenched over the past five decades.

Currently, the only acceptable terminology is borderline tumor, whereas other diagnoses historically utilized for these lesions, such as "atypical proliferative tumor" and "tumor of LMP," are no longer favored.

SBTs comprise about 50% of all borderline tumors. The vast majority of non-SBTs are of the mucinous type. Borderline endometrioid, seromucinous, clear cell, and Brenner tumors are very rare. In contrast to SBTs, non-SBTs are not associated with peritoneal implants. Details on borderline tumors are discussed later (see "Serous Borderline Tumor," "Mucinous Borderline Tumor," "Endometrioid Borderline Tumors," "Seromucinous Borderline Tumor," "Clear Cell Cystadenomas/Adenofibromas and Clear Cell Borderline Tumors" "Borderline Brenner Tumors" sections).

PRIMARY VERSUS METASTATIC OVARIAN CARCINOMAS

The ovaries are the most common site for metastases within the gynecologic tract, with metastatic disease comprising 5% to 30% of malignant neoplasms involving the ovary. Indeed, ovarian metastasis may represent the first manifestation of an extraovarian primary, as these lesions are often significantly larger than the associated primary tumor. These are often cystic, mimicking primary ovarian carcinomas by imaging, and exhibit deceptive bland or discordant microscopic morphology (24). The most common sources of ovarian metastases are the colon, endometrium, breast, appendix, and stomach (25).

Mucinous Metastases

Distinction between a primary ovarian mucinous neoplasm and ovarian metastasis with mucinous differentiation represents one of the most challenging scenarios for pathologists when evaluating

mucinous lesions within the ovary. With awareness of deceptive patterns and strict application of refined criteria, primary ovarian mucinous carcinomas prove to be rare compared to metastatic mucinous carcinomas.

Metastatic mucinous carcinomas typically exhibit at least two of the following features: bilaterality, size smaller than 10 to 12 cm, involvement of the ovarian surface, multiple tumor nodules within the ovarian parenchyma, and a haphazard infiltrative pattern of stromal invasion. Still, a minority of metastases from the colorectum, pancreaticobiliary tract, appendix, and endocervix can exhibit gross and microscopic features simulating a primary ovarian mucinous or endometrioid tumor (11,12,26,27). Of note, large, unilateral, and multicystic metastases do exist and can be misinterpreted as primary ovarian MBTs with intraepithelial carcinoma or well-differentiated mucinous or endometrioid carcinomas. Some of these metastases display highly differentiated areas adjacent to invasive areas, simulating benign lesions or MBT. In general, the possibility of metastatic mucinous carcinoma should always be considered when a mucinous carcinoma is identified in the ovary, particularly if extraovarian disease is also present.

IHC can be of value in this distinction. In general, primary ovarian mucinous tumors are positive for cytokeratin (CK) 7 and variably positive for CK20, whereas most GI carcinomas are negative for CK7 and positive for CK20. CDX-2 and SATB2 are IHC markers of colorectal differentiation, which can be focally positive in primary ovarian mucinous lesions with GI phenotype (albeit usually less diffuse than metastatic GI tumors). p16 IHC stain and molecular tests for HPV are useful in identifying cases of metastatic endocervical adenocarcinoma. PAX-8, ER, and PR staining are often of limited utility, because these are negative in a significant number of primary ovarian mucinous neoplasms.

Clinical evaluation is usually required to exclude a clinically occult extraovarian source. Many investigators consider a mucinous carcinoma in the ovary metastatic until proven otherwise (28). In cases of ovarian tumors demonstrating an extraovarian phenotype, without demonstrable primary disease elsewhere, the possibility of a somatic malignancy arising from an ovarian teratoma must be considered. The morphology and immunophenotype of these somatic malignancies are indistinguishable from that of their eutopic counterparts, and identification of a background teratomatous component in these cases is the most relevant feature to confirm a teratomatous ovarian origin. In these cases, the tumors are staged as primary ovarian.

Mucinous Tumors Associated With Pseudomyxoma Peritonei

PMP is a clinicopathologic syndrome in which mucoid peritoneal nodules and/or mucinous ascites are present. The pools of extracellular mucin are typically accompanied by neoplastic mucinous epithelium, but the degree of cellularity and atypia may vary. Morphologic, IHC, and molecular genetic studies have shown that PMP virtually always derives from GI (usually appendiceal) low-grade mucinous neoplasms, whereas the ovarian involvement is secondary (11,29). Extra-appendiceal primary sites are less common and include pancreatic mucinous neoplasms, as well as colorectal, urachal, and gallbladder mucinous adenocarcinomas (30,31). Thus, in the setting of PMP, appendectomy and thorough examination of the GI and pancreaticobiliary tracts should be performed. It is important to note that a macroscopically normal appendix very rarely harbors a neoplastic lesion (32), but when removed, the appendix should be submitted entirely for microscopic examination.

Similarly to the scenario described earlier, the possibility of somatic transformation from a teratoma must be considered in cases in which thorough clinical and radiologic workup fail to demonstrate a primary lesion, particularly when there is evidence of teratoma in the background ovarian tissue. Characteristically, mucinous tumors arising in ovarian teratomas might present with mucinous ascites and exhibit prominent—the so-called dissecting—mucin extravasation in the stroma. Although limited data are available, mucinous tumors arising in teratomas do not seem to be associated with adverse outcomes, even when extraovarian involvement is present (11,33,34).

Nonmucinous Metastases

Nonmucinous metastases commonly originate from breast cancer or endometrial endometrioid carcinomas (25). Endometrioid carcinomas synchronously detected in the ovaries and the endometrium present a unique problem in gynecologic pathology. Recent data suggest that these synchronous tumors are clonally related to the majority of cases and thus represent metastasis from one location to the other, usually endometrium to ovaries (35,36). Given the observed indolent behavior of these low-grade endometrioid tumors, these have been suggested to be classified as "FIGO stage IIIA–simulating independent primary tumors" (37).

SEROUS TUMORS

Benign Serous Cystadenoma and Adenofibroma

Benign serous tumors including cystadenomas and adenofibromas are common and account for two-thirds of benign ovarian epithelial tumors and the majority of ovarian serous tumors. They are equally distributed among unilocular cysts, multilocular cysts, and cystadenofibromas and generally display a serous epithelial lining lacking proliferation. The finding of polyclonality in the epithelium of most serous cystadenomas suggests that the epithelial component is not neoplastic (38), and molecular data evaluating the stromal component in serous cystadenofibromas suggest that the stromal component may indeed represent the neoplastic component of these lesions (39). Accordingly, most serous cystadenomas and adenofibromas are probably not true epithelial neoplasms but ovarian fibromas coincidentally presenting with a dilated epithelial inclusion cyst (40).

Cystadenomas are generally lined by pseudostratified, tubal-type epithelium, containing the characteristic secretory and ciliated cells, but can occasionally demonstrate a single layer of flattened to cuboidal epithelial cells with uniform basal nuclei, particularly in larger lesions, in which the increased intracystic pressure may cause epithelial attenuation. Mitoses and atypia are generally absent, and dystrophic calcifications may be seen in the stroma underlying the epithelium.

Some degree of epithelial proliferation can be seen in a subset of benign serous tumors, manifested by epithelial pseudostratification and papillae formation, which occasionally demonstrate detachment of cell clusters, similar to that seen in SBT. Differentiating benign serous tumors with areas of epithelial proliferation from SBT is based primarily on the extent of the epithelial proliferation. As such, if the proliferation is focal and involves less than 10% of the overall epithelium, a diagnosis of serous cystadenoma with focal epithelial proliferation should be rendered—these lesions are not classified as SBT. Conversely, serous lesions in which the proliferation encompasses more than 10% of the total epithelium should be regarded as SBT.

Serous Borderline Tumor

SBTs comprise about 50% of all borderline ovarian tumors. A remarkable aspect of SBTs is their association with peritoneal implants in the absence of invasive disease. Molecular data suggest that in primary ovarian SBT, peritoneal implants derive from the ovarian lesion. In a study evaluating 62 primary ovarian SBT-implant pairs, 59 (95%) cases demonstrated identical KRAS or BRAF mutations (41). This study included both "noninvasive" and "invasive implants"; thus, some of these cases were truly LGSC according to the current terminology (see "College of American Pathologists, 2020 World Health Organization, and International Collaboration on Cancer Reporting Guidelines" section). Another unusual aspect of SBT includes the fact that tumor microinvasion and the presence of associated lymph node lesions, which occur in a minority of cases, do not negatively influence patient outcomes (42).

Historically, an attempt was made to further classify SBTs based on microscopic architecture, with the aim to improve risk stratification for patients. Tumors with more complex architecture characterized by nonhierarchical branching of delicate micropapillae were proposed to be classified as micropapillary SBT or noninvasive (micropapillary) LGSCs (noninvasive MPSC/noninvasive LGSC). Micropapillary pattern was reported to be significantly associated with the presence of "invasive implants," progression to LGSC, and worse prognosis (43). This concept has been subject to significant debate over the past decades, with the general consensus being that the presence of invasive peritoneal disease determines patient outcomes, whereas the architecture of the primary tumor has less impact on prognosis (44-46).

Current recommendations define invasive serous proliferations of the peritoneal surfaces as LGSCs of either the ovary or the peritoneum, and the term "borderline tumor with invasive implant" is no longer recommended. The remainder of tumors still classified as micropapillary/cribriform SBTs are reported to be a risk factor for subsequent transition to LGSC but show no association with adverse outcomes (45,46). As a result, the terms "noninvasive MPSC" and "noninvasive LGSC" are no longer recommended by the WHO, and the term *micropapillary/cribriform SBT* should be used instead. The clinical features of patients with SBTs are similar to those for serous cystadenomas, with the mean age at diagnosis being 50 years (47). Approximately one-third of SBTs are bilateral (46).

Gross and Microscopic Findings

Grossly, SBTs generally demonstrate a predominantly cystic lesion with intracystic excrescences and/or exophytic papillae, reflecting ovarian surface involvement.

Fine, friable, and exuberant papillary projections are typically present on the internal surface of the cysts and may also be observed on the external surface. Although SBTs with their papillary projections are easily distinguished from the smooth inner and outer surfaces of serous cystadenomas, thorough sampling for histologic examination is required to rule out invasion. As a general rule, two sections per cm are necessary to accurately diagnose these lesions (48).

SBT is characterized by hierarchically branching papillae lined by stratified epithelium with tufting and detachment of cells and cell clusters. Stratification and budding involving at least 10% of the epithelium warrant a diagnosis of SBT (**Figure 8.7-2**). Similarly, foci of nonhierarchical branching with fine elongated micropapillae (defined as being at least 5 times long as they are wide) emanating directly from large central papillae—commonly referred to as Medusa head appearance—may be present. Fusion of the epithelial buds creates a Roman bridge or cribriform appearance (**Figure 8.7-3**). Currently, the definition of micropapillary/cribriform subtype requires an area larger than 5 mm in diameter consisting purely of micropapillary/cribriform structures. When the micropapillary/cribriform component is less than 5 mm in diameter, the diagnosis of SBT with micropapillary/cribriform features is rendered.

Ciliated cells resembling fallopian tube epithelium are present in about one-third of tumors. Nuclei display mild atypia and tend to be ovoid or rounded, occasionally containing prominent nucleoli. Mitoses are not common, and psammoma bodies may be seen in up to half of SBTs.

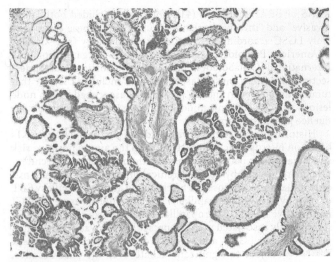

Figure 8.7-2. Serous borderline tumor displaying a complex papillary pattern with detachment of atypical cell clusters at the tips of the papillae.

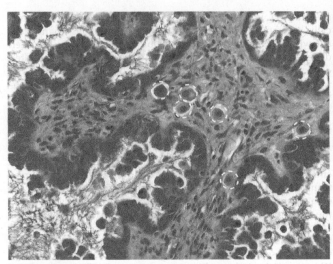

Figure 8.7-4. Microinvasion in a serous borderline tumor. Individual cells with abundant eosinophilic cytoplasm are present in the stromal core of a papillary structure as highlighted by dashed lines.

Microinvasion in Serous Borderline Tumor versus Microinvasive Low-Grade Serous Carcinoma

It is important to note that microinvasion in SBT and microinvasive LGSC have to be distinguished carefully. Two distinct types of "microinvasion" have been defined in association with serous tumors. The eosinophilic type of microinvasion accounts for the vast majority of reported cases, characterized by individual cells and small clusters of cells with abundant eosinophilic cytoplasm, which appear to be budding into the superficial stromal cores of the papillae (**Figure 8.7-4**). The lesion can be multifocal, but each focus must be smaller than 5 mm. Reportedly, microinvasion is quite common and may be found in 25% or more of SBTs (48). A study evaluating these eosinophilic cells showed loss of expression of conventional IHC markers, a lower proliferation index, and other findings, suggesting that these represent terminally differentiated cells, some of which are undergoing senescence/apoptosis (49).

The second type of microinvasion occurs less commonly and displays the destructive pattern of invasion seen in LGSC. This pattern is characterized by a haphazard infiltration of small solid cell nests and micropapillae. The epithelial structures are often

surrounded by a clear space and associated with an identifiable stromal response. When this pattern of invasion is detected in one or more foci, but importantly, each of these foci is smaller than 5 mm in greatest dimension, the lesion is best classified as microinvasive LGSC.

Although more data are necessary to determine the clinical significance of this finding from a prognosis and management perspective, microinvasion in SBT does not appear to have immediate clinical relevance (42). Whether or not staging is needed for a woman with microinvasive LGSC remains unclear. Follow-up or any treatment does not appear to influence recurrence or survival.

Associated Peritoneal Lesions: Endosalpingiosis and "Implants"

SBTs are often associated with serous lesions involving the peritoneum. Endosalpingiosis, or benign glandular inclusions, may involve the peritoneal surfaces in patients with or without benign or malignant serous ovarian tumors and are found in 40% of patients with SBT. These glands are typically lined by simple columnar epithelium, which displays tubal differentiation. The epithelium may display minor degrees of atypia and form simple papillary structures; psammoma bodies are often present and may persist after degeneration of the epithelium. This would need to be a new paragraph, preceded and followed by enter, like this: "[...] psammoma bodies are often present and may persist after degeneration of the epithelium.

A population-based series in Denmark reported 14% of patients with SBT with implants (47). In addition, 21.7% of SBTs had implants, according to a large multi-institutional study in Germany (50). In these two studies, 83% of implants were classified as "noninvasive implants" and 17% as "invasive implants." Using current terminology and diagnostic criteria, the latter would now qualify as LGSC. Implants (of the type previously known as "noninvasive") have two morphologic forms: epithelial and desmoplastic. Epithelial implants are papillary, their morphology resembling the ovarian SBT [...]" Implants (of the type previously known as "noninvasive") have two morphologic forms: epithelial and desmoplastic. Epithelial implants are papillary, their morphology resembling the ovarian SBT (**Figure 8.7-5**). The fibrovascular cores of the papillae are covered by mildly atypical cells. Mitoses are usually absent, but psammomatous calcifications are common and may be extensive.

Desmoplastic implants, on the other hand, are plaque-like thickenings that can extend into the septae along omental lobules, giving them a low-power appearance that mimics invasion

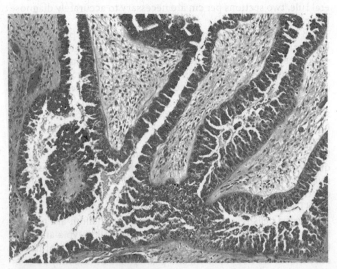

Figure 8.7-3. Micropapillary growth in a serous borderline tumor. There is no invasion of underlying stroma.

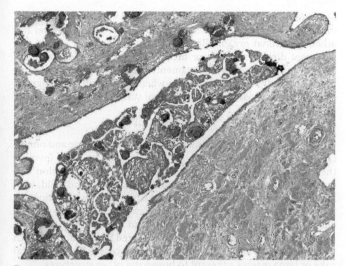

Figure 8.7-5. Epithelial peritoneal implant associated with serous borderline tumor. The implant displays a papillary architecture with psammomatous calcification. Note there is no invasion of adjacent peritoneum at the top right and bottom left.

(**Figure 8.7-6**). They are associated with an exuberant granulation tissue–like fibroblastic proliferation, characterized by edematous fascicles of plump fibroblasts and small vessels, surrounding the neoplastic cells, which may demonstrate gland-like or papillary structures and are lined by mildly atypical epithelial cells. Psammoma bodies are often identified. Mitotic figures are usually absent. Distinction of these lesions from foci of extraovarian LGSC can be extremely challenging, particularly for pathologists who may be unfamiliar with these rare lesions. Importantly, the diagnosis of SBT with peritoneal implant requires the exclusion of invasion.

Lymph Nodes

Nodal endosalpingiosis, or benign glandular inclusions, is found in 45% of patients with SBT in whom lymph nodes are examined, in comparison to about 10% of women who have nodes removed for other reasons. Lymph node involvement by SBT might present as single cells, and papillary or glandular structures, and is identified in up to 42% of patients (42). Although these lesions were earlier referred to as "metastases," it is preferable to use the term *lymph node involvement* by SBT as they have no adverse effect on prognosis. Still, according to the WHO

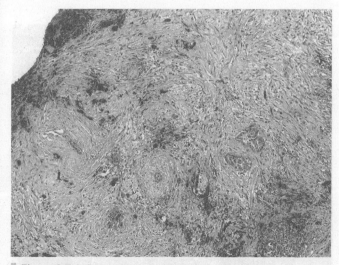

Figure 8.7-6. Desmoplastic peritoneal implant displays an abundant granulation tissue–like spindle cell stroma with rare scattered glands lined by minimally atypical, slightly stratified epithelium.

recommendations, SBTs with lymph node involvement are to be staged as N1 disease. The presence of endosalpingiosis alone does not warrant higher stage.

Clinical Behavior

The prognosis of SBT—with or without implants—is excellent without the need of additional therapy, although patients may develop complications due to adhesions. In six prospective randomized trials including 373 patients with SBTs followed for a mean of 6.7 years, the survival was 100% (51), and large studies (some population based) in the United States, Korea, and Sweden have shown a 10-year survival of 96% to 100% (52-54). Similarly, a population-based Danish study did not identify any significant difference between the survival of patients with stage I SBT and the expected survival of the general population (47).

Nonetheless, clinical follow-up may be of value as long-term data now indicate that a small but significant proportion of SBT with implants will progress to invasive LGSC (55). Micropapillary/cribriform pattern and advanced disease stage are reported risk factors for subsequent development of LGSC. A recent study including 942 women with SBT diagnosed between 1978 and 2002 with a median follow-up period of 15 years demonstrated that 4% of typical SBT and 11% of micropapillary SBT progressed to LGSC. The diagnosis of LGSC occurred after a median of 10 years (ranging 0.6-25 years) following the original diagnosis of SBT (46). Uzan and associates followed 168 women with advanced-stage SBT and observed a recurrence rate of 26.8% (45/168), in which 37 were noninvasive and seven invasive recurrences (56). This study also reported a 25% incidence of progression to invasive disease within the subset of patients with a first noninvasive peritoneal recurrence and a primary diagnosis of typical SBT. The survival for patients with lymph node involvement, microinvasion, or microinvasive carcinoma unassociated with peritoneal metastases is also nearly 100%.

Low-Grade Serous Carcinoma

LGSC is a rather uncommon, distinct subtype of invasive carcinoma comprising only about 2.5% of malignant epithelial tumors of the ovary (**Table 8.7-2**). LGSC is currently believed to arise from SBTs and does not represent simply a low-grade version of the more common HGSC, as the two entities are fundamentally different in clinical presentation, pathogenesis, molecular drivers, and outcomes.

Until the 2020 WHO classification of female genital tumors (1), the term "noninvasive LGSC" was used interchangeably with what is now referred to as micropapillary/cribriform SBT. In addition, the previously utilized "invasive implant" terminology has now been eliminated, and these are now known as metastases of primary ovarian LGSC or foci of primary peritoneal LGSC, depending on the presence of ovarian involvement by SBT or LGSC. These are major changes in the interpretation and terminology utilized to describe what essentially remains the same phenomenon. Importantly, comparing literature data on SBT and LGSC published at different points in time requires careful consideration of the definitions used in each publication.

Gross and Microscopic Findings

The mean age of patients is 45 years, and LGSCs often present with bilateral ovarian involvement. The mean tumor size is 11 cm, and surface involvement is present in approximately half of the cases. Like SBT, LGSC has a cystic and papillary gross appearance and, unlike HGSC, generally does not demonstrate necrosis. LGSC might display multiple growth patterns, including nests, gland-like structures, papillae, or micropapillae, often surrounded by clear spaces or clefts (**Figure 8.7-7**). Psammoma bodies are common. The tumor cells tend to be rounded with scant cytoplasm and exhibit mild or moderate nuclear atypia, often with prominent small nucleoli. Mitotic activity tends to be low, usually 3 to 5 mitoses/10 high-power field (HPF) (1).

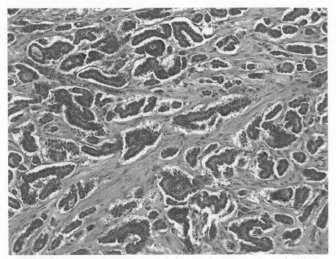

Figure 8.7-7. Low-grade serous carcinoma characterized by small papillae consisting of mildly atypical tumor cells and surrounded by clear spaces.

An exophytic pattern displaying micropapillary growth is most common, but a confluent or cribriform glandular pattern may be present. The characteristic architectural feature of invasion is an infiltrative growth pattern, in which micropapillae and small solid nests are haphazardly arranged and embedded in a fibrous stroma (**Figure 8.7-7**) (57). Invasive foci often display only mild cytologic atypia, but occasional moderate atypia may be present. If severe atypia is present, the diagnosis of HGSC should be considered, and p53 IHC staining should be performed. The presence of invasive peritoneal foci warrants rendering the diagnosis of LGSC, even in the absence of ovarian invasion.

Clinical Behavior

The natural history of LGSC includes slow, indolent growth and resistance to carboplatin and Taxol chemotherapy. Recurrences typically maintain the well-differentiated histologic appearance of the primary tumor, even when occurring decades later. Although the patterns of spread are similar to ordinary HGSC, stage III LGSC is more likely to be stage IIIA as compared to HGSC, which nearly always presents at the advanced FIGO stage IIIC. When disease is confined to the ovary, the prognosis is excellent, whereas patients with FIGO stage II-IV disease have significantly worse prognosis, with median PFS of 28.1 months and median OS of 101.7 months (58). In general, advanced LGSC is incurable but grows slow and has late recurrences. Rare instances of transformation to HGSC have been described.

High-Grade Serous Carcinoma of Ovarian, Tubal, and Peritoneal Origin

HGSC is the most common ovarian carcinoma and accounts for approximately 70% of OC cases (**Table 8.7-2**). Alterations leading to loss of p53 function and frequent copy number alterations are the molecular hallmarks of HGSC (59). HGSC probably arises from tubal-type epithelium, most commonly at the fimbriated end of the fallopian tube, or alternatively from ovarian or peritoneal epithelial inclusion cysts lined by tubal-type epithelium. For practical purposes, the clinical and pathologic features of tubal, ovarian, and peritoneal HGSCs are indistinguishable.

Clinical and Operative Findings

HGSC typically presents in the sixth and seventh decades, with a mean age at diagnosis being 63 years for advanced-stage tumors. At the time of diagnosis, the tumor is usually disseminated throughout the pelvic and abdominal cavities. The vast majority

of advanced-stage ovarian carcinomas involve peritoneal surfaces, including the pelvic peritoneum and the surfaces of the bowel and other abdominal organs. Both pelvic and abdominal spread can represent direct extension or metastasis. For example, direct extension to the bowel, broad ligament, or uterus can occur by contiguous growth, or by metastasis when exfoliation of malignant cells results in seeding of the peritoneal surfaces.

Gross Findings

The tumor size varies from microscopic to a large pelvic and omental mass by more than 20 cm. The dominant mass often involves the appendix and ovary on the right and the sigmoid colon and ovary on the left. It is typically multilocular, cystic, and solid, with soft, friable papillae protruding into the cyst cavities; occasionally, the tumor may be completely solid, demonstrating a pink to gray cut surface, with areas of hemorrhage and necrosis. Omental and other peritoneal metastases are characterized by firm nodules with white or gray cut surfaces, which may coalesce to form an omental cake or large masses adherent to bowel and other structures.

Sometimes, the ovaries are of normal in size, the ovarian surfaces often display a varying degree of papillary excrescences. The appearance of the fallopian tubes is variable and may appear normal, be adherent to the ovarian tumor, or, occasionally, be entirely replaced by carcinoma. In some instances, a tumorous papillary outgrowth of the fimbriae constitutes the largest pelvic tumor. Rarely, the fallopian tube is dilated and filled with neoplastic cells; in the past, these were the only cases classified as being of tubal origin. When no clear tubal involvement is appreciated on gross examination, the tubes are to be entirely submitted for histologic evaluation according to the SEE-FIM protocol (see "Recommendations Regarding Gross Examination" section) for appropriate primary site assignment. Microscopic tumor foci are identified within a grossly normal-appearing omentum in 22% of cases. Thus, it is recommended that at least 10 random sections of the omentum are submitted for histologic examination in cases in which gross involvement of the omentum is not apparent (see "Recommendations Regarding Gross Examination" section).

Microscopic Findings

HGSCs display complex papillary and solid growth patterns and marked cytologic atypia. Frequently, they display a lace-like or labyrinthine pattern characterized by extensive bridging and coalescence of papillae, resulting in slit-like spaces (**Figures 8.7-8 and 8.7-9**). Coexistence of several architectural patterns is characteristic of HGSC, and areas of solid growth, glandular, and cribriform patterns are commonly present. A distinct combination of solid,

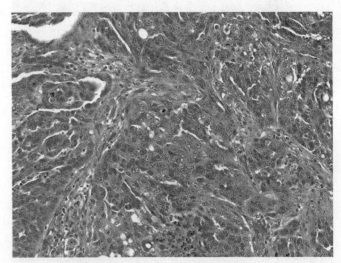

Figure 8.7-8. High-grade serous carcinoma displaying solid and papillary growth patterns and slit-like spaces.

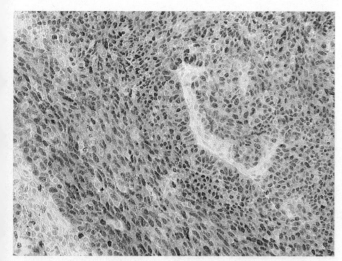

Figure 8.7-9. High-grade serous carcinoma is positive for PAX8 immunostaining.

pseudoendometrioid, and transitional-like (SET) growth patterns has been described, often associated with *BRCA1* and *BRCA2* mutations. HRD tumors often also exhibit prominent intratumoral lymphocytic infiltrates and geographical necrosis (60,61).

Nearly all cases display areas of large, pleomorphic nuclei with prominent red nucleoli and may even demonstrate tumor giant cells (**Figure 8.7-8**). Mitoses, including abnormal mitotic figures, are numerous, and necrosis is often extensive. Psammoma bodies are present in the majority of cases. Although cytoplasmic clearing may occur, they lack the characteristic architectural patterns of clear cell carcinomas, and the presence of cytoplasmic clearing, in isolation, should not be interpreted as a component of clear cell carcinoma.

The fallopian tube mucosa displays STIC in a substantial proportion of cases (**Figure 8.7-10**) (62,63). Because these are typically very small lesions, on the order of 1 to 3 mm or less, they may be easily overlooked (64). STIC is usually, but not always, confined to the fimbriae, and complete histologic evaluation of the fallopian tube increases the diagnostic yield of STIC. Accordingly, the

fallopian tubes should be meticulously examined and entirely embedded for microscopic examination in all extrauterine HGSCs, as per the mentioned SEE-FIM protocol (see "Recommendations Regarding Gross Examination" section). Deeper sections need to be obtained if foci of atypia are to be identified histologically. Foci of in situ or invasive occult carcinoma may be very subtle and are often less than 1 mm in maximum diameter.

The WHO and CAP recommend using the following criteria for primary site assignment in extrauterine HGSC: When an STIC is present, or when the fimbriated end of the fallopian tube is not separable for a tubo-ovarian mass, the assigned primary site is the fallopian tube. An ovarian primary site is only considered when both the fallopian tubes are separable from the tumor mass and no STIC can be detected upon extensive examination of the fallopian tubes. Primary peritoneal HGSCs are exceedingly rare, and this diagnosis requires that both the ovaries and the fallopian tubes have been entirely submitted for histologic evaluation and found to be free of invasive or in situ lesions associated with HGSC. The term *tubo-ovarian primary* is only recommended to be used in the setting of small biopsies, when complete sectioning of ovaries and fallopian tubes is not feasible (65).

A prospective study using current criteria and in toto examination of the fallopian tube fimbriae found that 83% of chemonaïve HGSCs and 76% of post-treatment HGSCs were assigned as fallopian tube primaries. In the same study, ovarian primaries comprised 17% and 12% and primary peritoneal HGSC comprised 0% and 7% of chemonaïve and postadjuvant therapy tumors, respectively (66). Foci of carcinoma that remain after neoadjuvant chemotherapy often display extensive fibrosis, lymphohistiocytic infiltrates, and psammomatous calcification with scant carcinomatous epithelium. STIC may persist after neoadjuvant chemotherapy (67).

The CRS has been developed to assess histopathologic response to neoadjuvant therapy in interval debulking specimens for advanced-stage (IIIC and IV) disease. CRS stratifies patients into three groups: CRS 1 corresponds to no or minimal response, CRS 2 to residual tumor with signs of response, and CRS 3 to near-complete or complete tumor response (**Figure 8.7-11**). Importantly, CRS is based on omental assessment, as scoring applied to adnexal tumor masses did not prove to be a biomarker of prognosis (68). Since its proposal in 2015, the CRS system has been shown to have high interobserver reproducibility and has been validated in multiple studies (69). A recent meta-analysis including

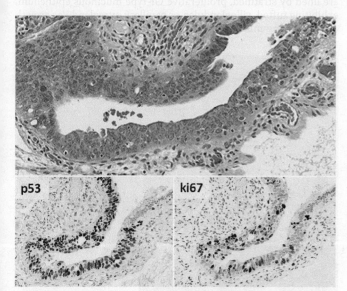

Figure 8.7-10. Serous tubal intraepithelial carcinoma displays a stratified layer of markedly atypical tubal epithelium without invasion of the underlying lamina propria of the fallopian tube mucosa. Tumor cells show an aberrant pattern of p53 staining. Ki67 expression is increased in the neoplastic epithelium.

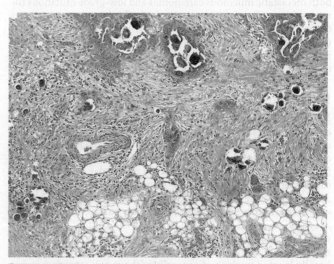

Figure 8.7-11. Omental metastasis of high-grade serous carcinoma showing moderate therapy response (CRS 2). Nests of viable tumor cells are present. Prominent fibrosis and associated lymphohistiocytic inflammatory infiltrate are also appreciated, representing the histologic correlates of response to chemotherapy. Psammoma bodies within the fibroinflammatory reaction indicate sites of previous tumor.

data on 877 individual patients found CRS to be significantly associated with both PFS and OS in multivariate models (16). The reported HR for PFS was 0.55 (95% CI, 0.45-0.66) when comparing CRS 1/2 versus CRS 3 patients. CRS remained significantly associated with PFS in a subgroup analysis only including patients with R0 debulking surgery.

MUCINOUS TUMORS

Primary ovarian mucinous tumors include cystadenomas, MBTs, and carcinomas (intraepithelial and invasive). Cystadenomas and MBTs are noninvasive and are distinguished primarily by the degree of architectural complexity. There is a quantitative spectrum of epithelial proliferation in mucinous tumors that includes mucinous cystadenomas with focal epithelial proliferation, MBTs, and MBTs with intraepithelial carcinoma and/or microinvasion, providing evidence that these tumors constitute a biologic spectrum with individual types representing successive steps in the sequence of ovarian mucinous carcinogenesis. The majority of lesions within this spectrum harbor KRAS mutations or other alterations leading to RAS pathway activation, with CDKN2A alterations also commonly shared between mucinous lesions (70,71). The genomic events involved in progression to invasive disease include *TP53* alterations and amplification of the 9p13 chromosome region (72). Importantly, mural nodules can be present in all primary ovarian mucinous tumors. These areas have been classified as reactive/sarcoma-like, anaplastic carcinoma, or true sarcomatous nodules. The presence and histologic subtype of these nodules play a significant role in clinical outcomes.

Mucinous tumors may arise in association with other ovarian neoplasms, namely, Brenner tumors and teratomas (73). In cases of mucinous lesions arising in associated with teratomas, both components share the genomic alterations typical of germ cell tumors (74-76). It is important to note that mucinous lesions arising from teratomas demonstrate IHC staining patterns, which are indistinguishable from the teratomatous epithelium from which they arise; hence, distinguishing a primary ovarian mucinous lesion arising as somatic transformation in a teratoma from a true metastatic mucinous carcinoma to the ovary can be diagnostically very challenging, requiring clinical correlation and extensive tumor sampling.

The other types of mucinous tumors seen in the ovary include metastatic mucinous carcinomas, most commonly from the GI tract or endocervix, as well as low-grade mucinous tumors of appendiceal origin secondarily involving the ovary (11). Importantly, both metastatic mucinous carcinomas and low-grade mucinous tumors of appendiceal origin can simulate primary ovarian mucinous tumors, usually MBT and primary ovarian mucinous carcinoma (29). It is now clear that primary ovarian mucinous carcinoma are much less common than previously believed, and most mucinous carcinomas within the ovary prove to be metastatic (77).

Mucinous Cystadenoma and Adenofibroma

Mucinous cystadenomas comprise about 15% of benign ovarian epithelial neoplasms and approximately 80% of all primary mucinous tumors of the ovary, whereas mucinous adenofibromas are far less common. Mean patient age at presentation is around 50 years. Mucinous cystadenomas are unilocular or multilocular tumors of variable size, ranging from a few centimeters to over 30 cm, with a mean size of approximately 10 cm, and are unilateral in more than 95% of cases. The outer surface of the capsule is typically smooth and white, whereas the content is generally thick and gelatinous. Histologically, they are composed of glands and cysts lined by simple nonstratified mucinous epithelium with basally located nuclei and generally without any cytologic atypia (**Figure 8.7-12**). When epithelial atypia or proliferation resembling MBT is present, this feature is generally focal. Cystadenomas with less than 10% of epithelial proliferation are categorized as mucinous cystadenoma with focal epithelial proliferation (78).

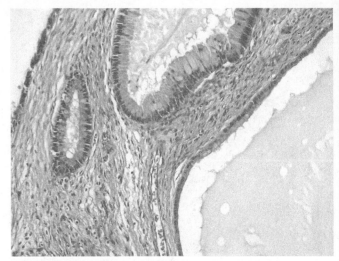

Figure 8.7-12. Mucinous cystadenoma shows a single layer of columnar epithelium with small basal nuclei and abundant mucin-rich cytoplasm.

Nodules composed of transitional cells, also referred to as a Brenner tumor component, are present in up to 18% of mucinous cystadenomas (**Figure 8.7-13**).

Mucinous Borderline Tumor

According to the 2020 WHO recommendations, mucinous borderline tumor is defined as a noninvasive mucinous lesion exhibiting architecturally complex GI-type epithelium. Seromucinous lesions earlier included in the MBT category as "endocervical like" or "Müllerian" subtype of MBT are no longer regarded as a subtype of mucinous tumors, but rather represent a separate category within endometriosis-associated ovarian lesions and are termed *seromucinous borderline tumors* (see "Seromucinous Tumors" section).

MBTs are typically large, multicystic tumors with a smooth capsule, with median size of 20 to 22 cm, demonstrating unilateral ovarian involvement in more than 95% of cases (29,79,80). The locules of the tumor are usually filled with thick gelatinous to mucoid material, and the lining appears smooth, generally without grossly evident papillary excrescences. Microscopically, the cysts are lined by stratified, proliferative GI-type mucinous epithelium, exhibiting tufted, villoglandular, or papillary intraglandular growth and displaying mild-to-moderate nuclear atypia; stromal invasion

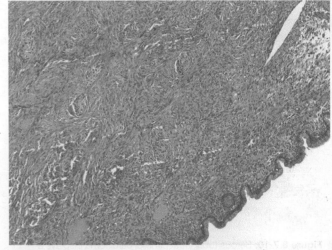

Figure 8.7-13. Mixed mucinous-Brenner tumor with several Brenner-type (transitional) nests within the stroma toward the top left and a single layer of mucinous epithelium at the bottom right.

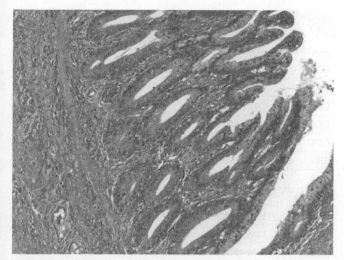

Figure 8.7-14. Mucinous borderline tumor. The glandular structures are lined by stratified, mildly atypical cells.

is, by definition, absent (**Figure 8.7-14**). Given the high degree of heterogeneity in these lesions, it is recommended to submit one section per cm for mucinous tumors smaller than 10 cm, and two sections per cm for tumors larger than 10 cm. Solid areas of the tumor are to be sampled preferentially, as these are the areas that most likely represent either invasive carcinoma or prognostically relevant mural nodules.

Review of the literature on tumors meeting the diagnostic criteria for MBT reveals a generally benign behavior. Rare reports of recurrence of well-sampled tumors diagnosed by experts are generally attributed to incomplete resection due to adhesions and/or cystectomy (81). The majority of reported "advanced-stage MBTs" most likely represent unrecognized mucinous metastases to the ovary, particularly in the setting of PMP (see "Mucinous Tumors Associated with Pseudomyxoma Peritonei" section). With the notable exception of MBT with anaplastic carcinomatous or sarcomatous nodules, which behave aggressively, and after removal of tumors with PMP-like extraovarian spread (which likely represent metastatic disease to the ovaries), most MBT consist of stage I tumors with benign behavior. There is no reliable documentation of peritoneal implants associated with true primary ovarian MBT.

Mucinous Borderline Tumors With Intraepithelial Carcinoma

Noninvasive mucinous tumors with areas of marked nuclear atypia are classified as MBT with intraepithelial carcinoma. When confined to the ovaries, MBTs with intraepithelial carcinoma have excellent prognosis, with close to 100% survival. A small number of so-called "advanced-stage intraepithelial mucinous carcinomas" have been reported, with few tumor deaths. Because metastatic mucinous carcinomas might mimic MBT with intraepithelial carcinoma, it is possible that some seemingly advanced-stage cases with poor outcomes are metastases from concealed extraovarian tumors or represent MBT with intraepithelial carcinoma in which an area of invasive carcinoma was failed to be sampled during pathologic evaluation.

Mucinous Borderline Tumors With Microinvasion

Microinvasion in MBT has been defined as small foci of stromal invasion characterized by single cells or small clusters of mucinous epithelial cells that show the same degree of cytologic atypia as the MBT component. The microinvasive foci may be multiple but should not exceed 5 mm in greatest dimension. However, data available regarding the prognostic impact of microinvasion are very limited and heterogeneous in terms of definitions used and sampling protocols.

Mucinous Carcinoma

Clinical and Operative Findings

Primary ovarian mucinous carcinomas are rare and comprise 3% of all ovarian epithelial malignancies (**Table 8.7-2**). They typically present as large unilateral ovarian masses without ovarian surface involvement or extraovarian disease, with more than 90% of these tumors being diagnosed as FIGO stage I.

Gross Findings

The gross findings are similar to MBTs in that the tumors are typically large, unilateral, multicystic mucus-containing tumors with smooth white capsules, having mean and median size of 18 to 22 cm, respectively. Solid areas as well as foci of necrosis or hemorrhage may be present.

Microscopic Findings

Mucinous carcinomas display a variety of growth patterns, with most tumors containing areas of MBT adjacent to areas of carcinoma. The pattern of invasion might be infiltrative/destructive or expansile/confluent. In the expansile/confluent pattern, the glandular epithelium is markedly crowded and interconnected, with little intervening stroma, but cytologic atypia is usually not pronounced (**Figure 8.7-15**). The infiltrative/destructive pattern of invasion consists of irregular nests of tumor cells exhibiting marked cytologic atypia, with an associated desmoplastic response. Although these two patterns might coexist, the expansile/confluent pattern is more common and generally more indolent. Areas of destructive invasion in an MBT should measure more than 5 mm in greatest dimension in order to render a diagnosis of invasive carcinoma. As mentioned earlier, the presence of infiltrative invasion should raise concern for metastatic disease, and the possibility of an extraovarian primary should always be considered (see "Primary versus Metastatic Ovarian Carcinomas" section).

Clinical Behavior

Patients with stage IA/B mucinous carcinomas have a 5-year survival of about 84%, similar to comprehensively staged 2013 FIGO stage IA/B patients with the other cell types of ovarian carcinoma (82). For patients with MBT with microinvasion and/or intraepithelial carcinoma, a staging procedure is unlikely to yield positive findings, but no data are available to address its value. Carcinomas with expansile/confluent pattern of invasion are associated with significantly better patient outcomes compared to infiltrative/destructive type of invasion (83,84). Bona fide advanced-stage

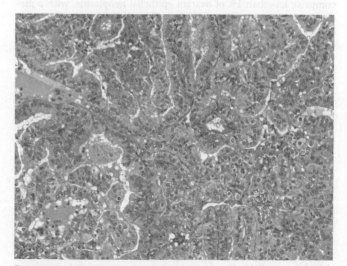

Figure 8.7-15. Mucinous carcinoma with confluent glandular pattern of invasion manifested by complex and interconnected epithelial proliferation lacking stroma.

mucinous ovarian carcinomas have a poor prognosis, their 5-year survival appears to be significantly worse than that for HGSCs (82).

Mural Nodules in Mucinous Tumors

On rare occasions, primary ovarian mucinous tumors contain mural nodules. While these occur most commonly in association to MBT, they may also be encountered in a small subset of mucinous cystadenomas and mucinous carcinomas. Mural nodules have been subclassified into sarcoma-like, anaplastic carcinomatous, and sarcomatous nodules based on morphologic and IHC properties. The most common are the anaplastic carcinomatous nodules, which contain large, pleomorphic epithelioid cells and intermixed spindle and/or rhabdoid cells. Necrosis and brisk mitotic activity are often present. Sarcomatous nodules are the least common form of mural nodules and are characterized by high-grade, undifferentiated cells and necrotic areas. Sarcoma-like mural nodules contain a heterogeneous cell population of spindled and round mononuclear cells, inflammatory infiltrate, and osteoclast-type giant cells (85).

IHC for CK assists in the distinction between carcinomatous, sarcoma-like, or sarcomatous nodules. Malignant mural nodules and the underlying mucinous component have been shown to share the same molecular alterations in the majority of cases, providing evidence that mural nodules probably represent a dedifferentiated subclone of the originating mucinous lesion (86,87). Strikingly, a recent study has reported that not only malignant nodules but also sarcoma-like mural nodules—although previously considered reactive lesions—are clonally related to the underlying mucinous lesion (88). Anaplastic carcinomatous nodules have been reported to show aggressive behavior, typically in the subset of cases that are stage IB and above (89). Very limited follow-up data are available in sarcomatous and sarcoma-like nodules.

ENDOMETRIOID TUMORS

The overwhelming majority of endometrioid ovarian lesions are carcinomas. Endometrioid adenofibromas and endometrioid borderline tumors (EBTs) are diagnosed quite infrequently. Endometrioid ovarian carcinomas display both similarities with and differences from their uterine counterparts in their common molecular alterations. Ovarian endometrioid lesions are frequently associated with endometriosis.

Benign Endometrioid Adenofibromas

Endometrioid adenofibromas are uncommon benign tumors that comprise less than 1% of ovarian epithelial neoplasms, with a median age at presentation of 57 year. These lesions are unilateral in 83% of cases, and the mean tumor size is 10 cm. The lesions typically exhibit a smooth external surface, whereas the cut surface is densely fibrotic, often containing scattered cystic foci, creating a honeycomb appearance. Microscopically, the stromal component is fibromatous but lacks endometrial-type stroma. The epithelial element, often resembling proliferative-type endometrium, demonstrates tubular glands or cysts. Foci of background endometriosis are common.

Endometrioid Borderline Tumors

EBTs are rare, comprising only about 0.2% of ovarian epithelial neoplasms. Historically, a variety of terms, including "proliferative endometrioid tumor," "atypical endometrioid adenofibroma," and "endometrioid tumor of LMP," have been employed for these tumors, but currently, the accepted WHO terminology is that of EBT (Table 8.7-3).

EBTs typically present in the fifth or sixth decade and are usually unilateral and confined to the ovary; however, 5% of EBTs present at FIGO stage II-III. Many patients have a history of endometriosis, or have coexisting endometrial hyperplasia or endometrial endometrioid carcinoma; therefore, patients with EBT should undergo endometrial sampling or a hysterectomy (90).

■ TABLE 8.7-3. Abbreviations Used in This Section

AGUS	Atypical glandular cells of undetermined significance
EBT	Endometrioid borderline tumors
CAP	College of American Pathologists
CK	Cytokeratin
CCBT	Clear cell borderline tumor
CCC	Clear cell carcinoma of the ovary
EBT	Endometrioid borderline tumor
FNA	Fine-needle aspiration
FATWO	Female adnexal tumor of Wolffian origin
HGSC	High-grade serous carcinoma
LAMN	Low-grade appendiceal mucinous neoplasm
LGSC	Low-grade serous carcinoma
MLAC	Mesonephric-like adenocarcinoma
MBT	Mucinous borderline tumor
PMP	Pseudomyxoma peritonei
SMBT	Seromucinous borderline tumor
SBT	Serous borderline tumor
SEE-FIM	Sectioning and extensively examining the fimbriated end
STIC	Serous tubal intraepithelial carcinoma
STIL	Serous tubal intraepithelial lesion
WHO	World Health Organization

The two characteristic architectural appearances of EBT are adenofibromatous and intracystic. In the adenofibromatous variant, crowded, irregularly shaped glands are arranged in a vaguely lobular architecture, within a fibromatous stroma (**Figure 8.7-16**). In the intracystic pattern, simple papillary structures protrude into an endometriotic cyst. The epithelium can show varying degrees of architectural complexity and glandular crowding. Confluent glandular growth should be interpreted as an area of invasive carcinoma and is designated microinvasion if the confluent area measures less than 5 mm. When the confluent epithelial focus exceeds 5 mm in diameter, or there is evidence of destructive stromal invasion, a diagnosis of carcinoma is warranted. However, areas of squamous or

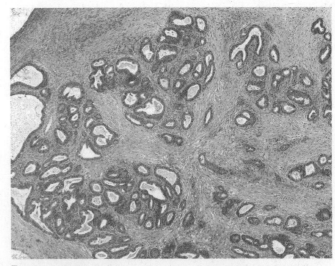

Figure 8.7-16. Endometrioid borderline tumor with endometrioid glands embedded in fibrous stroma and intracystic papillary growth. Glands in the upper middle area exhibit squamous metaplasia.

morular metaplasia, which are often present in the adenofibromatous form, should not be regarded as confluent proliferation. The prognosis of EBT is excellent. Among 134 reported EBTs with a mean follow-up of approximately 5 years, there were no cases with malignant behavior identified (28,91). Stromal microinvasion does not affect prognosis (90).

Endometrioid Carcinoma

Endometrioid carcinomas account for 10% to 15% of ovarian carcinomas (**Table 8.7-2**). Most endometrioid carcinomas arise from endometriosis, whereas a smaller subset progress from endometrioid adenofibromas. Ovarian endometrioid carcinomas commonly harbor alterations in the WNT/β-catenin, PI3K, and MAPK pathways and often show loss of ARID1A (92). Molecular subtypes of ovarian endometrioid carcinoma have been proposed and are analogous to those originally identified in endometrial endometrioid carcinomas. The ultramutated/POLE exonuclease domain–mutated subtype accounts for 5%, the hypermutated/MMRd subtype for 13%, *TP53* mutated for 9% to 13%, whereas the no specific molecular profile (NSMP) subtype constitutes 69% to 73% of cases (93,94). The molecular subgroups stratify patients into significantly different prognostic groups (95,96). Clear cell cancer and endometrioid OC are overrepresented in women with Lynch syndrome (97); hence, universal screening for MMRd is recommended in endometrioid and mixed endometrioid/clear cell histologies (98,99).

Clinical and Operative Findings

Ovarian endometrioid carcinomas are most common in the fifth and sixth decades, with a mean patient age at diagnosis of 55 years. Tumors are usually unilateral, with their size ranging from 12 to 20 cm (mean of 11 cm). The stage distribution differs significantly from serous carcinomas, with a significant proportion of endometrioid carcinomas typically being diagnosed in early stages; in a recently published series, stage I/II tumors constituted 83% of all cases (100). Evidence of endometriosis, either in the ipsilateral or contralateral ovary, within the tumor itself, or even at extraovarian sites, is found in up to 71% of the cases (94). Importantly, up to 25% of the patients have concurrent endometrial hyperplasia or endometrial endometrioid carcinoma (35,36,101).

Gross Findings and Microscopic Findings

Endometrioid carcinomas have a smooth outer surface. On cut section, these tumors are generally solid and cystic, with the cysts containing friable tissue and bloody, mucoid, or greenish fluid. Solid tumors exhibiting extensive hemorrhage and necrosis occur less commonly. The gross appearance of tumors arising from endometriosis is generally cystic, with the cystic content being dark brown fluid, whereas the invasive lesion presents as a solitary or multiple solid nodules or papillary excrescences protruding from the cyst wall.

Endometrioid carcinomas show significant morphologic heterogeneity. Most commonly, a confluent glandular epithelial proliferation exceeding 5 mm (the limit for microinvasion) is present. This pattern is characterized by extensive glandular branching, budding, true cribriform architecture, and highly complex papillary proliferations (**Figure 8.7-17**), with the predominant pattern of invasion being confluent glandular growth. Less commonly, a destructive and infiltrative growth pattern is observed. This pattern is characterized by angulated glands, irregularly spaced and unevenly shaped tumor nests, and solid sheets with jagged edges surrounded by desmoplastic stroma.

Architecturally, well-differentiated endometrioid adenocarcinoma accounts for the majority of cases and are characterized by a confluent or cribriform proliferation of glands lined by tall, stratified columnar epithelium with sharp luminal borders (**Figure 8.7-18**). A villoglandular growth pattern might also be observed. Squamous differentiation and squamous morules are present in up to 50% of cases, and foci of mucinous differentiation, secretory changes, or

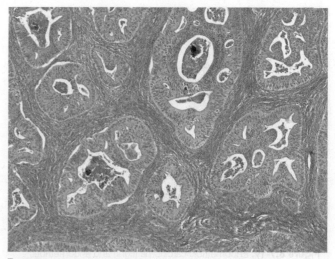

Figure 8.7-17. Endometrioid adenocarcinoma displaying an infiltrative pattern of cellular islands containing endometrioid-type epithelium with a cribriform pattern.

a trabecular growth pattern resembling sex cord-stromal elements may also be seen. In the majority of cases, a component of endometriosis, endometrioid adenofibroma, or EBT can be identified in the background. Grading of endometrioid carcinomas is a required item for reporting by most guidelines, and the most commonly used grading system is the FIGO system, which is based on the amount of solid glandular growth present, with the cutoff values of 5% and 50% being used to stratify tumors into three grades (102).

The majority of bona fide endometrioid carcinomas can be shown to be associated with endometriosis when extensive histologic sampling and meticulous searching for the histologic features of endometriosis are performed. However, direct continuity between endometriosis and carcinoma can only be demonstrated in a subset of cases, most commonly within the lining of an endometriotic cyst, which contains papillary excrescences, or nodules of carcinoma protruding into the cyst (**Figure 8.7-19**). The mean age of women with endometrioid carcinoma associated with endometriosis is 5 to 10 years younger than for women whose endometrioid tumors are unassociated with endometriosis. Endometriosis-associated ovarian endometrioid carcinomas, and particularly tumors arising in an endometriotic cyst, are most commonly low grade and stage I, and therefore, the prognosis is excellent.

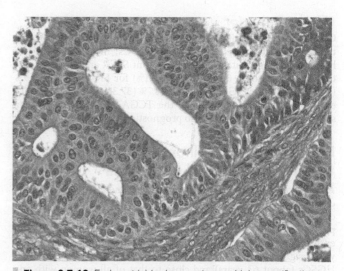

Figure 8.7-18. Endometrioid adenocarcinoma, high magnification (same case as Figure 23.37) showing tall columnar epithelium with sharply punched-out glandular spaces and mild-to-moderate cytologic atypia.

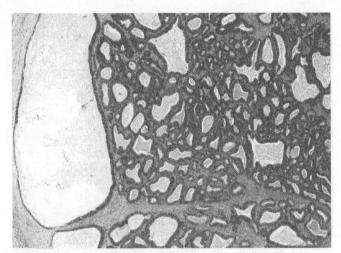

Figure 8.7-19. Endometrioid carcinoma (right) and endometriotic cyst (left).

It is to note that glandular, cribriform, and solid patterns are common in HGSC (103,104). A significant proportion of ovarian carcinomas earlier classified as endometrioid histotype, in fact, represented pseudoendometrioid areas in what we now know as SET features of HGSC (see "High-Grade Serous Carcinoma of Ovarian, Tubal, and Peritoneal Origin" section). When adhering to current diagnostic criteria, bona fide high-grade endometrioid carcinomas result to be rare. Foci of squamous differentiation, secretory change, background endometriosis, or endometrioid adenofibroma can be of value in supporting the diagnosis of endometrioid carcinoma.

Endometrioid Carcinoma, Seromucinous Type

Historically, ovarian carcinomas exhibiting seromucinous differentiation were termed "endocervical-type mucinous carcinoma" and later reclassified as seromucinous carcinoma. Invasive seromucinous tumors are now regarded as a subtype of endometrioid ovarian carcinoma with a mixture of serous and endocervical-type mucinous epithelium (105). As in other endometrioid neoplasms, clear cell changes and areas of squamous differentiation are often present (106).

Clinical Behavior

Overall, endometrioid carcinomas of the ovary have a substantially better prognosis than typical HGSCs, in part due to the high proportion of stage I cases. A recent SEER analysis reported the 5-year OS to be 87.1% (83.6%-90.1%) for FIGO IA-IB, 83.9% (79.3%-87.5%) for FIGO IC-II, and 44.7% (37.3%-51.9%) for III disease (82). As mentioned earlier, the TCGA analogous molecular subgroups stratify patients into prognostic groups (95,96).

Endometrioid Carcinoma Associated With Uterine Endometrial Carcinoma

Approximately 14% of women with endometrioid ovarian carcinoma are found to have concurrent endometrial endometrioid carcinoma, often with associated background endometrial hyperplasia. The median age of women who present with simultaneous endometrial and ovarian endometrioid carcinomas is about 50 years, significantly lower than the median age of presentation for HGSCs (about 63 years) and close to that of all women with endometrioid carcinomas (55-58 years). The median ovarian tumor size in these cases is about 9 cm, and the tumors in both sites are generally well-differentiated carcinomas.

Historically, the distinction between these representing synchronous independent primary tumors versus metastatic disease from the endometrium to the ovary has guided clinical management and thus required careful evaluation of the clinicopathologic features. The features favoring synchronous primaries included histologic dissimilarity between the two tumors, the presence of atypical endometrial hyperplasia, absent or only superficial myometrial invasion, lack of lymphatic invasion, unilateral ovarian tumor involving ovarian parenchyma, the presence of background endometriosis, and lack of distant spread of either tumors (107).

Recently, it has been established that the overwhelming majority of synchronous endometrioid carcinomas detected in the endometrium and the ovary are clonally related (35,36). However, despite their metastatic origin, these tumors exhibit an indolent behavior (108). Hence, when both tumors are low grade, the myometrial invasion comprises less than 50%, and extensive lymphovascular invasion or involvement of other sites is absent, it is now recommended that these tumors be managed as independent synchronous tumors (109).

SEROMUCINOUS TUMORS

Seromucinous tumors are characterized by an admixture of different Müllerian-derived epithelial cells, containing varying proportions of tubal-type epithelial cells and endometrioid epithelium with endocervical-type mucinous and/or squamous differentiation.

These lesions have previously been termed *endocervical-type/Müllerian mucinous tumors*. However, recent studies revealed that these often arise from endometriosis and share morphologic features, hormone receptor positivity, and molecular alterations (including ARID1A mutations) with endometrioid lesions (110). Thus, seromucinous tumors are no longer regarded as a subtype of mucinous ovarian lesions.

In the 2020 edition of the WHO classification (Table 8.7-1), seromucinous cystadenomas/adenofibromas and SMBTs represent a separate subcategory within endometriosis-associated neoplasms. Meanwhile, seromucinous carcinoma is no longer a separate entity but is currently regarded as a variant of endometrioid carcinoma of the ovary (105).

Seromucinous Cystadenoma and Adenofibroma

There are limited data available in the literature, with the largest series on benign seromucinous tumors comprising 22 cases. In this study, the mean patient age was 62 years, the range being 32 to 83 years. The majority of tumors were unilateral, with a mean size of 9 cm (range between 0.7 and 30 cm) (111). The lesional glands are embedded in a fibromatous stroma. The glandular structures are lined by cytologically bland, Müllerian-type epithelium containing a broad variety of cells, including hobnail and ciliated cells, endocervical-type mucinous cells, or, less commonly, goblet cells and endometrioid-type epithelium. The latter commonly shows mucinous or squamous differentiation. The different morphologies might be sharply demarcated or admixed. It is to note that the distinction between seromucinous cystadenoma and endometriotic cyst or endometrioid cystadenoma/adenofibroma exhibiting tubal or mucinous metaplasia might be arbitrary (85).

Seromucinous Borderline Tumor

SMBTs are rare but more common than benign seromucinous lesions. SMBT is characterized by an admixture of Müllerian-type epithelia and architectural complexity comprising more than 10% of the tumor volume. Both loss of ARID1A expression and KRAS mutations are common (110,112). These tumors present in patients of a wide age range. Up to 40% of tumors are bilateral, their mean size being 9 to 10 cm. In 30% to 50% of SMBTs, a background of endometriosis is noted (113).

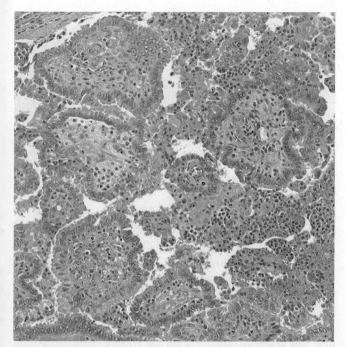

Figure 8.7-20. Seromucinous borderline tumor characterized by edematous papillae and neutrophilic infiltrates. The lining contains an admixture of endocervical-type mucinous, eosinophilic, and endometrioid epithelial cells.

Microscopically, SMBTs are composed of complex, hierarchically branching papillae (**Figure 8.7-20**). The papillae often have edematous stroma containing numerous neutrophils, or may occasionally be more fibrotic, and are lined by an admixture of Müllerian cell types, as described earlier in "Seromucinous Cystadenoma and Adenofibroma" section. The epithelium is cytologically bland but often shows stratification and/or tufting. Microinvasion, lymph node involvement, and peritoneal implants have been described in the literature; however, frank malignant behavior has not been reported (114,115). One study reported three cases of SMBTs coexisting with clear cell carcinoma and one case coexisting with a clear cell borderline adenofibroma, suggesting that extensive sampling of SMBTs is needed to detect potential associated high-grade neoplasms (116). Endometrioid malignancies have also been associated with SMBT (115). Seromucinous carcinomas are now classified as a subtype of endometrioid carcinoma, discussed in "Endometrioid Carcinoma, Seromucinous Type" section.

CLEAR CELL OVARIAN TUMORS

The vast majority of clear cell neoplasms of the ovaries are carcinomas, and these comprise about 8% of ovarian carcinomas (**Table 8.7-2**). Clear cell adenofibromas and clear cell borderline tumors (CCBTs) are vanishingly rare. The cells with clear cytoplasm contain glycogen.

Clear Cell Cystadenomas/Adenofibromas and Clear Cell Borderline Tumors

These are among the rarest of the ovarian epithelial tumors, with only four cases diagnosed as such in a series of 472 clear cell neoplasms (117). Importantly, caution is advised when rendering a diagnosis of clear cell adenofibroma, as it is likely that these represent an inadequately sampled, unusual, or subtle clear cell carcinoma.

CCBTs are exceedingly rare, comprising less than 1% of all ovarian borderline tumors (118). The characteristic molecular events in CCBT are ARID1A loss and PIK3CA mutations, similarly to clear cell carcinoma and to other endometriosis-associated ovarian neoplasms (119). Macroscopically, the majority are mixed solid and

cystic. Microscopically, CCBT shows glandular crowding, epithelial stratification, and mild atypia but, definitionally, lack stromal invasion.

Distinction of a CCBT from clear cell carcinoma is often difficult. The presence of markedly crowded glands, papillary or tubulocystic structures, or marked nuclear atypia excludes the diagnosis of CCBT, and a diagnosis of clear cell carcinoma should be rendered. Neither microinvasion nor intraepithelial carcinoma is defined for this entity. Peritoneal "implants" have not been described in association with these tumors, and the presence of extraovarian disease should be interpreted as metastatic carcinoma, making the primary lesion an ovarian clear cell carcinoma. Among the limited reported CCBTs, there is no reported recurrence or tumor death.

Clear Cell Carcinomas

Clear cell carcinomas (CCC) represent approximately 5% to 12% of all ovarian epithelial malignancies in North America and Europe (82,120). CCC is more common in Asia, particularly Japan, and in Asian Americans as compared to Caucasians (121-123). In a 2019 study involving a Japanese patient cohort, CCC accounted for 27% of all epithelial ovarian carcinomas, and in patients under the age of 50, CCC was the most common ovarian malignancy (124). Characteristic molecular alterations include loss of ARID1A function, often coexisting with PIK3CA mutations (125,126); in addition, TERT promoter mutations occur in up to 16% of CCC cases. MMRd is a rare occurrence in CCC, present in 2% to 6% of the cases (94,127,128). Still, clear cell morphology is overrepresented in women with Lynch syndrome, and routine screening for MMRd should be considered, especially in patients under the age of 53 years (99,129). Similarly to ovarian endometrioid and endometrial carcinomas, the TCGA molecular classification stratifies patients with ovarian CCC into prognostic groups (130).

Clinical and Operative Findings

The mean age of patients with CCC is 56 years (100). Symptoms related to the presence of a pelvic or abdominal mass are frequent. CCC is the most common epithelial ovarian neoplasm to be associated with vascular thrombosis (131) and paraneoplastic hypercalcemia (132). Among all histologic subtypes of ovarian carcinoma, the association with endometriosis is strongest for CCC. Endometriosis—in either close proximity to the tumor or elsewhere in the pelvis or abdomen—is detected in 55% to 74% of the cases (94,127). Approximately 35% of CCCs present as FIGO stage IA-IB and 38% in stage IC-II, whereas only 27% are diagnosed in higher stages (III-IV) (82). The higher frequency of surface involvement seems to correlate with the observed higher risk of intraoperative tumor rupture likely due to the extent and inherent difficulty in dissecting adhesions associated with endometriosis (133).

Gross Findings

Tumors are typically unilateral, with tumor size up to 30 cm (mean diameter of 12-15 cm). They may be solid and fibrous, with a honeycomb cut surface resembling adenofibromatous lesions. Other characteristic gross presentations of CCC include thick-walled unilocular cysts, with multiple nodules protruding into the lumen, and multiloculated cystic masses. The content of the cysts varies from watery or mucinous to a viscous chocolate brown fluid, typically associated with endometriotic cysts. Cystic CCCs are significantly more likely to be associated with endometriosis and atypical endometriosis as compared to the adenofibromatous type (134).

Microscopic Findings

CCCs display several different architectures—most commonly papillary, tubulocystic, and solid patterns—that often co-occur in the same lesion (**Figures 8.7-21-8.7-23**). A prominent adenofibromatous component might also be present in a subset of cases. The solid pattern of CCC is characterized by sheets of large

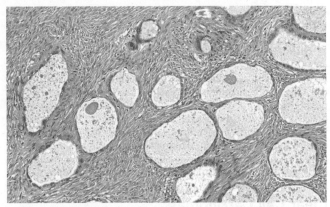

Figure 8.7-21. Clear cell carcinoma, tubulocystic pattern. The cystic and glandular spaces are lined by deceptively bland, benign-appearing, flattened to cuboidal epithelium.

polyhedral cells demonstrating abundant, clear to eosinophilic cytoplasm, separated by delicate fibrovascular septae or densely fibrotic stroma. The papillary pattern consists of papillae with prominent stromal hyalinization and/or myxoid stroma. The tubulocystic pattern is characterized by tubules and cysts of varying sizes. Despite its name, many of the cells comprising CCC may not demonstrate cytoplasmic clearing and may instead demonstrate eosinophilic cytoplasm. The nuclei vary from small, rounded, or angulated nuclei to large and pleomorphic nuclei with prominent red nucleoli, with a significant proportion of cases demonstrating a combination of both. In the tubulocystic and papillary patterns, the epithelial lining might be flattened and deceptively bland. Careful scrutiny is needed to reveal cells with high-grade nuclei elsewhere in these cases.

CCC is considered high grade in all cases. Although several grading systems have been proposed, none has had consistent and reproducible correlations with stage-independent prognosis. The distinction of CCC from HGSC and endometrioid carcinoma is occasionally problematic, as the latter may contain areas of clear cell change. CCCs are typically negative for ER, PR, and WT1 and demonstrate variable positivity for HNF-1β, Napsin A, and AMACR (135,136).

Clinical Behavior

Stage is the most important prognostic factor in CCC. For FIGO stage IA/B tumors, the reported 5-year survival rate is 87% to 92%, with this figure decreasing to 70% to 75% and 24% to 29% for stage IC/II and III/IV carcinomas, respectively (82,137). Tumor rupture does not seem to have a prognostic impact, and several studies, including a series of 193 patients with stage I CCC in which intraoperative tumor rupture occurred in 36% of cases, have not demonstrated a negative survival impact (133).

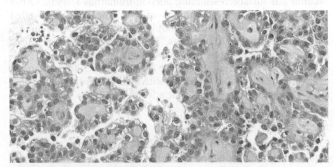

Figure 8.7-22. Clear cell carcinoma, papillary pattern. Tumor cells are arranged around fibrovascular cores that show characteristic hyalinization and myxoid changes.

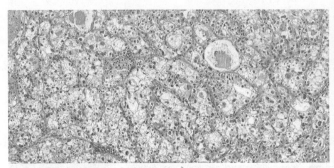

Figure 8.7-23. Clear cell carcinoma, solid and glandular pattern with severe cytologic atypia.

BRENNER TUMORS

Brenner tumors comprise 5% to 10% of ovarian epithelial tumors. Nearly all of these are benign Brenner tumors, whereas borderline and malignant Brenner tumors are very uncommon. The tumors are characterized by nests of stratified epithelium resembling urothelium. It is no longer recommended to use the historical terms benign or borderline transitional cell tumor, or transitional cell carcinoma, to diagnose these entities. Brenner tumors exhibit true urothelial differentiation and are thought to derive from Walthard nests (138). According to our current definition of malignant Brenner tumor, the presence of a benign and/or borderline Brenner tumor component is required. A substantial subset of tumors earlier diagnosed as transitional cell carcinoma without a precursor component actually represent transitional-like differentiation in HGSCs with SET features (139,140).

Benign Brenner Tumor

The mean patient age at diagnosis is 56 years. These are commonly incidentally found microscopic tumors, with most tumors being 2 cm or smaller, although larger tumors measuring more than 10 cm in greatest dimension have been described. Benign Brenner tumors are well circumscribed and exhibit a firm and rubbery consistency, whereas the serosal surface is generally smooth or slightly bosselated. The cut surfaces are typically solid and may be whorled or lobulated; less commonly, a cystic component might also be present. Microscopically, the characteristic feature is sharply demarcated nests of transitional-appearing epithelium within a densely fibrous stroma (**Figure 8.7-24**). Mucinous metaplasia is often present, with mucinous cells typically lining cystic spaces within the nests of transitional-like epithelium. Hyalinized areas of the stroma are common, and dystrophic calcifications are observed in approximately half of the cases (73).

The combined presence of Brenner and mucinous components appears to be more frequent than previously reported (**Figure 8.7-13**). Approximately 25% of benign ovarian epithelial tumors with a mucinous component also demonstrate a benign Brenner component, whereas 16% of tumors with a benign Brenner component also exhibit a mucinous component. A metaplastic mucinous component may occasionally form the dominant part of the tumor and accounts for the association of Brenner tumors with mucinous cystadenomas. Some authors suggest that the majority of nonteratomatous mucinous tumors of the ovary actually represent benign Brenner tumors, exhibiting an overgrowth of the mucinous component (73). Supporting this notion is the fact that mucinous and Brenner components of mixed tumors have been reported to be clonal, exhibiting highly concordant somatic mutations (141,142).

Borderline Brenner Tumors

These rare neoplasms are thought to arise from benign Brenner tumors. Alterations of CDKN2A, KRAS, and PIK3CA have been reported (143). Patients present at a mean age of 59 years. Borderline Brenner tumors are always unilateral and confined to the

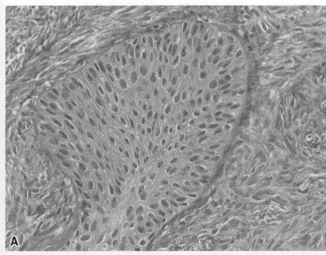
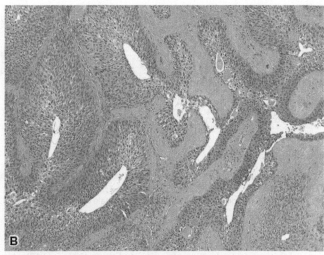

Figure 8.7-24. A: Brenner tumor. The transitional cell type is characterized by ovoid to spindled nuclei with prominent nuclear grooves, which resembles urothelium. B: Borderline Brenner tumor with expansile proliferation of transitional-type epithelium displaying mild-to-moderate cytologic atypia.

ovary. They usually demonstrate a prominent cystic component and are much larger than their benign counterparts, usually measuring 10 to 28 cm, with a mean diameter of 18 cm. The borderline component typically presents as papillary or polypoid projections within the cysts. Nearly all cases display an adjacent benign Brenner tumor component that presents as solid and fibrous lesion on cut surface. Microscopically, the intracystic papillae are lined by transitional-type epithelium that resembles low-grade noninvasive papillary transitional cell neoplasms of the urinary tract. Mucinous and squamous metaplasia are common. An uncommon pattern is characterized by solid nests of transitional epithelium crowding within the cyst wall (Figure 8.7-25). Occasionally, significant atypia and increased mitotic activity might be present, but the presence of stromal invasion excludes the diagnosis of borderline Brenner tumor. Local recurrences are rare, and no malignant behavior has been reported.

Malignant Brenner Tumors

The definition of malignant Brenner tumor requires the presence of benign and/or borderline Brenner component. By using these more restrictive criteria, cases of HGSC with transitional-like features have been removed from this category. The remaining bona fide malignant Brenner tumors lack *TP53* alterations and harbor *PIK3CA* mutations and *MDM2* amplification, even though a key

driver event has not yet been identified (144). Malignant Brenner tumors comprise 0.3% of ovarian carcinomas and occur at a mean age of 61 years (Table 8.7-2). They have a mean size of 10 cm but have been described to be as large as 25 cm and are typically unilateral (145). In malignant Brenner tumors, the benign Brenner component may be identifiable as a solid fibrous nodule within a cyst wall, although sometimes malignant Brenner tumors are completely solid. The characteristic microscopic feature of malignant Brenner tumor is the presence of thick, blunt, and often elongated papillary folds with fibrovascular cores, lined by markedly atypical transitional-type epithelium, although a predominantly solid pattern can be seen in up to half of the cases (Figure 8.7-25). Stromal invasion is present and characterized by haphazard infiltrative growth of epithelium at the base of the papillae into the cyst wall, or extensive areas of solid epithelial proliferation with scant or no fibrovascular support. Rarely, scattered angulated invasive nests appear to arise directly from a benign Brenner tumor without a borderline component. Malignant Brenner tumors are mostly diagnosed in early stage. The stage distribution is as follows: stage IA/B, 57%; stage IC/II, 26%; and stage III/IV, 17%. Five-year survival rates are approximately 90% for localized disease, 56% with regionally advanced disease, and 29% when distant metastases are present (82).

MIXED EPITHELIAL OVARIAN TUMORS

It is well known that many high-grade carcinomas may demonstrate overlapping morphologic and IHC features of various histologic types (Table 8.7.4). Historically, mixed epithelial carcinomas were frequently diagnosed; however, the majority of these cases are now regarded as HGSC with heterogeneous/variant morphology (146). Currently, mixed ovarian carcinomas are thought to be rare, representing less than 1% of all ovarian carcinomas (147). The 2020 WHO definition of a bona fide mixed carcinoma requires the presence of two or more histotypes clearly distinguishable on hematoxylin and eosin (H&E)-stained slides and preferably exhibiting distinct IHC profiles, or unequivocal differences shown by ancillary testing. When these diagnostic criteria are applied and collision tumors are excluded, the combination of endometrioid and CCCs proves to be the most common mixed tumor (146).

CARCINOSARCOMA

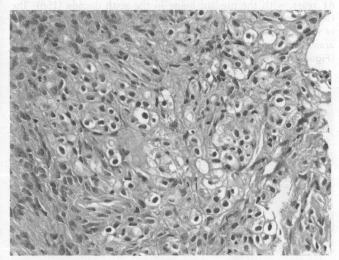

Figure 8.7-25. Malignant Brenner tumor characterized by small variably sized nests of transitional-type cells with an infiltrative pattern.

Carcinosarcomas are biphasic tumors, exhibiting carcinomatous (usually high-grade) and sarcomatous elements, and comprise about 5% of ovarian carcinomas in the United States (82).

■ **TABLE 8.7-4. Immunohistochemical Markers Commonly Used in the Diagnosis of Epithelial Ovarian Tumors**

	Proportion of Cases Showing Positive Immunohistochemical Staining				
	PAX8 (%)	WT1 (%)	Abnormal p53 (%)[a]	Napsin A (%)	PR (%)
High-grade serous carcinoma	95	97	94-98	1	37-42
Low-grade serous carcinoma	87-100	98-100	0	0	59-60
Endometrioid carcinoma	82	10-14	14-15	3-8	81-85
Clear cell carcinoma	95	1	11-12	92	5-7
Mucinous carcinoma	39-47	0-1	61-66	0-3	0-4

[a]Abnormal p53 expression refers to strong nuclear reaction in >80% of tumor cell nuclei, complete absence of staining in tumor cell nuclei with retained internal control, or cytoplasmic expression.

Based on the 5th Edition of WHO Classification of Female Genital Tumors. Vol. 4. 5th ed. WHO International Agency for Research on Cancer; 2020.

From IARC 2020

Carcinosarcomas are considered variants of epithelial malignancies exhibiting metaplastic sarcomatous differentiation (147). As such, the two components are clonally related, most commonly harboring concordant alterations of the *TP53* gene (148,149). In addition to *TP53*, other frequently altered genes include *PIK3CA*, *PPP2R1A*, *KRAS*, *PTEN*, *CHD4*, and *BCOR* (150). The mean age at diagnosis is 65 years, which is slightly higher than that for HGSC. Tumor size typically ranges from 15 to 20 cm, with a stage distribution similar to that of HGSC. The characteristic microscopic feature is an intimate admixture of malignant epithelial and mesenchymal elements (**Figure 8.7-26**). The malignant epithelial element is most commonly an HGSC, but other histotypes have also been observed. The sarcoma component is usually homologous and consists of sheets of rounded to spindled cells with marked nuclear atypia and a high mitotic index. When present, heterologous elements are most commonly chondrosarcoma, osteosarcoma, or rhabdomyosarcoma. There is no minimum volume of sarcomatous element required for rendering the diagnosis of carcinosarcoma. Occasionally, a tumor that is otherwise a typical carcinoma may demonstrate a small focus of sarcoma; although the prognostic

significance of this finding is unclear, these tumors are currently classified as carcinosarcomas.

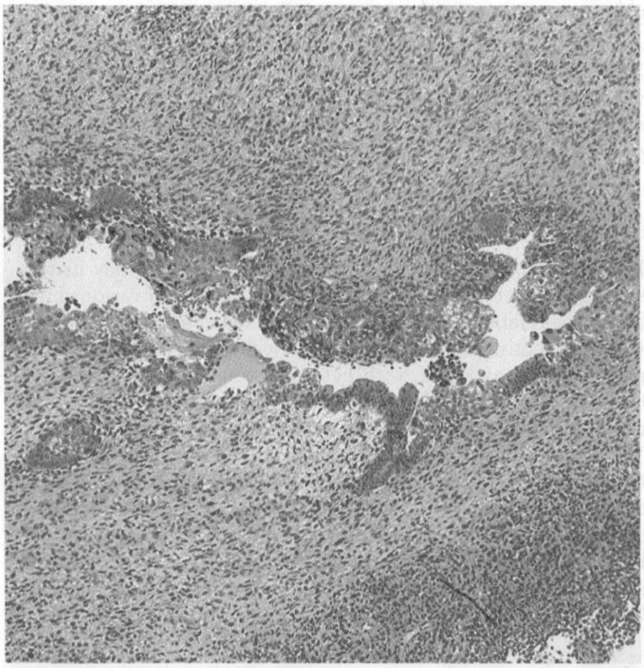

Most carcinosarcomas are diagnosed at an advanced stage (III/IV), and only 5% of these are ovary confined. When stratified for stage, disease-specific survival of carcinosarcoma is much worse than that for HGSC. In a recent study, the 5-year survival for stage IA/B was reported as 71%, decreasing to 39% and 16% for stages IC/II and III/IV, respectively (82). The presence of heterologous elements and the histologic subtype of the carcinoma component do not appear to influence prognosis (151).

MESONEPHRIC-LIKE ADENOCARCINOMA

MLAC has been included in the 2020 WHO classification as a distinct entity. MLACs frequently harbor KRAS mutations; in KRAS wild-type cases, NRAS or BRAF mutations are often identified (152). While mesonephric adenocarcinomas of the lower gynecologic tract have been shown to originate from mesonephric remnants, such association has not been established for the morphologically similar tumors arising in the upper gynecologic tract. Hence, these are termed *mesonephric-like adenocarcinomas*. Recent studies suggest a Müllerian origin of at least a subset of MLAC based on their relatively frequent association with other Müllerian lesions, such as endometriosis, adenoma/adenofibroma, SBT, or LGSC. In three reported cases of MLAC presenting concurrently with LGSC, as well as in one case of MLAC arising in an SBT, both components harbored identical point mutations in either the *KRAS* or *NRAS* genes and shared other characteristic genomic alterations (153-155).

Patients' age at the time of diagnosis ranges between 29 and 81 years, with the median being in the sixth decade (156). The tumors are usually unilateral and variable in size. Their cut surface is solid, or solid and cystic (152,157,158). MLAC might contain areas of glandular, ductal, tubular, papillary, or solid architecture (**Figure 8.7-27**). Tubular structures might contain eosinophilic

Figure 8.7-26. Carcinosarcoma. The carcinomatous component shows glandular and squamous differentiation. The sarcomatous component consists of bland, spindled cells in a pale eosinophilic extracellular matrix and round, hyperchromatic cells representing rhabdomyosarcomatous differentiation (lower right corner).

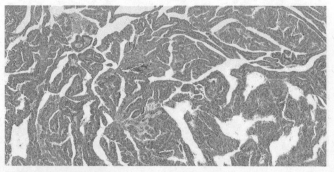

Figure 8.7-27. Mesonephric-like adenocarcinoma displaying ductal and papillary architecture.

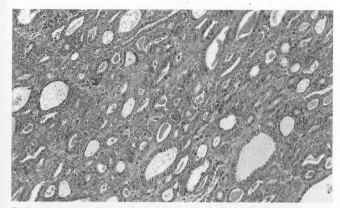

Figure 8.7-28. Mesonephric-like adenocarcinoma. Tubular structures containing eosinophilic intraluminal material are characteristic of mesonephric differentiation.

colloid-like material in the lumen (**Figure 8.7-28**). Nuclei show characteristic vesicular chromatine with clearing, inconspicuous nucleoli and crowding similar to the nuclei seen in papillary thyroid carcinomas. The typical IHC profile of MLAC consists of GATA3, TTF1 and PAX8 positivity, luminal CD10 reactivity, and negative reaction with ER, PR, and WT1.

OTHER OVARIAN TUMORS

Undifferentiated and Dedifferentiated Carcinoma

Although undifferentiated carcinomas are regarded as malignant epithelial tumors, these do show no readily identifiable feature of any line of differentiation. Dedifferentiated carcinomas are biphasic tumors, composed of a well-differentiated and an undifferentiated component. When strict pathologic criteria are employed for the diagnoses, these comprise less than 1% of ovarian carcinomas. Similar to their endometrial counterparts, key genetic alterations inactivate components of the SWI/SNF chromatin remodeling complex, such as ARID1A/B or SMARCA4/2/B1 (159). MMRd is also common (160). The mean age at presentation is 53 years, and nearly all patients are diagnosed in stages III and IV (120). Undifferentiated areas are composed of solid sheets of discohesive cells with monotonous nuclei (**Figure 8.7-29**). Geographic necrosis, brisk mitotic activity, and prominent lymphocytic infiltrates are commonly appreciated. In cases of dedifferentiated carcinomas, the well-differentiated component is commonly a FIGO grade I-II endometrioid carcinoma (161). It is important to detect the presence of an undifferentiated component, as it indicates aggressive clinical behavior. Solid sheets of undifferentiated carcinoma and the solid pattern of endometrioid carcinoma have to be distinguished. Loss of expression of MMR and SWI/SNF complex proteins and focal reactivity only to CK18 and EMA are characteristics for undifferentiated

carcinomas. Other markers of epithelial differentiation are typically negative (160). When considering a diagnosis of undifferentiated carcinoma, it is important to exclude the possibility of a metastasis from a lung primary. The differential diagnosis also includes small cell carcinoma of the ovary, hypercalcemic type; small cell neuroendocrine carcinoma; as well as sarcomas and lymphomas.

Small Cell Carcinoma of the Ovary, Hypercalcemic Type

Small cell carcinoma of the ovary, hypercalcemic type, is an undifferentiated malignant tumor with poor prognosis, which does not exhibit any marker of epithelial differentiation; however, it is mentioned in this subchapter for its differential diagnostic relevance. This rare neoplasm occurs in young women with a mean age of 25 years. The characteristic microscopic pattern displays sheets of small cells with interspersed follicle-like spaces. Genomically, it is characterized by deleterious germline or somatic mutations in a single gene, *SMARCA4*, in almost all cases (162).

TUMORS OF THE FALLOPIAN TUBES

Benign Fallopian Tube Tumors

The most common benign tumor of the fallopian tube is the adenomatoid tumor, which is a neoplasm of mesothelial origin. These are nearly always incidental findings within the mesosalpinx or wall of the fallopian tube, typically measuring 1 to 2 cm. They are firm and yellowish on cut section. Microscopically, they display interanastomosing tubules and glands without atypia or mitotic activity. The cytoplasm is eosinophilic and vacuolated. Of note, a small biopsy of a peritoneal mesothelioma can have an identical histologic appearance. Recent studies suggest that TRAF7 mutations drive the activation of the NF-κB signaling pathway in adenomatoid tumors (163). Loss of BAP1 function has not been detected in these lesions. Benign papillomas, serous adenofibromas, and SBTs can arise from the tubal mucosa, and leiomyomas may arise from the smooth muscle component of the mesosalpinx. Occasional examples of tubal adenomyomas probably represent endometriosis with an associated prominent smooth muscle hyperplasia. Mesothelial/peritoneal inclusion cysts may also arise from the serosal surface of the fallopian tube. Although multiloculated peritoneal cysts are generally benign, these can recur in up to 50% of cases (164).

Wolffian tumors—also commonly termed *female adnexal tumor of probable Wolffian origin* (FATWO)—are rare epithelial neoplasms usually found within the broad ligament but have also been reported in the ovary. As the name suggests, these tumors probably arise from mesonephric remnants. Wolffian tumors are generally benign; however, recurrences and metastases have been reported in rare cases (165). Rare pathogenic mutations detected involve the genes *STK11*, *APC*, and *MBD4* (166).

Malignant Fallopian Tube Tumors

The overwhelming majority of ovarian and peritoneal HGSCs arise from STIC (see "High-Grade Serous Carcinoma of Ovarian, Tubal, and Peritoneal Origin" section). There are very rare reports of CCC and endometrioid carcinomas of the fallopian tube. Because these tumors often arise from endometriosis, it is conceivable that tubal primaries also arise in endometriosis. Thorough sampling of the endometrium might reveal a primary—or less commonly synchronous—endometrial endometrioid carcinoma or CCC (167). Metastases to the fallopian tube might originate from the endometrium or the uterine cervix, whereas nongynecologic primaries include colon, stomach, biliary, appendiceal, and breast carcinomas (168). Metastases might involve any layer of the fallopian tube. Importantly, a metastasis involving the tubal epithelium might mimic STIC (169). Depending on the primary tumor, these lesions can also exhibit an aberrant p53 IHC pattern (170,171).

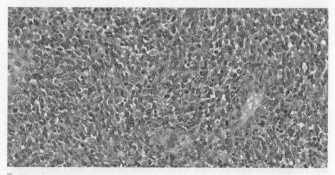

Figure 8.7-29. Undifferentiated carcinoma composed of solid sheets of discohesive, relatively monotonous, hyperchromatic tumor cells. Note the brisk mitotic activity.

References

1. World Health Organization (WHO). *Female Genital Tumors.* Vol 4. 5th ed. WHO International Agency for Research on Cancer; 2020.

2. Kommoss S, Gilks CB, du Bois A, Kommoss F. Ovarian carcinoma diagnosis: the clinical impact of 15 years of change. *Br J Cancer.* 2016;115(8):993-999.

3. Sung PL, Chang YH, Chao KC, Chuang CM, Task Force on Systematic Review and Meta-analysis of Ovarian Cancer. Global distribution pattern of histological subtypes of epithelial ovarian cancer: a database analysis and systematic review. *Gynecol Oncol.* 2014;133(2):147-154.

4. Buza N. Frozen section diagnosis of ovarian epithelial tumors: diagnostic pearls and pitfalls. *Arch Pathol Lab Med.* 2019;143(1):47-64.

5. Tornos C, Soslow RA, eds. *Frozen Section of Ovarian Lesions.* Springer; 2011.

6. Heatley MK. A systematic review of papers examining the use of intraoperative frozen section in predicting the final diagnosis of ovarian lesions. *Int J Gynecol Pathol.* 2012;31(2):111-115.

7. Ratnavelu ND, Brown AP, Mallett S, et al. Intraoperative frozen section analysis for the diagnosis of early stage ovarian cancer in suspicious pelvic masses. *Cochrane Database Syst Rev.* 2016;3(3):CD010360.

8. Huang Z, Li L, Li C, et al. Diagnostic accuracy of frozen section analysis of borderline ovarian tumors: a meta-analysis with emphasis on misdiagnosis factors. *J Cancer.* 2018;9(16):2817-2824.

9. Moore L, Gajjar K, Jimenez-Linan M, Crawford R. Prevalence of appendiceal lesions in appendicectomies performed during surgery for mucinous ovarian tumors: a retrospective study. *Int J Gynecol Cancer.* 2016;26(8):1386-1389.

10. Rosendahl M, Haueberg Oester LA, Høgdall CK. The importance of appendectomy in surgery for mucinous adenocarcinoma of the ovary. *Int J Gynecol Cancer.* 2017;27(3):430-436.

11. Stewart CJ, Ardakani NM, Doherty DA, Young RH. An evaluation of the morphologic features of low-grade mucinous neoplasms of the appendix metastatic in the ovary, and comparison with primary ovarian mucinous tumors. *Int J Gynecol Pathol.* 2014;33(1):1-10.

12. Ackroyd SA, Goetsch L, Brown J, Houck K, Wang C, Hernandez E. Pancreaticobiliary metastasis presenting as primary mucinous ovarian neoplasm: a systematic literature review. *Gynecol Oncol Rep.* 2019;28:109-115.

13. Hu J, Khalifa RD, Roma AA, Fadare O. The pathologic distinction of primary and metastatic mucinous tumors involving the ovary: a re-evaluation of algorithms based on gross features. *Ann Diagn Pathol.* 2018;37:1-6.

14. Akbarzadeh-Jahromi M, Aslani FS, Raeisi H, Momtahan M, Taheri N. Comparison of frozen and permanent section diagnosis in ovarian neoplasms: analysis of factors affecting accuracy. *Int J Gynecol Pathol.* 2022;41(4):327-336.

15. Shih KK, Garg K, Soslow RA, Chi DS, Abu-Rustum NR, Barakat RR. Accuracy of frozen section diagnosis of ovarian borderline tumor. *Gynecol Oncol.* 2011;123(3):517-521.

16. Cohen PA, Powell A, Böhm S, et al. Pathological chemotherapy response score is prognostic in tubo-ovarian high-grade serous carcinoma: a systematic review and meta-analysis of individual patient data. *Gynecol Oncol.* 2019;154(2):441-448.

17. Gilks CB, Selinger CI, Davidson B, et al. Data set for the reporting of ovarian, fallopian tube and primary peritoneal carcinoma: recommendations from the International Collaboration on Cancer Reporting (ICCR). *Int J Gynecol Pathol.* 2022;41:S119-S142.

18. Singh N, Gilks CB, Hirschowitz L, et al. Primary site assignment in tubo-ovarian high-grade serous carcinoma: consensus statement on unifying practice worldwide. *Gynecol Oncol.* 2016;141(2):195-198.

19. Singh N, McCluggage WG, Gilks CB. High-grade serous carcinoma of tubo-ovarian origin: recent developments. *Histopathology.* 2017;71(3):339-356.

20. Skala SL, Hagemann IS. Optimal sampling of grossly normal omentum in staging of gynecologic malignancies. *Int J Gynecol Pathol.* 2015;34(3):281-287.

21. Allen VA, Takashima Y, Nayak S, Manahan KJ, Geisler JP. Assessment of false-negative ascites cytology in epithelial ovarian carcinoma: a study of 313 patients. *Am J Clin Oncol.* 2017;40(2):175-177.

22. Davidson W, Madan R, O'Neil M, Tawfik OW, Fan F. Utility of peritoneal washing cytology in staging and prognosis of ovarian and fallopian tube neoplasms: a 10-year retrospective analysis. *Ann Diagn Pathol.* 2016;22:54-57.

23. Rush SK, Swisher EM, Garcia RL, et al. Pathologic findings and clinical outcomes in women undergoing risk-reducing surgery to prevent ovarian and fallopian tube carcinoma: a large prospective single institution experience. *Gynecol Oncol.* 2020;157(2):514-520.

24. Lobo J, Machado B, Vieira R, Bartosch C. The challenge of diagnosing a malignancy metastatic to the ovary: clinicopathological characteristics vary and morphology can be different from that of the corresponding primary tumor. *Virchows Arch.* 2017;470(1):69-80.

25. Bruls J, Simons M, Overbeek LI, Bulten J, Massuger LF, Nagtegaal ID. A national population-based study provides insight in the origin of malignancies metastatic to the ovary. *Virchows Arch.* 2015;467(1):79-86.

26. Ronnett BM, Yemelyanova AV, Vang R, et al. Endocervical adenocarcinomas with ovarian metastases: analysis of 29 cases with emphasis on minimally invasive cervical tumors and the ability of the metastases to simulate primary ovarian neoplasms. *Am J Surg Pathol.* 2008;32(12):1835-1853.

27. Zhang W, Tan C, Xu M, Wu X. Appendiceal mucinous neoplasm mimics ovarian tumors: challenges for preoperative and intraoperative diagnosis and clinical implication. *Eur J Surg Oncol.* 2019;45(11):2120-2125.

28. Seidman JD, Cho KR, Ronnett BM. Surface epithelial tumors of the ovary. In: Kurman RJ, Ellenson LH, Ronnett BM, eds. *Blaustein's Pathology of the Female Genital Tract 6th.* Springer; 2011:679-784.

29. Ronnett BM, Kajdacsy-Balla A, Gilks CB, et al. Mucinous borderline ovarian tumors: points of general agreement and persistent controversies regarding nomenclature, diagnostic criteria, and behavior. *Hum Pathol.* 2004;35(8):949-960.

30. Shelekhova KV, Zhuravlev AS, Krylova DD, Konstantinov AS, Shtan LV, Kheinshtein VA. Pseudomyxoma peritonei as a first manifestation of kras-mutated urachal mucinous cystadenocarcinoma of the bladder: a case report. *Int J Surg Pathol.* 2017;25(6):563-566.

31. Hackeng WM, de Guerre LEVM, Kuypers KC, et al. Pseudomyxoma peritonei after a total pancreatectomy for intraductal papillary mucinous neoplasm with colloid carcinoma in lynch syndrome. *Pancreas.* 2019;48(1):135-138.

32. Lin JE, Seo S, Kushner DM, Rose SL. The role of appendectomy for mucinous ovarian neoplasms. *Am J Obstet Gynecol.* 2013;208(1):46.e1-46.e464.

33. Vang R, Gown AM, Zhao C, et al. Ovarian mucinous tumors associated with mature cystic teratomas: morphologic and immunohistochemical analysis identifies a subset of potential teratomatous origin that shares features of lower gastrointestinal tract mucinous tumors more commonly encountered as secondary tumors in the ovary. *Am J Surg Pathol.* 2007;31(6):854-869.

34. McKenney JK, Soslow RA, Longacre TA. Ovarian mature teratomas with mucinous epithelial neoplasms: morphologic heterogeneity and association with pseudomyxoma peritonei. *Am J Surg Pathol.* 2008;32(5):645-655.

35. Anglesio MS, Wang YK, Maassen M, et al. Synchronous endometrial and ovarian carcinomas: evidence of clonality. *J Natl Cancer Inst.* 2016;108(6):djv428.

36. Schultheis AM, Ng CK, De Filippo MR, et al. Massively parallel sequencing-based clonality analysis of synchronous endometrioid endometrial and ovarian carcinomas. *J Natl Cancer Inst.* 2016;108(6):djv427.

37. Casey L, Singh N. Metastases to the ovary arising from endometrial, cervical and fallopian tube cancer: recent advances. *Histopathology.* 2020;76(1):37-51.

38. Cheng EJ, Kurman RJ, Wang M, et al. Molecular genetic analysis of ovarian serous cystadenomas. *Lab Invest.* 2004;84(6):778-784.

39. Hunter SM, Anglesio MS, Sharma R, et al. Copy number aberrations in benign serous ovarian tumors: a case for reclassification? *Clin Cancer Res.* 2011;17(23):7273-7282.

40. Hunter SM, Dall GV, Doyle MA, et al. Molecular comparison of pure ovarian fibroma with serous benign ovarian tumours. *BMC Res Notes.* 2020;13(1):349.

41. Ardighieri L, Zeppernick F, Hannibal CG, et al. Mutational analysis of BRAF and KRAS in ovarian serous borderline (atypical proliferative) tumours and associated peritoneal implants. *J Pathol.* 2014;232(1):16-22.

42. McKenney JK, Balzer BL, Longacre TA. Lymph node involvement in ovarian serous tumors of low malignant potential (borderline tumors): pathology, prognosis, and proposed classification. *Am J Surg Pathol.* 2006;30(5):614-624.

43. Burks RT, Sherman ME, Kurman RJ. Micropapillary serous carcinoma of the ovary. A distinctive low-grade carcinoma related to serous borderline tumors. *Am J Surg Pathol.* 1996;20(11):1319-1330.

44. Eichhorn JH, Bell DA, Young RH, Scully RE. Ovarian serous borderline tumors with micropapillary and cribriform patterns: a study of 40 cases and comparison with 44 cases without these patterns. *Am J Surg Pathol.* 1999;23(4):397-409.

45. McCluggage WG. Ovarian borderline tumours: a review with comparison of serous and mucinous types. *Diagnostic Histopathology.* 2014;20(9):333-350.

46. Vang R, Hannibal CG, Junge J, Frederiksen K, Kjaer SK, Kurman RJ. Long-term behavior of serous borderline tumors subdivided into atypical proliferative tumors and noninvasive low-grade carcinomas: a population-based clinicopathologic study of 942 cases. *Am J Surg Pathol.* 2017;41(6):725-737.

47. Hannibal CG, Vang R, Junge J, et al. A nationwide study of serous "borderline" ovarian tumors in Denmark 1978-2002: centralized pathology review and overall survival compared with the general population. *Gynecol Oncol.* 2014;134(2):267-273.

48. Seidman JD, Kraus JA, Yemelyanova A, et al. Ovarian low grade serous neoplasms: evaluation of sampling recommendations based on tumors expected to have invasion (those with peritoneal invasive low grade serous carcinoma (invasive implants). *Modern Pathol.* 2009;22(Suppl 1):236.

49. Maniar KP, Wang Y, Visvanathan K, Shih IeM, Kurman RJ. Evaluation of microinvasion and lymph node involvement in ovarian serous borderline/atypical proliferative serous tumors: a morphologic and immunohistochemical analysis of 37 cases. *Am J Surg Pathol.* 2014;38(6):743-755.

50. du Bois A, Ewald-Riegler N, de Gregorio N, et al. Borderline tumours of the ovary: a cohort study of the Arbeitsgmeinschaft Gynakologische Onkologie (AGO) study group. *Eur J Cancer.* 2013;49(8):1905-1914.

51. Seidman JD, Kurman RJ. Ovarian serous borderline tumors: a critical review of the literature with emphasis on prognostic indicators. *Hum Pathol.* 2000;31(5):539-557.

52. Sherman ME, Mink PJ, Curtis R, et al. Survival among women with borderline ovarian tumors and ovarian carcinoma: a population-based analysis. *Cancer.* 2004;100(5):1045-1052.

53. Akeson M, Zetterqvist BM, Dahllof K, Jakobsen AM, Brannstrom M, Horvath G. Population-based cohort follow-up study of all patients operated for borderline ovarian tumor in western Sweden during an 11-year period. *Int J Gynecol Cancer.* 2008;18(3):453-459.

54. Park JY, Kim DY, Kim JH, Kim YM, Kim YT, Nam JH. Surgical management of borderline ovarian tumors: the role of fertility-sparing surgery. *Gynecol Oncol.* 2009;113(1):75-82.

55. Chui MH, Xing D, Zeppernick F, et al. Clinicopathologic and molecular features of paired cases of metachronous ovarian serous borderline tumor and subsequent serous carcinoma. *Am J Surg Pathol.* 2019;43(11):1462-1472.

56. Uzan C, Zanini-Grandon AS, Bentivegna E, et al. Outcome of patients with advanced-stage borderline ovarian tumors after a first peritoneal noninvasive recurrence: impact on further management. *Int J Gynecol Cancer.* 2015;25(5):830-836.

57. Bell KA, Smith Sehdev AE, Kurman RJ. Refined diagnostic criteria for implants associated with ovarian atypical proliferative serous tumors (borderline) and micropapillary serous carcinomas. *Am J Surg Pathol.* 2001;25(4):419-432.

58. Gershenson DM, Sun CC, Lu KH, et al. Clinical behavior of stage II-IV low-grade serous carcinoma of the ovary. *Obstet Gynecol.* 2006;108(2):361-368.

59. Shih IM, Wang Y, Wang TL. The origin of ovarian cancer species and precancerous landscape. *Am J Pathol.* 2021;191(1):26-39.

60. Soslow RA, Han G, Park KJ, et al. Morphologic patterns associated with BRCA1 and BRCA2 genotype in ovarian carcinoma. *Mod Pathol.* 2012;25(4):625-636.

61. Ritterhouse LL, Nowak JA, Strickland KC, et al. Morphologic correlates of molecular alterations in extrauterine müllerian carcinomas. *Mod Pathol.* 2016;29(8):893-903.

62. Dubeau L. The cell of origin of ovarian epithelial tumors and the ovarian surface epithelium dogma: does the emperor have no clothes? *Gynecol Oncol.* 1999;72(3):437-442.

63. Piek JM, van Diest PJ, Zweemer RP, et al. Dysplastic changes in prophylactically removed fallopian tubes of women predisposed to developing ovarian cancer. *J Pathol.* 2001;195(4):451-456.

64. Bogaerts JMA, Steenbeek MP, van Bommel MHD, et al. Recommendations for diagnosing STIC: a systematic review and meta-analysis. *Virchows Arch.* 2022;480(4):725-737.

65. Singh N, Benson JL, Gan C, et al. Disease distribution in low-stage tubo-ovarian high-grade serous carcinoma (HGSC): implications for assigning primary site and FIGO stage. *Int J Gynecol Pathol.* 2018;37(4):324-330.

66. Singh N, Gilks CB, Wilkinson N, McCluggage WG. Assessment of a new system for primary site assignment in high-grade serous carcinoma of the fallopian tube, ovary, and peritoneum. *Histopathology.* 2015;67(3):331-337.

67. Colon E, Carlson JW. Evaluation of the fallopian tubes after neoadjuvant chemotherapy: persistence of serous tubal intraepithelial carcinoma. *Int J Gynecol Pathol.* 2014;33(5):463-469.

68. Böhm S, Faruqi A, Said I, et al. Chemotherapy response score: development and validation of a system to quantify histopathologic response to neoadjuvant chemotherapy in tubo-ovarian high-grade serous carcinoma. *J Clin Oncol.* 2015;33(22):2457-2463. doi:10.1200/JCO.2014.60.5212

69. Said I, Böhm S, Beasley J, et al. The Chemotherapy Response Score (CRS): interobserver reproducibility in a simple and prognostically relevant system for reporting the histologic response to neoadjuvant chemotherapy in tuboovarian high-grade serous carcinoma. *Int J Gynecol Pathol.* 2017;36(2):172-179.

70. Hunter SM, Gorringe KL, Christie M, Rowley SM, Bowtell DD, Campbell IG. Pre-invasive ovarian mucinous tumors are characterized by CDKN2A and RAS pathway aberrations. *Clin Cancer Res.* 2012;18(19):5267-5277.

71. Mackenzie R, Kommoss S, Winterhoff BJ, et al. Targeted deep sequencing of mucinous ovarian tumors reveals multiple overlapping RAS-pathway activating mutations in borderline and cancerous neoplasms. *BMC Cancer.* 2015;15:415. doi:10.1186/s12885-015-1421-8

72. Cheasley D, Wakefield MJ, Ryland GL, et al. The molecular origin and taxonomy of mucinous ovarian carcinoma. *Nat Commun.* 2019;10(1):3935.

73. Seidman JD, Khedmati F. Exploring the histogenesis of ovarian mucinous and transitional cell (brenner) neoplasms and their relationship with Walthard cell nests: a study of 120 tumors. *Arch Pathol Lab Med.* 2008;132(11):1753-1760.

74. Kerr SE, Flotte AB, McFalls MJ, Vrana JA, Halling KC, Bell DA. Matching maternal isodisomy in mucinous carcinomas and associated ovarian teratomas provides evidence of germ cell derivation for some mucinous ovarian tumors. *Am J Surg Pathol.* 2013;37(8):1229-1235.

75. Fujii K, Yamashita Y, Yamamoto T, et al. Ovarian mucinous tumors arising from mature cystic teratomas—a molecular genetic approach for understanding the cellular origin. *Hum Pathol.* 2014;45(4):717-724.

76. Snir OL, Buza N, Hui P. Mucinous epithelial tumours arising from ovarian mature teratomas: a tissue genotyping study. *Histopathology.* 2016;69(3):383-392.

77. Seidman JD, Kurman RJ, Ronnett BM. Primary and metastatic mucinous adenocarcinomas in the ovaries: incidence in routine practice with a new approach to improve intraoperative diagnosis. *Am J Surg Pathol.* 2003;27(7):985-993.

78. Seidman JD, Soslow RA, Vang R, et al. Borderline ovarian tumors: diverse contemporary viewpoints on terminology and diagnostic criteria with illustrative images. *Hum Pathol.* 2004;35(8):918-933.

79. Riopel MA, Ronnett BM, Kurman RJ. Evaluation of diagnostic criteria and behavior of ovarian intestinal-type mucinous tumors: atypical proliferative (borderline) tumors and intraepithelial, microinvasive, invasive, and metastatic carcinomas. *Am J Surg Pathol.* 1999;23(6):617-635.

80. Yemelyanova AV, Vang R, Judson K, Wu LS, Ronnett BM. Distinction of primary and metastatic mucinous tumors involving the ovary: analysis of size and laterality data by primary site with reevaluation of an algorithm for tumor classification. *Am J Surg Pathol.* 2008;32(1):128-138.

81. Irving JA, Clement PB. Recurrent intestinal mucinous borderline tumors of the ovary: a report of 5 cases causing problems in diagnosis, including distinction from mucinous carcinoma. *Int J Gynecol Pathol.* 2014;33(2):156-165.

82. Peres LC, Cushing-Haugen KL, Kobel M, et al. Invasive epithelial ovarian cancer survival by histotype and disease stage. *J Natl Cancer Inst.* 2019;111(1):60-68.

83. Khunamornpong S, Settakorn J, Sukpan K, Suprasert P, Siriaunkgul S. Primary ovarian mucinous adenocarcinoma of intestinal type: a clinicopathologic study of 46 cases. *Int J Gynecol Pathol.* 2014;33(2):176-185.

84. Gouy S, Saidani M, Maulard A, et al. Characteristics and prognosis of stage I ovarian mucinous tumors according to expansile or infiltrative type. *Int J Gynecol Cancer.* 2018;28(3):493-499.

85. Talia KL, Parra-Herran C, McCluggage WG. Ovarian mucinous and seromucinous neoplasms: problematic aspects and modern diagnostic approach. *Histopathology.* 2022;80(2):255-278.

86. Desouki MM, Khabele D, Crispens MA, Fadare O. Ovarian mucinous tumor with malignant mural nodules: dedifferentiation or collision? *Int J Gynecol Pathol.* 2015;34(1):19-24.

87. Mesbah Ardakani N, Giardina T, Amanuel B, Stewart CJ. Molecular profiling reveals a clonal relationship between ovarian mucinous tumors and corresponding mural carcinomatous nodules. *Am J Surg Pathol.* 2017;41(9):1261-1266.

88. Chapel DB, Lee EK, Da Silva AFL, et al. Mural nodules in mucinous ovarian tumors represent a morphologic spectrum of clonal neoplasms: a morphologic, immunohistochemical, and molecular analysis of 13 cases. *Mod Pathol.* 2021;34(3):613-626.

89. Provenza C, Young RH, Prat J. Anaplastic carcinoma in mucinous ovarian tumors: a clinicopathologic study of 34 cases emphasizing the crucial impact of stage on prognosis, their histologic spectrum, and overlap with sarcomalike mural nodules. *Am J Surg Pathol.* 2008;32(3):383-389.

90. Ricotta G, Maulard A, Candiani M, et al. Endometrioid borderline ovarian tumor: clinical characteristics, prognosis, and managements. *Ann Surg Oncol.* 2022;29(9):5894-5903.

91. Roth LM, Emerson RE, Ulbright TM. Ovarian endometrioid tumors of low malignant potential: a clinicopathologic study of 30 cases with comparison to well-differentiated endometrioid adenocarcinoma. *Am J Surg Pathol.* 2003;27(9):1253-1259.

92. McConechy MK, Ding J, Senz J, et al. Ovarian and endometrial endometrioid carcinomas have distinct CTNNB1 and PTEN mutation profiles. *Mod Pathol.* 2014;27(1):128-134.

93. Hoang LN, McConechy MK, Köbel M, et al. Polymerase epsilon exonuclease domain mutations in ovarian endometrioid carcinoma. *Int J Gynecol Cancer.* 2015;25(7):1187-1193.

94. Bennett JA, Pesci A, Morales-Oyarvide V, Da Silva A, Nardi V, Oliva E. Incidence of mismatch repair protein deficiency and associated clinicopathologic features in a cohort of 104 ovarian endometrioid carcinomas. *Am J Surg Pathol.* 2019;43(2):235-243.

95. Parra-Herran C, Lerner-Ellis J, Xu B, et al. Molecular-based classification algorithm for endometrial carcinoma categorizes ovarian endometrioid carcinoma into prognostically significant groups. *Mod Pathol.* 2017;30(12):1748-1759.

96. Krämer P, Talhouk A, Brett MA, et al. Endometrial cancer molecular risk stratification is equally prognostic for endometrioid ovarian carcinoma. *Clin Cancer Res.* 2020;26(20):5400-5410.

97. Niskakoski A, Pasanen A, Porkka N, et al. Converging endometrial and ovarian tumorigenesis in lynch syndrome: shared origin of synchronous carcinomas. *Gynecol Oncol.* 2018;150(1):92-98.

98. Rambau PF, Duggan MA, Ghatage P, et al. Significant frequency of MSH2/MSH6 abnormality in ovarian endometrioid carcinoma supports histotype-specific Lynch syndrome screening in ovarian carcinoma. *Histopathology.* 2016;69(2):288-297.

99. Leskela S, Romero I, Cristobal E, et al. Mismatch repair deficiency in ovarian carcinoma: frequency, causes, and consequences. *Am J Surg Pathol.* 2020;44(5):649-656.

100. Rambau PF, Vierkant RA, Intermaggio MP, et al. Association of p16 expression with prognosis varies across ovarian carcinoma histotypes: an ovarian tumor tissue analysis consortium study. *J Pathol Clin Res.* 2018;4(4):250-261.

101. Kelemen LE, Rambau PF, Koziak JM, Steed H, Köbel M. Synchronous endometrial and ovarian carcinomas: predictors of risk and associations with survival and tumor expression profiles. *Cancer Causes Control.* 2017;28(5):447-457.

102. Prat J, FIGO Committee on Gynecologic Oncology. Staging classification for cancer of the ovary, fallopian tube, and peritoneum. *Int J Gynaecol Obstet.* 2014;124(1):1-5.

103. McCluggage WG. My approach to and thoughts on the typing of ovarian carcinomas. *J Clin Pathol.* 2008;61(2):152-163.

104. Soslow RA. Histologic subtypes of ovarian carcinoma: an overview. *Int J Gynecol Pathol.* 2008;27(2):161-174.

105. Rambau PF, McIntyre JB, Taylor J, et al. Morphologic reproducibility, genotyping, and immunohistochemical profiling do not support a category of seromucinous carcinoma of the ovary. *Am J Surg Pathol.* 2017;41(5):685-695.

106. Taylor J, McCluggage WG. Ovarian seromucinous carcinoma: report of a series of a newly categorized and uncommon neoplasm. *Am J Surg Pathol.* 2015;39(7):983-992.

107. Scully RE, Young RH, Clement PB. *Tumors of the Ovary, Maldeveloped Gonads, Fallopian Tube and Broad Ligament.* Armed Forces Institute of Pathology; 1998.

108. Heitz F, Amant F, Fotopoulou C, et al. Synchronous ovarian and endometrial cancer—an international multicenter case-control study. *Int J Gynecol Cancer.* 2014;24(1):54-60.

109. Blake Gilks C, Singh N. Synchronous carcinomas of endometrium and ovary: a pragmatic approach. *Gynecol Oncol Rep.* 2018;27:72-73.

110. Wu CH, Mao TL, Vang R, et al. Endocervical-type mucinous borderline tumors are related to endometrioid tumors based on mutation and loss of expression of ARID1A. *Int J Gynecol Pathol.* 2012;31(4):297-303.

111. Ben-Mussa A, McCluggage WG. Ovarian seromucinous cystadenomas and adenofibromas: first report of a case series. *Histopathology.* 2021;78(3):445-452.

112. Kim KR, Choi J, Hwang JE, et al. Endocervical-like (Müllerian) mucinous borderline tumours of the ovary are frequently associated with the KRAS mutation. *Histopathology.* 2010;57(4):587-596.

113. Nagamine M, Mikami Y. Ovarian seromucinous tumors: pathogenesis, morphologic spectrum, and clinical issues. *Diagnostics (Basel).* 2020;10(2):77.

114. Shappell HW, Riopel MA, Smith Sehdev AE, Ronnett BM, Kurman RJ. Diagnostic criteria and behavior of ovarian seromucinous (endocervical-type mucinous and mixed cell-type) tumors: atypical proliferative (borderline) tumors, intraepithelial, microinvasive, and invasive carcinomas. *Am J Surg Pathol.* 2002;26(12):1529-1541.

115. Rodriguez IM, Irving JA, Prat J. Endocervical-like mucinous borderline tumors of the ovary: a clinicopathologic analysis of 31 cases. *Am J Surg Pathol.* 2004;28(10):1311-1318.

116. Vroobel KM, McCluggage WG. Ovarian clear cell tumors associated with seromucinous borderline tumor: a case series. *Int J Gynecol Pathol.* 2022;41(1):76-81.

117. Zhao C, Wu LS, Barner R. Pathogenesis of ovarian clear cell adenofibroma, atypical proliferative (borderline) tumor, and carcinoma: clinicopathologic features of tumors with endometriosis or adenofibromatous components support two related pathways of tumor development. *J Cancer.* 2011;2:94-106.

118. Uzan C, Dufeu-Lefebvre M, Fauvet R, et al. Management and prognosis of clear cell borderline ovarian tumor. *Int J Gynecol Cancer.* 2012;22(6):993-999.

119. Yamamoto S, Tsuda H, Takano M, Tamai S, Matsubara O. Loss of ARID1A protein expression occurs as an early event in ovarian clear-cell carcinoma development and frequently coexists with PIK3CA mutations. *Mod Pathol.* 2012;25(4):615-624.

120. Köbel M, Kalloger SE, Huntsman DG, et al. Differences in tumor type in low-stage versus high-stage ovarian carcinomas. *Int J Gynecol Pathol.* 2010;29(3):203-211.

121. Yahata T, Banzai C, Tanaka K, Niigata Gynecological Cancer Registry. Histology-specific long-term trends in the incidence of ovarian cancer and borderline tumor in Japanese females: a population-based study from 1983 to 2007 in Niigata. *J Obstet Gynaecol Res.* 2012;38(4):645-650.

122. Chiang YC, Chen CA, Chiang CJ, et al. Trends in incidence and survival outcome of epithelial ovarian cancer: 30-year national population-based registry in Taiwan. *J Gynecol Oncol.* 2013;24(4):342-351.

123. Fuh KC, Shin JY, Kapp DS, et al. Survival differences of Asian and Caucasian epithelial ovarian cancer patients in the united states. *Gynecol Oncol.* 2015;136(3):491-497.

124. Machida H, Matsuo K, Yamagami W, et al. Trends and characteristics of epithelial ovarian cancer in Japan between 2002 and 2015: a JSGO-JSOG joint study. *Gynecol Oncol.* 2019;153(3):589-596.

125. Wu RC, Ayhan A, Maeda D, et al. Frequent somatic mutations of the telomerase reverse transcriptase promoter in ovarian clear cell carcinoma but not in other major types of gynaecological malignancy. *J Pathol.* 2014;232(4):473-481.

126. Huang HN, Chiang YC, Cheng WF, Chen CA, Lin MC, Kuo KT. Molecular alterations in endometrial and ovarian clear cell carcinomas: clinical impacts of telomerase reverse transcriptase promoter mutation. *Mod Pathol.* 2015;28(2):303-311.

127. Parra-Herran C, Bassiouny D, Lerner-Ellis J, et al. p53, Mismatch repair protein, and pole abnormalities in ovarian clear cell carcinoma: an outcome-based clinicopathologic analysis. *Am J Surg Pathol.* 2019;43(12):1591-1599.

128. Ge H, Xiao Y, Qin G, et al. Mismatch repair deficiency is associated with specific morphological features and frequent loss of ARID1A expression in ovarian clear cell carcinoma. *Diagn Pathol.* 2021;16(1):12.

129. Vierkoetter KR, Ayabe AR, VanDrunen M, Ahn HJ, Shimizu DM, Terada KY. Lynch syndrome in patients with clear cell and endometrioid cancers of the ovary. *Gynecol Oncol.* 2014;135(1):81-84.

130. Similä-Maarala J, Soovares P, Pasanen A, et al. TCGA molecular classification in endometriosis-associated ovarian carcinomas: novel data on clear cell carcinoma. *Gynecol Oncol.* 2022;165(3):577-584.

131. Duska LR, Garrett L, Henretta M, Ferriss JS, Lee L, Horowitz N. When 'never-events' occur despite adherence to clinical guidelines: the case of venous thromboembolism in clear cell cancer of the ovary compared with other epithelial histologic subtypes. *Gynecol Oncol.* 2010;116(3):374-377.

132. Lim D, Oliva E. Gynecological neoplasms associated with paraneoplastic hypercalcemia. *Semin Diagn Pathol.* 2019;36(4):246-259.

133. Suh DH, Park JY, Lee JY, et al. The clinical value of surgeons' efforts of preventing intraoperative tumor rupture in stage I clear cell carcinoma of the ovary: a Korean multicenter study. *Gynecol Oncol.* 2015;137(3):412-417.

134. Veras E, Mao TL, Ayhan A, et al. Cystic and adenofibromatous clear cell carcinomas of the ovary: distinctive tumors that differ in their pathogenesis and behavior: a clinicopathologic analysis of 122 cases. *Am J Surg Pathol.* 2009;33(6):844-853.

135. Fadare O, Zhao C, Khabele D, et al. Comparative analysis of Napsin A, Alpha-Methylacyl-Coenzyme A Racemase (AMACR, P504S), and hepatocyte nuclear factor 1 beta as diagnostic markers of ovarian clear cell carcinoma: an immunohistochemical study of 279 ovarian tumours. *Pathology.* 2015;47(2):105-111.

136. Pors J, Segura S, Cheng A, et al. Napsin-A and AMACR are superior to HNF-1β in distinguishing between mesonephric carcinomas and clear cell carcinomas of the gynecologic tract. *Appl Immunohistochem Mol Morphol.* 2020;28(8):593-601.

137. Bennett JA, Dong F, Young RH, Oliva E. Clear cell carcinoma of the ovary: evaluation of prognostic parameters based on a clinicopathological analysis of 100 cases. *Histopathology.* 2015;66(6):808-815.

138. Roma AA, Masand RP. Ovarian Brenner tumors and Walthard nests: a histologic and immunohistochemical study. *Hum Pathol.* 2014;45(12):2417-2422.

139. Ali RH, Seidman JD, Luk M, Kalloger S, Gilks CB. Transitional cell carcinoma of the ovary is related to high-grade serous carcinoma and is distinct from malignant brenner tumor. *Int J Gynecol Pathol.* 2012;31(6):499-506.

140. Karnezis AN, Aysal A, Zaloudek CJ, Rabban JT. Transitional cell-like morphology in ovarian endometrioid carcinoma: morphologic, immunohistochemical, and behavioral features distinguishing it from high-grade serous carcinoma. *Am J Surg Pathol.* 2013;37(1):24-37.

141. Wang Y, Wu RC, Shwartz LE, et al. Clonality analysis of combined Brenner and mucinous tumours of the ovary reveals their monoclonal origin. *J Pathol.* 2015;237(2):146-151.

142. Tafe LJ, Muller KE, Ananda G, et al. Molecular genetic analysis of ovarian brenner tumors and associated mucinous epithelial neoplasms: high variant concordance and identification of mutually exclusive ras driver mutations and myc amplification. *Am J Pathol.* 2016;186(3):671-677.

143. Kuhn E, Ayhan A, Shih IeM, Seidman JD, Kurman RJ. The pathogenesis of atypical proliferative brenner tumor: an immunohistochemical and molecular genetic analysis. *Mod Pathol.* 2014;27(2):231-237.

144. Pfarr N, Darb-Esfahani S, Leichsenring J, et al. Mutational profiles of brenner tumors show distinctive features uncoupling urothelial carcinomas and ovarian carcinoma with transitional cell histology. *Genes Chromosomes Cancer.* 2017;56(10):758-766.

145. Nasioudis D, Sisti G, Holcomb K, Kanninen T, Witkin SS. Malignant brenner tumors of the ovary; a population-based analysis. *Gynecol Oncol.* 2016;142(1):44-49.

146. Mackenzie R, Talhouk A, Eshragh S, et al. Morphologic and molecular characteristics of mixed epithelial ovarian cancers. *Am J Surg Pathol.* 2015;39(11):1548-1557.

147. McCluggage WG, Singh N, Gilks CB. Key changes to the world health organization (WHO) classification of female genital tumours introduced in the 5th edition (2020). *Histopathology.* 2022;80(5):762-778.

148. Jin Z, Ogata S, Tamura G, et al. Carcinosarcomas (malignant mullerian mixed tumors) of the uterus and ovary: a genetic study with special reference to histogenesis. *Int J Gynecol Pathol.* 2003;22(4):368-373.

149. Gotoh O, Sugiyama Y, Takazawa Y, et al. Clinically relevant molecular subtypes and genomic alteration-independent differentiation in gynecologic carcinosarcoma. *Nat Commun.* 2019;10(1):4965.

150. Zhao S, Bellone S, Lopez S, et al. Mutational landscape of uterine and ovarian carcinosarcomas implicates histone genes in epithelial-mesenchymal transition. *Proc Natl Acad Sci U S A.* 2016;113(43):12238-12243.

151. Hollis RL, Croy I, Churchman M, et al. Ovarian carcinosarcoma is a distinct form of ovarian cancer with poorer survival compared to tubo-ovarian high-grade serous carcinoma. *Br J Cancer.* 2022;127(6):1034-1042.

152. Mirkovic J, McFarland M, Garcia E, et al. Targeted genomic profiling reveals recurrent KRAS mutations in mesonephric-like adenocarcinomas of the female genital tract. *Am J Surg Pathol.* 2018;42(2):227-233.

153. Chapel DB, Joseph NM, Krausz T, Lastra RR. An ovarian adenocarcinoma with combined low-grade serous and mesonephric morphologies suggests a müllerian origin for some mesonephric carcinomas. *Int J Gynecol Pathol.* 2018;37(5):448-459.

154. Dundr P, Gregová M, Němejcová K, et al. Ovarian mesonephric-like adenocarcinoma arising in serous borderline tumor: a case report with complex morphological and molecular analysis. *Diagn Pathol.* 2020;15(1):91.

155. McCluggage WG, Vosmikova H, Laco J. Ovarian combined low-grade serous and mesonephric-like adenocarcinoma: further evidence for a mullerian origin of mesonephric-like adenocarcinoma. *Int J Gynecol Pathol.* 2020;39(1):84-92.

156. Koh HH, Park E, Kim HS. Mesonephric-like adenocarcinoma of the ovary: clinicopathological and molecular characteristics. *Diagnostics (Basel).* 2022;12(2):326.

157. McFarland M, Quick CM, McCluggage WG. Hormone receptor-negative, thyroid transcription factor 1-positive uterine and ovarian adenocarcinomas: report of a series of mesonephric-like adenocarcinomas. *Histopathology.* 2016;68(7):1013-1020.

158. Silva EM, Fix DJ, Sebastiao APM, et al. Mesonephric and mesonephric-like carcinomas of the female genital tract: molecular characterization including cases with mixed histology and matched metastases. *Mod Pathol.* 2021;34(8):1570-1587.

159. Coatham M, Li X, Karnezis AN, et al. Concurrent ARID1A and ARID1B inactivation in endometrial and ovarian dedifferentiated carcinomas. *Mod Pathol.* 2016;29(12):1586-1593.

160. Tafe LJ, Garg K, Chew I, Tornos C, Soslow RA. Endometrial and ovarian carcinomas with undifferentiated components: clinically aggressive and frequently underrecognized neoplasms. *Mod Pathol.* 2010;23(6):781-789.

161. Silva EG, Deavers MT, Bodurka DC, Malpica A. Association of low-grade endometrioid carcinoma of the uterus and ovary with undifferentiated carcinoma: a new type of dedifferentiated carcinoma? *Int J Gynecol Pathol.* 2006;25(1):52-58.

162. Witkowski L, Goudie C, Foulkes WD, McCluggage WG. Small-Cell carcinoma of the ovary of hypercalcemic type (malignant rhabdoid tumor of the ovary): a review with recent developments on pathogenesis. *Surg Pathol Clin.* 2016;9(2):215-226.

163. Goode B, Joseph NM, Stevers M, et al. Adenomatoid tumors of the male and female genital tract are defined by TRAF7 mutations that drive aberrant NF-kB pathway activation. *Mod Pathol.* 2018;31(4):660-673.

164. Rapisarda AMC, Cianci A, Caruso S, et al. Benign multicystic mesothelioma and peritoneal inclusion cysts: are they the same clinical and histopathological entities? A systematic review to find an evidence-based management. *Arch Gynecol Obstet.* 2018;297(6):1353-1375.

165. Sinha R, Bustamante B, Tahmasebi F, Goldberg GL. Malignant female adnexal tumor of probable wolffian origin (FATWO): a case report and review for the literature. *Gynecol Oncol Rep.* 2021;36:100726.

166. Bennett JA, Ritterhouse LL, Furtado LV, et al. Female adnexal tumors of probable Wolffian origin: morphological, immunohistochemical, and molecular analysis of 15 cases. *Mod Pathol.* 2020;33(4):734-747.

167. Kolin DL, Nucci MR. Fallopian tube neoplasia and mimics. *Surg Pathol Clin.* 2019;12(2):457-479.

168. Na K, Kim HS. Clinicopathological characteristics of fallopian tube metastases from primary endometrial, cervical, and nongynecological malignancies: a single institutional experience. *Virchows Arch.* 2017;471(3):363-373.

169. Rabban JT, Vohra P, Zaloudek CJ. Nongynecologic metastases to fallopian tube mucosa: a potential mimic of tubal high-grade serous carcinoma and benign tubal mucinous metaplasia or nonmucinous hyperplasia. *Am J Surg Pathol.* 2015;39(1):35-51.

170. Kommoss F, Faruqi A, Gilks CB, et al. Uterine serous carcinomas frequently metastasize to the fallopian tube and can mimic serous tubal intraepithelial carcinoma. *Am J Surg Pathol.* 2017;41(2):161-170.

171. Singh R, Cho KR. Serous tubal intraepithelial carcinoma or not? Metastases to fallopian tube mucosa can masquerade as in situ lesions. *Arch Pathol Lab Med.* 2017;141(10):1313-1315.

CHAPTER **8.8**

Epithelial Ovarian Cancer: Prognostic Factors

Kathryn A. Mills and Ernst Lengyel

TUMOR STAGE

The OC FIGO staging system (**Table 8.6-1**) was updated in 2014. Although there continues to be variability in outcomes for patients with the same stage of disease, which reflects both the importance of the completeness of staging (particularly for early-stage disease) and the differing biology of the histologic subtypes of OC, stage itself remains one of the most important prognostic factors. U.S. SEER data from 2011 to 2017 show a 5-year relative survival of 93% for patients with stage I disease, 75% for those with stage II disease, and 30% for distant disease (stages III and IV) (1,2). Data from the United Kingdom in the Million Women study similarly demonstrate that those with advanced-stage disease (FIGO stage III/IV) had the poorest OS at a dismal 12% and 7%, respectively (3) (**Table 8.8-1**).

AGE

Older women have a much worse prognosis. In the Million Women study, each 5-year incremental increase in age was associated with

a 19% increased risk of death from OC (3). This is in part because they have an increased incidence of high-stage and high-grade disease at the time of diagnosis (**Table 8.8-2**) (4). Moreover, they may be less able to tolerate aggressive therapy. Interestingly, the impact of age may become less critical as time from diagnosis and treatment increases (3).

PROGNOSTIC VARIABLES IN EARLY-STAGE DISEASE

About one-quarter of patients present with stage I or II EOC (**Table 8.8-3**) (5), and for this cohort, prognostic factors may help inform whether or not chemotherapy should be administered (**Figure 8.9-1**). A multivariable analysis for recurrence from GOG trials 95 and 157, both of which enrolled surgically staged volunteers with "high-risk early-stage" disease (ie, 1988 FIGO stage IA/B grade 3, stage IC or II any grade, stage I or II clear cell), identified four independent predictors of worse prognosis: age greater than 60 years (HR 1.57), stage II (HR 2.7 vs stage IA or IB), grade 2 (HR

■ **TABLE 8.8-1. 1-, 5-, and 10-Year Survival, Overall and by Tumor Stage at Diagnosis and Histologic Type in the Prospective U.K. Million Women Study**

| Ovarian Cancer Type | Cases | % Survival at Timepoint (95% CI) | | |
		1 Year	5 Years	10 Years
All ovarian cancer	13,085	76 (75-77)	38 (37-39)	29 (28-30)
Fully malignant ovarian cancer (excluding borderline tumors)	11,954	74 (73-74)	33 (32-34)	23 (22-24)
Stage at diagnosis				
Stage I	1,853	97 (97-98)	87 (86-89)	81 (79-83)
Stage II	515	88 (85-91)	62 (58-67)	47 (42-52)
Stage III	3,705	76 (74-77)	26 (24-27)	12 (11-14)
Stage IV	1,758	61 (58-63)	14 (13-16)	7 (5-8)
Unknown	5,254	72 (71-73)	36 (35-38)	28 (27-30)
Ovarian cancer histotypes				
Serous borderline tumor	514	99 (98-100)	95 (93-97)	92 (89-95)
Mucinous borderline tumor	617	99 (98-100)	97 (95-98)	96 (94-97)
Serous carcinoma	6,060	80 (79-81)	31 (30-32)	18 (17-19)
Mucinous carcinoma	575	81 (77-84)	63 (59-67)	57 (53-61)
Endometrioid carcinoma	797	93 (91-94)	69 (65-72)	59 (55-63)
Clear cell carcinoma	517	85 (82-88)	54 (50-59)	47 (42-51)
Carcinosarcoma	376	60 (55-65)	21 (17-25)	17 (13-21)
Other/Unspecified	3,629	56 (55-58)	21 (20-23)	15 (13-16)

Table shows ovarian cancer–specific survival at 1, 5, and 10 yrs from diagnosis, calculated using a lifetable approach, for all Million Women study participants diagnosed with ovarian cancer, after exclusion of 137 cases diagnosed at death (*N* = 13,085). The above crude survival data are unadjusted for age, stage, or other factors.

From Gaitskell KR, Hermon C, Barnes I, et al. Ovarian cancer survival by stage, histotype, and pre-diagnostic lifestyle factors, in the prospective UK Million Women Study. *Cancer Epidemiol.* 2022;76:102074.

■ TABLE 8.8-2. SEER Data 1975 to 2001

	Incidence of Stage by Age Group		
Age Group (n)	Stage I, n (%)	Stage II, n (%)	Stage III-IV, n (%)
<20 (628)	388 (62)	46 (7)	194 (31)
20-49 (10,243)	4,340 (42)	773 (8)	5,130 (50)
50-59 (10,788)	2,830 (26)	833 (8)	7, 125 (66)
60-69 (12,201)	2,162 (18)	767(6)	9,272 (76)
70-79 (10,259)	1,409 (14)	636 (6)	8,214 (80)
80+ (3,813)	707 (12)	389 (69)	4,717 (81)
Total 47,932	11,836 (24.6)	3,444 (7.2)	34,652 (72.3)
5-yr relative survival by age group and stage			
20-49	0.93	0.87	0.38
50-59	0.91	0.68	0.31
60-69	0.94	0.61	0.23
70-79	0.77	0.51	0.14
80+	0.69	0.11	0.03

AFP, α-fetoprotein; CA-125, cancer antigen 125; CRP, C-reactive protein; DHEAS, dehydroepiandrosterone sulfate; FSH, follicle-stimulating hormone; GnRH, gonadotropin-releasing hormone; GO, gonorrhea; hCG, human chorionic gonadotropin; LDH, lactic dehydrogenase; LLQ, left lower quadrant; OCP, oral contraceptive pill; PID, pelvic inflammatory disease; RLQ, right lower quadrant; SEER, Surveillance, Epidemiology, and End Results.

Adapted from Wright JD, Chen L, Tergas AI, et al. Trends in relative survival for ovarian cancer from 1975 to 2011. *Obstet Gynecol.* 2015;125(6):1345-1352.

1.84 vs grade 1) or grade 3 (HR 2.47 vs grade 1), and positive cytology (HR 1.72) (6).

Malignant ascites is associated with worse outcomes and is incorporated into stage. Although capsular rupture should be avoided where possible, the data on the prognostic significance of capsular rupture are conflicting, likely because there are several confounding variables, including time of rupture (preoperative vs intraoperative) and cause of rupture (spontaneous vs iatrogenic). The current 2013 FIGO staging system (**Table 8.6-1**) separates out these categories, which were previously all lumped together as stage IC. Tumor size is not prognostic in stage I disease; low-grade early-stage tumors may be very large.

Uncertainty remains regarding adhesions. Adherence is judged to be dense if a sharp dissection is required to mobilize the tumor, when a raw area is left in the place of adherence, or when cyst rupture results from dissecting the adhesions free. The staging is more straightforward when the surgeon encounters discrete implants separate from the primary tumor or when solid tumor is found invading adjacent structures. However, more often, there is apparently benign adherence of an ovarian tumor to adjacent structures in the absence of metastatic implants or obvious direct tumor extension. Older literature suggests that such "benign" adhesions, when dense—the tumor attached to the pelvic sidewall or the sigmoid colon, are associated with a relapse risk equivalent to stage II

■ TABLE 8.8-3. Distribution of 562 Invasive Ovarian Carcinomas by Cell Type, Washington Hospital Center, 1991 to 2013

	Stage I	Stage II	Stage III	Stage IV	Total (%)
High-grade serous	11	18	248	94	371 (66.0)
Low-grade serous	2	0	22	5	29 (5.2)
Endometrioid	21	8	10	2	41 (7.3)
Clear cell	24	8	10	3	45 (8.0)
Mucinous	13	1	1	0	15 (2.7)
Transitional	6	0	0	0	6 (1.1)
Carcinosarcoma	1	5	21	7	34 (6.0)
Seromucinous	4	1	0	0	5 (0.9)
Mixed	4	3	4	2	13 (2.3)
Undifferentiated	0	1	1	0	2 (0.4)
Squamous	0	0	0	1	1 (0.2)
Total (%)	86 (15.3)	45 (8.0)	317 (56.4)	114 (20.3)	562

High-grade serous includes those of peritoneal and tubal origin. Transitional cell carcinomas (other than malignant Brenner tumors) are classified as high-grade serous carcinoma (see text).

From Seidman JD, Vang R, Ronnett BM, et al. Distribution and case-fatality ratios by cell type for ovarian carcinomas: a 22 year series of 562 patients with uniform, current histological classification. *Gynecol Oncol.* 2015;136:336-340.

(7). However, a review from 2015 did not identify dense adhesions as an independent prognostic factor (5).

Histologic Subtype

The distribution of cell types in early-stage disease is very different from the distribution in advanced-stage disease. Most advanced-stage cancers are of high-grade serous histology, whereas less than a quarter of early-stage cancers are serous. Endometrioid and clear cell cancers tend to present at an early stage (Table 8.8-3). Serous histology has been reported to be a poor prognostic factor in stage I disease, especially in patients who have not been comprehensively staged (1). From 4% to 25% of patients with apparent stage I OC will have nodal involvement when lymph nodes are pathologically examined; the risk for lymph node involvement correlates with histology (high risk with high-grade serous and clear cell tumors) and grade (higher risk with higher grade). In addition, ovarian carcinosarcoma portends a dismal diagnosis, even at early stage, with only 60% of all patients diagnosed alive at 1 year (1,3). In early stage, locoregional diseases clear cell cancers have a better prognosis than HGSCs (1). While patients with advanced-stage mucinous tumors also fare poorly, stage I mucinous tumors are generally low grade and have a good prognosis (Figure 8.9-2A,B).

When reading older series regarding the importance of tumor histology, it should be remembered that diagnostic criteria for the major cell types of ovarian carcinoma have undergone significant shifts over the past two decades. Serous carcinomas have been more clearly distinguished from endometrioid carcinoma and clear cell carcinomas with which they have often been confused. Serous carcinoma has been divided into two distinct groups, the more common high grade and the less common low grade, which are no longer considered different grades of the same tumor, but rather biologically different tumor entities.

Grade

Analyzing tumor grade as a prognostic factor, in general, in stage I disease is problematic because of the interplay between histologic subtype and grade and because of issues with reproducibility of grade. Three of the five types of carcinomas, HGSOC, LGSOC, and clear cell carcinoma, already have a designated grade by definition. In studies that do not separately analyze tumors by cell type, grade is associated not only with the likelihood of lymph node involvement in apparent stage I disease but also with the likelihood of recurrence in fully staged patients with stage I disease. Once cell type is determined, grade adds information primarily for endometrioid and mucinous cell types. From FIGO data for surgically staged stage I disease (8), the 5-year OS is 92%, 85%, and 79% for grade 1, 2, and 3 tumors, respectively. Stage IA and IB grade 1 carcinomas have disease-specific survival rates as high as 97% in the absence of any adjuvant therapy.

CA-125 Levels in Early-Stage Disease

A report analyzing data from 600 surgically staged (including lymphadenectomy) patients with FIGO stage I EOC found preoperative serum CA-125 30 U/mL or higher to be an independent predictor of decreased survival (HR 2.7) (9). Clear cell and mucinous tumors had somewhat lower preoperative CA-125 levels. The only independent predictive factor other than CA-125 was age greater than 70 years (HR 2.6).

PROGNOSTIC VARIABLES IN STAGE III/IV DISEASE

Volume of Residual Disease After Surgery

The volume of residual disease following cytoreduction surgery is consistently and directly correlated with survival for both stage III and stage IV diseases (Figure 8.6-5). Most series have focused on the size of the largest residual mass and not the total number of lesions, but the number of residual masses may be an important prognostic factor as well. There is, of course, a correlation between volume of disease before surgery and residual disease remaining after surgery (10). While patients with stage IIIC disease who are without residual disease after surgery do better than patients with stage IIIC disease who have macroscopic residual disease, they still have a significantly worse prognosis than patients with stage IIIA disease (who are more likely to have low-grade tumors). The surgical aspects of OC management are covered in Section 6.

Histologic Subtype and Grade in Advanced Disease

In advanced-stage disease, mucinous and clear cell histologies are associated with a significantly worse prognosis than HGSCs, likely because of chemotherapy resistance (1). Advanced-stage endometrioid tumors are associated with a better prognosis than advanced-stage serous tumors (Figure 8.9-2A,B). The prognostic importance of histology holds even in stage IV disease; a study from Japan reported that women with serous or endometrioid tumors had a median OS of 3.1 versus 0.9 years for those with clear cell or mucinous tumors (11).

When reviewing 12 GOG studies, the PFS (HR 0.69; CI 0.5-0.96) was longer in clear cell cancer than in HGSC with a trend toward improved OS (HR 0.76; CI 0.53-1.09) in early stages (I and II) (12). However, in advanced stage, clear cell cancer had worse PFS and OS (HR1.66, CI 1.43-1.91) (Figure 8.8.1).

It must be remembered that grade, cell type, and stage are confounded; the grade is contained in the definition of three of the five cell types of ovarian carcinoma. LGSCs are more likely to be stage IIIA or IIIB as compared to HGSCs, which nearly always presents as stage IIIC or IV disease. In addition, LGSCs occur in younger women who tend to have less comorbidity.

An analysis of tumors of women treated on GOG #158 (which included only women with optimally debulked stage III disease) found that 8.7% of women with LGSC had a median PFS of 45 versus 19.8 months for the women with high-grade disease (13). Median OS was 126 months for those with LGSC versus 67.6% for those with HGSC. In GOG #182, which included patients with optimal and suboptimally cytoreduced stage III-IV disease, women with LGSC and no gross residual disease after surgery ($n = 47$) had the best outcomes, with a median OS of 97 versus 77 months for those with HGSC and no gross residual disease ($n = 358$) (14). On the other hand, women with LGSC and gross residual disease did not fare much better than their counterparts with HGSC and residual disease. Median OS was 42 months for those with LGSC and gross residual disease versus 38 months for those with HGSC and gross residual disease.

CA-125 Levels in Advanced Disease

Although not all patients with advanced OC have an elevated serum CA-125 level, serum levels of CA-125 generally reflect volume of disease in women with initially elevated levels. Postoperative (prechemotherapy) CA-125 levels have prognostic significance. Decline of CA-125 with chemotherapy is also prognostic. In one study, normalization of CA-125 (level <35 U/mL) after the third cycle of treatment was associated with a median OS of 42 months compared to a median OS of 22 months for those whose CA-125 did not normalize. This association held true even within the subgroup of optimal microscopically debulked patients (15). Patients with premaintenance baseline CA-125 values 10 U/mL or less have a superior PFS compared to those with higher levels, even if in the normal CA-125 range (16).

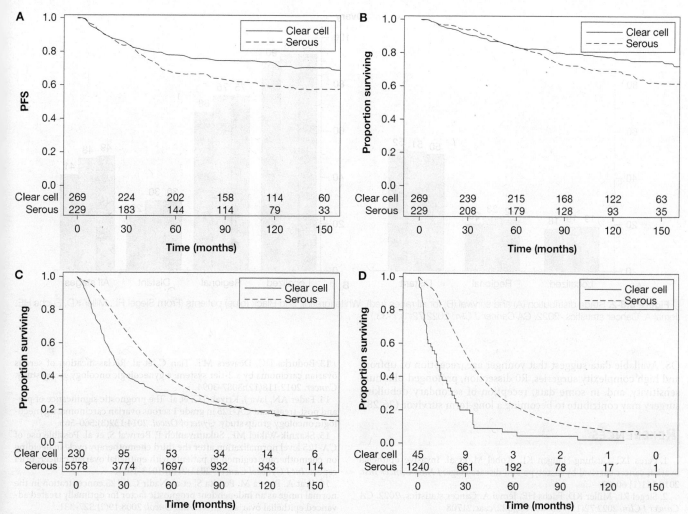

Figure 8.8-1. PFS and OS in patients with early-stage clear cell ovarian cancer. OS, overall survival; PFS, progression-free survival.(From Oliver KE, Brady WE, Birrer M, et al. An evaluation of progression free survival and overall survival of ovarian cancer patients with clear cell carcinoma versus serous carcinoma treated with platinum therapy: an NRG Oncology/Gynecologic Oncology Group experience. *Gynecol Oncol.* 2017;147(2):243-249.)

Other Prognostic Factors

Poor performance status and an increased number of patient-reported symptoms, particularly lower extremity edema, are associated with worse outcomes. Increased BMI at the time of diagnosis has not been previously associated with increased mortality in most studies, but a recent study did show a modest decrease in survival with higher prediagnostic BMI of 30 or above (3). A prediagnosis history of vigorous exercise was shown in the WHI to be associated with a 26% lower risk of OC-specific mortality, though this has not always been true in available studies (17). Perioperative infection has been reported to be an independent risk factor for poor outcomes, with an associated decrease in median OS by nearly 2 years (18). Thrombocytosis has been reported to be associated with advanced disease and shortened survival (19) as has perioperative venous thromboembolism (VTE) (20). VTE is more common in women with clear cell carcinomas, but the poor prognosis was independent of histology. In a recent retrospective study of 227 patients with clear cell carcinoma, those with VTE had decreased optimal cytoreduction and decreased OS (21).

In the United States, African American race is associated with worse outcomes, and this disparity has been increasing over time; differences in access to care may account for a large portion of this finding, as studies at single institutions with consistent treatment of patients or on clinical trials do not show significant differences

in outcomes by race (22). However, on a national level, social determinants of health do affect OC survival. Despite having no difference in the genetic makeup of the cancer and similar clinical stage distribution, African American patients have a significantly lower survival (**Figure 8.8-2**) (2,23). A Black woman has a 41% chance of surviving 5 years from the time of her diagnosis, whereas a White woman has a 48% chance, indicating Black women account for none of the survival gains in OC seen over the past 20 years. One factor contributing to this disparity in survival includes less access to an experienced, high-volume gynecologic oncologist. Indeed, being Black was associated with a decrease likelihood of a hysterectomy, and colon and lymph node resection (24). Another factor is adjuvant treatment; a Black woman is less likely to be treated according to guidelines and receive timely adjuvant chemotherapy (25). While some of this might be accounted for by higher comorbidity scores and economic factors of Black patients, institutionalized racism may also be a factor.

Long-Term Survivors

Investigators have sought to understand the patients with advanced-stage disease who go on to become long-term survivors. These are generally defined as patients who survive greater than 7 to 10 years after diagnosis, and at most, 10% to 15% of patients will fall into this category. Unfortunately, OC is still an incurable disease, and most novel treatments improve PFS, but not

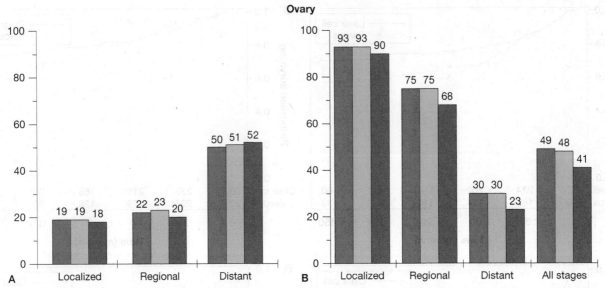

Figure 8.8-2. Stage distribution (A) and survival (B) for all races (red), White (green), and Black (blue) patients (From Siegel RL, Miller KD, Fuchs HE, Jemal A. Cancer statistics, 2022. *CA Cancer J Clin.* 2022;72(1):7-33.)

OS. Available data suggest that younger age, reception of upfront and high complexity surgeries, R0 dissection, prolonged platinum sensitivity, and, in some data, reception of secondary debulking surgery may contribute to becoming a long-term survivor (26-28).

REFERENCES

1. Peres LC, Cushing-Haugen KL, Kobel M, et al. Invasive epithelial ovarian cancer survival by histotype and disease stage. *J Natl Cancer Inst.* 2019;111(1):60-68.

2. Siegel RL, Miller KD, Fuchs HE, Jemal A. Cancer statistics, 2022. *CA Cancer J Clin.* 2022;72(1):7-33. doi:10.3322/caac.21708

3. Gaitskell K, Hermon C, Barnes I, et al. Ovarian cancer survival by stage, histotype, and pre-diagnostic lifestyle factors, in the prospective UK million women study. *Cancer Epidemiol.* 2022;76:102074. doi:10.1016/j.canep.2021.102074

4. Wright AA, Cronin A, Milne D, et al. Effect of intraperitoneal chemotherapy on survival for ovarian cancer in clinical practice and frequency of use. *J Clin Oncol.* 2014;32:5576. Accessed November 27, 2014. https://ascopubs.org/doi/10.1200/jco.2014.32.15_suppl.5576

5. Seidman JD, Vang R, Ronnett BM, Yemelyanova A, Cosin JA. Distribution and case-fatality ratios by cell-type for ovarian carcinomas: a 22-year series of 562 patients with uniform current histological classification. *Gynecol Oncol.* 2015;136(2):336-340.

6. Chan JK, Tian C, Monk BJ, et al. Prognostic factors for high-risk early-stage epithelial ovarian cancer: a gynecologic oncology group study. *Cancer.* 2008;112(10):2202-2210.

7. Dembo AJ, Davy M, Stenwig AE, Berle EJ, Bush RS, Kjorstad K. Prognostic factors in patients with stage I epithelial ovarian cancer. *Obstet Gynecol.* 1990;75(2):263-273.

8. Heintz AP, Odicino F, Maisonneuve P, et al. Carcinoma of the ovary. FIGO 26th annual report on the results of treatment in gynecological cancer. *Int J Gynaecol Obstet.* 2006;95(Suppl. 1):S161-S192. doi:10.1016/S0020-7292(06)60033-7

9. Obermair A. Preoperative serum CA125 in surgical stage 1 epithelial ovarian cancer. *Gynecol Oncol.* 2007;107(2):357-358.

10. Horowitz NS, Miller A, Rungruang B, et al. Does aggressive surgery improve outcomes? Interaction between preoperative disease burden and complex surgery in patients with advanced-stage ovarian cancer: an analysis of GOG 182. *J Clin Oncol.* 2015;33(8):937-943.

11. Mizuno M, Kajiyama H, Shibata K, et al. Prognostic value of histological type in stage IV ovarian carcinoma: a retrospective analysis of 223 patients. *Br J Cancer.* 2015;112(8):1376-1383.

12. Oliver KE, Brady WE, Birrer M, et al. An evaluation of progression free survival and overall survival of ovarian cancer patients with clear cell carcinoma versus serous carcinoma treated with platinum therapy: an NRG oncology/gynecologic oncology group experience. *Gynecol Oncol.* 2017;147(2):243-249.

13. Bodurka DC, Deavers MT, Tian C, et al. Reclassification of serous ovarian carcinoma by a 2-tier system: a gynecologic oncology group study. *Cancer.* 2012;118(12):3087-3094.

14. Fader AN, Java J, Krivak TC, et al. The prognostic significance of pre- and post-treatment CA-125 in grade 1 serous ovarian carcinoma: a gynecologic oncology group study. *Gynecol Oncol.* 2014;132(3):560-565.

15. Skaznik-Wikiel ME, Sukumvanich P, Beriwal S, et al. Possible use of CA-125 level normalization after the third chemotherapy cycle in deciding on chemotherapy regimen in patients with epithelial ovarian cancer: brief report. *Int J Gynecol Cancer.* 2011;21(6):1013-1017.

16. Prat A, Parera M, Peralta S, et al. Nadir CA-125 concentration in the normal range as an independent prognostic factor for optimally treated advanced epithelial ovarian cancer. *Ann Oncol.* 2008;19(2):327-331.

17. Zhou Y, Chlebowski R, LaMonte MJ, et al. Body mass index, physical activity, and mortality in women diagnosed with ovarian cancer: results from the women's health initiative. *Gynecol Oncol.* 2014;133(1):4-10.

18. Matsuo K, Prather CP, Ahn EH, et al. Significance of perioperative infection in survival of patients with ovarian cancer. *Int J Gynecol Cancer.* 2012;22(2):245-253.

19. Stone RL, Nick AM, McNeish IA, et al. Paraneoplastic thrombocytosis in ovarian cancer. *N Engl J Med.* 2012;366(7):610-618.

20. Gunderson CC, Thomas ED, Slaughter KN, et al. The survival detriment of venous thromboembolism with epithelial ovarian cancer. *Gynecol Oncol.* 2014;134(1):73-77.

21. Ye S, Yang J, Cao D, et al. Characteristic and prognostic implication of venous thromboembolism in ovarian clear cell carcinoma: a 12-year retrospective study. *PLoS One.* 2015;10(3):e0121818.

22. Terplan M, Temkin S, Tergas A, Lengyel E. Does equal treatment yield equal outcomes? The impact of race on survival in epithelial ovarian cancer. *Gynecol Oncol.* 2008;111(2):173-178.

23. Somasegar S, Weiss AS, Norquist BM, et al. Germline mutations in black patients with ovarian, fallopian tube and primary peritoneal carcinomas. *Gynecol Oncol.* 2021;163(1):130-133.

24. Bristow RE, Zahurak ML, Ibeanu OA. Racial disparities in ovarian cancer surgical care: a population-based analysis. *Gynecol Oncol.* 2011;121(2):364-368.

25. Chen F, Bailey CE, Alvarez RD, Shu XO, Zheng W. Adherence to treatment guidelines as a major determinant of survival disparities between black and white patients with ovarian cancer. *Gynecol Oncol.* 2021;160(1):10-15. doi:10.1016/j.ygyno.2020.10.040

26. Hoppenot C, Eckert MA, Tienda SM, Lengyel E. Who are the long-term survivors of high grade serous ovarian cancer? *Gynecol Oncol.* 2018;148(1):204-212.

27. Clarke CL, Kushi LH, Chubak J, et al. Predictors of long-term survival among high-grade serous ovarian cancer patients. *Cancer Epidemiol Biomarkers Prev.* 2019;28(5):996-999.

28. Javellana M, Hoppenot C, Lengyel E. The road to long-term survival: surgical approach and longitudinal treatments of long-term survivors of advanced-stage serous ovarian cancer. *Gynecol Oncol.* 2019;152(2):228-234.

CHAPTER **8.9**

Management of Early-Stage Ovarian Cancer

Katherine C. Kurnit and Gini F. Fleming

MANAGEMENT OF EARLY-STAGE (I AND II) OVARIAN CANCER

Approximately 25% of women with ovarian carcinoma present with stage I or II disease. An algorithm for standard management of early-stage disease is shown in **Figure 8.9-1**. Unlike advanced-stage OCs, which are usually HGSCs, early-stage tumors are more often of mucinous, clear cell, or endometrioid histology (**Table 8.7-2**).

Surgical Therapy for Early-Stage Ovarian Carcinoma

Surgical management of newly diagnosed OC, including consideration of fertility-sparing approaches, is covered in Chapter 8.6.

Postoperative Therapy for Stage I Ovarian Carcinoma

Patients with stage IA and IB grade 1 carcinomas have disease-specific survival rates as high as 97% in the absence of any postoperative therapy and hence adjuvant therapy is not recommended (**Figure 8.9-2**) (1,2). Support for this comes from GOG trials conducted in the 1990s, which showed that overall, patients with stage IA or IB and grade 1 or 2 disease had a 5-year DFS rate of 91% and a 5-year OS rate of 94% with surgery alone (3). Beyond this, other patients with early-stage disease have a risk of recurrence sufficiently high enough to warrant adjuvant therapy,

although the benefit of such treatment has been difficult to ascertain because the number of patients with higher grade early-stage disease is small (so trials are difficult to complete) and the overall risk of recurrence is small (so large trials are needed). Published trials have included multiple histologic types with very different biology and variable staging and generally have lacked the power to show interactions between treatment and grade or histologic subtype. In addition, treatment at recurrence may be curative for a small number of patients who did not receive initial adjuvant treatment.

Chemotherapy for Early-Stage High-Grade Serous Cancers

As shown in **Figure 8.9-1**, postoperative chemotherapy is usually recommended for patients with high-grade stage IA or IB tumors and most tumors of stage IC or higher. But it must be appreciated that we do not have good evidence that such treatment improves OS (**Table 8.9-1**). Most are older trials, have patients with variably staged tumors, and included patients with OC of multiple different histologic subtypes. Despite this, although individual trial results vary somewhat, as a group they have shown consistent improvement in DFS for postoperative chemotherapy versus observation or radiotherapy. The only clear demonstration of an OS benefit in the treatment of early-stage OC comes from a joint analysis of two large European trials, which together randomized 923 patients with early-stage disease (over 90% stage I) to receive either platinum-based chemotherapy or no initial adjuvant treatment

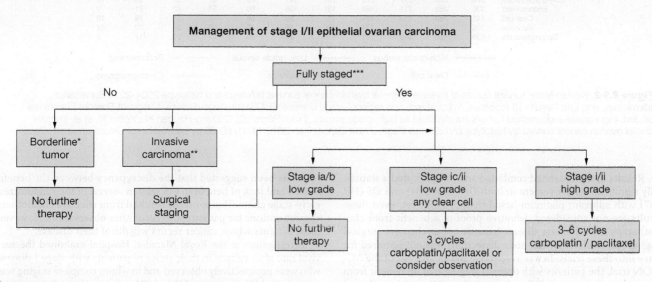

Figure 8.9-1. Management of stage I/II epithelial ovarian carcinoma.

*For unstaged borderline tumors that have intraepithelial carcinoma, micropapillary architecture >5 mm, or microinvasion, consider staging using a minimally invasive approach.

**some data suggest that the risk of nodal metastases in expansile mucinous tumors is low enough that further staging is not warranted; in some situations, uterus and contralateral ovary may be preserved.

***full staging includes removal of the affected ovary and tube, omentectomy, lymph node dissection, possible appendectomy.

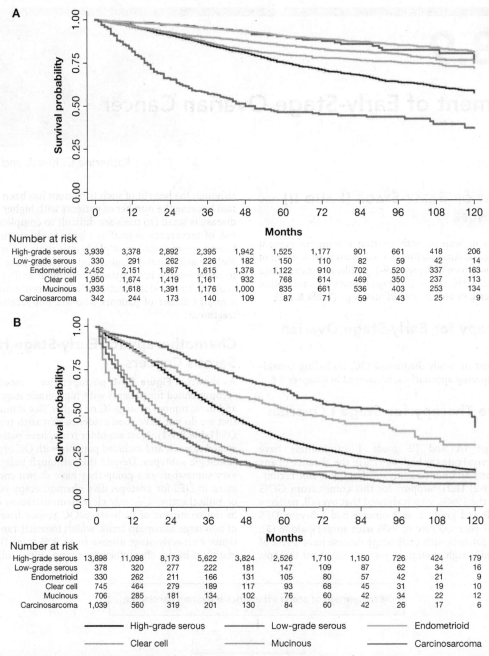

Number at risk										
High-grade serous	3,939	3,378	2,892	2,395	1,942	1,525	1,177	901	661	418	206
Low-grade serous	330	291	262	226	182	150	110	82	59	42	14
Endometrioid	2,452	2,151	1,867	1,615	1,378	1,122	910	702	520	337	163
Clear cell	1,950	1,674	1,419	1,161	932	768	614	469	350	237	113
Mucinous	1,935	1,618	1,391	1,176	1,000	835	661	536	403	253	134
Carcinosarcoma	342	244	173	140	109	87	71	59	43	25	9

Number at risk										
High-grade serous	13,898	11,098	8,173	5,622	3,824	2,526	1,710	1,150	726	424	179
Low-grade serous	378	320	277	222	181	147	109	87	62	34	16
Endometrioid	330	262	211	166	131	105	80	57	42	21	9
Clear cell	745	464	279	189	117	93	68	45	31	19	10
Mucinous	706	285	181	134	102	76	60	42	34	22	12
Carcinosarcoma	1,039	560	319	201	130	84	60	42	26	17	6

Figure 8.9-2. Kaplan-Meier survival curves of invasive epithelial ovarian cancer survival by stage and histotype 2004-2014 Surveillance, Epidemiology, and End Results 18 registries. A: Localized- and regional-stage disease. B: Distant-stage disease. Malignant Brenner tumors are excluded. High-grade endometrioid tumors are classified as high-grade serous. (From Peres LC, Cushing-Haugen KL, Kobel M, et al. Invasive epithelial ovarian cancer survival by histotype and disease stage. *J Natl Cancer Inst*. 2019;111(1):60-68.by permission of Oxford University Press)

(4). Results of a preplanned combined analysis indicated a statistically significant improvement in both DFS (HR 0.64) and OS (HR 0.67) with adjuvant platinum-based therapy (4,5). Yet, even these results are not considered definitive proof of a benefit from chemotherapy in early-stage disease because comprehensive surgical staging (particularly lymph node dissection) was not required for entry into these trials. In a retrospective subset analysis of the ACTION trial, the patients with optimal staging had no benefit from chemotherapy, suggesting that the overall positive results reflected the benefit of chemotherapy in women with low-volume stage III disease. However, only 151 patients (of variable histology) were optimally staged, which is too few to provide statistical power for firm conclusions about the benefit of chemotherapy in this subgroup (Figure 8.9-3).

It has been suggested that the discrepancy between the benefit in DFS and lack of benefit in OS seen in several of the randomized early-stage chemotherapy trials resulted from effective chemotherapeutic options for patients who recur after observation. However, most patients whose cancer recurs will die of their disease.

Investigators at the Royal Marsden Hospital examined the survival rate after relapse in their series of patients with stage I disease who were prospectively observed and in whom complete staging was not required (6). Sixty-one (31%) of 194 patients relapsed at a median of 17 months (range, 6 months to 15.7 years), and 55 of them received platinum-based chemotherapy at the time of relapse. PFS at 5 years after relapse was only 24%. In an updated analysis, the authors compared patients with relapsed stage I disease to patients with stage IIIC disease and found similar disease-specific survival outcomes (7).

■ TABLE 8.9-1. Randomized Trials of Platinum-Based Chemotherapy in Early-Stage Ovarian Carcinoma

Author (yr)	N	Eligibility	Arms	Outcome
Chiara (1994)	70	Stage IA/B Gr 3, any IC, II	WAR vs cisplatin/cyclophosphamide	5-yr OS 53% vs 71% RFS 50% vs 74% P = NS Only 67% of patients completed WAR
Bolis (1995)	83	Stage IA/B Gr 2/3	Observation vs cisplatin	5-yr DFS 65% vs 83% 5-yr OS 82% vs 88%
Trope (2000)	162	Stage I Gr 2/3 or Gr 1 aneuploid/clear cell	Observation vs carboplatin	5-yr DFS 80% vs 85% 5-yr OS 70% vs 71% P = NS
ICON1 (2003)	477	Physician uncertain about the need for chemotherapy	Observation vs platinum-based chemotherapy	5-yr RFS 62% vs 73% P = .01 5-yr OS 70% vs 79% P = .03
ACTION (2003)	448	Stage IA/B Gr 2-3 All IC, IIA, and clear cell	Observation vs platinum-based chemotherapy	5-yr RFS 68% vs 76% P = .02 5-yr OS 78% vs 85% P = NS
Bell (2006)	427	Stage IA/B Gr 3 or clear cell All IC, II	Carboplatin/paclitaxel three cycles vs six cycles	HR RFS 0.761 P = NS 5-yr OS no difference
Mannel (2011)	542	Stage IA/B Gr 3 or clear cell, IC, II	Carboplatin/paclitaxel three cycles followed by observation vs followed by weekly paclitaxel × 26	5-yr RFS 77% vs 80% P = NS

DFS, disease-free survival; Gr, grade; HR, hazard ratio; NS, not significant; OS, overall survival; RFS, relapse-free survival; WAR, whole abdominal radiotherapy. From Fleming G, Seidman JD, Lengyel E. Epithelial ovarian cancer. In: Barakat RR, Berchuck A, Markmann M, et al, eds. *Principles and Practice of Gynecologic Oncology*. 6th ed. Lippincott Williams & Wilkins; 2013:757-847.

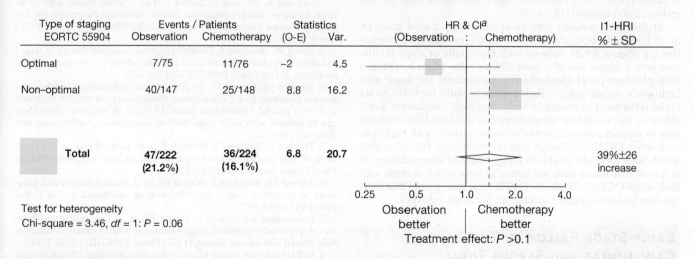

Figure 8.9-3. Forest plots of the interaction between the two staging categories (optimal and nonoptimal) versus treatment effect (adjuvant chemotherapy better vs observation better) for cancer-specific survival (CSS). Solid squares = hazard ratios (HRs) for CSS (with the area of the square being proportional to the variance of the estimated effect); length of the horizontal line through the square = 95% confidence interval (CI); open diamond = HR (middle of the diamond); horizontal points of the diamond = 95% CI for the combined data; EORTC, European Organization of Research and Treatment of Cancer; O-E, number of events observed minus number of events expected under the null hypothesis; SD, standard deviation; Var., variance of 1 divided by the logarithm of the HR. Linear trends and heterogeneity of the HRs to detect differences in relative size of treatment effect were assessed by a chi-square test for interaction. All statistical tests were two sided. (From Trimbos B, Timmers P, Pecorelli S, et al. Surgical staging and treatment of early ovarian cancer: long-term analysis from a randomized trial. *J Natl Cancer Inst.* 2010;102(13):982-987.)

Duration of Chemotherapy for Early-Stage Disease

The GOG #157 trial randomized 427 eligible patients with early-stage disease and unfavorable prognostic markers (stage IA or IB grade 3, clear cell, stage IC, and completely resected stage II) to receive either three or six cycles of carboplatin (area under the curve [AUC] 7.5)/paclitaxel (175 mg/m^2) chemotherapy (8). Surgical staging was required, although 29% of patients had surgical procedures that were considered inadequate or inadequately documented. A 5-year OS did not differ by treatment arm (HR 1.02). Adjusting for initial FIGO stage and tumor grade, the recurrence rate was 24% lower for patients getting six cycles, but this difference was not statistically significant (relative hazard 0.761, 95% CI, 0.512-1.13). There was a slightly lower estimated benefit of six cycles of chemotherapy in the completely staged group (HR 0.66 for incompletely staged vs 0.796 for completely staged patients), but there was no significant evidence of heterogeneity in treatment effect. Toxicity was increased with six cycles of chemotherapy; in particular, the rate of grade 3 or 4 neurotoxicity was 11% versus only 2% with three cycles. A subsequent exploratory analysis suggested that for the 97 women with serous tumors, the risk of recurrence was significantly lower after six versus three cycles of chemotherapy (83% vs 60%; HR 0.33; CI, 0.14-0.77, $P = .04$), whereas for those with nonserous tumors, including clear cell carcinomas, no benefit was seen (9). The 5-year OS for women with serous carcinomas was 86% for those receiving six cycles of therapy and 73% for those receiving three cycles of therapy; this difference did not reach statistical significance.

The GOG conducted a subsequent trial (GOG #175) in the same patient-population randomizing 542 eligible women to either three cycles of carboplatin (AUC 6)/paclitaxel (175 mg/m^2) with or without maintenance therapy with weekly paclitaxel 40 mg/m^2 for 24 weeks (10). No significant difference in recurrence-free interval (HR 0.807) or OS was seen. Only 29% of subjects had serous histology, and their results did not differ from those of the overall population who had as expected a high percentage of clear cell and endometrioid tumors (HR 0.822).

At this time, patients with comprehensively staged stage IA or IB low-grade EOC should not undergo postoperative chemotherapy (**Figure 8.9-2**). Patients with high-grade or stage IC disease have a relapse risk of at least 20%, and this might be reduced with platinum-based chemotherapy, particularly for those with high-grade serous tumors. Paclitaxel/carboplatin for three to six cycles is the usual treatment for early-stage high-risk disease, and it is further supported by a systematic review that found the strongest data to support adjuvant chemotherapy in patients with high-risk, early-stage OC (11), although data remain weaker for identifying which patients might be able to forego adjuvant chemotherapy. It is hoped that future data will better address which women with early-stage OCs actually derive benefit from therapy and that therapy may be better targeted to different histologic subtypes.

EARLY-STAGE FALLOPIAN TUBE CARCINOMAS AND SEROUS TUBAL INTRAEPITHELIAL CARCINOMAS

A small number of patients present with obvious early-stage disease in the fallopian tubes, which is frequently incidentally detected after surgery for a nononcologic indication such as incontinence or after prophylactic salpingo-oophorectomy performed for cancer prevention in women with a *BRCA* mutation. For these patients, we recommend comprehensive surgical staging (see Chapter 8.6).

Most fallopian tube carcinomas are of high-grade serous histology. Prognosis has been reported to be dependent on the depth of invasion of the tumor into the fallopian tube. When controlled for stage and grade, early-stage fallopian tube cancers appear to have a prognosis similar to that of early-stage cancers appearing to arise

from the ovary (12). Older FIGO data suggest that patients with stage I fallopian tube cancers have a 5-year OS of 81% (13).

There is considerable uncertainty regarding the treatment of isolated STIC lesions. Steenbeek et al conducted a systematic review that included 38 patients with STIC lesions (14). The cytology from IP washings was positive for malignant cells in four (10.5%) cases. A variety of surgical operations were performed on the majority of patients with STIC, but no patient had evidence of invasive carcinoma or peritoneal carcinomatosis, nor did either develop during follow-up. However, if an STIC is present at the time of RRSO for a pathologic variant of BRCA1/2 mutation, the 5- and 10-year risks of peritoneal carcinomatosis were high at 10.5% and 27.5% respectively. For women without a STIC lesion, it was 0.3% and 0.9%, respectively. Another systematic review found that three (4.5%) of 67 *BRCA* mutation carriers in their cohort with STIC lesions were diagnosed with primary peritoneal cancer during follow-up (15). When no invasive carcinoma is seen, management options include observation (with or without CA-125 testing) or subsequent surgical staging, with the decision about chemotherapy based upon the presence or absence of invasive carcinoma on the final surgical pathology. Overall, there are insufficient data to support full staging in patients with STIC lesions, but given the risk of developing peritoneal carcinomatosis, it is a reasonable choice. There are insufficient data regarding prognostic importance of isolated positive washings in patients with STIC lesions and insufficient data regarding benefit of chemotherapy in these situations. Some consensus guidelines do encourage consultation with a gynecologic oncologist after diagnosis of an STIC lesion who will be able to discuss the implications of an STIC diagnosis and the pros and cons of staging surgery.

REFERENCES

1. Peres LC, Cushing-Haugen KL, Kobel M, et al. Invasive epithelial ovarian cancer survival by histotype and disease stage. *J Natl Cancer Inst.* 2019;111(1):60-68.
2. Gaitskell K, Hermon C, Barnes I, et al. Ovarian cancer survival by stage, histotype, and pre-diagnostic lifestyle factors, in the prospective UK Million Women Study. *Cancer Epidemiol.* 2022;76:102074. doi:10.1016/j.canep.2021.102074
3. Young RC, Walton LA, Ellenberg SS, et al. Adjuvant therapy in stage I and stage II epithelial ovarian cancer. Results of two prospective randomized trials. *N Engl J Med.* 1990;322(15):1021-1027.
4. Trimbos JB, Parmar M, Vergote I, et al. International collaborative ovarian neoplasm trial 1 and adjuvant chemotherapy in ovarian neoplasm trial: two parallel randomized phase III trials of adjuvant chemotherapy in patients with early-stage ovarian carcinoma. *J Natl Cancer Inst.* 2003;95(2):105-112.
5. Trimbos B, Timmers P, Pecorelli S, et al. Surgical staging and treatment of early ovarian cancer: long-term analysis from a randomized trial. *J Natl Cancer Inst.* 2010;102(13):982-987.
6. Ahmed FY, Wiltshaw E, A'Hern RP, et al. Natural history and prognosis of untreated stage I epithelial ovarian carcinoma. *J Clin Oncol.* 1996;14(11):2968-2975.
7. Kolomainen DF, A'Hern R, Coxon FY, et al. Can patients with relapsed, previously untreated, stage I epithelial ovarian cancer be successfully treated with salvage therapy? *J Clin Oncol.* 2003;21(16):3113-3118.
8. Bell J, Brady MF, Young RC, et al. Randomized phase III trial of three versus six cycles of adjuvant carboplatin and paclitaxel in early stage epithelial ovarian carcinoma: a Gynecologic Oncology Group study. *Gynecol Oncol.* 2006;102(3):432-439. doi:10.1016/j.ygyno.2006.06.013
9. Chan JK, Tian C, Fleming GF, et al. The potential benefit of 6 vs. 3 cycles of chemotherapy in subsets of women with early-stage high-risk epithelial ovarian cancer: an exploratory analysis of a Gynecologic Oncology Group study. *Gynecol Oncol.* 2010;116(3):301-306.
10. Mannel RS, Brady MF, Kohn EC, et al. A randomized phase III trial of IV carboplatin and paclitaxel × 3 courses followed by observation versus weekly maintenance low-dose paclitaxel in patients with early-stage ovarian carcinoma: a Gynecologic Oncology Group study. *Gynecol Oncol.* 2011;122(1):89-94.
11. Lawrie TA, Winter-Roach BA, Heus P, Kitchener HC. Adjuvant (post-surgery) chemotherapy for early stage epithelial ovarian cancer. *Cochrane Database Syst Rev.* 2015;2015(12):CD004706.

12. Vaysse C, Touboul C, Filleron T, et al. Early stage (IA-IB) primary carcinoma of the fallopian tube: case-control comparison to adenocarcinoma of the ovary. *J Gynecol Oncol*. 2011;22(1):9-17.

13. Heintz A, Odicino F, Maisonneuve P, et al. Carcinoma of the ovary. FIGO 26th annual report on the results of treatment in gynecological cancer. *Int J Gynaecol Obstet*. 2006;95(Suppl 1):S161-S192. doi:10.1016/S0020-7292(06)60033-7

14. Steenbeek MP, van Bommel MHD, Bulten J, et al. Risk of peritoneal carcinomatosis after risk-reducing salpingo-oophorectomy: a systematic review and individual patient data meta-analysis. *J Clin Oncol*. 2022;40(17):1879-1891.

15. Patrono MG, Iniesta MD, Malpica A, et al. Clinical outcomes in patients with isolated serous tubal intraepithelial carcinoma (STIC): a comprehensive review. *Gynecol Oncol*. 2015;139(3):568-572.

CHAPTER **8.10**

Management of Borderline Tumors and Low-Grade Serous Tumors

Katherine C. Kurnit and Gini F. Fleming

INTRODUCTION

Borderline ovarian malignancies (previously called tumors of LMP) comprise 10% to 20% of OCs, and most are serous or mucinous. They were first described by Taylor in 1929 and recognized by FIGO in 1971 as a distinct histologic subtype. Their histology is reviewed in detail in Section 7. In general, patients with borderline tumors present at a younger age (on average 10 years younger) and have earlier stage disease than women with invasive ovarian carcinomas; over 75% of borderline ovarian tumors are stage I at the time of diagnosis (1).

SBTs are precursors to LGSCs, and MBTs are precursors to invasive mucinous tumors. SBTs are much more common than MBTs in the United States; in Asia, the rate of MBTs has been reported to be similar or higher than that of SBTs (2).

Nearly all MBTs are stage I at the time of diagnosis. Even when women with SBTs present with more advanced-stage disease, survival is prolonged. The very long natural history of borderline tumors makes accurate collection of outcomes and performing clinical trials challenging. Because these tumors are particularly likely to affect young women, decisions regarding fertility sparing, egg retrieval, and surgical menopause in the treatment of early-stage disease are often pertinent.

EARLY-STAGE BORDERLINE TUMORS

Surgery

Issues of surgical management of an ovarian mass, including borderline tumors, are covered in Section 6. Most often, this involves an initial minimally invasive surgical approach, removing the mass intact. Surgery is the cornerstone of the treatment for early-stage borderline ovarian tumors. It is often not known preoperatively whether an ovarian mass will prove to be a borderline tumor, and the accuracy of frozen section in the diagnosis of ovarian tumors has been reported to be low; 20% to 30% of ovarian tumors diagnosed as borderline at the time of frozen section examination prove to be invasive carcinomas on further sampling (3).

A full staging of borderline tumors along with salpingo-oophorectomy and omentectomy has historically been recommended, and the large (950 patients), prospective cohort study reported that incomplete staging was an independent risk factor for recurrence (1). However, as lymph node involvement in SBTs does not appear to affect prognosis, and as current guidelines recommend no systemic adjuvant therapy for women with implants, upstaging would not have therapeutic implications, and the inferior prognosis for unstaged patients may simply be a result of stage shift (4).

As such, the role of restaging borderline tumors not fully staged at the time of initial surgery remains controversial. In one retrospective multicenter study, the rate of upstaging was 15% for serous tumors; it is lower for mucinous tumors (5-7). The most relevant situation for restaging appears to be in women with apparent stage I SBT with microinvasion or micropapillary histology, which has the highest risk of invasive implants. Still, it is widely accepted that the majority of patients can be followed without additional surgery after obtaining a baseline abdominopelvic CT scan and CA-125 (serous) or CEA (mucinous) tumor marker (2). Of note, the German study discussed earlier reported that elevated CA-125 was associated with peritoneal implants of any type, but was not independently predictive of future relapse (8).

Because many women with borderline tumors are in their childbearing years, the efficacy and safety of conservative surgery for early-stage disease are important. There is no evidence that fertility-sparing surgery has an adverse effect on OS in patients with stage I borderline tumors, although it is tied to increased recurrence rates. A meta-analysis of 39 studies including 5,105 women concluded that for women with unilateral tumors, recurrence rates were 25.3% for women undergoing cystectomy versus 12.5% for those undergoing unilateral salpingo-oophorectomy (9). For women with bilateral tumors, the recurrence rate was 25.6% for bilateral cystectomy and 26.1% for unilateral cystectomy plus contralateral cystectomy. The cumulative pregnancy rate was 45.4% for unilateral salpingo-oophorectomy and 40.3% for unilateral cystectomy; however, survival was not different. There is no evidence of additional benefit from prophylactic hysterectomy when childbearing is completed; however, at the time of recurrence, most surgeons will perform a hysterectomy and remove the contralateral ovary, especially if a woman has completed childbearing.

For women with recurrent mucinous tumors, cystectomy for mucinous borderline lesions is not advisable, and, in general, every effort should be made to remove mucinous tumors surgically intact without spillage. The appendix should be evaluated intraoperatively to exclude an appendiceal tumor, and if there is any question of abnormality, it should be removed. In patients who present with stage II borderline tumors, a total abdominal hysterectomy and BSO with appropriate staging of the peritoneal cavity is usually recommended.

Prognosis and Therapy of Early-Stage Serous and Mucinous Borderline Tumors

In general, survival outcomes for early-stage SBT are excellent (10). However, recurrences from early-stage SBTs can present very late, 10 to 15 years after the initial diagnosis. In one representative report of 160 stage I SBTs, 11 patients developed recurrent tumor at a median of 16 years after initial surgery (range, 7-39 years), and eight died of the disease (11). Neither microinvasion nor micropapillary growth pattern appears to impact recurrence rates (1). Similarly, a meta-analysis of 42 studies suggested that lethal recurrence rates were 18.3% for early-stage typical SBTs, 16.8% for micropapillary serous tumors, and 10.7% for borderline tumors with microinvasion (9). Recurrences may still be borderline tumors or may have transformed into invasive cancers. These invasive cancers are more often, but not always, of low grade and carry a significantly worse prognosis than recurrences where the tumor remains noninvasive (**Figure 8.10-1**).

MBTs tend to be large, and areas of microinvasion can easily be missed if they are not sampled thoroughly. However, the clinical relevance of this is unclear, as microinvasion does not have clear prognostic significance. A review of eight series including 116 patients with mucinous ovarian tumors and stromal microinvasion reported that none developed an invasive recurrence (12). However, median follow-up in a number of these series was under 5 years. Intraepithelial cancer may also occur in MBTs, and although this is usually benign, there are occasional reports of malignant behavior.

In general, although the overall prognosis of early-stage MBTs is excellent, they can occasionally recur and may recur late. Uzan et al reported that although MBTs relapsed less often than SBTs, the recurrences are much more likely to be invasive (13). Patients with invasive recurrences, like those with other advanced-stage mucinous tumors, do poorly.

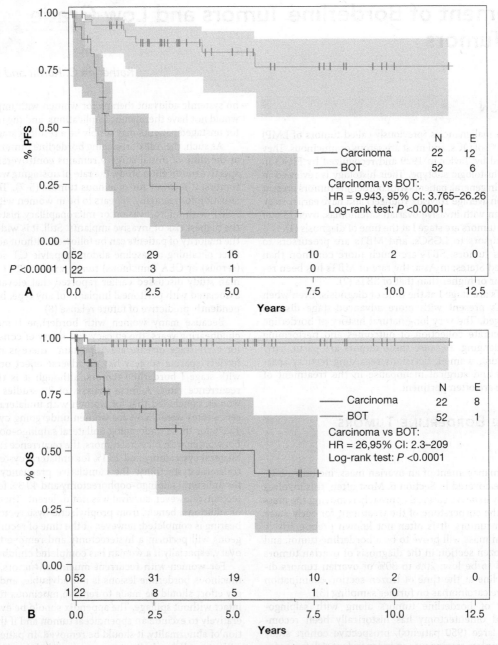

Figure 8.10-1. (A) Progression-free survival (PFS) and (B) overall survival (OS) after relapse of a borderline ovarian tumor—relapse as invasive carcinoma versus relapse as borderline ovarian tumor (BOT). CI, confidence interval; HR, hazard ratio.(From du Bois, Ewald-Riegler N, de Gregorio N, et al. Borderline tumours of the ovary: a cohort study of the Arbeitsgemeinschaft Gynäkologische Onkologie (AGO) study group. *Eur J Cancer.* 2013;49(8):1905-1914)

ADVANCED-STAGE SEROUS BORDERLINE TUMORS

Surgery

Chemotherapy does not appear to have a role in the treatment of borderline tumors, regardless of stage, histology, or the presence of microinvasion; hence, surgery is the primary treatment. Retrospective studies suggest that the proportion of patients achieving optimal cytoreductive surgery is stage-for-stage higher for patients with serous LMP tumors and LGSCs than for those with serous EOC. Residual disease is an important prognostic factor for both recurrence-free survival and OS.

Prognosis and Adjuvant Systemic Therapy

Residual disease after surgery, the presence of advanced disease before surgery, and invasive implants showing clear stromal invasion are poor prognostic factors. Seidman and Kurman reported on a review of 97 publications including 4,129 patients and noted that after 7.4 years of follow-up, the survival of patients with noninvasive peritoneal implants was 95.3% as compared with 66% for those with invasive implants (the latter would currently be classified as invasive LGSCs) (14). Lymph node involvement did not confer a poor prognosis and was associated with a 98% survival rate at 6.5 years. Finally, a 2014 meta-analysis also reported no benefit of adjuvant systemic therapy for any subset of advanced-stage borderline tumors (4). Adjuvant therapy is, therefore, not recommended.

THERAPY FOR ADVANCED-STAGE LOW-GRADE SEROUS CANCERS AND INVASIVE RECURRENCES OF SEROUS BORDERLINE TUMORS

As shown in **Figure 8.10-1**, noninvasive recurrences of borderline tumors continue to have a relatively good prognosis and should be treated with surgical resection. Shvartzman et al identified 112 patients with de novo LGSCs and 41 with invasive recurrences of borderline tumors. There were no statistically significant differences between the two groups in median age (42.7 vs 45.4 years [at relapse]), PFS (19.5 vs 25 months), or OS (81.8 vs 82.8 months) (15). Age less than 35 years has been reported to be a poor prognostic factor among patients with advanced-stage LGSC (16). A 2020 study also suggested that increased sampling may detect microinvasive disease more readily, which may account for subsequent invasion in previously diagnosed SBTs (17).

The recommendation for newly diagnosed LGSC remains surgical removal of all tumor followed by adjuvant therapy (18). However, this paradigm is no longer limited to cytotoxic chemotherapy, and some consensus guidelines have recently been adjusted to reflect these evolving approaches in light of the acknowledgment that LGSC is considered a relatively chemotherapy-resistant disease.

In a combined analysis of four frontline chemotherapy trials, the Arbeitsgemeinschaft Gynäkologische Onkologie (AGO) reported that the response rate for LGSC was only 23.1% versus 90.1% for HGSC (19). Even lower response rates to neoadjuvant therapy have been reported, and the use of neoadjuvant therapy for LGSC is rarely advised if the disease appears unresectable (20).

A retrospective cohort study published in 2017 reported an improvement in PFS for patients who received maintenance hormonal therapy, with a median PFS of 64.9 months compared with 26.4 months for patients who had observation only (21). Although no difference in OS was seen, maintenance hormonal therapy in frontline treatment of LGSC is frequently used.

Given the promise of hormonal therapy in the setting of low chemotherapy response rates, the question of whether any cytotoxic chemotherapy is necessary in the frontline setting has been posed. A 2016 abstract presented results of a very small retrospective series of women with advanced-stage LGSC treated with cytoreductive surgery followed by adjuvant hormonal therapy (AHT) (mostly aromatase inhibitors) and no chemotherapy (22). When compared to a control group of patients treated with chemotherapy, there was no difference in PFS. However, CA-125 measurements have been shown to decline with adjuvant chemotherapy for advanced-stage LGSC with normalization of CA-125 after one of first three cycles being associated with better outcomes, suggesting a degree of chemotherapy sensitivity for some patients (23). Some consensus guidelines now include AHT as an option. In addition, a phase III clinical trial continues to enroll as of 2022, which evaluates the use of cytotoxic chemotherapy followed by maintenance letrozole versus letrozole alone. These results are eagerly anticipated.

Treatment of progressive unresectable LGSC remains challenging. Gershenson et al reported a retrospective review of 108 chemotherapy regimens administered to 58 patients with low-grade serous ovarian tumors (24). There was an ORR of 3.7%, with one complete and three partial responses. The median time to progression was 29 weeks. Two series reported the activity of bevacizumab combined with various chemotherapies and reported response rates ranging from 40% to 50% (25,26).

Most LGSCs are ER/PR positive, and there are case reports of major responses to tamoxifen, leuprolide, and anastrozole. The MD Anderson group retrospectively reviewed outcomes of 219 hormonal therapy regimens in 133 women with recurrent LGSCs of the ovary or peritoneum (27). The ORR was 9%, with six complete and two partial responses (to anastrozole, letrozole, and tamoxifen). Median time to progression was 7.4 months.

Given the high frequency of *KRAS* and *BRAF* mutations in LGSCs, targeted therapies for these pathways have been explored. A trial of selumetinib, which inhibits MEK-1/2 (downstream signaling effectors of KRAS/BRAF activating mitogenic signaling) in women with LGSCs, was performed first (28). The majority of participants had at least three prior cytotoxic regimens. There was a 15% response rate with a median PFS of 11 months. Of patients from whom sufficient tumor material was available, 6% had tumors with *BRAF* mutations, and 41% had tumors with *KRAS* mutations. No correlation between response and mutation status was observed. In contrast, the results of the phase III study of binimetinib (a different MEK inhibitor) compared with physician's choice chemotherapy were published in 2020 and showed no statistically significant difference between the two arms (9.1 months for binimetinib vs 10.6 months for physician's choice) (29). As a result, the trial was stopped early. A subsequent subset analysis of patients in the binimetinib arm reported an improvement in response rate for patients whose tumors had *KRAS* mutations compared with those whose tumors were *KRAS* wild type (44% vs 19%, P = .004).

GOG 281 was a randomized trial that compared treatment with trametinib to physician's choice treatment. Median PFS in the trametinib group was 13.0 months compared with 7.2 months in the standard-of-care group (HR 0.48, 95% CI 0.36-0.64; $P <$ .0001) (30). The most frequent grade 3 or 4 adverse events in the trametinib group were skin rash (13%), anemia (13%), hypertension (12%), diarrhea (10%), nausea (9%), and fatigue (8%). There was no evidence that mutation status was predictive for PFS. More major responses were seen with trametinib than standard-of-care therapy in mutation (KRAS, BRAF, or NRAS)-positive patients (11 [50%] of 22 vs two [9%] of 22), which was not the case in mutation-negative patients (four [8%] of 48 vs three [7%] of 42), although this did not reach statistical significance (multiple comparison adjusted P = .11, test for interaction). The use of trametinib has now been incorporated into some consensus guidelines for platinum-resistant, recurrent LGSC.

The role of *KRAS* mutations and other predictive biomarkers in selecting targeted therapies for patients with LGSC will likely be an area for future investigation, as will newer agents targeting this pathway. For example, GOG 3052 is a phase 2 study of VS-6766 (dual RAF/MEK inhibitor) either alone and in combination with defactinib (FAK inhibitor) in women with recurrent LGSC.

REFERENCES

1. Bois A, Ewald-Riegler N, Gregorio N, et al. Borderline tumours of the ovary: a cohort study of the Arbeitsgemeinschaft Gynakologische Onkologie (AGO) study group. *Eur J Cancer.* 2013;49(8):1905-1914.

2. Morice P, Uzan C, Fauvet R, Gouy S, Duvillard P, Darai E. Borderline ovarian tumour: pathological diagnostic dilemma and risk factors for invasive or lethal recurrence. *Lancet Oncol.* 2012;13(3):103-115.

3. Song T, Choi CH, Kim HJ, et al. Accuracy of frozen section diagnosis of borderline ovarian tumors. *Gynecol Oncol.* 2011;122(1):127-131.

4. Harter P, Gershenson D, Lhomme C, et al. Gynecologic Cancer Inter-Group (GCIG) consensus review for ovarian tumors of low malignant potential (borderline ovarian tumors). *Int J Gynecol Cancer.* 2014;24(9 Suppl 3):S5-S8.

5. Zapardiel I, Rosenberg P, Peiretti M, et al. The role of restaging borderline ovarian tumors: single institution experience and review of the literature. *Gynecol Oncol.* 2010;119(2):274-277.

6. Trillsch F, Mahner S, Vettorazzi E, et al. Surgical staging and prognosis in serous borderline ovarian tumours (BOT): a subanalysis of the AGO ROBOT study. *Br J Cancer.* 2015;112(4):660-666.

7. Decker K, Speth S, Brugge HGT, et al. Staging procedures in patients with mucinous borderline tumors of the ovary do not reveal peritoneal or omental disease. *Gynecol Oncol.* 2017;144(2):285-289.

8. Fotopoulou C, Sehouli J, Ewald-Riegler N, et al. The value of serum CA125 in the diagnosis of borderline tumors of the ovary: a subanalysis of the prospective multicenter ROBOT study. *Int J Gynecol Cancer.* 2015;25(7):1248-1252.

9. Vasconcelos I, Sousa Mendes M. Conservative surgery in ovarian borderline tumours: a meta-analysis with emphasis on recurrence risk. *Eur J Cancer.* 2015;51(5):620-631.

10. Gaitskell K, Hermon C, Barnes I, et al. Ovarian cancer survival by stage, histotype, and pre-diagnostic lifestyle factors, in the prospective UK million women study. *Cancer Epidemiol.* 2022;76:102074. doi:10.1016/j.canep.2021.102074

11. Silva EG, Tornos C, Zhuang Z, Merino MJ, Gershenson DM. Tumor recurrence in stage I ovarian serous neoplasms of low malignant potential. *Int J Gynecol Pathol.* 1998;17(1):1-6.

12. Vasconcelos I, Darb-Esfahani S, Sehouli J. Serous and mucinous borderline ovarian tumours: differences in clinical presentation, high-risk histopathological features, and lethal recurrence rates. *BJOG.* 2016;123(4):498-508.

13. Uzan C, Nikpayam M, Ribassin-Majed L, et al. Influence of histological subtypes on the risk of an invasive recurrence in a large series of stage I borderline ovarian tumor including 191 conservative treatments. *Ann Oncol.* 2014;25(7):1312-1319.

14. Seidman JD, Kurman RJ. Ovarian serous borderline tumors: a critical review of the literature with emphasis on prognostic indicators. *Hum Pathol.* 2000;31(5):539-557.

15. Shvartsman HS, Sun CC, Bodurka DC, et al. Comparison of the clinical behavior of newly diagnosed stages II-IV low-grade serous carcinoma of the ovary with that of serous ovarian tumors of low malignant potential that recur as low-grade serous carcinoma. *Gynecol Oncol.* 2007;105(3):625-629.

16. Gershenson DM, Bodurka DC, Lu KH, et al. Impact of age and primary disease site on outcome in women with low-grade serous carcinoma of the ovary or peritoneum: results of a large single-institution registry of a rare tumor. *J Clin Oncol.* 2015;33(24):2675-2682.

17. Seidman JD, Savage J, Krishnan J, Vang R, Kurman RJ. Intratumoral heterogeneity accounts for apparent progression of noninvasive serous tumors to invasive low-grade serous carcinoma: a study of 30 low-grade serous tumors of the ovary in 18 patients with peritoneal carcinomatosis. *Int J Gynecol Pathol.* 2020;39(1):43-54.

18. Slomovitz B, Gourley C, Carey MS, et al. Low-grade serous ovarian cancer: state of the science. *Gynecol Oncol.* 2020;156(3):715-725.

19. Grabowski JP, Harter P, Heitz F, et al. Operability and chemotherapy responsiveness in advanced low-grade serous ovarian cancer. An analysis of the AGO study group metadatabase. *Gynecol Oncol.* 2016;140(3):457-462.

20. Cobb LP, Sun CC, Iyer R, et al. The role of neoadjuvant chemotherapy in the management of low-grade serous carcinoma of the ovary and peritoneum: further evidence of relative chemoresistance. *Gynecol Oncol.* 2020;158(3):653-658.

21. Gershenson DM, Bodurka DC, Coleman RL, Lu KH, Malpica A, Sun CC. Hormonal maintenance therapy for women with low-grade serous cancer of the ovary or peritoneum. *J Clin Oncol.* 2017;35(10):1103-1111.

22. Fader AN, Jernigan AM, Bergstrom J, et al. Primary cytoreductive surgery and adjuvant hormone therapy in women with advanced low-grade serous carcinoma: reducing overtreatment without compromising survival? *Gynecol Oncol.* 2016;141:29-30.

23. Fader AN, Java J, Krivak TC, et al. The prognostic significance of pre- and post-treatment CA-125 in grade 1 serous ovarian carcinoma: a gynecologic oncology group study. *Gynecol Oncol.* 2014;132(3):560-565.

24. Gershenson DM, Sun CC, Bodurka D, et al. Recurrent low-grade serous ovarian carcinoma is relatively chemoresistant. *Gynecol Oncol.* 2009;114(1):48-52.

25. Grisham RN, Iyer G, Sala E, et al. Bevacizumab shows activity in patients with low-grade serous ovarian and primary peritoneal cancer. *Int J Gynecol Cancer.* 2014;24(6):1010-1014.

26. Dalton HJ, Fleming ND, Sun CC, Bhosale P, Schmeler KM, Gershenson DM. Activity of bevacizumab-containing regimens in recurrent low-grade serous ovarian or peritoneal cancer: a single institution experience. *Gynecol Oncol.* 2017;145(1):37-40.

27. Gershenson DM, Sun CC, Iyer RB, et al. Hormonal therapy for recurrent low-grade serous carcinoma of the ovary or peritoneum. *Gynecol Oncol.* 2012;125(3):661-666.

28. Farley J, Brady WE, Vathipadiekal V, et al. Selumetinib in women with recurrent low-grade serous carcinoma of the ovary or peritoneum: an open-label, single-arm, phase 2 study. *Lancet Oncol.* 2013;14(2):134-140.

29. Monk BJ, Grisham RN, Banerjee S, et al. MILO/ENGOT-ov11: binimetinib versus physician's choice chemotherapy in recurrent or persistent low-grade serous carcinomas of the ovary, fallopian tube, or primary peritoneum. *J Clin Oncol.* 2020;38(32):3753-3762.

30. Gershenson DM, Miller A, Brady WE, et al. Trametinib versus standard of care in patients with recurrent low-grade serous ovarian cancer (GOG 281/LOGS): an international, randomised, open-label, multicentre, phase 2/3 trial. *Lancet.* 2022;399(10324):541-553.

CHAPTER **8.11**

Management of Advanced-Stage Ovarian Cancer

Katherine C. Kurnit and Gini F. Fleming

SURGERY

A simplified algorithm for the management of advanced-stage disease is shown in **Figure 8.11-1**. Surgery for advanced-stage disease as well as the timing of surgery (upfront vs after three or more cycles of neoadjuvant therapy) is covered in Section 6.

Upfront surgery for definitive diagnosis and removal of as much tumor as possible has long been the standard in OC therapy. However, neoadjuvant chemotherapy is increasingly being used in situations where a complete gross resection is not expected, or the patient is frail as multiple prospective, randomized trials have not found neoadjuvant chemotherapy to be inferior to primary debulking procedures (1,2).

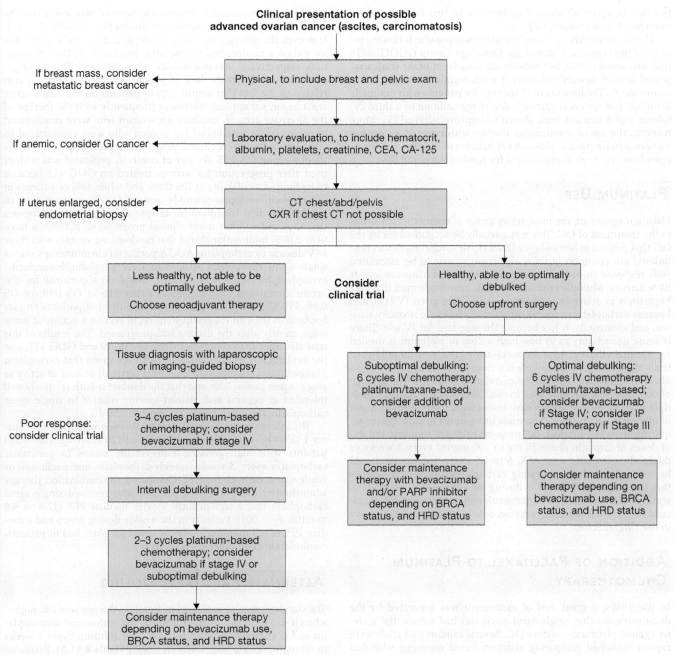

Figure 8.11-1. Upfront management of advanced ovarian cancer. CT, computed tomography; CXR, chest x-ray; GI, gastrointestinal; IP, intraperitoneal; IV, intravenous; HRD, homologous recombination deficiency.

Owing to the criticisms of several of those studies, neoadjuvant chemotherapy is considered to be most appropriate for patients who are medically unfit for primary debulking surgery, or those whose tumors are not felt to be susceptible to optimal cytoreduction at the time of diagnosis (3). It is clear that women whose disease is successfully surgically debulked to minimal or no residual disease have an improved survival, although how much of this is a direct result of the surgical effort and how much reflects initial tumor volume and unknown biologic/genetic, social, or health factors in patients who have debulkable disease remains unclear.

CHEMOTHERAPY

The majority of women with advanced-stage OC have HGSC, and women with this tumor type have predominated in the trials of advanced disease. Hence, the trials discussed in this section may be assumed to apply primarily to HGSC.

Adjuvant (or neoadjuvant) treatment is rarely curative for women with advanced-stage EOC, even when there is no residual disease after cytoreductive surgery (see **Figure 8.6-4**). Approximately 50% to 70% of patients with measurable disease after surgery will have a complete or partial response to platinum-based first-line postoperative therapy (4). In trials including patients who underwent both an optimal and suboptimal cytoreduction, at least half will generally have a complete clinical response to platinum-based regimens, with disappearance of all disease on imaging and normalization of CA-125. Unfortunately, even among women with complete clinical remission, the majority eventually develops recurrent disease.

The most common frontline therapy in the United States is currently six cycles of IV paclitaxel/carboplatin. Some physicians administer eight or nine cycles of therapy, particularly when interval debulking is performed. However, three small randomized trials that investigated the benefit of prolonging duration of treatment beyond six cycles all showed an increase in toxicity, but no improvement in outcomes (5-7).

The use of weekly paclitaxel regimens was popular following results of the Japanese Gynecologic Oncology Group (JGOG) 3016 trial discussed earlier, but subsequent data from other trials suggested limited benefit and every 3 week regimens are now more common (8). The benefits of IP therapy for patients with optimally debulked tumors are controversial, and the addition of a third cytotoxic agent has not been shown to improve survival (9). More recently, the use of maintenance therapy with targeted agents has increased in frequency, although OS benefits to maintenance strategies have not been demonstrated for most of the population.

PLATINUM USE

Platinum agents are the most active group of chemotherapy drugs in the treatment of OC. This may partially be accounted for by the fact that defects in homologous DNA repair (including *BRCA* mutations) are common in OCs, and these appear to be associated with response to platinum therapy. A variety of platinum agents have activity. Multiple randomized trials have confirmed that carboplatin is as active as cisplatin when both are given IV (10), and because carboplatin produces substantially less neurotoxicity, nausea, and ototoxicity, it has become the standard for IV use. There is some uncertainty as to how high a dose of platinum is needed for optimal efficacy. An older meta-analysis of over 60 published trials showed a correlation between dose intensity of cisplatin and observed response rate, but the correlation held only over a range of doses lower than those used in clinical practice today (11). Multiple trials of varying design have tested higher versus lower doses of platinum agents, including trials using doses of carboplatin requiring stem cell support, but no good evidence supports the use of doses of cisplatin above 50 mg to 100 mg/m^2 every 3 weeks or doses of carboplatin over AUC 5 to 7.5 every 3 weeks. It should be recognized when comparing carboplatin dosing across trials that there may be variation in dosing for a given AUC depending, among other things, on how glomerular filtration rate (GFR) is calculated. AUC 6 is the most common dose used for first-line therapy in the United States.

ADDITION OF PACLITAXEL TO PLATINUM CHEMOTHERAPY

In the 1980s, a great deal of excitement was generated by the demonstration that single-agent paclitaxel had substantial activity against platinum-resistant OC. Several randomized trials were rapidly launched comparing platinum-based regimens with and without taxane in the first-line treatment of OC.

The results of the first two of these trials (GOG 111 [12] and OV-10 [13]) clearly demonstrated that combination chemotherapy with paclitaxel and cisplatin prolonged both PFS and OS compared with cyclophosphamide/cisplatin. In GOG 111, which included 386 women with suboptimally debulked or stage IV disease, the median OS was 37 months for those treated with paclitaxel (135 mg/m^2 over 24 hours) and cisplatin as compared to 25 months for those receiving cyclophosphamide and cisplatin (12). Similar results were found in the more inclusive (stages IIB-IV) European OV-10 trial, which reported a median OS of 36 months for the paclitaxel-containing arm (175 mg/m^2 over 3 hours) versus 26 months for the cyclophosphamide-containing arm (13).

The other two trials did not as clearly support the addition of paclitaxel to frontline therapy. The three arms of GOG 132 were single-agent paclitaxel (200 mg/m^2 over 24 hours), single-agent cisplatin (100 mg/mg^2), and the combination of cisplatin 75 mg/m^2 plus paclitaxel 135 mg/m^2 over 24 hours (380) (14). Six hundred fourteen women with suboptimally debulked or stage IV disease were treated. The response rate to single-agent paclitaxel in

patients with measurable disease was significantly lower than to either of the platinum-containing regimens (42% vs 67%, $P < .01$). However, the difference in median OS (30.2, 25.9, and 26.3 months for patients randomized to cisplatin, paclitaxel, or the combination, respectively) was not statistically significant. The investigators speculated that the lack of benefit for the combination arm related to the fact that almost 50% of patients on the single-agent arms began subsequent treatment (frequently with the therapy of the alternate arm, ie, cisplatin for women who were randomized to paclitaxel and paclitaxel for women who were randomized to cisplatin) before overt clinical progression, presumably on the basis of a rising CA-125. By way of contrast, paclitaxel was seldom used after progression for women treated on GOG 111 because of its limited availability at the time, and while 48% of patients in the cisplatin/cyclophosphamide arm of OV-10 crossed over to paclitaxel as first treatment for relapse or progression, it appears that they did so after overt clinical progression. ICON3, a large ($n = 2,075$) multinational trial that randomized women with stage I-IV disease to carboplatin AUC 6/paclitaxel chemotherapy versus single-agent carboplatin AUC 6 or CAP (cisplatin/doxorubicin/cyclophosphamide) chemotherapy, found no superiority for the taxane-containing combination in either PFS or OS (HR for OS 0.98; 95% CI, 0.87-1.10) (15). About one-third of patients on carboplatin in the control group went on to receive a taxane at some stage, mostly after the disease had progressed. The results of this trial also appear to contradict those of OV-10 and GOG 111, and the explanation remains unclear. However, given that carboplatin plus paclitaxel combination therapy is certainly at least as active as single-agent carboplatin and that the doublet is both relatively well tolerated in general and platelet-sparing relative to single-agent carboplatin, the combination became standard.

The international phase II Elderly Women with Ovarian Cancer 1 (EWOC-1) trial randomly assigned 120 older-age (age >70) patients with high geriatric vulnerability scores to paclitaxel/carboplatin every 3 weeks, weekly carboplatin and paclitaxel, or single-agent carboplatin (16). Compared to combination therapy administered every 3 weeks, patients who received single-agent carboplatin had a significantly shorter median PFS (12.5 vs 4.8 months, $P < .001$). Patients in the weekly dosing group had a median PFS of 8.3 months. Therefore, even for older less fit patients, combination chemotherapy is preferred.

ALTERNATE PACLITAXEL DOSING

The standard dose of paclitaxel in frontline therapy was 135 mg/m^2 when it was used as a 24-hour infusion in combination with cisplatin and is currently 175 mg/m^2 as 3-hour infusion every 3 weeks or 80 mg/m^2 as a 1-hour infusion weekly (**Table 8.11-1**). Paclitaxel was historically administered as a 24-hour infusion to minimize hypersensitivity reactions and to diminish neurotoxicity when it was administered in combination with cisplatin.

Attempts at escalating the every 3-week paclitaxel dose have been made. A prospective, randomized trial in previously untreated patients with advanced OC compared two different doses of paclitaxel (175 vs 225 mg/m^2), with all patients receiving carboplatin at an AUC of 5 (17). No improvement in survival was reported for the higher dose regimen. Subsequently, based on data in women with metastatic breast cancer that weekly paclitaxel was superior to every 3-week paclitaxel in terms of response and survival, the JGOG randomly assigned 637 women with stages II to IV OC, primary peritoneal cancer, or fallopian tube cancer to six cycles of either standard therapy with carboplatin AUC 6 plus paclitaxel 180 mg/m^2 over 3 hours every 21 days or dose-dense therapy with carboplatin AUC 6 every 21 days plus paclitaxel 80 mg/m^2 on days 1, 8, and 15 of a 21-day cycle (18). Patients with measurable disease who had a major response received three additional cycles of chemotherapy. Interval or secondary debulking surgery was permitted. The dose-dense regimen was superior in terms of both median PFS (28.2 vs

■ TABLE 8.11-1. Selected Trials Testing Taxane Variations in Frontline Therapy

Trials	Eligibility Criteria	Arms	PFS	OS
SCOTROC (23)	1077 IC-IV	Carbo AUC 5 + paclitaxel 175 mg/m^2 q3wk vs Carbo AUC 5 + docetaxel 75 mg/m^2 q3wk	14.8 mo vs 15 mo	2 yr 69% vs 2 yr 64%
Bolis et al. (17)	502 IIB-IV	Carbo AUC 6 + paclitaxel 175 mg/m^2 vs Carbo AUC 6 + paclitaxel 225 mg/m^2	4 yr PFS 41.5% vs 4 yr PFS 39.2%	4 yr OS 46.2% vs 4 yr OS 47.3%
GOG 162 (64)	324 III or IV suboptimal	Cisplatin 75 mg/m^2 + paclitaxel 135 mg/m^2/24 hr vs Cisplatin 75 mg/m^2 + paclitaxel 135 mg/m^2/96 hr	1.03 yr vs 1.05 yr	2.49 yr vs 2.54 yr
JOG3016 (18)	637 II-IV	Carbo AUC 6 q3wk + paclitaxel 180 mg/m^2 q3wk vs Carbo AUC 6 q3 wk + paclitaxel 80 mg/m^2/wk	17.5 mo vs 28.2 mo	62.2 mo vs 100.5 mo
GOG 262 (19)	692 III-IV (580 w/bev; 112 w/o bev)	Carbo AUC 6 q3wk + paclitaxel 175 mg/m^2 q3wk vs Carbo AUC 6 q3wk + paclitaxel 80 mg/m^2/wk	No Bev 10.3 mo Bev 14.7 mo vs No Bev 14.2 mo Bev 14.9 mo	No OS difference between arms
MITO-7 (20)	822 IC-IV	Carbo AUC 6 q3wk + paclitaxel 175 mg/m^2 q3wk vs Carbo AUC 2 q1wk + paclitaxel 60 mg/m^2/wk	17.3 mo vs 18.3 mo	2 yr OS 78.9% vs 2 yr OS 77.3%
ICON8 (8,22)	IC-IV	Carbo AUC 5 q3wk + paclitaxel 175 mg/m^2 q3wk vs Carbo AUC 5 q3wk + paclitaxel 80 mg/m^2/wk vs Carbo AUC 2 q1wk + paclitaxel 80 mg/m^2/wk	23.9 mo vs 25.3 mo vs 24.8 mo	47.4 mo vs 54.8 mo vs 53.4 mo

AUC, area under the curve; carbo, carboplatin; OS, overall survival; PFS, progression-free survival; q, every.

From Bolis G, Scarfone G, Polverino G, et al. Paclitaxel 175 or 225 mg per meters squared with carboplatin in advanced ovarian cancer: a randomized trial. *J Clin Oncol*. 2004;22(4):686-690.

From Chan JK, Brady MF, Penson RT, et al. Weekly vs. every-3-week paclitaxel and carboplatin for ovarian cancer. *N Engl J Med*. 2016;374(8):738-748.

From Clamp AR, James EC, McNeish IA, et al. Weekly dose-dense chemotherapy in first-line epithelial ovarian, fallopian tube, or primary peritoneal cancer treatment (ICON8): overall survival results from an open-label, randomised, controlled, phase 3 trial. *Lancet Oncol*. 2022;23(7):919-930.

From Clamp AR, James EC, McNeish IA, et al. Weekly dose-dense chemotherapy in first-line epithelial ovarian, fallopian tube, or primary peritoneal carcinoma treatment (ICON8): primary progression free survival analysis results from a GCIG phase 3 randomised controlled trial. *Lancet*. 2019;394(10214):2084-2095.

From Katsumata N, Yasuda M, Isonishi S, et al. Long-term results of dose-dense paclitaxel and carboplatin versus conventional paclitaxel and carboplatin for treatment of advanced epithelial ovarian, fallopian tube, or primary peritoneal cancer (JGOG 3016): a randomised, controlled, open-label trial. *Lancet Oncol*. 2013;14(10): 1020-1026.

From Pignata S, Scambia G, Katsaros D, et al. Carboplatin plus paclitaxel once a week versus every 3 weeks in patients with advanced ovarian cancer (MITO-7): a randomised, multicentre, open-label, phase 3 trial. *Lancet Oncol*. 2014;15(4):396-405.

From Spriggs DR, Brady MF, Vaccarello L, et al. Phase III randomized trial of intravenous cisplatin plus a 24- or 96-hour infusion of paclitaxel in epithelial ovarian cancer: a Gynecologic Oncology Group Study. *J Clin Oncol*. 2007;25(28):4466-4471.

From Vasey PA, Jayson GC, Gordon A, et al. Phase III randomized trial of docetaxel-carboplatin versus paclitaxel-carboplatin as first-line chemotherapy for ovarian carcinoma. *J Natl Cancer Inst*. 2004;96:1682-1691.

17.5 months; HR 0.76; 95% CI, 0.62-0.91) and median OS (100.5 vs 62.2 months, HR 0.79; 95% CI, 0.63-0.90). All subgroups (age, stage, residual disease) appeared to benefit, except for women with clear cell or mucinous tumors. The dose-dense regimen was more myelotoxic than standard therapy and required an increased number of dose delays and reductions.

The GOG performed a confirmatory trial (GOG 262) using carboplatin AUC 6 with weekly paclitaxel 80 mg/m^2 compared to carboplatin AUC 6 with every 3-week paclitaxel 175 mg/m^2 (19). Bevacizumab 15 mg/kg every 3 weeks, given with chemotherapy and then until progression, was optional but was selected by 84% ($n = 580$) of patients. Overall, there was no difference between the arms for PFS (14.7 vs 14.0 months, $P = .18$), but in the subset ($n = 112$) that did not receive bevacizumab, PFS was significantly improved (14.2 vs 10.3 months, $P = .03$). Anemia and neuropathy were increased on the weekly paclitaxel arm. The mechanism by which bevacizumab might potentially obscure a benefit of weekly paclitaxel remains uncertain.

The Multicenter Italian Trials in ovarian cancer 7 (MITO-7) trial used a regimen of weekly paclitaxel at a somewhat lower dose that the JGOG trial: 60 mg/m^2 and combined it with weekly carboplatin AUC 2 (20). The control arm was every 3-week paclitaxel 175 mg/m^2 plus carboplatin AUC 6 given every 3 weeks. There was no difference in PFS between the arms (18.3 months for weekly and 17.3 months for every 3 weeks), but there was decreased toxicity, including febrile neutropenia, thrombocytopenia, renal toxicity, and neuropathy, as well as significantly better QoL in the weekly arm.

ICON8 was a three-arm trial of 1,566 women evaluating standard therapy with carboplatin every 3 weeks plus paclitaxel every 3 weeks (group 1), a regimen of carboplatin every 3 weeks plus weekly paclitaxel (group 2), and a regimen in which both carboplatin and paclitaxel are given weekly (group 3) (8,21). No bevacizumab was used, which addressed some of the limitations of GOG 262. There were no differences in median PFS across the three groups: 17.7 versus 20.8 versus 21.0 months in groups 1, 2, and 3 ($P > .05$). Grade 3 and 4 toxicities were increased with weekly treatment, although a subsequent QoL analysis showed no significant differences between the groups at 9 months after treatment (22). Based on the totality of these data, the use of weekly paclitaxel regimens has subsequently declined in the United States and Europe.

ALTERNATE TAXANES

The Scottish Gynaecological Cancer Trials Group tested the incorporation of docetaxel into frontline therapy (23). One thousand seventy-seven women with stage IC to IV OC or primary peritoneal carcinoma were randomized to six cycles of carboplatin AUC 5 and either docetaxel 75 mg/m^2 or paclitaxel 175 mg/m^2. At a median follow-up of 23 months, there was no difference in PFS (15 months for docetaxel, 14.8 months for paclitaxel) or OS (2-year OS 64% for docetaxel and 69% for paclitaxel). This was confirmed in a subsequent report with longer follow-up. Docetaxel was associated with less neurotoxicity (11% vs 30% grade ≥2 neurosensory toxicity) and more myelotoxicity (11 patients vs 3 patients with neutropenic fever).

Albumin-bound paclitaxel has been shown to have activity in OC, although it has not been formally compared to paclitaxel in a randomized trial. Despite this, it is clinically used when patients have developed a hypersensitivity reaction to paclitaxel (24).

ADDITION OF A THIRD CYTOTOXIC AGENT TO FRONTLINE CHEMOTHERAPY

There are no data that addition of any third cytotoxic agent to frontline chemotherapy of OC improves outcomes, despite an immense amount of investigation of this strategy. Multiple randomized phase III trials testing the addition of doxorubicin, epirubicin, gemcitabine, and topotecan to a platinum/taxane backbone either sequentially or all at the same time have all been negative. An international multiarm randomized study, GOG 182/ICON5, randomized 4,312 patients with advanced-stage OC to carboplatin/paclitaxel or carboplatin/paclitaxel combined with either gemcitabine, liposomal doxorubicin, or topotecan (9). PFS ranged from 15.4 to 17.5 months across the four treatment arms, with an HR of 0.94 to 1.07, which was not statistically different among any of the combination regimens studied.

SUBSTITUTION OF AN ALTERNATE CYTOTOXIC AGENT FOR PACLITAXEL

A randomized phase III trial substituting gemcitabine for paclitaxel as frontline therapy showed inferior OS for women on the gemcitabine-containing arm (25). Results with liposomal doxorubicin have been more interesting. The phase III MITO-2 trial randomly assigned 820 chemotherapy-naive patients with stage IC to IV OC to carboplatin AUC 5 plus paclitaxel 175 mg/m^2 or to carboplatin AUC 5 plus liposomal doxorubicin 30 mg/m^2, every 3 weeks for six cycles (26). The primary end point was PFS. Median PFS was 19.0 and 16.8 months with carboplatin/liposomal doxorubicin and carboplatin/paclitaxel, respectively (HR, 0.95; 95% CI, 0.81-1.13; P = .58). Median OS times were 61.6 and 53.2 months with carboplatin/liposomal doxorubicin and carboplatin/paclitaxel, respectively (HR, 0.89; 95% CI, 0.72-1.12; P = .32). Carboplatin/liposomal doxorubicin produced less neurotoxicity and alopecia but more hematologic adverse effects. There was no relevant difference in global QoL after three and six cycles. This regimen may be an option for patients with severe neuropathy or taxane allergies.

ADDITION OF BEVACIZUMAB TO PRIMARY CHEMOTHERAPY

Bevacizumab is a humanized monoclonal antibody targeting VEGF. Elevated VEGF or VEGF-A expression occurs in all stages of OC and is associated with poor prognosis, including shorter survival. Bevacizumab as a single agent produced response rates in the range of 15% to 20% in the setting of recurrent OC (27). Two large randomized trials testing the addition of bevacizumab in the upfront setting have shown an improvement in PFS, but no improvement in OS in primary analyses (**Table 8.11-2**).

GOG 218 was a placebo-controlled three-arm study in women with stage III (incompletely resected) and stage IV disease (27). This trial compared a control group receiving carboplatin AUC 6/paclitaxel 175 mg/m^2 to carboplatin/paclitaxel with concomitant bevacizumab (15 mg/kg every 3 weeks) and to carboplatin/paclitaxel with concomitant bevacizumab followed by maintenance bevacizumab for an additional 16 doses (once every 3 weeks). In groups receiving bevacizumab, it was not started until cycle 2, to avoid postoperative wound healing problems. Median PFS for the three arms was 10.3, 11.2, and 14.1 months, respectively, but there were no significant differences in OS between the groups. The experimental regimen was tolerable; bowel perforation or fistula requiring medical intervention occurred in 1.2% of patients in the control arm, 2.8% of patients in the concomitant-only bevacizumab arm, and 2.6% of patients in the concomitant plus maintenance bevacizumab arm. As the primary end point of the study was PFS, the blind was not maintained after progression, and the authors noted that the end point of OS could have been contaminated by effect of postprogression therapy. The most recent published update of GOG 218 showed no differences in OS between the bevacizumab throughout, bevacizumab concurrent, or placebo groups (median OS 43.4 vs 40.8 vs 41.1 months, P = .34) (28). Various retrospective subset analyses of this trial have been published. Because blocking VEGF inhibits the formation of ascites in preclinical studies, one study examined whether the presence of ascites might affect the benefit from bevacizumab (29). Patients with no ascites (n = 221) had no improvement with bevacizumab in either PFS (aHR 0.81) or OS (aHR 0.94), whereas those with ascites had significantly improvement in both PFS (aHR 0.71) and OS (aHR 0.82) (29). In a separate exploratory analysis of patients with stage IV disease, those who received bevacizumab throughout had an HR 0.75 (95% CI 0.59-0.95) relative to the placebo group (28).

A second trial, ICON7, was led by European investigators and had only two arms: carboplatin/paclitaxel and carboplatin/paclitaxel with concomitant and 12 additional cycles of consolidation every 3-week bevacizumab) (4). There was no placebo, the bevacizumab dose used was lower, 7.5 mg/kg every 3 weeks rather than the 15 mg/kg used in the North American GOG 218 trial, and women with both high-risk early-stage and with more advanced disease were eligible to participate. The restricted mean PFS for the control group and the group receiving bevacizumab were similar at 20.3 versus 21.8 months; restricted mean OS times were also not different at 44.6 versus 45.5 months. Restricted means were used for analysis because there was evidence of nonproportional hazards. In an exploratory analysis of a predefined subgroup of 502 patients with poor prognosis disease (stage IV or stage III with over 1.0 cm residual disease; similar to the population of GOG 218 as a whole), a significant difference in restricted mean OS was observed: 34.5 months for standard therapy versus 39.3 months with bevacizumab (30). A subsequent retrospective analysis of the ICON7 demonstrated that patients with a slow CA-125 clearance (CA-125 elimination rate constant K [KELIM] <1) had the greatest benefit in terms of OS from bevacizumab (31). KELIM as a predictor of benefit to bevacizumab was confirmed when applying the algorithm to the GOG 218 phase III trial (32). Taken together, these subanalyses suggest that the subset of patients with the poorest prognosis seems to have the greatest benefit from receipt of bevacizumab.

The most important increase in toxicity with the addition of bevacizumab in the ICON7 study was the risk of grade 2 or higher hypertension (18% with bevacizumab and 2% with standard therapy) and the risk for grade 3 or higher thromboembolic events (7% with bevacizumab vs 3% with standard therapy). The primary QoL end point in the ICON7 trial was global QoL as assessed by the EORTC QoL questionnaire-core 30 at week 54 (33). At week 54 (approximately just at the end of bevacizumab therapy), the mean

▪ TABLE 8.11-2. Randomized Trials in Epithelial Ovarian Cancer With or Without Bevacizumab

Trial Name	Population	Arms	Results Median PFS/OS	
Frontline setting				
GOG 218 (27,28)	Stage III-IV first line	Bev + carbo + paclitaxel →bev vs Bev + carbo + paclitaxel →placebo vs Placebo + carbo + paclitaxel →placebo	14.1 mo/43.4 mo 11.2 mo/40.8 mo 10.3 mo/41.1 mo	PFS: *P* < .001 for bev throughout vs placebo throughout OS: NS
ICON7 (4,30)	Stage IIB-IV first line Stage I-IIA if gr3 or clear cell	Bev + carbo + paclitaxel →bev vs Carbo + paclitaxel	19 mo/45.5 mo 17.3 mo/44.6 mo	NS
Recurrent setting				
OCEANS (65,66)	Platinum-sensitive first recurrence	Gem + carbo + bev→bev vs Gem + carbo + placebo → placebo	12.4 mo/33.6 mo 8.4 mo/32.9 mo	*P* < .0001 for PFS; *P* = .65 for OS
AURELIA (67) (Pujade-Lauraine, 2014)	Platinum-resistant, 1-2 prior regimens	Chemotherapy + bev→bev Chemotherapy (crossover at progression) Chemotherapy = PLD, topotecan, or weekly paclitaxel	6.7 mo/16.6 mo 3.4 mo/13.3 mo	*P* < .001 for PFS; *P* = .17 for OS
GOG 213 (68) (Coleman, 2017)[a]	Platinum-sensitive first recurrence	Carbo + paclitaxel + bev → bev vs Paclitaxel + carbo	13.8 mo/42.2 mo 10.4 mo/37.3 mo	*P* < .0001 for PFS; *P* = .056 for OS

Bev, bevacizumab; carbo, carboplatin; gr, grade; NS, not statistically significant; OS, overall survival; PFS, progression-free survival; PLD, pegylated liposomal doxorubicin.

[a]OS reported as immature.

From Aghajanian C, Goff B, Nycum LR, Wang YV, Husain A, Blank SV. Final overall survival and safety analysis of OCEANS, a phase 3 trial of chemotherapy with or without bevacizumab in patients with platinum-sensitive recurrent ovarian cancer. *Gynecol Oncol.* 2015;139(1):10-16.

From Aghajanian C, Sill MW, Darcy KM, et al. Phase II trial of bevacizumab in recurrent or persistent endometrial cancer: a Gynecologic Oncology Group study. *J Clin Oncol.* 2011;29(16):2259-2265.

From Burger RA, Brady MF, Bookman MA, et al. Incorporation of bevacizumab in the primary treatment of ovarian cancer. *N Engl J Med.* 2011;365(26): 2473-2483.

From Coleman RL, Brady MF, Herzog TJ, et al. Bevacizumab and paclitaxel-carboplatin chemotherapy and secondary cytoreduction in recurrent, platinum-sensitive ovarian cancer (NRG Oncology/Gynecologic Oncology Group study GOG-0213): a multicentre, open-label, randomised, phase 3 trial. *Lancet Oncol.* 2017;18(6):779-791

From Oza AM, Cook AD, Pfisterer J, et al. Standard chemotherapy with or without bevacizumab for women with newly diagnosed ovarian cancer (ICON7): overall survival results of a phase 3 randomised trial. *Lancet Oncol.* 16(8):928-936.

From Perren TJ, Swart AM, Pfisterer J, et al. A phase 3 trial of bevacizumab in ovarian cancer. *N Engl J Med.* 2011;365(26):2484-2496.

From Pujade-Lauraine E, Hilpert F, Weber B, et al. Bevacizumab combined with chemotherapy for platinum-resistant recurrent ovarian cancer: the AURELIA open-label randomized phase III trial. *J Clin Oncol.* 2014;32(13):1302-1308.

From Tewari KS, Burger RA, Enserro D, et al. Final overall survival of a randomized trial of bevacizumab for primary treatment of ovarian cancer. *J Clin Oncol.* 2019;37(26):2317-2328.

score was 6.4 points lower in the bevacizumab arm (*P* < .0001). By week 76, global QoL was not significantly different between arms.

Based on the results of GOG 218 and ICON7, the European Medicines Agency approved the use of bevacizumab in combination with paclitaxel plus carboplatin for the frontline treatment of advanced OC with at least stage IIIB disease in the EU. Subsequently, bevacizumab became FDA approved in the United States for frontline use in OC. However, its use upfront is not universal, in large part due to the lack of OS benefit seen with bevacizumab in the overall population in either study as well as the high cost of the drug. These discussions have been further complicated by alternative maintenance therapy approaches described later.

The appropriate duration of bevacizumab therapy has also been debated. Because the PFS curves for both GOG 218 and ICON7, which administered bevacizumab only for a fixed period of time after completion of chemotherapy, appear to converge at some point after discontinuation of bevacizumab (nonproportional hazards), it was hypothesized that bevacizumab benefit is dependent on continued administration. However, phase III data showed no difference in PFS or OS in patients treated with 30 months of bevacizumab compared with those treated for the standard 15 months (median PFS 26.0 vs 24.2 months) (34). Thus, limiting maintenance treatment to 15 months duration is appropriate. Results from MITO-16/MANGO2b trial suggest that retreatment with bevacizumab following progression in the platinum-sensitive setting may still be beneficial (35).

INTRAPERITONEAL CHEMOTHERAPY

IP chemotherapy provides a means by which high concentrations of drugs and long durations of tissue exposure can be attained at the peritoneal surface. IP progression of disease remains the major source of morbidity and mortality in OC, and many chemotherapeutic agents including cisplatin, carboplatin, topotecan, and paclitaxel have been tested for feasibility with IP administration. Larger or less water-soluble molecules will stay longer in the peritoneal cavity and have a higher peritoneal cavity-to-plasma concentration ratio (sometimes referred to as "pharmacologic advantage"), but may not get into the bloodstream. The direct penetration of chemotherapy agents into tumor masses is limited to 1 to 2 mm from the tumor surface. Early work by Los et al, using a rat IP tumor model, found that the concentration of cisplatin at the periphery of tumor nodules was higher after IP administration of cisplatin, but the concentration at the center of the nodules was identical after IP and IV administration (36). Hence, (a) the theoretical benefit is only for very small tumor volumes, and (b) agents that do not reach therapeutic systemic levels when given by the IP route need to be administered IV as well. Cisplatin has a 10- to 20-fold pharmacologic advantage when given IP. For a given dose of cisplatin, peak concentrations are higher with IV cisplatin, and this has resulted in somewhat decreased toxicity in a randomized comparison of the same doses of cisplatin given IP versus IV, including less hearing loss and neuromuscular toxicity. However, the amount of cisplatin recovered in the urine, reflecting total systemic exposure, is similar, regardless of whether the administration is IV or IP. Similarly, carboplatin given IP at an AUC of 6 has been shown to produce an AUC in the peritoneal cavity about 17 times higher than that of carboplatin given IV while producing a very similar serum AUC (37). Paclitaxel, on the other hand, has a pharmacologic advantage of about 1,000, and significant levels persist in the peritoneal cavity 1 week after drug administration. However, the dose that can be given is limited by abdominal pain, and serum paclitaxel concentrations detected in patients treated with IP paclitaxel at feasible doses are low (38). Administration of IP chemotherapy can be technically challenging, and catheter-related issues are common.

Clinical Use of Intraperitoneal Therapy for Ovarian Cancer

In January 2006, the NCI issued a clinical alert supporting the use of IP cisplatin chemotherapy in women with optimally surgically debulked OC. A 2006 meta-analysis of eight trials comparing IP

to IV platinum-based chemotherapy (all but one used cisplatin) showed an average 21.6% decrease in the risk of death (HR 0.79; 95% CI, 0.70-0.89) with IP therapy (39). Because the expected median duration of survival for women with optimally debulked OC receiving standard treatment is approximately 4 years, this size reduction in the death rate was estimated to translate into about a 12-month increase in median OS. The power of this analysis was based primarily on the survival benefits for IP chemotherapy observed in the first three randomized trials summarized in **Table 8.11-3** (40-42). However, none of these trials used a modern carboplatin/weekly paclitaxel IV arm, and all of them used IP cisplatin at 100 mg/m^2, which has been deemed unacceptably toxic. In GOG 172, only 42% of patients on the IP arm received the six planned cycles of IP therapy due to either cisplatin-related toxicities or catheter problems.

Significant effort was put into developing a more tolerable IP regimen, by either dose reducing the cisplatin or substituting IP carboplatin for IP cisplatin. These less toxic regimens were compared with an all IV weekly paclitaxel/every 3-week carboplatin regimen in GOG 252 (43). The three arms of GOG 252 included the all IV carboplatin plus dose-dense paclitaxel regimen published

■ **TABLE 8.11-3. Selected Randomized Trials of Intraperitoneal versus Intravenous Chemotherapy in Primarily Debulked Ovarian Cancer**

References	N	Regimens	Median PFS	Median OS	Comments
SWOG 8501/ GOG104 Alberts et al. (40)	546	IV cyclophosphamide 600 mg/m^2 + IP cisplatin 100 mg/m^2 × 6 vs IV cyclophosphamide 600 mg/m^2 + IP cisplatin 100 mg/m^2 × 6	N/A	49 mo vs 41 mo P = .02	<2 cm residual disease permitted; 58% of patients in both groups completed 6 cycles of cisplatin
GOG 114/SWOG 9227 Markman et al (69)	462	IV carboplatin AUC 9 × 2 followed by IV paclitaxel 135 mg/m^2/24 hr + IP cisplatin 100 mg/m^2 × 6 vs IV paclitaxel 135 mg/m^2/24 hr + IV cisplatin 75 mg/m^2 × 6	28 mo vs 22 mo P = .01	63 mo vs 52 mo P = .05	18% of patients on IP arm got ≤2 cycles of IP therapy
GOG 172 Armstrong et al. (42)	416	D1 IV paclitaxel 135 mg/m^2/24 hr + D2 IP cisplatin 100 mg/m^2 + D8 IP paclitaxel 60 mg/m^2 vs D1 IV cisplatin 75 mg/m^2 + D1 IV paclitaxel 135 mg/m^2/24 hr	24 mo vs 19 mo	67 mo vs 50 mo	49% of patients received ≤3 cycles of IP therapy
GOG 252 Walker et al. (43,70)	1,560	D1 IV carboplatin AUC 6 + D1,8,15 IV paclitaxel 80 mg/m^2 vs D1 IP carboplatin AUC 6 + D1, 8, 15 IV paclitaxel 80 mg/m^2 vs D1 IV paclitaxel 135 mg/m^2/3 hr + D2 IP cisplatin 75 mg/m^2 + D8 IP paclitaxel 60 mg/m^2	24.9 mo 27.4 mo 26.2 mo	75.5 78.9 72.9	Bevacizumab 15 mg/kg IV D1 given on all arms
iPocc Fujiwara et al. (44)	655^a	D1 IV carboplatin AUC 6 + D1, 8, 15 IV paclitaxel 80 mg/m^2 vs D1 IP carboplatin AUC 6 + D1, 8, 15 IV paclitaxel 80 mg/m^2	20.7 mo 23.5 mo P = .04	67.0 mo 64.9 mo P = .04	Included patients with suboptimal debulkings: 1-2 cm residual (5%) and >2 cm residual (55%) disease 6-8 cycles administered No maintenance therapy allowed

IP, intraperitoneal; IV, intravenous; OS, overall survival; PFS, progression-free survival.

^{a}Intention-to-treat population. Results for intention-to-treat population are listed.

From Alberts DS, Liu PY, Hannigan E, et al. Intraperitoneal cisplatin plus intravenous cyclophosphamide versus intravenous cisplatin plus intravenous cyclophosphamide for stage III ovarian cancer. *N Engl J Med.* 1996;335(26):1950-1954.

From Armstrong DK, Bundy B, Wenzel L, et al. Intraperitoneal cisplatin and paclitaxel in ovarian cancer. *N Engl J Med.* 2006;353:34-43.

From Fujiwara KN, Yamamoto S, Tanabe K, et al. A randomized phase 3 trial of intraperitoneal versus intravenous carboplatin with dose-dense weekly paclitaxel in patients with ovarian, fallopian tube, or primary peritoneal carcinoma (a GOTIC-001/JGOG-3019/GCIG, iPocc Trial) (LBA 3). *Gynecol Oncol.* 2022;166:S49-S50.

From Markman M, Bundy B, Alberts DS, et al. Phase III trial of standard-dose intravenous cisplatin plus paclitaxel versus moderately high-dose carboplatin followed by intravenous paclitaxel and intraperitoneal cisplatin in small-volume stage III ovarian carcinoma: an intergroup study of the Gynecologic Oncology Group, Southwestern Oncology Group, and Eastern Cooperative Oncology Group. *J Clin Oncol.* 2001;19:1001-1007.

From Walker JL, Brady MF, Wenzel L, et al. Randomized trial of intravenous versus intraperitoneal chemotherapy plus bevacizumab in advanced ovarian carcinoma: an NRG Oncology/Gynecologic Oncology Group Study. *J Clin Oncol.* 2019;37(16):1380-1390.

From Walker JL, Brady MF, Wenzel L. A phase II trial of bevacizumab with IV versus IP chemotherapy for ovarian, fallopian tube, and peritoneal carcinoma: an NRG Oncology Study. *Gynecol Oncol.* 2016. Late Breaking Abstract.

From Fujiwara K, Nagao S, Yamamoto K, et al. A randomized phase 3 trial of intraperitoneal versus intravenous carboplatin with dose-dense weekly paclitaxel in patients with ovarian, fallopian tube, or primary peritoneal carcinoma (a GOTIC-001/JGOG-3019/GCIG, iPocc Trial) (LBA 3). *Gynecol Oncol.* 2022;166:S49-S50.

by the JGOG, the identical regimen with the carboplatin administered IP instead of IV, and a modification of the regimen used in GOG 172 with paclitaxel 135 mg/m^2 IV over 3 hours day 1, cisplatin 75 mg/m^2 IP on day 2, and paclitaxel 60 mg/m^2 IP on day 8. All three arms were combined with bevacizumab, which was administered every 3 weeks and continued for 22 cycles. Final results of this trial were published in 2019 and showed no difference between the three arms, with a median PFS of 24.9 months for the all IV arm, 27.4 months for the IP carboplatin arm, and 26.2 months for the IP cisplatin arm. It has been hypothesized that the use of bevacizumab may have obscured the benefits of IP therapy, as it is postulated to have obscured the benefits of weekly paclitaxel in GOG 262. Most recently, the GOTIC-001/JGOG-3019/GCIG, iPocc trial was presented at the 2022 Society for Gynecologic Oncology annual meeting (44). A notable difference from prior studies was that patients with suboptimal debulking surgery were included, with a large subset of patients having suboptimally debulked disease. In addition, IP and IV carboplatin were compared with no other differences between the regimens. Although a PFS benefit was seen, there was no OS benefit. With these more recent largely negative results, especially in the context of newer upfront maintenance therapies as well as the toxicity and inconvenience of IP regimens, IP chemotherapy for frontline OC is rarely used.

CONSOLIDATION/MAINTENANCE

Many women with OC have an excellent response to first-line chemotherapy, but most will nonetheless relapse and die of their disease. Approximately two-thirds of patients with advanced OC will achieve a clinical complete remission following chemotherapy, that is, have no evidence of disease on physical examination or in radiographic studies together with a serum CA-125 in the normal range.

Multiple maintenance strategies are now available, including bevacizumab, as discussed earlier, and PARPi (discussed later). Discussions around which, if any, improve OS are ongoing and important to consider. In addition, increasing use of biomarker-selected subgroups suggests that the idea of a single approach for all patients with newly diagnosed, advanced OC is no longer appropriate.

Consolidative/Maintenance Chemotherapy

As is the case for use of a third cytotoxic agent in frontline combination therapy, use of a third cytotoxic agent such as topotecan or epirubicin for consolidation/maintenance therapy has failed to improve outcomes (45-47). Two small prospective trials of consolidation with high-dose chemotherapy with hematopoietic stem cell support were also both negative (48,49).

Before the advent of targeted therapy, the most promising trial of maintenance therapy to date had been a Southwest Oncology Group (SWOG)/GOG trial randomizing women in clinical complete remission to either three or 12 cycles of IV paclitaxel 175 mg/m^2 every 4 weeks (50). The trial was halted by its data and safety monitoring board after a planned interim efficacy analysis at a point when there was a statistically significant improvement in time to progression but no difference in OS between the treatment arms (PFS 28 vs 21 months, one-sided $P = .0035$) and subsequent survival comparisons were not possible due to study logistics. An unplanned retrospective subgroup analysis suggested a trend toward survival benefit in the group of patients who started maintenance therapy with a CA-125 level of less than 10 (50). A subsequent Italian study group randomized 200 patients with stages IIb to IV disease who were in clinical or pathologic complete response after six courses of paclitaxel/platinum-based chemotherapy to either observation or six consolidation courses of paclitaxel 175 mg/m^2 every 3 weeks (51). Grade 2 or greater sensory neurotoxicity was reported in 28.0% of the paclitaxel-arm patients. Two-year PFS rate was 54% and 59% (P = not significant) in the control and maintenance arms, respectively. Corresponding 2-year OS rate was 90% and 87% (P = not significant). GOG 212 randomized women in clinical complete remission after primary therapy for stage III or

IV disease to maintenance paclitaxel poliglumex, maintenance paclitaxel, or observation, and results demonstrated no difference in OS, although PFS may have been modestly improved (52).

Maintenance With Poly(ADP-Ribose) Polymerase Inhibitors

The use of maintenance PARPi has been the biggest change in primary treatment for advanced OC in the past 5 years. In general, PARPi impairs a cell's ability to repair single-stranded DNA breaks (53,54). In cells that already lack homologous recombination repair, such as those with *BRCA1* or *BRCA2* mutations, this results in an accumulation of double-stranded DNA breaks. Without homologous recombination repair, cells are forced to use nonhomologous end-joining, which has higher rates of errors. This synthetic lethality seen in tumors with HRD is the basis for many of the trials that have been done to date.

There are now three different FDA approvals involving PARPi maintenance therapy in the frontline setting: maintenance olaparib as a single agent, maintenance niraparib as a single agent, and the combination of olaparib and bevacizumab. Each approval is for a slightly different subgroup of patients with advanced OC as summarized in **Table 8.11-4**.

First, in 2018, olaparib was FDA approved for patients with germline or somatic BRCA mutations, with advanced EOC following response to frontline platinum-based chemotherapy. This approval was based on data from SOLO1, which enrolled 391 patients with stage III or IV, newly diagnosed HGSC or endometrioid OC who had a germline or somatic *BRCA1* or *BRCA2* mutation (55). Patients must have had a partial or complete response to primary platinum-based chemotherapy and were randomly assigned to olaparib 300 mg twice daily orally or placebo. Treatment was continued for 2 years, and the primary end point was PFS. Patients who received olaparib maintenance had a significant improvement in PFS (HR 0.30, 95% CI 0.23-0.41). These data were updated in 2021 to show a median PFS of 56 months in the olaparib group compared with 13.8 months in the placebo group, demonstrating a persistent improvement even after discontinuation at 24 months (**Figure 8.11-2**) (56).

Next, in April 2020, niraparib was FDA approved for all patients with advanced EOC who have had a complete or partial response to frontline platinum-based chemotherapy, regardless of biomarker status. This was based on data from PRIMA, which enrolled 733 patients with newly diagnosed stage III or IV HGSC or endometrioid OC who had completed six to nine cycles of platinum-based chemotherapy and had a complete or partial response (57). All tumors had HRD testing using a commercially available HRD score that incorporated LOH, telomeric-allelic imbalance, and large-scale state transitions. Tumors were considered to be HRD if there was a BRCA mutation, and/or if the commercially available HRD score was at least 42. Patients were randomly assigned to niraparib 300 mg orally once daily (later amended to allow for dose reduction to 200 mg for weight <77 kg or platelet count <150,000) or placebo. This study showed that patients who received niraparib had a significant improvement in PFS (HR 0.43, 95% CI 0.31-0.59). However, this difference was most notable in patients with BRCA mutations (HR 0.40, 95% CI 0.24-0.62) and more modest in patients with homologous recombination–proficient tumors (HR 0.68, 95% CI 0.49-0.94).

Shortly thereafter, in May 2020, the combination of olaparib and bevacizumab was FDA approved for patients with advanced OC whose tumors had a complete or partial response to frontline platinum-based chemotherapy plus bevacizumab and whose tumors demonstrate HRD. This was based on data from PAOLA-1, which enrolled 806 patients with stage III or IV HGSC or endometrioid OC, regardless of biomarker status, or patients with other EOC who also had a germline *BRCA* mutation (58). Patients whose tumors had a complete or partial response to platinum-based chemotherapy in combination with bevacizumab were randomly assigned to olaparib 300 mg orally twice daily or placebo to be given concurrently with bevacizumab maintenance therapy. Treatment was continued for 2 years. Those who received

■ TABLE 8.11-4. Summary of Frontline PARP Inhibitor Maintenance Trials and Their Resultant Indications

Trial	Eligibility Criteria	Arms	Findings	Resultant FDA Approval
SOLO1	• High-grade serous or endometrioid • Germline or somatic *BRCA1* or *BRCA2* mutation • Stage III or IV • Complete or partial response to chemotherapy • Received platinum-based chemotherapy without bevacizumab • Required tumor debulking if stage III; required tumor debulking or primary biopsy if stage IV	Olaparib Placebo	**Median progression-free survival** (olaparib vs placebo): Overall cohort (germline or somatic *BRCA* mutations): Not reached vs 13.8 mo (HR 0.30, 95% CI 0.23-0.41, *P* < .001) Updated analysis (2021): 56 vs 13.8 mo (HR 0.33, 95% CI 0.25-0.43)	First-line maintenance therapy for patients with germline or somatic BRCA mutated, advanced epithelial ovarian cancer following partial or complete response to frontline platinum-based chemotherapy.
PRIMA	• High-grade serous or endometrioid • Subgroup with homologous recombination deficiency (HRD) (*BRCA* mutation or score >42 on myChoice test); other subgroup included those with proficient or unknown HRD status • Stage III or IV • Complete or partial response to chemotherapy • Received at least 6-9 cycles of chemotherapy • Required to have had residual disease after surgery, received neoadjuvant therapy, or be inoperable if stage III, or any stage IV	Niraparib Placebo	**Median progression-free survival** (niraparib vs placebo): HRD cohort: 21.9 vs 10.4 mo (HR 0.43, 95% CI 0.31-0.59, *P* < .001) Overall cohort: 13.8 vs 8.2 mo (HR 0.62, 95% CI 0.50-0.76, *P* < .001)	First-line maintenance therapy for patients with advanced epithelial ovarian cancer following partial or complete response to frontline platinum-based chemotherapy, regardless of HRD status.
PAOLA-1	• High-grade serous or endometrioid, or other nonmucinous epithelial histology with germline *BRCA* mutation • Any *BRCA* mutation status, any HRD status • Stage III or IV • Complete or partial response to chemotherapy • Received bevacizumab as part of treatment • Not required to have had tumor debulking; any debulking outcome allowed	Olaparib, bevacizumab maintenance Placebo, bevacizumab maintenance	**Median progression-free survival** (olaparib vs placebo): Overall cohort: 22.1 vs 16.6 mo (HR 0.59, 95% CI 0.49-0.72, *P* < .001) Somatic *BRCA* mutation cohort: 37.2 vs 21.7 mo (HR 0.31, 95% CI 0.20-0.47) Somatic *BRCA* wild-type cohort: 18.9 vs 16.0 mo (HR 0.71, 95% CI 0.58-0.88) HRD cohort (score ≥42): 37.2 vs 17.7 mo (HR 0.33, 95% CI 0.25-0.45) HRD positive, wild-type somatic *BRCA* cohort: 28.1 vs 16.6 mo (HR 0.43, 95% CI 0.28-0.66) HRD-negative or unknown cohort: 16.9 vs 16.0 mo (HR 0.92, 95% CI 0.72-1.17)	First-line maintenance therapy in combination with bevacizumab for patients with advanced epithelial ovarian cancer whose tumors demonstrate HRD, following partial or complete response to frontline platinum-based chemotherapy.
VELIA	• High-grade serous • Any *BRCA* mutation status, any HRD status • Stage III or IV • Enrolled before chemotherapy • 6 cycles of chemotherapy • Required to have had tumor debulking	Carboplatin, paclitaxel, veliparib with veliparib maintenance Carboplatin, paclitaxel, veliparib with placebo maintenance *NOTE:* This arm was not included in the primary analysis Carboplatin, paclitaxel, placebo with placebo maintenance	**Median progression-free survival** (veliparib throughout vs placebo throughout): Germline *BRCA* mutation: 34.7 vs 22.0 mo (HR 0.44, 95% CI 0.28-0.68, *P* < .001) HRD tumors (score ≥33): 31.9 vs 20.5 mo (HR 0.57, 95% CI 0.43-0.76, *P* < .001) Overall cohort (intention to treat): 23.5 vs 17.3 mo (HR 0.68, 95% CI 0.56-0.83, *P* < .001)	None

CI, confidence interval; FDA, Food and Drug Administration; HR, hazard ratio. From Kurnit KC, Fleming GF, Lengyel E. Updates and new options in advanced epithelial ovarian cancer treatment. *Obstet Gynecol.* 2021;137(1):108-121.

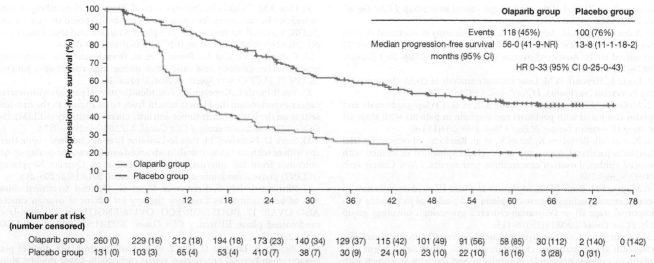

Figure 8.11-2. Long-term progression-free survival with maintenance olaparib treatment for patients with newly diagnosed advanced ovarian cancer and a BRCA mutation (SOLO1/GOG 3004) phase III trial. CI, confidence interval; HR, hazard ratio. (Figure 3A from Banerjee S, Moore KN, Colombo N, et al. Maintenance olaparib for patients with newly diagnosed advanced ovarian cancer and a BRCA mutation (SOLO1/GOG 3004): 5-year follow-up of a randomised, double-blind, placebo-controlled, phase 3 trial. *Lancet Oncol.* 2021;22(12):1721-1731.)

olaparib in combination with bevacizumab had a longer PFS (HR 0.59, 95% CI 0.49-0.72). This difference was most notable in patients with HRD tumors using the commercially available HRD score and including those with BRCA mutations (HR 0.33, 95% CI 0.25-0.45). There was no difference in PFS for the patients who had homologous recombination–proficient tumors, or whose HRD status was unknown (HR 0.92, 95% CI 0.72-1.17).

Two other PARPi have been evaluated in the primary maintenance setting in phase III randomized controlled trials. Although both rucaparib (59) and veliparib (60) demonstrated some survival benefit, neither is approved in this setting at the time of this writing.

Based on these data, PARPi maintenance therapy in the frontline setting has become more widespread. Data are strongest and it is considered standard of care for those patients with *BRCA* mutations, but even those patients without *BRCA* mutations whose tumors show HRD might benefit in PFS. The subgroup of patients whose tumors are homologous recombination proficient are where the benefit of PARPi therapy is less consistent. It is also important to note that, to date, OS data are limited/immature. The OS data from SOLO1 (BRCA mutation carriers) showed a "clinically meaningful albeit not statistically significant" OS benefit: At 7 years, 67.0% of olaparib patients versus 46.5% of placebo patients were alive (61). Thus, it is important that all discussion around maintenance therapy include a discussion of QoL considerations. Although these drugs are generally well tolerated in the primary setting, they can cause cytopenias, nausea, and significant fatigue. Other complications include anemia and, in rare instances, myelodysplastic syndrome/acute myeloid leukemia (MDS/AML) (55,57). After the initial treatment and completion of adjuvant therapy, this may be the only significant period of time that many patients with advanced OC are off of treatment and thus discussions should weigh the potential side effects and risks against benefit in this context.

Maintenance with Immune Checkpoint Inhibitors

More recently, immunotherapy, specifically immune checkpoint inhibitor therapy, has been evaluated in the primary maintenance setting. Although there was a great deal of excitement about these agents, current data are disappointing. JAVELIN Ovarian 100 was a phase 3 trial of patients with stage III or IV EOC who were randomized to chemotherapy (carboplatin and paclitaxel) plus avelumab concurrently and as maintenance, versus chemotherapy with avelumab maintenance, versus

chemotherapy alone (62). The study was stopped early when no PFS benefit was seen at the planned interim analysis (avelumab throughout: HR 1.14, 95% CI 0.86-1.56; avelumab maintenance: HR 1.43, 95% CI 1.05-1.95). IMagyn050/GOG 3015/ENGOT-OV39 was a phase III trial of patients with stage III or IV OC who were randomized to chemotherapy (carboplatin and paclitaxel) plus bevacizumab, with or without atezolizumab concurrently for 22 cycles (63). As in the JAVELIN trial, there was no PFS benefit seen with the addition of atezolizumab (HR 0.92, 95% CI 0.79-1.07). Therefore, immunotherapy in the frontline setting is not currently standard of care. However, many other trials with other agents and combinations are currently ongoing. Still at this time, there is insufficient evidence to use checkpoint inhibitor as adjuvant therapy.

REFERENCES

1. Vergote I, Tropé CG, Amant F, et al. Neoadjuvant chemotherapy or primary surgery in stage IIIC or IV ovarian cancer. *N Engl J Med.* 2010;363(10):943-953. doi:10.1056/NEJMoa0908806

2. Kehoe S, Hook J, Nankivell M, et al. Primary chemotherapy versus primary surgery for newly diagnosed advanced ovarian cancer (CHORUS): an open-label, randomised, controlled, non-inferiority trial. *Lancet.* 2015;386(9990):249-257. doi:10.1016/S0140-6736(14)62223-6

3. Wright AA, Bohlke K, Armstrong DK, et al. Neoadjuvant chemotherapy for newly diagnosed, advanced ovarian cancer: society of gynecologic oncology and American society of clinical oncology clinical practice guideline. *Gynecol Oncol.* 2016;143(1):3-15. doi:10.1016/j.ygyno.2016.05.022

4. Perren TJ, Swart AM, Pfisterer J, et al. A phase 3 trial of bevacizumab in ovarian cancer. *N Engl J Med.* 2011;365(26):2484-2496. doi:10.1056/NEJMoa1103799

5. Hakes TB, Chalas E, Hoskins WJ, et al. Randomized prospective trial of 5 versus 10 cycles of cyclophosphamide, doxorubicin, and cisplatin in advanced ovarian carcinoma. *Gynecol Oncol.* 1992;45(3):284-289.

6. Bertelsen K, Jakobsen A, Stroyer J, et al. A prospective randomized comparison of 6 and 12 cycles of cyclophosphamide, adriamycin, and cisplatin in advanced epithelial ovarian cancer: a Danish ovarian study group trial (DACOVA). *Gynecol Oncol.* 1993;49(1):30-36.

7. Lambert HE, Rustin GJ, Gregory WM, Nelstrop AE. A randomized trial of five versus eight courses of cisplatin or carboplatin in advanced epithelial ovarian carcinoma. A North Thames ovary group study. *Ann Oncol.* 1997;8(4):327-333.

8. Clamp AR, James EC, McNeish IA, et al. Weekly dose-dense chemotherapy in first-line epithelial ovarian, fallopian tube. *Lancet.* 2019;394(10214):2084-2095.

9. Bookman MA, Brady MF, McGuire WP, et al. Evaluation of new platinum-based treatment regimens in advanced-stage ovarian

cancer: a phase III trial of the gynecologic cancer intergroup. *J Clin Oncol.* 2009;27(9):1419-1425.

10. Aabo K, Adams M, Adnitt P, et al. Chemotherapy in advanced ovarian cancer: four systematic meta-analyses of individual patient data from 37 randomized trials. Advanced ovarian cancer trialists' group. *Br J Cancer.* 1998;78(11):1479-1487.

11. Levin L, Hryniuk WM. Dose intensity analysis of chemotherapy regimens in ovarian carcinoma. *J Clin Oncol.* 1987;5(5):756-767.

12. McGuire WP, Hoskins WJ, Brady MF, et al. Cyclophosphamide and cisplatin compared with paclitaxel and cisplatin in patients with stage III and stage IV ovarian cancer. *N Engl J Med.* 1996;334(1):1-6.

13. Piccart MJ, Bertelsen K, James K, et al. Randomized intergroup trial of cisplatin-paclitaxel versus cisplatin-cyclophosphamide in women with advanced epithelial ovarian cancer: three-year results. *J Natl Cancer Inst.* 2000;92(9):699-708.

14. Muggia FM, Braly PS, Brady MF, et al. Phase III randomized study of cisplatin versus paclitaxel versus cisplatin and paclitaxel in patients with suboptimal stage III or IV ovarian cancer: a gynecologic oncology group study. *J Clin Oncol.* 2000;18(1):106-115.

15. International Collaborative Ovarian Neoplasm Group. Paclitaxel plus carboplatin versus standard chemotherapy with either single-agent carboplatin or cyclophosphamide, doxorubicin, and cisplatin in women with ovarian cancer: the ICON3 randomised trial. *Lancet.* 2002;360(9332):505-515. doi:10.1016/S0140-6736(02)09738-6

16. Falandry, C., et al. Efficacy and safety of first-line single-agent carboplatin vs carboplatin plus paclitaxel for vulnerable older adult women with ovarian cancer: A GINECO/GCIG randomized clinical trial. *JAMA Oncol.* 2021;7(6):853-861.

17. Bolis G, Scarfone G, Polverino G, et al. Paclitaxel 175 or 225 mg per meters squared with carboplatin in advanced ovarian cancer: a randomized trial. *J Clin Oncol.* 2004;22(4):686-690.

18. Katsumata N, Yasuda M, Isonishi S, et al. Long-term results of dose-dense paclitaxel and carboplatin versus conventional paclitaxel and carboplatin for treatment of advanced epithelial ovarian, fallopian tube, or primary peritoneal cancer (JGOG 3016): a randomised, controlled, open-label trial. *Lancet Oncol.* 2013;14(10):1020-1026. doi:10.1016/S1470-2045(13)70363-2

19. Chan JK, Brady MF, Penson RT, et al. Weekly vs. every-3-week paclitaxel and carboplatin for ovarian cancer. *N Engl J Med.* 2016;374(8):738-748. doi:10.1056/NEJMoa1505067

20. Pignata S, Scambia G, Katsaros D, et al. Carboplatin plus paclitaxel once a week versus every 3 weeks in patients with advanced ovarian cancer (MITO-7): a randomised, multicentre, open-label, phase 3 trial. *Lancet Oncol.* 2014;15(4):396-405. doi:10.1016/S1470-2045(14)70049-X

21. Clamp AR, James EC, McNeish IA, et al. Weekly dose-dense chemotherapy in first-line epithelial ovarian, fallopian tube, or primary peritoneal cancer treatment (ICON8): overall survival results from an open-label, randomised, controlled, phase 3 trial. *Lancet Oncol.* 2022;23(7):919-930. doi:10.1016/S1470-2045(22)00283-2

22. Blagden SP, Cook AD, Poole C, et al. Weekly platinum-based chemotherapy versus 3-weekly platinum-based chemotherapy for newly diagnosed ovarian cancer (ICON8): quality-of-life results of a phase 3, randomised, controlled trial. *Lancet Oncol.* 2020;21(7):969-977.

23. Vasey PA, Jayson GC, Gordon A, et al. Phase III randomized trial of docetaxel-carboplatin versus paclitaxel-carboplatin as first-line chemotherapy for ovarian carcinoma. *J Natl Cancer Inst.* 2004;96:1682-1691.

24. Parisi A, Palluzzi E, Cortellini A, et al. First-line carboplatin/nab-paclitaxel in advanced ovarian cancer patients, after hypersensitivity reaction to solvent-based taxanes: a single-institution experience. *Clin Transl Oncol.* 2020;22(1):158-162.

25. Gordon AN, Teneriello M, Janicek MF, et al. Phase III trial of induction gemcitabine or paclitaxel plus carboplatin followed by paclitaxel consolidation in ovarian cancer. *Gynecol Oncol.* 2011;123(3):479-485.

26. Pignata S, Scambia G, Ferrandina G, et al. Carboplatin plus paclitaxel versus carboplatin plus pegylated liposomal doxorubicin as first-line treatment for patients with ovarian cancer: the MITO-2 randomized phase III trial. *J Clin Oncol.* 2011;29(27):3628-3635.

27. Burger RA, Brady MF, Bookman MA, et al. Incorporation of bevacizumab in the primary treatment of ovarian cancer. *N Engl J Med.* 2011;365(26):2473-2483. doi:10.1056/NEJMoa1104390

28. Tewari KS, Burger RA, Enserro D, et al. Final overall survival of a randomized trial of bevacizumab for primary treatment of ovarian cancer. *J Clin Oncol.* 2019;37(26):2317-2328.

29. Ferriss JS, Java JJ, Bookman MA, et al. Ascites predicts treatment benefit of bevacizumab in front-line therapy of advanced epithelial ovarian, fallopian tube and peritoneal cancers: an NRG oncology/GOG study. *Gynecol Oncol.* 2015;139(1):17-22.

30. Oza AM, Cook AD, Pfisterer J, et al. Standard chemotherapy with or without bevacizumab for women with newly diagnosed ovarian cancer (ICON7): overall survival results of a phase 3 randomised trial. *Lancet Oncol.* 2015;16(8):928-936. doi:10.1016/S1470-2045(15)00086-8

31. Colomban O, Tod M, Peron J, et al. Bevacizumab for newly diagnosed ovarian cancers: best candidates among high-risk disease patients (ICON-7). *JNCI Cancer Spectr.* 2020;4(3):pkaa026.

32. You B, Purdy C, Copeland LJ, et al. Identification of patients with ovarian cancer experiencing the highest benefit from bevacizumab in the first-line setting on the basis of their tumor-intrinsic chemosensitivity (KELIM): the GOG-0218 validation study. *J Clin Oncol.* 2022;40(34):3965-3974.

33. Stark D, Nankivell M, Pujade-Lauraine E, et al. Standard chemotherapy with or without bevacizumab in advanced ovarian cancer: quality-of-life outcomes from the International Collaboration on Ovarian Neoplasms (ICON7) phase 3 randomised trial. *Lancet Oncol.* 2013;14(3):236-243.

34. Pfisterer J, Joly F, Kristensen G, et al. Optimal treatment duration of bevacizumab as front-line therapy for advanced ovarian cancer: AGO-OVAR 17 BOOST/GINECO OV118/ENGOT Ov-15 open-label randomized phase III trial. *J Clin Oncol.* 2023;41:893-902. doi:10.1200/JCO.22.01010

35. Pignata S, Lorusso D, Joly F, et al. Carboplatin-based doublet plus bevacizumab beyond progression versus carboplatin-based doublet alone in patients with platinum-sensitive ovarian cancer: a randomised, phase 3 trial. *Lancet Oncol.* 2021;22(2):267-276.

36. Los G, Ruevekamp M, Bosnie N, De Graaf PW, McVie JG. Intraperitoneal tumor growth and chemotherapy in a rat model. *Eur J Cancer Clin Oncol.* 1989;25(12):1857-1866.

37. Miyagi Y, Fujiwara K, Kigawa J, et al. Intraperitoneal carboplatin infusion may be a pharmacologically more reasonable route than intravenous administration as a systemic chemotherapy. A comparative pharmacokinetic analysis of platinum using a new mathematical model after intraperitoneal vs. intravenous infusion of carboplatin—a Sankai Gynecology Study Group (SGSG) study. *Gynecol Oncol.* 2005;99(3):591-596. doi:10.1016/j.ygyno.2005.06.055

38. Fujiwara K, Armstrong D, Morgan M, Markman M. Principles and practice of intraperitoneal chemotherapy for ovarian cancer. *Int J Gynecol Cancer.* 2007;17(1):1-20.

39. Jaaback K, Johnson N. Intraperitoneal chemotherapy for the initial management of primary epithelial ovarian cancer. *Cochrane Database Syst Rev.* 2006;(1):CD005340. doi:10.1002/14651858.CD005340.pub2

40. Alberts DS, Liu PY, Hannigan EV, et al. Intraperitoneal cisplatin plus intravenous cyclophosphamide versus intravenous cisplatin plus intravenous cyclophosphamide for stage III ovarian cancer. *N Engl J Med.* 1996;335(26):1950-1955.

41. Markman M. Intraperitoneal chemotherapy in the management of malignant disease. *Expert Rev Anticancer Ther.* 2001;1(1):142-148. doi:10.1586/14737140.1.1.142

42. Armstrong DK, Bundy B, Wenzel L, et al. Intraperitoneal cisplatin and paclitaxel in ovarian cancer. *N Engl J Med.* 2006;354(1):34-43. doi:10.1056/NEJMoa052985

43. Walker JL, Brady MF, Wenzel L, et al. Randomized trial of intravenous versus intraperitoneal chemotherapy plus bevacizumab in advanced ovarian carcinoma: an NRG oncology/gynecologic oncology group study. *J Clin Oncol.* 2019;37(16):1380-1390. doi:10.1200/JCO.18.01568

44. Fujiwara K, Nagao S, Yamamoto K, et al. A randomized phase 3 trial of intraperitoneal versus intravenous carboplatin with dose-dense weekly paclitaxel in patients with ovarian, fallopian tube, or primary peritoneal carcinoma (a GOTIC-001/JGOG-3019/GCIG, iPocc Trial) (LBA 3). *Gynecol Oncol.* 2022;166:S49-S50.

45. Placido S, Scambia G, Vagno G, et al. Topotecan compared with no therapy after response to surgery and carboplatin/paclitaxel in patients with ovarian cancer: multicenter Italian trials in ovarian cancer (MITO-1) randomized study. *J Clin Oncol.* 2004;22(13):2635-2642.

46. Bolis G, Danese S, Tateo S, et al. Epidoxorubicin versus no treatment as consolidation therapy in advanced ovarian cancer: results from a phase II study. *Int J Gynecol Cancer.* 2006;16(Suppl. 1):74-78.

47. du Bois A, Weber B, Rochon J, et al. Addition of epirubicin as a third drug to carboplatin-paclitaxel in first-line treatment of advanced ovarian cancer: a prospectively randomized gynecologic cancer intergroup trial by the arbeitsgemeinschaft gynaekologische onkologie ovarian cancer study group and the groupe d'Investigateurs nationaux pour l'Etude des cancers ovariens. *J Clin Oncol.* 2006;24(7):1127-1135. doi:10.1200/JCO.2005.03.2938

48. Pujade-Lauraine E, Cure H, Battista C, et al. High dose chemotherapy in ovarian cancer. *Int J Gynecol Cancer.* 2001;11(Suppl. 1):64-67.

49. Papadimitriou C, Dafni U, Anagnostopoulos A, et al. High-dose melphalan and autologous stem cell transplantation as consolidation treatment in patients with chemosensitive ovarian cancer: results of a single-institution randomized trial. *Bone Marrow Transplant.* 2008;41(6):547-554.

50. Markman M, Liu PY, Moon J, et al. Impact on survival of 12 versus 3 monthly cycles of paclitaxel (175 mg/m^2) administered to patients with advanced ovarian cancer who attained a complete response to primary platinum-paclitaxel: follow-up of a southwest oncology group and gynecologic oncology group phase 3 trial. *Gynecol Oncol.* 2009;114(2):195-198.

51. Pecorelli S, Favalli G, Gadducci A, et al. Phase III trial of observation versus six courses of paclitaxel in patients with advanced epithelial ovarian cancer in complete response after six courses of paclitaxel/platinum-based chemotherapy: final results of the after-6 protocol. *J Clin Oncol.* 2009;27:4642-4648.

52. Copeland LJ, Brady MF, Burger RA, et al. Phase III randomized trial of maintenance taxanes versus surveillance in women with advanced ovarian/tubal/peritoneal cancer: a gynecologic oncology group 0212: NRG oncology study. *J Clin Oncol.* 2022;40:4119-4128. doi:10.1200/JCO.22.00146

53. Plummer R. Perspective on the pipeline of drugs being developed with modulation of DNA damage as a target. *Clin Cancer Res.* 2010;16(18):4527-4531.

54. Helleday T. The underlying mechanism for the PARP and BRCA synthetic lethality: clearing up the misunderstandings. *Mol Oncol.* 2011;5(4):387-393.

55. Moore K, Colombo N, Scambia G, et al. Maintenance olaparib in patients with newly diagnosed advanced ovarian cancer. *N Engl J Med.* 2018;379(26):2495-2505. doi:10.1056/NEJMoa1810858

56. Banerjee S, Moore KN, Colombo N, et al. Maintenance olaparib for patients with newly diagnosed advanced ovarian cancer and a BRCA mutation (SOLO1/GOG 3004): 5-year follow-up of a randomised, double-blind, placebo-controlled, phase 3 trial. *Lancet Oncol.* 2021;22:1721-1731.

57. González-Martín A, Pothuri B, Vergote I, et al. Niraparib in patients with newly diagnosed advanced ovarian cancer. *N Engl J Med.* 2019;381(25):2391-2402. doi:10.1056/NEJMoa1910962

58. Ray-Coquard I, Pautier P, Pignata S, et al. Olaparib plus bevacizumab as first-line maintenance in ovarian cancer. *N Engl J Med.* 2019;381(25):2416-2428.

59. Monk BJ, Parkinson C, Lim MC, et al. A randomized, phase III trial to evaluate rucaparib monotherapy as maintenance treatment in patients with newly diagnosed ovarian cancer (ATHENA-MONO/GOG-3020/ENGOT-ov45). *J Clin Oncol.* 2022;40(34):3952-3964. doi:10.1200/JCO.22.01003

60. Coleman RL, Fleming GF, Brady MF, et al. Veliparib with first-line chemotherapy and as maintenance therapy in ovarian cancer. *N Engl J Med.* 2019;381:2403-2415. doi:10.1056/NEJMoa1909707

61. DiSilvestro P, Banerjee S, Colombo N, et al. Overall survival with maintenance olaparib at a 7-year follow-up in patients with newly diagnosed advanced ovarian cancer and a BRCA mutation: the SOLO1/GOG 3004 trial. *J Clin Oncol.* 2023;41:609-617. doi:10.1200/JCO.22.01549

62. Monk BJ, Colombo N, Oza AM, et al. Chemotherapy with or without avelumab followed by avelumab maintenance versus chemotherapy alone in patients with previously untreated epithelial ovarian cancer (JAVELIN ovarian 100): an open-label, randomised, phase 3 trial. *Lancet Oncol.* 2021;22(9):1275-1289.

63. Moore KN, Bookman M, Sehouli J, et al. Atezolizumab, bevacizumab, and chemotherapy for newly diagnosed stage III or IV ovarian cancer: placebo-controlled randomized phase III trial (IMagyn050/GOG 3015/ENGOT-OV39). *J Clin Oncol.* 2021;39(17):1842-1855. doi:10.1200/JCO.21.00306

64. Spriggs DR, Brady MF, Vaccarello L, et al. Phase III randomized trial of intravenous cisplatin plus a 24- or 96-hour infusion of paclitaxel in epithelial ovarian cancer: a Gynecologic Oncology Group Study. *J Clin Oncol.* 2007;25(28):4466-4471.

65. Aghajanian C, Sill MW, Darcy KM, et al. Phase II trial of bevacizumab in recurrent or persistent endometrial cancer: a Gynecologic Oncology Group study. *J Clin Oncol.* 2011;29(16):2259-2265.

66. Aghajanian C, Goff B, Nycum LR, Wang YV, Husain A, Blank SV. Final overall survival and safety analysis of OCEANS, a phase 3 trial of chemotherapy with or without bevacizumab in patients with platinum-sensitive recurrent ovarian cancer. *Gynecol Oncol.* 2015;139(1):10-16.

67. Pujade-Lauraine E, Hilpert F, Weber B, et al. Bevacizumab combined with chemotherapy for platinum-resistant recurrent ovarian cancer: the AURELIA open-label randomized phase III trial. *J Clin Oncol.* 2014;32(13):1302-1308.

68. Coleman RL, Brady MF, Herzog TJ, et al. Bevacizumab and paclitaxel-carboplatin chemotherapy and secondary cytoreduction in recurrent, platinum-sensitive ovarian cancer (NRG Oncology/Gynecologic Oncology Group study GOG-0213): a multicentre, open-label, randomised, phase 3 trial. *Lancet Oncol.* 2017;18(6):779-791.

69. Markman M, Bundy B, Alberts DS, et al. Phase III trial of standard-dose intravenous cisplatin plus paclitaxel versus moderately high-dose carboplatin followed by intravenous paclitaxel and intraperitoneal cisplatin in small-volume stage III ovarian carcinoma: an intergroup study of the gynecologic oncology group, southwestern oncology group, and eastern cooperative oncology group. *J Clin Oncol.* 2001;19:1001-1007.

70. Walker JL, Brady MF, Wenzel L. A phase II trial of bevacizumab with IV versus IP chemotherapy for ovarian, fallopian tube, and peritoneal carcinoma: an NRG Oncology Study. *Gynecol Oncol.* 2016. Late Breaking Abstract.

CHAPTER

8.12

Approach to Advanced and Recurrent Clear Cell, Mucinous, or Endometrioid Cancer

Katherine C. Kurnit and Gini F. Fleming

TREATMENT CONSIDERATIONS FOR ADVANCED OR RECURRENT CLEAR CELL, MUCINOUS, AND ENDOMETRIOID OVARIAN CANCER

Historically, clinical trials for EOC included all histologic subtypes together. It has become obvious that this is not optimal and that the different histologic subtypes are both biologically and clinically distinct. Because high-grade serous tumors make up about two-thirds of advanced-stage disease, there has been little power to draw conclusions about the relative benefit of the treatment under study to less common subtypes. However, sensitivity to standard cytotoxic chemotherapy differs across histology, and in this section, we review data to support this and how it might inform management.

Endometrioid Ovarian Cancer

Endometrioid OC is an endometriosis-associated malignancy, much like clear cell carcinoma (2), and it is overrepresented among the histologies for women with Lynch syndrome. On average, endometrioid OC presents at a younger age than HGSC of the ovary, and a high proportion of cases are diagnosed in early-stage FIGO I (3). Most reports include only grade 1 and 2 tumors in the category of endometrioid OC (1); both early-stage and advanced-stage grade 1/2 endometrioid tumors have better outcomes than any other OC subtype, except LGSC. Molecular characterization of endometrioid OC using the four TCGA subtypes seen in endometrial cancer (*POLE* mutated [*POLE*mut], MMRd, p-53 abnormal [p-53abn], and no specific molecular profile [NSMP]) has been used to categorize endometrioid OC (4). A review of four studies found that 5% of endometrioid OCs were *POLE*mut, 14.6% were

MMRd, 14% were p53abnormal, and 66.4% had NSMP. The *PO-LE*mut tumors did uniformly well, and the p-53abn group had the worst prognosis, with 2.8-fold increased risk of death compared to the NSMP group. There was little difference in outcomes between the NSMP and MMRd groups.

All women with recurrent endometrioid OC should have their tumors tested for MSI or MMRd, as single-agent checkpoint therapy may be effective in the setting of these alterations. ER and PR positivity is often seen, and endocrine therapy with aromatase inhibitors or tamoxifen may be attempted (5-6).

Clear Cell Ovarian Carcinoma

Depending on geographic and ethnic risk factors, clear cell carcinoma represents 5% to 25% of ovarian carcinomas, with the highest rates among Asian women. Clear cell carcinoma tends to present in younger women and more often at an early stage than HGSOC. Endometriosis is a risk factor; only about 6% of clear cell OCs are BRCA1/2 related. Clear cell carcinomas are associated with a high incidence of thrombosis; hypercalcemia is also seen more frequently than in the other epithelial histologies (7).

Early-stage clear cell OC has a relatively good prognosis (**Figure 8.9-1**) (1), whereas advanced-stage disease carries a worse prognosis than HGSC. One single institution experience including 110 FIGO stage I clear cell cancers found that 3-year PFS was 93%, 90%, and 56% for women with stage IA disease (56% of the cohort), those with stage IC disease based solely on rupture (28%), and those with stage IC based on surface involvement and/or positive cytology (8) (**Figure 8.12-1**). For those with advanced clear cell carcinoma, poorer outcomes are attributed to the lower response rates seen with platinum/taxane treatment than those with HGSC. Unfortunately, there is no other chemotherapy regimen that has been shown to be more effective and, as such, carboplatin/paclitaxel remains the standard (neo)adjuvant therapy for advanced disease.

The benefit of adjuvant chemotherapy in early-stage disease is controversial. Some consensus guidelines note that both adjuvant chemotherapy and observation are reasonable options for stage IA clear cell carcinoma. Beyond that, chemotherapy is recommended for higher stage disease. On the other hand, the ESMO guidelines suggest chemotherapy for those with FIGO stage IC2-3 disease, but not earlier disease, especially if comprehensively staged (7).

Response rates to standard chemotherapy in women with relapsed disease, whether or not it falls in a classic platinum-sensitive timeframe, are low. Investigational approaches aim to take advantage of known molecular alterations in clear cell carcinoma. For example, approximately 15% of clear cell OCs are MMRd, raising interest in immunotherapy as an option. The phase II NRG

GY003 trial enrolled people with recurrent or persistent disease who had received up to three cytotoxic regimens and randomly assigned them to nivolumab or nivolumab plus ipilimumab (9). In an exploratory analysis, those who had clear cell carcinoma ($N = 12$) had a 5-fold higher odds of response compared to other tumor types. These treatments are now under investigation in a clinical trial exclusively enrolling people with extrarenal clear cell carcinoma (NCT03355976).

Mucinous Ovarian Tumors

Mucinous ovarian carcinoma is a rare tumor, representing about 1% to 3% of EOCs, and it presents both diagnostic and therapeutic difficulties for oncologists. It is seen in younger women than other EOCs; 26% of mucinous tumors are diagnosed in women under the age of 44 years. The difficulties in distinguishing it from metastatic GI tract tumors are discussed in "Pathology" section (Chapter 8.7). It is not associated with germline BRCA1/2 mutations; the only clinical risk factor that has been identified is smoking (10).

Sixty-five to 80% of mucinous OCs are diagnosed in stage I, at which time they have a good prognosis (see **Figure 8.9-2**) (1); however, subtypes seem to be important, with infiltrative subtypes appearing to carry a worse prognosis than the expansile subtype (11). When diagnosed at an advanced stage III/IV, the median OS is only 12 to 33 months. As these cancers are not usually chemotherapy sensitive, complete surgical resection is important, and the size of residual disease has been shown to be significantly associated with OS and event-free survival (11).

An international frontline trial (mEOC/GOG 0241) for stage II-IV (or recurrent after stage I disease) mucinous OCs randomly assigned women to carboplatin/paclitaxel with or without bevacizumab versus a regimen used in GI malignancies, capecitabine/oxaliplatin with or without bevacizumab (12). Unfortunately, this trial was closed owing to poor enrollment after only 50 patients were enrolled. No OS benefit was seen for the addition of bevacizumab (HR 1.04). OS HR was 0.78 ($P = 0.48$) for capecitabine/oxaliplatin versus carboplatin/paclitaxel. Response rate was 27% for capecitabine/oxaliplatin and 22% for carboplatin/paclitaxel. Retrospective pathology review revealed that only 45% (18/40) of cases with available material had confirmed primary mucinous OC. However, there was no clear evidence that patients with confirmed primary mucinous OC had different outcomes from those considered to have metastatic disease. Because there were no firm conclusions, several retrospective studies attempted to address the question of whether GI regimens may be beneficial. One small case series showed no difference between regimens (13). In contrast, a second, larger retrospective cohort study reported an OS benefit when GI-directed chemotherapy regimen was used (14).

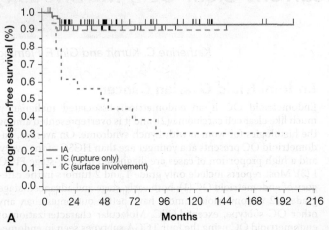

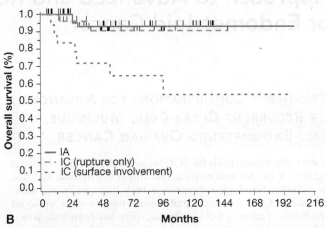

Figure 8.12-1. Kaplan-Meier survival analysis for ovarian clear cell carcinoma stratified by stage I breakdown—progression-free survival (A) and overall survival (B). (From Shu CA, Zhou Q, Jotwani AR, et al. Ovarian clear cell carcinoma, outcomes by stage: the MSK experience. *Gynecol Oncol.* 2015;139(2):236-241.)

Genomic alterations in mucinous carcinomas have been reported (10). Between 20% and 38% of mucinous tumors have been reported to be *HER2* amplified, and an additional 2% to 12% have *HER2* or *HER3* mutations and 15% to 20% have been reported to be MMRd. As such, women with advanced disease should have their tumors evaluated for these molecular abnormalities, which may provide treatable targets.

REFERENCES

1. Peres LC, Cushing-Haugen KL, Kobel M, et al. Invasive epithelial ovarian cancer survival by histotype and disease stage. *J Natl Cancer Inst.* 2019;111(1):60-68.

2. Anglesio MS, Yong PJ. Endometriosis-associated ovarian cancers. *Clin Obstet Gynecol.* 2017;60(4):711-727.

3. Nonneville A, Zemmour C, Frank S, et al. Clinicopathological characterization of a real-world multicenter cohort of endometrioid ovarian carcinoma: analysis of the French national ESME-unicancer database. *Gynecol Oncol.* 2021;163(1):64-71.

4. D'Alessandris N, Travaglino A, Santoro A, et al. TCGA molecular subgroups of endometrial carcinoma in ovarian endometrioid carcinoma: a quantitative systematic review. *Gynecol Oncol.* 2021;163(2):427-432.

5. Bowman A, Gabra H, Langdon SP, et al. CA125 response is associated with estrogen receptor expression in a phase II trial of letrozole in ovarian cancer: identification of an endocrine-sensitive subgroup. *Clin Cancer Res.* 2002;8(7):2233-2239.

6. McLaughlin PMJ, Klar M, Zwimpfer TA, et al. Maintenance therapy with aromatase inhibitor in epithelial ovarian cancer (MATAO): study protocol of a randomized double-blinded placebo-controlled multi-center phase III trial. *BMC Cancer.* 2022;22(1):508.

7. Gadducci A, Multinu F, Cosio S, Carinelli S, Ghioni M, Aletti GD. Clear cell carcinoma of the ovary: epidemiology, pathological and biological features, treatment options and clinical outcomes. *Gynecol Oncol.* 2021;162(3):741-750.

8. Shu CA, Zhou Q, Jotwani AR, et al. Ovarian clear cell carcinoma, outcomes by stage: the MSK experience. *Gynecol Oncol.* 2015;139(2):236-241.

9. Zamarin D, Burger RA, Sill MW, et al. Randomized phase II Trial of nivolumab versus nivolumab and ipilimumab for recurrent or persistent ovarian cancer: an NRG oncology study. *J Clin Oncol.* 2020;38(16):1814-1823.

10. Morice P, Gouy S, Leary A. Mucinous ovarian carcinoma. *N Engl J Med.* 2019;380(13):1256-1266.

11. Colombo N, Sessa C, Bois AD, et al. ESMO-ESGO consensus conference recommendations on ovarian cancer: pathology and molecular biology, early and advanced stages, borderline tumours and recurrent disease. *Int J Gynecol Cancer.* 2019;29(4):728-760.

12. Gore M, Hackshaw A, Brady WE, et al. An international, phase III randomized trial in patients with mucinous epithelial ovarian cancer (mEOC/GOG 0241) with long-term follow-up: and experience of conducting a clinical trial in a rare gynecological tumor. *Gynecol Oncol.* 2019;153(3):541-548.

13. Schlappe BA, Zhou QC, O'Cearbhaill R, et al. A descriptive report of outcomes of primary mucinous ovarian cancer patients receiving either an adjuvant gynecologic or gastrointestinal chemotherapy regimen. *Int J Gynecol Cancer.* 2019;29:904-909..

14. Kurnit KC, Sinno AK, Fellman BM, et al. Effects of gastrointestinal-type chemotherapy in women with ovarian mucinous carcinoma. *Obstet Gynecol.* 2019;134(6):1253-1259.

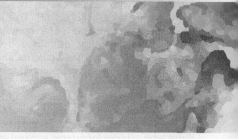

CHAPTER **8.13**

Treatment of Ovarian Carcinosarcoma

Katherine C. Kurnit and Gini F. Fleming

OVARIAN CARCINOSARCOMA

Ovarian carcinosarcomas make up 4.9% of EOCs. They occur at a slightly older age and have a generally worse prognosis overall than EOC, with an estimated 5-year survival of 66% for women diagnosed with localized ovarian carcinosarcoma (vs 82% for HGSC) and 17% for those diagnosed with distant disease (vs 32% with HGSC) (1). The presence of homologous (fibrosarcoma or leiomyosarcoma) versus heterologous (chondrosarcoma, rhabdomyosarcoma, osteosarcoma, or liposarcoma) elements has not been consistently found to have any clear influence on outcomes (2). Optimal cytoreduction is associated with improved outcomes, and it is generally recommended that primary management of these tumors resemble that of HGSC.

There have been few trials specifically in ovarian carcinosarcoma, largely due to the rarity of this disease. Thigpen et al evaluated cisplatin as first-line treatment in a phase 2 trial that included 136 volunteers (3). The overall response rate was 20%, with only one complete response. Median PFS was 5.2 months, and median OS was 11.7 months. Given the rarity of ovarian carcinosarcoma, contemporary trials have evaluated these patients in trials that also included those diagnosed with uterine carcinosarcoma. In GOG 261, women with stage I-IV ovarian or uterine carcinosarcomas were randomly assigned to frontline therapy with either paclitaxel plus carboplatin or ifosfamide plus paclitaxel (4). Among the 90 eligible women with ovarian carcinosarcoma (only 15% had stage I or II disease), those receiving paclitaxel plus carboplatin had longer OS (30 vs 25 months) and PFS (15 months vs 10 months), although differences were not statistically significant.

REFERENCES

1. Peres LC, Cushing-Haugen KL, Kobel M, et al. Invasive epithelial ovarian cancer survival by histotype and disease stage. *J Natl Cancer Inst.* 2019;111(1):60-68.

2. del Carmen MG, Birrer M, Schorge JO. Carcinosarcoma of the ovary: a review of the literature. *Gynecol Oncol.* 2012;125(1):271-277.

3. Tate Thigpen J, Blessing JA, DeGeest K, Look KY, Homesley HD, Gynecologic Oncology Group. Cisplatin as initial chemotherapy in ovarian carcinosarcomas: a gynecologic oncology group study. *Gynecol Oncol.* 2004;93(2):336-339. doi:10.1016/j.ygyno.2004.01.007

4. Walker JL, Brady MF, Wenzel L, et al. Randomized trial of intravenous versus intraperitoneal chemotherapy plus bevacizumab in advanced ovarian carcinoma: an NRG oncology/gynecologic oncology group study. *J Clin Oncol.* 2019;37(16):1380-1390. doi:10.1200/JCO.18.01568

CHAPTER **8.14**

Ovarian Cancer: Survivorship Issues

Katherine C. Kurnit and Gini F. Fleming

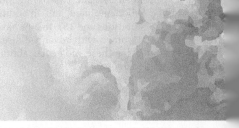

SURVIVORSHIP AFTER A DIAGNOSIS OF OVARIAN CANCER

There are relatively few studies of long-term effects of therapy for OC. A systematic review of studies examining QoL in patients who survived OC after treatment (in the days before widespread use of maintenance therapies) found that QoL is generally good compared to healthy women, but fear of recurrence, sexual problems, and treatment sequelae, particularly neuropathy, persist (1). Aspects of sexual distress include desire, physical arousal (sensation and lubrication), enjoyment, orgasm, dyspareunia/pain, and the overall partner relationship. The psychological and sociocultural factors affecting sexuality after a cancer diagnosis often involve anxiety and depression, coping with an altered body image, and decreased sexual satisfaction in both partners. Addressing body image and sexuality becomes especially important if surgery involves a new ostomy, or leads to leg lymphedema, large scars, and abdominal adhesions. This often requires a consult with a clinical psychologist who can discuss psychosexual interventions, such as cognitive behavioral therapy (2). Treatments may include multimodal pelvic floor therapy, which can improve sexual satisfaction, and other therapeutics, including self-stimulation, vaginal lubricants, local estrogen, vaginal dilators, and vibrators (3). Hyaluronic acid, available as a vaginal suppository, may hydrate the mucosa and facilitate tissue repair (3).

In premenopausal women with OC, the removal of the ovaries results in premature menopause. Consequently, women suffer from symptoms, including hot flashes and vaginal dryness, and those who achieve long-term survival are at increased risk for osteoporosis. There has historically been some concern about prescribing HT to OC survivors because (a) epidemiologic evidence suggests that estrogen replacement therapy slightly increases the risk of developing OC de novo and (b) most OCs express ERs, and antiestrogens, such as tamoxifen, may produce tumor shrinkage in a small subset of women with advanced OC. However, long-term results of the AHT trial that enrolled 150 women showed that HT is safe for the majority of OC survivors (4). In this trial, women with any stage OC were randomized to HRT or no HRT, where HRT selection was according to treating physician preference. At a median follow-up of 19 years for living patients, OS was significantly improved in patients receiving HRT (HR 0.63, $P = .011$). No statistically significant difference in adverse events was seen between groups. A 2015 meta-analysis examining the role of HRT on survival confirmed the absence of any negative effect on OC outcomes (5). Indeed, a clinical practice statement from the SGO supports the safety of HRT in survivors who have HGSOC (6). Low-dose estrogen replacement therapy using rings or creams has minimal systemic side effects but has shown to be efficient in improving vaginal dryness and atrophy.

Neuropathy is a symptom flagged in most surveys of OC survivors (2) and is more common in older patients, patients with diabetes, and in Black patients. An Italian retrospective review queried 120 women who received carboplatin AUC 5 plus paclitaxel 175 mg/m^2 every 3 weeks for six cycles and remained in clinical remission (7). Fifty four percent had some neurologic toxicity during chemotherapy (42% grade 1, 11% grade 2, and 1% grade 3). The probability of residual neurotoxicity after the end of chemotherapy was 15% at 6 months and 11% at 2 years. Rates of neuropathy are higher with dose-dense weekly paclitaxel regimens and with cisplatin-containing regimens. Although agents such as duloxetine and gabapentin can provide some symptomatic alleviation for neuropathy, and exercise and acupuncture may sometimes improve symptoms (2), it is best prevented by timely dose reduction when it becomes apparent. Patients should be questioned about numbness and tingling in their hands and feet at each visit during treatment, and agent substitution (eg, docetaxel for paclitaxel, carboplatin for cisplatin) or dose modification should be considered before neuropathy becomes severe, particularly in patients whose QoL might be significantly affected by even less severe neuropathy (eg, musicians).

Risks of second primaries, particularly for patients with a *BRCA* mutation or Lynch syndrome, should be kept in mind. Despite recommendations for genetic testing upfront, estimates indicate that a significant proportion of people with OC are not tested. In one retrospective cohort study that included almost 29,000 people deemed to have high-risk breast, ovarian, pancreatic, and prostate cancers diagnosed from 2013 to 2019 in the Seattle-Puget Sound area, only 17% underwent testing (8). Although people with OC had the highest testing rate, it was only 40%. Increased testing rates was associated with White race, commercial insurance, urban residence, family history of cancer, and a diagnosis of triple-negative breast cancer. National consensus guideline–concordant testing was only 44% as well. These data point out disparities in access to genetic testing that still need to be addressed. As such, the issue should be reconsidered during follow-up visits for all patients to not only ensure they are tested but also that their family members are offered the opportunity to be screened if indicated.

Other issues are common to many cancer survivors and are not limited to patients with OC, including sleep disturbances, anxiety, fear of recurrence, lymphedema, and financial toxicity (2). Many of these issues can be addressed with expert consultation with psychotherapy or other support services available on an institutional or community level. It is important that these and other QoL-related concerns are addressed at regular follow-up visits.

Follow-up of Patients in Remission

National consensus guidelines for follow-up of patients with OC who enter a clinical complete remission include a history and clinical examination every 2 to 4 months for 2 years, then every 3 to 6 months for 3 years, then annually after 5 years (Table 8.14-1). Monitoring CA-125 or other tumor markers at every visit if initially elevated should be discussed with the patient, but imaging should only be done as clinically indicated. Pelvic examination should be performed periodically. A rise in CA-125 in patients with a history of HGSC is fairly specific for recurrence, particularly if the pretreatment CA-125 was significantly elevated and a second

■ **TABLE 8.14-1. Regular Monitoring of Patients With Epithelial Ovarian Cancer**

FIGO (2014) Stage I-IV epithelial ovarian cancer	Visits every 2–4 mo for 2 yr, then 3–6 mo for 3 yr, then annually after 5 yr
	Physical examination including pelvic examination
	Chest/abdominal/pelvic CT, MRI, PET/CT, or PET (skull base to mid-thigh) as clinically indicated (no routine imaging)
	CBC and chemistry profile as indicated
	CA-125 or other tumor markers if initially elevated or persistent after the end of adjuvant chemotherapy
	Refer patient and family member for genetic risk evaluation, if not previously done
	Regular mammogram
	Regular health care: blood pressure monitoring, vaccinations, weight management
	Long-term wellness care: exercise, nutrition, mental health, sexual health, bone health

CBC, complete blood count; CT, computed tomography; FIGO, International Federation of Gynaecology and Obstetrics; MRI, magnetic resonance imaging; PET, positron emission tomography.

confirmatory CA-125 shows that the titer is continuing to rise. The CA-125 may rise before any evidence of disease on imaging, and in about one-third of all women over 6 months will elapse between the initial CA-125 rise and the time they develop symptoms. Recurrent OC is not curable, and it is not clear that earlier detection can improve either survival or QoL. The Medical Research Council (OV-05) and the EORTC 55955 conducted a phase 3 trial in which 1,442 women with a clinical complete remission after first-line platinum-containing therapy were followed with serial CA-125 levels followed by random assignment ($N = 529$) to either initiate treatment at the time of biochemical recurrence (defined as a CA-125 exceeding twice the upper limit of normal) or wait until the time of clinical evidence of recurrence (9). Twenty percent of women had a rise in CA-125 within 6 months of completing primary chemotherapy, 33% between 6 and 12 months, and 45% after 12 months or more. Treatment at the time of CA-125 rise resulted in starting chemotherapy 4.8 months earlier compared to patients treated only at the time of clinical recurrence. However, survival (defined as survival from the time of CA-125 rise) did not differ between the two groups, at 25.7 months for women assigned to early treatment and 27.1 months for those assigned to delayed treatment. Most importantly, women receiving early treatment had a worse QoL as measured by a shorter time to deterioration of the global health score on the EORTC QLQ-C30 questionnaire.

Issues concerning the use of CA-125 as part of follow-up should be discussed with patients. Detection of disease, although not symptomatic, may allow patients more opportunity to participate in trials of new agents or allow for secondary debulking of lower volume disease, but it cannot be claimed to improve survival, and some women may opt for less aggressive monitoring.

Uses of CA-125 During Ovarian Cancer Treatment

Tumor markers to diagnose OC are discussed in Section 5. CA-125 is widely used to monitor for cancer recurrence in patients with complete remission after frontline therapy, but as described earlier, this has not been shown to improve survival. For women with a high CA-125 at baseline, the marker correlates with volume

of disease and is often checked with each cycle of chemotherapy. Multiple studies have shown that the rapidity of CA-125 normalization and depth of CA-125 nadir after completion of primary therapy have prognostic value. For example, one group found median PFS and OS for women with stage III or IV OC who achieved a value of less than 35 U/mL after the third cycle to be 18 and 42 months, respectively, compared to 9 and 22 months for patients whose tumor marker did not normalize ($P < .001$) (10). The authors suggested that in future trials, women whose CA-125 does not normalize after the third cycle should be switched to an alternate regimen. At this time, there are no clear, clinical interventions known to improve outcomes for those women who do not show the desired decline in CA-125.

A number of CA-125 response definitions, such as 50% or 75% decline, have been developed. Caution should be used when relying on CA-125 to assess response to therapy, particularly in women with heavily pretreated disease, because major discordance may develop (ie, the cancer progresses while the CA-125 value declines). In addition, there may be a "marker flare" after the first cycle of chemotherapy. For example, Sabbatini et al reported that only half of the patients who eventually had a CA-125 decline with liposomal doxorubicin therapy had a decline before the second cycle of therapy (11). More recently, reanalysis of the AURELIA study found that progression of disease in patients with platinum-resistant OC was detected earlier by imaging criteria than by CA-125 levels (12). Thus, use of imaging as well as evaluation of symptoms and the clinical examination in the platinum-resistant setting remain important.

REFERENCES

1. Ahmed-Lecheheb D, Joly F. Ovarian cancer survivors' quality of life: a systematic review. *J Cancer Surv.* 2016;10(5):789-801.

2. Emery J, Butow P, Lai-Kwon J, Nekhlyudov L, Rynderman M, Jefford M. Management of common clinical problems experienced by survivors of cancer. *Lancet.* 2022;399(10334):1537-1550.

3. Rizzuto I, Oehler MK, Lalondrelle S. Sexual and psychosexual consequences of treatment for gynaecological cancers. *Clin Oncol (R Coll Radiol).* 2021;33(9):602-607.

4. Eeles RA, Morden JP, Gore M, et al. Adjuvant hormone therapy may improve survival in epithelial ovarian cancer: results of the AHT randomized trial. *J Clin Oncol.* 2015;33(35):4138-4144. doi:10.1200/JCO.2015.60.9719

5. Li D, Ding CY, Qiu LH. Postoperative hormone replacement therapy for epithelial ovarian cancer patients: a systematic review and meta-analysis. *Gynecol Oncol.* 2015;139(2):355-362. doi:10.1016/j.ygyno.2015.07.109

6. Sinno AK, Pinkerton J, Febbraro T, et al. Hormone therapy (HT) in women with gynecologic cancers and in women at high risk for developing a gynecologic cancer: a Society of Gynecologic Oncology (SGO) clinical practice statement: this practice statement has been endorsed by the North American menopause society. *Gynecol Oncol.* 2020;157(2):303-306.

7. Pignata S, De Placido S, Biamonte R, et al. Residual neurotoxicity in ovarian cancer patients in clinical remission after first-line chemotherapy with carboplatin and paclitaxel: the multicenter Italian trial in ovarian cancer (MITO-4) retrospective study. *BMC Cancer.* 2006;6:5.

8. Clark NM, Roberts EA, Fedorenko C, et al. Genetic testing among patients with high-risk breast, ovarian, pancreatic, and prostate cancers. *Ann Surg Oncol.* 2023;30:1312-1326. doi:10.1245/s10434-022-12755-y

9. Rustin GJ, van der Burg ME, Griffin CL, Guthrie D, Lamont A, Jayson GC. Early versus delayed treatment of relapsed ovarian cancer (MRC OV05/EORTC 55955): a randomised trial. *Lancet.* 2010;376(9747):1155-1163.

10. Skaznik-Wikiel ME, Sukumvanich P, Beriwal S, et al. Possible use of CA-125 level normalization after the third chemotherapy cycle in deciding on chemotherapy regimen in patients with epithelial ovarian cancer: brief report. *Int J Gynecol Cancer.* 2011;21(6):1013-1017.

11. Sabbatini P, Mooney D, Iasonos A, et al. Early CA-125 fluctuations in patients with recurrent ovarian cancer receiving chemotherapy. *Int J Gynecol Cancer.* 2007;17(3):589-594.

12. Lindemann K, Kristensen G, Mirza MR, et al. Poor concordance between CA-125 and RECIST at the time of disease progression in patients with platinum-resistant ovarian cancer: analysis of the AURELIA trial. *Ann Oncol.* 2016;27(8):1505-1510.

CHAPTER **8.15**

Treatment of Persistent and Recurrent Ovarian Cancer and Palliative Care

Katherine C. Kurnit and Gini F. Fleming

TREATMENT OF PERSISTENT/RECURRENT DISEASE

Of women diagnosed with FIGO stage III or IV OC, more than 70% will have a recurrence of their disease within the first 5 years (1) and less than 10% are long-term survivors (2). Recurrent disease is generally not curable. Of those who are not cured by primary therapy, about 10% will progress on or within 1 month of completion of primary platinum treatment and are traditionally described as having disease that is "primary platinum refractory," about 15% will progress 1 to 6 months after completion of completion of primary therapy and are said to have "primary platinum-resistant" disease, and 75% have disease that recurs more than 6 months after primary therapy, which is termed (potentially) "platinum sensitive." Historically, the disease in women with recurrence between 6 and 12 months after surgery has been referred to as "partially platinum sensitive."

These groupings are prognostic: A European retrospective review of patients receiving antitumor therapy at first recurrence showed median OS to be 43 months for women with platinum-sensitive disease, 20.5 months in women with partially platinum-sensitive disease, 12.7 months for platinum-resistant disease, and 9.8 months for platinum-refractory disease (3).

Timing of Treatment Initiation

As recurrent OC is not generally curable, maintaining QoL needs to be considered in choice of therapy and timing of therapy for recurrent disease. As discussed in Section 14, there was no survival advantage for early institution of chemotherapy for a rise in CA-125 in asymptomatic patients in one randomized controlled trial (4). It is, therefore, reasonable to elect close follow-up or continuation of current maintenance (if maintenance therapy is being employed) for women with a rise in tumor marker but no symptoms and no or minimal disease on imaging.

Secondary Cytoreductive Surgery

Surgery in the treatment of recurrent OC is covered in detail in Section 6.10, and as discussed, it is generally considered for women with platinum-sensitive recurrence in combination with chemotherapy when the recurrent disease is expected to be completely resectable.

Second-Line Chemotherapy

In 1991, Markman et al published an influential retrospective review of 72 patients who had responded to initial platinum-based therapy and were subsequently retreated with a platinum-based regimen defining the concept of "platinum sensitivity" for EOC treatment (5). The response rates were 27% for women with a "platinum-free interval" of 5 to 12 months, 33% for those with a platinum-free interval of 13 to 24 months, and 59% for those with a platinum-free interval of over 24 months, showing that platinum-free interval is predictive of response to platinum-based therapy as well as prognostic for OS.

Platinum-free interval is predictive of response to most chemotherapies, not just platinum-based therapies. In women with platinum-resistant disease, response rates to a variety of standard chemotherapeutic agents range from 10% to 25% and duration of response is typically less than 6 months. By comparison, response rates are usually over 30% and duration of response over 8 months for women with platinum-sensitive disease. This appears to be true for noncytotoxic agents as well as cytotoxic agents. For example, a trial of single-agent cediranib (an antiangiogenic tyrosine kinase inhibitor) yielded a 26% response rate in subjects with platinum-sensitive disease versus no responders in the platinum-resistant cohort (6). Other factors, in particular tumor volume (lower response rates for larger tumor volumes), response to initial therapy, and histology, are also predictive of response to subsequent therapy.

Choice of second-line therapies will need to adjust as frontline therapy shifts. For example, it has become clear that women whose cancer progresses on PARPi maintenance have less benefit from further platinum therapy than women whose cancer recurs after observation alone. In the SOLO2/ENGOT Ov-21 trial (which tested maintenance olaparib against placebo in patients with platinum-sensitive relapsed OC), time to second progression (TTSP) for women receiving subsequent platinum-based therapy was 14.3 months for subjects who had received placebo, but only 7 months for those who had received olaparib (7). For subjects receiving subsequent nonplatinum chemotherapy, TTSP was 8.3 and 5.5 months, respectively.

Platinum-Sensitive Disease

Although the definition of platinum-sensitive recurrent OC is, as noted earlier, somewhat arbitrary, in recent years, it has traditionally been used for women whose cancer returns more than 6 months after their most recent dose of platinum-based chemotherapy. For most women with platinum-sensitive OC, a retrial of platinum-based therapy has historically provided the best outcomes, even if the time to recurrence was not over a year. The MITO-8 trial in patients whose disease had recurred between 6 and 12 months after primary platinum-based therapy randomly assigned participants to platinum-based doublet therapy versus non–platinum-based therapy (8). PFS was significantly shorter in the nonplatinum arm (median 12.8 vs 16.4 months, $P = .025$); OS was numerically worse (21.8 vs 24.5 months, $P = .06$). To what extent this remains true for women whose disease progresses while they are on PARPi therapy is unclear.

Single Agent versus Combination Cytotoxic Therapy in Platinum-Sensitive Disease

There have been several randomized trials comparing platinum-based combination cytotoxic therapy to single-agent platinum therapy in women with platinum-sensitive recurrent OC (**Table 8.15-1**). In general, these show consistently superior response rates

■ **TABLE 8.15-1. Selected Trials of Combination Cytotoxic Therapy in Women With First Recurrence of Platinum-Sensitive Recurrent Ovarian Cancer**

Study (yr)	N	Regimen	RR	Median PFS	Median OS
Comparisons of Different Cytotoxic agents					
ICON4/AGO-OVAR 2.2 (2003) (Parmar et al. 2003)	802	Platinum[a] vs platinum + paclitaxel	54% vs 66% $P = .06$	10 mo vs 13 mo HR 0.76 (0.66-0.89)	24 mo vs 29 mo HR 0.82 (0.69-0.97)
AGO-OVAR2.5 (2006) (Pfisterer et al. 2006)	356	Carbo vs carbo+gemcitabine	31% vs 47% $P = .0016$	5.8 mo 8.6 mo $P = .0031$	17.3 mo 18 mo $P = NS$
CALYPSO (2010) (Pujade-Lauraine et al. 2010, Wagner et al. 2012)	976	Carbo+PLD vs carbo+paclitaxel	N/A	11.3 mo vs 9.4 mo HR 0.82 (0.72-0.94)	30.7 mo vs 33 mo $P = NS$
HECTOR (2016) (Sehouli et al. 2016)	550	Carbo+topo vs standard therapy[b]	73.1% vs 75.1% $P = NS$	10 mo vs 10 mo	25 mo vs 31 mo $P = NS$
AGO-OVAR 2.21 (2020) (Pfisterer et al. 2020)	682	Carbo+PLD+BEV vs carbo+gem+BEV	N/A	13.3 mo vs 11.6 mo HR 0.81 (0.68-0.96)	31.9 mo vs 27.8 mo HR 0.81 (0.67-0.98).
Addition of Bevacizumab					
OCEANS (2012) (Aghajanian et al. 2012, Aghajanian et al. 2015)	484	Carbo+gem vs carbo+gem+BEV	78.5% vs 57.4% $P < .001$	8.4 mo vs 12.4 mo HR 0.484 (0.38-0.61)	32.9 mo vs 33.6 mo $P = NS$
GOG 213 (2017) (Coleman et al. 2017)	674	Carbo+paclitaxel vs carbo+paclitaxel+BEV	59% vs 78% $P < .001$	10.4 mo vs 18.8 mo HR 0.63 (0.53-0.74)	37.3 mo vs 42.2 mo HR 0.83 (0.68-1.005)[c]
MITO16b/MANGO-OV2/ ENGOT-ov17 (2021) (Pignata et al. 2021) All patients had prior BEV	406	Platinum doublet vs doublet+BEV	N/A	8.8 mo vs 11.8 mo HR 0.51 (0.41-0.65)	26.7 mo vs 27.1 mo $P = NS$

[a]Control arm CAP or single-agent carboplatin.

[b]Investigator choice of carbo+paclitaxel, carbo+gemcitabine (selected by 191 patients), carbo+PLD.

[c]Incorrect TFI stratification for 45 patients; adjustment after audited treatment-free interval gives adjusted HR of 0.823 (0.68-0.996).

BEV, bevacizumab; carbo, carboplatin; gem, gemcitabine; HR, hazard ratio; NS, not significant; OS, overall survival; PFI, platinum-free interval; PFS, progression-free survival; PLD, pegylated liposomal doxorubicin; RR, response rate; topo, topotecan.

From Aghajanian C, Blank SV, Goff BA, et al. OCEANS: a randomized, double-blind, placebo-controlled phase III trial of chemotherapy with or without bevacizumab in patients with platinum-sensitive recurrent epithelial ovarian, primary peritoneal, or fallopian tube cancer. *J Clin Oncol*. 2012;30(17):2039-2045.

From Aghajanian C, Goff B, Nycum LR, Wang YV, Husain A, Blank SV. Final overall survival and safety analysis of OCEANS, a phase 3 trial of chemotherapy with or without bevacizumab in patients with platinum-sensitive recurrent ovarian cancer. *Gynecol Oncol*. 2015;139(1):10-16.

From Coleman RL, Brady MF, Herzog TJ, et al. Bevacizumab and paclitaxel-carboplatin chemotherapy and secondary cytoreduction in recurrent, platinum-sensitive ovarian cancer (NRG Oncology/Gynecologic Oncology Group study GOG-0213): a multicentre, open-label, randomised, phase 3 trial. *Lancet Oncol*. 2017;18(6):779-791. From Parmar MK, Ledermann JA, Colombo N, et al. Paclitaxel plus platinum-based chemotherapy versus conventional platinum-based chemotherapy in women with relapsed ovarian cancer: the ICON4/AGO-OVAR-2.2 trial. *Lancet*. 2003;361(9375):2099-2106.

From Pfisterer J, Plante M, Vergote I, et al. Gemcitabine plus carboplatin compared with carboplatin in patients with platinum-sensitive recurrent ovarian cancer: an intergroup trial of the AGO-OVAR, the NCIC CTG, and the EORTC GCG. *J Clin Oncol*. 2006;24(29):4699-4707.

From Pfisterer J, Shannon CM, Baumann K, et al. Bevacizumab and platinum-based combinations for recurrent ovarian cancer: a randomised, open-label, phase 3 trial. *Lancet Oncol*. 2020;21(5):699-709.

From Pignata S, Lorusso D, Joly F, et al. Carboplatin-based doublet plus bevacizumab beyond progression versus carboplatin-based doublet alone in patients with platinum-sensitive ovarian cancer: a randomised, phase 3 trial. *Lancet Oncol*. 2021;22(2):267-276.

From Pujade-Lauraine E, Wagner U, Aavall-Lundqvist E, et al. Pegylated liposomal doxorubicin and carboplatin compared with paclitaxel and carboplatin for patients with platinum-sensitive ovarian cancer in late relapse. *J Clin Oncol*. 2010;28(20):3323-3329.

From Sehouli J, Chekerov R, Reinthaller A, et al. Topotecan plus carboplatin versus standard therapy with paclitaxel plus carboplatin (PC) or gemcitabine plus carboplatin (GC) or pegylated liposomal doxorubicin plus carboplatin (PLDC): a randomized phase III trial of the NOGGO-AGO-study group-AGO Austria and GEICO-ENGOT-GCIG intergroup study (HECTOR). *Ann Oncol*. 2016;27(12):2236-2241.

From Wagner U, Marth C, Largillier R, et al. Final overall survival results of phase III GCIG CALYPSO trial of pegylated liposomal doxorubicin and carboplatin vs paclitaxel and carboplatin in platinum-sensitive ovarian cancer patients. *Br J Cancer*. 2012;107(4):588-591.

and superior PFS, but not superior OS with combination therapy. In one historical exception that did show an OS benefit to combination therapy, the ICON-4 trial, which randomly assigned participants to single-agent platinum versus paclitaxel/platinum-based combination therapy, most patients had not had prior taxane (9). Despite the lack of any OS benefit and the generally increased toxicity with combination therapy, platinum-based combination regimens have become usual treatment for women with disease recurring over 12 months after completion of primary chemotherapy. Combination therapy consistently increases complete response rates, which can sometimes allow a second period off therapy with no evidence of disease.

Choice of the second cytotoxic agent between paclitaxel, gemcitabine, and pegylated liposomal doxorubicin seems to make little difference in cancer outcomes and has tended to depend on toxicity. For example, for patients with significant residual neurotoxicity, paclitaxel is a less attractive choice, whereas for those who prefer to travel less frequently for infusion, pegylated doxorubicin is more attractive as it is given on an every 4 week schedule. A trial comparing carboplatin, pegylated liposomal doxorubicin, and bevacizumab to the combination of carboplatin, gemcitabine, and bevacizumab in women with first disease recurrence over 6 months after completion of frontline therapy showed a slight benefit to the liposomal doxorubicin arm: PFS 13.3 versus 11.6 months (HR 0.81, 0.68-0.96); OS 31.9 versus 27.8 months (HR 0.81, 0.67-0.98) (10).

Repeated courses of carboplatin therapy place patients at risk for hypersensitivity reactions. Such reactions rarely occur with the first treatment; rather, they are associated with cumulative dose and have been reported to occur in up to 27% of women receiving more than seven cycles of carboplatin. These reactions usually occur during drug infusion and are associated with flushing, nausea, hypertension, and bronchoconstriction. They may be severe and/or fatal (11). Atypical hypersensitivity reactions, occurring after drug infusion, have also been described. However, patients with OC, as discussed earlier, may derive substantial benefit from retreatment with platinum-based therapy, and an attempt at continuation of platinum therapy may be the best option. A number of desensitization protocols have been published and appear to be generally effective (12-15); they often involve premedication with steroids and antihistamines and starting dilute infusions very slowly and then gradually increasing the concentration and rate over 4 to 24 hours. Moreover, not all patients allergic to carboplatin will be allergic to cisplatin, so switching to a different platinum might be an option.

Patients with a complete response to second-line platinum therapy will usually have a shorter time to recurrence after the second treatment regimen than after the first, and recurrent OCs eventually become resistant to platinum and all other chemotherapy agents.

Addition of Bevacizumab to Cytotoxic Therapy for Women With Platinum-Sensitive Recurrence

Bevacizumab added to platinum-based chemotherapy and continued as maintenance after cessation of chemotherapy has been shown to improve PFS, and it had a small OS benefit in one study, but generally does not improve OS in the setting of recurrent disease (16-18) (**Table 8.15-1**). The OCEANS trial excluded women with prior bevacizumab (16), but GOG 213 allowed prior maintenance bevacizumab if it had been discontinued at least 6 months before documentation of recurrent disease (18). Only 10% of participants on GOG 213 had prior bevacizumab, but results appeared to be consistent, regardless of prior bevacizumab use. The MITO16b-MANGO-OV2-ENGOT-ov17 trial specifically enrolled women who received frontline therapy that included bevacizumab and had disease recurrence more than 6 months after last platinum dose. Participants were randomly assigned to receive a platinum-based doublet or a platinum-based doublet with the addition of bevacizumab (no placebo). Chemotherapy was continued for six cycles; for those assigned to bevacizumab, bevacizumab continued thereafter as maintenance. 72% of participants' disease had progressed after completion of bevacizumab maintenance. Median PFS was improved by 3 months; there was no difference in OS. There was no apparent difference in PFS benefit for those who were still on bevacizumab at the time of disease progression.

PARP Inhibitor Maintenance After Second-line Therapy

In the era before frontline use of PARPi maintenance therapy, four randomized trials evaluated the use of PARPi (niraparib, olaparib, rucaparib) as maintenance therapy after induction of response with second-line platinum-based therapy, and all showed a PFS benefit, most dramatic for those with germline or tumor BRCA mutation (19-22).

The SOLO2 trial randomly assigned 295 participants with germline or somatic BRCA1 or BRCA2 mutation to maintenance therapy with olaparib or placebo. Median PFS was 19.1 months with olaparib versus 5.5 months with placebo (HR 0.30, 0.22-0.41) (21). Median OS in SOLO2 also appeared to be improved: 51.7 months with olaparib and 38.8 months with placebo (HR 0.74, 0.54-1.00). For those without a germline or tumor BRCA mutation, there may not be any OS benefit (23). For example, in the ENGOT-OV16/NOVA study, PFS for those with no germline BRCA mutation was 9.3 months with niraparib versus 3.9 months with placebo (HR 0.45, 0.34-0.61), but OS was not different for those receiving niraparib (31.1 months for niraparib vs 36.5 months for placebo; HR 1.1, 0.831-1.459) (24).

All maintenance therapies have some toxicity and, given their lack of survival benefit in most cases, should be administered in shared decision-making with the patient. PARPi cause cytopenias and can cause nausea. Their potential to cause MDS and secondary leukemia (AML) remains a concern but seems less frequent than originally feared. This risk has been suggested to be higher in older women and in women carrying a germline BRCA1/2 mutation (25). On the SOLO2 trial, MDS or AML occurred in 16 (8%) of participants receiving olaparib and four (4%) of those receiving placebo, mostly in the post-treatment period (23).

Single-agent PARPi therapy as treatment (rather than maintenance) for recurrent disease is no longer recommended, because OS has been reported to be lower with such treatment than with standard chemotherapy despite promising response rates with PARPi therapy. The SOLO3 trial randomly assigned women with germline BRCA-mutated OC recurrent less than 12 months after most recent platinum chemotherapy dose to single-agent olaparib or physicians choice of nonplatinum single-agent chemotherapy and found an ORR of 72% with olaparib versus 51% with chemotherapy (26). Similarly, the ARIEL4 trial randomized women with BRCA1- or BRCA2-mutated OC and two or more prior chemotherapy regimens to oral rucaparib or chemotherapy (27). Patients 0 to 12 months from their most recent platinum-based chemotherapy received weekly paclitaxel as the control arm; those 12 or more months from most recent platinum-based therapy received a platinum-based regimen as control. However, based on reports of detrimental OS in these trials, they are no longer available for use in the recurrent disease setting (28). In the latter part of 2022, all three available PARPi were withdrawn from the market as later line treatment for recurrent OC associated with a BRCA mutation (olaparib and rucaparib) or HRD (niraparib).

Currently, PARPi therapy is widely used as frontline maintenance therapy, which raises the question of whether it is of benefit as maintenance in the recurrent setting for those patients who received prior PARPi therapy. The phase III OReO/ENGOT Ov-38 trial attempted to address this question (29). Subjects enrolled (N = 220) had received prior PARPi maintenance therapy and were in complete or partial response to platinum-based therapy. The duration of PARPi must have been at least 18 months for *BRCA* mutation carriers and 12 months for noncarriers if it were following first-line therapy (patients who progressed after only a short duration of i maintenance therapy were not eligible). In the preliminary abstract, median PFS was reported to be improved from 2.8 months with placebo to 4.3 months in those randomized to rechallenge with olaparib among the cohort with BRCA-mutant OC (HR 0.57, 0.37-0.87) and from 3.8 to 5.3 months in non–*BRCA*-mutant cohort (HR 0.43, 0.26-0.71). It will be interesting to see if duration since prior PARPi therapy is also predictive (as duration since prior platinum therapy is predictive of response to future platinum).

In summary, for most women with OC who initially responded well to platinum-based therapy and recur more than 6 months after most recent platinum therapy, a platinum-based combination is standard. Time till subsequent progression will be shorter for women who have received PARPi maintenance therapy. The addition of bevacizumab (with subsequent maintenance bevacizumab) can improve PFS, even in the setting of prior bevacizumab, but appears to have little impact on OS. It may be an attractive option for those whose disease has progressed on PARPi therapy. PARPi maintenance therapy may extend PFS (and OS for *BRCA* mutation carriers), particularly if they have not had prior PARPi therapy. Exactly which patients who do receive primary PARPi therapy will derive major benefit from a second round of PARPi maintenance remains to be seen.

Platinum-Resistant Disease

In general, tumors resistant to platinum are more resistant to any cytotoxic agent. Response rates to conventional single-agent therapy in this group of women are in the range of 10% to 15%, median PFS is about 3 to 4 months, and median OS is 9 to 12 months. Agents used in this setting are pegylated liposomal doxorubicin, gemcitabine, topotecan, bevacizumab, and weekly paclitaxel. As combination of cytotoxic agents has not been shown to be superior to single-agent therapy, sequential treatment with single agents is the usual approach. Significant differences in terms of response rate or survival between various agents in platinum-resistant disease are not usually seen, and treatment selection will often be based on toxicity or convenience (30). For example, in randomized comparisons of gemcitabine versus liposomal doxorubicin, gemcitabine causes more cytopenia, and liposomal doxorubicin more mucositis and palmar-plantar dysesthesia (31).

Unlike the addition of a second cytotoxic agent, the addition of bevacizumab to cytotoxic therapy in the setting of platinum-resistant disease is of benefit. The open-label phase III AURELIA trial randomly assigned participants with platinum-resistant OC to standard single-agent therapy (investigator choice of weekly paclitaxel, liposomal doxorubicin, or topotecan) with or without bevacizumab (32). PFS was almost doubled (from 3.4 to 6.7 months; HR 0.48, $P < .001$), and response rate (27.3% vs 11.8%) was also improved. OS prolongation did not reach significant (13.3 vs 16.6 months; HR 0.85, $P = .17$). In an exploratory analysis, the largest benefit seen with bevacizumab was combined with weekly paclitaxel (PFS improved from 3.9 to 10.4 months) (30).

Women with recurrent OC who show minimal or no benefit (with prolonged disease stabilization considered a benefit) from two different therapies in a row have a very poor prognosis. Palliative care is paramount in this setting.

REFERENCES

1. Kurnit KC, Fleming GF, Lengyel E. Updates and new options in advanced epithelial ovarian cancer treatment. *Obstet Gynecol.* 2021;137(1):108-121.

2. Javellana M, Hoppenot C, Lengyel E. The road to long-term survival: surgical approach and longitudinal treatments of long-term survivors of advanced-stage serous ovarian cancer. *Gynecol Oncol.* 2019;152(2):228-234.

3. Freyer G, Ray-Coquard I, Fischer D, et al. Routine clinical practice for patients with recurrent ovarian carcinoma: results from the TROCADERO study. *Int J Gynecol Cancer.* 2016;26(2):240-247.

4. Rustin GJ, van der Burg ME, Griffin CL, et al. Early versus delayed treatment of relapsed ovarian cancer (MRC OV05/EORTC 55955): a randomised trial. *Lancet.* 2010;376(9747):1155-1163. doi:10.1016/S0140-6736(10)61268-8

5. Markman M, Rothman R, Hakes T, et al. Second-line platinum therapy in patients with ovarian cancer previously treated with cisplatin. *J Clin Oncol.* 1991;9(3):389-393.

6. Hirte H, Lheureux S, Fleming GF, et al. A phase 2 study of cediranib in recurrent or persistent ovarian, peritoneal or fallopian tube cancer: a trial of the Princess Margaret, Chicago and California phase II consortia. *Gynecol Oncol.* 2015;138(1):55-61.

7. Frenel JS, Kim JW, Berton-Rigaud D, et al. 813MO Efficacy of subsequent chemotherapy for patients with BRCA1/2 mutated platinum-sensitive recurrent epithelial ovarian cancer (EOC) progressing on olaparib vs placebo: the SOLO2/ENGOT Ov-21 trial. *Ann Oncol.* 2020;31:S615.

8. Pignata S, Scambia G, Bologna A, et al. Randomized controlled trial testing the efficacy of platinum-free interval prolongation in advanced ovarian cancer: the MITO-8, MaNGO, BGOG-Ov1, AGO-Ovar2.16, ENGOT-Ov1, GCIG study. *J Clin Oncol.* 2017;35(29):3347-3353. doi:10.1200/JCO.2017.73.4293

9. Parmar MK, Ledermann JA, Colombo N, et al. Paclitaxel plus platinum-based chemotherapy versus conventional platinum-based chemotherapy in women with relapsed ovarian cancer: the ICON4/AGO-OVAR-2.2 trial. *Lancet.* 2003;361(9375):2099-2106.

10. Pfisterer J, Shannon CM, Baumann K, et al. Bevacizumab and platinum-based combinations for recurrent ovarian cancer: a randomised, open-label, phase 3 trial. *Lancet Oncol.* 2020;21(5):699-709. doi:10.1016/S1470-2045(20)30142-X

11. Dizon DS, Sabbatini PJ, Aghajanian C, Hensley ML, Spriggs DR. Analysis of patients with epithelial ovarian cancer or fallopian tube carcinoma retreated with cisplatin after the development of a carboplatin allergy. *Gynecol Oncol.* 2002;84(3):378-382. doi:10.1006/gyno.2001.6519

12. O'Malley DM, Vetter MH, Cohn DE, Khan A, Hays JL. Outpatient desensitization in selected patients with platinum hypersensitivity reactions. *Gynecol Oncol.* 2017;145(3):603-610. doi:10.1016/j.ygyno.2017.03.015

13. Lee CW, Matulonis UA, Castells MC. Carboplatin hypersensitivity: a 6-h 12-step protocol effective in 35 desensitizations in patients with gynecological malignancies and mast cell/IgE-mediated reactions. *Gynecol Oncol.* 2004;95(2):370-376. doi:10.1016/j.ygyno.2004.08.002

14. Lee CW, Matulonis UA, Castells MC. Rapid inpatient/outpatient desensitization for chemotherapy hypersensitivity: standard protocol effective in 57 patients for 255 courses. *Gynecol Oncol.* 2005;99(2):393-399. doi:10.1016/j.ygyno.2005.06.028

15. Otani IM, Wong J, Banerji A. Platinum chemotherapy hypersensitivity: prevalence and management. *Immunol Allergy Clin North Am.* 2017;37(4):663-677. doi:10.1016/j.iac.2017.06.003

16. Aghajanian C, Blank SV, Goff BA, et al. OCEANS: a randomized, double-blind, placebo-controlled phase III trial of chemotherapy with or without bevacizumab in patients with platinum-sensitive recurrent epithelial ovarian, primary peritoneal, or fallopian tube cancer. *J Clin Oncol.* 2012;30(17):2039-2045. doi:10.1200/JCO.2012.42.0505

17. Aghajanian C, Goff B, Nycum LR, Wang YV, Husain A, Blank SV. Final overall survival and safety analysis of OCEANS, a phase 3 trial of chemotherapy with or without bevacizumab in patients with platinum-sensitive recurrent ovarian cancer. *Gynecol Oncol.* 2015;139(1):10-16.

18. Coleman RL, Brady MF, Herzog TJ, et al. Bevacizumab and paclitaxel-carboplatin chemotherapy and secondary cytoreduction in recurrent, platinum-sensitive ovarian cancer (NRG Oncology/Gynecologic Oncology Group study GOG-0213): a multicentre, open-label, randomised, phase 3 trial. *Lancet Oncol.* 2017;18(6):779-791.

19. Ledermann J, Harter P, Gourley C, et al. Olaparib maintenance therapy in patients with platinum-sensitive relapsed serous ovarian cancer: a preplanned retrospective analysis of outcomes by BRCA status in a randomised phase 2 trial. *Lancet Oncol.* 2014;15(8):852-861.

20. Mirza MR, Monk BJ, Herrstedt J, et al. Niraparib maintenance therapy in platinum-sensitive, recurrent ovarian cancer. *N Engl J Med.* 2016;375(22):2154-2164. doi:10.1056/NEJMoa1611310

21. Pujade-Lauraine E, Ledermann JA, Selle F, et al. Olaparib tablets as maintenance therapy in patients with platinum-sensitive, relapsed ovarian cancer and a BRCA1/2 mutation (SOLO2/ENGOT-Ov21): a double-blind, randomised, placebo-controlled, phase 3 trial. *Lancet Oncol.* 2017;18(9):1274-1284. doi:10.1016/S1470-2045(17)30469-2

22. Swisher EM, Lin KK, Oza AM, et al. Rucaparib in relapsed, platinum-sensitive high-grade ovarian carcinoma (ARIEL2 Part 1): an international, multicentre, open-label, phase 2 trial. *Lancet Oncol.* 2017;18(1):75-87. doi:10.1016/S1470-2045(16)30559-9

23. Poveda A, Floquet A, Ledermann JA, et al. Olaparib tablets as maintenance therapy in patients with platinum-sensitive relapsed ovarian cancer and a BRCA1/2 mutation (SOLO2/ENGOT-Ov21): a final analysis of a double-blind, randomised, placebo-controlled, phase 3 trial. *Lancet Oncol.* 2021;22(5):620-631.

24. Matulonis U, Herrstedt J, Oza A, et al. Long-term safety and secondary efficacy endpoints in the ENGOT-OV16/NOVA phase III trial of niraparib in recurrent ovarian cancer. *Gynecol Oncol.* 2021;162(S1):S24-S25.

25. Trillsch F, Mahner S, Ataseven B, et al. Efficacy and safety of olaparib according to age in BRCA1/2-mutated patients with recurrent platinum-sensitive ovarian cancer: analysis of the phase III SOLO2/ENGOT-Ov21 study. *Gynecol Oncol.* 2022;165(1):40-48.

26. Penson RT, Valencia RV, Cibula D, et al. Olaparib versus nonplatinum chemotherapy in patients with platinum-sensitive relapsed ovarian cancer and a germline BRCA1/2 mutation (SOLO3): a randomized phase III trial. *J Clin Oncol.* 2020;38(11):1164-1174. doi:10.1200/JCO.19.02745

27. Kristeleit R, Lisyanskaya A, Fedenko A, et al. Rucaparib versus standard-of-care chemotherapy in patients with relapsed ovarian cancer and a deleterious BRCA1 or BRCA2 mutation (ARIEL4): an international, open-label, randomised, phase 3 trial. *Lancet Oncol.* 2022;23(4):465-478. doi:10.1016/S1470-2045(22)00122-X

28. Tew WP, Lacchetti C, Kohn EC; PARP Inhibitors in the Management of Ovarian Cancer Guideline Expert Panel. Poly(ADP-Ribose) polymerase inhibitors in the management of ovarian cancer: ASCO guideline rapid recommendation update. *J Clin Oncol.* 2022;40(33):3878-3881.

29. Pujade-Lauraine E, Selle F, Scambia G, et al. LBA33 maintenance olaparib rechallenge in patients (pts) with ovarian carcinoma (OC) previously treated with a PARP inhibitor (PARPi): phase IIIb OReO/ENGOT Ov-38 trial. *Ann Oncol.* 2021;32(Suppl 5):1308-1309.

30. Pujade-Lauraine E, Banerjee S, Pignata S. Management of platinum-resistant, relapsed epithelial ovarian cancer and new drug perspectives. *J Clin Oncol.* 2019;37(27):2437-2448.

31. Mutch DG, Orlando M, Goss T, et al. Randomized phase III trial of gemcitabine compared with pegylated liposomal doxorubicin in patients with platinum-resistant ovarian cancer. *J Clin Oncol.* 2007;25(19):2811-2818.

32. Pujade-Lauraine E, Hilpert F, Weber B, et al. Bevacizumab combined with chemotherapy for platinum-resistant recurrent ovarian cancer: the AURELIA open-label randomized phase III trial. *J Clin Oncol.* 2014;32(13):1302-1308.

CHAPTER **8.16**

New Therapeutics

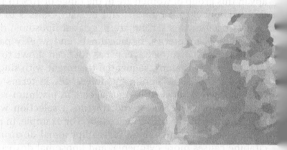

Katherine C. Kurnit and Gini F. Fleming

ANTIBODY-DRUG CONJUGATES

Antibody-drug conjugates (ADCs), in which a toxic chemotherapy agent is linked to a targeting monoclonal antibody, have been remarkably effective in multiple tumor types, and mirvetuximab soravtansine-gynx, an ADC in which the maytansinoid DM4, a potent tubulin-binding agent, is linked to a folate receptor-α (FRα)-binding antibody, was granted accelerated approval by the FDA in November 2022 (1). It is indicated for the treatment of adults with platinum-resistant OC with tumor FRα expression by an approved companion assay and one to three prior regimens. FRα is a transmembrane glycoprotein that facilitates the transport of folate into cells. Elevated expression may be associated with more poorly differentiated, aggressive malignancies (2). Approval of mirvetuximab was based on a single-arm trial of 106 patients that reported a confirmed ORR of 31.7% (3). Adverse reactions include fatigue, transaminitis, cytopenias, and ocular toxicity; product labeling includes a box warning for ocular toxicity.

Other ADCs have also shown promising preliminary results in the therapy of OC. STRO-002 is a second ADC targeting FRα, which received a fast-track designation by the FDA in August 2021 for use in patients with platinum-resistant OC (4). Another target of relevance is NaPi2b, a sodium diphosphate transporter (5). Although an ADC targeting NaPi2b was not successful (6), upifitamab rilsodotin (XMT-1536) remains under investigation based on promising responses in a phase I trial (7).

CELL CYCLE CHECKPOINT KINASE INHIBITORS

As one method of protecting themselves from DNA damage, cells can activate cell cycle checkpoints, which arrest the cell cycle and allow time for repair of damaged DNA. HGSOC is characterized by universal *TP53* mutations, which cause dysfunction of the G1/S checkpoint, making HGSOC more heavily reliant on G2-checkpoint arrest to facilitate DNA damage repair. Cell cycle checkpoint inhibitors leverage the high replicative stress seen in HGSOC and may be most active in combination with cytotoxic

chemotherapy (8). Wee-1 kinase is one example; it is integral for the G2 checkpoint. Adavosertib is an oral Wee-1 inhibitor that was tested in combination with gemcitabine versus gemcitabine alone in women with platinum-resistant or refractory HGSOC (9). PFS was longer with the combination (4.6 vs 3.0 months), but the drug is no longer being developed. A second oral Wee-1 inhibitor, ZN-c3, produced a PR in a patient with OC during phase I testing (10) and is being tested in multiple clinical trials.

Given that LGSOC and invasive ductal breast cancer are often both ER positive, the CDK4/6 inhibitors (palbociclib, abemaciclib, or ribociclib) (10) might be effective in the treatment of LGSOC. Several studies are underway.

GAS6/AXL PATHWAY

AXL and its activating ligand, growth arrest specific 6 (GAS6), are expressed in HGSOC, but not in normal ovarian tissue. Their expression is associated with poor prognosis, resistance to treatment, and poor survival (12). AVB-500 is a recombinant fusion protein dimer that acts as a decoy, trapping GAS6 with an affinity about 200-fold higher than wild-type AXL, and thus potentially inhibiting downstream signaling of many cancer-related processes. It was tested in combination with paclitaxel or pegylated liposomal doxorubicin in a phase I trial of women with platinum-resistant OC; the paclitaxel-containing combination was reported to have a response rate of 34.8% (13). A phase III trial assessing the combination of AVB-500 plus paclitaxel versus paclitaxel alone in women with platinum-resistant OCs is underway as of 2022.

IMMUNOLOGIC THERAPIES

In 2003, Zhang et al made the seminal observation that among patients in clinical complete remission, the presence of intratumoral T cells was a strongly favorable prognostic factor (14). However, OC appears to be "immunologically cold": response rates for single-agent PD-1/L1 inhibitors in OC are low, and numerous randomized trials of the addition of standard PD-1/L1 immune checkpoint inhibitors to chemotherapy for OC have been negative.

Some newer approaches involve the addition of a second immune checkpoint-acting agent, or use of a bispecific antibody that targets more than one immune checkpoint. For example, a randomized phase II trial of single-agent PD-1 inhibition with nivolumab versus nivolumab plus the CTLA-4 blocking antibody, ipilimumab, in women with OC and a platinum-free interval of less than 12 months found a 12.2% response rate for single-agent nivolumab versus a 31.4% response rate for the combination ($P = .034$) (15).

Bispecific antibodies that connect cytotoxic T cells to a tumor cell are one promising approach for multiple tumor types, and multiple trials for OC are underway. These agents have the limitation that they are restricted to patients of certain HLA types (generally HLA-A*02). Considerable other research into novel immunotherapeutic approaches for OC is ongoing, including trials of vaccines and cell-based therapies including adoptive transfer of autologous T cells that are expanded or genetically modified. There is reason for optimism that such approaches will prove effective in the near future.

REFERENCES

1. FDA gives nod to mirvetuximab soravtansine. *Cancer Discov.* 2023;13:8. doi:10.1158/2159-8290.CD-NB2022-0075

2. Birrer MJ, Betella I, Martin LP, Moore KN. Is targeting the folate receptor in ovarian cancer coming of age? *Oncologist.* 2019;24(4):425-429.

3. Matulonis UA, Lorusso D, Oaknin A, et al. Efficacy and safety of mirvetuximab soravtansine in patients with platinum-resistant ovarian cancer with high folate receptor alpha expression: results from the SORAYA study. Presented at Society of Gynecologic Oncology (SGO) Annual Meeting on Women's Cancer; March 19, 2022; Phoenix, AZ. Accessed December 2, 2022. https://investor.immunogen.com/node/20766/pdf

4. Sutro Biopharma Inc. Sutro Biopharma announces STRO-002 FDA fast track designation for patients with advanced ovarian cancer. 2021. https://prn.to/2UuhmLR

5. Nurgalieva AK, Popov VE, Skripova VS, et al. Sodium-dependent phosphate transporter NaPi2b as a potential predictive marker for targeted therapy of ovarian cancer. *Biochem Biophys Rep.* 2021;28:101104. doi:10.1016/j.bbrep.2021.101104

6. Banerjee S, Oza AM, Birrer MJ, et al. Anti-NaPi2b antibody-drug conjugate lifastuzumab vedotin (DNIB0600A) compared with pegylated liposomal doxorubicin in patients with platinum-resistant ovarian cancer in a randomized, open-label, phase II study. *Ann Oncol.* 2018;29(4):917-923.

7. Tolcher AW, Ulahannan SV, Papadopoulos KP, et al. Phase 1 dose escalation study of XMT-1536, a novel NaPi2b-targeting antibody-drug conjugate (ADC), in patients (pts) with solid tumors likely to express NaPi2b. *J Clin Oncol.* 2019;37(15_suppl):3010.

8. Lee J, Minasian L, Kohn EC. New strategies in ovarian cancer treatment. *Cancer.* 2019;125(24_suppl):4623-4629. doi:10.1002/cncr.32544. PMID: 31967682 PMCID: PMC7437367

9. Lheureux S, Cristea MC, Bruce JP, et al. Adavosertib plus gemcitabine for platinum-resistant or platinum-refractory recurrent ovarian cancer: a double-blind, randomised, placebo-controlled, phase 2 trial. *Lancet.* 2021;397(10271):281-292.

10. Tolcher A, Mamdami H, Chalasani P, et al. Clinical activity of single-agent ZN-c3, an oral WEE1 inhibitor, in a phase 1 dose-escalation trial in patients with advanced solid tumors. *Cancer Res.* 2021;81(13_Suppl):016.

11. Goel S, Bergholz JS, Zhao JJ. Targeting CDK4 and CDK6 in cancer. *Nat Rev Cancer.* 2022;22(6):356-372.

12. Rankin EB, Fuh KC, Taylor TE, et al. AXL is an essential factor and therapeutic target for metastatic ovarian cancer. *Cancer Res.* 2010;70(19):7570-7579.

13. Fuh KC, Bookman MA, Liu JF, et al. Phase 1b study of AVB-500 in combination with paclitaxel or pegylated liposomal doxorubicin platinum-resistant recurrent ovarian cancer. *Gynecol Oncol.* 2021;163(2):254-261.

14. Zhang L, Conejo-Garcia JR, Katsaros D, et al. Intratumoral T cells, recurrence, and survival in epithelial ovarian cancer. *N Engl J Med.* 2003;348(3):203-213.

15. Zamarin D, Burger RA, Sill MW, et al. Randomized phase II trial of nivolumab versus nivolumab and ipilimumab for recurrent or persistent ovarian cancer: an NRG oncology study. *J Clin Oncol.* 2020;38(16):1814-1823.

OVARIAN GERM CELL TUMORS

Ovarian Germ Cell Tumors: Introduction, Anatomy, Natural History, and Patterns of Spread

Dimitrios Nasioudis and Emily M. Ko

INTRODUCTION

Malignant ovarian germ cell tumors (MOGCTs) comprise a heterogeneous group of tumors arising from germ cells. The 2020 World Health Organization (WHO) classification of MOGCTs includes dysgerminoma, yolk sac tumor (YST), embryonal carcinoma, nongestational choriocarcinoma, mixed germ cell tumors (GCTs), teratomas (immature teratoma [IT]), mature teratoma, and various types of monodermal teratoma as well as somatic-type tumors arising from a dermoid cyst), and germ cell sex cord-stromal tumors (gonadoblastoma and unclassified mixed germ cell sex cord-stromal tumors) (Table 9.1-1) (1). This classification was updated from 2014, and differences include terminology (YST replaces endodermal sinus tumor) and inclusion of germ cell sex cord-stromal tumors as a distinct subtype.

Although mature teratomas are relatively common, representing approximately 20% of ovarian neoplasms, the malignant GCTs are less common and account for 2% to 3% of all ovarian cancers. The most common histologic subtypes of MOGCT are dysgerminoma, IT, YST, and mixed GCTs (2).

Significant improvement in outcomes has been achieved over the past several decades. The implementation of effective cisplatin-based chemotherapy (CBCT) regimens has yielded excellent survival rates, even for patients with advanced-stage disease. Modern research efforts focus on survivorship, fertility preservation, limitation of therapy, and treatment of refractory disease. Because most MOGCTs arise in adolescents and young women,

collaborative care involves coordination among different specialties (gynecologic oncology, medical oncology, pediatric oncology, pediatric surgery, pathology, and radiology).

ANATOMY

The relevant anatomy consists of the upper female genital tract and the lymphatic system. Malignant GCTs affect the ovary and are unilateral in over 90% of cases (3). Because these can be large, ranging from 4 to 38 cm in one series, the ipsilateral fallopian tube may be obliterated or distorted by the tumor (3), but the uterus is typically uninvolved.

As subsequently discussed, nodal metastasis may occur in approximately 10% of apparent early-stage cases (4), so the pelvic and para-aortic nodal anatomy should be appreciated, as discussed elsewhere for epithelial ovarian cancer. Omental and hepatic metastases may occur, so upper abdominal anatomy is relevant. Like epithelial ovarian cancer, an understanding of both pelvic and upper abdominal anatomy is critical to surgical staging and treatment.

NATURAL HISTORY

Because MOGCTs tend to be large and rapidly growing, most patients with MOGCT present with a palpable pelvic/abdominal mass associated with abdominal pain (80%). Less common presenting symptoms include abdominal distention (35%), ascites (20%), fever (10%), and vaginal bleeding (10%). Overall duration of symptoms is usually short (median 2-4 weeks). Approximately 10% of patients will present with an acute abdomen due to tumor rupture, intra-abdominal bleeding, or ovarian torsion (5,6).

Based on a systematic review of the literature identifying 102 cases, dysgerminoma (38.2%) and YST (30.4%) are the most common histotypes, and most patients presented with early-stage disease (76.4%) and large tumors (mean size 17.9 cm) (7).

Stage distribution is variable in the literature, but most patients are diagnosed with early-stage disease. A single center in India reported the distribution of stages I-IV MOGCT to be 15.4% (n = 6), 35.9% (n = 14), 46.2% (n = 18), and 2.6% (n = 1), respectively (8). In another series of 130 patients from Bangkok, 64% of patients were diagnosed with stages I-II disease (9). More commonly, unilateral, stage I disease is encountered, with most reports detailing at least 85% of patients with stages I-II disease (10,11).

Overall, outcomes are good. In one study of 89 patients who were evaluable for responses, four patients had progressive disease, whereas 85 had complete response. The 5-year progression-free survival (PFS) and overall survival (OS) were 82.4% (95% confidence interval [CI], 75.4%-89.5%) and 92.4% (95% CI, 87.6%-97.2%), respectively (9). Median OS was not reached at 5 years (8). In the RARECARE European database consisting of 19 contributing countries, GCTs had a 5-year relative survival of 85% (95% CI 83-87) (12). Within this group of 1,969 patients with MOGCT, the 5-year relative survival was slightly higher for patients with dysgerminomas (90%; 95% CI 88-93), compared to patients with YSTs

---

■ **TABLE 9.1-1. Classification of Ovarian Germ Cell Tumors**

Teratoma, benign
Immature teratoma, NOS
Dysgerminoma
Yolk sac tumor
Embryonal carcinoma
Choriocarcinoma, NOS
Mixed germ cell tumor
Monodermal teratomas and somatic type tumors arising from a
  dermoid cyst
Struma ovarii, NOS
Struma ovarii, malignant
Strumal carcinoid
Teratoma with malignant transformation
Cystic teratoma, NOS
Germ cell sex cord-stromal tumor
  Gonadoblastoma
    Dissecting gonadoblastoma
Undifferentiated gonadal tissue
Mixed germ cell sex cord-stromal tumor, unclassified

From WHO Classification of Tumours Editorial Board. *Female Genital Tumours: WHO Classification of Tumours.* Vol. 4. 5th ed. IARC; 2020.

NOS, not otherwise specified.

(86%; 95% CI 81%-90%), mixed GCTs (85%; 95% CI 74-91), ITs (83%; 95% CI 80-86), or other GCTs (63%; 95% CI 51%-73%) (13). Interestingly, the 5-year relative survival was 100% in 101 patients with dysgerminoma aged 14 years or below, compared to 29% in 24 patients over 64 years old. This pattern was consistent among all patients with GCTs, with survival declining with age. The AIRTUM Italian group reported over 95% of 1- and 5-year relative survival for all MOGCTs (14). Likewise, survival was excellent for a Korean group of 171 patients who underwent fertility-sparing surgery (FSS). Recurrent disease developed in 25 (14.6%) patients, and five (2.9%) patients died of disease during the median follow-up time of 86 months (range, 9-294 months). In total, the 5-year disease-free survival (DFS) and OS was 86% and 97%, respectively. When stratified by stage, the 5-year DFS was 84% for stage I and 89% for stages II-IV; the 5-year OS was 99% for stage I and 91% for stages II-IV patients (15).

In general, patients with early-stage disease and favorable prognostic factors have excellent outcomes. These patients are more commonly able to forego adjuvant chemotherapy and receive FSS and observation alone. Observation without chemotherapy has allowed evaluation of the natural history of these good prognosis tumors. The Multicenter Italian Trials in Ovarian cancer (MITO) group followed 31 patients with stage I dysgerminomas, IA-IC G2-G3 ITs, and IA mixed MOGCTs with YST component who received no adjuvant chemotherapy after surgery. Only one patient relapsed, and she was successfully treated with conservative surgery and adjuvant therapy (16).

Patients with YST, also known as endodermal sinus tumor, have historically experienced less favorable outcomes than patients with other histologic subtypes. In contrast to other histologic subtypes, YSTs can grow very rapidly, yielding a rapidly apparent mass upon presentation and extraovarian spread at diagnosis in approximately one-third of patients (17,18). These tumors are much more aggressive despite chemotherapy, have a higher recurrence rate, and have a lower DFS and OS. For example, Park et al compared yolk sac with non–yolk sac histologies and showed a 5-year PFS of 70% versus 88% ($P = .005$) and a 5-year OS of 87% versus 99% ($P = .003$) (15).

PATTERNS OF SPREAD

Stage distribution of MOGCT at diagnosis is different than that of patients with epithelial ovarian carcinoma. In an analysis of the Surveillance, Epidemiology, and End Results (SEER) database, 61% of patients presented with disease limited to the ovary (19). Similarly, among 1,649 patients with available staging information that were included in the National Cancer Database (NCDB), the majority (63.3%) had stage I disease, whereas 8.3% had stage II, 22.6% stage III, and only 5.8% had stage IV disease (20).

Lymphatic spread is relatively common for MOGCT, and rates of lymph node metastases vary by histology. In a retrospective database analysis that included 1,425 patients with apparent early-stage MOGCT who underwent lymph node sampling/dissection, overall rate of lymph node metastases was 10.3% (4). The highest rate was observed among patients with dysgerminoma (17.9%), whereas the lowest among those with IT (3.2%). For patients with YST and mixed GCTs, the rate of lymph node involvement was 7.6% and 7%, respectively (4). A systematic review of the literature that identified three studies with 2,436 patients reported a similar (10.9%) rate of lymph node involvement (21), whereas a slightly higher incidence (12.65%) was noted in a large retrospective study that included patients undergoing FFS (15). The main route of lymphatic drainage occurs along the ovarian veins to the para-aortic and paracaval lymph nodes; however, lymphatic drainage along the broad ligament to the internal and external iliac lymph nodes can occur. In a small cohort of 48 pediatric patients with pure dysgerminoma, a high rate (14.8%) of para-aortic lymph node involvement was found, mirroring data from testicular germ cell literature (22).

Like epithelial ovarian carcinoma, MOGCT can spread through direct seeding in the peritoneal cavity. A study evaluating the quality of staging procedures performed in 131 pediatric patients with MOGCT has elucidated the intraperitoneal patterns of spread of MOGCT (23). Among 100 patients who had samples of ascitic fluid or peritoneal washings, 23% were positive for malignant cells, where for five patients, there was no other evidence of extraovarian disease. Omental involvement was also common; among 77 patients who underwent omentectomy, 15.6% of grossly abnormal- and 4% of normal-appearing samples had malignant tumor deposits. Similarly, among 29 patients with suspicious peritoneal implants, 62% were positive for malignancy on final pathology (23).

Although MOGCTs are less likely to spread hematogenously, metastases to the liver, bone, brain, and lung have been reported and will upstage patients to stage IV disease. An analysis of the SEER database reported that 27.7% of patients with MOGCT diagnosed between 1978 and 2010 presented with distant metastases (20). Given the advancements in imaging techniques and earlier workup, the number of patients presenting with distant metastases at diagnosis is decreasing. In a retrospective study from Norway, the rate of distant metastases decreased from 39% for patients diagnosed between 1953 and 1980 to 20% for those diagnosed 1980 to 2009 (24). Similarly, lower incidence of distant metastases (10%-14%) has been reported in more modern cohorts (11,25).

REFERENCES

1. WHO Classification of Tumours Editorial Board. *Female Genital Tumours: WHO Classification of Tumours.* 5th ed. Vol. 4. IARC; 2020.
2. Matei D, Brown J, Frazier L. Updates in the management of ovarian germ cell tumors. *Am Soc Clin Oncol Educ Book.* Vol. 4, pp 1-3; 2013.
3. Safdar NS, Stall JN, Young RH. Malignant mixed germ cell tumors of the ovary: an analysis of 100 cases emphasizing the frequency and interrelationships of their tumor types. *Am J Surg Pathol.* 2021;45(6):727-741.
4. Nasioudis D, Ko EM, Haggerty AF, et al. Performance of lymphadenectomy for apparent early stage malignant ovarian germ cell tumors in the era of platinum-based chemotherapy. *Gynecol Oncol.* 2020;157(3):613-618.
5. Gershenson DM, Del Junco G, Copeland LJ, Rutledge FN. Mixed germ cell tumors of the ovary. *Obstet Gynecol.* 1984;64(2):200-206.
6. De Backer A, Madern GC, Oosterhuis JW, Hakvoort-Cammel FG, Hazebroek FW. Ovarian germ cell tumors in children: a clinical study of 66 patients. *Pediatr Blood Cancer.* 2006;46(4):459-464.
7. Kodama M, Grubbs BH, Blake EA, et al. Feto-maternal outcomes of pregnancy complicated by ovarian malignant germ cell tumor: a systematic review of literature. *Eur J Obstet Gynecol Reprod Biol.* 2014;181:145-156.
8. Lakshmanan M, Gupta S, Kumar V, et al. Germ cell tumor ovary: an institutional experience of treatment and survival outcomes. *Indian J Surg Oncol.* 2018;9(2):215-219.
9. Tangjitgamol S, Hanprasertpong J, Manusirivithaya S, Wootipoom V, Thavaramara T, Buhachat R. Malignant ovarian germ cell tumors: clinico-pathological presentation and survival outcomes. *Acta Obstet Gynecol Scand.* 2010;89(2):182-189.
10. Rungoutok M, Suprasert P. Oncology and reproductive outcomes over 16 years of malignant ovarian germ cell tumors treated by fertility sparing surgery. *World J Clin Oncol.* 2022;13(10):802-812.
11. Park M, Lim J, Lee JA, et al. Incidence and outcomes of malignant ovarian germ cell tumors in Korea, 1999-2017. *Gynecol Oncol.* 2021;163(1):79-84.
12. Ray-Coquard I, Trama A, Seckl MJ, et al. Rare ovarian tumours: epidemiology, treatment challenges in and outside a network setting. *Eur J Surg Oncol.* 2019;45(1):67-74.
13. Damjanov I, Amenta PS, Zarghami F. Transformation of an AFP-positive yolk sac carcinoma into an AFP-negative neoplasm. Evidence for in vivo cloning of the human parietal yolk sac carcinoma. *Cancer.* 1984;53(9):1902-1907.
14. AIRTUM Working Group, Busco S, Buzzoni C, et al. Italian cancer figures—report 2015: the burden of rare cancers in Italy. *Epidemiol Prev.* 2016;40(1 Suppl 2):1-120.
15. Park JY, Kim DY, Suh DS, et al. Analysis of outcomes and prognostic factors after fertility-sparing surgery in malignant ovarian germ cell tumors. *Gynecol Oncol.* 2017;145(3):513-518.

16. Mangili G, Giorda G, Ferrandina G, et al. Surveillance alone in stage I malignant ovarian germ cell tumors: a MITO (Multicenter Italian Trials in Ovarian cancer) prospective observational study. *Int J Gynecol Cancer.* 2021;31(9):1242-1247.

17. Young RH. The yolk sac tumor: reflections on a remarkable neoplasm and two of the many intrigued by it—Gunnar Teilum and Aleksander Talerman—and the bond it formed between them. *Int J Surg Pathol.* 2014;22(8):677-687.

18. Young RH, Wong A, Stall JN. Yolk Sac tumor of the ovary: a report of 150 cases and review of the literature. *Am J Surg Pathol.* 2022;46(3):309-325.

19. Solheim O, Gershenson DM, Tropé CG, et al. Prognostic factors in malignant ovarian germ cell tumours (The surveillance, epidemiology and end results experience 1978-2010). *Eur J Cancer.* 2014;50(11):1942-1950.

20. Hinchcliff E, Rauh-Hain JA, Clemmer JT, et al. Racial disparities in survival in malignant germ cell tumors of the ovary. *Gynecol Oncol.* 2016;140(3):463-469.

21. Kleppe M, Amkreutz LC, Van Gorp T, Slangen BF, Kruse AJ, Kruitwagen RF. Lymph-node metastasis in stage I and II sex cord stromal and malignant germ cell tumours of the ovary: a systematic review. *Gynecol Oncol.* 2014;133(1):124-127.

22. Duhil de Benaze G, Pacquement H, Faure-Conter C, et al. Paediatric dysgerminoma: results of three consecutive French germ cell tumours clinical studies (TGM-85/90/95) with late effects study. *Eur J Cancer.* 2018;91:30-37.

23. Billmire D, Vinocur C, Rescorla F, et al. Outcome and staging evaluation in malignant germ cell tumors of the ovary in children and adolescents: an intergroup study. *J Pediatr Surg.* 2004;39(3):424-429.

24. Solheim O, Kærn J, Tropé CG, et al. Malignant ovarian germ cell tumors: presentation, survival and second cancer in a population based Norwegian cohort (1953-2009). *Gynecol Oncol.* 2013;131(2):330-335.

25. Newton C, Murali K, Ahmad A, et al. A multicentre retrospective cohort study of ovarian germ cell tumours: evidence for chemotherapy de-escalation and alignment of paediatric and adult practice. *Eur J Cancer.* 2019;113:19-27.

CHAPTER **9.2**

Malignant Ovarian Germ Cell Tumors: Etiology, Epidemiology, Risk Factors, Genetics, and Molecular Biology

Dimitrios Nasioudis, Emily M. Ko, Koji Matsuo, and Anil K. Sood

ETIOLOGY

Biologically, MOGCTs, like testis cancer, are derived from primordial germ cells, which undergo defective meiosis. Based on their pluripotency, these germ cells can then differentiate into any of the extraembryonic or somatic tissue types, including ectoderm, mesoderm, and endoderm. The specific resultant abnormal tissue type characterizes the histology of the MOGCT (1,2).

Karyotypic abnormalities are common and include aneuploidy or chromosomal rearrangements (3). In contrast, mature teratomas commonly have a normal karyotype and rarely (7%) demonstrate chromosomal abnormalities (4,5). This finding of aneuploidy in GCTs is concordant with the hypothesis that the mitosis/meiosis switch is dysregulated, leading to abnormal chromosomal segregation and development of uncontrolled growth (6,7). Analysis of centromeric heteromorphism suggests that 65% to 70% of benign teratomas result from a post–meiosis I type error (homozygotes), whereas the remaining 30% to 35% are caused by defective meiosis I, as demonstrated by heterozygosity of centromeric markers (4). Among MOGCTs, aneuploidy and chromosomal translocations or truncations like those encountered in testicular carcinoma have been widely reported (3,8). The presence of an isochromosome 12p (i12p) has been noted in ovarian tumors (9), albeit less commonly than in testis cancer. Gains of 12p material may be present in 77% of dysgerminomas and lower percentages of other MOGCTs. Other chromosomal aberrations such as loss or gain in chromosomes 1, 11, 12, 16, and X can be identified (10). The association between dysgerminoma and dysgenetic gonads is well recognized and should be managed accordingly, as discussed later. MicroRNAs from the *miR-371-373* and *miR-302* clusters are overexpressed in all GCTs, anecdotally correlate with disease burden, and are the promising candidate biomarkers for disease monitoring and diagnosis (11).

KIT gene mutations appear to be amplified in dysgerminomas and may provide a clue as to the etiology of dysgerminomas. *KIT* mutations in exon 17 codon 816 lead to increased survival and proliferation of undifferentiated oogonia, potentially leading to dysgerminoma (1). Interestingly, *KIT* mutations have not been detected in ITs and are most common in unilateral dysgerminomas, suggesting late development—after migration to the gonadal ridges in embryonic development (12). In addition, this *KIT* alteration represents a potential therapeutic target (13). Other mutations in dysgerminomas have been occasionally identified, including *DICER1*, *TP53*, and *KRAS* (14). Protein expression and gene mutation studies of MOGCT have recently been reviewed, and overexpression of *POU5F1*, *KIT*, *NANOG*, *PDPN*, and *SOX2* is notable among the frequently overexpressed genes (14).

EPIDEMIOLOGY AND RISK FACTORS

The epidemiology of MOGCT is distinct from the more common epithelial ovarian cancer histologies and so is considered separately here.

MOGCT represents the most common group of nonepithelial ovarian neoplasms, accounting for approximately 3% of all ovarian tumors in the United States (15). These tumors disproportionately occur in children, adolescents, and young adults and represent 75% of malignant ovarian neoplasms in children (15-18).

The incidence of MOGCT varies according to geographic region and race **(Figure 9.2-1)**, appearing to be slightly higher in Eastern Asian and American Hispanic females. Worldwide, the incidence of MOGCT ranges from 0.2 to 0.5 per 100,000 females (15,19-22). An analysis of the National Cancer Institute's (NCI) SEER Program identified 1,262 cases of MOGCT diagnosed between 1973 and 2002, with an overall age-standardized incidence rate (ASR) of 0.338 per 100,000 women-years (19). This has remained essentially

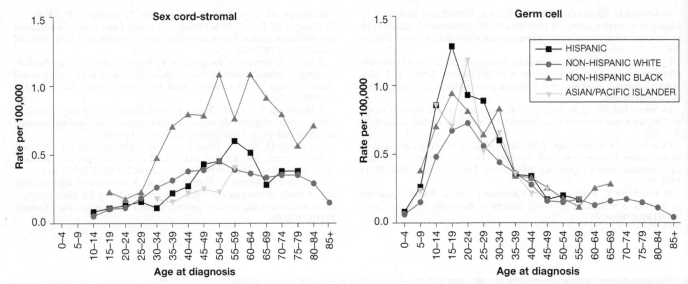

Figure 9.2-1. Age-specific malignant ovarian germ cell tumor incidence rate by race among U.S. women, Surveillance, Epidemiology, and End Results-18, 2003 to 2012. (From Torre LA, Trabert B, DeSantis CE, et al. Ovarian cancer statistics, 2018. *CA Cancer J Clin.* 2018;68(4):284-296)

stable since 1995, with 0.4 cases per 100,000 million women in the 2019 SEER database analysis (15). A lower incidence (ASR 0.13) was reported by the RARECAREnet database that covers 27 European countries (20). On the other hand, higher incidence of MOGCT has been observed among Eastern Asian patients (21,22). An analysis of the Korean Central Cancer Registry (KCCR) reported an ASR of 0.539 per 100,000 women-years with an overall increase annual percent change (APC) of 1.01%, especially in the less than 19-year age group (APC 1.96%) (22). A similar ASR was also observed in an analysis of the Osaka prefecture data (21).

Regarding differences in incidence pertaining to race, a 2006 analysis of the SEER database also revealed a marginally higher incidence among Asian/Pacific islander (ASR 0.43) compared to White women (ASR 0.35, $P = .059$) (19). An updated analysis of the SEER database revealed a higher incidence in Hispanics (0.5/100,000) and a lower incidence in American Indians/Alaska Natives (0.2/100,000). When viewed as percentage distribution of ovarian cancer cases by race/ethnicity, 7% of ovarian cancers in Hispanic females were GCTs, compared with 5% for Asian/Pacific Islander and non-Hispanic Black females and 2% for non-Hispanic White females (15). These findings also mirror a higher prevalence of central nervous system (CNS) GCTs observed in the Asian population.

MOGCT can arise during infancy, whereas their incidence increases sharply with the onset of puberty and peaks between 15 and 19 years. In an analysis of the European RARECAREnet database, the median age at diagnosis of an MOGCT was 27 years, with a peak ASR observed in the 15- 24-year-old group (0.305), whereas lower rates were noted in the less than 14 years (ASR 0.11), 25 to 64 (ASR 0.107), and 65 years or above (ASR 0.06) age groups (20). Based on 2,541 cases from the SEER database, median age at diagnosis was 22 years (19). Similarly, among 2,125 cases identified in the South Korea, 43.2% and 42.9% were diagnosed in patients aged 19 or above and 20 to 34 years, respectively (22). SEER database analysis also revealed a peak incidence for all histologies, except IT, among patients aged 15 to 19 years (19). On the contrary, among 752 cases of MOGCTs diagnosed between 1989 and 2015 in the Netherlands, 27% of patients were 19 years or below age group, whereas 35% were in 21 to 40 years (23).

The most recent SEER database analysis has evaluated incidence rates by age and race/ethnicity. A peak in the incidence of all MOGCT occurs at age 19 in Hispanic and Asian/Pacific Islander females, is slightly later at age 24 in White females, and is bimodal in Black females, occurring at ages 19 and 34 (**Figure 9.2-1**) (15).

Based on data extracted from the Cancer Incidence in 5 Continents (CI5) series that included cases spanning 25 years, the highest incidence of MOGCTs was observed for patients aged 10 to 19 years (ranging from 0.19 to 0.98 cases per 100,000 females based on geographic region) (18). Again, countries from East Asia and Central and North America reported the highest incidence of MOGCT, suggesting a possible genetic component. In addition, a small increase in the incidence of MOGCT was noted in regions with high and very high human development index (HDI), though it is unclear if this is related to health system changes. The highest increase was observed in Eastern Asian countries among patients aged 10 to 19 (average APC 4.37%) and 20 to 39 (average APC 4.84%) years (18).

Histology distribution may vary according to patient race. Data from the NCDB revealed that White patients were more likely to present with dysgerminoma whereas Blacks were more likely to be diagnosed with a teratoma or YSTs (24). Similarly, in an analysis of the SEER database, dysgerminoma rates were higher in Whites and other non-Whites compared to Black women (19). In addition, racial disparities exist in the survival of MOGCT with Black patients, especially those with advanced-stage disease experiencing worse oncologic outcomes (25).

Apart from disorders of sex development (conditions in which there is discordance between chromosomal, gonadal, and phenotypic sex), there are no strong epidemiologic risk factors for the development of MOGCT. Maternal hormonal factors, such as exogenous hormone use, high body mass index, age at index pregnancy less than 20 years, and oral contraception use, have been linked with an increased risk of MOGCT in the daughters (26,27). To date, there are no studies demonstrating a clear association between risk of MOGCT and family history of cancer. A recent study revealed a higher incidence of MOGCT than expected (3 vs 0.7) among 7,998 relatives of patients with MOGCT, though this association did not reach statistical significance (28). However, in a case-parent triad study, association between single-nucleotide polymorphisms in SPRY4, BAK1, and GAB2 and development of GCT was reported (29).

GENETICS

Unlike serous carcinomas of the ovary and fallopian tube, MOGCTs are not associated with *BRCA1, BRCA2*, Lynch syndrome, or any of the related mutations.

The impact of gonadal dysgenesis must be understood. Abnormal karyotypes containing Y chromosomal material are designated "dysgenetic gonads" and occur in phenotypic females with a 46,XY karyotype, mixed gonadal dysgenesis with a 45,X/46,XY karyotype, or complete androgen-insensitivity syndrome (AIS). Females with these dysgenetic gonads containing Y chromosomal material are at significant risk of developing gonadoblastoma and MOGCT, especially dysgerminoma. Gonadoblastoma by itself is considered a benign neoplasm containing both germ cells and sex cord-stromal cells, but it may predispose to the development of a MOGCT or serve as an in situ neoplasm, which could induce development of an MOGCT (30-34). In fact, when IT, mixed GCT, or dysgerminoma is detected bilaterally, up to 50% of cases have dysgenetic gonads (30,32,33). A recent review of 50 patients with MOGCT treated at a single institution showed that 14% had a 46,XY karyotype (six patients with dysgerminoma and one patient with mixed GCT). Of these seven patients, five had Swyer syndrome and two had complete AIS (30). Concurrent gonadoblastoma was found in five of the seven patients. Of the 21 patients with dysgerminoma, six had an XY karyotype (29%) (30).

The diagnosis of ovarian embryonal carcinoma may also prompt consideration of performing chromosomal analysis because some tumors may be associated with Y-chromosome–containing gonadal dysgenesis.

Bilateral adnexectomy should be performed in the setting of gonadal dysgenesis to remove the risk of subsequent MOGCT.

MOLECULAR BIOLOGY

MOGCTs originate from primordial germ cells, which undergo defective meiosis. High expression of transcription factors related to the embryonic stem cell–like pluripotency and undifferentiated state have been detected in MOGCTs, whereas bilateral tumors express more stem cell markers than unilateral cases (12).

MOGCTs are overall characterized by low mutational burden and high incidence of aneuploidy (2,35,36). Molecular and

chromosomal changes associated with MOGCTs are organized in **Table 9.2-1**. The first study to perform whole-exome sequencing on MOGCTs evaluated 24 samples matched with germline samples and performed somatic copy number aberration (CNA) profiles in 87 MOGCTs (35). These authors found a very low mutational frequency (average 0.05 mutations/Mb) compared with other cancer types and concluded that this was consistent with their embryologic origin.

Karyotypic abnormalities are common and include aneuploidy or chromosomal rearrangements arising from abnormal segregation of chromosomes during meiotic division or mitosis (1,3,35,37). The largest study to evaluate CNA profiles demonstrated multiple chromosomal deletions and gains, with a mean of 35% of the genome affected by CNAs (35). The average number of changes varied by histology, present in 52% of dysgerminomas, 44% of YSTs, and only 3% of ITs. Chromosomal gains of 12p, detected in all MOGCT except pure ITs, contain the *KRAS* gene, which can lead to aberrant activation of the *MAPK/ERK* pathway (35). Gain of chromosome 12p can be found in 82% of dysgerminomas, 58% of YSTs, and 43% of mixed MOGCTs (35,38).

Other chromosomal aberrations such as loss or gain may be identified, but chromosomal gain tends to be more common than chromosomal loss (10,35,39). Gain of genetic material has been described in chromosomes 1p, 6p, 12q, 15q, 20q, 21q, and 22q, and whole chromosomal gain has been reported in chromosomes 7, 8, 17, and 19 (39). Others have reported alterations in chromosomes 1, 11, 16, and X (10,35). Specific recurrent focal deletions may affect chromosomal regions 1p36.32, 2q11.1, 4q28.1, 5p15.33, 5q11.1, and 6q27 (35,36).

MicroRNAs from the miR-371-373 and miR-302 clusters are overexpressed in all GCTs, anecdotally correlate with disease burden, and appear to be promising candidate biomarkers for disease monitoring and diagnosis (11). Protein expression and gene mutation studies of MOGCT report overexpression of POU5F1, CASP8, CDH3, CXCL10, IL6R, NANOG, PLBD1, and PDPN (1).

TABLE 9.2-1. Molecular and Chromosomal Alterations in Specific Histologies of Malignant Ovarian Germ Cell Tumors

Histologic Subtype	Molecular Alteration	Estimated Prevalence (%)
Dysgerminoma	*KIT* mutation	30-50
	Gain of chromosome 12p (*KRAS*)	77-82
	DICER1, TP53, KRAS	Uncommon
	Y-chromosome gonadal dysgenesis	29
Immature teratoma	Loss of heterozygosity	100
	Very low mutational burden	
Yolk sac tumor	*PI3K/AKT/mTOR* amplification	40
	KIT mutation	10-55
	Gain of chromosome 12p (*KRAS*)	58
	KRAS mutation	10
	ARID1A mutation	10
	TGF-β/BMP	
	Wnt/bβ-catenin signaling	
Embryonal carcinoma	CD30 expression	80
	Y-chromosome gonadal dysgenesis	
	KRAS mutation	
Choriocarcinoma	Wnt/β-catenin signaling	
Gonadoblastoma	*KIT* mutation	>50
	Y-chromosome gonadal dysgenesis	
Mixed germ cell tumor	Gain of chromosome 12p (*KRAS*)	43
All histologies	Low tumor mutational burden	
	Significant aneuploidy	
	Chromosomal rearrangements	
	Overexpression of microRNA	

Dysgerminomas are characterized by a high incidence of *KIT* gene mutations (~30%-50%) in known hotspot domains (2,13,35,40). *KIT* mutations are associated with advanced-stage disease (13,41). *KIT* is a growth factor receptor pivotal for normal germ cell migration and development and can lead to activation of several intracellular pathways, such as *RAS/MEK, PI3K/mTOR*, and *JAK/STAT*, thereby representing a potential therapeutic target (2).

YSTs and ITs have a distinct molecular profile from ovarian dysgerminoma (**Table 9.2-1**) (1). A recent molecular analysis of 10 patients with YST identified molecular alterations in four (40%) patients, whereas three (33%) patients harbored a targetable oncogenic mutation in the *KRAS, KIT*, and *ARID1A* genes, respectively (42). In a larger analysis of 41 samples from 30 patients with YST, mutations in *KRAS* and *KIT* genes were identified, whereas *ARID1A* and *PARK2* gene deletions and *CDKN1B, ZNF217*, and *KRAS* gene amplifications were the most common copy number alterations (43). *KIT* and *KRAS* mutations have been confirmed by others (35,44). Microsatellite instability and *OVOL2* gene expression were associated with chemoresistance. None of the samples harbored a *TP53* mutation (43). YSTs are also characterized by amplifications of the *PIK3CA* and *AKT1* genes and activation of the TGF-β/BMP and Wnt/β-catenin pathways (1,35).

In the series by Van Nieuwenhuysen et al, two patients had *KRAS* mutations: one had embryonal carcinoma, and the other had a mixed dysgerminoma/YST. Both had an aggressive disease course and died of disease (35). In addition, embryonal carcinomas express CD30 in 80% of cases (45).

A recent multiregion whole-exome sequencing of 52 tumor components from 10 patients with IT revealed that ITs are molecularly characterized by 2N near-diploid genomes with extensive loss of heterozygosity, extremely low total mutation burden, and an absence of somatic nonsynonymous mutations or other known oncogenic variants (37). In addition, different tumor components were indistinguishable molecularly, indicating a shared clonal origin and transformation to malignant neoplasm secondary to epigenetic dysregulation.

With the incorporation of next-generation sequencing into routine clinical practice, genomic alterations that can be capitalized with targeted agents may be identified. An analysis of a large commercial database identified 43 patients with MOGCT who harbored actionable mutations, including *ARID1A* (42%), *PIK3CA* (19%), TMB-high (14%), *FBXW7* (11%), *PTEN* (10%), *CDKN2A* (9%), *NF1* (9%), and 17 other actionable mutations (<8% each) (46). Also notable are the identifications of several candidate driver mutations, including *FIP1L1, BUB1B, CASC5, AKT1*, and *PIK3CD* (35). Notably absent are mutations in *p53*.

These molecular findings may correlate with patient outcomes. A recent study examining paired primary and metastatic GCT demonstrated significant molecular heterogeneity, whereas TP53 pathway alterations (TP53 mutations and MDM2 amplification) were associated with cisplatin resistance (47). Higher mutational rate significantly correlated with death from disease (35). Low mutational rate may result in chemosensitivity and decreased development of chemoresistant clones, yielding a correlation with improved outcomes even in the setting of advanced disease.

REFERENCES

1. Kraggerud SM, Hoei-Hansen CE, Alagaratnam S, et al. Molecular characteristics of malignant ovarian germ cell tumors and comparison with testicular counterparts: implications for pathogenesis. *Endocr Rev.* 2013;34(3):339-376.

2. Maoz A, Matsuo K, Ciccone MA, et al. Molecular pathways and targeted therapies for malignant ovarian germ cell tumors and sex cord-stromal tumors: a contemporary review. *Cancers (Basel).* 2020;12(6):1398.

3. Baker BA, Frickey L, Yu IT, Hawkins EP, Cushing B, Perlman EJ. DNA content of ovarian immature teratomas and malignant germ cell tumors. *Gynecol Oncol.* 1998;71(1):14-18.

4. Surti U, Hoffner L, Chakravarti A, Ferrell RE. Genetics and biology of human ovarian teratomas. I. Cytogenetic analysis and mechanism of origin. *Am J Hum Genet.* 1990;47(4):635-643.

5. Deka R, Chakravarti A, Surti U, et al. Genetics and biology of human ovarian teratomas. II. Molecular analysis of origin of nondisjunction and gene-centromere mapping of chromosome I markers. *Am J Hum Genet.* 1990;47(4):644-655.

6. Looijenga LH, Van Agthoven T, Biermann K. Development of malignant germ cells—the environmental hypothesis. *Int J Dev Biol.* 2013;57(2-4):241-253.

7. Taylor-Weiner A, Zack T, O'Donnell E, et al. Genomic evolution and chemoresistance in germ-cell tumours. *Nature.* 2016;540(7631):114-118.

8. Murty VV, Dmitrovsky E, Bosl GJ, Chaganti RS. Nonrandom chromosome abnormalities in testicular and ovarian germ cell tumor cell lines. *Cancer Genet Cytogenet.* 1990;50(1):67-73.

9. Speleman F, De Potter C, Dal Cin P, et al. i(12p) in a malignant ovarian tumor. *Cancer Genet Cytogenet.* 1990;45(1):49-53.

10. Shen DH, Khoo US, Xue WC, Cheung AN. Ovarian mature cystic teratoma with malignant transformation. An interphase cytogenetic study. *Int J Gynecol Pathol.* 1998;17(4):351-357.

11. Murray MJ, Halsall DJ, Hook CE, Williams DM, Nicholson JC, Coleman N. Identification of microRNAs from the miR-371~373 and miR-302 clusters as potential serum biomarkers of malignant germ cell tumors. *Am J Clin Pathol.* 2011;135(1):119-125.

12. Hoei-Hansen CE, Kraggerud SM, Abeler VM, Kaern J, Rajpert-De Meyts E, Lothe RA. Ovarian dysgerminomas are characterised by frequent KIT mutations and abundant expression of pluripotency markers. *Mol Cancer.* 2007;6:12.

13. Cheng L, Roth LM, Zhang S, et al. KIT gene mutation and amplification in dysgerminoma of the ovary. *Cancer.* 2011;117(10):2096-2103.

14. Sever M, Jones TD, Roth LM, et al. Expression of CD117 (c-kit) receptor in dysgerminoma of the ovary: diagnostic and therapeutic implications. *Mod Pathol.* 2005;18(11):1411-1416.

15. Torre LA, Trabert B, DeSantis CE, et al. Ovarian cancer statistics, 2018. *CA Cancer J Clin.* 2018;68(4):284-296.

16. Testa U, Petrucci E, Pasquini L, Castelli G, Pelosi E. Ovarian cancers: genetic abnormalities, tumor heterogeneity and progression, clonal evolution and cancer stem cells. *Medicines (Basel).* 2018;5(1):16.

17. Matz M, Coleman MP, Sant M, et al. The histology of ovarian cancer: worldwide distribution and implications for international survival comparisons (CONCORD-2). *Gynecol Oncol.* 2017;144(2):405-413.

18. Hubbard AK, Poynter JN. Global incidence comparisons and trends in ovarian germ cell tumors by geographic region in girls, adolescents and young women: 1988-2012. *Gynecol Oncol.* 2019;154(3):608-615.

19. Smith HO, Berwick M, Verschraegen CF, et al. Incidence and survival rates for female malignant germ cell tumors. *Obstet Gynecol.* 2006;107(5):1075-1085.

20. Ray-Coquard I, Trama A, Seckl MJ, et al. Rare ovarian tumours: epidemiology, treatment challenges in and outside a network setting. *Eur J Surg Oncol.* 2019;45(1):67-74.

21. Ioka A, Tsukuma H, Ajiki W, Oshima A. Ovarian cancer incidence and survival by histologic type in Osaka, Japan. *Cancer Sci.* 2003;94(3):292-296.

22. Park M, Lim J, Lee JA, et al. Incidence and outcomes of malignant ovarian germ cell tumors in Korea, 1999-2017. *Gynecol Oncol.* 2021;163(1):79-84.

23. van der Hel OL, Timmermans M, van Altena AM, et al. Overview of non-epithelial ovarian tumours: incidence and survival in the Netherlands, 1989-2015. *Eur J Cancer.* 2019;118:97-104.

24. Hinchcliff E, Rauh-Hain JA, Clemmer JT, et al. Racial disparities in survival in malignant germ cell tumors of the ovary. *Gynecol Oncol.* 2016;140(3):463-469.

25. Bryant CS, Kumar S, Shah JP, et al. Racial disparities in survival among patients with germ cell tumors of the ovary—United States. *Gynecol Oncol.* 2009;114(3):437-441.

26. Poynter JN. *Epidemiology of Germ Cell Tumors.* Springer; 2014.

27. Walker AH, Ross RK, Haile RW, Henderson BE. Hormonal factors and risk of ovarian germ cell cancer in young women. *Br J Cancer.* 1988;57(4):418-422.

28. Poynter JN, Richardson M, Roesler M, Krailo M, Amatruda JF, Frazier AL. Family history of cancer in children and adolescents with germ cell tumours: a report from the Children's Oncology Group. *Br J Cancer.* 2018;118(1):121-126.

29. Marcotte EL, Pankratz N, Amatruda JF, et al. Variants in BAK1, SPRY4, and GAB2 are associated with pediatric germ cell tumors: a report from the Children's Oncology Group. *Genes Chromosomes Cancer.* 2017;56(7):548-558.

30. Lin KY, Bryant S, Miller DS, Kehoe SM, Richardson DL, Lea JS. Malignant ovarian germ cell tumor—role of surgical staging and gonadal dysgenesis. *Gynecol Oncol*. 2014;134(1):84-89.

31. Cools M, Drop SL, Wolffenbuttel KP, Oosterhuis JW, Looijenga LH. Germ cell tumors in the intersex gonad: old paths, new directions, moving frontiers. *Endocr Rev*. 2006;27(3):468-484.

32. Capito C, Arnaud A, Hameury F, et al. Dysgerminoma and gonadal dysgenesis: the need for a new diagnosis tree for suspected ovarian tumours. *J Pediatr Urol*. 2011;7(3):367-372.

33. Capito C, Leclair MD, Arnaud A, et al. 46,XY pure gonadal dysgenesis: clinical presentations and management of the tumor risk. *J Pediatr Urol*. 2011;7(1):72-75.

34. Robboy SJ, Jaubert F. Neoplasms and pathology of sexual developmental disorders (intersex). *Pathology*. 2007;39(1):147-163.

35. Van Nieuwenhuysen E, Busschaert P, Neven P, et al. The genetic landscape of 87 ovarian germ cell tumors. *Gynecol Oncol*. 2018;151(1):61-68.

36. Van Nieuwenhuysen E, Lambrechts S, Lambrechts D, Leunen K, Amant F, Vergote I. Genetic changes in nonepithelial ovarian cancer. *Expert Rev Anticancer Ther*. 2013;13(7):871-882.

37. Heskett MB, Sanborn JZ, Boniface C, et al. Multiregion exome sequencing of ovarian immature teratoma reveals 2N near-diploid genomes, paucity of somatic mutations, and extensive allelic imbalances shared across mature, immature, and disseminated components. *Mod Pathol*. 2020;33(6):1193-1206.

38. Cossu-Rocca P, Zhang S, Roth LM, et al. Chromosome 12p abnormalities in dysgerminoma of the ovary: a FISH analysis. *Mod Pathol*. 2006;19(4):611-615.

39. Kraggerud SM, Szymanska J, Abeler VM, et al. DNA copy number changes in malignant ovarian germ cell tumors. *Cancer Res*. 2000;60(11):3025-3030.

40. AACR Project GENIE Consortium. AACR Project GENIE: powering precision medicine through an international consortium. *Cancer Discov*. 2017;7(8):818-831.

41. Hersmus R, Stoop H, van de Geijn GJ, et al. Prevalence of c-KIT mutations in gonadoblastoma and dysgerminomas of patients with disorders of sex development (DSD) and ovarian dysgerminomas. *PLoS One*. 2012;7(8):e43952.

42. Hodroj K, Stevovic A, Attignon V, et al. Molecular characterization of Ovarian Yolk Sac Tumor (OYST). *Cancers (Basel)*. 2021;13(2):220.

43. Zong X, Zhang Y, Peng X, et al. Analysis of the genomic landscape of yolk sac tumors reveals mechanisms of evolution and chemoresistance. *Nat Commun*. 2021;12(1):3579.

44. Ichikawa Y, Yoshida S, Koyama Y, et al. Inactivation of p16/CDKN2 and p15/MTS2 genes in different histological types and clinical stages of primary ovarian tumors. *Int J Cancer*. 1996;69(6):466-470.

45. Leroy X, Augusto D, Leteurtre E, Gosselin B. CD30 and CD117 (c-kit) used in combination are useful for distinguishing embryonal carcinoma from seminoma. *J Histochem Cytochem*. 2002;50(2):283-285.

46. Brown J, Farley JH, Herzog TJ, et al. Feasibility of a platform trial based on molecular analysis in rare gynecologic cancers. *J Clin Oncol*. 2019;37:e14585.

47. Cheng ML, Donoghue MTA, Audenet F, et al. Germ cell tumor molecular heterogeneity revealed through analysis of primary and metastasis pairs. *JCO Precis Oncol*. 2020;4:PO.20.00166.

CHAPTER **9.3**

Ovarian Germ Cell Tumors: Clinical Presentation and Diagnostic Evaluation and Workup

Allison M. Puechl, Priya Bhosale, Dimitrios Nasioudis, Emily M. Ko, and Sara Stoneham

CLINICAL PRESENTATION

MOGCTs usually occur in prepubertal females and young females of reproductive age, with a median age of 16 to 22 years, depending on the histologic subtype (1-3) (see Section 9, Chapter 2). Most MOGCT are large and grow rapidly, so more than 80% of patients present with a palpable pelvic/abdominal mass and abdominal pain. Less common presenting symptoms include abdominal distention (35%), ascites (20%), fever (10%), and vaginal bleeding (10%). The overall duration of symptoms is usually short, with a median of 2 to 4 weeks. Approximately 10% of patients present with an acute abdomen due to tumor rupture, intra-abdominal bleeding, or ovarian torsion. This finding is somewhat more common in patients with endodermal sinus tumor or mixed GCTs and is frequently misdiagnosed as acute appendicitis (4-6). However, among adolescents with an adnexal mass, torsion is not associated with an increased risk of malignancy. Based on 180 pediatric and adolescent patients who presented with ovarian torsion and an adnexal mass, almost half underwent oophorectomy, and only 14% (*n* = 12) had a malignancy (7). Occasionally, β-human chorionic gonadotropin (β-hCG) production from tumor cells can cause isosexual precocious puberty, signs of pregnancy, or abnormal vaginal bleeding (4-6).

Most mature teratomas, however, are incidentally diagnosed at the time of imaging performed for a separate indication and are, therefore, small when diagnosed. Whether mature or immature, large teratomas can cause pelvic pain and pressure owing to their size. The rate of torsion varies in different series from 3% to 16%, increases based on size, and may be increased during pregnancy (8-10). These patients can present with peritoneal signs, including abdominal tenderness, guarding, vomiting, fever, and abnormal bleeding (11). Occasionally, teratomas can rupture and cause peritonitis and even chronic granulomatous peritonitis in the setting of a chronic leak, though this is very rare (8).

A very rare but important presentation of IT is paraneoplastic anti–*N*-methyl-D-aspartate receptor (NMDA) encephalitis (12,13). A young patient with a suspicious adnexal mass may present with memory problems, psychiatric symptoms, unresponsiveness, seizures, dyskinesias, autonomic instability, and/or hypoventilation. In these patients, auto-antibodies are generated against the extracellular N-terminal domain of the NR1 subunit. These can be detected by serology for NMDA antibody titers. Early diagnosis and treatment through surgery and immunotherapy yield a 75% chance of recovery (12,13).

Monodermal teratomas include struma ovarii and carcinoid. Struma ovarii can be either benign or malignant and consists of thyroid tissue. Patients with struma ovarii may present with hyperthyroidism (14,15). Carcinoids are another monodermal teratomas that can present with symptoms and signs due to serotonin release. These patients may present with carcinoid syndrome, with flushing, hypertension, diarrhea, bronchospasm, heart disease, and right heart failure (11,16).

MOGCTs can occur during pregnancy or the immediate post-partum period and are the most common type of ovarian cancer diagnosed during pregnancy (6,17). In the series reported by Gordon, 20 of 158 patients with dysgerminoma were diagnosed during pregnancy or after delivery (18). Nondysgerminomatous ovarian tumors occur less frequently during pregnancy, but rare cases have been reported (19-22). Based on a systematic review of the literature identifying 102 cases, dysgerminoma (38.2%) and YST (30.4%) are the most common histologic subtypes, and most patients present with early-stage disease (76.4%) and large tumors (mean size 17.9 cm) (23). A marked increase in α-fetoprotein (AFP) may herald the presence of a GCT with a yolk sac component. Therefore, a significant AFP or lactic dehydrogenase (LDH) elevation during pregnancy in the presence of an adnexal mass should raise suspicion of an MOGCT.

Patients with OGCTs diagnosed during pregnancy can usually be treated successfully without compromising the health of the fetus. Surgical resection of tumors and computed tomography (CT) have been performed safely in the second and third trimesters. Chemotherapy administration (bleomycin, etoposide, cisplatin) following the first trimester does not appear to increase the risk of congenital malformations (17,23). However, rapid disease progression and/or pregnancy termination/miscarriage have been recorded, especially for nondysgerminomatous tumors (24). In addition, pregnancies affected by MOGCT have an increased rate of intrauterine growth restriction (IUGR) (22.8%) and preterm birth (43.2%) (17,23).

Choriocarcinoma is a rare malignant tumor that can be gestational or nongestational. Gestational choriocarcinoma is discussed separately. Nongestational choriocarcinoma of the ovary is very rare but occurs in children and women of reproductive age with precocious puberty, abnormal vaginal bleeding, and elevated β-hCG levels. Nongestational choriocarcinoma of the ovary can mimic ectopic pregnancy due to the β-hCG production (25).

DIAGNOSTIC EVALUATION/WORKUP

Biologic Markers

GCTs produce biologic markers that can be detected in patient's serum. The development of specific and sensitive radioimmunoassay techniques to measure β-hCG and AFP led to dramatic improvements in patient surveillance. Serial measurements of serum markers can aid in the diagnosis and, more importantly, are used to monitor response to treatment and detect subclinical recurrences. Table 9.3-1 illustrates typical findings in the sera of patients with various tumor histologic types. YST and choriocarcinoma produce AFP and β-hCG, respectively. Embryonal carcinoma can secrete both β-hCG and AFP but, most commonly, produces β-hCG. Mixed tumors may produce either, both, or none of the markers, depending on the type and quantity of histologic elements present. Dysgerminoma is commonly devoid of hormonal production, although a small percentage of tumors produce low levels of β-hCG, if multinucleated syncytiotrophoblastic giant cells are present. It should be noted that an elevated level of AFP or high level of β-hCG (>100 units/mL) denotes the presence of tumor elements

other than dysgerminoma, and therapy should be adjusted accordingly. Although ITs do not uniformly secrete any biomarkers, up to 59% have elevated CA-19-9 levels, up to 23% have elevated CA-125 levels, and occasional tumors can produce AFP (11,26-28). An additional tumor marker is LDH that is frequently elevated in patients with MOGCTs, especially dysgerminomas. Unfortunately, it is less specific than β-hCG or AFP, because it may be increased secondary to a variety of medical conditions, thus limiting its clinical utility. CA-125 can also be nonspecifically elevated in patients with MOGCTs and may be associated with poor outcomes (29,30).

Monodermal teratomas can secrete hormones based on the tissue in the tumor. Patients with struma ovarii may have a low thyroid-stimulating hormone (TSH) with elevated free triiodothyronine (T3) and thyroxine (T4) levels (31). Thyroid-stimulating immunoglobulins have been reported in the setting of Graves disease resulting from thyroid hormone secretion (32). Carcinoid tumors may secrete hormones, including serotonin, intestinal hormone peptide YY, insulin, glucagon, gastrin, adrenocorticotropic hormone (ACTH), and β-endorphin (11,33,34).

If the history and physical examination suggest gonadal dysgenesis in a premenarchal female, a preoperative karyotype should be performed. If the karyotype returns with dysgenetic gonads containing Y-chromosome material, both ovaries should be removed at the time of primary surgery, as MOGCTs commonly arise within dysgenetic gonads (35,36). Approximately 1% of patients aged 0 to 18 years with MOGCT have XY gonadal dysgenesis (Swyer syndrome); although rare, it is essential to diagnose this to avoid subsequent development of MOGCT (37).

Imaging

The goals of imaging in the evaluation of the young female with a pelvic mass are to predict benign versus malignant histology, determine the site of origin, and assess for metastatic disease (38). Ovarian origin can be suggested by the presence of a "claw" of normal ovarian tissue surrounding an ovarian mass, by separation from surrounding structures, and by tracing the gonadal vessels to the mass (38,39). There are advantages and disadvantages to each imaging modality. Ultrasound is widely available and low cost, but optimal pelvic visualization requires a transvaginal probe, which may be problematic in a young virginal patient. Ultrasound can detect vascularity but does not assess adequately for metastatic disease (40). It remains the first-line diagnostic imaging modality (38). CT reliably detects calcium and fat within a mass and provides evaluation of metastatic disease, but anatomic delineation of adnexal structures is limited, and it utilizes ionizing radiation, which is problematic in young premenarchal or reproductive-aged female patients. Magnetic resonance imaging (MRI) has excellent contrast resolution that delineates pelvic structures well, and T1-weighted imaging demonstrates fat, hemorrhage, tumor vasculature, and fibrous stroma. It does not utilize ionizing radiation but is limited by motion artifact. MRI is often employed in the setting of a nondiagnostic ultrasound (41).

Imaging features differ based on histology and often allow a presumptive diagnosis based on these characteristics (11,38,42). The combination of imaging characteristics and serum markers provides a specific diagnostic framework (Figure 9.3-1).

TABLE 9.3-1. Serum Tumor Markers That Characterize Malignant Ovarian Germ Cell Tumors

Histology	α-Fetoprotein (AFP)	β-hCG	Lactate Dehydrogenase (LDH)	CA-125	CA-19-9
Dysgerminoma	Normal	Sometimes increased	Increased	Variable	Normal
Immature teratoma	Sometimes increased	Normal	Normal	Sometimes increased	Sometimes increased
Yolk sac tumor	Increased	Normal	Sometimes increased	Variable	Normal
Embryonal carcinoma	Increased	Increased	Increased	Variable	Normal
Choriocarcinoma	Normal	Increased	Normal	Variable	Normal

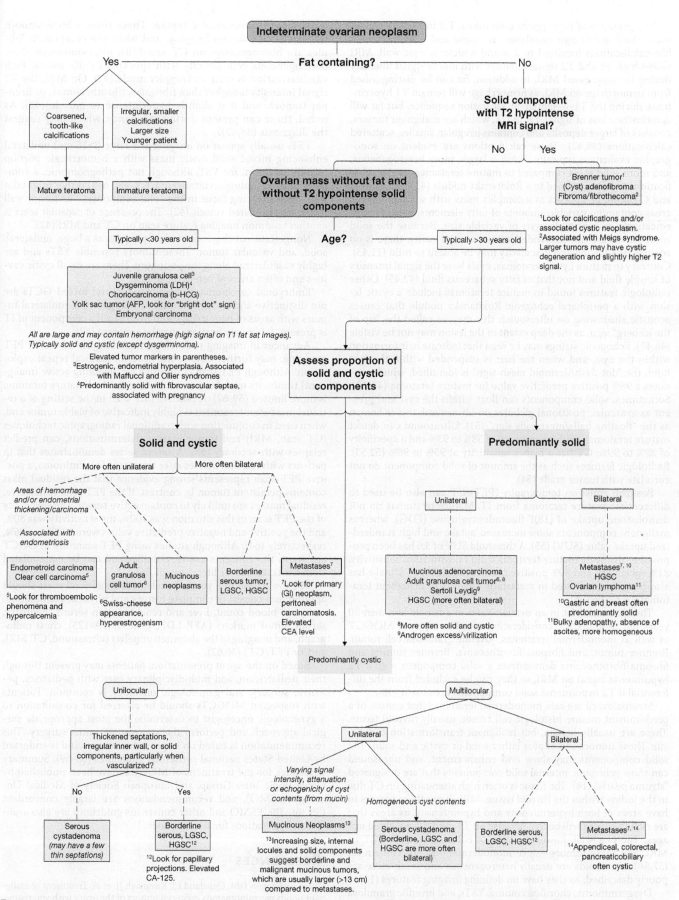

Figure 9.3-1. Flowchart of an algorithmic approach to ovarian neoplasms. (Used with permission of Radiological society of North America, from Taylor EC, Irshaid L, Mathur M. Multimodality imaging approach to ovarian neoplasms with pathologic correlation. *Radiographics*. 2021;41(1): 289-315. doi:10.1148/rg.2021200086; permission conveyed through Copyright Clearance Center, Inc)

The presence of fat suggests a teratoma. Fat in mature teratomas, which are benign neoplasms, is coarse and contains tooth-like calcifications localized to a mural nodule or cyst wall. MRI shows high T1 and T2 signal intensity with loss of signal intensity during fat-suppressed MRI. In addition, fat can be distinguished from hemorrhage on MRI, as hemorrhage will remain T1 hyperintense during the T1-weighted fat-saturation sequence, but fat will demonstrate loss of signal. Fat in ITs, which are malignant tumors, consists of larger deposits and contains irregular, smaller, scattered calcifications (38,42). These calcifications are evident on sonographic evaluation typically within a larger, more heterogeneous, and more solid mass compared to mature teratomas, as the calcifications are not confined to a Rokitansky nodule (43,44). On MRI and CT scan, IT appears as a complex mass with solid and cystic areas containing variable amounts of fatty elements, irregular calcifications, and multiple cysts of variable size. Because the solid components are not suspended within a cystic cavity, there is no acoustic shadowing and vascularity may be absent to mild (11,43). Contrary to mature cystic teratomas, cysts have the signal intensity of simple fluid and not that of fatty sebaceous fluid (42,45). Other radiologic features found in mature teratomas include a cystic lesion with a peripheral echogenic Rokitansky nodule that causes acoustic shadowing on ultrasound; this may be called the "tip of the iceberg" sign, as the deep extent of the lesion may not be visible (46,47). Echogenic strings may be seen that indicate hair formation within the cyst, and when the hair is suspended within the cyst fluid, the "dot-dash/dermoid mesh sign" is identified, which connotes a 98% positive predictive value for mature teratoma (48-50). Sometimes, solid components can float within the cyst and present as avascular, positional globules on ultrasound; this is known as the "floating balls/meat balls sign" (51). Ultrasound can detect mature teratomas, with a sensitivity of 58% to 93% and a specificity of 88% to 99%; CT has a higher sensitivity at 93% to 98% (52,53). Radiologic features such as the amount of solid component do not correlate with tumor grade (54).

Positron emission tomography (PET)/CT can also be used to differentiate mature teratoma from IT. Mature teratomas do not demonstrate uptake of (18)F-fluorodeoxyglucose (FDG), whereas malignant components show increased uptake and high standardized uptake value (SUV) (55). A threshold SUV of 3.6 has been proposed to delineate mature teratoma from IT, with 100% sensitivity, 81% specificity, and 89% positive predictive value (56). Uptake has also been demonstrated in metastatic deposits of malignant teratomatous tissue (56).

The absence of fat in an ovarian mass in a female less than 30 years old prompts the consideration of other types of MOGCT as well as monodermal teratomas, juvenile granulosa cell tumor, Brenner tumor, and fibroma/fibrothecoma. Brenner tumors and fibroma/fibrothecoma demonstrate a solid component with a T2 hypointense signal on MRI, so they can be excluded from the differential if T2 hypointense solid components are absent (38).

Struma ovarii are rare monodermal teratomas that consist of a predominant mature histologic cell tumor, usually thyroid tissue. These are usually benign, but malignant transformation can occur. These tumors can appear either solid or cystic and solid. The solid components may show avid enhancement, and ultrasound can show echogenic internal solid components that are designated "struma pearls" (14). The tissue is often high attenuating on CT due to the iodine within the thyroid tissue. MRI shows these tumors to have areas of both hyperintensity and hypointensity, as areas that are rich in colloid will be hypointense on T1- and T2-weighted images. The cyst wall, however, does not enhance on either CT or MRI, and these tumors—since monodermal—do not contain fat (57,58). Carcinoids are usually heterogeneous and solid; these are poorly described, so they have no defining imaging features (11).

Dysgerminoma, choriocarcinoma, YSTs, and juvenile granulosa cell tumors are all often large and may contain areas of hemorrhage, which manifest as high signal on T1-weighted images on MRI (38).

Dysgerminomas on ultrasound usually appear as large (>10 cm), purely solid masses that are divided into component lobules with fibrovascular septae. These tumors have smooth lobulated contours on imaging, and while the component lobules are homogeneous on CT and MRI, ultrasound can show heterogeneous echogenicity with speckled calcifications. Rich vascularization is seen on Doppler mode (42). On MRI, the T2 signal intensity is higher than fibromas, fibrothecomas, or Brenner tumors, and it is slightly hyperintense to muscle (42). As noted, these can present during pregnancy, which may suggest the diagnosis (38,42).

YSTs usually appear on imaging as a large (>15 cm) unilateral enhancing mixed solid/cystic mass with a hemorrhagic portion (42). In addition, for YST, although not pathognomonic, a common imaging finding on ultrasound, CT, and MRI is the "bright dot sign," an enhancing focus in the solid components or tumor wall representing dilated vessels (42). The presence of capsular tears is another common imaging feature seen on CT and MRI (42).

Nongestational choriocarcinoma presents as a large, unilateral, solid, and vascular tumor. These tumors resemble YSTs and are highly vascularized along the periphery. There are small cystic cavities and often areas of hemorrhage (25).

Embryonal carcinoma, polyembryoma, and mixed GCTs are not distinctive and usually present with large, solid, unilateral tumors with areas of hemorrhage and necrosis. If a component of IT is present, fat or calcifications may be apparent (42).

Advances in imaging technology, including the advent of PET scanning, may further obviate the need for surgical repeat exploration. Although PET scan is sensitive for detecting active (malignant) tumor, its usefulness in evaluating residual mature teratoma is more limited (59-62). A positive PET scan in the setting of a residual mass after treatment is highly indicative of viable tumor and, when used in conjunction with traditional radiographic techniques (CT scan, MRI) and tumor marker determinations, can predict relapses with accuracy (63). A recent series demonstrates that in patients with residual masses after treatment for seminoma, a positive PET scan represents strong evidence that the residual mass contains persistent tumor. In contrast, if the PET scan is negative, residual masses are unlikely to contain active tumor. The specificity of the PET scan in this situation was 100%, the sensitivity was 80%, and the positive and negative predictive values were 100% and 95%, respectively (64). Although studies using PET scanning in OGCT are scant, the concepts are very similar and can be extrapolated from the testis cancer literature (65,66).

The evaluation of a young female with an adnexal mass should at minimum consist of complete history and physical examination, complete blood count, liver and renal function serum chemistry, serum tumor markers (AFP, LDH, β-hCG, CA-125), chest radiograph, and imaging of the abdomen or pelvis (ultrasound, CT, MRI, and/or PET/CT) (36,67).

Based on the age at presentation, patients may present through their pediatrician, and multidisciplinary care with pediatrics, pediatric surgery, and gynecologic oncology is common. Patients with suspected MOGCTs should be referred for consultation to a gynecologic oncologist to determine the most appropriate surgical approach and perform the appropriate initial surgery. This recommendation is based on improved outcomes and is endorsed by United States national consensus guidelines (68-69). Summary guidelines for the treatment of MOGCT have been published by Gynecologic Inter-Group, and European Society of Medical Oncology (ESMO), and recommendations are largely concordant (35,36). The ESMO and other consensus guidelines are also available in applications for smartphones.

REFERENCES

1. Gershenson DM, Copeland LJ, Kavanagh JJ, et al. Treatment of malignant nondysgerminomatous germ cell tumors of the ovary with vincristine, dactinomycin, and cyclophosphamide. *Cancer.* 1985;56(12):2756-2761.

2. Solheim O, Gershenson DM, Tropé CG, et al. Prognostic factors in malignant ovarian germ cell tumours (The surveillance, epidemiology and end results experience 1978-2010). *Eur J Cancer.* 2014;50(11):1942-1950.

3. Mikus M, Benco N, Matak L, et al. Fertility-sparing surgery for patients with malignant ovarian germ cell tumors: 10 years of clinical experience from a tertiary referral center. *Arch Gynecol Obstet*. 2020;301(5):1227-1233.

4. Gershenson DM, Del Junco G, Copeland LJ, Rutledge FN. Mixed germ cell tumors of the ovary. *Obstet Gynecol*. 1984;64(2):200-206.

5. De Backer A, Madern GC, Oosterhuis JW, Hakvoort-Cammel FG, Hazebroek FW. Ovarian germ cell tumors in children: a clinical study of 66 patients. *Pediatr Blood Cancer*. 2006;46(4):459-464.

6. Asadourian LA, Taylor HB. Dysgerminoma. An analysis of 105 cases. *Obstet Gynecol*. 1969;33(3):370-379.

7. Lawrence AE, Fallat ME, Hewitt G, et al. Factors associated with torsion in pediatric patients with ovarian masses. *J Surg Res*. 2021;263:110-115.

8. Comerci JT Jr, Licciardi F, Bergh PA, Gregori C, Breen JL. Mature cystic teratoma: a clinicopathologic evaluation of 517 cases and review of the literature. *Obstet Gynecol*. 1994;84(1):22-28.

9. Caruso PA, Marsh MR, Minkowitz S, Karten G. An intense clinicopathologic study of 305 teratomas of the ovary. *Cancer*. 1971;27(2):343-348.

10. Peterson WF, Prevost EC, Edmunds FT, Hundley JM Jr, Morris FK. Benign cystic teratomas of the ovary; a clinico-statistical study of 1,007 cases with a review of the literature. *Am J Obstet Gynecol*. 1955;70(2):368-382.

11. Saleh M, Bhosale P, Menias CO, et al. Ovarian teratomas: clinical features, imaging findings and management. *Abdom Radiol (NY)*. 2021;46(6):2293-2307.

12. Park SB, Kim JK, Kim KR, Cho KS. Imaging findings of complications and unusual manifestations of ovarian teratomas. *Radiographics*. 2008;28(4):969-983.

13. Dalmau J, Gleichman AJ, Hughes EG, et al. Anti-NMDA-receptor encephalitis: case series and analysis of the effects of antibodies. *Lancet Neurol*. 2008;7(12):1091-1098.

14. Zalel Y, Caspi B, Tepper R. Doppler flow characteristics of dermoid cysts: unique appearance of struma ovarii. *J Ultrasound Med*. 1997;16(5):355-358.

15. Devaney K, Snyder R, Norris HJ, Tavassoli FA. Proliferative and histologically malignant struma ovarii: a clinicopathologic study of 54 cases. *Int J Gynecol Pathol*. 1993;12(4):333-343.

16. Chaowalit N, Connolly HM, Schaff HV, Webb MJ, Pellikka PA. Carcinoid heart disease associated with primary ovarian carcinoid tumor. *Am J Cardiol*. 2004;93(10):1314-1315.

17. Korenaga TK, Tewari KS. Gynecologic cancer in pregnancy. *Gynecol Oncol*. 2020;157(3):799-809.

18. Gordon A, Lipton D, Woodruff JD. Dysgerminoma: a review of 158 cases from the Emil Novak Ovarian Tumor Registry. *Obstet Gynecol*. 1981;58(4):497-504.

19. Christman JE, Teng NN, Lebovic GS, Sikic BI. Delivery of a normal infant following cisplatin, vinblastine, and bleomycin (PVB) chemotherapy for malignant teratoma of the ovary during pregnancy. *Gynecol Oncol*. 1990;37(2):292-295.

20. Farahmand SM, Marchetti DL, Asirwatham JE, Dewey MR. Ovarian endodermal sinus tumor associated with pregnancy: review of the literature. *Gynecol Oncol*. 1991;41(2):156-160.

21. Horbelt D, Delmore J, Meisel R, Cho S, Roberts D, Logan D. Mixed germ cell malignancy of the ovary concurrent with pregnancy. *Obstet Gynecol*. 1994;84(4 Pt 2):662-664.

22. Rajendran S, Hollingworth J, Scudamore I. Endodermal sinus tumour of the ovary in pregnancy. *Eur J Gynaecol Oncol*. 1999;20(4):272-274.

23. Kodama M, Grubbs BH, Blake EA, et al. Feto-maternal outcomes of pregnancy complicated by ovarian malignant germ cell tumor: a systematic review of literature. *Eur J Obstet Gynecol Reprod Biol*. 2014;181:145-156.

24. Bakri YN, Ezzat A, Akhtar M, Dohami H, Zahrani A. Malignant germ cell tumors of the ovary. Pregnancy considerations. *Eur J Obstet Gynecol Reprod Biol*. 2000;90(1):87-91.

25. Bazot M, Cortez A, Sananes S, Buy JN. Imaging of pure primary ovarian choriocarcinoma. *AJR Am J Roentgenol*. 2004;182(6):1603-1604.

26. Sinha NK. Struma ovarii with elevated CA-125 levels and ascites mimicking advanced ca ovary. *J Clin Diagn Res*. 2014;8(3):140-141.

27. Kikkawa F, Nawa A, Tamakoshi K, et al. Diagnosis of squamous cell carcinoma arising from mature cystic teratoma of the ovary. *Cancer*. 1998;82(11):2249-2255.

28. Marina NM, Cushing B, Giller R, et al. Complete surgical excision is effective treatment for children with immature teratomas with or without malignant elements: a Pediatric Oncology Group/Children's Cancer Group Intergroup Study. *J Clin Oncol*. 1999;17(7):2137-2143.

29. Kim JH, Park JY, Kim JH, Kim YM, Kim YT, Nam JH. The role of preoperative serum cancer antigen 125 in malignant ovarian germ cell tumors. *Taiwan J Obstet Gynecol*. 2018;57(2):236-240.

30. Sekiya S, Seki K, Nagai Y. Rise of serum CA 125 in patients with pure ovarian yolk sac tumors. *Int J Gynaecol Obstet*. 1997;58(3):323-324.

31. Young RH. New and unusual aspects of ovarian germ cell tumors. *Am J Surg Pathol*. 1993;17(12):1210-1224.

32. Teale E, Gouldesbrough DR, Peacey SR. Graves' disease and co-existing struma ovarii: struma expression of thyrotropin receptors and the presence of thyrotropin receptor stimulating antibodies. *Thyroid*. 2006;16(8):791-793.

33. Yaegashi N, Tsuiki A, Shimizu T, et al. Ovarian carcinoid with severe constipation due to peptide YY production. *Gynecol Oncol*. 1995;56(2):302-306.

34. Sporrong B, Falkmer S, Robboy SJ, et al. Neurohormonal peptides in ovarian carcinoids: an immunohistochemical study of 81 primary carcinoids and of intraovarian metastases from six mid-gut carcinoids. *Cancer*. 1982;49(1):68-74.

35. Ray-Coquard I, Morice P, Lorusso D, et al. Non-epithelial ovarian cancer: ESMO Clinical Practice Guidelines for diagnosis, treatment and follow-up. *Ann Oncol*. 2018;29(Suppl 4):iv1-iv18.

36. Brown J, Friedlander M, Backes FJ, et al. Gynecologic Cancer Intergroup (GCIG) consensus review for ovarian germ cell tumors. *Int J Gynecol Cancer*. 2014;24(9 Suppl 3):S48-S54.

37. Calaminus G, Schneider DT, von Schweinitz D, et al. Age-dependent presentation and clinical course of 1465 patients aged 0 to less than 18 years with ovarian or testicular germ cell tumors; data of the MAKEI 96 protocol revisited in the light of prenatal germ cell biology. *Cancers (Basel)*. 2020;12(3):611.

38. Taylor EC, Irshaid L, Mathur M. Multimodality imaging approach to ovarian neoplasms with pathologic correlation. *Radiographics*. 2021;41(1):289-315.

39. Saksouk FA, Johnson SC. Recognition of the ovaries and ovarian origin of pelvic masses with CT. *Radiographics*. 2004;24(Suppl 1):S133-S146.

40. Expert Panel on Women's Imaging, Atri M, Alabousi A, et al. ACR Appropriateness Criteria((R)) clinically suspected adnexal mass, no acute symptoms. *J Am Coll Radiol*. 2019;16(5S):S77-S93.

41. Spencer JA, Ghattamaneni S. MR imaging of the sonographically indeterminate adnexal mass. *Radiology*. 2010;256(3):677-694.

42. Shaaban AM, Rezvani M, Elsayes KM, et al. Ovarian malignant germ cell tumors: cellular classification and clinical and imaging features. *Radiographics*. 2014;34(3):777-801.

43. Buy JN, Ghossain MA, Moss AA, et al. Cystic teratoma of the ovary: CT detection. *Radiology*. 1989;171(3):697-701.

44. Jung SE, Lee JM, Rha SE, Byun JY, Jung JI, Hahn ST. CT and MR imaging of ovarian tumors with emphasis on differential diagnosis. *Radiographics*. 2002;22(6):1305-1325.

45. Ueno T, Tanaka YO, Nagata M, et al. Spectrum of germ cell tumors: from head to toe. *Radiographics*. 2004;24(2):387-404.

46. Beller MJ. The "tip of the iceberg" sign. *Radiology*. 1998;209(2):395-396.

47. Quinn SF, Erickson S, Black WC. Cystic ovarian teratomas: the sonographic appearance of the dermoid plug. *Radiology*. 1985;155(2):477-478.

48. Sheth S, Fishman EK, Buck JL, Hamper UM, Sanders RC. The variable sonographic appearances of ovarian teratomas: correlation with CT. *AJR Am J Roentgenol*. 1988;151(2):331-334.

49. Patel MD, Feldstein VA, Lipson SD, Chen DC, Filly RA. Cystic teratomas of the ovary: diagnostic value of sonography. *AJR Am J Roentgenol*. 1998;171(4):1061-1065.

50. Vyas B, Dyer RB. The "dot-dash" sign. *Abdom Imaging*. 2015;40(7):2901-2902.

51. Tongsong T, Wanapirak C, Khunamornpong S, Sukpan K. Numerous intracystic floating balls as a sonographic feature of benign cystic teratoma: report of 5 cases. *J Ultrasound Med*. 2006;25(12):1587-1591.

52. Mais V, Guerriero S, Ajossa S, Angiolucci M, Paoletti AM, Melis GB. Transvaginal ultrasonography in the diagnosis of cystic teratoma. *Obstet Gynecol*. 1995;85(1):48-52.

53. Friedman AC, Pyatt RS, Hartman DS, Downey EF Jr, Olson WB. CT of benign cystic teratomas. *AJR Am J Roentgenol*. 1982;138(4):659-665.

54. Yamaoka T, Togashi K, Koyama T, et al. Immature teratoma of the ovary: correlation of MR imaging and pathologic findings. *Eur Radiol*. 2003;13(2):313-319.

55. Yamanaka Y, Tateiwa Y, Miyamoto H, et al. Preoperative diagnosis of malignant transformation in mature cystic teratoma of the ovary. *Eur J Gynaecol Oncol*. 2005;26(4):391-392.

56. Yokoyama T, Takehara K, Yamamoto Y, et al. The usefulness of 18F-FDG-PET/CT in discriminating benign from malignant ovarian teratomas. *Int J Clin Oncol*. 2015;20(5):960-966.

57. Matsuki M, Kaji Y, Matsuo M, Kobashi Y. Struma ovarii: MRI findings. *Br J Radiol*. 2000;73(865):87-90.

58. Jung SI, Kim YJ, Lee MW, Jeon HJ, Choi JS, Moon MH. Struma ovarii: CT findings. *Abdom Imaging*. 2008;33(6):740-743.

59. Albers P, Bender H, Yilmaz H, Schoeneich G, Biersack HJ, Mueller SC. Positron emission tomography in the clinical staging of patients with Stage I and II testicular germ cell tumors. *Urology.* 1999;53(4):808-811.

60. Hain SF, O'Doherty MJ, Timothy AR, Leslie MD, Harper PG, Huddart RA. Fluorodeoxyglucose positron emission tomography in the evaluation of germ cell tumours at relapse. *Br J Cancer.* 2000;83(7): 863-869.

61. Kollmannsberger C, Oechsle K, Dohmen BM, et al. Prospective comparison of [18F]fluorodeoxyglucose positron emission tomography with conventional assessment by computed tomography scans and serum tumor markers for the evaluation of residual masses in patients with nonseminomatous germ cell carcinoma. *Cancer.* 2002;94(9):2353-2362.

62. Sanchez D, Zudaire JJ, Fernandez JM, et al. 18F-fluoro-2-deoxyglucose-positron emission tomography in the evaluation of nonseminomatous germ cell tumours at relapse. *BJU Int.* 2002;89(9):912-916.

63. Sugawara Y, Zasadny KR, Grossman HB, Francis IR, Clarke MF, Wahl RL. Germ cell tumor: differentiation of viable tumor, mature teratoma, and necrotic tissue with FDG PET and kinetic modeling. *Radiology.* 1999;211(1):249-256.

64. Becherer A, Mitterbauer M, Jaeger U, et al. Positron emission tomography with [18F]2-fluoro-D-2-deoxyglucose (FDG-PET) predicts relapse of malignant lymphoma after high-dose therapy with stem cell transplantation. *Leukemia.* 2002;16(2):260-267.

65. Murphy JJ, Tawfeeq M, Chang B, Nadel H. Early experience with PET/CT scan in the evaluation of pediatric abdominal neoplasms. *J Pediatr Surg.* 2008;43(12):2186-2192.

66. Basu S, Rubello D. PET imaging in the management of tumors of testis and ovary: current thinking and future directions. *Minerva Endocrinol.* 2008;33(3):229-256.

67. Gershenson DM. Current advances in the management of malignant germ cell and sex cord-stromal tumors of the ovary. *Gynecol Oncol.* 2012;125(3):515-517.

68. Giede KC, Kieser K, Dodge J, Rosen B. Who should operate on patients with ovarian cancer? An evidence-based review. *Gynecol Oncol.* 2005;99(2):447-461.

69. Earle CC, Schrag D, Neville BA, et al. Effect of surgeon specialty on processes of care and outcomes for ovarian cancer patients. *J Natl Cancer Inst.* 2006;98(3):172-180.

CHAPTER **9.4**

Surgery for Ovarian Germ Cell Tumors

Giorgia Mangili, Deborah Billmire, Dimitrios Nasioudis, and Emily M. Ko

GOAL OF PRIMARY SURGERY

The goals of primary surgery for MOGCTs are to obtain an accurate diagnosis, remove all visible tumor, and determine the extent of disease to provide prognostic information and guide postoperative management. Appropriate treatment in patients with reproductive potential must balance the oncologic outcomes of the patient with her fertility desires, all within the bounds of safety. Thus, surgical decision-making differs based on the age of the patient, extent of disease, reproductive desires, and specific histology.

OPERATIVE FINDINGS

Malignant GCTs of the ovary tend to be quite large. In the MD Anderson Cancer Center (MDACC) series, these tumors ranged in size from 7 to 40 cm, with a median size of 16 cm (1). Predominance of right-sided over left-sided involvement was noted. Bilaterality of tumor involvement (especially true stage IB disease) appears to be exceedingly rare, except for dysgerminoma, as bilateral involvement occurs in 10% to 15% of patients with dysgerminoma (2-5). For nondysgerminomatous tumors, bilateral involvement signifies either advanced disease with metastatic spread to the contralateral ovary or the presence of a mixed GCT with a prominent dysgerminoma component. Ascites is noted in approximately 20% of cases. Rupture of tumors, either preoperatively or intraoperatively, occurs in approximately 20% of cases. Torsion of the ovarian pedicle was documented in 5% of patients in the MDACC series (1).

Benign cystic teratoma is associated with malignant GCTs in 5% to 10% of cases. These coexistent teratomas may occur in the ipsilateral ovary, in the contralateral ovary, or bilaterally. Likewise, a preexisting gonadoblastoma may be noted in association with dysgerminoma and dysgenetic gonads related to a 46,XY karyotype (6-9). Malignant GCTs generally spread along the peritoneal surface or through lymphatic dissemination. Although the relative frequency of these two principal mechanisms of dissemination is difficult to discern, it is generally accepted that these neoplasms more commonly metastasize to lymph nodes than epithelial tumors. The high prevalence of inadequate staging procedures makes the true incidence of lymph node involvement uncertain. Although uncommon, MOGCTs have a somewhat greater predilection than epithelial tumors to undergo hematogenous metastasis to the liver or lung parenchyma.

The stage distribution is also very different from that of epithelial tumors. In most large series, approximately 60% to 70% of tumors are stage I (2). The next most common stage is stage III, accounting for 25% to 30% of tumors. Stages II and IV are relatively uncommon.

Determination of the exact diagnosis at the time of primary surgery may be challenging, related to the unreliability of intraoperative frozen section diagnosis. In a Children's Oncology Group (COG) study, 38% of intraoperative frozen sections were not concordant with the final pathology, and the institutional pathology diagnosis differed from central pathology review in 24% of patients (10). In both adult and pediatric practice, patients are often assumed to have a benign GCT based on imaging, and proper staging is not done. In a previous review of imaging appearance in a trial for nongerminoma malignant GCTs, just over half of the patients had mixed tumors containing benign teratoma elements. This often results in a preoperative presumption of benign pathology (11). Conversely, a study in the Netherlands found that premenarchal females underwent oophorectomy more commonly than other age groups (12). This uncertainty provides a significant challenge to the surgeon and underscores the need for planned fertility preservation in most young patients with suspected malignant GCTs, because fertility cannot be regained once the gynecologic organs are removed.

ROUTE OF PRIMARY SURGERY

When considering the route of primary surgery, the surgeon should base their choice of minimally invasive surgery (MIS) versus laparotomy versus on their surgical experience and the intent to avoid tumor rupture.

When laparotomy is the selected approach, a vertical midline laparotomy is the incision that allows appropriate access to the upper abdomen. Although a transverse incision is cosmetically superior, it is usually insufficient to provide adequate exposure for evaluation, staging biopsies, and resection of large pelvic tumors or metastatic disease in the upper abdomen.

MIS, whether conventional laparoscopic or robot assisted, is the preferred approach for primary surgery and staging when feasible. Although trials specific to this approach for MOGCTs have not been performed, this approach is considered preferable to open surgery when the same surgical outcomes can be obtained. Minimally invasive techniques can be employed for select patients if the quality of staging is not compromised and the surgical specimen can be extracted intact without capsule rupture or spill, utilizing contained extraction and/or minilaparotomy. Evidence on the role and safety of MIS for ovarian cancer staging derives from small retrospective studies (13). In a recent analysis of the NCDB, one in three patients with apparent early-stage MOGCT underwent MIS. Although these patients were less likely to undergo omentectomy or lymphadenectomy compared to those who had laparotomy, they had superior perioperative outcomes with shorter inpatient stay and lower unplanned 30-day readmission rate, whereas 3-year OS rates were comparable (14).

EXTENT OF PRIMARY SURGERY AND SURGICAL STAGING

Surgical staging is both therapeutic and diagnostic, aiming to remove macroscopic disease and determine the extent of disease spread. This information is prognostic and can guide postoperative management. A meticulous approach is important for every patient, but it is of critical importance for those patients with early clinical disease to detect the presence of occult or microscopic metastases and provide chemotherapy in those situations. Staging of OGCTs follows the same principles applicable to epithelial ovarian tumors, as described by the International Federation of Gynaecology and Obstetricians (FIGO) (see **Table 9.4-1**) (15). Proper surgical staging procedures are summarized in **Table 9.4-2**.

Primary Surgery

The type of primary operative procedure depends on the surgical findings. Because many of these patients are young women for whom preservation of fertility is a priority, minimizing the surgical resection while ensuring removal of tumor bulk must be thoughtfully balanced. Because bilateral involvement is rare, except in pure dysgerminoma and advanced disease, fertility-sparing unilateral salpingo-oophorectomy with preservation of the contralateral ovary and of the uterus is usually the procedure of choice. Ovarian cystectomy as the sole treatment is not recommended (16-18). If the contralateral ovary appears grossly normal on careful inspection, it should be left undisturbed. Random sampling of the contralateral ovary is discouraged in patients with unilateral ovarian involvement, based on the increased risk of postoperative adhesions, infertility, and premature ovarian failure.

■ TABLE 9.4-1. Staging of Malignant Ovarian Germ Cell Tumors

Stage	Description
I	Tumor limited to ovaries
IA	Tumor limited to one ovary, no ascites, intact capsule
IB	Tumor limited to both ovaries, no ascites, intact capsule
IC	Tumor either stage IA or IB, but with ascites present containing malignant cells or with ovarian capsule involvement or rupture or with positive peritoneal washings
II	Tumor involving one or both ovaries with extension to the pelvis
IIA	Extension to uterus or tubes
IIB	Involvement of both ovaries with pelvic extension
IIC	Tumor either stage IIA or IIB, but with ascites present containing malignant cells or with ovarian capsule involvement or rupture or with positive peritoneal washings
III	Tumor involving one or both ovaries with tumor implants outside the pelvis or with positive retroperitoneal or inguinal lymph nodes. Superficial liver metastases qualify as stage III
IIIA	Tumor limited to the pelvis with negative nodes but with microscopic seeding of the abdominal peritoneal surface
IIIB	Negative nodes, tumor implants in the abdominal cavity <2 cm
IIIC	Positive nodes or tumor implants in the abdominal cavity >2 cm
IV	Distant metastases present

Adapted from Kehoe S. FIGO staging in ovarian carcinoma and histological subtypes. *J Gynecol Oncol.* 2020;31(4):e70.

■ TABLE 9.4-2. Surgical Staging Procedure for Adult Malignant Ovarian Germ Cell Tumors

1. Ascites, if present, is evacuated and submitted for cytologic analysis before manipulation of any intraperitoneal organs. If no peritoneal fluid is noted, cytologic washings of the pelvis and bilateral paracolic gutters is performed before manipulation of the intraperitoneal contents.
2. The entire peritoneal cavity and its structures are carefully inspected and palpated in a methodical manner, starting with the subphrenic spaces and moving caudad toward the pelvis. The subdiaphragmatic areas, omentum, colon, all peritoneal surfaces, the entire retroperitoneum, and small intestinal serosa and mesentery are evaluated. Any suspicious areas are submitted for biopsy or excised. When using minimally invasive surgery, visual inspection and instrument palpation are utilized to achieve the same evaluation.
3. Next, the primary ovarian tumor and pelvis are examined. Both ovaries are carefully assessed for size, presence of obvious tumor involvement, capsular rupture, external excrescences, or adherence to surrounding structures.
4. If the disease seems to be limited to the ovary or localized to the pelvis, then random staging biopsies of structures at risk are performed. These sites include the omentum (with generous biopsies from multiple areas) and the peritoneal surfaces (bilateral paracolic gutters, cul-de-sac, lateral pelvic walls, vesicouterine reflection, and subdiaphragmatic areas). Any adhesions are generously sampled. Biopsy of normal-appearing tissues in the pediatric population is typically not performed.
5. The para-aortic and bilateral pelvic lymph node–bearing areas are carefully palpated. Any suspicious nodes are excised or sampled. If no suspicious areas are detected, a bilateral pelvic and para-aortic lymphadenectomy is performed in the adult population; this is not performed in the pediatric population. Currently, there is no evidence that a complete para-aortic and/or pelvic lymphadenectomy yields better oncologic outcomes.
6. If obvious gross metastatic disease is present, it is excised if feasible. If it cannot be excised, it is sampled to document disease extent. Cytoreductive surgery is discussed below. The use of minimally invasive surgery in the setting of metastatic disease has not been extensively studied.

Extent of Surgical Staging

Surgical staging of MOGCT has been extrapolated from the management of epithelial ovarian carcinoma (19). However, data from the pediatric literature suggest that less extensive staging with preservation of grossly normal organs may not compromise oncologic outcomes. In the pediatric intergroup study POG 9048/CCG 8891 (Pediatric Oncology Group 9048 and Children's Cancer Group 8891), although adherence to surgical guidelines occurred in only one out of 56 patients with MOGCT, 95% of patients were long-term survivors (20). Similarly, in another cohort of 131 pediatric patients with MOGCT, although only three patients underwent complete staging with lymphadenectomy, OS rates were excellent (21).

At present, the surgical approach for adult patients with MOGCTs includes comprehensive surgical staging. A thorough determination of the disease extent by inspection and palpation should be made. If the disease appears confined to one or both ovaries, comprehensive staging biopsies should be performed in adult patients. Regardless of the extent of staging, the use of a synoptic report in all circumstances is encouraged to remove ambiguity and compensate for details that might be subjectively overlooked in individual operative reports, thereby informing future study and guideline formation.

In the absence of a grossly abnormal omentum, routine omentectomy can be omitted and replaced by multiple omental biopsies. An analysis of SEER database that included 2,238 patients younger than 40 years observed a decreasing trend in the performance of omentectomy and no impact on cancer-specific survival (22). Similarly, in another retrospective study, among 223 patients, 74% underwent omentectomy; 10-year OS was comparable between patients who did and did not undergo omentectomy (92% and 97.9%, respectively, $P = .34$) (23). The number of omental sections does correlate with sensitivity; in patients with IT and other ovarian tumors, the sensitivity increased from 82% to 95% when the number of blocks increased from 5 to 10 (24). Therefore, it would be advisable to take enough biopsies to result in 10 sections of omentum.

The benefit of lymphadenectomy is controversial. Approximately 25% of patients with MOGCTs have lymph node metastases (25). Any enlarged or suspicious lymph nodes identified on preoperative imaging should be removed. Pelvic and para-aortic lymph nodes should be examined and palpated, and any grossly abnormal lymph nodes should be removed. Routine systemic lymphadenectomy, although historically performed, may be unnecessary because MOGCTs are exquisitely sensitive to chemotherapy. Chan et al performed a SEER database analysis of the impact of lymphadenectomy for women with stage I ovarian cancer, and while lymphadenectomy generally impacted survival in patients with ovarian cancer, the subset of patients with MOGCT showed no difference in outcomes (26). A single-institution retrospective study of 50 patients showed that lack of surgical staging was independently associated with disease recurrence, but OS was no different (27). A recent analysis of the NCDB that included 2,774 patients did not demonstrate an OS benefit among patients who underwent lymph node sampling/dissection (hazard ratio [HR] 1.33, 95% CI: 0.82, 2.14) (28). Similarly, a SEER database analysis that included 1,083 patients with apparent stage I disease demonstrated that lymphadenectomy was not associated with improved OS on multivariate analysis (HR 1.26, 95% CI: 0.62, 2.58) (29). However, oncologic safety and outcomes related to omitting routine lymphadenectomy as part of staging have not been prospectively evaluated in patients who do not receive adjuvant chemotherapy. Lymphadenectomy in adult patients with MOGCT continues to be recommended for adult patients with apparent early-stage MOGCT, as nodal involvement would necessitate chemotherapy, when it would otherwise be avoided.

Bilateral Ovarian Involvement

Patients with bilateral ovarian lesions and the desire for future fertility represent a challenge. Risk of relapse, tumor histology, and sensitivity to chemotherapy should be balanced with the risk of premature ovarian failure and desire for fertility preservation. Bilateral ovarian involvement in MOGCTs is rare (4%-6%), except for dysgerminomas (10%-15%) (29-31). Bilateral malignant GCTs are also rare in pediatric/adolescent patients, and clinicians should be aware of the increased risk of previously unrecognized gonadal dysgenesis in this subset of patients. If both ovaries have large tumors, the opportunity to recognize that one of them is a streak ovary is lost (32).

Several studies have examined the options of neoadjuvant chemotherapy (NACT) followed by FSS, or by removal of the worst-appearing ovary with contralateral ovarian biopsy followed by chemotherapy. There are no data regarding the ability of chemotherapy to eradicate a primary ovarian tumor. In testis cancer, there are presumptive data suggesting that tumor may persist after chemotherapy in the gonad and that the testis may be a drug sanctuary. In exceptional situations, it may be reasonable to preserve an involved ovary in a patient who will be receiving chemotherapy. However, it is conceivable that ovarian preservation could increase the risk for recurrence in these selected cases. The decision to preserve an involved ovary is difficult and must be made carefully considering patients' wishes.

In one study, 21 (91%) of 23 patients with unresectable or bulky disease treated with NACT responded; 18 of these patients underwent interval unilateral salpingo-oophorectomy, omentectomy, and lymphadenectomy. Only five of these patients had residual disease, and they received two more cycles of chemotherapy. After a mean follow-up of 74 months, all 23 patients were alive and without evidence of disease (33). Other case series report similar findings (21,34,35). Sigismondi et al reported on two patients who had good results after removal of the worst-appearing ovary with biopsy and preservation of the lesser affected ovary (30).

If normal ovarian tissue can be identified in patients with bilateral macroscopic ovarian involvement, unilateral salpingo-oophorectomy and contralateral cystectomy are preferred. However, if both ovaries are completely replaced by tumor, removal of the largest tumor mass and biopsy of the contralateral ovary could be considered for patients with only dysgerminoma, but this is based on limited evidence (30,36). If frozen examination reveals a dysgenetic gonad, then bilateral salpingo-oophorectomy is indicated (37). However, because this is a difficult diagnosis on frozen section and castration carries significant sequelae, this determination should preferably be made by karyotypic analysis, optimally performed in the preoperative setting where appropriate counseling can be performed.

A benign cystic teratoma of the contralateral ovary may be present in 5% to 10% of patients with MOGCT (30). In this setting, contralateral ovarian cystectomy of the mature teratoma with preservation of remaining normal ovarian tissue is recommended.

The advent of in vitro fertilization technology also has an impact on operative management (38). Convention has dictated that if a bilateral salpingo-oophorectomy is necessary, a hysterectomy should also be performed. However, with current assisted reproduction technologies (ARTs) involving donor oocyte and hormonal support, a woman without ovaries can sustain a normal intrauterine pregnancy. Similarly, if the uterus and one ovary are resected because of tumor involvement, current techniques provide the opportunity for oocyte retrieval from the remaining ovary, in vitro fertilization with sperm from her male partner, and embryo implantation into a surrogate's uterus. As the field of ART is evolving, traditional guidelines concerning surgical treatment in young patients with gynecologic tumors must be thoughtfully adapted to individual circumstances.

CYTOREDUCTIVE SURGERY

In adult patients with widespread tumor encountered at initial surgery, maximal cytoreductive surgery is performed, similar to the surgical management of advanced epithelial ovarian cancer. The surgeon should remove the maximum amount of tumor, within safe and practical limits, because the amount of residual tumor after surgery does influence OS and is the most important prognostic factor (39-45). Patients cannot always be salvaged, so primary debulking with maximal effort is essential in patients with advanced disease (46). Because most MOGCTs are detected at an earlier stage, data surrounding cytoreductive surgery in MOGCTs are limited. The utility of cytoreductive surgery is supported by an early study of the Gynecologic Oncology Group (GOG), which found that 15 (28%) of 54 patients with completely resected disease at primary surgery failed a combination of vincristine, dactinomycin, and cyclophosphamide (VAC), compared to 15 (68%) of 22 patients with incompletely resected disease treated with the same regimen (47). In this study, a higher percentage of patients with bulky postoperative residual disease (82%) failed chemotherapy compared to patients with minimal residual disease (55%). A subsequent GOG study evaluated patients with MOGCT who received the combination regimen of cisplatin, vinblastine, and bleomycin (PVB). Patients with nondysgerminomatous tumors and clinically nonmeasurable disease after surgery had a greater likelihood of remaining progression free than those with measurable disease (65% vs 34%) (48). In addition, patients who had been surgically debulked to optimal disease had an outcome intermediate between patients with suboptimal disease and those with optimal disease without debulking.

While surgical debulking is standard in adult patients with widespread disease, the pediatric approach favors neoadjuvant platinum-based chemotherapy, except for pure IT. The pediatric perspective is that IT is not sensitive to chemotherapy, so those patients are not reflective of the other malignant germ cell histologies and should be considered separately. In pediatric patients with widespread IT, a more aggressive surgical approach is felt to be indicated.

Important principles for surgical decision-making in the setting of MOGCT include resection of the primary tumor with a unilateral salpingo-oophorectomy (not cystectomy), consideration of FSS in most cases, recognition that routine lymphadenectomy is controversial, and the need for thoughtful and mature intraoperative judgment in the setting of widespread disease, carefully weighing the risks of cytoreductive maneuvers in the setting of chemosensitive tumors. Even in the face of extensive metastatic disease, it may be possible to perform a fertility-sparing procedure with preservation of a normal contralateral ovary, though outcomes data are lacking.

FERTILITY PRESERVATION

Patients who have not completed childbearing with certainty should retain their uterus and contralateral normal-appearing ovary. Unilateral salpingo-oophorectomy with careful removal of the affected ovary to avoid tumor spillage is performed. Although the safety of FSS for MOGCT has not been prospectively evaluated, large retrospective studies have reported excellent oncologic and reproductive outcomes with retention of ovarian function and frequent conception (22,46,49-53). Weinberg et al demonstrated that all patients who underwent FSS resumed normal menstrual function within 1 year of completing chemotherapy, and 80% achieved spontaneous pregnancy (49).

MANAGING THE UNSTAGED PATIENT

Unfortunately, many patients are frequently diagnosed with an MOGCT following the removal of a presumed benign adnexal mass (due to limitations of preoperative imaging and frozen section) and do not undergo complete staging. Incomplete staging has been associated with a higher risk of relapse, but no change in OS in an adult population. A multivariate analysis of 144 patients with stage I MOGCTs by MITO showed that incomplete surgical staging was associated with higher risk of tumor recurrence (odds ratio

[OR] 2.37, 95% CI 1.04, 5.44) (54). In another report, incomplete staging surgery (absence of peritoneal and lymph node evaluation) in 171 patients was independently associated with worse DFS (HR 2.68, 95% CI 1.22, 5.91) (55). Nevertheless, incomplete staging was not associated with worse OS in either study. This reflects the exquisite chemosensitivity of MOGCTs, which allows high salvage rates at the time of recurrence. One case series of five patients showed no benefit to a second staging operation, as these procedures showed negative findings, small residual tumors that did not change stage, or advanced cancer where additional cytoreductive surgery was not technically feasible; in addition, all these patients required adjuvant chemotherapy (56). Therefore, the benefit of a second surgery to achieve complete staging is limited.

Because the management of incompletely staged patients is complex, patients with MOGCT should promptly be referred to specialized cancer centers. If the decision is made to administer adjuvant chemotherapy based on tumor characteristics such as histology, tumor grade, the presence of capsule invasion, and/or rupture, the performance of staging surgery is unlikely to provide any additional survival benefit. However, if the decision is made to omit adjuvant chemotherapy, surgical staging could reduce the risk of relapse by identifying the subset of patients with otherwise unrecognized advanced disease who would benefit from adjuvant chemotherapy. An alternative to a second surgery includes careful radiologic examination of the lymphatic beds and evaluation of serum markers; patients with favorable initial histologic findings and no suspicious imaging or serologic findings can undergo surveillance. Such patients must be counseled on the increased risk of relapse and the rare possibility of a nonsalvageable recurrence leading to death.

SECOND-LOOK SURGERY

Since 1960, second-look laparotomy was included in the routine management of patients with epithelial ovarian cancer to assess disease status after a fixed interval of chemotherapy. This approach was extrapolated to the management of patients with OGCTs. In a review of the MDACC experience with second-look laparotomy, findings were negative in 52 of 53 patients (57). The one patient with positive findings at second-look laparotomy had an elevated AFP level before surgery, which accurately predicted residual disease. This patient received subsequent chemotherapy with PVB and entered a prolonged remission. Of the patients with negative findings, one woman relapsed 9 months after the negative second-look surgery and subsequently died. Thirteen patients in this series had biopsy-proven evidence of residual mature teratoma (the so-called "chemotherapeutic retroconversion") at second-look laparotomy; treatment was discontinued in all patients, and none developed recurrence. Thus, in this series, second-look surgery did not add prognostic information or alter the therapeutic management of patients. The role of second-look surgery is further obscured in the setting of advancement in imaging techniques (CT scanning, PET, and MRI) and in an era where tumor marker measurements are part of routine care of patients with GCTs.

The GOG experience with second-look laparotomy in OGCTs has been reviewed (58). One hundred and seventeen patients who were enrolled prospectively on GOG protocols using cisplatin-based chemotherapy after initial surgical staging and cytoreduction (GOG protocols #45, 78, and 90) underwent second-look surgical procedures. Of these, 45 surgical procedures were performed in patients who received three courses of cisplatin, etoposide, and bleomycin (BEP) after complete tumor resection. In this subgroup, 38 patients had negative findings, two patients had IT, and five patients had mature teratoma. One of the patients with residual IT received further chemotherapy, and one did not. Both women with residual IT and the rest of the patients remained disease free. One patient with negative second-look surgery findings subsequently relapsed and succumbed to disease. Hence, there is no benefit to second-look surgery in the subgroup of patients with completely resected primary OGCTs. In contrast, 72 patients in this series treated with similar chemotherapy had advanced incompletely resected tumors before beginning adjuvant treatment. In this subgroup, 48 patients did not have teratoma elements in their primary tumor. At second-look surgery, 45 patients had no residual tumor, and three patients displayed persistent endodermal sinus tumor or embryonal carcinoma. All three of the latter patients died despite further treatment. Five patients with negative second laparotomies recurred, of which only one was salvaged with chemotherapy. Thus, the value of second-look surgery in patients with incompletely resected GCTs, not containing teratoma, is arguably minimal. However, in the subgroup of patients with incompletely resected tumors containing teratoma elements (total of 24 patients), second-look surgery had an impact on subsequent management. Of these patients, 16 were found to have mature teratoma at second look, which was bulky or progressive in seven cases. Four additional patients were found to have residual IT. Fourteen of the total 16 patients with teratoma and six of the seven women with bulky residual tumor remained disease free after surgical resection. Therefore, although second-look laparotomy is not indicated for patients with tumor completely resected primarily or in those patients with initially incompletely resected tumor not containing teratoma, there may be a clinical benefit to second-look surgery in patients with incompletely resected primary tumor with elements of teratoma.

SECONDARY CYTOREDUCTION

The value of secondary cytoreductive surgery in the management of OGCTs is even less clear than that of primary cytoreductive surgery. Although secondary cytoreduction is of questionable benefit for patients with refractory epithelial ovarian cancer (59,60), GCTs are relatively more chemosensitive than epithelial tumors and are more likely to respond to second-line therapy. Therefore, if a patient has an isolated focus of persistent tumor after first-line chemotherapy in an area such as the lung, liver, retroperitoneum, or brain, then surgical extirpation should be considered before changing chemotherapy regimens. Although this clinical situation is extremely rare, it has been encountered in other situations involving chemosensitive tumors, such as gestational trophoblastic disease and testicular cancer.

Unlike testicular cancer, the finding of a residual mass after completion of chemotherapy is less common in patients with OGCTs because these women are likely to have considerable tumor debulking at the time of the diagnostic surgical procedure and thus enter chemotherapy with significantly less tumor burden. At completion of chemotherapy, men with nonseminomatous tumors or seminoma may have persistent mature teratoma or desmoplastic fibrosis. In patients with bulky dysgerminoma, residual masses after chemotherapy are very likely to represent desmoplastic fibrosis. Although persistent mature teratoma may remain in some patients with pure ovarian ITs or mixed GCTs at the completion of chemotherapy as documented by second-look laparotomy, most patients are left with multiple small peritoneal implants rather than with a dominant mass (58). However, it is now recognized that occasional patients who have received chemotherapy for ITs or mixed GCTs containing teratoma will have bulky residual teratoma after chemotherapy. The natural history or biologic implications of these findings are not clear. In testicular cancer, patients with bulky residual teratoma may experience slow progression of tumor or may develop overtly malignant tumors over time (61,62). There are similar anecdotal reports of progressive mature teratoma in patients with OGCT after chemotherapy (63-65). Considering this information, it seems appropriate to resect persistent masses in patients with negative markers after chemotherapy for GCTs containing IT. If viable neoplasm is found, additional chemotherapy should be considered. However, if only mature teratoma is resected, observation is generally recommended.

In pediatric and adolescent patients, residual or new masses with negative markers should be biopsied. These may be new secondary somatic malignancies, such as primitive neuroectodermal tumor (PNET), sarcoma, or IT. PNET or sarcoma would need alternate chemotherapy, and IT would require resection, so these are important to detect (66,67).

DIFFERENCES IN PEDIATRIC AND ADULT PARADIGMS

Significant differences exist between the traditional surgical management of pediatric and adult patients with MOGCT. Management of pediatric patients with MOGCT does not include omentectomy, routine biopsies of normal-appearing tissue, or routine lymphadenectomy, and decisions always emphasize FSS. Although the management of adult patients has historically involved a complete staging procedure with omentectomy, multiple staging biopsies, a complete pelvic, and para-aortic lymphadenectomy, it is shifting to reflect less aggressive staging and an approach that is more like the pediatric population. Patients with widespread disease are managed differently, as adults favor debulking but the pediatric approach favors neoadjuvant platinum-based chemotherapy, except for pure IT.

Universal support exists for fertility-sparing approaches in women of reproductive age who have not definitively completed childbearing. Future studies will provide guidance on appropriate limitations of therapy.

REFERENCES

1. Gershenson DM, Del Junco G, Copeland LJ, Rutledge FN. Mixed germ cell tumors of the ovary. *Obstet Gynecol.* 1984;64(2):200-206.
2. Gordon A, Lipton D, Woodruff JD. Dysgerminoma: a review of 158 cases from the Emil Novak Ovarian Tumor Registry. *Obstet Gynecol.* 1981;58(4):497-504.
3. Ayhan A, Tuncer ZS, Yanik F, Bükülmez O, Yanik A, Küçükali T. Malignant germ cell tumors of the ovary: Hacettepe hospital experience. *Acta Obstet Gynecol Scand.* 1995;74(5):384-390.
4. Santoni R, Cionini L, D'Elia F, Scarselli GF, Branconi F, Savino L. Dysgerminoma of the ovary: a report on 29 patients. *Clin Radiol.* 1987;38(2):203-206.
5. Bjorkholm E, Lundell M, Gyftodimos A, Silfverswärd C. Dysgerminoma. The Radiumhemmet series 1927-1984. *Cancer.* 1990;65(1):38-44.
6. Shen DH, Khoo US, Xue WC, Cheung AN. Ovarian mature cystic teratoma with malignant transformation. An interphase cytogenetic study. *Int J Gynecol Pathol.* 1998;17(4):351-357.
7. Berg FD, Kürzl R, Hinrichsen MJ, Zander J. Familial 46,XY pure gonadal dysgenesis and gonadoblastoma/dysgerminoma: case report. *Gynecol Oncol.* 1989;32(2):261-267.
8. Kingsbury AC, Frost F, Cookson WO. Dysgerminoma, gonadoblastoma, and testicular germ cell neoplasia in phenotypically female and male siblings with 46 XY genotype. *Cancer.* 1987;59(2):288-291.
9. Fisher RA, Salm R, Spencer RW. Bilateral gonadoblastoma/dysgerminoma in a 46 XY individual: case report with hormonal studies. *J Clin Pathol.* 1982;35(4):420-424.
10. Dicken BJ, Billmire DF, Rich B, et al. Utility of frozen section in pediatric and adolescent malignant ovarian nonseminomatous germ cell tumors: a report from the children's oncology group. *Gynecol Oncol.* 2022;166(3):476-480.
11. Billmire D, Dicken B, Rescorla F, et al. Imaging appearance of nongerminoma pediatric ovarian germ cell tumors does not discriminate benign from malignant histology. *J Pediatr Adolesc Gynecol.* 2021;34(3):383-386.
12. Hermans AJ, Kluivers KB, Janssen LM, et al. Adnexal masses in children, adolescents and women of reproductive age in the Netherlands: a nationwide population-based cohort study. *Gynecol Oncol.* 2016;143(1):93-97.
13. Gremeau AS, Bourdel N, Jardon K, et al. Surgical management of non-epithelial ovarian malignancies: advantages and limitations of laparoscopy. *Eur J Obstet Gynecol Reprod Biol.* 2014;172:106-110.
14. Nasioudis D, Minis E, Chapman-Davis E, et al. Minimally invasive staging of apparent stage I malignant ovarian germ cell tumors: prevalence and outcomes. *J Minim Invasive Gynecol.* 2019;26(3):471-476.
15. Kehoe S. FIGO staging in ovarian carcinoma and histological subtypes. *J Gynecol Oncol.* 2020;31(4):e70.
16. Schwartz PE. Surgery of germ cell tumours of the ovary. *Forum (Genova).* 2000;10(4):355-365.

17. Gershenson DM. Fertility-sparing surgery for malignancies in women. *J Natl Cancer Inst Monogr*. 2005;(34):43-47.

18. Peccatori FA, Azim HA Jr, Orecchia R, et al. Cancer, pregnancy and fertility: ESMO clinical practice guidelines for diagnosis, treatment and follow-up. *Ann Oncol*. 2013;24(Suppl 6):vi160-vi170.

19. Gershenson DM. Update on malignant ovarian germ cell tumors. *Cancer*. 1993;71(4 Suppl):1581-1590.

20. Rogers PC, Olson TA, Cullen JW, et al. Treatment of children and adolescents with stage II testicular and stages I and II ovarian malignant germ cell tumors: a Pediatric Intergroup Study—Pediatric Oncology Group 9048 and Children's Cancer Group 8891. *J Clin Oncol*. 2004;22(17):3563-3569.

21. Billmire D, Vinocur C, Rescorla F, et al. Outcome and staging evaluation in malignant germ cell tumors of the ovary in children and adolescents: an intergroup study. *J Pediatr Surg*. 2004;39(3):424-429.

22. Nasioudis D, Mastroyannis SA, Latif NA, Ko EM. Trends in the surgical management of malignant ovarian germcell tumors. *Gynecol Oncol*. 2020;157(1):89-93.

23. Qin B, Xu W, Li Y. Are omentectomy and lymphadenectomy necessary in patients with apparently early-stage malignant ovarian germ cell tumors? *Int J Gynecol Cancer*. 2019;29(2):398-403.

24. Skala SL, Hagemann IS. Optimal sampling of grossly normal omentum in staging of gynecologic malignancies. *Int J Gynecol Pathol*. 2015;34(3):281-287.

25. Kumar S, Shah JP, Bryant CS, et al. The prevalence and prognostic impact of lymph node metastasis in malignant germ cell tumors of the ovary. *Gynecol Oncol*. 2008;110(2):125-132.

26. Chan JK, Urban R, Hu JM, et al. The potential therapeutic role of lymph node resection in epithelial ovarian cancer: a study of 13918 patients. *Br J Cancer*. 2007;96(12):1817-1822.

27. Lin KY, Bryant S, Miller DS, Kehoe SM, Richardson DL, Lea JS. Malignant ovarian germ cell tumor—role of surgical staging and gonadal dysgenesis. *Gynecol Oncol*. 2014;134(1):84-89.

28. Nasioudis D, Ko EM, Haggerty AF, et al. Performance of lymphadenectomy for apparent early stage malignant ovarian germ cell tumors in the era of platinum-based chemotherapy. *Gynecol Oncol*. 2020;157(3):613-618.

29. Mahdi H, Swensen RE, Hanna R, et al. Prognostic impact of lymphadenectomy in clinically early stage malignant germ cell tumour of the ovary. *Br J Cancer*. 2011;105(4):493-497.

30. Sigismondi C, Scollo P, Ferrandina G, et al. Management of bilateral malignant ovarian germ cell tumors: a MITO-9 retrospective study. *Int J Gynecol Cancer*. 2015;25(2):203-207.

31. Roychoudhuri R, Putcha V, Moller H. Cancer and laterality: a study of the five major paired organs (UK). *Cancer Causes Control*. 2006;17(5):655-662.

32. Hennes E, Zahn S, Lopes LF, et al. Molecular genetic analysis of bilateral ovarian germ cell tumors. *Klin Padiatr*. 2012;224(6):359-365.

33. Talukdar S, Kumar S, Bhatla N, Mathur S, Thulkar S, Kumar L. Neo-adjuvant chemotherapy in the treatment of advanced malignant germ cell tumors of ovary. *Gynecol Oncol*. 2014;132(1):28-32.

34. Bafna UD, Umadevi K, Kumaran C, Nagarathna DS, Shashikala P, Tanseem R. Germ cell tumors of the ovary: is there a role for aggressive cytoreductive surgery for nondysgerminomatous tumors? *Int J Gynecol Cancer*. 2001;11(4):300-304.

35. Raveendran A, Gupta A, Bagga R, et al. Advanced germ cell malignancies of the ovary: should neo-adjuvant chemotherapy be the first line of treatment? *J Obstet Gynaecol*. 2010;30(1):53-55.

36. Zhao T, Liu Y, Jiang H, Zhang H, Lu Y. Management of bilateral malignant ovarian germ cell tumors: experience of a single institute. *Mol Clin Oncol*. 2016;5(2):383-387.

37. Jonson AL, Geller MA, Dickson EL. Gonadal dysgenesis and gynecologic cancer. *Obstet Gynecol*. 2010;116(Suppl 2):550-552.

38. Saunders DM, Kemp JF, Smith DH. In vitro fertilization and the surgeon. *Aust N Z J Surg*. 1983;53(1):53-55.

39. Lai CH, Chang TC, Hsueh S, et al. Outcome and prognostic factors in ovarian germ cell malignancies. *Gynecol Oncol*. 2005;96(3):784-791.

40. Lee CW, Song MJ, Park ST, et al. Residual tumor after the salvage surgery is the major risk factors for primary treatment failure in malignant ovarian germ cell tumors: a retrospective study of single institution. *World J Surg Oncol*. 2011;9:123.

41. Gershenson DM. Management of ovarian germ cell tumors. *J Clin Oncol*. 2007;25(20):2938-2943.

42. Ghaemmaghami F, Hasanzadeh M, Karimi Zarchi M, Fallahi A. Nondysgerminomatous ovarian tumors: clinical characteristics, treatment, and outcome. A case-controlled study. *Int J Surg*. 2008;6(5):382-386.

43. Li J, Yang W, Wu X. Prognostic factors and role of salvage surgery in chemorefractory ovarian germ cell malignancies: a study in Chinese patients. *Gynecol Oncol*. 2007;105(3):769-775.

44. Cicin I, Eralp Y, Saip P, et al. Malignant ovarian germ cell tumors: a single-institution experience. *Am J Clin Oncol*. 2009;32(2):191-196.

45. Karalok A, Comert GK, Kilic C, et al. Cytoreductive surgery in advanced stage malignant ovarian germ cell tumors. *J Gynecol Obstet Hum Reprod*. 2019;48(7):461-466.

46. Ertas IE, Taskin S, Goklu R, et al. Long-term oncological and reproductive outcomes of fertility-sparing cytoreductive surgery in females aged 25 years and younger with malignant ovarian germ cell tumors. *J Obstet Gynaecol Res*. 2014;40(3):797-805.

47. Slayton RE, Park RC, Silverberg SG, Shingleton H, Creasman WT, Blessing JA. Vincristine, dactinomycin, and cyclophosphamide in the treatment of malignant germ cell tumors of the ovary. A Gynecologic Oncology Group Study (a final report). *Cancer*. 1985;56(2):243-248.

48. Williams SD, Blessing JA, Moore DH, Homesley HD, Adcock L. Cisplatin, vinblastine, and bleomycin in advanced and recurrent ovarian germ-cell tumors. A trial of the Gynecologic Oncology Group. *Ann Intern Med*. 1989;111(1):22-27.

49. Weinberg LE, Lurain JR, Singh DK, Schink JC. Survival and reproductive outcomes in women treated for malignant ovarian germ cell tumors. *Gynecol Oncol*. 2011;121(2):285-289.

50. Chan JK, Tewari KS, Waller S, et al. The influence of conservative surgical practices for malignant ovarian germ cell tumors. *J Surg Oncol*. 2008;98(2):111-116.

51. Johansen G, Dahm-Kähler P, Staf C, Flöter Rådestad A, Rodriguez-Wallberg KA. Fertility-sparing surgery for treatment of non-epithelial ovarian cancer: oncological and reproductive outcomes in a prospective nationwide population-based cohort study. *Gynecol Oncol*. 2019;155(2):287-293.

52. Bercow A, Nitecki R, Brady PC, Rauh-Hain JA. Outcomes after fertility-sparing surgery for women with ovarian cancer: a systematic review of the literature. *J Minim Invasive Gynecol*. 2021;28(3):527-536.e1.

53. Zamani N, Rezaei Poor M, Ghasemian Dizajmehr S, Alizadeh S, Modares Gilani M. Fertility sparing surgery in malignant ovarian Germ cell tumor (MOGCT): 15 years experiences. *BMC Womens Health*. 2021;21(1):282.

54. Mangili G, Sigismondi C, Lorusso D, et al. The role of staging and adjuvant chemotherapy in stage I malignant ovarian germ cell tumors (MOGTs): the MITO-9 study. *Ann Oncol*. 2017;28(2):333-338.

55. Park JY, Kim DY, Suh DS, et al. Analysis of outcomes and prognostic factors after fertility-sparing surgery in malignant ovarian germ cell tumors. *Gynecol Oncol*. 2017;145(3):513-518.

56. Tangjitgamol S, Hanprasertpong J, Manusirivithaya S, Wootipoom V, Thavaramara T, Buhachat R. Malignant ovarian germ cell tumors: clinico-pathological presentation and survival outcomes. *Acta Obstet Gynecol Scand*. 2010;89(2):182-189.

57. Gershenson DM, Copeland LJ, del Junco G, Edwards CL, Wharton JT, Rutledge FN. Second-look laparotomy in the management of malignant germ cell tumors of the ovary. *Obstet Gynecol*. 1986;67(6):789-793.

58. Williams SD, Blessing JA, DiSaia PJ, Major FJ, Ball HG 3rd, Liao SY. Second-look laparotomy in ovarian germ cell tumors: the gynecologic oncology group experience. *Gynecol Oncol*. 1994;52(3):287-291.

59. Scarabelli C, Campagnutta E, Zarrelli A, et al. [Second surgery in the management of ovarian cancer]. *Minerva Ginecol*. 1994;46(1-2):5-13.

60. Parazzini F, Raspagliesi F, Guarnerio P, Bolis G. Role of secondary surgery in relapsed ovarian cancer. *Crit Rev Oncol Hematol*. 2001;37(2):121-125.

61. Andre F, Fizazi K, Culine S, et al. Peritoneal carcinomatosis in germ-cell tumor: relations with retroperitoneal lymph node dissection. *Am J Clin Oncol*. 2000;23(5):460-462.

62. Chen YS, Kuo JY, Chin TW, et al. Prepubertal testicular germ cell tumors: 25-year experience in Taipei Veterans General Hospital. *J Chin Med Assoc*. 2008;71(7):357-361.

63. Vartanian RK, McRae B, Hessler RB. Sebaceous carcinoma arising in a mature cystic teratoma of the ovary. *Int J Gynecol Pathol*. 2002;21(4):418-421.

64. Ronnett BM, Seidman JD. Mucinous tumors arising in ovarian mature cystic teratomas: relationship to the clinical syndrome of pseudomyxoma peritonei. *Am J Surg Pathol*. 2003;27(5):650-657.

65. Shen X, Fan Y, Cao S. Primary malignant melanoma arising in an ovarian cystic teratoma. *Melanoma Res*. 2017;27(6):601-606.

66. Terenziani M, D'Angelo P, Bisogno G, et al. Teratoma with a malignant somatic component in pediatric patients: the Associazione Italiana Ematologia Oncologia Pediatrica (AIEOP) experience. *Pediatr Blood Cancer*. 2010;54(4):532-537.

67. Ehrlich Y, Beck SDW, Ulbright TM, et al. Outcome analysis of patients with transformed teratoma to primitive neuroectodermal tumor. *Ann Oncol*. 2010;21(9):1846-1850.

CHAPTER **9.5**

Ovarian Germ Cell Tumors: Pathology and Prognostic Factors

Elizabeth Euscher and Robert Tucker Burks

PATHOLOGY

The 2020 WHO classification of OGCTs includes dysgerminoma, teratomas (IT, mature teratoma, and various types of monodermal teratoma as well as somatic-type tumors arising from a dermoid cyst), YST, embryonal carcinoma, nongestational choriocarcinoma, mixed GCTs, and germ cell sex cord-stromal tumors (gonadoblastoma and unclassified mixed germ cell sex cord-stromal tumors) (see Section 9, Chapter 1, **Table 9.1-1**) (1). Although mature teratomas are relatively common, representing approximately 20% of ovarian neoplasms, the malignant GCTs are less common and account for 2% to 3% of all ovarian cancers. MOGCTs are considered to arise analogous to most examples of postpubertal GCTs of the testis, with frequent i(12p) and possible 12p amplification. Ovarian mature teratoma and IT that arise in association with other GCT elements are likely derived from the latter, as in postpubertal testes. Conversely, pure mature teratoma and IT develop from benign germ cells between meiosis I and meiosis II, via a parthenogenetic-like mechanism, and lack i(12p) or other evidence of 12p amplification (2). This chapter reviews each of the more commonly identified GCTs and provides the gross, histologic, and most salient immunohistochemical (IHC) characteristics of each, as well as the differential diagnosis for each entity.

Teratomas

Ovarian teratomas are GCTs that typically contain tissue derived from two or three embryonic layers; however, monodermal teratomas with tissue of only one type, such as thyroid (struma ovarii), carcinoid tumor, or PNET, also exist (3). Teratomas represent approximately 95% of OGCTs. Teratomas are subclassified according to whether immature neuroectodermal tissue is present (IT) or absent (mature teratoma).

Mature teratomas have a wide age distribution and are bilateral in approximately 10% of cases. Most teratomas are mature cystic teratomas that contain differentiated tissue components, such as skin, glandular epithelium, glial tissue, cartilage, and bone (**Figure 9.5-1**). Any tissue type present in adults may be represented in teratomas. Frequently, a collection of mixed tissue types will be found in a nodule in the wall of the cyst, called a Rokitansky nodule. Microscopically, mature teratoma is characterized by the presence of mature somatic tissues with the organization and morphology identical to their eutopic location, so cystic areas can be lined by different types of epithelium. While mature cystic teratomas are benign neoplasms, in rare cases, they may contain a somatic malignancy, such as squamous cell carcinoma (**Figure 9.5-2**), papillary thyroid carcinoma, sarcoma, small cell carcinoma, or other non-GCT (4). Such secondary malignant transformation is seen in older patients and occurs in 0.2% to 1.4% of mature teratomas. A rare, but potentially life-threatening clinical manifestation of ovarian mature teratomas is autoimmune encephalitis associated with antibodies to the NMDA receptor (5,6). The encephalitis may present with psychiatric symptoms and is typically responsive to surgical removal of the teratoma.

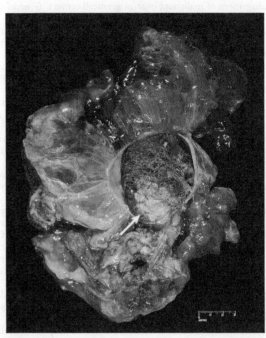

Figure 9.5-1. Ovarian mature cystic teratoma, gross image; note mass of hair filling a cystic space (arrow).

ITs in adult women, in contrast to mature cystic teratomas, are uncommon tumors. They represent about 3% of all ovarian teratomas, but ITs are the third most common form of MOGCTs, accounting for 15% to 20% of all MOGCTs. Most immature ovarian teratomas (90%) are unilateral neoplasms. ITs are predominantly large solid tumors, but they may contain some cystic areas that are irregular and multiloculated (**Figure 9.5-3**). The cut surface of ITs is soft and fleshy or encephaloid in appearance (**Figure 9.5-7**). Areas of hemorrhage and necrosis are common. Microscopically, these tumors contain a variety of mature and immature tissue components. However, the hallmark feature is the presence of tissues in embryonic stages of development. The immature elements almost always consist of immature neural tissue (neuroectodermal origin). Rarely, immature elements may also originate from immature cartilage (mesodermal origin) and gut epithelium (endodermal origin). Nevertheless, tumor grade is based only on the immature neuroectoderm that microscopically appears as primitive-like small round blue cells focally organized into rosettes and tubules, or cellular aggregates of mitotically active glial tissue (**Figure 9.5-3**). Embryoid bodies in small numbers may also be found, whereas mature tissues can also be encountered. Neuroectoderm elements stain positive for neural markers such as GFRa-1 synaptophysin, S100, and NSE, as well as SOX2 (more specific marker for immature neural tissue), Ki-67m and cyclin D1 (5).

There is a correlation between disease prognosis and the degree of immaturity in the teratoma. The three-tier grading system is still

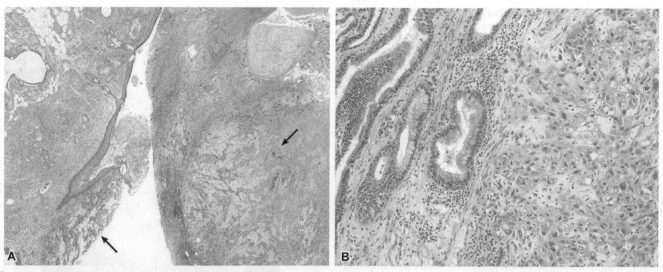

Figure 9.5-2. Malignant transformation in an ovarian mature cystic teratoma: (A) mature ectodermal elements (skin and sebaceous glands) have an abrupt transition to squamous cell carcinoma (arrows); (B) squamous cell carcinoma is adjacent to endodermal elements (intestinal glands, left).

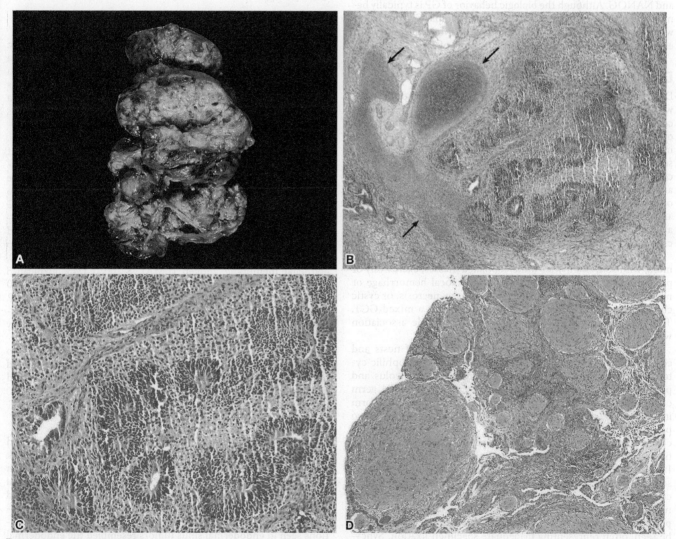

Figure 9.5-3. (A) Immature teratoma, gross image; (B) low-power H&E image showing immature neuroectoderm adjacent to cartilage (arrows); (C) high-power H&E image depicting rosettes and primitive tubules; (D) nodules of mature glial tissue in peritoneal tissue. H&E, hematoxylin and eosin.

most often used (1). Grade 1 ITs display some immaturity, but the immature neural tissue does not exceed, in estimated visual aggregate, the area of one low-power field (40× total magnification) on any single slide. Grade 2 ITs contain immature neural tissue in one to three low-power fields on any slide. Grade 3 ITs contain immature neural tissue in greater than three low-power fields in at least one slide. Some authors prefer classifying ITs as either low (grade 1)- or high (grades 2 and 3)-grade teratomas because the latter classification has better interobserver performance. The amount of immature neuroepithelium for purposes of grading is evaluated per single slide rather than as an aggregate over multiple slides. Overgrowth of immature neuroectodermal tissue in an extensive, confluent mass represents PNET that has a poor prognosis. In patients whose neoplasm has disseminated beyond the ovary, the grade of the tumor metastasis is important to predict survival and determine treatment.

Occasionally, peritoneal, omental, or lymph node implants containing only mature glial tissue may be found (gliomatosis peritonei [GP]) (**Figure 9.5-3**). These deposits may be multiple and small (<3 mm). Molecular data suggest that mature glial implants are genetically unrelated to the associated teratoma and may represent a metaplastic phenomenon likely induced by the teratoma in a paracrine manner (7,8). However, recent genomic data support another theory, suggesting that glial implants derive from intraperitoneal dissemination of IT that differentiates into mature glial cells (3). Glial implants stain positive for SOX2 and negative for OCT4 and NANOG. Although the biologic behavior of GP is typically benign, they can rarely progress to high-grade glioma. Given possible widespread dissemination, it is important to sample peritoneal disease thoroughly to identify any coexisting foci of IT.

Dysgerminoma

Dysgerminoma shares common biologic and pathologic features with testicular seminoma. Although dysgerminoma is the most common MOGCT, it represents only 1% to 2% of all malignant ovarian tumors (1). The mean patient age at presentation is approximately 22 years. A small percentage of these tumors arise in the setting of disorders of sexual development with a Y-chromosome–containing karyotype (such as pure 46,XY and mixed 45/45,XY) and may be associated with gonadoblastoma. Approximately 20% of dysgerminomas are bilateral (about 10% on gross examination and an additional 10% microscopically). Dysgerminoma that are associated with gonadoblastoma and gonadal dysgenesis have increased risks of bilateral involvement.

On gross examination, dysgerminomas are usually large tumors, with soft, fleshly tan-white, lobulated masses, exclusively or predominantly solid that have very limited focal hemorrhage or necrosis (**Figure 9.5-4**). Prominent hemorrhage, necrosis, or cystic changes are not expected and, if present, suggest a mixed GCT. The presence of calcifications may suggest possible association with gonadoblastoma.

Microscopically, dysgerminomas are composed of nests and cords of primitive germ cells, with clear to pale eosinophilic cytoplasm, a central large nucleus with prominent nucleolus and prominent cytoplasmic borders that resemble primordial germ cells (**Figure 9.5-5**). Nuclei are enlarged but are relatively uniform in size, may be rounded or have flat sides, and contain one or two prominent nucleoli. Numerous mitotic figures are usually appreciated. The nests of tumor cells are separated by bands of fibrous tissue rich in lymphocytes and sometimes epithelioid histiocytes. Lymphocytes can extend beyond septa and involve tumor nests obscuring the neoplastic cells. Occasionally, in approximately 20% of cases, a granulomatous reaction may be found with the presence of noncaseating granulomas that may also obscure underlying neoplastic cells. Small cysts or pseudoglandular spaces may sometimes be seen, often representing inadequate specimen fixation. Syncytiotrophoblastic cells can be present in about 3% of dysgerminomas and are usually found around vessels or any areas of hemorrhage. It

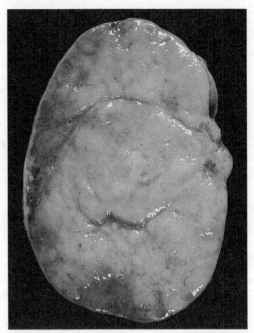

Figure 9.5-4. Dysgerminoma, gross image; cut surface shows a "fish-flesh" appearance.

should be underscored that the presence of syncytiotrophoblastic cells in the absence of cytotrophoblastic cells does not indicate a mixed GCT. These tumors have been designated dysgerminoma with syncytiotrophoblastic giant cells but have the same prognosis as dysgerminomas (9). They might, however, be associated with a detectable increase in serum hCG levels. Luteinized stromal cells may also be found and may be account for hormone excess, especially in cases of tumors that produce hCG.

Dysgerminomas contain abundant cytoplasmic glycogen that can be visualized using the periodic acid-Schiff (PAS) stain. Membranous immunoreactivity for placenta-like alkaline phosphatase (PLAP), c-kit (CD117), LIN28, and podoplanin (D2-40) is also commonly observed (10). Nuclear stem cell markers NANOG and SALL4 are also positive. The most helpful IHC stain is the nuclear transcription factor OCT3/4, which is highly sensitive and specific for dysgerminoma and embryonal carcinoma as a group (11) (**Figure 9.5-5**). Dysgerminomas lack IHC expression of CD30, epithelial membrane antigen (EMA), S-100, CD45, glypican-3 (GPC3), and SOX2, whereas embryonal carcinomas express CD30 and SOX2. In contrast to YST, dysgerminoma is negative for AFP. Syncytiotrophoblastic cells, if present as described earlier, will display hCG, GPC3, and CK7 staining (12). Dysgerminoma is the only OGCT that stains positive for c-kit. While 25% to 50% of dysgerminomas have c-kit mutations, this does not connote sensitivity to imatinib (13-15). A summary of IHC stains that might be utilized in the evaluation of dysgerminoma and other OGCTs is provided in **Table 9.5-1**.

Yolk Sac Tumor

YSTs, formerly known as endodermal sinus tumors, are the second most common MOGCT and account for 20% of cases, with a peak incidence at 19 years of age, rarely occurring after age 40. Teilum described these tumors in the 1940s, when he identified several unique features of YST. He recognized that despite being included with clear cell carcinomas (CCCs) as "mesonephroma ovarii," endodermal sinus tumors were distinct. Because the papillary formations seen in endodermal sinus tumors resembled the endodermal sinuses seen in the rat placenta, he labeled these tumors "endodermal sinus tumors" and published defining characteristics in 1959

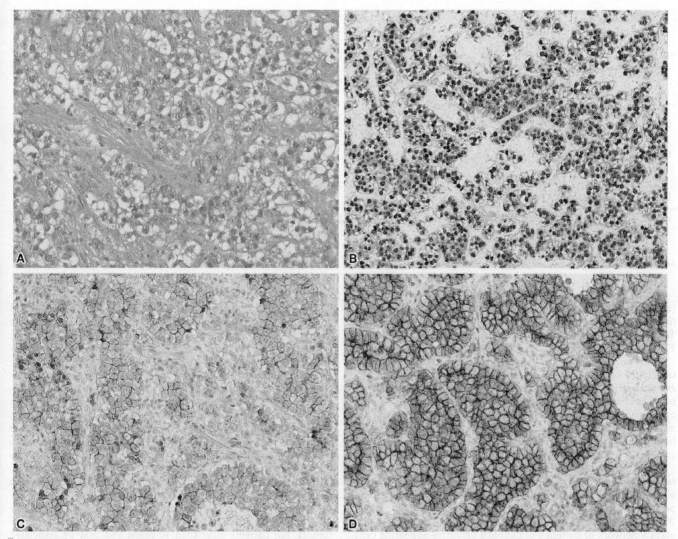

Figure 9.5-5. (A) Hematoxylin and eosin image of dysgerminoma at high power showing nests of large, polygonal cells with clear cytoplasm; nuclei have a prominent nucleolus; nests are separated by collagenous bands; (B) OCT3/4 stain has diffuse, nuclear staining; (C) membranous staining for CD117; (D) membranous and cytoplasmic staining for D2-40.

■ TABLE 9.5-1. Diagnostic Immunohistochemical Markers Used for Ovarian Germ Cell Tumors

Marker	Description	Yolk Sac Tumor	Dysgerminoma	Embryonal Carcinoma	Choriocarcinoma	Immature Teratoma
SALL-4	Ubiquitous marker of germ cell differentiation; not specific to type of OGCT; nuclear staining	+	+	+	+/− (staining in mononuclear cells)	+ (variable intensity)
AFP	Granular cytoplasmic staining; often patchy or focal; considered specific for yolk sac tumor but not as sensitive as glypican-3	+	Rarely focal staining	−	−	−
Glypican 3	Cytoplasmic staining; more sensitive than AFP with good specificity for yolk sac tumor versus other germ cell subtype but can be expressed in somatic carcinomas	+	−	−	+/−	−
OCT4	Nuclear staining	−	+	+ (may be lost after chemotherapy)	−	−

(continued)

■ **TABLE 9.5-1. Diagnostic Immunohistochemical Markers Used for Ovarian Germ Cell Tumors (***continued***)**

Marker	Description	Yolk Sac Tumor	Dysgerminoma	Embryonal Carcinoma	Choriocarcinoma	Immature Teratoma
CD117	Membranous staining	+/− (some solid pattern tumors express)	>85% +	−	−	−
D2-40	Membranous and cytoplasmic staining	+/− (rare tumors express)	+	+/−	−	−
CD30	Membranous staining	−	−	+ (may be lost after chemotherapy)	−	−
SOX2	Nuclear staining pattern	−	−	+	−	+
hCG	Cytoplasmic staining	−	− (will stain syncytiotrophoblast cells when present)	−	+ (syncytiotrophoblast)	−

AFP, α-fetoprotein; OGCTs, ovarian germ cell tumors.

(16). Subsequently, Talerman recognized that endodermal sinus tumors could be seen as part of mixed GCTs (17). Interestingly, Teilum and Talerman became close friends due to their interest in YSTs (18).

Ovarian YSTs are typically large and unilateral, although metastasis to the opposite ovary may occur. These tumors have a smooth external surface unless rupture or invasion into surrounding structures has occurred. On sectioning, these neoplasms are solid and cystic and tan to gray in color, commonly with hemorrhage and necrosis. The cut surface may appear mucoid or gelatinous with honeycomb appearance (**Figure 9.5-6**). The honeycomb appearance is associated with a polyvesicular-vitelline component (19).

YSTs are distinctive for displaying a myriad of histologic patterns, a characteristic that is exploited in the differential of some somatic carcinomas. The most common microscopic pattern in primary ovarian tumors is the reticular or microcystic pattern (**Figure 9.5-7**). The tumor has a loose mesh-like pattern, and it displays a network of flattened or cuboidal primitive-appearing cells with varying degrees of atypia. The endodermal sinus (festoon)

pattern contains Schiller-Duval bodies (**Figure 9.5-7**) that have a central elongated capillary surrounded by connective tissue and a peripheral layer of primitive columnar cells. These structures are situated in cavities lined by YST cells. When present, Schiller-Duval bodies may be a helpful diagnostic feature, but they are present in approximately 20% of all YSTs (20).

Other less common patterns of YST include polyvesicular-vitelline, enteric, solid, parietal, glandular, tubular, endometrioid-like, hepatoid, and mesenchymal patterns (21) (**Figure 9.5-7**). Most patterns of YST may contain eosinophilic hyaline globules that are PAS positive, do not contain AFP, and are diastase resistant; however, this feature is nonspecific because these globules may be found in non-GCTs.

Some types of YST, particularly glandular and hepatoid pattern YST, may closely resemble endometrioid, clear cell, or other adenocarcinomas. Age is an important and distinctive factor, because OGCTs usually occur in younger patients than epithelial ovarian tumors. For patients older than 40 years, YST may be associated with endometriosis or a somatic epithelial tumor (most common endometrioid carcinoma). When associated with a somatic epithelial component, the yolk sac element is thought to represent dedifferentiation from carcinoma; these tumors are biologically different from pure YSTs and are less responsive to chemotherapy.

AFP is the traditional marker for YSTs, as these tumors usually demonstrate cytoplasmic staining for keratin and AFP. However, AFP staining may be focal or weak, especially for tumors with a glandular pattern, and can be negative for tumors with parietal and mesenchymal-like patterns. In addition, AFP-negative parietal pattern YST may be seen following chemotherapy treatment (22). Lack of staining for cytokeratin (CK) 7 and EMA supports a diagnosis of YST (23). GPC-3 is more sensitive as a YST marker, but it is not entirely specific as staining is seen in embryonal carcinoma, hepatocellular carcinoma (HCC), and CCC (ref—Young 2022 would work for the CCC part of this, maybe HCC). Another recent biomarker more sensitive and specific than AFP for YSTs is ZBTB16 (24). The pluripotency marker SALL4 can also be useful for the diagnosis of YST because of the limited sensitivity of the AFP IHC stain, but it is also expressed in other GCTs and, rarely, in other tumors such as urothelial and gastric tumors (25). Other positive markers include LIN28, α-1-antitrypsin, and villin, whereas endodermal tumor elements may stain positive for their corresponding tissue marker (eg, intestinal components for CK20, CDX2, or CEA and hepatic components for hepatocyte paraffin antigen 1) (**Figure 9.5-8**). YSTs are usually negative for OCT3/4, CD117, SOX2, D2-40, and CD30. CCC can also sometimes be confused for YST, particularly during intraoperative frozen section examination. CCC, which is also characterized by distinctive architectural features (papillary,

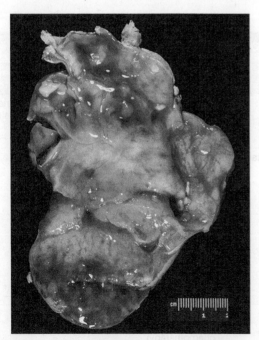

Figure 9.5-6. Yolk sac tumor, gross image.

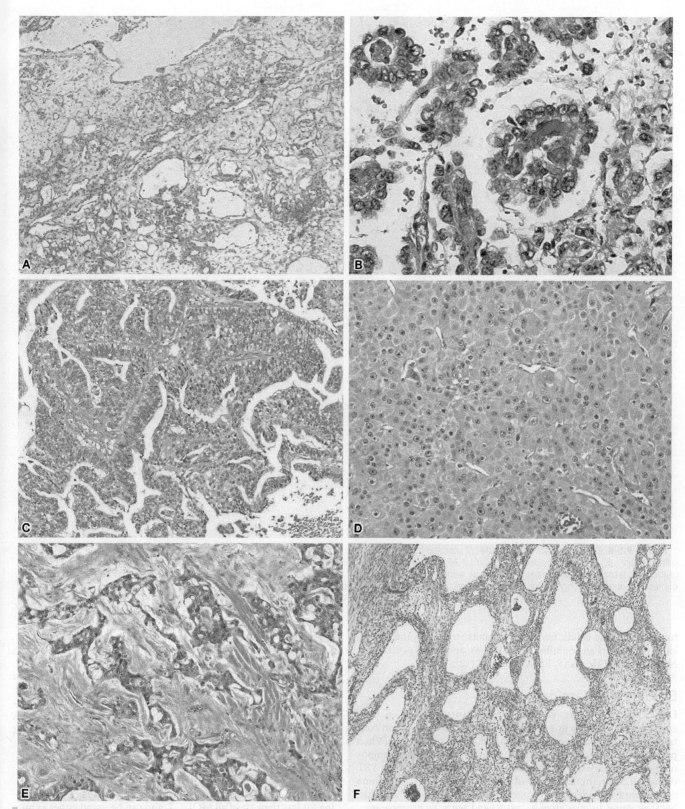

Figure 9.5-7. Microscopic hematoxylin and eosin images of yolk sac tumor: (A) microcystic/reticular pattern with characteristic loose meshwork appearance; (B) Schiller-Duval body; (C) glandular pattern: subnuclear vacuoles, lack of nuclear polarity, and interconnecting glandular spaces help to distinguish from endometrioid carcinoma; (D) hepatoid pattern; (E) parietal patter: note basement membrane–like material between islands of neoplastic cells; (F) polyvesicular-vitelline pattern.

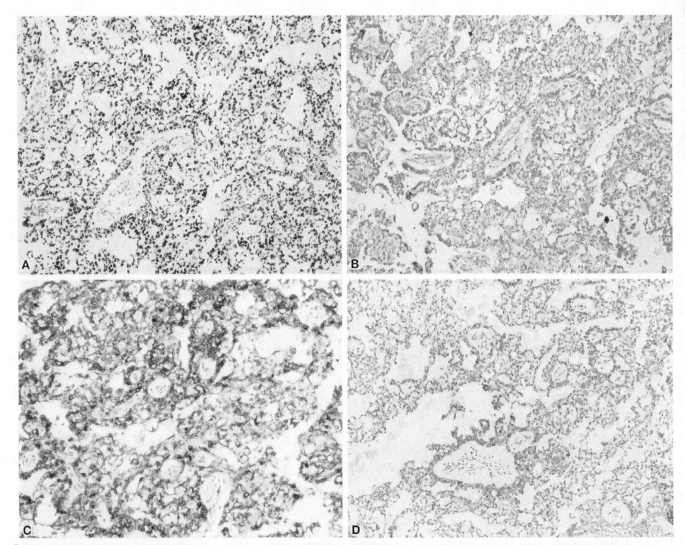

Figure 9.5-8. Immunohistochemical profile of yolk sac tumor: (A) diffuse, nuclear staining for SALL4, a nonspecific marker of germ cell differentiation; (B) patchy cytoplasmic staining for AFP, a specific but not always sensitive marker for yolk sac tumor; (C) cytoplasmic staining for glypican-3, a more sensitive marker for yolk sac tumor though less specific than AFP; (D) patchy staining for keratin 20: more differentiated areas may express markers reflecting the line of differentiation, such as intestinal differentiation. AFP, α-fetoprotein.

tubulocystic, and solid), frequently exhibits stromal hyalinization, lacks microcysts and Schiller-Duval bodies, and stains positive for Napsin A, HNF1b, PAX8, EMA, and CK7 (12).

Embryonal Carcinoma

Embryonal carcinoma is rare in the ovary, either as pure embryonal carcinoma or as a component of a mixed GCT, in contrast to its frequent presence in testicular mixed GCTs (26). When present, ovarian embryonal carcinoma is usually a minor component of a mixed GCT and associated, often intimately, with YST (**Figure 9.5-9**). The diagnosis of ovarian embryonal carcinoma can prompt consideration of performing chromosomal analysis, because some tumors may be associated with Y-chromosome–containing gonadal dysgenesis (9).

On gross examination, embryonal carcinoma is unilateral, solid, and large with extensive areas of hemorrhage and necrosis. Microscopically, this tumor demonstrates rudimentary epithelial differentiation and is composed of very crowded sheets and nests of large primitive cells with high nucleus-to-cytoplasm ratio, enlarged and pleomorphic irregularly contoured nuclei with prominent nucleoli, and ample mitotic figures and apoptotic bodies (27). Tumor cells grow in sheets or nests and focal glandular, solid,

and papillary patterns may be seen. Vascular invasion is common. Embryonal carcinoma stains for PLAP, keratin AE1/AE3, CD30, SALL4, LIN28, and OCT3/4. SOX2 is variably positive (~50%), whereas EMA, CD177, and GPC are negative (26,28). In contrast to dysgerminoma, embryonal carcinoma seldom stains for c-kit. Syncytiotrophoblast-like tumor cells (usually found at the periphery or within hemorrhagic foci) staining positive for hCG and CK may be present. If it is accompanied by cytotrophoblastic cells, that may indicate the presence of a choriocarcinoma component.

Choriocarcinoma

Primary nongestational ovarian choriocarcinoma is rare, accounting for less than 1% of all MOGCT, and can be found either as pure choriocarcinoma or as a component of a mixed OGCT. Choriocarcinomas are macroscopically unilateral, solid, and friable and display abundant hemorrhage and necrosis (**Figure 9.5-10**). Microscopically, these neoplasms show a plexiform pattern composed of an admixture of syncytiotrophoblastic and mononucleated cytotrophoblastic cells (**Figure 9.5-10**). Syncytiotrophoblastic giant cells may form syncytial knots and have abundant eosinophilic to amphophilic cytoplasm containing vacuoles and are characterized by multiple atypical, hyperchromatic nuclei. Cytotrophoblastic

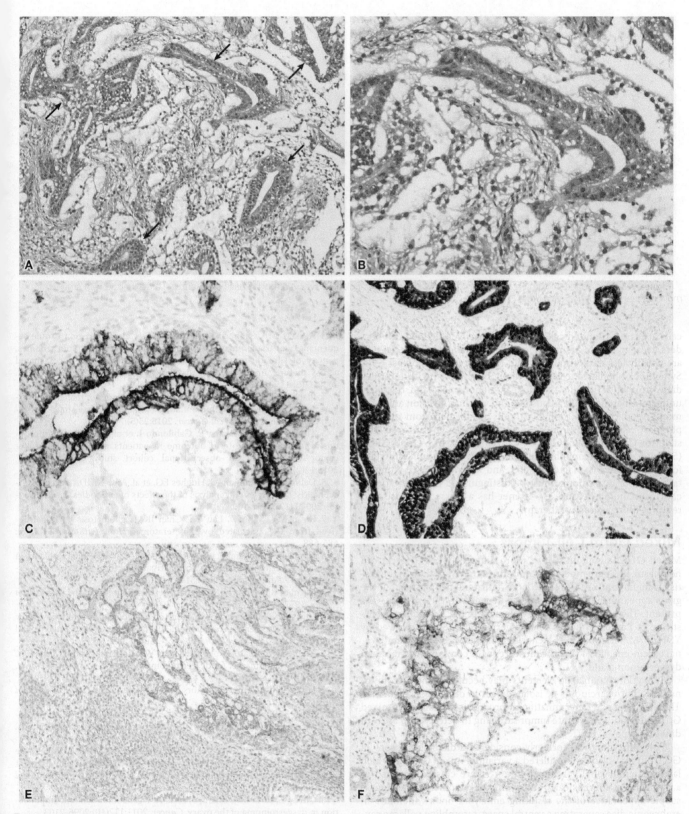

■ **Figure 9.5-9.** Embryonal carcinoma admixed with yolk sac tumor: (A) atypical glands (arrows) are surrounded by yolk sac tumor displaying the microcystic/reticular pattern; (B) at high power, cells of embryonal carcinoma have large nuclei and prominent nucleoli with conspicuous mitotic activity; CD30 (C) and OCT3/4 (D) highlight embryonal carcinoma (yolk sac component negative). Yolk sac component is highlighted by α-fetoprotein (E) and glypican-3 (F).

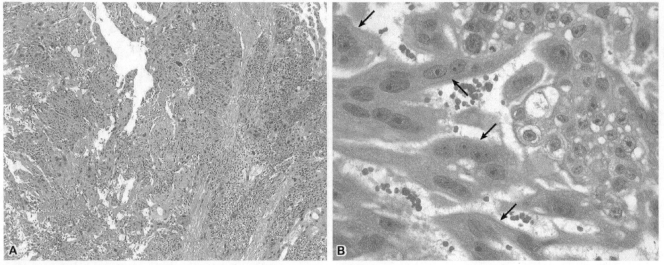

Figure 9.5-10. Choriocarcinoma at low (A) and high (B) power; multinucleated syncytiotrophoblastic cells (arrows) are admixed with smaller, mononuclear cytotrophoblastic cells.

cells are large, rounded cells and often have well-defined cell borders, clear to lightly eosinophilic cytoplasm, and single nuclei that are usually less darkly staining than the syncytiotrophoblast cells. Syncytiotrophoblastic cells may rarely be admixed with intermediate trophoblastic cells that appear mononuclear and relatively uniform. Dilated vascular sinusoids and vascular invasion are commonly seen. Syncytiotrophoblast cells are formed from cytotrophoblast cells and do produce hCG. All cells of choriocarcinoma stain for CK, α-inhibin, GATA3, CD10, SALL4, EMA, and GPC3 (5). Intermediate trophoblastic cells within the tumor will stain for human placental lactogen, p63, and inhibin (29,30). Nongestational choriocarcinoma must be distinguished from gestational choriocarcinoma because the former has a worse prognosis and requires more aggressive therapy.

Mixed Germ Cell Tumors

Mixed OGCTs contain two or more different types of germ cell neoplasm. They are much less common in the ovary than in the testis. Malignant mixed GCTs are large, unilateral neoplasms, but the gross appearance on the cut surface depends on the type of GCTs present. The most common GCT element in the Armed Forces Institute of Pathology series was dysgerminoma (80%), followed by YST (70%), teratoma (53%), choriocarcinoma (20%), and embryonal carcinoma (13%) (2). The most frequent combination has been dysgerminoma and YST.

Syncytiotrophoblastic elements may occur as either a component of choriocarcinoma or isolated cells in other GCT elements. The diagnosis and determination of prognosis of malignant mixed GCTs depend on adequate tumor sampling to detect small areas of different types of GCT.

Polyembryoma was formerly considered a distinct category of GCT but may also be considered a variant of mixed GCT in which layers of embryonal carcinoma and YST are closely arranged in a pattern that mimics early embryonic development. The microscopic appearance of the resulting embryoid bodies includes an embryonic disc separating a ventral space, resembling yolk sac cavity and a dorsal space resembling amniotic cavity. Teratoma is also present in most cases.

References

1. WHO Classification of Tumours Editorial Board. *Female Genital Tumours: WHO Classification of Tumours.* 5th ed. Vol 4. IARC; 2020.

2. Poulos C, Cheng L, Zhang S, Gersell DJ, Ulbright TM. Analysis of ovarian teratomas for isochromosome 12p: evidence supporting a dual histogenetic pathway for teratomatous elements. *Mod Pathol.* 2006;19:766-771.

3. Heskett MB, Sanborn JZ, Boniface C, et al. Multiregion exome sequencing of ovarian immature teratomas reveals 2N near-diploid genomes, paucity of somatic mutations, and extensive allelic imbalances shared across mature, immature, and disseminated components. *Mod Pathol.* 2020;33(6):1193-1206.

4. Black JD, Roque DM, Pasternak MC, et al. A series of malignant ovarian cancers arising from within a mature cystic teratoma: a single institution experience. *Int J Gynecol Cancer.* 2015;25(5):792-797.

5. Titulaer MJ, McCracken L, Gabilondo I, et al. Treatment and prognostic factors for long-term outcome in patients with anti-NMDA receptor encephalitis: an observational cohort study. *Lancet Neurol.* 2013;12(2):157-165.

6. Dalmau J, Gleichman AJ, Hughes EG, et al. Anti-NMDA-receptor encephalitis: case series and analysis of the effects of antibodies. *Lancet Neurol.* 2008;7(12):1091-1098.

7. Kwan MY, Kalle W, Lau GT, Chan JK. Is gliomatosis peritonei derived from the associated ovarian teratoma? *Hum Pathol.* 2004;35(6):685-688.

8. Ferguson AW, Katabuchi H, Ronnett BM, Cho KR. Glial implants in gliomatosis peritonei arise from normal tissue, not from the associated teratoma. *Am J Pathol.* 2001;159(1):51-55.

9. Kurman RJ, Norris HJ. Malignant germ cell tumors of the ovary. *Hum Pathol.* 1977;8(5):551-564.

10. Ulbright TM. Germ cell tumors of the gonads: a selective review emphasizing problems in differential diagnosis, newly appreciated, and controversial issues. *Mod Pathol.* 2005;18(Suppl 2):S61-S79.

11. Cheng L, Thomas A, Roth LR, Zheng W, Michael H, Abdul Karim FW. OCT4: a novel biomarker for dysgerminoma of the ovary. *Am J Surg Pathol.* 2004;28(10):1341-1346.

12. Euscher ED. Germ cell tumors of the female genital tract. *Surg Pathol Clin.* 2019;12(2):621-649.

13. Sever M, Jones TD, Roth LM, et al. Expression of CD117 (c-kit) receptor in dysgerminoma of the ovary: diagnostic and therapeutic implications. *Mod Pathol.* 2005;18(11):1411-1416.

14. Hoei-Hansen CE, Kraggerud SM, Abeler VM, Kaern J, Rajpert-De Meyts E, Lothe RA. Ovarian dysgerminomas are characterised by frequent KIT mutations and abundant expression of pluripotency markers. *Mol Cancer.* 2007;6:12.

15. Cheng L, Roth LM, Zhang S, et al. KIT gene mutation and amplification in dysgerminoma of the ovary. *Cancer.* 2011;117(10):2096-2103.

16. Teilum G. Endodermal sinus tumors of the ovary and testis. Comparative morphogenesis of the so-called mesoephroma ovarii (Schiller) and extraembryonic (yolk sac-allantoic) structures of the rat's placenta. *Cancer.* 1959;12:1092-1105.

17. Talerman A. The incidence of yolk sac tumor (endodermal sinus tumor) elements in germ cell tumors of the testis in adults. *Cancer.* 1975;36(1):211-215.

18. Young RH. The yolk sac tumor: reflections on a remarkable neoplasm and two of the many intrigued by it-Gunnar Teilum and Aleksander Talerman-and the bond it formed between them. *Int J Surg Pathol.* 2014;22(8):677-687.

19. Young RH, Wong A, Stall JN. Yolk Sac tumor of the ovary: a report of 150 cases and review of the literature. *Am J Surg Pathol.* 2022;46(3):309-325.

20. Kurman RJ, Norris HJ. Endodermal sinus tumor of the ovary: a clinical and pathologic analysis of 71 cases. *Cancer.* 1976;38(6):2404-2419.

21. Roth LM. Variants of yolk sac tumor. *Pathol Case Rev.* 2004;10:186-192.

22. Damjanov I, Amenta PS, Zarghami F. Transformation of an AFP-positive yolk sac carcinoma into an AFP-negative neoplasm. Evidence for in vivo cloning of the human parietal yolk sac carcinoma. *Cancer.* 1984;53(9):1902-1907.

23. Ramalingam P, Malpica A, Silva EG, Gershenson DM, Liu JL, Deavers MT. The use of cytokeratin 7 and EMA in differentiating ovarian yolk sac tumors from endometrioid and clear cell carcinomas. *Am J Surg Pathol.* 2004;28(11):1499-1505.

24. Xiao GQ, Li F, Unger PD, et al. ZBTB16: a novel sensitive and specific biomarker for yolk sac tumor. *Mod Pathol.* 2016;29(6):591-598.

25. Cao D, Humphrey PA, Allan RW. SALL4 is a novel sensitive and specific marker for metastatic germ cell tumors, with particular utility in detection of metastatic yolk sac tumors. *Cancer.* 2009;115(12):2640-2651.

26. Kurman RJ, Norris HJ. Embryonal carcinoma of the ovary: a clinicopathologic entity distinct from endodermal sinus tumor resembling embryonal carcinoma of the adult testis. *Cancer.* 1976;38(6):2420-2433.

27. Roth LM, Talerman A. Recent advances in the pathology and classification of ovarian germ cell tumors. *Int J Gynecol Pathol.* 2006;25(4):305-320.

28. Cheng L, Zhang S, Talerman A, Roth LM. Morphologic, immunohistochemical, and fluorescence in situ hybridization study of ovarian embryonal carcinoma with comparison to solid variant of yolk sac tumor and immature teratoma. *Hum Pathol.* 2010;41(5):716-723.

29. Beck JS, Fulmer HF, Lee ST. Solid malignant ovarian teratoma with "embryoid bodies" and trophoblastic differentiation. *J Pathol.* 1969;99(1):67-73.

30. Vance RP, Geisinger KR. Pure nongestational choriocarcinoma of the ovary. Report of a case. *Cancer.* 1985;56(9):2321-2325.

CHAPTER **9.6**

Therapy for Ovarian Germ Cell Tumors: Radiation, Chemotherapy, Targeted Therapy, Immunotherapy, and Other New and Novel Agents

Brenna E. Swift, Dimitrios Nasioudis, and Allan Covens

EVOLUTION OF CHEMOTHERAPY

One of the great triumphs of cancer treatment in the 1970s and 1980s has been the development of effective chemotherapy for testicular cancer (1,2). The lessons learned from prospective, randomized trials in testicular cancer were subsequently applied to OGCTs. Presently, the overwhelming majority of patients with OGCTs survive their disease with the judicious use of surgery and cisplatin-based combination chemotherapy. There are many similarities, but a few important differences between testicular cancer and OGCTs.

Historically, the first regimens used successfully for women with OGCTs were VAC or VAC-type regimens. Such treatments had curative potential, especially for early-stage disease. However, among patients with advanced disease, the number of long-term survivors after VAC therapy remained under 50%. In the series reported from the MDACC, although 86% of patients with stage I tumors were cured with VAC, the efficacy of the regimen was significantly lower for patients with advanced disease (3). Only 57% of stage II patients and 50% of stage III patients achieved long-term control. The two patients with stage IV tumors in this series succumbed to the disease. Similarly, in a GOG study, only seven out of 22 patients with incompletely resected OGCTs achieved long-term disease control after VAC, as compared with 39 of 54 patients with completely resected tumors (4). In that report, 11 of 15 patients with stage III and both patients with stage IV disease progressed within 12 months. These data suggest that VAC chemotherapy was insufficient for the treatment of advanced-stage and/or incompletely resected OGCTs.

Owing to the experience gained from the treatment of testicular tumors demonstrating the superiority of cisplatin-based regimens, new platinum-based regimens were tested in patients with OGCTs as summarized in **Table 9.6-1**. Gershenson et al reported the efficacy of PVB in a small series of patients treated at the MDACC (5). Among 15 patients, seven received PVB in the adjuvant setting and eight received the combination at the time of recurrence. Six

of seven patients treated with PVB upfront became long-term survivors. Among them, three women had optimally debulked stage III disease (5).

Subsequently, the PVB combination was evaluated prospectively in GOG protocol #45 (6). In this study, 47 (53%) of 89 patients with nondysgerminomatous ovarian tumors were disease free, with a median follow-up of 52 months. The latest treatment failure occurred at 28 months. Eight other patients had durable remissions with second-line therapy, and a few other patients had nonprogressive or slowly progressive IT. Thus, the 4-year OS was approximately 70%. Of note, 29% of patients enrolled in this trial had received prior radiation or chemotherapy, which might have negatively affected the overall outcome. Histologic type and marker elevation before treatment were not associated with adverse outcome. However, even among patients with nonmeasurable and presumably small-volume disease, and without prior treatment, eight of 30 patients treated with PVB ultimately failed.

In testicular cancer, subsequent experience has documented that etoposide is at least equivalent to vinblastine and produces improved survival in patients with high tumor volume (2). Furthermore, the use of etoposide in place of vinblastine led to reduced neurologic toxicity, abdominal pain, and constipation. The latter two adverse effects are particularly important for patients with OGCTs, as many have had recent abdominal surgery. These observations led to the evaluation of the combination of BEP (**Table 9.6-2**) in patients with OGCTs. In a series from the MDACC, long-term remissions were recorded in 25 of 26 patients treated with BEP (7). The only patient who succumbed to disease had been noncompliant with treatment, monitoring, and follow-up. In this series, four patients with measurable disease after surgery had complete remissions after BEP treatment. This led to a prospective GOG study evaluating BEP in patients with OGCTs (8). The regimen was highly effective, 91 of 93 enrolled patients being free of disease at follow-up. On the basis of these data, although BEP and VAC have not been prospectively compared, BEP emerged as the

■ **TABLE 9.6-1. Platinum-Based Chemotherapy in Ovarian Germ Cell Tumors**

Institution	Histology	Stage	Regimen	Progression Free/Total
MD Anderson (5)	Nondysgerminoma	I-IV	PVB	10/15
GOG 45 (8)	Nondysgerminoma	II-IV	PVB and/or VAC or EP	47/89
Australia (10)	All	I-IV	Multiple	53/58
Hospital 12 de Octubre (9)	All	I-IV	Multiple	80/108
MD Anderson (7)	All	I-III	BEP	25/26
GOG 78 (8)	Nondysgerminoma	I-III	BEP	89/93
The United Kingdom (12)	All	I-IV	JEB	43/48
GOG (13)	Dysgerminoma	IB-III	Carbo-etoposide	37/37
Greece (16)	All	I-IV	3-d BEP	46/48
Taiwanese GOG (17)	All	I-IV	3-d BEP	192/204
Australia (67)	All (majority testicular)	Metastatic	Accelerated BEP	35/43
GOG (65)	IT	I-IV	BEP	70/81
Italy (71)	All	I	BEP	64/73

BEP, bleomycin, etoposide, and cisplatin; GOG, Gynecologic Oncology group; JEB, carboplatin, etoposide, and bleomycin; PVB, cisplatin, vinblastine, and bleomycin

preferred regimen for patients with OGCTs. The inclusion of cisplatin in the treatment of ovarian tumors resulted in an improvement in survival and disease control, as shown by the results of GOG studies, as well as by other clinical series (9-11).

As a result of increased neurotoxicity, ototoxicity, and nephrotoxicity from cisplatin, substitution of carboplatin has been evaluated in treatment of GCTs. The carboplatin, etoposide, and bleomycin (JEB) regimen (etoposide 120 mg/m^2 on days 1 through 3, carboplatin 600 mg/m^2 on day 2, and bleomycin 15 mg/m^2 on day 3) was evaluated in patients aged 0 to 16 years with recurrent stage 1 and advanced-stage testicular and OGCTs. In 137 patients treated with a median of five cycles (range 3-8) of JEB, the 5-year OS was 90.9% (95% CI, 83.9%-95.0%) and the event-free survival (EFS) was 87.8% (95% CI, 81.1%-92.4%) (12). Owing to the chemosensitivity of dysgerminomas, the GOG evaluated adjuvant carboplatin and etoposide (carboplatin 400 mg/m^2 on day 1 plus etoposide 120 mg/m^2 on days 1, 2, and 3 every 4 weeks for three courses) for completely resected stage IB-III diseases. There were no recurrences of dysgerminoma in 39 patients treated with this regimen (13). Although highly active in these studies, the dose of carboplatin is high (area under the curve [AUC] 7-9), and this regimen is not routinely recommended because of significantly less experience accumulated with its use and the concern that this regimen is not as effective in tumors containing nondysgerminomatous elements. The accrual closed early for this ovarian germ cell study, owing to a concern that carboplatin was less efficacious compared to cisplatin in testicular GCTs. However, the dose of carboplatin was 350 to 500 mg/m^2 and AUC 5 in these two testicular cancer studies, which was lower than the study in ovarian dysgerminoma (14,15).

An abbreviated 3-day BEP regimen was evaluated in 48 patients, the majority with stage I disease (65%) and complete resection

■ **TABLE 9.6-2. BEP Regimen**

Cisplatin	20 mg/m^2 days 1-5
Etoposide	100 mg/m^2 days 1-5
Bleomycin	30 units intravenously weekly

Three courses given at 21-day intervals.
BEP, bleomycin, etoposide, and cisplatin.

From Williams S, Blessing JA, Liao SY, Ball H, Hanjani P. Adjuvant therapy of ovarian germ cell tumors with cisplatin, etoposide, and bleomycin: A trial of the Gynecologic Oncology Group. *J Clin Oncol.* 1994;12(4):701-706. doi:10.1200/JCO.1994.12.4.701

(67%). All patients with stage I or II disease and all dysgerminomas did not have a disease recurrence. Patients presenting with stage III or IV nondysgerminomas had 20% progressive disease (16). In a Taiwanese GOG study, an abbreviated 3-day BEP regimen was safe and effective for 204 patients with OGCT, including all histologies and stages. The EFS was 94%, with seven patients experiencing grade 3/4 hematologic toxicity (17).

Immediate Toxicity of Chemotherapy

Acute adverse effects of chemotherapy can be substantial, and these patients should be treated by physicians experienced in their management. About 25% of patients develop febrile neutropenic episodes during chemotherapy and require hospitalization and broad-spectrum antibiotics. Cisplatin can be associated with nephrotoxicity and neurotoxicity. This can be mitigated by ensuring adequate hydration during and immediately after chemotherapy and by avoidance of aminoglycoside antibiotics. Bleomycin can cause pulmonary fibrosis. Pulmonary function testing is frequently used to follow these patients. However, the value of carbon monoxide diffusion capacity to predict early lung disease has been challenged (18). The most effective method for monitoring patients with GCTs is careful physical examination of the chest. Findings of early bleomycin lung disease are a lag or diminished expansion of one hemithorax or fine bibasilar rales that do not clear with cough. These findings can be very subtle, but if present, immediate discontinuation of bleomycin should be mandated. It is important to note that randomized trials in good prognosis testicular cancer have suggested that bleomycin is an important component of the treatment regimen, particularly if only three courses of therapy are given (19,20). However, evaluation of etoposide and cisplatin (EP) in eight patients with all stages of OGCTs showed an EFS of 87.5% (21).

Patients with advanced OGCTs should receive three to four courses of treatment given in full dose and on schedule. There is presumptive evidence in testicular cancer that the timeliness of chemotherapy may be associated with outcome. Thus, treatment is given, regardless of hematologic parameters on the scheduled day of treatment. Because most patients will not develop neutropenic sepsis, hematopoietic growth factors are not routinely necessary (22). It is reasonable to use hematopoietic growth factors to avoid dose reductions for patients with previous episodes of neutropenic sepsis or in unusually ill patients who are at a higher risk of myelosuppressive complications or those who received prior radiotherapy (RT). Modern antiemetic therapy, an example of which is shown in **Table 9.6-3**, has greatly lessened chemotherapy-induced

▪ TABLE 9.6-3. Antiemetic Regimen
Granisetron 1 mg IV 30 min before cisplatin daily for 5 d OR
Ondansetron 0.15 mg/kg IV daily 30 min prior and 4 hr after cisplatin daily for 5 d PLUS
Dexamethasone 20 mg IV 30 min before cisplatin on days 1 and 2 PLUS Aprepitant 125 mg PO on day 1 and 80 mg PO on days 2 and 3, before cisplatin infusion

IV, intravenous; PO, by mouth.

emesis. By following these guidelines and providing supportive care as indicated, virtually all patients can be treated on schedule, in full or nearly full dose. Chemotherapy-related mortality should be less than 1%. In GOG protocol #78, there were no toxic deaths among 93 patients treated (8).

Sequelae of Chemotherapy

The evolutionary development and refinement of combination chemotherapy have resulted in the cure of a high percentage of patients with chemosensitive tumors, such as lymphomas, testicular cancer, gestational trophoblastic disease, and MOGCTs. Within the past few years, several reports have described the long-term effects of chemotherapy in cancer survivors. As expected, most reports refer to the more common lymphomas and testicular cancers.

A recognized effect of chemotherapy used for the treatment of GCTs is the risk of secondary malignancies. Etoposide is associated with the development of acute myelogenous leukemia (AML) with certain morphologic and cytogenetic features (23-27). This treatment complication appears to be cumulative dose (23,25) and schedule dependent (27). Of 138 patients with OGCTs treated with NACT or adjuvant chemotherapy, one patient died of acute lymphoblastic leukemia 2 years after surgery and adjuvant JEB (28). Of 348 patients with male GCT receiving three to four courses of BEP as first-line therapy at the Indiana University, two developed etoposide-related leukemia. None of the 67 patients who received only three courses developed AML (23). Similarly, in the study reported by Pedersen-Bjergaard et al (23), five out of 212 patients developed acute leukemia or myelodysplastic syndrome after etoposide therapy. However, all patients who developed AML received more than 2,000 mg/m^2 of etoposide. None of the 130 patients who received less than this dose developed AML. Morphologically, these leukemias are monocytic or myelomonocytic (M4 or M5). Characteristic chromosomal translocations (mostly involving the 11q23 region) are frequently, but not always, present. Leukemia after etoposide treatment occurs within 2 to 3 years compared with alkylating agent–induced AML, which has a longer latency period. Late occurrence of chronic myelogenous leukemia after treatment of testicular cancer was reported (24). In the GOG protocol testing the efficacy of BEP in women with OGCTs, one case of AML was recorded among 91 patients treated (8). An additional case of lymphoma was diagnosed during follow-up in this series, yet a correlation between chemotherapy and lymphoproliferative disorders has not been reported to date. Taking these issues into account, most clinicians consider BEP as the chemotherapy regimen of choice. The incidence of second neoplasms is quite low, particularly in patients receiving low cumulative etoposide doses. The continued use of etoposide over vinblastine is based on its superior efficacy demonstrated in testis cancer (2). Furthermore, vinblastine-induced abdominal pain and ileus are troublesome for some patients, particularly for those who underwent abdominal surgery, such as women with OGCTs. The risk/benefit ratio continues to favor etoposide over vinblastine.

Platinum-based chemotherapy has also shown an increased relative risk of developing secondary leukemia (4.0, 95% CI; 1.4-11.4). A dose response was observed with relative risk of 7.6 at doses over 1,000 mg of platinum ($P < .001$) (29). The overall risk of developing

a secondary cancer was 1.6- to 2.1-fold after two or more cycles of cisplatin for testicular cancer. Small intestine, bladder, kidney, and lung cancers had a 2.0- to 3.7-fold increased risk after cisplatin treatment, compared to no increased risk of these secondary cancers in patients with testicular cancer treated with surgery alone (30). At a median of 20 years after platinum-based chemotherapy for testicular cancer, platinum levels remain significantly elevated for patients treated with cisplatin compared to carboplatin or surgery alone. The serum levels were higher in patients treated with a higher cumulative dose of cisplatin (31). This long-term retention of platinum in human tissues is possibly related to late toxicity (32).

There also continues to be considerable focus on the long-term effects of chemotherapy on gonadal function. Studies of patients with a variety of cancers suggest that, although ovarian dysfunction or failure is a risk of chemotherapy, the majority of survivors can anticipate normal menstrual and reproductive function (33-38). Factors such as old age at initiation of therapy, greater cumulative drug dose (39), and longer duration of therapy (35) have an adverse effect on future gonadal function, including earlier age of menopause, reduction in antral follicle count, and anti-Müllerian hormone. Successful pregnancies after treatment with combination chemotherapy have been well documented in other types of malignancies, including Hodgkin disease, non-Hodgkin lymphomas, and leukemia. There are similar reports in patients with MOGCTs (36-38,40-43). In a review of the MDACC series (41), 27 (68%) of 40 patients who had retained a normal contralateral ovary and uterus maintained regular menses consistently after completion of chemotherapy, and 33 (83%) were having regular menses at the time of follow-up. Of 16 patients who had attempted to become pregnant, 12 were successful. One patient underwent an elective first-trimester abortion, and the other 11 patients bore 22 healthy infants over time, none of which had a major birth defect. In a series from Milan, among 169 patients with OGCTs, 138 underwent FSS, and of those, 81 underwent adjuvant chemotherapy (44). After treatment, all but one woman recovered menstrual function, and 55 conceptions were recorded. Forty normal full-term babies were delivered. There were four babies with congenital malformations, one in a patient who did not receive chemotherapy and three in women who had received chemotherapy (the difference was not statistically significant). A multi-institutional retrospective cohort study described 42 of 45 patients who desired pregnancy were able to conceive. There were a total of 65 pregnancies and 56 live births born to 40 women (37).

The GOG evaluated the quality of life and psychosocial characteristics of survivors of OGCTs compared with matched controls. In this analysis, the survivors appeared to be well adjusted, were able to develop strong relationships, and were free of significant depression (45). The impact on fertility was modest or none in patients undergoing FSSs (46). OGCT survivors appeared to be free of any major physical illnesses at a median follow-up of 10 years, as compared with matched controls. The only differences were higher rates of reported hypertension (17% vs 8%, $P = .02$), hypercholesterolemia (9.8% vs 4.4%, $P = .09$), and hearing loss (5.3% vs 1.5%, $P = .09$) compared with controls (47). Among chronic functional problems, numbness, tinnitus, nausea elicited by reminders of chemotherapy (vs general nausea triggers for controls), and Raynaud symptoms were reported more frequently by survivors. Interestingly, late effects of treatment are more pronounced among children receiving treatment for GCTs (48). Specifically, neurotoxicity, growth abnormalities, pulmonary toxicity, and gastrointestinal toxicity have been reported in a higher proportion than in adult patients. In a multicenter retrospective study of 138 patients with OGCT, other chronic treatment-related toxicities were kidney injury ($N = 2$), cardiac failure ($N = 1$), tinnitus/hearing loss ($N = 9$), bleomycin lung ($N = 4$), and peripheral neuropathy ($N = 11$) (28). Other long-term sequelae after treatment with cisplatin include cardiovascular disease, neurotoxicity, ototoxicity, nephrotoxicity, pulmonary complications, avascular necrosis, and suicide (49,50). As OGCTs often effect young women and have good prognosis, consideration of treatment side effects is important as the paradigm shifts to increased observation in early-stage disease.

PREVIOUS USE OF RADIATION THERAPY IN DYSGERMINOMA

In the past, many patients with stage I dysgerminoma and all patients with higher stage dysgerminoma tumors received RT (51). Radiation was delivered to the ipsilateral hemipelvis (with shielding of the contralateral ovary and the head of the femur) and to the para-aortic nodes. A single field with the upper limit at T10 to T11 and the lower limit at L4 to L5 level was used. For stage III retroperitoneal disease, curative RT used an additional field for mediastinum and supraclavicular nodes. In the presence of peritoneal involvement, the whole abdomen and pelvis, mediastinum, and supraclavicular nodes were irradiated. Typically, 30 Gy (7.5-9 Gy/week) was given as prophylactic irradiation for stage I tumors. For curative irradiation of stage III disease, 35 to 40 Gy total dose was given to the pelvis, and a boost (10 Gy) was delivered to the involved nodes.

When irradiating above the diaphragm, De Palo et al gave 30 additional Gy 3 to 6 weeks after completion of irradiation below the diaphragm. When irradiating the entire abdominal cavity, the fields were similar to those used for epithelial tumors (52-55). The results of RT were excellent. De Palo et al (51) reported that all 13 stage I patients (12 stage IA and one with stage IB) treated with RT were alive and free of disease, with a median follow-up of 77 months. The 5-year relapse-free survival (RFS) for 12 stage III patients was 61.4%, and the OS was 89.5%. Lawson and Adler (53) reported that 10 of 14 stage I-III patients were alive, with a median follow-up of 54 months. In this small series, there was no correlation between survival and stage of disease or the size of the primary tumor. Others reported similar results, with overall progression-free rates varying between 70% and 90% (56,57).

However, despite the remarkable radiosensitivity of dysgerminoma, RT is currently rarely performed, as chemotherapy is equally/more effective, less toxic, and less likely to compromise gonadal function. Given that most patients are cured with either surgery alone or combined surgery and chemotherapy, and the young age at the time of diagnosis, consideration should also be given to the delayed carcinogenic effects of intermediate-dose radiation. Review of the SEER database shows that 10 (13%) of 70 patients who received RT for an MOGCT developed a second cancer, significantly higher than patients who did not receive RT (58).

Sequelae of Radiation Therapy

There is limited information about the late effects of RT in patients with dysgerminoma. In a review of the late effects of RT in patients receiving abdominal therapy for ovarian dysgerminoma at the MDACC, there was a small increase in reported dyspareunia and the number of bowel movements (59). Somewhat surprisingly, at a median follow-up of 12 years, none of the 43 patients treated with RT developed small bowel obstruction. No other significant intestinal or bladder problems were recorded. As expected, none of the patients treated with radiation conceived (60). A recent review of the SEER database indicates an increased risk of secondary malignancy in patients

who received radiation for an MOGCT. In this study, 10 (10%) of 70 patients who received RT for an MOGCT developed a second cancer, significantly higher than in patients who did not receive RT (58). In practice, RT is currently rarely administered, as chemotherapy is effective and preservation of ovarian function is preferred (61).

ADJUVANT TREATMENT BY RISK AND HISTOLOGY

Current national consensus guidelines recommend observation for stage I dysgerminomas and grade 1 ITs in adult women. Adjuvant chemotherapy is recommended for other histologies and advanced-stage disease. However, the ESMO guidelines suggest active surveillance is an option for stage IA/IB, grade 2 and 3 ITs and stage IA/IB YSTs (62). This is discrepant from pediatrics where observation is recommended for all stages of completely resected IT (63,64). As a result of toxicities from chemotherapy and high salvage rates at the time of recurrence, there is increasing evidence for observation rather than adjuvant chemotherapy in most stage I OGCTs as shown in **Table 9.6-4**. In a large database study of stage 1 GCTs, yolk sac was the only histology with improved outcomes with adjuvant chemotherapy (65). An ongoing, large collaborative trial (AGCT1531) between the COG and the NCI aims to assess whether stage I nondysgerminoma and stage I, grade 2 and 3 IT can be followed by active surveillance. This trial also aims to assess the role of bleomycin and etoposide with either carboplatin or cisplatin in patients under age 25 with nondysgerminoma and advanced-stage disease. In poor-risk disease, adjuvant chemotherapy with an accelerated BEP regimen repeated every 2 weeks (instead of 3) for four cycles with a maximum of 12 doses of bleomycin has shown feasibility and tolerability in a phase 2 trial (66). This regimen is currently being investigated in a phase 3 trial (ANZUP P3BEP or COG-AGCT1532). The changing paradigm for adjuvant treatment of GCTs is summarized in **Table 9.6-5**.

Dysgerminoma

The majority of patients with dysgerminoma present with stage I disease. These patients can be treated with unilateral salpingo-oophorectomy and can be observed carefully with regular pelvic examinations, abdominopelvic CT, and tumor markers, including LDH and hCG. Lymphadenectomy has not been associated with improved survival (67). Fifteen to 25% of patients observed will experience recurrence and will require chemotherapy. In patients with more advanced disease, the risk of recurrence is significant enough to warrant adjuvant treatment.

Dysgerminoma is very responsive to cisplatin-based chemotherapy (7,9). Since 1984, patients with advanced dysgerminoma were eligible for GOG protocols. Patients enrolled on these studies received three to four courses of PVB or BEP. In a combined analysis, 20 patients were evaluated (68). All had stage III or IV disease, and most of them had suboptimal (>2 cm) residual tumor. With a median follow-up of 26 months, 19 of the 20 women were disease free. Among 11 patients

■ **TABLE 9.6-4. Active Surveillance for Adult Stage I Ovarian Germ Cell Tumors**

Institution	Histology	Stage	Progression Free/Total	Overall Survival/Total
Italy (78)	IT	I-II	20/22	22/22
The United Kingdom (77)	All	I	16/24	23/24
The United Kingdom (82)	Nondysgerminoma	I	8/9	9/9
The United Kingdom (83)	All	IA	21/31	30/31
Korea (84)	All	I	24/31	30/31
Italy (70)	All	I	57/71	68/71
Italy and the United Kingdom (81)	IT	I	72/81	80/81
Italy (71)	Dysgerminoma, IT, mixed	I	30/31	31/31

■ TABLE 9.6-5. Risk Stratification and Adjuvant Treatment for OGCTs

	Histology	Stage	COG Stage	Current Adjuvant Treatment	Future Directions
Low risk	Dysgerminoma	FIGO IA/IB		Observation	Observation
		FIGO IC		BEP ×3	Observation (71,84)
	IT	FIGO IA/IB	I	Grade 1—Observation Grade 2/3—BEP ×3	All grades—Observation (65,71,84) AGCT1531 (NCT03067181)
	IT grades 1-3	IC		BEP	?Observation (70,71,84) AGCT1531 (NCT03067181)
	Nondysgerminoma (YST/mixed/other)	FIGO IA/IB		BEP ×3	Observation (65,84) YST—BEP ×3 (65,70) AGCT1531 (NCT03067181)
Standard risk	Dysgerminoma	FIGO II-IV	COG II-IV <11 y COG II-III ≥11 y	BEP ×3-4 or EP-Carbo (69,85)	BEP vs BEC AGCT1531 (NCT03067181)
	IT	II-III		BEP ×3-4	?Observation (28)
	Nondysgerminoma (YST/mixed/other)	FIGO IC-III		BEP ×3-4	BEP vs BEC (histology specific) AGCT1531 (NCT03067181)
Poor risk	Nondysgerminoma (YST/mixed/other)	FIGO IV	COG IV ≥11 y	BEP ×4	BEP vs accelBEP (66) vs histology specific

BEC, bleomycin, etoposide, and carboplatin; BEP, bleomycin, etoposide, and cisplatin; COG, Children's Oncology Group; EP, etoposide and cisplatin; FIGO, International Federation of Gynaecology and Obstetrics; OGCTs, ovarian germ cell tumors; YST, yolk sac tumor.

Adapted and modified from Marks RD, Underwood PB, Othersen HB, Wallace KM, Moore TN. Dysgerminoma-100% control with combined therapy in six consecutive patients with advanced disease. *Int J Radiat Oncol Biol Phys.* 1978;4(5):453-456. doi:10.1016/0360-3016(78)90078-0

with clinically measurable tumor, 10 had complete responses to chemotherapy. Fourteen patients who underwent second-look laparotomy had completely negative results. Thus, it appears that nearly all patients with advanced dysgerminoma treated with chemotherapy will be durable complete responders (68). There is no evidence for debulking in GCTs owing to their chemosensitivity.

Radiation is rarely considered initial treatment and only then in unusual circumstances, such as in older patients or in those with serious concomitant illness that preclude the use of systemic chemotherapy. For most, the preferred adjuvant therapy is BEP. This regimen almost invariably reduces recurrence in nondysgerminomatous tumors as well as dysgerminoma. Most patients treated with BEP will retain fertility. An alternative regimen tested by the GOG consists of a 3-day regimen with carboplatin and etoposide. On this protocol, all 39 patients with pure dysgerminoma remained free of disease at a median follow-up of 7.8 years (13). The Malignant Germ Cell Tumor International Consortium (MaGIC) pooled data from six international pediatric and gynecologic oncology trials in GCTs. There were 126 eligible patients (56 received carboplatin-based and 70 received cisplatin-based chemotherapy). The 5-year EFS and OS were similar for carboplatin- (5-year EFS = 0.96 [95% CI, 0.85-0.99], 5-year OS = 0.96 [95% CI, 0.85-0.99]) and cisplatin-based (5-year EFS = 0.93 [95% CI, 0.83-0.97], 5-year OS = 0.96 [95% CI, 0.87-0.99]) regimens (69).

The implications of elevated hCG or AFP levels in patients with dysgerminoma should be emphasized. These tumor markers are usually increased in patients with nondysgerminomatous tumors. Therefore, AFP elevation denotes the presence of elements other than dysgerminoma, and treatment should be tailored accordingly. An elevated hCG level can be seen in pure dysgerminoma. This finding should not alter therapy, but it should prompt reexamination of the tumor specimen to determine whether nongestational trophoblastic cells are present or if the tumor contains nondysgerminomatous elements.

Nondysgerminoma

GOG 78 included 93 patients with stage I-III surgically resected nondysgerminoma (two choriocarcinomas, 25 YSTs, 42ITs, 24 mixed GCTs). All patients received adjuvant treatment with three

cycles of BEP. Only two of 93 patients developed recurrent disease (both IT), with a median follow-up of 38.6 months. However, two patients developed a secondary hematologic malignancy (8). This trial established three cycles of BEP as standard of care for nondysgerminoma.

Other studies have suggested adjuvant chemotherapy may be overtreatment for stage I nondysgerminoma. In AGCT0132, 25 female children (mean age 12) with stage I primarily YSTs were followed with active surveillance after surgery. Eleven of 12 received successful salvage chemotherapy, and this strategy avoided chemotherapy in half of patients (4-year EFS = 52%; 95% CI, 31%-69%; 4-year OS = 96%; 95% CI, 74%-99%). All patients had elevated AFP at the time of recurrence (46). An NCDB study of 497 patients with stage IA/IB GCTs showed no difference in OS with adjuvant chemotherapy in grade 2 (P = .35) and grade 3 (P = .47) ITs and mixed GCTs (P = .55). Patients with stage IA/IB YSTs had improved 5-year OS with adjuvant chemotherapy (92.7% vs 79.6%, P = .019) (65). Similarly, in a multicenter retrospective study, there was no difference in OS with or without adjuvant chemotherapy for stage I dysgerminoma and IT (70). These findings were confirmed in an observation prospective study with no recurrences in 22 stage IA/IB patients with IT and mixed GCTs followed by active surveillance (71). These findings support surveillance to stage IA/IB nondysgerminoma tumors. The ongoing AGCT1531 trial (NCT03067181) aims to assess active surveillance for stage I nondysgerminoma tumors.

The current standard of care for advanced-stage nondysgerminoma tumors is three to four cycles of BEP. Carboplatin has been used for pediatric GCTs in the U.K. regimen with similar clinical outcomes and less toxicity (12). The MaGIC compared previous trials with cisplatin-based therapy in 620 patients and carboplatin based in 163 patients with pediatric extracranial malignant GCTs. The overall multivariate model showed no significant difference in EFS (cisplatin: 4-year EFS = 86%; 95% CI, 83%-89% vs carboplatin: 4-year EFS = 86%; 95% CI, 79%-90%; P = .87) (72). The ongoing AGCT1531 trial aims to assess bleomycin, etoposide, and either carboplatin or cisplatin in women under age 25 with advanced-stage GCTs.

Immature Teratoma

The situation of patients with IT is more complex. Our current treatment strategy for adults with ITs is based on a retrospective analysis of 58 patients, in which higher grade correlated with worse prognosis. Specifically, only one of 14 patients with grade 1 IT recurred, but there was an 18% recurrence rate for grade 2 tumors and a 70% recurrence rate for grade 3 tumors (73). These data were further informed by a report of 41 patients with IT by Gershenson et al (74), in which 94% of patients treated with surgery only recurred, compared with 14% of patients treated with surgery and chemotherapy. These studies set the current standard of care for women with IT, which is surveillance for stage I grade 1 IT and adjuvant chemotherapy with three courses of BEP for all other patients. This recommendation has come into question based on the probable underestimation of tumor stage in the Norris report and multiple studies in the pediatric and adult population, suggesting that observation may be a viable approach in a subset of these patients (63). Although surgery followed by adjuvant therapy may cure most patients with localized high-grade teratoma, it is possible that the risk of relapse is sufficiently low in a defined population of well-staged patients, to warrant clinical observation with careful follow-up, such that relapsing patients would be diagnosed with small-volume tumor and cured with subsequent salvage chemotherapy.

Studies supporting surgery without chemotherapy in the pediatric population include the POG/CCG Intergroup Study (INT) 0106, which reported on 44 female children with completely resected ovarian IT who were observed closely without adjuvant chemotherapy. In this series, 26 patients had grade 2 or 3 IT, and 13 patients had microscopic foci of YST. At 4 years, the EFS was 97.7% with only one recurrence, which was salvaged with BEP; the OS rate was thus 100%. The authors concluded that surgery alone is curative for children with completely resected ovarian IT (75,76). In addition, investigators at Mount Vernon and Charing Cross Hospitals in England have observed 15 patients with stage IA tumors after initial surgical treatment (77). Of these, nine patients had grade 2 or 3 IT and six had elements of endodermal sinus tumor. There were three recurrences in this series, one of nine in the pure IT group and two of six in the mixed histology group. Two of these patients were salvaged with chemotherapy, and one patient died of pulmonary embolus. Of note is that the patient who died became pregnant 4 months after diagnosis and could not be followed adequately because of her pregnancy. Investigators at the University of Milan have also reported the clinical outcomes of 32 patients with pure ovarian IT followed prospectively (78). In this group, nine patients had grade 2 and 3 stage IA ITs and were treated with surgery and intensive surveillance. Only two recurrences were noted in this group. They consisted of one case of mature teratoma and one case of gliosis. The mature teratoma was resected, and the patient with gliosis was followed without treatment. Both patients are alive and well and never received chemotherapy. Furthermore, among four patients with stage IC tumors treated with surgical resection and surveillance, there was one case of gliosis and one recurrence with mature tissue, which was resected (no chemotherapy). All patients are currently free of disease. Subsequently, Mann et al (79) reported on the outcomes of 54 pediatric patients in the United Kingdom with ovarian IT after complete surgical resection and no adjuvant chemotherapy. The EFS and OS rates were 85.9% and 95.1%, respectively, also supporting primary surgical treatment for completely resected ovarian ITs in pediatric patients. Similarly, in testicular teratoma, surgery is the primary treatment as chemoresistance is common (80).

Most recently, the MaGIC and the GOG published outcomes on pediatric and adult patients with ovarian ITs to establish a uniform treatment approach across all age groups (64). Of 179 patients included (98 pediatric, 81 adult), 90 pediatric patients had surgery alone, whereas all adult patients had adjuvant chemotherapy. The 5-year EFS and OS rates were 91% and 99% among pediatric patients and 87% and 93% among adults, respectively. Grade was the most important risk factor for relapse, suggesting that surgery alone was sufficient for patients with grade 1 tumors across all ages and all stages. Because postoperative chemotherapy did not decrease relapses in the pediatric cohort, the authors suggest that high-grade recurrent disease in the pediatric patient is not chemosensitive. A collaborative retrospective cohort study in stage I IT found similar rates of recurrence in patients who underwent

surveillance compared to adjuvant chemotherapy (9/81 vs 2/27; $P = .72$) (81). Similarly, chemotherapy reduced future relapse and progression in all histologies of OGCTs, except for IT, and there were no radiologic responses to chemotherapy in IT (28). Adult patients with higher grade tumors may do well with observation alone, using chemotherapy or second surgery in the event of relapse. Although this concept is supported by evidence derived from the pediatric literature and limited information in adults, it is currently being evaluated in a large prospective trial, AGCT1531 (NCT03067181), which aims to inform best practice for adult adjuvant treatment.

TARGETED THERAPY, IMMUNOTHERAPY, AND OTHER NEW AND NOVEL AGENTS

Targeted therapy, immunotherapy, and other new and novel agents are not currently utilized in the upfront setting. Consideration of these modalities is limited to the recurrent or refractory setting and is discussed in Chapter 9.7.

REFERENCES

1. Einhorn LH, Donohue J. Cis-diamminedichloroplatinum, vinblastine, and bleomycin combination chemotherapy in disseminated testicular cancer. *J Urol*. 2002;167(2):928-932. doi:10.1016/S0022-5347(02)80301-9
2. Williams SD, Birch R, Einhorn LH, Irwin L, Greco FA, Loehrer PJ. Treatment of disseminated germ-cell tumors with cisplatin, bleomycin, and either vinblastine or etoposide. *N Engl J Med*. 1987;316(23):1435-1440. doi:10.1056/NEJM198706043162302
3. Gershenson DM, Copeland LJ, Kavanagh JJ, et al. Treatment of malignant nondysgerminomatous germ cell tumors of the ovary with vincristine, dactinomycin, and cyclophosphamide. *Cancer*. 1985;56(12):2756-2761. doi:10.1002/1097-0142(19851215)56:12<2756::AID-CNCR2820561206>3.0.CO;2-6
4. Slayton RE, Park RC, Silverberg SG, et al. Tumors, including endometriosis: vincristine, dactinomycin, and cyclophosphamide in the treatment of malignant germ cell tumors of the ovary. *Obstet Gynecol Surv*. 1986;41(2):117. doi:10.1097/00006254-198602000-00020
5. Gershenson DM, Kavanagh JJ, Copeland LJ, et al. Treatment of malignant nondysgerminomatous germ cell tumors of the ovary with vinblastine, bleomycin, and cisplatin. *Cancer*. 1986;57(9):1731-1737. doi:10.1002/1097-0142(19860501)57:9<1731::AID-CNCR2820570904>3.0.CO;2-R
6. Williams SD, Blessing JA, Moore DH, Homesley HD, Adcock L. Cisplatin, vinblastine, and bleomycin in advanced and recurrent ovarian germ-cell tumors. A trial of the Gynecologic Oncology Group. *Ann Intern Med*. 1989;111(1):22-27. doi:10.7326/0003-4819-111-1-22
7. Gershenson DM, Morris M, Cangir A, et al. Treatment of malignant germ cell tumors of the ovary with bleomycin, etoposide, and cisplatin. *J Clin Oncol*. 1990;8(4):715-720. doi:10.1200/JCO.1990.8.4.715
8. Williams S, Blessing JA, Liao SY, Ball H, Hanjani P. Adjuvant therapy of ovarian germ cell tumors with cisplatin, etoposide, and bleomycin: a trial of the Gynecologic Oncology Group. *J Clin Oncol*. 1994;12(4):701-706. doi:10.1200/JCO.1994.12.4.701
9. Culine S, Lhomme C, Kattan J, Michel G, Duvillard P, Droz JP. Cisplatin-based chemotherapy in the management of germ cell tumors of the ovary: the Institut Gustave Roussy Experience. *Gynecol Oncol*. 1997;64(1):160-165. doi:10.1006/gyno.1996.4547
10. Segelov E, Campbell J, Ng M, et al. Cisplatin-based chemotherapy for ovarian germ cell malignancies: the Australian experience. *J Clin Oncol*. 1994;12(2):378-384. doi:10.1200/JCO.1994.12.2.378
11. Dimopoulos MA, Papadopoulou M, Andreopoulou E, et al. Favorable outcome of ovarian germ cell malignancies treated with cisplatin or carboplatin-based chemotherapy: a Hellenic Cooperative Oncology Group Study. *Gynecol Oncol*. 1998;70(1):70-74. doi:10.1006/gyno.1998.5047
12. Mann JR, Raafar F, Robinson K, et al. The United Kingdom Children's Cancer Study Group's second germ cell tumor study: carboplatin, etoposide, and bleomycin are effective treatment for children with malignant extracranial germ cell tumors, with acceptable toxicity. *J Clin Oncol*. 2000;18(22):3809-3818.
13. Williams SD, Kauderer J, Burnett AF, Lentz SS, Aghajanian C, Armstrong DK. Adjuvant therapy of completely resected dysgerminoma with carboplatin and etoposide: a trial of the Gynecologic Oncology Group. *Gynecol Oncol*. 2004;95(3):496-499. doi:10.1016/j.ygyno.2004.07.044
14. Bajorin DF, Sarosdy MF, Pfister DG, et al. Randomized trial of etoposide and cisplatin versus etoposide and carboplatin in patients

with good-risk germ cell tumors: a multiinstitutional study. *J Clin Oncol.* 1993;11(4):598-606.

15. Horwich A, Sleijfer DT, Fossa SD, et al. Randomized trial of bleomycin, etoposide, and cisplatin compared with bleomycin, etoposide, and carboplatin in good-prognosis metastatic nonseminomatous germ cell cancer: a Multiinstitutional Medical Research Council/European Organization for Research and Treatment of Cancer Trial. *J Urol.* 1998;159:1099-1100. doi:10.1016/s0022-5347(01)63845-x

16. Dimopoulos MA, Papadimitriou C, Hamilos G, et al. Treatment of ovarian germ cell tumors with a 3-day bleomycin, etoposide, and cisplatin regimen: a prospective multicenter study. *Gynecol Oncol.* 2004;95(3):695-700. doi:10.1016/j.ygyno.2004.08.018

17. Chen CA, Lin H, Weng CS, et al. Outcome of 3-day bleomycin, etoposide and cisplatin chemotherapeutic regimen for patients with malignant ovarian germ cell tumours: a Taiwanese Gynecologic Oncology Group study. *Eur J Cancer.* 2014;50(18):3161-3167. doi:10.1016/j.ejca.2014.10.006

18. McKeage MJ, Evans BD, Atkinson C, Perez D, Forgeson GV, Dady PJ. Carbon monoxide diffusing capacity is a poor predictor of clinically significant bleomycin lung. New Zealand Clinical Oncology Group. *J Clin Oncol.* 1990;8(5):779-783.

19. Loehrer PJ, Johnson D, Elson P, et al. Importance of bleomycin in favorable-prognosis disseminated germ cell tumors: an Eastern Cooperative Oncology Group trial. *J Clin Oncol.* 1995;13(2):470-476.

20. de Wit R, Stoter G, Kaye SB, et al. Importance of bleomycin in combination chemotherapy for good-prognosis testicular nonseminoma: a randomized study of the European Organization for Research and Treatment of Cancer Genitourinary Tract Cancer Cooperative Group. *J Clin Oncol.* 1997;15:1837-1843.

21. Linasmita V, Wilailak S, Srisupundit S. Cis-platinum-based chemotherapy in management of malignant ovarian germ cell tumors. *Int J Gynecol Obstet.* 1998;61:69-71.

22. American Society of Clinical Oncology. Recommendations for the use of hematopoietic colony-stimulating factors: evidence-based, clinical practice guidelines. *J Clin Oncol.* 1994;12(11):2471-2508.

23. Pedersen-Bjergaard J, Daugaard G, Hansen SW, Rørth M, Philip P, Larsen SO. Increased risk of myelodysplasia and leukaemia after etoposide, cisplatin, and bleomycin for germ-cell tumours. *Lancet.* 1991;338(8763):359-363. doi:10.1016/0140-6736(91)90490-G

24. Pedersen-Bjergaard J, Brøndum-Nielsen K, Karle H, Johansson B. Chemotherapy-related—and late occurring—Philadelphia chromosome in AML, ALL and CML. Similar events related to treatment with DNA topoisomerase II inhibitors? *Leukemia.* 1997;11(9):1571-1574. doi:10.1038/sj.leu.2400769

25. Pui CH. Epipodophyllotoxin-related acute myeloid leukaemia. *Lancet.* 1991;338(8780):1468. doi:10.1016/0140-6736(91)92779-2

26. Pui CH, Ribeiro RC, Hancock ML, et al. Acute Myeloid Leukemia in children treated with epipodophyllotoxins for acute lymphoblastic leukemia. *N Engl J Med.* 1991;325(24):1682-1687. doi:10.1056/NEJM199112123252402

27. Ratain MJ, Kaminer LS, Bitran JD, et al. Acute nonlymphocytic leukemia following etoposide and cisplatin combination chemotherapy for advanced non-small-cell carcinoma of the lung. *Blood.* 1987;70(5):1412-1417. doi:10.1182/blood.V70.5.1412.1412

28. Newton C, Murali K, Ahmad A, et al. A multicentre retrospective cohort study of ovarian germ cell tumours: evidence for chemotherapy de-escalation and alignment of paediatric and adult practice. *Eur J Cancer.* 2019;113:19-27. doi:10.1016/j.ejca.2019.03.001

29. Travis LB, Holowaty EJ, Bergfeldt K, et al. Risk of leukemia after platinum-based chemotherapy for ovarian cancer. *N Engl J Med.* 1999;340(5):351-357. doi:10.1056/nejm199902043400504

30. Hellesnes R, Kvammen Ø, Myklebust T, et al. Continuing increased risk of second cancer in long-term testicular cancer survivors after treatment in the cisplatin era. *Int J Cancer.* 2020;147(1):21-32. doi:10.1002/ijc.32704

31. Hjelle LV, Gundersen PO, Oldenburg J, et al. Long-term platinum retention after platinum-based chemotherapy in testicular cancer survivors: a 20-year follow-up study. *Anticancer Res.* 2015;35(3):1619-1625.

32. Tothill P, Klys HS, Matheson LM, McKay K, Smyth JF. The long-term retention of platinum in human tissues following the administration of cisplatin or carboplatin for cancer chemotherapy. *Eur J Cancer.* 1992;28(8-9):1358-1361. doi:10.1016/0959-8049(92)90519-8

33. Byrne J, Mulvihill JJ, Myers MH, et al. Effects of treatment on fertility in long-term survivors of childhood or adolescent cancer. *N Engl J Med.* 1987;317(21):1315-1321. doi:10.1056/NEJM198711193172104

34. Siris ES, Leventhal BG, Vaitukaitis JL. Effects of childhood leukemia and chemotherapy on puberty and reproductive function in girls. *N Engl J Med.* 1976;294(21):1143-1146. doi:10.1056/NEJM197605202942102

35. Nicosia SV, Matus-Ridley M, Meadows AT. Gonadal effects of cancer therapy in girls. *Cancer.* 1985;55(10):2364-2372. doi:10.1002/1097-0142(19850515)55:10<2364::AID-CNCR2820551011>3.0.CO;2-E

36. Ju UC, Kang WD, Kim SM. Oncologic and reproductive outcomes after fertility-sparing surgery in young women with malignant ovarian germ cell tumors. *Eur J Gynaecol Oncol.* 2021;42(5):832-837. doi:10.31083/j.ejgo4205127

37. Tamauchi S, Kajiyama H, Yoshihara M, et al. Reproductive outcomes of 105 malignant ovarian germ cell tumor survivors: a multicenter study. *Am J Obstet Gynecol.* 2018;219(4):385.e1-385.e7. doi:10.1016/j.ajog.2018.07.021

38. Zamani N, Rezaei Poor M, Ghasemian Dizajmehr S, Alizadeh S, Modares Gilani M. Fertility sparing surgery in malignant ovarian Germ cell tumor (MOGCT): 15 years experiences. *BMC Womens Health.* 2021;21(1):1-7. doi:10.1186/s12905-021-01437-8

39. Gershenson DM. Menstrual and reproductive function after treatment with combination chemotherapy for malignant ovarian germ cell tumors. *J Clin Oncol.* 1988;6(2):270-275.

40. Gershenson DM, Miller AM, Champion VL, et al. Reproductive and sexual function after platinum-based chemotherapy in long-term ovarian germ cell tumor survivors: a Gynecologic Oncology Group Study. *J Clin Oncol.* 2007;25(19):2792-2797.

41. Brewer M, Gershenson DM, Herzog CE, et al. Outcome and reproductive function after chemotherapy for ovarian dysgerminoma. *J Clin Oncol.* 1999;17(9):2670-2675.

42. Rustin GJ, Pektasides D, Bagshawe KD, Newlands ES, Begent RH. Fertility after chemotherapy for male and female germ cell tumours. *Int J Androl.* 1987;10(1):389-392. doi:10.1111/j.1365-2605.1987.tb00208.x

43. Pektasides D, Rustin GJS, Newlands ES. Fertility after chemotherapy for ovarian germ cell tumours. *Int J Gynecol Obstet.* 1988;26(2):333. doi:10.1016/0020-7292(88)90301-3

44. Zanetta G, Bonazzi C, Cantu M, et al. Survival and reproductive function after treatment of malignant germ cell ovarian tumors. *J Clin Oncol.* 2001;19(4):1015-1020.

45. Champion V, Williams SD, Miller A, et al. Quality of life in long-term survivors of ovarian germ cell tumors: a Gynecologic Oncology Group Study. *Gynecol Oncol.* 2007;105(3):687-694. doi:10.1016/j.ygyno.2007.01.042

46. Billmire DF, Cullen JW, Rescorla FJ, et al. Surveillance after initial surgery for pediatric and adolescent girls with stage I ovarian germ cell tumors: report from the Children's Oncology Group. *J Clin Oncol.* 2014;32(5):465-470. doi:10.1200/JCO.2013.51.1006

47. Matei D, Miller AM, Monahan P, et al. Chronic physical effects and health care utilization in long-term ovarian germ cell tumor survivors: a Gynecologic Oncology Group study. *J Clin Oncol.* 2009;27(25):4142-4149.

48. Hale GA, Marina NM, Jones-Wallace D, et al. Late effects of treatment for germ cell tumors during childhood and adolescence. *J Pediatr Hematol Oncol.* 1999;21(2):115-122. doi:10.1097/00043426-199903000-00007

49. Fung C, Dinh P, Ardeshir-Rouhani-Fard S, Schaffer K, Fossa SD, Travis LB. Toxicities associated with cisplatin-based chemotherapy and radiotherapy in long-term testicular cancer survivors. *Adv Urol.* 2018;2018:8671832. doi:10.1155/2018/8671832

50. Hellesnes R, Myklebust TÅ, Fosså SD, et al. Testicular cancer in the cisplatin era: causes of death and mortality rates in a population-based cohort. *J Clin Oncol.* 2021;39(32):3561-3573. doi:10.1200/jco.21.00637

51. De Palo G, Lattuada A, Kenda R, et al. Germ cell tumors of the ovary: the experience of the National Cancer Institute of Milan. I. Dysgerminoma. *Int J Radiat Oncol Biol Phys.* 1987;13(6):853-860. doi:10.1016/0360-3016(87)90099-X

52. Krepart G, Smith JP, Rutledge F, Delclos L. The treatment for dysgerminoma of the ovary. *Cancer.* 1978;41(3):986-990. doi:10.1002/1097-0142(197803)41:3<986::AID-CNCR2820410328>3.0.CO;2-P

53. Lawson AP, Adler GF. Radiotherapy in the treatment of ovarian dysgerminomas. *Int J Radiat Oncol Biol Phys.* 1988;14(3):431-434. doi:10.1016/0360-3016(88)90256-8

54. Freed JH, Cassir JF, Pierce VK, et al. Dysgerminoma of the ovary. *Cancer.* 1979;43(3):798-805.

55. Marks RD, Underwood PB, Othersen HB, Wallace KM, Moore TN. Dysgerminoma-100% control with combined therapy in six consecutive patients with advanced disease. *Int J Radiat Oncol Biol Phys.* 1978;4(5):453-456. doi:10.1016/0360-3016(78)90078-0

56. Björkholm E, Gyftodimos A, Lundell M, Silfverswärd C. Dysgerminoma. The Radiumhemmet series 1927-1984. *Cancer.* 1990;65(1):38-44. doi:10.1002/1097-0142(19900101)65:1<38::AID-CNCR2820650110>3.0.CO;2-U

57. Santoni R, Cionini L, D'Elia F, Scarselli GF, Branconi F, Savino L. Dysgerminoma of the ovary: a report on 29 patients. *Clin Radiol.* 1987;38(2):203-206. doi:10.1016/S0009-9260(87)80038-7

58. Solheim O, Gershenson DM, Tropé CG, et al. Prognostic factors in malignant ovarian germ cell tumours (The surveillance, epidemiology and end results experience 1978-2010). *Eur J Cancer.* 2014;50(11):1942-1950. doi:10.1016/j.ejca.2014.03.288

59. Howell S, Shalet S. Gonadal damage from chemotherapy and radiotherapy. *Endocrinol Metab Clin North Am.* 1988;27(4):927-943.

60. Casey AC, Bhodauria S, Shapter A, Nieberg R, Berek JS, Farias-Eisner R. Dysgerminoma: the role of conservative surgery. *Gynecol Oncol.* 1996;63(3):352-357. doi:10.1006/gyno.1996.0335

61. Ayhan A, Bildirici I, Gunalp S, et al. Pure dysgerminoma of the ovary: a review of 45 well staged cases. *Eur J Gynaecol Oncol.* 2000;21(1):98-101.

62. Ledermann JA, Raja FA, Fotopoulou C, Gonzalez-Martin A, Colombo N, Sessa C. Newly diagnosed and relapsed epithelial ovarian carcinoma: ESMO clinical practice guidelines for diagnosis, treatment and follow-up. *Ann Oncol.* 2013;24(suppl 6):vi24-vi32. doi:10.1093/annonc/mdt333

63. Faure-Conter C, Pashankar F. Immature ovarian teratoma: when to give adjuvant therapy? *J Pediatr Hematol Oncol.* 2017;39(7):487-489. doi:10.1097/MPH.0000000000000950

64. Pashankar F, Hale JP, Dang H, et al. Is adjuvant chemotherapy indicated in ovarian immature teratomas? A combined data analysis from the Malignant Germ Cell Tumor International Collaborative. *Cancer.* 2016;122(2):230-237. doi:10.1002/cncr.29732

65. Nasioudis D, Frey MK, Chapman-Davis E, Caputo TA, Holcomb KM. Surveillance only for high-risk FIGO stage IA/IB malignant ovarian germ cell tumors: results from a National Cancer Database. *Am J Clin Oncol.* 2021;44(5):195-199. doi:10.1097/COC.0000000000000805

66. Grimison PS, Stockler MR, Chatfield M, et al. Accelerated BEP for metastatic germ cell tumours: a multicenter phase II trial by the Australian and New Zealand Urogenital and Prostate Cancer Trials Group (ANZUP). *Ann Oncol.* 2014;25(1):143-148. doi:10.1093/annonc/mdt369

67. Mahdi H, Swensen RE, Hanna R, et al. Prognostic impact of lymphadenectomy in clinically early stage malignant germ cell tumour of the ovary. *Br J Cancer.* 2011;105(4):493-497. doi:10.1038/bjc.2011.267

68. Williams SD, Blessing JA, Hatch KD, et al. Chemotherapy of advanced dysgerminoma: trials of the Gynecologic Oncology Group. *J Clin Oncol.* 1991;9(11):1950-1955.

69. Shah R, Xia C, Krailo M, et al. Is carboplatin-based chemotherapy as effective as cisplatin-based chemotherapy in the treatment of advanced-stage dysgerminoma in children, adolescents and young adults? *Gynecol Oncol.* 2018;150(2):253-260. doi:10.1016/j.ygyno.2018.05.025

70. Mangili G, Sigismondi C, Lorusso D, et al. The role of staging and adjuvant chemotherapy in stage I malignant ovarian germ cell tumors (MOGTs): the MITO-9 study. *Ann Oncol.* 2017;28(2):333-338. doi:10.1093/annonc/mdw563

71. Mangili G, Giorda G, Ferrandina G, et al. Surveillance alone in stage i malignant ovarian germ cell tumors: a MITO (Multicenter Italian Trials in Ovarian cancer) prospective observational study. *Int J Gynecol Cancer.* 2021;31(9):1242-1247. doi:10.1136/ijgc-2021-002575

72. Frazier AL, Stoneham S, Rodriguez-Galindo C, et al. Comparison of carboplatin versus cisplatin in the treatment of paediatric extracranial malignant germ cell tumours: a report of the Malignant Germ Cell International Consortium. *Eur J Cancer.* 2018;98:30-37. doi:10.1016/j.ejca.2018.03.004

73. Norris HJ, Zirkin HJ, Benson WL. Immature (malignant) teratoma of the ovary: a clinical and pathologic study of 58 cases. *Cancer.* 1976;37(5):2359-2372.

74. Gershenson DM, del Junco G, Silva EG, et al. Immature teratoma of ovary. *Obstet Gynecol.* 1986;68:624-629.

75. Cushing B, Giller R, Ablin A, et al. Surgical resection alone is effective treatment for ovarian immature teratoma in children and adolescents: a report of the Pediatric Oncology Group and the Children's Cancer Group. *Am J Obstet Gynecol.* 1999;181(2):353-358. doi:10.1016/S0002-9378(99)70561-2

76. Marina NM, Cushing B, Giller R, et al. Complete surgical excision is effective treatment for children with immature teratomas with or without malignant elements: a Pediatric Oncology Group/Children's Cancer Intergroup Study. *J Clin Oncol.* 1999;17(7):2137-2143.

77. Dark GG, Bower M, Newlands ES, Paradinas F, Rustin GJ. Surveillance policy for stage I ovarian germ cell tumors. *J Clin Oncol.* 1997;15(2):620-624. doi:10.1200/JCO.1997.15.2.620

78. Bonazzi C, Peccatori F, Colombo N, Lucchini V, Cantu MG, Mangioni C. Pure ovarian immature teratoma, a unique and curable disease: 10 years' experience of 32 prospectively treated patients. *Obstet Gynecol.* 1994;84(4):598-604.

79. Mann JR, Gray ES, Thornton C, et al. Mature and immature extracranial teratomas in children: the UK Children's Cancer Study Group experience. *J Clin Oncol.* 2008;26:3590-3597.

80. Wetherell D. Mature and immature teratoma: a review of pathological characteristics and treatment options. *Med Surg Urol.* 2014;3(1):1-5. doi:10.4172/2168-9857.1000124

81. Bergamini A, Sarwar N, Ferrandina G, et al. Response to letter entitled: re: can we replace adjuvant chemotherapy with surveillance for stage IA-C immature ovarian teratomas of any grade? An international multicenter analysis. *Eur J Cancer.* 2021;152:257-258. doi:10.1016/j.ejca.2021.05.002

82. Mitchell PL, Al-Nasiri N, A'Hern R, et al. Treatment of nondysgerminomatous ovarian germ cell tumors: an analysis of 69 cases. *Cancer.* 1999;85(10):2232-2244. doi:10.1002/(SICI)1097-0142(19990515)85:10<2232::AID-CNCR19>3.0.CO;2-4

83. Patterson DM, Murugaesu N, Holden L, Seckl MJ, Rustin GJS. A review of the close surveillance policy for stage I female germ cell tumors of the ovary and other sites. *Int J Gynecol Cancer.* 2008;18(1):43-50. doi:10.1111/j.1525-1438.2007.00969.x

84. Park JY, Kim DY, Suh DS, et al. Outcomes of surgery alone and surveillance strategy in young women with stage I malignant ovarian germ cell tumors. *Int J Gynecol Cancer.* 2016;26(5):859-864. doi:10.1097/IGC.0000000000000702

85. Storey DJ, Rush R, Stewart M, et al. Endometrioid epithelial ovarian cancer: 20 years of prospectively collected data from a single center. *Cancer.* 2008;112(10):2211-2220. doi:10.1002/cncr.23438

CHAPTER **9.7**

Treatment of Persistent and Recurrent Ovarian Germ Cell Tumors

Brenna E. Swift and Allan Covens

MANAGEMENT OF RESIDUAL OR RECURRENT DISEASE

The large majority of patients with OGCTs are cured with surgery and platinum-based chemotherapy. However, a small percentage of patients have persistent or progressive disease during treatment or recur after completion of treatment. Like in testicular cancer, these treatment failures are categorized as platinum resistant (progression during or within 4-6 weeks of completing treatment) or platinum sensitive (recurrence beyond 6 weeks from platinum-based therapy). In a series from MDACC, 42 treatment failures were identified among 160 patients with OGCTs treated between 1970 and 1990 (1). Treatment failure in these patients was attributed to inadequate surgery in 14 patients, inadequate radiation in five patients, inadequate chemotherapy in 16 patients (underdosing and noncompliance), treatment-related toxicity in one patient, and unidentifiable causes in six patients. A significant number of patients included in this series had received VAC-based chemotherapy, which accounted for the higher-than-expected rate of recurrence.

Given the high curability rate of OGCTs with primary treatment, the management of recurrent disease represents a complex and often difficult issue and preferably should be performed in a specialized center. Data to guide the management of patients with recurrent OGCTs are scant and largely extrapolated from the clinical experience with testicular cancer. The single most important prognostic factor in patients with testicular cancer is whether or not they are refractory to cisplatin. The likelihood of cure with high-dose salvage therapy in patients who relapse from a complete remission after initial therapy is as high as 60% or more. On the other hand, in patients who are truly cisplatin refractory, the likelihood of long-term survival and cure is significantly less. However, up to 30% to 40% of these patients can become long-term survivors. Approximately 30% of patients with recurrent platinum-sensitive testicular cancer can be salvaged with second-line chemotherapy (vinblastine, ifosfamide, platinum) (2). High-dose therapy with carboplatin, etoposide with or without cyclophosphamide or ifosfamide, and stem cell rescue has been shown to be highly active in this setting (3,4).

Generally, in patients who are not cisplatin refractory, one course of standard-dose therapy, usually cisplatin, vinblastine, and ifosfamide, is given. If an initial response is seen, then two subsequent courses of high-dose chemotherapy (HDCT) with carboplatin and etoposide and stem cell rescue are undertaken (5). A report from the Indiana University describes this approach among 184 patients with recurrent testicular cancer. At a median follow-up of 48 months, 116 patients were in complete remission. Remarkably, of the subgroup of 40 patients who were platinum refractory, 18 became disease free after HDCT (6). Although this approach has not been prospectively tested in women with recurrent platinum-sensitive OGCTs, because of the rarity of such patients, the concepts are very similar and support the use of high-dose therapy in this setting. A retrospective analysis on the use of HDCT for recurrent OGCTs at the Indiana University revealed that patients with recurrent OGCTs tend to be referred late and have worse outcomes compared with their male counterparts (7). Of 13 women treated with HDCT for recurrent OGCTs, 11 had YSTs and eight were platinum refractory. In this series, four achieved long-term survival; however, only five received HDCT as second-line therapy, the rest being referred late in the course of their disease (7). Similarly, six patients received HDCT with autologous hematopoietic stem cell transplantation (ASCT) as first-line salvage regimen, with four achieving long-term EFS. HDCT was attempted in seven patients as a subsequent salvage treatment, but two patients did not have sufficient stem cells for ASCT, and of the five who completed treatment, only one achieved long-term EFS (8). It is, therefore, important to consider early referral to a specialized center for the management of recurrent disease to maximize chances of cure. An ongoing Alliance phase III clinical trial (NCT02375204) is comparing standard-dose salvage chemotherapy with paclitaxel, ifosfamide, and cisplatin versus a high-dose regimen with paclitaxel and ifosfamide followed by high-dose carboplatin and etoposide, with stem cell rescue as first salvage regimen for relapsed GCTs. The results of the study will set the definitive approach for the management of recurrent GCTs.

Active agents in the setting of recurrence after HDCT include ifosfamide, taxanes, gemcitabine, and oxaliplatin (9-12). In a phase II trial from the Indiana University, the combination of gemcitabine and paclitaxel induced objective responses in 10 of 31 patients who had recurred after HDCT. Of those, five patients were free of disease 2 years after treatment (6). The combination of gemcitabine and oxaliplatin induced a 46% response rate in a group of 31 patients with recurrent GCTs. Over 60% of these patients were platinum resistant or refractory (12).

TARGETED THERAPY, IMMUNOTHERAPY, AND OTHER NEW AND NOVEL AGENTS

For patients with platinum-resistant OGCTs, novel and targeted agents are needed.

The most common mutations detected in OGCTs were KIT and KRAS (13), similar to testicular GCTs (14). *KIT* gene mutations were found in 24% to 44% of dysgerminomas (13,15,16). Amplification of chromosome 12p, which contains the oncogene KRAS, was found in 82% of dysgerminomas, 58% of YSTs, and 43% of mixed GCTs, but not in ITs (13). In 33.3% of patients with YSTs, targetable oncogenic mutations in KRAS, KIT, and ARID1A were identified, including 66.7% of patients with relapsed disease (17).

Imatinib has shown success as a KIT-targeted treatment in GIST (18) and chronic myelogenous leukemia (19). In metastatic testicular seminoma, results are mixed with a complete response reported in one patient (20) followed by limited effectiveness in a small phase 2 trial of six patients (21). These mixed results may be related to the type of mutation in the *KIT* gene (22). Other potential therapies targeting KRAS mutations include MEK inhibitors, such as trametinib and cobimetinib, in colorectal and low-grade serous ovarian cancers (23,24). Preclinical results have shown tumors with ARID1A mutation are more susceptible to PARP inhibitors (25).

There have been limited studies in immunotherapy in OGCTs (25). Male GCTs have shown expression of programmed death ligand-1 (PD-L1) (26), but preliminary results of immune checkpoint inhibitors, including pembrolizumab and avelumab, in male GCTs showed no response (27,28). Two of seven platinum-refractory male germ cell patients with relapse after HDCT and ASCT had a long-term response to nivolumab and pembrolizumab. Both patients had high expression of PD-L1 (29). An ongoing trial is assessing dual checkpoint blockade with durvalumab, a PD-L1 inhibitor, and tremelimumab, a cytotoxic T lymphocyte–associated protein 4 (CTLA-4) inhibitor, in relapsed and refractory male GCTs (NCT03158064). Novel treatments for recurrent, refractory OGCTs are needed, and referral for treatment with investigational agents is appropriate.

REFERENCES

1. Messing MJ, Gershenson DM, Morris M, Burke TW, Kavanagh JJ, Wharton JT. Primary treatment failure in patients with malignant ovarian germ cell neoplasms. *Int J Gynecol cancer*. 1992;2(6):295-300. doi:10.1046/j.1525-1438.1992.02060295.x

2. Einhorn LH. Salvage therapy for germ cell tumors. *Semin Oncol*. 1994;21(4 suppl 7):47-51.

3. Broun ER, Nichols CR, Turns M, et al. Early salvage therapy for germ cell cancer using high dose chemotherapy with autologous bone marrow support. *Cancer*. 1994;73(6):1716-1720. doi:10.1002/1097-0142(19940315)73:6<1716::AID-CNCR2820730627>3.0.CO;2-L

4. Broun ER, Nichols CR, Gize G, et al. Tandem high dose chemotherapy with autologous bone marrow transplantation for initial relapse of testicular germ cell cancer. *Cancer*. 1997;79(8):1605-1610. doi:10.1002/(SICI)1097-0142(19970415)79:8<1605::AID-CNCR25>3.0.CO;2-0

5. Lotz J, André T, Donsimoni R, et al. High dose chemotherapy with ifosfamide, carboplatin, and etoposide combined with autologous bone marrow transplantation for the treatment of poor-prognosis germ cell tumors and metastatic trophoblastic disease in adults. *Cancer*. 1995;75(3):874-885. doi:10.1002/1097-0142(19950201)75:3<874::AID-CNCR2820750320>3.0.CO;2-Q

6. Einhorn LH, Williams SD, Chamness A, Brames MJ, Perkins SM, Abonour R. High-dose chemotherapy and stem-cell rescue for metastatic germ-cell tumors. *N Engl J Med*. 2007;357(4):340-348. doi:10.1056/NEJMoa067749

7. Ammakkanavar NR, Matei D, Abonour R, et al. High-dose chemotherapy for recurrent ovarian germ cell tumors. *J Clin Oncol*. 2015;33(2):226-227.

8. Meisel JL, Woo KM, Sudarsan N, et al. Development of a risk stratification system to guide treatment for female germ cell tumors. *Gynecol Oncol*. 2015;138(3):566-572. doi:10.1016/j.ygyno.2015.06.029

9. Loehrer PJ, Gonin R, Nichols CR, et al. Vinblastine plus ifosfamide plus cisplatin as initial salvage therapy in recurrent germ cell tumor. *J Clin Oncol*. 1998;16(7):2500-2504.

10. Hinton S, Catalano P, Einhorn LH, et al. Phase II study of paclitaxel plus gemcitabine in refractory germ cell tumors (E9897): a trial of the Eastern Cooperative Oncology Group. *J Clin Oncol.* 2002;20(7):1859-1863.

11. Einhorn LH, Brames MJ, Juliar B, et al. Phase II study of paclitaxel plus gemcitabine salvage chemotherapy for germ cell tumors after progression following high-dose chemotherapy with tandem transplant. *J Clin Oncol.* 2007;25(5):513-516.

12. Kollmannsberger C, Beyer J, Liersch R, et al. Combination chemotherapy with gemcitabine plus oxaliplatin in patients with intensively pretreated or refractory germ cell cancer: a study of the German Testicular Cancer Study Group. *J Clin Oncol.* 2004;22(1):108-114.

13. Van Nieuwenhuysen E, Busschaert P, Neven P, et al. The genetic landscape of 87 ovarian germ cell tumors. *Gynecol Oncol.* 2018;151(1):61-68. doi:10.1016/j.ygyno.2018.08.013

14. Shen H, Wang L, Bowlby R, et al. Integrated molecular characterization of testicular germ cell tumors. *Cell Rep.* 2018;23(11):3392-3406. doi:10.1016/j.celrep.2018.05.039

15. Cheng L, Roth LM, Zhang S, et al. KIT gene mutation and amplification in dysgerminoma of the ovary. *Cancer.* 2011;117(10):2096-2103. doi:10.1002/cncr.25794

16. Hoei-Hansen CE, Kraggerud SM, Abeler VM, Kærn J, Rajpert-De Meyts E, Lothe RA. Ovarian dysgerminomas are characterised by frequent KIT mutations and abundant expression of pluripotency markers. *Mol Cancer.* 2007;6(1):12. doi:10.1186/1476-4598-6-12

17. Hodroj K, Stevovic A, Attignon V, et al. Molecular characterization of ovarian yolk sac tumor (OYST). *Cancers (Basel).* 2021;13(2):1-9. doi:10.3390/cancers13020220

18. Corless CL, Barnett CM, Heinrich MC. Gastrointestinal stromal tumours: origin and molecular oncology. *Nat Rev Cancer.* 2011;11(12):865-878. doi:10.1038/nrc3143

19. Eiring AM, Khorashad JS, Morley K, Deininger MW. Advances in the treatment of chronic myeloid leukemia. *BMC Med.* 2011;9(1):99. doi:10.1186/1741-7015-9-99

20. Pedersini R, Vattemi E, Mazzoleni G, Graiff C. Complete response after treatment with imatinib in pretreated disseminated testicular seminoma with overexpression of c-KIT. *Lancet Oncol.* 2007;8(11):1039-1040. doi:10.1016/S1470-2045(07)70344-3

21. Einhorn LH, Brames MJ, Heinrich MC, Corless CL, Madani A. Phase II study of imatinib mesylate in chemotherapy refractory germ cell tumors expressing KIT. *Am J Clin Oncol.* 2006;29:12-13.

22. Jen JY, Routh ED, Rubinas T, et al. KRAS/BRAF mutation status and ERK1/2 activation as biomarkers for MEK1/2 inhibitor therapy in colorectal cancer. *Mol Cancer Ther.* 2009;8(4):834-843. doi:10.1158/1535-7163.MCT-08-0972

23. Gershenson DM. A randomized phase II/III study to assess the efficacy of trametinib in patients with recurrent or progressive low-grade serous ovarian or peritoneal cancer. *Gynecol Oncol.* 2020;159:22. doi:10.1016/j.ygyno.2020.06.045

24. Park Y, Chui MH, Suryo Rahmanto Y, et al. Loss of ARID1A in tumor cells renders selective vulnerability to combined ionizing radiation and PARP inhibitor therapy. *Clin Cancer Res.* 2019;25(18):5584-5593. doi:10.1158/1078-0432.CCR-18-4222

25. Maoz A, Matsuo K, Ciccone MA, et al. Molecular pathways and targeted therapies for malignant ovarian germ cell tumors and sex cord–stromal tumors: a contemporary review. *Cancers (Basel).* 2020;12(6):1-24. doi:10.3390/cancers12061398

26. Fankhauser CD, Curioni-Fontecedro A, Allmann V, et al. Frequent PD-L1 expression in testicular germ cell tumors. *Br J Cancer.* 2015;113(3):411-413. doi:10.1038/bjc.2015.244

27. Adra N, Einhorn LH, Althouse SK, et al. Phase II trial of pembrolizumab in patients with platinum refractory germ-cell tumors: a Hoosier Cancer Research Network Study GU14-206. *Ann Oncol.* 2018;29(1):209-214. doi:10.1093/annonc/mdx680

28. Mego M, Svetlovska D, Chovanec M, et al. Phase II study of avelumab in multiple relapsed/refractory germ cell cancer. *Invest New Drugs.* 2019;37(4):748-754. doi:10.1007/s10637-019-00805-4

29. Zschäbitz S, Lasitschka F, Hadaschik B, et al. Response to anti-programmed cell death protein-1 antibodies in men treated for platinum refractory germ cell cancer relapsed after high-dose chemotherapy and stem cell transplantation. *Eur J Cancer.* 2017;76:1-7. doi:10.1016/j.ejca.2017.01.033

CHAPTER **9.8**

Ovarian Germ Cell Tumors: Special Conditions

Dan Wang and Bradley R. Corr

Two clinical conditions that affect patients with GCTs warrant specific discussion, including GP and growing teratoma syndrome (GTS).

GLIOMATOSIS PERITONEI

GP is a rare, benign condition characterized by mature glial tissue implants that are widespread throughout the peritoneum (1). GP is most often associated with IT, but various primary ovarian tumors have been described (2,3). There is a paucity of data in the literature about this condition, and therefore, its pathogenesis is poorly understood.

GP appears grossly as firm, gray to white miliary nodularity dispersed throughout the peritoneum and omentum. GP is often diagnosed on IHC staining using hematoxylin and eosin, demonstrating mature glial tissue (**Figure 9.8-1**). Neural IHC markers, such as glial fibrillary acidic protein (GFAP), aid in diagnosis and

are used to differentiate GP from low-grade ovarian epithelial tumor (**Figure 9.8-2**).

The exact pathogenesis of GP is unknown. One theory hypothesizes that the mature glial implants occur as a result of tumor rupture during initial surgery or as a result of angiolymphatic spread (4). This theory is supported by case reports demonstrating glial tissue in the omentum and retroperitoneal lymph nodes (1,5). A separate theory considers that GP is genetically unrelated to ovarian teratoma and instead derives from stem cells (2,6). In a case series of 21 patients, Liang et al found that all tumors expressed SOX2, but not OCT4 or NANOG, supporting a stem cell origin (3).

The prognosis of GP is generally considered favorable (4). It is a benign condition and is considered grade 0 by the WHO. Yoon et al reported a higher recurrence rate in patients with primary IT and concurrent GP compared to patients without GP, but OS was no different. Furthermore, all relapses were composed of mature glial tissue at the time of subsequent surgical removal (2). In patients

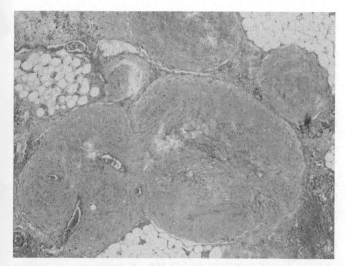

Figure 9.8-1. Hematoxylin and eosin stain, ×40 Peritoneal gliomatosis showing a discrete nodule of mature glial tissue, which is surrounded by fibroadipose tissue of the peritoneum.

in which GP was found at the time of initial surgery, Wang et al reported on 8 patients and found that even with residual disease after surgery, all patients were asymptomatic and alive (7). Although multiple case series have demonstrated favorable outcomes, long-term follow-up continues to be recommended for these patients, because recurrence and malignant transformation have been reported. The validity of malignant transformation has been challenged (4,9).

IT with GP often occurs in young patients, and fertility-sparing treatment should be considered in such patients who wish to preserve fertility. Complete resection of GP is often not feasible due to the extensive miliary distribution. Wang et al describe eight patients with GP who were treated with FSS; all but one had residual disease postoperatively. All patients were alive, with a median follow-up of 60.5 (3-144) months, and 3 patients experienced spontaneous pregnancy (7). Similarly, Bentivegna et al reported on 6 patients with GP treated with conservative surgery, of which only one had complete macroscopic resection. No patients died of their disease, with a median follow-up of 39 months (range 6-114) (10). These case series suggest that GP can be quiescent for extended periods of time without impacting survival. Therefore, a conservative surgical approach may be considered in these patients after exclusion of the rare coexistence of metastatic IT.

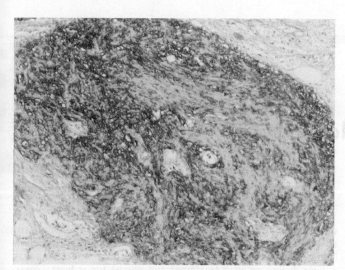

Figure 9.8-2. Positive immunohistochemical staining of the mature glial tissue with glial fibrillary acidic protein, ×100.

GROWING TERATOMA SYNDROME

GTS is a rare clinical entity that presents as an enlarging mass either during or after chemotherapy in up to 40% of patients with IT (11). GTS most commonly occurs in patients with ovarian ITs or mixed OGCTs who have received adjuvant chemotherapy, but it has also been described in men with testicular germ cell cancers. The incidence of GTS in MOGCTs varies from 12% to 40% (11). To date, less than 200 cases are reported in the literature.

The diagnosis of GTS requires benign tumor growth during or after adjuvant chemotherapy, normal serum tumor markers, and pathologic demonstration of mature teratoma in the resected specimen (12).

Owing to the rarity of GTS, the etiology and clinical behaviors are still poorly understood. The two hypotheses surrounding pathogenesis of GTS include (1) transformation of malignant cells into benign mature elements and (2) selective elimination of malignant elements by chemotherapy leaving residual mature, chemotherapy-resistant components (13). Ultimately, these different descriptions describe a similar process whereby malignant tumor components are eliminated (14). It is important to note that IT does have the potential to recur as mature elements, even without prior adjuvant chemotherapy.

Several authors have suggested risk factors for GTS. André et al suggest that risk factors for the development of GTS in nonseminomatous germ cell tumors (NSGCTs) include (1) the presence of mature elements in the primary tumor, (2) no tumor reduction of size during chemotherapy, and (3) the presence of mature elements in postchemotherapy residual masses (15). Kikawa et al describe risk factors for GTS as incomplete resection of primary tumor, the presence of high-grade IT in primary tumor, and advanced stage (16). Additional risk factors include the presence of neuroectodermal tumor and involvement of primary peritoneum (17). Wang et al comprehensively evaluated 175 patients with ovarian IT, of whom 35 developed GTS. Residual disease at initial surgery and the presence of GP were found to be independent risk factors. In their study, 38.9% of patients with GP developed GTS during subsequent follow-up (18). This has prompted some to consider GP as a subtype of GTS (10). Therefore, clinicians should be aware that patients with IT and GP may develop subsequent GTS and that evidence of clinical recurrence requires biopsy to differentiate benign GTS or GP from malignant disease.

Contrary to NSGCT, which is highly chemosensitive, GTS is resistant to both chemotherapy and RT. Therefore, surgery is the cornerstone of the treatment for GTS. Surgical debulking with complete resection is the primary treatment, and histology should confirm the diagnosis. Complete resection is essential, as the recurrence rate for partial resection is 72% to 83%, compared with 0% to 12.7% for complete resection (19). Wang et al demonstrated that only one of 18 patients developed a GTS recurrence after a complete resection, compared to 10 of 17 patients after an incomplete resection. The presence of residual disease after GTS surgery was a risk factor for recurrence (18). Similarly, André et al described 30 patients with GTS who underwent residual tumor resection. The recurrence rate for patients with an incomplete resection was 84%, compared with 4% after a complete resection (15). In a literature review of 48 patients with GTS, Kikawa et al found that four patients who underwent incomplete resection recurred (16). Based on these data, complete surgical resection should be the goal for every patient with GTS.

GTS is most commonly confined to the pelvis, abdomen, and retroperitoneum, but rare distant metastatic sites such as lung and mediastinum have also been described (20). GTS usually recurs as multiple large metastases in the peritoneal cavity that compress adjacent vascular, hepatic, urologic, and gastrointestinal structures. Owing to this large size and the complexity of surgery, the treatment often involves a multidisciplinary surgical approach and should be performed at a tertiary referral center (18). The complexity of the surgery has up to an 11% reported mortality (19).

FSS is an option for women of childbearing potential with mixed OGCTs, but limited data exist surrounding FSS in patients with GTS. Bentivegna et al have reported the largest surgical outcomes series after primary debulking surgery for ovarian GTS (N = 38).

Twenty of these patients underwent conservative surgical treatment. Six patients desired future fertility; of these six patients, four patients conceived spontaneously and one patient conceived with assisted reproductive technology (21). Wang et al describe 27 of 35 patients with GTS who underwent FSS after the diagnosis of GTS. During follow-up, FSS was not associated with an increased risk of GTS recurrence compared with radical surgery. Four of seven patients with desired fertility conceived, resulting in five singleton pregnancies. At a median follow-up of 73 months (range 11-401), three patients were alive with no evidence of disease, and one was alive with disease (18). Based on these data, FSS is feasible in young patients with desired fertility, as the overall prognosis of GTS is favorable, and spontaneous pregnancy after the treatment of GTS is possible.

Patients with GTS should continue surveillance, as GTS has a variable growth rate and unpredictable clinical behavior. GTS usually develops within 24 months of initial surgery, but development up to 19 years later has been reported (22). It is crucial to differentiate between recurrent malignant IT and GTS, as the treatment strategy and prognosis are markedly different. Patients with recurrent malignant IT require complete resection followed by adjuvant chemotherapy; patients with GTS require complete resection to relieve compression and reduce the risk of recurrence, but adjuvant chemotherapy is not indicated.

The overall prognosis of GTS is excellent, with a low but present risk of malignant transformation to sarcoma, adenocarcinoma, and carcinoid tumor (20,23). The 5-year OS after GTS is 89%; reported deaths were attributed to postoperative complications (19). Prolonged follow-up with tumor markers and imaging should be considered.

REFERENCES

1. Robboy SJ, Scully RE. Ovarian teratoma with glial implants on the peritoneum. An analysis of 12 cases. *Hum Pathol.* 1970;1(4):643-653.

2. Yoon NR, Lee JW, Kim BG, et al. Gliomatosis peritonei is associated with frequent recurrence, but does not affect overall survival in patients with ovarian immature teratoma. *Virchows Arch.* 2012;461(3):299-304.

3. Liang L, Zhang Y, Malpica A, et al. Gliomatosis peritonei: a clinicopathologic and immunohistochemical study of 21 cases. *Mod Pathol.* 2015;28(12):1613-1620.

4. Nielsen SN, Scheithauer BW, Gaffey TA. Gliomatosis peritonei. *Cancer.* 1985;56(10):2499-2503.

5. Kim NR, Lim S, Jeong J, Cho HY. Peritoneal and nodal gliomatosis with endometriosis, accompanied with ovarian immature teratoma: a case study and literature review. *Korean J Pathol.* 2013;47(6):587-591.

6. Ferguson AW, Katabuchi H, Ronnett BM, Cho KR. Glial implants in gliomatosis peritonei arise from normal tissue, not from the associated teratoma. *Am J Pathol.* 2001;159(1):51-55.

7. Wang D, Jia CW, Feng RE, Shi HH, Sun J. Gliomatosis peritonei: a series of eight cases and review of the literature. *J Ovarian Res.* 2016;9(1):45.

8. Wang D, Zhu S, Jia C, Cao D, Yang J, Xiang Y. Oncological and reproductive outcomes of cystectomy compared with unilateral salpingo-oophorectomy as fertility-sparing surgery in patients with apparent early stage pure immature ovarian teratomas. *Ann Surg Oncol.* 2021;28(11):6684-6693.

9. Dadmanesh F, Miller DM, Swenerton KD, Clement PB. Gliomatosis peritonei with malignant transformation. *Mod Pathol.* 1997;10(6):597-601.

10. Bentivegna E, Gonthier C, Uzan C, et al. Gliomatosis peritonei: a particular entity with specific outcomes within the growing teratoma syndrome. *Int J Gynecol Cancer.* 2015;25(2):244-249.

11. Van Nguyen JM, Bouchard-Fortier G, Ferguson SE, Covens A. How common is the growing teratoma syndrome in patients with ovarian immature teratoma? *Int J Gynecol Cancer.* 2016;26(7):1201-1206.

12. Logothetis CJ, Samuels ML, Trindade A, Johnson DE. The growing teratoma syndrome. *Cancer.* 1982;50(8):1629-1635.

13. DiSaia PJ, Saltz A, Kagan AR, Morrow CP. Chemotherapeutic retroconversion of immature teratoma of the ovary. *Obstet Gynecol.* 1977;49(3):346-350.

14. Amsalem H, Nadjari M, Prus D, Hiller N, Benshushan A. Growing teratoma syndrome vs chemotherapeutic retroconversion: case report and review of the literature. *Gynecol Oncol.* 2004;92(1):357-360.

15. André F, Fizazi K, Culine S, et al. The growing teratoma syndrome: results of therapy and long-term follow-up of 33 patients. *Eur J Cancer.* 2000;36(11):1389-1394.

16. Kikawa S, Todo Y, Minobe S, Yamashiro K, Kato H, Sakuragi N. Growing teratoma syndrome of the ovary: a case report with FDG-PET findings. *J Obstet Gynaecol Res.* 2011;37(7):926-932.

17. Zagame L, Pautier P, Duvillard P, Castaigne D, Patte C, Lhommé C. Growing teratoma syndrome after ovarian germ cell tumors. *Obstet Gynecol.* 2006;108(3 pt 1):509-514.

18. Wang D, Zhu S, Jia C, et al. Diagnosis and management of growing teratoma syndrome after ovarian immature teratoma: a single center experience. *Gynecol Oncol.* 2020;157(1):94-100.

19. Saso S, Galazis N, Iacovou C, et al. Managing growing teratoma syndrome: new insights and clinical applications. *Future Sci OA.* 2019;5(9):FSO419.

20. Djordjevic B, Euscher ED, Malpica A. Growing teratoma syndrome of the ovary: review of literature and first report of a carcinoid tumor arising in a growing teratoma of the ovary. *Am J Surg Pathol.* 2007;31(12):1913-1918.

21. Bentivegna E, Azaïs H, Uzan C, et al. Surgical outcomes after debulking surgery for intraabdominal ovarian growing teratoma syndrome: analysis of 38 cases. *Ann Surg Oncol.* 2015;22(suppl 3):S964-S970.

22. Tantitamit T, U'Wais A, Huang KG. An ultralate female growing teratoma syndrome: 19 years after aggressive treatment for advanced ovarian immature teratoma. *Gynecol Minim Invasive Ther.* 2020;9(3):150-153.

23. Kato N, Uchigasaki S, Fukase M. How does secondary neoplasm arise from mature teratomas in growing teratoma syndrome of the ovary? A report of two cases. *Pathol Int.* 2013;63(12):607-610.

CHAPTER **9.9**

Ovarian Germ Cell Tumors: Follow-Up and Survivorship Issues

Olesya Solheim and David M. Gershenson

SURVIVORSHIP

Based on the excellent survival outcomes of most patients with malignant ovarian germ cell tumors (MOGCTs) when treated according to modern therapeutic principles and the long life expectancy of survivors, the prevention and eventual treatment of long-term adverse effects has become an important issue. The designation "long-term effects" refers to adverse events or complications that appear during or after treatment and persist for at least 1 year, whereas "late effects" are those that become clinically important

1 year or later after the termination of treatment (1). Long-term toxicities may remain constant over time or may decrease or increase after treatment. Long-term adverse effects that impact well-being of patients with malignant GCTs have been reported in multiple studies of testicular cancer survivors (2,3). These effects include treatment-induced peripheral neurotoxicity and ototoxicity, and increased risk of cardiovascular disease, metabolic syndrome, Raynaud phenomenon, hypogonadism, infertility, and second cancers. Though the incidence and development of late effects might be lower in woman than in men with GCTs, very few studies have assessed long-term effects in MOGCT survivors.

Neurotoxicity

Peripheral neurotoxicity is one of the most common long-term effects of treatment with cisplatin-based chemotherapy (CBCT) (4-6). The neurotoxic effects of CBCT are often limited to sensory functions; they do usually not impair motor functions (4). Although axonal damage has been related to CBCT, the principal pathophysiologic effect is due to degeneration of the dorsal nerve ganglion, where this drug accumulates (6-8). Clinical, electrophysiologic, morphologic, and toxicologic studies have demonstrated that neuropathy occurs early in CBCT (9). Further studies have suggested that peripheral neuropathy usually progresses for approximately 3 to 6 months after CBCT and eventually subsides in most patients, although recovery is often incomplete. The development, incidence, and severity of cisplatin-induced neuropathy and its relative clinical symptoms depend not only on individual risk factors but also on the cumulative dose, treatment duration, and, probably, also dose intensity (4-11). In testicular cancer survivors, the degree of self-reported, long-term neuropathy has been associated with serum cisplatin level, which is detectible within a median of 11 years after CBCT (12). About half of the MOGCT survivors reported "overall neuropathy" after their CBCT, but only 10% of them had severe pathologic, neurologic, or neurophysiologic findings with impact on daily living (5).

Ototoxicity

Cisplatin-induced ototoxicity represents a distinct feature of neurotoxicity, presumably caused by selective damage to the outer hair cells (13). Cisplatin-induced ototoxicity may be experienced during or after CBCT; it typically manifests as tinnitus or a high-frequency hearing loss and shows large interindividual variations (14-16). Depending on the number of chemotherapy cycles and the type of schedule applied, approximately 20% to 30% of long-term testicular cancer survivors experience neuro/ototoxicity following CBCT (15,16).

Raynaud Phenomenon

Raynaud phenomenon is an abnormal vasospastic response to low temperatures or emotional stress that causes reduced blood supply to the fingers and toes. As a result, hypoxia with a marked white or blue discoloration of fingers and toes appears, paired with coldness, stiffness, and numbness during the attacks. Both bleomycin and cisplatin are believed to contribute to cold-induced vasospasms (17,18). RT can also lead to Raynaud phenomenon (19). Twenty to 40% of testicular cancer survivors report Raynaud phenomenon after chemotherapy (4,11). Matei et al reported a higher prevalence of Raynaud phenomenon in long-term MOGCT survivors compared to age-matched controls (20).

Cardiovascular Disease and Metabolic Syndrome

The development of premature cardiovascular disease has become a growing concern in long-term testicular cancer survivors in whom cisplatin is believed to lead to endothelial dysfunction and development of premature atherosclerosis combined with the increase in dyslipidemia, hypertension, and increased body mass index (BMI) (21-24). The relative risk for subsequent myocardial infarction in 5-year testicular cancer survivors is nearly doubled after CBCT (24). The development of premature cardiovascular disease seems to be reflected in increased serum C-reactive protein levels 10 to 15 years before a serious cardiovascular event (myocardial infarction, stroke) (25). Smoking increases cisplatin-related risks of cardiovascular disease (21). In general, women have a lower risk of cardiovascular disease than men, so findings from testicular cancer survivors cannot be assumed to apply females with certainty.

Metabolic syndrome is characterized by a group of metabolic risk factors occurring in one person. These risk factors include abdominal obesity, dyslipidemia, hypertension, and insulin resistance. Several reports on testicular cancer survivors have suggested that metabolic syndrome is associated with the cumulative dose of chemotherapy (21-26). A study of long-term MOGCT survivors by the GOG reported a higher likelihood of hypertension in patients treated with CBCT (20). However, this study did not analyze other risk factors for metabolic syndrome or the association with cumulative dose of cisplatin. So far, only one study has reported on clinical and biochemical factors that are accepted risk factors for cardiovascular disease in long-term survivors of ovarian malignancies after CBCT (27). This study comprised only 21 patients, so larger, updated studies are needed.

Second Cancers

One of the most serious late effects of cytotoxic treatment, particularly for young survivors, is the significant risk of a second cancer compared to age-matched controls from the general population. Non–germ cell cancers can be induced by RT, chemotherapy, or both. In testicular cancer survivors, the development of a second solid cancer (10-30 years after testicular cancer diagnosis) represents a major life-threatening late effect, which is most probably related to RT and chemotherapy (1,2,25,28). For patients with testicular cancer treated with RT alone, second cancers are typically located within the radiation field. These cancers most often occur in the kidney, urinary bladder, pancreas, and stomach (2).

Chemotherapy for MOGCT is usually based on cisplatin combined with etoposide, the substance which is associated with the development of AML. Etoposide-induced AML occurs within 2 to 5 years of exposure and is cumulative dose dependent (29,30). In protocol 78 of the GOG, which tested the regimen of BEP, there was one case of AML among the 91 included patients (31). An additional case of lymphoma was diagnosed among survivors from that study, but the relationship between that occurrence and the BEP regimen was uncertain, as a correlation between chemotherapy and lymphoproliferative disorders has not been established. Solheim et al reported that 13% of 10-year MOGCT survivors who had received cytotoxic treatment developed at least one second solid cancer compared with 0% in those treated by surgery only (32).

A review of the SEER database indicates an increased risk of secondary malignancy in patients who received radiation for an MOGCT. In this study, 10 (10%) of 70 patients who received RT for an MOGCT developed a second cancer, significantly higher than in patients who did not receive RT (33). In practice, RT is rarely administered, because chemotherapy is effective and preservation of ovarian function is preferred (31,33).

Gonadal Function and Fertility

Gonadal Function

In females, the term "gonadal function" describes the endocrine and exocrine function of the ovaries. Oocyte maturation and ovulation depend on ovarian production of progesterone and estrogen (primarily estradiol), which is, in turn, stimulated by pituitary production of LH and FSH. At birth, the ovaries contain 1 to 2 million immature oocytes, which are encapsulated in early-stage, or primordial, follicles. These follicles are progressively lost throughout life until menopause. Maturing primordial follicles are required for the development of sexual characteristics, like breast growth, for menarche, and for pregnancy.

Premature ovarian failure is a syndrome characterized by persistent amenorrhea, decreased estradiol and progesterone serum levels, and increased FSH and LH serum levels before the age of 40 years. Premature ovarian failure is preceded by loss of fertility and irregular menses (32,34). Most types of chemotherapy and RT of the ovaries lead to an irreversibly diminished reserve of primordial follicles in girls and adolescents (**Figure 9.9-1**) (35). The residual reserve determines the remaining duration of the survivor's ovarian function and fertility. Alkylating agents such as procarbazine and cyclophosphamide are viewed as the most powerful drugs leading to loss of follicles (36). Factors including older age at treatment initiation, greater cumulative drug dose, and longer treatment duration favor premature ovarian failure (32,34-38).

In a review of the MDACC series, 27 (68%) of 40 patients who had retained a normal contralateral ovary and uterus maintained regular menses consistently after completion of chemotherapy, and 33 (83%) were having regular menses at the time of follow-up (39).

Although dysgerminoma is extremely radiosensitive, gonadal dysfunction, sterility, and RT-related adverse effects such as fibrosis in the genital tract make RT less desirable than BEP in most patients. In a review of the late effects of RT in patients receiving abdominal therapy for ovarian dysgerminoma, there was a small increase in reported dyspareunia and the number of bowel movements (40). Somewhat surprisingly, at a median follow-up of 12 years, none of the 43 patients treated with RT developed small bowel obstruction. No other significant intestinal or bladder problems were recorded. As expected, none of the patients treated with radiation conceived (41).

Major abdominal surgery may lead to pelvic fibrosis, in turn leading to distortion or even stenosis in the passage of the ovum, thereby reducing the chance of pregnancy. Therefore, meticulous surgical technique and avoidance of unnecessary operative maneuvers (eg, biopsy of a normal contralateral ovary) are required for preventing future complications (42-44). Another cause of infertility in this population is unnecessary bilateral salpingo-oophorectomy and hysterectomy because FSS is possible in nearly all patients with MOGCT, and long-term outcomes including pregnancy are excellent. In a series from Milan, among 55 patients treated with FSS, without further chemotherapy, 12 out of 12 patients who attempted conception became pregnant and 12 normal deliveries were recorded (45). Two additional pregnancies occurred in this group and resulted in termination, one of which was because of in-uterus detection of fetal malformation. In GOG 9901, among

132 survivors of OGCTs treated with surgery and platinum-based chemotherapy, 71 patients had fertility-sparing procedures (45). Of those fertile survivors, 62 (87.3%) maintained menstrual periods and 24 survivors reported 37 successful pregnancies. Although the survivors reported increased incidence of gynecologic problems and diminished sexual pleasure, they also tended to have stronger, more positive relationships with their significant others (46).

Fertility

Fertility refers to a woman's ability to have a child, whereas the terms "parenthood" and "reproduction" reflect whether a woman has ever initiated a pregnancy. Post-cancer fertility is an important dimension of cancer survivors' quality of life (47). Most studies of MOGCT survivors treated with FSS and chemotherapy suggest that these methods have little to no impact on fertility or teratogenicity (32,42,43,45,48). In a series of 40 patients who underwent FSS, 16 patients attempted to conceive and 12 were successful (39). One patient underwent an elective first-trimester abortion, and the other 11 patients bore 22 healthy infants over time, none of which had a major birth defect. In a series from Milan, among 169 patients with OGCTs, 138 underwent FSS, and of those, 81 underwent adjuvant chemotherapy (44). After treatment, all but one woman recovered menstrual function, and 55 conceptions were recorded. Forty normal full-term babies were delivered. There were four babies with congenital malformations, one in a patient who did not receive chemotherapy and three in women who had received chemotherapy. The difference was not statistically significant.

Although these successful pregnancy outcomes after CBCT have been documented, chemotherapy-induced infertility has been described in 18% of patients. This appears unrelated to the cumulative dose of cisplatin (49). Regular menses resume in more than 80% of MOGCT survivors, but recovery of menstrual function may not prove fertility (42,43,45,48).

There is limited support for the fertility-preserving role of gonadotropin-releasing hormone agonist during chemotherapy, and most experts would not endorse its routine use (50). In addition, oocyte harvesting before chemotherapy may delay treatment and may be unnecessary, except in older patients with limited ovarian reserve. Other techniques to preserve ovarian tissue remain experimental.

Subsequent Ovarian Cysts

As with any group of patients with a history of pelvic surgery, patients with OGCTs may develop functional cysts in the residual ovary. Muram et al reported the experience with 27 patients with OGCTs who underwent unilateral salpingo-oophorectomy and

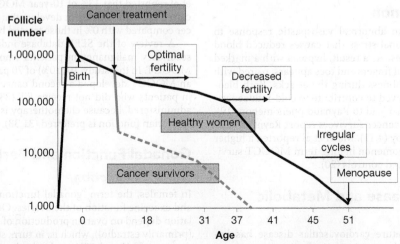

Figure 9.9-1. Schematic display of the reduction of the number of ovarian follicles during aging of females, both with (red line) and without (black line) previous cytotoxic treatment. (Modified from Hamre H. Thesis, Faculty of Medicine, University of Oslo, 2013.)

were followed for 12 to 215 months after completion of therapy. Of the 18 patients who maintained ovarian function, 13 (72%) developed functional cysts during follow-up (51). A trial of oral contraceptives and serial ovarian surveillance with sonography is helpful is distinguishing functional cysts from tumor recurrence.

Quality of Life

The GOG evaluated the quality of life and psychosocial characteristics of survivors of OGCTs compared with matched controls. In this analysis, the survivors appeared to be well adjusted, were able to develop strong relationships, and were free of significant depression (52). The impact on fertility was modest or none in patients undergoing FSSs (46). OGCT survivors appeared to be free of any major physical illnesses at a median follow-up of 10 years, as compared with matched controls. The only differences were higher rates of reported hypertension (17% vs 8%, $P = .02$), hypercholesterolemia (9.8% vs 4.4%, $P = .09$), and hearing loss (5.3% vs 1.5%, $P = .09$) compared with controls (53). Chronic functional problems including numbness, tinnitus, nausea, and Raynaud symptoms were reported by survivors after chemotherapy. Interestingly, late effects of treatment are more pronounced among children receiving treatment for GCTs (54). Specifically, neurotoxicity, growth abnormalities, pulmonary toxicity, and gastrointestinal toxicity have been reported in a higher proportion than in adult patients. Despite persistence of a few sequelae of treatment, in general, OGCT survivors enjoy a healthy life comparable to that of controls, justifying administration of curative treatment in full and timely dosing.

REFERENCES

1. Aziz NM. Cancer survivorship research: challenge and opportunity. *J Nutr.* 2002;132(11 suppl):3494S-3503S.

2. Travis LB, Fosså SD, Schonfeld SJ, et al. Second cancers among 40,576 testicular cancer patients: focus on long-term survivors. *J Natl Cancer Inst.* 2005;97(18):1354-1365.

3. Travis LB, Beard C, Allan JM, et al. Testicular cancer survivorship: research strategies and recommendations. *J Natl Cancer Inst.* 2010;102(15):1114-1130.

4. Hausheer FH, Schilsky RL, Bain S, Berghorn EJ, Lieberman F. Diagnosis, management, and evaluation of chemotherapy-induced peripheral neuropathy. *Semin Oncol.* 2006;33(1):15-49.

5. Solheim O, Skalleberg J, Warncke T, Ørstavik K, Tropé C, Fosså SD. Long-term neurotoxicity and Raynaud's phenomenon in patients treated with cisplatin-based chemotherapy for malignant ovarian germ cell tumor. *Acta Obstet Gynecol Scand.* 2019;98(2):240-249.

6. Meijer C, de Vries EG, Marmiroli P, Tredici G, Frattola L, Cavaletti G. Cisplatin-induced DNA-platination in experimental dorsal root ganglia neuronopathy. *Neurotoxicology.* 1999;20(6):883-887.

7. McKeage MJ, Hsu T, Screnci D, Haddad G, Baguley BC. Nucleolar damage correlates with neurotoxicity induced by different platinum drugs. *Br J Cancer.* 2001;85(8):1219-1225.

8. McDonald ES, Randon KR, Knight A, Windebank AJ. Cisplatin preferentially binds to DNA in dorsal root ganglion neurons in vitro and in vivo: a potential mechanism for neurotoxicity. *Neurobiol Dis.* 2005;18(2):305-313.

9. Thompson SW, Davis LE, Kornfeld M, Hilgers RD, Standefer JC. Cisplatin neuropathy. Clinical, electrophysiologic, morphologic, and toxicologic studies. *Cancer.* 1984;54(7):1269-1275.

10. Ekborn A, Laurell G, Andersson A, Wallin I, Eksborg S, Ehrsson H. Cisplatin-induced hearing loss: influence of the mode of drug administration in the guinea pig. *Hear Res.* 2000;140(1-2):38-44.

11. Osanto S, Bukman A, Van Hoek F, Sterk PJ, De Laat JA, Hermans J. Long-term effects of chemotherapy in patients with testicular cancer. *J Clin Oncol.* 1992;10(4):574-579.

12. Sprauten M, Darrah TH, Peterson DR, et al. Impact of long-term serum platinum concentrations on neuro- and ototoxicity in Cisplatin-treated survivors of testicular cancer. *J Clin Oncol.* 2012;30(3):300-307.

13. Bauer CA, Brozoski TJ. Cochlear structure and function after round window application of ototoxins. *Hear Res.* 2005;201(1-2):121-131.

14. Skalleberg J, Solheim O, Fosså SD, et al. Long-term ototoxicity in women after cisplatin treatment for ovarian germ cell cancer. *Gynecol Oncol.* 2017;145(1):148-153.

15. Bokemeyer C, Berger CC, Hartmann JT, et al. Analysis of risk factors for cisplatin-induced ototoxicity in patients with testicular cancer. *Br J Cancer.* 1998;77(8):1355-1362.

16. Oldenburg J, Kraggerud SM, Cvancarova M, Lothe RA, Fossa SD. Cisplatin-induced long-term hearing impairment is associated with specific glutathione s-transferase genotypes in testicular cancer survivors. *J Clin Oncol.* 2007;25(6):708-714.

17. Oldenburg J, Kraggerud SM, Brydøy M, Cvancarova M, Lothe RA, Fossa SD. Association between long-term neuro-toxicities in testicular cancer survivors and polymorphisms in glutathione-s-transferase-P1 and -M1, a retrospective cross sectional study. *J Transl Med.* 2007;5:70.

18. Teutsch C, Lipton A, Harvey HA. Raynaud's phenomenon as a side effect of chemotherapy with vinblastine and bleomycin for testicular carcinoma. *Cancer Treat Rep.* 1977;61(5):925-926.

19. Vogelzang NJ, Bosl GJ, Johnson K, Kennedy BJ. Raynaud's phenomenon: a common toxicity after combination chemotherapy for testicular cancer. *Ann Intern Med.* 1981;95(3):288-292.

20. Westbury CB, Harrington KJ, Rhys-Evans P, et al. Raynaud's phenomenon after radical radiotherapy for tumours of the head and neck. *Postgrad Med J.* 2003;79(929):176-177.

21. Haugnes HS, Aass N, Fosså SD, et al. Components of the metabolic syndrome in long-term survivors of testicular cancer. *Ann Oncol.* 2007;18(2):241-248.

22. Haugnes HS, Wethal T, Aass N, et al. Cardiovascular risk factors and morbidity in long-term survivors of testicular cancer: a 20-year follow-up study. *J Clin Oncol.* 2010;28(30):4649-4657.

23. Meinardi MT, Gietema JA, van der Graaf WT, et al. Cardiovascular morbidity in long-term survivors of metastatic testicular cancer. *J Clin Oncol.* 2000;18(8):1725-1732.

24. van den Belt-Dusebout AW, de Wit R, Gietema JA, et al. Treatment-specific risks of second malignancies and cardiovascular disease in 5-year survivors of testicular cancer. *J Clin Oncol.* 2007;25(28):4370-4378.

25. Wethal T, Haugnes HS, Kjekshus J, et al. C-reactive protein; a potential marker of second cancer and cardiovascular disease in testicular cancer survivors? *Eur J Cancer.* 2010;46(18):3425-3433.

26. van den Belt-Dusebout AW, Nuver J, de Wit R, et al. Long-term risk of cardiovascular disease in 5-year survivors of testicular cancer. *J Clin Oncol.* 2006;24(3):467-475.

27. Wethal T, Kjekshus J, Røislien J, et al. Treatment-related differences in cardiovascular risk factors in long-term survivors of testicular cancer. *J Cancer Surviv.* 2007;1(1):8-16.

28. de Vos FY, Nuver J, Willemse PH, et al. Long-term survivors of ovarian malignancies after cisplatin-based chemotherapy; cardiovascular risk factors and signs of vascular damage. *Eur J Cancer.* 2004;40(5):696-700.

29. Murbraech K, Solheim O, Aulie HM, Fossa SD, Aakhus S. The impact of cisplatinum-based chemotherapy on ventricular function and cardiovascular risk factors in female survivors after malignant germ cell cancer. *ESC Heart Fail.* 2015;2(3):142-149.

30. Howard R, Gilbert E, Lynch CF, et al. Risk of leukemia among survivors of testicular cancer: a population-based study of 42,722 patients. *Ann Epidemiol.* 2008;18(5):416-421.

31. Nichols CR, Breeden ES, Loehrer PJ, Williams SD, Einhorn LH. Secondary leukemia associated with a conventional dose of etoposide: review of serial germ cell tumor protocols. *J Natl Cancer Inst.* 1993;85(1):36-40.

32. Solheim O, Kærn J, Tropé CG, et al. Malignant ovarian germ cell tumors: presentation, survival and second cancer in a population based Norwegian cohort (1953-2009). *Gynecol Oncol.* 2013;131(2):330-335.

33. Solheim O, Gershenson DM, Tropé CG, et al. Prognostic factors in malignant ovarian germ cell tumours (The surveillance, epidemiology and end results experience 1978-2010). *Eur J Cancer.* 2014;50(11):1942-1950.

34. Kokcu A. Premature ovarian failure from current perspective. *Gynecol Endocrinol.* 2010;26(8):555-562.

35. Nicosia SV, Matus-Ridley M, Meadows AT. Gonadal effects of cancer therapy in girls. *Cancer.* 1985;55(10):2364-2372.

36. Brydoy M, Fosså SD, Dahl O, Bjøro T. Gonadal dysfunction and fertility problems in cancer survivors. *Acta Oncol.* 2007;46(4):480-489.

37. Byrne J, Mulvihill JJ, Myers MH, et al. Effects of treatment on fertility in long-term survivors of childhood or adolescent cancer. *N Engl J Med.* 1987;317(21):1315-1321.

38. Siris ES, Leventhal BG, Vaitukaitis JL. Effects of childhood leukemia and chemotherapy on puberty and reproductive function in girls. *N Engl J Med.* 1976;294(21):1143-1146.

39. Brewer M, Gershenson DM, Herzog CE, Mitchell MF, Silva EG, Wharton JT. Outcome and reproductive function after chemotherapy for ovarian dysgerminoma. *J Clin Oncol.* 1999;17(9):2670-2675.

40. Howell S, Shalet S. Gonadal damage from chemotherapy and radiotherapy. *Endocrinol Metab Clin North Am*. 1998;27(4):927-943.

41. Casey AC, Bhodauria S, Shapter A, Nieberg R, Berek JS, Farias-Eisner R. Dysgerminoma: the role of conservative surgery. *Gynecol Oncol*. 1996;63(3):352-357.

42. Low JJ, Perrin LC, Crandon AJ, Hacker NF. Conservative surgery to preserve ovarian function in patients with malignant ovarian germ cell tumors. A review of 74 cases. *Cancer*. 2000;89(2):391-398.

43. Kanazawa K, Suzuki T, Sakumoto K. Treatment of malignant ovarian germ cell tumors with preservation of fertility: reproductive performance after persistent remission. *Am J Clin Oncol*. 2000;23(3):244-248.

44. Zanetta G, Bonazzi C, Cantù M, et al. Survival and reproductive function after treatment of malignant germ cell ovarian tumors. *J Clin Oncol*. 2001;19(4):1015-1020.

45. Gershenson DM, Miller AM, Champion VL, et al. Reproductive and sexual function after platinum-based chemotherapy in long-term ovarian germ cell tumor survivors: a Gynecologic Oncology Group Study. *J Clin Oncol*. 2007;25(19):2792-2797.

46. Billmire D, Vinocur C, Rescorla F, et al. Outcome and staging evaluation in malignant germ cell tumors of the ovary in children and adolescents: an intergroup study. *J Pediatr Surg*. 2004;39(3):424-429.

47. Cousineau TM, Domar AD. Psychological impact of infertility. *Best Pract Res Clin Obstet Gynaecol*. 2007;21(2):293-308.

48. Perrin LC, Low J, Nicklin JL, Ward BG, Crandon AJ. Fertility and ovarian function after conservative surgery for germ cell tumours of the ovary. *Aust N Z J Obstet Gynaecol*. 1999;39(2):243-245.

49. Gaffan J, Holden L, Newlands ES, et al. Infertility rates following POMB/ACE chemotherapy for male and female germ cell tumours—a retrospective long-term follow-up study. *Br J Cancer*. 2003;89(10):1849-1854.

50. Sun X, Dongol S, Jiang J, Kong B. Protection of ovarian function by GnRH agonists during chemotherapy: a meta-analysis. *Int J Oncol*. 2014;44(4):1335-1340.

51. Muram D, Gale CL, Thompson E. Functional ovarian cysts in patients cured of ovarian neoplasms. *Obstet Gynecol*. 1990;75(4):680-683.

52. Champion V, Williams SD, Miller A, et al. Quality of life in long-term survivors of ovarian germ cell tumors: a Gynecologic Oncology Group study. *Gynecol Oncol*. 2007;105(3):687-694.

53. Matei D, Miller AM, Monahan P, et al. Chronic physical effects and health care utilization in long-term ovarian germ cell tumor survivors: a Gynecologic Oncology Group study. *J Clin Oncol*. 2009;27(25):4142-4149.

54. Hale GA, Marina NM, Jones-Wallace D, et al. Late effects of treatment for germ cell tumors during childhood and adolescence. *J Pediatr Hematol Oncol*. 1999;21(2):115-122.

CHAPTER **9.10**

Ovarian Germ Cell Tumors: Future Directions

Isabelle Ray-Coquard and Lindsay Frazier

In contrast to many other ovarian malignancies, MOGCTs are associated with an excellent prognosis, limited toxicity, and a reproductive-age patient demographic. Virtually, all patients with early-stage, completely resected OGCTs survive after appropriate management with surgery and adjuvant therapy. In addition, up to 80% of patients with incompletely resected or advanced tumors are expected to be long-term survivors. Therefore, future research in OGCTs focuses on refining and limiting surgical and systemic therapy in order to maintain this excellent prognosis while minimizing toxicity and preserving fertility.

SURGERY AND STAGING

Surgery continues to have a pivotal role in the management of all patients with OGCTs, but the extent of surgical staging is debatable. Although the guidelines for adult females with MOGCTs include full surgical staging with biopsies of the peritoneum and omentum and a pelvic and para-aortic lymphadenectomy, this is not performed in the pediatric population unless gross disease is identified. Clarification of differences in biology and effective treatment between the adult and pediatric populations is important, and efforts are underway to harmonize surgical recommendations and staging systems across groups.

As outlined in previous chapters, MIS is a viable option for many patients with MOGCT. This operative technique decreases morbidity and improves perioperative outcomes, but publications are limited to small retrospective case series. Additional data are anticipated to inform recommendations surrounding the surgical approach.

The utility of NACT with interval cytoreductive surgery is also an important consideration in patients who have extensive disease at the time of diagnosis. This may allow an increased opportunity for FSS and MIS.

MOLECULAR TESTING

The era of personalized medicine has informed treatment decisions for many types of cancers. Because most patients with MOGCTs are cured with surgery and adjuvant chemotherapy when appropriate, it is unlikely that molecular profiling will change treatment recommendations in the upfront setting. However, the management of recurrent or refractory disease may be informed by results of molecular profiling. This has not been well studied to date.

Investigators are evaluating the presence of p16 expression in MOGCTs to determine the utility of studying CDK inhibitors. All patients have been accrued to this study (1).

ADJUVANT THERAPY

The role of surveillance in low-risk patients is expanding. Current studies seek to identify the cohort of low-risk patients who can safely be observed rather than treated. Investigations are also underway to define regimens with decreased toxicity instead of the conventional combination of BEP. Current trials are designed to determine whether carboplatin can be substituted for cisplatin as a less toxic alternative.

The COG is conducting a large trial of 2,059 participants in collaboration with the NRG Oncology Group entitled, "A Phase 3 study of active surveillance for low risk and a randomized trial of carboplatin vs. cisplatin for standard risk pediatric and adult patients with germ cell tumors" (2). The low-risk cohort in this trial includes patients who have stage I grade 2 to 3 ovarian ITs or stage

I nonseminoma or seminoma malignant GCTs. These patients undergo observation to determine whether a strategy of complete surgical resection followed by surveillance can maintain an OS rate of at least 95.7% at 2 years for pediatric, adolescent, and adult patients with stage I (low-risk) malignant GCTs, and at least 95% for patients with ovarian pure IT. The standard risk cohort in this trial includes patients aged 11 to less than 25 years who have newly diagnosed metastatic OGCT of FIGO stages IC, II, and III (COG stages II and III) that contain at least one of the following: YST, embryonal carcinoma, or choriocarcinoma. Patients in this arm are randomized to BEP or bleomycin, etoposide, and carboplatin.

Caution should be exercised in evaluating open trials, as some trials listed as GCTs are instead accruing patients with sex cord-stromal tumors, and these are very different entities (3).

There are also different recommendations for upfront treatment for adult and pediatric patients, and cooperative groups and research groups seek to harmonize these differences.

In addition, the search for optimal chemotherapeutic drugs and combinations in recurrent and refractory disease is ongoing. Current and completed studies include paclitaxel, ifosfamide, and cisplatin (TIP); paclitaxel and gemcitabine; temozolomide; docetaxel; and autologous peripheral blood stem cell transplant for both adult and pediatric patients (4). Some phase I studies allow patients with GCTs to enroll, and these represent options for patients with disease that does not respond to more conventional agents (5,6). Vaccine trials and immunotherapy trials, including immunotherapy using tumor-infiltrating lymphocytes, are also underway and allow for accrual of patients with MOGCTs (7-10).

Surveillance

Gaps in knowledge include the most efficient surveillance schedule related to imaging techniques and frequency of follow-up. Quality of life assessments are ongoing to evaluate the long-term effects of treatment, including chronic fatigue (11,12).

Strategies for Research

International collaborative trials among specialties investigating these rare tumors, even though challenging, are one of the safest ways to address some of the unknown aspects of this disease. The MaGIC is a global consortium of pediatric oncologists, gynecologic oncologists, testicular cancer specialists, surgeons, pathologists, epidemiologists, statisticians, bioinformaticists, and biomedical scientists united to develop more effective treatments for GCTs through scientific inquiry (13). Areas of investigation include clinical research, basic and translational research, and the development and running of clinical trials. The Gynecologic Cancer Intergroup (GCIG) functions as a collaborative research body

for all gynecologic cancers and has published consensus guidelines on OGCTs (14). In addition, the NRG Oncology Group and the COG are cooperative groups with active investigations into the optimal management of MOGCTs.

References

1. ClinicalTrials.gov. Immunohistochemical evaluation of protein P16 expression in ovarian germ cell tumors. https://clinicaltrials.gov/ct2/show/NCT04283773?term=germ+cell&cond=Ovary+Cancer&draw=2&rank=2

2. ClinicalTrials.gov. Active surveillance, bleomycin, etoposide, carboplatin or cisplatin in treating pediatric and adult patients with germ cell tumors. https://clinicaltrials.gov/ct2/show/NCT03067181?term=germ+cell&recrs=ad&cond=ovarian+cancer&draw=2&rank=7

3. ClinicalTrials.gov. TC or BEP in treating patients with malignant ovarian germ cell tumors (MOGCT-01). https://clinicaltrials.gov/ct2/show/NCT02429687?term=germ+cell&cond=Ovary+Cancer&draw=2&rank=1

4. ClinicalTrials.gov. Autologous peripheral blood stem cell transplant for germ cell tumors. https://clinicaltrials.gov/ct2/show/NCT00432094?term=germ+cell&cond=Ovary+Cancer&draw=2&rank=8

5. ClinicalTrials.gov. https://clinicaltrials.gov/ct2/results?cond=ovarian+cancer&term=germ+cell&type=&rslt=&recrs=a&recrs=d&age_v=&gndr=&intr=&titles=&outc=&spons=&lead=&id=&cntry=&state=&city=&dist=&locn=&rsub=&strd_s=&strd_e=&prcd_s=&prcd_e=&sfpd_s=&sfpd_e=&rfpd_s=&rfpd_e=&lupd_s=&lupd_e=&sort=

6. ClinicalTrials.gov. A study of SGN-ALPV in advanced solid tumors. https://clinicaltrials.gov/ct2/show/NCT05229900?term=germ+cell&recrs=ad&cond=ovarian+cancer&draw=2&rank=8

7. ClinicalTrials.gov. Vaccine therapy with sargramostim (GM-CSF) in treating patients with her-2 positive stage III-IV breast cancer or ovarian cancer. https://clinicaltrials.gov/ct2/show/NCT00436254?term=germ+cell&recrs=ad&cond=ovarian+cancer&draw=2&rank=6

8. ClinicalTrials.gov. https://clinicaltrials.gov/ct2/show/NCT02834013?term=germ+cell&recrs=ad&cond=ovarian+cancer&draw=2&rank=9

9. ClinicalTrials.gov. Secured access to pembrolizumab for patients with selected rare cancer types (AcSé). https://clinicaltrials.gov/ct2/show/NCT03012620?term=germ+cell&recrs=ad&cond=ovarian+cancer&draw=2&rank=10

10. ClinicalTrials.gov. Quality-of-life study of patients with previously treated ovarian cancer. https://clinicaltrials.gov/ct2/show/NCT00003794?term=germ+cell&cond=Ovary+Cancer&draw=2&rank=3

11. ClinicalTrials.gov. Immunotherapy using tumor infiltrating lymphocytes for patients with metastatic cancer. https://clinicaltrials.gov/ct2/show/NCT01174121?term=germ+cell&recrs=ad&cond=ovarian+cancer&draw=2&rank=33

12. ClinicalTrials.gov. Living after a rare cancer of the ovary: chronic fatigue, quality of life and late effects of chemotherapy (VIVROVAIRE TR). https://clinicaltrials.gov/ct2/show/NCT03418844?term=germ+cell&cond=Ovary+Cancer&draw=2&rank=10

13. Malignant Germ Cell International Consortium. Accessed February 5, 2023. https://magicconsortium.com

14. Brown J, Friedlander M, Backes FJ, et al. Gynecologic Cancer Intergroup (GCIG) consensus review for ovarian germ cell tumors. *Int J Gynecol Cancer*. 2014;24(9 suppl 3):S48-S54. doi:10.1097/IGC.0000000000000223

OVARIAN SEX CORD-STROMAL TUMORS

Ovarian Sex Cord-Stromal Tumors: Introduction, Anatomy, Natural History, and Patterns of Spread

R. Tyler Hillman and Carrie Langstraat

INTRODUCTION

The adult ovary is composed of four developmentally distinct components that can each give rise to benign and malignant tumors: the ovarian surface epithelium, germ cells, connective tissue stroma, and the hormonally active sex cords. The connective tissue stroma and sex cords comprise the supporting structure for the survival and maturation of germ cells, all of which are covered by the surface epithelium. Granulosa cells and Sertoli cells, generally considered to be homologous, are derived from the sex cord cells, whereas the pluripotent mesenchymal cells are the precursors of theca cells, Leydig cells, and fibroblasts. The cell type composition of the mature male or female gonad is genetically controlled, and an initially bipotential gonad begins to differentiate early in human embryonic development. In individuals with XY karyotype, male gonadal sex and Sertoli cell development are induced by expression of the Y-chromosome–encoded transcription factor *SRY* and its downstream target *SOX9*. Conversely, in XX karyotype individuals who normally lack *SRY* expression, β-catenin pathway signaling induced by *WNT4* and *RSPO1* expression specifies the earliest steps in female gonad development. Subsequent expression of *FOXL2*, a gene critical to the pathogenesis of adult-type granulosa cell tumors (AGCTs), is required to maintain adult ovary function in mice (1,2). Germline loss-of-function mutations of the human *FOXL2* gene cause premature ovarian failure as part of the autosomal dominant blepharophimosis/ptosis/epicanthus inversus syndrome (BPES) (3). The neoplastic transformation of gonadal cellular constituents, either singly or in various combinations collectively, results in benign and malignant tumors that are collectively termed sex cord-stromal tumors (SCSTs).

The classification of the SCSTs provides the template by which this chapter endeavors to stratify and define these tumor entities according to their morphologic characteristics (**Table 10.1-1**). Overall, the majority of SCSTs are benign and are associated with a favorable long-term prognosis. In addition, a significant proportion of SCSTs are diagnosed in patients younger than age 40 years, and these have the potential to produce a variety of steroid hormones. Hence, adequate knowledge of the natural history of each of these tumors is imperative in diagnosing and individualizing definitive surgical and adjuvant therapy.

SCSTs are rare entities, which has led to significant knowledge gaps regarding optimal management strategies. Recent advances in techniques of genomic analysis have clarified the molecular pathogenesis of many SCST subtypes, but as of now this has not translated into novel therapeutic options. The recently reported completion of two prospective clinical trials of therapeutic interventions in recurrent SCST (4,5) generates renewed optimism that evidence-based evaluation of important clinical questions is feasible in these diseases. It is hoped that increased multidisciplinary and multinational research efforts will gradually fill in remaining gaps and ultimately improve outcomes for patients diagnosed with SCSTs.

■ **TABLE 10.1-1. Classification of Sex Cord-Stromal Tumors of the Ovary**

Sex Cord-Stromal Tumors

Pure stromal tumors

- Fibroma
- Cellular fibroma
- Thecoma
- Luteinized thecoma associated with sclerosing peritonitis
- Fibrosarcoma
- Sclerosing stromal tumor
- Signet-ring stromal tumor
- Microcystic stromal tumor
- Leydig cell tumor
- Steroid cell tumor
- Steroid cell tumor, malignant

Pure sex cord tumors

- Adult granulosa cell tumor
- Juvenile granulosa cell tumor
- Sertoli cell tumor
- Sex cord tumor with annular tubules

Mixed sex cord-stromal tumors

- Sertoli-Leydig cell tumor
  - Well differentiated
  - Moderately differentiated
    - With heterologous elements
  - Poorly differentiated
    - With heterologous elements
  - Retiform
    - With heterologous elements
- Sex cord-stromal tumors, not otherwise specified

REFERENCES

1. Uhlenhaut NH, Jakob S, Anlag K, et al. Somatic sex reprogramming of adult ovaries to testes by FOXL2 ablation. *Cell*. 2009;139:1130-1142.

2. Uda M, Ottolenghi C, Crisponi L, et al. Foxl2 disruption causes mouse ovarian failure by pervasive blockage of follicle development. *Hum Mol Genet*. 2004;13:1171-1181.

3. Crisponi L, Deiana M, Loi A, et al. The putative forkhead transcription factor FOXL2 is mutated in blepharophimosis/ptosis/epicanthus inversus syndrome. *Nat Genet*. 2001;27:159-166.

4. Banerjee SN, Tang M, O'Connell RL, et al. A phase 2 study of anastrozole in patients with oestrogen receptor and/progesterone receptor positive recurrent/metastatic granulosa cell tumours/sex-cord stromal tumours of the ovary: the PARAGON/ANZGOG 0903 trial. *Gynecol Oncol*. 2021;163:72-78.

5. Ray-Coquard I, Harter P, Lorusso D, et al. Effect of weekly paclitaxel with or without bevacizumab on progression-free rate among patients with relapsed ovarian sex cord-stromal tumors: the ALIENOR/ENGOT-ov7 randomized clinical trial. *JAMA Oncol*. 2020;6:1923-1930.

Ovarian Sex Cord-Stromal Tumors: Etiology, Epidemiology, Risk Factors, Genetics, and Molecular Biology

R. Tyler Hillman

INCIDENCE AND MORTALITY

SCSTs are estimated to account for approximately 2% of all malignant ovarian neoplasms (1,2). The incidence rate of SCSTs in the United States has been estimated to be approximately 0.2 to 0.5 per 100,000 using large cancer registries (1,2) but may be an underestimate owing to misclassification of early-stage disease as nonmalignant. For example, one historical, non–age-adjusted estimate for the incidence rate of granulosa cell tumors (GCTs) alone in Israel between 1960 and 1975 was 0.9 per 100,000 (3). Whether demographic or environmental factors have led to changes in SCST, incidence over time is a key area of epidemiologic investigation. A large longitudinal cohort study conducted in Scandinavia between 1953 and 2012 found that the incidence rate for GCTs remained constant at 0.6 to 0.8 per 100,000 despite substantial social shifts in lifestyle and hormonal therapy usage during the study period (4). Collectively, some evidence suggests SCSTs are identified more frequently in Black patients compared to patients of other racial/ethnic backgrounds (1,5). Investigators using data from the National Cancer Institute's Surveillance, Epidemiology, and End Results (SEER) program found that between 2010 and 2014, the rate of SCST diagnosis in Black patients (0.5/100,000) was approximately 5 times the rate of diagnosis in Asian/Pacific Islanders (0.1/100,000), the group with the lowest incidence among those examined (1). Although SCSTs account for a decreasing proportion of all ovarian malignancies with advancing age, the annual age-related incidence continues to increase through the sixth decade of life (1,6).

The overall age-related incidence of SCST obscures significant differences among histologic subtypes. AGCTs account for 90% of all SCSTs and have a median diagnosis age of around 45 to 50 years, with most occurring in the fourth to fifth decades of life (7-9). Juvenile-type granulosa cell tumors (JGCTs) incidence peaks in adolescence, with reported median diagnosis age of 7 to 8 years (10,11). The median patient age at diagnosis for Sertoli-Leydig cell tumors (SLCTs) has been reported to be between 25 and 35 years (12,13), with 75% of the tumors occurring before age 30 and less than 10% after age 50. Patients with well-differentiated SLCTs present at an average age of 35 years, or 10 years later than patients with intermediate or poorly differentiated lesions. Conversely, tumors with retiform patterns are generally detected 10 years earlier than the intermediate and poorly differentiated tumors (12-14). Ovarian sex cord tumor with annular tubules (SCTATs) was first described in 1970s (15), and single-institution studies report that this rare entity accounts for approximately 1% to 6% of SCSTs, with a median age of diagnosis around 22 years (16,17). Thecomas and fibromas are benign SCSTs with peak incidence of diagnosis after the fifth decade of life, although these rarely can be seen in patients under age 30 (18-20). Gynandroblastoma is an extremely rare SCST (if strict morphologic criteria are followed to establish the diagnosis), with case reports describing diagnosis predominantly in premenopausal patients although with wide variability (21-24).

The great majority of SCSTs are unilateral stage I lesions, for which survival outcomes are generally excellent. SEER data demonstrate that the 5-year disease-specific survival in the United States between 2007 and 2013 was 98% for stage I SCST (1). However, the potential for patients with AGCTs to experience a first recurrence many years after initial diagnosis may make 5-year disease-specific survival an underestimate of long-term disease mortality. For example, one series of 97 patients with AGCT and a median follow-up period of 88 months reported that 47% of recurrences occurred more than 5 years after diagnosis and that early-stage disease showed an increased proclivity for very late recurrence (25).

ETIOLOGY AND RISK FACTORS

There are no known environmental risk factors for the development of SCSTs. The question of whether reproductive factors, including the use of fertility-promoting agents and oral contraceptives, increase the risk of GCT has been extensively studied. Unkila-Kallio et al examined a possible link between fertility-promoting agents and GCTs using the nationwide Finnish Cancer Registry (26). They analyzed the occurrence of GCTs in Finland from 1965 to 1994 against sales statistics for ovulation inducers. The incidence of GCTs declined by nearly 40% from 1965 to 1969 and 1985 to 1994 despite a 13-fold increase in the use of clomiphene citrate and a 200-fold increase in human menopausal gonadotropin use; oral contraceptive use increased 5-fold. As mentioned earlier, a subsequent larger cohort study conducted across Finland, Iceland, Norway, and Sweden between 1953 and 2012 found a stable incidence rate for GCTs, casting further doubt on the hypothesis that fertility-promoting agents or oral contraceptives have a significant causative role in the etiology of this disease (4). Although informative about broad social trends in the exposures of interest, strictly speaking these large epidemiologic studies are unable to evaluate a causal link because they lack ascertainment of hormonal agent usage on a per-patient level.

A case-control study examined risk factors in 72 patients with GCT compared to both the general population and epithelial ovarian cancer control patients (27). Among other findings, diagnosis of GCT was significantly more likely in patients with body mass index (BMI) greater than 30 kg/m^2 (odds ratio [OR] 5.80) and significantly less likely in patients who smoked (OR 0.46), used oral contraceptive pills (OR 0.32), or had higher parity when compared to the general population. These data are consistent with a hypothesis that modulators of lifetime estrogen exposure such as obesity and smoking may influence GCT risk. A separate population-based case-control study by Bryk et al examined associations between patients with AGCT in the Finnish Cancer Registry and purchases of prescription postmenopausal hormone therapies (28), finding no increased risk of AGCT in users of either estradiol-only or estrogen-progestin hormone therapy. Owing to their rarity, much less is known about environmental or lifestyle risk factors for less common SCST types.

GENETICS

Genetic evidence indicates that germline mutations may increase the risk for developing certain subtypes of SCST. Although AGCTs sharing a similar molecular pathogenesis and pedigree have been described with multiple affected close relatives (29,30), there are no known monogenic germline predisposition syndromes associated with this disease. Somatic missense mutations in the RNase IIIb domain of the gene coding for the microRNA processing enzyme *DICER1* are frequently found in SLCT. This most often affects one of five codons involved in metal binding that are critical to the catalytic microRNA cleavage function of the encoded enzyme (31,32). In contrast, germline *DICER1* mutations are less common in patients with SLCT and tend to be truncating, loss-of-function alleles (31,33). Evidence from noncancer exome sequencing data sets indicates that approximately one in 10,000 individuals carry a deleterious germline *DICER1* mutation, representing a Mendelian cancer risk syndrome associated with an increased risk of SLCT, gynandroblastoma, pediatric pleuropulmonary blastoma, and other malignancies (34). No precise estimate is available for the penetrance of SLCT in patients carrying pathogenic germline *DICER1* mutations. SLCT surveillance recommendations in this population are based on expert opinion and include periodic physical examination and pelvic ultrasound (every 6-12 months) (32). In contrast to similar surveillance approaches in patients with more common hereditary breast and ovarian cancer risk syndromes, consideration should be given to initiating screening in childhood among *DICER1* mutation carriers because peripubertal diagnosis of both SLCT and gynandroblastoma has been described. Screening recommendations for extraovarian conditions associated with *DICER1* germline mutations can be found elsewhere (32).

The association between SCTAT and Peutz-Jeghers syndrome (PJS) was known from the time this tumor type was first described in 1970 (15). Germline pathogenic mutations in the *STK11* gene, the causative lesion of PJS, account for approximately one-third of all cases of SCTAT (35). In contrast, *STK11* mutations are rare in sporadic SCTATs (36).

MOLECULAR BIOLOGY

Our current knowledge regarding various autocrine and endocrine regulatory mechanisms influencing ovarian function, the overexpression of inhibin in several SCSTs, the alterations in ovarian steroidogenesis, and the changes in circulating gonadotropin levels in SCSTs provides clues regarding the pathogenesis of these tumors. Investigations to date exploring the interactive regulatory mechanisms of inhibin, activin, follistatin, and follicle-stimulating hormone (FSH) have predominantly included the more common GCTs. FSH provides a fundamental regulatory role in the differentiation of granulosa cells during the early stages of follicle development. Specifically, FSH stimulates cell proliferation, increases the availability of cell surface prolactin and luteinizing hormone (LH) receptors, and induces aromatase activity, resulting in increased estradiol production. Other growth regulatory factors such as insulin-like growth factor (IGF) and epidermal growth factor modulate these actions, including the enhancement of the mitogenic effects of FSH. In addition, FSH secretion from the anterior pituitary is modulated in part by the serum levels of inhibin, activin, estrogens, and/or androgens.

Inhibin, a heterodimeric glycoprotein hormone composed of an α-subunit and one of two β-subunits, is secreted by the granulosa cells of the ovary (37). Inhibin A consists of αA and βA; inhibin B consists of αB and βB. Petraglia et al demonstrated that serum inhibin B was dramatically increased in eight of nine patients with GCTs, whereas inhibin A was slightly increased in

all patients (38). The major physiologic function of inhibin is to inhibit the secretion of FSH by the anterior pituitary gland. Inhibin is expressed in excessive quantities by GCTs. Although it maintains its regulatory function pertaining to FSH suppression, it appears to be ineffective in controlling estrogen production and cell proliferation within the gonad. Inhibin B levels in particular have been shown to correlate well with disease status in patients with AGCT (39).

Activin, also a peptide hormone of ovarian granulosa cell origin, is composed of two β-subunits that are identical to those of inhibin. In contrast to inhibin, activin stimulates the secretion of FSH and induces the production of estradiol, while having a negative impact on progesterone production and promoting granulosa cell differentiation (40). Lin et al (41) performed comparative genomic hybridization of a set of 37 AGCTs (36 primaries, one recurrence) obtained from five hospitals in Taiwan. All patients had stage I disease, except for one stage III patient with limited disease at initial diagnosis. Twenty-two (61%) of the 36 primary tumors had chromosomal imbalances. The nonrandom changes included loss of 22q in 31% of tumors, gain of chromosome 14 in 25% of tumors, and gain of chromosome 12 in 14% of tumors. Monosomy 22 frequently coexisted with trisomy 14. High-level amplification, as can be seen in many aggressive carcinomas, was not detected in any of these GCTs. More recent whole-exome sequencing of 24 primary and recurrent AGCTs identified focal deletion of 21q22.3 (9/24 tumors) and 3p29 (7/24 tumors) as recurrent copy number variants in this disease (42).

Shah and colleagues (43) performed whole-transcriptome paired-end RNA sequencing on four GCTs. They discovered a missense mutation, c.C402G (p.Cys134Trp), in *FOXL2*, a member of the forkhead-winged helix family of transcription factors. This gene is known to be involved in ovarian differentiation and is required for the normal development of granulosa cells in humans (44) and mice (45,46). *FOXL2* c.C402G mutations are present in over 95% of AGCTs, but a small minority of JGCTs (47). These results support a molecular basis for the disparate clinical course observed between JGCTs and AGCTs and provide a means to improve diagnosis in difficult cases. Although mutant *FOXL2* is likely an oncogene and key driver of AGCT pathogenesis, a lack of high-quality genetic model systems has hampered experimental efforts to determine the precise molecular alterations associated with this very specific mutation.

Previous molecular profiling studies have examined AGCTs using a variety of sequencing platforms, including whole-genome sequencing (48-50), exome sequencing (42,51), and targeted/panel sequencing (42,52,53). *TERT* promoter mutations, truncating *KMT2D* mutations, and pathogenic *TP53* mutations emerged as consensus recurrent events observed in multiple AGCT cohorts. More recently, a large series of 423 AGCTs analyzed using commercial tumor profiling was reported (54). No tumors in this series exhibited microsatellite instability, and none had high levels of genomic loss of heterozygosity, a marker of homologous recombination deficiency. Sixty-seven tumors were assessed for PD-L1 expression, and 94% were negative. Potentially actionable variants including *MTAP* deletion (5.8%) and activating *PIK3CA* mutations (5.4%) were identified. Most notably, this study identified *TP53*-mutated AGCT (8.3% of all cases) as having a higher tumor mutational burden and more extensive genomic loss of heterozygosity than *TP53* nonmutated tumors, suggesting a unique molecular pathogenesis for this subtype of AGCT.

Molecular studies of JGCTs are limited, but early investigations identified *AKT1* and *GNAS* mutations as recurrent and potentially driver events (55-57). More recently, multiplatform molecular analysis of a relatively large series of 31 JGCTs from 28 patients was reported (58). In this study, *AKT1* mutations were found in 29% of JGCTs, and most tumors were also found to have mutations in genes encoding enzymes with chromatin remodeling activity, including *KMT2C*, *KMT2D*, *ARID1A*, and *SETD2*. RNA sequencing of tumors in this same cohort identified *TERT* rearrangements, leading to in-frame fusion transcripts in a subset of JGCTs. Notably, genome-wide DNA methylation analysis revealed significant global differences between JGCT and AGCT, suggesting distinct epigenetic etiologies for these malignancies.

Normal granulosa cells are a source of estradiol during the follicular phase of the ovulatory cycle and express hormone receptors. The expression of estrogen receptor α (ERα) and progesterone receptor (PR) has been examined in SCST subtypes, predominantly GCTs. Farinola et al (59) examined expression in 41 AGCTs and 28 SLCTs, finding that expression of both receptors was frequent across both histologic subtypes. In total, these authors found expression of ERα in 66% of AGCTs and 79% of SLCTs, with PR expression identified in 98% and 86%, respectively. ERβ and PR were found to be detectable in all 56 primary stage I AGCTs studied by Hutton et al (60), with only 20% of tumors expressing ERα. Similar results were also reported by an independent group (61). There is clinical evidence that modulators of estrogen and progesterone pathway signaling are effective therapies for subsets of SCST (62). The prospective PARAGON trial of anastrozole monotherapy in patients with recurrent GCT used ER and/or PR expression in 10% of tumor cells as an inclusion criterion. The objective response rate was 10.5%, lower than anticipated from previously reported retrospective series. This suggests that ER/PR expression may at best be an imperfect predictive biomarker for response to hormonal deprivation in patients with GCT.

REFERENCES

1. Torre LA, Trabert B, DeSantis CE, et al. Ovarian cancer statistics, 2018. *CA Cancer J Clin.* 2018;68:284-296.

2. Quirk JT, Natarajan N. Ovarian cancer incidence in the United States, 1992–1999. *Gynecol Oncol.* 2005;97:519-523.

3. Ohel G, Kaneti H, Schenker JG. Granulosa cell tumors in Israel: a study of 172 cases. *Gynecol Oncol.* 1983;15:278-286.

4. Bryk S, Pukkala E, Martinsen J-I, et al. Incidence and occupational variation of ovarian granulosa cell tumours in Finland, Iceland, Norway and Sweden during 1953–2012: a longitudinal cohort study. *BJOG.* 2017;124:143-149.

5. Mink PJ, Sherman ME, Devesa SS. Incidence patterns of invasive and borderline ovarian tumors among white women and black women in the United States. Results from the SEER program, 1978–1998. *Cancer.* 2002;95:2380-2389.

6. Cramer DW, Devesa SS, Welch WR. Trends in the incidence of endometrioid and clear cell cancers of the ovary in the United States. *Am J Epidemiol.* 1981;114:201-208.

7. Sun HD, Lin H, Jao MS, et al. A long-term follow-up study of 176 cases with adult-type ovarian granulosa cell tumors. *Gynecol Oncol.* 2012;124:244-249.

8. Lee IH, Choi CH, Hong DG, et al. Clinicopathologic characteristics of granulosa cell tumors of the ovary: a multicenter retrospective study. *J Gynecol Oncol.* 2011;22:188-195.

9. Levin G, Zigron R, Haj-Yahya R, Matan LS, Rottenstreich A. Granulosa cell tumor of ovary: a systematic review of recent evidence. *Eur J Obstet Gynecol Reprod Biol.* 2018;225:57-61.

10. Vassal G, Flamant F, Caillaud JM, Demeocq F, Nihoul-Fekete C, Lemerle J. Juvenile granulosa cell tumor of the ovary in children: a clinical study of 15 cases. *J Clin Oncol.* 1988;6:990-995.

11. Calaminus G, Wessalowski R, Harms D, Göbel U. Juvenile granulosa cell tumors of the ovary in children and adolescents: results from 33 patients registered in a prospective cooperative study. *Gynecol Oncol.* 1997;65:447-452.

12. Young RH, Scully RE. Ovarian Sertoli-Leydig cell tumors. A clinicopathological analysis of 207 cases. *Am J Surg Pathol.* 1985;9:543-569.

13. Tavassoli FA, Norris HJ. Sertoli tumors of the ovary. A clinicopathologic study of 28 cases with ultrastructural observations. *Cancer.* 1980;46:2281-2297.

14. Roth LM, Anderson MC, Govan AD, Langley FA, Gowing NF, Woodcock AS. Sertoli-Leydig cell tumors: a clinicopathologic study of 34 cases. *Cancer.* 1981;48:187-197.

15. Scully RE. Sex cord tumor with annular tubules a distinctive ovarian tumor of the Peutz-Jeghers syndrome. *Cancer.* 1970;25:1107-1121.

16. Shen K, Wu PC, Lang JH, Huang RL, Tang MT, Lian LJ. Ovarian sex cord tumor with annular tubules: a report of six cases. *Gynecol Oncol.* 1993;48:180-184.

17. Qian Q, You Y, Yang J, et al. Management and prognosis of patients with ovarian sex cord tumor with annular tubules: a retrospective study. *BMC Cancer.* 2015;15:270.

18. Evans AT, III, Gaffey TA, Malkasian GD Jr, Annegers JF. Clinicopathologic review of 118 granulosa and 82 theca cell tumors. *Obstet Gynecol.* 1980;55:231-238.

19. Björkholm E, Silfverswärd C. Theca-cell tumors. Clinical features and prognosis. *Acta Radiol Oncol.* 1980;19:241-244.

20. Chechia A, Attia L, Temime RB, Makhlouf T, Koubaa A. Incidence, clinical analysis, and management of ovarian fibromas and fibrothecomas. *Am J Obstet Gynecol.* 2008;199:473.e1-473.e4.

21. Yamada Y, Ohmi K, Tsunematu R, et al. Gynandroblastoma of the ovary having a typical morphological appearance: a case study. *Jpn J Clin Oncol.* 1991;21:62-68.

22. Limaïem F, Lahmar A, Ben Fadhel C, Bouraoui S, M'zabi-Regaya S. Gynandroblastoma. Report of an unusual ovarian tumour and literature review. *Pathologica.* 2008;100:13-17.

23. Novak ER. Gynandroblastoma of the ovary: review of 8 cases from the ovarian tumor registry. *Obstet Gynecol.* 1967;30:709-715.

24. Chivukula M, Hunt J, Carter G, Kelley J, Patel M, Kanbour-Shakir A. Recurrent gynandroblastoma of ovary—a case report: a molecular and immunohistochemical analysis. *Int J Gynecol Pathol.* 2007;26:30-33.

25. Mangili G, Ottolina J, Gadducci A, et al. Long-term follow-up is crucial after treatment for granulosa cell tumours of the ovary. *Br J Cancer.* 2013;109:29-34.

26. Unkila-Kallio L, Leminen A, Tiitinen A, Ylikorkala O. Nationwide data on falling incidence of ovarian granulosa cell tumours concomitant with increasing use of ovulation inducers. *Hum Reprod.* 1998;13:2828-2830.

27. Boyce EA, Costaggini I, Vitonis A, et al. The epidemiology of ovarian granulosa cell tumors: a case-control study. *Gynecol Oncol.* 2009;115:221-225.

28. Bryk S, Katuwal S, Haltia U-M, Tapper J, Tapanainen JS, Pukkala E. Parity, menopausal hormone therapy, and risk of ovarian granulosa cell tumor—a population-based case-control study. *Gynecol Oncol.* 2021;163:593-597.

29. Roze JF, Kutzera J, Koole W, et al. Familial occurrence of adult granulosa cell tumors: analysis of whole-genome germline variants. *Cancers.* 2021;13(10):2430. doi:10.3390/cancers13102430

30. Stevens TA, Brown J, Zander DS, Bevers MW, Gershenson DM, Ramondetta LM. Adult granulosa cell tumors of the ovary in two first-degree relatives. *Gynecol Oncol.* 2005;98:502-505.

31. Heravi-Moussavi A, Anglesio MS, Cheng S-WG, et al. Recurrent somatic DICER1 mutations in nonepithelial ovarian cancers. *N Engl J Med.* 2012;366:234-242.

32. Schultz KAP, Williams GM, Kamihara J, et al. Dicer1 and associated conditions: identification of at-risk individuals and recommended surveillance strategies. *Clin Cancer Res.* 2018;24:2251-2261.

33. Conlon N, Schultheis AM, Piscuoglio S, et al. A survey of DICER1 hotspot mutations in ovarian and testicular sex cord-stromal tumors. *Mod Pathol.* 2015;28:1603-1612.

34. Kim J, Field A, Schultz KAP, Hill DA, Stewart DR. The prevalence of DICER1 pathogenic variation in population databases. *Int J Cancer.* 2017;141:2030-2036.

35. Young RH, Welch WR, Dickersin GR, Scully RE. Ovarian sex cord tumor with annular tubules: review of 74 cases including 27 with Peutz-Jeghers syndrome and four with adenoma malignum of the cervix. *Cancer.* 1982;50:1384-1402.

36. Connolly DC, Katabuchi H, Cliby WA, Cho KR. Somatic mutations in the STK11/LKB1 gene are uncommon in rare gynecological tumor types associated with Peutz-Jegher's syndrome. *Am J Pathol.* 2000;156:339-345.

37. Makanji Y, Zhu J, Mishra R, et al. Inhibin at 90: from discovery to clinical application, a historical review. *Endocr Rev.* 2014;35:747-794.

38. Petraglia F, Luisi S, Pautier P, et al. Inhibin B is the major form of inhibin/activin family secreted by granulosa cell tumors. *J Clin Endocrinol Metab.* 1998;83:1029-1032.

39. Mom CH, Engelen MJA, Willemse PHB, et al. Granulosa cell tumors of the ovary: the clinical value of serum inhibin A and B levels in a large single center cohort. *Gynecol Oncol.* 2007;105:365-372.

40. Namwanje M, Brown CW. Activins and inhibins: roles in development, physiology, and disease. *Cold Spring Harb Perspect Biol.* 2016;8:a021881. doi:10.1101/cshperspect.a021881

41. Lin Y-S, Eng H-L, Jan Y-J, et al. Molecular cytogenetics of ovarian granulosa cell tumors by comparative genomic hybridization. *Gynecol Oncol.* 2005;97:68-73.

42. Hillman RT, Celestino J, Terranova C, et al. KMT2D/MLL2 inactivation is associated with recurrence in adult-type granulosa cell tumors of the ovary. *Nat Commun.* 2018;9:2496.

43. Shah SP, Köbel M, Senz J, et al. Mutation of FOXL2 in granulosa-cell tumors of the ovary. *N Engl J Med.* 2009;360:2719-2729.

44. Crisponi L, Deiana M, Loi A, et al. The putative forkhead transcription factor FOXL2 is mutated in blepharophimosis/ptosis/epicanthus inversus syndrome. *Nat Genet.* 2001;27:159-166.

45. Schmidt D, Ovitt CE, Anlag K, et al. The murine winged-helix transcription factor Foxl2 is required for granulosa cell differentiation and ovary maintenance. *Development.* 2004;131:933-942.

46. Uda M, Ottolenghi C, Crisponi L, et al. Foxl2 disruption causes mouse ovarian failure by pervasive blockage of follicle development. *Hum Mol Genet.* 2004;13:1171-1181.

47. Goulvent T, Ray-Coquard I, Borel S, et al. DICER1 and FOXL2 mutations in ovarian sex cord-stromal tumours: a GINECO Group study. *Histopathology.* 2016;68:279-285.

48. Pilsworth JA, Cochrane DR, Xia Z, et al. TERT promoter mutation in adult granulosa cell tumor of the ovary. *Mod Pathol.* 2018;31:1107-1115.

49. Roze J, Monroe G, Kutzera J, et al. Whole genome analysis of ovarian granulosa cell tumors reveals tumor heterogeneity and a high-grade TP53-specific subgroup. *Cancers.* 2020;12:1-22.

50. Wang YK, Bashashati A, Anglesio MS, et al. Genomic consequences of aberrant DNA repair mechanisms stratify ovarian cancer histotypes. *Nat Genet.* 2017;49:856-865.

51. Alexiadis M, Rowley SM, Chu S, et al. Mutational landscape of ovarian adult granulosa cell tumors from whole exome and targeted TERT promoter sequencing. *Mol Cancer Res.* 2019;17:177-185.

52. Da Cruz Paula A, da Silva EM, Segura SE, et al. Genomic profiling of primary and recurrent adult granulosa cell tumors of the ovary. *Mod Pathol.* 2020;33:1606-1617.

53. Pilsworth JA, Cochrane DR, Neilson SJ, et al. Adult-type granulosa cell tumor of the ovary: a FOXL2-centric disease. *J Pathol Clin Res.* 2021;7:243-252.

54. Hillman RT, Lin DI, Lawson B, Gershenson DM. Prevalence of predictive biomarkers in a large cohort of molecularly defined adult-type ovarian granulosa cell tumors. *Gynecol Oncol.* 2021;162(3):728-734.

55. Auguste A, Bessière L, Todeschini A-L, et al. Molecular analyses of juvenile granulosa cell tumors bearing AKT1 mutations provide insights into tumor biology and therapeutic leads. *Hum Mol Genet.* 2015;24:6687-6698.

56. Bessière L, Todeschini AL, Auguste A, et al. A hot-spot of in-frame duplications activates the oncoprotein AKT1 in juvenile granulosa cell tumors. *EBioMedicine.* 2015;2:421-431.

57. Kalfa N, Ecochard A, Patte C, et al. Activating mutations of the stimulatory G protein in juvenile ovarian granulosa cell tumors: a new prognostic factor? *J Clin Endocrinol Metab.* 2006;91:1842-1847.

58. Vougiouklakis T, Zhu K, Vasudevaraja V, et al. Integrated analysis of ovarian juvenile granulosa cell tumors reveals distinct epigenetic signatures and recurrent TERT rearrangements. *Clin Cancer Res.* 2022;28(8):1724-1733. doi:10.1158/1078-0432.CCR-21-3394

59. Farinola MA, Gown AM, Judson K, et al. Estrogen receptor α and progesterone receptor expression in ovarian adult granulosa cell tumors and Sertoli-Leydig cell tumors. *Int J Gynecol Pathol.* 2007;26:375-382.

60. Hutton SM, Webster LR, Nielsen S, Leung Y, Stewart CJR. Immunohistochemical expression and prognostic significance of oestrogen receptor-alpha, oestrogen receptor-beta, and progesterone receptor in stage 1 adult-type granulosa cell tumour of the ovary. *Pathology.* 2012;44:611-616.

61. Ciucci A, Ferrandina G, Mascilini F, et al. Estrogen receptor β: potential target for therapy in adult granulosa cell tumors? *Gynecol Oncol.* 2018;150:158-165.

62. Van Meurs HS, Van Lonkhuijzen LRCW, Limpens J, Van Der Velden J, Buist MR. Hormone therapy in ovarian granulosa cell tumors: a systematic review. *Gynecol Oncol.* 2014;134:196-205.

CHAPTER **10.3**

Ovarian Sex Cord-Stromal Tumors: Clinical Presentation, Diagnostic Evaluation, and Workup

Carrie Langstraat

CLINICAL PRESENTATION

SCSTs account for nearly 90% of all functioning ovarian neoplasms (1). Apart from fibromas, the clinical presentation of patients with SCSTs is frequently governed by the clinical manifestations resulting from estrogen and androgen production (2-4). Although GCT, theca cell, and Sertoli cell tumors are generally considered to be estrogenic, and SLCTs and steroid cell tumors (SCTs) are predominantly androgenic, the functional endocrinologic manifestations of these tumors are variable. In addition, any ovarian tumor including those not in the SCST family may be hormonally active if their stroma is stimulated to undergo luteinization.

Patients with AGCT often present with one or more of the following clinical symptoms: abnormal vaginal bleeding, abdominal distention, amenorrhea, and abdominal pain (3-9). In addition to clinical signs related to hormone production, a large unilateral mass, often exceeding 10 cm in diameter, is the most common radiographic finding (3,7,10). In contrast to epithelial ovarian cancer, patients with GCT commonly present with stage I disease, with only 10% to 15% of patients presenting with ascites or advanced disease (5,11). Atypical adenomatous hyperplasia (42%), adenocarcinoma in situ (5%), and invasive adenocarcinoma (22%) are frequently observed in association with unopposed estrogen production (12). Many other investigators have corroborated the high prevalence of glandular hyperplasia and have reported adenocarcinoma frequencies ranging from 3% to 27% (2-4,6,7,9,10,13-15). Selective ovarian venous catheterizations during surgery have documented hormonal production, including the secretion of large quantities of estrogen from the ovary harboring the GCT. The return of serum estrogen to physiologic levels after surgical resection has also been demonstrated. Occasionally, patients with GCTs present with endometrial changes (decidual reaction of the stroma or secretory characteristics of the glands), consistent with tumor production of progesterone (16). Rarely, virilizing changes such as oligomenorrhea, hirsutism, and other masculinizing signs may accompany GCTs (17-19).

JGCTs account for 5% of all GCTs and may demonstrate a distinct tumor morphology and biology from the typical AGCT (20). In a clinicopathologic analysis of 125 cases of JGCT, 44% occurred before age 10, and only 3% after the third decade of life (21). Clinical evidence of isosexual precocious pseudopuberty is common (21-25). Rarely, a patient will harbor an androgen-secreting JGCT accompanied by virilization (21,23,24). Although the signs of either precocious pseudopuberty or virilization are dramatic, the most consistent clinical sign at presentation in patients with JGCTs is increasing abdominal girth. Young et al indicated that in only two of 113 nonpregnant patients with JGCTs was the treating physician unable to palpate a mass on abdominal, pelvic, and/or rectal examination (21). Similar to AGCTs, JGCTs are most often unilateral, and the majority of patients present with early-stage disease (21,23-25). Extraovarian spread is infrequently encountered at exploration, whereas rupture of the tumor is noted in approximately 10% of cases. Ascites contributes to the abdominal distention in 10% to 36% of cases (21,23-25).

Thecomas are among the most hormonally active SCSTs and, compared to granulosa tumors, present most frequently in the sixth and seventh decades of life and are generally benign. Thecomas are unilateral in 98% of patients and range from less than 1 to 40 cm in diameter (26-28). Abnormal bleeding is common (27,28). In the series reported by Evans et al (2), endometrial hyperplasia was observed in 37% of evaluable patients, and adenocarcinoma consistent with an unopposed estrogen effect was documented in an additional 27%.

Fibromas are the most common SCSTs. They are hormonally inactive, rarely malignant, and present in size ranging from microscopic to extremely large masses. Ascites is detected in association with 10% to 15% of ovarian fibromas that exceed a diameter of 10 cm (29). Furthermore, 1% of patients develop a hydrothorax in addition to the hydroperitoneum (Meigs syndrome) (30).

Sclerosing stromal cell tumors (SSTs) are benign neoplasms within the thecoma-fibroma family of ovarian tumors, which present during the second and third decades of life (31-34). In contrast to thecomas, SSTs are usually inactive endocrinologically (31,35). However, in a limited number of cases, steroidogenic activity has been demonstrated, even including androgenic manifestations, particularly if the patient is pregnant (31,35-39).

Sertoli cell tumors are rare tumors, which produce estrogen in approximately two-thirds of reported cases and present with hormonally associated signs as discussed earlier (40). Excessive renin production, refractory hypertension, and hypokalemia have been observed in patients with Sertoli cell tumors (41). Sertoli cell tumors have arisen in patients with PJS (41,42). These tumors are most commonly benign; however, features such as large size (>5 cm), necrosis, nuclear atypia, and high mitotic index suggest a higher risk of recurrence (40).

The presentation of SLCTs is related to the degree of histologic differentiation, the presence of a retiform pattern, and/or heterologous elements. SLCTs are rarely bilateral and present most commonly during the second and third decades of life (43-45). Frank virilization occurs in 35% of the patients with SLCTs, and another 10% to 15% have some clinical manifestations consistent with androgen excess. Signs of masculinization include amenorrhea, voice deepening, hirsutism, breast atrophy, clitorimegaly, loss of female contour, and temporal hair recession (44).

SCTATs present in the third to fourth decades of life with abnormal vaginal bleeding and one in three SCTATs occur in patients with PJS (46-52). PJS-associated SCTATs are often not detected via clinical examination. These tumors are typically small (many microscopic), multifocal, calcified, and bilateral and found incidentally at the time of surgery. The non-PJS tumors are considerably larger, seldom multifocal or calcified, and invariably unilateral. Assessment of circulating steroid levels has confirmed the presence of excessive estrogen in essentially all SCTAT cases, and expected clinical consequences as reviewed earlier are commonly seen (47,48,53,54). In contrast to PJS-associated tumors, elevated progesterone levels have been documented in patients with non-PJS (47,53,54).

Gynandroblastoma is an extremely rare tumor. In a recent review of the world literature, Martin-Jimenez et al (55) were able to identify only 17 authenticated cases of gynandroblastoma. These tumors demonstrate readily identifiable (at least 10%) granulosa cells, and tubules of Sertoli cells and theca and/or Leydig cells may also be present in varying degrees. The rarity of such cases makes generalizations about clinical presentation impossible, but signs and symptoms are typically related to size or hormonal activity of the tumor. Regardless of the associated hormonal activity, gynandroblastomas are considered benign (55,56).

Leydig cell tumors are rare, small, unilateral tumors, which typically present after menopause and are frequently not detectable via clinical examination or pelvic imaging. Most patients will demonstrate one or more of the following related to a hyperandrogenic state: hirsutism, acne, deepening of the voice, breast atrophy, clitorimegaly, and male pattern baldness. In contrast to the frequently dramatic onset and progression of virilization witnessed with SLCTs, ovarian Leydig cell tumors are generally characterized by a more indolent course. Paraskevas and Scully (57) reported an interval of 7 years between recognized onset of signs and symptoms of androgen excess and diagnosis.

Neoplasms identified as SCTs but lacking the specific characteristics of Leydig cell tumors are collectively classified as steroid cell tumors, not otherwise specified (SCTNOS). The average age at presentation of SCTNOS is 4, ranging from early childhood to the ninth decade of life (58,59). These generally solid yellow tumors are usually larger and more frequently bilateral than Leydig cell tumors. Hayes and Scully (58) reported that 81% of cases were localized (stage I), 6% were stage II, and 13% were stage III or IV. Clinical signs and/or symptoms of androgen excess are common. Approximately 10% to 15% of patients are asymptomatic, with tumors detected incidentally during routine pelvic examination or at the time of pelvic surgery. The steroid hormone–secreting capacities of SCTNOS are more diverse than those of most SCSTs and include cortisol excess (58-65). While elevated plasma levels of corticosteroids are typically observed in conjunction with SCTNOS, the number of overt presentations with Cushing syndrome is limited (60,63,65). However, 17% of the clinically malignant tumors reported by Hayes and Scully (58) were associated with Cushing syndrome. The serum testosterone and androstenedione levels are invariably elevated, as are urinary 17-ketosteroids; presumably, the latter reflect the level of excess androstenedione production.

EVALUATION/WORKUP

The workup of patients with SCST is dependent on the histologic type as well as the presenting symptoms. Patients presenting with precocious puberty should undergo a thorough evaluation by a pediatric endocrinologist. If an ovarian mass is identified on imaging, preoperative imaging, including a magnetic resonance imaging (MRI) or computed tomography (CT) of the abdomen and pelvis, should be considered before surgery to assess for metastatic disease and to allow for surgical planning. Patients presenting with abnormal uterine bleeding or postmenopausal bleeding should undergo age-dependent workup, which may include thyroid-stimulating hormone (TSH), FSH, LH, estradiol, pelvic ultrasound, and endometrial biopsy. Additional imaging in these patients will be dependent on findings on ultrasound. Most SCSTs will appear as a unilateral, hypoechoic solid lesion on ultrasound (66). Once malignant SCST is diagnosed, patients should undergo imaging, including a CT of the chest, abdomen, and pelvis, to assess for metastatic disease. In addition, tumor markers may be present in some malignant SCSTs.

Tumor Markers

The majority of patients presenting with advanced GCTs will recur. Identification of a specific serum tumor marker(s) would facilitate early detection of recurrent disease and monitoring of treatment effectiveness (2,3,7,10). As noted earlier, serum estrogens are generally produced by GCTs and have been utilized as an indicator of disease status (50). Unfortunately, serum estradiol levels are occasionally normal and more frequently are only marginally increased, making them less than ideal for monitoring in most patients. Several proteins derived from granulosa cells, including inhibin, follicle-regulating protein, and anti-Müllerian hormone (AMH, or Müllerian-inhibiting substance), are useful markers (67-75). In a prospective evaluation of 27 patients with GCTs, Jobling et al (69) demonstrated that serum inhibin levels are typically elevated 7-fold above normal follicular-phase levels before primary surgical management. In a comparative investigation of serum inhibin B and AMH, elevations in both were noted in 123 patients with primary and recurrent GCTs. The area under the curve of each was greater than 0.90 and somewhat higher when used in combination (76). Mom et al (77) showed that inhibin B was the predominant form of inhibin secreted by these tumors, with a sensitivity and specificity of 89% and 100%, respectively, compared with 67% and 100% for inhibin A. Elevations in inhibin B were present in 85% of recurrences, and predated clinical evidence of recurrence by a median of 11 months. Both inhibin and calretinin have become useful immunohistochemical markers to assist in the diagnosis of GCTs and other SCSTs (20). Although information specific to JGCTs is limited, the various tumor markers discussed earlier for AGCTs would appear to be applicable to JGCTs for monitoring of recurrent disease.

REFERENCES

1. Tavassoli FA. Ovarian tumors with functioning manifestations. *Endocr Pathol*. 1994;5(3):137-148.

2. Evans AT III, Gaffey TA, Malkasian GD, Annegers JF. Clinicopathologic review of 118 granulosa and 82 theca cell tumors. *Obstet Gynecol*. 1980;55(2):231-238.

3. Malmström H, Högberg T, Risberg B, Simonsen E. Granulosa cell tumors of the ovary: prognostic factors and outcome. *Gynecol Oncol*. 1994;52(1):50-55.

4. Ohel G, Kaneti H, Schenker JG. Granulosa cell tumors in Israel: a study of 172 cases. *Gynecol Oncol*. 1983;15(2):278-286.

5. Cronjé HS, Niemand I, Bam RH, Woodruff JD. Review of the granulosa-theca cell tumors from the Emil Novak ovarian tumor registry. *Am J Obstet Gynecol*. 1999;180(2 Pt 1):323-327.

6. Pankratz E, Boyes DA, White GW, Galliford BW, Fairey RN, Benedet JL. Granulosa cell tumors. A clinical review of 61 cases. *Obstet Gynecol*. 1978;52(6):718-723.

7. Piura B, Nemet D, Yanai-Inbar I, Cohen Y, Glezerman M. Granulosa cell tumor of the ovary: a study of 18 cases. *J Surg Oncol*. 1994;55(2):71-77.

8. Schumer ST, Cannistra SA. Granulosa cell tumor of the ovary. *J Clin Oncol*. 2003;21(6):1180-1189.

9. Schweppe KW, Beller FK. Clinical data of granulosa cell tumors. *J Cancer Res Clin Oncol*. 1982;104(1-2):161-169.

10. Stenwig JT, Hazekamp JT, Beecham JB. Granulosa cell tumors of the ovary. A clinicopathological study of 118 cases with long-term follow-up. *Gynecol Oncol*. 1979;7(2):136-152.

11. Levin G, Zigron R, Haj-Yahya R, Matan LS, Rottenstreich A. Granulosa cell tumor of ovary: A systematic review of recent evidence. *Eur J Obstet Gynecol Reprod Biol*. 2018;225:57-61.

12. Gusberg SB, Kardon P. Proliferative endometrial response to theca-granulosa cell tumors. *Am J Obstet Gynecol*. 1971;111(5):633-643.

13. Björkholm E, Silfverswärd C. Prognostic factors in granulosa-cell tumors. *Gynecol Oncol*. 1981;11(3):261-274.

14. Chen VW, Ruiz B, Killeen JL, Coté TR, Wu XC, Correa CN. Pathology and classification of ovarian tumors. *Cancer*. 2003;97(10 suppl):2631-2642.

15. Stuart GC, Dawson LM. Update on granulosa cell tumours of the ovary. *Curr Opin Obstet Gynecol*. 2003;15(1):33-37.

16. Young RH, Oliva E, Scully RE. Luteinized adult granulosa cell tumors of the ovary: a report of four cases. *Int J Gynecol Pathol*. 1994;13(4):302-310.

17. Nakashima N, Young RH, Scully RE. Androgenic granulosa cell tumors of the ovary. A clinicopathologic analysis of 17 cases and review of the literature. *Arch Pathol Lab Med*. 1984;108(10):786-791.

18. Norris HJ, Taylor HB. Virilization associated with cystic granulosa tumors. *Obstet Gynecol*. 1969;34(5):629-635.

19. Zanagnolo V, Pasinetti B, Sartori E. Clinical review of 63 cases of sex cord stromal tumors. *Eur J Gynaecol Oncol*. 2004;25(4):431-438.

20. McCluggage WG, Young RH. Immunohistochemistry as a diagnostic aid in the evaluation of ovarian tumors. *Semin Diagn Pathol*. 2005;22(1):3-32.

21. Young RH, Dickersin GR, Scully RE. Juvenile granulosa cell tumor of the ovary. A clinicopathological analysis of 125 cases. *Am J Surg Pathol*. 1984;8(8):575-596.

22. Lack EE, Perez-Atayde AR, Murthy AS, Goldstein DP, Crigler JF, Vawter GF. Granulosa theca cell tumors in premenarchal girls: a clinical and pathologic study of ten cases. *Cancer*. 1981;48(8):1846-1854.

23. Plantaz D, Flamant F, Vassal G, et al. Granulosa cell tumors of the ovary in children and adolescents. Multicenter retrospective study in 40 patients aged 7 months to 22 years. *Arch Fr Pédiatr*. 1992;49(9):793-798.

24. Vassal G, Flamant F, Caillaud JM, Demeocq F, Nihoul-Fekete C, Lemerle J. Juvenile granulosa cell tumor of the ovary in children: a clinical study of 15 cases. *J Clin Oncol*. 1988;6(6):990-995.

25. Zaloudek C, Norris HJ. Granulosa tumors of the ovary in children: a clinical and pathologic study of 32 cases. *Am J Surg Pathol*. 1982;6(6):503-512.

26. Barrenetxea G, Schneider J, Centeno MM, et al. Pure theca cell tumors. A clinicopathologic study of 29 cases. *Eur J Gynaecol Oncol*. 1990;11(6):429-432.

27. Björkholm E, Silfverswärd C. Theca-cell tumors. Clinical features and prognosis. *Acta Radiol Oncol*. 1980;19(4):241-244.

28. Burandt E, Young RH. Thecoma of the ovary: a report of 70 cases emphasizing aspects of its histopathology different from those often portrayed and its differential diagnosis. *Am J Surg Pathol*. 2014;38(8):1023-1032.

29. Samanth KK, Black WC III. Benign ovarian stromal tumors associated with free peritoneal fluid. *Am J Obstet Gynecol*. 1970;107(4):538-545.

30. Meigs JV. Fibroma of the ovary with ascites and hydrothorax; Meigs' syndrome. *Am J Obstet Gynecol*. 1954;67(5):962-985.

31. Chalvardjian A, Scully RE. Sclerosing stromal tumors of the ovary. *Cancer*. 1973;31(3):664-670.

32. Gee DC, Russell P. Sclerosing stromal tumours of the ovary. *Histopathology*. 1979;3(5):367-376.

33. Lam RM, Geittmann P. Sclerosing stromal tumor of the ovary. A light, electron microscopic and enzyme histochemical study. *Int J Gynecol Pathol*. 1988;7(3):280-290.

34. Roth LM, Gaba AR, Cheng L. On the pathogenesis of sclerosing stromal tumor of the ovary: a neoplasm in transition. *Int J Gynecol Pathol*. 2014;33(5):449-462.

35. Suit PF, Hart WR. Sclerosing stromal tumor of the ovary. An ultrastructural study and review of the literature to evaluate hormonal function. *Cleve Clin J Med*. 1988;55(2):189-194.

36. Bennett JA, Oliva E, Young RH. Sclerosing stromal tumors with prominent luteinization during pregnancy: a report of 8 cases emphasizing diagnostic problems. *Int J Gynecol Pathol*. 2015;34(4):357-362.

37. Cashell AW, Cohen ML. Masculinizing sclerosing stromal tumor of the ovary during pregnancy. *Gynecol Oncol*. 1991;43(3):281-285.

38. Ismail SM, Walker SM. Bilateral virilizing sclerosing stromal tumours of the ovary in a pregnant woman with Gorlin's syndrome: implications for pathogenesis of ovarian stromal neoplasms. *Histopathology*. 1990;17(2):159-163.

39. Katsube Y, Iwaoki Y, Silverberg SG, Fujiwara A. Sclerosing stromal tumor of the ovary associated with endometrial adenocarcinoma: a case report. *Gynecol Oncol*. 1988;29(3):392-398.

40. Oliva E, Alvarez T, Young RH. Sertoli cell tumors of the ovary: a clinicopathologic and immunohistochemical study of 54 cases. *Am J Surg Pathol*. 2005;29(2):143-156.

41. Korzets A, Nouriel H, Steiner Z, et al. Resistant hypertension associated with a renin-producing ovarian Sertoli cell tumor. *Am J Clin Pathol*. 1986;85(2):242-247.

42. Ferry JA, Young RH, Engel G, Scully RE. Oxyphilic Sertoli cell tumor of the ovary: a report of three cases, two in patients with the Peutz-Jeghers syndrome. *Int J Gynecol Pathol*. 1994;13(3):259-266.

43. Roth LM, Anderson MC, Govan AD, Langley FA, Gowing NF, Woodcock AS. Sertoli-Leydig cell tumors: a clinicopathologic study of 34 cases. *Cancer*. 1981;48(1):187-197.

44. Tavassoli FA, Norris HJ. Sertoli tumors of the ovary. A clinicopathologic study of 28 cases with ultrastructural observations. *Cancer*. 1980;46(10):2281-2297.

45. Young RH, Scully RE. Ovarian Sertoli-Leydig cell tumors. A clinicopathological analysis of 207 cases. *Am J Surg Pathol.* 1985;9(8):543-569.

46. Ahn GH, Chi JG Lee SK. Ovarian sex cord tumor with annular tubules. *Cancer.* 1986;57(5):1066-1073.

47. Benagiano G, Bigotti G, Buzzi M, D'Alessandro P, Napolitano C. Endocrine and morphological study of a case of ovarian sex-cord tumor with annular tubules in a woman with Peutz-Jeghers syndrome. *Int J Gynaecol Obstet.* 1988;26(3):441-452.

48. Hart WR, Kumar N, Crissman JD. Ovarian neoplasms resembling sex cord tumors with annular tubules. *Cancer.* 1980;45(9):2352-2363.

49. Podczaski E, Kaminski PF, Pees RC, Singapuri K, Sorosky JI. Peutz-Jeghers syndrome with ovarian sex cord tumor with annular tubules and cervical adenoma malignum. *Gynecol Oncol.* 1991;42(1):74-78.

50. Shen K, Wu PC, Lang JH, Huang RL, Tang MT, Lian LJ. Ovarian sex cord tumor with annular tubules: a report of six cases. *Gynecol Oncol.* 1993;48(2):180-184.

51. Solh HM, Azoury RS, Najjar SS. Peutz-Jeghers syndrome associated with precocious puberty. *J Pediatr.* 1983;103(4):593-595.

52. Young RH, Welch WR, Dickersin GR, Scully RE. Ovarian sex cord tumor with annular tubules: review of 74 cases including 27 with Peutz-Jeghers syndrome and four with adenoma malignum of the cervix. *Cancer.* 1982;50(7):1384-1402.

53. Crain JL. Ovarian sex cord tumor with annular tubules: steroid profile. *Obstet Gynecol.* 1986;68(3 suppl):75S-79S.

54. Jenne DE, Reimann H, Nezu J, et al. Peutz-Jeghers syndrome is caused by mutations in a novel serine threonine kinase. *Nat Genet.* 1998;18(1):38-43.

55. Martin-Jimenez A, Condom-Munró E, Valls-Porcel M, Giné-Martin L, Del Amo E, Balagueró-Lladó L. Gynandroblastoma of the ovary. Review of the literature. *J Gynecol Obstet Biol Reprod (Paris).* 1994;23(4):391-394.

56. Novak ER. Gynandroblastoma of the ovary: review of 8 cases from the ovarian tumor registry. *Obstet Gynecol.* 1967;30(5):709-715.

57. Paraskevas M, Scully RE. Hilus cell tumor of the ovary. A clinicopathological analysis of 12 Reinke crystal-positive and nine crystal-negative cases. *Int J Gynecol Pathol.* 1989;8(4):299-310.

58. Hayes MC, Scully RE. Ovarian steroid cell tumors (not otherwise specified). A clinicopathological analysis of 63 cases. *Am J Surg Pathol.* 1987;11(11):835-845.

59. Sharma R, Goel RK, Rana A, Sachdev R. Ovarian steroid cell tumor, not otherwise specified. *Pathologica.* 2018;110(2):121-122.

60. Adeyemi SD, Grange AO, Giwa-Osagie OF, Elesha SO. Adrenal rest tumour of the ovary associated with isosexual precocious pseudopuberty and cushingoid features. *Eur J Pediatr.* 1986;145(3):236-238.

61. Clement PB, Young RH, Scully RE. Clinical syndromes associated with tumors of the female genital tract. *Semin Diagn Pathol.* 1991;8(4):204-233.

62. Dengg K, Fink FM, Heitger A, et al. Precocious puberty due to a lipid-cell tumour of the ovary. *Eur J Pediatr.* 1993;152(1):12-14.

63. Donovan JT, Otis CN, Powell JL, Cathcart HK. Cushing's syndrome secondary to malignant lipoid cell tumor of the ovary. *Gynecol Oncol.* 1993;50(2):249-253.

64. Taylor HB, Norris HJ. Lipid cell tumors of the ovary. *Cancer.* 1967;20(11):1953-1962.

65. Young RH, Scully RE. Ovarian steroid cell tumors associated with Cushing's syndrome: a report of three cases. *Int J Gynecol Pathol.* 1987;6(1):40-48.

66. Javadi S, Ganeshan DM, Jensen CT, Iyer RB, Bhosale PR. Comprehensive review of imaging features of sex cord-stromal tumors of the ovary. *Abdom Radiol (NY).* 2021;46(4):1519-1529.

67. Boggess JF, Soules MR, Goff BA, Greer BE, Cain JM, Tamimi HK. Serum inhibin and disease status in women with ovarian granulosa cell tumors. *Gynecol Oncol.* 1997;64(1):64-69.

68. Gustafson ML, Lee MM, Asmundson L, MacLaughlin DT, Donahoe PK. Müllerian inhibiting substance in the diagnosis and management of intersex and gonadal abnormalities. *J Pediatr Surg.* 1993;28(3):439-444.

69. Jobling T, Mamers P, Healy DL, et al. A prospective study of inhibin in granulosa cell tumors of the ovary. *Gynecol Oncol.* 1994;55(2):285-289.

70. Lane AH, Lee MM, Fuller AF, Kehas DJ, Donahoe PK, MacLaughlin DT. Diagnostic utility of Müllerian inhibiting substance determination in patients with primary and recurrent granulosa cell tumors. *Gynecol Oncol.* 1999;73(1):51-55.

71. Lappöhn RE, Burger HG, Bouma J, Bangah M, Krans M. Inhibin as a marker for granulosa cell tumor. *Acta Obstet Gynecol Scand Suppl.* 1992;155:61-65.

72. Lappöhn RE, Burger HG, Bouma J, Bangah M, Krans M, de Bruijn HW. Inhibin as a marker for granulosa-cell tumors. *N Engl J Med.* 1989;321(12):790-793.

73. Rey RA, Lhommé C, Marcillac I, et al. Antimüllerian hormone as a serum marker of granulosa cell tumors of the ovary: comparative study with serum alpha-inhibin and estradiol. *Am J Obstet Gynecol.* 1996;174(3):958-965.

74. Rodgers KE, Marks JF, Ellefson DD, et al. Follicle regulatory protein: a novel marker for granulosa cell cancer patients. *Gynecol Oncol.* 1990;37(3):381-387.

75. Sluijmer AV, Heineman MJ, Evers JL, de Jong FH. Peripheral vein, ovarian vein and ovarian tissue levels of inhibin in a postmenopausal patient with a granulosa cell tumour. *Acta Endocrinol (Copenh).* 1993;129(4):311-314.

76. Färkkilä A, Koskela S, Bryk S, et al. The clinical utility of serum anti-Müllerian hormone in the follow-up of ovarian adult-type granulosa cell tumors—a comparative study with inhibin B. *Int J Cancer.* 2015;137(7):1661-1671.

77. Mom CH, Engelen MJ, Willemse PH, et al. Granulosa cell tumors of the ovary: the clinical value of serum inhibin A and B levels in a large single center cohort. *Gynecol Oncol.* 2007;105(2):365-372.

CHAPTER **10.4**

Surgery for Ovarian Sex Cord-Stromal Tumors

Carrie Langstraat

The definitive management of SCSTs is dependent on surgical stage, histologic subtype, patient's age, and desire for fertility preservation. Surgical resection alone is sufficient for benign SCSTs. Adjuvant therapy should be considered for patients with advanced-stage GCT or SLCTs with poor differentiation or with mesenchymal heterologous elements and is discussed separately (1).

Surgery remains the cornerstone for the treatment for patients with SCSTs. Following sampling of peritoneal washings for cytologic assessment, inspection of peritoneal surfaces and abdominal viscera is conducted to detect macroscopic disease. Resection of the ovarian tumor constitutes sufficient therapy for the essentially benign neoplasms, including thecomas, fibromas, gynandroblastomas, stromal luteomas, Leydig cell, sclerosing stromal, Sertoli cell, and well-differentiated SLCTs. Furthermore, SCTATs associated with PJS are also considered benign and can be similarly managed, but it is imperative that the endocervix be evaluated and subsequently monitored for the potential development of adenoma malignum of the cervix (ACM). If the uterus is preserved, a thorough curettage must be performed in all patients with estrogen-producing tumors whether they are considered to be benign or potentially malignant (2).

Upon histologic confirmation of GCTs, intermediate or poorly differentiated SLCTs, SCSTs with annular tubules independent of PJS, and sex cord tumor not otherwise specified (SCTNOS), surgical staging is required. This includes peritoneal biopsies, omentectomy, and resection of grossly suspicious pelvic or para-aortic lymph nodes. Careful inspection of the peritoneum and nodal basin is critical because residual disease is strongly correlated with recurrence. The role of routine lymphadenectomy in the absence of grossly suspicious lymph nodes is debatable, and current guidelines support omission of a formal lymphadenectomy. This recommendation is based on the low frequency of lymph node metastasis and low incidence of isolated nodal recurrence. In three recent series of 1,706 patients with GCT who underwent lymphadenectomy, 58 (3.1%) harbored lymph node metastases (3-5). Risk of lymph node metastases is associated with stage, with 25% of patients with stage IV disease having lymph node metastasis (3-5). In the absence of suspicious lymphadenopathy, lymphadenectomy does not appear to improve survival in GCT or SLST. Furthermore, isolated retroperitoneal recurrences are rare. In 34 patients with recurrent GCTs, two recurred in the retroperitoneum only, two in the pelvis and retroperitoneum, and one in the pelvis, abdomen, and retroperitoneum (6). In another series of 87 patients, only two of 18 recurrences were isolated to the retroperitoneum (7). Overall, approximately 10% to 15% of first recurrences involve the retroperitoneum.

Fertility preservation may be considered in patients with malignant SCST with early-stage disease. In a review of the 1988 to 2001 SEER database, Zhang et al identified 376 patients with ovarian SCST (8). The survival for the group of 110 patients with stage I-II diseases who underwent conservative surgery without hysterectomy was similar to patients who underwent standard surgery. The Japanese Gynecologic Oncology Group (GOG) reported outcomes on 243 patients younger than 49 years with stage I disease. In this population, there was no difference in cause-specific survival in patients undergoing fertility-preserving therapy (3). For older patients or those with advanced-stage disease or bilateral ovarian involvement, abdominal hysterectomy and bilateral salpingo-oophorectomy are usually indicated. Others have reported conservative management for patients with advanced JGCTs treated with cytoreduction and chemotherapy, leading to prolonged disease-free intervals and multiple pregnancies (2).

Although no randomized evidence exists pertaining to the efficacy of cytoreduction in malignant SCSTs, based on the benefits observed with their epithelial counterparts, we endorse an aggressive maximum effort at primary surgery if metastatic disease is encountered. In a multivariate analysis of 176 patients with GCTs, only residual disease after primary surgery and tumor size were predictive of recurrence (9). Furthermore, in a series of 86 patients with advanced-stage disease, residual disease, but not adjuvant chemotherapy, was associated with recurrence and survival (3).

The value of secondary cytoreduction continues to be controversial but appears to be meritorious for the more indolent tumor types, such as GCTs and SCTATs not associated with PJS. Repeat cytoreduction frequently affords these patients extended palliation and should be considered the cornerstone for the treatment of recurrent disease. Recently, cytoreductive surgery with heated intraperitoneal chemotherapy has been suggested as a treatment option for patients with recurrent GCT (10).

References

1. Gershenson DM, Copeland LJ, Kavanagh JJ, Stringer CA, Saul PB, Wharton JT. Treatment of metastatic stromal tumors of the ovary with cisplatin, doxorubicin, and cyclophosphamide. *Obstet Gynecol.* 1987;70(5):765-769.

2. Powell JL, Kotwall CA, Shiro BC. Fertility-sparing surgery for advanced juvenile granulosa cell tumor of the ovary. *J Pediatr Adolesc Gynecol.* 2014;27(4):e89-e92.

3. Ebina Y, Yamagami W, Kobayashi Y, et al. Clinicopathological characteristics and prognostic factors of ovarian granulosa cell tumors: a JSGO-JSOG joint study. *Gynecol Oncol.* 2021;163(2):269-273.

4. Kuru O, Boyraz G, Uckan H, et al. Retroperitoneal nodal metastasis in primary adult type granulosa cell tumor of the ovary: can routine lymphadenectomy be omitted? *Eur J Obstet Gynecol Reprod Biol.* 2017;219:70-73.

5. Seagle BL, Ann P, Butler S, Shahabi S. Ovarian granulosa cell tumor: a National Cancer Database study. *Gynecol Oncol.* 2017;146(2):285-291.

6. Gershenson DM. Chemotherapy of ovarian germ cell tumors and sex cord stromal tumors. *Semin Surg Oncol.* 1994;10(4):290-298.

7. Abu-Rustum NR, Restivo A, Ivy J, et al. Retroperitoneal nodal metastasis in primary and recurrent granulosa cell tumors of the ovary. *Gynecol Oncol.* 2006;103(1):31-34.

8. Zhang M, Cheung MK, Shin JY, et al. Prognostic factors responsible for survival in sex cord stromal tumors of the ovary—an analysis of 376 women. *Gynecol Oncol.* 2007;104(2):396-400.

9. Sun HD, Lin H, Jao MS, et al. A long-term follow-up study of 176 cases with adult-type ovarian granulosa cell tumors. *Gynecol Oncol.* 2012;124(2):244-249.

10. Al-Badawi IA, Abu-Zaid A, Azzam A, AlOmar O, AlHusaini H, Amin T. Cytoreductive surgery and hyperthermic intraperitoneal chemotherapy for management of recurrent/relapsed ovarian granulosa cell tumor: a single-center experience. *J Obstet Gynaecol Res.* 2014;40(9):2066-2075.

CHAPTER **10.5**

Ovarian Sex Cord-Stromal Tumors: Pathology and Prognostic Factors

Robert H. Young and Barrett Lawson

Introduction

Adult Granulosa Cell Tumor

Pathology

AGCTs have an average diameter of approximately 12 cm, but a subset, 10% to 15%, of cases are small and not appreciated on pelvic examination (1). Most characteristically, they are solid and cystic, with the locules filled with fluid or clotted blood and separated by solid tissue (**Figure 10.5-1**), or they are uniformly solid. The solid tissue may be gray white or yellow and soft or firm; hemorrhage is occasionally seen and may be striking. Rarely, AGCTs are cystic, usually thin walled, but occasionally thick walled, and may be multilocular or unilocular (2).

Microscopic examination reveals an almost exclusive population of granulosa cells or, more often, an additional component of fibroblasts, theca cells, or both. The granulosa cells grow in a wide

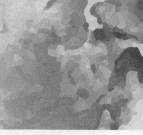

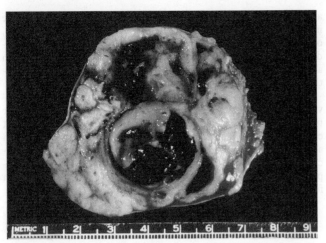

Figure 10.5-1. Granulosa cell tumor, adult type. The sectioned surface is solid and cystic. The cysts contain blood and the solid tissue is yellow to white.

variety of patterns. Commonly, the histologic features are that of solid sheets of round blue cells with scant cytoplasm, with variably prominent epithelial patterns including (in rough order of frequency): cords, trabeculae, nests, microfollicles, and macrofollicles. The microfollicular pattern is characterized by numerous small cavities (Call-Exner bodies) (**Figure 10.5-2**) that may contain eosinophilic fluid, one or a few degenerating nuclei, hyalinized basement membrane material, or, rarely, basophilic fluid. Call-Exner bodies, although touted as the hallmark of AGCTs, are uncommon and may be mimicked in various other neoplasms. The microfollicles are typically separated by well-differentiated granulosa cells that contain scanty cytoplasm and pale, angular, or oval, often-grooved nuclei arranged haphazardly in relation to one another and to the follicles. The uncommon macrofollicular pattern is characterized by cysts lined by well-differentiated granulosa cells beneath which theca cells are present. The majority of AGCTs are actually characterized in greater part, sometimes uniformly, by a relatively diffuse growth of cells with scant cytoplasm with epithelial patterns of growth either absent or only focal, and often only seen after careful scrutiny. The corded-trabecular and insular forms of GCTs are characterized by cords, thicker bands, and islands of granulosa cells often separated by a fibrothecomatous stroma. Rare tumors have a watered silk (moire silk) or gyriform pattern, in which cords

have picturesque regular arrangements captured by the noted designation. Most AGCTs have cells with scant cytoplasm, but in some, the neoplastic cells have moderate-to-abundant amount of eosinophilic cytoplasm; the term *luteinized granulosa cell tumor* is appropriate when such cells predominate (3). Some other tumors have appreciable cytoplasm, which is pale and resembles the cytoplasm of typical thecoma cells; such tumors often have a nodular growth pattern. In these cases, a reticulin stain may be helpful in disclosing the epithelial nature of the background tumor and hence the diagnosis of GCT rather than thecoma (4). The cells in GCTs usually have round to oval, pale, and often-grooved nuclei (**Figure 10.5-2**), but rarely, the cells are spindle shaped, resembling a cellular fibroma or low-grade fibrosarcoma; mitotic figures (MFs) may be numerous but are rarely atypical. There is usually only mild nuclear atypia, but approximately 2% of tumors contain mononucleate and multinucleate cells with large, bizarre, hyperchromatic nuclei, the presence of which does not appear to worsen prognosis (5). Rare tumors transform to foci of anaplasia with adverse prognostic significance (6). Fashedemi et al described four stage IA neoplasms, one of which developed widespread disease 17 months after initial diagnosis (6).

Although the histologic appearance of AGCTs is usually easily recognized, supplemental immunohistochemical studies may help facilitate diagnosis in difficult cases. Inhibin, calretinin, and SF1 are typically positive, whereas reticulin highlights nests or groups of cells rather than individual, pericellular staining as previously mentioned (4).

Prognostic Factors

The staging system for GCTs is the same as that used for epithelial ovarian cancer. It was revised in 2014 (International Federation of Gynaecology and Obstetrics [FIGO]). Surgical stage has been recognized as the most important prognostic factor for GCTs, whereas the impact of tumor size, histologic subtype, nuclear atypia, and mitotic activity on outcome is less clear; larger, well-characterized series are necessary to clarify existing discrepancies (7-9). GCTs are prone to rupture, which appears to adversely impact survival and be a predictive factor for recurrence in stage I patients, justifying stratification as stage IC (10-12). In a series of 240 patients, treated before 1984, age greater than 60 years, tumor size greater than 10 cm, advanced stage, residual tumor, and use of hormonal therapy were associated with GCT-related death. However, on multivariate analysis only stage remained significant for survival (13). The presence of residual tumor following initial debulking surgery has been shown to be a significant adverse prognostic factor (14). Tumor size has been variably associated with risk of death (14-18). Increasing degrees of nuclear atypia and increasing mitotic frequency per 10 high-power fields (HPFs) have been correlated inversely with prognosis, but older series, in particular, may contain tumors that by present-day criteria would not be accepted as GCTs. Specimens from patients with more advanced disease tend to demonstrate higher grade of atypia and/or more MFs (10,15-17). Despite its somewhat subjective assessment, nuclear grade has reportedly been a reliable prognostic indicator in stage I cases, but the authors are personally dubious about this finding (10,17). High-grade transformation, also referred to as sarcomatous transformation, has been described and is suspected as having a more aggressive clinical course; however, such cases are rare (6). The significance of histologic subtypes has been debated, and they appear to be of minimal value. Several investigative groups have failed to confirm Kottmeier's report of the prognostic importance of histologic patterns alone in GCTs (10,15,16,19-21). Similarly, the results of investigations utilizing flow cytometric analysis of DNA content have been inconsistent. Klemi et al reported a significant survival advantage for patients with tumors demonstrating normal ploidy and/or an S-phase fraction (SPF) of less than 6% (22). However, other investigators have suggested that nondiploid GCTs are infrequently encountered (23,24). Another investigation of 20 GCTs

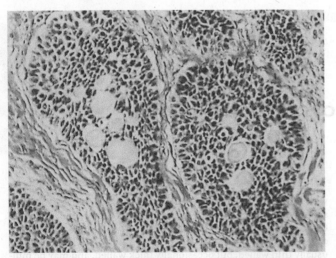

Figure 10.5-2. Granulosa cell tumor, adult type, microfollicular pattern. Several nests of granulosa cells with small oval and angular nuclei enclose multiple Call-Exner bodies.

found that the degree of nuclear atypia, mitotic count, Ki-67 index, and DNA aneuploidy were not predictive of tumor recurrence (11). Chadha et al reported that three of five aneuploid tumors from a total population of 43 GCTs were vimentin negative but positive for cytokeratin and epithelial membrane antigen and, therefore, cautioned that such highly aneuploid tumors may represent undifferentiated carcinomas (23). Indeed, it is clear, as alluded to already, that some series of GCTs in the literature include undifferentiated carcinomas not otherwise specified, or recently recognized entities such as the small cell carcinoma of hypercalcemic type. Therefore, series with unusually large numbers of late-stage or poor prognosis cases should be evaluated cautiously.

Investigators have analyzed several potential molecular markers, including p53 status, telomerase, Ki-67, c-myc, HER2/neu, and vascular endothelial growth factor (VEGF) in GCTs (25-31). To date, no molecular marker provides additional prognostic information for GCTs beyond what is known from stage and histopathologic parameters.

Ala-Fossi et al stained 30 GCTs for the inhibin subunit. All 24 stage I and II tumors were positive, whereas four of six stage II-IV tumors were negative (32). Those that were negative were poorly differentiated and exhibited rapid disease progression. Whether other observers would have accepted these tumors as valid GCTs is a concern. Stage was the sole independent prognostic factor.

Juvenile Granulosa Cell Tumor

Pathology

The gross appearances of JGCTs are similar to the adult form, with a solid and cystic neoplasm commonly containing hemorrhagic fluid (33-35). Uniformly solid and uniformly cystic neoplasms are also encountered; the latter may be multilocular or, in rare instances, unilocular (2). The solid component is typically yellow tan or gray and, occasionally, exhibits extensive necrosis, hemorrhage, or both.

Microscopic examination typically reveals a predominantly solid cellular tumor with focal follicle formation, but occasionally, a uniformly solid or a uniformly follicular pattern is seen. In the solid areas, the neoplastic cells may be arranged diffusely or as multiple nodules of various sizes. The follicles typically vary in size and shape; Call-Exner bodies are rarely encountered, and the follicles rarely reach the large size of those in the macrofollicular AGCT. The follicular lumens in the juvenile tumor contain eosinophilic or basophilic fluid, which stains with mucicarmine in approximately two of three cases.

The two characteristic cytologic features of the neoplastic juvenile granulosa cells that distinguish them from those of AGCT are their generally rounded, hyperchromatic nuclei, which almost always lack grooves, and their almost invariable moderate-to-abundant eosinophilic or vacuolated (luteinized) cytoplasm (Figure 10.5-3). Nuclear atypia in JGCTs varies from minimal to marked; in approximately 13% of the cases, severe degrees are present. The mitotic rate also varies greatly but is generally higher than that seen in AGCTs, often being five or more per 10 HPFs (33). In cases with severe nuclear atypia, the normal balanced follicular and solid patterns of these tumors is still usually retained, but occasionally, it is lost with a more diffuse pattern of growth and extensive necrosis, a picture that causes concern prognostically. However, follow-up information on these rare cases does not exist currently, but we comment on the concerning morphology on a case-by-case basis.

Prognostic Factors

Young et al noted that surgical stage represented the most reliable prognostic indicator (33). Tumor size, mitotic activity, and nuclear atypia were significant predictors only when analyzed without regard to stage. In that series, rupture did not correlate with outcome. Schneider et al reported on a group of 54 SCSTs in children and adolescents from Germany (45 JGCTs and nine others) (36).

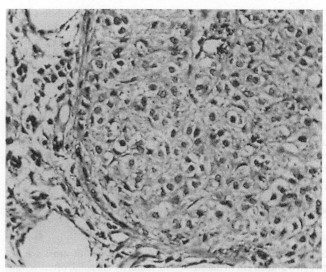

Figure 10.5-3. Granulosa cell tumor, juvenile type. A nodule of tumor is composed of large cells with abundant cytoplasm and slightly pleomorphic, hyperchromatic nuclei.

They addressed the outcome of patients with "accidental" stage IC disease, defined as violation of the tumor capsule during surgery, versus "natural" stage IC tumors, with preoperative rupture or malignant ascites. Among 12 patients with accidental stage IC disease, there were no recurrences. In contrast, five of the nine patients with natural stage IC disease recurred ($P = 0.001$). Assessment of DNA content via flow cytometry in JGCTs demonstrated nondiploid patterns in nearly half (37,38). However, Jacoby et al were unable to correlate DNA ploidy or SPF with either stage of disease or prognosis in patients with localized disease (37). In the series by Schneider et al, mitotic activity correlated with prognosis (36). There were no relapses in 35 patients whose tumors exhibited low or moderate mitotic activity. Among those with high mitotic activity (>19 mitoses per 10 HPFs), approximately half recurred. As noted earlier, although objective proof is not available, there are rare cases in which severe atypia, extensive necrosis, and the absence of the usual balanced architecture of these tumors cause concern.

Fibroma

Pathology

Fibromas histologically are composed of intersecting fascicles of cells with bland, spindled to ovoid nuclei and scant cytoplasm with variable collagenous or hyalinized stroma (39). Some tumors are intensely cellular (39). Rare cases containing eosinophilic hyaline globules or melanin pigment have been reported (40,41).

Prognostic Factors

The prognosis for patients diagnosed with cellular fibromas is generally favorable. Recurrences of these tumors, which we consider of low malignant potential, are generally correlated with adherent disease, rupture, or incomplete removal at the time of primary resection (39,42). In contrast, fibrosarcomas have a higher likelihood of recurrence but fortunately are rare (42).

Sertoli Cell Tumor

Pathology

On gross examination, these rare tumors are typically solid, lobulated, and yellow and sometimes demonstrate variable hemorrhage and necrosis (43,44).

Microscopic examination shows hollow or solid tubules lined by cells that usually exhibit relatively bland cytologic features, but rare tumors exhibit moderate-to-severe nuclear atypia. In most of these tumors, a tubular pattern predominates, but occasionally, a diffuse pattern is conspicuous.

Prognostic Factors

The great majority of these rare tumors have been unilateral stage I lesions. The majority of Sertoli cell tumors are well differentiated and are rarely malignant (43). Oliva et al reported that in patients with known stage and adverse outcomes, 71% had moderate-to-severe nuclear atypia and 85% had a mitotic count of 5 or higher per 10 HPFs (43).

Sertoli-Leydig Cell Tumor

Pathology

SLCTs vary in size from small to huge masses, but most are between 5 and 15 cm in diameter. The majority are solid, often yellow, and lobulated (**Figure 10.5-4**), but many are solid and cystic. Pure cystic tumors are rare, in contrast to GCTs. Poorly differentiated tumors tend to be larger than more differentiated tumors and more frequently contain areas of hemorrhage and necrosis (45,46). Tumors with heterologous or retiform components are more often cystic than other tumors in this category (47-50). The heterologous tumors occasionally simulate mucinous cystic tumors on gross examination, and retiform tumors may contain large edematous intracystic papillae, resembling serous papillary tumors, or may be soft and spongy, with varying degrees of cyst formation (49,51).

Well-differentiated SLCTs are characterized by a predominantly tubular pattern (52). On low-power examination, a nodular architecture is often conspicuous, with fibrous bands intersecting lobules composed of small, round, hollow, or, less often, solid tubules lined by well-differentiated cells and separated by variable numbers of Leydig cells. Rarely, the tubules appear pseudoendometrioid (53).

SLCTs of intermediate and poor differentiation form a continuum characterized by a variety of patterns and combinations of cell types (45,46,54). Some tumors exhibit intermediate differentiation

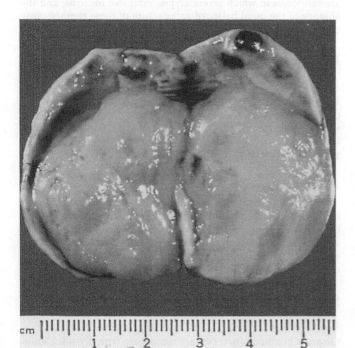

Figure 10.5-4. Sertoli-Leydig cell tumor. The sectioned surface of the tumor is focally lobulated and was yellow in the fresh state.

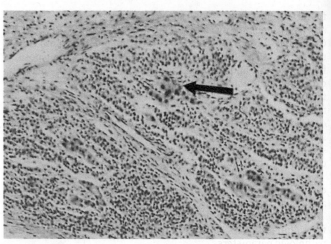

Figure 10.5-5. Sertoli-Leydig cell tumor, intermediate differentiation. Nests of large Leydig cells (arrow) lie among bands of immature Sertoli cells. (Reprinted with permission from Morris JM, Scully RE. *Endocrine Pathology of the Ovary.* Mosby; 1958;82-96.)

in some areas and poor differentiation in others; less commonly, tumors of intermediate differentiation contain well-differentiated foci. Both the Sertoli cells and the Leydig cells may exhibit varying degrees of immaturity. In tumors of intermediate differentiation, immature Sertoli cells have small, round, oval, or angular nuclei, generally scanty cytoplasm, and are arranged typically in ill-defined masses, often creating a lobulated appearance on low power; solid and hollow tubules, nests, broad columns of Sertoli cells, and, most characteristically, thin cords resembling the sex cords of the embryonic testis are often present (**Figure 10.5-5**). These structures are separated by stroma, which ranges from fibromatous to densely cellular to edematous, and typically contains clusters of well-differentiated Leydig cells (**Figure 10.5-5**). Cysts containing eosinophilic secretion may be present, creating a thyroid-like appearance, and follicle-like spaces are encountered rarely (55). These spaces can impart a focal resemblance to juvenile granulosa cell tumor. The Sertoli cell and Leydig cell elements, singly or in combination, may contain varying and sometimes large amounts of lipid, in the form of small or large droplets. When a significant amount of the tumor is composed of immature cellular mesenchymal tissue with high mitotic activity resembling a nonspecific sarcoma, the tumor is poorly differentiated.

Fifteen percent of SLCTs have a substantial retiform component and are so designated because they are composed of a network of elongated tubules and cysts, both of which may contain papillae, resembling the rete testis (46). This pattern is usually accompanied by other patterns of SLCTs, but sometimes, an entire tumor has a retiform pattern.

Heterologous elements occur in approximately 20% of SLCTs (49). About 20% contain glands and cysts lined by well to moderately-differentiated intestinal-type epithelium (49,50). Mesenchymal heterologous elements, encountered in 5% of tumors, include islands of cartilage arising on a sarcomatous background, areas of embryonal rhabdomyosarcoma, or both (56).

Prognostic Factors

Stage is the most important predictor of outcome in SLCTs. Fortunately, 97% of SLCTs are stage I at diagnosis, and less than 20% of these localized tumors become clinically malignant. The most cogent phenotypic prognostic determinant for stage I SLCTs is the degree of histologic differentiation (45,49). Approximately one-half of the reported SLCTs are of intermediate differentiation, 10% are well differentiated, 20% are heterologous, and the remainder are poorly differentiated. No extraovarian spread or subsequent recurrences were encountered by Young and Scully among

23 well-differentiated SLCTs (52). However, approximately 10% of intermediate and 60% of poorly differentiated tumors, as well as 20% of heterologous tumors, demonstrated clinically malignant behavior (49). The heterologous tumors contain either endodermal elements such as gastrointestinal epithelium and carcinoids or mesenchymal elements including skeletal muscles and/or cartilage. The endodermal elements are typically associated with intermediately differentiated homologous elements and represent 75% of the heterologous SLCTs. Their corresponding prognosis parallels that of the intermediately differentiated homologous tumors. In contrast, heterologous tumors containing mesenchymal elements account for 5% of all SLCTs and invariably coexist with a poorly differentiated homologous component. The clinically aggressive malignant behavior of poorly differentiated heterologous tumors is evident by the extremely low rates of survival (45,49).

SLCTs harboring a retiform pattern are associated with a 20% rate of malignancy, significantly higher than the 12% rate in nonretiform SLCTs. Young and Scully noted that 14 of 25 retiform cases were of intermediate differentiation, with one demonstrating poorly differentiated homologous histology and 10 exhibiting heterologous elements (three intermediate and seven poorly differentiated) (46,49). The less favorable prognosis likely reflects the frequency of associated heterologous and/or poorly differentiated homologous lesions. This concept is supported by the finding that the majority of the metastatic lesions do not contain retiform patterns (49). Although only four of over 100 reported intermediately differentiated SLCTs were clinically malignant, three of the four contained retiform patterns (46,49).

Tumor size, mitotic activity, and rupture have been reported to influence prognosis (45,49). The size, mitotic index, and rupture frequency appear to increase as histologic dedifferentiation increases. Notwithstanding these associations, substratification of intermediate and poorly differentiated lesions according to these parameters is the most significant prognostic feature.

Sex Cord Tumor With Annular Tubules

Pathology

These tumors may be associated or unassociated with PJS. Grossly, the PJS-associated tumors (when visible, as many are microscopic) are small, solid, and yellow and are frequently bilateral. The non–PJS-associated neoplasms, which are almost always grossly visible, may be similar but, in some cases, are solid and cystic or mostly cystic. This tumor is characterized microscopically by the presence of simple and complex annular tubules (**Figure 10.5-6**). The simple

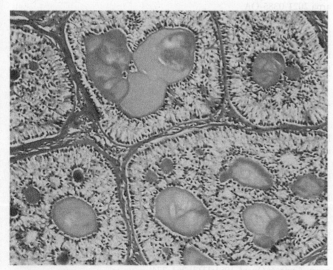

Figure 10.5-6. Sex cord tumor with annular tubules. Numerous rounded tubules encircle multiple hyaline bodies.

tubules have the shape of a ring, with the nuclei oriented around the periphery and around a central hyalinized body composed of basement membrane–like material; an intervening anuclear cytoplasmic zone forms the major component of the ring. The more numerous complex tubules are rounded structures comprising intercommunicating rings revolving around multiple hyaline bodies. In patients with PJS, the tumors are typically multifocal and exhibit calcification.

Prognostic Factors

Notwithstanding their histologic similarities, the differences in the natural history and long-term prognosis for SCTATs associated with or independent of PJS are readily apparent. Those detected in women with PJS are benign, as expected given their small size. Important in the management of this entity, however, is the recognition that approximately 15% of these patients develop gastric-type endocervical adenocarcinoma, previously referred to as adenoma malignum (57). In addition, there are rare exceptions to the rule of usual good outcome. Barker et al reported a 54-year-old woman with SCTAT and PJS demonstrating aggressive malignant behavior, with multiple recurrences (58). In their review of the literature, the authors identified two previous such patients. Because of delayed declaration of symptoms, the diagnosis of adenoma malignum is frequently made following examination of the hysterectomy specimen. In a review by Srivatsa et al, the prognosis for patients with PJS with SCTAT and adenoma malignum is ominous, due to the aggressive and often deep invasion of the cervical cancer, which is refractory to treatment (59).

Based on the compiled data from four reported series including 63 patients with SCTATs and without clinically apparent PJS, the rate of malignancy was approximately 20% (57,60-62). Primary extraovarian extension and/or frequency of recurrence have been correlated with the original tumor size and mitotic activity. The tumor characteristically has a relatively long doubling time, a propensity for lymphatic dissemination, and is apt to remain lateralized. Because the primary ovarian lesion is invariably unilateral, the lymphatic metastases are invariably ipsilateral, extending within the confines from the para-aortic region to the supraclavicular area. The nature of retroperitoneal metastases generally facilitates surgical resection and repeat cytoreduction. This tumor's indolent growth pattern, coupled with the relative ease of resection, affords patients extended palliation.

Leydig Cell Tumors

Pathology

Histologically, Leydig cell tumors are typically composed of a monotonous proliferation of cells with abundant eosinophilic cytoplasm, and they less often have pale foamy lipid-rich cells than other SCTs (see later). The cells are predominantly cytologically bland, but bizarre nuclear atypia may be encountered; this is almost always unassociated with mitotic activity and should not lead to concern for malignancy. Roth and Sternberg subdivided these tumors according to location and possibly the cell of origin, namely, Leydig cell tumors of hilar type versus nonhilar type (63). Whereas the latter presumably arise from ovarian stromal cells and are extremely rare, the former tumors are located in the hilus of the ovary and encroach on or extend into the ovarian stroma to varying degrees. Other features of Leydig cell tumors (including location in the ovarian hilus or adjacent to nonmedullated nerve fibers, association with hilar cell hyperplasia, fibrinoid vascular changes in the tumor, and clustering of cells around vessels) indicate that tumors lacking crystals of Reinke should likely be considered Leydig cell tumors (63).

Prognostic Factors

In a review of the English literature through 1988, 38 Reinke-positive cases were accrued, and only a single case of a clinically malignant lesion was identified (64,65). Based on tumor size (15 cm) alone, this sole example might be considered an outlier. Hence, ovarian Leydig cell tumors are essentially benign neoplasms.

Steroid Cell Tumor, Not Otherwise Specified

Pathology

These tumors are typically solid, well circumscribed, occasionally lobulated (**Figure 10.5-7**) and, on average, measure 8.4 cm in diameter (66). Approximately 5% are bilateral. They are typically yellow or orange but are occasionally red, dark brown, or black. Necrosis, hemorrhage, and cystic degeneration are occasionally observed.

On microscopic examination, the tumor cells are typically arranged diffusely but occasionally grow in nests, irregular clusters, thin cords, and columns. A fibrous and somewhat hyalinized stroma is notable in occasional tumors. The polygonal to rounded tumor cells have distinct cell borders, central nuclei, and moderate-to-abundant amounts of cytoplasm varying from eosinophilic and granular to vacuolated and spongy (**Figure 10.5-8**). In approximately 60% of the cases, nuclear atypia is absent or minimal and mitotic activity is low (<2 MFs per 10 HPFs) (66). In the remaining cases, grades 1 to 3 nuclear atypia are present, usually associated with an increase in mitotic activity (up to 15 MFs per 10 HPFs). Occasional small SCTs (formally placed in the stromal luteoma category) are associated with hyperthecosis, which may contribute to the androgenic manifestations in such cases.

Prognostic Factors

In contrast to the benign natural history of Leydig cell tumors, SCTNOS is associated with an appreciable rate of clinical malignancy (although there may be a reporting bias). In the largest series in the literature, 43% of patients with follow-up of 3 years or more demonstrated extraovarian disease, either at primary surgery or during subsequent follow-up (66). Multiple factors appear to correlate with the frequency of disseminated disease, including age, stage, tumor size, mitotic activity, tumor necrosis, hemorrhage, and symptoms of Cushing syndrome. The average age of patients with spread is 16 years older than patients without metastatic disease. No clinically malignant cases have been reported to date in patients younger than 15 years. All malignant SCTNOS were reported to measure 7 cm or more in greatest diameter; 78% of all tumors 7 cm or larger were malignant, whereas

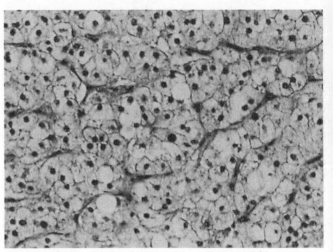

Figure 10.5-8. Steroid cell tumor. The tumor cells are large and rounded and laden with lipid vacuoles. (Reprinted with permission from Hayes MC, Scully RE. Ovarian steroid cell tumors not otherwise specified [lipid cell tumors]: a clinicopathologic analysis of 63 cases. *Am J Surg Pathol.* 1987;11:835-845.)

only 21% of benign tumors exceeded this dimension (66). The most cogent determinant correlating with malignant potential was mitotic activity, with 92% of malignant tumors displaying 2 or more MFs per 10 HPFs. Similarly, in the presence of necrosis, 86% were malignant; if hemorrhage was present, 77% were malignant. In addition, three of four patients (17% of all malignant cases) with recognizable Cushing syndrome harbored clinically malignant disease (66).

Although the majority of recurrences become clinically manifest within 3 years of diagnosis, Hayes and Scully reported that 22% of recurrences occurred after 3 years, usually after 5 years; the longest interval was 19 years (66). Therefore, the duration of post-treatment surveillance should be essentially lifelong.

REFERENCES

1. Fathalla MF. The occurrence of granulosa and theca tumours in clinically normal ovaries. A study of 25 cases. *J Obstet Gynaecol Br Commonw.* 1967;74(2):278-282.

2. Boyraz B, Watkins JC, Soubeyran I, et al. Cystic granulosa cell tumors of the ovary: an analysis of 80 cases of an often diagnostically challenging entity. *Arch Pathol Lab Med.* 2022;146(12):1450-1459. doi:10.5858/arpa.2021-0385-OA

3. Young RH, Oliva E, Scully RE. Luteinized adult granulosa cell tumors of the ovary: a report of four cases. *Int J Gynecol Pathol.* 1994;13(4):302-310.

4. Stall JN, Young RH. Granulosa cell tumors of the ovary with prominent thecoma-like foci: a report of 16 cases emphasizing the ongoing utility of the reticulin stain in the modern era. *Int J Gynecol Pathol.* 2019;38(2):143-150.

5. Young RH, Scully RE. Ovarian sex cord–stromal tumors with bizarre nuclei: a clinicopathologic analysis of 17 cases. *Int J Gynecol Pathol.* 1983;1(4):325-335.

6. Fashedemi Y, Coutts M, Wise O, et al. Adult granulosa cell tumor with high-grade transformation: report of a series with FOXL2 mutation analysis. *Am J Surg Pathol.* 2019;43(9):1229-1238.

7. Schumer ST, Cannistra SA. Granulosa cell tumor of the ovary. *J Clin Oncol.* 2003;21(6):1180-1189.

8. Miller BE, Barron BA, Wan JY, Delmore JE, Silva EG, Gershenson DM. Prognostic factors in adult granulosa cell tumor of the ovary. *Cancer.* 1997;79(10):1951-1955.

9. Fujimoto T, Sakuragi N, Okuyama K, et al. Histopathological prognostic factors of adult granulosa cell tumors of the ovary. *Acta Obstet Gynecol Scand.* 2001;80(11):1069-1074.

10. Bjorkholm E, Silfversward C. Prognostic factors in granulosa-cell tumors. *Gynecol Oncol.* 1981;11(3):261-274.

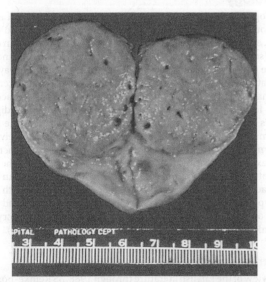

Figure 10.5-7. Steroid cell tumor, unclassified. The sectioned surface of the tumor is lobulated and was yellow orange in the fresh state. This tumor was from a 9-year-old virilized girl.

11. Wilson MK, Fong P, Mesnage S, et al. Stage I granulosa cell tumours: a management conundrum? Results of long-term follow up. *Gynecol Oncol.* 2015;138(2):285-291.

12. Bryk S, Färkkilä A, Bützow R, et al. Characteristics and outcome of recurrence in molecularly defined adult-type ovarian granulosa cell tumors. *Gynecol Oncol.* 2016;143(3):571-577.

13. Bryk S, Färkkilä A, Bützow R, et al. Clinical characteristics and survival of patients with an adult-type ovarian granulosa cell tumor: a 56-year single-center experience. *Int J Gynecol Cancer.* 2015;25(1):33-41.

14. Sun HD, Lin H, Jao MS, et al. A long-term follow-up study of 176 cases with adult-type ovarian granulosa cell tumors. *Gynecol Oncol.* 2012;124(2):244-249.

15. Malmstrom H, Hogberg T, Risberg B, Simonsen E. Granulosa cell tumors of the ovary: prognostic factors and outcome. *Gynecol Oncol.* 1994;52(1):50-55.

16. Fox H, Agrawal K, Langley FA. A clinicopathologic study of 92 cases of granulosa cell tumor of the ovary with special reference to the factors influencing prognosis. *Cancer.* 1975;35(1):231-241.

17. Stenwig JT, Hazekamp JT, Beecham JB. Granulosa cell tumors of the ovary. A clinicopathological study of 118 cases with long-term follow-up. *Gynecol Oncol.* 1979;7(2):136-152.

18. Bjorkholm E, Silfversward C. Granulosa- and theca-cell tumors. Incidence and occurrence of second primary tumors. *Acta Radiol Oncol.* 1980;19(3):161-167.

19. Evans AT, Gaffey TA, Malkasian GD Jr, Annegers JF. Clinicopathologic review of 118 granulosa and 82 theca cell tumors. *Obstet Gynecol.* 1980;55(2):231-238.

20. Bjorkholm E. Granulosa cell tumors: a comparison of survival in patients and matched controls. *Am J Obstet Gynecol.* 1980;138(3):329-331.

21. Kottmeier HL. *Carcinoma of the Female Genitalia.* Williams & Wilkins; 1953.

22. Klemi PJ, Joensuu H, Salmi T. Prognostic value of flow cytometric DNA content analysis in granulosa cell tumor of the ovary. *Cancer.* 1990;65(5):1189-1193.

23. Chadha S, Cornelisse CJ, Schaberg A. Flow cytometric DNA ploidy analysis of ovarian granulosa cell tumors. *Gynecol Oncol.* 1990;36(2):240-245.

24. Evans MP, Webb MJ, Gaffey TA, Katzmann JA, Suman VJ, Hu TC. DNA ploidy of ovarian granulosa cell tumors. Lack of correlation between DNA index or proliferative index and outcome in 40 patients. *Cancer.* 1995;75(9):2295-2298.

25. Ala-Fossi SL, Maenpaa J, Aine R, Koivisto P, Koivisto AM, Punnonen R. Prognostic significance of p53 expression in ovarian granulosa cell tumors. *Gynecol Oncol.* 1997;66(3):475-479.

26. Kappes S, Milde-Langosch K, Kressin P, et al. p53 mutations in ovarian tumors, detected by temperature-gradient gel electrophoresis, direct sequencing and immunohistochemistry. *Int J Cancer.* 1995;64(1):52-59.

27. Villella J, Herrmann FR, Kaul S, et al. Clinical and pathological predictive factors in women with adult-type granulosa cell tumor of the ovary. *Int J Gynecol Pathol.* 2007;26(2):154-159.

28. King LA, Okagaki T, Gallup DG, Twiggs LB, Messing MJ, Carson LF. Mitotic count, nuclear atypia, and immunohistochemical determination of Ki-67, c-myc, p21-ras, c-erbB2, and p53 expression in granulosa cell tumors of the ovary: mitotic count and Ki-67 are indicators of poor prognosis. *Gynecol Oncol.* 1996;61(2):227-232.

29. Liu FS, Ho ES, Lai CR, et al. Overexpression of p53 is not a feature of ovarian granulosa cell tumors. *Gynecol Oncol.* 1996;61(1):50-53.

30. Dowdy SC, O'Kane DJ, Keeney GL, Boyd J, Podratz KC. Telomerase activity in sex cord–stromal tumors of the ovary. *Gynecol Oncol.* 2001;82(2):257-260.

31. Färkkilä A, Anttonen M, Pociuviene J, et al. Vascular endothelial growth factor (VEGF) and its receptor VEGFR-2 are highly expressed in ovarian granulosa cell tumors. *Eur J Endocrinol.* 2011;164(1):115-122.

32. Ala-Fossi SL, Aine R, Punnonen R, Mäenpää J. Is potential to produce inhibins related to prognosis in ovarian granulosa cell tumors? *Eur J Gynaecol Oncol.* 2000;21(2):187-189.

33. Young RH, Dickersin GR, Scully RE. Juvenile granulosa cell tumor of the ovary. A clinicopathological analysis of 125 cases. *Am J Surg Pathol.* 1984;8(8):575-596.

34. Lack EE, Perez-Atayde AR, Murthy AS, Goldstein DP, Crigler JF, Vawter GF. Granulosa theca cell tumors in premenarchal girls: a clinical and pathologic study of ten cases. *Cancer.* 1981;48(8):1846-1854.

35. Zaloudek C, Norris HJ. Granulosa tumors of the ovary in children: a clinical and pathologic study of 32 cases. *Am J Surg Pathol.* 1982;6(6):503-512.

36. Schneider DT, Calaminus G, Wessalowski R, et al. Ovarian sex cord–stromal tumors in children and adolescents. *J Clin Oncol.* 2003;21(12):2357-2363.

37. Jacoby AF, Young RH, Colvin RB, et al. DNA content in juvenile granulosa cell tumors of the ovary: a study of early- and advanced-stage disease. *Gynecol Oncol.* 1992;46(1):97-103.

38. Swanson SA, Norris HJ, Kelsten ML, Wheeler JE. DNA content of juvenile granulosa tumors determined by flow cytometry. *Int J Gynecol Pathol.* 1990;9(2):101-109.

39. Prat J, Scully RE. Cellular fibromas and fibrosarcomas of the ovary: a comparative clinicopathologic analysis of seventeen cases. *Cancer.* 1981;47(11):2663-2670.

40. Michal M, Kacerovska D, Mukensnabl P, et al. Ovarian fibromas with heavy deposition of hyaline globules: a diagnostic pitfall. *Int J Gynecol Pathol.* 2009;28(4):356-361.

41. Taylor J, McCluggage WG. Ovarian sex cord-stromal tumors with melanin pigment: report of a previously undescribed phenomenon. *Int J Gynecol Pathol.* 2019;38(1):92-96.

42. Irving JA, Alkushi A, Young RH, Clement PB. Cellular fibromas of the ovary: a study of 75 cases including 40 mitotically active tumors emphasizing their distinction from fibrosarcoma. *Am J Surg Pathol.* 2006;30(8):929-938.

43. Oliva E, Alvarez T, Young RH. Sertoli tumors of the ovary: a clinicopathologic and immunohistochemical study of 54 cases. *Am J Surg Pathol.* 2005;29(2):143-156.

44. Tavassoli FA, Norris HJ. Sertoli tumors of the ovary. A clinicopathologic study of 28 cases with ultrastructural observations. *Cancer.* 1980;46(10):2281-2297.

45. Roth LM, Anderson MC, Govan AD, Langley FA, Gowing NF, Woodcock AS. Sertoli-Leydig cell tumors: a clinicopathologic study of 34 cases. *Cancer.* 1981;48(1):187-197.

46. Young RH, Scully RE. Ovarian Sertoli-Leydig cell tumors with a retiform pattern: a problem in histopathologic diagnosis. A report of 25 cases. *Am J Surg Pathol.* 1983;7(8):755-771.

47. Roth LM, Slayton RE, Brady LW, Blessing JA, Johnson G. Retiform differentiation in ovarian Sertoli-Leydig cell tumors. A clinicopathologic study of six cases from a Gynecologic Oncology Group study. *Cancer.* 1985;55(5):1093-1098.

48. Talerman A. Ovarian Sertoli-Leydig cell tumor (androblastoma) with retiform pattern. A clinicopathologic study. *Cancer.* 1987;60(12):3056-3064.

49. Young RH, Scully RE. Ovarian Sertoli-Leydig cell tumors. A clinicopathological analysis of 207 cases. *Am J Surg Pathol.* 1985;9(8):543-569.

50. Young RH, Prat J, Scully RE. Ovarian Sertoli-Leydig cell tumors with heterologous elements. I. Gastrointestinal epithelium and carcinoid: a clinicopathologic analysis of thirty-six cases. *Cancer.* 1982;50:2448-2456.

51. Young RH. Sertoli-Leydig cell tumors of the ovary: review with emphasis on historical aspects and unusual variants. *Int J Gynecol Pathol.* 1993;12(2):141-147.

52. Young RH, Scully RE. Well-differentiated ovarian Sertoli-Leydig cell tumors: a clinicopathological analysis of 23 cases. *Int J Gynecol Pathol.* 1984;3(3):277-290.

53. McCluggage WG, Young RH. Ovarian Sertoli-Leydig cell tumors with pseudoendometrioid tubules (pseudoendometrioid Sertoli-Leydig cell tumors). *Am J Surg Pathol.* 2007;31(4):592-597.

54. Zaloudek C, Norris HJ. Sertoli-Leydig tumors of the ovary. A clinicopathologic study of 64 intermediate and poorly differentiated neoplasms. *Am J Surg Pathol.* 1984;8(6):405-418.

55. Ordulu Z, Young RH. Sertoli-Leydig cell tumors of the ovary with follicular differentiation often resembling juvenile granulosa cell tumor: a report of 38 cases including comments on sex cord-stromal tumors of mixed forms (so-called gynandroblastoma). *Am J Surg Pathol.* 2021;45(1):59-67.

56. Prat J, Young RH, Scully RE. Ovarian Sertoli-Leydig cell tumors with heterologous elements. II. Cartilage and skeletal muscle: a clinicopathologic analysis of twelve cases. *Cancer.* 1982;50(11):2465-2475.

57. Young RH, Welch WR, Dickersin GR, Scully RE. Ovarian sex cord tumor with annular tubules: review of 74 cases including 27 with Peutz-Jeghers syndrome and four with adenoma malignum of the cervix. *Cancer.* 1982;50(7):1384-1402.

58. Barker D, Sharma R, McIndoe A, et al. An unusual case of sex cord tumor with annular tubules with malignant transformation in a patient with Peutz-Jeghers syndrome. *Int J Gynecol Pathol.* 2010;29(1):27-32.

59. Srivatsa PJ, Keeney GL, Podratz KC. Disseminated cervical adenoma malignum and bilateral ovarian sex cord tumors with annular tubules associated with Peutz-Jeghers syndrome. *Gynecol Oncol.* 1994;53(2):256-264.

60. Shen K, Wu PC, Lang JH, Huang RL, Tang MT, Lian LJ. Ovarian sex cord tumor with annular tubules: a report of six cases. *Gynecol Oncol.* 1993;48(2):180-184.

61. Hart WR, Kumar N, Crissman JD. Ovarian neoplasms resembling sex cord tumors with annular tubules. *Cancer.* 1980;45(9):2352-2363.

62. Ahn GH, Chi JG, Lee SK. Ovarian sex cord tumor with annular tubules. *Cancer.* 1986;57:1066-1073.

63. Roth LM, Sternberg WH. Ovarian stromal tumors containing Leydig cells. II. Pure Leydig cell tumor, non-hilar type. *Cancer.* 1973;32(4):952-960.

64. Paraskevas M, Scully RE. Hilus cell tumor of the ovary. A clinicopathological analysis of 12 Reinke crystal-positive and nine crystal-negative cases. *Int J Gynecol Pathol.* 1989;8(4):299-310.

65. Dunnihoo DR, Grieme DL, Woolf RB. Hilar-cell tumors of the ovary. Report of 2 new cases and a review of the world literature. *Obstet Gynecol.* 1966;27(5):703-713.

66. Hayes MC, Scully RE. Ovarian steroid cell tumors (not otherwise specified). A clinicopathological analysis of 63 cases. *Am J Surg Pathol.* 1987;11(11):835-845.

CHAPTER **10.6**

Therapy for Ovarian Sex Cord-Stromal Tumors: Radiation, Chemotherapy, Targeted Therapy, Immunotherapy, and Other New and Novel Agents

R. Tyler Hillman

CHEMOTHERAPY—ADJUVANT TREATMENT

The decision to use adjuvant systemic treatment for SCSTs following primary surgery is based on recurrence risk as estimated from surgical stage and histologic subtype, often incorporating information about patient age and desire for future fertility. Most patients with stage I GCTs have an excellent prognosis after surgery alone and do not require adjuvant therapy. For those patients with stage IC disease, consideration should be given to adjuvant therapy on an individualized basis acknowledging that high-quality, prospective data are lacking in this area. One key factor to consider is that patients with stage IC GCT probably have worse outcomes than those with stage IA disease. In a study of 104 patients with stage I GCTs, Wilson et al (1) observed higher relapse rates (43% vs 24%; $P = .02$) and shorter time to relapse (10.2 years vs 16.2 years; $P = .007$) in patients with stage IC versus stage IA disease.

The question of whether chemotherapy reduces the risk of recurrence with stage IC disease is controversial and remains an active area of investigation. The MITO-9 investigators looked at whether patients with stage IC GCTs benefitted from adjuvant chemotherapy (paclitaxel/carboplatin or bleomycin/etoposide/cisplatin [BEP]) (2). Of 40 patients included in this retrospective study, 23% received adjuvant chemotherapy, and there was no statistically significant difference in survival outcomes when comparing patients who received adjuvant chemotherapy to those who did not (5-year disease-free survival 27% and 50%, respectively; $P = .4$). Epidemiologic studies have also not shown a survival benefit with adjuvant chemotherapy in early-stage GCT. Nasioudis et al (3) examined patients with stage IC GCT diagnosed between 2004 and 2015 in the National Cancer Database (NCDB). Of 492 patients included in this study, 33.7% received adjuvant chemotherapy. After adjusting for patient age, tumor size, and performance of lymphadenectomy, the authors found that chemotherapy for stage IC GCT was not associated with a survival benefit (hazard ratio [HR] 1.07, 95% confidence interval [CI] 0.52-2.21). National consensus guidelines continue to include both adjuvant chemotherapy and surveillance as options for the management of stage IC SCSTs. Although paclitaxel/carboplatin given every 21 days is the preferred regimen, the optimal duration of chemotherapy has not

been established. Given the lack of conclusive data for a survival benefit with adjuvant chemotherapy for stage IC GCT, treatment approaches in this setting should be individualized.

Stage I well-differentiated SLCTs have very low risk of recurrence following surgery, whereas those tumors with intermediate differentiation may recur in 11% and poorly differentiated tumors in 59% of cases (4). Other histologic features such as the presence of heterologous (eg, gastrointestinal) elements or a retiform pattern have also been linked to a poor prognosis (4,5). The MITO-9 group has reported their experience with 21 patients with SLCTs (6). Five patients received adjuvant chemotherapy—platinum-based chemotherapy in four (BEP in two and paclitaxel/carboplatin in two), and one received the combination of methotrexate, 5-fluorouracil, and cyclophosphamide. Three of the five patients subsequently died of disease. Seven patients (one stage IA grade 1, three stage IA grade 2, one stage IC grade 2, and two stage IIIC grade 3) relapsed, four of whom had stage IA disease and did not receive adjuvant chemotherapy. Five of these patients were treated with surgery plus chemotherapy, one received chemotherapy alone, and one received palliation only. All six patients who received chemotherapy were treated with platinum-based regimens—either BEP or paclitaxel/carboplatin. At the time of the report, two patients—one with stage IA grade 1 and one with stage IA grade 2—were clinically disease free, and the other five died of disease. Gui et al (7) reported 40 cases of stage IA or IC ovarian SLCTs seen at Peking Union Medical College Hospital in Beijing, China, between 1966 and 2009. Of 34 cases with intermediate or poor differentiation, 23 received adjuvant chemotherapy (17 platinum-based chemotherapy; six non–platinum-based chemotherapy) following surgery. None of the 23 patients relapsed, whereas two of 11 patients who did not receive adjuvant chemotherapy relapsed. Although no high-quality data indicate that adjuvant chemotherapy for SLCTs with high-risk pathologic features reduces recurrence risk, published guidelines and expert opinion support the use of adjuvant chemotherapy for advanced-stage disease or in the presence of high-risk histologic features.

Less data exist regarding the postoperative management of rarer SCST subtypes. Calaminus et al (8) reported the outcome of 33 patients with JGCTs—24 treated with surgery alone and nine with surgery and cisplatin-based chemotherapy. The authors reported six relapses with 60 months median follow-up: two of 20 stage IA, two of eight stage IC, and two of five stages IIC-IIIC. Three patients with stage IIC-IIIC diseases treated with adjuvant cisplatin-based therapy remained disease free at 46 to 66 months after diagnosis. German investigators published their 15-year experience (1985-2000) with 54 SCSTs in children and adolescents (9). Forty-five were JGCTs. Twelve received adjuvant chemotherapy for stages IC-IIIC disease. BEP and cisplatin/etoposide/ifosfamide were the most used regimens. Six patients remained in remission after adjuvant chemotherapy 15 to 106 months later. A seventh developed a contralateral JGCT 10 years after her initial primary tumor. Five of the 12 have recurred, three of whom died 16 to 28 months from diagnosis. A more recent retrospective series of 17 patients with early-stage JGCT included four with stage IC disease (10), with most patients undergoing fertility-sparing surgery and only two receiving adjuvant chemotherapy. After a median follow-up period of 80 months, no recurrences were noted. Together these results suggest that although adjuvant chemotherapy has a role in the upfront management of advanced-stage JGCT, the approach in stage I disease should be individualized, given excellent outcomes with surveillance alone.

CHEMOTHERAPY—ADVANCED-STAGE DISEASE

Most patients presenting with advanced-stage (stages II-IV) SCST should receive chemotherapy, either postoperatively or as primary systemic therapy, with appropriate consideration given to individual characteristics, such as performance status and comorbidities. The GOG has reported the largest series of patients with ovarian SCSTs treated with chemotherapy (11). Using a single-arm design, eligible patients with incompletely resected stages II-IV or recurrent disease were administered four cycles of BEP. The primary outcome was the frequency of negative second-look surgery. Seventy-five patients entered, but 18 were ineligible because of incorrect histology or disease status. Of the 57 eligible patients, 41 had recurrent disease and 16 had advanced-stage primary disease. Thirty-nine had gross residual disease following surgery. Forty-eight had GCTs, seven had SLCTs, one had a malignant thecoma, and one had an unclassified SCST. Based on these results, BEP was established as an active regimen, with 37% of patients undergoing second-look surgery having negative findings. In addition, 11 of 16 primary disease patients and 21 of 41 recurrent disease patients remained progression free at a median follow-up of 3 years. The regimen was toxic, with two bleomycin-related fatalities among the first six patients treated with the initial bleomycin dose of 20 U/m^2 (maximum 30 U) weekly for 9 weeks. The bleomycin dose was then reduced (20 U/m^2 every 3 weeks × 4 cycles), with no further toxicity. Grade 4 myelotoxicity occurred in 61% of the patients.

Owing to the toxicity of BEP especially in older patients, subsequent efforts have explored alternative chemotherapy regimens for advanced-stage or high-risk disease. In 1995, a case report documented a dramatic response to paclitaxel in a patient with a GCT 2 years following cessation of platinum-based therapy (12). Subsequently, Brown et al (13) reported a retrospective review of taxane therapy in 44 patients with newly diagnosed or recurrent SCSTs. Eleven patients received paclitaxel and a platinum drug for newly diagnosed SCSTs; all were alive at the time of the report, with a median follow-up of 52 months. Of 37 patients treated with a taxane for recurrent SCST, seven had no measurable disease after secondary cytoreductive surgery, and 30 had measurable disease. The response rate in the latter cohort was 42%. In a follow-up study, the same group of investigators retrospectively compared the efficacy and side effects of taxanes, with or without platinum, with the combination of BEP (14). The outcomes of the two groups were similar, but the side effects associated with the BEP regimen appeared to be greater. The authors concluded that taxane and platinum chemotherapy warrants further investigation in SCSTs. A subsequent

collaborative multicenter prospective randomized trial (GOG-264) comparing BEP to paclitaxel/carboplatin for advanced or recurrent SCSTs was closed early after 63 patients were enrolled, following an interim futility analysis in 2020. Owing to similar activity and improved toxicity profile, paclitaxel/carboplatin has largely supplanted BEP for first-line treatment of SCSTs.

Given the overall experience with chemotherapy for SCSTs over the past 3+ decades, it appears that these neoplasms are only moderately chemosensitive. In a report of 27 patients with chemotherapy-naïve GCTs who received BEP, nine patients had measurable disease and were evaluable for response (15). One of these patients had a complete response, and one had a partial response, for an overall response rate of 22%. The question of whether chemotherapy improves outcomes in SCST has also been examined using large administrative databases. For example, two separate epidemiologic studies conducted using the SEER registry and NCDB both failed to show an improvement in disease-free survival associated with the use of adjuvant chemotherapy in the treatment of stages II-IV GCT (16,17). A retrospective series of 118 patients with GCT between 1996 and 2003 also failed to show a benefit in disease-free recurrence with the use of adjuvant chemotherapy (18). In contrast, an analysis of NCDB examining a small number of advanced-stage non-GCT SCSTs, more than 70% of which were SLCTs found a survival benefit with the use of adjuvant chemotherapy (3).

The collective experience with systemic therapy for SCTATs is scant. Their endocrine activities suggest that the tumors may retain responsiveness to perturbation of gonadotropin levels. A case report documents a complete response to BEP in a patient with recurrent SCTAT (19). A more recent report of 13 patients with SCTAT noted that six (46.2%) patients experienced 14 recurrences (20). Two of these patients achieved a complete response without further recurrence after secondary cytoreductive surgery and chemotherapy with BEP or platinum, vinblastine, and bleomycin. Three patients achieved a partial response and were alive with disease at the time of the report after surgery and/or radiation. Another report describes complete response in a 44-year-old patient with recurrent SCTAT treated with docetaxel, carboplatin, and bevacizumab after having a partial response to BEP (21).

RADIATION

Whereas some investigators have reported improved outcomes in patients with SCST treated with adjuvant radiation therapy, other investigators have found no clear benefit (22-26). Because of the rarity of GCT, it is difficult to conduct prospective trials in these patients. Several retrospective series provide some data on the use of radiation therapy. Savage et al (26) reviewed the outcomes of 62 patients treated for AGCTs from 1969 to 1995. Thirty-eight (61%) had stage I disease. Eleven of the stage I patients had adjuvant pelvic radiation. The 10-year disease-free survival of these patients was 77% versus 78% for stage I patients treated with surgery alone. Unfortunately, neither complete surgical staging information nor the features that led to the selection of patients for adjuvant radiation were provided. For eight patients with inoperable disease (or residual disease postoperatively), radiation resulted in complete responses in four (50%) that lasted 16 months to 5 years. Wolf et al (24) reported on 34 patients with GCTs, 14 of whom had measurable disease. Six (43%) of the 14 had a clinical complete response. Three of the responders were alive without evidence of disease 10 to 21 years after radiation. More recently, investigators reviewed patients with GCT treated between 1961 and 2006 (25). In this series, 31 of 103 patients received adjuvant radiation, and this was associated with an improvement in disease-free survival (251 months vs 112 months; unadjusted $P = .02$). Because prospective data are lacking and retrospective studies are heterogeneous in both inclusion criteria and outcomes, adjuvant radiation therapy in the primary treatment of SCSTs cannot be routinely recommended.

REFERENCES

1. Wilson MK, Fong P, Mesnage S, et al. Stage l granulosa cell tumours: a management conundrum? Results of long-term follow up. *Gynecol Oncol.* 2015;138:285-291.

2. Mangili G, Ottolina J, Cormio G, et al. Adjuvant chemotherapy does not improve disease-free survival in FIGO stage IC ovarian granulosa cell tumors: the MITO-9 study. *Gynecol Oncol.* 2016;143:276-280.

3. Nasioudis D, Ko EM, Haggerty AF, et al. Role of adjuvant chemotherapy in the management of stage IC ovarian granulosa cell tumors. *Gynecol Oncol Rep.* 2019;28:145-148.

4. Young RH, Scully RE. Ovarian Sertoli-Leydig cell tumors with a retiform pattern: a problem in histopathologic diagnosis. A report of 25 cases. *Am J Surg Pathol.* 1983;7:755-771.

5. Young RH, Scully RE. Ovarian Sertoli-Leydig cell tumors. A clinicopathological analysis of 207 cases. *Am J Surg Pathol.* 1985;9:543-569.

6. Sigismondi C, Gadducci A, Lorusso D, et al. Ovarian Sertoli-Leydig cell tumors. A retrospective MITO study. *Gynecol Oncol.* 2012;125: 673-676.

7. Gui T, Cao D, Shen K, et al. A clinicopathological analysis of 40 cases of ovarian Sertoli-Leydig cell tumors. *Gynecol Oncol.* 2012;127: 384-389.

8. Calaminus G, Wessalowski R, Harms D, Göbel U. Juvenile granulosa cell tumors of the ovary in children and adolescents: results from 33 patients registered in a prospective cooperative study. *Gynecol Oncol.* 1997;65:447-452.

9. Schneider DT, Calaminus G, Wessalowski R, et al. Ovarian sex cord-stromal tumors in children and adolescents. *J Clin Oncol.* 2003;21:2357-2363.

10. Bergamini A, Ferrandina G, Candotti G, et al. Stage I juvenile granulosa cell tumors of the ovary: a multicentre analysis from the MITO-9 study. *Eur J Surg Oncol.* 2021;47:1705-1709.

11. Homesley HD, Bundy BN, Hurteau JA, Roth LM. Bleomycin, etoposide, and cisplatin combination therapy of ovarian granulosa cell tumors and other stromal malignancies: a gynecologic oncology group study. *Gynecol Oncol.* 1999;72:131-137.

12. Tresukosol D, Kudelka AP, Edwards CL, Charnsangavej C, Narboni N, Kavanagh JJ. Recurrent ovarian granulosa cell tumor: a case report of a dramatic response to Taxol. *Int J Gynecol Cancer.* 1995;5: 156-159.

13. Brown J, Shvartsman HS, Deavers MT, Burke TW, Munsell MF, Gershenson DM. The activity of taxanes in the treatment of sex cord-stromal ovarian tumors. *J Clin Oncol.* 2004;22:3517-3523.

14. Brown J, Shvartsman HS, Deavers MT, et al. The activity of taxanes compared with bleomycin, etoposide, and cisplatin in the treatment of sex cord-stromal ovarian tumors. *Gynecol Oncol.* 2005;97:489-496.

15. Van Meurs HS, Buist MR, Westermann AM, Sonke GS, Kenter GG, Van Der Velden J. Effectiveness of chemotherapy in measurable granulosa cell tumors: a retrospective study and review of literature. *Int J Gynecol Cancer.* 2014;24:496-505.

16. Oseledchyk A, Gennarelli RL, Leitao MM, et al. Adjuvant chemotherapy in patients with operable granulosa cell tumors of the ovary: a surveillance, epidemiology, and end results cohort study. *Cancer Med.* 2018;7:2280-2287.

17. Seagle B-LL, Ann P, Butler S, Shahabi S. Ovarian granulosa cell tumor: a National Cancer Database study. *Gynecol Oncol.* 2017;146:285-291.

18. Meisel JL, Hyman DM, Jotwani A, et al. The role of systemic chemotherapy in the management of granulosa cell tumors. *Gynecol Oncol.* 2015;136:505-511.

19. Puls LE, Hamous J, Morrow MS, Schneyer A, MacLaughlin DT, Castracane VD. Recurrent ovarian sex cord tumor with annular tubules: tumor marker and chemotherapy experience. *Gynecol Oncol.* 1994;54:396-401.

20. Qian Q, You Y, Yang J, et al. Management and prognosis of patients with ovarian sex cord tumor with annular tubules: a retrospective study. *BMC Cancer.* 2015;15:270.

21. Sho T, Yanazume S, Fukuda M, Togami S, Kamio M, Kobayashi H. Impact of taxane plus bevacizumab for ovarian sex cord tumor with annular tubules. *J Obstet Gynaecol Res.* 2019;45:1423-1428.

22. Taira Y, Hirakawa M, Nagayama C, Ikemiyagi K, Touma T, Tokashiki M. Successful treatment of adult-type granulosa cell tumor of the ovary by palliative radiotherapy. *J Obstet Gynaecol Res.* 2012;38:461-465.

23. Choan E, Samant R, Fung MFK, Le T, Hopkins L, Senterman M. Palliative radiotherapy for recurrent granulosa cell tumor of the ovary: a report of 3 cases with radiological evidence of response. *Gynecol Oncol.* 2006;102:406-410.

24. Wolf JK, Mullen J, Eifel PJ, Burke TW, Levenback C, Gershenson DM. Radiation treatment of advanced or recurrent granulosa cell tumor of the ovary. *Gynecol Oncol.* 1999;73:35-41.

25. Hauspy J, Beiner ME, Harley I, et al. Role of adjuvant radiotherapy in granulosa cell tumors of the ovary. *Int J Radiat Oncol Biol Phys.* 2011;79:770-774.

26. Savage P, Constenla D, Fisher C, et al. Granulosa cell tumours of the ovary: demographics, survival and the management of advanced disease. *Clin Oncol (R Coll Radiol).* 1998;10:242-245.

CHAPTER **10.7**

Treatment of Persistent or Recurrent Sex Cord-Stromal Tumors

R. Tyler Hillman

SECONDARY CYTOREDUCTIVE SURGERY

SCSTs as a group often have an indolent course, and disease at first recurrence is frequently oligometastatic and confined to the abdomen and pelvis. For example, in a series of 35 patients with a first recurrence of GCT reported by the MITO-9 group, none presented with distant disease (1), and the median time to first recurrence was 53.2 months. The surgical accessibility of recurrent disease combined with long disease-free intervals makes secondary tumor-reductive surgery an attractive management option for recurrent GCT, and this is borne out by current practice patterns.

In the aforementioned MITO-9 cohort, 33 (94%) of 35 patients underwent tumor-reductive surgery as a treatment for recurrent disease. Surgery is also frequently employed in the treatment of recurrent SLCTs. In a recent review summarizing the treatment course of patients with recurrent SLCT identified across 33 separate publications, distant recurrences were uncommon, and 49 (86%) of 57 patients with detailed treatment information underwent tumor-reductive surgery for first recurrence (2). The use and type of adjuvant chemotherapy was heterogeneous in this series, making it difficult to draw firm conclusions regarding survival outcomes and treatment modalities. Although no prospective data have demonstrated the superiority of surgery compared to systemic treatment alone, expert opinion and fundamental oncologic principles nevertheless support the use of secondary tumor-reductive surgery for many patients with a first recurrence of GCT or SLCT.

A separate question is how best to identify patients with recurrent SCST as the candidates for tumor-reductive surgery. There is currently no evidence as to whether the levels of serum tumor markers (eg, inhibin A/B) inversely correlate with cytoreductive success. Formal predictors of cytoreductive success such as the iMODEL (3,4) and Arbeitsgemeinschaft Gynaekologische Onkologie (AGO) score (5,6) were developed specifically for the management of epithelial ovarian cancer and are not validated for use in SCST. In general, patients with a first recurrence of GCT or SLCT with disease confined to the abdomen and pelvis should be evaluated for surgery, with appropriate consideration given to performance status, organ function, and likelihood of an optimal resection. Even in patients with a locoregional recurrence, the extent of disease can impact the likelihood of successful tumor-reductive surgery. Patients with focal disease implants will be more amenable to resection than those with diffuse carcinomatosis. Scant data exist regarding the surgical management of less common SCST subtypes in the recurrent setting, although individual cases with successful outcomes have been reported (7). Most surgery for recurrent SCST is probably best accomplished through a laparotomy incision to allow full exploration of the abdominal cavity. However, case reports have described successful SCST cytoreductive surgery using a minimally invasive approach (8,9). For the treatment of a second recurrence and beyond, additional tumor-reductive surgeries can be considered on an individualized basis.

Chemotherapy

Approaches to the use of chemotherapy in the treatment of recurrent SCST are similar to those employed for advanced-stage disease (see Chapter 10.6). Most patients treated with surgery alone in the upfront setting, such as for early-stage disease, should receive platinum-based chemotherapy as a component of treatment for a first recurrence. One approach to recurrent GCT commonly employed at MD Anderson Cancer Center is to perform secondary tumor-reductive surgery if feasible, followed by six adjuvant cycles of paclitaxel/carboplatin chemotherapy. This is based in part on data from a series published by Brown et al (10) that included 30 patients with recurrent SCST and measurable disease treated with taxanes (mostly paclitaxel). In this study, 17 patients received taxane without platinum and 13 patients received platinum-containing taxane regimens. The response rate to platinum-containing taxane regimens was 54%, consistent with historical response rates reported for BEP in recurrent disease and with less toxicity (11). For patients previously treated with chemotherapy, approaches to systemic therapy for a first GCT recurrence could include retreatment with the prior regimen, use of an alternative chemotherapy regimen (eg, taxane-containing regimen for a patient who previously received BEP), or hormonal therapy. There are no high-quality data to support one strategy over another, but treatment with additional chemotherapy is generally favored for patients with a long disease-free interval following upfront treatment. For those unusual patients with a short disease-free interval or progression during primary treatment, a decision regarding treatment strategy will depend on many factors, including hormone receptor expression status, performance status, and patient goals of care.

There are fewer data regarding the comparative effectiveness of different chemotherapy regimens in the treatment of rarer SCST subtypes. One case report documented a complete response to BEP in a patient with recurrent SCTAT (12). Conversely, another case report of a patient with recurrent SCTAT documented partial response to BEP, followed by complete response to docetaxel/carboplatin/bevacizumab (13). Several groups have reported on the use of hyperthermic intraperitoneal chemotherapy (HIPEC)

employed at the time of tumor-reductive surgery for recurrent GCT. For example, one series in 2014 reported on six patients with recurrent GCT who received cisplatin (50 mg/m^2) and doxorubicin (15 mg/m^2) applied to the abdomen for 90 minutes at the time of secondary tumor-reductive surgery (14). Although all patients were alive and disease free at a median follow-up interval of 27 months, two (33%) experienced grade 3-4 toxicities. Subsequently, results from a prospective registry of patients with rare ovarian cancers treated with HIPEC were published in 2018, including 37 patients with GCTs and eight patients with Leydig cell tumors who were treated with a wide range of HIPEC regimens (15). Although outcomes for the GCT subgroup were good, with a median disease-free survival of 34.6 months, the registry design meant there was no comparator group to allow the contribution of HIPEC to be assessed objectively. Overall HIPEC for recurrent SCST should only be considered at high-volume referral centers with extensive experience in this procedure, and ideally, treatment should occur as part of a clinical trial.

ENDOCRINE THERAPY

Hormonal therapy has been best studied in the treatment of AGCT, both because these tumors are more common than other SCST subtypes and also because AGCTs frequent express ER or PR (16,17). There is a mechanistic basis for estrogen-dependent AGCT growth as the gene encoding aromatase (the enzyme responsible for estrogen synthesis) is regulated by the *FOXL2* transcription factor (18,19). Until recently, all data describing the use of hormonal therapies in GCT were from retrospective case series and may be affected by selection bias leading to overly optimistic estimates of efficacy. Moreover, considerable heterogeneity exists in the types of hormonal agents used to treat GCT, including aromatase inhibitors, progestins, gonadotropin hormone–releasing hormone (GnRH) agonists/antagonists, and selective ER modulators. In a systematic review of 415 investigations, van Meurs et al (20) identified 19 eligible studies that included 31 patients with GCTs treated with 38 evaluable hormonal therapies. Overall, the authors reported a 25.8% complete response rate and a 45.2% partial response rate. Four patients had stable disease, and five had disease progression. Median progression-free survival (PFS) was 18 (range 0-60) months. Although sample sizes were small, five different regimens were reported to have 100% response rates, including anastrozole, letrozole, alternating medroxyprogesterone acetate/tamoxifen, and diethylstilbestrol.

Although retrospective studies report high GCT response rates to aromatase inhibitors, this has recently been called into question after the first prospective trial of anastrozole in SCSTs was reported. The PARAGON/ANZGOG 0903 trial (21) was a single-arm, multicenter study designed to evaluate anastrozole in postmenopausal patients with ER- and/or PR-positive gynecologic cancers and included an arm for recurrent GCT/SCSTs in the basket trial design. Eligibility for this study included at least 10% of tumor cells staining positive for ER and/or PR. A total of 41 patients with GCT/SCSTs were enrolled, and it is notable that most (61%) had not received prior chemotherapy. The clinical benefit rate at 12 weeks (primary outcome) was 78.9%. However, only a single patient in this group had an objective response, with the rest having stable disease. Therefore, the partial response rate at 12 weeks with anastrozole in this trial was 2.6%; the investigators noted that additional partial responses were identified after the initial 12-week assessment. Several points about this study deserve mention. First, clinical benefit rate as a study outcome, which includes stable disease, may overestimate therapeutic effectiveness in GCT, which often has an indolent pattern of growth even in the recurrent setting. Second, PARAGON/ANZGOG 0903 provides an appropriate lens through which to view prior retrospective series examining the effectiveness of aromatase inhibitors in GCT, as objective response rates are likely far lower than had been previously thought.

Considered broadly, it seems probable that reports of exceptionally high response rates to other endocrine therapies should also be interpreted with caution.

Angiogenesis Inhibitors

Färkkilä et al (22) found that VEGF and VEGF-2 were highly expressed in primary and recurrent GCTs. In addition, although VEGF protein expression was not predictive of tumor recurrence in this series, high levels of circulating VEGF were found in the serum of patients with primary GCTs. Tao et al (23) reported on eight patients with recurrent GCTs (seven adult and one juvenile) who were treated with bevacizumab. One patient had a complete response, and two had a partial response. The GOG conducted a phase 2 trial of bevacizumab in 36 patients with recurrent SCSTs (24). The majority (32 patients) had GCTs, and four had unclassified SCSTs. These 36 patients received a total of 491 cycles of bevacizumab, with a median of nine treatment cycles per patient. Six (16.7%) patients had a partial response, and 28 (77.8%) had stable disease. The median PFS was 9.3 months. Based on this, single-agent bevacizumab is considered an active agent in the treatment of recurrent SCST.

More recently, European investigators have reported the results of a randomized, prospective trial (ALIENOR/ENGOT-ov7) to determine the efficacy of six cycles of weekly paclitaxel 80 mg/m^2 with or without bevacizumab in recurrent SCST (25). The primary outcome was 6-month PFS, and patients who had received at least one prior platinum-based chemotherapy were eligible. Weekly paclitaxel alone was associated with 6-month PFS of 71% (95% CI, 55%-84%), identifying this as an active regimen. Although response rates were higher in the combination group (44% vs 25%), the addition of bevacizumab did not result in improved PFS. Nearly half of the patients in this trial had received prior treatment with a "platinum-based combination," presumably including a taxane in many cases, so these results may also support weekly paclitaxel as efficacious in patients with SCST previously treated with taxane chemotherapy.

Other Agents

Garcia-Donas et al (26) have suggested that ketoconazole (a CYP17 inhibitor) may have benefit in metastatic GCTs, reporting on a patient with recurrent GCT who remained progression free for 10 months while on the drug. Experience with this approach is limited, and since the publication of this case report in 2013, no additional reports of ketoconazole treatment in GCT have appeared. In 2018, a case report of a patient with recurrent AGCT treated with letrozole and metformin was published (27), describing the achievement of long-term disease control on this regimen. Because retrospective data suggest that aromatase inhibitors have single-agent activity in the treatment of AGCT and no other reports of metformin alone have been published, these results must be interpreted with appropriate caution.

REFERENCES

1. Mangili G, Sigismondi C, Frigerio L, et al. Recurrent granulosa cell tumors (GCTs) of the ovary: a MITO-9 retrospective study. *Gynecol Oncol.* 2013;130:38-42.
2. Nef J, Huber DE. Ovarian Sertoli-Leydig cell tumours: a systematic review of relapsed cases. *Eur J Obstet Gynecol Reprod Biol.* 2021;263:261-274.
3. Shi T, Zhu J, Feng Y, et al. Secondary cytoreduction followed by chemotherapy versus chemotherapy alone in platinum-sensitive relapsed ovarian cancer (SOC-1): a multicentre, open-label, randomised, phase 3 trial. *Lancet Oncol.* 2021;22:439-449.
4. Tian W-J, Chi DS, Sehouli J, et al. A risk model for secondary cytoreductive surgery in recurrent ovarian cancer: an evidence-based proposal for patient selection. *Ann Surg Oncol.* 2012;19:597-604.
5. Harter P, Sehouli J, Vergote I, et al. Randomized trial of cytoreductive surgery for relapsed ovarian cancer. *N Engl J Med.* 2021;385:2123-2131.
6. Harter P, Sehouli J, Reuss A, et al. Prospective validation study of a predictive score for operability of recurrent ovarian cancer: the Multicenter Intergroup Study DESKTOP II. A project of the AGO Kommission OVAR, AGO Study Group, NOGGO, AGO-Austria, and MITO. *Int J Gynecol Cancer.* 2011;21:289-295.
7. Powell JL, Connor GP, Henderson GS. Management of recurrent juvenile granulosa cell tumor of the ovary. *Gynecol Oncol.* 2001;81:113-116.
8. García Pineda V, Hernández A, Cabanes M, Siegrist J, Gracia M, Zapardiel I. Tertiary cytoreductive surgery by laparoscopy in granulosa cell tumor recurrence. *Int J Gynecol Cancer.* 2020;30:1844-1845.
9. Tinelli R, Stomati M, Trojano G, et al. Laparoscopic treatment of ovarian granulosa cells tumor developed in the pelvic anterior preperitoneal space 20 years after laparotomic salpingo-oophorectomy: case report and review of literature. *Gynecol Endocrinol.* 2020;36:926-928.
10. Brown J, Shvartsman HS, Deavers MT, Burke TW, Munsell MF, Gershenson DM. The activity of taxanes in the treatment of sex cord-stromal ovarian tumors. *J Clin Oncol.* 2004;22:3517-3523.
11. Homesley HD, Bundy BN, Hurteau JA, Roth LM. Bleomycin, etoposide, and cisplatin combination therapy of ovarian granulosa cell tumors and other stromal malignancies: a gynecologic oncology group study. *Gynecol Oncol.* 1999;72:131-137.
12. Puls LE, Hamous J, Morrow MS, Schneyer A, MacLaughlin DT, Castracane VD. Recurrent ovarian sex cord tumor with annular tubules: tumor marker and chemotherapy experience. *Gynecol Oncol.* 1994;54:396-401.
13. Sho T, Yanazume S, Fukuda M, Togami S, Kamio M, Kobayashi H. Impact of taxane plus bevacizumab for ovarian sex cord tumor with annular tubules. *J Obstet Gynaecol Res.* 2019;45:1423-1428.
14. Al-Badawi IA, Abu-Zaid A, Azzam A, AlOmar O, AlHusaini H, Amin T. Cytoreductive surgery and hyperthermic intraperitoneal chemotherapy for management of recurrent/relapsed ovarian granulosa cell tumor: a single-center experience. *J Obstet Gynaecol Res.* 2014;40:2066-2075.
15. Mercier F, Bakrin N, Bartlett DL, et al. Peritoneal carcinomatosis of rare ovarian origin treated by cytoreductive surgery and hyperthermic intraperitoneal chemotherapy: a multi-institutional cohort from PSOGI and BIG-RENAPE. *Ann Surg Oncol.* 2018;25:1668-1675.
16. Farinola MA, Gown AM, Judson K, et al. Estrogen receptor α and progesterone receptor expression in ovarian adult granulosa cell tumors and Sertoli-Leydig cell tumors. *Int J Gynecol Pathol.* 2007;26:375-382.
17. Chadha S, Rao BR, Slotman BJ, van Vroonhoven CCJ, van der Kwast TH. An immunohistochemical evaluation of androgen and progesterone receptors in ovarian tumors. *Hum Pathol.* 1993;24(1):90-95.
18. Fleming NI, Knower KC, Lazarus KA, Fuller PJ, Simpson ER, Clyne CD. Aromatase is a direct target of FOXl2: C134W in granulosa cell tumors via a single highly conserved binding site in the ovarian specific promoter. *PLoS One.* 2010;5:e14389.
19. Wang D-S, Kobayashi T, Zhou L-Y, et al. Foxl2 up-regulates aromatase gene transcription in a female-specific manner by binding to the promoter as well as interacting with ad4 binding protein/steroidogenic factor 1. *Mol Endocrinol.* 2007;21:712-725.
20. Van Meurs HS, Van Lonkhuijzen LRCW, Limpens J, Van Der Velden J, Buist MR. Hormone therapy in ovarian granulosa cell tumors: a systematic review. *Gynecol Oncol.* 2014;134:196-205.
21. Banerjee SN, Tang M, O'Connell RL, et al. A phase 2 study of anastrozole in patients with oestrogen receptor and/progesterone receptor positive recurrent/metastatic granulosa cell tumours/sex-cord stromal tumours of the ovary: the PARAGON/ANZGOG 0903 trial. *Gynecol Oncol.* 2021;163:72-78.
22. Färkkilä A, Anttonen M, Pociuviene J, et al. Vascular endothelial growth factor (VEGF) and its receptor VEGFR-2 are highly expressed in ovarian granulosa cell tumors. *Eur J Endocrinol.* 2011;164:115-122.
23. Tao X, Sood AK, Deavers MT, et al. Anti-angiogenesis therapy with bevacizumab for patients with ovarian granulosa cell tumors. *Gynecol Oncol.* 2009;114:431-436.
24. Brown J, Brady WE, Schink J, et al. Efficacy and safety of bevacizumab in recurrent sex cord-stromal ovarian tumors: results of a phase 2 trial of the Gynecologic Oncology Group. *Cancer.* 2014;120:344-351.
25. Ray-Coquard I, Harter P, Lorusso D, et al. Effect of weekly paclitaxel with or without bevacizumab on progression-free rate among patients with relapsed ovarian sex cord-stromal tumors: the ALIENOR/ENGOT-ov7 randomized clinical trial. *JAMA Oncol.* 2020;6(12):1-9.
26. Garcia-Donas J, Hurtado A, García-Casado Z, et al. Cytochrome P17 inhibition with ketoconazole as treatment for advanced granulosa cell ovarian tumor. *J Clin Oncol.* 2013;31:e165-e166.
27. Rush SK, Goff BA. Treatment of recurrent granulosa cell tumor with metformin and letrozole: a case report. *Gynecol Oncol Rep.* 2018; 25:60-62.

CHAPTER **10.8**

Ovarian Sex Cord-Stromal Tumors: Special Conditions

Carrie Langstraat

SCSTs often coexist with genetic conditions, including PJS, Ollier disease, and Maffucci syndrome. The association of these conditions with SCSTs seems more than chance alone. Here we discuss some of these conditions and their association with SCST.

PJS is an autosomal dominant disorder characterized by multiple gastrointestinal hamartomas and mucocutaneous pigmentations. The *PJS* gene was mapped to chromosome 19p13.3 (1) and was later identified as a novel serine-threonine kinase, STK11 (2). *STK11* is a tumor suppressor gene acting through multiple pathways, most classically through AMP-activated protein kinase–mediated inhibition of the rapamycin signaling pathway. Patients with PJS are at increased risk of gynecologic malignancy, specifically SCTAT and AMC (3). Approximately 36% of SCTATs are observed in patients with PJS. Furthermore, 15% of PJS-associated SCTATs also develop AMC, a neoplasm that defies early diagnosis and is associated with a relatively high mortality rate (4-6). Patients with PJS have a lifetime risk of ovarian cancer of 18% to 21%, adenoma malignum of 10%, and uterine cancer of 9% (3). Data on risk-reducing strategies and on surveillance for malignancy are lacking. Based on expert opinion, children with PJS should be examined annually starting at age 8 for signs of precocious. Cervical cancer screening should start between ages 18-20 (7). Some experts also recommend annual pelvic ultrasounds starting at age 25 (8).

JGCTs have been reported in association with enchondromatosis alone (Ollier disease) or concomitantly with hemangiomas (Maffucci syndrome) (9-12). Individuals with these relatively uncommon mesodermal dysplasias generally present before puberty and frequently develop secondary neoplasms, most commonly sarcomas, after the second decade of life. JGCTs are the next most frequent tumor associated with these disorders and become evident during the first and second decades of life. These observations appear to imply more than coincidental occurrences and suggest a generalized mesodermal dysplasia, perhaps contributing to the pathogenesis of these neoplastic processes. In addition, congenital bilateral JGCTs of the ovary have been reported in leprechaunism, a disease characterized by insulin resistance resulting from an insulin receptor defect (13).

A hereditary pattern, as well as coexistence of thyroid disease, cervical embryonal rhabdomyosarcoma, and pleuropulmonary blastoma (PPB) has been chronicled in patients with SLCTs (14,15). In 2009, DICER1 mutations were described in familial PPB (16), which has been further demonstrated in patients with SLCT (17). Additional details on DICER1 mutations and need for surveillance can be reviewed in Section 10.2.

Gorlin syndrome (nevoid basal cell carcinoma syndrome) is a rare inherited multisystem disorder. Gorlin syndrome is associated with an inherited predisposition to the development of ovarian fibromas along with several other abnormalities, the most frequent of which is the appearance of basal cell nevi at an early age (18).

REFERENCES

1. Hemminki A, Tomlinson I, Markie D, et al. Localization of a susceptibility locus for Peutz-Jeghers syndrome to 19p using comparative genomic hybridization and targeted linkage analysis. *Nat Genet.* 1997;15(1):87-90.
2. Jenne DE, Reimann H, Nezu J, et al. Peutz-Jeghers syndrome is caused by mutations in a novel serine threonine kinase. *Nat Genet.* 1998;18(1):38-43.
3. Boardman LA, Thibodeau SN, Schaid DJ, et al. Increased risk for cancer in patients with the Peutz-Jeghers syndrome. *Ann Intern Med.* 1998;128(11):896-899.
4. Podczaski E, Kaminski PF, Pees RC, Singapuri K, Sorosky JI. Peutz-Jeghers syndrome with ovarian sex cord tumor with annular tubules and cervical adenoma malignum. *Gynecol Oncol.* 1991;42(1):74-78.
5. Shen K, Wu PC, Lang JH, Huang RL, Tang MT, Lian LJ. Ovarian sex cord tumor with annular tubules: a report of six cases. *Gynecol Oncol.* 1993;48(2):180-184.
6. Solh HM, Azoury RS, Najjar SS. Peutz-Jeghers syndrome associated with precocious puberty. *J Pediatr.* 1983;103(4):593-595.
7. Latchford A, Cohen S, Auth M, et al. Management of Peutz-Jeghers Syndrome in Children and Adolescents: A position paper form the ESPGHAN polyposis working group. *J Pediatr Gastroenterol Nutr.* 2019;68(3):442-452.
8. Tacheci I, Kopacova M, Bures J. Peutz-Jeghers syndrome. *Curr Opin Gastroenterol.* 2021;37(3):245-254.
9. Asirvatham R, Rooney RJ, Watts HG. Ollier's disease with secondary chondrosarcoma associated with ovarian tumour. A case report. *Int Orthop.* 1991;15(4):393-395.
10. Tamimi HK, Bolen JW. Enchondromatosis (Ollier's disease) and ovarian juvenile granulosa cell tumor. *Cancer.* 1984;53(7):1605-1608.
11. Tanaka Y, Sasaki Y, Nishihira H, Izawa T, Nishi T. Ovarian juvenile granulosa cell tumor associated with Maffucci's syndrome. *Am J Clin Pathol.* 1992;97(4):523-527.
12. Young RH, Dickersin GR, Scully RE. Juvenile granulosa cell tumor of the ovary. A clinicopathological analysis of 125 cases. *Am J Surg Pathol.* 1984;8(8):575-596.
13. Brisigotti M, Fabbretti G, Pesce F, et al. Congenital bilateral juvenile granulosa cell tumor of the ovary in leprechaunism: a case report. *Pediatr Pathol.* 1993;13(5):549-558.
14. Schultz KA, Pacheco MC, Yang J, et al. Ovarian sex cord-stromal tumors, pleuropulmonary blastoma and DICER1 mutations: a report from the International pleuropulmonary blastoma registry. *Gynecol Oncol.* 2011;122(2):246-250.
15. Schultz KA, Yang J, Doros L, et al. DICER1-pleuropulmonary blastoma familial tumor predisposition syndrome: a unique constellation of neoplastic conditions. *Pathol Case Rev.* 2014;19(2):90-100.
16. Hill DA, Ivanovich J, Priest JR, et al. DICER1 mutations in familial pleuropulmonary blastoma. *Science.* 2009;325(5943):965.
17. Schultz KAP, Harris AK, Finch M, et al. DICER1-related Sertoli-Leydig cell tumor and gynandroblastoma: clinical and genetic findings from the International ovarian and testicular stromal tumor registry. *Gynecol Oncol.* 2017;147(3):521-527.
18. Raggio M, Kaplan AL, Harberg JF. Recurrent ovarian fibromas with basal cell nevus syndrome (Gorlin syndrome). *Obstet Gynecol.* 1983;61(3 suppl):95s-96s.

CHAPTER **10.9**

Ovarian Sex Cord-Stromal Tumors: Follow-Up and Survivorship Issues

Carrie Langstraat

Surveillance strategies for patients with SCST are dependent on histologic diagnosis and stage of disease. Patients with benign SCSTs need no additional follow-up. Patients with malignant SCST should be followed at regular intervals, every 3 to 6 months, with pelvic examination and tumor markers (1). AGCT and JGCT can often demonstrate an increase in inhibin B, and this is often used as a tumor marker for these patients. Androgen-secreting tumors can be followed with testosterone levels. Imaging is reserved for patients with clinical signs and symptoms of recurrence. Patients should be given resources to assist in coping with fatigue related to chemotherapy, menopausal symptoms, and healthy lifestyle choices. An ongoing study will better define the challenges facing our survivors of SCST (2).

Malignant SCST are often diagnosed in premenopausal patients. Patients undergoing bilateral oophorectomy as part of their treatment should undergo counseling regarding hormone replacement therapy (HRT). There are currently no data to support the safety of HRT in these patients. Furthermore, the response of some SCST (in particular AGCT) to antiestrogen therapy suggests that HRT might be contraindicated in this particular patient population. Additional research is needed to define the safety and role of HRT in these young patients.

REFERENCES

1. Salani R, Khanna N, Rimer M, et al. An update on post-treatment surveillance and diagnosis or recurrence in women with gynecologic malignancies: Society of Gynecologic Oncology (SGO) recommendations. *Gynecol Oncol.* 2017;146:3-10.

2. Gernier F, Ahmed-Lecheheb D, Pautier P, et al. Chronic fatigue, quality of life and long-term side-effects of chemotherapy in patients treated for non-epithelial ovarian cancer: national case-control protocol study of the GINECO-Vivrovaire rare tumors INCa French network for rare malignant ovarian tumors. *BMC Cancer.* 2021;21(1):1147.

CHAPTER **10.10**

Ovarian Sex Cord-Stromal Tumors: Future Directions

R. Tyler Hillman

INTRODUCTION

Gaps in Knowledge

Owing in large part to the rarity of SCST subtypes, there are significant gaps in our knowledge regarding many aspects of molecular pathogenesis and optimal treatment strategies. Several specific clinical situations deserve special focus in future research efforts. First, it will be important to further refine definitions of high-risk, early-stage disease, including the identification of biomarkers and clinical characteristics that best correlate with benefit from adjuvant chemotherapy in the upfront setting. Second, following the publication of the PARAGON/ANZGOG 0903 trial (1) showing lower-than-expected response rates to anastrozole monotherapy in recurrent GCT, new strategies are needed for the prioritization of hormonal therapies, including novel predictive biomarkers beyond ER and PR expression. Third, although significant progress has been made recently in the molecular characterization of AGCT (2-4) and SLCT (5), continued collaborative work is needed to improve our understanding of the molecular drivers of rarer SCST subtypes. Lastly, recognizing the prolonged course for patients with recurrent disease, additional data are needed to clarify the role of cytoreductive surgery in the second line and beyond, as well as whether hyperthermic intraperitoneal chemotherapy has a role in the treatment of SCSTs.

Molecular Insights

Recent years have seen a dramatic increase in data regarding the driver mutation landscape of SCSTs, largely owing to the decreasing costs and increasing availability of massively parallel sequencing platforms. In some cases, observational data have suggested that certain recurrent somatic mutations may have prognostic importance or otherwise identify unique molecular disease subtypes. For example, separate reports have suggested that *TERT* promoter mutations (4) or *KMT2D* mutations (2) may be associated with increased recurrence risk in AGCT. In addition, *TP53* mutation seems to identify a subset of AGCT with increased somatic mutation rate and genome instability (3). A critical next step will be to prospectively evaluate relationships between molecular driver events, treatment response, recurrence risk, and survival outcomes. Such efforts may take the form of a disease-specific registry, likely requiring cross-discipline and cross-institution collaboration to catalogue molecular alterations and track outcomes over time. Compared to AGCT, less is known about the molecular landscape of rarer SCSTs, although there has been recent progress better understanding genetic alterations underlying JGCT (6-8). Collaborative approaches will be necessary in order to describe the molecular landscape of rarer SCSTs because pooling of biospecimen resources held by multiple institutional tumor banks will likely be necessary to catalogue the driver mutation landscape.

Genetic Model Systems

There are few experimental model systems available to study SCST pathogenesis in a laboratory setting. For example, only a single well-characterized immortalized AGCT cell line known to carry the *FOXL2* c.C402G hotspot mutation exists (9). Given recent insights into the molecular heterogeneity of AGCT, it is unlikely that a single culture-adapted cell line recapitulates disease biology with high fidelity. Moreover, additional model systems will be needed to fully capture the role played by diverse human genetic backgrounds on disease pathogenesis. Although experimental methods exist for the isolation and immortalization of sex cord components from the male and female gonads, there are few, if any, cell culture models for rarer forms of SCST that have endogenous fidelity to the molecular genetics of these tumor types. Recent advances in the development of primary organoid cultures from epithelial ovarian cancers (10) will hopefully spur similar efforts to develop conditions for the primary culture of SCSTs, an important first step in developing a platform for studying the genetic and phenotypic diversity of these diseases. Robust primary tumor culture systems will also accelerate the development of rational clinical trial designs for the treatment of SCSTs, by facilitating the generation of reproducible and genotype-informed preclinical data.

The development of novel, clinically relevant animal models of SCST subtypes must be a key focus for future translational research. Heterogeneous approaches to the development of a mouse GCT model have been reported, but to date, there does not yet exist a genetically engineered mouse model of the human *FOXL2* c.C402G mutation, and it is not known if an equivalent missense mutation causes cancer in mice. GCT mouse models reported to date rely on ectopic expression of powerful oncogenes (eg, SV40) (11) or inactivation of genes such as *PTEN* or *CTNNB1* (12,13) that are not frequently affected in AGCT (3). Overexpression of constitutively active TGF-β receptor 1 has also been shown to induce tumor formation in mouse granulosa cells (14). As the molecular driver landscape of GCT becomes better understood, it is hoped that this knowledge will be operationalized to develop new animal disease models that more closely recapitulate the genetic landscape of the human disease. The development of in vivo model systems for rarer SCST subtypes has been considerably more limited and remains an important area for future research.

Clinical Trials

The recent publication of two prospective clinical trials in SCST (1,15) supports an optimistic outlook on the feasibility of creating an evidence-based approach to the treatment of these diseases. Nevertheless, significant questions remain regarding the optimal use of systemic therapy in the recurrent setting, and treatment strategies do not yet incorporate emerging data regarding driver mutations or molecular biomarkers. As disease-specific mutational landscapes become better defined, there is hope that patients with SCSTs harboring relevant biomarkers will more frequently be able to access appropriate basket trials. Improvements in the fidelity and availability of *in vitro* and *in vivo* SCST model systems will spur novel trial designs while also creating opportunities for biomarker-based translational outcomes to be incorporated into future trial concepts. Collaboration across institutions and disciplines will be necessary to improve treatment outcomes in these rare and oftentimes difficult-to-treat diseases.

REFERENCES

1. Banerjee SN, Tang M, O'Connell RL, et al. A phase 2 study of anastrozole in patients with oestrogen receptor and/progesterone receptor positive recurrent/metastatic granulosa cell tumours/sex-cord stromal tumours of the ovary: the PARAGON/ANZGOG 0903 trial. *Gynecol Oncol.* 2021;163:72-78.

2. Hillman RT, Celestino J, Terranova C, et al. KMT2D/MLL2 inactivation is associated with recurrence in adult-type granulosa cell tumors of the ovary. *Nat Commun.* 2018;9:2496.

3. Hillman RT, Lin DI, Lawson B, Gershenson DM. Prevalence of predictive biomarkers in a large cohort of molecularly defined adult-type ovarian granulosa cell tumors. *Gynecol Oncol.* 2021;162(3): 728-734.

4. Pilsworth JA, Cochrane DR, Xia Z, et al. TERT promoter mutation in adult granulosa cell tumor of the ovary. *Mod Pathol.* 2018;31:1107-1115.

5. Heravi-Moussavi A, Anglesio MS, Cheng S-WG, et al. Recurrent somatic DICER1 mutations in nonepithelial ovarian cancers. *N Engl J Med.* 2012;366:234-242.

6. Auguste A, Bessière L, Todeschini A-L, et al. Molecular analyses of juvenile granulosa cell tumors bearing AKT1 mutations provide insights into tumor biology and therapeutic leads. *Hum Mol Genet.* 2015;24:6687-6698.

7. Vougiouklakis T, Zhu K, Vasudevaraja V, et al. Integrated analysis of ovarian juvenile granulosa cell tumors reveals distinct epigenetic signatures and recurrent TERT rearrangements. *Clin Cancer Res.* 2022;28(8):1724-1733. doi:10.1158/1078-0432.CCR-21-3394

8. Bessière L, Todeschini AL, Auguste A, et al. A hot-spot of in-frame duplications activates the oncoprotein AKT1 in juvenile granulosa cell tumors. *EBioMedicine.* 2015;2:421-431.

9. Nishi Y, Yanase T, Mu Y, et al. Establishment and characterization of a steroidogenic human granulosa-like tumor cell line, KGN, that expresses functional follicle-stimulating hormone receptor. *Endocrinology.* 2001;142:437-445.

10. Kopper O, de Witte CJ, Löhmussaar K, et al. An organoid platform for ovarian cancer captures intra- and interpatient heterogeneity. *Nat Med.* 2019;25:838-849.

11. Garson K, Macdonald E, Dubé M, Bao R, Hamilton TC, Vanderhyden BC. Generation of tumors in transgenic mice expressing the SV40 T antigen under the control of ovarian-specific promoter 1. *J Soc Gynecol Investig.* 2003;10:244-250.

12. Laguë M-N, Paquet M, Fan H-Y, et al. Synergistic effects of Pten loss and WNT/CTNNB1 signaling pathway activation in ovarian granulosa cell tumor development and progression. *Carcinogenesis.* 2008;29:2062-2072.

13. Boerboom D, Paquet M, Hsieh M, et al. Misregulated Wnt/beta-catenin signaling leads to ovarian granulosa cell tumor development. *Cancer Res.* 2005;65:9206-9215.

14. Gao Y, Vincent DF, Davis AJ, Sansom OJ, Bartholin L, Li Q. Constitutively active transforming growth factor β receptor 1 in the mouse ovary promotes tumorigenesis. *Oncotarget.* 2016;7:40904-40918.

15. Ray-Coquard I, Harter P, Lorusso D, et al. Effect of weekly paclitaxel with or without bevacizumab on progression-free rate among patients with relapsed ovarian sex cord-stromal tumors: the ALIENOR/ENGOT-ov7 randomized clinical trial. *JAMA Oncol.* 2020;6(12):1-9.

BREAST CANCER

CHAPTER 11.1

Breast Cancer: Introduction

Theresa A. Graves

Breast cancer is the most common cancer diagnosed in women in both the developed and less developed countries of the world, globally constituting one in four of all cancers in women.

As a complex compilation of diseases for which detection, diagnosis, and multidisciplinary management strategies are continually evolving, the management of breast cancer is more complicated than cancers of many of the other disease sites. Treatment paradigms are constantly modified based on systematic research and

with each improvement to the standards of care, new questions, challenges, and controversies arise.

The predictive and prognostic factors identified in the tumor biology of breast cancer have been instrumental in designing new treatment strategies. This chapter provides insight into the multidisciplinary care of patients with breast cancer, highlighting the essential information to assist in the understanding and treatment of breast cancer, while emphasizing the current data and future developments.

CHAPTER 11.2

Breast Cancer: Epidemiology, Risk Factors, Anatomy, and Natural History

Michelle E. Wakeley

EPIDEMIOLOGY

Nearly 290,000 women and 3,000 men are diagnosed with breast cancer each year in the United States. Breast cancer remains the most common cancer in women, comprising 31% of all new cancer diagnoses, and represents the second most lethal malignancy in women. It accounts for 15% of all cancer-related deaths annually, and nearly 44,000 Americans die from breast cancer each year (1). While the incidence of breast cancer has been steadily increasing by a rate of 0.5% per year since the mid-2000s, breast cancer–associated mortality peaked in 1989 and has since declined by 42%, currently 12.9%. Reflecting advancements in detection and treatment, breast cancer mortality continues to decline, at a rate of 1.1% annually from 2013 to 2019. The rate of decline in breast cancer mortality is slowing, noting a decrease of 3.3% annually from 1995 to 1998 and 1.9% annually from 1998 to 2013 (1).

Globally, breast cancer incidence reflects access to mammography as well as risk factors, with the highest incidence in North America, New Zealand, Australia, and Northern and Western Europe. Worldwide, breast cancer is estimated to account for 1.7 million cases and over 500,000 deaths annually (2).

RISK FACTORS

Risk factors associated with breast cancer have been well characterized by a number of high-quality studies, and a number of risk calculator models have sought to quantify and convey their cumulative effects. Factors that increase estrogen exposure, including

female gender, parity, early menarche or late menopause, and late age of first pregnancy, all are associated with an increased risk. When examining the effects of more direct estrogen exposure, however, the impact of estrogen is less clear.

The use of oral contraceptive pills has been examined in detail, including subgroup analyses of the many different formulations of oral contraceptives, with no increased risk for breast cancer identified (3). A 2015 review of nearly 210,000 women undergoing hormonal infertility treatments also found no association between these treatments and breast cancer risk, best demonstrated in women undergoing in vitro fertilization therapy (4). The Women's Health Initiative, a randomized controlled trial in the 1990s, however, found that combined estrogen plus progestin therapy for menopausal hormonal treatment was associated with an increase in both total and invasive breast cancer diagnoses when compared to placebo, but that estrogen-only treatment was not (5).

Contemporary studies have identified familial and genetic risk factors for breast cancer. Pathogenic mutations of the *BRCA-1* gene have been well characterized as breast cancer genetic risk factors, with multiple mutations in the tumor suppressor localized to 17q21. BRCA-1 pathogenic mutations are linked to significantly higher rates of both breast and ovarian cancer (6). Similarly, mutations involving the *BRCA-2* gene, localized to 13q12-13, increases breast cancer risk (7). Mutations in both *BRCA* genes are inherited in an autosomal dominant manner and are associated with lifetime breast cancer risks as high as 90%, with an odds ratio (OR) of 7.62 for BRCA-1 and 5.23 for BRCA-2 (8,9).

BRCA mutations were originally felt to account for 45% of families with increased incidence of breast cancer and 80% of families with early-onset breast and ovarian cancer. However, more up-dated analysis suggests these mutations account for between 12% and 31% of breast cancer risk in these families (10). Additional familial risk factors for breast cancer include Li-Fraumeni syndrome (P53 mutation), hereditary diffuse gastric cancer (CDH1), *CHEK2* and *PALB2* genes involved in checkpoint function and DNA repair, Cowden syndrome (PTEN), and Peutz-Jeghers syndrome (STK11) (9,10). We continue to increase our understanding of epigenetic modifications, such as BRCA-1 methylation, and how these findings may impact our ability to predict an individual's risk. Widespread adoption of these prediction tools is currently hampered by an inability to generalize these data (11). Indeed, genetic and genomic information not only increased our understanding of breast cancer risk but, as discussed elsewhere, also plays an integral part of personalized treatment (12).

Extensive mammographic density is associated with a substantial increase in the risk of invasive breast cancer. The percentage of mammographic imaging occupied by dense breast tissue is associated with variations in the number of epithelial and nonepithelial cells within the breast, and women with more than 75% of breast occupied with dense tissue are at increased risk of breast cancer compared with those women with 10% or less dense tissue, with an OR of 4.7 (13,14). This has led to multiple initiatives to identify and quantify the density of tissue in individuals, with studies demonstrating that combining Breast Imaging Reporting and Data System (BI-RADS) breast density rating with automatic breast density rating systems allowing for better identification of women at increased risk. In addition, the understanding of the genetics and biologic basis of breast density as a risk factor is under investigation (15,16).

The impact of modifiable risk factors on breast cancer development has been more difficult to delineate. Obesity is often cited as a risk factor for breast cancer, owing to adipose tissue's ability to serve as a source of extragonadal estrogen. But in a large-scale prospective study, obesity in premenopausal women was not associated with an increased risk for developing breast cancer; in postmenopausal women, however, increased body mass index (BMI) was associated with an increased risk (17). Detailed review of the Women's Health Initiative data demonstrated that BMI may not be an adequate surrogate of this risk, and that more specifically, a high relative body fat percentage was directly correlated with increased risk of invasive breast cancer (18). Dietary habits have also been associated with modest impacts on breast cancer risk, most significantly in the postmenopausal population (19). Alcohol consumption's impact on the risk of breast cancer has not been consistently demonstrated; however, a meta-analysis of available studies demonstrates a slight increase in relative risk (RR) with an increasing number of drinks per day (20).

Environmental exposures also seem to contribute to the risk of breast cancer. Night shift work has been suspected of altering breast cancer risk in women, and a large meta-analysis demonstrated that any exposure to night shift work had an RR of 1.19; in addition, the risk of breast cancer increased by 3% with every 5 years of consistent night shift work completed (21). This correlation has been echoed in other similar works; however, a large national database study from the Netherlands in the early 2000s failed to demonstrate the same impact (22,23). The mechanism behind breast cancer risk after night shift work has been linked to circadian rhythm disruption and associated alterations in melatonin-driven pathways, including both estrogen production and estrogen receptor (ER) binding.

The relationship between radiation and chemical exposure and increases in breast cancer risk has also been consistently seen. Survivors of Hodgkin lymphoma are at increased risk for developing treatment-related secondary solid tumors up to 40 years following radiation treatment. Women younger than 30 years, and particularly younger than 20 years, at the time of mantle radiation for Hodgkin disease are at significant risk for developing breast cancer

(24). Actuarial calculation predicted a 34% risk of developing breast cancer at 25 years following radiation treatment in the youngest patients less than 20 years, 22.3% risk in those 20 to 29 years of age, and 3.5% risk for those aged 30 years or above at the time of treatment (25).

Chemical exposure impact was quantified by the Long Island Breast Cancer Study project in the 1990s, where common pollutants in the Long Island area including common pesticides and their breakdown products failed to demonstrate a clear impact on breast cancer risk (26,27).

Our understanding of the impact of race and ethnicity on risk of breast cancer remains incomplete, but current data indicate disparities exist on, both linked to and independent from, screening and treatment access (28). A Surveillance, Epidemiology, and End Results (SEER) database study of women with breast cancer, age 68 years and above, demonstrated African American women to have significantly worse survival than White women. Adjusting for predictor variables, such as tumor characteristics, screening, biologic markers, treatments, and comorbidities, did reduce this difference in survival, but did not eliminate it (28). Racial differences have also been detected in 21-gene recurrence score (RS) assays completed on non-Hispanic White (NHW) and non-Hispanic Black (NHB) patients in an urban population. Even when controlling age, clinical stage, tumor grade, and histologic characteristics, NHB women remained more likely to have high-risk lesions on RS testing (29). At least one international study demonstrated that mortality related to breast cancer is quite variable globally, but these differences are closely linked to access to early detection programs and treatment facilities (30).

Specific subsets of patients with benign breast disease have been noted to have an increased risk of breast cancer. In a cohort of over 9,000 patients followed from the Mayo Clinic after a diagnosis of benign breast disease, the RR of breast cancer when compared to the general population was 1.56. Risk was greatest in those where atypia is identified (RR 4.24) and in those with proliferative lesions without atypia (RR 1.88) (31,32).

Risk factors for male breast cancer do differ from female breast cancer risks. Similar to female breast cancer, the most significant risk factors for the development of breast cancer in men are genetic predisposition and familial. Whereas female breast cancer consistently demonstrates an association between hormone receptor (HR) expression and overall survival (OS), male breast cancer does not. More specifically, male breast cancer demonstrates no correlation between progesterone or HER2 HR expression and OS (33).

The combined risk of many of the factors discussed throughout this section is quantified by a number of risk calculator models, including the Cuzick, Gail, and Claus models. The Gail model was created as a widely applicable general calculator. However, it was designed based on data from a nearly all White female population and has been subsequently modified to better approximate the risk of African American and Hispanic women as well (34). Alternatively, the Claus model was designed to correct shortcomings of the Gail model, including accounting for more distant familial impacts and accounting for other hormonally responsive malignancies. The inclusion of these factors makes the Claus model best suited for higher risk patients, specifically those with a first-degree relative with breast cancer (34).

ANATOMY

The breast is a modified sweat gland composed of branching ducts and glandular lobules and is situated between the subdermal adipose tissue and the superficial pectoral fascia. The mammary gland consists of the tissue overlying the pectoralis major muscle, extending vertically from the second to sixth ribs and horizontally from the sternum to the midaxillary line. The gland extends more laterally from the chest wall as the axillary tail, to join the axilla and form the breast.

The breast parenchyma is composed of 15 to 20 sections, or lobes, each composed of multiple smaller lobules. Lobules make up the glandular milk forming unit and drain through a complex series of ducts, which increase in diameter as they traverse from the lobule to the nipple. Most peripherally, the terminal ductal lobular units (TDLUs) empty into the subsegmental ducts. These then coalesce with others to form segmental ducts and, eventually, lactiferous ducts, which then drain through the nipple complex. This complex drainage system exists intermixed with blood vessels, nerves, and lymphatics throughout the breast parenchyma. Likely reflective of their high metabolic activity, the lobule has been implicated as the origin of most breast pathology, including fibrocystic disease, and most carcinomas including ductal carcinoma in situ (DCIS) and lobular carcinoma in situ (LCIS), with the notable exception being papilloma's (35).

The glandular tissue of the breast is supported by a complex fascial support system. Cooper ligaments serve as the suspensory ligaments of the breast; they are fibrous bands extending perpendicularly from the dermis to the breast tissue. The breast parenchyma itself is encircled in a three-dimensional ring of fibrous fascial tissue, which fuses anteriorly with Cooper ligaments and posteriorly to the chest wall, providing a scaffold within which the remainder of the breast tissue is structured (36).

The retromammary bursa, positioned between the posterior aspect of the breast's circumferential fascia and the pectoralis major muscle, allows for movement of breast tissue on the chest wall and consists of loose areolar tissue. Within this tissue lies a dense system of lymphatics, which, together with a complex network of lymphatic drainage from the skin of the neck, chest, and abdomen, constitutes the lymphatic drainage of the breast. Lymphatic drainage originates in the breast lobules and traverses intramammary nodes before exiting through one of three major channels to the bilateral subclavian veins and thoracic duct. The axillary, or lateral, pathway is the dominate drainage pathway for the breast, carrying more than 75% of breast lymphatic drainage from the lateral quadrants to the axilla. The internal mammary pathway can drain the medial or lateral breast through the intercostal spaces to the parasternal nodes. Finally, the retromammary pathway drains the deep portions of the breast to the subclavicular plexus.

NATURAL HISTORY OF BREAST CANCER

The term *breast cancer* encompasses a diverse group of tumor biology, and although important differences exist, there are several behavioral patterns shared by this family of disease. A majority of breast pathology originates within the lobule and progresses outward through the ducts (35). Invasive disease occurs when, rather than growing along the natural path of the duct, malignant cells erode through the basement membrane and involve surrounding structures. Following erosion, invasive disease can then be found involving the adjacent lobules, or traveling along the associated lymphatics, nerves, and vasculature. The three primary lymphatic drainage channels for the breast, the axillary, internal mammary, and retromammary pathways, produce the most common routes of continued spread. More lateral based lesions tend to metastasize via the axillary pathway, whereas medial lesions traverse the internal mammary pathway (37). Increasing size of a primary tumor directly correlates with the risk of both nodal positivity and bone marrow positivity (38). Involvement of the dermal lymphatics leads to the characteristic erythematous and edematous skin known as peau d'orange.

Less commonly, locally advanced disease can occur when malignant cells invade skin, pectoralis or intercostal muscle, or surrounding osseous structures, including the clavicle or rib. Metastatic disease from breast cancer most commonly presents in the lung, bone, lymph node (LN), liver, and pleura, as identified by Lee in a 1983 review of more than 2,000 autopsies of women who died of breast cancer (39). Additional common sites of metastasis included the adrenal glands and the brain. Recurrent disease following breast cancer treatment is often identified in a similar distribution, with bone being the most common site, accounting for 40% to 60% of recurrence, followed by lung, accounting for an additional 20% (40). More contemporary reviews have linked patterns for metastatic disease to characteristics of tumor biology, especially hormonal expression. ER and progesterone receptor positive (PR+) lesions have demonstrated the best overall prognosis, with a propensity for late osseous metastasis, whereas HER2-expressing lesions are more likely to present with remote central nervous system metastases. Finally, tumors without any hormonal positivity, or triple-negative breast cancers (TNBCs), are commonly the most locally aggressive but are also most likely to present with central nervous system metastases early, within the first 5 years of diagnosis (41).

Location of disease origin within the breast remains an important prognostic factor, with studies demonstrating significantly worse breast cancer–specific survival and OS rates for primary tumors located in the inner quadrant of the breast compared to those of the outer quadrant (37). This is thought to be related to the difference in primary lymphatic drainage, as inner quadrant disease tends to drain more occultly into the internal mammary pathway. Left-sided breast cancer has also been demonstrated to be approximately 13% more common than right-sided breast cancer, when lesions are unilateral (42). Although an exact understanding of this left-sided predilection is unclear, some evidence suggests that epigenetic profiles of the right and left breast differ. These epigenetic changes result in variable methylation of ion channels and, therefore, differences in metabolic activity, which could account for variable oncologic risk (43). Predictive features for breast cancers more likely to metastasize, and characteristic patterns of metastasis, remain topics of ongoing study. Whole-exome sequencing and tissue microarray–based data continually demonstrate the complexity of clonal expansion linked to metastasis but provide promising avenues for future prognostication (38,44).

REFERENCES

1. Siegel RL, Miller KD, Fuchs HE, Jemal A. Cancer statistics, 2022. *CA Cancer J Clin.* 2022;72(1):7-33.
2. Torre LA, Bray F, Siegel RL, Ferlay J, Lortet-Tieulent J, Jemal A. Global cancer statistics, 2012. *CA Cancer J Clin.* 2015;65(2):87-108.
3. Marchbanks PA, Curtis KM, Mandel MG, et al. Oral contraceptive formulation and risk of breast cancer. *Contraception.* 2012;85(4):342-350.
4. Gennari A, Costa M, Puntoni M, et al. Breast cancer incidence after hormonal treatments for infertility: systematic review and meta-analysis of population-based studies. *Breast Cancer Res Treat.* 2015;150(2):405-413.
5. Chlebowski RT, Hendrix SL, Langer RD, et al. Influence of estrogen plus progestin on breast cancer and mammography in healthy postmenopausal women: the Women's Health Initiative Randomized Trial. *JAMA.* 2003;289(24):3243-3253.
6. Miki Y, Swensen J, Shattuck-Eidens D, et al. A strong candidate for the breast and ovarian cancer susceptibility gene BRCA1. *Science.* 1994;266(5182):66-71.
7. Wooster R, Neuhausen SL, Mangion J, et al. Localization of a breast cancer susceptibility gene, BRCA2, to chromosome 13q12-13. *Science.* 1994;265(5181):2088-2090.
8. Walker-Smith TL, Peck J. Genetic and genomic advances in breast cancer diagnosis and treatment. *Nurs Womens Health.* 2019;23(6):518-525.
9. Hu C, Hart SN, Gnanaolivu R, et al. A population-based study of genes previously implicated in breast cancer. *N Engl J Med.* 2021;384(5):440-451.
10. Scalia-Wilbur J, Colins BL, Penson RT, Dizon DS. Breast cancer risk assessment: moving beyond BRCA 1 and 2. *Semin Radiat Oncol.* 2016;26(1):3-8.
11. Wong EM, Southey MC, Terry MB. Integrating DNA methylation measures to improve clinical risk assessment: are we there yet? The case of BRCA1 methylation marks to improve clinical risk assessment of breast cancer. *Br J Cancer.* 2020;122(8):1133-1140.
12. Kalinsky K, Barlow WE, Gralow JR, et al. 21-Gene assay to inform chemotherapy benefit in node-positive breast cancer. *N Engl J Med.* 2021;385(25):2336-2347.

13. Boyd NF, Guo H, Martin LJ, et al. Mammographic density and the risk and detection of breast cancer. *N Engl J Med.* 2007;356(3):227-236.

14. Boyd NF, Martin LJ, Yaffe MJ, Minkin S. Mammographic density and breast cancer risk: current understanding and future prospects. *Breast Cancer Res.* 2011;13(6):223.

15. Kerlikowske K, Ma L, Scott CG, et al. Combining quantitative and qualitative breast density measures to assess breast cancer risk. *Breast Cancer Res.* 2017;19(1):97.

16. Wanders JOP, Holland K, Karssemeijer N, et al. The effect of volumetric breast density on the risk of screen-detected and interval breast cancers: a cohort study. *Breast Cancer Res.* 2017;19(1):67.

17. Tretli S. Height and weight in relation to breast cancer morbidity and mortality. A prospective study of 570,000 women in Norway. *Int J Cancer.* 1989;44(1):23-30.

18. Iyengar NM, Arthur R, Manson JE, et al. Association of body fat and risk of breast cancer in postmenopausal women with normal body mass index: a secondary analysis of a randomized clinical trial and observational study. *JAMA Oncol.* 2019;5(2):155-163.

19. Thomson CA. Diet and breast cancer: understanding risks and benefits. *Nutr Clin Pract.* 2012;27(5):636-650.

20. Ellison RC, Zhang Y, McLennan CE, Rothman KJ. Exploring the relation of alcohol consumption to risk of breast cancer. *Am J Epidemiol.* 2001;154(8):740-747.

21. Wang F, Yeung KL, Chan WC, et al. A meta-analysis on dose-response relationship between night shift work and the risk of breast cancer. *Ann Oncol.* 2013;24(11):2724-2732.

22. Schernhammer ES, Kroenke CH, Laden F, Hankinson SE. Night work and risk of breast cancer. *Epidemiology.* 2006;17(1):108-111.

23. Koppes LL, Geuskens GA, Pronk A, Vermeulen RC, de Vroome EM. Night work and breast cancer risk in a general population prospective cohort study in the Netherlands. *Eur J Epidemiol.* 2014;29(8):577-584.

24. Schaapveld M, Aleman BM, van Eggermond AM, et al. Second cancer risk up to 40 years after treatment for Hodgkin's lymphoma. *N Engl J Med.* 2015;373(26):2499-2511.

25. Aisenberg AC, Finkelstein DM, Doppke KP, Koerner FC, Boivin JF, Willett CG. High risk of breast carcinoma after irradiation of young women with Hodgkin's disease. *Cancer.* 1997;79(6):1203-1210.

26. Gammon MD, Wolff MS, Neugut AI, et al. Environmental toxins and breast cancer on Long Island. II. Organochlorine compound levels in blood. *Cancer Epidemiol Biomarkers Prev.* 2002;11(8):686-697.

27. Schoenfeld ER, O'Leary ES, Henderson K, et al. Electromagnetic fields and breast cancer on Long Island: a case-control study. *Am J Epidemiol.* 2003;158(1):47-58.

28. Curtis E, Quale C, Haggstrom D, Smith-Bindman R. Racial and ethnic differences in breast cancer survival: how much is explained by screening, tumor severity, biology, treatment, comorbidities, and demographics? *Cancer.* 2008;112(1):171-180.

29. Holowatyj AN, Cote ML, Ruterbusch JJ, et al. Racial differences in 21-gene recurrence scores among patients with hormone receptor-positive, node-negative breast cancer. *J Clin Oncol.* 2018;36(7):652-658.

30. Rivera-Franco MM, Leon-Rodriguez E. Delays in breast cancer detection and treatment in developing countries. *Breast Cancer (Auckl).* 2018;12:1178223417752677.

31. Hartmann LC, Sellers TA, Frost MH, et al. Benign breast disease and the risk of breast cancer. *N Engl J Med.* 2005;353(3):229-237.

32. Louro J, Román M, Posso M, et al. Differences in breast cancer risk after benign breast disease by type of screening diagnosis. *Breast.* 2020;54:343-348.

33. Yao N, Shi W, Liu T, et al. Clinicopathologic characteristics and prognosis for male breast cancer compared to female breast cancer. *Sci Rep.* 2022;12(1):220.

34. Singletary SE. Rating the risk factors for breast cancer. *Ann Surg.* 2003;237(4):474-482.

35. Wellings SR, Jensen HM, Marcum RG. An atlas of subgross pathology of the human breast with special reference to possible precancerous lesions. *J Natl Cancer Inst.* 1975;55(2):231-273.

36. Rehnke RD, Groening RM, Van Buskirk ER, Clarke JM. Anatomy of the superficial fascia system of the breast: a comprehensive theory of breast fascial anatomy. *Plast Reconstr Surg.* 2018;142(5):1135-1144.

37. Gaffney DK, Tsodikov A, Wiggins CL. Diminished survival in patients with inner versus outer quadrant breast cancers. *J Clin Oncol.* 2003;21(3):467-472.

38. Klevesath MB, Pantel K, Agbaje O, et al. Patterns of metastatic spread in early breast cancer. *Breast.* 2013;22(4):449-454.

39. Lee YT. Patterns of metastasis and natural courses of breast carcinoma. *Cancer Metastasis Rev.* 1985;4(2):153-172.

40. Lee YT. Breast carcinoma: pattern of recurrence and metastasis after mastectomy. *Am J Clin Oncol.* 1984;7(5):443-449.

41. Chikarmane SA, Tirumani SH, Howard SA, Jagannathan JP, DiPiro PJ. Metastatic patterns of breast cancer subtypes: what radiologists should know in the era of personalized cancer medicine. *Clin Radiol.* 2015;70(1):1-10.

42. Tulinius H, Sigvaldason H, Olafsdóttir G. Left and right sided breast cancer. *Pathol Res Pract.* 1990;186(1):92-94.

43. Masuelli S, Real S, Campoy E, et al. When left does not seem right: epigenetic and bioelectric differences between left- and right-sided breast cancer. *Mol Med.* 2022;28(1):15.

44. Avigdor BE, Cimino-Mathews A, DeMarzo AM, et al. Mutational profiles of breast cancer metastases from a rapid autopsy series reveal multiple evolutionary trajectories. *JCI Insight.* 2017;2(24):e96896

CHAPTER **11.3**

Breast Cancer: Clinical Presentation

Julia Tassinari

INTRODUCTION

Breast cancer presents as a range of clinical scenarios. For the majority of people presenting with a new diagnosis, breast cancer is an asymptomatic entity identified after abnormal screening mammography. Effective screening tests aim to identify breast cancer before symptoms, providing a greater scope of therapeutic options and improved survival outcomes. This hypothesis has been studied, and recent evaluation in the UK Age Trial has demonstrated reduced mortality with the addition of annual screening mammogram for women in the decade before age 50 (1). Although short diagnostic interval mammographic screening commencement at age 40 is shown to reduce breast cancer mortality, many women continue to experience long diagnostic intervals between recommended screening. This is concerning as longer intervals to diagnosis are associated with lower 5-year survival of patients with breast cancer (2).

For people who present with symptoms, a palpable breast mass is the most common presentation of local disease, often as a hard mass with irregular borders. Additional abnormal findings on self- or clinical breast examination can also establish a diagnosis.

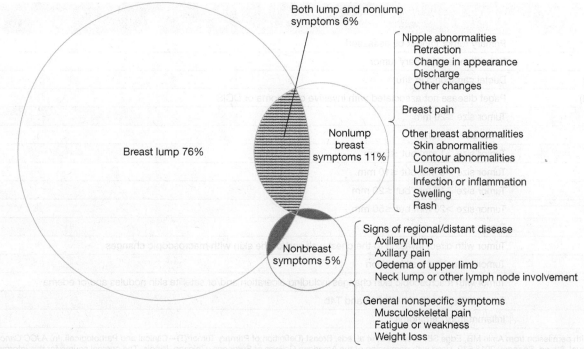

Figure 11.3-1. Presenting signs and symptoms for women newly diagnosed with breast cancer. (From Koo MM, von Wagner C, Abel GA, McPhail S, Rubin GP, Lyratzopoulos G. Typical and atypical presenting symptoms of breast cancer and their associations with diagnostic intervals: evidence from a national audit of cancer diagnosis. *Cancer Epidemiol.* 2017;48:140-146.)

These include skin changes (peau d'orange, dimpling, erythema, retractions), breast swelling and new asymmetry, nipple discharge, inversion/retraction, or skin changes (scaling/crusting nipple rash). Axillary lymphadenopathy can be evidence of locally advanced disease and may present as the only site of disease without evidence of a primary cancer (occult breast carcinoma). Although it is a less typical presentation, patients presenting with complaints of abdominal pain (liver metastases), skeletal pain or pathologic fractures (bone metastases), and shortness of breath (lung metastases) can lead to a diagnosis of metastatic breast cancer. At the time of diagnosis, 64% of patients have local stage breast cancer, 27% have regional involvement, and 6% have metastatic disease (3).

One audit of 2,316 women presenting with breast cancer in the United Kingdom investigated the variation in the length of the patient interval (time from symptom onset to presentation to medical attention) and the primary care interval (time from presentation to specialist referral) across symptom groups using descriptive analyses and quantile regression. In all, 56 presenting symptoms were described: Breast lump was the most frequent (83%), followed by nonlump breast symptoms of nipple abnormalities (7%) and breast pain (6%), followed by nonbreast symptoms, such as back pain (1%) and weight loss (0.3%). About one in six women with breast cancer present with a large spectrum of symptoms other than a breast lump. Women who present with nonlump breast symptoms tend to delay seeking help (**Figure 11.3-1**) (4).

Other external factors can influence clinical presentation. During the COVID pandemic and with decreased access to screening and routine breast examinations, an increase in locally advanced breast cancers (LABCs) were identified, even in regions with screening capabilities (5). Women in childbearing years can present later, as diagnosis can be delayed when breast changes are thought to be benign processes associated with breastfeeding, dense breast tissue, and pregnancy-associated breast changes.

PHYSICAL EXAMINATION

For people being evaluated for possible breast cancer, the physical examination includes examination of the breasts and assessment of the LN basins of the chest wall, supraclavicular, cervical, and axillae bilaterally. Examination should be completed with the patient in both the upright and supine positions. Inspection should reveal any skin changes, dimpling, nipple inversion, or gross asymmetry between the breasts. Breast palpation involves a bimanual examination. Whether circular movements are utilized or more linear palpation, the breasts must be examined systematically from the sternum medially, to the axillary tail and chest wall laterally, the clavicle superiorly, and the intramammary fold inferiorly, to achieve a comprehensive examination.

With arms placed in a dependent position or extended forward, the tension on the intercostal brachial fascia is decreased, allowing better palpable access to the nodal basins to assess for axillary lymphadenopathy. Supraclavicular and cervical lymphadenopathy should also be assessed.

STAGING

Breast cancer is staged using both the American Joint Committee on Cancer (AJCC) and the International Union for Cancer Control classification system based on tumor size, LN status, and the presence or absence of metastatic disease (tumor-node-metastasis, TNM). Stage is established first clinically and then pathologically using the histopathologic data from the surgical specimen.

Emerging data, and targeted breast cancer treatment advancements, suggest that combining anatomic staging and tumor biology yields a predictive synergy for determining breast cancer prognosis. In response to a deeper understanding of breast cancer genomics and tumor biology, the *AJCC Staging Manual*, eighth edition, created significant changes and new staging guidelines in 2018. The stage changes vary by tumor histology, receptor status, tumor grade, and Oncotype Dx scores (all *P* < .0001). Overall, the transition to the eighth edition is expected to provide better disease understanding, clinical care, individualized treatment recommendations, and future research avenues (6,7). The staging systems are provided in **Tables 11.3-1 through 11.3-4.**

■ TABLE 11.3-1. Tumor Staging of Breast Cancer

Tx	Primary tumor cannot be assessed
T0	No evidence of primary tumor
Tis (DCIS)	Ductal carcinoma in situ
Tis (Paget)	Paget disease not associated with invasive carcinoma or DCIS
T1	Tumor size ≤20 mm
T1mi	Timor size ≤1 mm
T1a	Tumor size >1 mm but ≤5 mm
T1b	Tumor size >5 mm but ≤10 mm
T1c	Tumor size >10 mm but ≤20 mm
T2	Tumor size >20 mm but ≤50 mm
T3	Tumor size >50 mm
T4	Tumor with direct invasion to the chest wall and/or the skin with macroscopic changes
T4a	Tumor with chest wall invasion
T4b	Tumor with macroscopic skin changes including ulceration and/or satellite skin nodules and/or edema
T4c	Tumor with criteria of both T4a and T4b
T4d	Inflammatory carcinoma

Reprinted with permission from Amin MB, Edge SB, Greene FL, et al, eds. Breast (Definition of Primary Tumor (T)—Clinical and Pathological). In: *AJCC Cancer Staging Manual*. 8th ed. Springer; 2018:619. Used with permission of the American College of Surgeons, Chicago, Illinois. The original source for this information is the AJCC Cancer Staging System (2023).

■ TABLE 11.3-2. Nodal Staging of Breast Cancer

	Clinical Classification	Pathologic Classification
NX	Regional lymph nodes cannot be assessed (eg, previously removed)	Regional lymph nodes cannot be assessed
N0	No regional lymph node metastases (by imaging or examination)	No regional lymph node metastasis identified
N1	Metastasis to movable ipsilateral level I and II axillary lymph nodes	Micrometastases or metastases in one to three axillary lymph nodes and/or clinically negative internal mammary nodes with micrometastases or macrometastases detected by sentinel lymph node biopsy
N1mi	Micrometastases (~200 cells, >0.2 mm but none >2 mm)	Micrometastases (~200 cells, >0.2 mm but none >2 mm) pN1a—Metastases in one to three axillary lymph nodes, with at least one metastasis > 2 mm pN1b—Metastases in ipsilateral internal mammary sentinel nodes pN1c—pN1a and pN1b combined
N2	Metastasis to ipsilateral level I and II axillary lymph nodes that are clinically fixed or matted; or in ipsilateral internal mammary nodes in the absence of clinically evidence axillary node metastases	Metastases in four to nine axillary lymph nodes or positive ipsilateral internal mammary lymph nodes by imaging in the absence of axillary lymph node metastases
N2a	Metastasis to ipsilateral level I and II axillary lymph nodes fixed to one another (matted) or to other structures	Metastases in four to nine axillary lymph nodes (at least one tumor deposit > 2 mm)
N2b	Metastasis only in ipsilateral internal mammary nodes and in the absence of clinically evidence axillary node metastases	Metastasis only in clinically detected internal mammary nodes with or without microscopic confirmation, with pathologically negative axillary nodes
N3	Metastases in ipsilateral infraclavicular (level III axillary) lymph nodes with or without level I and II axillary lymph nodes involvement; or in ipsilateral supraclavicular lymph node with or without axillary or internal mammary lymph node involvement	Metastases in 10+ axillary lymph nodes, or in infraclavicular (level III) lymph nodes, or in ipsilateral internal mammary lymph nodes by imaging in the presence of one or more positive level I and II axillary lymph nodes, or in more than three axillary lymph nodes and in internal mammary lymph nodes with micrometastases or macrometastases detected by sentinel lymph node biopsy but not clinically detected, or in ipsilateral supraclavicular lymph nodes
N3a	Metastasis to ipsilateral infraclavicular lymph nodes	Metastases in 10+ axillary lymph nodes (at least one tumor deposit >2 mm) or metastases to the infraclavicular (level III axillary) lymph nodes
N3b	Metastasis to ipsilateral internal mammary lymph nodes and axillary lymph nodes	pN1a or pN2a in the presence of cN2b (positive internal mammary nodes by imaging) or pN2a in the presence of pN1b
N3c	Metastasis in ipsilateral supraclavicular lymph nodes	Metastases in ipsilateral supraclavicular lymph nodes

Reprinted with permission from Amin MB, Edge SB, Greene FL, et al, eds. Breast (Definition of Regional Lymph Nodes—Clinical (cN)). In: *AJCC Cancer Staging Manual*. 8th ed. Springer; 2018:619. Used with permission of the American College of Surgeons, Chicago, Illinois. The original source for this information is the AJCC Cancer Staging System (2023).

■ TABLE 11.3-3. Clinical Staging of Breast Cancer

TNM	Grade	HER2	ER	PR	Clinical Prognostic Stage
TisN0M0	Any	Any	Any	Any	0
T1N0M0	G1	Positive	Positive	Positive	IA
T0N1miM0				Negative	IA
T1N1miM0					
			Negative	Positive	IA
				Negative	IA
		Negative	Positive	Positive	IA
				Negative	IA
			Negative	Positive	IA
				Negative	IB
T1N0M0	G2	Positive	Positive	Positive	IA
T0N1miM0				Negative	IA
T1N1miM0					
			Negative	Positive	IA
				Negative	IA
		Negative	Positive	Positive	IA
				Negative	IA
			Negative	Positive	IA
				Negative	IB
T1N0M0	G3	Positive	Positive	Positive	IA
T0N1miM0				Negative	IA
T1N1miM0					
			Negative	Positive	IA
				Negative	IA
		Negative	Positive	Positive	IA
				Negative	IB
			Negative	Positive	IB
				Negative	IB
T0N1M0	G1	Positive	Positive	Positive	IB
T1N1M0				Negative	IIA
T2N0M0					
			Negative	Positive	IIA
				Negative	IIA
		Negative	Positive	Positive	IB
				Negative	IIA
			Negative	Positive	IIA
				Negative	IIA
T0N1M0	G2	Positive	Positive	Positive	IB
T1N1M0				Negative	IIA
T2N0M0					
			Negative	Positive	IIA
				Negative	IIA
		Negative	Positive	Positive	IB
				Negative	IIA
			Negative	Positive	IIA
				Negative	IIB
T0N1M0	G3	Positive	Positive	Positive	IB
T1N1M0				Negative	IIA
T2N0M0					
			Negative	Positive	IIA
				Negative	IIA
		Negative	Positive	Positive	IIA
				Negative	IIB
			Negative	Positive	IIB
				Negative	IIB
T2N1M0	GI	Positive	Positive	Positive	IB
T3N0M0				Negative	IIA
			Negative	Positive	IIA
				Negative	IIB
		Negative	Positive	Positive	IIA
				Negative	IIB
			Negative	Positive	IIB
				Negative	IIB
T2N1M0	G2	Positive	Positive	Positive	IB
T3N0M0				Negative	IIA
			Negative	Positive	IIA
				Negative	IIB
		Negative	Positive	Positive	IIA
				Negative	IIB
			Negative	Positive	IIB
				Negative	IIIB

(continued)

■ TABLE 11.3-3. Clinical Staging of Breast Cancer (*continued*)

TNM	Grade	HER2	ER	PR	Clinical Prognostic Stage
T2N1M0	G3	Positive	Positive	Positive	IB
T3N0M0				Negative	IIB
			Negative	Positive	IIB
				Negative	IIB
		Negative	Positive	Positive	IIB
				Negative	IIIA
			Negative	Positive	IIIA
				Negative	IIIB
T0N2M0	G1	Positive	Positive	Positive	IIA
T1N2M0				Negative	IIIA
T2N2M0			Negative	Positive	IIIA
T3N1M0				Negative	IIIA
T3N2M0		Negative	Positive	Positive	IIA
				Negative	IIIA
			Negative	Positive	IIIA
				Negative	IIIB
T0N2M0	G2	Positive	Positive	Positive	IIA
T1N2M0				Negative	IIIA
T2N2M0			Negative	Positive	IIIA
T3N1M0				Negative	IIIA
T3N2M0		Negative	Positive	Positive	IIA
				Negative	IIIA
			Negative	Positive	IIIA
				Negative	IIIB
T0N2M0	G3	Positive	Positive	Positive	IIB
T1N2M0				Negative	IIIA
T2N2M0			Negative	Positive	IIIA
T3N1M0				Negative	IIIA
T3N2M0		Negative	Positive	Positive	IIIA
				Negative	IIIB
			Negative	Positive	IIIB
				Negative	IIIC
T4N0M0	G1	Positive	Positive	Positive	IIIA
T4N1M0				Negative	IIIB
T4N2M0			Negative	Positive	IIIB
AnyTN3M0				Negative	IIIB
		Negative	Positive	Positive	IIIB
				Negative	IIIB
			Negative	Positive	IIIB
				Negative	IIIC
T4N0M0	G2	Positive	Positive	Positive	IIIA
T4N1M0				Negative	IIIB
T4N2M0			Negative	Positive	IIIB
AnyTN3M0				Negative	IIIB
		Negative	Positive	Positive	IIIB
				Negative	IIIB
			Negative	Positive	IIIB
				Negative	IIIC
T4N0M0	G3	Positive	Positive	Positive	IIIB
T4N1M0				Negative	IIIB
T4N2M0			Negative	Positive	IIIB
AnyTN3M0				Negative	IIIB
		Negative	Positive	Positive	IIIB
				Negative	IIIC
			Negative	Positive	IIIC
				Negative	IIIC
AnyT AnyN M1	Any	Any	Any	Any	IV

ER, estrogen receptor; PR, progesterone receptor; HER2, human epidermal growth factor receptor 2; TNM, tumor-node-metastasis.

Reprinted with permission from Amin MB, Edge SB, Greene FL, et al, eds. Breast (AJCC Prognostic Stage Groups). In: *AJCC Cancer Staging Manual*. 8th ed. Springer; 2018:621. Used with permission of the American College of Surgeons, Chicago, Illinois. The original source for this information is the AJCC Cancer Staging System (2023).

▪ TABLE 11.3-4. Pathologic Staging of Breast Cancer

TNM	Grade	HER2	ER	PR	Pathologic Prognostic Stage
TisN0M0	Any	Any	Any	Any	0
T1N0M0 T0N1miM0 T1N1miM0	G1	Positive	Positive	Positive	IA
				Negative	IA
			Negative	Positive	IA
				Negative	IA
		Negative	Positive	Positive	IA
				Negative	IA
			Negative	Positive	IA
				Negative	IA
T1N0M0 T0N1miM0 T1N1miM0	G2	Positive	Positive	Positive	IA
				Negative	IA
			Negative	Positive	IA
				Negative	IA
		Negative	Positive	Positive	IA
				Negative	IA
			Negative	Positive	IA
				Negative	IB
T1N0M0 T0N1miM0 T1N1miM0	G3	Positive	Positive	Positive	IA
				Negative	IA
			Negative	Positive	IA
				Negative	IA
		Negative	Positive	Positive	IA
				Negative	IA
			Negative	Positive	IA
				Negative	IB
T0N1M0 T1N1M0 T2N0M0	G1	Positive	Positive	Positive	IA
				Negative	IB
			Negative	Positive	IB
				Negative	IIA
		Negative	Positive	Positive	IA
				Negative	IB
			Negative	Positive	IB
				Negative	IIA
T0N1M0 T1N1M0 T2N0M0	G2	Positive	Positive	Positive	IA
				Negative	IB
			Negative	Positive	IB
				Negative	IIA
		Negative	Positive	Positive	IA
				Negative	IIA
			Negative	Positive	IIA
				Negative	IIA
T0N1M0 T1N1M0 T2N0M0	G3	Positive	Positive	Positive	IA
				Negative	IIA
			Negative	Positive	IIA
				Negative	IIA
		Negative	Positive	Positive	IB
				Negative	IIA
			Negative	Positive	IIA
				Negative	IIA
T2N1M0 T3N0M0	GI	Positive	Positive	Positive	IA
				Negative	IIB
			Negative	Positive	IIB
				Negative	IIB
		Negative	Positive	Positive	IA
				Negative	IIB
			Negative	Positive	IIB
				Negative	IIB
T2N1M0 T3N0M0	G2	Positive	Positive	Positive	IB
				Negative	IIB
			Negative	Positive	IIB
				Negative	IIB
		Negative	Positive	Positive	IB
				Negative	IIB
			Negative	Positive	IIB
				Negative	IIB

(continued)

■ TABLE 11.3-4. Pathologic Staging of Breast Cancer (*continued*)

TNM	Grade	HER2	ER	PR	Pathologic Prognostic Stage
T2N1M0 T3N0M0	G3	Positive	Positive	Positive	IB
				Negative	IIB
			Negative	Positive	IIB
				Negative	IIB
		Negative	Positive	Positive	IIA
				Negative	IIB
			Negative	Positive	IIB
				Negative	IIIA
T0N2M0 T1N2M0 T2N2M0 T3N1M0 T3N2M0	G1	Positive	Positive	Positive	IB
				Negative	IIIA
			Negative	Positive	IIIA
				Negative	IIIA
		Negative	Positive	Positive	IB
				Negative	IIIA
			Negative	Positive	IIIA
				Negative	IIIA
T0N2M0 T1N2M0 T2N2M0 T3N1M0 T3N2M0	G2	Positive	Positive	Positive	IB
				Negative	IIIA
			Negative	Positive	IIIA
				Negative	IIIA
		Negative	Positive	Positive	IB
				Negative	IIIA
			Negative	Positive	IIIA
				Negative	IIIB
T0N2M0 T1N2M0 T2N2M0 T3N1M0 T3N2M0	G3	Positive	Positive	Positive	IIA
				Negative	IIIA
			Negative	Positive	IIIA
				Negative	IIIA
		Negative	Positive	Positive	IIB
				Negative	IIIA
			Negative	Positive	IIIA
				Negative	IIIC
T4N0M0 T4N1M0 T4N2M0 AnyTN3M0	G1	Positive	Positive	Positive	IIIA
				Negative	IIIB
			Negative	Positive	IIIB
				Negative	IIIB
		Negative	Positive	Positive	IIIA
				Negative	IIIB
			Negative	Positive	IIIB
				Negative	IIIB
T4N0M0 T4N1M0 T4N2M0 AnyTN3M0	G2	Positive	Positive	Positive	IIIA
				Negative	IIIB
			Negative	Positive	IIIB
				Negative	IIIB
		Negative	Positive	Positive	IIIA
				Negative	IIIB
			Negative	Positive	IIIB
				Negative	IIIC
T4N0M0 T4N1M0 T4N2M0 AnyTN3M0	G3	Positive	Positive	Positive	IIIB
				Negative	IIIB
			Negative	Positive	IIIB
				Negative	IIIB
		Negative	Positive	Positive	IIIB
				Negative	IIIC
			Negative	Positive	IIIC
				Negative	IIIC
AnyT AnyN M1	Any	Any	Any	Any	IV

ER, estrogen receptor; PR, progesterone receptor; HER2, human epidermal growth factor receptor 2; TNM, tumor-node-metastasis.

Reprinted with permission from Amin MB, Edge SB, Greene FL, et al, eds. *AJCC Cancer Staging Manual*. 8th ed. Springer; 2018; Used with permission of the American College of Surgeons, Chicago, Illinois. The original source for this information is the AJCC Cancer Staging System (2023).

REFERENCES

1. Duffy SW, Vulkan D, Cuckle H, et al. Effect of mammographic screening from age 40 years on breast cancer mortality (UK Age trial): final results of a randomised, controlled trial. *Lancet Oncol.* 2020;21:1165-1172.

2. Webber C, Jiang L, Grunfeld E, Groome PA. Identifying predictors of delayed diagnoses in symptomatic breast cancer: a scoping review. *Eur J Cancer Care (Engl).* 2017;26:e12483.

3. American Cancer Society. Breast cancer: facts and figures. 2019. https://www.cancer.org/content/dam/cancer-org/research/cancer-facts-and-statistics/breast-cancer-facts-and-figures/breast-cancer-facts-and-figures-2019-2020.pdf

4. Koo MM, von Wagner C, Abel GA, McPhail S, Rubin GP, Lyratzopoulos G. Typical and atypical presenting symptoms of breast cancer and their associations with diagnostic intervals: evidence from a national audit of cancer diagnosis. *Cancer Epidemiol.* 2017;48:140-146.

5. Alagoz O, Lowry KP, Kurian AW, et al. Impact of the COVID-19 pandemic on breast cancer mortality in the US: estimates from collaborative simulation modeling. *J Natl Cancer Inst.* 2021;113:1484-1494.

6. Giuliano AE, Connolly JL, Edge SB, et al. Breast cancer-major changes in the American Joint Committee on Cancer eighth edition cancer staging manual: updates to the AJCC breast TNM staging system: the 8th edition. *CA Cancer J Clin.* 2017;67:290-303.

7. Amin MB, Edge SB, Greene FL, et al., eds. *AJCC (American Joint Committee on Cancer) Cancer Staging Manual.* Springer; 2018.

CHAPTER **11.4**

Breast Imaging

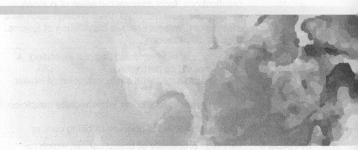

Martha B. Mainiero and Robert C. Ward

Breast imaging can be performed as a screening tool in asymptomatic women to detect early cancer or as a diagnostic examination in women with symptoms, abnormal screening examinations, or previously treated for breast cancer. Mammography remains the most widely used technique for screening. Digital breast tomosynthesis (DBT) is a mammography technique used in both screening and diagnostic mammography. Other modalities such as ultrasound (US) and magnetic resonance imaging (MRI) serve as adjunct tools in the diagnostic setting or in high-risk screening.

SCREENING GUIDELINES

The efficacy of mammography for average-risk women was established by multiple randomized controlled trials that demonstrated absolute mortality reduction, achieved by mammography's ability to detect both DCIS and invasive breast cancer at a smaller size and earlier stage than in unscreened women. A 2012 meta-analysis performed by the Independent UK Panel on Breast Cancer Screening that included 11 randomized trials and a 2015 systematic review of 90 studies confirmed that screening with mammography results in a 20% reduction in breast cancer mortality (1,2). Randomized controlled trials enrolled women aged 40 to 74 years, so there is no direct evidence of mortality reduction in patients below age 40 or over age 74.

Consensus guidelines regarding which age to begin screening and how frequently to screen women at average risk vary, based upon the perceived relative importance of its benefits, which include less invasive treatment options as well as mortality reduction and its risks, which include false positives and the possibility of overdiagnosis. As the rate of breast cancer significantly increases in the second half of a woman's 40s, the American Cancer Society (ACS) recommends that women have the opportunity to begin screening mammography at age 40 and recommends routine annual screening at age 45 to 54 years (with the option of annual or biennial screening starting at age 55), continuing as long as the woman is in good health and expected to live another 10 years (3). The U.S. Preventive Services Task Force (USPSTF) review found adequate evidence that mammography screening reduces breast cancer mortality in women aged 40 to 74 years but noted that the least mortality benefit is in women aged 40 to 49 years with no family history. The USPSTF, therefore, recommends biennial screening in women aged 50 to 74 years and

recommends that the decision to start screening at age 40 should be an individual one (4). This is in contrast to the recommendations of other organizations, including the American College of Obstetricians and Gynecologists, the American College of Radiology (ACR), and the American Society of Breast Surgeons (ASBrS), all of which continue to offer routine screening beginning at age 40 (5-7).

MAMMOGRAPHY AND DIGITAL BREAST TOMOSYNTHESIS

Not all cancers will be found by mammography as overlapping breast tissue, especially in dense breasts, can obscure cancer. DBT is a mammography technique that is typically performed in the same acquisition as the digital mammography examination. The patient is positioned, and the breast is compressed as in a standard mammogram. With DBT, the x-ray tube moves to obtain multiple low-dose images. From these images, reconstructed slices through the breast tissue are displayed, improving the visualization of breast cancer. When these slices are interpreted along with the planar digital mammography images, the sensitivity and specificity of the examination is increased (8). A systematic review and meta-analysis of 16 studies showed an increase in sensitivity of 69% to 86% and 84% to 90% when DBT is added to digital mammography in women with dense breasts (9). With newer DBT software, both tomographic slices and a synthesized digital mammogram can now be performed at the same radiation dose as a standard (two-dimensional [2D]) digital mammogram while maintaining the improved performance of DBT performed in addition to digital mammography (10). Between 2015 and 2017, the percentage of screening mammograms in the United States performed with tomosynthesis increased from 12.9% to 43.2% (11).

In a screening population, approximately 10% of patients will be "recalled" either for additional imaging with additional mammographic views as a diagnostic mammogram or for US. The cancer detection rate in screening mammography averages 3 to 8 per 1,000 women screened. Of positive screening examinations, 3% to 8% will have a diagnosis of cancer, with 20% to 40% of biopsies recommended positive for cancer (12). The rates of positive biopsy are higher in patients presenting with a palpable lump.

Unlike screening mammography, diagnostic mammography requires direct supervision and is performed in patients who

■ TABLE 11.4-1. BI-RADS Assessment Categories

Categorization of Breast Density	
BI-RADS 0	Examination is not complete. Often means additional workup is needed (eg, spot compression, US)
BI-RADS 1	No change in examination from prior; no abnormal findings appreciated
BI-RADS 2	Benign finding, detected at routine screening. This includes breast cyst, fibroadenoma, fatty densities, surgical scar, scattered microcalcifications, and the presence of breast implants
BI-RADS 3	*Probably* benign finding; typically, a 6-mo follow-up will be needed. Findings included are tiny clusters of calcifications, focal asymmetric areas of nonpalpable fibroglandular densities, focal findings such as a dilated duct, and generalized distribution of lesions, such as calcifications
BI-RADS 4 4A 4B 4C	Suspicious or indeterminate findings identified. A biopsy should be performed. Finding associated with a **low** suspicion of breast cancer Finding associated with an **intermediate** suspicion of breast cancer Finding of **moderate** concern of being cancer
BI-RADS 5	Very high probability of breast cancer, which requires immediate action
BI-RADS 6	Imaging of a known cancer, proven by biopsy
Almost entirely fatty	
Few areas of fibroglandular density identified	
Heterogeneous density, which may obscure a small mass	
Extreme density, associated with a lower sensitivity of mammography	

BI-RADS, Breast Imaging Reporting and Data System; US, ultrasound.

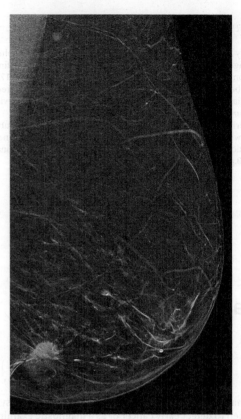

Figure 11.4-1. Breast Imaging Reporting and Data System category 5 finding on mammography. Left mediolateral oblique projection from digital breast tomosynthesis demonstrates a high-density spiculated mass near the inframammary fold. This is highly suspicious for malignancy and warranted biopsy, which demonstrated invasive ductal carcinoma.

have signs or symptoms of breast disease, abnormal screening mammography, or who are undergoing imaging surveillance for a breast finding. Medicare also pays for diagnostic mammography in women with a personal history of breast cancer.

Mammography Regulations and Reporting

The Breast Imaging Reporting and Data System (BI-RADS), first published in 1993, is a lexicon developed by the ACR to standardize terminology used in reporting findings on breast imaging studies (13). It includes terms for describing features of masses (shapes and margins) and calcifications (morphology and distribution). It defines final assessment categories to describe the radiologist's level of suspicion to comply with the federally mandated Mammography Quality Standards Act (MQSA) regulations. All mammograms must be assessed with a final BI-RADS category of 0 to 6 (**Table 11.4-1**). **Figure 11.4-1** gives a representative picture of a BI-RADS 5 mammographic image using digital tomosynthesis.

The report must include the date of comparison films; the indication for the examination (screening, recall, clinical finding, or follow-up); an assessment of overall breast composition to indicate the relative possibility that a lesion may be hidden by normal tissue, limiting the sensitivity of the examination; a description of any significant findings; and an overall summary impression.

BREAST ULTRASOUND

US is an essential component of the diagnostic evaluation of clinically and mammographically detected findings and helps characterize masses as benign, probably benign, or suspicious based upon characteristics such as shape and margins (**Figure 11.4-2**). In these settings, US is typically performed as a limited or targeted examination. Complete breast US not only can be performed as an

adjunct to mammography in screening women with dense breasts but also substantially increases the false-positive rate. In a randomized controlled multicenter trial of women with dense breast tissue, the cancer detection rate of mammography alone was 7.6 per 1,000 women screened and increased to 11.8 per 1,000 women screened with the addition of US, but the positive predictive value decreased from 22.6% for mammography alone to 8.9% for the combined examination (14). Therefore, US for screening women with dense breasts is a decision made at the individual patient level.

Breast Magnetic Resonance Imaging

Contrast-enhanced breast MRI is the most sensitive modality in the detection and staging of breast cancer. Unlike mammography and US that rely on anatomic changes, breast MRI, through the intravenous injection of gadolinium-based contrast, also images the physiologic changes of tumor angiogenesis and surrounding tissue permeability associated with breast cancer. However, there is overlap between the contrast enhancement pattern of benign and malignant processes, which lowers the specificity of breast MRI. Lower specificity and higher cost limit the use of MRI to high-risk screening, preoperative evaluation of patients with breast cancer, and additional evaluation of imaging or clinical findings in selected situations.

Recommended parameters for breast MRI are set by the ACR for proper imaging, interpretation, and accreditation. MRI of the breast should be performed with a dedicated breast coil, using at least a 1.5-T magnet, and imaging parameters should be instituted to optimize high spatial and temporal resolution (15). Standard breast MRI is performed as a dynamic contrast-enhanced examination in which multiple postcontrast images are obtained to characterize the rapidity with which a lesion enhances and washes out with contrast.

Breast MR reporting is standardized based on the ACR BI-RADS MR lexicon, which, similar to mammography, incorporates

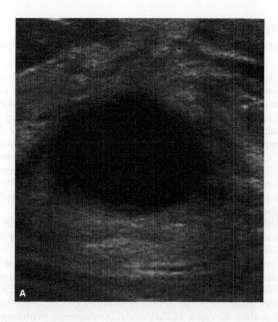

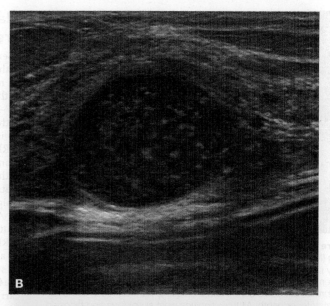

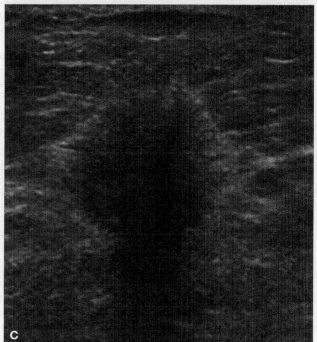

Figure 11.4-2. Ultrasound features of benign, probably benign, and suspicious masses. A: Benign. Oval circumscribed anechoic mass with an imperceptible wall and posterior acoustic enhancement, consistent with a benign cyst. B: Probably benign. Oval circumscribed mass with internal echoes, suggestive of a complicated cyst or fibroadenoma. Ultrasound follow-up was recommended to document 2 years of stability, indicating benignity. C: Suspicious or highly suspicious. Irregular hypoechoic mass with spiculated margins, suspicious or highly suspicious for malignancy, warranting biopsy, demonstrating invasive ductal carcinoma.

terminology and specific descriptors of breast MRI findings, in addition to assigning a final BI-RADS category in the assessment (16). Descriptors of breast MRI findings include focus, mass, and nonmass enhancement (NME). By definition, a focus is less than 5 mm, and any space-occupying lesion 5 mm or larger constitutes a mass. Masses are evaluated based on shape, margin characteristics, internal enhancement, and kinetic analysis. The most characteristic appearance of an invasive breast cancer on MRI is an irregular mass with heterogeneous or rim enhancement, and rapid wash-in and washout kinetics. NME can be focal, linear, segmental, regional, or diffuse. The most characteristic MRI appearance of DCIS is NME in a linear or segmental distribution. **Figure 11.4-3** provides an example of suspicious findings on MRI.

Screening Breast Magnetic Resonance Imaging

Ample data support the higher sensitivity and cancer detection rate of MRI over all other breast screening modalities, including mammography and US, especially in high-risk populations where the sensitivity of mammography is lowest. Kuhl et al in a 5-year surveillance study that included more than 500 women at high risk for breast cancer found that MRI was far more sensitive than either mammography or US (91% vs 33% and 40%) (17). MRI and mammography combined have the highest sensitivity, usually because mammography can detect calcifications in DCIS that MRI does not. In a high-risk population, MRI and mammography combined performed higher than US and mammography combined (92.7% vs 52%) (18). The performance of breast MRI in high-risk women is the same after negative digital mammography or negative DBT, with a cancer detection rate of 11 per 1,000 women screened with MRI after digital mammography and 16 per 1,000 women screened with MRI after DBT (19). Therefore, in high-risk populations, screening with both mammography (digital or DBT) and MRI is recommended.

In 2007, the ACS published guidelines for high-risk screening with MRI based on scientific evidence and expert opinion and is in the process of reviewing the newer literature and updating these

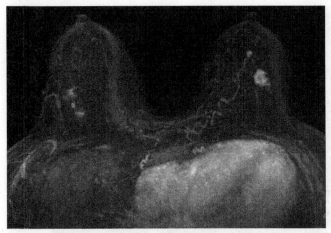

Figure 11.4-3. Suspicious findings on magnetic resonance imaging (MRI). Axial subtracted post–contrast-enhanced maximum intensity projection image from MRI demonstrates clumped nonmass enhancement in the right breast at posterior depth, an irregular mass in the left breast at middle depth, and a unique enhancing focus in the left breast at anterior depth. All three findings were suspicious and biopsied, each demonstrating primary breast malignancy.

guidelines (3,20). Current recommendations for screening breast MRI as an adjunct to mammography include women with certain genetic mutations and syndromes, lifetime risk more than 20% based upon family history, or a history of Hodgkin disease with radiation to the chest under age 30 (**Table 11.4-2**). Because those guidelines were published in 2007, there has been additional evidence that women with a personal history of breast cancer may benefit as much from screening with MRI as much other high-risk groups for whom screening breast MRI is recommended (21-23). For example, Lehman et al found a similar cancer detection rate of 17 to 18 per 1,000 and higher specificity (94% vs 86%) for MRI in women with a personal history of breast cancer compared to women with family history or genetic risk factors. However, other studies have confirmed a higher cancer detection rate of MRI compared to mammography in this population (10.8 vs 8.2 per 1,000) but a lower specificity (61.4% vs 70%) (24). Therefore, although it is promising that MRI can aid in the detection of breast cancer in this subset of women at increased risk, there is no clear consensus on when to use screening MRI in this population. Certain subgroups of these women, such as those diagnosed with breast cancer before 65 and especially before age 50 and those with dense breasts, are most likely to benefit (25).

In an effort to reduce the time and cost of MRI so that it might be more accessible for screening, abbreviated MRI protocols have been developed, which include only the first postcontrast imaging with no kinetic information. In a randomized controlled trial of abbreviated MRI versus DBT in women with dense breasts, abbreviated MRI detected significantly more breast cancers (11.8/1,000 women) compared to DBT (4.8/1,000 women), with a much higher sensitivity (95.7% vs 39.1%) albeit with slightly lower specificity (86.75 vs 97.4%) (26).

TABLE 11.4-2. Criteria for the Use of Annual Screening MRI

Known BRCA mutation
First-degree relative of a known BRCA mutation carrier (but otherwise not tested)
Personal risk of breast cancer exceeds 20% (using risk prediction models)
Prior radiation to the chest before the age of 30
Known familial genetic syndrome with an increased risk of breast cancer (eg, Li-Fraumeni)

MRI, magnetic resonance imaging.

Magnetic Resonance Imaging for the Preoperative Evaluation of Breast Cancer

There are multiple clinical trials demonstrating that in patients with breast cancer, MRI detects additional disease not identified on mammography or US, with additional cancer rate 16% to 20% in the ipsilateral breast and 4.1% to 5.5% in the contralateral breast (27-29). However, the use of MRI in the preoperative setting is not without controversy. Two randomized controlled trials have shown no improvement in reexcision rates with or without preoperative MRI (30,31). A third randomized controlled trial of women less than 56 years showed a significantly reduced rate of reoperation, with no change in the final number of mastectomies (32). In a meta-analysis, preoperative MRI was shown to be associated with a higher ipsilateral and contralateral mastectomy rate (33).

Although the ASBrS recommends not ordering breast MRI routinely in all patients with breast cancer, preoperative breast MRI is used by 41% of breast surgeons in daily practice (34,35). In a survey, breast surgeons responded that they are most likely to select patients with breast cancer for breast MRI if they have the following characteristics (in decreasing likelihood): *BRCA* gene carriers, family or personal history of breast cancer, dense breasts, age less than 40 years, axillary nodal involvement, mammographically occult disease, multifocal or multicentric disease, invasive lobular histology, triple-negative cancer, T2-T3 stages, candidates for mastectomy who request breast conservation, and radiologists discretion (36). There is conflicting evidence about which patients benefit most from breast MRI, and additional trials are underway to address these questions (37).

Breast Magnetic Resonance Imaging: Other Roles

MRI is useful in determining response to neoadjuvant chemotherapy (NACT), with a meta-analysis showing a sensitivity of 84% and a specificity of 83% for quantitative, dynamic contrast-enhanced MRI in comprehensively evaluating response to NACT (38). Recurrence following breast-conservation therapy (BCT) is also better detected and sized more accurately by MRI, and MRI can be useful in postoperative patients in whom conventional imaging is challenging (39-41).

For women presenting with suspicious clinical findings of breast cancer and negative conventional imaging tests, MRI of the breast can add value. This includes women with metastatic axillary LNs but no mammographically detected primary cancer, pathologic unilateral nipple discharge, suspicious palpable mass, or Paget disease in the setting of a negative mammogram and US. Evaluation of mammographic calcifications or other mammographic or sonographic abnormalities is discouraged, and suspicious findings should undergo core biopsy.

EMERGING MODALITIES IN BREAST IMAGING

Other methods of imaging that take advantage of vascular physiologic changes associated with breast cancer have been developed as alternatives to breast MRI for diagnostic evaluation but are not as widely accepted or available. Molecular breast imaging (MBI) is a nuclear medicine technique in which a radioactive tracer, usually Tc-99m sestamibi, is injected intravenously. This technique requires a specialized gamma camera that images the breast over approximately 40 minutes while the patient is seated, gently compressing the breast in positions similar to mammography (42). The sensitivity and specificity are high and comparable to MRI, but as the examination requires radiation exposure to the whole body, it is not indicated for screening even high-risk women (25). Contrast-enhanced mammography (CEM) uses intravenous iodinated contrast injection and combines the anatomic information of mammography with the vascular physiologic information of contrast enhancement. In a meta-analysis and systematic review using a hierarchical summary receiver operating characteristic (HSROC) model, the area under the curve was 0.94, with CEM having a sensitivity of 95% and a specificity of 78% for the detection of breast cancer in dense breasts (43). Therefore, CEM is a promising newer diagnostic technique that can provide the benefits of MRI at lower cost.

REFERENCES

1. Independent UK Panel on Breast Cancer Screening. The benefits and harms of breast cancer screening: an independent review. *Lancet.* 2012;380:1778-1786.

2. Myers ER, Moorman P, Gierisch JM, et al. Benefits and harms of breast cancer screening: a systematic review. *JAMA.* 2015;314(15):1615-1634.

3. Smith RA, Andrews KS, Brooks D, et al. Cancer screening in the United States, 2019: a review of current American Cancer Society guidelines and current issues in cancer screening. *CA Cancer J Clin.* 2019;69(3):184-210.

4. Siu AL, U.S. Preventive Services Task Force. Screening for breast cancer: U.S. preventive services task force recommendation statement. *Ann Intern Med.* 2016;164(4):279-296.

5. American College of Obstetricians and Gynecologists. Breast cancer risk assessment and screening in average-risk women. July 2017. Accessed January 18, 2022. https://www.acog.org/clinical/clinical-guidance/practice-bulletin/articles/2017/07/breast-cancer-risk-assessment-and-screening-in-average-risk-women

6. Expert Panel on Breast Imaging, Mainiero MB, Moy L, et al. ACR appropriateness criteria® breast cancer screening. *J Am Coll Radiol.* 2017;14(11S):S383-S390.

7. Breast Surgeons. The American Society of Breast Surgeons position statement on screening mammography. Accessed January 18, 2022. https://www.breastsurgeons.org/docs/statements/Position-Statement-on-Screening-Mammography.pdf

8. Rafferty EA, Park JM, Philpotts LE, et al. Assessing radiologist performance using combined digital mammography and breast tomosynthesis compared with digital mammography alone: results of a multicenter, multireader trial. *Radiology.* 2013;266(1):104-113.

9. Phi XA, Tagliafico A, Houssami N, Greuter MJW, de Bock GH. Digital breast tomosynthesis for breast cancer screening and diagnosis in women with dense breasts—a systematic review and meta-analysis. *BMC Cancer.* 2018;18(1):380.

10. Zeng B, Yu K, Gao L, Zeng X, Zhou Q. Breast cancer screening using synthesized two-dimensional mammography: a systematic review and meta-analysis. *Breast.* 2021;59:270-278.

11. Richman IB, Hoag JR, Xu X, et al. Adoption of digital breast tomosynthesis in clinical practice. *JAMA Intern Med.* 2019;179(9):1292-1295.

12. D'Orsi CJ. The clinically relevant breast imaging audit. *J Breast Imaging.* 2020;2(1):2-6.

13. D'Orsi CJ, Sickles EA, Mendelson EB, et al. *ACR BI-RADS® Atlas, Breast Imaging Reporting and Data System.* American College of Radiology; 2013.

14. Berg WA, Blume JD, Cormack JB, et al. Combined screening with ultrasound and mammography vs mammography alone in women at elevated risk of breast cancer. *JAMA.* 2008;299(18):2151-2163.

15. American College of Radiology (ACR). ACR Practice parameter for the performance of contrast enhanced magnetic resonance imaging (MRI) of the breast. Accessed January 18, 2022. https://www.acr.org/-/media/ACR/Files/Practice-Parameters/MR-Contrast-Breast.pdf

16. Morris EA, Comstock CE, Lee CH, et al. ACR BI-RADS® magnetic resonance imaging. In: D'Orsi CJ, Sickles EA, Mendelson EB, et al, eds. *ACR BI-RADS®Atlas, Breast Imaging Reporting and Data System.* American College of Radiology; 2013.

17. Kuhl CK, Schrading S, Leutner CC, et al. Mammography, breast ultrasound, and magnetic resonance imaging for surveillance of women at high familial risk for breast cancer. *J Clin Oncol.* 2005;23:8469-8476.

18. Berg WA, Zhang Z, Lehrer D, et al. Detection of breast cancer with addition of annual screening ultrasound or a single screening MRI to mammography in women with elevated breast cancer risk. *JAMA.* 2012;307:1394-1404.

19. Roark AA, Dang PA, Niell BL, Halpern EF, Lehman CD. Performance of screening breast MRI after negative full-field digital mammography versus after negative digital breast tomosynthesis in women at higher than average risk for breast cancer. *AJR Am J Roentgenol.* 2019;212(2):271-279.

20. Saslow D, Boetes C, Burke W, et al. American Cancer Society guidelines for breast screening with MRI as an adjunct to mammography. *CA Cancer J Clin.* 2007;57:75-89.

21. Lehman CD, Lee JM, DeMartini WB, et al. Screening MRI in women with a personal history of breast cancer. *J Natl Cancer Inst.* 2016;108(3):djv349.

22. Brennan S, Liberman L, Dershaw DD, Morris E. Breast MRI screening of women with a personal history of breast cancer. *AJR Am J Roentgenol.* 2010;195(2):510-516.

23. Destounis S, Arieno A, Morgan R. Personal history of premenopausal breast cancer as a risk factor for referral to screening breast MRI. *Acad Radiol.* 2016;23(3):353-357.

24. Wernli KJ, Ichikawa L, Kerlikowske K, et al. Surveillance breast MRI and mammography: comparison in women with a personal history of breast cancer. *Radiology.* 2019;292(2):311-318.

25. Monticciolo DL, Newell MS, Moy L, Niell B, Monsees B, Sickles EA. Breast cancer screening in women at higher-than-average risk: recommendations from the ACR. *J Am Coll Radiol.* 2018;15:408-414.

26. Comstock CE, Gatsonis C, Newstead GM, et al. Comparison of abbreviated breast MRI vs digital breast tomosynthesis for breast cancer detection among women with dense breasts undergoing screening. *JAMA.* 2020;323(8):746-756.

27. Houssami N, Ciatto S, Macaskill P, et al. Accuracy and surgical impact of magnetic resonance imaging in breast cancer staging: systematic review and meta-analysis in detection of multifocal and multicentric cancer. *J Clin Oncol.* 2008;26(19):3248-3258.

28. Brennan ME, Houssami N, Lord S, et al. Magnetic resonance imaging screening of the contralateral breast in women with newly diagnosed breast cancer: systematic review and meta-analysis of incremental cancer detection and impact on surgical management. *J Clin Oncol.* 2009;27(33):5640-5649.

29. Plana MN, Carreira C, Muriel A, et al. Magnetic resonance imaging in the preoperative assessment of patients with primary breast cancer: systematic review of diagnostic accuracy and meta-analysis. *Eur Radiol.* 2012;22(1):26-38.

30. Turnbull L, Brown S, Harvey I, et al. Comparative effectiveness of MRI in breast cancer (COMICE) trial: a randomised controlled trial. *Lancet.* 2010;375:563-571.

31. Peters NH, van Esser S, van den Bosch MA, et al. Preoperative MRI and surgical management in patients with nonpalpable breast cancer: the MONET-randomised controlled trial. *Eur J Cancer.* 2011;47:879-886.

32. Gonzalez V, Sandelin K, Karlsson A, et al. Preoperative MRI of the breast (POMB) influences primary treatment in breast cancer: a prospective, randomized, multicenter study. *World J Surg.* 2014;38(7):1685-1693.

33. Houssami N, Turner RM, Morrow M. Meta-analysis of pre-operative magnetic resonance imaging (MRI) and surgical treatment for breast cancer. *Breast Cancer Res Treat.* 2017;165(2):273-283.

34. Choosing Wisely. Don't routinely order breast MRI in new breast cancer patients. Released June 27, 2016. Accessed January 29, 2022. https://www.choosingwisely.org/clinician-lists/breast-surgeons-mris-in-new-breast-cancer-patients/

35. Parker A, Schroen AT, Brenin DR. MRI utilization in newly diagnosed breast cancer: a survey of practicing surgeons. *Ann Surg Oncol.* 2013;20:2600-2606.

36. Lee J, Tanaka E, Eby PR et al. Preoperative breast MRI: surgeons' patient selection patterns and potential bias in outcomes analyses. *AJR Am J Roentgenol.* 2017;208:923-932.

37. Sardanelli F, Trimboli RM, Houssami N, et al. Solving the preoperative breast MRI conundrum: design and protocol of the MIPA study. *Eur Radiol.* 2020;30(10):5427-5436.

38. Jun W, Cong W, Xianxin X, Daqing J. Meta-analysis of quantitative dynamic contrast-enhanced MRI for the assessment of neoadjuvant chemotherapy in breast cancer. *Am Surg.* 2019;85(6):645-653.

39. Belli P, Costantini M, Romani M, Marano P, Pastore G. Magnetic resonance imaging in breast cancer recurrence. *Breast Cancer Res Treat.* 2002;73:223-235.

40. Walstra CJEF, Schipper RJ, Winter-Warnars GA, et al. Local staging of ipsilateral breast tumor recurrence: mammography, ultrasound, or MRI? *Breast Cancer Res Treat.* 2020;184(2):385-395.

41. Kim MY, Suh YJ, An YY. Imaging surveillance for the detection of ipsilateral local tumor recurrence in patients who underwent oncoplastic breast-conserving surgery with acellular dermal matrix: abbreviated MRI versus conventional mammography and ultrasonography. *World J Surg Oncol.* 2021;19(1):290.

42. Hunt KN. Molecular breast imaging: a scientific review. *J Breast Imaging.* 2021;3(4):416-426.

43. Cozzi A, Magni V, Zanardo M, Schiaffino S, Sardanelli F. Contrast-enhanced mammography: a systematic review and meta-analysis of diagnostic performance. *Radiology.* 2022;302(3):568-581. doi:10.1148/radiol.21142

CHAPTER **11.5**

Breast Pathology

Yihong Wang and Evgeny Yakirevich

BENIGN EPITHELIAL CHANGES

A normal breast is composed of ducts, lobules, and stroma (**Figure 11.5-1**). The TDLUs are the basic functional units of the breast that are microscopically composed of two cell layers: an inner luminal cell layer with secretory function and outer myoepithelial layer providing support and contractile function (**Figure 11.5-2**).

The breast ducts and lobules can show a wide range of benign alterations, including *fibrocystic changes, usual ductal hyperplasia* (UDH), *radial scar, complex sclerosing lesion,* and *atypical hyperplasia. Fibrocystic changes* encompass a group of nonproliferative benign lesions that are not associated with an increased risk of breast cancer. Clinically, patients with *fibrocystic changes* may present with "lumpy-bumpy" breasts on palpation and dense breasts with cysts on imaging. Microscopically, fibrocystic changes show benign histology, including cysts, apocrine metaplasia, fibrosis, and adenosis (**Figure 11.5-3**). Cysts frequently rupture, releasing secretory material into the adjacent stroma. The resulting chronic inflammation and fibrosis can contribute to palpable nodularity of the breast.

Proliferative changes without atypia include *UDH, sclerosing adenosis, radial scar, radial/complex sclerosing lesion,* and *papilloma* and are often coexist. They are associated with a slight increase in the risk of subsequent development of breast cancer (1-3). *UDH* is an architecturally, cytologically, and molecularly heterogeneous proliferation of benign epithelial cells with haphazard orientation and irregular luminal spaces (**Figure 11.5-4**).

Sclerosing adenosis, radial scar, and *radial/complex sclerosing lesion* show distortion of normal breast architecture by fibrous or fibroelastotic connective tissue. This irregular gland pattern may mimic an invasive carcinoma on imaging (**Figures 11.5-5 and 11.5-6**). These benign proliferations maintain a normal myoepithelial cell layer, highlighted by immunohistochemical (IHC) stains.

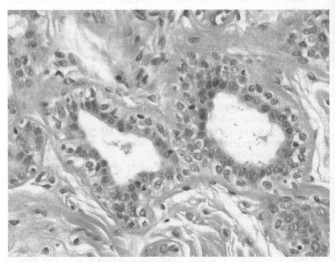

Figure 11.5-2. Normal breast ducts and lobules are composed of two cell layers. The inner luminal layer is surrounded by the outer myoepithelial cell layer.

An *intraductal papilloma* comprises arborizing fronds with well-developed fibrovascular cores lined by myoepithelial cells and covered with one or more layers of epithelial cells (**Figure 11.5-7**). *Papillomas* involving large ducts may cause bloody nipple discharge. Benign epithelial lesions usually do not cause symptoms but can present as calcifications or densities on imaging or incidental findings on surgical excision. Proliferative changes without atypia carry a 1.5- to 2-fold increased risk of developing breast cancer (1-3).

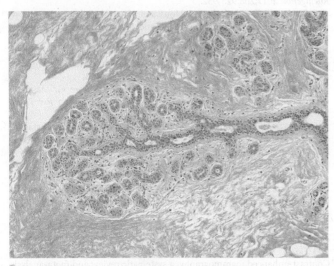

Figure 11.5-1. Normal breast terminal duct lobular unit.

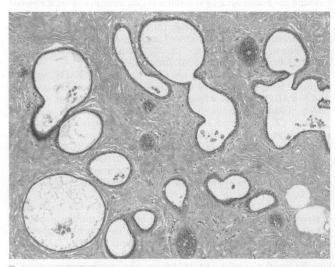

Figure 11.5-3. Fibrocystic changes. Variable-sized cysts are lined by cuboidal to columnar epithelium in a fibrous stroma. The cysts may contain secretory debris and calcifications.

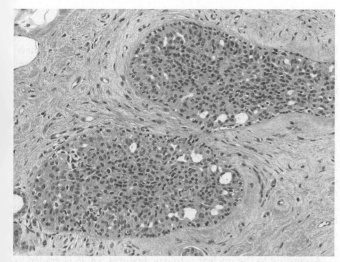

Figure 11.5-4. Usual ductal hyperplasia. Expanded ducts are filled with cytologically benign heterogeneous epithelial cells varying in size, shape, and orientation. Irregular fenestrations are prominent at the periphery.

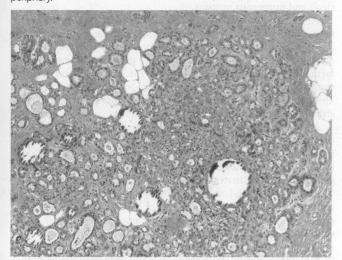

Figure 11.5-5. Sclerosing adenosis. Enlarged lobular unit with increased irregular compressed glands in fibrous stroma may be mistaken as malignancy in core needle biopsy. Several calcifications are present.

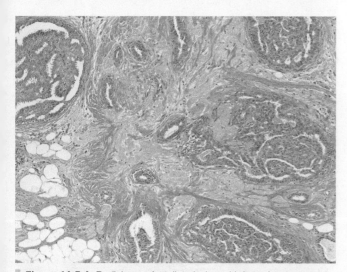

Figure 11.5-6. Radial scar. A stellate lesion with irregular ducts and lobules radiating from the fibroelastotic center. At periphery, epithelium shows usual ductal hyperplasia. The entrapped glands in the center may mimic an invasive ductal carcinoma.

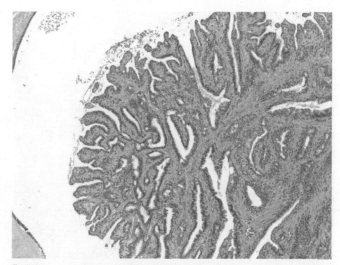

Figure 11.5-7. Intraductal papilloma. A well-circumscribed papillary proliferation fills a dilated duct. The fibrovascular cores are covered by an inner myoepithelial cell layer and an outer epithelial cell layer.

Atypical hyperplasia is a clonal proliferation having some, but not all, of the histologic features of carcinoma in situ. It is associated with a 4- to 5-fold increased risk of developing breast cancer. *Atypical hyperplasia* is divided into *atypical ductal hyperplasia* (ADH) and *atypical lobular hyperplasia* (ALH). *ADH* is recognized by its cytologic and architectural features similar to low-grade *DCIS*. It consists of a relatively monomorphic proliferation of regularly spaced cells, sometimes forming arches, rigid bridges, bulbous micropapillae, or cribriform polarized spaces (**Figure 11.5-8**) (4). *ADH* is distinguished from *DCIS* in that it only partially fills involved ducts. *ALH* consists of cells identical to LCIS (described later), but the cells do not fill or distend more than 50% of the acini within a lobule. *ADH* and *ALH* express high ER levels, have a low rate of proliferation, and may have acquired chromosomal aberrations, such as losses of 16q and 17p or gains of 1q, which are features also found in low-grade *DCIS* and ER-positive invasive breast cancer. Reproducibility of *ADH* diagnosis is still problematic, but more uniform criteria are now used by most pathologists (4). There is still controversy about whether size criteria should be used to separate *ADH* from low-grade *DCIS* (two completely involved ducts or 2 mm in contiguous extent). *ADH* can also involve radial scar, intraductal papilloma, or fibroadenoma (FA).

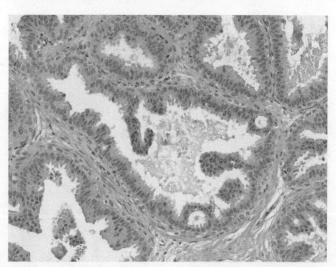

Figure 11.5-8. Atypical ductal hyperplasia (ADH). An intraductal epithelial proliferation of monotonous low-grade neoplastic cells. ADH exhibits architectural atypia in the form of "roman arches" and "club-shaped" micropapillae.

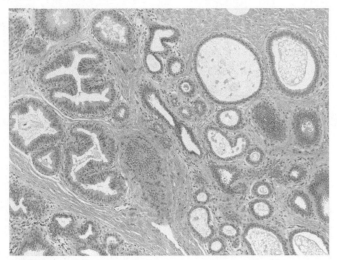

Figure 11.5-9. Columnar cell lesion (CCL). On the right, columnar cell change reveals a transformation of the terminal duct lobular unit from a cuboidal to the columnar epithelium lining cystically dilated acini. On the left, columnar cell hyperplasia demonstrates variably dilated acini with irregular contours and an epithelial thickening or "piling up." CCLs are frequently associated with luminal secretions and calcifications.

Columnar cell lesions (CCLs) encompass a spectrum of benign to atypical entities, including *columnar cell change* (CCC), *columnar cell hyperplasia* (CCH), and *flat epithelial atypia* (FEA). *CCLs* are clonal alterations of TDLUs characterized by enlarged variably dilated acini lined by columnar epithelial cells; some may have apical snouts (5). *CCLs* with epithelial cell lining of one to two cells thick are referred to as *CCC*; those with epithelial thickening greater than two cell layers are recognized as *CCH* (**Figure 11.5-9**). They commonly contain luminal secretions or calcifications, which are detected on mammography. *FEA* is characterized by dilated acini with round contours and is lined by one to several layers of low-grade monomorphic cuboidal to columnar cells (**Figure 11.5-10**). Molecular studies indicate a logical continuum from *CCLs/FEA* to *ADH* and low-grade *DCIS* (6). Limited data from epidemiologic studies suggest that *CCLs* are associated with a very low risk of breast cancer progression (RR ~1.5-fold) (7).

Carcinoma in Situ

Carcinoma in situ is the earliest form of breast cancer. The neoplastic cells grow within the ducts and lobules with intact basement membrane and myoepithelial cell layer without invasion into the surrounding tissue. Carcinoma in situ may involve the ductal-lobular system or extend into sclerosing (sclerosing adenosis), papillary, or fibroepithelial lesions.

Ductal Carcinoma in Situ

DCIS is a noninvasive proliferation of cohesive neoplastic cells confined within the ductal system, but it can extend to the lobules (lobular involvement or lobular cancerization). *DCIS* encompasses a heterogeneous group of nonobligate precursor lesions to invasive breast carcinoma. The current classification system is based on nuclear grade (stronger predictor of outcome), architectural pattern, and the presence or absence of necrosis (8).

According to the nuclear cytologic features, *DCIS* is graded as low, intermediate, and high nuclear grade (9,10). Low-grade *DCIS* is characterized by small monomorphic nuclei, whereas high-grade DCIS is composed of large pleomorphic nuclei with prominent nucleoli and numerous mitoses.

Architectural patterns of *DCIS* include *solid, cribriform, papillary,* and *micropapillary*. Combinations of these patterns are not uncommon in a biopsy. The *cribriform, papillary, micropapillary,* or, less often, *solid* patterns of *DCIS* are usually composed of uniform low-grade or intermediate-grade nuclei. *Cribriform* patterns show smooth, rounded, "punched-out" spaces (**Figure 11.5-11**). The *papillary DCIS* contains fibrovascular cores, whereas the *micropapillary* pattern lacks fibrovascular cores.

Necrosis in association with *DCIS* may be punctate or comedo. On gross examination, lactiferous ducts with comedo necrosis are filled with a yellow paste–like material, resembling small skin plugs (comedones). Histologically, the ducts contain central eosinophilic granular necrotic material with nuclear debris (**Figure 11.5-12**). The necrotic material often becomes calcified. These coarse calcifications have a distinctive linear and/or branching mammographic appearance. Usually, comedo necrosis is associated with high-grade solid *DCIS*, and some systems categorize such cases as *comedo-type DCIS*. However, comedo necrosis can be seen in low-grade lesions in rare cases. Periductal fibrosis and inflammation are common in *comedo-type DCIS*. They can be a diagnostic problem, as they

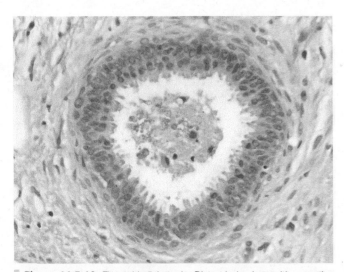

Figure 11.5-10. Flat epithelial atypia. Distended acinus with smooth contour lined by several layers of mildly atypical cells with apical snouts and contains luminal secretions and calcifications. The nuclei of the neoplastic cells are round and uniform and have inconspicuous nucleoli.

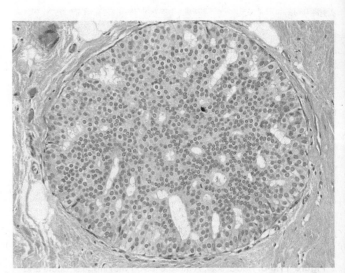

Figure 11.5-11. Low-grade ductal carcinoma in situ. The expanded duct is filled with low-grade neoplastic cells forming rigid cribriform microlumens, resembling "punched-out" spaces.

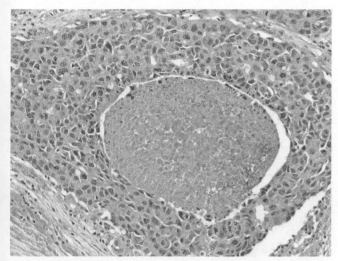

Figure 11.5-12. High-grade ductal carcinoma in situ (DCIS). DCIS shows a solid architectural pattern with associated calcification and comedo-type necrosis.

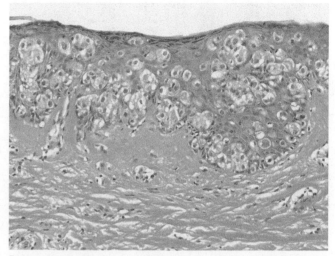

Figure 11.5-13. Paget disease. Nipple section with intraepidermal large round cells with abundant pale cytoplasm and large nuclei with prominent nucleoli. Paget cells are seen singly and in clusters and replace the keratinocytes.

might obscure microinvasion (defined as invasive carcinoma <1 mm), which is more frequently associated with *comedo-type DCIS* than other patterns (11). In some cases, high-grade *DCIS* grows in one layer of atypical cells called clinging *DCIS*.

Lesion size is often problematic by pathologic evaluation, as most *DCIS* are not mass-forming lesions. When feasible, all tissue from an excisional specimen should be submitted sequentially for histologic evaluation. If this is not possible, at least the entire area of the targeted lesion should be examined microscopically. Margin width is most easily measured microscopically in perpendicular sections, which requires the presence of colored inks for the unique identification of each margin.

The American Society of Clinical Oncology (ASCO)/College of American Pathologists (CAP) recommends testing of *DCIS* for ER to determine the potential benefit of endocrine therapies (ETs) to reduce the risk of future breast cancer (12).

Paget Disease of the Nipple

Paget disease of the nipple reflects the direct extension of high-grade *DCIS* into the lactiferous ducts and adjacent skin. Clinically, the nipple appears excoriated. The *DCIS* may or may not be accompanied by invasive carcinoma. The Paget cells are large round cells with prominent nucleoli and pale cytoplasm. They occur singly within the epidermis or form groups at the dermal-epidermal junction, mimicking malignant melanoma (**Figure 11.5-13**). Lesional cells of Paget disease are often positive by IHC for cytokeratin 7 (CK7), HER2, and GATA3.

Lobular Carcinoma In Situ

Lobular carcinoma in situ (LCIS) is defined as a noninvasive neoplastic proliferation of dyscohesive cells originating in the TDLUs. The cells may extend into the adjacent duct, growing beneath the normal ductal epithelium, a pattern known as "pagetoid spread." Loss of E-cadherin and cytoplasmic expression of p120 catenin by IHC can help diagnose *LCIS*. Currently, *LCIS* is considered both a risk factor for and a nonobligate precursor of invasive breast carcinoma. Three clinically relevant histologic subtypes of *LCIS* include *classic*, *florid*, and *pleomorphic* (13).

Classic LCIS is a multicentric and often bilateral lesion, with no identifying features on gross or radiographic evaluation, and is often found as an incidental finding in biopsies performed for another reason. In *classic LCIS*, more than 50% of the lobule is distended by a monomorphic population of small uniform cells with round nuclei and scant cytoplasm (**Figure 11.5-14**). The term

"lobular neoplasia" is often used to encompass both *LCIS* and *ALH*, which have identical cytologic features but minor architectural differences. *Classic LCIS* is typically ER and PR positive and HER2 negative. Positive margins in *classic LCIS* are not clinically relevant and are not recorded.

Pleomorphic LCIS and *florid LCIS* are unifocal and continuous in distribution. *Pleomorphic LCIS* is composed of large dyscohesive cells with marked nuclear pleomorphism, equivalent to high-grade nuclei of *DCIS* (**Figure 11.5-15**). *Florid LCIS* is defined as confluent mass-like classic LCIS with minimal intervening stroma (**Figure 11.5-16**). Both *pleomorphic LCIS* and *florid LCIS* are more frequently associated with comedo-type necrosis and microcalcifications and detected on screening mammography. The *florid LCIS* is typically ER positive, whereas *pleomorphic LCIS* may be ER negative and HER2 overexpressed. These morphologic subtypes are often associated with invasive carcinoma, and therefore, excision is recommended when these lesions are diagnosed on core needle biopsy (CNB). The relevance of margin status in *pleomorphic* and *florid LCIS* is not well established (13).

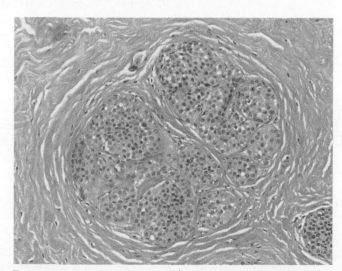

Figure 11.5-14. Classic lobular carcinoma in situ. Expanded acini are markedly distended by a monomorphic population of small uniform dyscohesive cells. The underlying lobular architecture is still recognizable.

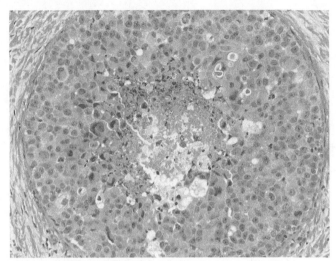

Figure 11.5-15. Pleomorphic lobular carcinoma in situ. The solid proliferation of large dyscohesive cells with marked nuclear pleomorphism, prominent nucleoli, and increased mitotic activity is similar to high-grade ductal carcinoma in situ. Comedo necrosis is seen in the center.

INVASIVE BREAST CARCINOMA

Invasive carcinoma of the breast is defined by the presence of stromal invasion, usually manifested by a fibrotic, desmoplastic stromal reaction around the invading tumor cells. Breast carcinoma has a wide variety of morphologic appearances. The majority of invasive carcinomas (75%) have no specific histologic features and are designated as *invasive breast carcinoma of no special type* (IBC-NST) or traditionally as *invasive ductal carcinoma* (IDC).

Invasive carcinoma is graded according to the Nottingham Histologic Score, reflecting the tumor aggressiveness. Tumors are scored for tubule formation, nuclear pleomorphism, and mitotic rate. Grade 1 carcinomas grow in a tubular or cribriform pattern and have small uniform nuclei and a low mitotic activity (**Figure 11.5-17**). Grade 2 carcinomas have solid clusters or single infiltrating cells and show greater nuclear pleomorphism and higher proliferation. Grade 3 carcinomas grow in nests or solid sheets with tumor necrosis, marked nuclear hyperchromasia and pleomorphism, and a high mitotic activity (**Figure 11.5-18**) (**Table 11.5-1**) (14,15).

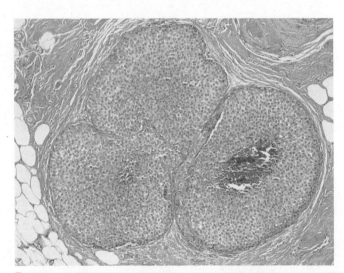

Figure 11.5-16. Florid lobular carcinoma in situ (LCIS). Acini are markedly expanded (>40-50 cells in diameter) with minimal intervening stroma, calcifications, and necrosis. Cytologic features are similar to classic LCIS.

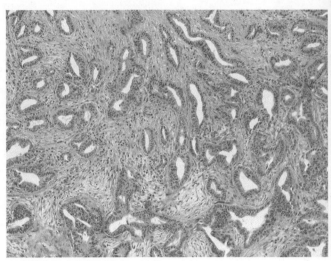

Figure 11.5-17. Invasive ductal carcinoma, grade 1. This invasive tumor shows tubule and gland formation in >75% of the tumor, has small uniform nuclei, and low mitotic activity.

The immune infiltrate associated with the tumors is referred to as tumor-infiltrating lymphocytes (TILs). TILs are mononuclear lymphocytes associated with tumor cells and the surrounding stroma. They reflect the host immune response against the tumor. TILs are gaining importance as a prognostic marker, as dense TILs have been shown to be associated with a better outcome and better response to neoadjuvant treatment (16,17).

Special Types

About 25% of the invasive breast carcinomas have varying morphologic patterns, which lead to several subclassifications. Special histologic types of breast cancer often harbor unique genetic aberrations, sometimes have distinct gene signatures, and frequently show associations with specific morphologic features, clinical behavior, and prognosis.

Invasive Lobular Carcinoma

The most common breast cancer of a specific type is *invasive lobular carcinoma* (ILC). It comprises approximately 10% of all breast

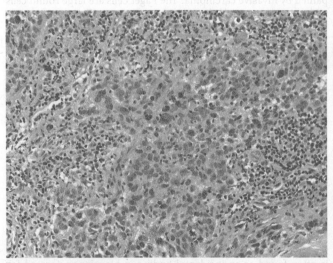

Figure 11.5-18. Invasive ductal carcinoma, grade 3. The tumor shows little to no tubule or gland formation, marked nuclear pleomorphism, and high mitotic activity. This high-grade tumor is associated with dense tumor-infiltrative lymphocytes.

Score	Feature		
	Tubule/Gland formation		
1	>75% of the tumor		
2	10%-75% of tumor		
3	<10% of tumor		
	Nuclear pleomorphism		
1	Small, regular, uniform cells		
2	Moderately increased in size and variability		
3	Marked variation		
	Mitotic count per 10 high-power fields, depend on microscope field diameter (mm)/ field area (mm²)		
1	≤8 (0.55 mm/0.237 mm²)		
2	9-17 (0.55 mm/0.237 mm²)		
3	≥18 (0.55 mm/0.237 mm²)		
Total Score	**Final Grading (add the scores for gland formation, nuclear pleomorphism, and mitotic count)**		
3-5	Grade 1		
6 or 7	Grade 2		
8 or 9	Grade 3		

■ TABLE 11.5-1. Semiqualitative Method for Assessing Histologic Grade for Invasive Breast Tumors

cancers. Like *LCIS*, most cases show biallelic loss of expression of *CDH1*, the gene that encodes E-cadherin (18). The *classic* form of *ILC* is composed of small monotonous tumor cells growing as single cells or in linear columns, often in concentric (targetoid) patterns around normal ducts (**Figure 11.5-19**). *ILC* often does not form a discrete tumor mass. It is diffusely infiltrative without eliciting a stromal desmoplastic response. The tumors are frequently upstaged after surgery (19).

Other clinically relevant patterns of *ILC* composed of the same monomorphic small cells include *solid* with sheets of tumor cells, *alveolar* with tumor cells arranged in globular aggregates, and *tubulolobular* with an admixture of invasive lobular and tubular carcinoma growth patterns with low-grade nuclei. The mixed architectural pattern of *tubulolobular* carcinoma parallels the expression of markers of ductal and lobular differentiation, and these tumors appear to have a good prognosis.

Another variant is *pleomorphic lobular carcinoma* (PLC), in which large neoplastic cells show marked nuclear atypia and pleomorphism, similar to *pleomorphic LCIS*. PLC can show *apocrine*, *histiocytoid*, or *signet-ring cell* differentiation. Classic *ILC* is almost always ER positive and HER2 negative, whereas *PLC* can be HER2 amplified.

The prognosis of patients with *ILC* is associated with histologic patterns. The outcomes are controversial; however, the long-term survival appears to be worse compared with *IDC* (20). The patterns of metastatic disease are different, with *ILC* having a propensity to metastasize to peritoneal and pleural surfaces, meninges, bones, skin, gastrointestinal (GI) tract, uterus, and ovaries, while relatively sparing regional LNs and lungs (21,22).

Tubular Carcinoma

Tubular carcinoma is a low-grade invasive carcinoma with more than 90% of the tumor composed of small glands or tubules that can be difficult to distinguish from benign lesions, especially radial scars. Tubular carcinomas are small, usually less than 1 cm, and are frequently detected by screening mammography. The tubules are arranged haphazardly, often within a fibrous stroma. They are round to ovoid or angular with open lumens and are lined by a single layer of monomorphic epithelial cells (**Figure 11.5-20**). Myoepithelial cells are absent. IHC for myoepithelial markers (smooth muscle myosin heavy chain, p63, and calponin) helps confirm the diagnosis on needle biopsy. *Tubular carcinoma* is often associated with CCLs, mainly FEA, ADH/DCIS, and lobular neoplasia (23). Tubular carcinoma is almost always ER positive and HER2 negative.

Cribriform Carcinoma

Invasive cribriform carcinoma is a low-grade carcinoma with more than 90% of the tumor composed of epithelial nests with cribriform (sieve-like) spaces similar to cribriform DCIS (**Figure 11.4-21**). In contrast to DCIS, tumor islands lack a myoepithelial cell layer. Invasive cribriform carcinomas are typically ER/PR positive HER2 negative. The prognosis of patients with this subtype is excellent, similar to invasive tubular carcinoma (24).

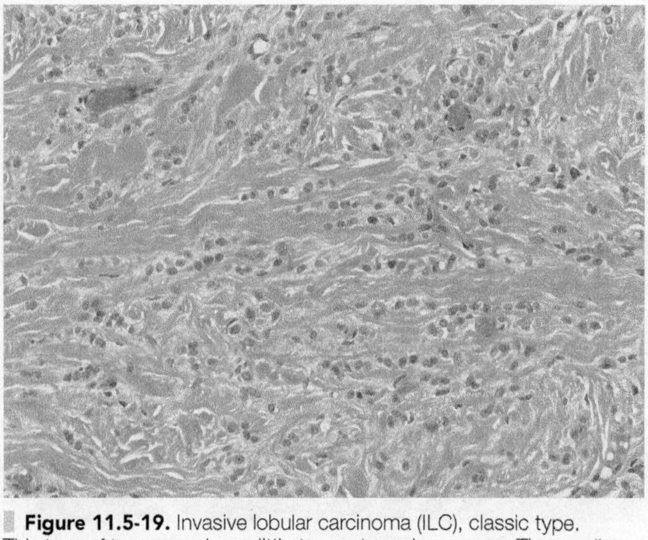

■ Figure 11.5-19. Invasive lobular carcinoma (ILC), classic type. This type of tumor produces little to no stromal response. The small uniform tumor cells of this classic ILC are found scattered or arranged in single-file linear cords.

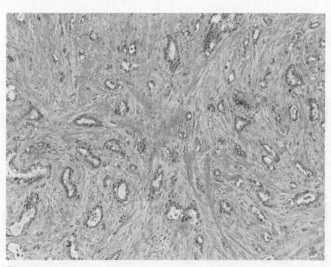

■ Figure 11.5-20. Tubular carcinoma. The haphazard proliferation of angulated glands composed of a single layer of monomorphic tumor cells in a fibrous stroma with desmoplasia.

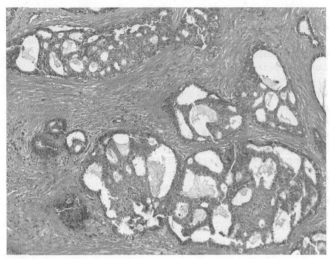

Figure 11.5-21. Cribriform carcinoma. The tumor is composed of infiltrative nests with cribriform architecture that is similar to cribriform ductal carcinoma in situ; however, the myoepithelial cell layer is absent.

Mucinous Carcinoma

Mucinous (or colloid) carcinoma usually occurs in postmenopausal women. The tumor is well circumscribed and may have a gelatinous gross appearance. Microscopically, more than 90% of the tumor is composed of nests of uniform small cells surrounded by pools of mucin (**Figure 11.4-22**). The in situ component is minimal but may also show intraductal mucin production. Pure mucinous tumors are low grade and have an excellent prognosis, with a low risk of LN metastasis (25). In some cases, *mucinous carcinoma* may have *micropapillary* features referred to as *mucinous micropapillary carcinoma*. This pattern is associated with lymphovascular invasion and LN metastases (26).

In rare cases of *mucinous cystadenocarcinoma*, mucin accumulates in cystic spaces; and the lining cells contain abundant intracytoplasmic mucin. In contrast to mucinous carcinoma, these tumors are ER negative, PR negative, and HER2 negative, although most reported cases had a relatively good prognosis.

Papillary Carcinoma

Papillary carcinoma is characterized by fibrovascular stalks covered by neoplastic epithelium. Several different entities are

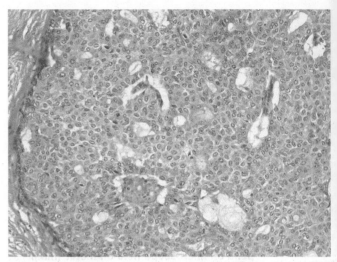

Figure 11.5-23. Papillary carcinoma. This solid papillary carcinoma is composed of uniform population of round to spindled neoplastic cells growing in a solid pattern with fibrovascular stalks. Papillary carcinomas lack the myoepithelial cell layer.

encompassed within this terminology. *Solid papillary carcinoma* and *encapsulated papillary carcinoma* have indolent behavior like a *DCIS*, although they lack surrounding myoepithelial cells (**Figure 11.5-23**) (27). Encapsulated papillary carcinoma forms a well-circumscribed mass surrounded by a fibrous capsule. *Frank invasion* is defined as the spread of irregular infiltrative glands beyond the capsule, usually in the form of *IDC*. *Invasive papillary carcinomas* have frankly invasive growth patterns with destructive stromal invasion.

Invasive Micropapillary Carcinoma

Invasive micropapillary carcinoma is characterized by reversely polarized (inside-out) growth of tumor clusters with no fibrovascular cores and surrounded by clear spaces in more than 90% of the tumor (**Figure 11.5-24**). Despite small tumor size, most tumors have intermediate to high nuclear grade, lymphatic space invasion, and positive axillary LNs at presentation (28). Therefore, this type is associated with a worse prognosis than IDC. Most tumors are ER positive and PR positive. HER2 can display a unique basolateral staining pattern in positive cases (29).

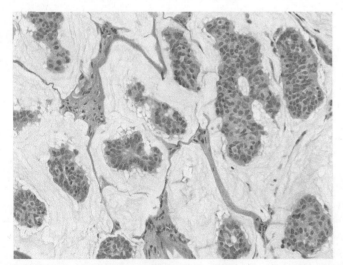

Figure 11.5-22. Mucinous carcinoma. The tumor is composed of nests of uniform cells with low- to intermediate-grade nuclei surrounded by mucin pools, rendering a gross gelatinous appearance.

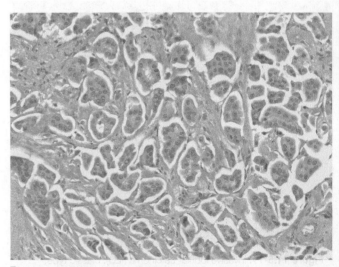

Figure 11.5-24. Invasive micropapillary carcinoma. Small clusters of intermediate-grade neoplastic cells with no fibrovascular cores lie within clear spaces that mimic tumor cells in angiolymphatic spaces.

Carcinoma With Apocrine Differentiation

Carcinoma with apocrine differentiation (or *apocrine carcinoma*) is characterized by large tumor cells with abundant eosinophilic granular cytoplasm, distinct cell borders, and prominent nucleoli (**Figure 11.5-25**). These features are present in more than 90% of the tumor. The majority of apocrine carcinomas are positive for androgen receptor (AR) and GCDFP-15, although AR testing is not performed routinely. Apocrine carcinomas are ER negative, PR negative, and HER2 positive in about 50% of cases. Triple-negative apocrine carcinomas have a more favorable prognosis than other TNBCs.

Secretory Carcinoma

Rare histologic types of TNBC have a favorable prognosis compared to other tumors in this molecular group and include *adenoid cystic carcinoma* and *secretory carcinoma*. *Secretory carcinoma* is composed of epithelial cells with intracytoplasmic and extracellular secretions and is associated with *ETV6-NTRK3* gene fusions (**Figure 11.5-26**). These tumors have an indolent clinical course and rarely metastasize.

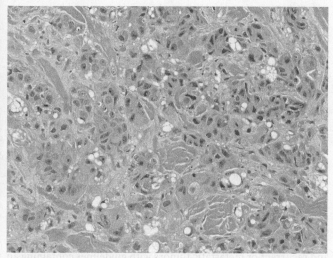

Figure 11.5-25. Carcinoma with apocrine differentiation. The pleomorphic tumor cells have abundant granular eosinophilic cytoplasm and prominent nucleoli.

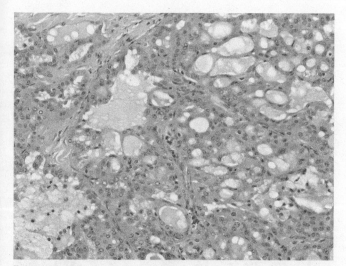

Figure 11.5-26. Secretory carcinoma. The tumor is composed of acini and microcysts filled with eosinophilic secretions. Secretory carcinomas harbor characteristic *ETV6-NTRK3* gene fusions.

OTHER TUMORS

Fibroepithelial Lesions

Fibroepithelial lesions are biphasic neoplasms composed of stromal (mesenchymal) and epithelial components. This group includes FAs and *phyllodes tumors* (PTs). FAs are the most common benign breast tumors. They are usually less than 3 cm in size and most common in young women, especially under 30 years. *FAs* may grow in a pericanalicular pattern with stromal cells growing around open ducts and/or intracanalicular with stromal compression of ducts into clefts (**Figure 11.5-27**). *Cellular FAs* and *juvenile FAs* exhibit a mild-to-moderate increase in stromal cellularity; however, they lack other features of *PT*. *Complex FAs* are defined by the presence of cysts greater than 3 mm, sclerosing adenosis, epithelial calcifications, and papillary apocrine metaplasia. *Complex FAs* do not confer increased breast cancer risk if adjustments are made for other categories of benign breast disease and lobular involution (30).

PTs are biphasic tumors similar to FAs with a spectrum of morphology and biologic behavior. The median age at diagnosis is 45, which is several decades later than *FA*. These tumors are grossly well circumscribed but are infiltrative on microscopic examination. *PTs* are distinguished from *FAs* based on higher stromal cellularity, leaf-like architecture, higher mitotic rate, nuclear pleomorphism, stromal overgrowth, and infiltrative border (**Figure 11.5-28**). The spectrum of *PTs* includes a *benign PT* that resembles *FA* but is more cellular and mitotically active, *borderline PT*, and *malignant PT* that may be difficult to distinguish from sarcoma. Local recurrence may be seen with all types of *PTs*; therefore, complete excision of the lesion is the primary goal. Both *FA* and *PT* are driven by somatic mutations in *MED12*, a component of a complex protein called mediator complex subunit 12 that links RNA polymerase II to specific DNA-binding transcription factors. Malignant *FTs* harbor mutations in additional genes, such as *TERT*.

Metaplastic Carcinoma

The term *metaplastic carcinoma* describes tumors with distinct morphologic patterns different from invasive ductal and lobular carcinoma and different outcomes. This group encompasses epithelial tumors (carcinomas) showing squamous, spindle cell, and/or mesenchymal/matrix producing differentiation. *Metaplastic squamous cell carcinomas* are usually cystic and should be distinguished from primary cutaneous or metastatic squamous cell carcinomas. *Spindle cell carcinomas* express at least focally

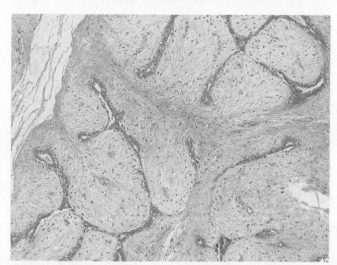

Figure 11.5-27. Fibroadenoma. The lesion is composed of both stromal and epithelial components. The border is well circumscribed. The intracanalicular growth pattern shows stromal compression of ducts, forming slit-like spaces.

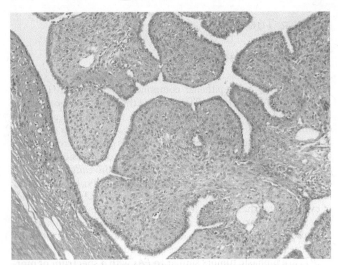

Figure 11.5-28. Phyllodes tumor (PT). PT has a leaf-like growth pattern and increased stromal cellularity. The stromal cells exhibit nuclear pleomorphism, higher mitotic rate, and infiltrative border.

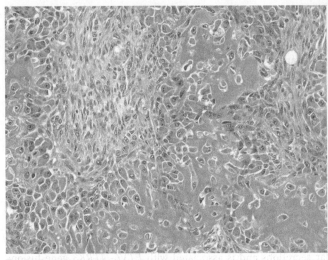

Figure 11.5-30. Metaplastic carcinoma. An example of metaplastic carcinoma with osseous heterologous mesenchymal differentiation.

epithelial markers (cytokeratins) and p63 despite their spindle cell morphology and are aggressive tumors with a high rate of extranodal metastases (**Figure 11.5-29**) (31). *Metaplastic carcinoma with heterologous mesenchymal differentiation* may contain cartilage or bone (**Figure 11.5-30**). The majority of *metaplastic carcinomas* are triple negative. Two histologic patterns with more favorable prognosis are important to recognize, such as *low-grade adenosquamous carcinoma* and *fibromatosis-like metaplastic carcinoma*.

Inflammatory Carcinoma

Inflammatory carcinoma is a clinical term for LABC characterized by erythema, edema, warmth, and tenderness of the mammary skin, resulting in a "peau d'orange" skin. Biopsies of the skin from such patients often show tumor thrombi in dermal lymphatic channels (**Figure 11.5-31**), but this is not true in every case.

Angiosarcoma

Angiosarcoma is the most common primary sarcoma of the breast that may be spontaneous or associated with previous radiation therapy (RT) for breast cancer. The tumors are composed of

anastomosing vascular channels lined by endothelial cells, which range from mildly atypical to frankly malignant (**Figure 11.5-32**). The distinction between a benign *hemangioma* and a low-grade *angiosarcoma* can be difficult on a small biopsy. High-level *MYC* amplification is a genomic hallmark of radiation-induced sarcoma.

BREAST CANCER BIOMARKERS

Several approaches have been used to subclassify breast cancer into clinically meaningful subtypes. Based on gene expression profiling, breast cancers cluster into three main groups: "luminal" (predominantly ER positive/HER2 negative), "HER2 enriched" (HER2 positive), and "basal like" (ER negative/HER2 negative). These molecular subtypes correlate reasonably well with ER, PR, and HER2 protein expression, which is easily assessed by standard clinical assays. The ASCO and CAP recommend that ER, PR, and HER2 testing be done on all primary invasive breast carcinomas and recurrent or metastatic tumors with guidelines containing an algorithm for testing, interpretation, reporting, and requirements for standardization and validation of testing techniques (12,31).

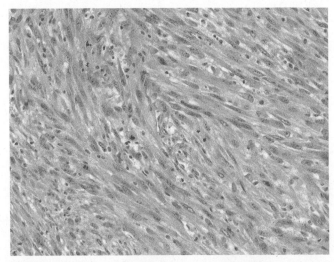

Figure 11.5-29. Metaplastic carcinoma. This metaplastic carcinoma is composed of spindle cells with pleomorphic nuclei and increased mitoses. These tumors express at least focally epithelial markers (keratins) and p63.

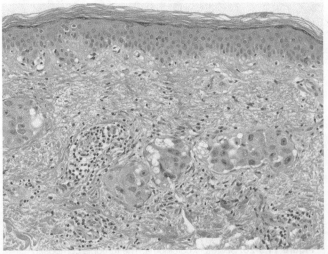

Figure 11.5-31. Inflammatory carcinoma. A punch biopsy of the breast skin shows tumor emboli in dilated dermal lymphatics.

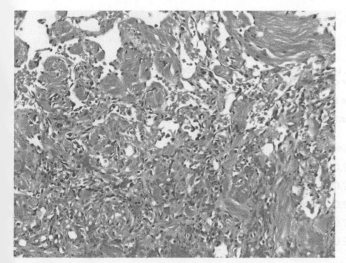

Figure 11.5-32. Angiosarcoma. The tumor consists of anastomosing vascular spaces lined by atypical endothelial cells.

HORMONAL RECEPTORS

About 75% to 80% of invasive breast cancers are HR positive, and studies have shown a substantial survival benefit from ET among patients with ER-positive tumors (12). Measurement of ER and PR in breast cancers is performed to predict clinical benefits from ET. PR expression tends to vary more than ER expression, which helps account for PR's effectiveness in stratifying ER-positive cases into prognostic categories. ER, and PR status is determined in formalin-fixed, paraffin-embedded tissue sections by IHC. A *positive result* is equal to or greater than 1% of cell nuclei staining positive (**Figure 11.5-33**). The percentage of cells with nuclear positivity for ER and PR may be reported as a specific number or a range. Invasive carcinomas with 1% to 10% of cells staining for ER (not PR) are reported as "low positive" according to the 2020 update (12). There are limited data on the overall benefit of ETs for patients with low-level (1%-10%) ER expression, but it is still recommended for these patients.

HER2

HER2, or ERBB2, is a membrane receptor tyrosine kinase that promotes cell proliferation, development, and survival. Cancers with HER2 protein overexpression are usually due to gene amplification. HER2-positive tumors constitute approximately 20% of all breast cancers and may be ER positive or ER negative. Clinically, HER2 amplification is detected by IHC for protein overexpression (**Figure 11.5-34**) or in situ hybridization (ISH) for gene amplification, such as fluorescence in situ hybridization (FISH) or chromogenic in situ hybridization (CISH) (**Figure 11.5-35**). The ASCO and CAP have issued recommendations for reporting the results of HER2 testing by IHC with updated revision in 2018 (32) (**Table 11.5-2**).

HER2 testing by FISH or CISH determines the presence or absence of gene amplification. Most assays include a chromosome enumeration probe (CEP17) to determine the ratio of HER2 signals to copies of chromosome 17. Either the number of HER2 signals or the ratio of HER2 to CEP17 can be used to determine the presence of

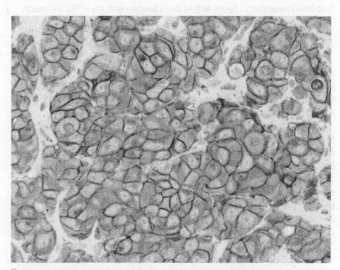

Figure 11.5-34. HER2-positive breast cancer detected by immunohistochemistry (IHC). HER2 protein overexpression in tumor cells is detected by IHC with antibodies specific for HER2. Positive HER2 (3+) shows strong membrane immunoreactivity.

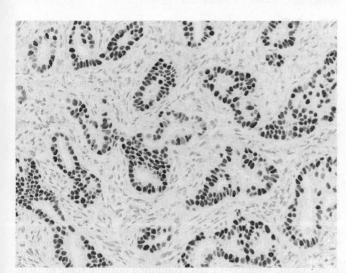

Figure 11.5-33. Estrogen receptor (ER) expression in invasive ductal carcinoma detected by immunohistochemistry with antibodies specific for ER. This ER-positive tumor shows strong nuclear immunoreactivity in 90% of the tumor cells.

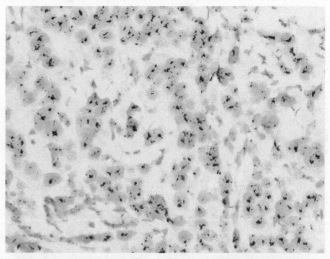

Figure 11.5-35. HER2-positive breast cancer identified by HER2 chromogenic in situ hybridization. The *HER2* gene copy number increase is detected using a *HER2*-specific probe (black signal), which is typically co-hybridized to tumor cell nuclei with a second probe specific to the centromeric region of chromosome 17 (red signal).

■ **TABLE 11.5-2. HER2 Testing by Immunohistochemistry (IHC) and Dual-Probe ISH Reporting**

Test Type	Score/Group	Interpretation	Scoring Criteria (ASCO/CAP 2018)
IHC	Score 0	Negative	No staining observed, or membrane staining that is incomplete and faint/barely perceptible and in ≤10% of tumor cells
	Score 1+	Negative	Incomplete membrane staining that is faint/barely perceptible and in >10% of tumor cells
	Score 2+	Equivocal	Weak-to-moderate complete membrane staining in >10% of tumor cells. Must order reflex test with ISH
	Score 3+	Positive	Circumferential membrane staining that is complete, intense, and in >10% of tumor cells
ISH	Group 1	Positive	HER2/CEP17 ratio ≥2.0; average HER2 signals/cell ≥4.0
	Group 2	Negative[a]	HER2/CEP17 ratio ≥2.0; average HER2 signals/cell <4.0
	Group 3	Positive[a]	HER2/CEP17 ratio <2.0; average HER2 signals/cell ≥6.0
	Group 4	Negative[a]	HER2/CEP17 ratio <2.0; average HER2 signals/cell ≥4.0 and <6.0
	Group 5	Negative	HER2/CEP17 ratio <2.0; average HER2 signals/cell <4.0

ISH, in situ hybridization.

[a]The final interpretation needs to take consideration with the HER2 IHC result.

amplification. In the majority of carcinomas, both methods provide the same result. Groups 1 and 5 are the most common. For groups 2 to 4, final ISH results are based on a concurrent review of IHC, with a second reviewer recounting the ISH test if IHC is 2+.

About 60% of HER2-negative metastatic breast cancers express low levels of HER2, defined as an HER2 ISH negative with HER2 IHC 1+ or 2+ (32). Currently available HER2-directed therapies have been ineffective in patients with these "HER2 low" cancers. However, ongoing clinical trials in the metastatic setting of new therapeutic agents may change how we approach HER2 testing in the future. The new generation of HER2-targeted drugs, such as trastuzumab-duocarmazine (SYD-985) and trastuzumab-deruxtecan (DS-8201), has shown favorable outcomes in HER2 "low" breast cancers (31-32). If this becomes standard, the often-subtle distinction between an HER2 IHC 0 and IHC 1+ result will become a critical treatment threshold.

Ki-67

Ki-67 is a nuclear protein and a marker of cell proliferation. The MIB-1 monoclonal antibody is used to assess Ki-67 (**Figure 11.5-36**).

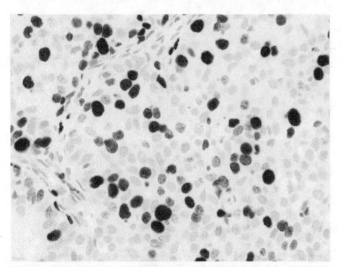

■ **Figure 11.5-36.** Ki-67 in breast cancer by immunohistochemistry. Nuclear stain highlights Ki-67–positive tumor cells. In this case, the Ki-67 proliferation index is estimated as 35%.

The percentage of Ki-67–positive tumor cells determined by IHC is often used to (1) estimate prognosis in early-stage disease regarding whether further adjuvant chemotherapy is warranted, (2) predict whether chemotherapy may or may not be active, and (3) monitor patients during or after neoadjuvant endocrine therapy (NAET) or chemotherapy to determine whether the regimen chosen is working or an alternative should be considered.

The monarchE clinical trial also established the benefit of a CDK4/6 inhibitor for adjuvant treatment of adult patients with HR-positive, HER2-negative, node-positive, early-stage breast cancer at high risk of recurrence and a Ki-67 score 20% and more (33). With a lack of consensus regarding the definition of low versus high expression or an appropriate cut-point for positivity, the evaluation of Ki-67 expression is not currently recommended by either ASCO or other national consensus guidelines. However, The International Ki67 in Breast Cancer Working Group (IKWG) has established and recommended adopting a standardized visual scoring method for clinical assessment (34).

OTHER MARKERS

PD-L1 Expression

Predictive biomarkers for immune checkpoint inhibitors therapies in breast cancer currently include tumor mutational burden and PD-L1 expression by IHC. The phase 3 IMpassion130 trial on metastatic TNBC led to the Food and Drug Administration (FDA) accelerated approval of atezolizumab, a monoclonal anti–PD-L1 antibody in 2019, which demonstrated a statistically significant benefit to progression-free survival (PFS) with the exploratory regimen versus placebo/chemotherapy in PD-L1 immune cell–positive patients (35). However, the subsequent IMpassion131 trial failed to meet the primary end point of PFS superiority in patients with PD-L1 positivity in the frontline treatment. It led to the withdrawal of FDA approval in 2021 (36). The results from another clinical trial—KEYNOTE-355 on PD-L1 expression and pembrolizumab—on untreated metastatic TNBC found that pembrolizumab plus chemotherapy showed a significant and clinically meaningful improvement in PFS versus placebo chemotherapy among patients with metastatic TNBC with PD-L1 IHC combined positive score of 10 or more. This study suggests a role in adding pembrolizumab to standard chemotherapy for the first-line treatment of metastatic TNBC (37).

GENOMIC STUDIES AND BREAST CANCER SUBTYPES

Molecular techniques have shown that breast cancer is a heterogeneous disease. Early transcriptome studies classified breast cancers into distinct molecular subtypes based on the expression of distinct "intrinsic" genes that differed in clinical outcome (38). Luminal A tumors show high expression of ER and related genes, with low proliferation. Luminal B tumors also show expression of ER but have high proliferation and show variable expression of PR and HER2. The HER2-enriched group of tumors expresses the HER2 oncoprotein and related genes, with variable expression of HRs. Basal-like tumors express basal markers such as cytokeratin 5/6 and epidermal growth factor receptor (EGFR), and they typically lack expression of ER, PR, and HER2 (triple-negative tumors). This subgroup of tumors is the most frequent type found in BRCA1-associated breast cancer.

Gene expression signatures are also used for chemotherapy decision-making in ER-positive, HER2-negative breast cancer. There are a variety of prognostic assays, such as Oncotype Dx, MammaPrint, Prosigna (PAM50), EndoPredict, Breast Cancer Index, and Genomic Grade Index. Oncotype Dx (21-gene panel) and MammaPrint (70-gene panel) are most widely used. Although both these assays contain many genes in their panels, their recurrence risk scores are weighted by the receptor status and proliferation-related genes.

More recent pan-genomic studies based on DNA copy number, DNA methylation, exome sequencing, messenger RNA arrays, microRNA sequencing, and protein arrays provided further categorization by demonstrating different molecular profiles for each group (39). Luminal A subtype is enriched in specific mutations in *GATA3*, *PIK3CA*, and *MAP3K1*, whereas basal-like tumors are enriched in *TP53* mutations. Potentially targetable genomic alterations in breast cancer include *ERBB2 (HER2)* gene amplification, neurotrophic receptor tyrosine kinase (*NTRK*) fusions, and *PIK3CA*, *AKT1*, and *PTEN* mutations. Genomic alterations in metastatic breast cancer associated with resistance to ET include *ESR1-* and *ERBB2*-activating mutations, *NF1* loss-of-function mutations, alterations in other MAPK pathway genes, and ER transcriptional regulators (40).

Comprehensive genomic profiling (CGP) based on next-generation sequencing detects a high frequency of therapeutically targetable alteration in clinical samples of patients with primary and metastatic breast cancer (41). Several CGP platforms, including FoundationOne, Caris Molecular Intelligence, and Tempus xT, detect tumor mutational burden (TMB), microsatellite instability (MSI), and all classes of genomic alterations, including substitutions, insertions/deletions, gene fusions, and copy number alterations.

CONCLUSION

Breast cancers represent complex networks of malignant cells and their associated microenvironment. ER, PR, and HER2 are the most common biomarkers in clinical practice to evaluate prognosis and predict response to therapy. Recent advancements have led to the approval of a growing list of personalized therapies and corresponding biomarkers, including tumor-infiltrating lymphocytes, Ki-67, and PD-L1. Pathologic evaluation is critical in determining patient diagnoses, guiding management decisions, providing prognostic information, and helping optimize patient care in the era of precision breast cancer medicine.

REFERENCES

1. Dupont WD, Page DL. Risk factors for breast cancer in women with proliferative breast disease. *N Engl J Med*. 1985;312:146-151.

2. Santen RJ, Mansel R. Benign breast disorders. *N Engl J Med*. 2005;353:275-285.

3. Azzopardi JG. Benign and malignant proliferative epithelial lesions of the breast; a review. *Eur J Cancer Clin Oncol*. 1983;19:1717-1720.

4. Schnitt SJ, Connolly JL, Tavassoli FA, et al. Interobserver reproducibility in the diagnosis of ductal proliferative breast lesions using standardized criteria. *Am J Surg Pathol*. 1992;16:1133-1143.

5. Fraser JL, Raza S, Chorny K, Connolly JL, Schnitt SJ. Columnar alteration with prominent apical snouts and secretions: a spectrum of changes frequently present in breast biopsies performed for microcalcifications. *Am J Surg Pathol*. 1998;22:1521-1527.

6. Dabbs DJ, Carter G, Fudge M, Peng Y, Swalsky P, Finkelstein S. Molecular alterations in columnar cell lesions of the breast. *Mod Pathol*. 2006;19:344-349.

7. Aroner SA, Collins LC, Schnitt SJ, Connolly JL, Colditz GA, Tamimi RM. Columnar cell lesions and subsequent breast cancer risk: a nested case-control study. *Breast Cancer Res*. 2010;12:R61.

8. Pinder SE, Collins LC, Fox SB, eds. Ductal carcinoma in situ. In: *WHO Classification of Tumors Editorial Board. Breast Tumours*. International Agency for Research on Cancer; 2019:76-81.

9. Wells WA, Carney PA, Eliassen MS, Grove MR, Tosteson AN. Pathologists' agreement with experts and reproducibility of breast ductal carcinoma-in-situ classification schemes. *Am J Surg Pathol*. 2000;24:651-659.

10. Lester SC, Bose S, Chen YY, et al. Protocol for the examination of specimens from patients with ductal carcinoma in situ of the breast. *Arch Pathol Lab Med*. 2009;133:15-25.

11. de Mascarel I, MacGrogan G, Mathoulin-Pélissier S, Soubeyran I, Picot V, Coindre JM. Breast ductal carcinoma in situ with microinvasion: a definition supported by a long-term study of 1248 serially sectioned ductal carcinomas. *Cancer*. 2002;94:2134-2142.

12. Allison KH, Hammond MEH, Dowsett M, et al. Estrogen and Progesterone receptor testing in Breast Cancer: ASCO/CAP guideline update. *J Clin Oncol*. 2020;38:1346-1366.

13. Sokolova A, Lakhani SR. Lobular carcinoma in situ: diagnostic criteria and molecular correlates. *Mod Pathol*. 2021;34:8-14.

14. Elston CW, Ellis IO. Pathological prognostic factors in breast cancer. I. The value of histological grade in breast cancer: experience from a large study with long-term follow-up. *Histopathology*. 1991;19:403-410.

15. Bane AL, Tjan S, Parkes RK, Andrulis I, O'Malley FP. Invasive lobular carcinoma: to grade or not to grade. *Mod Pathol*. 2005;18:621-628.

16. Adams S, Gray RJ, Demaria S, et al. Prognostic value of tumor-infiltrating lymphocytes in triple-negative breast cancers from two phase III randomized adjuvant breast cancer trials: ECOG 2197 and ECOG 1199. *J Clin Oncol*. 2014;32:2959-2966.

17. Denket C, Minckwitz G, Brase JC, et al. Tumor-infiltrating lymphocytes and response to neoadjuvant chemotherapy with or without carboplatin in human epidermal growth factor receptor 2-positive and triple-negative primary breast cancers. *J Clin Oncol*. 2015;33:983-991.

18. Ciriello G, Gatza ML, Beck AH, et al. Comprehensive molecular portraits of invasive lobular breast cancer. *Cell*. 2015;163:506-519.

19. Arpino G, Bardou VJ, Clark GM, Elledge RM. Infiltrating lobular carcinoma of the breast: tumor characteristics and clinical outcome. *Breast Cancer Res*. 2004;6:R149-R156.

20. Pestalozzi BC, Zahrieh D, Mallon E, et al. Distinct clinical and prognostic features of infiltrating lobular carcinoma of the breast: combined results of 15 International Breast Cancer Study Group clinical trials. *J Clin Oncol*. 2008;26:3006-3014.

21. Moatamed NA, Apple SK. Extensive sampling changes T-staging of infiltrating lobular carcinoma of breast: a comparative study of gross versus microscopic tumor sizes. *Breast J*. 2006;12:511-517.

22. Ferlicot S, Vincent-Salomon A, Médioni J, et al. Wide metastatic spreading in infiltrating lobular carcinoma of the breast. *Eur J Cancer*. 2004;40:336-341.

23. Abdel-Fatah TM, Powe DG, Hodi Z, Lee AH, Reis-Filho JS, Ellis IO. High frequency of coexistence of columnar cell lesions, lobular neoplasia, and low grade ductal carcinoma in situ with invasive tubular carcinoma and invasive lobular carcinoma. *Am J Surg Pathol*. 2007;31:417-426.

24. Page DL, Dixon JM, Anderson TJ, Lee D, Stewart HJ. Invasive cribriform carcinoma of the breast. *Histopathology*. 1983;7:525-536.

25. Diab SG, Clark GM, Osborne CK, Libby A, Allred DC, Elledge RM. Tumor characteristics and clinical outcome of tubular and mucinous breast carcinomas. *J Clin Oncol*. 1999;17:1442-1448.

26. Barbashina V, Corben AD, Akram M, Vallejo C, Tan LK. Mucinous micropapillary carcinoma of the breast: an aggressive counterpart to conventional pure mucinous tumors. *Hum Pathol*. 2013;44:1577-1585.

27. Collins LC, Carlo VP, Hwang H, Barry TS, Gown AM, Schnitt SJ. Intracystic papillary carcinomas of the breast: a reevaluation using a panel of myoepithelial cell markers. *Am J Surg Pathol.* 2006;30:1002-1007.

28. Pettinato G, Manivel CJ, Panico L, Sparano L, Petrella G. Invasive micropapillary carcinoma of the breast: clinicopathologic study of 62 cases of a poorly recognized variant with highly aggressive behavior. *Am J Clin Pathol.* 2004;121:857-866.

29. Zhou S, Yang F, Bai Q, et al. Intense basolateral membrane staining indicates HER2 positivity in invasive micropapillary breast carcinoma. *Mod Pathol.* 2020;33:1275-1286.

30. Nassar A, Visscher DW, Degnim AC, et al. Complex fibroadenoma and breast cancer risk: a mayo clinic benign breast disease cohort study. *Breast Cancer Res Treat.* 2015;153:397-405.

31. Carter MR, Hornick JL, Lester S, Fletcher CD. Spindle cell (sarcomatoid) carcinoma of the breast: a clinicopathologic and immunohistochemical analysis of 29 cases. *Am J Surg Pathol.* 2006;30:300-309.

32. Wolff AC, Hammond MEH, Allison KH, et al. HER2 testing in breast cancer: American Society of Clinical Oncology/College of American Pathologists clinical practice guideline focused update. *Arch Pathol Lab Med.* 2018;142:1364-1382.

33. Johnston SRD, Harbeck N, Hegg R, et al. Abemaciclib combined with endocrine therapy for the adjuvant treatment of HR+, HER2-, node-positive, high-risk, early breast cancer (monarchE). *J Clin Oncol.* 2020;38:3987-3998.

34. Nielsen TO, Leung SCY, Rimm DL, et al. Assessment of Ki67 in breast cancer: updated recommendations from the international Ki67 in breast cancer working group. *J Natl Cancer Inst.* 2021;113:808-819.

35. Schmid P, Rugo HS, Adams S, et al. Atezolizumab plus nab-paclitaxel as first-line treatment for unresectable, locally advanced or metastatic triple-negative breast cancer (IMpassion130): updated efficacy results from a randomised, double-blind, placebo-controlled, phase 3 trial. *Lancet Oncol.* 2020;21:44-59.

36. Miles D, Gligorov J, André F, et al. Primary results from IMpassion131, a double-blind, placebo-controlled, randomised phase III trial of first-line paclitaxel with or without atezolizumab for unresectable locally advanced/metastatic triple-negative breast cancer. *Ann Oncol.* 2021;32:994-1004.

37. Cortes J, Cescon DW, Rugo HS, et al. Pembrolizumab plus chemotherapy versus placebo plus chemotherapy for previously untreated locally recurrent inoperable or metastatic triple-negative breast cancer (KEYNOTE-355): a randomised, placebo-controlled, double-blind, phase 3 clinical trial. *Lancet.* 2020;396:1817-1828.

38. Perou CM, Sørlie T, Eisen MB, et al. Molecular portraits of human breast tumours. *Nature.* 2000;406:747-752.

39. Cancer Genome Atlas Network. Comprehensive molecular portraits of human breast tumours. *Nature.* 2012;490:61-70.

40. Ross DS, Pareja F. Molecular pathology of breast tumors: diagnostic and actionable genetic alterations. *Surg Pathol Clin.* 2021;14:455-471.

41. Vasan N, Yelensky R, Wang K, et al. A targeted next-generation sequencing assay detects a high frequency of therapeutically targetable alterations in primary and metastatic breast cancers: implications for clinical practice. *Oncologist.* 2014;19:453-458.

CHAPTER **11.6**

Surgical Management of the Breast

Doreen L. Wiggins and Theresa A. Graves

Surgical management of breast cancer has evolved into a multidisciplinary, evidence-based specialty, which requires coordinated care alongside medical oncology, radiation oncology, and genetics. The surgical approach has advanced in parallel with our evolving understanding of tumor biology, evolving over time, from the radical mastectomy proposed by Halsted to breast-conservation surgery (BCS), guided by Fisher and colleagues of the National Surgical Adjuvant Breast and Bowel Project (NSABP), to personalized treatment paradigms based on the data indicating that breast cancer is a highly heterogeneous disease.

IN SITU DISEASE

Despite the adoption of conservative surgery for invasive disease, surgical management of DCIS of the breast lagged. As DCIS can present with a diffuse pattern and/or skipped lesions, it was potentially less likely to achieve negative surgical margins with breast conservation, and thus mastectomy was standard of care. However, the movement to adopt less aggressive surgery mirrored the approach to early invasive breast cancer. Although no phase 3 trials evaluated mastectomy versus BCT, the seminal NSABP-17 trial was informative. This trial, launched in 1985, enrolled women with localized DCIS=-098 who were randomly assigned to compare lumpectomy only (LO) to lumpectomy followed by radiation therapy (L-RT), with the end point of the ipsilateral breast tumor recurrence (IBTR) rate (1). At 5 years, women treated by L-RT had a 60% lower risk of IBTR compared with those treated by LO. Subsequent updates continue to demonstrate a considerable benefit for L-RT compared with LO (2). A second prospective randomized DCIS trial (NSABP B-24) investigated the addition of tamoxifen (TAM) to L-RT (L-RT + TAM). Women treated with L-RT + TAM experienced a 31% reduction in the risk of IBTR compared with those treated by L-RT and a 53% reduction in the risk of contralateral breast tumors (3). Retrospective studies and a meta-analysis show that between 25% and 40% are ultimately identified as having an invasive carcinoma and upstaged at excision (4,5).

Despite breast conservation being the standard surgical treatment for DCIS, some will require mastectomy. Widely accepted indications for this include persistent positive margins after wide local reexcision, multicentric disease, a sizeable tumor-to-breast size ratio for which BCS would result in a less-than-desirable cosmetic outcome, and previous ipsilateral radiation (or any other contraindication for RT) (6). A sentinel lymph node biopsy (SLNB) should be performed at the time of mastectomy based on the 25% to 40% upstage to invasive disease identified at the time of excision and the subsequent inability to perform an SLNB following mastectomy. Current research aims to perform an SLNB more judiciously among this group of people. As an example, the SentiNOT study evaluated the use of an iron oxide nanoparticle tracer before surgery for women with DCIS, and at interim analysis that included volunteers undergoing 189 mastectomies, invasive breast cancer was found in 47 specimens. With the ability to identify the tracer in an SLN weeks after injection, delayed SLNB was performed in 41, indicating that 78% of this group avoided SLNB (7). The use of the

■ TABLE 11.6-1. Current Randomized Clinical Trials for DCIS. All Evaluate Immediate Surgery Versus Active Surveillance

Eligibility	LORIS[a] n = 932	COMET[b] n = 1,200	LORD[c] n = 1,240	LORETTA[d] n = 340
Age range (y)	>45	40 and older	45 and older	40 and older
DCIS nuclear grade	1 or 2	1	1 or 2	1 or 2
Comedo-necrosis allowed?	No	Yes	No	No
ER positivity?	NA	Positive	NA	Positive
HER2 status	NA	If checked, must be negative	NA	Negative
Size	NA	Any	Any	Up to 2.5 cm
Endocrine therapy allowed	No	Yes	No	Yes (mandatory)

ER, estrogen receptor; DCIS, ductal carcinoma in situ.

[a]Gaunt C. A phase III trial of surgery versus active monitoring for LOw RISk Ductal Carcinoma in Situ (DCIS). doi:10.1186/ISRCTN27544579

[b]Comparing an Operation to Monitoring, With or Without Endocrine Therapy (COMET) Trial For Low Risk DCIS (COMET). https://clinicaltrials.gov/ct2/show/NCT02926911

[c]Management of Low-risk (Grade I and II) DCIS (LORD). https://clinicaltrials.gov/ct2/show/NCT02492607

[d]From Gaunt, C. A Phase III Trial of Surgery versus Active Monitoring for LOw RISk Ductal Carcinoma in Situ (DCIS). doi:10.1186/ISRCTN27544579; 2. Comparing an Operation to Mon-itoring, With or Without Endocrine Therapy (COMET) Trial For Low Risk DCIS (COMET). https://clinicaltrials.gov/ct2/show/NCT02926911; 3. Management of Low-risk (Grade I and II) DCIS (LORD). https://clinicaltrials.gov/ct2/show/NCT02492607; 4. Single-arm confirmatory trial of endocrine therapy alone for estrogen receptor-positive, low-risk ductal carcinoma in situ of the breast (JCOG1505, LORETTA trial). https://center6.umin.ac.jp/cgi-open-bin/ctr_e/ctr_view.cgi?recptno=R000032260.

nanoparticle tracer plus blue dye also significantly outperformed isotope and blue dye in detection of the sentinel node (40/40 vs 26/40, $P < .001$).

Although sentinel node biopsy is standard for women with DCIS undergoing mastectomy, it is not entirely clear if it plays a role in BCT. In the largest series looking at this issue, nodal involvement was seen in only 5% of cases; however, 70% of these metastases were detected only by IHC staining (8). While lymphatic mapping for women undergoing BCT was considered in patients with a span of DCIS greater than 4 cm, those who present with a mass on mammography, women with palpable DCIS, high-grade DCIS on core biopsy, and the presence (or question of) microinvasion, the only current indication is for those patients with DCIS undergoing mastectomy.

A large meta-analysis aimed to identify predictors of an invasive breast cancer recurrence (IBCR) after treatment of DCIS with BCT. Six factors were statistically significant: Black race (pooled estimate [ES], 1.43; 95% confidence interval [CI], 1.15-1.79), premenopausal status (ES, 1.59; 95% CI, 1.20-2.11), palpable mass (ES, 1.84; 95% CI, 1.47-2.29), involved margins (ES, 1.63; 95% CI, 1.14-2.32), high histologic grade (ES, 1.36; 95% CI, 1.04-1.77), and high p16 expression (ES, 1.51; 95% CI, 1.04-2.19) (9). Contemporary randomized trials are accruing patients to determine optimal treatment, and to prevent overtreatment, for low (± intermediate) nuclear grade DCIS (Table 11.6-1).

EARLY INVASIVE DISEASE

Early invasive breast cancer is typically defined by a tumor size of 2 cm or less. These lesions are identified by breast screening modalities, mammogram, US, or breast MRI and diagnosed by CNB. BCS is offered as standard of care if the primary breast tumor can be resected with clear margins and a cosmetically acceptable result. Image detected lesions are typically identified using radiology localization techniques, including, but not limited to, the wire localization, magnetic seeds, radiofrequency tags, or intraoperative US localization. Such techniques are typically not necessary for people who present with a palpable mass. Relative contraindications to breast conservation include multicentricity and clinical contraindications to RT (pregnancy, prior breast RT, collagen-vascular disease, and nonaccessibility).

At the time of definitive surgery, intraoperative specimen radiograph and pathologic gross margin analysis are essential to ensure an adequate resection was performed. The reexcision lumpectomy

rate (RELR) is highly variable among surgeons and reflects the difficulty in balancing acceptable cosmetic outcome with the need to obtain negative margins; it is often influenced by patient factors, such as tumor-to-breast size ratio. Incision placement along Langer lines, periareolar, and inframammary positions are preferred for optimal cosmetic outcome without compromise to adequate resection and margin status. Typically, the surgical margins are oriented by the surgeon at the time of surgery using ink or sutures to assist with pathologic evaluation of margin status. If skin or fascia form anatomic boundaries, this should be indicated in the operative report to assist with planning of further treatment because reexcision may not be necessary for involved anterior and posterior margins in this setting. An oncoplastic closure should be performed in conjunction with plastic surgery, if needed, to preserve the shape of the breast.

For women undergoing BCS, margin status is one of several components impacting local recurrence. A meta-analysis of 33 studies, with over 28,000 patients, showed that positive margins increased the incidence of an IBTR by 2-fold compared to negative margins (10). Interestingly, the width of a negative margin was not associated with reductions in the risk of an IBTR. This analysis formed the basis of a 2014 consensus statement supported by both the Society of Surgical Oncologists (SSO) and the American Society of Therapeutic Radiation Oncology (ASTRO), which adopts an adequate margin when there is pathologically no evidence of invasive tumor at the surgically inked margin (10).

In 2015, Chagpar et al reported the results of a randomized trial evaluating the role of resecting additional tissue circumferentially around the tumor cavity (called cavity-shaved margins) on outcomes in more than 200 women undergoing BCS (ie, partial mastectomy) for stages 0 to III breast cancer (11). The median age of the patients was 61 years (range, 33-94). Of those enrolled, 23%, 19%, and 53% had invasive cancer, DCIS alone, or both, respectively. Compared to those who did not undergo shaved margins, shave margins resulted in a significantly lower rate of positive margins (19% vs 34%, $P = .01$) and less women underwent second surgical procedures (10% vs 21%, $P = .02$).

LOCALLY ADVANCED BREAST CANCER

LABC is a heterogeneous collection of presentations that include advanced-stage primary tumors, nodal involvement, and inflammatory breast cancers (IBCs). Presentations may span tumor size T2-T4 with involvement of chest wall or skin ulceration, skin satellites, or nodal involvement. The definition of LABC may include other characteristics, such as large, operable breast tumors.

Systemic therapy for early-stage breast cancer has provided significant improvement in operability of breast cancer, and primary systemic therapy (neoadjuvant) is equivalent to adjuvant therapy in OS and disease-free survival (DFS). For those patients with operable but large tumors that would require total mastectomy for definitive surgery, neoadjuvant therapy (NT) facilitates conversion to BCT in as many as 25% of people with LABC, without compromising OS and DFS, increasing surgical complications, or delaying adjuvant therapy. For those presenting with clinically involved axillary nodes, NACT may also allow the opportunity to proceed with an SLNB rather than the standard complete axillary dissection; there is a 30% to 40% decrease in nodal positivity and 20% pathologic complete response (pCR) (12).

Pretherapy evaluation of the axillary LNs with clinical examination and US before the initiation of NACT may be utilized to stage the axilla with fine-needle aspiration (FNA) (13).

For people presenting with ER-positive LABC, the role of the 21-gene RS to guide treatment with neoadjuvant hormone therapy (NHT) versus NACT was evaluated in one randomized trial (14). NHT was found to be convert volunteers from mastectomy to BCS among those with an RS up to 25. The conversion rate to BCS among people with RS less than 11 or RS 11 to 25, both of which received NHT, was over 70%; however, for those with RS 11 to 25 or 26 or higher who received NACT, conversion rate to BCS was 63.6% and 57.1%, respectively. These results were particularly useful during the 2019-2021 COVID-19 pandemic because it provided the ability to identify candidates for NHT for whom surgery could be delayed without compromise in the long-term outcome while minimizing immunosuppression and viral exposure (15).

SURGERY FOR INFLAMMATORY BREAST CANCER

IBC occurs in 1% to 6% of all breast cancer and is clinically characterized by erythema and edema of at least one-third of the breast. It is treated as a specific breast cancer subtype, and guidance came from an international panel on IBC, convened in 2018 at the Morgan Welch Inflammatory Breast Cancer Research Program Conference. Highlights of the recommendations are noted in Recommendations for the management of IBC and are summarized in **Table 11.6-2** (16).

ONCOPLASTIC BREAST SURGERY

Discussions with the patient regarding surgery should include considerations for mastectomy versus breast conservation. For those undergoing mastectomy, the role of skin- (SSM) and nipple-sparing mastectomy (NSM), the options and timing of reconstructive surgery (none, implant based [**Figure 11.6-1**], and autologous tissue transfer), staging of the axilla, and the role/timing of systemic therapy and RT are also important points that must be covered and are best done within the context of a multidisciplinary consultation, including, if appropriate, the primary surgeon, plastic surgeon, medical oncologist, and radiation oncologist.

At the time of mastectomy, surgical incisions should be planned with the reconstructive surgeon to allow for optimal cosmesis but with the goal of thin flaps to remove all breast tissue and minimize the risk of local recurrence. A separate axillary incision can be created if necessary for more extensive nodal surgery to preserve the vascularity of the flaps or improve surgical access. For patients undergoing NSM, all ductal tissue beneath the nipple should be removed; this specimen should be separately sent to pathology to evaluate adequacy of the nipple margin. If the nipple margin

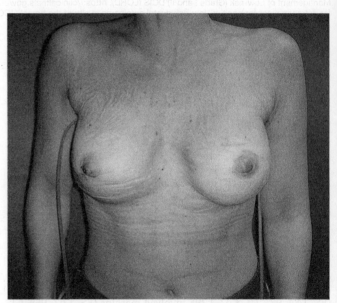

Figure 11.6-1. Bilateral skin- and nipple-sparing mastectomy with immediate implant-based plastic reconstructive surgery.

▪ TABLE 11.6-2. Recommendations on the Management of Inflammatory Breast Cancer
Photographs should be taken at diagnosis to document findings and shared in the medical record for members of the multidisciplinary oncology.
Breast MRI should be performed to evaluate the primary lesion and to evaluate for multicentric disease.
PET-CT scans should be performed to evaluate for metastatic disease.
A skin punch biopsy should be performed to evaluate for dermal lymphatic invasion, a pathognomonic sign of IBC. However, skin biopsy is not mandated to make the diagnosis of IBC.
All patients with stage III or de novo stage IV IBC should receive systemic therapy, including chemotherapy with or without targeted treatment. Decisions regarding medical, surgical, or radiation therapy require a multidisciplinary approach.
The only guideline-concordant surgical option for IBC is a modified radical mastectomy with delayed reconstruction.
Preoperative radiotherapy (or chemoradiation) may be necessary to obtain negative surgical margins.
Contralateral prophylactic mastectomy should be deferred to ensure that complications related to this nononcologic surgery do not delay radiotherapy or adjuvant chemotherapy administration.

IBC, inflammatory breast cancer; MRI, magnetic resonance imaging; PET-CT, positron emission tomography-computed tomography.

returns positive for malignancy, the patient should undergo a resection of the nipple-areolar complex (NAC).

Oncoplastic breast surgery (OBS), including both SSM (**Figure 11.6-2**) and NSM, is an oncologically safe option. OBS is cosmetic focused and is often a collaborative surgical procedure with breast and plastic surgery. The goal of OBS is to improve scar orientation/placement, sensation, and breast symmetry (17). No randomized controlled trials have compared oncologic outcomes in traditional (simple) mastectomy to OBS. Initial studies comparing conservative mastectomy to SSM and NSM were based on patients in a single institution and, therefore, difficult to generalize to a broader population. As a result, national consensus guidelines includes the option for NSM with caveats for patient inclusion: early-stage, biologically favorable invasive breast cancer, or DCIS; no nipple involvement on imaging; and confirmation that disease is at least 2 cm from the nipple. Pathologic nipple discharge, or evidence of Paget disease, serves as contraindication to NSM.

A 2019 meta-analysis reported that outcomes for SSM and NSM do not differ from those for standard mastectomy and that recurrence rates in the NAC after NSM are acceptably low (0%-3.7%) (18). NSM is also associated with high patient satisfaction and good psychological adjustment (19) and with significantly better body image, satisfaction with nipple appearance, satisfaction with nipple sensitivity, and decreased feeling of mutilation compared to SSM (20). NSM, however, carries an inherently greater risk of NAC and mastectomy flap complications and necrosis, which are reportedly as high as 30% (21). Risk factors for postoperative ischemic complications have been studied at length. Intrinsic or patient-specific

factors include BMI and breast morphology (breast size, mastectomy weight, and ptosis), patient age, and smoking (22). Extrinsic influences such as radiation, incision pattern, mastectomy flap thickness, and the type of reconstruction also contribute to postoperative ischemic complications (23).

Although implant-based procedures remain the most used techniques for NSM and SSM reconstruction, the number of flap-based options has increased significantly in recent years. In addition to pedicle transverse rectus abdominis musculocutaneous (PTRAM), free TRAM (FTRAM), and latissimus dorsi (LD) flaps, patients and surgeons now have newer perforator procedures, such as deep inferior epigastric perforator (DIEP) and superficial inferior epigastric perforator (SIEA) flaps, from which to choose.

Funded by the National Cancer Institute (NCI) in 2011, the Mastectomy Reconstruction Outcomes Consortium (MROC) was a prospective cohort study of selected practices in the United States and Canada with high volumes of breast reconstruction (24). Study participants were women undergoing first-time reconstruction following mastectomy for breast cancer treatment or prophylaxis. Patients receiving first-time immediate or delayed reconstruction were eligible for study participation. Surgical options evaluated in this analysis included single and two-staged implant-based techniques; combination LD flap/implant procedures, PTRAM flaps, FTRAM flaps, and DIEP flaps. For any complication, implant-based procedures were associated with the lowest rate (24.7%), whereas DIEP flaps were the highest (46.9%). For major complications, both implant-based and LD flap procedures had lower rates compared with PTRAM, FTRAM, and DIEP flaps. The multivariate analyses

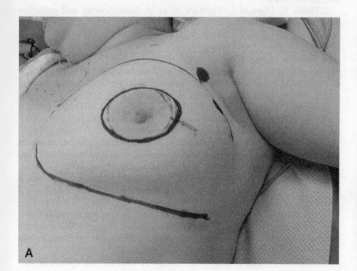

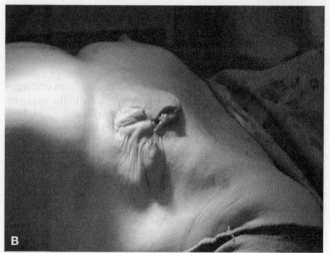

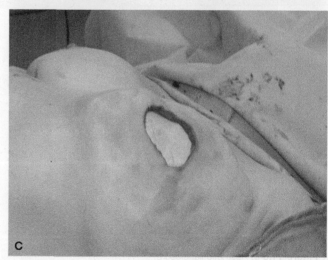

Figure 11.6-2. Skin-sparing mastectomy. A: Surgical marking for purposes of reconstruction. B: Completed skin-sparing mastectomy flaps. C: Intraoperative transverse rectus abdominis musculocutaneous flap.

also identified several patient-level characteristics that were significant predictors of complications. For any complication, older age was associated with a higher risk among those aged 45 to 54.9 years (OR 1.68, $P = .03$), 55 to 64.9 years (OR 1.96, $P = .009$), and 65 years and above (OR 2.30, $P = .007$), compared with patients under age 35 years. Women with BMI of 30.0 to 34.9 kg/m^2 (OR 1.54, $P = .005$) and 35 kg/m^2 or greater (OR 2.29, $P < .001$) were at significantly greater risk, compared with patients with normal BMI (between 18.5 and 25 kg/m^2). Additional risk factors for any complication included immediate reconstruction (OR 1.82, $P = .017$), bilateral reconstruction (OR 1.52, $P < .0001$), and RT during or after reconstruction (OR 1.50, $P = .014$).

AESTHETIC FLAT CLOSURE AND CONTRALATERAL PROPHYLACTIC MASTECTOMY

A patient-directed social movement of "Going or Living Flat" aims to increase awareness and acceptance for mastectomy without reconstruction as an active surgical option. The motivation driving this patient preference, also known as aesthetic flat closure (**Figure 11.6-3**), is reported to include a desire to reduce the risk of recurrence and to avoid radiation, postdiagnosis radiologic imaging, and the issues inherent in reconstruction (eg, multiple surgeries, foreign-material placement, and an increased risk of infection and other complications). A national survey reported 22% of women experienced a low level of surgeon support for going flat, and this strongly predicted patient dissatisfaction (25). Most patients undergoing mastectomy alone are satisfied with their surgical outcome. Surgeons may optimize the patient experience by recognizing and supporting a patient's decision to omit BCS or reconstruction (25). Patients' surgical preferences regarding definitive surgery and reconstruction should represent a shared decision-making process.

A consensus statement from the ASBrS recommends that women with unilateral breast cancer who are at average risk and negative for a gene mutation should be discouraged from undergoing a contralateral prophylactic mastectomy (CPM). The majority of these women will not obtain a survival benefit, and CPM doubles the risk of surgical complications (26). Among women with breast cancer, the absolute risk of developing contralateral breast cancer (CBC) exceeds that of the general population and is approximately 0.6% per year in historic series. Because systemic adjuvant chemotherapy reduces the risk of CBC by 20%, TAM 50%, and aromatase inhibitors (AIs) 60%, the contemporary risk of developing a CBC is predicted to be approximately 0.2% to 0.5% per year for those undergoing adjuvant therapies (27).

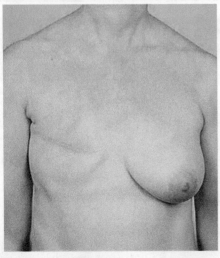

Figure 11.6-3. Aesthetic flat closure.

Palliative Mastectomy

Palliative mastectomy refers to expedient surgical management of a fungating, bleeding breast cancer encompassing the breast and chest wall and performed as a palliative procedure with noncurative intent. Operative intent may be considered to alleviate patient's suffering and optimize local control. Surgical management should be discussed with multidisciplinary providers, coordinating surgical, medical, and radiation oncology planning to optimize care. The rationale for palliative mastectomy is to relieve the patient of a bulky cancerous breast and to avoid bleeding, infection, or odor from an open necrotizing mass.

Although the mastectomy intent is not curative, alleviating symptoms caused by local tumefaction can bring relief to the patient. Factors limiting the ability to pursue surgical intervention include the patient's overall physical condition; the ability to achieve negative tumor resection margins, including the posterior or chest wall margins; and known direct extension of the tumor to underlying viscera. Primary closure, split-thickness skin grafting, or a more complex reconstructive procedure may be necessary and dependent on the disease burden. Preoperative RT is effective in the reduction of tumor burden and control of tumor hemorrhage.

REFERENCES

1. Wapnir IL, Dignam JJ, Fisher B, et al. Long-term outcomes of invasive ipsilateral breast tumor recurrences after lumpectomy in NSABP B-17 and B-24 randomized clinical trials for DCIS. *J Natl Cancer Inst.* 2011;103:478-488.

2. Fisher B, Dignam J, Wolmark N, et al. Lumpectomy and radiation therapy for the treatment of intraductal breast cancer: findings from national surgical adjuvant breast and bowel project B-17. *J Clin Oncol.* 1998;16:441-452.

3. Fisher B, Land S, Mamounas E, Dignam J, Fisher ER, Wolmark N. Prevention of invasive breast cancer in women with ductal carcinoma in situ: an update of the national surgical adjuvant breast and bowel project experience. *Semin Oncol.* 2001;28:400-418.

4. Miller-Ocuin JL, Howard-McNatt M, Levine EA, Chiba A. Is sentinel lymph node biopsy necessary for ductal carcinoma in situ patients undergoing mastectomy? *Am Surg.* 2020;86:955-957.

5. Brennan ME, Turner RM, Ciatto S, et al. Ductal carcinoma in situ at core-needle biopsy: meta-analysis of underestimation and predictors of invasive breast cancer. *Radiology.* 2011;260:119-128.

6. Van Cleef A, Altintas S, Huizing M, Papadimitriou K, Van Dam P, Tjalma W. Current view on ductal carcinoma in situ and importance of the margin thresholds: a review. *Facts Views Vis ObGyn.* 2014;6:210-218.

7. Karakatsanis A. Hersi AF, Pistiolis L, et al. Effect of preoperative injection of superparamagnetic iron oxide particles on rates of sentinel lymph node dissection in women undergoing surgery for ductal carcinoma in situ (SentiNot study). *Br J Surg.* 2019;106:720-728.

8. Wilkie C, White L, Dupont E, Cantor A, Cox CE. An update of sentinel lymph node mapping in patients with ductal carcinoma in situ. *Am J Surg.* 2005;190:563-566.

9. Visser LL, Groen EJ, van Leeuwen FE, Lips EH, Schmidt MK, Wesseling J. Predictors of an invasive breast cancer recurrence after DCIS: a systematic review and meta-analyses. *Cancer Epidemiol Biomarkers Prev.* 2019;28:835-845.

10. Moran MS, Schnitt SJ, Giuliano AE, et al. Society of surgical oncology-American society for radiation oncology consensus guideline on margins for breast-conserving surgery with whole-breast irradiation in stages I and II invasive breast cancer. *Int J Radiat Oncol Biol Phys.* 2014;88:553-564.

11. Chagpar AB, Killelea BK, Tsangaris TN, et al. A randomized, controlled trial of cavity shave margins in breast cancer. *N Engl J Med.* 2015;373:503-510.

12. Mamounas EP. Impact of neoadjuvant chemotherapy on locoregional surgical treatment of breast cancer. *Ann Surg Oncol.* 2015;22:1425-1433.

13. Mainiero MB. Regional lymph node staging in breast cancer: the increasing role of imaging and ultrasound-guided axillary lymph node fine needle aspiration. *Radiol Clin North Am.* 2010;48:989-997.

14. Bear HD, Wan W, Robidoux A, et al. Using the 21-gene assay from core needle biopsies to choose neoadjuvant therapy for breast cancer: a multicenter trial. *J Surg Oncol.* 2017;115:917-923.

15. Dietz JR, Moran MS, Isakoff SJ, et al. Recommendations for prioritization, treatment, and triage of breast cancer patients during the COVID-19 pandemic. The COVID-19 pandemic breast cancer consortium. *Breast Cancer Res Treat.* 2020;181:487-497.

16. Ueno NT, Espinosa Fernandez JR, Cristofanilli M, et al. International consensus on the clinical management of inflammatory breast cancer from the Morgan Welch inflammatory breast cancer research program 10th anniversary conference. *J Cancer.* 2018;9:1437-1447.

17. Santos G, Urban C, Edelweiss MI, et al. Long-term comparison of aesthetical outcomes after oncoplastic surgery and lumpectomy in breast cancer patients. *Ann Surg Oncol.* 2015;22:2500-2508.

18. Wu ZY Kim HJ, Lee JW, et al. Breast cancer recurrence in the nipple-areola complex after nipple-sparing mastectomy with immediate breast reconstruction for invasive breast cancer. *JAMA Surg.* 2019;154:1030-1037.

19. Lanitis S, Tekkis PP, Sgourakis G, Dimopoulos N, Al Mufti R, Hadjiminas DJ. Comparison of skin-sparing mastectomy versus non-skin-sparing mastectomy for breast cancer: a meta-analysis of observational studies. *Ann Surg.* 2010;251:632-639.

20. Didier F, Radice D, Gandini S, et al. Does nipple preservation in mastectomy improve satisfaction with cosmetic results, psychological adjustment, body image and sexuality? *Breast Cancer Res Treat.* 2009;118:623-633.

21. Endara M, Chen D, Verma K, Nahabedian MY, Spear SL. Breast reconstruction following nipple-sparing mastectomy: a systematic review of the literature with pooled analysis. *Plast Reconstr Surg.* 2013;132: 1043-1054.

22. Paprottka FJ, Schlett CL, Luketina R, et al. Risk factors for complications after skin-sparing and nipple-sparing mastectomy. *Breast Care.* 2019;14:289-297.

23. Salibian AA, Frey JD, Bekisz JM, Karp NS, Choi M. Ischemic complications after nipple-sparing mastectomy: predictors of reconstructive failure in implant-based reconstruction and implications for decision-making. *Plast Reconstr Surg Glob Open.* 2019;7:e2280.

24. Wilkins EG, Hamill JB, Kim HM, et al. Complications in post-mastectomy breast reconstruction: one-year outcomes of the Mastectomy Reconstruction Outcomes Consortium (MROC) study. *Ann Surg.* 2018;267:164-170.

25. Baker JL, Dizon DS, Wenziger CM, et al. "Going Flat" after mastectomy: patient-reported outcomes by online survey. *Ann Surg Oncol.* 2021;28:2493-2505.

26. Boughey JC, Attai DJ, Chen SL, et al. Contralateral Prophylactic Mastectomy (CPM) consensus statement from the American Society of Breast Surgeons: data on CPM outcomes and risks. *Ann Surg Oncol.* 2016;23:3100-3105.

27. Early Breast Cancer Trialists' Collaborative Group. Effects of chemotherapy and hormonal therapy for early breast cancer on recurrence and 15-year survival: an overview of the randomised trials. *Lancet.* 2005;365:1687-1717.

CHAPTER **11.7**

Surgical Management of the Axilla

Charu Taneja

MANAGEMENT OF THE CLINICALLY AND PATHOLOGICALLY NEGATIVE AXILLA

Historically, axillary dissection was used to stage the axilla as well as to provide regional control, but this procedure was associated with significant morbidity. With decreasing tumor size at diagnosis, less than 30% of clinically node-negative patients had pathologic axillary involvement; this led to the development of the less invasive and significantly less morbid procedure of SLNB (1). Indeed, compared to full axillary lymph node dissection (ALND), sentinel node biopsy is associated with lower complication rates, including sensory loss, lymphedema, mobility restriction, and infection (2), and has been validated in large multicenter trials (3,4). The largest trial, NSABP B-32, evaluated the impact of sentinel node biopsy with or without ALND in more than 5,600 women, almost 4,000 of whom had pathologically node-negative disease (5). This study showed no differences between the two groups in locoregional recurrence (LRR), DFS, or OS at 10-year follow-up (6). This allowed surgeons to safely omit axillary dissection in patients with negative sentinel node biopsy. **Figure 11.7-1** provides an algorithm to approach the axilla for people with early-stage breast cancer (7).

Management of Clinically Node-Negative, SLN+ Patient

Initially, all patients with a positive SLNB underwent a completion ALND. However, the NSABP B-04 trial demonstrated that 40% of people who were clinically node negative but were found to have nodal involvement on pathologic examination experienced no differences in their long-term outcome whether the axilla was observed, treated surgically, or radiated (8). This raised the question of whether axillary dissection could be omitted in patients with a clinically negative axilla, but SLN+ at surgery.

The American College of Surgeons Oncology Group (ACOSOG) Z0011 study (Z11 study) was designed to determine whether the performance of completion ALND affected survival or local control in women with T1-T2 breast cancer undergoing BCS with clinically negative axillae and one to two positive SLNs (2). All study volunteers received whole-breast irradiation and adjuvant systemic therapy, and the study excluded patients with T3 tumors, clinically node-positive patients, patients undergoing neoadjuvant systemic therapy or mastectomy, or those with greater than three positive SLNs or nodes with gross extranodal extension. Patients with one to two positive sentinel nodes identified at surgery were randomized to undergo ALND or no further treatment. With a median follow-up of 6.3 years, the OS rate was 91.8% in the ALND group versus 92.5% in the sentinel node biopsy group alone. The rate of nodal recurrence in both arms was less than 1%. On 10-year follow-up, there was no significant difference in OS or LRR between the two groups, despite a 27% rate of pathologic node involvement among the group who underwent ALND (9,10). Similarly, the International Breast Cancer Study Group (IBCSG) 23-01 trial evaluated whether ALND might be overtreatment in patients who have micrometastases (0.2-2 mm) only in the sentinel node (11,12). There was no difference in DFS or OS between patients followed by SLNB alone versus those undergoing completion ALND, despite finding an additional 13% positive non–sentinel nodes in those who underwent ALND.

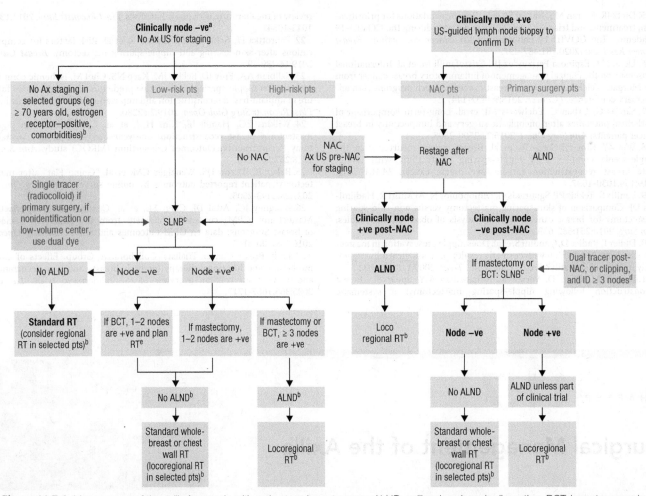

Figure 11.7-1. Management of the axilla for people with early-stage breast cancer. ALND, axillary lymph node dissection; BCT, breast-conserving therapy; NAC, neoadjuvant chemotherapy; pts, patients; RT, radiotherapy; SLNB, sentinel lymph node biopsy; US, ultrasound. (Brackstone M, Baldassarre FG, Perera FE, et al. Management of the axilla in early-stage breast cancer: Ontario Health (Cancer Care Ontario) and ASCO guideline. *J Clin Oncol.* 2021;39:3056-3082. doi:10.1200/JCO.21.00934)

[a]Refers to all patients with no palpable axillary nodes on physical examination, including those who might have had an US that was equivocal, abnormal, or even biopsy-proven positive.

[b]Decision making should be made on a case-by-case basis and include a patient-centered approach, that is, consider and discuss pros and cons of various options in light of patient's specific circumstances, values, and preferences.

[c]Do not recommend SLNB prechemotherapy except in special circumstances after multidisciplinary discussion.

[d]Evidence supports the use of dual localizing tracer (blue dye and radioisotope) and harvesting ≥ 3 nodes or else perform ALND to minimize FNR; any clipped positive nodes should be localized for surgery.

[e]In rare circumstances (eg, a small T1aN1), it is possible to avoid radiation (see Justification and Recommendation 3D).

+ve, positive; -ve negative; ALND, axillary lymph node dissection; Ax, axillary; CVT, breast-conserving therapy; Dx, diagnosis; ER, estrogen receptor; FNR, false-negative rate HT, hormonal therapy; NAC, neoadjuvant chemotherapy; pts, patients; RT, radiation treatment; SLNB, sentinel lymph node biopsy; US, ultrasound.

From Muriel Brackstone M, Baldassarre FG, Perera FE, et al. Management of the axilla in early-stage breast cancer: Ontario health (Cancer Care Ontario) and ASCO guideline. *J Clin Oncol.* 2021;39(27):3056-3082. doi:10.1200/JCO.21.00934

The evaluation of axillary surgery versus radiation for people with a positive SLN was evaluated in the European Organization for Research and Treatment of Cancer (EORTC) 10981-22023 AMAROS (After mapping of the Axilla: Radiotherapy or Surgery) trial (13). The results showed no significant difference between the two groups (ALND vs axillary RT) in 5-year axillary recurrence, DFS, and OS. However, there was a higher incidence of lymphedema in the group undergoing axillary dissection. Similar results were also seen in the Optimal Treatment Of the Axillar – Surgery Or Radiotherapy (OTOASOR) (14) and the Agència d'Avaluació de Tecnologies i Recerca Mèdiques (AATRM) 048/13/2000 (15) trials. Although the ACOSOG Z0011 trial had excluded patients undergoing mastectomy, 17% of patients in the AMAROS trial, they were not excluded in IBCSG 23-01, OTOASOR, or AATRM, where 18%, 16%, and 12%, respectively, underwent mastectomy. Therefore, the totality of the data supports the omission of ALND

for people undergoing mastectomy, even if the SLN is positive (1). Controversy continues with regard to the extent of regional nodal radiation in the patient with a positive SLN, as well as the role of surgery when the patient presents with a clinically negative node but is found to have suspicious nodes on radiologic examination. In these patients, management is based on planned surgery, tumor burden in the nodes, and planned adjuvant therapy.

Role of Sentinel Node Biopsy Following Neoadjuvant Systemic Therapy for Node-Positive Patients

Sentinel node biopsy followed by axillary dissection in clinically node-negative patients undergoing NACT was studied in the NSABP B-27 trial and has been found to be reliable with a sentinel node identification rate of 85% and a false-negative rate of 11% (16). In contemporary meta-analyses, the false-negative rate for SLNB after NACT was as low as 6% to 8% (17,18). Hence, the performance of sentinel node biopsy before NACT is not recommended if the patient is clinically and radiologically node negative. If suspicious nodes are identified before initiation of NACT, a biopsy of these nodes can be performed percutaneously (either FNA or CNB) to determine nodal status.

NACT is used to facilitate breast conservation and potentially de-escalate axillary surgery; 30% to 40% of patients undergoing NACT will have complete eradication of the nodal disease. Three prospective clinical studies ACOSOG Z1071 (19), SENTINA (20), and SN FNAC (21) have elucidated the role of SLNB after NACT. In the ACOSOG Z1071 trial, all patients with biopsy-proven axillary metastasis underwent NACT, followed by SLNB with immediate ALND (19). The false-negative rate for SLNB was 12.6% but decreased with the use of dual tracers and clipping of the node at the time of initial biopsy (targeted axillary surgery). In 7% of patients, the sentinel node could not be identified. Similarly, the false-negative rate was 14% in the SENTINA trial (20) and 8.4% to 13.3% in the SN FNAC trial (21).

Modalities to decrease this false-negative rate are under investigation, but the current recommendation is the use of dual tracers and identification of two to three nodes with removal of the previously biopsied node. A concern raised by these trials was the risk of nodal recurrence among patients converted from node positive to node negative who did not undergo an axillary dissection and to address this; most were offered axillary radiation. For women with persistently positive sentinel nodes, a sign of chemoresistant disease, an axillary dissection is still recommended. However, axillary recurrences appear to happen rarely. This was shown in one single tertiary center study that included 610 patients undergoing NACT for cN1 disease. They reported that 91% converted to cN0 and underwent SLNB. Of these, 234 (42%) patients had three negative sentinel nodes and did not undergo any further axillary surgery, 88% received adjuvant radiation, and no axillary recurrences were seen in these patients (22).

While the role of NACT in de-escalating axillary surgery continues to be studied, the role of NAET in patients presenting with one to two positive nodes is also starting to be better defined. In one study, omission of axillary dissection or radiation on women with low-volume axillary nodal disease after NAET was not associated with nodal recurrence (23). These questions will be further answered by ongoing clinical trials.

Inflammatory Breast Cancer

SLNB is not recommended for patients with IBC. It is postulated that obstruction of the dermal lymphatics by cancer results in abnormal patterns of lymphatic flow and may result in a high false-negative rate of 18% to 25%. It has also been noted that over 80% of patients with IBC who do not map to a sentinel node had residual nodal disease. A 2018 feasibility study included 16 women with IBC who underwent post-NACT SLNB followed by ALND (24). It demonstrated that the sentinel node could only be identified in four of 16 patients and supports the recommendation for continued axillary dissection in these patients (25). The accepted indications for ALND are provided in **Table 11.7-1**.

■ TABLE 11.7-1. Indications for Axillary Lymph Node Dissection (ALND)

Inflammatory breast cancer
Clinical stage T4 breast cancer
Failed sentinel node mapping during surgery (relative indication in the era of Oncotype Dx)
Axillary recurrence after prior breast cancer treatment

Sentinel Node Biopsy in Patients With Ductal Carcinoma In Situ

Traditionally, patients at high risk of having invasive cancer on excision, including those with high-risk or large lesions and patients with DCIS presenting with a palpable mass, underwent SLNB at the time of their primary breast surgery. Recent studies have demonstrated the low risk of sentinel node positivity and an upgrade to an invasive cancer with the use of larger biopsy samples. A study from the European Institute of Oncology Study that included 854 patients undergoing SLNB for pure DCIS without evidence of microinvasion on pathologic examination found a 1.9% rate of SLN positivity (26). The authors reported that the sentinel node was found to be the only positive node if an axillary dissection was performed. In another study based on data from the National Cancer Database, 18% of women with DCIS undergoing BCS had SLNB, and of these, metastatic nodes were seen in only 0.9% women (27). Similarly in a UK study of 26,696 women with screen detected DCIS on core biopsy, 21% were upgraded to invasive cancer on excision; and of these women, 12% had positive nodes (28). For women with a final pathology result of DCIS, positive sentinel nodes were identified only in 0.2%. Results such as these have led to a "Do Not Do" recommendation by the United Kingdom's National Institute for Health and Care of Excellence (NICE) (29). Similarly, a Danish population-based study demonstrated that in patients with DCIS undergoing SLNB, 94.5% were pN0, 3% were pN1mic and 2.5% were pN1a (30). Patients undergoing mastectomy were more likely to be SLN positive than those undergoing breast conservation (7% vs 3.5%, nonsignificant). The upgrade rate from DCIS to invasive cancer was 16.7%. In conclusion, the authors suggest that SLNB only be performed in patients with DCIS undergoing mastectomy. If breast-conserving resection demonstrated invasive cancer, an SLNB can be performed as a second procedure.

Patients With Ductal Carcinoma In Situ Undergoing Contralateral Prophylactic Mastectomy

The rate of occult breast cancer diagnosed at the time of CPM is 3% to 5%, of which half are DCIS. Modeled data suggest that 73 SLNs were required to avoid one ALND postmastectomy and that the complications per breast cancer detected are higher with routine SLNB as compared to directed ALND, unless the risk of occult breast cancer approaches 28%, at which point it is equal (31). When preoperative MRI was used before CPM in a single-institution study, four (1%) of 393 patients undergoing routine SLNB were spared ALND. In this study, all patients with occult cancer had an abnormal MRI (32). Although data do not support routine use of SLNB in CPM, the risk should be discussed with patients at risk of contralateral axillary metastases, for example, patients with a germline mutation in a breast cancer susceptibility gene.

Sentinel Node Biopsy in Older Patients: The Choosing Wisely Campaign

Although the incidence of breast cancer in women older than 65 years is increasing, the rate of nodal positivity decreases, and most older women will have early-stage HR-positive cancer. The CALGB 9343 study was designed to test the hypothesis that women over 70 years could forgo radiation after BCS (33). In this trial, 60% of volunteers did not have nodal evaluation, and at 10-year follow-up, the axillary recurrence rate was 3% in women treated with TAM and 0% in the TAM and XRT group, suggesting that nodal evaluation was not necessary. Other prospective randomized trials have demonstrated that the omission of axillary surgery in older women treated with ET is safe and that these women have equivalent disease-specific mortality with or without axillary surgery (34,35). The omission of axillary staging is supported by the SSO as part of its Choosing Wisely campaign (36), although it may be useful

■ **TABLE 11.7-2. Scenarios Where Axillary Staging Can Be Omitted**

TABLE 11.7-2. Scenarios Where Axillary Staging Can Be Omitted
DCIS treated with lumpectomy
Contralateral prophylactic mastectomy
Patients >70 years with early-stage ER (+), HER2-negative breast cancer

DCIS, ductal carcinoma in situ; ER, estrogen receptor.

if it will impact decision-making for chemotherapy or radiation. **Table 11.7-2** provides scenarios where axillary evaluation (SLNB or ALND) can be omitted (37).

TECHNIQUE OF AXILLARY LYMPH NODE DISSECTION

In the United States, standard practice for ALND requires removal of level I and level II LNs. Level I is defined as nodal tissue lateral to the pectoralis minor muscle, and level II is defined as nodal tissue posterior to the pectoralis minor muscle. Level III nodes (nodal tissue medial to the pectoralis minor muscle) are generally not included in the dissection owing to increased morbidity. Retrieval of level III nodes requires transection of the pectoralis minor muscle. Interpectoral nodes (Rotter nodes) should be removed if suspicious. At minimum, 10 nodes should be retrieved during the procedure. The axilla is bounded by the axillary vein superiorly, the serratus anterior muscle medially, the LD muscle laterally, the subscapularis muscle posteriorly, and the clavipectoral fascia anteriorly. The thoracodorsal nerve to the latissimus muscle and the long thoracic nerve to the serratus anterior muscle are preserved. Preservation of the main trunk of the intercostobrachial nerve decreases the risk of arm paresthesia. The risk of lymphedema with axillary dissection ranges from 6% to 50% and increases with increased BMI and receipt of regional nodal radiation in addition to axillary dissection (38,39).

Sentinel Lymph Node Biopsy

The SLNB is performed using radioactive colloid material (technetium 99), blue dye (methylene blue or lymphazurin blue), or a combination of both radioactive and blue dyes. Using dual-tracer techniques increases the identification rate of sentinel nodes to 95% to 99%. The SLN identification rate with a periareolar/subareolar injection of the radiocolloid and blue dye injection is higher than that with a peritumoral injection (40). The radioactive colloid is typically injected in the nuclear medicine department, and a lymphoscintigram, which shows the lymphatic drainage pattern of the tumor, is obtained. Because in the majority of patients, drainage is seen in the ipsilateral axilla, it has been recommended that the radioactive isotope can be injected reliably after the induction of anesthesia with avoidance of preoperative lymphoscintigraphy (41). During the surgery, a separate axillary incision is made to perform the procedure. The axilla is interrogated with a handheld gamma probe to identify sentinel node(s). The sentinel node can be "hot," "blue," or "hot and blue." Each sentinel node is excised and counted over 10 seconds. For SLN identification with radioactivity, nodes with counts greater than 10% of the most radioactive node are excised. If blue dye is used, any blue node or node with an adjacent, blue-stained lymphatic is a sentinel node. Before completion of the procedure, the axilla is palpated for any grossly abnormal nodes, as false negativity can occur when nodes are replaced by tumor.

Patients undergoing SLNB have lymphedema incidence as high as 8% and other associated morbidities, such as chronic pain (15%-56%), loss of strength (5%-35%), and axillary web syndrome (12%-20%) (42). Newer anatomic descriptions of the axilla by Clough and Li divide the axilla into zones based on the relationship

of the sentinel node to the lateral thoracic vein and second intercostobrachial nerve, with the goal of decreasing the disruption of the arm lymphatics and potentially decreasing arm lymphedema following axillary surgery for breast cancer (43,44) Clough et al divided the axilla into four zones, separated by the lateral thoracic vein and the second intercostal brachial nerve (44). In this scheme, in 242 patients with stage I/II breast cancer, the sentinel node was identified medial to the vein at 98.2% of the time, usually below the nerve (86.8%). The upper lateral zone, adjacent to the lymphatic drainage of the arm, never contained the sentinel node. The procedure of axillary reverse mapping (ARM) uses the injection of blue dye into the upper arm while injecting radioactive dye into the breast and thus hoping to avoid injury to the lymphatics of the arm (45). However, in 0% to 28% of cases, the axillary node draining the arm is also the sentinel node and cannot be spared owing to oncologic concerns.

Intraoperative identification of the arm nodes and lymphatics also allows for a Lymphatic Microsurgical Preventive Healing Approach (LYMPHA)—which aims to decrease lymphedema by creating a bypass to restore lymphatic flow. In a recent analysis of published data, it is noted that the addition of LYMPHA decreased the rate of lymphedema from 33.4% for patients undergoing ALND and regional nodal radiation to 10%; and for those patients undergoing axillary dissection alone, the lymphedema rate decreased from 14.1% to 2.1% with the addition of LYMPHA (46). While lymphatic mapping to the internal mammary (IM) chain has been performed, its impact on outcome remains unclear (47).

Intraoperative assessment of SLNs using touch imprints and routine IHC staining can be used to enable an immediate therapeutic lymphadenectomy if indicated, thus sparing the patient from a second procedure. However, intraoperative assessment may have unacceptable rates of false-negative results, ranging from 36% to 71% (48). Intraoperative assessment of the SLN has been largely abandoned in clinically node-negative patients undergoing upfront sentinel node biopsy.

Future Directions on Lymphatic Surgery

In addition to prevention of lymphedema by lymphatic venous bypass, other modalities include limiting the role of nodal evaluation in personalizing management of breast cancer. These include assessing the role of biologic factors such as grade, receptor status, and Oncotype Dx RS as evidenced by the AJCC eighth edition staging. This is paralleled by decreasing tumor size at diagnosis and decreasing SLN positivity rate to 13% to 17% (49). The omission of axillary staging is being studied in multiple randomized trials, and results should help more selectively approach people with breast cancer in an individualized manner.

REFERENCES

1. Mittendorf EA, Bellon JR, King TA. Regional nodal management in patients with clinically node-negative breast cancer undergoing upfront surgery. *J Clin Oncol.* 2020;38:2273-2280.

2. Giuliano AE, Hunt KK, Ballman KV, et al. Axillary dissection vs no axillary dissection in women with invasive breast cancer and sentinel node metastasis: a randomized clinical trial. *JAMA.* 2011;305:569-575.

3. Giuliano AE, Haigh PI, Brennan MB, et al. Prospective observational study of sentinel lymphadenectomy without further axillary dissection in patients with sentinel node-negative breast cancer. *J Clin Oncol.* 2000;18:2553-2559.

4. Veronesi U, Paganelli G, Viale G, et al. A randomized comparison of sentinel-node biopsy with routine axillary dissection in breast cancer. *N Engl J Med.* 2003;349:546-553.

5. Krag DN, Anderson SJ, Julian TB, et al. Sentinel-lymph-node resection compared with conventional axillary-lymph-node dissection in clinically node-negative patients with breast cancer: overall survival findings from the NSABP B-32 randomised phase 3 trial. *Lancet Oncol.* 2010;11:927-933.

6. Julian TB, Anderson SJ, Krag DN, et al. 10-yr follow-up results of NSABP B-32, a randomized phase III clinical trial to compare sentinel

node resection (SNR) to conventional axillary dissection (AD) in clinically node-negative breast cancer patients. *J Clin Oncol.* 2013;31:1000.

7. Brackstone M, Baldassarre FG, Perera FE, et al. Management of the axilla in early-stage breast cancer: Ontario health (Cancer Care Ontario) and ASCO guideline. *J Clin Oncol.* 2021;39:3056-3082.

8. Fisher B, Jeong JH, Anderson S, Bryant J, Fisher ER, Wolmark N. Twenty-five-year follow-up of a randomized trial comparing radical mastectomy, total mastectomy, and total mastectomy followed by irradiation. *N Engl J Med.* 2002;347:567-575.

9. Giuliano AE, Ballman K, McCall L, et al. Locoregional recurrence after sentinel lymph node dissection with or without axillary dissection in patients with sentinel lymph node metastases: long-term follow-up from the American College of Surgeons Oncology Group (Alliance) ACOSOG Z0011 randomized trial. *Ann Surg.* 2016;264:413-420.

10. Giuliano AE, Ballman KV, McCall L, et al. Effect of axillary dissection vs no axillary dissection on 10-year overall survival among women with invasive breast cancer and sentinel node metastasis: the ACOSOG Z0011 (Alliance) randomized clinical trial. *JAMA.* 2017;318:918-926.

11. Galimberti V, Cole BF, Zurrida S, et al. Axillary dissection versus no axillary dissection in patients with sentinel-node micrometastases (IBCSG 23-01): a phase 3 randomised controlled trial. *Lancet Oncol.* 2013;14:297-305.

12. Galimberti V, Cole BF, Viale G, et al. Axillary dissection versus no axillary dissection in patients with breast cancer and sentinel-node micrometastases (IBCSG 23-01): 10-year follow-up of a randomised, controlled phase 3 trial. *Lancet Oncol.* 2018;19:1385-1393.

13. Donker M, van Tienhoven G, Straver ME, et al. Radiotherapy or surgery of the axilla after a positive sentinel node in breast cancer (EORTC 10981-22023 AMAROS): a randomised, multicentre, open-label, phase 3 non-inferiority trial. *Lancet Oncol.* 2014;15:1303-1310.

14. Sávolt Á, Péley G, Polgár C, et al. Eight-year follow up result of the OTOASOR trial: the optimal treatment of the Axilla—Surgery or Radiotherapy after positive sentinel lymph node biopsy in early-stage breast cancer: a randomized, single centre, phase III, non-inferiority trial. *Eur J Surg Oncol.* 2017;43:672-679.

15. Solá M, Alberro JA, Fraile M, et al. Complete axillary lymph node dissection versus clinical follow-up in breast cancer patients with sentinel node micrometastasis: final results from the multicenter clinical trial AATRM 048/13/2000. *Ann Surg Oncol.* 2013;20:120-127.

16. Mamounas EP, Brown A, Anderson S, et al. Sentinel node biopsy after neoadjuvant chemotherapy in breast cancer: results from national surgical adjuvant breast and bowel project Protocol B-27. *J Clin Oncol.* 2005;23:2694-2702.

17. Kelly AM, Dwamena B, Cronin P, Carlos RC. Breast cancer sentinel node identification and classification after neoadjuvant chemotherapy-systematic review and meta analysis. *Acad Radiol.* 2009;16:551-563.

18. Geng C, Chen X, Pan X, Li J. The feasibility and accuracy of sentinel lymph node biopsy in initially clinically node-negative breast cancer after neoadjuvant chemotherapy: a systematic review and meta-analysis. *PloS One.* 2016;11:e0162605.

19. Boughey JC, Suman VJ, Mittendorf EA, et al. Sentinel lymph node surgery after neoadjuvant chemotherapy in patients with node-positive breast cancer: the ACOSOG Z1071 (Alliance) clinical trial. *JAMA.* 2013;310:1455-1461.

20. Schwentner L, Helms G, Nekljudova V, et al. Using ultrasound and palpation for predicting axillary lymph node status following neoadjuvant chemotherapy—results from the multi-center SENTINA trial. *Breast.* 2017;31:202-207.

21. Boileau JF, Poirier B, Basik M, et al. Sentinel node biopsy after neoadjuvant chemotherapy in biopsy-proven node-positive breast cancer: the SN FNAC study. *J Clin Oncol.* 2015;33:258-264.

22. Barrio AV, Montagna G, Mamtani A, et al. Nodal recurrence in patients with node-positive breast cancer treated with sentinel node biopsy alone after neoadjuvant chemotherapy—a rare event. *JAMA Oncol.* 2021;7:1851-1855.

23. Murphy BM, Hoskin TL, Degnim AC, Boughey JC, Hieken TJ. Surgical management of axilla following neoadjuvant endocrine therapy. *Ann Surg Oncol.* 2021;28:8729-8739.

24. DeSnyder SM, Mittendorf EA, Le-Petross C, et al. Prospective feasibility trial of sentinel lymph node biopsy in the setting of inflammatory breast cancer. *Clin Breast Cancer.* 2018;18:e73-e77.

25. American Society of Breast Surgeons. Consensus guideline on axillary management for patients with in-situ and invasive breast cancer: a concise overview. 2022. https://www.breastsurgeons.org/docs/statements/Consensus-Guideline-on-the-Management-of-the-Axilla-Concise-Overview.pdf

26. Intra M, Rotmensz N, Veronesi P, et al. Sentinel node biopsy is not a standard procedure in ductal carcinoma in situ of the breast: the experience of the European institute of oncology on 854 patients in 10 years. *Ann Surg.* 2008;247:315-319.

27. James TA, Palis B, McCabe R, et al. Evaluating the role of sentinel lymph node biopsy in patients with DCIS treated with breast conserving surgery. *Am J Surg.* 2020;220:654-659.

28. Nicholson S, Hanby A, Clements K, et al. Variations in the management of the axilla in screen-detected ductal carcinoma in situ: evidence from the UK NHS breast screening programme audit of screen detected DCIS. *Eur J Surg Oncol.* 2015;41:86-93.

29. National Institute for Health and Care Excellence. Early and locally advanced breast cancer. 2009. https://www.nice.org.uk/guidance/ng101/chapter/Recommendations#surgery-to-the-axilla

30. van Roozendaal LM, Goorts B, Klinkert M, et al. Sentinel lymph node biopsy can be omitted in DCIS patients treated with breast conserving therapy. *Breast Cancer Res Treat.* 2016;156:517-525.

31. Boughey JC, Cormier JN, Xing Y, et al. Decision analysis to assess the efficacy of routine sentinel lymphadenectomy in patients undergoing prophylactic mastectomy. *Cancer.* 2007;110:2542-2550.

32. McLaughlin SA, Stempel M, Morris EA, Liberman L, King TA. Can magnetic resonance imaging be used to select patients for sentinel lymph node biopsy in prophylactic mastectomy? *Cancer.* 2008;112:1214-1221.

33. Hughes KS, Schnaper LA, Berry D, et al. Lumpectomy plus tamoxifen with or without irradiation in women 70 years of age or older with early breast cancer. *N Engl J Med.* 2004;351:971-977.

34. International Breast Cancer Study Group, Rudenstam CM, Zahrieh D, et al. Randomized trial comparing axillary clearance versus no axillary clearance in older patients with breast cancer: first results of International Breast Cancer Study Group trial 10-93. *J Clin Oncol.* 2006;24:337-344.

35. Martelli G, Boracchi P, Ardoino I, et al. Axillary dissection versus no axillary dissection in older patients with T1N0 breast cancer: 15-year results of a randomized controlled trial. *Ann Surg.* 2012;256:920-924.

36. Society of Surgical Oncology. Choosing wisely. Don't routinely use sentinel node biopsy in clinically node negative women ≥70 years of age with early stage hormone receptor positive, HER2 negative invasive breast cancer. 2016. https://www.choosingwisely.org/clinician-lists/sso-sentinel-node-biopsy-in-node-negative-women-70-and-over/

37. Hersh EH, King TA. De-escalating axillary surgery in early-stage breast cancer. *Breast.* 2022;62(Suppl 1):S43-S49.

38. Petrek JA, Heelan MC. Incidence of breast carcinoma-related lymphedema. *Cancer.* 1998;83:2776-2781.

39. Petrek JA, Senie RT, Peters M, Rosen PP. Lymphedema in a cohort of breast carcinoma survivors 20 years after diagnosis. *Cancer.* 2001;92:1368-1377.

40. Chagpar A, Martin RC 3rd, Chao C, et al. Validation of subareolar and periareolar injection techniques for breast sentinel lymph node biopsy. *Arch Surg.* 2004;139:614-618; discussion 618-620.

41. Johnson CB, Boneti C, Korourian S, Adkins L, Klimberg VS. Intraoperative injection of subareolar or dermal radioisotope results in predictable identification of sentinel lymph nodes in breast cancer. *Ann Surg.* 2011;254:612-618.

42. Verbelen H, Gebruers N, Eeckhout FM, Verlinden K, Tjalma W. Shoulder and arm morbidity in sentinel node-negative breast cancer patients: a systematic review. *Breast Cancer Res Treat.* 2014;144:21-31.

43. Li J, Zhang Y, Zhang W, et al. Intercostobrachial nerves as a novel anatomic landmark for dividing the axillary space in lymph node dissection. *ISRN Oncol.* 2013;2013:279013.

44. Clough KB, Nasr R, Nos C, Vieira M, Inguenault C, Poulet B. New anatomical classification of the axilla with implications for sentinel node biopsy. *Br J Surg.* 2010;97:1659-1665.

45. Thompson M, Korourian S, Henry-Tillman R, et al. Axillary Reverse Mapping (ARM): a new concept to identify and enhance lymphatic preservation. *Ann Surg Oncol.* 2007;14:1890-1895.

46. Johnson AR, Kimball S, Epstein S, et al. Lymphedema incidence after axillary lymph node dissection: quantifying the impact of radiation and the lymphatic microsurgical preventive healing approach. *Ann Plast Surg.* 2019;82:S234-S241.

47. Caudle AS, Smith BD. Do internal mammary nodes matter? *Ann Surg Oncol.* 2019;26:930-932.

48. Van Diest PJ, Torrenga H, Borgstein PJ, et al. Reliability of intraoperative frozen section and imprint cytological investigation of sentinel lymph nodes in breast cancer. *Histopathology.* 1999;35:14-18.

49. Magnoni F, Galimberti V, Corso G, Intra M, Sacchini V, Veronesi P. Axillary surgery in breast cancer: an updated historical perspective. *Semin Oncol.* 2020;47:341-352.

CHAPTER **11.8**

Endocrine Therapy for Breast Cancer

Mary Anne Fenton

Approximately 70% of breast cancers are HR+ (1), and treatments that target the ER pathway are a mainstay of treatment. These agents act by various means, including the suppression of estrogen production (gonadotropin-releasing hormone [GnRH] analogs), inhibition of the conversion of peripheral estrogen from androgens (AIs), competitive binding to the ER (selective estrogen receptor modulators [SERMs]), or degradation of the ER (selective estrogen receptor downregulators) (Table 11.8-1).

Estrogen, a steroid hormone, is a transcription factor that binds to intracellular ERs in the form of estradiol, which activates a conformational change and initiates estradiol-dependent gene transcription through interactions with coactivators and corepressors of cell proliferation and differentiation pathways (2). The ASCO/CAP guidelines define breast cancer as ER+ and PR+ with 1% to 100% tumor nuclei positivity by validated IHC testing (3). While ER tumor expression is prognostic for recurrence and survival and predictive of response to ET, PR is primarily prognostic. Of note, 2% to 3% of all breast cancers are ER low, with 1% to 10% tumor nuclei ER staining, and whereas ET is typically recommended, the benefits of treatment are likely not as significant compared to those that have higher levels of ER expression (4).

In DCIS, ER positivity is predictive of a benefit to treatment as chemoprevention—with reductions in the risk of recurrence (for DCIS or as an invasive breast cancer) and on new primary breast cancer events; it has no impact on OS (5). The Early Breast Cancer Trialist' Collaborative Group (EBCTCG) meta-analysis of patient-level data, with long-term follow-up, addresses therapeutic benefits of cancer therapies. These analyses consistently affirm that antiestrogen therapy reduces breast cancer recurrence by up to 50% and breast cancer mortality by 31% for HR+ breast cancer (6).

ENDOCRINE THERAPY FOR NEWLY DIAGNOSED HORMONE RECEPTOR–POSITIVE DISEASE

Omitting Chemotherapy for People With HR+ Disease: Role of Genomic Expression Profiling

GEP divides HR+ HER2-negative breast cancer into intrinsic subtype, prognostic of systemic recurrence and predictive of response to chemotherapy (7). The luminal A subtype, when described using traditional IHC features, typically has a high ER/PR, low grade, and low Ki-67 proliferation index and, in clinical setting, is associated with high disease control with adjuvant ET alone. In contrast, luminal B breast cancer is typically high grade, relatively high Ki-67 proliferation index, and has low ER/PR expression by IHC (8). GEPs validated for HR+ HER2-negative breast cancer for prognosis include the Amsterdam 70-gene prognostic profile and the 21-gene RS assay (9,10); another that uses a 50-gene signature requires further clinical validation (11).

The Trial Assigning Individualized Options for Treatment (TAILORx) was a seminal phase III trial of 6,711 surgically staged volunteers with HR+ HER2-negative node-negative breast cancer (stage pT1-2pN0) (10,12). Treatments were stratified based on the RS: for those with RS 10 or less received ET, those with RS over 25 received chemotherapy, and those with RS 11 to 25 were randomly assigned to ET or chemotherapy. Volunteers over age 50 with RS 25 or less and those aged 50 years or below with RS 15 or less had no additional benefit in invasive disease-free survival (IDFS), distant relapse-free survival (DRFS), and OS, with the addition of

TABLE 11.8-1. Endocrine Therapy Agents Used in the Treatment of ER+ Breast Cancer

Type	Chemoprevention	Adjuvant or Neoadjuvant	Metastatic
Selective estrogen receptor modulator	Tamoxifen		
Aromatase inhibitor (steroidal)	Exemestane		
Aromatase inhibitor (nonsteroidal)	Anastrozole Letrozole		
GnRH analogs		Leuprorelin Goserelin Triptorelin	
CDK4/6 inhibitors (used in combination with ET)		Abemaciclib	Abemaciclib Ribociclib Palbociclib
Selective estrogen receptor downregulators			Fulvestrant

ER, estrogen receptor; ET, endocrine therapy; GnRH, gonadotropin-releasing hormone agonist.

■ TABLE 11.8-2. Randomized Trials of Genome Expression Profiles in HR+ HER2-Negative Breast Cancer

	Main outcome: 9-y Distant Recurrence-Free Rate (DRF)				
Trial (n)	Patient Group	Treatment	9-y DRF (%)		
TAILORx (10) (9,719)	Low risk (RS ≤10)	ET	96.8		
	Intermediate risk (RS 11-25)	ET vs ET + chemotherapy	94.5 95.0	Age <50, RS 11-15	93 94
				Age <50, RS 16-20	93 95
				Age <50, RS 21-25	82 90
	High risk (RS ≥26)	ET + chemotherapy	86.8		
RxPONDER (13) (5,018, N1 disease, RS ≤25)	Main outcome: 5-y Invasive Disease-Free Survival				
	ET vs ET + chemotherapy	Premenopause: 89% vs 94%		Postmenopause: 92% vs 91%	
MINDACT (9,14) (6,693, Clinical risk based on Adjuvant! Online; Genomic risk based on 70-gene signature)	5-y Distant Metastasis-Free Survival (%)				
	High clinical/low genomic risk	ET vs ET + chemotherapy	94 96		
	Low clinical/high genomic risk		95 96		

ET, endocrine therapy; RS, Recurrence Score.

chemotherapy to ET. In contrast, volunteers aged 50 years or below with an RS 16 to 20 or 21 to 25 had a significant improvement in distant disease-free survival (DDFS) with chemotherapy followed by ET. At 9 years, the improvement was 1.6% for RS 16 to 20 and 6.5% for RS 21 to 25. How clinically meaningful these reductions in DDFS are for patients has been called into question, as well as how much of the benefit is related to ovarian function suppression (OFS) from chemotherapy. As such, for patients aged 50 years or below with RS between 16 and 25, we recommend engaging in shared decision-making.

The subsequent prospective phase III Clinical Trial RX for Positive Node, Endocrine Responsive Breast Cancer (RxPONDER) addressed the question of chemotherapy benefit for HR+ HER2 negative with one to three positive axillary LNs after surgical staging (stage N1). Volunteers with an RS 0 to 25 were randomly assigned either ET alone or ET and chemotherapy combined (13). In volunteers over age 50, there was no benefit in the addition of adjuvant chemotherapy to ET. In patients aged 50 years or less, IDFS at 5 years was 93.9% with chemotherapy followed by ET compared to 89% with ET alone (HR 0.60, 95% CI 0.43-0.83).

Finally, the MINDACT trial enrolled over 6,000 women with early-stage breast cancer who were assigned a risk profile based on clinical risk (using an online risk calculator) and genomic risk (using a 70-gene expression profile). For this trial, those with low clinical/low genomic risk (41%) were treated with ET only; those with high clinical/high genomic risk (27%) were treated with chemotherapy and ET; those with discordant results were randomly assigned to ET with or without adjuvant chemotherapy. Among those with high clinical/low genomic risk, compared to no adjuvant chemotherapy, chemotherapy was associated with a slightly improved 5-year survival rate without distant metastases (5yDMFR, 95.9% vs 94.4%; HR 0.78, 95% CI 0.50-1.21). Among those with low clinical/high genomic risk, the 5yDMFR was 95.8% versus 95% (HR 1.17, 95% CI 0.59-2.28) (9). These results were confirmed with 9-year follow-up, although it suggested that women under 50 years may have a clinically significant advantage with chemotherapy if they had high clinical/low genomic risk (8yDMFR, 93.6% vs 88.6%) without chemotherapy (9). Of note, an updated analysis profiled those with an ultralow-risk 70-gene signature (n = 1,000), 14% who

received chemotherapy plus ET. The 8yDMFR was 97%, and breast cancer–specific survival was 99.6% (14). These trials are summarized in Table 11.8-2.

The lack of consistent benefits for adjuvant chemotherapy by age may reflect a more aggressive phenotype in younger patients that is not captured in current GEPs, the weighted benefit of chemotherapy-induced ovarian suppression on outcomes, or perhaps, the decreased efficacy of ET. Of note, in The Suppression of Ovarian Function Trial (SOFT), the addition of OFS to ET among patients receiving both OFS and chemotherapy, OFS plus chemotherapy reduced recurrence further compared to OFS plus ET alone, which may reflect the patients' clinical risk. It remains unclear if OFS can replace chemotherapy.

AGENTS AND THE DURATION OF TREATMENT IN THE ADJUVANT SETTING

Adjuvant ET for 5 years reduces the risk of local recurrence, new primary breast cancer, systemic recurrence, and mortality from breast cancer. The EBCTCG meta-analysis reported that the proportional benefit of ET is constant between breast cancer stages and that although the absolute benefit fluctuates based on the estimated risk of systemic recurrence, the reduction in recurrence lasts out to 15 years (4). For people with node-negative HR+ disease, the risk of systemic recurrence at 10 years approximates 34.8%. With TAM treatment for 5 years, the risk of systemic recurrence is 19.1% at 10 years, translating into an absolute risk reduction of 15%. For people with node-positive disease, the benefits of ET are larger because they have a higher risk of systemic recurrence.

TAM, an SERM, was the first adjuvant ET shown in randomized clinical trials to reduce systemic recurrence, CBC, and mortality from breast cancer (6). TAM has differential effects on various tissues, through competitive binding to the ER. TAM, like estrogen, improves bone mineral density in postmenopausal women, but because it exerts an agonistic effect on endometrial tissue, it may contribute to the development of endometrial polyps, higher rates of postmenopausal bleeding, and rarely, if not addressed, a greater risk of uterine cancer, particularly in postmenopausal women. It is recommended that women on TAM report any menstrual changes, dysfunctional uterine bleeding, or other symptoms to their gynecologist and medical oncologist; however, routine pelvic USs are not indicated in the absence of symptoms because of its high false-positive rate, which may expose people to more invasive procedures (15). Other potential side effects of TAM include hot flashes, weight gain, mood changes, increased vaginal discharge, cataracts, and, rarely, retinal abnormalities. The EBCTCG meta-analysis also reported a slight numeric increase in mortality from pulmonary emboli associated with TAM (4). Because TAM can increase ovarian stimulation, premenopausal women should be prescribed appropriate contraception, as it is possible to become pregnant. Of note, TAM is considered a teratogen, and it should not be taken if one is breastfeeding.

Seminal-extended ET trials have completed accrual (**Table 11.8-3**). In the NCI of Canada-led MA.17 trial, TAM followed by letrozole significantly improved DFS compared to TAM alone (93% vs 87%, $P \le .001$) and was associated with an improvement in OS (96% vs 93.6%, $P = .25$) (16). In the Adjuvant Tamoxifen: Longer Against Shorter (ATLAS) trial, among volunteers receiving TAM for 10 years, there was a significant reduction in recurrence of 18% versus 20.8% with 5 years (RR 0.84) and breast cancer mortality of 9.7% versus 11.5% (17). The Adjuvant Tamoxifen Treatment Offer More (aTTom) trial was of similar study design to ATLAS, and results were presented in abstract form, showing that compared to 5 years, 10 years of TAM reduced breast cancer recurrence and mortality (18). The TAM extension trial long-term follow-up is of particular interest for global breast cancer specialists, particularly where access to AI treatment is limited.

There are several other extension trials of TAM followed by AI. In the Extended Adjuvant Aromatase Inhibition after Sequential Endocrine Therapy (DATA), HR+ postmenopausal volunteers who completed 5 years of ET were randomly assigned to an additional 3 to 6 years; compared to an additional 3 years, there was no benefit in DFS to 6 years of treatment (19). Similar findings were noted in the Investigation on the Duration of Extended Letrozole (IDEAL) trial; after 5 years of ET, volunteers were randomly assigned to 2.5 or 5 years of letrozole, and no difference in DFS was observed (20). The Secondary Adjuvant Long-Term Study with Anastrozole (SALSA) was conducted by the Austrian Breast and Colorectal Cancer Study Group as a prospective phase III trial of postmenopausal HR+ stages I-III patients who completed 5 years of ET (TAM 51%, AI 7.3%, or both 41.7%) and evaluated extended treatment for 2 versus 5 years (21). At a median follow-up of 10 years, patients on longer duration therapy had a higher risk of bone fractures (HR 1.35), and there was no difference in DFS or OS reported. The Italian GIM4 phase III trial of HR+ postmenopausal stages I-III volunteers who completed 2 to 3 years of TAM were randomized to 2 to 3 years further of letrozole (total, 5 years; control group) or 5 years of extended therapy (total, 10 years) (22). At 12 years of follow-up, a significant improved DFS was seen in

extended therapy, with DFS 67% for 7 years of ET compared with 62% for 5 years of therapy (HR 0.78, 95% CI 0.65-0.93). Of note, ET discontinuation was 19% in the control and 37% in the extended therapy arm, with the main reasons for drug discontinuation being arthralgias/myalgias.

AIs prevent conversion of androgens, such as androstenedione to estrogens, by the enzyme aromatase. The resulting decrease in circulating estrogen is effective treatment for HR+ breast cancer in postmenopausal women. Compared to TAM, the AIs provide additional reduction in recurrence and mortality with a greater benefit in higher stage breast cancer. Of the three commercially available AIs, anastrozole and letrozole are nonsteroidal, and exemestane is steroidal. However, there are no demonstrable differences in efficacy or toxicity between them. Toxicities of AIs commonly include hot flashes, joint or muscle aches, vaginal dryness, elevation of cholesterol, hair thinning, accelerated loss of bone density, sexual dysfunction, and possible cardiac events. In a large adjuvant trial, the most common reason for patients to stop AIs was arthralgias described in studies as AI-associated musculoskeletal syndrome (AIMSS), management strategies of AIMSS, and other side effects, which are discussed in the survivorship section of this chapter. Informed decision-making is necessary to tailor a treatment approach for the individual patient (23)

Nonadherence to adjuvant ET is common, and this appears to be associated with an increased risk of systemic recurrence. The BIG 1-98 was a large international four-arm double-blind phase III trial of 5 years total of ET for HR+ postmenopausal patients consisting of either TAM alone, letrozole alone, TAM for 2.5 years followed by letrozole for 2.5 years, or letrozole for 2.5 years followed by TAM for 2.5 years (24). Less than 90% adherence to the treatment and early study withdrawal were associated with decreased DFS. This was also demonstrated in the CANTO/NCT01993498 French trial of adjuvant ET trial for HR+ premenopausal stages I-III volunteers prescribed with adjuvant TAM and/or luteinizing hormone-releasing hormone (LHRH) agonist. Serum TAM levels were measured in over 1,000 patients 1 year after prescription, and 16% were noted to have a serum TAM below threshold level, indicating nonadherence (25). At a median follow-up of 2.4 years, this was associated with shorter DDFS compared to those whose blood levels indicated they were taking the drug (HR 2.31, 95% CI 1.05-5.06) corresponding to 89.5% and 95.4% of volunteers alive without a distant recurrence at 3 years in those deemed nonadherent and adherent, respectively.

In population studies, higher nonadherence is noted in younger and minority patients, in part due to the side effects and barriers to care. The Carolina Breast Cancer Study, a longitudinal population study of 2,988 female patients with stages II and III breast cancer, reported that barriers included habit, risk-benefit tradeoff (side effects), and resource barriers (26). Resource barriers were noted to be higher in younger, minority patients, or patients uninsured or on public insurance.

■ TABLE 11.8-3. Seminal Trials of Adjuvant Endocrine Therapy Evaluating Extended Treatment							
Trial	N	Arms	Disease-Free Survival	P-Value	Overall Survival	P-Value	Follow-Up (Years)
MA.17 (55,56)[a]	5,169[b]	T→L	93%	≤0.001	96%	0.25	5.3
		T→P	87%	≤0.001	93.6%	≤0.001	
		HR – 0.52			HR – 0.061		
ATLAS (17)	6,846[c]	T × 5 y	79%	−0.002	79%	−0.01	7.5
		T × 10 y	82%		81%		
aTTom (18)	6,953[d]	T × 5 y	81%	−0.003	73.9%	−0.1	4.2
		T × 10 y	83%		75.5%		

ER, estrogen receptor; L, letrozole; P, placebo; T, tamoxifen.
[a]Adjusted for crossover.
[b]Postmenopausal, ER positive, node positive, and node negative.
[c]Premenopausal, ER positive, node positive, and node negative.
[d]Premenopausal and postmenopausal, ER positive and unknown, node positive, and node negative.

Adjuvant ET counseling should follow the model of patient-centered care to include discussion with patients of risks of recurrence, absolute reduction in recurrence over time, and medication recommendation, including discussion of common and rare side effects. Reassurance that the practitioner is available for ongoing management of side effects and a source of assistance with financial barriers to care should be conveyed. In our practice, patient navigators, social work, and financial counselors screen patients for social determinants of health and distress, including financial distress, and assist patients with insurance and copay issues. All members of the multidisciplinary team (surgery, radiation, medical oncology) discuss at every visit why the patient is prescribed their adjuvant ET and discuss patient concerns and management of side effects.

OVARIAN ABLATION OR SUPPRESSION

Ovarian ablation or ovarian suppression (collectively "ovarian function suppression" [OFS]) is therapeutic option for premenopausal women with higher risk HR+ breast cancer, clinically defined as having received adjuvant chemotherapy. In premenopausal females, the ovaries are the major source for estrogen, and silencing the ovaries via surgical oophorectomy, RT, or the use of a GnRHa analog (goserelin, leuprolide, or triptorelin) may reduce breast cancer recurrence at the cost of an increase in side-effect profile.

The IBCSG coordinated two prospective phase III trials to evaluate the benefit of ovarian suppression in high-risk premenopausal HR+ patients. Patients were considered premenopausal based on biochemical parameters. In the SOFT, volunteers underwent either surgery alone or surgery and chemotherapy combined (physician/patient choice) within 8 months of enrollment, premenopausal status was verified biochemically, and volunteers were assigned to TAM alone, TAM plus OFS, or exemestane plus OFS (27). The Tamoxifen and Exemestane Trial (TEXT) companion study was composed of 2,600 premenopausal volunteers randomly assigned to TAM and OFS or exemestane and OFS following surgery and adjuvant chemotherapy, if indicated (28). In an 8-year analysis of the SOFT, OFS significantly improved DFS (78.9% vs 83.2% with TAM and OFS) and OS (83.2% and 85.9%, $P = .009$) (29). Side effects were higher in OFS groups, including osteoporosis and arthralgias. In the combined SOFT and TEXT 9-year follow-up exemestane and OFS versus TAM and OFS, a 2% absolute improvement over TAM and OFS in DFS was noted for exemestane and OFS (30). The EBCTCG conducted a meta-analysis of four randomized trials, including the SOFT and TEXT that included 7,000 HR+ premenopausal patients on OFS randomized to TAM or AI (31). The 10-year DFS favored the AI treatment, with absolute DFS of 18% versus 15% (RR = 0.79, 95% CI 0.69-0.90).

Young women as a group appear to have a higher risk of breast cancer recurrence and achieve a modest benefit from ovarian suppression and AI therapy to maximally suppress estrogen levels. What is missing in the equation are biomarkers for who is most at risk and who will benefit from maximal endocrine suppression. Risks of endocrine suppression in young women include detriments in their overall quality of life, increased risk of osteoporotic fractures, sexual dysfunction, and early-onset coronary artery disease (32).

CYCLIN-DEPENDENT KINASE INHIBITORS

Dysregulation of the cell cycle by the acquisition of genetic mutations is a common feature of cancer cells, providing a selective growth advantage. Cyclin-dependent kinases (CDKs) have a critical role in regulating cell cycle kinetics. CDK 4 and 6 inhibitors (CDK4/6i) in combination with ET improve PFS and OS in postmenopausal women as well as premenopausal women and men on LHRH agonists with de novo stage IV or metastatic HR+

HER2-negative breast cancer. With the success in the metastatic setting, trials exploring CDK4/6i in early-stage disease were conducted and likely, due to different patient populations, showed varying results.

MonarchE is an open-label phase III trial of over 5,000 volunteers (men and premenopausal and postmenopausal women) who had completed all primary treatment (surgery with or without chemotherapy) and randomly assigned them to adjuvant ET either alone or in combination with abemaciclib (150 mg orally twice daily for 2 years) (33,34). At an interim analysis of 27 months, IDFS at 3 years was 89% versus 83% (HR 0.70, 95% CI 0.59-0.82) and DRFS 90% versus 86% (HR 0.69, 95% CI 0.57-0.83). Longer follow-up is required to assess for an impact on OS. Toxicity of grade 3 or higher adverse event (AE) with abemaciclib (50% vs 16%) was primarily diarrhea. Based on monarchE, abemaciclib is FDA approved for adjuvant therapy in combination with ET in people with high-risk disease, defined as node-positive HR+ HER2-negative breast cancer with Ki-67 20 or higher or those with N1 disease and either size 5 cm or larger, high grade, or four or more positive LNs (35).

Other trials looking at adjuvant CDK4/6i have not shown benefit. The PENELOPE-B trial looked at 1 year of adjuvant palbociclib added to ET after NACT and did not show improved IDFS in volunteers with residual disease after NACT (36). In the PALLAS trial, volunteers were randomly assigned to ET with or without palbociclib for 2 years; there was no improvement in IDFS with the addition of palbociclib (37). Differences in eligibility may have had an impact on these results, although cross-trial comparisons are difficult to justify.

NEOADJUVANT ENDOCRINE THERAPY

NAET is an option for select patients with HR+ HER2-negative postmenopausal patients who otherwise would require mastectomy (38). Clinical trials demonstrate tumor shrinkage by clinical and radiographic examination and breast preservation similar to NACT (39-41). Biomarkers such as high ER expression by IHC (luminal A) predict a clinical response to NAET (42), although pCRs are rare. Clinical response and breast preservation rates are higher with neoadjuvant AI versus TAM (39,40,43).

GEPs, such as the 21-gene RS, are predictive and prognostic of benefit in adjuvant ET, and small retrospective trials of women who are not the candidates for BCS showed that those with the lowest RS were most likely to benefit from NAET (RS 0-11 75%, RS 11-25 57%). Patient selection of NAET versus NACT may be aided by GEP on tumor biopsy specimen. Conversely, patient tumors with high GEP (luminal B) are more likely to respond to NACT (40,42-44).

In our multidisciplinary breast cancer clinic that includes breast surgery, medical oncology, radiation oncology, cancer genetics, navigation, pathology, and radiology with an embedded tumor board, the members discuss NAET for select postmenopausal HR+/HER2− low-grade breast cancer when breast preservation cannot be achieved, and clinical staging suggests low-volume LN disease or LN-negative disease. If NAET is considered, it is our practice to order a GEP on the breast tumor biopsy specimen, such as the 21-gene RS, for an RS 0 to 11, we discuss the option of 4 to 6 months of NAET with an AI, and subsequent BCS if surgically feasible. Following BCS to negative margins and axillary staging, residual disease in the breast is expected and is not an indication for adjuvant chemotherapy. A pCR is not expected and not necessary for BCS, and prognostic value is unknown compared to NACT. Nodal pCR is extremely low at 13%, and ALND is the standard of care for clinically node-positive patients upfront or those with residual nodal disease. We do not recommend NAET with premenopausal patients because of the absence of data. The use of NAET may be expanded during times of crisis, as experienced globally during the COVID-19 pandemic both to optimize patient safety and to improve workflow management (45-47).

ENDOCRINE THERAPY FOR RISK REDUCTION

Risk factors for developing invasive breast cancer include increasing age, family history of breast cancer particularly in first-degree relatives, ADH, LCIS, and DCIS. The Breast Cancer Risk Assessment Tool (modified Gail model) is a useful tool to estimate an individual patient's risk of developing breast cancer. The tool is not designed to assess high-risk groups, such as previous history of invasive breast cancer, DCIS, LCIS, previous chest radiation for Hodgkin lymphoma, personal history of a mutation associated with an elevated risk of breast cancer, or family history concerning for such mutation. The Breast Cancer Risk Assessment Tool consists of patient age, race/ethnicity, age at first menses, age at first live birth, history of benign breast biopsies, and the number of first-degree relatives with breast cancer to identify patients at increased risk for breast cancer. Patients aged 35 years or above with a modified Gail model of 1.7% or more 5-year risk for breast cancer may benefit from pharmacologic therapy with SERMs or AIs.

A meta-analysis of the seminal SERM prevention trials utilizing TAM in normal or higher risk women showed a 38% reduction in the incidence of HR+ invasive breast cancer (48). TAM was compared directly to the SERM raloxifene in the NSABP-P2 prevention trial for high-risk postmenopausal women (49). Raloxifene is less effective than TAM in the prevention of invasive breast cancer (RR 1.24) and similar in reducing the risk of DCIS (RR 1.22). Raloxifene was associated with a reduced incidence of endometrial cancer (RR 0.55) and thromboembolic events (RR 0.75) compared to TAM. Long-term raloxifene retains 76% of the effectiveness of TAM as a chemoprevention drug and, as such, continues to have an important role.

"Low-dose" TAM is a therapeutic option based on a small placebo-controlled trial of 500 women with 5.1-year follow-up (50). Volunteers aged 75 years or below with intraepithelial neoplasia (atypical hyperplasia or in situ cancer) were randomized to TAM 5 mg once daily orally for 3 years compared to placebo. At 5 years follow-up, there were 14 breast cancer events with TAM and 28 with placebo (11.6 vs 23.9 per 1,000 person-years; HR, 0.48; 95% CI, 0.26-0.92; $P = .02$). There were 12 serious AEs reported with TAM and 16 with placebo, including one deep vein thrombosis and one stage I endometrial cancer with TAM and one pulmonary embolism with placebo. Of note, TAM is not available in 5 mg in the United States, and options would include 10 mg every other day or utilizing a pill cutter.

Several data sets also demonstrate the efficacy of AIs for prevention in postmenopausal women with increased risk of breast cancer, including the International Breast Intervention Study-II (IBIS-II) randomized placebo-controlled trial of anastrozole (51) and MAP.3 randomized placebo-controlled trial of exemestane (52). **Table 11.8-4** reviews the seminal trials in this space.

Patients with DCIS are at higher risk for new breast cancer events, such as local recurrence, new primary DCIS, or invasive breast cancer. In NSABP-B24, chemoprevention with TAM was demonstrated in women with DCIS who underwent surgery and radiation (53). Volunteers were subsequently randomized to TAM or placebo; the TAM group had a 37% reduction in breast cancer events. In a subset analysis, the volunteers with ER+ DCIS, TAM reduced breast cancer events by 51%; of note, no risk reduction was seen for the ER− patients (5). In the IBIS-II DCIS phase III double-blind randomized trial of postmenopausal women with a history of HR+ DCIS status post (s/p) surgical resection (not all patients received radiation), anastrozole was similar to TAM in risk reduction for local recurrence (54).

REFERENCES

1. Howlader N, Altekruse SF, Li CI, et al. US incidence of breast cancer subtypes defined by joint hormone receptor and HER2 status. *J Natl Cancer Inst.* 2014;106:dju055.

2. McDonnell DP, Wardell SE, Chang C-Y, Norris JD. Next-generation endocrine therapies for breast cancer. *J Clin Oncol.* 2021;39:1383-1388.

3. Allison KH, Hammond MEH, Dowsett M, et al. Estrogen and progesterone receptor testing in breast cancer: ASCO/CAP guideline update. *J Clin Oncol.* 2020;38:1346-1366.

4. Early Breast Cancer Trialists' Collaborative Group (EBCTCG). Relevance of breast cancer hormone receptors and other factors to the efficacy of adjuvant tamoxifen: patient-level meta-analysis of randomised trials. *Lancet.* 2011;378:771-784.

5. Allred DC, Anderson SJ, Paik S, et al. Adjuvant tamoxifen reduces subsequent breast cancer in women with estrogen receptor–positive ductal carcinoma in situ: a study based on NSABP protocol B-24. *J Clin Oncol.* 2012;30:1268-1273.

6. Early Breast Cancer Trialists' Collaborative Group (EBCTCG). Effects of chemotherapy and hormonal therapy for early breast cancer on recurrence and 15-year survival: an overview of the randomised trials. *Lancet.* 2005;365:1687-1717.

7. Perou CM, Sørlie T, Eisen MB, et al. Molecular portraits of human breast tumours. *Nature.* 2000;406:747-752.

8. Ades F, Zardavas D, Bozovic-Spasojevic I, et al. Luminal B breast cancer: molecular characterization, clinical management, and future perspectives. *J Clin Oncol.* 2014;32:2794-2803.

9. Cardoso F, van't Veer LJ, Bogaerts J, et al. 70-gene signature as an aid to treatment decisions in early-stage breast cancer. *N Engl J Med.* 2016;375:717-729.

10. Sparano JA, Gray RJ, Makower DF, et al. Prospective validation of a 21-gene expression assay in breast cancer. *N Engl J Med.* 2015;373:2005-2014.

11. Liu MC, Pitcher BN, Mardis ER, et al. PAM50 gene signatures and breast cancer prognosis with adjuvant anthracycline- and taxane-based chemotherapy: correlative analysis of C9741 (Alliance). *NPJ Breast Cancer.* 2016;2:15023.

12. Sparano JA, Gray RJ, Makower DF, et al. Adjuvant chemotherapy guided by a 21-gene expression assay in breast cancer. *N Engl J Med.* 2018;379(2):111-121. doi:10.1056/NEJMoa1804710

13. Kalinsky K, Barlow WE, Gralow JR, et al. 21-gene assay to inform chemotherapy benefit in node-positive breast cancer. *N Engl J Med.* 2021;385:2336-2347.

▪ TABLE 11.8-4. Seminal Trials of Endocrine Therapy for Risk Reduction

Trial	N	Arms	Cumulative Rate of Invasive Breast Cancer (per 1,000)	P-Value	Cumulative Rate of Noninvasive Breast Cancer (per 1,000)	P-Value	Follow-up (Years)
NSABP-P1 (57)	13,207	T	24.8	<0.001	10.2	−0.008	7
		P	42.5		15.8		
IBIS-I (58)	7,154	T	61.8	<0.001	10.1	−0.047	16
		P	80.9		16.1		
MAP3 (49)	4,560	E	4.8	−0.002	3.9	−0.31	2.9
		P	14.1		6.2		
IBIS-II (51)	3,864	A	16.7	−0.001	3.1	−0.009	5
		P	32.9		10.3		

A, anastrozole; E, exemestane; P, placebo; T, tamoxifen.

14. Lopes Cardozo JMN, Drukker CA, Rutgers EJT, et al. Outcome of patients with an ultralow-risk 70-gene signature in the MINDACT trial. *J Clin Oncol*. 2022;40:1335-1345.

15. Gerber B, Krause A, Müller H, et al. Effects of adjuvant tamoxifen on the endometrium in postmenopausal women with breast cancer: a prospective long-term study using transvaginal ultrasound. *J Clin Oncol*. 2000;18:3464-3470.

16. Goss PE, Ingle JN, Martino S, et al. A randomized trial of letrozole in postmenopausal women after five years of tamoxifen therapy for early-stage breast cancer. *N Engl J Med*. 2003;349:1793-1802.

17. Davies C, Pan H, Godwin J, et al. Long-term effects of continuing adjuvant tamoxifen to 10 years versus stopping at 5 years after diagnosis of oestrogen receptor-positive breast cancer: ATLAS, a randomised trial. *Lancet*. 2013;381:805-816.

18. Gray RG, Rea DW, Handley K, et al. aTTom: Long-term effects of continuing adjuvant tamoxifen to 10 years versus stopping at 5 years in 6,953 women with early breast cancer. *J Clin Oncol*. 2013;31:5-5.

19. Tjan-Heijnen VCG, van Hellemond IEG, Peer PGM, et al. Extended adjuvant aromatase inhibition after sequential endocrine therapy (DATA): a randomised, phase 3 trial. *Lancet Oncol*. 2017;18:1502-1511.

20. Blok EJ, Kroep JR, Kranenbarg EMK, et al. Optimal duration of extended adjuvant endocrine therapy for early breast cancer; results of the Ideal trial (BOOG 2006-05). *J Natl Cancer Inst*. 2018;110:40-48.

21. Gnant M, Fitzal F, Rinnerthaler G, et al. Duration of adjuvant aromatase-inhibitor therapy in postmenopausal breast cancer. *N Engl J Med*. 2021;385:395-405.

22. Del Mastro L, Mansutti M, Bisagni G, et al. Extended therapy with letrozole as adjuvant treatment of postmenopausal patients with early-stage breast cancer: a multicentre, open-label, randomised, phase 3 trial. *Lancet Oncol*. 2021;22:1458-1467.

23. Graff SL. Treatment of premenopausal women: finding the right-sized endocrine therapy. *JCO Oncol Pract*. 2022;18:217-220.

24. Chirgwin JH, Giobbie-Hurder A, Coates AS, et al. Treatment adherence and its impact on disease-free survival in the Breast International Group 1-98 Trial of tamoxifen and letrozole, alone and in sequence. *J Clin Oncol*. 2016;34:2452-2459.

25. Pistilli B, Paci A, Ferreira AR, et al. Serum detection of nonadherence to adjuvant tamoxifen and breast cancer recurrence risk. *J Clin Oncol*. 2020;38:2762-2772.

26. Wheeler SB, Spencer J, Pinheiro LC, et al. Endocrine therapy nonadherence and discontinuation in black and white women. *J Natl Cancer Inst*. 2019;111:498-508.

27. Francis PA, Regan MM, Fleming GF, et al. Adjuvant ovarian suppression in premenopausal breast cancer. *N Engl J Med*. 2015;372:436-446.

28. Pagani O, Regan MM, Francis PA, et al. Adjuvant exemestane with ovarian suppression in premenopausal breast cancer. *N Engl J Med*. 2014;371:107-118.

29. Pan K, Bosserman LD, Chlebowski RT. Ovarian suppression in adjuvant endocrine therapy for premenopausal breast cancer. *J Clin Oncol*. 2019;37:858-861.

30. Francis PA, Pagani O, Fleming GF, et al. Tailoring adjuvant endocrine therapy for premenopausal breast cancer. *N Engl J Med*. 2018;379:122-137.

31. Early Breast Cancer Trialists' Collaborative Group (EBCTCG). Aromatase inhibitors versus tamoxifen in premenopausal women with oestrogen receptor-positive early-stage breast cancer treated with ovarian suppression: a patient-level meta-analysis of 7030 women from four randomised trials. *Lancet Oncol*. 2022;23:382-392.

32. Honigberg MC, Zekavat SM, Aragam K, et al. Association of premature natural and surgical menopause with incident cardiovascular disease. *JAMA*. 2019;322:2411-2421.

33. Johnson SRD, Harbeck N, Hegg R, et al. Abemaciclib combined with endocrine therapy for the adjuvant treatment of HR+, HER2−, node-positive, high-risk, early breast cancer (monarchE). *J Clin Oncol*. 2020;38:3987-3998.

34. Harbeck N, Rastogi P, Martin M, et al. Adjuvant abemaciclib combined with endocrine therapy for high-risk early breast cancer: updated efficacy and Ki-67 analysis from the monarchE study. *Ann Oncol*. 2021;32:1571-1581.

35. Royce M, Osgood C, Mulkey F, et al. FDA approval summary: abemaciclib with endocrine therapy for high-risk early breast cancer. *J Clin Oncol*. 2022;40:1155-1162.

36. Loibl S, Marmé F, Martin M, et al. Palbociclib for residual high-risk invasive HR-positive and HER2-negative early breast cancer—the PENELOPE-B trial. *J Clin Oncol*. 2021;39:1518-1530.

37. Gnant M, Dueck AC, Frantal S, et al. Adjuvant palbociclib for early breast cancer: the PALLAS trial results (ABCSG-42/AFT-05/BIG-14-03). *J Clin Oncol*. 2022;40:282-293.

38. Sella T, Weiss A, Mittendorf EA, et al. Neoadjuvant endocrine therapy in clinical practice: a review. *JAMA Oncol*. 2021;7:1700-1708.

39. Eiermann W, Paepke S, Appfelstaedt J, et al. Preoperative treatment of postmenopausal breast cancer patients with letrozole: a randomized double-blind multicenter study. *Ann Oncol*. 2001;12:1527-1532.

40. Smith IE, Dowsett M, Ebbs SR, et al. Neoadjuvant treatment of postmenopausal breast cancer with anastrozole, tamoxifen, or both in combination: the Immediate Preoperative Anastrozole, Tamoxifen, or Combined with Tamoxifen (IMPACT) multicenter double-blind randomized trial. *J Clin Oncol*. 2005;23:5108-5116.

41. Cataliotti L, Buzdar AU, Noguchi S, et al. Comparison of anastrozole versus tamoxifen as preoperative therapy in postmenopausal women with hormone receptor-positive breast cancer: the Pre-Operative "Arimidex" Compared to Tamoxifen (PROACT) trial. *Cancer*. 2006;106:2095-2103.

42. Gianni L, Zambetti M, Clark K, et al. Gene expression profiles in paraffin-embedded core biopsy tissue predict response to chemotherapy in women with locally advanced breast cancer. *J Clin Oncol*. 2005;23(29):7265-7277. doi:10.1200/JCO.2005.02.0818

43. Whitworth P, Beitsch P, Mislowsky A, et al. Chemosensitivity and endocrine sensitivity in clinical luminal breast cancer patients in the prospective Neoadjuvant Breast Registry Symphony Trial (NBRST) predicted by molecular subtyping. *Ann Surg Oncol*. 2017;24:669-675.

44. Ueno T, Masuda N, Yamanaka T, et al. Evaluating the 21-gene assay recurrence score° as a predictor of clinical response to 24 weeks of neoadjuvant exemestane in estrogen receptor-positive breast cancer. *Int J Clin Oncol*. 2014;19:607-613.

45. Park KU, Gregory M, Bazan J, et al. Neoadjuvant endocrine therapy use in early stage breast cancer during the Covid-19 pandemic. *Breast Cancer Res Treat*. 2021;188:249-258.

46. Martí C, Sánchez-Méndez JI. Neoadjuvant endocrine therapy for luminal breast cancer treatment: a first-choice alternative in times of crisis such as the COVID-19 pandemic. *Ecancermedicalscience*. 2020;14:1027.

47. Thompson CK, Lee MK, Baker JL, Attai DJ, DiNome ML. Taking a second look at neoadjuvant endocrine therapy for the treatment of early stage estrogen receptor positive breast cancer during the COVID-19 outbreak. *Ann Surg*. 2020;272:e96-e97.

48. Cuzick J, Powles T, Veronesi U, et al. Overview of the main outcomes in breast-cancer prevention trials. *Lancet*. 2003;361:296-300.

49. Vogel VG, Costantino JP, Wickerham DL, et al. Update of the National Surgical Adjuvant Breast and Bowel Project Study of Tamoxifen and Raloxifene (STAR) P-2 trial: preventing breast cancer. *Cancer Prev Res (Phila)*. 2010;3:696-706.

50. DeCensi A, Puntoni M, Guerrieri-Gonzaga A, et al. Randomized placebo controlled trial of low-dose tamoxifen to prevent local and contralateral recurrence in breast intraepithelial neoplasia. *J Clin Oncol*. 2019;37:1629-1637.

51. Cuzick J, Sestak I, Forbes JF, et al. Anastrozole for prevention of breast cancer in high-risk postmenopausal women (IBIS-II): an international, double-blind, randomised placebo-controlled trial. *Lancet*. 2014;383:1041-1048.

52. Goss PE, Ingle JN, Alés-Martínez JE, et al. Exemestane for breast-cancer prevention in postmenopausal women. *N Engl J Med*. 2011;364:2381-2391.

53. Fisher B, Dignam J, Wolmark N, et al. Tamoxifen in treatment of intraductal breast cancer: National surgical adjuvant breast and bowel project B-24 randomised controlled trial. *Lancet*. 1999;353:1993-2000.

54. Forbes JF, Sestak I, Howell A, et al. Anastrozole versus tamoxifen for the prevention of locoregional and contralateral breast cancer in postmenopausal women with locally excised ductal carcinoma in situ (IBIS-II DCIS): a double-blind, randomised controlled trial. *Lancet*. 2016;387:866-873. doi:10.1016/S0140-6736(15)01129-0

55. Goss PE, Ingle JN, Martino S, et al. A randomised trial of letrozole in postmenopausal women after five years of tamoxifen therapy for early-stage breast cancer. *N Engl J Med*. 2003;349(19):1793-1802.

56. Jin H, Tu D, Zhao N, et al. Longer-term outcomes of letrozole versus placebo after 5 years of tamoxifen in the NCIC CTG MA.17 trial: analyses adjusting for treatment crossover. *J Clin Oncol*. 2012;30(7):718-721.

57. Fisher B, Land S, Mamounas E, et al. Prevention of invasive breast cancer in women with ductal carcinoma in situ: an update of the National Surgical Adjuvant Breast and Bowel Project experience. *Semin Oncol*. 2001;28:400-418.

58. Cuzick J, Sestak I, Cawthorn S, et al. Tamoxifen for prevention of breast cancer: extended long-term follow-up of the IBIS-I breast cancer prevention trial. *Lancet Oncol*. 2015;16(1):67-75.

CHAPTER 11.9

Approaches to Systemic Therapy for Breast Cancer: Neoadjuvant and Adjuvant Management

Stephanie L. Graff

Systemic therapy outside the endocrine pathway includes cytotoxic chemotherapy, immune checkpoint inhibitors, and targeted antibody therapy, including antibody-drug conjugates (ADCs). Factors that drive decision-making with these agents include stage of disease, biomarkers, other prognostic tests, and/or evidence of disease resistance. Concepts that often arise in the discussion of chemotherapy are detailed in Table 11.9-1. In addition, commonly used agents in the adjuvant setting for breast cancer are listed in Table 11.9-2.

NEOADJUVANT CHEMOTHERAPY

Preoperative or neoadjuvant (NACT) is the standard treatment for patients with locally advanced, unresectable breast cancers or with large breast tumors who would require a mastectomy but desire an attempt at BCS, unless the patient is too old or frail to tolerate chemotherapy. Increasingly, NACT is also utilized in HER2-positive breast cancer (HER2+) and TNBC because the presence or absence of a pCR offers important prognostic information, which can help tailor subsequent treatments or identify appropriate clinical trials (1).

For patients with resectable breast cancer, a 2005 meta-analysis of studies that compared preoperative with identical postoperative chemotherapy demonstrated equivalent DFS and OS and a significant increase in the percentage of patients able to undergo BCS (2). Updated results from two neoadjuvant trials conducted by the NSABP (B-18 and B-27) reported a trend toward improvement in DFS favoring preoperative chemotherapy, particularly in patients under the age of 50 (3). Although intriguing, these results should be considered more as hypothesis generating than for treatment guidance.

TABLE 11.9-1. Concepts Around Systemic Therapy for Breast Cancer

Dose intensity	For many chemotherapeutic agents, higher drug concentrations result in increased killing of cancer cells in vitro (or a dose-response curve). However, it is not entirely clear that increasing dose improves outcomes in breast cancer. For example, high-dose therapy with autologous hematopoietic stem cell transplantation appeared promising in early trials, but this was not borne out in randomized trials and has since been abandoned.
Dose density	The administration of similar or lower doses of one or more agents more frequently. This often allows administration of a higher overall dose of a drug with less toxicity and also may increase the drug's cytotoxic effects by increasing the likelihood of catching a higher proportion of cancer cells in the most vulnerable phases of their cell cycle.
Non–cross-resistant drug combinations	Using agents, either concurrently or sequentially, with different mechanisms of action, different mechanisms of drug resistance, and, when possible, nonoverlapping toxicities. Switching to a non–cross-resistant drug or regimen may improve response, even when the patient is responding to the initial regimen.

TABLE 11.9-2. Systemic Agents Used in the Neoadjuvant or Adjuvant Treatment of Breast Cancer

Anthracycline-containing regimens Doxorubicin + cyclophosphamide (AC) Epirubicin + cyclophosphamide (EC) AC or EC followed by paclitaxel (Pac) Docetaxel + AC (TAC)	**Non–anthracycline-containing regimens** Cyclophosphamide, methotrexate, 5-fluorouracil (CMF) Docetaxel + cyclophosphamide (TC) Carboplatin + Pac or T
HER2-directed combinations AC followed by Pac/T + trastuzumab AC followed by Pac/T + H + pertuzumab TC + trastuzumab (TCH) TCH + pertuzumab (TCHP) Pac + trastuzumab Pact + trastuzumab + pertuzumab	**Immunotherapy containing (triple-negative breast cancer only)** Carboplatin + Pac + pembrolizumab followed by AC/EC + pembrolizumab
Extended treatment Olaparib (BRCA mutation + only) Trastuzumab (HER2 + only) Pembrolizumab (TNBC only) Endocrine therapy (HR+ only)	**Post-NACT treatment (if residual disease is present)** Capecitabine Trastuzumab emtansine (HER2+ only)

NACT, neoadjuvant chemotherapy; TNBC, triple-negative breast cancer.

Evaluating Response to Neoadjuvant Chemotherapy

In patients with visible or palpable disease, response (or lack thereof) can often be assessed on physical examination. Sequential imaging studies (discussed earlier) can usually indicate whether or not a patient is responding, though occasionally clinically "stable" tumors will prove to be largely or totally replaced with fibrous tissue. However, imaging can be relatively insensitive for assessing the breast and axilla for microscopic disease following resolution of any visible tumor mass or abnormal nodes.

The NSABP utilized a definition of pCR that required the absence of invasive disease in the breast, irrespective of the presence of any residual disease in the axillary nodes (breast-only pCR) (3). In addition, others have reported that the presence of residual DCIS in the breast, in the absence of residual invasive disease, had no impact on survival outcomes (4). Despite these reports, it has become clear that persistent disease in the axillary nodes is associated with higher recurrence rates, whereas conversion from node-positive to node-negative disease with NACT indicates a good prognosis (5). Based on these findings, most contemporary U.S. studies use the absence of invasive disease in the breast and axilla (ypT0/isN0) as their definition of pCR.

Other investigators suggest that the extent of residual disease after NACT may be prognostic in the absence of a pCR. European investigators have used a number of scoring systems, the best known of which is the Miller/Payne grading system, to assess post-NACT pathologic specimens for both residual disease and chemotherapy response, and the results of which have been shown to correlate with DFS and OS (6). In the United States, Symmans and colleagues reported that the size and cellularity of residual invasive disease in the breast and the number and size of metastatic deposits in the axillary nodes predicted distant recurrence (7). These variables are incorporated into a formula called the residual cancer burden (RCB). RCB analyses have been incorporated into a number of NACT studies, both to stratify non-pCR responses and to validate this methodology. In the 2005 meta-analysis comparing identical NACT versus adjuvant chemotherapy regimens, pCR was associated with 52% improvements in both DFS and OS (2). Similarly, in the I-Spy2 trial, which has a platform adaptive neoadjuvant clinical trial design across all subsets of breast cancer (HR+, HER2+, and TNBC), event-free survival (EFS) at 3 years was directly correlated with the degree of RCB and highest EFS was among those achieving a pCR (1). In summary, although the optimal way to assess response to NACT remains controversial, the prognostic implication of response to NACT, particularly pCR, is striking.

Neoadjuvant Chemotherapy Considerations

A general principle regarding NACT regimens is that chemotherapeutic agents that have proven effectiveness in the adjuvant setting should have similar efficacy against disease in the breast and axillary nodes as well as occult metastatic disease in the neoadjuvant setting. Thus, there is no reason to use different regimens based on sequence of chemotherapy in respect to surgery. The choice of specific chemotherapy drugs and regimens should be based on our understanding of therapy response as related to tumor biology and patient subsets and is similar to the considerations on the approach to adjuvant treatment.

What to do for patients who are not responding to NACT is unknown. In one trial, patients not responding after four cycles of the anthracycline-based regimen were switched to docetaxel, and while 55% had a clinical response to the taxane, their pCR rate was only 2% and their 3-year survival was markedly inferior to those who respond to treatment (8). In the GeparTrio trial, patients who did not respond with at least a 50% reduction in tumor size after two cycles of docetaxel plus AC (doxorubicin plus cyclophosphamide) (TAC) were randomly assigned to either four more cycles

of TAC or four cycles of vinorelbine and capecitabine (NX) every 21 days (9). Although both groups of patients had similar clinical response (51%) and pCR (5%-6%) rates, a recent update of the trial reported that patients switched to NX demonstrated significant (41%) improvement in DFS compared to patients who continued on TAC. Meanwhile, patients responding after two cycles of TAC were randomized to four or six more cycles of the same regimen, and although the longer treatment duration had only a modest impact on the pCR rate (24% vs 21%), it did result in significant improvement in DFS.

Treatment for patients who go to surgery after NACT and are found to have significant residual disease is based on their tumor type. While patients with HR+ breast cancer continue on to receive the adjuvant endocrine therapy that was planned regardless of response, patients with HER2+ or TNBC may be eligible for adaptive plans based on the presence of residual disease identified within the surgical pathology. These approaches are discussed in the subsequent section.

CHEMOTHERAPY REGIMENS

HER2-Negative Disease (HR+ or Triple-Negative Breast Cancer)

In HER2-negative disease, tumor biology continues to be a driving force in the decision for adjuvant versus NACT. As discussed in the section on endocrine therapy, for people with HR+ breast cancer, many patients undergo upfront surgery for definitive pathologic staging followed by GEP to characterize the risk of distant cancer recurrence and benefit of chemotherapy. In contrast, people with TNBC who are clinically LN negative may still be offered NACT, given the more biologically aggressive nature of the disease, which indicates a higher likelihood of pCR, compared to those with ER+ disease and data supporting response-adapted treatments for those who do not achieve pCR.

The backbone of adjuvant chemotherapy and NACT in HER2-negative disease remains cyclophosphamide in combination with taxanes and/or anthracyclines. The data supporting adjuvant chemotherapy (vs no treatment), including anthracycline- and taxane-based approaches, come from the EBCTCG (10). As compared to no treatment, anthracycline-based chemotherapy reduced breast cancer mortality from 36% to 29% (RR 0.79) and decreased overall mortality by 5% (RR 0.84). Chemotherapy regimens that included six cycles of cyclophosphamide with standard doses of either of the common anthracyclines, doxorubicin or epirubicin, and 5-fluorouracil (CAF or CEF) resulted in larger relative improvements in OS (36%) than regimens in which patients received just four cycles of standard-dose doxorubicin or epirubicin with cyclophosphamide (AC or EC, 22%). Compared to nonchemotherapy controls, administration of cyclophosphamide, methotrexate, and 5-fluorouracil (CMF) was associated with a 30% relative reduction in breast cancer recurrence (29.6% vs 39.8%), which resulted in a 6.2% improvement in breast cancer mortality and a 4.7% improvement in overall mortality. These results were highly statistically significant owing to the large numbers of patients involved (8,575 patients in the anthracycline-based trials, 5,253 in the CMF trials). The difference in the outcomes for the control groups likely reflects different patient populations, with only 18% of patients treated on the anthracycline-based trials having node-negative cancers compared to 66% on the CMF trials. Benefits from chemotherapy were essentially equivalent across multiple patient subgroups, including age, node status, HR status, and tumor grade, and administration of adjuvant ET (TAM) did not reduce the benefit of receiving adjuvant chemotherapy. And these benefits are seen without the modern overlay of HER2 testing and HER2-directed therapy or molecular profiling to better predict benefit from chemotherapy, suggesting larger benefits if these trials were to be repeated in the selected populations treated today.

EBCTCG also provides the evidence for anthracycline-taxane–based treatments (10). In patients administered standard-dose anthracyclines as compared to CMF, risk of recurrence (41% vs 42%), breast cancer mortality (32% vs 33%), and overall mortality (33% vs 35%) were similar at 10 years. Regarding the benefits of adding a taxane to anthracycline-based adjuvant chemotherapy, in trials where the same number of cycles of anthracyclines was used in the control arm as the experimental arm, the addition of taxanes resulted in a reduction in the risk of recurrence of breast cancer (35%-30%, RR 0.84), breast cancer mortality (24%-21%, RR 0.86) and overall mortality (27%-24%, RR 0.90). The aggregate results were consistent across age groups, nodal status, and HR status. In the majority of studies included in this 2012 meta-analysis, the taxane (whether paclitaxel or docetaxel) was administered q3weeks, thus potentially underestimating the benefits of dose-dense q2week or weekly paclitaxel.

Several contemporary clinical trials have broadened the options for adjuvant chemotherapy in persons deemed to be at sufficient risk of recurrence. The U.S. Oncology Trial 9735 enrolled more than 1,000 volunteers (>50% with node-positive disease and >70% with ER-positive disease) and randomly assigned treatment with AC or docetaxel and cyclophosphamide (TC) every 3 weeks for four cycles (11). At a median follow-up of 7 years, TC remained superior to AC, with a 26% improvement in DFS, which translated into a 6% absolute increase, and a 31% rise in OS (5% absolute benefit). The DFS benefit was apparent, independent of age, nodal status, and HR status (though not statistically significant in the subgroups). Short-term toxicities were comparable across the two arms of the study, but four patients on the AC arm have died of possible late complications of treatment, one with congestive heart failure and three with leukemia or myelodysplasia. Though of relatively modest size, this study has had a major impact on the treatment of patients with low- to intermediate-risk disease in the United States, presumably due to the appeal of avoiding exposure to an anthracycline without sacrificing efficacy. In the NSABP-B38 trial, almost 5,000 patients with node-positive, early-stage breast cancer were randomly assigned to one of three regimens: dose-dense AC followed by dose-dense paclitaxel (AC-T), dose-dense AC followed by paclitaxel plus gemcitabine (AC-TG), or a three-drug combination of TAC (12). There were no significant differences in either DFS or OS at 5 years between any of the regimens. However, TAC was associated with significantly higher rates of febrile neutropenia (9% vs 3% with AC-T and AC-TG). The regimens with paclitaxel, on the other hand, were associated with higher rates of chemotherapy-induced peripheral neuropathy (CIPN). A 2016 meta-analysis exploring the three largest trials comparing TC to anthracyclines in combination with taxanes (TaxAC) showed that among the 2,125 patients randomized, TaxAC was superior (13). Four-year IDFS was 88.2% for TC and 90.7% for TaxAC. Subgroup analysis suggested that patients with LN-negative, HR+ breast cancer may remain reasonable candidates for TC chemotherapy, reflected in the ITT populations of the TAILORx and RxPONDER trials where 56% and 42%, respectively, were treated with TC chemotherapy (14,15).

In 2021, results of the KEYNOTE 522 trial led to the approval of the use of immunotherapy with pembrolizumab for patients with stage II or stage III TNBC (16). Patients were randomized to neoadjuvant weekly paclitaxel and carboplatin (administer either weekly or every 3 weeks) followed by doxorubicin/epirubicin and cyclophosphamide every 3 weeks either with or without pembrolizumab through the duration every 3 weeks and then continuing adjuvant pembrolizumab for 1 year (17). Addition of pembrolizumab improved pCR from 51% to 65%, and results were independent of PD-L1 expression. Pembrolizumab also improved 3-year EFS (84% vs 77%). While questions remain about optimal chemotherapy backbone and duration of checkpoint inhibitor, this represents the current standard of care for stage II/III TNBC.

For patients' tumors treated with NACT that do not have a pCR, response-adapted adjuvant therapy may be appropriate.

The CREATE-X trial assigned 900 patients with HER2 negative, including TNBC and HR+ breast cancer, who did not have pCR after NACT to eight cycles of adjuvant chemotherapy versus no further chemotherapy (18). Patients receiving capecitabine had a higher 5-year DFS (74% vs 68%, HR 0.70) and OS (89% vs 84%, HR 0.59), but much of that improvement was likely driven by the TNBC population (5-year DFS 70% vs 56%, HR 0.58). Based on this subset analysis, consensus guidelines recommend limiting use of adjuvant capecitabine to patients with TNBC (19). Criticisms of the CREATE-X study, however, are worth noting. First, patients in CREATE-X were treated with anthracycline-taxane–based chemotherapy, so for patients otherwise receiving checkpoint inhibitors, PARP inhibitors, or platinums, there is no evidence to support the addition of capecitabine. Next, CREATE-X enrolled an Asian patient population, which could affect the generalizability of results on Western patient populations. Based on these criticisms, we are limited in our utilization of capecitabine but recognize it as an option for high-risk, residual disease after NACT. Two further randomized trials raise questions as to whether there is a survival benefit for adjuvant capecitabine after NACT. In a Spanish trial tested capecitabine after standard NACT in a phase 3 trial that enrolled over 800 volunteers, 74% of whom had a basal phenotype (20). At a median follow-up of 7.3 years, there was no difference in DFS with capecitabine or observation (HR 0.82, 95% CI 0.63-1.06). In a trial conducted by the Eastern Cooperative Group and the American College of Radiology Intergroup (ECOG-ACRIN EA 1,131) that included 410 volunteers with clinical stage II or III TNBC who had 1 cm or larger residual disease after NACT, 3-year IDFS was 42% with platinum (carboplatin or cisplatin) and only 49% with capecitabine, which was far lower than what was statistically expected (21).

Approximately 5% of unselected patients with breast cancer will have a germline BRCA1 or BRCA2 pathogenic variant (previously "mutation"). These pathogenic variants predispose the associated tumors that develop to deficiencies in homologous recombination repair, rendering them sensitive to inhibition of poly(adenosine diphosphate-ribose) polymerase (PARP). This ultimately contributes to synthetic lethality, sometimes described as "double hit" leading to cell death. In the phase 3 OlympiA trial, 1 year of the oral PARP inhibitor, olaparib, was compared to placebo for the adjuvant treatment of HER2-negative, germline BRCA pathogenic variant breast cancer (22). Among those with HR+ disease, they were required to have four or more positive LNs or, if treated with NACT, no pCR and a high clinical/pathologic risk score as described elsewhere (23). Among those with TNBC, they needed to have ≥T2 or ≥N1 disease, or if treated with NACT, no pCR. In this genetically selected, high-risk population, the addition of adjuvant olaparib improved IDFS 8.8% (77.1% placebo vs 85.9% olaparib, HR 0.58). This represents an important improvement in outcome and a compelling reason to consider genetic counseling and testing for patients diagnosed with breast cancer.

HER2-Positive Disease

With the rapid growth kinetics of HER2+ breast cancers, it is not surprising that a significant percentage of patients with these cancers present with large tumors or locally advanced disease, making them ideal candidates for NT. While the percentage of patients with HER2+ cancers who achieve a pCR with NACT alone is relatively high, especially those with HR-negative/HER2+ disease, blocking HER2 signaling clearly enhances the chemosensitivity and chemoresponse of HER2+ breast cancers. Thus, HER2-directed therapy is now widely indicated in the adjuvant context based on seminal results from three randomized trials that consistently demonstrated substantial improvements in DFS and OS with the addition of trastuzumab during or after standard adjuvant chemotherapy (Table 11.9-3) (24-28). In the neoadjuvant context, an analysis of two randomized trials demonstrated significant improvements in pCR rates with the addition of trastuzumab to chemotherapy versus chemotherapy alone (RR 2.07, 95% CI 1.41-3.03) (27). Combining trastuzumab with chemotherapy was also associated with a reduction in the relapse rate (26% vs 39%, 95% CI 0.48-0.94) and a trend toward improvement in the risk of death (13% vs 20% mortality rate).

For the earliest-stage HER2+ breast cancer, clinical T1b or T1c and clinical N0 breast cancers, treatment with adjuvant trastuzumab-containing chemotherapy is appropriate. Tolaney et al demonstrated a high 7-year DFS (93%) and OS (95%) when patients were treated with 12 doses of weekly paclitaxel and trastuzumab, followed by completion of 1 year of adjuvant trastuzumab (29). Small numbers of patients with N1 mic (1.5%) and T2 tumors (8.9%) were included in the study population as well; 64% were co-positive for ER and HER2 (29).

Given concerns about the incidence of cardiotoxicity seen in patients with HER2+ who received both an anthracycline and trastuzumab, and the demonstrated synergy between trastuzumab and a variety of chemotherapeutic agents in vitro, the Breast Cancer International Research Group (BCIRG) 006 trial was designed to test the efficacy and toxicity of a non–anthracycline-based chemotherapy regimen plus trastuzumab against a standard anthracycline-based chemotherapy regimen with or without trastuzumab (**Table 11.9-3**) (24). The use of carboplatin alongside docetaxel and trastuzumab (TCH) was associated with a lower rate of congestive heart failure (0.4%) compared to arms containing doxorubicin (0.4% vs 0.7% and 2% with AC→docetaxel or AC→docetaxel/trastuzumab) and was also associated with a lower likelihood of a sustained drop in left ventricular ejection fraction (9.4% vs 11.2% and 18.6%) (24). In addition to reducing cardiac toxicity, dropping the anthracycline reduced vomiting and mucositis and appeared to markedly reduce, if not eliminate, the small but real risk (0.33% in patients on AC-T or AC-TH) of developing a treatment-related leukemia. This regimen represents another reasonable option for early-stage HER2+ breast cancer, particularly LN-negative disease.

For patients with larger primary tumors (T2, T3, T4) or clinically positive LNs, two large prospective trials have shown the addition of pertuzumab, a HER2 monoclonal antibody that binds to a different epitope than trastuzumab blocking HER2-HER3 dimerization, to a trastuzumab-containing NACT regimen improved pCR (30,31). The NeoSPHERE trial was an open-label randomized phase II trial that enrolled 417 patients with operable, locally advanced, or inflammatory HER2+ breast cancer and randomly assigned them to 12 weeks of treatment using one of four regimens: docetaxel (100 mg/m^2 every 3 weeks for four cycles) plus trastuzumab (group A), docetaxel plus trastuzumab

and pertuzumab (group B), pertuzumab plus trastuzumab alone (group C), or docetaxel plus pertuzumab (group D) (30). After surgery, patients on the docetaxel arms received three cycles of 5-fluorouracil, epirubicin, and cyclophosphamide (FEC) and completed a year of trastuzumab, whereas patients in group C received both docetaxel and FEC followed by trastuzumab. The pCR rates were 29%, 46%, 17%, and 24% in groups A, B, C, and D, respectively. Compared to patients with HR-positive disease, the pCR rates were generally higher in those with HR-negative tumors. Serious (grade 3/4) AEs in patients treated with docetaxel (groups A, B, and D) included neutropenia, febrile neutropenia, and diarrhea. The addition of pertuzumab to the docetaxel plus trastuzumab combination did not appear to increase toxicity, including cardiac AEs. These results are fascinating, not only because of the higher pCR rate seen on the chemotherapy plus trastuzumab and pertuzumab arm but also because of the frequency of pCRs associated with dual HER2-targeted therapy alone, raising the intriguing possibility that there may be a subset of HER2+ patients who can be effectively treated without the toxic effects of chemotherapy, a hypothesis still being explored in ongoing trials. The second study, TRYPHAENA, compared two anthracycline-containing arms, FEC with trastuzumab and pertuzumab (HP) followed by docetaxel with HP (arm A) versus FEC (without HP) followed by docetaxel with HP (arm B), versus an arm that notably spared anthracyclines, consisting of docetaxel, carboplatin, trastuzumab, and pertuzumab (TCHP, arm C) (33). pCR was reported for 61.6% (arm A), 57.3% (arm B), and 66.2% (arm C) of patients (31). The TRAIN-2 study demonstrated that anthracycline-sparing regimens resulted in no difference in EFS or OS as compared to regimens that utilized anthracyclines (32). However, the anthracycline-containing arm resulted in a clinically significant reduction in cardiac ejection fraction in twice as many patients (7.7% as compared to 3.2%, $P = .04$). Therefore, our standard approach is an anthracycline-sparing regimen in HER2+ breast cancer. All patients receiving trastuzumab, with or without anthracycline, should have cardiac function evaluated before starting chemotherapy and before starting trastuzumab, after which cardiac monitoring should be individualized based on patient age, baseline ejection fraction, and risk factors for developing cardiac dysfunction. At our institution, we utilize echocardiograms for this purpose. Consensus guidelines can be used to modify or hold treatment based on changes to cardiac function (33).

It is important to remember that following surgery and/or completion of adjuvant chemotherapy, all patients should then continue HER2 biologic treatment to complete a full year. For patients who received only trastuzumab, continuing the single

■ TABLE 11.9-3. Adjuvant Trials in HER2-Positive Breast Cancer

Trial	Regimens	N	DFS (vs Control)	OS
NCCTG 9831 NSABP B-31	Chemotherapy[a] + Tr vs chemotherapy alone	4,045[b]	HR = 0.69 (95% CI, 0.57-0.85)	HR = 0.67 (95% CI, 0.48-0.93)
HERA	Chemotherapy[c] followed by Tr[d] (1 y) vs chemotherapy alone	5,090	HR = 0.76 (95% CI, 0.43-0.67)	HR = 0.76 (95% CI, 0.47-1.23)[e]
BCIBU 006[f]	ACR→D Tr vs carboplatin + D + Tr vs AC→D	3,222	HR = 0.61 (95% CI, 0.43-0.76) HR = 0.67 (95% CI, 0.54-0.83)	HR = 0.59 (95% CI, 0.42-0.85) HR = 0.66 (95% CI, 0.47-0.93)

BCIRG, Breast Cancer International Research Group; CI, confidence interval; D, docetaxel; HERA, Herceptin Adjuvant trial; HR, hazard ratio; NCCTG, North Central Clinical Trials Group; NSABP, National Surgical Breast and Bowel Project; Tr, trastuzumab.

[a]In both studies, treatment was administered for 52 weeks. All patients received four cycles of doxorubicin 60 mg/m^2 and cyclophosphamide 600 mg/m^2 (AC) every 3 weeks followed by paclitaxel (T). Administered at 80 mg/m^2 weekly for 12 weeks (NCCTG), or either 80 mg/m^2 weekly for 12 weeks or 175 mg/m^2 every 3 weeks for four cycles (NSABP). All patients on NSABP B-31 started Tr **concurrent** with paclitaxel; one-third of patients on NCCTG study started trastuzumab concurrent with paclitaxel, the rest started it **sequentially**, after completing paclitaxel.
[b]The results were reported as a joint analysis of both studies.
[c]In HERA, <25% received both an anthracycline and a taxane.
[d]Patients randomly assigned to Tr were further randomly assigned to 1 vs 2 years of therapy There was no difference between 1 and 2 years of trastuzumab therapy.
[e]Results are reported with Tr for 1 year. They are confounded by crossover; 52% of patients on observation ultimately were treated with Tr.
[f]Results of the second interim analysis are presented.

agent is appropriate. For patients who received both pertuzumab and trastuzumab, the evidence-based approach is to continue the doublet.

HER2+ breast cancer also has options for response-adapted treatment after NACT, similar to the response-adapted approach discussed earlier with TNBC based on the CREATE-X trial. Notably, for patients with HER2+ breast cancer treated with NACT who did not achieve pCR, there is evidence to support transition from the initial HER2 biologic to ado-trastuzumab emtansine (T-DM1), which is an ADC of trastuzumab and the cytotoxic emtansine. In the KATHERINE trial, patients treated with neoadjuvant taxane- and trastuzumab-based therapy were randomized to continue trastuzumab or switch to TDM-1 (34). Switch therapy was ultimately shown to improve DFS (88% vs 77%, HR 0.50) with acceptable differences in toxicity, where side effects leading to discontinuation of TDM-1 included thrombocytopenia (4.2%), increased bilirubin (2.6%), increased aspartate transaminase (AST) or alanine transaminase (ALT) (1%-2%), peripheral sensory neuropathy (1.5%), and decreased ejection fraction (1.2%). Newer generations of HER2-directed therapies are being explored to potentially improve the response seen in KATHERINE, including tucatinib and trastuzumab-deruxtecan.

REFERENCES

1. Symmans WF, Yau C, Chen YY, et al. Assessment of residual cancer burden and event-free survival in neoadjuvant treatment for high-risk breast cancer: an analysis of data from the I-SPY2 randomized clinical trial. *JAMA Oncol.* 2021;7:1654-1663.

2. Mauri D, Pavlidis N, Ioannidis JPA. Neoadjuvant versus adjuvant systemic treatment in breast cancer: a meta-analysis. *J Natl Cancer Inst.* 2005;97:188-194.

3. Rastogi P, Anderson SJ, Bear HD, et al. Preoperative chemotherapy: updates of national surgical adjuvant breast and bowel project protocols B-18 and B-27. *J Clin Oncol.* 2008;26:778-785.

4. Mazouni C, Peintinger F, Wan-Kau S, et al. Residual ductal carcinoma in situ in patients with complete eradication of invasive breast cancer after neoadjuvant chemotherapy does not adversely affect patient outcome. *J Clin Oncol.* 2007;25:2650-2655.

5. Rouzier R, Extra JM, Klijanienko J, et al. Incidence and prognostic significance of complete axillary downstaging after primary chemotherapy in breast cancer patients with T1 to T3 tumors and cytologically proven axillary metastatic lymph nodes. *J Clin Oncol.* 2002;20:1304-1310.

6. Ogston KN, Miller ID, Payne S, et al. A new histological grading system to assess response of breast cancers to primary chemotherapy: prognostic significance and survival. *Breast.* 2003;12:320-327.

7. Symmans WF, Peintinger F, Hatzis C, et al. Measurement of residual breast cancer burden to predict survival after neoadjuvant chemotherapy. *J Clin Oncol.* 2007;25:4414-4422.

8. Heys SD, Hutcheon AW, Sarkar TK, et al. Neoadjuvant docetaxel in breast cancer: 3-year survival results from the Aberdeen trial. *Clin Breast Cancer.* 2002;3(Suppl 2):S69-S74.

9. Huober J, von Minckwitz G, Denkert C, et al. Effect of neoadjuvant anthracycline-taxane-based chemotherapy in different biological breast cancer phenotypes: overall results from the GeparTrio study. *Breast Cancer Res Treat.* 2010;124:133-140.

10. Early Breast Cancer Trialists' Collaborative Group (EBCTCG), Peto R, Davies C, et al. Comparisons between different polychemotherapy regimens for early breast cancer: meta-analyses of long-term outcome among 100,000 women in 123 randomised trials. *Lancet.* 2012;379:432-444.

11. Jones S, Holmes FA, O'Shaughnessy J, et al. Docetaxel with cyclophosphamide is associated with an overall survival benefit compared with doxorubicin and cyclophosphamide: 7-year follow-up of US oncology research trial 9735. *J Clin Oncol.* 2009;27:1177-1183.

12. Swain SM, Tang G, Geyer CE Jr, et al. Definitive results of a phase III adjuvant trial comparing three chemotherapy regimens in women with operable, node-positive breast cancer: the NSABP B-38 trial. *J Clin Oncol.* 2013;31:3197-3204.

13. Blum JL, Flynn PJ, Yothers G, et al. Anthracyclines in early breast cancer: the ABC Trials-USOR 06-090, NSABP B-46-I/USOR 07132, and NSABP B-49 (NRG oncology). *J Clin Oncol.* 2017;35:2647-2655.

14. Sparano JA, Gray RJ, Makower DF, et al. Adjuvant chemotherapy guided by a 21-gene expression assay in breast cancer. *N Engl J Med.* 2018;379:111-121.

15. Kalinsky K, Barlow WE, Gralow JR, et al. 21-gene assay to inform chemotherapy benefit in node-positive breast cancer. *N Engl J Med.* 2021;385:2336-2347.

16. Schmid P, Cortes J, Dent R, et al.; KEYNOTE-522 Investigators. Event-free survival with pembrolizumab in early triple-negative breast cancer. *N Engl J Med.* 2022;386(6):556-567. doi:10.1056/NEJMoa2112651

17. Cortes J, Cescon DW, Rugo HS, et al. Pembrolizumab plus chemotherapy versus placebo plus chemotherapy for previously untreated locally recurrent inoperable or metastatic triple-negative breast cancer (KEYNOTE-355): a randomised, placebo-controlled, double-blind, phase 3 clinical trial. *Lancet.* 2020;396:1817-1828.

18. Masuda N, Lee SJ, Ohtani S, et al. Adjuvant capecitabine for breast cancer after Preoperative Chemotherapy. *N Engl J Med.* 2017;376:2147-2159.

19. Denduluri N, Somerfield MR, Chavez-MacGregor M, et al. Selection of optimal adjuvant chemotherapy and targeted therapy for early breast cancer: ASCO guideline update. *J Clin Oncol.* 2021;39(6):685-693. doi:10.1200/JCO.20.02510

20. Lluch A, Barrios CH, Torrecillas L, et al. Phase III trial of adjuvant capecitabine after standard neo-/adjuvant chemotherapy in patients with early triple-negative breast cancer (GEICAM/2003-11_CIBOMA/2004-01). *J Clin Oncol.* 2020;38:203-213.

21. Mayer IA, Zhao F, Arteaga CL, et al. Randomized phase III postoperative trial of platinum-based chemotherapy versus capecitabine in patients with residual triple-negative breast cancer following neoadjuvant chemotherapy: ECOG-ACRIN EA1131. *J Clin Oncol.* 2021;39:2539-2551.

22. Tutt ANJ, Garber JE, Kaufman B, et al. Adjuvant olaparib for patients with BRCA1- or BRCA2-mutated breast cancer. *N Engl J Med.* 2021;384:2394-2405.

23. Mittendorf EA, Jeruss JS, Tucker SL, et al. Validation of a novel staging system for disease-specific survival in patients with breast cancer treated with neoadjuvant chemotherapy. *J Clin Oncol.* 2011;29:1956-1962.

24. Slamon D, Eiermann W, Robert N, et al. Adjuvant trastuzumab in HER2-positive breast cancer. *N Engl J Med.* 2011;365:1273-1283.

25. Goldhirsch A, Gelber RD, Piccart-Gebhart MJ, et al. 2 years versus 1 year of adjuvant trastuzumab for HER2-positive breast cancer (HERA): an open-label, randomised controlled trial. *Lancet.* 2013;382:1021-1028.

26. Gianni L, Dafni U, Gelber RD, et al. Treatment with trastuzumab for 1 year after adjuvant chemotherapy in patients with HER2-positive early breast cancer: a 4-year follow-up of a randomised controlled trial. *Lancet Oncol.* 2011;12:236-244.

27. Perez EA, Romond EH, Suman VJ, et al. Four-year follow-up of trastuzumab plus adjuvant chemotherapy for operable human epidermal growth factor receptor 2-positive breast cancer: joint analysis of data from NCCTG N9831 and NSABP B-31. *J Clin Oncol.* 2011;29:3366-3373.

28. Romond EH, Perez EA, Bryant J, et al. Trastuzumab plus adjuvant chemotherapy for operable HER2-positive breast cancer. *N Engl J Med.* 2005;353:1673-1684.

29. Tolaney SM, Barry WT, Dang CT, et al. Adjuvant paclitaxel and trastuzumab for node-negative, HER2-positive breast cancer. *N Engl J Med.* 2015;372:134-141.

30. Gianni L, Pienkowski T, Im YH, et al. Efficacy and safety of neoadjuvant pertuzumab and trastuzumab in women with locally advanced, inflammatory, or early HER2-positive breast cancer (NeoSphere): a randomised multicentre, open-label, phase 2 trial. *Lancet Oncol.* 2012;13:25-32.

31. Schneeweiss A, Chia S, Hickish T, et al. Pertuzumab plus trastuzumab in combination with standard neoadjuvant anthracycline-containing and anthracycline-free chemotherapy regimens in patients with HER2-positive early breast cancer: a randomized phase II cardiac safety study (TRYPHAENA). *Ann Oncol.* 2013;24:2278-2284.

32. van der Voort A, van Ramshorst MS, van Werkhoven ED, et al. Three-year follow-up of neoadjuvant chemotherapy with or without anthracyclines in the presence of dual ERBB2 blockade in patients with ERBB2-positive breast cancer: a secondary analysis of the TRAIN-2 randomized, phase 3 trial. *JAMA Oncol.* 2021;7:978-984.

33. Armenian SH, Lacchetti C, Barac A, et al. Prevention and monitoring of cardiac dysfunction in survivors of adult cancers: American Society of Clinical Oncology clinical practice guideline. *J Clin Oncol.* 2017;35(8):893-911. doi:10.1200/JCO.2016.70.5400

34. von Minckwitz G, Huang CS, Mano MS, et al. Trastuzumab emtansine for residual invasive HER2-positive breast cancer. *N Engl J Med.* 2019;380:617-628.

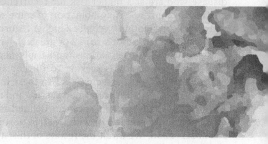

CHAPTER 11.10

Radiation Therapy for Breast Cancer

Jaroslaw T. Hepel and Chelsea Miller

RT is an important and well-established treatment modality for women with breast cancer. Many women are candidates for BCT, which includes postoperative RT. In addition, select women undergoing mastectomy who have locally advanced disease or high-risk features also benefit from postoperative RT. In these settings, radiation has been shown to reduce the risk of local and regional recurrence. Importantly, this reduction in local failure has been shown to translate into improved OS with long-term follow-up (1).

BREAST-CONSERVING THERAPY

BCT, which consists of BCS followed by adjuvant RT, has been a major advance in the treatment of breast cancer. This approach affords women equal oncologic outcomes while avoiding removal of the entire breast (mastectomy) with the associated negative impact on functional, cosmetic, self-image, and emotional outcomes. This approach is substantiated by level 1 evidence and is the standard approach for most women diagnosed with breast cancer today. To be a candidate for BCT, a patient must be a candidate for BCS with removal of all clinically evident disease identified by physical examination and imaging. In addition, the patient must be a candidate for adjuvant RT. Relative contraindications to RT include some connective tissue disorders (eg, scleroderma and lupus) and prior breast irradiation.

Although one of the earliest trials evaluating BCT showed inferior results compared with mastectomy, this trial used insufficient radiation doses by modern standards. Subsequent trials conducted in both Europe and North America have all shown equivalent DFS and OS between BCT and mastectomy. The largest of these trials was NSABP B06, which randomly assigned 1,851 patients to one of three arms: total mastectomy, lumpectomy alone, or lumpectomy with radiation. At 20 years follow-up, there was no difference between total mastectomy versus lumpectomy with radiation in DFS (36% and 35%, respectively; $P = .26$), DDFS (49% and 46%, respectively; $P = .34$), or OS (47% and 46%, respectively; $P = .57$) (2). In addition, the IBTR was 39% with BCS alone and 14% with BCS and RT.

The impact of RT on survival was addressed in the EBCTCG meta-analysis, which evaluated data from greater than 10,000 women from 17 randomized trials of radiation versus no radiation following BCS (3). They found that the addition of RT reduced the 10-year risk of any first recurrence (locoregional or distance) from 35% to 19% ($P < .0001$). Most importantly, this translated into an OS benefit at 15-years follow-up, with an absolute reduction in overall mortality of 3.8% ($P = .0005$).

POSTMASTECTOMY RADIATION THERAPY

For women who undergo a mastectomy and are deemed to be at moderate-to-high risk for local recurrence, RT to the chest wall and regional lymphatics is indicated. The criteria that define "moderate" and "high" risk have evolved over time and continue to do so, as our understanding of the important factors related to local and regional recurrence grows.

Early trials of postmastectomy RT showed a decrease in local recurrence, but no apparent benefit in OS (1). However, the trials varied greatly in radiation technique and dose, as well as including some patients who did not receive systemic therapy. There have since been three contemporary trials that have evaluated the benefit of postmastectomy RT. The Danish Breast Cancer Cooperative group (DBCCG) conducted one trial evaluating of 1,708 premenopausal women with pathologic stage II or III breast cancer treated with mastectomy and CMF chemotherapy who were randomly assigned to observation or to treatment with RT to the chest wall and regional nodes (4). RT was associated with a significant reduction in local-regional recurrence compared to chemotherapy alone (9% vs 32%, $P < .001$). It was also associated with a significant survival benefit at 10 years (54% vs 45%, $P < .001$). A second DBCCG trial looked at more than 1,300 postmenopausal women with stage II-III breast cancer treated with mastectomy and TAM (30 mg/d for 1 year) who were randomly assigned to treatment with RT or no RT (5). With a median follow-up of over 10 years, RT was associated with a significant reduction in local-regional recurrence compared to TAM alone (8% vs 35%, $P < .001$) and a significant improvement in OS (45% vs 36%, $P = .03$). These two studies have been criticized for the low number of axillary LNs removed on axillary dissection and higher-than-expected axillary recurrent rates in the control groups. The British Columbia Trial also addressed the question of postmastectomy RT by randomizing more than 300 women to CMF chemotherapy with or without RT (6). This trial also showed a local-regional control benefit, as well as an OS benefit to RT. Unlike the Danish trials, a median of 11 LNs was removed with ALND, which is considered appropriate. At 20 years follow-up, isolated recurrence was 10% versus 26% and OS was 47% versus 37% in favor of postmastectomy RT. The relative magnitude of benefit from RT was similar in women with one to three positive nodes (HR 0.76, 95% CI 0.50-1.15) compared to those with four or more positive nodes (HR 0.70, 95% CI 0.46-1.06).

The EBCTCG performed a meta-analysis of individual patient data from randomized trials of postmastectomy RT (1). This analysis included 8,500 women, and for those with any involved axillary nodes, RT resulted in a 17% absolute reduction in 5-year local recurrence (6% vs 23%) and a 4.4% absolute improvement in 15-year OS (40.2% vs 35.8%). An update of this analysis showed that the reduction in local-regional recurrence and breast cancer mortality is evident not only in patients with four or more involved axillary LNs but also in those with one to three involved axillary nodes (7). In these women with one to three positive axillary nodes, the addition of postmastectomy RT reduced the risks of local-regional recurrence from 20.3% to 3.8% at 10 years, any recurrence (local or distant) from 45.7% to 34.2% at 10 years, and breast cancer mortality from 47.0% to 37.9% at 15 years.

Postmastectomy RT, therefore, is recommended for all patients with locally advanced disease (T4 or four or more positive nodes). RT is also generally recommended to patients with one to three positive nodes or involved surgical margins, as these patients are also at moderate-to-high risk for local recurrence. The use of postmastectomy RT in patients with T1-2 N0 disease with high-risk features is controversial, but a subset of patients with node-negative disease who are at a higher risk for recurrence may benefit from postmastectomy RT. A combination of some of the following risk factors has been found to confer a higher recurrence risk, including young age, larger tumor size (T2 or greater), lymphovascular space invasion (LVSI), close margins, and triple-negative disease (8,9). The SUPREMO study is seeking to further answer the question of the need for postmastectomy RT in these intermediate-risk patients (10). This study has finished accrual and randomized women with intermediate-risk breast cancer, defined as pT1-2 N1, pT3 N0, or pT2 N0 if also grade 3 or with LVSI, to postmastectomy RT versus observation. We await the results of this study to have further guidance with regard to the role of postmastectomy RT in this population of women.

RADIATION THERAPY TO THE REGIONAL LYMPH NODES

RT improves not only the likelihood of tumor control in the breast or along the chest wall but also regional control in the draining LN basins for patients at risk for harboring micrometastatic disease at these sites. The role of RT in axillary management has been looked at in several clinical trials. The ACOSOG Z0011 trial (discussed earlier) has suggested that RT to the axillary LNs may not be necessary, particularly for those felt to be at low risk for recurrence (11). However, it should be noted that all patients in this trial received breast irradiation and that there was no central review of the radiation fields, which is important for quality control. The importance of the latter point was shown in a retrospective review of the radiation fields used in this trial, which revealed that 19% of patients were treated with regional nodal irradiation (RNI) targeting the axilla and supraclavicular fossa (SCF), and an additional 50% of patient were treated with "high" tangents targeting the level I/II axilla (12). Therefore, the majority of patients on this trial in fact had RT to at least a portion of the regional LNs. The EORTC AMAROS trial enrolled women who had a clinically negative axilla but had one to three positive LNs on sentinel node biopsy and randomized them to ALND versus RT to the axillary (levels I-III) and supraclavicular LNs (13). The rates of axillary recurrence were noninferior with the use of axillary RT, and recurrence was rare in both arms. The rate of axillary recurrence was 0.41% versus 1.04% at 5 years and 0.93% versus 1.82% at 10 years ($P = .37$). Importantly, the rates of arm lymphedema were significantly higher with ALND compared to axillary RT, with 40% versus 22% at 1 year and 28% versus 14% at 5 years. There was no difference in DFS or OS between the two arms. Taking these two trials together, ALND can be safely omitted, with a corresponding lower risk of arm lymphedema, in women with low tumor burden (clinically node negative) and one to three positive axillary LNs, provided that axillary RT is administered.

The management of LNs beyond the axilla was evaluated in two additional trials. In both trials, all patients had breast surgery and ALND and then were randomly assigned to undergo RNI (targeting the high axillary, supraclavicular, and IM LNs) versus breast or chest wall RT alone. In the NCI of Canada—Clinical Trials Group (NCIC-CTG) MA.20 trial, 1,832 women with node-positive or high-risk node-negative disease were included (14). At 10 years, RNI resulted in significant improvements in DFS (HR 0.76, $P = .01$), isolated locoregional DFS (HR 0.59, $P = .0009$), and DDFS (HR 0.76, $P = .03$). There was no corresponding statistically significant difference in OS. In the EORTC 22922/10925 trial, 4,004 women with node-positive or centrally and medially located node-negative disease were enrolled (15). At 10 years, RNI again resulted in significant improvements in DFS (HR 0.89, $P = .04$) and DDFS (HR 0.86, $P = .02$). In addition, there was a significant reduction in breast cancer mortality (HR 0.82, $P = .02$), although only a trend was noted toward improvement in OS (HR 0.82, $P = .06$). These trials demonstrate that for high-risk patients, RNI not only improves regional disease control but also impacts risk of metastatic disease and breast cancer mortality.

The inclusion of the IM nodes in RNI has been controversial. Classic surgical data have shown that the risk of IM node involvement can be as high as 20% to 40%, particularly for patients who have medially located tumors and involved axillary LNs (16,17). In addition, retrospective data have suggested that RT to the IM chain may confer a survival benefit (18,19). Conversely, clinical relapse in the IM chain even in these patients is rare, with estimates placing this at less than 1% (20). In addition, RT to the IM LNs is not without consequence, increasing both heart and lung radiation doses, which can contribute to pulmonary toxicity and late cardiac morbidity.

To evaluate the benefits of IM nodal irradiation, Hennequin et al randomized women with positive axillary LNs or those with centrally/medically located tumors irrespective of nodal status to breast and supraclavicular irradiation with or without IM nodal irradiation (21). At 10 years, there was no difference in the primary end point of OS. Despite these results, some have criticized this trial because it included patients who were at a relatively low risk for recurrence, thus underpowering the primary end point. The DBCCG-IMN study evaluated RT to the IM nodes in a trial that included 3,089 volunteers (19). Given concerns over risk of cardiac toxicity with the use of both anthracyclines and IM nodal irradiation, women with left-sided breast cancer received RNI to axillary and supraclavicular LNs only, whereas women with right-sided breast cancer received RNI that included the IM nodes. At 8 years follow-up, OS was improved with IM nodal irradiation from 72.2% to 75.9% ($P = .005$). Cardiac deaths were equal in both groups, but again IM nodal irradiation was only administered to right-sided breast cancers. Therefore, the decision to add IM nodal irradiation to RNI should be considered for patients at higher risk of IM nodal involvement. However, the risk of additional cardiac toxicity based on radiation technique and the patient's specific anatomy needs to be factored into this decision.

RADIATION THERAPY AFTER NEOADJUVANT CHEMOTHERAPY AND SURGERY

NACT for LABC or for biologically aggressive breast cancer subtypes (triple negative or her2neu positive) provides valuable prognostic information based on tumor response and results in downstaging of disease for responders. This later benefit allows for some patients who were initially not candidates for BCT to be able to undergo breast preservation. NSABP B18 randomized 1,523 patients to NACT or the same chemotherapy given postoperatively (22). Both DFS and OS were not different between the two arms. However, the rate of BCT increased from 60% to 68% with NACT. For patients who were initially not candidates for BCT, this represents a 20% increase. The rate of IBTR in patients who underwent BCT was not different between NACT and adjuvant chemotherapy (7.9% and 5.8%, respectively, $P = .23$). Long-term follow-up has confirmed that BCT following NACT remains appropriate with a low risk of recurrence (23).

Achieving a pCR to NACT has been shown to be a favorable prognostic factor in terms of OS (22,23). However, achieving a pCR does not necessarily confer a low risk of local recurrence after surgery. Patients who have a pCR after NACT and undergo BCS remain at high risk of recurrence without RT. Therefore, whole-breast RT (WBRT) remains an important part of BCT for these patients (22). In addition, patients who have high-risk, locally advanced disease (T4 or N2 or greater) treated with mastectomy, despite achieving pCR, remain at high risk for local-regional recurrence and still benefit from adjuvant chest wall RT and RNI (24). In some patients with moderate-risk disease, who normally would benefit from postmastectomy RT, achieving a pCR with NACT may confer a lower risk of recurrence. Pooled subset analysis of the NSABP B18 and B27 trials was performed looking at local and regional recurrence following NACT and mastectomy without RT (25). Patients with initial cT1-2 N1 disease had a rate of local recurrence of 0%, 11%, and 17% when achieving a pCR in both LNs and the breast, a pCR in the nodes but not the breast, and no pCR in either the nodes or the breast, respectively. These data would suggest some patients who achieve a pCR are at low risk for local and regional recurrence after mastectomy and may not require adjuvant RT; this is being evaluated in ongoing clinical trials.

RADIATION THERAPY FOR IN SITU BREAST DISEASE

Approximately 20% to 30% of patients treated with local excision alone for DCIS have a recurrence, with about half of these recurrences being invasive cancer. As a result, radiation is often delivered as a means of local recurrence risk reduction. Several randomized trials have compared wide local excision followed by WBRT versus observation alone, and all have demonstrated decreased rates of local recurrence with the addition of RT by 38% to 62% (26).

In addition, an EBCTCG meta-analysis found that the absolute magnitude of the 10-year risk reduction with addition of radiation was 15%. Local recurrence reduction was seen across all risk groups, with the largest absolute benefit seen in patients with high-risk factors including size greater than 2 cm, high grade, the presence of comedo necrosis, and positive resection margins. However, there was no significant difference in breast cancer–specific mortality or OS with the use of RT for DCIS (26).

Attempts at identifying subgroups of patients at low risk for recurrence following excision alone have met with limited success. Wong et al prospectively evaluated a series of patients treated with wide resection margins of at least 1 cm and still reported a 5-year recurrence rate of 12% (27). A prospective trial run by the Eastern Oncology Cooperative Group (ECOG) evaluated omission of RT for patients with high-grade tumors but less than 1 cm in size (28). Local recurrence was 15.3% at 5 years despite a mean tumor size of only 5 mm. The Radiation Therapy Oncology Group (RTOG) 9804 trial compared observation to RT in more than 600 women who were felt to have particularly low-risk DCIS (29). This favorable-risk group was defined as DCIS that was mammogram detected measuring 2.5 cm or less pathologically, nuclear grade 1 to 2, with negative margins by 3 mm. Local recurrence was 0.9% versus 6.7% at 7 years for RT versus observation ($P < .001$). Unfortunately, with continued follow-up, the risk of local recurrence increases by approximately 1% per year with surgery alone. At 15 years, the risk of local recurrence was 7.1% versus 15.1% for RT versus observation ($P < .001$) (30). Although RT again resulted in a statistically significant reduction in local recurrence, the absolute benefit of RT in patients with favorable-risk DCIS is smaller. Thus, omission of radiation can be considered after discussion with the patient and the understanding that this approach carries a higher recurrence risk. Genomic assays to help stratify which patients with DCIS have the lowest benefit from radiation have been developed, including Oncotype-DCIS and DCISionRT (31,32). However, independent prospective validation of these assays is still needed to best define their role.

DE-ESCALATION OF RADIATION THERAPY

Escalation of therapy for high-risk breast cancers has resulted in improved outcomes and survival. However, equally important is de-escalation of therapy for patient with low-risk breast cancers with the goal of maintaining a high rate of cure but limiting treatment-related toxicity and morbidity. From a radiation perspective, this has been accomplished by reducing the number of daily treatments (hypofractionation), reducing the volume of treatment (partial breast irradiation [PBI]), and omitting radiation entirely for appropriately selected patients.

Hypofractionation

Standard fractionated RT for breast cancer is defined as radiation delivered in 1.8 to 2.0 Gy per fraction (or treatment session), once daily, 5 days per week, over 5 to 7 weeks. Whelan et al reported 10-year results of the Canadian study that randomized more than 1,200 women to either standard WBRT (50 Gy in 25 fractions) or a hypofractionated regimen (42.5 Gy in 16 fractions) (33). The IBTR rate at 10 years was similar: 6.7% for standard fractionation and 6.2% for hypofractionation. Good-to-excellent cosmetic outcome was also similar (71.3% and 69.8%, respectively). Long-term outcomes from the United Kingdom START trials have also been published (34). START-B enrolled 2,215 women and randomized them to receive either 50 Gy in 25 fractions or 40 Gy in 15 fractions. At 10 years, the local-regional recurrence rate was not statistically different: 5.5% for standard versus 4.3% for hypofractionation. The side effects of RT, including breast shrinkage, telangiectasia, and breast edema, were notably less common with hypofractionation, and cosmetic outcomes were not different between the two treatment schedules. These trials provided robust, level 1 evidence that hypofractionation is safe and equally effective. Although there are some limitations to whom hypofractionation whole-breast irradiation can be applied, many women can now be offered this more convenient treatment option (35). For the future, the UK FAST-Forward trial is evaluating an even shorter WBRT schedule of 26 Gy in 5 fractions delivered over just 1 week (36). Preliminary 5-year data show comparable outcomes; however, mature 10-year data are needed before this regimen can be recommended for routine use.

Partial Breast Irradiation

The concept of partial breast RT arose out of the realization that the majority of recurrences for early-stage breast cancers occur at or near the region of the lumpectomy site (37,38). Thus, only the breast tissue surrounding the tumor bed needs radiation treatment. This approach is called either PBI or accelerated partial breast irradiation (APBI). Limiting RT to a smaller portion of the breast results in two major advantages. First, there is a reduction in the volume of irradiated tissue, thereby preserving these tissues from potential deleterious radiation effects. This includes minimal-to-no dose exposure to the heart and lung. Second, by reducing the volume of treatment, the overall treatment time can be safely accelerated to deliver the entire course of radiation, often, within 1 week. Multiple techniques have been developed for the delivery of APBI. These are discussed in more detail in "Radiation Therapy Techniques." This treatment approach was initially guided by multiple single- and multi-institutional phase II trials, which have demonstrated the comparable efficacy of PBI (39). There are now seven contemporary phase III randomized trials that evaluated WBRT and PBI. The Groupe Européen de Curiethérapie of European Society for Radiotherapy and Oncology (GEC-ESTRO) enrolled 1,184 women with early-stage breast cancer treated with BCS and were randomly assigned to treatment using standard WBRT or APBI (using an interstitial multicatheter technique) (40). At 5 years follow-up, there was no statistically significant difference in IBTR (1.4% vs 0.9%), DFS, OS, or late toxicity. The IMPORT-LOW trial is a particularly important study that enrolled 2,018 patients into three randomized arms (41). The two relevant arms for this discussion compared WBRT and PBI. WBRT was delivered using tangential photon fields with field-in-field dose modulation. PBI was delivered using reduced volume "mini-tangents" with field-in-field dose modulation. The delivered dose was 40 Gy in 15 fractions for both arms. Therefore, the only variable changed between the two treatment arms was the irradiated volume, thus fundamentally evaluating the concept of PBI without other confounding variables. At 5 years, the IBTR was noninferior (1.1% vs 0.5%). OS was also the same (95% vs 96.3%, $P = .693$). Both acute toxicity and late toxicity were improved with PBI. Cosmetic outcome was not different. The Canadian RAPID trial randomized 2,135 patients to WBRT or APBI using an external beam, 3D conformal radiation technique (42). At 8 years, IBTR was 2.8% with WBRT and 3.0% with APBI. This met noninferiority criteria. OS was also not different. The NSABP B39/RTOG 9413 trial enrolled 4,216 patients who were randomized to WBRT versus APBI using either external beam

■ **TABLE 11.10-1. Guidelines for Appropriate Patient Selection for PBI**

ASTRO "Suitable" Criteria
Patient factors
  Age ≥ 50 yr
  BRCA1/2 mutation not present
Pathologic factors
  Histology: Invasive ductal or other favorable invasive subtypes or DCIS (grade 1-2 only)
  Tumor size ≤ 2 cm
  T stage: T1
  Grade: any (invasive); 1-2 (DCIS)
  No LVSI
  ER positive
  Margins negative by at least 2 mm
  Unicentric and unifocal
Nodal factors
  N stage: pN0 (i−, i+)
  Nodal surgery: SN Bx or ALND
Treatment factors
  Neoadjuvant therapy not allowed

American Brachytherapy Society
  Age ≥ 50 yr
  Invasive carcinoma (any histology) or DCIS
  Tumor size ≤ 3 cm
  Margins negative (no tumor at inked margin)
  ER + or −
  No LVSI
  Lymph node negative by SN Bx or ALND (pN0)

American Society of Breast Surgeons
  Age ≥ 45 yr
  Invasive ductal carcinoma or DCIS
  Tumor size ≤ 3 cm
  Margins negative by at least 2 mm
  Lymph node negative by SN Bx or ALND (pN0)

ALND, axillary lymph node dissection; ASTRO, American Society for Radiation Oncology; DCIS, ductal carcinoma in situ; ER, estrogen receptor; LVSI, lymphovascular space invasion; PBI, partial breast irradiation.

3D conformal radiation, interstitial multicatheter brachytherapy (IMB), or intracavitary brachytherapy (43). This trial used an ambitious equivalence design, assuming 90% CI that the HR would be between 0.667 and 1.5. At a median follow-up of 10 years, the IBTR was 3.9% with WBRT and 4.6% with APBI (HR 1.22; 90% CI 0.94-1.58). Although the trial did not meet statistical equivalence as the 90% CI of the HR exceeded 1.5, there was no clinically meaningful difference in IBTR. The absolute difference in IBTR was only 0.7% at 10 years. OS was not different. Three additional smaller phase III trials also showed no difference in IBTR between WBRT and APBI (44-46). Based on this robust level 1 evidence, PBI is an appropriate option for many women with early-stage breast cancer and should be considered as preferred options (47). Criteria for appropriate selection of patients for PBI should be based on the inclusion criteria of the abovementioned phase III clinical trials and on guidelines published by the American Brachytherapy Society (ABS), ASBrS, and ASTRO (**Table 11.10-1**) (48-50).

Omission of Radiation Therapy

Although the benefits of RT have been effectively established, ongoing work is aiming to better elucidate who may *not* benefit from RT, thus sparing them from the inconvenience and potential toxicities of treatment. Patients with early-stage, node-negative breast cancer with tumors 2 cm or less (T1a-c N0), which are both ER positive and her2neu negative, are considered to be a lower risk group. However, initial evaluation of omission of RT in unselected patients in this group resulted in an unacceptably high rate of local recurrence. This was examined in the NSABP B-21 trial, which evaluated over 1,000 women (51). Women of all ages with tumors

1 cm or less and ER-positive, LN-negative disease were included. Patients underwent BCS and were randomly assigned to adjuvant treatment with TAM alone versus RT alone versus both RT and TAM. The primary end points were IBTR and incidence of CBC. As reported, TAM was not as effective in preventing IBTR as RT alone, and the combination of both resulted in the best outcomes. The incidence of IBTR at 8 years on TAM alone, RT alone, and the combination was 16.5%, 9.3%, and 2.8%, respectively.

A subgroup felt to be at particularly low risk of recurrence is older patients, as they tend to have more indolent tumor biology. The Cancer and Leukemia Group B (CALGB) 9343 trial evaluated omission of RT in women aged 70 years or above treated with BCS (52,53). These women had tumors 2 cm or larger in size and were ER positive and LN negative. The rate of IBTR was 5% versus 1% at 5 years (*P* < .001) and 10% versus 2% at 10 years (*P* < .001) for ET alone versus ET and RT. The rate of salvage mastectomy and OS were not different between the two arms. The Postoperative Radiotherapy In Minimal-risk Elderly (PRIME) II trial also evaluated omission of RT following BCS in women aged 65 years or above with T1-2 (≤3 cm), node-negative breast cancers that were ER positive, randomizing more than 1,300 patients (54). At 5 years, the IBTR rate was 4.1% versus 1.2% with ET alone versus ET and RT. While the rate of local recurrence was higher in both of these trials among women who did not receive radiation, the absolute benefit of radiation was small, suggesting that it may be reasonable for older women with small tumors to forego RT, provided they are candidates for ET (55). In these trials, older age was used as a surrogate to identify patients with less aggressive tumor biology. Ongoing trials are evaluating the use of genomic-based assays to define less aggressive tumor biology where the value of radiation may be small. These trials may identify a subset of younger women and better select older women for omission of RT.

RADIATION THERAPY: OTHER INDICATIONS

For patients who experience locally recurrent breast cancer, local therapy with surgery and/or radiation may be an option. For some, cure can be achieved, and in most, RT can help reduce the risk of significant morbidity of uncontrolled, local disease.

Oligometastatic disease is a transitional state between localized disease and widespread systemic disease, where the volume and number of metastatic deposits is limited, and local therapy (with or without systemic therapy) is an option. Although only a small percentage of these patients can have long-term DFS, this is in distinct contrast to patients with widespread metastatic disease in whom cure is not possible. Although such tumor biology is considered rare in breast cancer, aggressive local therapy with radiation and/or surgery should be considered for select patients. Stereotactic body RT or stereotactic radiosurgery is an ideal method of RT for these patients. With this method, high ablative doses of radiation are delivered in a highly conformal manner with extreme precision. This is typically done in just one to five treatments or fractions and can be applied not just to the brain but almost any part of the body. The large radiation doses result in a high probability of local disease control, and the conformality and precision allows for a low risk of side effects and complications (48,56).

For patients with widespread metastatic disease, RT can be used effectively for palliation of lesions involving the chest wall, regional lymphatics, bone, brain, lung, and liver, among other areas. Indication for radiation in this setting includes palliation of symptomatic lesions not responding or unlikely to respond to systemic therapy and prevention of complications of local disease progression, such as impending pathologic fracture from bone metastasis, impingement of the spinal cord or nerve roots from spine metastasis, or neurologic sequelae from brain metastases. Palliative radiation courses range from a one-time 8-Gy treatment to a 2- to 3-week course of daily treatments of 2.5 to 3 Gy per fraction for a total dose of 30 to 37.5 Gy.

RADIATION THERAPY TECHNIQUES

Radiation treatment planning and delivery has dramatically evolved since the inception of BCT, from low-energy Cobalt units using indiscriminate en face treatment fields, to high-energy linear accelerators with rudimentary 2D planning, and now to modern CT-based, 3D treatment planning with sophisticated dose modulation. This is important to understand, as we have come a long way in our ability to spare normal tissues, and this needs to be considered when evaluating long-term toxicity data from obsolete techniques that are clearly inferior and posed substantially higher risk to underlying organs compared to modern methods.

For modern radiation treatment planning, the process begins with the "simulation." This is a session at which the patient position for treatment is established. For breast cancer, this is typically in the supine position with the ipsilateral arm or both arms up, although other treatment positions are sometimes used to optimize target and normal tissue geometry including prone positioning on a specialized breast board. Appropriate immobilization devices are used to ensure the stability and reproducibility of the patient position during daily treatments. Tattoos are placed to allow for precise positioning with aid of in-room targeting lasers. A CT scan is obtained in the established treatment position. This data set is used to design treatment portals and to perform dose calculations. This allows for tailoring the treatment fields to the specific anatomy of the patient and allows for optimization of target doses and normal tissue sparing. Once an appropriate treatment plan is generated, the virtual plan is verified on the patient via imaging through the treatment portals and/or CT imaging on the treatment machine. The whole process undergoes rigorous quality assurance procedures to ensure the utmost accuracy in all facets of treatment delivery.

Intact Breast

Following BCS, the entire residual breast tissue is included in the irradiated volume with or without regional LN groups depending on the risk of subclinical disease spread to these regions. Treatment portals are oriented tangential to the breast to avoid lung and heart irradiation. Photon energies of 6 to 10 MV are preferred to treat the breast. Energies greater than 6 to 10 MV may underdose superficial tissue beneath the skin surface but may be helpful in decreasing hot spots for patients with large breasts. Dose modulation with wedges, tissue compensators, electronic compensation (field-in-field techniques), or intensity-modulated radiation therapy (IMRT) is used to optimize dose distribution and dose homogeneity across the target volumes. Typical prescription doses are 45 to 50.4 Gy in 1.8 to 2.0 Gy per fraction for 25 to 28 treatments given 5 days/week over 5 to 6 weeks using standard fractionation and 40 to 42.5 Gy in 2.66 to 2.67 Gy per fraction for 15 to 16 treatments over 3 weeks using hypofractionation. This is followed by a boost to the tumor bed consisting of 10 to 16 Gy in 1.8 to 2.5 Gy per fraction over an additional 1 to 1.5 weeks. This results in a total cumulative dose of 60 to 66 Gy or 50 to 52.5 Gy for standard fractionation and hypofractionation, respectively.

The tumor bed has the highest risk of harboring subclinical or microscopic disease, and clinical evidence has shown that it is the site at highest risk for recurrence. The value of adding a tumor bed boost was evaluated by two randomized trials. The EORTC 22881-10882 trial involved more than 5,300 women with stage I or II breast cancer who were randomly assigned to whole-breast treatment with or without a tumor bed boost of 16 Gy (57). With a median follow-up of 17 years, there was no difference in 20-year OS between the boost and the no-boost group (60% vs 61%, HR 1.05, 95% CI 0.92-1.19). However, the rate of IBTR favored those who underwent a boost (9% vs 13%, HR 0.65, 99% CI 0.52-0.81). A separate randomized trial from Lyon, France, also showed a reduction in local relapse with a 10-Gy boost (58). The boost targets the lumpectomy cavity with an appropriate margin. Planning

should be performed using CT-based simulation to ensure appropriate target coverage and can be delivered using one of several techniques, including en face electrons, three-dimensional conformal RT (3D-CRT), IMRT, Accuboost, or other brachytherapy techniques (59,60).

Chest Wall

For women at high risk for local or regional recurrence following mastectomy, RT is delivered to the chest wall and regional lymphatics. Similar to intact breast treatment, a 3D-CRT technique using tangentially oriented beams or IMRT is used. Typically, tissue-equivalent bolus material is used on the chest wall surface, for at least a portion of the treatment, to increase dose build-up in superficial chest wall tissues. Other techniques such as en face electrons fields or mixed electron and photon fields can also be used to target the tissues at risk. The typical prescription dose is 45 to 50.4 Gy in 1.8 to 2.0 Gy per fraction for 25 to 28 treatments over 5 to 6 weeks. This can be followed by a boost to the mastectomy scar/operative bed to a total dose of 60 to 66 Gy. A hypofractionation RT schedule may also be appropriate.

For patients undergoing mastectomy, reconstructive options are an important consideration for most women. The plastic surgeon should be involved early in the multidisciplinary management of these patients, as many factors can have significant implications on the ultimate cosmetic outcome. Among these factors are the type of reconstruction used and sequencing of reconstruction and postmastectomy radiation.

Regional Lymphatics

From a radiation oncology perspective, the regional lymphatics are divided into four anatomic groups: low axilla (level I and lower level II), high axilla (high level II and level III), SCF, and IM chain. Each of these regions can be targeted based on the risk of subclinical disease involvement.

For patients with node-negative disease, the risk of a recurrence in the axilla or SCF is uncommon, and inclusion of these nodal regions is not necessary. For patients with involved axillary LNs, and particularly those with four or more involved nodes, the SCF is at risk and should be treated. The SCF is typically treated with a single anterior oblique field that is matched to the tangential breast fields. The matching technique is crucial to prevent beam overlap and thus significant dose hot spots at the beam junctions. For women with involved axillary LNs who undergo a completion axillary dissection, treatment of the lower dissected axilla is generally not necessary, as the risk of failure after an en bloc resection is not common. Avoiding irradiation of the lower axilla in these patients is desirable, as irradiation increases the risk of arm lymphedema following axillary dissection. Thus, treatment of the lower axilla is typically reserved for patients at high risk of subsequent axillary failure. This includes patients who do not undergo axillary evaluation but are at risk for axillary LN involvement, patients with positive SLNs who do not undergo a completion dissection, and patients with involved axillary LNs who undergo dissection but have high-risk factors. The axilla is typically treated by extending the oblique SCF field laterally. Often, a posterior field, posterior axillary boost (PAB), is added to supplement dose to the posterior portion of the axilla. Alternatively, IMRT can be employed.

The IM nodes are located in the first five intercostal spaces adjacent to the IM vessels, just lateral to the sternum. The first three intercostal spaces are typically targeted for treatment as these represent the highest-risk region. Several techniques can be used to treat the IM nodes. The most common methods are either IMRT or modification of the whole-breast tangential beams using deep or partial-wide fields.

Regional LNs are treated to a total dose of 45 to 50.4 Gy in 1.8 to 2.0 Gy per fraction over 5 to 6 weeks. A hypofractionation RT schedule may also be considered.

Accelerated Partial Breast Irradiation

Numerous techniques for the delivery of APBI have been employed involving both external beam and brachytherapy techniques. The most common techniques are IMB, intracavitary balloon brachytherapy (IBB), 3D-CRT, and IMRT. IMB is characterized by the percutaneous placement of multiple catheters into and surrounding the lumpectomy cavity in such a manner as to deliver the prescription dose to the tumor bed with a margin of 1.0 to 2.0 cm. This technique is versatile and can conform to the most complex tumor bed geometry. IBB was developed as a simplification of the IMB technique. IBB involves the percutaneous placement of a single catheter applicator into the lumpectomy cavity. This is performed either at the time of surgery under direct visualization with an open cavity or postoperatively under US and/or CT guidance. Once the end of the applicator is positioned within the lumpectomy cavity, the balloon at the end of the applicator is inflated to conform to the cavity. Dose is prescribed to a 1-cm distance from the balloon surface to encompass the tumor bed with an appropriate margin. Several balloon and balloon-like catheters are commercially available, including Mammosite, Contura, and SAVI. A prescription dose of 34.0 Gy in 10 fractions given twice daily over 1 week is used for IMB and IBB (43). APBI using 3D-CRT is an external beam technique that employs four to five noncoplanar, tangential oriented beams targeted to the lumpectomy cavity. To account for breast motion, respiratory motion, patient motion, and setup error, a larger margin of 2.5 cm is used with this technique. A prescription dose of 38.5 Gy in 10 fractions given twice daily over 1 week is used for APBI using 3D-CRT (42,43). IMRT is a technique using either multiple fixed beams or arc therapy with precisely planned dose modulation to deliver a very conformal dose distribution to the target volume. This technique was used in the Florence randomized APBI trial with favorable outcomes in terms of acute toxicity, late toxicity, and cosmetic outcome (46). A dose of 30 Gy in 5 fractions given on alternating days over 1.5 weeks is prescribed with this technique.

REFERENCES

1. Clarke M, Collins R, Darby S, et al. Effects of radiotherapy and of differences in the extent of surgery for early breast cancer on local recurrence and 15-year survival: an overview of the randomised trials. *Lancet.* 2005;366(9503):2087-2106. doi:10.1016/S0140-6736(05)67887-7

2. Fisher B, Anderson S, Bryant J, et al. Twenty-year follow-up of a randomized trial comparing total mastectomy, lumpectomy, and lumpectomy plus irradiation for the treatment of invasive breast cancer. *N Engl J Med.* 2002;347(16):1233-1241. doi:10.1056/NEJMoa022152

3. Early Breast Cancer Trialists' Collaborative Group (EBCTCG), Darby S, McGale P, et al. Effect of radiotherapy after breast-conserving surgery on 10-year recurrence and 15-year breast cancer death: meta-analysis of individual patient data for 10,801 women in 17 randomised trials. *Lancet.* 2011;378(9804):1707-1716. doi:10.1016/S0140-6736(11)61629-2

4. Overgaard M, Christensen JJ, Johansen H, et al. Evaluation of radiotherapy in high-risk breast cancer patients: report from the Danish Breast Cancer Cooperative Group (DBCG 82) trial. *Int J Radiat Oncol Biol Phys.* 1990;19(5):1121-1124.

5. Overgaard M, Jensen MB, Overgaard J, et al. Postoperative radiotherapy in high-risk postmenopausal breast-cancer patients given adjuvant tamoxifen: Danish Breast Cancer Cooperative Group DBCG 82c randomised trial. *Lancet.* 1999;353(9165):1641-1648. doi:10.1016/S0140-6736(98)09201-0

6. Ragaz J, Olivotto IA, Spinelli JJ, et al. Locoregional radiation therapy in patients with high-risk breast cancer receiving adjuvant chemotherapy: 20-year results of the British Columbia randomized trial. *J Natl Cancer Inst.* 2005;97(2):116-126. doi:10.1093/jnci/djh297

7. Early Breast Cancer Trialists' Collaborative Group (EBCTCG), McGale P, Taylor C, et al. Effect of radiotherapy after mastectomy and axillary surgery on 10-year recurrence and 20-year breast cancer mortality: meta-analysis of individual patient data for 8135 women in 22 randomised trials. *Lancet.* 2014;383(9935):2127-2135. doi:10.1016/S0140-6736(14)60488-8

8. Jagsi R, Raad RA, Goldberg S, et al. Locoregional recurrence rates and prognostic factors for failure in node-negative patients treated with mastectomy: implications for postmastectomy radiation. *Int J Radiat Oncol Biol Phys.* 2005;62(4):1035-1039. doi:10.1016/j.ijrobp.2004.12.014

9. Wang J, Shi M, Ling R, et al. Adjuvant chemotherapy and radiotherapy in triple-negative breast carcinoma: a prospective randomized controlled multi-center trial. *Radiother Oncol.* 2011;100(2):200-204. doi:10.1016/j.radonc.2011.07.007

10. Velikova G, Williams LJ, Willis S, et al. Quality of life after postmastectomy radiotherapy in patients with intermediate-risk breast cancer (SUPREMO): 2-year follow-up results of a randomised controlled trial. *Lancet Oncol.* 2018;19(11):1516-1529. doi:10.1016/S1470-2045(18)30515-1

11. Giuliano AE, Hunt KK, Ballman KV, et al. Axillary dissection vs no axillary dissection in women with invasive breast cancer and sentinel node metastasis: a randomized clinical trial. *JAMA.* 2011;305(6):569-575. doi:10.1001/jama.2011.90

12. Jagsi R, Chadha M, Moni J, et al. Radiation field design in the ACOSOG Z0011 (Alliance) trial. *J Clin Oncol.* 2014;32(32):3600-3606. doi:10.1200/JCO.2014.56.5838

13. Donker M, van Tienhoven G, Straver ME, et al. Radiotherapy or surgery of the axilla after a positive sentinel node in breast cancer (EORTC 10981-22023 AMAROS): a randomised, multicentre, open-label, phase 3 non-inferiority trial. *Lancet Oncol.* 2014;15(12):1303-1310. doi:10.1016/S1470-2045(14)70460-7

14. Whelan TJ, Olivotto IA, Levine MN. Regional nodal irradiation in early-stage breast cancer. *N Engl J Med.* 2015;373(19):1878-1879. doi:10.1056/NEJMc1510505

15. Poortmans PM, Collette S, Kirkove C, et al. Internal mammary and medial supraclavicular irradiation in breast cancer. *N Engl J Med.* 2015;373(4):317-327. doi:10.1056/NEJMoa1415369

16. Morrow M, Foster RS. Staging of breast cancer: a new rationale for internal mammary node biopsy. *Arch Surg.* 1981;116(6):748-751.

17. Veronesi U, Cascinelli N, Bufalino R, et al. Risk of internal mammary lymph node metastases and its relevance on prognosis of breast cancer patients. *Ann Surg.* 1983;198(6):681-684.

18. Chang JS, Park W, Kim YB, et al. Long-term survival outcomes following internal mammary node irradiation in stage II-III breast cancer: results of a large retrospective study with 12-year follow-up. *Int J Radiat Oncol Biol Phys.* 2013;86(5):867-872. doi:10.1016/j.ijrobp.2013.02.037

19. Thorsen LBJ, Offersen BV, Danø H, et al. DBCG-IMN: a population-based cohort study on the effect of internal mammary node irradiation in early node-positive breast cancer. *J Clin Oncol.* 2016;34:314-320. doi:10.1200/JCO.2015.63.6456

20. Freedman GM, Fowble BL, Nicolaou N, et al. Should internal mammary lymph nodes in breast cancer be a target for the radiation oncologist? *Int J Radiat Oncol Biol Phys.* 2000;46(4):805-814.

21. Hennequin C, Bossard N, Servagi-Vernat S, et al. Ten-year survival results of a randomized trial of irradiation of internal mammary nodes after mastectomy. *Int J Radiat Oncol Biol Phys.* 2013;86(5):860-866. doi:10.1016/j.ijrobp.2013.03.021

22. Fisher B, Brown A, Mamounas E, et al. Effect of preoperative chemotherapy on local-regional disease in women with operable breast cancer: findings from national surgical adjuvant breast and bowel project B-18. *J Clin Oncol.* 1997;15(7):2483-2493.

23. Wolmark N, Wang J, Mamounas E, Bryant J, Fisher B. Preoperative chemotherapy in patients with operable breast cancer: nine-year results from national surgical adjuvant breast and bowel project B-18. *J Natl Cancer Inst Monogr.* 2001;(30):96-102. doi:10.1093/oxfordjournals.jncimonographs.a003469

24. Buchholz TA, Tucker SL, Masullo L, et al. Predictors of local-regional recurrence after neoadjuvant chemotherapy and mastectomy without radiation. *J Clin Oncol.* 2002;20(1):17-23. doi:10.1200/JCO.2002.20.1.17

25. Mamounas EP, Anderson SJ, Dignam JJ, et al. Predictors of locoregional recurrence after neoadjuvant chemotherapy: results from combined analysis of national surgical adjuvant breast and bowel project B-18 and B-27. *J Clin Oncol.* 2012;30(32):3960-3966. doi:10.1200/JCO.2011.40.8369

26. Early Breast Cancer Trialists' Collaborative Group (EBCTCG), Correa C, McGale P, et al. Overview of the randomized trials of radiotherapy in ductal carcinoma in situ of the breast. *J Natl Cancer Inst Monogr.* 2010;2010(41):162-177. doi:10.1093/jncimonographs/lgq039

27. Wong JS, Kaelin CM, Troyan SL, et al. Prospective study of wide excision alone for ductal carcinoma in situ of the breast. *J Clin Oncol.* 2006;24(7):1031-1036. doi:10.1200/JCO.2005.02.9975

28. Hughes LL, Wang M, Page DL, et al. Local excision alone without irradiation for ductal carcinoma in situ of the breast: a trial of the

eastern cooperative oncology group. *J Clin Oncol*. 2009;27(32):5319-5324. doi:10.1200/JCO.2009.21.8560

29. McCormick B, Winter K, Hudis C, et al. RTOG 9804: a prospective randomized trial for good-risk ductal carcinoma in situ comparing radiotherapy with observation. *J Clin Oncol*. 2015;33(7):709-715. doi:10.1200/JCO.2014.57.9029

30. McCormick B, Winter KA, Woodward W, et al. Randomized phase III trial evaluating radiation following surgical excision for good-risk ductal carcinoma in situ: long-term report from NRG Oncology/RTOG 9804. *J Clin Oncol*. 2021;39(32):3574-3582. doi:10.1200/JCO.21.01083

31. Rakovitch E, Nofech-Mozes S, Hanna W, et al. Multigene expression assay and benefit of radiotherapy after breast conservation in ductal carcinoma in situ. *J Natl Cancer Inst*. 2017;109(4):djw256. doi:10.1093/jnci/djw256

32. Bremer T, Whitworth PW, Patel R, et al. A biological signature for breast ductal carcinoma in situ to predict radiotherapy benefit and assess recurrence risk. *Clin Cancer Res*. 2018;24(23):5895-5901. doi:10.1158/1078-0432.CCR-18-0842

33. Whelan TJ, Pignol JP, Levine MN, et al. Long-term results of hypofractionated radiation therapy for breast cancer. *N Engl J Med*. 2010;362(6):513-520. doi:10.1056/NEJMoa0906260

34. Haviland JS, Owen JR, Dewar JA, et al. The UK standardisation of breast radiotherapy (START) trials of radiotherapy hypofractionation for treatment of early breast cancer: 10-year follow-up results of two randomised controlled trials. *Lancet Oncol*. 2013;14(11):1086-1094. doi:10.1016/S1470-2045(13)70386-3

35. Smith BD, Bellon JR, Blitzblau R, et al. Radiation therapy for the whole breast: executive summary of an American Society for Radiation Oncology (ASTRO) evidence-based guideline. *Pract Radiat Oncol*. 2018;8(3):145-152. doi:10.1016/j.prro.2018.01.012

36. Murray Brunt A, Haviland JS, Wheatley DA, et al. Hypofractionated breast radiotherapy for 1 week versus 3 weeks (FAST-Forward): 5-year efficacy and late normal tissue effects results from a multicentre, non-inferiority, randomised, phase 3 trial. *Lancet*. 2020;395(10237):1613-1626. doi:10.1016/S0140-6736(20)30932-6

37. Veronesi U, Marubini E, Mariani L, et al. Radiotherapy after breast-conserving surgery in small breast carcinoma: long-term results of a randomized trial. *Ann Oncol*. 2001;12(7):997-1003.

38. Vicini FA, Kestin LL, Goldstein NS. Defining the clinical target volume for patients with early-stage breast cancer treated with lumpectomy and accelerated partial breast irradiation: a pathologic analysis. *Int J Radiat Oncol Biol Phys*. 2004;60(3):722-730. doi:10.1016/j.ijrobp.2004.04.012

39. Hepel JT, Wazer DE. A comparison of brachytherapy techniques for partial breast irradiation. *Brachytherapy*. 2012;11(3):163-175. doi:10.1016/j.brachy.2011.06.001

40. Strnad V, Ott OJ, Hildebrandt G, et al. 5-year results of accelerated partial breast irradiation using sole interstitial multicatheter brachytherapy versus whole-breast irradiation with boost after breast-conserving surgery for low-risk invasive and in-situ carcinoma of the female breast: a randomised, phase 3, non-inferiority trial. *Lancet*. 2016;387:229-238. doi:10.1016/S0140-6736(15)00471-7

41. Coles CE, Griffin CL, Kirby AM, et al. Partial-breast radiotherapy after breast conservation surgery for patients with early breast cancer (UK IMPORT LOW trial): 5-year results from a multicentre, randomised, controlled, phase 3, non-inferiority trial. *Lancet*. 2017;390(10099):1048-1060. doi:10.1016/S0140-6736(17)31145-5

42. Whelan TJ, Julian JA, Berrang TS, et al. External beam accelerated partial breast irradiation versus whole breast irradiation after breast conserving surgery in women with ductal carcinoma in situ and node-negative breast cancer (RAPID): a randomised controlled trial. *Lancet*. 2019;394(10215):2165-2172. doi:10.1016/S0140-6736(19)32515-2

43. Vicini FA, Cecchini RS, White JR, et al. Long-term primary results of accelerated partial breast irradiation after breast-conserving surgery for early-stage breast cancer: a randomised, phase 3, equivalence trial. *Lancet*. 2019;394(10215):2155-2164. doi:10.1016/S0140-6736(19)32514-0

44. Polgár C, Major T, Takácsi-Nagy Z, Fodor J. Breast-conserving surgery followed by partial or whole breast irradiation: twenty-year results of a phase 3 clinical study. *Int J Radiat Oncol Biol Phys*. 2021;109(4):998-1006. doi:10.1016/j.ijrobp.2020.11.006

45. Rodríguez N, Sanz X, Dengra J, et al. Five-year outcomes, cosmesis, and toxicity with 3-dimensional conformal external beam radiation therapy to deliver accelerated partial breast irradiation. *Int J Radiat Oncol Biol Phys*. 2013;87(5):1051-1057. doi:10.1016/j.ijrobp.2013.08.046

46. Meattini I, Marrazzo L, Saieva C, et al. Accelerated partial breast irradiation compared with whole-breast irradiation for early breast cancer: long-term results of the randomized phase III APBI-IMRT-Florence trial. *J Clin Oncol*. 2020;38(35):4175-4183. doi:10.1200/JCO.20.00650

47. Hepel JT, Wazer DE. Partial breast irradiation is the preferred standard of care for a majority of women with early-stage breast cancer. *J Clin Oncol*. 2020;38(20):2268-2272. doi:10.1200/JCO.19.02594

48. Rusthoven KE, Kavanagh BD, Cardenes H, et al. Multi-institutional phase I/II trial of stereotactic body radiation therapy for liver metastases. *J Clin Oncol*. 2009;27(10):1572-1578. doi:10.1200/JCO.2008.19.6329

49. Shah C, Vicini F, Shaitelman SF, et al. The American Brachytherapy Society consensus statement for accelerated partial-breast irradiation. *Brachytherapy*. 2018;17(1):154-170. doi:10.1016/j.brachy.2017.09.004

50. Correa C, Harris EE, Leonardi MC, et al. Accelerated partial breast irradiation: executive summary for the update of an ASTRO evidence-based consensus statement. *Pract Radiat Oncol*. 2017;7(2):73-79. doi:10.1016/j.prro.2016.09.007

51. Fisher B, Bryant J, Dignam JJ, et al. Tamoxifen, radiation therapy, or both for prevention of ipsilateral breast tumor recurrence after lumpectomy in women with invasive breast cancers of one centimeter or less. *J Clin Oncol*. 2002;20(20):4141-4149.

52. Hughes KS, Schnaper LA, Berry D, et al. Lumpectomy plus tamoxifen with or without irradiation in women 70 years of age or older with early breast cancer. *N Engl J Med*. 2004;351(10):971-977. doi:10.1056/NEJMoa040587

53. Hughes KS, Schnaper LA, Bellon JR, et al. Lumpectomy plus tamoxifen with or without irradiation in women age 70 years or older with early breast cancer: long-term follow-up of CALGB 9343. *J Clin Oncol*. 2013;31(19):2382-2387. doi:10.1200/JCO.2012.45.2615

54. Kunkler IH, Williams LJ, Jack WJL, Cameron DA, Dixon JM; PRIME II investigators. Breast-conserving surgery with or without irradiation in women aged 65 years or older with early breast cancer (PRIME II): a randomised controlled trial. *Lancet Oncol*. 2015;16(3):266-273. doi:10.1016/S1470-2045(14)71221-5

55. Hepel JT, Wazer DE. Should a woman age 70 to 80 years receive radiation after breast-conserving surgery? *J Clin Oncol*. 2013;31(19):2377-2381. doi:10.1200/JCO.2012.48.3875

56. Wang XS, Rhines LD, Shiu AS, et al. Stereotactic body radiation therapy for management of spinal metastases in patients without spinal cord compression: a phase 1-2 trial. *Lancet Oncol*. 2012;13(4):395-402. doi:10.1016/S1470-2045(11)70384-9

57. Bartelink H, Maingon P, Poortmans P, et al. Whole-breast irradiation with or without a boost for patients treated with breast-conserving surgery for early breast cancer: 20-year follow-up of a randomised phase 3 trial. *Lancet Oncol*. 2015;16(1):47-56. doi:10.1016/S1470-2045(14)71156-8

58. Romestaing P, Lehingue Y, Carrie C, et al. Role of a 10-Gy boost in the conservative treatment of early breast cancer: results of a randomized clinical trial in Lyon, France. *J Clin Oncol*. 1997;15(3):963-968.

59. Hepel JT, Evans SB, Hiatt JR, et al. Planning the breast boost: comparison of three techniques and evolution of tumor bed during treatment. *Int J Radiat Oncol Biol Phys*. 2009;74(2):458-463. doi:10.1016/j.ijrobp.2008.08.051

60. Leonard KL, Hepel JT, Styczynski JR, Hiatt JR, Dipetrillo TA, Wazer DE. Breast boost using noninvasive image-guided breast brachytherapy vs. external beam: a 2:1 matched-pair analysis. *Clin Breast Cancer*. 2013;13(6):455-459. doi:10.1016/j.clbc.2013.08.005

CHAPTER 11.11

Multidisciplinary Approach to Breast Cancer Care

Theresa A. Graves, Stephanie L. Graff, and Jaroslaw T. Hepel

A multidisciplinary team approach is crucial for optimal workup and treatment of all cancer patients, especially those with breast cancer. Success cannot be achieved without integration of all team members. The key components of the multidisciplinary breast cancer care team are pathology, radiology, surgery, medical oncology, and radiation oncology. The "tumor board" is the venue where all team members can come together for discussion of specific patient cases. At the tumor board, patient cases are presented prospectively. Each patient's history and physical examination, radiologic imaging, and pathology are presented and reviewed. Additional workup and treatment decision can then be discussed and made specific to the patient's individual case. The tumor board facilitates decision-making for key aspects of breast cancer care, such as whether a patient is a candidate for BCT, sequencing of chemotherapy and surgery, and need for adjuvant therapies. The tumor board is considered a key quality metric in any breast cancer program.

Even more robust multidisciplinary care can be provided via the multidisciplinary clinic (MDC) with an embedded multidisciplinary tumor board as provided in our institution. In a breast cancer MDC, patients can see different subspecialty physicians in one place and optimally during the same visit. This greatly facilitates interdisciplinary care integration and leads to improved patient satisfaction. In addition, important ancillary services can be integrated through the MDC, including nutritional services, physical and lymphedema therapy, genetic counseling, social work/emotional support services, and palliative care services. These ancillary services and an integrated nurse navigation program can be crucial in helping patients through the different and sometimes challenging aspects of cancer care as well as to address treatment-related side effects and quality of life.

Algorithms to our approach for ER-positive (**Figure 11.11-1**), TNBC (**Figure 11.11-2**), and HER2/neu-positive breast cancer (**Figure 11.11-3**) show our general approach to people with newly diagnosed disease. At each step, a discussion between the multiple providers involved in the care of the patient occurs, most notably at points where critical decisions are made. Importantly, these algorithms do not replace the need and importance of the multidisciplinary patient conference, which lies at the center of our approach to breast cancer.

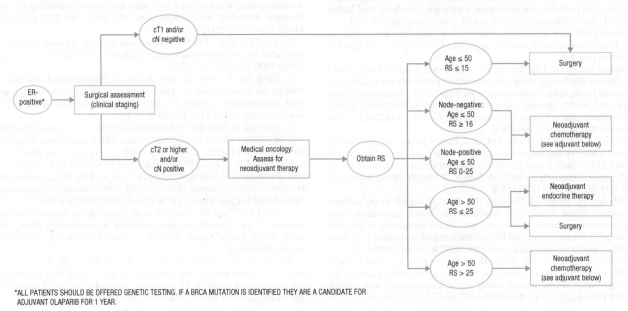

*ALL PATIENTS SHOULD BE OFFERED GENETIC TESTING. IF A BRCA MUTATION IS IDENTIFIED THEY ARE A CANDIDATE FOR ADJUVANT OLAPARIB FOR 1 YEAR.

Figure 11.11-1. Approach to newly diagnosed estrogen receptor (ER)-positive breast cancer. pCR, pathologic complete response; RS, Recurrence Score.

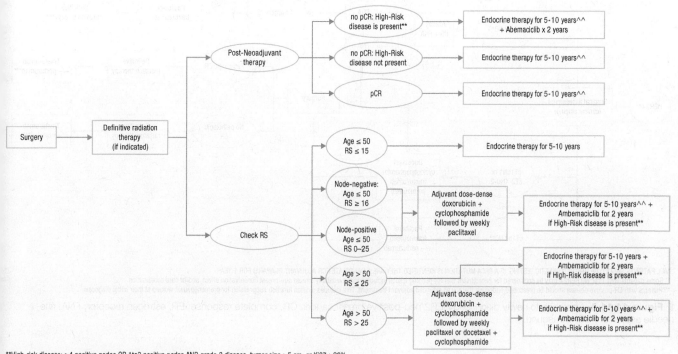

**High-risk disease: ≥4 positive nodes OR 1to3 positive nodes AND grade 3 disease, tumor size ≥5 cm, or Ki67 ≥20%
^^ Ovarian function suppression is indicated in premenopausal women who received chemotherapy for breast cancer treatment

Figure 11.11-1. (continued)

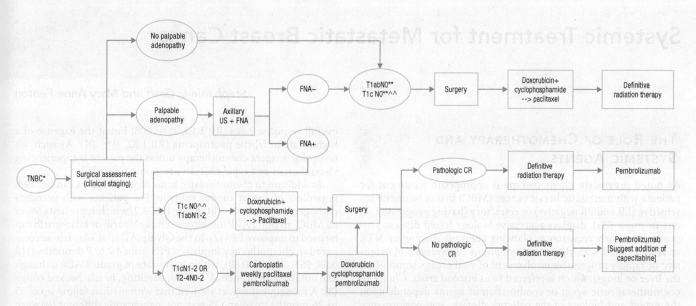

*ALL PATIENTS SHOULD BE OFFERED GENETIC TESTING. IF A BRCA MUTATION IS IDENTIFIED THEY ARE A CANDIDATE FOR ADJUVANT OLAPARIB FOR 1 YEAR.
** Some patients with T1bc N0 TNBC may be considered for neoadjuvant therapy pending issues including trial availability, breast size/breast conservation effect, and/or care coordination.
^^T1c N0 patients may be considered for either neoadjuvant or adjuvant approaches, again, pending issues including trial availability, breast size/breast conservation effect, and/or care coordination.

Figure 11.11-2. Approach to newly diagnosed triple-negative breast cancer (TNBC). CR, complete response; FNA, fine-needle aspiration; US, ultrasound.

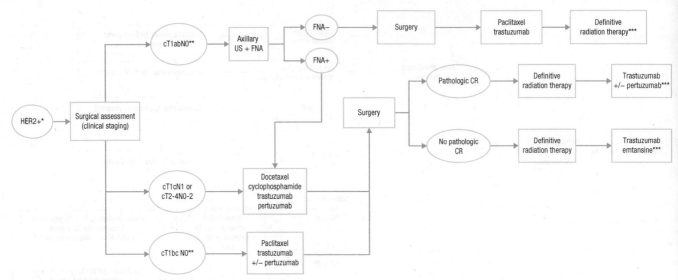

*ALL PATIENTS SHOULD BE OFFERED GENETIC TESTING. IF A BRCA MUTATION IS IDENTIFIED THEY ARE A CANDIDATE FOR ADJUVANT OLAPARIB FOR 1 YEAR.
** Some patients with T1bc N0 HER2+ may be considered for neoadjuvant therapy pending issues including trial availability, breast size/breast conservation effect, and/or care coordination.
***Patients with ER-positive disease should be prescribed endocrine therapy as extended adjuvant treatment. This includes ovarian function suppression for premenopausal women at their initial diagnosis.

Figure 11.11-3. Approach to newly diagnosed HER2/neu-positive breast cancer. CR, complete response; ER, estrogen receptor; FNA, fine-needle aspiration; US, ultrasound.

CHAPTER **11.12**

Systemic Treatment for Metastatic Breast Cancer

Stephanie L. Graff and Mary Anne Fenton

THE ROLE OF CHEMOTHERAPY AND SYSTEMIC AGENTS

As noted previously, chemotherapy is appropriate treatment for patients with metastatic breast cancer (MBC) that is hormone insensitive (ER and PR negative) or refractory (having progressed on one or more ETs), displays aggressive biology (rapid disease progression or early recurrence following adjuvant therapy or NT), or is associated with significant symptoms or evidence of extensive or rapidly progressive involvement of vital organs (most often the liver or lungs), which is referred to as *visceral crisis*. Choice of chemotherapeutic agent or combination of agents depends upon the extent and biology of the patient's disease, age, performance status and comorbid medical conditions, the timing and extent of prior treatment, and shared decision-making between patient and physician balancing benefits of treatment and toxicities of therapy. Common agents used in MBC are listed in **Table 11.12-1**.

A 2013 meta-analysis compared combination versus single-agent chemotherapy in this setting and found that there was no difference in OS associated with either approach, even when analyzed by line of chemotherapy, schema of treatment, and dose intensity (1). Interestingly, in an analysis for PFS (eight trials, 866 patients), combination therapy was significantly associated with a higher risk of progression compared to single-agent treatment (HR 1.16, P = .01). Combination therapy resulted in significantly higher overall response rates (RR 1.13, P = .008) but at the expense of a higher rate of febrile neutropenia (RR 1.32, P = .01). As such, we favor single-agent chemotherapy unless the patient is experiencing visceral crisis and rapid objective response is needed.

In addition to chemotherapy, some targeted agents can be used, regardless of breast cancer subtype. For patients with germline pathogenic variants in BRCA1 or BRCA2, which represents 5% of all MBC, an oral PARP inhibitor such as olaparib or talazoparib can be used to improve PFS (2). In the OlympiAD trial, olaparib as compared to chemotherapy improved PFS from 4.2 to 7.0 months (HR 0.58, 95% CI 0.43-0.80), with a lower rate of grade 3 AEs, although still notable risk of anemia, nausea, vomiting, headache, and cough (3). A subsequent report showed that with median follow-up of 25 to 26 months, median OS was not significantly different between the two arms (19.3 months with olaparib vs 17.1 months with treatment of physicians' choice [TPC]; HR 0.90, 95% CI 0.66-1.23) (4). A separate trial called EMBRACA evaluated talazoparib compared to chemotherapy. Like OlympiAD, talazoparib results in an improved median PFS of 8.6 versus 5.6 months (HR 0.54, 95% CI 0.41-0.71), with similar toxicity profile to olaparib (5). As seen with olaparib, there was no significant impact on OS; at a median follow-up of 44.9 months with talazoparib and 36.8 months with chemotherapy, the median OS was 19.3 and 19.5 months, respectively (HR 0.848, 95% CI 0.670-1.073) (6). Fam-trastuzumab deruxtecan (T-DXd), an ADC that targets HER2, also showed activity in breast cancers, regardless of HER2 expression. In the phase 2 DAISY study, 179

■ **TABLE 11.12-1. Agents Used in the Treatment of Metastatic Breast Cancer**

Anthracyclines
  Doxorubicin
  Epirubicin
  Liposomal doxorubicin

Taxanes/Microtubules-targeted agents
  Paclitaxel
  Docetaxel
  nAb-paclitaxel
  Eribulin
  Vinorelbine
  Ixabepilone

Cyclophosphamide

Platinum salts
  Cisplatin
  Carboplatin

Gemcitabine

Etoposide

Antiestrogens
  Tamoxifen
  Anastrozole
  Letrozole
  Exemestane
  Fulvestrant
  GnRH analogs

HER2-directed agents
  Trastuzumab
  Pertuzumab
  Ado-trastuzumab emtansine
  Lapatinib
  Trastuzumab deruxtecan
  Tucatinib
  Margetuximab

CDK4/6 inhibitors
  Abemaciclib
  Ribociclib
  Palbociclib

Everolimus

Sacituzumab govitecan

GnRH, gonadotropin hormone-releasing hormone.

study volunteers (almost 40% who had received six or more prior lines of treatment) were included: 68 were HER2 positive, 73 were HER2 low (defined as HER2 IHC 2+ ISH negative or HER2 IHC 1+), and 38 were HER2 negative (HER2 IHC 0). The objective response rate with T-DXd was 71%, 37.5%, and 30%, with median PFS of 11.1, 6.7, and 4.2 months, respectively (7). In DESTINY-06, almost 600 volunteers with previously treated metastatic HER2 low breast cancer (89% with ER-positive disease) were randomly assigned to trastuzumab or standard chemotherapy (8). Compared to chemotherapy, T-DXd improved PFS (9.9 vs 5.1 months, HR 0.50, 95% CI 0.40-0.63) and OS (23.4 vs 16.8 months, HR 0.64, 95% CI 0.49-0.84).

Immunotherapy also has a role in the treatment of MBC. In the United States, the FDA has granted a tissue-agnostic approval to pembrolizumab for tumors that express high TMB (≥10 mutations/Mb) or are microsatellite instability high or mismatch repair deficient (9). These signatures are thought to occur more commonly in TNBC, but certainly can be seen in any breast cancer treatment type and represent an option to expand treatment for patients with MBC. Specifically, in TNBC, immunotherapy with pembrolizumab is also approved for tumors that express PD-L1, defined as a combined positive score (CPS) 10 or higher (the percentage of total cells [tumor cells, lymphocytes, macrophages] that stain for

PD-L1), based on the KEYNOTE 355 study (10,11). In KEYNOTE 355, over 800 volunteers were randomized to nab-paclitaxel, paclitaxel, or gemcitabine/carboplatin with or without pembrolizumab, with stratification by CPS. In those with CPS greater than 10, the addition of pembrolizumab improved OS (23.0 vs 16.1 months, HR 0.73), with anticipated increased in immune-related AEs in the pembrolizumab arm.

Lastly, a trophoblastic cell surface antigen (TROP2) ADC is approved for the treatment of metastatic TNBC in patients who have received at least two prior lines of therapy, with at least one of those in the metastatic setting. Sacituzumab govitecan-hziy is an ADC composed of a highly specific TROP2 antibody, bound to a cytotoxic "payload" in the form of SN-38, which is more potent than its parent compound, irinotecan, via a hydrolyzable linker that allows the drug to be released in the tumor microenvironment (12). In ASCENT, 468 patients randomized to sacituzumab govitecan-hziy versus chemotherapy TPC had an improvement in OS from 6.7 to 12.1 months (HR 0.48), with significant grade 3 toxicity in neutropenia (51%), diarrhea (10%), and anemia (8%) (13).

HER2-Directed Therapy

For people with HER2+ MBC, the optimal first-line regimen is currently trastuzumab, pertuzumab, and docetaxel, although that is being challenged in numerous clinical trials, given the recent rapid expansion of available and highly effective agents targeting HER2 in the second- and third-line setting. In the phase III CLEOPATRA study, the addition of pertuzumab to trastuzumab and docetaxel (THP) improved OS (57 vs 41 months, 8-year survival rate 37% vs 23%, HR 0.69) (14,15). As such, THP has become the standard for frontline therapy in HER2+ MBC. However, given the toxicity profile (67% rate of diarrhea, 53% risk of neutropenia including 14% G3/4 febrile neutropenia) and the low percentage of patients accrued to the trial who had previously received trastuzumab (10%) and pertuzumab, it is unclear that THP will remain the standard as newer generations of HER2-targeted therapies including the ADCs are tested in frontline MBC trials. Alternative frontline approaches include substituting paclitaxel, or, for patients who are both HER2+ and HR+ treating with ET (TAM or an AI) in combination with trastuzumab and pertuzumab, paclitaxel is a reasonable option (16,17). Similarly, if the patient progressed within 6 months of adjuvant therapy, it is reasonable to move to the next line of therapy: If adjuvant trastuzumab/pertuzumab, trastuzumab emtansine (TDM-1) is an option.

TDM-1 has been shown in both the TH3RESA trial and the EMILIA trial to be better than lapatinib and capecitabine or chemotherapy TPC and trastuzumab. In TH3RESA, patients were randomized to TDM-1 versus chemotherapy TPC in combination with trastuzumab (18). Compared to chemotherapy, TDM-1 improved PFS (6.2 vs 3.3 months, HR 0.52) and OS (22.7 vs 15.8 months). EMILIA compared TMD-1 to lapatinib plus capecitabine, and patients receiving TDM-1 experienced an improved in PFS (10 vs 6 months, HR 0.65, 95% CI 0.55-0.77) and median OS (31 vs 25 months, HR 0.68, 95% CI 0.55-0.85) and a lower rate of grade 3/4 toxicity (41% vs 57%) (19). Both of these trials were before the advent of adjuvant TDM-1 for patients with residual disease after NACT. It remains unknown how prior exposure to TDM-1 in the adjuvant setting will affect the response in the metastatic setting.

Following TDM-1, numerous options now exist, all of which are currently being evaluated in a variety of earlier line settings, including first line and neoadjuvant. In a phase II trial of T-DXd in patients who had previously been treated with TDM-1, the overall response rate was 60.9%, with the median duration of response of 14.8 months and median PFS 16.4 months (20). Common AEs included neutropenia (20.7%), anemia (8.7%), and nausea (7.6%), and on independent review, as many as 13.6% of patients experienced interstitial lung disease (ILD), including G3-4 (0.5%) and fatal (2.2%) events. T-DXd was compared directly to T-DM1 in 524 volunteers with HER2-positive breast cancer who had previously been treated with trastuzumab and a taxane (21). Compared to T-DM1, T-DXd resulted in a higher overall response rate (79.7% vs 34.2%) and higher survival rates at 12 months, including PFS (75.8% vs 34.1%, HR 0.28, 95% CI 0.22-0.37) and OS (94.1% vs 85.9%, HR 0.55, 95% CI 0.36-0.86). Still, the rate of ILD was reported at 10.5% in those treated with T-DXd compared to 1.9% with TDM-1.

Tucatinib is an oral tyrosine kinase selective for the kinase domain of HER2. In the phase 3 HER2CLIMB trial, conducted in the third line after progression on trastuzumab, pertuzumab, and TDM-1, the addition of tucatinib to trastuzumab and capecitabine was shown to significantly improve PFS (1-year PFS 33.1% with tucatinib vs 12.3% with placebo, HR 0.54, median PFS 7.8 vs 5.6 months) (22). This study was unique in design in that it allowed volunteers with untreated brain metastasis to participate, which is important given the prevalence of brain metastases among those with HER2+ MBC. The 1-year PFS rate was 24.9% in the tucatinib arm and 0% in the placebo arm, with median PFS 7.6 versus 5.4 months. AEs included diarrhea, palmar-plantar erythrodysesthesia (PPE) syndrome, nausea, fatigue, vomiting, and elevated AST/ALT. Many of these AEs are common with capecitabine. In comparing to the control arm, the addition of tucatinib increased G3 diarrhea (12.9% vs 8.6%), PPE syndrome (13.1% vs 9.1%), stomatitis (2.5% vs 0.5%), and AST/ALT (4.5%/5.4% vs 0.5%/0.5%).

Other options for HER2+ MBC include lapatinib, margetuximab, and trastuzumab in combinations with cytotoxic chemotherapy. Lapatinib is a tyrosine kinase inhibitor that has been studied both in combination with trastuzumab, an appealing option for patients who are not candidates for cytotoxic therapy, and in combination with capecitabine, which postprogression on the HER2CLIMB regimen may have less relevance in the emerging treatment paradigm. When utilized as dual-HER2 blockade with trastuzumab, lapatinib was shown to improve median PFS and OS, as compared to trastuzumab alone (median PFS 11 vs 8 weeks [HR = 0.74], OS 14 vs 10 months [HR 0.74]) (23).

Margetuximab is an Fc-engineered anti–HER2-receptor monoclonal antibody used in combination with chemotherapy in the phase 3 SOPHIA trial (24). Margetuximab, as compared to trastuzumab, in combination with chemotherapy (included cytotoxics were capecitabine, eribulin, gemcitabine, and vinorelbine), improved median PFS (5.8 vs 4.9 months, HR 0.76, 95% CI 0.59-0.98). Beyond margetuximab, treatment with the control arm of the SOPHIA study remains a reasonable option for patients who continue to have a good performance status.

Endocrine Therapy in Metastatic Breast Cancer

In 2022 for the first time, patients with HR+ HER2-negative metastatic breast cancer (HR+MBC) treated up front with endocrine-based therapy (including a CDK4/6i) had a median OS of greater than 5 years, a hopeful sign of progress in treating HR+MBC (25). Presentation with HR+MBC may occur beyond 10 years after initial diagnosis (26) and typically presents with bone, liver, lung, and/or LN metastasis; lobular histology may spread to GI tract, pleura, and mesentery. Biopsy of a new metastasis is the standard of care to confirm metastasis and verify ER, PR, and HER2 status and to obtain next-generation sequencing for detection of actionable mutations and selection of therapies. Up to 15% of metastasis may have an ER status different than the primary cancer (27). Hormonal-directed therapy is optimal initial therapy in the setting of stage IV HR+ HER2-negative breast cancer unless an impending visceral crisis mandates chemotherapy to maximize time to response and avert impending organ failure.

The current standard of care for the first-line treatment of HR+MBC is ET in combination with CDK4/6i therapy, although many options for combination exist. In a meta-analysis of phases 2 and 3 randomized controlled trials of postmenopausal women with HR+MBC, no single-agent ET or chemotherapy was better than CDK4/6 inhibitor in combination with hormonal therapy for

PFS, with a similar HR for outcomes between palbociclib, ribociclib, and abemaciclib (28). At the 2022 ASCO Annual Meeting, the final results of the phase III PALOMA-2 trial were presented (29). This study evaluated letrozole with or without palbociclib as first-line treatment. Although it did meet its primary end point of improvement in PFS (median 27.6 vs 1.45 months, HR 0.56, 95% CI 0.46-0.69), the median OS was not changed (53.9 months with palbociclib and 51.2 months with placebo, HR 0.956, 95% CI 0.777-1.1777). Seminal trials of CDK4/6 inhibitors in advanced and metastatic breast cancer are detailed in **Table 11.12-2**.

Premenopausal women with OFS were included in Paloma-3 and MONALEESA-7 and derive a similar benefit in PFS. ET with and without a CDK4/6i offers PFS benefit even with visceral disease and in premenopausal women (30). In an FDA pooled analysis, efficacy of CDK4/6i was similar in patients on prior ET, as first- or second-line therapy, and in combination with AI or fulvestrant (31). Predictable toxicities of CDK4/6i include cytopenia, GI distress, and, rarely, interstitial pneumonitis. QT prolongation seems to be a unique AE with ribociclib.

The endocrine partner for CDK4/6i therapy for HR+MBC includes TAM, AIs, and the selective estrogen receptor downregulator (SERD), fulvestrant. In premenopausal women and men with HR+MBC, OFS may need to be added. For patients who received and were adherent with prior hormonal therapy, the interval between last dose of hormonal therapy and time of recurrence are indicators of subsequent response to the same hormonal agent; for example, if a patient has completed adjuvant AI therapy more than 1 year before systemic recurrence, the patient may again be responsive to an AI, particularly in combination with other agents, such as CDK4/6 inhibitors. Fulvestrant, a monthly intramuscular injection, is approved for use in the postmenopausal setting and is also effective in premenopausal patients with OFS.

The addition of an mTOR inhibitor everolimus, as compared to placebo, to second-line ET with exemestane, demonstrated a significant improvement in PFS from 3 to 7 months in favor of everolimus in the phase III BOLERO trial, conducted before the advent of CDK4/6i (32). Given the paucity of data for treatment with everolimus after treatment with a CDK4/6i and the small improvement in PFS, this drug is falling out of use.

Next-generation sequencing for specific actionable mutations of metastatic sites or circulating tumor DNA (ctDNA) can direct next lines of systemic anticancer therapy. The phosphatidylinositol 3-kinase (PIK3) pathway mutations occur in approximately 40% of HR+ HER2-negative breast cancers. In a planned subset analysis of the phase III SOLAR-1 trial looking at only those patients whose tumors had activating PIK3 (p110 α) mutations (specific activating mutations E542K, E545X, and H1047X), patients randomized to PIK3-α inhibitor alpelisib (33) plus fulvestrant compared to fulvestrant alone had prolonged PFS of 5.7 versus 11.0 months ($P <$ .001). Significant toxicity included rash (9.9%), diarrhea (6.7%), and hyperglycemia (36.6%).

Mechanisms of resistance to hormonal therapy includes mutations in ER-alfa receptor, ligand-independent activation of growth pathways, and activation of alternative growth pathways, including MAP kinase pathways (34), and ongoing investigation of mechanisms of resistance will contribute to targeted therapy development. ESR1 mutations can be detected on tumor or ctDNA. Small trials suggest reduced efficacy of AI as compared to fulvestrant in patients with ESR1 mutations. Currently, data are insufficient to recommend routine testing for ESR mutation to guide decision-making.

Selection of first-line HR+MBC therapy depends on shared decision-making with the patient, prior treatment history, and treatment side-effect profile. The authors' practice at the diagnosis of systemic relapse is to discuss options of oral therapy for first-line treatment with an AI and CDK4/6i, if the patient had received an AI within the preceding 12 months, consider fulvestrant and CDK4/6. After progression on CDK4/6i, PIK3CA mutation status informs treatment, and if present, we consider alpelisib and fulvestrant. If

■ **TABLE 11.12-2. Seminal Phase II and III Trials of CDK4/6 Inhibitor in Combination With Endocrine Therapy**

CDK4/6	Trial	Design	Intervention	Control	PFS (months)	ORR (%)	OS (months)
Abemaciclib	MONARCH-1 (37)	Phase 2/later line	Abemaciclib	NA	6	19.7	17.7
	MONARCH-2 (38)	Phase 3/second line	Fulvestrant/abemaciclib	Fulvestrant	16.4 vs 9.3 mo (HR 0.55, 95% 0.45-0.68)	48 vs 21	Not reported
	MONARCH-3 (39)	Phase 3/first line	Abemaciclib/AI	AI	NR vs 14.7 mo (HR 0.54, 95% CI 0.41-0.72)	59 vs 44	Not reported
Palbociclib	PALOMA-1 (40)	Phase 2/first line	Palbociclib/letrozole	Letrozole	20.2 vs 10.2 mo (HR 0.49, 95% CI 0.32-0.75)	55 vs 39	37.5 vs 34.5 (HR 0.90, 95% CI 0.62-1.29)
	PALOMA-2 (41)	Phase 3/first line	Palbociclib/letrozole	Letrozole	24.8 vs 14.5 mo (HR 0.58, 95% CI 0.46-0.72)	53 vs 44	Not reported
	PALOMA-3 (42)	Phase 3/second line	Palbociclib/fulvestrant	Fulvestrant	9.5 vs 4.6 mo (HR 0.46, 95% CI 0.36-0.59)	25 vs 15	35 vs 28 mo (NR 0.81, 95% CI 0.55-0.94)
Ribociclib	MONALEESA-2 (43)	Phase 3/first line	Ribociclib/letrozole	Letrozole	25 vs 16 mo (HR 0.568, 95% CI 0.46-0.70)	43 vs 29	Not reported
	MONALEESA-3 (44)	Phase 3/up to 1 prior line	Ribociclib/fulvestrant	Fulvestrant	21 vs 13 (HR 0.59, 95% CI 0.48-0.73)	58 vs 46	54 vs 42 mo (HR 0.73, 95% CI 0.59-0.90)
	MONALEESA-7 (45)	Phase 3/first line, pre-/perimenopausal	Ribociclib/goserelin/AI or tamoxifen	Goserelin/AI or tamoxifen	24 vs 13 mo (HR 0.55, 95% CI 0.44-0.69)	51 vs 36	Not reported

AI, aromatase inhibitor; CI, confidence interval; HR, hazard ratio; PFS, progression-free survival; OS, overall survival.

no activating PIK3CA mutation, we consider single-agent fulvestrant or everolimus in combination with exemestane. Clinical trial participation is appropriate at any point in the treatment of MBC, and early consultation and regular follow-up with a palliative and supportive care expert is appropriate.

Oral anticancer therapies have significant benefit in terms of quality of life and PFS, yet neither patient nor practitioner should underestimate difficulties with oral therapy, including side effects, financial toxicity, and barriers to compliance. Oral anticancer therapy management requires patient education, follow-up for toxicity and compliance, as well as active advocation of the provider throughout the prior authorization, patient assistance with copays, and patient assistance programs.

DURATION OF TREATMENT IN METASTATIC DISEASE

The optimal duration of treatment with chemotherapy in MBC is unknown. In general, studies of more prolonged administration of chemotherapy have demonstrated prolongation of time to peak (TTP) but little or no improvement in OS, often associated with increased toxicity and inferior quality of life. A meta-analysis of 11 trials, which compared fixed duration chemotherapy with treatment to disease progression, confirmed prolongation of PFS, with a modest increase in OS. In practice, treatment is often administered until a response plateau is reached (based on imaging studies or tumor marker), development of cumulative toxicities, or shared decision-making between patient and physician leads to a drug holiday. In patients with HR+ disease, an effort to delay disease progression by initiating some novel (to the patient) form of ET is reasonable, though this is not supported by any objective data.

In HER2+ disease, continuation of the HER2-directed therapy without cytotoxic or resumption of trastuzumab alone is reasonable (35). Whether to resume chemotherapy as soon as there is evidence of disease progression or to wait until the patient begins to have symptoms is not known, and again, shared decision-making should be employed. In accordance with guidelines, early integration with palliative and/or supportive care teams for patients with metastatic disease is appropriate to collaboratively manage goals of care, as well as symptoms and distress (36).

REFERENCES

1. Dear RF, McGeechan K, Jenkins MC, Barratt A, Tattersall MHN, Wilcken N. Combination versus sequential single agent chemotherapy for metastatic breast cancer. *Cochrane Database Syst Rev.* 2013;2013(12):CD008792. doi:10.1002/14651858.CD008792.pub2

2. Fasching PA, Yadav S, Hu C, et al. Mutations in BRCA1/2 and other panel genes in patients with metastatic breast cancer—association with patient and disease characteristics and effect on prognosis. *J Clin Oncol.* 2021;39(15):1619-1630. doi:10.1200/JCO.20.01200

3. Robson M, Im SA, Senkus E, et al. Olaparib for metastatic breast cancer in patients with a germline BRCA mutation. *N Engl J Med.* 2017;377(6):523-533. doi:10.1056/NEJMoa1706450

4. Robson ME, Tung N, Conte P, et al. OlympiAD final overall survival and tolerability results: olaparib versus chemotherapy treatment of physician's choice in patients with a germline BRCA mutation and HER2-negative metastatic breast cancer. *Ann Oncol.* 2019;30(4):558-566. doi:10.1093/annonc/mdz012

5. Litton JK, Rugo HS, Ettl J, et al. Talazoparib in patients with advanced breast cancer and a germline BRCA mutation. *N Engl J Med.* 2018;379(8):753-763. doi:10.1056/NEJMoa1802905

6. Litton JK, Hurvitz SA, Mina LA, et al. Talazoparib versus chemotherapy in patients with germline BRCA1/2-mutated HER2-negative advanced

breast cancer: final overall survival results from the EMBRACA trial. *Ann Oncol.* 2020;31(11):1526-1535. doi:10.1016/j.annonc.2020.08.2098

7. Mosele MF, Lusque A, Dieras V, et al. LBA1—unraveling the mechanism of action and resistance to Trastuzumab deruxtecan (T-DXd): biomarker analyses from patients from DAISY trial. *Ann Oncol.* 2022; 33(suppl 3):S123-S147. doi:10.1016/j.annonc.2022.03.277

8. Modi S, Jacot W, Yamashita T, et al. Trastuzumab deruxtecan in previously treated HER2-low advanced breast cancer. *N Engl J Med.* 2022;387(1):9-20. doi:10.1056/NEJMoa2203690

9. Alva AS, Mangat PK, Garrett-Mayer E, et al. Pembrolizumab in patients with metastatic breast cancer with high tumor mutational burden: results from the Targeted Agent and Profiling Utilization Registry (TAPUR) study. *J Clin Oncol.* 2021;39(22):2443-2451. doi:10.1200/JCO.20.02923

10. Cortes J, Cescon DW, Rugo HS, et al. Pembrolizumab plus chemotherapy versus placebo plus chemotherapy for previously untreated locally recurrent inoperable or metastatic triple-negative breast cancer (KEYNOTE-355): a randomised, placebo-controlled, double-blind, phase 3 clinical trial. *Lancet.* 2020;396(10265):1817-1828. doi:10.1016/S0140-6736(20)32531-9

11. Cortes J, Rugo HS, Cescon DW, et al. Pembrolizumab plus chemotherapy in advanced triple-negative breast cancer. *N Engl J Med.* 2022;387(3):217-226. doi:10.1056/NEJMoa2202809

12. Goldenberg DM, Cardillo TM, Govindan SV, Rossi EA, Sharkey RM. Trop-2 is a novel target for solid cancer therapy with sacituzumab govitecan (IMMU-132), an antibody-drug conjugate (ADC). *Oncotarget.* 2015;6(26):22496-22512. doi:10.18632/oncotarget.4318

13. Bardia A, Hurvitz SA, Tolaney SM, et al. Sacituzumab govitecan in metastatic triple-negative breast cancer. *N Engl J Med.* 2021;384(16): 1529-1541. doi:10.1056/NEJMoa2028485

14. Baselga J, Cortés J, Kim SB, et al. Pertuzumab plus trastuzumab plus docetaxel for metastatic breast cancer. *N Engl J Med.* 2012;366(2):109-119. doi:10.1056/NEJMoa1113216

15. Swain SM, Baselga J, Kim SB, et al. Pertuzumab, trastuzumab, and docetaxel in HER2-positive metastatic breast cancer. *N Engl J Med.* 2015;372(8):724-734. doi:10.1056/NEJMoa1413513

16. Bachelot T, Ciruelos E, Schneeweiss A, et al. Preliminary safety and efficacy of first-line pertuzumab combined with trastuzumab and taxane therapy for HER2-positive locally recurrent or metastatic breast cancer (PERUSE). *Ann Oncol.* 2019;30(5):766-773. doi:10.1093/annonc/mdz061

17. Rimawi M, Ferrero JM, de la Haba-Rodriguez J, et al. First-line trastuzumab plus an aromatase inhibitor, with or without pertuzumab, in human epidermal growth factor receptor 2-positive and hormone receptor-positive metastatic or locally advanced breast cancer (PERTAIN): a randomized, open-label phase II trial. *J Clin Oncol.* 2018;36(28):2826-2835. doi:10.1200/JCO.2017.76.7863

18. Krop IE, Kim SB, Martin AG, et al. Trastuzumab emtansine versus treatment of physician's choice in patients with previously treated HER2-positive metastatic breast cancer (TH3RESA): final overall survival results from a randomised open-label phase 3 trial. *Lancet Oncol.* 2017;18(6):743-754. doi:10.1016/S1470-2045(17)30313-3

19. Verma S, Miles D, Gianni L, et al. Trastuzumab emtansine for HER2-positive advanced breast cancer. *N Engl J Med.* 2012;367(19): 1783-1791. doi:10.1056/NEJMoa1209124

20. Modi S, Saura C, Yamashita T, et al. Trastuzumab deruxtecan in previously treated HER2-positive breast cancer. *N Engl J Med.* 2020;382(7): 610-621. doi:10.1056/NEJMoa1914510

21. Cortés J, Kim SB, Chung WP, et al. Trastuzumab deruxtecan versus trastuzumab emtansine for breast cancer. *N Engl J Med.* 2022;386(12): 1143-1154. doi:10.1056/NEJMoa2115022

22. Murthy RK, Loi S, Okines A, et al. Tucatinib, trastuzumab, and capecitabine for HER2-positive metastatic breast cancer. *N Engl J Med.* 2020;382(7):597-609. doi:10.1056/NEJMoa1914609

23. Blackwell KL, Burstein HJ, Storniolo AM, et al. Overall survival benefit with lapatinib in combination with trastuzumab for patients with human epidermal growth factor receptor 2-positive metastatic breast cancer: final results from the EGF104900 study. *J Clin Oncol.* 2012;30(21):2585-2592. doi:10.1200/JCO.2011.35.6725

24. Rugo HS, Im SA, Cardoso F, et al. Efficacy of margetuximab vs trastuzumab in patients with pretreated ERBB2-positive advanced breast cancer: a phase 3 randomized clinical trial. *JAMA Oncol.* 2021;7(4):573-584. doi:10.1001/jamaoncol.2020.7932

25. Hortobagyi GN, Stemmer SM, Burris HA, et al. Overall survival with ribociclib plus letrozole in advanced breast cancer. *N Engl J Med.* 2022;386(10):942-950. doi:10.1056/NEJMoa2114663

26. Pan H, Gray R, Braybrooke J, et al. 20-year risks of breast-cancer recurrence after stopping endocrine therapy at 5 years. *N Engl J Med.* 2017;377(19):1836-1846. doi:10.1056/NEJMoa1701830

27. Lindström LS, Karlsson E, Wilking UM, et al. Clinically used breast cancer markers such as estrogen receptor, progesterone receptor, and human epidermal growth factor receptor 2 are unstable throughout tumor progression. *J Clin Oncol.* 2012;30(21):2601-2608. doi:10.1200/JCO.2011.37.2482

28. Mauri D, Pavlidis N, Polyzos NP, Ioannidis JPA. Survival with aromatase inhibitors and inactivators versus standard hormonal therapy in advanced breast cancer: meta-analysis. *J Natl Cancer Inst.* 2006;98(18):1285-1291. doi:10.1093/jnci/djj357

29. Finn RS, Rugo HS, Dieras VC, et al. Overall survival (OS) with first-line palbociclib plus letrozole (PAL+LET) versus placebo plus letrozole (PBO+LET) in women with estrogen receptor–positive/human epidermal growth factor receptor 2–negative advanced breast cancer (ER+/HER2−ABC): analyses from PALOMA-2. *J Clin Oncol.* 2022;40(17 suppl):LBA1003. doi:10.1200/JCO.2022.40.17_suppl.LBA1003

30. Giuliano M, Schettini F, Rognoni C, et al. Endocrine treatment versus chemotherapy in postmenopausal women with hormone receptor-positive, HER2-negative, metastatic breast cancer: a systematic review and network meta-analysis. *Lancet Oncol.* 2019;20(10):1360-1369. doi:10.1016/S1470-2045(19)30420-6

31. Gao JJ, Cheng J, Bloomquist E, et al. CDK4/6 inhibitor treatment for patients with hormone receptor-positive, HER2-negative, advanced or metastatic breast cancer: a US Food and Drug Administration pooled analysis. *Lancet Oncol.* 2020;21(2):250-260. doi:10.1016/S1470-2045(19)30804-6

32. Baselga J, Campone M, Piccart M, et al. Everolimus in postmenopausal hormone-receptor–positive advanced breast cancer. *N Engl J Med.* 2012;366(6):520-529. doi:10.1056/NEJMoa1109653

33. André F, Ciruelos E, Rubovszky G, et al. Alpelisib for *PIK3CA*-mutated, hormone receptor–positive advanced breast cancer. *N Engl J Med.* 2019;380(20):1929-1940. doi:10.1056/NEJMoa1813904

34. Fan P, Jordan VC. New insights into acquired endocrine resistance of breast cancer. *Cancer Drug Resist.* 2019;2(2):198-209. doi:10.20517/cdr.2019.13

35. von Minckwitz G, du Bois A, Schmidt M, et al. Trastuzumab beyond progression in human epidermal growth factor receptor 2-positive advanced breast cancer: a German breast group 26/breast international group 03-05 study. *J Clin Oncol.* 2009;27(12):1999-2006. doi:10.1200/JCO.2008.19.6618

36. Ferrell BR, Temel JS, Temin S, et al. Integration of palliative care into standard oncology care: American Society of Clinical Oncology Clinical Practice Guideline Update. *J Clin Oncol.* 2017;35(1):96-112.

37. Dickler MN, Tolaney SM, Rugo HS, et al. MONARCH 1, A Phase II study of abemaciclib, a CDK4 and CDK6 inhibitor, as a single agent, in patients with refractory HR+/HER2− metastatic breast cancer. *Clin Cancer Res.* 2017;23(17):5218-5224. doi:10.1158/1078-0432.CCR-17-0754

38. Sledge GW, Toi M, Neven P, et al. MONARCH 2: abemaciclib in combination with fulvestrant in women with HR+/HER2− advanced breast cancer who had progressed while receiving endocrine therapy. *J Clin Oncol.* 2017;35(25):2875-2884. doi:10.1200/JCO.2017.73.7585

39. Goetz MP, Toi M, Campone M, et al. MONARCH 3: abemaciclib as initial therapy for advanced breast cancer. *J Clin Oncol.* 2017;35(32):3638-3646. doi:10.1200/JCO.2017.75.6155

40. Finn RS, Crown JP, Lang I, et al. The cyclin-dependent kinase 4/6 inhibitor palbociclib in combination with letrozole versus letrozole alone as first-line treatment of oestrogen receptor-positive, HER2-negative, advanced breast cancer (PALOMA-1/TRIO-18): a randomised phase 2 study. *Lancet Oncol.* 2015;16(1):25-35.

41. Finn RS, Martin M, Rugo HS, et al. Palbociclib and letrozole in advanced breast cancer. *N Engl J Med.* 2016;375(20):1925-1936. doi:10.1056/NEJMoa1607303

42. Turner NC, Slamon DJ, Ro J, et al. Overall survival with palbociclib and fulvestrant in advanced breast cancer. *N Engl J Med.* 2018;379(20):1926-1936. doi:10.1056/NEJMoa1810527

43. Hortobagyi GN, Stemmer SM, Burris HA, et al. Updated results from MONALEESA-2, a phase III trial of first-line ribociclib plus letrozole versus placebo plus letrozole in hormone receptor-positive, HER2-negative advanced breast cancer. *Ann Oncol.* 2018;29(7):1541-1547. doi:10.1093/annonc/mdy155

44. Slamon DJ, Neven P, Chia S, et al. Ribociclib plus fulvestrant for postmenopausal women with hormone receptor-positive, human epidermal growth factor receptor 2-negative advanced breast cancer in the phase III randomized MONALEESA-3 trial: updated overall survival. *Ann Oncol.* 2021;32(8):1015-1024. doi:10.1016/j.annonc.2021.05.353

45. Tripathy D, Im SA, Colleoni M, et al. Ribociclib plus endocrine therapy for premenopausal women with hormone-receptor-positive, advanced breast cancer (MONALEESA-7): a randomised phase 3 trial. *Lancet Oncol.* 2018;19(7):904-915. doi:10.1016/S1470-2045(18)30292-4

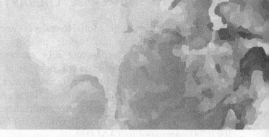

CHAPTER 11.13

Breast Cancer in the Older Patient

Theresa A. Graves and Mary Anne Fenton

Older age is the most common risk for breast cancer. Approximately 50% of breast cancer patients diagnosed in United States are over age 65 (1). Compared to younger women, older women are more likely to have breast cancers that are HR+ and HER2 negative, well or moderately differentiated, with a low proliferation index. In contrast, tumor size and nodal involvement have been shown to increase with age, likely in part due to the decline in mammogram screening in patients over the age of 70 years.

Despite the high prevalence of breast cancer in older women, they are less likely to receive standard care and may have worse outcomes as a result. In addition, women over age 70 are underrepresented in clinical trials. In a cancer registry retrospective cohort study in the United Kingdom, increasing age was associated with lower surgical rates, less frequent use of radiation, and increased use of primary ET (2). In a SEER-Medicare data set from 1992 to 2003, in patients with stage I and II breast cancer aged 67 to 79 years, compared to those aged 80 years and above, the tumor characteristics were similar for tumor grade and HR status. Patients aged 80 years and above were more likely to die of breast cancer than patients aged 67 to 79 years, in part due to less aggressive therapy including less chemotherapy (3).

An older patient diagnosed with an HR+ HER2-negative stage I breast cancer, treated with surgery and ET, is unlikely to have life expectancy impacted by breast cancer. In contrast, an older patient with a luminal B, triple-negative, or HER2-positive stage II and III breast cancer has a significant risk of systemic recurrence within 5 years and may have survival benefit from systemic chemotherapy, although this depends on factors such as their natural life expectancy and the presence of other comorbidities. Recommendations regarding systemic therapy should be based on tumor clinical features and risk of recurrence, within the reference of comorbidities, life expectancy, and patient preference.

There are tools available to assist practitioners in life expectancy, systemic treatment morbidity, and treatment benefit and toxicities for the individual patient. Patient assessment of life expectancy may be calculated with an online geriatric prognostic tool, such as ePrognosis (4) and PredictUK (5).

Geriatric assessments (GAs) also provide additional information to practitioners and patients of chemotherapy risks and toxicities based on individual patient variables. GA evaluates vulnerabilities in the geriatric population not typically addressed in usual patient assessment and provides an opportunity to attenuate toxicities through dose modifications and additional supportive care (6). The Cancer and Aging Research Group-Breast Cancer (CARG-BC) score was developed and validated for patients with early-stage breast cancer aged 65 years and above, to predict risk of grades 3 to 5 toxicity using the National Cancer Institute Common Terminology Criteria for Adverse Events (NCI-CTCAE) (7). The CARG-BC tool is composed of eight clinical and geriatric variables, such as physical function, comorbid medical conditions, falls, depression, social activity and support, cognition, nutritional status, and medication review. The ASCO Guidelines for Geriatric Oncology recommend a GA in patients aged 65 years or above with a plan for chemotherapy to identify risks for toxicities in older patients (6).

ADJUVANT CHEMOTHERAPY

Both providers and older patients forgo chemotherapy over concerns of worsening comorbidities and potentially negative impacts on independence, including risks of neuropathy, fatigue, and infection. Retrospective analyses from SEER cancer registries, which link patient's tumor stage and Medicare claims, represent a real-world experience. In one study of over 5,000 women aged 66 years and above diagnosed with HR-negative early-stage breast cancer, only 34% of patients received chemotherapy (8). Of this cohort, 52% of patients aged 62 to 69 years received chemotherapy compared to 5% of those aged 85 years or above. This same study reported that chemotherapy use was associated with a mortality reduction of 15%, with the greatest benefit seen in node-positive compared to node-negative disease. Another study looked at over 16,000 patients older than 65 years with stage I-III TNBC (9). The 5-year estimated OS was significantly different based on treatment patterns; it was 69% for patients receiving chemotherapy, 61% for patients recommended but not given chemotherapy, and 54% for patients not recommended chemotherapy and not given chemotherapy (P <.0001). After stratification, the benefit of chemotherapy persisted in those with node-negative disease (HR 0.80, 95% CI 0.66-0.97) and node-positive disease (HR 0.76, 95% CI 0.64-0.91). Another study was a SEER-Medicare linked analysis of patients with early-stage ER-negative, node-positive breast cancer aged 65 years and above (10). Chemotherapy significantly reduced breast cancer mortality (HR 0.72; 95% CI 0.54-0.96), with a similar benefit in the aged 70 or above subset (HR 0.74; 95% CI 0.56-0.97).

Chemotherapy benefit for ER-positive, HER2-negative breast cancer may not be significant, even for older patients with node-positive breast cancer. In the phase III TAILORx randomized trial, node-negative postmenopausal patients with RS 0 to 25 derived no benefit from adjuvant chemotherapy (11). The subsequent phase III RxPONDER of women with HR+ HER2-negative results show HR+ HER2-negative postmenopausal women with 1 to 3 positive LNs with RS 0 to 25 derive no benefit from adjuvant chemotherapy (12). Of note, only 11.5% of participants enrolled in RxPONDER were over age 70, and there was no chemotherapy benefit in the subset of patients aged 65 years and above.

Chemotherapy options for adults with breast cancer include adriamycin/cyclophosphamide (AC), adriamycin/cyclophosphamide followed by paclitaxel, or docetaxel/cyclophosphamide (TC). The option of TC may attenuate the cardiac toxicity risk of the AC regimen. The TC regimen was shown to be superior to AC in a phase III randomized trial for patients with stage I-III breast cancer, which included 16% of volunteers aged 65 years and above (13). In a subsequent retrospective observational study of women over age 70 prescribed TC, 91% of patients completed four cycles (14).

HER2-positive breast cancer has a significant risk of systemic recurrence within a short time of diagnosis similar to TNBC. In a systemic review of prospective randomized trials HER2-positive breast cancer in patients over age 60, there was a 47% RR reduction in systemic recurrence for patients receiving chemotherapy plus trastuzumab compared to chemotherapy alone (pooled HR 0.53; 95% CI, 0.36-0.77), and incidence of cardiac events was only 5% (15).

ADJUVANT ENDOCRINE THERAPY

The benefit of adjuvant hormonal therapy for endocrine-responsive breast cancers is of relevance to older patients, with approximately 80% of older women expressing ER+ cancers. Consistent with national guidelines, we discuss the benefits of adjuvant ET to all people with ER-positive breast cancers greater than 0.5 cm, with the aim to reduce systemic recurrence, local recurrence, new primary breast cancer, and breast cancer mortality. AIs demonstrate a slightly lower risk of recurrence in women over age 70 (14% vs 17%, RR 0.78) compared to TAM (16).

SURGICAL MANAGEMENT AND RADIATION ONCOLOGY IN THE OLDER PATIENT

Surgery remains the primary component for curative therapy in older patients, like their younger counterparts, with early-stage breast cancer. Data from a Cochrane meta-analysis concluded that primary hormonal treatment with TAM remains inferior to surgery with or without hormonal therapy for both local control and PFS in those older patients who are candidates for surgical intervention (17). Careful patient selection and comprehensive GA aid in the treatment decision-making process for older patients. These carefully selected patients tolerate breast surgery well, with low morbidity and mortality rates, which range from 0% to 2%. Selective surgical procedures in those older patients with significant comorbid illnesses may also be conducted under local anesthesia. Additional considerations must be given to alterations in short-term cognitive impairment associated with general anesthesia in the older patients (18).

The International Society of Geriatric Oncology (SIOG) task force and the European Society of Breast Cancer Specialists (EUSOMA) issued updated guidance for the diagnosis and treatment of breast cancer in older patients (19). Women over the age of 70 should be offered the same surgical options as younger women as well as postoperative radiation with early breast cancer. Postoperative RT following breast conservation, in combination with systemic therapy, has been shown to reduce 5-year recurrence, as well as 15-year breast cancer mortality risk, regardless of age.

Standard fractionation with boost to the lumpectomy cavity is considered a standard component for BCT with newer alternatives that have demonstrated excellent results, including hyperfractionated RT schedules, more rapid fractionation, and partial breast radiation (20). There has been recent emphasis on de-escalation of care in the older patients to avoid overtreatment of early-stage breast cancer with favorable biology. This has been directed by guidelines from the Choosing Wisely campaign and other consensus guidelines.

Choosing Wisely is an initiative of the American Board of Internal Medicine (ABIM) Foundation that promotes patient-physician discussions about benefits, risks and effectiveness of services as well as establishing unnecessary medical tests and procedures. This initiative was launched in 2012, prompting societies of specialty care to establish care practices that may not be necessary. The patient safety and quality committee of the ASBrS, in conjunction with the guidance of the Choosing Wisely campaign foundation, solicited the candidates from the general and quality control membership to produce a list of five care practices of breast care that may not be necessary (21). Initial and subsequent measures have included omission of axillary evaluation in patients older than 65 to 70 years with low-risk breast cancer. Work regarding the outcomes after SLNB and RT in older patients with early-stage ER-positive breast cancer has been evaluated in order to validate that overtreatment of early-stage breast cancer with favorable tumor biology in older patients may be harmful without affecting recurrence or survival. Evaluating women aged 70 years or above with ER-positive, HER2/neu-negative, clinically node-negative breast cancer between the years 2010 and 2018, noted 65.3% received SLNB and 54.4% received adjuvant RT. The SLNB rate increased 1%/year despite the adoption of the Choosing Wisely guidelines in 2016. The rates of RT did decrease 3.4%/year. A subsequent publication from 2021 showed there was no association between SLNB or RT for either local recurrence-free survival or DFS for older people with ER-positive clinically node-negative breast cancer (22).

Omitting postoperative WBRT has been directed by consensus guidelines based on a series of trials aimed at omitting postoperative WBRT in many women over the age of 65 with low-risk, clinically node-negative, HR-positive breast cancer. One of the earliest trials, CALGB 9343, enrolled women with low-risk HR-positive breast cancer over the age of 70 treated with breast conservation plus TAM with or without radiation. An updated review of the data revealed a 10-year local recurrence rate of 2% with radiation and 9% without and no significant difference in disease-specific mortality (23,24).

Subsequent studies of women over aged 65 included the PRIME trials, first initiated in 1997 to evaluate the effectiveness of WBRT in women with favorable HR-positive cancers. The PRIME I trial showed that WBRT was well tolerated in the older population and did not negatively impact quality of life (25). The PRIME II trial, like CALGB 9343, noted significant reduction in local recurrence from 4.1% to 1.3% in the low-risk older population treated without or with WBRT in the initial 5-year results (26). This represented an absolute risk reduction of only 2.8%, which would be considered modest.

The most recent evaluation of the PRIME II data at 10 years notes that the majority of patients had tumors smaller than 20 mm (T1), were grade 1 to 2, and were node negative (27). The 10-year incidence of ipsilateral breast recurrence with WBRT was 0.9% versus 9.8% without radiation. WBRT reduced the incidence of regional recurrence from 2.3% to 0.5%. There was no difference in distant recurrence, contralateral breast recurrence, and new (nonbreast) cancer. The difference in actuarial 10-year OS between receiving WBRT and no radiation was 81% versus 80.4%. Of note, most deaths were not linked to the breast cancer recurrence and not influenced by the use of RT, with breast-specific survival 98.2% in the no RT group and 97.8% in the radiation group. Overall, there was no difference in secondary end points of distant metastasis, CBC, or OS, while noting a small but significant difference in regional recurrence. There was a cautionary note in the most recent evaluation of the PRIME II data regarding the omission of RT in patients demonstrating low ER-positive tumors.

Studies of older women have found that they prefer BCT to mastectomy and that BCT is often associated with better quality of life (28). Surgical consideration should include estimates of the patient's life expectancy with and without cancer treatment as well as the impact of the disease and its treatment on the patient's quality of life. The treatment decision-making process should involve a multidisciplinary team with consideration of using a GA. It is important that this process adequately consider the preferences of the patient and the impact of other significant factors in the patient's life following comprehensive multidisciplinary consideration.

REFERENCES

1. DeSantis CE, Ma J, Gaudet MM, et al. Breast cancer statistics, 2019. *CA Cancer J Clin.* 2019;69(6):438-451. doi:10.3322/caac.21583

2. Lavelle K, Todd C, Moran A, Howell A, Bundred N, Campbell M. Non-standard management of breast cancer increases with age in the UK: a population based cohort of women > or = 65 years. *Br J Cancer.* 2007;96(8):1197-1203. doi:10.1038/sj.bjc.6603709

3. Schonberg MA, Marcantonio ER, Li D, Silliman RA, Ngo L, McCarthy EP. Breast cancer among the oldest old: tumor characteristics, treatment choices, and survival. *J Clin Oncol.* 2010;28(12):2038-2045. doi:10.1200/JCO.2009.25.9796

4. ePrognosis. Calculators. Accessed February 4, 2022. https://eprognosis.ucsf.edu/calculators/

5. Predict Breast Cancer. What is predict? Accessed February 9, 2022. https://breast.predict.nhs.uk/

6. Mohile SG, Dale W, Somerfield MR, et al. Practical assessment and management of vulnerabilities in older patients receiving chemotherapy: ASCO guideline for geriatric oncology. *J Clin Oncol.* 2018;36(22):2326-2347. doi:10.1200/JCO.2018.78.8687

7. Magnuson A, Sedrak MS, Gross CP, et al. Development and validation of a risk tool for predicting severe toxicity in older adults receiving chemotherapy for early-stage breast cancer. *J Clin Oncol.* 2021;39(6):608-618. doi:10.1200/JCO.20.02063

8. Elkin EB, Hurria A, Mitra N, Schrag D, Panageas KS. Adjuvant chemotherapy and survival in older women with hormone receptor–negative breast cancer: assessing outcome in a population-based, observational cohort. *J Clin Oncol.* 2006;24(18):2757-2764. doi:10.1200/JCO.2005.03.6053

9. Crozier JA, Pezzi TA, Hodge C, et al. Addition of chemotherapy to local therapy in women aged 70 years or older with triple-negative breast cancer: a propensity-matched analysis. *Lancet Oncol.* 2020;21(12):1611-1619. doi:10.1016/S1470-2045(20)30538-6

10. Giordano SH, Duan Z, Kuo YF, Hortobagyi GN, Goodwin JS. Use and outcomes of adjuvant chemotherapy in older women with breast cancer. *J Clin Oncol.* 2006;24(18):2750-2756. doi:10.1200/JCO.2005.02.3028

11. Sparano JA, Gray RJ, Makower DF, et al. Adjuvant chemotherapy guided by a 21-gene expression assay in breast cancer. *N Engl J Med.* 2018;379(2):111-121. doi:10.1056/NEJMoa1804710

12. Kalinsky K, Barlow WE, Gralow JR, et al. 21-Gene assay to inform chemotherapy benefit in node-positive breast cancer. *N Engl J Med.* 2021;385(25):2336-2347. doi:10.1056/NEJMoa2108873

13. Jones S, Holmes FA, O'Shaughnessy J, et al. Docetaxel with cyclophosphamide is associated with an overall survival benefit compared with doxorubicin and cyclophosphamide: 7-year follow-up of US oncology research TRIAL 9735. *J Clin Oncol.* 2009;27(8):1177-1183. doi:10.1200/JCO.2008.18.4028

14. Freyer G, Campone M, Peron J, et al. Adjuvant docetaxel/cyclophosphamide in breast cancer patients over the age of 70: results of an observational study. *Crit Rev Oncol Hematol.* 2011;80(3):466-473. doi:10.1016/j.critrevonc.2011.04.001

15. Brollo J, Curigliano G, Disalvatore D, et al. Adjuvant trastuzumab in elderly with HER-2 positive breast cancer: a systematic review of randomized controlled trials. *Cancer Treat Rev.* 2013;39(1):44-50. doi:10.1016/j.ctrv.2012.03.009

16. Dowsett M, Cuzick J, Ingle J, et al. Meta-analysis of breast cancer outcomes in adjuvant trials of aromatase inhibitors versus tamoxifen. *J Clin Oncol.* 2010;28(3):509-518. doi:10.1200/JCO.2009.23.1274

17. Fennessy M, Bates T, MacRae K, Riley D, Houghton J, Baum M. Late follow-up of a randomized trial of surgery plus tamoxifen versus tamoxifen alone in women aged over 70 years with operable breast cancer. *Br J Surg.* 2004;91(6):699-704. doi:10.1002/bjs.4603

18. Audisio RA. The surgical risk of elderly patients with cancer. *Surg Oncol.* 2004;13(4):169-173. doi:10.1016/j.suronc.2004.09.012

19. Biganzoli L, Battisti NML, Wildiers H, et al. Updated recommendations regarding the management of older patients with breast cancer: a joint paper from the European Society of Breast Cancer Specialists (EUSOMA) and the International Society of Geriatric Oncology (SIOG). *Lancet Oncol.* 2021;22(7):e327-e340. doi:10.1016/S1470-2045(20)30741-5

20. Smith BD, Gross CP, Smith GL, Galusha DH, Bekelman JE, Haffty BG. Effectiveness of radiation therapy for older women with early breast cancer. *J Natl Cancer Inst.* 2006;98(10):681-690. doi:10.1093/jnci/djj186

21. Landercasper J, Bailey L, Berry TS, et al. Measures of appropriateness and value for breast surgeons and their patients: the American Society of Breast Surgeons Choosing Wisely® Initiative. *Ann Surg Oncol.* 2016;23(10):3112-3118. doi:10.1245/s10434-016-5327-8

22. Carleton N, Zou J, Fang Y, et al. Outcomes after sentinel lymph node biopsy and radiotherapy in older women with early-stage, estrogen receptor-positive breast cancer. *JAMA Netw Open.* 2021;4(4):e216322. doi:10.1001/jamanetworkopen.2021.6322

23. Hughes KS, Schnaper LA, Berry D, et al. Lumpectomy plus tamoxifen with or without irradiation in women 70 years of age or older with early breast cancer. *N Engl J Med.* 2004;351(10):971-977. doi:10.1056/NEJMoa040587

24. Hughes KS, Schnaper LA, Bellon JR, et al. Lumpectomy plus tamoxifen with or without irradiation in women age 70 years or older with early breast cancer: long-term follow-up of CALGB 9343. *J Clin Oncol.* 2013;31(19):2382-2387. doi:10.1200/JCO.2012.45.2615

25. Prescott RJ, Kunkler IH, Williams LJ, et al. A randomised controlled trial of postoperative radiotherapy following breast-conserving surgery in a minimum-risk older population. The PRIME trial. *Health Technol Assess.* 2007;11(31):1-149, *iii-iv.* doi:10.3310/hta11310

26. Kunkler IH, Williams LJ, Jack WJL, Cameron DA, Dixon JM; PRIME II investigators. Breast-conserving surgery with or without irradiation in women aged 65 years or older with early breast cancer (PRIME II): a randomised controlled trial. *Lancet Oncol.* 2015;16(3):266-273. doi:10.1016/S1470-2045(14)71221-5

27. Kunkler IH, Williams LJ, Jack WJL, et al. PRIME II randomized trial (postoperative radiotherapy in minimum risk elderly): wide local excision and adjuvant hormonal therapy whole breast irradiation in women greater than or equal to 65 years with early invasive cancer: 10-year results. Presented at: 2020 San Antonio Breast Cancer Symposium; December 9, 2020. Abstract GS2-03.

28. Pierga JY, Girre V, Laurence V, et al. Characteristics and outcome of 1755 operable breast cancers in women over 70 years of age. *Breast.* 2004;13(5):369-375. doi:10.1016/j.breast.2004.04.012

CHAPTER **11.14**

Pregnancy-Associated Breast Cancer

Rani Bansal

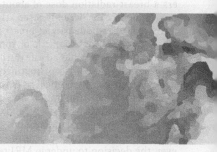

BACKGROUND AND EPIDEMIOLOGY OF PREGNANCY-ASSOCIATED BREAST CANCER

Human and animal models have demonstrated that pregnancy confers a protective effect on mammary tissues through differentiation. Nulliparous women and women delaying childbirth retain a high concentration of epithelial cells that are targets for carcinogens and are, therefore, suspectable to neoplastic transformation. *Pregnancy-associated breast cancer* (PABC) is defined as cancer diagnosed either during pregnancy or up to 12 months postpartum, and breast cancer is among the most diagnosed cancers encountered in pregnant women. The incidence of PABC ranges from 0.02% to 0.1%, and 17 to 100 per 100,000 pregnancies may be affected (1). It is felt that the incidence may increase in the future owing to the increased age at first pregnancy (2). For example, data from Sweden showed that between 1963 and 2002, the incidence increased from 16 to 37.4 per 100,000 deliveries, with an additional increase in breast cancer seen between the first and second year after delivery, from 10.6 to 15 per 100,000 deliveries. PABC accounts for up to 6.9% of all breast cancers in women younger than 45 years and in women below the age of 35, with the proportion of PABC increases up to 15.6% (3,4).

Risk Factors for Pregnancy-Associated Breast Cancer

A family history of breast cancer is one of the most known risk factors for the development of breast cancer and holds true for women who develop PABC. One study of about 1,700 premenopausal women found an association between a family history of breast cancer and PABC, with OR of 3.28 (5).

Age has also been suggested as a risk factor for PABC. One study of about 1,200 women showed that among parous women, there was a 5.3% increased risk annually in odds of breast cancer during first pregnancy after the age of 25 (6). Early menarche, BMI 23 kg/m^2 or higher, and late age at first delivery (age >30 years) were also shown to have a significant association with PABC (7).

Some studies have suggested that women with BRCA1/BRCA2 mutations had a greater risk of developing breast cancer by age 40 than nulliparous women with these mutations (8). One study also showed an increased incidence of PABC in patients with BRCA1 mutation compared to BRCA2 mutation cases (9). However, it is important to note that these were small studies, and thus it is still unclear regarding the influence of BRCA mutation during pregnancy.

Diagnosis/Imaging

Most women diagnosed with PABC present with a painless breast mass. However, benign lesions such as FAs and lactating adenomas are more common than PABC (10). Breast US is safe during pregnancy because of the lack of ionizing radiation and thus is the initial imaging recommended for diagnostic evaluation of a breast mass during pregnancy (11). US of the breast has shown high sensitivity for malignant abnormalities such as PABC, with sensitivity and negative predictive value approaching 100% (12).

Fetuses are most susceptible to dose-dependent teratogenic effects of imaging during organogenesis, which takes place between 2 and 20 weeks of gestational age, predominantly during the first trimester. Guidelines from the ACR suggest that fetal doses of up to 100 mGy are likely too subtle to be clinically detectable, regardless of gestational age (13). In general, conventional two-view mammography is considered safe during pregnancy as it delivers a breast radiation dose of about 3 mGy (14). However, mammography is considered less sensitive in pregnant women owing to increased radiodensity of breast tissue during pregnancy (15). US-guided CNB, stereotactic or tomosynthesis CNB, and needle localization are considered safe during pregnancy.

In contrast, MRI is not routinely recommended during pregnancy because of theoretical risks to the fetus, such as heat deposition, altered cell migration and proliferation, and damage to developing auditory nerves secondary to high acoustic noise. Per the ACR guidelines, data have not conclusively documented deleterious effects of MRI exposure on the developing fetus; however, the decision to undergo MRI testing needs to be determined based on the risks and benefits of such testing. MRI contrast agents should not be provided to pregnant patients as contrast agents can cross the placenta and have effects on the developing fetus (16). Contrast-enhanced MRI can be considered after delivery or in the case of pregnancy termination and is recommended to fully evaluate and stage locoregional disease as studies have shown that breast MRI can detect greater extent of disease than was evident on mammogram and breast US (17).

The use of other imaging modalities should be limited to those required for treatment planning. If a workup for metastatic disease is necessary, acceptable evaluations during pregnancy include chest radiographs, abdominal/liver US, and, if necessary, noncontrast skeletal MRI (18).

TREATMENT APPROACH TO PREGNANCY-ASSOCIATED BREAST CANCER

Determining the best therapeutic options in the treatment of PABC is challenging because of potential conflicts between maternal and fetal well-being. However, treatment can be safely delivered to pregnant women with breast cancer. Treatment strategies are determined by tumor biology, stage, gestational age, and patient/family wishes. Guidelines for pregnant women essentially follow those set forth for nonpregnant women, with the exception of RT, which is not performed while a person has a viable pregnancy and is further discussed in the subsequent section.

Pregnancy termination is rarely indicated for the treatment of PABC and should be reserved for aggressive tumors diagnosed early in the first trimester in which an aggressive treatment strategy is recommended, or in situations where the woman desires this before treatment.

A multidisciplinary approach is essential to providing optimal care, allowing for cooperation between medical, surgical and radiation oncology, radiology, obstetrics, and neonatology.

Anesthesia and Surgery

Physiologic adaptations during pregnancy must be considered for the safe conduct of anesthesia and surgery. Maternal changes include a 20% increase in oxygen consumption, a 20% reduction in pulmonary functional residual capacity, and 40% to 50% increase in blood volume and cardiac output. One significant consideration is the increase in swelling and friability of oropharyngeal tissues, with the loss of airway control representing the most common cause of anesthesia-related maternal mortality (19). Overall, observation studies have not shown any anesthetic drug to be dangerous to the fetus.

The safety of surgical intervention at any stage in the pregnancy is well established and should follow the same guidelines as those for nonpregnant women (20). Traditionally, a modified radical mastectomy has been considered the standard of care as this approach usually eliminates the need for irradiation and allows optimal control of disease within the axilla. However, BCS is increasingly seen as a reasonable alternative for pregnant women, particularly if the diagnosis is made in the later second and third trimesters as many women with PABC will receive neoadjuvant or adjuvant systemic therapy. This sequence of chemotherapy delays the timing for which RT is administered; therefore, treatment can be safely given after delivery.

LN staging remains a crucial part of breast cancer care, especially in women with PABC who tend to have a high percentage of axillary metastases (21). SLNB should be offered to women with early-stage PABC and can be safely performed during pregnancy. Studies have shown the feasibility of lymphoscintigraphy during pregnancy with a radiation dose of 1.67 µGy, which is significantly lower than that which would cause fetal teratogenesis (22). As in nonpregnant patients, axillary US and image-guided FNA of suspicious nodes may be helpful in diagnosing those patients with locally advanced disease. This is of relevance to patients for whom NT is being considered. The use of blue dye such as iso-sulfan blue and methylene blue should not be using during pregnancy as their safety has not been tested and can cause AEs, such as anaphylaxis, intestinal atresia, and fetal demise (23). SLNB is considered safe and accurate from a maternal perspective, with only one unsuccessful mapping and one recurrence among 97 patients with PABC (24).

Radiation Therapy

Therapeutic RT during pregnancy is contraindicated, and if indicated, it is typically delayed until the postpartum period. However, this has been challenged by some who feel that the risks of radiation to the fetus are overestimated, and exposure can be reduced sufficiently by proper shielding, resulting in fetal exposure doses that fall below accepted threshold levels (25). The lack of prospective data and the option of mastectomy for patients with PABC, however, continue to make the use of RT during PABC contraindicated.

Systemic Therapy

Chemotherapy

As in nonpregnant women, chemotherapy often plays a crucial role in both the adjuvant and neoadjuvant treatment in women with PABC. The effects of chemotherapy on fetal development and growth vary, depending on gestational age at the time of exposure; however, pregnancy is not an absolute contraindication to the use of systemic chemotherapy for breast cancer. In general, many studies have shown that OS of patients with breast cancer diagnosed during pregnancy does not differ significantly from that of nonpregnant patients with breast cancer (26).

When administered during the first trimester or period of organogenesis (about 3-12 weeks of gestation), chemotherapy has the potential to cause congenital malformations and fetal loss. Retrospective data have shown a rate of 14% to 20% of fetal malformations when chemotherapy was given during the first trimester (26). However, this rate significantly decreases to about 3% when chemotherapy is given after the first trimester and is consistent with the rate of birth deficits in the general population of infants born in the United States (27,28).

Anthracycline-based regimens are the preferred treatment choice in PABC. Studies have shown that different regimens and schedules that include anthracyclines can be used, such as 3-week cycles of FAC, FEC, AC, EC, or weekly epirubicin as monotherapy (29-31). Some studies suggest preference for doxorubicin rather than epirubicin due to increased fetal cardiac toxicities reported with epirubicin (32). The use of taxanes in pregnancy is likely safe; however, there are limited data to provide a more definitive statement. A review of 40 case reports of taxane administration during the second and third trimesters showed feasibility and safety with minimal fetal, maternal, or neonatal toxicity (33). As paclitaxel has been shown to have less placental transport, its use is favored over docetaxel (18); it may be a safe alternative for pregnant patients who are not otherwise candidates for anthracycline-containing regimens. Regarding dose-dense scheduling, there are limited data regarding the use of granulocyte colony–stimulating factor during pregnancy; thus, it is not recommended (34). It is important to note that chemotherapy dosages should not differ between pregnant and nonpregnant patients and that the dosage should be calculated using the actual body surface area. Chemotherapy has been shown to be as active in pregnant patients as in nonpregnant patients (35).

Timing of chemotherapy is critical, and it is contraindicated in the first trimester. Chemotherapy administration is also not recommended after 34 weeks of gestation because of the risk of spontaneous deliver during the hematologic nadir period (35). Treating PABC involves a multidisciplinary approach, careful consideration of all supportive care medication, and close observation with fetal monitoring and strict adherence to maternal blood pressure control during systemic therapy.

The developmental impact of chemotherapy on children has also been evaluated. Most recently, Amant and colleagues (36) documented the outcomes of 129 children exposed to chemotherapy during pregnancy, matched to 129 controls consisting of children whose mothers were not exposed during pregnancy. There were no differences among the groups regarding cognitive, cardiac, or general development of children during early childhood. However, children exposed to chemotherapy in utero were more frequently born premature. Although prematurity was associated with cognitive impairment in this study, the association was independent of whether their mothers received cancer treatment. This stresses the importance of avoiding iatrogenic premature delivery whenever possible and to deliver patients as near full-term if possible.

Anti-HER2 Therapy

Monoclonal antibody HER2-directed therapy, trastuzumab, is associated with oligohydramnios or anhydramnios as the ERBB2/neu receptor is involved in fetal organogenesis (37). While pertuzumab, TDM-1, and lapatinib have not been studied in PABC, the same contraindication applies. Thus, it is currently recommended that these patients receive chemotherapy and reserve anti-HER2 therapy to follow delivery. In response to the lack of data, the U.S. MotHER registry was created in 2008 to prospectively gather data on HER2-directed therapy in pregnancy (38).

Endocrine Therapy

TAM is contraindicated in pregnancy as the risk of birth defects can be high (39, 40). There are no long-term data available on children following exposure to TAM or an AI in utero. However, animal and preclinical data suggest that TAM is teratogenic, and as such, it (and by extrapolation, AIs) is best reserved until completion of the pregnancy. Thus, the recommendation currently is to avoid ET during pregnancy.

Immunotherapy

Anti–PD-1 (programmed death 1) agents have emerged in the landscape of oncology and are increasingly valuable agents for breast cancer treatment, particularly in TNBC. These agents have not been extensively studied in pregnancy; however, as PD-1 plays a critical role in the negative immune regulation that allows for maternal tolerance of pregnancy, it is of concern that these agents would have deleterious effects (41). There have been case reports of pregnant patients with malignancy, such as melanoma, receiving immunotherapy and the incidence of prematurity, intrauterine growth restriction, and congenital hypothyroidism in the fetus (42).

OUTCOMES FOR PATIENTS WITH PREGNANCY-ASSOCIATED BREAST CANCER

Historically, PABC carried a dismal prognosis, with survival rates of less than 20% at 5 years. However, it is likely that the prognosis is not directly attributable to the onset of cancer during pregnancy. Rather it reflects poor prognostic features of breast cancer when diagnosed in pregnant women compared to age-matched nonpregnant counterparts, including larger tumors that are frequently node positive (43). These cancers are more commonly infiltrating ductal adenocarcinomas, often high grade, HR negative, and HER2/neu positive, with associated lymphovascular invasion (44, 45).

Available data on the overall prognosis of women with PABC are conflicting. A meta-analysis of 30 publications (3,628 cases and 37,100 controls) showed PABC was associated with a poorer OS, especially in women diagnosed in the postpartum period (46). It is important to note that the meta-analysis included data derived from publications as early as 1965, when less effective treatment options were available, and included postpartum patients, though poorer outcomes in PABC diagnosed in the postpartum period have been corroborated by other studies (47). More recent data published in 2021 showed a cohort of 41 patients with PABC had a similar median OS when compared to matched controlled non-PABC patients at 82.2 versus 80.1 months. This study did find that more aggressive histology was found in the PABC group with a greater percentage of these patients with low PR expression and TNBC (48).

PREGNANCY AFTER BREAST CANCER TREATMENT

For women who become pregnant after breast cancer treatment, there appears to be no negative impact on survival outcomes. A study by Azim et al (49), which included 333 patients with 686 matched nonpregnant controls, showed that pregnancy after breast cancer was not detrimental to their risk of recurrence. This has been termed the "healthy-mother effect," suggesting that only healthy women give birth, and those who are sick in relation to their breast cancer will not (50). For women treated with BCT, breastfeeding may still be an option. Higgins and Haffty (51) reported on 11 patients who subsequently experienced 13 pregnancies. Following delivery, lactation was possible in the treated breast in four patients, but not possible in six. In three women, lactation was pharmacologically suppressed. In the majority of cases, lactation was possible in the untreated breast. The time interval from initial treatment did not appear to impact successful lactation. In four instances where lactation was not successful, a circumareolar incision was performed, suggesting that lactation may be less likely to occur in the case of centrally located lesions where the anatomy of central ducts may be altered. There are no strict guidelines to support the optimal timing for when to attempt pregnancy after breast cancer. There are no available data to inform whether prognosis is impacted based on the extent of time from treatment to subsequent pregnancy. Furthermore, women with prior breast cancer may develop recurrent disease many years following treatment, and waiting a period of 2 years does not guarantee avoidance of future recurrence.

For women of childbearing age who develop breast cancer, fertility should be discussed with patients, preferably before adjuvant treatment to determine if the patient wishes to preserve her fertility for future pregnancy. This is in keeping with clinical practice guidelines published by the ASCO for fertility preservation in patients diagnosed with cancer (52).

REFERENCES

1. National Toxicology Program. NTP monograph: developmental effects and pregnancy outcomes associated with cancer chemotherapy use during pregnancy. *NTP Monogr.* 2013;2(2):i-214.

2. Alfasi A, Ben-Aharon I. Breast cancer during pregnancy—current paradigms, paths to explore. *Cancers.* 2019;11:1669.

3. Andersson TM, Johansson ALV, Hsieh CC, Cnattingius S, Lambe M. Increasing incidence of pregnancy-associated breast cancer in Sweden. *Obstet Gynecol.* 2009;114(3):568-572.

4. Beadle BM, Woodward WA, Middleton LP, et al. The impact of pregnancy on breast cancer outcomes in women < or = 35 years. *Cancer.* 2009;115(6):1174-1184.

5. Hou N, Ogundiran T, Ojengbede O, et al. Risk factors for pregnancy-associated breast cancer: a report from the Nigerian Breast Cancer Study. *Ann Epidemiol.* 2013;23:551-557.

6. Robertson C, Primic-Zakelj M, Boyle P, Hsieh CC. Effect of parity and age at delivery on breast cancer risk in Slovenian women aged 25-54 years. *Int J Cancer.* 1997;73:1-9.

7. Kim YG, Jeon YW, Ko BK, et al. Clinicopathologic characteristics of pregnancy-associated breast cancer: results of analysis of a nationwide breast cancer registry database. *J Breast Cancer.* 2017;20:264-269.

8. Jernström H, Lerman C, Ghadirian P, et al. Pregnancy and risk of early breast cancer in carriers of BRCA1 and BRCA2. *Lancet.* 1999;354:1846-1850.

9. Johannsson O, Loman N, Borg A, Olsson H. Pregnancy-associated breast cancer in BRCA1 and BRCA2 germline mutation carriers. *Lancet.* 1998;352:1359-1360.

10. Kieturakis AJ, Wahab RA, Vijapura C, Mahoney MC. Current recommendations for breast imaging of the pregnant and lactating patient. *AJR Am J Roentgenol.* 2021;216(6):1462-1475.

11. Vashi R, Hooley R, Butler R, Geisel J, Philpotts L. Breast imaging of the pregnant and lactating patient: physiologic changes and common benign entities. *AJR Am J Roentgenol.* 2013;200:329-336.

12. Robbins J, Jeffries D, Roubidoux M, Helvie M. Accuracy of diagnostic mammography and breast ultrasound during pregnancy and lactation. *AJR Am J Roentgenol.* 2011;196:716-722.

13. McCollough CH, Schueler BA, Atwell TD, et al. Radiation exposure and pregnancy: when should we be concerned? *RadioGraphics.* 2007;27:909-917; discussion, 917-918.

14. Behrman RH, Homer MJ, Yang WT, Whitman GJ. Mammography and fetal dose. *Radiology.* 2007;243:605; author reply, 605-606.

15. Vashi R, Hooley R, Butler R, Geisel J, Philpotts L. Breast imaging of the pregnant and lactating patient: imaging modalities and pregnancy-associated breast cancer. *AJR Am J Roentgenol.* 2013;200:321-328.

16. Expert Panel on MR Safety, Kanal E, Barkovich AJ, et al. ACR guidance document on MR safe practices: 2013. *J Magn Reson Imaging.* 2013;37:501-530.

17. Myers KS, Green LA, Lebron L, Morris EA. Imaging appearance and clinical impact of preoperative breast MRI in pregnancy-associated breast cancer. *AJR Am J Roentgenol.* 2017;209(3):W177-W183.

18. Amant F, Loibl S, Neven P, Van Calsteren K. Breast cancer in pregnancy. *Lancet.* 2012;379:570-579.

19. Hawkins JL, Chang J, Palmer SK, Gibbs CP, Callaghan WM. Anesthesia-related maternal mortality in the United States: 1979-2002. *Obstet Gynecol.* 2011;117:69-74.

20. Peccatori FA, Azim HA Jr, Orecchia R, et al. Cancer, pregnancy and fertility: ESMO clinical practice guidelines for diagnosis, treatment and follow-up. *AnnOncol* 2013;24(suppl 6):vi160-vi170.

21. Padmagirison R, Gajjar K, Spencer C. Management of breast cancer during pregnancy. *Obstet Gynecol.* 2010;12:186-192.

22. Gentilini O, Cremonesi M, Trifirò G, et al. Safety of sentinel node biopsy in pregnant patients with breast cancer. *Ann Oncol.* 2004;15:1348-1351.

23. Pruthi S, Haakenson C, Brost BC, et al. Pharmacokinetics of methylene blue dye for lymphatic mapping in breast cancer—implications for use in pregnancy. *Am J Surg.* 2011;201:70-75.

24. Gropper AB, Calvillo KZ, Dominici L, et al. Sentinel lymph node biopsy in pregnant women with breast cancer. *Ann Surg Oncol.* 2014;21:2506-2511.

25. Kal HB, Struikmans H. Radiotherapy during pregnancy: fact and fiction. *Lancet Oncol.* 2005;6:328-333.

26. Ploquin A, Pistilli B, Tresch E, et al. 5-year overall survival after early breast cancer diagnosed during pregnancy: a retrospective case-control multicentre French study. *Eur J Cancer.* 2018;95:30-37.

27. Ring AE, Smith IE, Jones A, Shannon C, Galani E, Ellis PA. Chemotherapy for breast cancer during pregnancy: an 18-year experience from five London teaching hospitals. *J Clin Oncol.* 2005;23:4192-4197.

28. Centers for Disease Control and Prevention. National Center for Health and Statistics. Birth defects: data and statistics. July 23, 2018. https://www.cdc.gov/ncbddd/birthdefects/data.html

29. Hahn KM, Johnson PH, Gordon N, et al. Treatment of pregnant breast cancer patients and outcomes of children exposed to chemotherapy in utero. *Cancer.* 2006;107:1219-1226.

30. Loibl S, Han SN, von Minckwitz G, et al. Treatment of breast cancer during pregnancy: an observational study. *Lancet Oncol.* 2012;13:887-896.

31. Peccatori FA, Azim HA Jr, Scarfone G, et al. Weekly epirubicin in the treatment of gestational breast cancer (GBC). *Breast Cancer Res Treat.* 2009;115:591-594.

32. Framarino-Dei-Malatesta M, Perrone G, Giancotti A, et al. Epirubicin: a new entry in the list of fetal cardiotoxic drugs? Intrauterine death of one fetus in a twin pregnancy. Case report and review of literature. *BMC Cancer.* 2015;15:951.

33. Mir O, Berveiller P, Goffinet F, et al. Taxanes for breast cancer during pregnancy: a systematic review. *Ann Oncol.* 2010;21:425-426.

34. Peccatori FA, Lambertini M, Scarfone G, Del Pup L, Codacci-Pisanelli G. Biology, staging, and treatment of breast cancer during pregnancy: reassessing the evidences. *Cancer Biol Med.* 2018;15:6-13.

35. Loibl S, Schmidt A, Gentilini O, et al. Breast cancer diagnosed during pregnancy: adapting recent advances in breast cancer care for pregnant patients. *JAMA Oncol.* 2015;1:1145-1153.

36. Amant F, Vandenbroucke T, Verheecke M, et al. Pediatric outcome after maternal cancer diagnosed during pregnancy. *N Engl J Med.* 2015;373:1824-1834.

37. Azim HA Jr, Azim H, Peccatori FA. Treatment of cancer during pregnancy with monoclonal antibodies: a real challenge. *Expert Rev Clin Immunol.* 2010;6:821-826.

38. The MotHER Pregnancy Registry. http://clinicaltrials.gov/ct2/show/NCT00833963

39. Cullins SL, Pridjian G, Sutherland CM. Goldenhar's syndrome associated with tamoxifen given to the mother during gestation. *JAMA.* 1994;271:1905-1906.

40. Isaacs RJ, Hunter W, Clark K. Tamoxifen as systemic treatment of advanced breast cancer during pregnancy—case report and literature review. *Gynecol Oncol.* 2001;80:405-408.

41. Meggyes M, Miko E, Szigeti B, Farkas N, Szereday L. The importance of the PD-1/PD-L1 pathway at the maternal-fetal interface. *BMC Pregnancy Childbirth.* 2019;19:74.

42. Xu W, Moor RJ, Walpole ET, Atkinson VG. Pregnancy with successful foetal and maternal outcome in a melanoma patient treated with nivolumab

in the first trimester: case report and review of the literature. *Melanoma Res.* 2019;29:333-337.

43. Middleton LP, Chen V, Perkins GH, Pinn V, Page D. Histopathology of breast cancer among African-American women. *Cancer.* 2003;97(1 suppl):253-257.

44. Amant F, von Minckwitz G, Han SN, et al. Prognosis of women with primary breast cancer diagnosed during pregnancy: results from an international collaborative study. *J Clin Oncol.* 2013;31:2532-2539.

45. Murphy CG, Mallam D, Stein S, et al. Current or recent pregnancy is associated with adverse pathologic features but not impaired survival in early breast cancer. *Cancer.* 2012;118:3254-3259.

46. Azim HA Jr, Santoro L, Russell-Edu W, Pentheroudakis G, Pavlidis N, Peccatori FA. Prognosis of pregnancy-associated breast cancer: a meta-analysis of 30 studies. *Cancer Treat Rev.* 2012;38:834-842.

47. Callihan EB, Gao D, Jindal S, et al. Postpartum diagnosis demonstrates a high risk for metastasis and merits an expanded definition of pregnancy-associated breast cancer. *Breast Cancer Res Treat.* 2013;138:549-559.

48. Zhang R, Liu X, Huang W, et al. Clinicopathological features and prognosis of patients with pregnancy-associated breast cancer: a matched case control study. *Asia Pac J Clin Oncol.* 2021;17(4):396-402.

49. Azim HA Jr, Kroman N, Paesmans M, et al. Prognostic impact of pregnancy after breast cancer according to estrogen receptor status: a multicenter retrospective study. *J Clin Oncol.* 2013;31:73-79.

50. Sankila R, Heinävaara S, Hakulinen T. Survival of breast cancer patients after subsequent term pregnancy: "healthy mother effect." *Am J Obstet Gynecol.* 1994;170:818-823.

51. Higgins S, Haffty BG. Pregnancy and lactation after breast-conserving therapy for early stage breast cancer. *Cancer.* 1994;73:2175-2180.

52. Loren AW, Mangu PB, Beck LN, et al. Fertility preservation for patients with cancer: American Society of Clinical Oncology clinical practice guideline update. *J Clin Oncol.* 2013;31:2500-2510.

CHAPTER 11.15

Breast Cancer: Survivorship Issues

Christine Duffy and Don S. Dizon

Survival rates for breast cancer are 90% at 5 years, and even among those with metastatic disease, more than a quarter can expect to live 5 years (1). Despite the high survival rates, breast cancer treatment can result in short- and long-term health risks that can affect a survivor's quality of life (QoL) and risk for other chronic medical conditions. Survivors must also be monitored for recurrence and secondary cancers and encouraged to engage in healthy lifestyle practices. Both oncologists and primary care providers (PCPs) play an important role in caring for breast cancer survivors.

The Office of Cancer Survivorship and the National Coalition of Cancer Survivorship define cancer survivorship from the time of diagnosis through the balance of a person's life. Decisions made during initial diagnosis, such as surgical, chemotherapy, and hormonal treatments, may be crucial to long-term physical and mental health, yet only a minority of patients report feeling fully informed when making these decisions (2-5). Survivors with distant spread can live for many years but must cope with the sequelae of extended treatment. Redefining "survivorship" in this way helps shift away from a focus primarily at the end of initial cancer treatment, to one that includes the entire spectrum of a person's cancer journey.

The challenges survivors face change as the patients move through their cancer diagnosis and treatment, but many challenges (fear of recurrence, reconstruction issues) can surface at any time, and others (hormonal symptoms) may wax and wane over time. Although the section topics begin with early survivorship issues, we recognize that division into early and late is somewhat arbitrary (Table 11.15-1).

SURVEILLANCE

Breast cancer survivors must be monitored for both local and distant recurrence and new primary breast cancers and receive age-appropriate screening for other cancers. Surveillance includes a detailed cancer-related history and physical examination every 3 to 6 months for the first 3 years after primary therapy, then every 6 to 12 months for the next 2 years, and annually thereafter (6). Second primary breast cancer develops in approximately one in 20 survivors, with higher rates among women with genetic predisposition (7-9). The use of MRI for screening should be restricted to those who meet high-risk criteria (lifetime risk >20%) (6). Bone, liver, and lung are the most common sites of metastatic disease, and the risk of recurrence persists up to 30 years from diagnosis (10). Although breast cancer survivors are more likely to develop other new cancers (11,12), current guidelines recommend age-specific screening (6). There is no role for routine laboratory tests or imaging for surveillance in women treated with curative intent, as studies on surveillance including regular scans and labs showed no impact on survival and increased patient anxiety (6).

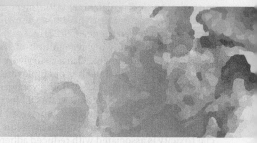

TABLE 11.15-1. Components of Survivorship

Prevention of recurrent and subsequent primary cancers
Screening for cancer recurrence or a new primary cancer
Addressing late physical and psychosocial effects of treatment
Addressing medical problems resulting from cancer or its treatment, including: • Lymphedema • Sexual dysfunction • Pain and fatigue • Psychological distress
Assisting with employment, insurance, and disability concerns
Care coordination between oncologist and primary care providers

Institute of Medicine and National Research Council. From *Cancer Patient to Cancer Survivor: Lost in Transition.* The National Academies Press; 2006. https://doi.org/10.17226/11468

Psychosocial Issues

Depression and anxiety are more prevalent among breast cancer survivors (13), and screening and appropriate referral to mental health providers are essential in those who report elevated scores on validated screening tools, such as the PHQ-9 and GAD-7 (6). Fear of recurrence is common and negatively affects QoL of survivors (14). These fears can resurface at times of surveillance visits and testing and, because breast cancer is prevalent, when friends, family, and co-workers are diagnosed. There is evidence that physical activity can help improve mental health and reduce worry (15,16). Cognitive behavioral therapies (CBTs) and mindfulness practices have been shown to improve QoL and depressive symptoms in breast cancer survivors (17,18). Pharmacologic treatment of depression and anxiety is similar as in the general population, with the caveat that patients on TAM should not be prescribed agents that are strong inhibitors of the cytochrome P450 2D6 (CYP2DC) (eg, paroxetine, fluoxetine, bupropion, duloxetine) and preference given to weak inhibitors (eg, escitalopram, sertraline mirtazapine, and venlafaxine) (19). Interventions that help survivors manage their anxiety have been shown to decrease both distress and fear of recurrence (20-22).

There is also growing recognition of the financial toxicity of cancer and its treatment. Cancer survivors are more likely to file for bankruptcy and report loss of employment or reduced employment after treatment (23,24). Being younger, non-White, of lower education and socioeconomic status all increase the risk of financial hardship (24,25). Screening survivors for financial concerns and referral to appropriate support systems are essential as financial toxicity is associated with reduced adherence to treatment (26) as well as increased risk of mortality (27).

Lifestyle Changes

Early survivorship is a crucial time for breast cancer survivors to make lifestyle changes, such as achieving a healthy weight and meeting physical activity recommendations. Weight gain after diagnosis has been linked to worse survival outcomes in patients with breast cancer (28,29). Exercise has a myriad of health benefits for breast cancer survivors and has been shown to improve anxiety, depression, fatigue, and overall physical function (30-32). Recommendations for exercise for cancer survivors mirror those for the general population with 150 minutes of moderate activity recommended per week (33). However, patients with breast cancer self-report low rates of receiving counseling advice regarding physical activity (34) or weight management (35,36). The data suggest that patients enrolled in weight loss or exercise programs, whose PCPs also provide counseling, have greater success (37,38). Common treatment-associated barriers to increased activity, such as neuropathy and fatigue, should be explored and mitigated when possible. As of date, no randomized controlled trials of dietary intervention have been shown to reduce breast cancer recurrence, but several meta-analyses suggest that a diet that is high in plant-based foods and low in animal fat, processed foods, and alcohol is associated with reduced risk (39-41). Maintaining a healthy well-balanced diet that is high in fruits and vegetables and whole grains and low in red and processed meat and limited alcohol is recommended by national cancer groups (6,42).

SIDE EFFECTS FROM ENDOCRINE THERAPY

ETs such as AIs, TAM, and ovarian suppression are the most widely used therapies in breast cancer. Rates of discontinuation of ETs are high owing to their adverse side effects (43,44); therefore, addressing adherence and side effects is essential. All of the ETs can cause hot flashes and vaginal dryness and can negatively affect QoL. Behavioral treatments for hot flashes include dressing in layers with natural fabrics, avoiding triggers such as hot liquids or spiced foods, exercise, and cognitive behavioral approaches to manage their perception of symptoms (45,46). Medications such as serotonin and norepinephrine reuptake inhibitors (SNRIs), serotonin reuptake inhibitors (SSRIs) (47), gabapentin, and pregabalin (48) are nonhormonal options to mitigate symptoms in survivors, with venlafaxine having the most convincing supportive data (49,50). SNRIs and SSRIs have significant side effects, including anorgasmia and GI symptoms, which can limit use. Gabapentin and pregabalin can cause weight gain and dizziness. Acupuncture has been shown to be effective as bupropion (51) and with few side effects. For vaginal dryness and dyspareunia, the use of glycerin or hyaluronic acid lubricants as vaginal moisturizers and using a lubricant during sex are beneficial. A pelvic examination is critical; if pain is localized to the vaginal entrance (ie, vestibular tenderness), 4% aqueous lidocaine is effective treatment, as shown in a randomized trial against a placebo preparation (52). There is no consistently documented increased risk of relapse in patients who use local estrogen therapy, although concerns have been raised regarding its effect on circulating estrogen levels in women on AIs (53). Providers can consider use if women have severe symptoms not controlled despite nonhormonal options (54). Most importantly, any patient with issues of sexual changes that cause distress should be referred for specialized counseling and an individualized treatment plan, which should include their partner (55).

Joint and muscle pain from AI can be quite disabling and contribute to nonadherence (43). Patients can switch AIs, and most will be able to tolerate a different AI with improved symptoms (56,57). Nonsteroidal anti-inflammatory medications (NSAIDs) can be effective, but kidney injury and GI bleeding risks limit long-term use, especially among older patients. Duloxetine has been shown to be effective for AI-induced pain (58) and can also treat mood disorders and hot flashes. Complementary approaches such as tart cherry extract (59) and acupuncture (60,61) have shown some efficacy as well. Data on physical activity interventions to reduce joint pain from AI is mixed but may help and has many other benefits for health (62,63).

TAM also carries the increased risk of venous thromboembolic disease (VTE), and AIs are associated with increased risk of cardiovascular disease, although the risk in AIs, compared with TAM, may be related to the cardioprotective effects of TAM (64). Survivors on TAM should be counseled on the warning signs of blood clots.

Bone Health

Chemotherapy-induced ovarian failure (COF), OFS, TAM in premenopausal women, and AIs in postmenopausal women are all associated with bone loss in breast cancer survivors (65). AI-induced bone loss is approximately 2% to 3% per year (66) compared to the 1% to 2% yearly loss seen in postmenopausal women (65). COF and ovarian suppressive therapy are associated with 7% to 8% bone loss (67,68), and the addition of an AI to ovarian suppressive therapy increases this to 11% (69).

TAM has a differential effect on bone loss based on menopausal status, with premenopausal women experiencing bone loss (1%-2% per year) whereas postmenopausal women gain bone density (1%-2% per year) (70,71). Current recommendations are to screen bone mineral density in those survivors who will be starting endocrine treatment known to accelerate bone loss. Therapy to ameliorate bone loss should be initiated in women with a T-score of −1.5 or lower who have risk factors and in all women with T-score of −2.0 or lower. All should be closely monitored with dual x-ray absorptiometry (DEXA) scan (minimum of every 2 years) for evidence of rapid bone loss (65,72). Bisphosphonate therapy (oral or IV) and denosumab (65,73) are both treatment options, but denosumab is associated with rebound bone loss and should be followed by bisphosphonate therapy (72), making bisphosphonates the preferred option. All survivors with osteopenia or osteoporosis should be screened and treated for vitamin D deficiency, counseled on adequate calcium intake based on menopausal status, and encouraged to engage in weight-bearing exercise (65).

Cardiovascular Health

The direct effects of radiation and chemotherapy on the heart are well documented (74). Anthracyclines can cause both an early-onset (≤1 year) and late-onset (>1 year) progressive cardiomyopathy causing reduced diastolic function and can appear up to 20 years post-treatment (75). Monoclonal antibodies (MABs), such as trastuzumab, also can cause cardiotoxicity, also in a dose-dependent manner. Most MAB cardiotoxicity occurs during treatment and dose reductions, or discontinuation may be required based on objective cardiac imaging. For patients with metastatic cancer, current recommendations include no specific interval for imaging but leave the decision to providers based on their clinical judgment and signs of heart failure (76). Risk of cardiotoxic effects is increased when anthracyclines and MABs are used together (77,78). RT is associated with increased risk for cardiovascular disease (79-81), particularly left-sided radiation (82). The risk of cardiotoxicity in cancer survivors makes post-treatment screening for signs and symptoms of ischemic heart disease and congestive heart failure essential throughout a survivor's lifetime as well as treatment of modifiable risk factors and counseling of lifestyle factors (76).

Fatigue

Fatigue is a common complaint among breast cancer survivors, with prevalence ranging from 7% to 52% (83) and can persistent even a decade after cancer treatment (84). On-treatment fatigue estimates range from 30% to 60% (85). The cytotoxic effects of chemotherapy and radiation treatments, as well as anxiety and depression are contributors to fatigue early in diagnosis. The etiology of fatigue that persists after active treatment is multifactorial, complex, and still poorly understood (86). Risk factors identified include younger age, higher BMI, smoking behavior, pretreatment fatigue, anxiety, insomnia, and pain (86,87). Treatment of fatigue requires a multifaceted approach—carefully reviewing sleep patterns, reviewing previous treatments, assessing cardiac and lung function, and screening and treatment of mood disorders. For survivors who have sleep disturbances, cognitive behavioral approaches to insomnia are both effective and carry minimal risk (88). Interventions such as yoga (89), acupuncture (90), and mindfulness (91,92) have been shown to improve fatigue in breast cancer survivors as well.

PAIN AND NEUROPATHY

Breast cancer survivors can experience pain as a result of surgical treatment, radiation, chemotherapy, and hormone therapy. Pain is highly prevalent among breast cancer survivors, and one in five long-term survivors reports moderately severe pain that negatively affects QoL (93). Nonpharmacologic options, which can be effective for all pain, and have low risk, include exercise, acupuncture, CBT, and mindfulness with coping skills training (94). Over-the-counter medications, such as lidocaine patches and menthol, can also be effective (95). NSAIDs can be effective, especially in musculoskeletal symptom (MSK) pain, but their use is limited owing to renal and GI toxicity. Pharmacologic options that have the most convincing data to support treatment for neuropathic pain include duloxetine, pregabalin, and opioids, although balance of benefits and harms of opioids for chronic pain should be weighed carefully and use reserved for those in whom symptom control with other treatments has not been successful (96).

Lymphedema

The reported overall incidence of breast cancer–related lymphedema (BCRL) varies based on measurement methods but ranges from 14% to 20% (97,98). ALND and receiving regional lymph node radiation (RLNR) increase risk, with combined ALND and RLNR treatment having the highest risk of 27% to 31% in 5-year follow-up (99,100). BMI over 30 at diagnosis, cellulitis, and a high number of positive LNs removed confer increased risk (99). Contrary to prior assumptions, resistance exercise does not increase the risk of lymphedema (101), and some data indicate it may confer protection (102,103). There is no evidence that blood pressure monitoring or air travel increases risk (104). Early surveillance and treatment are associated with reduced rates of chronic BCRL (98). For survivors who develop lymphedema, treatment is focused on manual lymphatic drainage (MLD), compressive garments, self-MLD exercises, and skin care (105).

Cancer-Related Cognitive Decline

Many breast cancer survivors self-report cognitive changes, although objective decline occurs in 15% to 25% (106,107). Cognitive decline as a result of breast cancer treatment includes mild-to-moderate declines in memory, attention, and executive function in patients after completion of chemotherapy (107,108). Depression, anxiety, and sleep disorders can all have a detrimental effect on cognition, and survivors with cognitive complaints should be evaluated and treated for these common conditions. Treatments shown as possibly effective include cognitive training, mindfulness, and physical activity, although the strength of the quality of evidence is low (109,110).

MOLECULAR-TARGETED THERAPIES

With innovations in treatment such as targeted therapies, and in immunomodulators, patients with MBC can live many years progression free from their cancer. However, these medications can also cause death and significant disabling side effects, such as colitis, hepatitis, neuropathies, skin disorders, and atypical infections (111). Effects can be protean and include inhibition of angiogenetic pathways, severe inflammatory syndromes, and autoimmune disorders (112). Patients may see their PCPs for seemingly simple illnesses when they could be experiencing life-threatening toxicities. PCPs consistently report knowledge gaps in caring for cancer survivors (113), and these patients may require the coordination and involvement of several specialists with expertise in identifying and managing these toxicities.

Fertility

For premenopausal women diagnosed with breast cancer, fertility concerns are among the most distressing (114). Counseling regarding fertility loss and preservation remains low in oncologists owing to concerns about increased risk of recurrence (115). Pregnancy itself does not appear to cause an increased risk of cancer recurrence (116), and current guidelines do not recommend against pursuing pregnancy in breast cancer survivors as long as adequate hormonal treatment has occurred for HR-positive tumors (114). Women should be referred to reproductive medicine if they are unable to conceive after 6 months, as many will have low ovarian reserves (6). For women who cannot conceive naturally, there are insufficient data regarding the safety of assisted reproductive technology (ART) (116), although small studies have not shown deleterious effects on survival (117). Most women under age 35 will resume menses after treatment, but menses does not indicate fertility; in addition, many women will stop menses, especially while on TAM therapy, but can still be fertile. Women should not become pregnant while on endocrine therapy. Decisions to temporarily interrupt endocrine therapy to conceive are nuanced and should be made in conjunction with their oncology team (118). For birth control, hormone-based methods are not recommended, regardless of hormone status, and alternatives include IUDs, barrier methods, and irreversible methods, such as tubal ligation or partner vasectomy for those who have completed childbearing.

Models of Care

Unfortunately, there is little consensus on what model of care delivery is best, and identifying outcome measures and supporting the development and evaluation of care models represent an important area for further research (119,120). Patients with cancer tend to prefer that oncologists screen for recurrence and late-effects monitoring (121), although no data suggest improved outcomes in terms of survival. Many wish to continue seeing their oncologist, breast surgeon, and radiation oncologists yearly. However, as our older population continues to age, the number of cancers diagnosed will increase and further stress our health care system, and access to cancer care. Most long-term survivors will resume care with their PCPs, who will provide the bulk of care (122), so coordination between PCPs and specialists is key. As we move toward a more integrated medical system, this may provide opportunities for enhanced communication and models of care.

For survivors to fully live their lives healthy and cancer free, regardless of who provides care, they need to turn their focus to the health behaviors that have been shown to prevent recurrence, new cancers, and death from chronic medical conditions such as cardiovascular disease, which remains a leading cause of death in breast cancer survivors (123,124). A network review of interventions for cancer survivors found that there were significant gaps in research related to management of chronic conditions in cancer survivors (125). In addition, screening for mood disorders, financial toxicity, and the sequelae of cancer treatment both short and long term is essential to ensure that survivors live their best life after a cancer diagnosis.

REFERENCES

1. Surveillance, Epidemiology, and End Results (SEER) Program. (www.seer.cancer.gov). SEER*Stat database: mortality—all COD, aggregated with state, total U.S. (1969-2018) <Katrina/Rita Population Adjustment>, National Cancer Institute, DCCPS, Surveillance Research Program, released May 2020. Underlying mortality data provided by NCHS. Accessed March 12, 2022. https://seer.cancer.gov/statfacts/html/breast.html

2. Banerjee R, Tsiapali E. Occurrence and recall rates of fertility discussions with young breast cancer patients. *Support Care Cancer.* 2016;24(1):163-171. doi:10.1007/s00520-015-2758-x

3. Mitchell S, Gass J, Hanna M. How well informed do patients feel about their breast cancer surgery options? Findings from a nationwide survey of women after lumpectomy and/or mastectomy. *J Am Coll Surg.* 2018;226(2):134-146.e3. doi:10.1016/j.jamcollsurg.2017.10.022

4. Lee CNH, Deal AM, Huh R, et al. Quality of patient decisions about breast reconstruction after mastectomy. *JAMA Surg.* 2017;152(8):741-748. doi:10.1001/jamasurg.2017.0977

5. Niemasik EE, Letourneau J, Dohan D, et al. Patient perceptions of reproductive health counseling at the time of cancer diagnosis: a qualitative study of female California cancer survivors. *J Cancer Surviv.* 2012;6(3):324-332. doi:10.1007/s11764-012-0227-9

6. Runowicz CD, Leach CR, Henry NL, et al. American Cancer Society/American Society of Clinical Oncology breast cancer survivorship care guideline. *J Clin Oncol.* 2016;34(6):611-635. doi:10.1200/JCO.2015.64.3809

7. Sung H, Freedman RA, Siegel RL, et al. Risks of subsequent primary cancers among breast cancer survivors according to hormone receptor status. *Cancer.* 2021;127(18):3310-3324. doi:10.1002/cncr.33602

8. Lee KD, Chen SC, Chan CH, et al. Increased risk for second primary malignancies in women with breast cancer diagnosed at young age: a population-based study in Taiwan. *Cancer Epidemiol Biomarkers Prev.* 2008;17(10):2647-2655. doi:10.1158/1055-9965.EPI-08-0109

9. Bernstein JL, Lapinski RH, Thakore SS, Doucette JT, Thompson WD. The descriptive epidemiology of second primary breast cancer. *Epidemiology.* 2003;14(5):552-558. doi:10.1097/01.ede.0000072105.39021.6d

10. Pedersen RN, Esen BÖ, Mellemkjær L, et al. The incidence of breast cancer recurrence 10-32 years after primary diagnosis. *J Natl Cancer Inst.* 2022;114(3):391-399. doi:10.1093/jnci/djab202

11. Bao S, Jiang M, Wang X, et al. Nonmetastatic breast cancer patients subsequently developing second primary malignancy: a population-based study. *Cancer Med.* 2021;10(23):8662-8672. doi:10.1002/cam4.4351

12. Cheng Y, Huang Z, Liao Q, et al. Risk of second primary breast cancer among cancer survivors: implications for prevention and screening practice. *PloS One.* 2020;15(6):e0232800. doi:10.1371/journal.pone.0232800

13. Carreira H, Williams R, Müller M, Harewood R, Stanway S, Bhaskaran K. Associations between breast cancer survivorship and adverse mental health outcomes: a systematic review [Erratum in: *J Natl Cancer Inst.* 2020;112(1):118]. *J Natl Cancer Inst.* 2018;110(12):1311-1327. doi:10.1093/jnci/djy177

14. Bergerot CD, Philip EJ, Bergerot PG, Siddiq N, Tinianov S, Lustberg M. Fear of cancer recurrence or progression: what is it and what can we do about it? *Am Soc Clin Oncol Educ Book.* 2022;42:1-10. doi:10.1200/EDBK_100031

15. Lahart IM, Metsios GS, Nevill AM, Carmichael AR. Physical activity for women with breast cancer after adjuvant therapy. *Cochrane Database Syst Rev.* 2018;1:CD011292. doi:10.1002/14651858.CD011292.pub2

16. Mishra SI, Scherer RW, Geigle PM, et al. Exercise interventions on health-related quality of life for cancer survivors. *Cochrane Database Syst Rev.* 2012;2012(8):CD007566. doi:10.1002/14651858.CD007566.pub2

17. Jassim GA, Whitford DL, Hickey A, Carter B. Psychological interventions for women with non-metastatic breast cancer. *Cochrane Database Syst Rev.* 2015;(5):CD008729. doi:10.1002/14651858.CD008729.pub2

18. Ye M, Du K, Zhou J, et al. A meta-analysis of the efficacy of cognitive behavior therapy on quality of life and psychological health of breast cancer survivors and patients. *Psychooncology.* 2018;27(7):1695-1703. doi:10.1002/pon.4687

19. Sideras K, Ingle JN, Ames MM, et al. Coprescription of tamoxifen and medications that inhibit CYP2D6. *J Clin Oncol.* 2010;28(16):2768-2776. doi:10.1200/JCO.2009.23.8931

20. Livingston PM, Russell L, Orellana L, et al. Efficacy and cost-effectiveness of an online mindfulness program (MindOnLine) to reduce fear of recurrence among people with cancer: study protocol for a randomised controlled trial. *BMJ Open.* 2022;12(1):e057212. doi:10.1136/bmjopen-2021-057212

21. Butow PN, Turner J, Gilchrist J, et al. Randomized trial of conquer-fear: a novel, theoretically based psychosocial intervention for fear of cancer recurrence. *J Clin Oncol.* 2017;35(36):4066-4077. doi:10.1200/JCO.2017.73.1257

22. Compen F, Bisseling E, Schellekens M, et al. Face-to-face and internet-based mindfulness-based cognitive therapy compared with treatment as usual in reducing psychological distress in patients with cancer: a multicenter randomized controlled trial. *J Clin Oncol.* 2018;36(23):2413-2421. doi:10.1200/JCO.2017.76.5669

23. Altice CK, Banegas MP, Tucker-Seeley RD, Yabroff KR. Financial hardships experienced by cancer survivors: a systematic review. *J Natl Cancer Inst.* 2016;109(2):djw205. doi:10.1093/jnci/djw205

24. Mols F, Tomalin B, Pearce A, Kaambwa B, Koczwara B. Financial toxicity and employment status in cancer survivors. A systematic literature review. *Support Care Cancer.* 2020;28(12):5693-5708. doi:10.1007/s00520-020-05719-z

25. Tangka FKL, Subramanian S, Jones M, et al. Insurance coverage, employment status, and financial well-being of young women diagnosed with breast cancer. *Cancer Epidemiol Biomarkers Prev.* 2020;29(3):616-624. doi:10.1158/1055-9965.EPI-19-0352

26. Knight TG, Deal AM, Dusetzina SB, et al. Financial toxicity in adults with cancer: adverse outcomes and noncompliance. *J Oncol Pract.* 2018;JOP1800120. doi:10.1200/JOP.18.00120

27. Ramsey SD, Bansal A, Fedorenko CR, et al. Financial insolvency as a risk factor for early mortality among patients with cancer. *J Clin Oncol.* 2016;34(9):980-986. doi:10.1200/JCO.2015.64.6620

28. Jung AY, Hüsing A, Behrens S, et al. Postdiagnosis weight change is associated with poorer survival in breast cancer survivors: a prospective population-based patient cohort study. *Int J Cancer.* 2021;148(1):18-27. doi:10.1002/ijc.33181

29. Playdon MC, Bracken MB, Sanft TB, Ligibel JA, Harrigan M, Irwin ML. Weight gain after breast cancer diagnosis and all-cause mortality: systematic review and meta-analysis. *J Natl Cancer Inst.* 2015;107(12):djv275. doi:10.1093/jnci/djv275

30. Buffart LM, Kalter J, Sweegers MG, et al. Effects and moderators of exercise on quality of life and physical function in patients with cancer: an individual patient data meta-analysis of 34 RCTs. *Cancer Treat Rev.* 2017;52:91-104. doi:10.1016/j.ctrv.2016.11.010

31. Swartz MC, Lewis ZH, Lyons EJ, et al. Effect of home- and community-based physical activity interventions on physical function among cancer survivors: a systematic review and meta-analysis. *Arch Phys Med Rehabil.* 2017;98(8):1652-1665. doi:10.1016/j.apmr.2017.03.017

32. Sweegers MG, Altenburg TM, Chinapaw MJ, et al. Which exercise prescriptions improve quality of life and physical function in patients with cancer during and following treatment? A systematic review and meta-analysis of randomised controlled trials. *Br J Sports Med.* 2018;52(8):505-513. doi:10.1136/bjsports-2017-097891

33. Campbell KL, Winters-Stone KM, Wiskemann J, et al. Exercise guidelines for cancer survivors: consensus statement from international multidisciplinary roundtable. *Med Sci Sports Exerc*. 2019;51(11):2375-2390. doi:10.1249/MSS.0000000000002116

34. Tarasenko YN, Miller EA, Chen C, Schoenberg NE. Physical activity levels and counseling by health care providers in cancer survivors. *Prev Med*. 2017;99:211-217. doi:10.1016/j.ypmed.2017.01.010

35. Arem H, Duan X, Ehlers DK, Lyon ME, Rowland JH, Mama SK. Provider discussion about lifestyle by cancer history: a nationally representative survey. *Cancer Epidemiol Biomarkers Prev*. 2021;30(2):278-285. doi:10.1158/1055-9965.EPI-20-1268

36. Jain R, Denlinger CS. Incorporating weight management into clinical care for cancer survivors: challenges, opportunities, and future directions. *Obesity (Silver Spring)*. 2017;25(Suppl 2):S27-S29. doi:10.1002/oby.22016

37. Grogg KA, Giacobbi PR, Blair EK, et al. Physical activity assessment and promotion in clinical settings in the United States: a scoping review. *Am J Health Promot*. 2022;36(4):714-737. doi:10.1177/08901171211051840

38. McVay M, Steinberg D, Askew S, Bennett GG. Provider counseling and weight loss outcomes in a primary care-based digital obesity treatment. *J Gen Intern Med*. 2019;34(6):992-998. doi:10.1007/s11606-019-04944-5

39. Schwingshackl L, Schwedhelm C, Galbete C, Hoffmann G. Adherence to Mediterranean diet and risk of cancer: an updated systematic review and meta-analysis. *Nutrients*. 2017;9(10):1063. doi:10.3390/nu9101063

40. Schwedhelm C, Boeing H, Hoffmann G, Aleksandrova K, Schwingshackl L. Effect of diet on mortality and cancer recurrence among cancer survivors: a systematic review and meta-analysis of cohort studies. *Nutr Rev*. 2016;74(12):737-748. doi:10.1093/nutrit/nuw045

41. Morze J, Danielewicz A, Przybyłowicz K, Zeng H, Hoffmann G, Schwingshackl L. An updated systematic review and meta-analysis on adherence to Mediterranean diet and risk of cancer. *Eur J Nutr*. 2021;60(3):1561-1586. doi:10.1007/s00394-020-02346-6

42. Ligibel JA, Basen-Engquist K, Bea JW. Weight management and physical activity for breast cancer prevention and control. *Am Soc Clin Oncol Educ Book*. 2019;39:e22-e33. doi:10.1200/EDBK_237423

43. Henry NL, Kim S, Hays RD, et al. Toxicity index, patient-reported outcomes, and early discontinuation of endocrine therapy for breast cancer risk reduction in NRG Oncology/NSABP B-35. *J Clin Oncol*. 2021;39(34):3800-3812. doi:10.1200/JCO.21.00910

44. Hershman DL, Shao T, Kushi LH, et al. Early discontinuation and non-adherence to adjuvant hormonal therapy are associated with increased mortality in women with breast cancer. *Breast Cancer Res Treat*. 2011;126(2):529-537. doi:10.1007/s10549-010-1132-4

45. Nonhormonal management of menopause-associated vasomotor symptoms: 2015 position statement of the North American Menopause Society. *Menopause*. 2015;22(11):1155-1172; quiz 1173-1174. doi:10.1097/GME.0000000000000546

46. Mann E, Smith MJ, Hellier J, et al. Cognitive behavioural treatment for women who have menopausal symptoms after breast cancer treatment (MENOS 1): a randomised controlled trial. *Lancet Oncol*. 2012;13(3):309-318. doi:10.1016/S1470-2045(11)70364-3

47. Shams T, Firwana B, Habib F, et al. SSRIs for hot flashes: a systematic review and meta-analysis of randomized trials. *J Gen Intern Med*. 2014;29(1):204-213. doi:10.1007/s11606-013-2535-9

48. Shan D, Zou L, Liu X, Shen Y, Cai Y, Zhang J. Efficacy and safety of gabapentin and pregabalin in patients with vasomotor symptoms: a systematic review and meta-analysis. *Am J Obstet Gynecol*. 2020;222(6):564.e12-579.e12. doi:10.1016/j.ajog.2019.12.011

49. Loprinzi CL, Kugler JW, Sloan JA, et al. Venlafaxine in management of hot flashes in survivors of breast cancer: a randomised controlled trial. *Lancet*. 2000;356(9247):2059-2063. doi:10.1016/S0140-6736(00)03403-6

50. Carpenter JS, Storniolo AM, Johns S, et al. Randomized, double-blind, placebo-controlled crossover trials of venlafaxine for hot flashes after breast cancer. *Oncologist*. 2007;12(1):124-135. doi:10.1634/theoncologist.12-1-124

51. Mao JJ, Bowman MA, Xie SX, Bruner D, DeMichele A, Farrar JT. Electroacupuncture versus gabapentin for hot flashes among breast cancer survivors: a randomized placebo-controlled trial. *J Clin Oncol*. 2015;33(31):3615-3620. doi:10.1200/JCO.2015.60.9412

52. Goetsch MF, Lim JY, Caughey AB. A practical solution for dyspareunia in breast cancer survivors: a randomized controlled trial. *J Clin Oncol*. 2015;33(30):3394-3400. doi:10.1200/JCO.2014.60.7366

53. Cold S, Cold F, Jensen MB, Cronin-Fenton D, Christiansen P, Ejlertsen B. Systemic or vaginal hormone therapy after early breast cancer: a Danish observational cohort study. *J Natl Cancer Inst*. 2022;114:1347-1354. doi:10.1093/jnci/djac112

54. Franzoi MA, Agostinetto E, Perachino M, et al. Evidence-based approaches for the management of side-effects of adjuvant endocrine

therapy in patients with breast cancer. *Lancet Oncol*. 2021;22(7):e303-e313. doi:10.1016/S1470-2045(20)30666-5

55. Dizon DS, Suzin D, McIlvenna S. Sexual health as a survivorship issue for female cancer survivors. *Oncologist*. 2014;19(2):202-210. doi:10.1634/theoncologist.2013-0302

56. Kadakia KC, Kidwell KM, Seewald NJ, et al. Prospective assessment of patient-reported outcomes and estradiol and drug concentrations in patients experiencing toxicity from adjuvant aromatase inhibitors. *Breast Cancer Res Treat*. 2017;164(2):411-419. doi:10.1007/s10549-017-4260-2

57. Briot K, Tubiana-Hulin M, Bastit L, Kloos I, Roux C. Effect of a switch of aromatase inhibitors on musculoskeletal symptoms in postmenopausal women with hormone-receptor-positive breast cancer: the ATOLL (articular tolerance of letrozole) study. *Breast Cancer Res Treat*. 2010;120(1):127-134. doi:10.1007/s10549-009-0692-7

58. Henry NL, Unger JM, Schott AF, et al. Randomized, multicenter, placebo-controlled clinical trial of duloxetine versus placebo for aromatase inhibitor-associated arthralgias in early-stage breast cancer: SWOG S1202. *J Clin Oncol*. 2018;36(4):326-332. doi:10.1200/JCO.2017.74.6651

59. Shenouda M, Copley R, Pacioles T, et al. Effect of tart cherry on Aromatase Inhibitor-Induced Arthralgia (AIA) in nonmetastatic hormone-positive breast cancer patients: a randomized double-blind placebo-controlled trial. *Clin Breast Cancer*. 2022;22(1):e30-e36. doi:10.1016/j.clbc.2021.06.007

60. Hershman DL, Unger JM, Greenlee H, et al. Effect of acupuncture vs sham acupuncture or waitlist control on joint pain related to aromatase inhibitors among women with early-stage breast cancer: a randomized clinical trial. *JAMA*. 2018;320(2):167-176. doi:10.1001/jama.2018.8907

61. Chen L, Lin CC, Huang TW, et al. Effect of acupuncture on aromatase inhibitor-induced arthralgia in patients with breast cancer: a meta-analysis of randomized controlled trials. *Breast*. 2017;33:132-138. doi:10.1016/j.breast.2017.03.015

62. Irwin ML, Cartmel B, Gross CP, et al. Randomized exercise trial of aromatase inhibitor-induced arthralgia in breast cancer survivors. *J Clin Oncol*. 2015;33(10):1104-1111. doi:10.1200/JCO.2014.57.1547

63. Roberts KE, Rickett K, Feng S, Vagenas D, Woodward NE. Exercise therapies for preventing or treating aromatase inhibitor-induced musculoskeletal symptoms in early breast cancer. *Cochrane Database Syst Rev*. 2020;1:CD012988. doi:10.1002/14651858.CD012988.pub2

64. Khosrow-Khavar F, Filion KB, Al-Qurashi S, et al. Cardiotoxicity of aromatase inhibitors and tamoxifen in postmenopausal women with breast cancer: a systematic review and meta-analysis of randomized controlled trials. *Ann Oncol*. 2017;28(3):487-496. doi:10.1093/annonc/mdw673

65. Shapiro CL, Van Poznak C, Lacchetti C, et al. Management of osteoporosis in survivors of adult cancers with nonmetastatic disease: ASCO clinical practice guideline. *J Clin Oncol*. 2019;37(31):2916-2946. doi:10.1200/JCO.19.01696

66. Eastell R, Hannon RA, Cuzick J, et al. Effect of an aromatase inhibitor on BMD and bone turnover markers: 2-year results of the Anastrozole, Tamoxifen, Alone or in Combination (ATAC) trial (18233230). *J Bone Miner Res*. 2006;21(8):1215-1223. doi:10.1359/jbmr.060508

67. Fogelman I, Blake GM, Blamey R, et al. Bone mineral density in premenopausal women treated for node-positive early breast cancer with 2 years of goserelin or 6 months of cyclophosphamide, methotrexate and 5-fluorouracil (CMF). *Osteoporos Int*. 2003;14(12):1001-1006. doi:10.1007/s00198-003-1508-y

68. Shapiro CL, Manola J, Leboff M. Ovarian failure after adjuvant chemotherapy is associated with rapid bone loss in women with early-stage breast cancer. *J Clin Oncol*. 2001;19(14):3306-3311. doi:10.1200/JCO.2001.19.14.3306

69. Gnant MF, Mlineritsch B, Luschin-Ebengreuth G, et al. Zoledronic acid prevents cancer treatment-induced bone loss in premenopausal women receiving adjuvant endocrine therapy for hormone-responsive breast cancer: a report from the Austrian Breast and Colorectal Cancer Study Group. *J Clin Oncol*. 2007;25(7):820-828. doi:10.1200/JCO.2005.02.7102

70. Love RR, Barden HS, Mazess RB, Epstein S, Chappell RJ. Effect of tamoxifen on lumbar spine bone mineral density in postmenopausal women after 5 years. *Arch Intern Med*. 1994;154(22):2585-2588.

71. Powles TJ, Hickish T, Kanis JA, Tidy A, Ashley S. Effect of tamoxifen on bone mineral density measured by dual-energy x-ray absorptiometry in healthy premenopausal and postmenopausal women. *J Clin Oncol*. 1996;14(1):78-84. doi:10.1200/JCO.1996.14.1.78

72. Hadji P, Aapro MS, Body JJ, et al. Management of aromatase inhibitor-associated bone loss (AIBL) in postmenopausal women with hormone sensitive breast cancer: joint position statement of the IOF, CABS, ECTS, IEG, ESCEO IMS, and SIOG. *J Bone Oncol*. 2017;7:1-12. doi:10.1016/j.jbo.2017.03.001

73. Reid DM, Doughty J, Eastell R, et al. Guidance for the management of breast cancer treatment-induced bone loss: a consensus position statement from a UK expert group. *Cancer Treat Rev.* 2008;34(Suppl 1):S3-S18. doi:10.1016/j.ctrv.2008.03.007

74. Bikiewicz A, Banach M, von Haehling S, Maciejewski M, Bielecka-Dabrowa A. Adjuvant breast cancer treatments cardiotoxicity and modern methods of detection and prevention of cardiac complications. *ESC Heart Fail.* 2021;8(4):2397-2418. doi:10.1002/ehf2.13365

75. Zamorano JL, Lancellotti P, Rodriguez Muñoz D, et al. 2016 ESC Position Paper on cancer treatments and cardiovascular toxicity developed under the auspices of the ESC committee for practice guidelines: the task force for cancer treatments and cardiovascular toxicity of the European Society of Cardiology (ESC). *Eur Heart J.* 2016;37(36):2768-2801. doi:10.1093/eurheartj/ehw211

76. Armenian SH, Lacchetti C, Barac A, et al. Prevention and monitoring of cardiac dysfunction in survivors of adult cancers: American Society of Clinical Oncology Clinical Practice guideline. *J Clin Oncol.* 2017;35(8):893-911. doi:10.1200/JCO.2016.70.5400

77. Swain SM, Ewer MS, Cortés J, et al. Cardiac tolerability of pertuzumab plus trastuzumab plus docetaxel in patients with HER2-positive metastatic breast cancer in CLEOPATRA: a randomized, double-blind, placebo-controlled phase III study. *Oncologist.* 2013;18(3):257-264. doi:10.1634/theoncologist.2012-0448

78. Perez EA, Suman VJ, Davidson NE, et al. Cardiac safety analysis of doxorubicin and cyclophosphamide followed by paclitaxel with or without trastuzumab in the North Central Cancer Treatment Group N9831 adjuvant breast cancer trial. *J Clin Oncol.* 2008;26(8):1231-1238. doi:10.1200/JCO.2007.13.5467

79. Koutroumpakis E, Deswal A, Yusuf SW, et al. Radiation-induced cardiovascular disease: mechanisms, prevention, and treatment. *Curr Oncol Rep.* 2022;24(5):543-553. doi:10.1007/s11912-022-01238-8

80. Cheng YJ, Nie XY, Ji CC, et al. Long-term cardiovascular risk after radiotherapy in women with breast cancer. *J Am Heart Assoc.* 2017;6(5):e005633. doi:10.1161/JAHA.117.005633

81. Darby SC, Ewertz M, McGale P, et al. Risk of ischemic heart disease in women after radiotherapy for breast cancer. *N Engl J Med.* 2013;368(11):987-998. doi:10.1056/NEJMoa1209825

82. Sardar P, Kundu A, Chatterjee S, et al. Long-term cardiovascular mortality after radiotherapy for breast cancer: a systematic review and meta-analysis. *Clin Cardiol.* 2017;40(2):73-81. doi:10.1002/clc.22631

83. Abrahams HJG, Gielissen MFM, Schmits IC, Verhagen CAHHVM, Rovers MM, Knoop H. Risk factors, prevalence, and course of severe fatigue after breast cancer treatment: a meta-analysis involving 12 327 breast cancer survivors. *Ann Oncol.* 2016;27(6):965-974. doi:10.1093/annonc/mdw099

84. Bower JE, Ganz PA, Desmond KA, et al. Fatigue in long-term breast carcinoma survivors: a longitudinal investigation. *Cancer.* 2006;106(4):751-758. doi:10.1002/cncr.21671

85. Bower JE. Cancer-related fatigue—mechanisms, risk factors, and treatments. *Nat Rev Clin Oncol.* 2014;11(10):597-609. doi:10.1038/nrclinonc.2014.127

86. Di Meglio A, Havas J, Soldato D, et al. Development and validation of a predictive model of severe fatigue after breast cancer diagnosis: toward a personalized framework in survivorship care. *J Clin Oncol.* 2022;40(10):1111-1123. doi:10.1200/JCO.21.01252

87. Ferreira AR, Di Meglio A, Pistilli B, et al. Differential impact of endocrine therapy and chemotherapy on quality of life of breast cancer survivors: a prospective patient-reported outcomes analysis. *Ann Oncol.* 2019;30(11):1784-1795. doi:10.1093/annonc/mdz298

88. Ma Y, Hall DL, Ngo LH, Liu Q, Bain PA, Yeh GY. Efficacy of cognitive behavioral therapy for insomnia in breast cancer: a meta-analysis. *Sleep Med Rev.* 2021;55:101376. doi:10.1016/j.smrv.2020.101376

89. Cramer H, Lauche R, Klose P, Lange S, Langhorst J, Dobos GJ. Yoga for improving health-related quality of life, mental health and cancer-related symptoms in women diagnosed with breast cancer. *Cochrane Database Syst Rev.* 2017;1:CD010802. doi:10.1002/14651858.CD010802.pub2

90. Zia FZ, Olaku O, Bao T, et al. The national cancer institute's conference on acupuncture for symptom management in oncology: state of the science, evidence, and research gaps. *J Natl Cancer Inst Monogr.* 2017;2017(52):lgx005. doi:10.1093/jncimonographs/lgx005

91. Chang YC, Yeh TL, Chang YM, Hu WY. Short-term effects of randomized mindfulness-based intervention in female breast cancer survivors: a systematic review and meta-analysis. *Cancer Nurs.* 2021;44(6):E703-E714. doi:10.1097/NCC.0000000000000889

92. Schell LK, Monsef I, Wöckel A, Skoetz N. Mindfulness-based stress reduction for women diagnosed with breast cancer. *Cochrane Database Syst Rev.* 2019;3:CD011518. doi:10.1002/14651858.CD011518.pub2

93. Manfuku M, Nishigami T, Mibu A, Tanaka K, Kitagaki K, Sumiyoshi K. Comparison of central sensitization-related symptoms and health-related quality of life between breast cancer survivors with and without chronic pain and healthy controls. *Breast Cancer.* 2019;26(6):758-765. doi:10.1007/s12282-019-00979-y

94. Syrjala KL, Jensen MP, Mendoza ME, Yi JC, Fisher HM, Keefe FJ. Psychological and behavioral approaches to cancer pain management. *J Clin Oncol.* 2014;32(16):1703-1711. doi:10.1200/JCO.2013.54.4825

95. Teoh D, Smith TJ, Song M, Spirtos NM. Care after chemotherapy: peripheral neuropathy, cannabis for symptom control, and mindfulness. *Am Soc Clin Oncol Educ Book.* 2018;38:469-479. doi:10.1200/EDBK_209437

96. Dowell D, Haegerich TM, Chou R. CDC guideline for prescribing opioids for chronic pain—United States, 2016. *MMWR Recomm Rep.* 2016;65(1):1-49. doi:10.15585/mmwr.rr6501e1

97. DiSipio T, Rye S, Newman B, Hayes S. Incidence of unilateral arm lymphoedema after breast cancer: a systematic review and meta-analysis. *Lancet Oncol.* 2013;14(6):500-515. doi:10.1016/S1470-2045(13)70076-7

98. Rafn BS, Christensen J, Larsen A, Bloomquist K. Prospective surveillance for breast cancer-related arm lymphedema: a systematic review and meta-analysis. *J Clin Oncol.* 2022;40(9):1009-1026. doi:10.1200/JCO.21.01681

99. McDuff SGR, Mina AI, Brunelle CL, et al. Timing of lymphedema after treatment for breast cancer: when are patients most at risk? *Int J Radiat Oncol Biol Phys.* 2019;103(1):62-70. doi:10.1016/j.ijrobp.2018.08.036

100. Naoum GE, Roberts S, Brunelle CL, et al. Quantifying the impact of axillary surgery and nodal irradiation on breast cancer-related lymphedema and local tumor control: long-term results from a prospective screening trial. *J Clin Oncol.* 2020;38(29):3430-3438. doi:10.1200/JCO.20.00459

101. Ammitzbøll G, Johansen C, Lanng C, et al. Progressive resistance training to prevent arm lymphedema in the first year after breast cancer surgery: results of a randomized controlled trial. *Cancer.* 2019;125(10):1683-1692. doi:10.1002/cncr.31962

102. Schmitz KH, Ahmed RL, Troxel AB, et al. Weight lifting for women at risk for breast cancer-related lymphedema: a randomized trial. *JAMA.* 2010;304(24):2699-2705. doi:10.1001/jama.2010.1837

103. Hasenoehrl T, Palma S, Ramazanova D, et al. Resistance exercise and breast cancer-related lymphedema-a systematic review update and meta-analysis. *Support Care Cancer.* 2020;28(8):3593-3603. doi:10.1007/s00520-020-05521-x

104. Ferguson CM, Swaroop MN, Horick N, et al. Impact of ipsilateral blood draws, injections, blood pressure measurements, and air travel on the risk of lymphedema for patients treated for breast cancer. *J Clin Oncol.* 2016;34(7):691-698. doi:10.1200/JCO.2015.61.5948

105. McLaughlin SA, Brunelle CL, Taghian A. Breast cancer-related lymphedema: risk factors, screening, management, and the impact of locoregional treatment. *J Clin Oncol.* 2020;38(20):2341-2350. doi:10.1200/JCO.19.02896

106. Ahles TA, Root JC, Ryan EL. Cancer- and cancer treatment-associated cognitive change: an update on the state of the science. *J Clin Oncol.* 2012;30(30):3675-3686. doi:10.1200/JCO.2012.43.0116

107. Lange M, Joly F, Vardy J, et al. Cancer-related cognitive impairment: an update on state of the art, detection, and management strategies in cancer survivors. *Ann Oncol.* 2019;30(12):1925-1940. doi:10.1093/annonc/mdz410

108. Janelsins MC, Heckler CE, Peppone LJ, et al. Longitudinal trajectory and characterization of cancer-related cognitive impairment in a nationwide cohort study. *J Clin Oncol.* 2018;36:JCO2018786624. doi:10.1200/JCO.2018.78.6624

109. Binarelli G, Joly F, Tron L, Lefevre Arbogast S, Lange M. Management of cancer-related cognitive impairment: a systematic review of computerized cognitive stimulation and computerized physical activity. *Cancers.* 2021;13(20):5161. doi:10.3390/cancers13205161

110. Treanor CJ, McMenamin UC, O'Neill RF, et al. Non-pharmacological interventions for cognitive impairment due to systemic cancer treatment. *Cochrane Database Syst Rev.* 2016;2016(8):CD011325. doi:10.1002/14651858.CD011325.pub2

111. Wang DY, Salem JE, Cohen JV, et al. Fatal toxic effects associated with immune checkpoint inhibitors: a systematic review and meta-analysis. *JAMA Oncol.* 2018;4(12):1721-1728. doi:10.1001/jamaoncol.2018.3923

112. Kroschinsky F, Stölzel F, von Bonin S, et al. New drugs, new toxicities: severe side effects of modern targeted and immunotherapy of cancer and their management. *Crit Care.* 2017;21(1):89. doi:10.1186/s13054-017-1678-1

113. Nekhlyudov L, O'malley DM, Hudson SV. Integrating primary care providers in the care of cancer survivors: gaps in evidence and future opportunities. *Lancet Oncol.* 2017;18(1):e30-e38. doi:10.1016/S1470-2045(16)30570-8

114. Paluch-Shimon S, Cardoso F, Partridge AH, et al. ESO-ESMO 4th international consensus guidelines for Breast Cancer in Young Women (BCY4). *Ann Oncol.* 2020;31(6):674-696. doi:10.1016/j.annonc.2020.03.284

115. Lambertini M, Di Maio M, Pagani O, et al. The BCY3/BCC 2017 survey on physicians' knowledge, attitudes and practice towards fertility and pregnancy-related issues in young breast cancer patients. *Breast.* 2018;42:41-49. doi:10.1016/j.breast.2018.08.099

116. Lambertini M, Blondeaux E, Bruzzone M, et al. Pregnancy after breast cancer: a systematic review and meta-analysis. *J Clin Oncol.* 2021;39(29):3293-3305. doi:10.1200/JCO.21.00535

117. Condorelli M, De Vos M, Lie Fong S, et al. Impact of ARTs on oncological outcomes in young breast cancer survivors. *Hum Reprod.* 2021;36(2):381-389. doi:10.1093/humrep/deaa319

118. Paluch-Shimon S, Cardoso F, Partridge AH, et al. ESO-ESMO 4th international consensus guidelines for breast cancer in young women (BCY4). *Ann Oncol.* 2020;31(6):674-696. doi:10.1016/j.annonc.2020.03.284

119. Leach CR, Alfano CM, Potts J, et al. Personalized cancer follow-up care pathways: a Delphi consensus of research priorities. *J Natl Cancer Inst.* 2020;112(12):1183-1189. doi:10.1093/jnci/djaa053

120. Nekhlyudov L, Mollica MA, Jacobsen PB, Mayer DK, Shulman LN, Geiger AM. Developing a quality of cancer survivorship care framework: implications for clinical care, research, and policy. *J Natl Cancer Inst.* 2019;111(11):1120-1130. doi:10.1093/jnci/djz089

121. Attai DJ, Katz MS, Streja E, et al. Patient preferences and comfort for cancer survivorship models of care: results of an online survey. *J Cancer Surviv.* 2023;17(5):1327-1337. doi:10.1007/s11764-022-01177-0

122. Smith TG, Strollo S, Hu X, Earle CC, Leach CR, Nekhlyudov L. Understanding long-term cancer survivors' preferences for ongoing medical care. *J Gen Intern Med.* 2019;34(10):2091-2097. doi:10.1007/s11606-019-05189-y

123. Afifi AM, Saad AM, Al-Husseini MJ, Elmehrath AO, Northfelt DW, Sonbol MB. Causes of death after breast cancer diagnosis: a US population-based analysis. *Cancer.* 2020;126(7):1559-1567. doi:10.1002/cncr.32648

124. Zaorsky NG, Churilla TM, Egleston BL, et al. Causes of death among cancer patients. *Ann Oncol.* 2017;28(2):400-407. doi:10.1093/annonc/mdw604

125. Kemp EB, Geerse OP, Knowles R, et al. Mapping systematic reviews of breast cancer survivorship interventions: a network analysis. *J Clin Oncol.* 2022;40(19):2083-2093. doi:10.1200/JCO.21.02015

SPECIAL TOPICS

Clinical Trials Methodology and Analysis

Jeffrey C. Miecznikowski, Austin Miller, and Michael W. Sill

Clinicians make treatment recommendations daily. These recommendations arise from culling information from standardized clinical guidelines, published reports, expert opinion, or personal experiences. The synthesis of information from these sources into a particular recommendation for an individual patient is based on a clinician's personal judgment. But what constitutes reliable and valid information worthy of consideration? It has long been recognized that properly planned and conducted clinical trials are important sources of empirical evidence for shaping clinical judgment. In this chapter, we describe a general system for classifying clinical study designs. We then present the components of a clinical trial and essential considerations for developing new trials. Because translational research (TR) objectives are incorporated into many modern cancer trials, some issues related to design and analyses of these components are also presented.

CLASSIFICATION OF STUDY DESIGNS

In general, a clinical study is any experiment involving human subjects, which evaluates an intervention that attempts to reduce the impact of a specific disease in a particular population. The term *clinical trial* is usually limited to prospective studies where individuals receive an intervention and then they are followed to access their health status. When an intervention is applied in order to prevent the onset of a particular disease, the trial is classified as a primary prevention trial. For example, a primary prevention trial may evaluate healthy lifestyles or a vitamin supplement in a population of individuals who are considered to be at risk of a particular disease. Secondary prevention trials evaluate interventions that are applied to individuals with early stages of a disease in order to reduce their risk of progressing to more advanced stages of the disease. Tertiary intervention trials are aimed at evaluating interventions that reduce the risk of morbidity or mortality due to a particular disease.

Clinical trials that evaluate methods for detecting disease in a preclinical state are called **screening trials**. Early detection may mean diagnosing a malignancy in an early stage (eg, the use of mammography in the detection of breast cancer) or in a premalignant state (eg, the use of Papanicolaou smear in the detection of cervical intraepithelial neoplasia). There are typically two types of interventions in a screening trial. The first intervention is the screening program (eg, annual mammograms), which involves individuals who appear to be free of the disease. However, once the disease is detected in an individual, a secondary intervention (eg, surgery) is performed in hopes of stopping the disease from progressing to more advanced stages. Consequently, screening trials require that *both* interventions are effective. An effective screening procedure is useless if the secondary intervention does not alter the course of the disease. On the other hand, an ineffective screening procedure would cause the secondary intervention to be applied indiscriminately or too late for the treatment to be effective.

An alternative to a clinical trial is a nonexperimental study (or **observational study**). In observational studies, individuals are observed and certain outcomes measured. Importantly, in contrast to clinical trials, no attempt is made to affect the outcome, for example, no treatment or drug is systematically administered. Observational studies have strengths and weaknesses when compared to clinical trials. Ethics may dictate that observational studies may be the only way for researchers to explore certain questions. For example, in exploring the link between maternal cigarette smoking in pregnant women and birth weight, it would be unethical to design a trial that randomizes pregnant women to smoking cigarettes. On the other hand, the results/conclusions from a randomized clinical trial (RCT) are considered stronger and have the potential to yield cause-and-effect conclusions unlike observational results. A full treatment of observational studies is outside the scope of this chapter. The remainder of this chapter focuses on the elements to consider in designing, implementing, and analyzing a clinical trial.

COMPONENTS OF A CLINICAL TRIAL

Objectives

In clinical oncology research, the ultimate purpose is to accomplish a defined objective, whether it be to develop a treatment plan that puts the patients into a disease-free state, reduce the risk of cancer recurrence, or allow patients to return to their normal lifestyle within a reasonable period of time. When it comes to a particular clinical trial, however, objectives need to be more precisely defined. In general, they typically incorporate three elements: the interventions to be evaluated, the "yardstick" to be used to measure treatment benefit (see section on "End Points"), and a brief description of the target population (see section on "Eligibility Criteria"). These three elements (ie, "what," "how," and "who") should be stated in the most precise, clear, and concise terms possible. An open dialogue among expert investigators remains the most effective approach for establishing the objectives of any clinical trial.

End Points

The end points of a trial typically consist of a measurable and reproducible entity in the patient's disease process that can be used to assess the efficacy of an intervention. A study may assess more than one end point, but in these instances, the end point of primary interest should be clearly specified or else the study design should carefully reflect the complexity of interpreting multiple outcomes. End points can also be a composite measure of multiple outcomes. For instance, some studies assessing health-related quality of life (QoL) aggregate patient-reported scores from several related items or domains that are all considered components of a larger concept called quality of life (QoL).

End points should be a valid (unbiased) measure of the treatment effect on the disease process. They should not be susceptible to a systematic error that favors one treatment, which would lead to biased estimates of the treatment's effect. For instance, trials assessing time to disease progression, in which the schedule for computed tomography (CT) imaging is different for each treatment group, are susceptible to assessment bias. Second, the measurement of an end point should be reliable and not susceptible to subjective interpretation. Third, end points that are directly relevant to the patient are preferable, although valid surrogate end points are considered indirectly relevant to the patient. Finally, end points that are not too expensive or inconvenient for the patient are preferred. It is not always possible for a single end point to exhibit all of these characteristics simultaneously. For example, avoiding death is very relevant to a patient with a lethal disease like advanced gynecologic cancer. Also, survival can usually be measured very reliably. However, most patients with cancer will not only receive the treatments prescribed by the study, but after exhibiting signs of disease progression, they often receive additional anticancer therapies. In this case, the validity of overall survival (OS) comparisons is suspect because they reflect not only the effects of the study treatment but also the effects of other therapies that are external to the study.

End points may be classified as categorical (eg, clinical response), continuous (eg, serum CA-125 values), or time to event (eg, survival time). A time-to-event end point includes both time (a continuous measure) and censoring status (categorical measure). The data type influences the methods of analysis.

Measurement Errors

The susceptibility of an outcome to measurement errors is an important consideration when choosing an end point. These can be characterized as random or systematic errors. *Random error* refers to variation occurring among measurements that is not predictable and appears to be due to chance alone. For example, a serum sample could be divided into 10 aliquots and submitted to the laboratory for CA-125 determination. If the laboratory returns nearly the same value for each aliquot, then the associated random error is low, and the measurement may be deemed reproducible. On the other hand, if the CA-125 values vary considerably among aliquots, perhaps due to inconsistent laboratory procedures, then individual values may be considered unreliable. In this case, taking the average CA-125 measurement across all 10 aliquots is expected to be a better estimate of the patient's true CA-125 value than any single measurement.

Deviations from the true value that occur in a regular manner are termed *systematic errors*, or *bias*. For example, suppose an investigator initiates a randomized trial comparing two treatments, with time to disease progression being the primary end point. The protocol indicates that the patient should be assessed after each cycle of therapy. However, suppose that a treatment cycle duration is 2 weeks for one treatment group and 4 weeks for the second treatment group. Using a more intense assessment schedule for the group being treated on 2-week cycles would tend to detect progressions earlier than in the group being treated every 4 weeks. Therefore, the time-to-failure comparison between treatments would systematically favor the treatment group with a longer interval between assessments.

When there are recognized sources of error, it is important that the study design implement procedures to avoid or minimize their effect. For example, random error in many cases can be accommodated by increasing either the number of individuals in the study (the sample size) or, in some cases, the number of assessments performed on each individual. Systematic measurement error cannot be addressed by increasing the sample size. In fact, increasing the sample size may exacerbate the problem, because small systematic errors in large comparative trials contribute to the chances of erroneously concluding that the treatment effect is statistically significant. The approaches to controlling sources of systematic error tend to be procedural. For example, treatment randomization is used to control selection bias, placebos are used to control observer bias, standardized assessment procedures and schedules are used to control measurement bias, and stratified analyses are used to control biases owing to confounding. For an extensive description of biases that can occur in analytic research, refer to a study by Sackett (1).

Surrogate End Points

Surrogate end points do not necessarily have direct clinical relevance to the patient. Instead, surrogate end points are often intermediate events in the etiologic pathway to other events that are directly relevant to the patient (2). The degree to which a treatment's effect on a surrogate end point predicts the treatment's effect on a clinically relevant end point is a measure of the surrogate's validity. The ideal surrogate end point is an observable event that is a necessary and sufficient precursor in the causal pathway to a clinically relevant event. In addition, the treatment's ability to alter the surrogate end point must be directly related to its impact on the true end point. It is important that the validity and reliability of a surrogate end point be established and not simply presupposed (3,4). Surrogate end points are sometimes justified on the basis of an analysis that demonstrates a statistical correlation between the surrogate event and a true end point. However, while such a correlation is a necessary condition, it is not a sufficient condition to justify using a particular surrogate as an end point in a clinical trial. For example, CA-125 levels following three cycles of treatment of ovarian cancer have been shown to be associated with OS (5). However, it has not (yet) been demonstrated that the degree to which any particular treatment reduces CA-125 levels reliably predicts its effects on clinically relevant end points, like OS.

Primary End Points in Gynecologic Oncology Treatment Trials

The U.S. Food and Drug Administration (FDA) organized a conference to consider end points for trials involving women diagnosed with advanced ovarian cancer (6). Meta-analyses were presented, which indicate that progression-free survival (PFS) can be considered a valid end point for trials involving women with advanced ovarian cancer. However, although the general validity of PFS for predicting OS has been established, PFS comparisons in a particular study can be biased because of differences in disease assessment schedules among treatment groups, either intentionally or unintentionally. In contrast, OS time is generally not susceptible to this source of bias.

The progression-free interval (PFI) may be a reasonable end point in trials involving patients with early or locally advanced cancer. The difference between PFI and PFS resides in how patients who die without any evidence of disease progression are handled in an analysis. Patients who die without evidence of progression are censored at the time of their death in a PFI analysis. That is, we consider that patient's PFI as unobserved, noting only that the PFI must be greater than the interval based on time of death. However, in a PFS analysis, these patients are considered an uncensored event, that is, their PFS is taken to be the interval based on time of death. If deaths due to non–cancer-related causes are common, then selecting PFI as the study end point will generally increase the study's sensitivity for detecting effective cancer treatments. In this case, however, the analysis needs to consider procedures that will account for treatment-related deaths, as well as deaths from competing causes, which may occur before disease recurrence. Simply censoring the time to recurrence in these cases can make a very toxic treatment appear more effective than it actually is.

In a number of gynecologic cancer trials, a new treatment increased the duration of PFS, but not OS. For example, OVAR 2.2, a second-line treatment trial involving patients with platinum-sensitive ovarian cancer, indicated that carboplatin and gemcitabine significantly decreased the hazard of first progression or death (PFS) by 28% (hazard ratio [HR] = 0.72, P = .003) when compared to carboplatin alone (7). However, there was no appreciable difference between the treatment groups with regard to the duration of OS (HR = 0.96, P = .735). Also, three trials evaluating maintenance bevacizumab for first- or second-line treatment of ovarian cancer reported significant prolongation of PFS (8-10), but no difference in OS. PFS may be a good surrogate for OS, but it appears to be susceptible to a small but not insignificant chance of false-positive prediction. Despite this, it is very rare for the results of an oncology trial to indicate that a new treatment prolongs OS but does not delay the onset of recurrence or progression.

It seems reasonable to expect that an anticancer treatment that prolongs survival should exert its influence by delaying the onset of new or increasing disease. This has prompted some investigators to recommend using both PFS and OS as trial end points (11-13). Specifically, trials involving patients with advanced-stage cancer are designed to assess OS in the final analysis, but PFS is monitored at scheduled interim analyses. If the trial's evolving evidence indicates that there is insufficient PFS benefit, then the trial may be stopped early with conclusion that the treatment has insufficient activity to warrant further investigation in the target population. This procedure tends to halt trials of inactive treatments early, but continue trials of active agents to completion.

To date, PFS has not been formally validated for use in trials involving patients with metastatic cervical, endometrial, or vulvar cancers. In the absence of a formally validated surrogate end point, OS and symptom relief remain reasonable end points. Because relief from symptoms is susceptible to assessment bias, trials utilizing these end points should use validated instruments (see section on "Measurement Errors") and consider blinding the study treatments whenever possible.

Response (disease status) assessed via reassessment laparotomy following treatment has been proposed for use as a study end point in ovarian cancer trials (14). The justification is that those patients with no pathologic evidence of disease are more likely to experience longer survival than those with evidence of disease. The principal drawback to this end point is that reassessment laparotomy is a very onerous procedure for the patient and that many patients refuse reassessment surgery or the surgery may become medically contraindicated. Even among patients of surgeons who are strong proponents of reassessment surgery, the percent of patients not reassessed is typically greater than 15%. These missing evaluations can significantly undermine the interpretability of the study.

In summary, the ideal primary end point provides valid and reliable evidence about the intervention's impact on the disease. It is, itself, either clinically relevant to the patient or a validated surrogate of a clinically relevant outcome. It should be convenient and cost-effective to measure. Unfortunately, in some trials, these features are not always available simultaneously. If a surrogate end point is used, then its validity should be established, not presumed.

Eligibility Criteria

The eligibility criteria serve two purposes in a clinical trial. The immediate purpose is to define those patients with a particular disease, clinical history, and personal and medical characteristics that may be considered for enrollment into the clinical trial. The subsequent purpose of eligibility criteria is typically evident after the clinical trial is completed and the results are available. At this time, physicians need to carefully consider to whom the results apply. Therefore, during study development, investigators should be cognizant of the generalizability of any results ultimately reported. A potentially useful approach for determining the necessity of a particular eligibility criterion is to clearly identify its function. In addition to defining the target population, there are four distinct functions that an eligibility criterion may serve: benefit-morbidity equipoise (safety), homogeneity of benefit (scientific), logistic, and regulatory (15).

Ideally, each patient who meets the eligibility criteria of a clinical trial would be asked to participate. However, this is seldom possible for multiple reasons. **Figure 12.1-1** displays common restrictions that can limit the entry of patients to a clinical trial. In

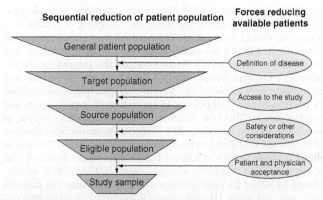

Figure 12.1-1. Sequential reduction of patient population.

particular, restricted access to the study may contribute to distorted sampling from the target population, which is called selection bias. For example, participating investigators at university hospitals might tend to enroll disproportionately more patients with cancer who have undergone more aggressive initial cytoreductive surgeries than their counterparts at community hospitals.

Eligibility criteria applied for safety are in place to eliminate patients for whom the risk of adverse effects from treatment is not commensurate with the potential for benefit. An example of this may be to restrict eligibility to patients with normal organ function based on concern that a trial therapeutic may be too toxic in such patients. Eligibility criteria may also be warranted when there is a scientific or biologic rationale for a variation in treatment benefit across patient subgroups, particularly if the effect of a new therapy may be expected to be dramatically inconsistent across the entire spectrum of the target population, so much so that statistical power can be compromised (15). One example of this type of exclusion criterion is found in Gynecologic Oncology Group (GOG) Protocol 152 (A phase 3 randomized study of cisplatin [NSC#119875] and taxol [paclitaxel] [NSC#125973] with interval secondary cytoreduction versus cisplatin and paclitaxel in patients with suboptimal stage III & IV epithelial ovarian carcinoma). This study was designed to assess the value of secondary cytoreductive surgery in patients with stage III ovarian cancer. All patients entered into this study were to receive three courses of cisplatin and paclitaxel. After completing this therapy, they were then randomized to either three additional courses of chemotherapy or interval secondary cytoreductive surgery, followed by three additional courses of chemotherapy. The eligibility criteria exclude those patients who had only microscopic residual disease following their primary cytoreductive surgery, because there is no scientific reason to expect interval cytoreduction would be of any value to patients with no gross residual disease. In addition, the desire to attain a study population with homogeneous prognosis is a common reason for eligibility criteria. In fact, eligibility criteria should be as broad as possible in order to enhance generalizability. Eligibility criteria based on regulatory considerations include those institutional and governmental regulations that require a signed and witnessed informed consent and study approval by the local Institutional Review Board. These restrictions are required in most research settings and are not subject to the investigator's discretion. Finally, they can be justified by logistic considerations. For example, a study that requires frequent clinic visits for proper evaluation or toxicity monitoring may restrict patients who are unable to arrange reliable transportation. The potential problem with such a restriction is how it is structured. A criterion requiring that the patient have a car at their disposal is probably too restrictive, because some patients from resource-poor areas may not have access to private transportation. Such a restriction tends to erode the generalizability of the trial by oversampling from resource-rich communities.

Many biostatisticians believe that eligibility criteria in oncology trials tend to be too restrictive and complicated (15,16). Overly restrictive or complex eligibility criteria hamper accrual, prolong the study's duration, and delay the reporting of results and, therefore, should be avoided. The Medical Research Council has demonstrated that it is possible to conduct trials with simple and few eligibility criteria (17). As an example, the International Collaborative Ovarian Neoplasms (ICON 3) trial compared standard carboplatin or a cisplatin-adriamycin-cyclophosphamide regimen to paclitaxel plus carboplatin in women with newly diagnosed ovarian cancer. This trial employed only six eligibility criteria, of which three were for safety (fit to receive chemotherapy; absence of sepsis, and bilirubin less than twice the normal level). This was in sharp contrast to GOG Protocol 162 (A phase 3 randomized trial of cisplatin [NSC #119875] with paclitaxel [NSC #125973] administered by either 24-hour infusion or 96-hour infusion in patients with selected stage III and stage IV epithelial ovarian cancer), which had 34 eligibility criteria.

PHASES OF THERAPEUTIC INTERVENTION TRIALS

The traditional approach to identifying and evaluating new drugs has relied on sequential evidence from phase 1, 2, and 3 clinical trials. Each of these study designs stem from very distinct study objectives. Phase 2 trials build on the evidence gathered from phase 1 trial results, and similarly, phase 3 trials build on phase 2 and phase 1 trial results. The investigation of a given treatment may be halted at any phase, due to either safety and/or efficacy issues. Depending upon the underlying investigation, the time from the initiation of a phase 1 trial for a given treatment to the completion of a phase 3 trial often spans several years. Trials can also include multiple phases. While this may cut down on the overall duration as compared to developing and running individual trials, additional up-front development time is increased with no guarantee that the additional phases will ever complete.

Phase 1 Trials

The purpose of a phase 1 trial is to determine an acceptable dose or schedule for a new therapy as determined by toxicity and/or pharmacokinetics. Owing to the limited number of patients involved in a phase 1 trial, outcome measures such as response and survival are not the primary interest in these studies. In general, the phase 1 trial marks the first use of a new experimental agent in humans. Most escalate dose or schedule of the new agent after either a prespecified number of consecutive patients have been successfully treated or within an individual as each dose is determined to be tolerable.

The usual phase 1 trial of a cytotoxic agent attempts to balance the delivery of the greatest dose intensity against an acceptable risk of dose-limiting toxicity (DLT). The conventional approach is to increase the dose of the new agent after demonstrating that a small cohort of consecutive patients (three to six) was able to tolerate the regimen. However, once an unacceptable level of toxicity occurs (eg, two or three patients experiencing DLT), the previously acceptable dose level is used to treat additional patients in order to provide further evidence that the current dose has an acceptable risk of DLT. If this dose is regarded as acceptable, it is called the recommended dose level (RDL) for further development. The RDL should not be confused with the maximum tolerated dose (MTD). The MTD is a theoretical concept used to design a phase 1 trials, whereas the RDL is an *estimate* of the MTD and may or may not be accurate.

Alternative strategies for estimating the MTD have been proposed. The primary motivation for these newer strategies is to reduce the number of patients treated at therapeutically inferior doses and to reduce the overall size of the study. One of these alternatives implements a Bayesian approach and is referred to as the continual reassessment method (CRM) (18). It has the attractive feature of determining the dose level for the next patient based

on statistically modeling the toxicity experience of the previously treated patients. While the traditional approach has been criticized for treating too many patients at subtherapeutic doses and providing unreliable estimates of the MTD, CRM has been criticized for tending to treat too many patients at doses higher than the MTD (19). Refinements to CRM have been proposed (20) and found to have good properties when compared to alternative dose-seeking strategies (21).

Another family of designs termed the *accelerated titration design* (ATD) allows doses to be escalated within each patient and incorporates toxicity or pharmacologic information from each course of therapy into the decision of whether or not to further escalate (22). Both the modified CRM and ATD designs can provide significant advantages over the conventional phase 1 design. Finally, phase I studies to identify doses for combinations of agents may require the consideration of potential pharmacokinetic or pharmacodynamic interactions (23).

More recently, a Bayesian phase I design has been proposed in clinical trials to simultaneously reduce the number of patients treated at subtherapeutic doses and overly toxic doses. These trials are called Bayesian Optimal INterval (BOIN) designs (24). The trial allows dose escalation, de-escalation, and continued administration at a particular dose if the evidence favors that decision. The Bayesian framework works as follows: (1) there are three hypotheses at each dose level being examined, one hypothesis corresponds to the dose level being at (or near) the targeted probability of a DLT (H_0), another hypothesis indicating the dose level is significantly less than the MTD (H_1), and the last stating that the dose level yields a significantly greater probability of DLTs than desired (H_2; the dose level is higher than the MTD); (2) after the data are collected, there are three possible decisions the study can take, which are continuing at the current dose ($\mathcal{R}$), escalating to the next dose level (ε), or deescalating to a lower dose level (D); and (3) the decision that minimizes the probability of making an error is taken. The error function to be minimized is given as follows:

$$\alpha = P(H_0)P(\bar{\mathcal{R}} \mid H_0) + P(H_1) P(\bar{\varepsilon} \mid H_1) + P(H_2)P(\bar{D} \mid H_2)$$

For the "local" BOIN design, the hypotheses specify specific point probabilities of DLT of interest (eg, that the dose level is below the targeted DLT rate such as 20%, at the targeted DLT rate say 30%, or above the targeted DLT rate like 40%). Then the distribution of the number of DLTs observed under each hypothesis is a simple binomial with their corresponding probability of having a DLT. When this methodology is utilized, the decision rules for escalating, continuing at the same dose, or de-escalating depend on the observed proportion of patients experiencing DLTs and two constants called λ_1 and λ_2 such that $0 \leq \lambda_1 < \lambda_2 \leq 1$, which, in turn, depend on the hypothesized DLT rates, the prior probability that a hypothesis is true, and the sample size. If the observed proportion of DLTs, $\hat{p} > \lambda_2$, then the trial de-escalates. If $\hat{p} < \lambda_1$, the trial escalates, and if $\lambda_1 < \hat{p} < \lambda_2$, then the trial continues at the same dose level. Patients are added to the dose levels according to these rules, and data collected until a sufficient number of patients are evaluated.

The determination of the recommended phase 2 dose would use an independent procedure with the data obtained in the trial. The authors suggested isotonic regression techniques but felt that many procedures are available for this task. The BOIN designs have been compared to the cumulative cohort design (CCD) in Ivanova et al (25), the modified toxicity probability interval (mTPI) design in Ji and Wang (26), and the CRM procedures in O'Quigley et al (18). There are two BOIN designs, local and global. The global BOIN design uses composite hypotheses (eg, where the probability of a DLT spans an interval rather than specific numbers). Simulation showed that the local BOIN design tended to better limit the number of patients assigned to highly toxic regimens and reduce the risk of a "poor allocation" of patients to dose levels. Other advantages are that targeted sample sizes do not have to be precisely met (flexible accrual), and accelerated titration like designs can be used by switching the targeted sample size from 1 to 3 after observing the first DLT. It is possible that BOIN design will become more commonly used in future phase 1 trials.

Other phase I study designs are often utilized for trials involving precision therapies. These studies often incorporate a biomarker end point that signals either the activation or deactivation of a targeted pathway. As the dose is increased for small cohorts of individuals, the biomarker is measured and toxicity monitored simultaneously. Then, statistical models are used to determine a safe dose where the targeted pathway is consistently activated or inhibited (27).

Even though the majority of phase 1 trials in cancer research follow what was described earlier, it should be mentioned that alternative phase 1 trials may arise in other settings, such as medical device trials, prevention trials, education intervention trials, and behavior modification trials, where the first phase of investigation may actually utilize healthy subjects, like studies interested determining the utility of a new educational intervention on smoking cessation. The phase 1 trial may simply be utilized as an approach toward gaining some experience with the intervention before moving forward to the next phase of investigation.

Phase 2 Trials

Once a dose and schedule for a new regimen has been determined, a reasonable next step is to seek evidence that the new regimen is worthy of further evaluation in a prespecified patient population. The principle goal of a phase 2 trial is to prospectively quantify the potential efficacy of the new therapy. Because a phase 2 trial treats more patients at the RDL than in a phase 1 trial, it also provides an opportunity to more reliably assess toxicities. A phase 2 trial is often referred to as a screening trial because it attempts to judiciously identify active treatments worthy of further study in much the same way a clinician screens patients for possibly a more extensive disease evaluation. The study should have adequate sensitivity to detect active treatments and adequate specificity for rejecting inactive treatments. A phase 2 trial may evaluate a single new treatment or incorporate randomization to evaluate several new therapies or treatment schedules simultaneously.

Traditionally, phase 2 trials have been designed as a single-arm trial, but the randomized phase 2 trial has been utilized with increasing frequency. However, investigators should consider several factors when designing the phase 2 trial as a single-arm or a multi-arm randomized trial. Although the required sample size is smaller for the single-arm trial, strong and sometimes unwarranted assumptions are required in the design (28). Single-arm trials assume that the probability of response to standard treatment in the target population is known with certainty, which is often suspect, because of unanticipated or unknown differences between the study sample and historical sample(s). For instance, there may be differences in the patients' prognoses unintentionally introduced by the study's eligibility criteria or changes in patient referral patterns. Differences in the response assessment schedule, the modalities for evaluation, or the definition of response may change over time and, therefore, distort comparisons with historical results. Therefore, whenever possible, we prefer the randomized controlled phase 2 design of a novel agent against an accepted standard treatment. However, when the probability of response to standard treatment is widely accepted to be very low (eg, <5%), a single-arm trial makes sense.

Phase 2 trials can have a single-stage or multistage design. In a single-stage design, a fixed number of patients are treated with the new therapy. The goal of the single-stage design is to achieve a predetermined level of precision in estimating the end point. Although precision is one important goal in cancer trials, investigators and trial experts aim to reduce the number of patients exposed to inferior (or inactive) therapies. For this reason, many phase 2 cancer trials use multistage designs. Multistage designs implement planned interim analyses of the data and apply predetermined rules to assess whether there is sufficient evidence to warrant continuing the trial. These rules are in place to stop accrual in trials with regimens having less than the desired activity, while allowing regimens having at least a minimally acceptable level of activity to proceed to completion. Two-stage designs that minimize the expected sample size when the new treatment has a clinically uninteresting level of activity have been proposed for single-arm studies (29) and multi-arm studies (30). In the cooperative group setting, there is often a need for flexibility in specifying exactly when the interim analysis will occur. This is due to the significant administrative and logistic overhead of coordinating the study in several clinics. Therefore, designs that do not require that the interim analyses occur after a precise number of patients are entered are useful particularly in the multi-institutional setting (31).

Regardless of the measure of treatment efficacy, toxicity is a secondary end point in phase 2 trials. This approach is not likely to be appropriate in phase 2 trials of very aggressive treatments in which stopping rules may explicitly consider both response and cumulative incidence of certain toxicities (32-34). Bayesian designs that permit continuous monitoring of both toxicity and response have also been proposed (35). Other designs account for simultaneous assessment of two outcomes (eg, response rate and survival), also referred to as a bivariate outcome (36).

The approach to clinical trials utilizing biomarker-driven selection and molecularly targeted therapies is discussed in the subsequent section.

Phase 3 Trials

The goal of a phase 3 trial is to prospectively and definitively determine the effects of a new therapy relative to a standard therapy in a well-defined patient population. Phase 3 trials are also used to determine an acceptable standard therapy when there is no prior consensus on the appropriate standard therapy. It is useful to distinguish phase 3 objectives as having an efficacy, equivalency, or noninferiority design consideration. An **efficacy** design is characterized by the search for an intervention strategy that provides a therapeutic advantage over the current standard of care. An **equivalency** trial seeks to demonstrate that two interventions can be considered sufficiently similar on the basis of outcome such that one can be reasonably substituted for the other. **Noninferiority** trials seek to identify new treatments that reduce toxicity, patient inconvenience, or treatment costs without significantly compromising efficacy.

Efficacy Trials

From the outset of efficacy trials, it is recognized that the benefit of a novel treatment (which is being evaluated) may be accompanied by an increased risk of toxicity, inconvenience, or financial cost, when compared to the standard of care. However, it is hoped that the benefits will be sufficiently large to offset these drawbacks. This is illustrated in **Figure 12.1-2**. Suppose treatment A is the standard of care for a particular target disease population. The quantitative *difference in efficacy* between treatments with respect to a particular outcome (B-A) can be described on a horizontal axis as in **Figure 12.1-2**. If we are reasonably certain that the difference between treatments is less than zero (left of 0), then we would consider treatment A to be better. On the other hand, if the treatment difference is greater than zero (right of 0), then we would conclude that the new treatment, B, is better. Furthermore, we can use dotted lines to demarcate on this graphic a region in which the difference between A and B is small enough to warrant no clinical preference for A or B. Consider the results from a trial expressed as the estimated *difference between treatments* and the corresponding 95% or 99% confidence interval (CI) superimposed on this graph. The CI depicts those values of the treatment difference that can be reasonably considered consistent with the data from the trial.

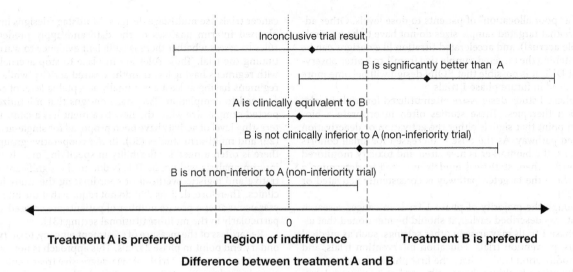

Figure 12.1-2. Graphical representation of the point estimates and confidence intervals describing the *difference* in efficacy between the standard treatment, A, and a new experimental regimen, B, from five hypothetical trials.

When the CIs are sufficiently broad that the data cannot distinguish between the treatments being tested, the trial is determined to be inconclusive (see **Figure 12.1-2**). This is a typical consequence of a small trial. On the other hand, if the CI entirely excludes the region where treatment A is better than treatment B, then we can conclude that treatment B is significantly better than treatment A (see **Figure 12.1-2**). Note that, in this case, the lower bound of the CI may extend into the region of clinical indifference, but the CI must exclude the region below (left of) 0 difference.

When an efficacy trial fails to demonstrate that a new experimental regimen is statistically superior to the control regimen, this should not be interpreted as demonstrating that these regimens are equally effective. Even though the estimated difference between two treatments may be near zero, the CI may not be able to rule out treatment differences that are clinically relevant. Therefore, we advocate cautious interpretation from efficacy studies, which conclude "therapeutic equivalency" when only a small difference between treatments with regard to the outcome is observed. Careful inspection of the CIs, like those in **Figure 12.1-2**, is appropriate, as well as where you personally consider the region of clinical indifference is located.

Equivalency Trials

The equivalency study design is perhaps a misnomer, because it is impractical to generate enough data from any trial to definitively claim that the two treatments are equivalent. Instead, an investigator typically defines the limits for treatment differences that can be interpreted as clinically irrelevant. If it is a matter of opinion for what differences in effect sizes can be considered clinically irrelevant, this issue can become a major source for controversy in the final interpretation of the trial results. Bioequivalence designs are occasionally conducted to demonstrate that two treatments exert similar influence on the expression of a biomarker. In this case, an investigator should have some notion about the acceptable range of biomarker expression that can be considered clinically equivalent. These studies are designed so that, within tolerable limits, the treatments can be considered as having similar biologic effects.

Noninferiority Trials

A noninferiority study design may be considered when the currently accepted standard treatment is associated with significant toxicity and a new and less toxic treatment becomes available. The goal of this type of study is to demonstrate that substituting the new treatment for the current standard treatment does not

compromise efficacy appreciably (37-40). Referring to **Figure 12.1-2**, the trial seeks to provide sufficient evidence to be reasonably certain that the difference between A and B lies above the lower boundary of the indifference region. This lower boundary is often called the "noninferiority margin." If the CI for the difference in efficacy fails to exclude the region where the standard regimen, A, is preferred, then there is insufficient evidence to conclude that the new regimen is not inferior to standard treatment.

The justification for the noninferiority margin selected in a particular study is often controversial. If this margin is set too low, then the study has an unacceptably high probability of recommending an inferior treatment. If it is too high, then the trial utilizes too many clinical and financial resources. In order to select an appropriate margin of noninferiority, it is important to recognize that even though a noninferiority trial may explicitly compare only two treatments, implicitly, there is a third treatment to be considered. For example, suppose that several historical studies indicate that treatment A is better than a placebo for treating a specific disease. In this case, the goal of a noninferiority study is to demonstrate that a new experimental treatment, B, does not significantly compromise efficacy when compared to currently accepted active standard treatment, A. However, it should also demonstrate that B would have been better than a placebo, if a placebo had been included in the current trial. In other words, the current trial will directly estimate the effectiveness of B relative to A, but it must also indirectly consider the effectiveness of B relative to the previous control treatment (placebo in this case). This indirect comparison relies on obtaining a reliable and unbiased estimate of the effectiveness of the current active control to the previous control from previous trials.

Sometimes, the margin of noninferiority is expressed as a proportion of the effectiveness of A relative to the previous standard treatment. For example, a noninferiority study could be designed to have a high probability of concluding that a new treatment retains at least 50% of the activity of the standard regimen, A. Note that an investigator may wish to be highly confident that none of the efficacy benefit of the current standard treatment be sacrificed. In this case, the margin of noninferiority is set at 0 (see **Figure 12.1-2**), and the design is the same as the efficacy trial. Indeed, an efficacy trial can be considered a study in which the investigator is willing to accept the new treatment B, only if the trial results indicate that B is statistically superior to A.

Obtaining reliable estimates for the activity of the currently accepted active standard treatment can be a very troublesome aspect of noninferiority oncology trials. For example, cisplatin 75 mg/m² and paclitaxel 135 mg/m² infused over 24 hours was the first platinum-taxane combination to demonstrate activity in the treatment of advanced ovarian cancer (41). Subsequently, several trials were conducted to assesses whether carboplatin could be safely substituted for cisplatin (42-44) or whether taxotere could be substituted for paclitaxel (45). However, there has been some controversy about the size of the benefit provided by paclitaxel (46). An investigator can reasonably ask: "What is the effect size of paclitaxel, and how much of this effect can I be reasonably certain is preserved by taxotere"?

Randomized Trials

There are several design features to consider when developing a phase 3 trial concept. One important feature to consider is treatment randomization. The RCT has several scientific advantages. First, both the known and unknown prognostic factors tend to be distributed similarly across the treatment groups when a trial implements randomized treatments. Second, a potential source of differential selection bias is eliminated. This bias could occur when there is an association between treatment choice and prognosis—it need not be intentional. When a physician's interest in a trial or a patient's decision to participate in the trial depends on the assigned treatment, a nonrandom association between treatment and prognosis can be introduced. Finally, randomization provides the theoretical underpinning for the significance test (47). In other words, the probability of a false-positive trial as stated in the study design is justified with randomization. It is important to recognize that these advantages, which are provided by randomizing the study treatments, are forfeited when all of the randomized patients are not included in the final analyses.

It is sometimes argued that because many factors that influence prognosis are known, perhaps other approaches to allocating treatments can be considered and statistical models should be used to adjust for any imbalances in prognosis. However, the conclusions from this type of trial must be conditioned on the completeness of knowledge about the disease and acceptability of the modeling assumptions. If the disease is moderately unpredictable with regard to the outcome, or the statistical model is inappropriate, then the conclusions are suspect.

Kunz and Oxman (48) have compared the results from overviews of RCT and non-RCT that evaluated the same intervention and reported that the nonrandomized studies tended to overestimate the treatment effect compared to randomized trials by 76% to 160%. Schulz et al (49) compared 33 RCTs that had inadequate concealment of the random treatment assignments to those studies that had adequate concealment. They found that even those with inadequate concealment tended to overestimate the treatment effect (relative odds) by 40%. Some investigators do not appreciate the importance of concealment and will go to considerable lengths to subvert it (50). When the randomization technique requires pregenerated random treatment assignments, one must guarantee that the investigators, who are enrolling patients, do not have access to the assignment lists.

It should be acknowledged that the patient-physician relationship can occasionally be challenged by introducing the concept of treatment randomization (51). Patients may prefer a sense of confidence from their physician regarding the "best" therapy for them. However, physicians involved in an RCT must honestly acknowledge that the best therapy is unknown and that an RCT is preferred to continued ignorance. One survey of 600 women seen in a breast clinic suggests that 90% of women prefer their doctor to admit uncertainty about the best treatment option, rather than give them false hope (52).

Randomization Techniques

The simplest approach to randomization is to assign treatments based on a coin flip, sequential digits from random number tables or computerized pseudo-random number generators. On average, each individual has a defined probability of being allocated to a particular study treatment, when they enter the study. Although this approach is simple, the statistical efficiency of the analyses can be enhanced by constraining the randomization so that each treatment is allocated an equal number of times. Permuted block randomization is sometimes used in order to promote equal treatment-group sizes. A block can be created by shuffling a fixed number of cards for each treatment and then assigning the patients according to the random order of the deck. After completing each block, there are an equal number of patients assigned to the treatment groups. For example, consider a trial comparing treatments A and B. There are six possible ways the block can be ordered when the block size is four: AABB, ABBA, BBAA, BABA, ABAB, and BAAB. A sufficient number of assignments for an RCT can be created by randomly selecting a series of blocks from the six distinct possibilities.

There are three features of blocked randomization to be considered. First, the probability of a particular treatment being allocated is not the same throughout the study, as in simple randomization. Taking the previous example, every fourth treatment is predetermined by the previous three allocations. Second, the use of small blocks in a single-clinic study may undermine concealment and allow an investigator to deduce the next treatment. This potential problem can be corrected by continually changing the block size throughout the assignment list. Third, large block sizes can undermine the benefits of blocking. As block sizes increase, the procedure resembles simple randomization.

The statistical efficiency of the study can be further enhanced by stratifying patients into groups with similar prognoses and using separate lists of blocked treatments for each stratum. This procedure is called stratified block randomization. It is worth noting that using simple randomization within stratum would defeat the purpose of stratification, because this is equivalent to using simple randomization for all patients. Likewise, trials that stratify on too many prognostic factors are likely to have many uncompleted treatment blocks at the end of the study, which also defeats the intent of blocking (53).

When it is desirable to balance on more than a few prognostic factors, an alternative is dynamic treatment allocation; one particular type being minimization. Whereas stratified block randomization will balance treatment assignments within each combination of the various factor levels, minimization tends to balance treatments within each level of the factor, separately. Each time a new patient is entered into the study, the number of individuals who share any of the prognostic characteristics of the new patient is tabulated. A metric, which measures the imbalance of these factors among the study treatments, is computed as if the new patient were allocated to each of the study treatments in turn. The patient is then allocated to the treatment that would favor the greatest degree of balance (54). In the event that the procedure indicates equal preference for two or more possible treatment allocations, simple randomization can be used to determine the individual's treatment assignment. Regardless of the degree of imbalance, however, this randomization process should not be deterministic. Instead, the treatments that restore the greatest degree of balance are more likely to be allocated.

Concealment during the randomization process refers to the procedure in which the assigned study treatment is not revealed to the patient or the investigator until after the subject has successfully enrolled onto the study. The purpose of concealment is to eliminate a bias that can arise from an individual's decision to participate in the study depending on the treatment assignment (55). Concealment is an essential component of RCTs.

Blinding is a procedure that prevents the patient or physician from knowing which treatment is being used. In a single-blinded study, the patient is unaware of which study treatments they are receiving. A double-blinded study results in a situation in which neither the patient nor the health care provider is aware of that information. One purpose of blinding is to avoid measurement bias, particularly differential measurement bias (see section on "End

Points"). This type of bias occurs when the value of a measurement is influenced by the knowledge of which treatment is being received. It can occur when the measurement of an end point is in part or totally subjective. Most methods for assessing pain are subjective and require treatment blinding in order to promote the study's validity.

Oncology trials frequently do not implement blinding for several reasons. It is rather difficult to blind treatments when various treatment modalities are used (eg, surgery vs radiation therapy, or intravenous [IV] vs oral administrations), when good medical practice is jeopardized (eg, special tests are required to monitor toxicity due to particular treatments), or when it is logistically difficult (eg, evaluating physician must be kept isolated from the treatment of patient). In the absence of blinding, care should be taken that the method of measuring the end point is precisely stated in the protocol and consistently applied to each patient uniformly. Trials that assess QoL or relief from symptoms should give serious consideration to treatment blinding. Schulz et al (56) have reviewed 110 RCTs published between 1990 and 1991 from four journals dedicated to obstetrics and gynecology. Thirty-one of these trials reported being double blinded. Schultz et al conclude that blinding should have been used more often, despite frequent impediments. Moreover, blinding seemed to have been compromised in at least three of the trials where it was implemented.

Placebos blind the patient and, usually the physician as well, to the knowledge of whether they are receiving an experimental or inert treatment. Placebos are frequently used in trials where there is no accepted standard treatment and the end point is susceptible to measurement bias. The use of a placebo is also important when the end point can be affected by the patient's psychological response to the knowledge of receiving therapy combined with a belief that the therapy is effective. This phenomenon is aptly named the "placebo effect." In such circumstances, the use of a placebo provides a treatment-to-control comparison that measures only the therapeutic effect. Note that the "placebo effect" is a distinctly different type of measurement bias from those that have been previously discussed. Careful ethical considerations must precede the use of a placebo or sham procedure in any clinical trial (57).

Trials With Historical Controls

The strict definition of a phase 3 trial does not necessarily require concurrent controls (ie, prospectively enrolled patients assigned the standard treatment) or randomization (ie, random treatment allocation). However, these two features are almost synonymous with phase 3 trials today.

The principal drawback from inferring treatment differences from a historically controlled trial is that the treatment groups may differ in a variety of characteristics that are not apparent. Differences in outcome, which are in fact due to differences in characteristics between the groups, may be erroneously attributed to the treatment. Although statistical models are often used to adjust for some potential biases, adjustments are possible for only factors that have been recorded accurately and consistently from both samples. Shifts in medical practice over time, differences in the definition of the disease, eligibility criteria, follow-up procedures, or recording methods can all contribute to a differential bias. Unlike random error, this type of error cannot be reduced by increasing the sample size. Moreover, the undesirable consequences of moderate biases may be exacerbated with larger sample sizes. When a trial includes *concurrent* controls, the definition of disease and the eligibility criteria can be applied consistently to both treatment groups. Also, the standard procedures for measuring the end point can be uniformly applied to all patients.

Factorial Designs

Factorial designs are used when several interventions are to be studied simultaneously. The term *factorial* arises from historical terminology in which the treatments were referred to as factors.

Each factor has corresponding levels, for example, an investigator may wish to compare a study agent administered at three dose levels: high dose, medium dose, and none. The total number of factor combinations being studied is the product of the number of levels for each factor or treatment. For example, a trial that evaluates treatment A at three levels and treatment B at two levels is called a 3-by-2 (denoted 3×2) factorial design. If the relative effects due to the various levels of treatment A are independent of the levels of B, the two treatments (A and B) can be evaluated simultaneously. The factorial design provides a significant reduction in the required sample size when compared to trials that study A and B separately. The key assumption necessary for a factorial design is that all treatments can be given simultaneously without interaction or interference.

The most commonly utilized factorial design is the 2×2 factorial design that includes two distinct treatment regimens at each of two factor levels. For example, suppose individuals entering a cancer prevention trial are randomly assigned to receive vitamin E (placebo-A or 50 mg/d) and β-carotene (placebo-B or 20 mg/d) in a study designed as a 2×2 factorial. In this case, the factors are vitamin E and β-carotene, whereas the respective factor levels are placebo-A or 50 mg/d for vitamin E and placebo-B or 20 mg/d for β-carotene. There are four treatment combinations. In a standard 2×2 design, the main effect of vitamin E can be ascertained by utilizing information from each of the four treatment groups. In some studies, however, the main effects may be of secondary importance as compared to the "interaction" between each factor. An interaction exists when the effect due to one of the factors (ie, treatment A) depends on the level of the other factor (treatment B). In drug discovery, a "positive" interaction may imply a synergistic effect of two drugs in combination, that is, the effect of the combination therapy is greater than the sum of the individual additive effects. Reliable tests of an interaction require a relatively large number of patients in each of the four treatment groups. If potential treatment interaction cannot reasonably ruled out or there is interest possible interactions, then attention to the statistical power of such tests is an important part of designing and interpreting the study results (58).

HYPOTHESIS TEST

A hypothesis is a conjecture based on prior experiences that leads to refutable predictions (59). A hypothesis is frequently framed in the context of either a null or an alternative hypothesis. In a therapeutic efficacy trial, a null hypothesis may postulate that a treatment does not influence patients' outcome. The alternative hypothesis is that a particular, well-defined treatment approach will influence the patients' outcome to a prespecified degree. These hypotheses cast the purpose of the trial into a clear framework. During the study design, the investigators select a test statistic from an appropriate statistical procedure (eg, an F-statistic from an analysis of variance, or a chi-square statistic from a logistic model) that evaluates the degree to which the study data support the null hypothesis. A type I error is committed when the null hypothesis is in fact true, but the test statistic leads the investigator to incorrectly conclude it is false. Committing the type I error would be disastrous if it means discontinuing the use of an active control treatment that is well tolerated and substituting an experimental therapy that is more toxic but, in reality, no better. A type II error is committed when the null hypothesis is not true, but the test statistic leads the investigator to erroneously conclude that it is true. Type II errors commonly occur in studies that involve too few subjects to reliably estimate clinically important treatment effects. Prospectively specifying the null hypothesis, the appropriate statistical method for the analysis, the test statistic, and quantifying the acceptable probabilities of type I error (ie, α-level) and type II error are essential elements for determining the appropriate design and sample size for a particular trial.

P-Value

At times, statisticians play the role of the conservative physician, cautiously prescribing a significance test only when it is appropriate. There is a general concern that the *P*-value is overused, even abused, and overemphasized. A common misconception is that the *P*-value is the probability that the null hypothesis is true. The null hypothesis is either true or false, and so it is not subject to a probability statement. It is the inference that an investigator makes, based on their data that are susceptible to error. The *P*-value is simply the probability that the test statistic would be as extreme or even more extreme, if the null hypothesis was in fact true (see section on "Hypothesis Test").

Misconceptions about the *P*-value may arise in part from a poor distinction between the *P*-value and α-level of a study (60). The α-level is the probability of the test statistic rejecting the null hypothesis when it is true. It is specified during the design phase of the study and is unaltered by the results obtained. The *P*-value results from a statistical test performed on the observed data.

Multiple Comparison Control for Clinical Trials

The previous section on hypothesis testing considers the type I and type II errors related to a single hypothesis test comparing the effects of two treatment arms on a single primary end point. For obvious reasons, agencies, practitioners, and patients are only willing to give up the tried-and-true standard in the face of strong evidence for a change. Randomized, single hypothesis trials designs can provide the strongest evidence possible. Generally, the hypothesis testing plan can be much more complex, with hypotheses related to multiple end points, primary and secondary hypothesis families, treatment arms, interim analyses, and population subgroups. Multiple hypothesis tests introduce the risk of hunting for significance, which undermines confidence in the final recommendation.

The so-called multiplicity problem (also referred to as multiple testing or multiple comparisons) arises when more than one hypothesis test could support the efficacy claim. Regulatory agencies aim to control the multiplicity problem among all the hypothesis tests included in the efficacy claim (61,62). To quantify the multiplicity problem, we define the family-wise type I error rate (FWER) (63,64) as the probability of at least one type I error in a family of hypothesis tests, regardless of the true null hypotheses. The family-wise control concept can apply to a single set of statistical hypotheses, to multiple hypothesis families within a study, or even across multiple studies. Without control, the FWER increases with the number of tests. A family of four tests, each with an α-level of 0.025, has an FWER of 0.096. Compared to the single test, this is a 5-fold increase in the risk of making a false efficacy claim (65).

The protocol can reduce the degree of multiplicity by limiting the number of objectives and prioritizing the end points into families based on clinical importance. End points directly supporting claims of clinical efficacy are included among the primary objectives. Secondary objectives include end points to show supporting evidence of efficacy.

Statistical methods for controlling the multiplicity effects start by specifying the maximum FWER allowed. Regulatory agencies generally target an FWER-α of 0.025 (one sided). A single hypothesis can use a test with an α-level equal to the FWER. If a hypothesis family includes two tests, a number of FWER controlling procedures are available. One option is to split the FWER-α between the two tests, such that FWER-α = 0.025 = $\alpha_1 + \alpha_2$ (62). For example, the Bonferroni correction (66) allocates the FWER-α equally to each test in the family ($\alpha_1 = \alpha_2 = 0.0125$). The Bonferroni method is a single-step method that divides the FWER-α equally among all the hypotheses in the family based on the number of hypotheses. With this procedure, rejection of one null hypothesis does not depend on any of the other tests, because the α-levels for all the hypotheses are specified a priori. Alternatively, stepwise methods

allocate the FWER-α based on *P*-values from the other tests in the family (67,68). These methods may reject more null hypotheses than the single-step procedures as a result of α-propagation. The α-propagation principle states that the α-level from a rejected hypothesis can be propagated to (or shared with) a null hypothesis that has not been rejected yet (69,70). However, stepwise methods are data driven and may not reflect the clinical relevance of the end points.

Hierarchical testing procedures require specifying the order of analysis for the hypotheses in a family before any data are analyzed. The ordering is subjective, with the most clinically relevant hypothesis tested first. In the most general case, the so-called Fallback procedures (71) allocate some of the FWER-α to each hypothesis in the family. The hypotheses are evaluated in a priori specified order. If a null hypothesis is rejected at its specified α level, that α can be propagated to hypotheses that have not been rejected, thereby increasing the α-levels of subsequent tests. The rules for α-propagation must be specified before data are analyzed. Graphical methods have been developed to effectively illustrate the α-propagation rules (72,73).

Consider a family of two ordered hypotheses, limiting the FWER-α to 0.025. First, the FWER-α is split arbitrarily between the two hypotheses, such that FWER-α = 0.025 = $\alpha_1 + \alpha_2$. For example, let $\alpha_1 = 0.005$ and $\alpha_2 = 0.02$. The hypotheses are tested in the prespecified order. If the first null hypothesis is rejected by an α_1 = 0.005 level test, then α_1 is propagated to the second hypothesis. This allows the second hypothesis to be assessed using an α-level of $\alpha_1 + \alpha_2 = 0.025$. If it is not rejected at its first test, the first null hypothesis is retained for possible future evaluation, and the second hypothesis is assessed using an $\alpha_2 = 0.02$ level test. If the second null hypothesis cannot be rejected, the testing sequence stops. If the second null hypothesis is rejected after the first hypothesis was not, the α_2 can be propagated back, allowing the first hypothesis to be retested using an α-level of $\alpha_1 + \alpha_2 = 0.025$.

The "fixed sequence" procedure is a special case in the hierarchical class of testing procedures. Once the hypothesis ordering is specified, all of FWER-α is allocated to the first null hypothesis. If the first null hypothesis is rejected, all the FWER-α is propagated to the second hypothesis, which is tested at the FWER-α level. No multiplicity adjustment is required. Once a test fails to reject a null hypothesis, the FWER-α is fully depleted, and the process stops. Subsequent hypotheses are not tested. Because compliance with this requirement is critical to maintaining FWER control, the ordering of the hypothesis tests should be carefully considered. Fixed sequence testing procedures work well when the first hypotheses have significant results. No statistical conclusions can be made for hypotheses ordered after the first test that fails.

The specific methods described earlier control the FWER within a single family of multiple hypothesis tests. In contrast, gatekeeping strategies control the FWER when transitions between families are required. For example, the trial design may include a primary objective family with two end points (PFS and OS), and a secondary objective family with several end points (response rate, response duration, toxicity rate, etc). Practically, the gap in time between maturity of the PFS and OS end points can be long enough to render this example infeasible.

A priori ordering of families is required. In this instance, the primary family must be successfully passed for the secondary family (74). The primary family may be classified as either a serial gatekeeper or parallel gatekeeper for the secondary family. A serial gatekeeping procedure requires rejection of all of the primary family null hypotheses before the secondary family is assessed. In the GYN Oncology setting, FWER in the primary end points is likely to be controlled using a fixed sequence procedure. Once the primary family is passed, any procedure for FWER control can be used in the secondary family.

A parallel gatekeeper allows testing of the secondary family if at least one null hypothesis is rejected in the primary family. These procedures must account for possibility that at least one primary null hypothesis does not reject. The computations become rather complex (75).

The FDA Guidance on Multiple Endpoints in Clinical Trials says, "As the number of end points analyzed in a single trial increases, the likelihood of making false conclusions about a drug's effects with respect to one or more of those end points becomes a concern if there is not appropriate adjustment for multiplicity" (62). The risk of false-positive findings rests on patients via the potential replacement of a proven effective standard-of-care therapy with a truly ineffective substitute. At the same time, the increasing cost and effort required to conduct a clinical trial leads to greater interest in having multiple ways to claim clinical efficacy. In response, a large number of procedures have been developed that control the risk of false-positive findings while accommodating multiple comparisons. The best procedure for a given clinical trial depends on the patients' condition, the objectives and end points, and the treatments available.

TRANSLATIONAL RESEARCH

Many modern clinical trials often involve the systematic collection and banking of biologic materials from the participants. The materials may include serum, plasma, urine, buccal cells, or tumor tissue, which are collected and stored in a biorepository. The biologic materials together with the clinical data can then be used to understand how a biologic effect translates into the treatment effect on the patient population. This translation gives rise to the concept of TR. In TR, discoveries in laboratory science are translated into practical applications. The flow of information from TR studies is a two-way street: (1) more complete understanding of tumor biology and (2) more effective treatments for patients.

The goal of this section is to provide clinical and laboratory scientists with some fundamental information needed to design, implement, and analyze the data from TR studies. The following sections develop the concepts for (1) biomarker discovery and verification and (2) biomarker validation. Insights are provided into what the goals and expectations a researcher can have when performing a biomarker study. With this knowledge at hand, the reader can avoid some of the mistakes, errors, and biases that have plagued TR and have led to false, misreported, or misleading reports.

It is important to understand that biomarkers can be used to diagnose a disease, to assess prognosis, to select appropriate treatments (predictive), or to assess treatment outcome (surrogate end point). Thus, biomarkers can be incorporated into many aspects of clinical practice and research once validated. There are two types of biomarker validation to consider: analytic and clinical validation. *Analytic validation* refers to obtaining evidence that the biomarker assay result is reproducible under a variety of conditions and that the assay is shown to accurately measure the intended analyte. This is essential before a biomarker can be clinically validated. Clinical validation involves demonstrating that the biomarker is "fit for purpose." That is, it functions properly for its intended use as a diagnostic, prognostic, treatment selective, or surrogate marker. The rigor needed to evaluate the clinical utility of a biomarker has recently been emphasized in light of several failed attempts at validating complex biomarkers (76-78).

Biospecimen Collection

The biologic specimens used in a study are typically gathered either prospectively or retrospectively. In the prospective approach, patients are identified and then followed forward in time. There are several advantages with the prospective approach. First, patient enrollment can focus on enrolling only individuals from the intended target population. Second, the procedures for collecting and preparing specimens can be tailored to the intended laboratory procedures. Third, the quality control procedures for collecting the clinical data can target those data items that are required for the specific study objectives. Fourth, the patient's treatment and follow-up assessments can be standardized and optimized in accordance with the goals of the study. When samples are retrospectively collected, the laboratory analysis is performed using previously archived specimens that may have been originally collected for another intended purpose. The investigator using a retrospective approach is a prisoner to the procedures that were set down before the current study goals were contemplated and, therefore, they may not be optimal for their intended objectives. For instance, the samples may have come from patients who are not representative of the target population. This reduces the generalizability of the study results. The specimens may have been obtained, prepared, or stored using outdated or less-than-optimal procedures for their laboratory tests. This could introduce biases in the measurements or reduce the power of the study.

Biomarker Development Process

A widely used definition of a biomarker is "a characteristic that is objectively measured and evaluated as an indicator of normal biologic processes, pathogenic processes, or pharmacologic responses to an intervention" (79). Biomarkers can be measurements of macromolecules (DNA, RNA, proteins, lipids), cells, or processes that describe a normal or abnormal biologic state in a patient. From the paradigm of TR described earlier, biomarkers can inform investigators on a patient's disease diagnosis, prognosis, prediction of response to therapy (ie, effect modifier), or prediction of a clinical outcome (ie, surrogate end point).

Generally speaking, biomarkers can be diagnostic, prognostic, or predictive. A diagnostic biomarker is designed to identify the presence of a disease or other condition, whereas a prognostic biomarker is an indicator that helps researchers in predicting the course of a patient's disease. Prognostic biomarkers are used to estimate the risk of a future clinical outcome and examples include state of the disease, histology of the tumor, or patient's performance status. A biomarker may also be deemed predictive, and as such, it can be used to modify the estimated risk of a future outcome but only when a particular type of treatment is taken. In patients with breast cancer, examples of predictive biomarkers are estrogen receptor status when the treatment is tamoxifen, or HER2/neu status when the treatment is trastuzumab. The phrase "treatment selection marker" may be preferable terminology for a predictive biomarker in order to avoid confusion with other uses of the word predictive. For immediate purposes here, predictive markers are viewed as a special class of prognostic markers, and we primarily focus on prognostic biomarker studies in general. Only in the section describing studies involving targeted therapies will the distinction be made.

In the following sections, a common biomarker development strategy is discussed that includes (1) biomarker discovery and (2) biomarker validation. In short, these steps are presented in **Figure 12.1-3** (discovery and test validation stage).

Discovery Phase

Regardless of whether the samples were retrospectively or prospectively collected, many studies are designed to discover biomarkers with clinical utility, from among many potentially useful biomarkers.

Since the invention of microarray technology and related high-throughput (HT) technologies, researchers have been able to compile large amounts information and an enormous pool of potential biomarkers. These so-called high-throughput platforms have become commonly used experimental platforms in the biologic realm (80). A HT platform is designed to measure large numbers (thousands or millions) of signatures in a biologic organism at a given time point. These platforms are a function of the postgenomic era and are often used to determine how genomic

Classifier Development Phase

- **Probe Discovery:** Identify a subset genes/proteins associated with the clinical outcome of interest.
- **Probe Verification:** Confirm measurements on selected genes/proteins using alternate laboratory techniques, like IHC or Rt-PCR.
- **Classifier Development:** Use the confirmed genes/proteins to develop a model (classifier) that appears to predict clinical outcome.

Classifier Verification Phase

- **Model Verification:** Confirm the model's properties using an small independent sample of individuals or cross-classification techniques.
- **Document Classifier:** Document the computational procedures and criteria for interpreting the lock-down model.

Classifier Validation

- **Validation:** Evaluate the model's predictive accuracy in a sample of individuals representative of the target population. Any changes to the procedures or the lock-down model to improve the classifier will require further validation.

For additional information see National Research Council. *Evolution of Translational Omics: Lessons Learned and the Path Forward* .Washington, DC: The National Academies Press, 2012.

Figure 12.1-3. Biomarker development for high-throughput technologies. (National Research Council. *Evolution of Translational Omics: Lessons Learned and the Path Forward*. The National Academies Press; 2012.) Used with permission of The National Academies Press, from National Research Council. *Evolution of Translational Omics: Lessons Learned and the Path Forward*. The National Academies Press; 2012; permission conveyed through Copyright Clearance Center, Inc.

expression is regulated or involved in biologic processes. The technologies in **Table 12.1-1** use hybridization and sequence-based platforms such as gene expression microarrays and RNA-Seq to obtain data matrices.

Several of the common HT assay platforms used in experiments designed for cancer diagnosis are listed in **Table 12.1-1**. These platforms were chosen to illustrate the diversity of platforms available for interrogating DNA, RNA, or proteins.

Preprocessing High-Throughput Platforms

In short, preprocessing algorithms are required in nearly all HT technologies listed in **Table 12.1-1**. This is due to the fact that HT platforms measure both biologic signal and technical signal. Therefore, the goal of preprocessing algorithms is removal of the technical signal. This technical signal can be considered in terms of background correction and normalization to adjust across experiments. The background corrections and normalization account for technical artifacts that can occur due to either the array construction or laboratory procedures that introduce systematic errors in the signal on individual arrays or across arrays. Often, these preprocessing techniques are specific to the platform employed (see, eg, Miecznikowski et al (81)); therefore, it is impractical to review all of the available preprocessing methods here.

Type I Error and Multiple Testing

The experiments performed in the HT discovery phase often have a goal of simply narrowing down the genome or proteome to a subset of potentially relevant biomarkers. In this sense, the scientists are performing a data reduction where the goal is to choose a subset of markers from the HT scope that are related to or associated with clinical outcome. The association with the outcome is assessed using a null hypothesis for each biomarker and summarizing "significance" with a P-value. In this case, the interpretation of each P-value differs slightly from a study with a single null hypothesis (see sections on "Hypothesis Test," "P-Value," and "Multiple Comparison Control for Clinical Trials").

When the type I error is limited to 5% for a single hypothesis, then there is only a 1-in-20 chance of rejecting that null hypothesis, if it is in fact true. This is a relatively uncommon occurrence. When there are 10,000 null hypotheses tested, as may be typical for some HT studies, even if all of the null hypotheses were true, one would expect 500 null hypotheses to be rejected at the 5% significance level. The chance of committing a type I error over the entire study should no longer be considered an uncommon occurrence.

Therefore, during the discovery phase of an HT experiment, the goal is to limit the type I error rate. That is, HT studies are designed to limit the number of false positives, denoted by V in

TABLE 12.1-1. Summary of Discovery Platforms, Material Analyzed in the Platform, and Recent Cancer Biomarker Discovery Studies Using the Given Platform

Platform	Material	Cancer Studies
aCGH microarray	DNA	Albertson et al (110), Hodgson et al (111), Pollack et al (112), Albertson (113), Albertson et al (114), Hackett et al (115), Garnis et al (116), Veltman et al (117), Pinkel and Albertson (118), Rossi et al (119), Idbaih et al (120).
Gene expression microarray	mRNA	Ramaswamy et al (121), Gordon et al (122), Tibshirani et al (123), Statnikov et al (124), Glas et al (125), Van't Veer et al (126), Sotiriou et al (127), Michiels et al (128), Barrier et al (129), Miecznikowski et al (130).
RNA-Seq	Transcriptomics	Levin et al (131), Pflueger et al (132).
DNA methylation	DNA	Portela and Esteller (133).
Mass spectrometry	Peptide/proteomics	Paweletz et al (134), Koopmann et al (135), Kolch et al (136), Diamandis (137,138), Lan et al (139).

aCGH, array comparative genomic hybridization.

■ TABLE 12.1-2A. Summary of Results From Analyzing Multiple Hypothesis Tests

	H_0 Retained	H_0 Rejected	Total
H_0 True	U	V	M_0
H_0 False	T	Q	M_1
	$M - R$	R	M

M_0 and M_1 are considered fixed (unknown) parameters representing the number of true nulls and the number of true alternatives, respectively. The random variables U and Q represent the number of the correct decisions, whereas the random variables T and V represent the number of incorrect decisions. V is the number of false positives.

■ TABLE 12.1-2B. Summaries of Type I Errors Using Random Variables Defined in Table 12.1-3

Abbreviation	Name	Quantity
FWER	Family-wise error rate	$Pr(V \geq 1)$
k-FWER	Generalized family-wise error rate	$Pr(V \geq k)$
FDR	False discovery rate	$E[V/R]$
k-FDR	Generalized false discovery rate	$E[VI(V \geq k)/(MAX(R,1))]$
PCER	Per comparison error rate	$E[V]/M$
TPPFP	Tail probabilities for the proportion of false positives	$Pr(V/R) > q$

See similar tables in Nichols T, Hayasaka S. Controlling the familywise error rate in functional neuroimaging: a comparative review. *Stat Methods Med Res.* 2003;12(5):419-446. doi:10.1191/0962280203sm341ra and Table 15.1 in Gentleman R, Huber W, Carey VJ, Irizarry RA, Dudoit S. *Bioinformatics and Computational Biology Solutions Using R and Bioconductor.* Springer; 2005:473 p. 128 illus. (HB).

Note I( ) in the equation for k-FDR denotes the indicator function and max( ) denotes the maximum operator. q in TPPFP should be determined before testing. Pr( ) denotes probability, and E[ ] denotes expectation.

Table 12.1-2a. Table 12.1-2b lists some alternative approaches to controlling the type I error rate during the discovery phase of the experiment. Statistically significant or interesting markers are determined from hypothesis testing in light of controlling one of the type I error rates listed in **Table 12.1-2b**.

Confirmation and Verification

In order to have reasonable power in light of multiple testing, the type I errors in **Table 12.1-2a** tend to be more liberal (more likely to reject null hypotheses) than standard scientific significance testing procedures. Thus, any markers from the discovery phase should be confirmed or verified using other methods, such as immunohistochemical (IHC) assays or reverse transcription polymerase chain reaction (RT-PCR). These verification platforms could use either the same samples from the discovery phase or a new independent set of samples. The goal for this step is to confirm that the biomarker signal from the discovery platform is accurately measuring the expression of the desired gene, protein, or RNA.

Including a confirmation step ensures researchers that their discovery markers can be confirmed using other platforms. This provides some reassurance in the ability of the markers to be confirmed on independent samples from possibly different institutions with, possibly, differing methods of assessment. Methods that describe how to correlate RT-PCR and IHC signals with their microarray counterparts can be found in the study by Press et al (82), van den Broek and van de Vijver (83), McShane et al (84), and Esteban et al (85).

In certain IHC assays, the results should be performed by, at least, two different observers who are blinded to the clinical data. This may alleviate the subjectivity in these experiments because IHC assays require selection of best regions to score and subjective measurements of staining intensity and percentage of stained cells.

Validation Phase

Various statistical models can be fit using the data in the discovery phase. At the end of the discovery phase, there should be a complete specification of the marker assay method and model and thorough documentation of the (final) lockdown model. The fully specified precise lockdown model will be evaluated using a validation data set. Note, for example, that this must include specifying all coefficients in the classification model and any of the rules for deciding the level of a biomarker.

Validation in biomarker experiments should always involve an independent data set, that is, data from patients that were not included in any of the discovery dataset(s). Note that internal validation procedures such as cross-validation, boot strapping, or other data resampling methods are useful to give insights into issues such as bias and variance of regression parameter estimates and stability of the model derived. In these internal validation procedures, some portion of the data are held out (test set), whereas a model is built on the remaining portion (training set). A limitation of these internal procedures is that there may be biases that affect the training and test sets equally. For example, if the set of specimens for confirmation are collected in the same laboratory, processed by the same technician, and run on the same equipment, then peculiarities of the data (equipment, lab, and technician) will be shared between the samples used to develop the model and the samples used to evaluate the model.

Even with the requirement of an independent data set, there may still be levels of validation evidence. For example, a lower level of validation evidence may be independent sets of specimens and clinical data collected at a single institution using carefully controlled protocols, with samples from the same patient population. Meanwhile, a higher level of validation evidence would be independent sets of specimens and clinical data collected at multiple institutions.

In addition, it should be stressed that the independent validation data set must be relevant to the intended use of the candidate biomarker test. Patients in the independent data set should have the same type of disease, the same stage, and same clinical setting for which the candidate test is intended to be used in the future. Ideally, the specimens for independent confirmation will have been collected at a different point in time, at different institutions, from a different patient population, with samples processed in a different laboratory to demonstrate that the test has broad applicability and is not overfit to any particular situation.

Publicly Available Data

Publicly available data sets can help with the development process, and furthermore, they can fill in gaps in the knowledge of systems biology, for example, provide the proteomics story when an individual investigation only generates genomic data. They can be used in an integrative analysis and a meta-analysis. These meta-analyses can strengthen the conclusions drawn from an individual researcher's study. They may also offer insights from other study populations. As DNA microarray technology has been widely applied to detect gene activity changes in many areas of biomedical research, development and curation of online microarray data repositories are at the forefront of research endeavors to use and reuse this mounting deluge of data. Several representative repositories of microarray data sets are available (see **Table 12.1-3**). A somewhat recent comparison of the available microarray databases was provided in Gardiner-Garden and Littlejohn (86). Computer programs like Anduril (Ovaska et al (87)) provide procedures for organizing, storing, and analyzing massive genomic data. Statistical packages in R have also been created that allows users to easily import data from database like Array Express into Bioconductor package (88).

Concordant with the development of online data repositories, researchers have developed specific data standards required for

■ **TABLE 12.1-3. Repositories of Microarray Datasets**

ArrayExpress: http://www.ebi.ac.uk/arrayexpress/

Gene Expression Omnibus (GEO): Edgar et al (140); http://www.ncbi.nlm.nih.gov/geo/

Center for Information Biology Gene Expression Database (CIBEX): Ikeo et al (92); http://cibex.nig.ac.jp/data/index.html

The Cancer Genome Atlas (TCGA): http://tcga-data.nci.nih.gov/tcga/tcgaHome2.jsp or https://gdc-portal.nci.nih.gov/

microarray analysis. The data standard concept describes the minimum information about a microarray experiment (MIAME) that is needed to enable the interpretation of the results of the experiment and to potentially reproduce the experiment (89). MIAME compliance will ensure that biologic properties of the samples and the phenotypes that were assayed were correctly recorded, thus ensuring that the data can be quickly assessed for its suitability in studying new questions. The public repositories including ArrayExpress (90), GEO (91), and CIBEX (92) are all designed to hold MIAME compliant microarray data.

Especially exciting for oncologists, multiple platforms of microarray data from The Cancer Genome Atlas (TCGA) are now available. The TCGA project is further described in Stratton et al (93), but, in short, represents one of the first large-scale attempts to study the multiple types of genetic mutations involved in multiple cancer types from different cohorts of patients. Initially, the pilot projects studied glioblastoma multiforme (GBM) and ovarian serous cystadenocarcinoma but have now expanded to cover roughly 25 different cancer types. For each cancer type, the patient cohorts (collected from different sites) include several hundred individuals, and the platform techniques include gene expression profiling, copy number variation profiling, single-nucleotide polymorphism (SNP) genotyping, methylation profiling, and microRNA profiling. These data have been made publicly available, making the TCGA data set a great resource for research using meta-analysis and integrative analysis techniques that were not previously available.

DEVELOPING TRANSLATIONAL RESEARCH STUDIES AND REPORTING RESULTS

Guidelines have been developed to promote accurate and complete reporting of results from biomarker studies. Throughout this section, the importance of having well-defined questions for the proposed data is stressed. In other words, serious thought, planning, and discussions among a team of scientists are necessary to successfully perform biomarker analysis, including discovery, verification, and validation.

In the discovery phase, it is important that the proposed technology has been validated; see, for example, technical replication studies in Strand et al (94), Callesen et al (95), Leyland-Jones et al (96), De Cecco et al (97), Hicks et al (98), Benton et al (99), Freidin et al (100), and Lawrie et al (101). During the discovery phase, it is also important to consider differences in material preparation, for example, frozen tissue samples versus paraffin-embedded tissues as discussed in Nowak et al (102), and Mittempergher et al (103). During the verification phase, these issues also may play a role; however, other concerns may arise, such as the level of concordance in signal necessary between the discovery platform and the verification platform. Ultimately, after discovery and verification, a "lockdown model" is carried forth to validation. The lockdown model can be interpreted in a decision theoretic setting; each future sample must be classified, or the outcome predicted based only on the model and a given sample signal from the intended technology.

In the validation phase, it is important to note that there is a major difference between answering a priori defined hypotheses and providing conclusions from exploratory analyses. Conclusions drawn from exploratory data analysis are descriptive results and typically need to be confirmed in a validation data set, whereas a priori hypothesis leads to stronger conclusions and does not necessarily need an external validation. Care should be given in reporting unanticipated significant effects as these are most likely due to chance and thus unlikely to be validated in other studies. Most importantly, researchers should keep in mind that, in the long term, the success of biomarker studies should be measured by the clinical improvement in patient outcomes.

A prodigious number of biomarker studies have been reported in the literature; however, a surprising number of these results are irreproducible. The reasons for these discrepancies may lie in differences in methodological procedures, inadequate control of false-positive findings, improper validation procedures, variability in the patient sampling, or any number of other differences in study design, conduct, or analytical procedures. Many published studies lack adequate information that would allow an evaluation of quality or comparability. In order to promote clear and complete reporting of biomarker studies, the REMARK guidelines have been developed (104). These guidelines make specific recommendations for preparing TR presentations, reports, and publications with regard to describing patient and sample characteristics, assay methodology, study design, methods of data analysis, and results. Although these recommendations have been distilled into bullets in **Table 12.1-4**, useful additional information can be found in the REMARK document (104).

■ **TABLE 12.1-4. REporting recommendations for tumor MARKer (REMARK) Prognostic Studies**

Introduction
1. State the marker examined, the study objectives, and any prespecified hypotheses.

Materials and methods
Patients
2. Describe the characteristics (eg, disease stage or comorbidities) of the study patients, including their source and inclusion and exclusion criteria.
3. Describe treatments received and how chosen (eg, randomized or rule based).

Specimen Characteristics
4. Describe type of biologic material used (including control samples) and methods of preservation and storage.

Assay methods
5. Specify the assay method used and provide (or reference) a detailed protocol, including specific reagents or kits used, quality control procedures, reproducibility assessments, quantitation methods, and scoring and reporting protocols. Specify whether and how assays were performed blinded to the study end point.

Study design
6. State the method of case selection, including whether prospective or retrospective and whether stratification or matching (eg, by stage of disease or age) was used. Specify the time period from which cases were taken, the end of the follow-up period, and the median follow-up time.
7. Precisely define all clinical end points examined.
8. List all candidate variables initially examined.
9. Give rationale for sample size; if the study was designed to detect a specific effect size, give the target power and effect size.

Statistical analysis methods
10. Specify all statistical methods, including details of any variable selection procedures and other model-building issues, how model assumptions were verified, and how missing data were handled.
11. Clarify how marker values were handled in the analyses; if relevant, describe methods used for cut point determination.

(continued)

■ **TABLE 12.1-4. REporting recommendations for tumor MARKer (REMARK) Prognostic Studies** (*continued*)

Results

Data

12. Describe the flow of patients through the study, including the number of patients included in each stage of the analysis (a diagram may be helpful) and reasons for dropout. Specifically, both overall and for each subgroup extensively examined, report the number of patients and the number of events.

13. Report distribution of basic demographic characteristics (at least age and sex), standard (disease-specific) prognostic variables, and tumor marker, including numbers of missing values.

Analysis and presentation

14. Show the relation of the marker to standard prognostic variables.

15. Present univariate analyses showing the relation between the marker and outcome, with the estimated effect (eg, HR and survival probability). Preferably provide similar analyses for all other variables being analyzed. For the effect of a tumor marker on a time-to-event outcome, a Kaplan-Meier plot is recommended.

16. For key multivariate analyses, report estimated effects (eg, HR) with confidence intervals for the marker and, at least for the final model, all other variables in the model.

17. Among reported results, provide estimated effects with confidence intervals from an analysis in which the marker and standard prognostic variables are included, regardless of their statistical significance.

18. If done, report results of further investigations, such as checking assumptions, sensitivity analyses, and internal validation.

Discussion

19. Interpret the results in the context of the prespecified hypotheses and other relevant study, including a discussion of limitations of the study.

20. Discuss implications for future research and clinical value.

REMARK criteria: Reprinted from McShane LM, Altman DG, Sauerbrei W, et al. REporting recommendations for tumor MARKer prognostic studies (REMARK). *J Natl Cancer Inst*. 2005;97(16):1180-1184

CLINICAL TRIALS INVOLVING TARGETED THERAPIES

A clinically useful biomarker can identify patients with diseases that are either resistant or sensitive to a specific targeted therapy. As such, they can be used to improve the efficiency of a study and provide more precise treatment for specific subgroups of patients. This concept is illustrated in **Table 12.1-5**. Suppose the probability of response to standard treatment is 20% in the general patient population. Furthermore, suppose that 20% of the individuals in the general patient population are very responsive to a new targeted treatment, such that, when the targeted agent is added to the standard treatment, the probability of response is 60% among this

sensitive subgroup, but unchanged in the nonsensitive subgroup. If the new treatment is combined with standard treatment in the general population, regardless of their sensitivity status, then the expected probability of response would only be 28% (ie, 20% of population have 60% response rate, and 80% have 20% response rate = 0.20 × 0.60 + 0.80 × 0.20 = 0.28). If a randomized trial was now designed to compare standard treatment versus standard treatment with the new agent, then over 1,000 patients would need to be enrolled in order to reliably detect this size of a treatment effect (**Table 12.1-5**). On the other hand, if the study used a perfectly accurate biomarker (sensitivity = 100% and specificity = 100%) to restrict enrollment to treatment-sensitive patients, then only 60 patients would be needed for the study (**Table 12.1-5**) and the expected number of patients needed to be screened would be about 300. In the real world, biomarkers are seldom perfect. Still, a biomarker with 80% sensitivity and 80% specificity could still be used to increase the prevalence of treatment-sensitive patients, for example, (**Figure 12.1-4**). In this case, the probability of response to the standard regimen with the new targeted agent in the enriched study population would be 40% (0.50 × 0.60 + 0.50 × 0.20 = 0.40). The two-arm trial designed with this imperfect biomarker to select sensitive patients would require 220 enrolled patients to reliably detect the difference in response rates (**Table 12.1-5**) and the expected number of patients needed to be screened would be about 688.

In any study design where a biomarker is used to enrich the study sample with individuals considered most likely to respond, it may not be possible to differentiate between an ineffective treatment and a clinically invalid biomarker. Misspecification of the treatment target and misclassification of the tumor state are fundamental reasons for study failure. There can be a mismatch between the agent and the patient selection process in an enrichment design owing to inadequate understanding of a potentially complex biologic pathway or the true target of the agent understudy or use of an invalid surrogate end point biomarker (**Figure 12.1-5**). A successful study depends on the degree to which the biomarker accurately measures the true state of the treatment's target(s). Ideally, measuring the agent's effect through the biomarker should measure the agent's effect through the targeted pathway (highlighted in indigo in **Figure 12.1-5**). If the treatment can influence the disease through pathways that are not captured by the biomarker, then the activity of the agent will be underestimated and potentially missed. For example, in ovarian cancer, mutations in the *BRCA1* and *BRCA2* genes identify tumors that are likely to respond to a class of agents referred to as poly (ADP-ribose) polymerase inhibitors (PARPi). However, responses to PARPi have been observed among patients with no *BRCA* mutations (105). This suggests that markers of other biologic pathways will be needed to identify PARPi-sensitive tumors, such as markers for methylation of the *BRCA* genes or other types of dysfunction in the homologous recombination mechanism. Therefore, if the biomarkers that are used to define PARPi sensitivity included only BRCA mutation status, then sensitivity is sacrificed. On the other hand, if the markers for determining PARPi sensitivity include inconsequential mutations in the *BRCA* genes, then specificity is diminished. In enrichment studies, loss of sensitivity and specificity decreases the predictive value of the marker, which, in turn, decreases the chances that a

	Probability of Response				Assumptions	
Patient Population	Standard Therapy (P_0)	Standard + Targeted Therapy (P_1)	Sample Size	Screen Size	Sensitivity	Specificity
Ideal target population	.20	.60	60	300	100	100
General population	.20	.28	1,022	1,022	–	–
Enriched population	.20	.40	220	688	80	80

■ **TABLE 12.1-5. Required Sample Size for a Randomized Trials With a Target Prevalence of 20%**

Design parameters: H_0: $P_0 \geq P_1$, $\alpha = 0.05$, $\beta = 0.10$.

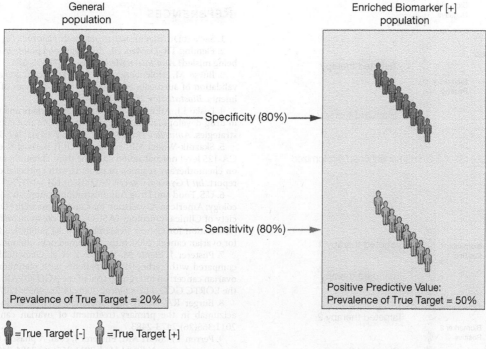

Figure 12.1-4. Hypothetical biomarker-based enrichment study.

study will identify active targeted agents (**Table 12.1-5 and Figure 12.1-4**). The schema for a biomarker-enriched randomized phase 2b or 3 trial is presented in **Figure 12.1-6**. The "umbrella design" generalizes this enrichment approach. In this case, multiple potentially predictive biomarkers are prioritized for study, and all of these biomarkers are assessed in each patient who is enrolled onto the study. If the patient's tumor expresses the biomarker with the highest priority, treatment is then randomly assigned to her as either an appropriate targeted therapy or standard therapy. If the patient's tumor does not express the biomarker with the highest priority, but does express the biomarker with the second highest priority, then treatment with another appropriate targeted therapy or standard treatment is randomly assigned to her. This process cascades sequentially through each of the biomarkers understudy in order of their priority. Individuals who do not express any of these biomarkers are either placed on a study involving a nontargeted therapy or considered off study. The schema for the umbrella design is depicted in **Figure 12.1-7**. It is important to recognize that these study designs cannot be used to demonstrate that the biomarker is, in fact, clinically predictive. For use in a phase 3 trial, this assumption of clinical predictiveness needs to be justified with data from external studies.

When it is necessary for a phase 3 study to demonstrate both that the biomarker is predictive and that the treatment is effective in the target population identified by the biomarker, there are several alternative designs (106). One approach randomizes treatment for all patients from the target population and prospectively stratifies the random treatment assignment based on discrete values of the biomarker value. This design assesses a treatment effect in each of the discrete biomarker levels. Other designs randomize between treatment strategies, such as assay-directed treatment versus standard therapy. These designs

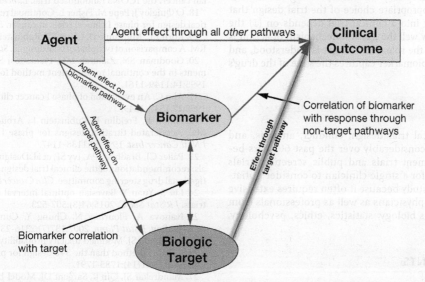

Figure 12.1-5. Schematic of the causal relationships and correlations between treatment, biomarker, biologic target, and clinical outcome.

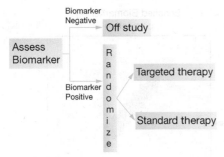

Figure 12.1-6. Phase 2b or 3 biomarker-enriched randomized treatment trial.

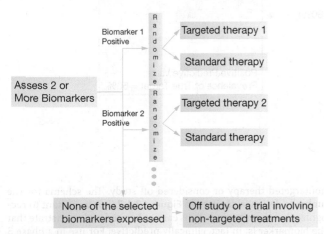

Figure 12.1-7. Phase 2b or 3 umbrella trial.

can be very inefficient and are generally not recommended (107). Study designs that adaptively modify the patient population when a planned interim analysis indicates that the biomarker identifies a subgroup of patients who are unlikely to respond or that utilize surrogate end points in a lead-in randomized phase 2 (seamless phase 2/3) study have also been proposed (108,109). Currently, adaptive designs for targeted therapies are an area of intense biostatistical research.

Careful planning is necessary for incorporating biomarkers into clinical trials. The appropriate choice of the trial design that incorporates a biomarker into a clinical trial depends on (1) the study's objectives, (2) how well the agent's mechanism of action is understood, (3) how well the role of the target is understood, and (4) how well the selected biomarker captures the state of the drug's true target(s).

CONCLUSION

The complexity of clinical trial design, conduct, analysis, and reporting has increased considerably over the past 60 years because randomized treatment trials and public screening trials first began. It is difficult for a single clinician to consider initiating a large-scale clinical study because it often requires extensive collaboration with other physicians as well as professionals from other disciplines, such as biology, statistics, ethics, psychology, and economics.

ACKNOWLEDGMENTS

Alan D. Hutson, PhD, Mark Brady, PhD, and Brian N. Bundy, PhD, contributed to prior editions of this chapter.

REFERENCES

1. Sackett DL. Bias in analytic research. *J Chronic Dis*. 1979;32(1-2):51-63.
2. Fleming TR, DeMets DL. Surrogate end points in clinical trials: are we being misled? *Ann Intern Med*. 1996;125(7):605-613.
3. Buyse M, Molenberghs G, Burzykowski T, Renard D, Geys H. The validation of surrogate endpoints in meta-analyses of randomized experiments. *Biostatistics*. 2000;1(1):49-67.
4. Lesko LJ, Atkinson AJ Jr. Use of biomarkers and surrogate endpoints in drug development and regulatory decision making: criteria, validation, strategies. *Annu Rev Pharmacol Toxicol*. 2001;41:347-366.
5. Skaznik-Wikiel ME, Sukumvanich P, Beriwal S, et al. Possible use of CA-125 level normalization after the third chemotherapy cycle in deciding on chemotherapy regimen in patients with epithelial ovarian cancer: brief report. *Int J Gynecol Cancer*. 2011;21(6):1013-1017.
6. U.S. Food and Drug Administration; American Society of Clinical Oncology; American Association for Cancer Research; FDA, the American Society of Clinical Oncology (ASCO), with co-sponsorship by the American Association for Cancer Research (AACR) public workshop on endpoints for ovarian cancer. 2006. https://pubmed.ncbi.nlm.nih.gov/17950384/
7. Pfisterer J, Plante M, Vergote I, et al. Gemcitabine plus carboplatin compared with carboplatin in patients with platinum-sensitive recurrent ovarian cancer: an intergroup trial of the AGO-OVAR, the NCIC CTG, and the EORTC GCG. *J Clin Oncol*. 2006;24(29):4699-4707.
8. Burger RA, Brady MF, Bookman MA, et al. Incorporation of bevacizumab in the primary treatment of ovarian cancer. *N Engl J Med*. 2011;365(26):2473-2483.
9. Perren TJ, Swart AM, Pfisterer J, et al. A phase 3 trial of bevacizumab in ovarian cancer. *N Engl J Med*. 2011;365(26):2484-2496.
10. Aghajanian C, Blank SV, Goff BA, et al. OCEANS: a randomized, double-blind, placebo-controlled phase III trial of chemotherapy with or without bevacizumab in patients with platinum-sensitive recurrent epithelial ovarian, primary peritoneal, or fallopian tube cancer. *J Clin Oncol*. 2012;30(17):2039-2045.
11. Royston P, Parmar MK, Qian W. Novel designs for multi-arm clinical trials with survival outcomes with an application in ovarian cancer. *Stat Med*. 2003;22(14):2239-2256.
12. Parmar MK, Barthel FM, Sydes M, et al. Speeding up the evaluation of new agents in cancer. *J Natl Cancer Inst*. 2008;100(17):1204-1214.
13. Oza AM, Castonguay V, Tsoref D, et al. Progression-free survival in advanced ovarian cancer: a Canadian review and expert panel perspective. *Curr Oncol*. 2011;18 Suppl 2:S20-S27.
14. Creasman WT. Second-look laparotomy in ovarian cancer. *Gynecol Oncol*. 1994;55(3 Pt 2):S122-S127.
15. George SL. Reducing patient eligibility criteria in cancer clinical trials. *J Clin Oncol*. 1996;14(4):1364-1370.
16. Begg CB, Engstrom PF. Eligibility and extrapolation in cancer clinical trials. *J Clin Oncol*. 1987;5(6):962-968.
17. International Collaborative Ovarian Neoplasm Group. Paclitaxel plus carboplatin versus standard chemotherapy with either single-agent carboplatin or cyclophosphamide, doxorubicin, and cisplatin in women with ovarian cancer: the ICON3 randomised trial. *Lancet*. 2002;360(9332):505-515.
18. O'Quigley J, Pepe M, Fisher L. Continual reassessment method: a practical design for phase I clinical trials in cancer. *Biometrics*. 1990;46:33-48.
19. Korn EL, Midthune D, Chen TT, Rubinstein LV, Christian MC, Simon RM. A comparison of two phase I trial designs. *Stat Med*. 1994;13:1799-1806.
20. Goodman SN, Zahurak ML, Piantadosi S. Some practical improvements in the continual reassessment method for phase I studies. *Stat Med*. 1995;14:1149-1161.
21. Ahn C. An evaluation of phase I cancer clinical trial designs. *Stat Med*. 1998;17:1537-1549.
22. Simon R, Freidlin B, Rubinstein L, Arbuck SG, Collins J, Christian MC. Accelerated titration designs for phase I clinical trials in oncology. *J Natl Cancer Inst*. 1997;89:1138-1147.
23. Paller CJ, Bradbury PA, Ivy SP, et al. Design of phase I combination trials: recommendations of the clinical trial design task force of the NCI investigational drug steering committee. *Clin Cancer Res*. 2014;20(16):4210-4217.
24. Liu S, Yuan Y. Bayesian optimal interval designs for phase I clinical trials. *J R Stat Soc C*. 2015;64(3):507-523.
25. Ivanova A, Flournoy N, Chung Y. Cumulative cohort design for dose-finding. *J Stat Plann*. 2007;137(7):2316-2327.
26. Ji Y, Wang SJ. Modified toxicity probability interval design: a safer and more reliable method than the 3+3 design for practical phase I trials. *J Clin Oncol*. 2013;31(14):1785-1791.
27. Mandrekar SJ, Qin R, Sargent DJ. Model-based phase I designs incorporating toxicity and efficacy for single and dual agent drug combinations: methods and challenges. *Stat Med*. 2010;29(10):1077-1083.

28. Mandrekar SJ, Sargent DJ. Randomized phase II trials: time for a new era in clinical trial design. *J Thorac Oncol.* 2010;5(7):932-934.

29. Simon R. Optimal two-stage designs for phase II clinical trials. *Control Clin Trials.* 1989;10:1-10.

30. Wieand S, Therneau T. A two-stage design for randomized trials with binary outcomes. *Control Clin Trials.* 1987;8:20-28.

31. Chen TT, Ng TH. Optimal flexible designs in phase II clinical trials. *Stat Med.* 1998;17:2301-2312.

32. Jennison C, Turnbull BW. Group sequential tests for bivariate response: Interim analyses of clinical trials with both efficacy and safety endpoints. *Biometrics.* 1993;49:741-752.

33. Bryant J, Day R. Incorporating toxicity considerations into the design of two-stage phase II clinical trials. *Biometrics.* 1995;51:1372-1383.

34. Conaway MR, Petroni GR. Designs for Phase II trials allowing for a trade-off between response and toxicity. *Biometrics.* 1996;52:1375-1386.

35. Thall P, Simon R, Estey E. New statistical strategy for monitoring safety and efficacy in single-arm clinical trials. *J Clin Oncol.* 1996;14(1):296-303.

36. Sill MW, Yothers G. A method for utilizing bivariate efficacy outcome measures to screen agents for activity in 2-stage phase II clinical trials. *Technical Report.* University of Buffalo; 2008:1-9.

37. Durrleman S, Simon R. Planning and monitoring of equivalence studies. *Biometrics.* 1990;46:329-336.

38. Senn S. Inherent difficulties with active control equivalence studies. *Stat Med.* 1993;12:2367-2375.

39. Wiens BL. Choosing an equivalence limit for noninferiority or equivalence studies. *Control Clin Trials.* 2002;23:2-14.

40. Rothmann M, Li N, Chen G, Chi GY, Temple R, Tsou HH. Design and analysis of non-inferiority mortality trials in oncology. *Stat Med.* 2003;22(2):239-264.

41. McGuire WP, Hoskins WJ, Brady MF, et al. A phase III trial comparing cisplatin/cytoxan and cisplatin/paclitaxel in advanced ovarian cancer. *Proc Am Soc Clin Oncol.* 1993;12:255.

42. Neijt JP, Engelholm SA, Tuxen MK, et al. Exploratory phase III study of paclitaxel and cisplatin versus paclitaxel and carboplatin in advanced ovarian cancer. *J Clin Oncol.* 2000;18(17):3084-3092.

43. du Bois A, Luck HJ, Meier W, et al. A randomized clinical trial of cisplatin/paclitaxel versus carboplatin/paclitaxel as first-line treatment of ovarian cancer. *J Natl Cancer Inst.* 2003;95(17):1320-1329.

44. Ozols RF, Bundy BN, Greer BE, et al. Phase III trial of carboplatin and paclitaxel compared with cisplatin and paclitaxel in patients with optimally resected stage III ovarian cancer: a Gynecologic Oncology Group study. *J Clin Oncol.* 2003;21(17):3194-3200.

45. Vasey PA. Role of docetaxel in the treatment of newly diagnosed advanced ovarian cancer. *J Clin Oncol.* 2003;21(10 suppl):136-144.

46. Sandercock J, Parmar MK, Torri V, Qian W. First-line treatment for advanced ovarian cancer: paclitaxel, platinum and the evidence. *Br J Cancer.* 2002;87(8):815-824.

47. Byar DP, Simon RM, Friedewald WT, et al. Randomized clinical trials. Perspectives on some recent ideas. *N Engl J Med.* 1976;295:74-80.

48. Kunz R, Oxman A. The unpredictability paradox: review of empirical comparisons of randomised and non-randomised clinical trials. *BMJ.* 1998;317:1185-1190.

49. Schulz KF, Chalmers I, Hayes RJ, Altman DG. Empirical evidence of bias. Dimensions of methodological quality associated with estimates of treatment effects in controlled trials. *JAMA.* 1995;273(5):408-412.

50. Schulz KF. Subverting randomization in controlled trials. *JAMA.* 1995;274(18):1456-1458.

51. Emanuel EJ, Patterson WB. Ethics of randomized clinical trials. *J Clin Oncol.* 1998;16(1):365-371.

52. Ellis PM, Coates AS. Ethics of randomized clinical trials. *J Clin Oncol.* 1998;16(7):2570.

53. Therneau TM. How many stratification factors are "too many" to use in a randomization plan? *Control Clin Trials.* 1993;14(2):98-108.

54. Pocock SJ, Simon R. Sequential treatment assignment with balancing for prognostic factors in the controlled clinical trial. *Biometrics.* 1975;31(1):103-115.

55. Schulz KF, Altman DG, Moher D. Allocation concealment in clinical trials. *JAMA.* 2002;288(19):2406-2407; author reply 2408-2409.

56. Schulz KF, Grimes DA, Altman DG, Hayes RJ. Blinding and exclusions after allocation in randomized controlled trials: survey of published parallel group trials in obstetrics and gynaecology. *BMJ.* 1996;312:742-744.

57. Rothman KJ, Michels KB. The continuing unethical use of placebo controls. *N Engl J Med.* 1994;331(6):394-398.

58. Green S, Liu PY, O'Sullivan J. Factorial design considerations. *J Clin Oncol.* 2002;20(16):3424-3430.

59. Last J, ed. *A Dictionary of Epidemiology.* Oxford University Press; 1995.

60. Goodman SN. p values, hypothesis tests, and likelihood: implications for epidemiology of a neglected historical debate. *Am J Epidemiol.* 1993;137(5):485-501.

61. Committee for Proprietary Medicinal Products. European agency for the evaluation of medicinal products points to consider on multiplicity issues in clinical trials. 2002. https://www.ema.europa.eu/en/documents/scientific-guideline/points-consider-multiplicity-issues-clinical-trials_en.pdf

62. U.S. Food and Drug Administration. Multiple endpoints in clinical trials guidance for industry. Center for Biologics Evaluation and Research. 2017. https://www.fda.gov/media/162416/download

63. Dmitrienko A, Tamhane AC, Bretz F, eds. Preface. In: *Multiple Testing Problems in Pharmaceutical Statistics.* CRC Press; 2010:Xi.

64. Alosh M, Bretz F, Huque M. Advanced multiplicity adjustment methods in clinical trials. *Stat Med.* 2014;33(4):693-713.

65. Li G, Taljaard M, Van den Heuvel ER, et al. An introduction to multiplicity issues in clinical trials: the what, why, when and how. *Int J Epidemiol.* 2017;46(2):746-755.

66. Hochberg Y. A sharper Bonferroni procedure for multiple tests of significance. *Biometrika.* 1988;75(4):800-802.

67. Holm, S. A simple sequentially rejective multiple test procedure. *Scand J Stat.* 1979;6(2):65-70.

68. Neuhauser M. How to deal with multiple endpoints in clinical trials. *Fundam Clin Pharmacol.* 2006;20(6):515-523.

69. Dmitrienko A, D'Agostino R. Traditional multiplicity adjustment methods in clinical trials. *Stat Med.* 2013;32(29):5172-5218.

70. Tamhane AC, Gou J. Advances in p-Value based multiple test procedures. *J Biopharm Stat.* 2018;28(1):10-27.

71. Wiens BL. A fixed sequence Bonferroni procedure for testing multiple endpoints. *Pharm Stat.* 2003;2(3):211-215.

72. Bretz F, Maurer W, Brannath W, Posch M. A graphical approach to sequentially rejective multiple test procedures. *Stat Med.* 2009;28(4):586-604.

73. Maurer W, Bretz F. A note on testing families of hypotheses using graphical procedures. *Stat Med.* 2014;33(30):5340-5346.

74. O'Neill RT. Secondary endpoints cannot be validly analyzed if the primary endpoint does not demonstrate clear statistical significance. *Control Clin Trials.* 1997;18(6):550-567.

75. Dmitrienko A, Offen WW, Westfall PH. Gatekeeping strategies for clinical trials that do not require all primary effects to be significant. *Stat Med.* 2003;22(15):2387-2400.

76. Ransohoff DF. Lessons from controversy: ovarian cancer screening and serum proteomics. *J Natl Cancer Inst.* 2005;97(4):315-319.

77. Institute of Medicine. *Evaluation of Biomarkers and Surrogate Endpoints in Chronic Disease.* National Academies Press; 2010. https://www.ncbi.nlm.nih.gov/books/NBK220297/

78. Goozner M. Duke scandal highlights need for genomics research criteria. *J Natl Cancer Inst.* 2011;103(12):916-917.

79. Biomarkers Definitions Working Group. Biomarkers and surrogate endpoints: preferred definitions and conceptual framework. *Clin Pharmacol Ther.* 2001;69(3):89-95.

80. Rajan S, Djambazian H, Dang HC, Sladek R, Hudson TJ. The living microarray: a high-throughput platform for measuring transcription dynamics in single cells. *BMC Genomics.* 2011;12:115.

81. Miecznikowski JC, Gaile DP, Liu S, Shepherd L, Nowak N. A new normalizing algorithm for BAC CGH arrays with quality control metrics. *J Biomed Biotechnol.* 2011;2011:860732.

82. Press MF, Hung G, Godolphin W, Slamon DJ. Sensitivity of HER-2/neu antibodies in archival tissue samples: potential source of error in immunohistochemical studies of oncogene expression. *Cancer Res.* 1994;54(10):2771-2777.

83. van den Broek LJ, van de Vijver MJ. Assessment of problems in diagnostic and research immunohistochemistry associated with epitope instability in stored paraffin sections. *Appl Immunohistochem Mol Morphol.* 2000;8(4):316-321.

84. McShane LM, Aamodt R, Cordon-Cardo C, et al. Reproducibility of p53 immunohistochemistry in bladder tumors. National Cancer Institute, Bladder Tumor Marker Network. *Clin Cancer Res.* 2000;6(5):1854-1864.

85. Esteban J, Baker J, Cronin M, et al. Tumor gene expression and prognosis in breast cancer: multi-gene RT-PCR assay of paraffin-embedded tissue. *Proc Am Soc Clin Oncol.* 2003;22:350.

86. Gardiner-Garden M, Littlejohn TG. A comparison of microarray databases. *Brief Bioinform.* 2001;2(2):143-158.

87. Ovaska K, Laakso M, Haapa-Paananen S, et al. Large-scale data integration framework provides a comprehensive view on glioblastoma multiforme. *Genome Med.* 2010;2(9):65.

88. Huber W, Carey VJ, Gentleman R, et al. Orchestrating high-throughput genomic analysis with bioconductor. *Nat Methods*. 2015;12(2):115-121.

89. Brazma A, Hingamp P, Quackenbush J, et al. Minimum information about a microarray experiment (MIAME)-toward standards for microarray data. *Nat Genet*. 2001;29(4):365-371.

90. European Bioinformatics Institute. ArrayExpress. 2012. http://www.ebi.ac.uk/arrayexpress/

91. National Center for Biotechnology Information. GEO: Gene Expression Omnibus. 2012. http://www.ncbi.nlm.nih.gov/geo/

92. Ikeo K, Ishi-I J, Tamura T, Gojobori T, Tateno Y. CIBEX: center for information biology gene expression database. *C R Biol*. 2003;326(10-11):1079-1082.

93. Stratton MR, Campbell PJ, Futreal PA. The cancer genome. *Nature*. 2009;458(7239):719-724.

94. Strand C, Enell J, Hedenfalk I, Ferno M. RNA quality in frozen breast cancer samples and the influence on gene expression analysis—a comparison of three evaluation methods using microcapillary electrophoresis traces. *BMC Mol Biol*. 2007;8:38.

95. Callesen AK, Vach W, Jorgensen PE, et al. Reproducibility of mass spectrometry based protein profiles for diagnosis of breast cancer across clinical studies: a systematic review. *J Proteome Res*. 2008;7(4):1395-1402.

96. Leyland-Jones BR, Ambrosone CB, Bartlett J, et al. Recommendations for collection and handling of specimens from group breast cancer clinical trials. *J Clin Oncol*. 2008;26(34):5638-5644.

97. De Cecco L, Musella V, Veneroni S, et al. Impact of biospecimens handling on biomarker research in breast cancer. *BMC Cancer*. 2009;9:409.

98. Hicks DG, Kushner L, McCarthy K. Breast cancer predictive factor testing: the challenges and importance of standardizing tissue handling. *J Natl Cancer Inst Monogr*. 2011;2011(42):43-45.

99. Benton P, Want E, Clayton T, et al. Intra-and inter-laboratory reproducibility of UPLC-TOF-MS for urinary metabolic profiling. *Anal Chem*. 2012;29(4):2424-2432.

100. Freidin MB, Bhudia N, Lim E, Nicholson AG, Cookson WO, Moffatt MF. Impact of collection and storage of lung tumor tissue on whole genome expression profiling. *J Mol Diagn*. 2012;14(2):140-148.

101. Lawrie CH, Ballabio E, Soilleux E, et al. Inter- and intra-observational variability in immunohistochemistry: a multicentre analysis of diffuse large B-cell lymphoma staining. *Histopathology*. 2012;61:18-25.

102. Nowak NJ, Miecznikowski J, Moore SR, et al. Challenges in array comparative genomic hybridization for the analysis of cancer samples. *Genet Med*. 2007;9(9):585-595.

103. Mittempergher L, de Ronde JJ, Nieuwland M, et al. Gene expression profiles from formalin fixed paraffin embedded breast cancer tissue are largely comparable to fresh frozen matched tissue. *PLoS One*. 2011;6(2):e17163.

104. McShane LM, Altman DG, Sauerbrei W, et al. REporting recommendations for tumor MARKer prognostic studies (REMARK). *Nat Clin Pract Oncol*. 2005;2(8):416-422.

105. Sessa C. Update on PARP1 inhibitors in ovarian cancer. *Ann Oncol*. 2011;22(suppl 8):viii72-viii76.

106. Simon R. Clinical trial designs for evaluating the medical utility of prognostic and predictive biomarkers in oncology. *Per Med*. 2010;7(1):33-47.

107. Freidlin B, McShane LM, Korn EL. Randomized clinical trials with biomarkers: design issues. *J Natl Cancer Inst*. 2010;102(3):152-160.

108. Wang SJ, O'Neill RT, Hung HM. Approaches to evaluation of treatment effect in randomized clinical trials with genomic subset. *Pharm Stat*. 2007;6(3):227-244.

109. Jenkins M, Stone A, Jennison C. An adaptive seamless phase II/III design for oncology trials with subpopulation selection using correlated survival endpoints. *Pharm Stat*. 2011;10:347-356.

110. Albertson DG, Ylstra B, Segraves R, et al. Quantitative mapping of amplicon structure by array CGH identifies CYP24 as a candidate oncogene. *Nat Genet*. 2000;25(2):144-146.

111. Hodgson G, Hager JH, Volik S, et al. Genome scanning with array CGH delineates regional alterations in mouse islet carcinomas. *Nat Genet*. 2001;29(4):459-464.

112. Pollack JR, Sorlie T, Perou CM, et al. Microarray analysis reveals a major direct role of DNA copy number alteration in the transcriptional program of human breast tumors. *Proc Natl Acad Sci U S A*. 2002;99(20):12963-12968.

113. Albertson DG. Profiling breast cancer by array CGH. *Breast Cancer Res Treat*. 2003;78(3):289-298.

114. Albertson DG, Collins C, McCormick F, Gray JW. Chromosome aberrations in solid tumors. *Nat Genet*. 2003;34(4):369-376.

115. Hackett CS, Hodgson JG, Law ME, et al. Genome-wide array CGH analysis of murine neuroblastoma reveals distinct genomic aberrations which parallel those in human tumors. *Cancer Res*. 2003;63(17):5266-5273.

116. Garnis C, Coe BP, Zhang L, Rosin MP, Lam WL. Overexpression of LRP12, a gene contained within an 8q22 amplicon identified by high-resolution array CGH analysis of oral squamous cell carcinomas. *Oncogene*. 2004;23(14):2582-2586.

117. Veltman JA, Fridlyand J, Pejavar S, et al. Array-based comparative genomic hybridization for genome-wide screening of DNA copy number in bladder tumors. *Cancer Res*. 2003;63(11):2872-2880.

118. Pinkel D, Albertson DG. Array comparative genomic hybridization and its applications in cancer. *Nat Genet*. 2005;37 Suppl:S11-S17.

119. Rossi MR, Conroy J, McQuaid D, Nowak NJ, Rutka JT, Cowell JK. Array CGH analysis of pediatric medulloblastomas. *Genes Chromosomes Cancer*. 2006;45(3):290-303.

120. Idbaih A, Marie Y, Lucchesi C, et al. BAC array CGH distinguishes mutually exclusive alterations that define clinicogenetic subtypes of gliomas. *Int J Cancer*. 2008;122(8):1778-1786.

121. Ramaswamy S, Tamayo P, Rifkin R, et al. Multiclass cancer diagnosis using tumor gene expression signatures. *Proc Natl Acad Sci U S A*. 2001;98(26):15149-15154.

122. Gordon GJ, Jensen RV, Hsiao LL, et al. Translation of microarray data into clinically relevant cancer diagnostic tests using gene expression ratios in lung cancer and mesothelioma. *Cancer Res*. 2002;62(17):4963-4967.

123. Tibshirani R, Hastie T, Narasimhan B, Chu G. Diagnosis of multiple cancer types by shrunken centroids of gene expression. *Proc Natl Acad Sci U S A*. 2002;99(10):6567-6572.

124. Statnikov A, Aliferis CF, Tsamardinos I, Hardin D, Levy S. A comprehensive evaluation of multicategory classification methods for microarray gene expression cancer diagnosis. *Bioinformatics*. 2005;21(5):631-643.

125. Glas AM, Floore A, Delahaye LJ, et al. Converting a breast cancer microarray signature into a high-throughput diagnostic test. *BMC Genomics*. 2006;7:278.

126. van 't Veer LJ, Dai H, van de Vijver MJ, et al. Gene expression profiling predicts clinical outcome of breast cancer. *Nature*. 2002;415(6871):530-536.

127. Sotiriou C, Neo SY, McShane LM, et al. Breast cancer classification and prognosis based on gene expression profiles from a population-based study. *Proc Natl Acad Sci U S A*. 2003;100(18):10393-10398.

128. Michiels S, Koscielny S, Hill C. Prediction of cancer outcome with microarrays: a multiple random validation strategy. *Lancet*. 2005;365(9458):488-492.

129. Barrier A, Boelle PY, Roser F, et al. Stage II colon cancer prognosis prediction by tumor gene expression profiling. *J Clin Oncol*. 2006;24(29):4685-4691.

130. Miecznikowski JC, Wang D, Liu S, Sucheston L, Gold D. Comparative survival analysis of breast cancer microarray studies identifies important prognostic genetic pathways. *BMC Cancer*. 2010;10:573.

131. Levin JZ, Berger MF, Adiconis X, et al. Targeted next-generation sequencing of a cancer transcriptome enhances detection of sequence variants and novel fusion transcripts. *Genome Biol*. 2009;10(10):R115.

132. Pflueger D, Rickman DS, Sboner A, et al. N-myc downstream regulated gene 1 (NDRG1) is fused to ERG in prostate cancer. *Neoplasia*. 2009;11(8):804-811.

133. Portela A, Esteller M. Epigenetic modifications and human disease. *Nat Biotechnol*. 2010;28(10):1057-1068.

134. Paweletz CP, Trock B, Pennanen M, et al. Proteomic patterns of nipple aspirate fluids obtained by SELDI-TOF: potential for new biomarkers to aid in the diagnosis of breast cancer. *Dis Markers*. 2001;17(4):301-307.

135. Koopmann J, Zhang Z, White N, et al. Serum diagnosis of pancreatic adenocarcinoma using surface-enhanced laser desorption and ionization mass spectrometry. *Clin Cancer Res*. 2004;10(3):860-868.

136. Kolch W, Neususs C, Pelzing M, Mischak H. Capillary electrophoresis-mass spectrometry as a powerful tool in clinical diagnosis and biomarker discovery. *Mass Spectrom Rev*. 2005;24(6):959-977.

137. Diamandis EP. Analysis of serum proteomic patterns for early cancer diagnosis: drawing attention to potential problems. *J Natl Cancer Inst*. 2004;96(5):353-356.

138. Diamandis EP. Mass spectrometry as a diagnostic and a cancer biomarker discovery tool: opportunities and potential limitations. *Mol Cell Proteomics*. 2004;3(4):367-378.

139. Lan KK, Rosenberger WF, Lachin JM. Sequential monitoring of survival data with the Wilcoxon statistic. *Biometrics*. 1995;51(3):1175-1183.

140. Edgar R, Domrachev M, Lash AE. Gene expression omnibus: NCBI gene expression and hybridization array data repository. *Nucleic Acids Res*. 2002;30(1):207-210.

CHAPTER **12.2**

Cost-Effective and Value-Based Gynecologic Cancer Care

Laura J. Havrilesky, Margaret I. Liang, Emeline M. Aviki, Shalini L. Kulasingam, Elizabeth L. Jewell, and David E. Cohn

OVERVIEW OF COST, QUALITY, AND VALUE IN HEALTH CARE

The cost of health care in the United States continues to rise; in 2020, health care spending encompassed 18% of the gross domestic product (GDP) (https://www.cms.gov/Research-Statistics-Data-and-Systems/Statistics-Trends-and-Reports/NationalHealth ExpendData/NHE-Fact-Sheet). Despite rising costs, there has not been a commensurate increase in the quality of care delivered in the United States. For this reason, there has been increasing pressure on health systems and providers to demonstrate "value," which is defined by high-quality and cost-effective care. In this chapter, we review the historical backdrop that has led to the current level of scrutiny being applied to health care providers to deliver value-based (high-quality and cost-conscious) care. We define value in health care and describe current and proposed methods to measure value. We present the concept of "financial toxicity," which measures the impact of the financial burden of cancer care at the patient rather than health system or societal level. Finally, we review the methodology of cost-effectiveness analyses (CEAs) and the current evidence regarding the cost-effectiveness of specific interventions in gynecologic cancers.

Cost and Comparative Effectiveness

Given that the ideal infrastructure for measuring value does not yet exist, how can we conduct outcomes-based research with the goal of improving health care quality? *Comparative effectiveness research* (CER) is defined by the National Academy of Medicine (NAM), previously named the Institute of Medicine (IOM), as "the generation and synthesis of evidence that compares the benefits and harms of alternative methods to prevent, diagnose, treat and monitor a clinical condition, or to improve the delivery of care."

As the field of CER has become integrated into health care policy and coverage decisions, there has concurrently been increasing concern that CER will lead to denial of certain health care interventions. As a result of concerns raised about resource rationing and the devaluation of life in health states with a high burden of disability, the Patient Protection and Affordable Care Act (ACA) of 2010 stated that "the Patient-Centered Outcomes Research Institute (PCORI)...shall not develop or employ a dollars-per-quality-adjusted life year (QALY) (or similar measure that discounts the value of a life because of an individual's disability) as a threshold to establish what type of health care is cost-effective or recommended" (1). This meant that PCORI, the institute that was created in response to concerns about the high cost of health care in the United States, was prohibited from sponsoring studies that included considerations of cost-effectiveness. Despite this, experts have argued that the funding of CER still provides quality evidence for employment in standard CEAs and will, therefore, ultimately inform the question of value in health care (2). In 2019, reauthorization legislation for PCORI clarified that in addition to relevant clinical outcomes, the economic burdens of the utilization of medical treatments, items, and services could be included as relevant patient-centered outcomes in funded research studies; formal CEA remains outside the scope of PCORI.

Summary

With increasing pressure to control the costs and improve the quality of health care, measurement of value will be an important means by which different treatments can be critically evaluated.

DEFINING AND MEASURING VALUE IN ONCOLOGY

Value can be defined broadly as the desirable health outcomes achieved per monetary unit spent (3). The United States is currently transitioning to a value-based reimbursement system. In March 2013, the National Commission on Physician Payment Reform published recommendations to transition to a blended payment system (4). These recommendations include elimination of stand-alone fee-for-service payment to medical practices and a transition to a payment model based on quality and value. These evolving changes in the reimbursement of medical care make it imperative that physicians understand the principles of defining quality and value in health care.

Status Quo Measurement of Value in Health Care

Health care quality measures have come into the spotlight on a national level as directed by the ACA, with the goal of understanding and optimizing the correlation between health care spending and quality care. To this end, mandatory reporting of quality measures was included in section 2701 of the ACA (1). However, the implementation of an effective and clinically relevant reporting system is limited by the complex process by which these quality measures are identified, vetted, and applied.

On April 16, 2015, the U.S. Senate passed legislation to repeal the sustainable growth rate (SGR) formula, which governed provider payment under Medicare's Physician Fee Schedule (5). In its place, the enactment of the Medicare Access and Children's Health Insurance Program Reauthorization Act (MACRA) of 2015 accelerated the movement toward value-based rather than volume-based payments. Starting in 2017, the Quality Payment Program created two pathways to link quality to payments: the Merit-Based Incentive Payment System (MIPS) and Advanced Alternative Payment Models (APMs). Under MIPS, four weighted categories (quality, resource use, clinical practice improvement activities, and meaningful use of electronic health record technology) are used to calculate an overall MIPS score, which is linked to provider payment adjustment based on performance. Providers can also opt out of MIPS by choosing to participate in an APM, which utilizes bundled payment arrangements for episodes of care and accountable care organizations to financially incentivize controlling cost growth while maintaining quality care over time.

In this context, the development of disease-specific APMs has necessarily gained traction. One example is the Centers for Medicare and Medicaid Services (CMS) Oncology Care Model (OCM), which is a demonstration project that launched in 2016 and invited oncology practices across the United States to voluntarily participate in an APM based on 6-month episodes of cancer care (6). The OCM utilizes two financial incentive strategies. First, in addition to traditional fee-for-service payments, OCM practices receive a $160 Monthly Enhanced Oncology Service (MEOS) fee from Medicare to support practice transformations focused on increasing 24/7 patient access, patient navigation, care plan documentation, and guideline-concordant care. Second, OCM practices have the opportunity to earn retrospective Performance-Based Payments (PBP) if they meet goals for Medicare spending as well as claims-based and patient-reported quality metrics. After five performance periods (July 2016 to January 2019), the OCM program resulted in a small reduction (1%) in total expenditures but ultimately a net loss to Medicare due to the two financial incentives (MEOS and PBP) (7). There was little evidence of value-oriented changes in chemotherapy drug regimens or radiation therapy, although some evidence of more cost-conscious use of costly supportive therapies (ie, white blood cell growth factors). In addition, there was no meaningful impact on emergency department (ED) visits, preventable hospitalizations, or hospice use at the end of life. With the OCM ending in 2022, forthcoming efforts from CMS that will affect gynecologic oncology care include the mandatory Radiation Oncology APM, a proposed successor to OCM called Oncology Care First, and the Acute Hospital at Home program (8).

In 2015, the Society of Gynecologic Oncology (SGO) began development of an Endometrial Cancer Alternative Payment (ECAP) model centered on the surgical management of endometrial cancer, which proposed management fees for four phases of endometrial cancer surgical care: (1) preoperative care, (2) surgery, (3) postoperative care weeks 0 to 2, and (4) postoperative care weeks 2 to 8 (9). Subsequent database modeling suggested that increasing the rate of minimally invasive surgery, reducing length of stay, and reducing readmissions and ED visits could result in savings through the proposed ECAP, while improving the quality of care (10). However, this exercise also demonstrated the complexities of fair attribution (establishing accountability for patient care and subsequent outcomes), risk adjustment (accounting for patient mix based on comorbidities or complexity of care delivered), and quality outcome measurement (gathering relevant data that are readily available and have enough granularity) (11). In addition, institutions and private payors have been engaged in various pilot testing of APMs centered around surgical care episodes.

Other potential opportunities to achieve value in health care may be related to the elimination of the use of therapies that are not cost-effective (eg, those that are more expensive, less effective, or both, than alternative treatments). Although there is no established agency in the United States that evaluates the cost-effectiveness of health care interventions, such models do exist in the United Kingdom, Canada, Australia, France and Germany through "value determination" reviews (12). An additional focus on value through the reduction in readmission rates has gained increasing attention; readmissions are a major contributor to health care costs and are estimated to account for approximately $17 billion annually (13); it is estimated that up to 75% of all readmissions are preventable (14). As such, the U.S. government has made reducing readmissions a priority to improve patient care and reduce health care spending, thereby increasing value. To address this goal, the Hospital Readmissions Reduction Program was established to limit reimbursements to hospitals with excess readmission ratios in six predefined conditions or procedures. In addition, the Bundled Payments for Care Improvement initiative was established to determine payments based upon episodes of care rather than for individual services using 48 predefined clinical diagnoses when patients are readmitted within 30 days of their index hospitalization (15-18).

Proposed Methods of Value Measurement in Oncology Care

In this section, we describe two innovative methods that have been proposed to assess value in oncology health care.

Value frameworks—tools to assess value in cancer care A high proportion of all health care spending occurs in oncology. Evidence indicates that patients with cancer want information about the comparative effectiveness of available treatments as well as information on their relative costs. The American Society of Clinical Oncology's (ASCO) Value in Cancer Care task force, first convened in 2007, has identified lists of common practices in oncology that were considered "low value" because of their expense and a lack of high-level evidence supporting their use (19,20). These lists, developed as part of the American Board of Internal Medicine Foundation's (ABIM) "Choosing Wisely" campaign, included avoidance of unnecessary imaging following an early-stage cancer diagnosis, avoidance of the provision of prophylactic antiemetic and bone marrow support regimens in low-risk settings, and avoidance of routine screening studies in patients with a low life expectancy. Of note, in 2013, the SGO published its own "top five" list of low-value interventions to avoid (1) the screening of asymptomatic, low-risk women for ovarian cancer; (2) the use of Pap smear as a surveillance strategy for endometrial cancer; (3) the performance of colposcopy for low-grade squamous intraepithelial lesion (LSIL) Pap smear results in patients with a history of cervical cancer; (4) the use of routine surveillance imaging in patients with a history of gynecologic cancer; and (5) the delay of palliative care for women with advanced or relapsed cancer (21).

ASCO Value Framework In 2015, the ASCO task force presented a Value Framework (version 1) for comparing the relative clinical benefit, toxicity, and cost of novel treatments in the medical oncology setting (21). An updated version (version 2) was published in 2016 based on comments received (22). The purpose of the framework is "to provide a standardized approach to assist physicians and patients in assessing the value of a new drug treatment for cancer as compared with one or several prevailing standards of care" and to provide oncologists with "information and physician-guided tools necessary to assess the relative value of cancer therapies as an element of shared decision making with their patients." The ASCO Value Framework was designed to define the value of medical interventions for the treatment of malignancy for which there exist phase III RCT data to inform outcomes. The framework provides the tools to calculate the net health benefit (NHB) score of a novel therapy compared with standard-of-care therapy for advanced or metastatic cancer using two criteria: (1) clinical benefit based on improvement in OS, PFS, or response rate and (2) toxicity differences. Bonus points are awarded for "tail" of the survival curve, palliation of symptoms, improvements in HRQoL, and treatment-free interval. The revised version favors the use of HRs over median OS or PFS, when available. Value snapshots are calculated differently for treatments with curative intent (maximum possible NHB score 100 points) as compared to those for metastatic disease (maximum possible NHB score 130 points). NHBs are intended to be presented alongside the drug-acquisition cost (DAC) and, if available, the patient's out-of-pocket cost for each therapy. **Figure 12.2-1** depicts an example of a value snapshot constructed using the ASCO format for the comparison of standard chemotherapy to chemotherapy plus bevacizumab for recurrent, platinum-resistant ovarian cancer, using the AURELIA clinical trial results (23,24).

Other efforts to develop tools to assess the value of cancer treatments include the European Society of Medical Oncology (ESMO) Magnitude of Clinical Benefit Scale (MCBS) (25), which has a broader purpose than the ASCO Value Framework not only to guide clinical decision-making but also to influence health policy and health technology assessment more broadly.

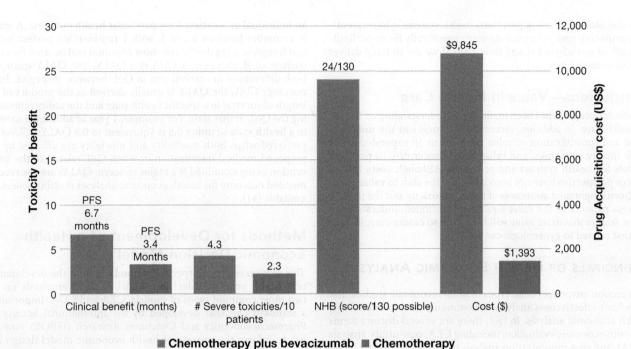

Figure 12.2-1. Value snapshot representing the benefits and costs of standard chemotherapy using weekly paclitaxel compared to standard chemotherapy plus bevacizumab for the treatment of platinum-resistant recurrent ovarian cancer. NHB, net health benefit.

The ESMO-MCBS assigns categorical benefit scores only to positive superiority or noninferiority RCTs. A recent collaboration between ASCO and ESMO found moderate concordance when comparing scores for 102 RCTs in the noncurative setting, with discordance mostly due to different approaches to scoring the relative and absolute gain of OS or PFS, tail of the curve, and including only high-grade versus all toxicities (26). These two value frameworks were utilized to evaluate FDA-approved treatments for platinum-sensitive recurrent ovarian cancer, including maintenance therapy with bevacizumab or PARPi and produced fairly concordant results (27).

The Porter value framework Harvard Business School economist Michael E. Porter argues that the definition and demonstration of value are integral to reining in costs and to overall health care reform. He states that "the absence of comprehensive and rigorous outcome and cost measurement is arguably the biggest weakness standing in the way of health care improvement" (3). He argues that surrogate measures of quality, such as the measurement of compliance to guidelines or even of patient satisfaction, do not necessarily indicate quality of care. To truly assess quality, the outcomes important to each disease must be defined and measured.

In an effort to begin defining high-quality outcomes, Porter has developed an idealized outcomes measures hierarchy, in which specific health outcomes are multitiered and defined for each disease. In oncology, the highest priority is assigned to survival, followed by functional status achieved, recovery times following treatment, effects of the treatment process on function and QoL, and sustainability of the cancer-free state. In the Porter value framework, costs are defined as they apply to a full optimal "cycle of care" for a given medical condition, usually representing periods of a year or more. Responsibility for outcomes and reimbursements are shared by all participating providers for a given heath condition.

Ultimately, Porter argues that "improving value requires either improving one or more outcomes without raising costs or lowering costs without compromising outcomes, or both" (28). Porter's strategic agenda for a high-value health care delivery system includes

six components: (1) organization of care into disease-related integrated practice units; (2) measurement of outcomes and costs for every patient; (3) bundled payments for care cycles; (4) integration of care delivery across facilities; (5) expansion of services across geography; and (6) building an enabling information technology platform.

Financial Toxicity—Costs From the Patient Perspective

The existing transformation to value-based care has unfortunately not led to a decrease in treatment costs for patients. While in the past, patients with insurance may have been shielded from the rising costs of cancer treatments, changes in insurance policy design have led to increased patient cost sharing. Estimates of the annualized net out-of-pocket costs among patients aged 65 years or above in the United States were recently reported for the various phases of cancer for medical services and prescription drugs: initial phase ($2,200 and $243), continuing phase ($466 and $127), and end-of-life phase ($3,823 and $448) (29). This review also provides estimates of patient time costs, which can include travel to care, waiting for care, and receiving care. Recently, there has been recognition that the financial burden of cancer care is another potential side effect of treatment, now coined "financial toxicity" (30). In an analysis of 4,655 patients with gynecologic cancer, 25% experienced payment issues as a result of cancer-related treatment costs (31). Importantly, in this patient sample, commercial insurance status was an independent risk factor for payment issues and higher financial distress. In gynecologic oncology, it is estimated that up to 50% of patients experience financial distress based on the Comprehensive Score for Financial Toxicity (COST) instrument, with more severe financial distress associated with increased use of cost-coping strategies and worse QoL (32-35). Financial hardship can be described in three domains: psychological response (ie, distress about the costs of care), material conditions (ie, out-of-pocket expenses, reduced income, medical debt), and coping behaviors (ie, skipping medication or delaying care owing to costs) (36). Therefore, in addition to controlling overall health care costs, all stakeholders including providers, health systems, pharmaceutical companies, and policymakers must specifically focus on limiting patient out-of-pocket and time costs if we are to truly deliver patient-centered care.

Conclusions—Value in Health Care

Significant progress has been made in the understanding of "value" in health care. In addition, recent developments in the measurement and quantification of value have led to an expanded effort to tie quality, outcomes, and value-based cancer care to payment models for health systems and providers. Although costs from a patient perspective have not been a focus of the shift to value, there has been heightened awareness of financial toxicity and the need to address patients in the value equation. Continued understanding of the factors that drive value will be critical to cancer care, including that related to gynecologic cancers.

PRINCIPALS OF HEALTH ECONOMIC ANALYSES

This section introduces basic types of health economic studies. The term "cost-effectiveness analysis" is commonly used to refer to any health economic analysis. In fact, there are several distinct forms of health economic evaluation, including CEA, cost-utility analysis (CUA), and cost-minimization analysis (CMA). CEA and CUA are the most frequently used health economic analyses. CEAs compare alternative interventions using a cost per unit of effectiveness such as a year of life gained (37). CUAs examine cost, effectiveness, and preferences for health outcomes. CMAs compare only cost (37).

Cost-effectiveness Analyses

Cost-effectiveness analysis (CEA) is defined by the United Kingdom's National Institute for Health and Clinical Excellence (NICE) as an economic study design in which the consequences of different interventions are measured using a single outcome (eg, years of life gained, deaths avoided) (38). A CEA is used to help prioritize the allocation of resources and to decide between two or more treatments or interventions. It compares a standard-of-care strategy to its more costly alternatives in terms of the additional cost per unit of effectiveness. Units of effectiveness in oncology CEA are most commonly expressed as additional survival time but may also be expressed in other terms; for example, the number of adverse events or additional procedures avoided or the number of cases of cancer prevented. This type of study is commonly used when a decision or health policymaker is operating within a given budget and is considering a limited range of options (37). When an intervention costs more and is also more effective than its alternative, the cost-effectiveness comparison is expressed as an incremental cost-effectiveness ratio (ICER), the ratio of the difference in costs to the difference in effectiveness between two strategies.

Cost-minimization Analyses

In some cases, alternative medical decisions have approximately equivalent effectiveness but potentially different costs. In such cases, the effectiveness component of a CEA may not be needed. CMAs assume comparable effectiveness between strategies and choose a preferred strategy based on the mean cost of each (39). For example, a decision analysis comparing the costs of three different surgical approaches to endometrial cancer staging assumed equal survival outcomes between strategies and, therefore, did not incorporate effectiveness (40).

Cost-utility Analyses

CUA is a form of CEA in which effectiveness is adjusted based on the QoL that is associated with each strategy. In CUAs, *utilities* are the measurement used for QoL and represent the preferences of an individual or a society for a particular health outcome. A utility is a number between 0 and 1, with 1 representing perfect health and 0 representing death. The most common metric used for comparison of strategies in a CUA is a QALY. The QALY quantifies both differences in survival and in QoL between strategies. In an oncology CUA, the QALY is usually derived as the product of the length of survival in a specific health state and the utility representing the QoL in that state. For example, 1 year of additional survival in a health state of utility 0.8 is equivalent to 0.8 QALYs. CUAs are preferred when both morbidity and mortality are affected by the proposed medical intervention or when QoL related to the intervention being examined is a major concern. QALYs are the recommended outcome for health economic analyses if utility scores are available (41).

Methods for Development of a Health Economic Decision Model

This section addresses specific methods used in the development of a health economic decision model, with an emphasis on the two most common types of models, CEA and CUA. Importantly, a standard checklist developed by the International Society for Pharmacoeconomics and Outcomes Research (ISPOR) now exists to inform the process of health economic model design and execution (42).

Define the model's perspective The perspective of a health economic model is the first important consideration as costs are calculated differently based on the perspective taken. Most CEAs are performed from a third-party payer or a societal perspective. In a third-party payer perspective model, costs assumed by an insurance company or by Medicare are incorporated. These may include professional fees for encounters and procedures, reimbursements to the hospital or ambulatory surgical center for postoperative care, or reimbursements for home health or rehabilitation care. A societal perspective is usually most appropriate as it accounts not only for all costs included from a third-party payer perspective but also for costs related to a patient's lost productivity and the caregiver's expense. For example, if one surgical approach results in a faster return to work, this will be associated with lower cost due to lost productivity. The use of the societal perspective has led to the recognition that minimally invasive surgery results in cost savings to society (40,43). Other perspectives of health economic models include the *patient* and *hospital* perspectives. A hospital perspective model might be used to inform the decision to purchase expensive equipment, such as robotic surgery platforms or an intraoperative radiotherapy facility.

Define the question Once the model's perspective has been determined, the clinical problem, standard approach, and any alternatives must be defined (44). The alternatives to the intervention of interest should always include a standard-of-care approach or even a "do nothing" approach. Next, a conceptual model for the analysis is developed, which outlines the possible consequences of each intervention. Decision models are often used as the conceptual framework for CEAs and have become an integral part of CEA studies.

Develop a decision tree A simple decision tree begins with a *decision node* representing the primary clinical decision being examined. Two or more strategies may be examined using one decision tree. The subsequent nodes in the tree are termed *chance nodes* and define the probability of each possible clinical event that follows from the initial decision. For example, if the decision node concerns the clinical question of whether to accept a blood transfusion, the first chance node may define the probability that the patient will be infected with a blood-borne infection such as HIV if they accept. Another chance node may define the risk of death if transfusion is refused (**Figure 12.2-2**). Probabilities defined at chance nodes are usually derived from the literature or from clinical trial data. At the end of each branch of a decision tree is the

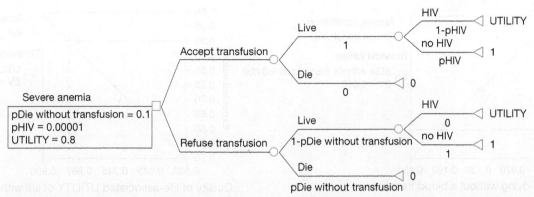

Figure 12.2-2. Simple decision tree representing the choice to accept or refuse a blood transfusion for severe anemia. The blue square is the decision node, green circles are chance nodes, and the red triangles are terminal nodes. Probabilities of events are depicted beneath each branch. Payoffs are listed to the right of terminal nodes. Three parameters are modeled as variables and have been given numeric values defined beneath the decision node: pHIV is the probability of being infected with HIV should the patient accept a transfusion. pDie without transfusion is the probability of death from severe anemia without a transfusion. UTILITY is the quality of life–related value of living with HIV, where 0 represents death and 1 represents perfect health.

terminal node, at which a payoff representing the effectiveness of that strategy occurs. In the blood transfusion example, the terminal nodes define three states: life, death, or life with a blood-borne infection such as HIV. The payoff for life is 1, for death is 0, and for infection is a utility representing a lifetime spent with the infection. The expected value of each strategy, or its effectiveness, is calculated as the weighted average of the probabilities and payoffs associated with each terminal branch of the tree. The strategy resulting in the highest expected value is said to be the most effective. Payoffs in an oncology decision model are usually survival time and QoL. In a CUA, the effectiveness might be the product of survival time and the QoL-based preference score, or utility.

Once all possible clinical events and their probabilities and payoffs have been defined by chance nodes, the costs of tests, treatments, and adverse events may be incorporated at each node. The cost associated with each strategy is calculated as a weighted average of the costs and probabilities associated with each branch of the tree.

Analysis of model After cost and effectiveness information have been collected and incorporated into the model, the analyses is performed. Results of cost-effectiveness models are expressed in terms of a comparison of two or more strategies. When one strategy is both more costly and less effective than an alternative strategy, it is said to be *dominated* and should not be considered. Likewise, a strategy that is both more effective and less costly is considered to be *dominant* and should be the treatment of choice. In these two cases, a numeric cost-effectiveness quantification is not needed. When one strategy is both more costly and more effective than an alternative, an ICER is calculated. This is expressed as the difference in the mean cost divided by the difference in mean effectiveness between strategies.

The ICER for comparison of intervention A and intervention B is defined as follows:

$$\text{ICER} = \frac{\text{Cost}_A - \text{Cost}_B}{\text{Effect}_A - \text{Effect}_B}$$

It is important to note that the ICER is *not* estimated by dividing the cost of one intervention by the measure of its own effectiveness. This average cost-effectiveness ratio is not comparable to the ICER and is not a useful metric in CEAs (45).

In the United States, an intervention was traditionally considered cost-effective relative to an alternative strategy if the ICER was less than $50,000 per year of life saved (YLS)/QALY (39).

Although ICER thresholds of $50,000/YLS are theoretically used in decision-making, they are not strictly applied. Social norms may raise this value such that interventions costing up to $100,000 or even greater per QALY have sometimes been considered cost-effective (46,47). The term "cost-effective" does not mean that a strategy saves money but rather that the additional cost of the intervention is worthwhile, usually from the perspective of society.

Sensitivity Analyses

Uncertainty in health economic analyses may exist about input parameters, such as cost, survival, or clinical probabilities. To assess the impact of such uncertainty on the findings of a decision model, a sensitivity analysis can be performed. The simplest form of sensitivity analysis is a one-way analysis. Estimates are varied one parameter at a time to evaluate the impact changes make on the outcome or conclusions of the model (48). For example, in the simple model describing the decision to accept or refuse a blood transfusion, varying the probability of death due to anemia or the utility related to QoL with HIV has an impact on the expected value of each decision (**Figure 12.2-3A,B**). Likewise, a two-way sensitivity analysis can be performed to evaluate the impact of varying two-model parameters simultaneously (**Figure 12.2-3C**). When variation in the key parameters of a model over their CIs or expected range of values does not change the model's results, the model is said to be insensitive to these variations and its conclusions can be more strongly interpreted. Models whose outcomes change significantly when key estimates are varied over a clinically reasonable range should be interpreted with caution.

Most clinical models are fairly complex and may warrant the use of multiple simultaneous sensitivity analyses. In a Monte Carlo probabilistic sensitivity analysis, each variable in the model can be sampled from a probability distribution representing its value (49). Sampling parameter values from probability distributions (rather than from a simple range of values) places greater weight on likely combinations of parameter values. Multiple sampling simulations of the model may then be run, each of which results in an individual cost-effectiveness comparison or estimate. Multiple simulations allow for construction of a cost-effectiveness scatterplot and the ability to express CIs around the ICER estimate (**Figure 12.2-4**), which effectively allows quantification of the total impact of uncertainty on the model and the confidence that can be placed in the analysis results.

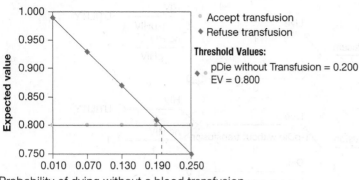

A

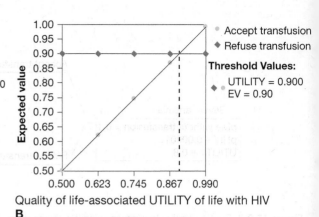

B

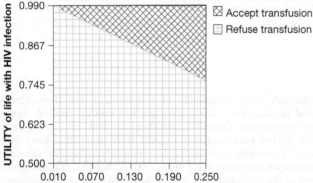

C

Figure 12.2-3. A: One-way sensitivity analysis on the probability of death from anemia without a blood transfusion. When the probability of death from anemia exceeds the threshold value of 0.2, the expected value (EV) of accepting the transfusion exceeds that of refusing transfusion and the correct choice is to accept the transfusion. **B:** One-way sensitivity analysis on the quality of life–related utility of living with HIV. When the utility exceeds the threshold value of 0.9, the EV of accepting the transfusion exceeds that of refusing transfusion and the correct choice is to accept the transfusion. **C:** Two-way sensitivity analysis in which the utility associated with HIV infection and the probability of death without transfusion are varied simultaneously. The blue-shaded area represents values for which acceptance of a transfusion results in the highest EV (payoff) and is the preferred choice. Green-shaded area represents combinations for which refusal of transfusion is the preferred choice.

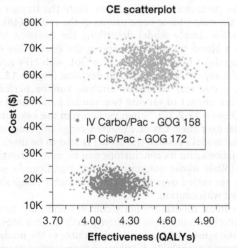

Figure 12.2-4. Cost-effectiveness (CE) scatterplot resulting from a Monte Carlo probabilistic sensitivity analysis for a model comparing intravenous (IV) carboplatin/paclitaxel to intraperitoneal (IP) cisplatin/paclitaxel and IV paclitaxel for advanced ovarian cancer. The simulation was repeated 10,000 times with sampling of key model parameters (cost, survival, probability of adverse events) from probability distributions. This simulation resulted in an estimate of 95% confidence intervals to surround the primary incremental CE ratio estimate. GOG, Gynecologic Oncology Group; QALYs, quality-adjusted life years. (Reprinted with permission. © 2008 American Society of Clinical Oncology. All rights reserved. Havrilesky L et al. *J Clin Oncol.* 2008;26(25):4144-4150.)

INPUT DEVELOPMENT FOR HEALTH ECONOMIC MODELS

The following section details methods for the development of input data for health economic models.

Estimation of Costs

Cost definitions The costs incorporated into a CEA depend on the study's perspective. The standard CEA or CUA is performed from a societal perspective (39). However, alternative perspectives include those of the patient, hospital, or a third-party payer. In a societal perspective analysis, the costs included are all of those borne by society and should, therefore, include both direct and indirect costs. Direct costs include direct medical costs (eg, professional and hospital costs, diagnostic tests and procedures) and direct nonmedical costs (such as travel to receive care). Indirect costs account for lost productivity due to time off work for illness, both for the patient and any caregivers. When a health economic model is performed from a nonsocietal perspective, the scope of the costs included may be narrower. For example, in an analysis performed from a third-party payer perspective, lost productivity would not be included.

Costs versus charges When performing a health economic analysis, it is important to distinguish costs from charges. Charges represent what the provider or hospital asks an individual to pay for a service and not the reimbursement provided by either a private third-party payer or Medicare. Because reimbursements by the CMS are generally considered to approximate the cost of providing a service, it is standard to use national Medicare reimbursements to approximate the costs of medical tests, procedures, or services in a health economic analysis (50). If a Medicare reimbursement is not available for a particular aspect of medical costs, charges may be used to calculate costs using a cost-charge ratio. Cost-charge ratios allow a calculation of the proportion of hospital charges that represent cost to the hospital. Cost-charge ratios are specific to individual hospital departments and may be available from CMS (http://www.cms.gov).

Surgical costs Health economic analyses in gynecologic oncology may include an estimate of the costs of surgical procedures. CMS reimbursements may be used to approximate these costs from a societal perspective. Direct surgical costs include professional fees (surgeon, anesthesiologist, pathologist), the cost of hospital recovery, and the costs of any tests or procedures performed in the postoperative period. Postoperative outpatient care is usually part of a global fee that includes the first 90 days of postoperative care and is, therefore, not included separately. Likewise, the reimbursement for recovery in the hospital or ambulatory surgery center is usually determined by a CMS code, and this reimbursement covers tests and inpatient care. However, additional procedures performed postoperatively are associated with additional professional fees.

Costs of hospitalization The cost of a hospitalization may be estimated for health economic models using the Diagnosis-Related Group (DRG), a CMS code that takes into account the primary diagnosis and the patient's comorbidities and is used to determine the reimbursement Medicare provides to the hospital. An alternative method for estimating the cost of an inpatient hospital stay is to use the Agency for Healthcare Research and Quality's (AHRQ) Healthcare Cost and Utilization Project (HCUP) Nationwide Inpatient Sample (NIS) (http://www.hcup-us.ahrq.gov/). This large all-payer public database provides inpatient data from a national sample of over 1,000 hospitals in 44 states and is released annually.

Outpatient treatment costs Outpatient treatments in gynecologic oncology often refer to chemotherapy. Cost tabulation should include the CMS reimbursements for the individual chemotherapy drugs and any other medications infused based on the designated J code for each drug. Tests performed routinely over the course of a cycle of treatment should also be included. Finally, the costs of infusion at an outpatient facility should be included using appropriate CPT codes.

Adverse events When two or more strategies are compared using a health economic model, it is critical that the adverse events associated with each strategy be accounted for. Specifically, when severe adverse events result in additional medical or nonmedical costs, these costs should be incorporated as well. For example, if one chemotherapy strategy results in a higher rate of febrile neutropenia, the cost of a hospitalization for this diagnosis should be incorporated into the cost of each strategy in proportion to the probability of the event in each treatment group. Adverse events whose frequencies are not significantly different between strategies or that do not generate additional cost (eg, grade 1 anemia) may reasonably be omitted from a CEA. However, models should adjust for QoL differences resulting from adverse events.

Cost collection as a component of phase III trials Although many cost-effectiveness studies are performed following completion of the clinical trials from which the data are derived, such analyses are ideally planned and executed in conjunction with prospective phase III trials. The ISPOR Task Force on Good Research Practices recommends that collection of health economic data should be fully integrated into phase III studies (50). In a phase III trial, prospective economic data are usually collected by accounting for differences in health resource utilization between treatment groups. Ideally, this might include an accounting of all health-related encounters in each treatment group. However, logistical considerations during trial planning often require prioritization as to which data elements will be collected. Therefore, it is often appropriate to choose to focus on "big ticket" items as well as resources that

are expected to differ between treatment arms. Resource utilization collection may be accomplished by means of subject diaries in which outpatient and inpatient encounters as well as travel and caregiver time may be recorded. National fee schedules and reimbursements are then generally used to assign costs to each element of resource utilization collected.

Modeling Effectiveness

Effectiveness in CEA should be reported in units of relevant clinical outcomes. For example, in oncology studies, effectiveness might be expressed as the number of cases of cancer prevented, the number of unnecessary surgical procedures avoided, or the number of cancer recurrences prevented. However, it is most common in oncology CEA to quantify effectiveness using survival. Thus, in CEAs, the comparison of alternative strategies might be described in terms of the cost per additional year of life, or QALY, saved. While OS is a standard outcome in both CEA and clinical trials, PFS may also be reported.

Modeling survival: Survival outcomes may be modeled in several ways. One simple method is to assign a survival time (eg, mean survival in years) to each relevant branch of a simple decision tree. Although this method accomplishes the assignment of a survival "value" to each branch of the model, it does not account for additional costs or changes in QoL that may need to be applied only to subjects who are still alive at a specific time. For example, it may be useful to apply the cost of additional cycles of treatment or adverse events to only those individuals remaining alive or progression free at a specific time point. An alternative, and more common, method is to use a modified Markov state transition model to represent survival. When a modified Markov approach is used, costs of events that are applied only if a subject is alive or has relapsed may be applied at each relevant time point. Likewise, changes in QoL during or after treatment may also be quantified. In the context of comparing effectiveness results of a prospective clinical trial, raw survival data can be used to model Kaplan-Meier survival curves directly (**Figure 12.2-5**).

Modeling Quality of Life

Medical interventions in oncology may improve QoL without extending life or may extend life but worsen quality during treatment. Economic analyses that are based only on cost and efficacy do not fully account for the value of many treatments and interventions. CUAs account for the morbidity, physical well-being, and emotional well-being associated with medical treatments. CUAs may be used when the interventions being considered affect both QoL and survival or when there is no expected difference in survival but a difference in QoL is anticipated (37).

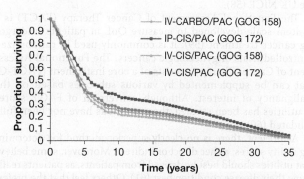

Figure 12.2-5. Survival curve output from a modified Markov state transition model designed to compare the cost-effectiveness of chemotherapy regimens studied in two randomized phase III trials. GOG, Gynecologic Oncology Group; IP, intraperitoneal; IV, intravenous. (Reprinted with permission. © 2008 American Society of Clinical Oncology. All rights reserved. Havrilesky L et al. *J Clin Oncol.* 2008;26(25):4144-4150.)

In CUAs, QoL is represented by a utility. A utility is a measure of the desirability or preference that individuals or societies place on a given health outcome (51,52). Utility scores are usually linked to judgments about the value of a particular health state. The anchor health states are 0 for death and 1 for perfect health. Applying utility scores to a cost-effectiveness model allows the outcome of the economic analysis, now the CUA, to be reported in QALYs.

Eliciting preferences for calculation of utility scores The use of utility scores in a cost-utility model requires a defined health state for each distinct outcome of the intervention and its alternative (53). For example, health states of interest in an ovarian cancer CUA may include (1) newly diagnosed ovarian cancer starting primary chemotherapy; (2) completed primary therapy, no evidence of disease; (3) progressive disease on treatment; or (4) end-stage ovarian cancer. Descriptions of health states are needed to derive utilities. The description of each health state includes information about the levels of physical health, emotional health, activities of daily living, and overall well-being (54). A rater provides preferences for each health state, and a utility score is created. Raters are selected according to the perspective of the study. For example, if a societal perspective is taken, then representatives of the general population should be used to score the preference (39). The preferences of individuals with conditions of interest (such as patients) or of physicians are important ancillary information that might be incorporated into studies performed from alternative perspectives, but these cannot be substituted for societal preferences when the model's perspective is societal (44). Several rigorous formal approaches to the direct measurement of preferences and calculation of utility scores for health states have been developed, of which the most commonly used are the standard gamble (SG) and the time-trade off (TTO) methods (55). Although there is some debate concerning consistency of results between the SG and TTO, they are both considered standard methods to elicit utilities (52,53,56).

Use of QoL instruments and health status classification systems to derive utilities for CER Measuring preferences for health outcomes using the direct SG and TTO methods is not a simple exercise and is beyond the scope of most clinical trials for which a CUA might be desirable. There exist a number of prescored health status classification systems to allow indirect assignment of utilities based on questionnaires and calibrated using prior studies of societal preferences. For example, EuroQoL-5D (EQ-5D) is a simple Likert scale questionnaire in which raters report no problem or some degree of problem in five dimensions: mobility, self-care, usual activities, pain/discomfort, anxiety, and depression (57). Based on mapping studies in representative populations, the dimension scores obtained from the EQ-5D may be directly converted to a utility score; this method is preferred by the UK NICE (58).

The Functional Assessment of Cancer Therapy (FACT) is a 33-item scale developed to measure QoL in patients undergoing cancer treatment (59). It is commonly used in randomized controlled trials of gynecologic cancers. The Functional Assessment of Cancer Therapy consists of a core instrument (FACT-G) that can be supplemented by various subscales based on the malignancy of interest. Although conversion of FACT scores to utilities has been studied, these methods have not been fully validated (60).

At present, there is no clearly superior method for determining utility scores, either direct or indirect. Moreover, some believe that utilities should best be derived from patients, as patients really know their disease condition best (61). Others feel that the preferences of the general public are most relevant because society as a whole must delegate distribution of its health care resources (62). As economic analyses evolve, the limitations of preference ratings should be examined and a consistent method of developing utility scores should be determined to allow for better comparisons to be made across cost-utility studies.

MODELING APPROACHES TO REDUCING MORTALITY FROM GYNECOLOGIC CANCERS

In the following section, methods for the development of cancer natural history models and their use in screening and prevention decision analyses are described. The current state of evidence for cervical and ovarian cancer screening and prevention as informed by the current literature as well as simulation modeling is be reviewed.

Modeling the Natural History of Cancer

In order to evaluate the effectiveness of a proposed cancer screening test or prevention strategy for which no phase III clinical trials have been completed, a model can be created that simulates the natural history of the disease with and without the intervention. The simplest model is a decision tree. Although decision trees are useful for modeling outcomes that occur over a short period of time, such as a year, they can become unwieldy when trying to model a disease that occurs over a longer period or that involves recurrent events, such as multiple episodes of screening or multiple cycles of treatment. Markov models are used for events that recur or occur in a predictable manner over time (63). They are particularly well suited to depicting the events associated with cancer, especially cancers that have a screening component.

Construction of a Markov natural history model For creation of a Markov model, the natural history of a cancer is broken up into a defined, mutually exclusive and exhaustive set of states. For cervical cancer, these states could include well, human papillomavirus (HPV) infection, preinvasive disease, undetected invasive cancer (stages I-IV), detected invasive cancer (stages I-IV), cancer death, and death from other causes. For high-grade serous ovarian cancer, natural history states might include well, serous intraepithelial serous carcinoma (STIC), undetected and detected invasive cancer (stages I-IV), cancer death, and death from other causes (**Figure 12.2-6**). Once the states have been defined, movement (referred to as "transition") between the states is defined to simulate the cancer's natural history. The probabilities of moving from one state to another over a fixed period of time are then used to populate the model. These are usually obtained from the epidemiologic literature, an analysis of an epidemiologic study, or expert opinion. Together, the states allowed transitions and probabilities constitute the model. Once programmed, the model can be used to calculate different outcomes, such as the lifetime risk of developing or dying from cancer. The outcomes are usually calculated for a cohort (or cohorts) of women who are assumed to enter the model at a given age and are then followed until death or a later age (eg, 100 years).

Calibration An important step in developing a natural history model is obtaining probabilities or estimates for key variables (referred to as *parameters*) from the literature. However, often, there are few or no available estimates for a given model parameter. The selection of a given clinical estimate is important because this affects the credibility of the model's aggregate result. Calibration is a process that involves comparing the model predicted results to observed data to ensure a reasonably good fit of one to the other. Model calibration involves several steps: (1) identification of calibration end points (for cancer, this usually means age-specific cancer incidence but can also include stage distribution and age-specific mortality curves); (2) establishment of criteria for determining how well the model predicted data fit the observed data. This may be visual inspection or using a statistical goodness-of-fit test; (3) adjustment of the set of model input parameters (ie, probabilities); and (4) comparison of model predicted outcomes to observed outcomes using the prespecified criteria and repeating steps 3 and 4 until a satisfactory calibration is achieved (64,65).

Validation Model validation (confirmation that the calibrated model predicts results that are consistent with observed results from clinical trials) can be achieved in a number of ways. The

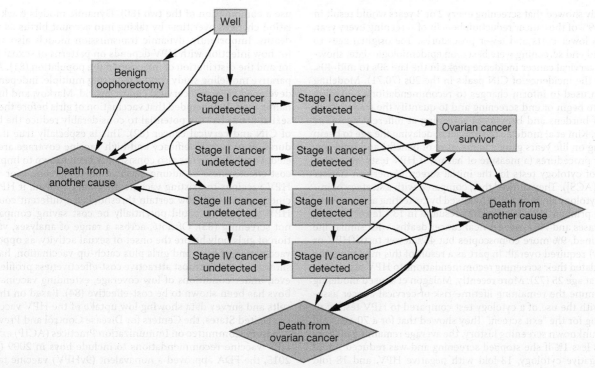

Figure 12.2-6. Influence diagram for models of the natural history of ovarian cancer. Arrows represent allowed transitions between health states. Diamonds represent terminal states. (From Havrilesky LJ, Sanders GD, Kulasingam S, et al. Development of an ovarian cancer screening decision model that incorporates disease heterogeneity: implications for potential mortality reduction. *Cancer.* 2011;117(3):545-553.)

most robust method is to compare model predicted outcomes with actual outcomes. For example, Havrilesky et al constructed a natural history model accounting for the observed heterogeneity of epithelial ovarian cancers. Validation was performed by simulating the prevalence screen phase of the UKCTOCS ovarian cancer screening trial. The model predicted the stage distribution of cancers detected by screening and the positive predictive value of the multimodality prevalence screen within their reported 95% CIs (66). To the degree that simulated results do not reproduce those observed in a clinical trial, the question arises whether there are key input parameters or model structural differences that affect the conclusions. A model can then be revised to determine whether the prediction is improved in an iterative process. When there exist no observed data to answer a given question, model validation may be achieved by comparing the results from models built by different, independent groups, to evaluate for similarity. This approach has been adopted by Cancer Intervention and Surveillance Modeling Network (CISNET), a consortium of National Cancer Institute (NCI)-sponsored investigators who use statistical modeling to study cancer control interventions in prevention, screening, and treatment and their effects on population trends in incidence and mortality. CISNET models are independently developed and have been calibrated to U.S. data. The results from comparative modeling studies conducted by members of the CISNET consortium have been used by the U.S. Preventive Services Task Force (USPSTF) to inform their recommendations for colorectal and breast cancer (67,68).

Simulation of Interventions

Markov models can be programmed to keep a count of the outcomes associated with diagnosis, treatment, and screening. Examples include the average number of false-positive or false-negative screening test results, the number of diagnostic procedures such as colposcopy or laparoscopy performed, number of preinvasive lesions detected, and treatments. Other important outcomes include

cancer incidence, stage distribution, and mortality. If the cohort of women is modeled over a sufficiently long period of time, the model can be used to calculate life expectancy, lifetime costs, and quality-adjusted life expectancy.

Cervical Cancer

For cervical cancer, modeling has played a particularly prominent role in informing decisions regarding which screening and triage tests to adopt, how frequently women should be screened, and whether the addition of vaccination to screening is cost-effective. This prominent role is due to the fact that trials of new screening tests include follow-up and treatment that often differ from clinical practice or are conducted in non–U.S. populations with different risk profiles and screening histories. Modeling studies can be used to project both short- and long-term results from trials. For example, although trials of HPV vaccines used cervical intraepithelial neoplasia (CIN) grade 2 or higher as primary outcomes, cancer incidence and death are more important outcomes for policymakers. Modeling has been used to project forward the results from the trials to estimate the long-term impact of vaccines, to estimate the potential cost-effectiveness of adding vaccination to screening, and to justify the expanded coverage of HPV vaccines to include boys. The following sections describe how models of HPV and cervical cancer have been used to enhance clinical data and inform recent policies regarding screening and vaccination for cervical cancer prevention.

QUESTIONS ADDRESSED BY CERVICAL CANCER MODELS

Appropriate age to begin/end and screening interval with cytology
In one of the earliest examples of a mathematical model of cervical cancer, in the 1980s, David Eddy examined the relationship between Pap smear screening interval and cancer incidence (69).

This study showed that screening every 2 or 3 years would result in 95% to 99% of the cancer reduction benefit of screening every year, but with lower costs and fewer procedures. The original ages to begin and end screening were based on epidemiologic data, showing that cervical cancer incidence peaks in the late 30s to mid-40s, but that the incidence of CIN peaks in the 20s (70,71). Modeling has been used to inform changes to recommendations regarding the age to begin or end screening and to quantify the trade-offs in terms of burdens and benefits of screening at different ages. For example, Kim et al modeled the impact of delaying the age to begin screening on life years gained (a measure of benefit) and total colposcopy procedures (a measure of harms) if HPV tests were used instead of cytology tests for the initial screen (American Cancer Society [ACS]). They showed that, compared with a strategy of initiating cytology alone at age 21 followed by co-testing at 30, screening with primary HPV testing at 25 resulted in 13% fewer cervical cancer cases and 7% fewer cervical cancer deaths, with similar life years gained, 9% more colposcopies but 45% fewer tests (HPV or cytology) required overall. In part as a result of this modeling, the ACS updated their screening recommendations to HPV testing beginning at age 25 (72). More recently, Malagon et al used modeling to determine the remaining lifetime risk of cervical cancer associated with the use of a cytology test compared to HPV testing or co-testing for the "exit screen." They showed that for a 70-year-old with an unknown screening history, the average remaining lifetime risk was less 1% if she stopped screening and was reduced 2-fold with negative cytology, 13-fold with negative HPV, and 18-fold with negative co-testing. These results suggest that an HPV test or co-test can provide greatest reassurance of a low remaining lifetime risk of cancer once screening ceases. Importantly, these studies illustrate how modeling can be used to examine issues related to age and screening interval that epidemiologic studies and clinical trials may not be able to answer (73).

Use of HPV testing in screening Modeling studies have examined the cost-effectiveness of adding HPV testing to screening programs (74). The strategy of HPV testing followed by triage based on cytology for women with positive results has shown particular promise (75,76); numerous large randomized trials of primary HPV testing have now confirmed the use of HPV testing as the primary screening test compared to co-testing with either cytology and HPV or cytology alone. For example, in the United States, the Addressing the Need for Advanced HPV Diagnostics (ATHENA) HPV study was a prospective 3-year cervical cancer screening trial that compared the performance of the cobas HPV test (Roche Molecular Diagnostics, Pleasanton, CA), which detects 12 HPV types and also provides separate results for HPV 16 and HPV 18, to cervical cytology and co-testing (77). An analysis restricted to women aged 25 years and above showed that primary screening with HPV, with genotyping and cytology to triage HPV-positive women, was more sensitive with a similar positive predictive value than cytology using an ASCUS cut point for referral to colposcopy. In the Human Papillomavirus for Cervical Cancer screening trial (HPV FOCAL) conducted in Canada, screening women aged 25 and 65 years with primary HPV testing resulted in significantly fewer CIN 2+ (risk ratio and 95% CI: 0.42 [0.25-0.69]) and CIN 3+ (risk ratio and 95% CI: 0.47 [0.34-0.67]) detected at 48 months compared to the control group (cytology with reflex HPV testing). Based on the results from these trials and prior modeling, in 2017, the USPSTF commissioned a systematic review and modeling study to determine whether screening with HPV as the primary test should be recommended. The results from the modeling study predicted that primary HPV testing strategies occurring at 5-year intervals were efficient (78). The USPSTF subsequently updated their recommendations in 2018 to include primary testing with HPV conducted every 5 years (79).

Quantifying the impact of HPV vaccination Two types of models have been used to explore HPV vaccine effectiveness: Markov state transition cohort models (described earlier) and dynamic transmission models, with a third category—hybrid models—that

use a combination of the two (80). Dynamic models track population changes over time by taking into account births as well as deaths. Importantly, dynamic transmission models also account for how infection with HPV depends on patterns of sexual behavior and the distribution of infection in the population (81). A comparative modeling study conducted using multiple, independently developed HPV and cervical cancer hybrid, Markov, and fully dynamic models concluded that vaccination of girls before the age of sexual debut has the potential to considerably reduce the burden of CIN and cervical cancer (82). This is especially true if a long duration of vaccine efficacy and high vaccine coverage are modeled. Vaccine price has also consistently been shown to impact the cost-effectiveness of adding vaccination to screening or adding HPV vaccines to existing vaccine programs. Indeed, if HPV vaccines are priced below certain thresholds for different countries, HPV vaccination could potentially be cost saving compared to not screening (83). Of note, across a range of analyses, vaccination of girls only before the onset of sexual activity, as opposed to vaccination of boys and girls plus catch-up vaccination, has been shown to have the most attractive cost-effectiveness profile. However, under conditions of low coverage, extending vaccination to boys has been shown to be cost-effective (84). Based on these results and survey data showing low uptake of the HPV vaccines in the United States, the Centers for Disease Control and Prevention Advisory Committee on Immunization Practices (ACIP) extended HPV vaccine recommendations to include boys in 2009 (85). In 2015, the FDA approved a nonavalent (9vHPV) vaccine targeted against seven high-risk and two low-risk HPV types associated with approximately 80% of cervical cancers. Modeling by Brisson was conducted to determine the impact of recommending this vaccine in a U.S. population and was included in the recommendation for use of this vaccine by the ACIP (86). This modeling study predicts that the use of the 9vHPV in both males and females will be cost saving when compared with 4vHPV if the cost of the new vaccine is at most $13 greater than the cost of the 4vHPV vaccine. The 9vHPV was cost saving in a number of scenarios, and the cost per QALY gained did not exceed $25,000 in any scenario across a range of assumptions about HPV natural history, cervical cancer screening, vaccine coverage, vaccine duration of protection, and health care costs.

In 2018, the FDA approved an expanded use for the 9vHPV vaccine up to age 45 in men and women (87). However, modeling conducted by five groups with independently developed models showed mixed results in terms of the benefits of vaccinating older age groups. In a summary of the modeling findings, the ACIP noted that expanding vaccination to adults through age 45 years compared to the existing vaccination program would produce relatively small additional health benefits and less favorable cost-effectiveness ratios. They noted that the incremental cost per QALY for also vaccinating adults through age 30 or 45 years exceeded $300,000 in four of five models (88). Based, in part, on the results of the modeling, the ACIP did not recommend routine vaccination up to age 45 but rather shared decision-making with a person's clinician to determine whether vaccination would be beneficial (88).

Screening in the era of HPV vaccines The issue of whether and how screening should change in the era of HPV vaccines is complex and depends on a number of factors. These include, but are not limited to, the performance of cytology and HPV tests in vaccinated women, the magnitude of reductions in CIN and cancer, and whether vaccination will affect screening behavior, in particular screening participation. In countries with early approval of the 4vHPV vaccine and high vaccine coverage, such as Australia, marked reductions in HPV prevalence and precancer have been demonstrated in vaccinated compared to unvaccinated cohorts (89,90). Although reductions in cancer have begun to be observed, the long time period between infection and cancer suggests that larger reductions should be expected in the coming decades (91,92). In vaccinated cohorts of women, cost-effective approaches to screening include strategies that use a less frequent screening interval, delayed age of first screening, and/or use of a strategy based on HPV DNA testing followed by cytology (75,93). Of note, modeling suggests that far fewer screens than currently recommended will be needed to continue to achieve significant reductions in cervical cancer (94,95).

Modeling has been used extensively in cervical cancer to inform how we should approach screening and add HPV vaccination programs to screening programs and will continue to play a key role in determining the most effective and cost-effective strategies for the prevention of cervical cancer.

Ovarian Cancer

Because the majority of ovarian cancers are diagnosed at an advanced stage, there has been considerable interest in designing screening strategies to diagnose and treat women earlier in the hopes of improving survival outcomes. Several key parameters may impact the success of any cancer screening program: (1) availability of effective treatment for screen positive individuals; (2) sufficiently high disease prevalence; (3) existence of an effective screening test; and (4) acceptable cost or cost-effectiveness of the screening program. Each of these parameters is addressed here in the context of development of a screening test for epithelial ovarian cancer.

Effectiveness of treatment Pathologic and genetic data now demonstrate that epithelial ovarian cancer is a heterogeneous disease, with a number of different precursor lesions. High-grade serous ovarian cancers primarily originate in the fallopian tubes, whereas some clear cell and endometrioid lesions appear to originate in endometriosis. Because there is no universal, clearly defined precursor lesion for all epithelial ovarian cancer, the target lesion for the screening tests that have been evaluated in the largest clinical trials is stage I disease. Women with stage I ovarian cancer with low-risk features may be cured without the need for adjuvant treatment, whereas those with higher risk stage I disease may still achieve excellent outcomes following three to six cycles of platin- and taxane-based chemotherapy (96).

Disease prevalence Perhaps, the biggest challenge to development of a successful ovarian cancer screening program is the low prevalence of this disease. The lifetime incidence of ovarian cancer in the United States is approximately 1.2%. In postmenopausal women, the most likely target population for a screening program, its prevalence is approximately 40 per 100,000 women. Disease prevalence has a direct impact on the achievable positive predictive value of a screening test, which defines the number of women undergoing diagnostic procedures or surgeries that would be required to diagnose one case of ovarian cancer. Given the invasive nature of ovarian biopsy or removal, expert opinion has suggested that the minimal acceptable positive predictive value for an ovarian cancer screening test should be 10%. To achieve this value in the postmenopausal population, a screening test needs to have a specificity exceeding 99.6%.

Effectiveness of screening test To date, no screening test for ovarian cancer has been proven effective in reducing mortality from this disease. Two large randomized trials have recently been performed to evaluate screening strategies utilizing the CA-125 serum test and transvaginal ultrasound. The Prostate, Lung, Colorectal and Ovarian (PLCO) screening trial randomized 78,216 women to either usual care or a combination of annual CA-125 for 6 consecutive years and annual transvaginal ultrasound for 4 consecutive years (97). After a median follow-up of 12.4 years, there was no difference in ovarian cancer mortality between the screened and unscreened groups. However, there was evidence of possible harm due to the screening intervention, in the form of a 15% rate of serious adverse events among women with false-positive screening tests who underwent surgical procedures. The authors concluded that simultaneous screening with CA-125 and ultrasound does not reduce ovarian cancer mortality and may introduce harms (98).

A second large screening trial, the UKCTOCS study, randomized 202,638 postmenopausal women to no intervention, annual transvaginal ultrasound, or a multimodality algorithm incorporating annual CA-125 and second-line transvaginal ultrasound. Although the stage distribution in the multimodality screening arm was shifted to favor early-stage cancers, ovarian cancer mortality was not statistically lower in this or a longer term follow-up study (99,100).

Comparative effectiveness of screening Several groups have used mathematical modeling to determine the likely success and cost-effectiveness of screening strategies. Skates and Singer designed the first reported stochastic simulation model of the natural history of ovarian cancer. This model suggested that screening using CA-125 could potentially save 3.4 years of life per case of cancer detected (101). Urban et al subsequently modified the Skates and Singer's model and performed a cost-effectiveness assessment of several screening strategies. The authors reported that multimodality screening with CA-125 followed by transvaginal ultrasound if CA-125 was abnormal was potentially cost-effective compared to single test strategies and no screening (102).

More recent screening models have incorporated new data about the pathophysiology and progression of ovarian cancer. Havrilesky et al constructed a natural history model that, based on the physical proximity of the ovaries to upper abdominal organs such as small bowel and omentum, allowed progression of stage I cancers either to stage II or directly to stage III (103). Disease incidence, mortality, and stage distribution were calibrated to reflect Surveillance, Epidemiology, and End Results (SEER) data. A modified version of this model was designed to account for the heterogeneity of ovarian cancer by modeling aggressive and indolent phenotypes with different rates of progression (66). These models highlighted factors that are important to the success of a screening program. For example, increasing the frequency of screening had a more favorable impact on reducing cancer mortality than increasing the sensitivity of the individual screening test. However, because of increased cost, increasing screening frequency actually reduced cost-effectiveness. Both models reinforced the important link between specificity and positive predictive value. An annual screening test with a sensitivity of 85% and specificity of less than 99% would have a positive predictive value not exceeding 4%. However, at a specificity of 99.9%, the positive predictive value for annual screening was excellent at 22%. Key factors in achieving a cost-effective screening test (defined as an ICER of <$50,000/YLS) were an inexpensive test, a very high test specificity, and infrequent (annual or less) testing. Screening appeared to be potentially most cost-effective when the test specificity was well above 99% and the testing interval was annually or less frequently (103).

These prior models confirm that very high test specificity is required to achieve acceptable positive predictive values, whereas mortality reduction is sensitive to screening frequency. However, given the ultimate failure of the two largest RCTs to prove the effectiveness of screening, natural history modeling may be best suited to examining potential combinations of ovarian cancer prevention and treatment as tools to reduce mortality.

Comparative effectiveness of salpingectomy as prevention The concept that most high-grade serous carcinomas of the ovary begin as serous tubal intraepithelial carcinoma in the fallopian tube (104-107) has led to increased availability of surgical specimens and data on incidence and prevalence of this precursor that can help inform our understanding of the natural history of ovarian cancer (108). Health policymakers and Obstetrics and Gynecology societies in Canada, the United States, and elsewhere formally recommend opportunistic salpingectomy as a preventive strategy (109,110), with favorable safety data in place and mortality data forthcoming (111). Based on retrospective data regarding the effect of salpingectomy on ovarian cancer incidence, several prevention approaches have been explored in cost-effectiveness modeling studies, including opportunistic salpingectomy at the time of tubal ligation, cesarean section, and hysterectomy. Analyses by Kwon et al and Dilley et al, performed without detailed natural history modeling, both found opportunistic salpingectomy to be dominant (less costly and more effective) when performed at the time of hysterectomy and cost-effective when performed at the time of elective surgical sterilization (112,113). Likewise, Venkatesh et al determined opportunistic salpingectomy at the time of cesarean delivery to be cost-effective compared to long-acting reversible contraception (114). In a subsequent, more granular Markov microsimulation model that incorporated population-based estimates of hysterectomy, ovarian cancer incidence, and death from other causes but did not fully model natural history, Naumann et al found that universal opportunistic salpingectomy at hysterectomy and sterilization would reduce ovarian cancer mortality by 6% and 8%, respectively, and result in substantial health care savings of $445 million annually in the United States (115). As population-based data on the mortality impacts of opportunistic salpingectomy programs begin to emerge (116), carefully developed models of the natural history of high-grade serous carcinomas will be an ideal tool for exploring the impact of changes in incidence due to such preventive approaches on treatment and other approaches to mortality reduction.

COST-EFFECTIVENESS OF THERAPEUTICS IN GYNECOLOGIC CANCERS

In the next section, an overview of the value and cost-effectiveness literature regarding therapeutic interventions for gynecologic malignancies is provided.

Ovarian Cancer

Chemotherapy for newly diagnosed ovarian cancer The standard treatment for ovarian cancer remains primary surgical staging with maximum possible cytoreduction followed by chemotherapy. However, prospective RCTs have demonstrated comparable OS and fewer surgical complications with neoadjuvant chemotherapy (NACT) with interval debulking surgery (IDS) (117,118). Cost-effectiveness modeling based on retrospectively collected SEER-Medicare data has suggested that primary debulking surgery (PDS) is cost-effective for women with stage IIIC ovarian cancer, with an ICER of $19,359/QALY (119). Conversely, a model based on RCT data found NACT to be a cost-saving treatment compared to PDS for patients with ovarian cancer greater than 65 years of age. However, in sensitivity analysis, assumptions of small increases in OS by 1.5 months or moderate declines in QoL with NACT resulted in PDS becoming a cost-effective option for this older population (120).

Introduction of taxanes The first cost-effectiveness studies in ovarian cancer chemotherapy were performed in response to the introduction of taxanes into the frontline chemotherapy regimen for this disease (121-123). When first introduced, paclitaxel-cisplatin was a more costly therapy than the old standard of cyclophosphamide-cisplatin. A number of cost-effectiveness investigations were performed using data from GOG 111. From the perspective of a U.S. oncology practice, the total drug costs for cisplatin plus paclitaxel were four times higher than those for cisplatin plus cyclophosphamide (US$9,918 vs US$2,527; year of costing not specified) (124). Compared with cisplatin plus cyclophosphamide, the incremental costs per year of life gained for cisplatin plus paclitaxel therapy were US$19,820 for inpatient treatment and US$21,222 for outpatient treatment. These incremental costs fall well within the generally accepted cost-effective range for new therapies. Carboplatin and paclitaxel are now both marketed as generics; older cost studies are, therefore, less applicable than when originally published. Given the current low cost of paclitaxel, any clinically superior regimen using this drug is also likely to be cost-effective.

Hyperthermic intraperitoneal chemotherapy (HIPEC) In the randomized open-label phase III OVHIPEC trial, the addition of HIPEC to IDS improved recurrence-free survival and OS in patients with stage III ovarian cancer (125). On the basis of the trial data, treatment with IDS and HIPEC in patients with stage III ovarian cancer was accompanied by a substantial gain in QALYs. Using U.S.-based costs, IDS and HIPEC was highly cost-effective, with an ICER of $2,436/QALY compared to IDS alone. In one-way sensitivity analyses, the probability of ostomy reversal and use of HIPEC at secondary cytoreduction did not substantially impact the cost-effectiveness of IDS and HIPEC (126).

Bevacizumab Bevacizumab is an anti-vascular endothelial growth factor (VEGF) inhibitor of angiogenesis and is FDA approved for the treatment of a number of different cancers, including platinum-resistant ovarian cancer. With regard to the primary treatment of ovarian cancer, the ICON 7 and GOG 218 phase III clinical trials of newly diagnosed ovarian cancer independently and simultaneously reported a small 2- to 6-month OS advantage to the addition of bevacizumab to primary combination carboplatin/paclitaxel, followed by 14 to 22 additional cycles of consolidation bevacizumab in the absence of progression (127,128). Even before the initial presentation of these data in ovarian cancer, questions were raised about the cost of universal bevacizumab. Cohn et al performed CEAs examining the likely clinical benefit of bevacizumab and the cost of the drug as well as its associated adverse events. These analyses demonstrated that there was no reasonable scenario under which bevacizumab could be considered cost-effective by existing measures (129,130). A subset analysis of the ICON 7 data revealed that the main benefit of bevacizumab appears to be confined to women with high-risk disease, such as those suboptimally cytoreduced and those with stage IV disease (127). Although, ideally, treatment of a smaller subset of women with ovarian cancer who are most likely to benefit would make this drug more cost-effective, attempts at modeling this scenario did not demonstrate this to be a cost-effective alternative (131).

Maintenance therapy Consolidation regimens that have been studied for ovarian cancer include paclitaxel, bevacizumab, and PARPi; all have a proven PFS benefit, but none has demonstrated an OS benefit in maintenance therapy following frontline chemotherapy. Lesnock et al performed a CEA of consolidation therapies following carboplatin/paclitaxel, comparing 12 months additional paclitaxel to 17 cycles additional bevacizumab. Clinical data were derived from the PFS results of GOG 178 and GOG 218. Consolidation therapy with paclitaxel was found to be cost-effective; bevacizumab consolidation was dominated (less effective and more costly) by paclitaxel consolidation (132). Gonzalez et al compared the cost of two frontline PARPi maintenance strategies, PARPi-for-all and biomarker-directed PARPi maintenance, using modified Markov decision models simulating the study designs of the PRIMA, VELIA, and, PAOLA-1 trials. PARPi-for-all was more costly and provided greater overall PFS benefit than a biomarker-directed PARPi strategy for each trial. However, the ICERs of PARPi-for-all compared to biomarker-directed PAPRi were $593,250/QA-PFY (PRIMA), $1,512,495/QA-PFY (VELIA), and $3,347,915/QA-PFY (PAOLA-1). At current drug pricing, there is no PFS improvement in a biomarker negative cohort that would make PARPi-for-all cost-effective compared to biomarker-directed maintenance (133).

Treatment of recurrent ovarian cancer Most women with ovarian cancer will achieve clinical remission following primary treatment but will eventually experience recurrence.

Platinum-sensitive recurrence Patients who experience recurrence more than 6 months after completing a first-line chemotherapy regimen are considered to have "platinum-sensitive" ovarian cancer and have an excellent response rate when retreated with platinum agents (134,135). Two large RCTs identified a PFS advantage for the combination regimens of gemcitabine plus carboplatin and paclitaxel plus platinum chemotherapy regimens (as well as an OS advantage for paclitaxel plus platinum) compared to platinum alone, and these regimens now constitute standard of care (136,137). The cost-effectiveness of chemotherapy for platinum-sensitive disease is highly dependent on drug cost at the time of the analysis. For example, in one Markov state transition model, paclitaxel plus carboplatin (both available as generics at analysis) had an ICER of $15,564 per additional progression-free year compared to single-agent carboplatin, whereas gemcitabine (not generic) plus carboplatin had a less attractive ICER of $278,388 per additional progression-free year compared to paclitaxel plus carboplatin (138). Given the current lower cost status of most standard chemotherapy agents, an individual's prior adverse event profile is likely to be the most important factor in chemotherapy agent decisions for recurrent ovarian cancer.

Similar to the frontline setting, PARPi are not cost-effective as maintenance therapy for platinum-sensitive recurrence, highlighting the need to control drug pricing in the United States. Even for patients with a germline BRCA1/2 mutation, Smith et al demonstrated that maintenance therapy with olaparib is not cost-effective, with an ICER of $258,864 per PF-LYS. To achieve an ICER of less than $50,000, the cost of olaparib should be $2,500 or less per month. For wild-type BRCA1/2 patients, maintenance therapy with olaparib is also not cost-effective (139). Zhong et al found similar cost concerns with PARPi niraparib and olaparib, which extend not only PFS in patients with platinum-sensitive recurrent ovarian cancer but are also associated with high DACs and ICERs at or above $250,000 per progression-free life year (PF-LY) in this model. Dottino et al similarly found that maintenance PARPi therapy for platinum-sensitive recurrent ovarian cancer is not cost-effective. Biomarker-directed treatment of patients with germline BRCA mutation or with HRD tumors is the preferred strategy compared with a treat-all strategy (140).

Platinum-resistant recurrence Ovarian cancer that recurs within 6 months of completing a first-line chemotherapy regimen has a poor prognosis, with cure being very unlikely. Rocconi et al performed a CEA of treatment options for recurrent platinum-resistant ovarian cancer and concluded that only best supportive care (no chemotherapy) was clearly cost-effective, whereas second-line monotherapy was possibly marginally cost-effective (ICER $64,104/YLS) as well (141). Even without incorporation of toxicity rates and costs, the authors found that combination chemotherapy regimens were never cost-effective for platinum-resistant disease because of unfavorable ICERs.

Bevacizumab is FDA approved for platinum-resistant recurrent ovarian cancer based on the results of the AURELIA trial, which demonstrated superior PFS when bevacizumab was added to standard-of-care single-agent chemotherapy (23). Two published cost-effectiveness studies are conflicting, do not include a "best supportive care" strategy, and are dependent on assumptions about subsequent bevacizumab use in this clinical setting (142,143).

Wolford et al examined the cost of niraparib, rucaparib, and olaparib for treatment in platinum-resistant, recurrent ovarian cancer and found the modest clinical benefit with costs of these novel therapies remains cost prohibitive (144).

Cervical Cancer

Primary treatment The standard treatment of cervical cancer has been established for very early-stage and locally advanced-stage disease. However, there is continued debate over the appropriate treatment of stage IB2 disease (145). Current options include primary surgery with radical hysterectomy and lymphadenectomy followed by tailored chemoradiation (CR), primary CR, and primary CR followed by simple hysterectomy. The choice of therapy depends on many factors, including available resources, costs, patient characteristics, and physician and patient preferences.

Two groups developed health economic models to inform the treatment of stage IB2 cervical cancer. Rocconi et al developed a decision model with a third-party payer perspective to compare three strategies: (1) radical hysterectomy followed by tailored therapy, (2) primary CR, and (3) NACT followed by simple hysterectomy. Radical hysterectomy was the least costly strategy per survivor at $41,212; CR and NACT followed by simple hysterectomy cost

$43,197 and $72,613 per survivor, respectively (146). The authors concluded that radical hysterectomy is the most cost-effective treatment for stage IB2 cervical cancer.

In a second analysis, Jewell et al used a modified Markov state transition decision model from a third-party payer perspective to compare primary CR to primary radical hysterectomy with tailored adjuvant therapy (RH+TA) for the treatment of stage IB2 cervical cancer. Patients undergoing completed radical hysterectomy were divided into three risk groups to determine adjuvant treatment based on surgical pathologic risk features. Adverse events and their costs were included. The model predicted 5-year OS of 79.6% in the RH+TA arm and 78.9% in the CR arm. The mean cost of RH+TA was $27,840 compared to $21,403 for CR. The ICER comparing RH+TA to CR was $63,689 per additional YLS (147). While Rocconi et al found RH+TA to be the least expensive option, Jewell et al found that RH+TA was the costlier treatment option in the base case. The difference in the outcomes of the two decision models may be related to differences in assumptions about the frequency of adjuvant radiotherapy and in cost estimates for radiotherapy. These studies demonstrate how the assumptions, inputs, and design of a model are critical to its results.

Use of radiation therapy in cervical cancer Intracavitary radiation treatment is recognized to play a significant and important role in the standard radiotherapy treatment of cervical carcinoma. The majority of centers worldwide use either low-dose rate (LDR) or high-dose rate (HDR) methods. Randomized trials have confirmed the apparent equivalence of HDR and LDR in terms of the incidence of adverse effects, tumor control, and survival (148). HDR is becoming more prevalent, possibly based on its outpatient nature, the ability to treat a greater number of patients, the ability to treat tumors at different sites, and the perceived cost savings to the health care system due mainly to the outpatient nature of the treatment. However, HDR treatment costs per insertion are frequently greater than LDR. Jones et al undertook a formal analysis of LDR versus HDR brachytherapy from a Canadian hospital perspective (149). Fixed and direct costs arising from equipment purchases, equipment maintenance fees, patient care, and operating costs including the staff, hospitalization, and operating room costs of LDR and HDR insertions were incorporated into a cost model. This study demonstrated that the LDR technique is less expensive when treating up to 80 patients per year. However, the ability to treat a significantly greater number of patients and the potential to treat other sites made the use of an HDR unit a more reasonable choice for high-volume centers where over 80 patients with cervical cancer are treated annually.

Recurrence and metastasis Following the publication of the phase 3 GOG 240 trial, which demonstrated a significant, 3.7-month OS advantage to incorporation of bevacizumab into the chemotherapy treatment of advanced and recurrent cervical cancer, several authors have assessed the economic impact of bevacizumab in cervical cancer treatment. Minion et al developed a Markov-based decision model and estimated the ICER of therapy with bevacizumab to be $295,164/QALY (150). Phippen et al performed a similar analysis, identifying an ICER of $155,000/QALY (151). Both groups identified the cost of bevacizumab as the main constraint on the cost-effectiveness of the new regimen.

Endometrial Cancer

Endometrial cancer is a disease in which outcomes research can be challenging; despite the high incidence of disease, the overall event rate (recurrence or death) is low. As such, RCTs for low- or intermediate-risk disease require a large number of subjects and long-term follow-up to demonstrate significance. CER approaches, therefore, may be quite relevant in endometrial cancer. CER in endometrial cancer spans aspects of surgical management, the use of adjuvant radiation and chemotherapy, surveillance for disease recurrence, and the evaluation and management of individuals at risk for or diagnosed with Lynch syndrome–associated cancers.

Preoperative testing The use of preoperative imaging in patients with clinical stage I endometrial cancer has, in certain circumstances, been demonstrated to identify disease that might not be amenable to resection. While certain authors supported the strategy of preoperative CT in patients planned to undergo surgery for endometrial cancer, others questioned the effectiveness and cost of this intervention. Bansal et al performed a study evaluating patients with endometrial cancer who underwent a preoperative CT of the abdomen and pelvis (152). In seven (3%) of 250 patients, the CT results led to an alteration of the surgical plan. In patients with high-risk histology (serous, clear cell, and sarcoma), the plan was changed in up to 13% of cases. When the cost of imaging was incorporated into their model, the authors estimated that more than $17,000 was expended to alter the management of one patient. As such, the authors argued that routine preoperative CT in patients with clinical stage I endometrial cancer was not cost-effective (see **Table 12.2-1**).

Laparotomy versus minimally invasive surgery Over the past few decades, minimally invasive surgery has been incorporated into the management of many malignancies, including endometrial cancer. Randomized trials of laparotomy versus laparoscopy were reported from the Netherlands (153), Australia (154), and the United States (155), all demonstrating similar oncologic outcomes between groups. These trials demonstrated that laparoscopy was associated with a modest improvement in QoL compared to laparotomy (156,157). Investigators from the Netherlands evaluated the cost of treatment relative to survival and QoL of subjects undergoing laparotomy or laparoscopic staging of their endometrial cancer (158). Despite a slightly increased cost for minimally invasive surgery (higher operative costs but lower hospital stay costs), total laparoscopic hysterectomy remained cost-effective because of the low rate of complications seen in the minimally invasive arm compared with laparotomy. This group also performed a meta-analysis of 12

trials of laparoscopic endometrial cancer surgery and reached the conclusion that laparoscopy was cost-effective compared to laparotomy (43).

Laparoscopy versus robot-assisted laparoscopy In 2006, the FDA cleared the first computer-aided (robotic) surgical system for hysterectomy. There has subsequently been a rapid incorporation of robotic surgery into gynecologic cancer practices, mainly for the treatment of endometrial cancer. Initial reports of this surgical approach demonstrated feasibility and acceptable toxicity. However, the initial purchase price of the robot (>$1 million), yearly maintenance contract (>$100,000 annually), and limited use of disposable instruments add a fixed cost to this procedure over laparoscopy or laparotomy. Given the expense of robotic surgery, analyses of the cost of robotic surgery have been published, often with differing conclusions. Initially, Bell et al described a series of patients who underwent abdominal, laparoscopic, or robotic staging for endometrial cancer, with the robotic approach being found less costly compared with laparotomy, but not significantly more expensive than laparoscopy (159). Subsequent to this report, other approaches have been utilized to assess the cost-effectiveness and comparative effectiveness of robotic surgery compared to other surgical approaches. Barnett et al utilized decision modeling from the perspectives of both society and the hospital (with and without the cost of the purchase of the robot incorporated) to assess the impact of surgical approach (laparotomy, laparoscopy, and robotic) for staging of endometrial cancer (40). These authors concluded that although laparoscopy is the least expensive approach, the decreased societal cost associated with an early return to normal function makes robotic surgery less expensive than laparotomy. In sensitivity analysis, when the costs of disposable instruments and equipment are minimized to less than one-half their current cost, robotic surgery becomes the least costly approach. The modeling approach with sensitivity analyses is critically important in helping to understand which factors drive cost in endometrial cancer surgery and to acknowledge that the perspective from which the analysis is taken significantly impacts the conclusions that can be drawn. In addition, a population-based CER analysis was undertaken by Wright et al describing more than 2,400 women who underwent minimally invasive surgery for endometrial cancer, 58% robotically and 42% laparoscopically (160). These authors found similar rates of complications but an increased cost with robotic surgery and concluded that longer term outcome data regarding robotic surgery are necessary before this approach should be considered standard for the management of endometrial cancer. Collectively, the data regarding robotic endometrial cancer surgery suggest an increased cost, decreased morbidity compared with laparotomy, and cost-effectiveness that varies based on the perspective from which the data are interpreted.

Lymphadenectomy for surgical staging Following two randomized trials suggesting that lymphadenectomy for unselected endometrial cancer does not improve survival outcomes (161,162), the role of this procedure in the routine management of endometrial cancer has undergone increased scrutiny. Various strategies have been proposed to identify patients who are at the highest risk for metastasis to the lymph nodes, generally incorporating tumor grade, depth of myometrial invasion, histology, and tumor size. Kwon et al found that as tumor grade increases, lymphadenectomy is more cost-effective than its omission, mainly due to the reduced rate of radiation in node-negative patients (163). Modeling of grade 3 endometrial cancer by Havrilesky et al demonstrated that lymph node dissection had an ICER of $40,183/QALY compared to no lymph node dissection (164). Cohn et al modeled grade 1 cancers and found that even in this group of patients at low risk for lymph node metastasis, routine lymphadenectomy was cost-effective compared to a strategy of selective lymphadenectomy, based on the assumption of a lower rate of adjuvant radiation in the surgically staged patients (165). Conversely, Lee et al demonstrated that when preoperative prediction models classified patients as low risk, selective lymphadenectomy was less costly

■ **TABLE 12.2-1. Utility Scores Elicited From Members of the Public and Cervical Cancer Survivors for Health States Related to the Treatment of Newly Diagnosed Cervical Cancer**

Rank	Treatment	Mean	95% Confidence Intervals
1	Minimally invasive radical hysterectomy No adjuvant treatment	0.94	0.89-0.99
2	Radical hysterectomy Low-risk features No adjuvant treatment	0.89	0.82-0.97
3	Radical hysterectomy Intermediate-risk features No adjuvant treatment	0.89	0.82-0.96
4	Radical hysterectomy Intermediate-risk features Adjuvant chemoradiation	0.80	0.72-0.89
5	Radical hysterectomy High-risk features Adjuvant chemoradiation High-dose rate brachytherapy	0.78	0.69-0.87
6	Primary chemoradiation	0.76	0.66-0.85
7	Aborted radical hysterectomy due to the extent of disease Primary chemoradiation	0.68	0.57-0.79

Reprinted from value in health, 14/4, Jewell, et al. Utility scores and treatment preferences for clinical early-stage cervical cancer, 582-586, with permission from Elsevier.

and more effective than routine lymphadenectomy (166). Havrilesky et al modeled a hypothetical test that could reliably predict lymph node metastasis, finding that such a test could be cost-effective as long as it was fairly inexpensive (167). Collectively, the cost-effectiveness data suggest that strategies to select a high-risk group for lymphadenectomy are more likely to be cost-effective. Sentinel lymph node mapping is a technique now adopted into routine endometrial cancer staging that reduces the number of lymph nodes removed while retaining sensitivity to identify metastatic disease (168). Suidan et al demonstrated that sentinel lymph node mapping compared with routine and selective lymphadenectomy has the lowest costs and highest quality-adjusted survival, making it the most cost-effective strategy in the management of low-risk endometrial carcinoma (169).

Surveillance for endometrial cancer recurrence Given that the OS of women with endometrial cancer is approximately 85%, investigators have challenged the notion that routine intermittent surveillance for pelvic examination and vaginal cytology (with or without chest imaging) is cost-effective or even necessary for most women with endometrial cancer. In support of the trend toward decreased intensity of surveillance, it has been estimated that the cost of routine vaginal cytology to identify a single asymptomatic recurrence is more than $44,000 (170). Whether the identification of these asymptomatic individuals leads to improved outcomes is even less certain (171).

Immunotherapy Immunotherapy regimens have emerged as a mainstay of treatment of endometrial cancer recurrence, with FDA-approved treatment regimens dependent on the microsatellite stability (MSS) or instability (MSI) of the tumor. A model to evaluate the cost-effectiveness of pembrolizumab compared to pegylated liposomal doxorubicin (PLD) or bevacizumab for the treatment of women with recurrent endometrial cancer after failing carboplatin and paclitaxel was created by Barrington et al For MSI-high patients, pembrolizumab was within cost-effective range compared to PLD, whereas bevacizumab was subjected to extended dominance. For patients with MSI-high recurrent endometrial cancers who have failed first-line chemotherapy, pembrolizumab is cost-effective relative to other single-agent drugs (172). In a subsequent analysis, the same authors found that the combination of pembrolizumab and lenvatinib is not cost-effective for MSS recurrences (173).

Lynch syndrome It is estimated that 2.3% of patients with endometrial cancer have Lynch syndrome as the cause of their disease (174). Given the relatively low prevalence of the disease, the ability to distinguish these patients from all those with sporadic disease would be enormously beneficial, as the probands and their families could be introduced to prevention and screening interventions that might decrease the risk of dying from Lynch-related malignancies. However, the clinical Amsterdam criteria are relatively insensitive and nonspecific in identifying Lynch syndrome. Thus, many institutions have begun utilizing IHC for the DNA mismatch repair genes as an initial screen for Lynch syndrome. Health economic studies of this strategy have demonstrated that utilizing IHC in patients with a first-degree relative with a Lynch-associated cancer is cost-effective (175). Other investigators have shown that the routine use of IHC with genetic testing for patients, with a triage to genetic testing based on a proband's age less than 60 years, is cost-effective compared to other screening strategies (176). In addition, the cost-effectiveness of strategies to prevent the disease in probands with known Lynch syndrome has been evaluated. Kwon et al demonstrated that in this population, annual surveillance with endometrial biopsy, pelvic ultrasound, and CA-125 at 30 years plus risk-reducing hysterectomy and oophorectomy at 40 years is the most effective strategy, though substantially more expensive than preventative surgery alone or screening alone, with an additional $194,000 spent per increase in year of survival compared to the next best strategy (177). The cost-effectiveness of risk-reducing surgery has also been confirmed by Yang et al, who demonstrated that this intervention is more cost-effective than either yearly examination or yearly invasive screening for malignancy (178).

CHAPTER SUMMARY

Gynecologic oncology provides a rich opportunity to investigate the cost-effectiveness and value of various diagnostic, therapeutic, screening, and preventative strategies. Although the field is still relatively young, substantial knowledge about these strategies has been gained through CER techniques and modeling. Continued investigation with refinement of tools for the investigation of value-based gynecologic cancer care is needed to advance the state of knowledge.

KEY POINTS

1. There is increasing pressure on health systems and providers in the United States to demonstrate "value," as defined by high-quality and cost-effective care.
2. CER provides the framework for studies that compare the potential harms and benefits of strategies to prevent, diagnose, or treat gynecologic malignancy.
3. Health economic studies, including CEA and CUA, compare medical interventions on the basis of their relative costs as well as their potential harms and benefits.
4. A key factor in the development of a cost-utility model is the incorporation of QoL, which requires a preference-based utility. The utility may be derived using a variety of QoL-related instruments. The use of the utility allows the results of a model to be expressed in QALYs, which are a standard effectiveness outcome.
5. The results of health economic decision models are highly dependent on their perspective and the assumptions made in their construction.
6. Uncertainty in health economic models is best described using multiple sensitivity analyses.
7. There is a growing body of evidence to guide clinical and resource allocation decisions in gynecologic oncology.

REFERENCES

1. United States Congress. Patient protection and affordable care act. 2009. https://www.congress.gov/111/plaws/publ148/PLAW-111publ148.pdf
2. Chandra A, Jena AB, Skinner JS. The pragmatist's guide to comparative effectiveness research. *J Econ Perspect.* 2011;25(2):27-46.
3. Porter ME. What is value in health care? *N Engl J Med.* 2010;363(26):2477-2481. doi:10.1056/NEJMp1011024
4. Society of General Internal Medicine (SGIM). Report of the National Commission on Physician Payment Reform. Accessed November 22, 2015. http://physicianpaymentcommission.org/wp-content/uploads/2013/03/physician_payment_report.pdf
5. United States Congress. Medicare access and CHIP reauthorization act of 2015. 2015. https://www.congress.gov/114/plaws/publ10/PLAW-114publ10.pdf
6. Abt Associates. Evaluation of the oncology care model: performance periods 1-5. 2021:1-5. https://innovation.cms.gov/data-and-reports/2021/ocm-evaluation-pp1-5
7. Keating NL, Jhatakia S, Brooks GA, et al. Association of participation in the oncology care model with Medicare payments, utilization, care delivery, and quality outcomes. *JAMA.* 2021;326(18):1829-1839. doi:10.1001/jama.2021.17642
8. Aviki EM, Schleicher SM, Boyd L, et al. The oncology care model and the future of alternative payment models: a gynecologic oncology perspective. *Gynecol Oncol.* 2021;162(3):529-531. doi:10.1016/j.ygyno.2021.07.014
9. Ko EM, Havrilesky LJ, Alvarez RD, et al. Society of gynecologic oncology future of physician payment reform task force report: the Endometrial Cancer Alternative Payment Model (ECAP). *Gynecol Oncol.* 2018;149(2):232-240. doi:10.1016/j.ygyno.2018.02.010
10. Wright JD, Havrilesky LJ, Cohn DE, et al. Estimating potential for savings for low risk endometrial cancer using the Endometrial Cancer Alternative Payment Model (ECAP): a companion paper to the society of gynecologic oncology report on the Endometrial Cancer Alternative

Payment Model. *Gynecol Oncol.* 2018;149(2):241-247. doi:10.1016/j.ygyno.2018.02.011

11. Liang MI, Aviki EM, Wright JD, et al. Society of gynecologic oncology future of physician payment reform task force: lessons learned in developing and implementing surgical alternative payment models. *Gynecol Oncol.* 2020;156(3):701-709. doi:10.1016/j.ygyno.2019.12.036

12. Schnipper LE, Davidson NE, Wollins DS, et al. American Society of Clinical Oncology Statement: a conceptual framework to assess the value of cancer treatment options. *J Clin Oncol.* 2015;33(23):2563-2577. doi:10.1200/JCO.2015.61.6706

13. Jencks SF, Williams MV, Coleman EA. Rehospitalizations among patients in the Medicare fee-for-service program. *N Engl J Med.* 2009;360(14):1418-1428. doi:10.1056/NEJMsa0803563

14. van Walraven C, Bennett C, Jennings A, Austin PC, Forster AJ. Proportion of hospital readmissions deemed avoidable: a systematic review. *CMAJ.* 2011;183(7):E391-E402. doi:10.1503/cmaj.101860

15. Centers for Medicare & Medicaid Services (US). Readmission reduction program. 2013. https://www.cms.gov/medicare/payment/prospective-payment-systems/acute-inpatient-pps/hospital-readmissions-reduction-program-hrrp

16. Centers for Medicare & Medicaid Services (US). Bundled Payments for Care Improvement (BPCI) initiative: general information. 2013. https://www.cms.gov/priorities/innovation/innovation-models/Bundled-Payments

17. Epstein AM. Revisiting readmissions—changing the incentives for shared accountability. *N Engl J Med.* 2009;360(14):1457-1459. doi:10.1056/NEJMe0901006

18. Hackbarth G, Reischauer R, Mutti A. Collective accountability for medical care—toward bundled Medicare payments. *N Engl J Med.* 2008;359(1):3-5. doi:10.1056/NEJMp0803749

19. Schnipper LE, Smith TJ, Raghavan D, et al. American society of clinical oncology identifies five key opportunities to improve care and reduce costs: the top five list for oncology. *J Clin Oncol.* 2012;30(14):1715-1724. doi:10.1200/JCO.2012.42.8375

20. Schnipper LE, Lyman GH, Blayney DW, et al. American society of clinical oncology 2013 top five list in oncology. *J Clin Oncol.* 2013;31(34):4362-4370. doi:10.1200/JCO.2013.53.3943

21. American Society of Clinical Oncology. Five things physicians and patients should question. ABIM Foundation. Updated October 31, 2013. Accessed January 6, 2015. https://www.surgonc.org/wp-content/uploads/2020/11/SSO-5things-List_2020-Updates-11-2020.pdf

22. Schnipper LE, Davidson NE, Wollins DS, et al. Updating the American society of clinical oncology value framework: revisions and reflections in response to comments received. *J Clin Oncol.* 2016;34:2925-2934. doi:10.1200/JCO.2016.68.2518

23. Pujade-Lauraine E, Hilpert F, Weber B, et al. Bevacizumab combined with chemotherapy for platinum-resistant recurrent ovarian cancer: the AURELIA open-label randomized phase III trial. *J Clin Oncol.* 2014;32(13):1302-1308. doi:10.1200/JCO.2013.51.4489

24. Foote J, Secord AA, Liang M, Cohn DE, Jewell E, Havrilesky LJ. ASCO value framework highlights the relative value of treatment options in ovarian cancer. *J Oncol Pract.* 2017;13(12):e1030-e1039. doi:10.1200/JOP.2017.025106

25. Cherny NI, Sullivan R, Dafni U, et al. A standardised, generic, validated approach to stratify the magnitude of clinical benefit that can be anticipated from anti-cancer therapies: the European Society for Medical Oncology Magnitude of Clinical Benefit Scale (ESMO-MCBS). *Ann Oncol.* 2015;26(8):1547-1573. doi:10.1093/annonc/mdv249

26. Cherny NI, de Vries EGE, Dafni U, et al. Comparative assessment of clinical benefit using the ESMO-magnitude of clinical benefit scale version 1.1 and the ASCO value framework net health benefit score. *J Clin Oncol.* 2019;37(4):336-349. doi:10.1200/JCO.18.00729

27. Foote JR, Secord AA, Liang MI, et al. Targeted composite value-based endpoints in platinum-sensitive recurrent ovarian cancer. *Gynecol Oncol.* 2019;152(3):445-451. doi:10.1016/j.ygyno.2018.11.028

28. Porter ME, Lee TH. The strategy that will fix health care. *Harvard Business Review* 91, 2013;10:50-70.

29. Yabroff KR, Mariotto A, Tangka F, et al. Annual report to the nation on the status of cancer, part 2: patient economic burden associated with cancer care. *J Natl Cancer Inst.* 2021;113(12):1670-1682. doi: 10.1093/jnci/djab192

30. Zafar SY, Abernethy AP. Financial toxicity, part I: a new name for a growing problem. *Oncology (Williston Park).* 2013;27(2):80-149.

31. Aviki EM, Manning-Geist BL, Sokolowski SS, et al. Risk factors for financial toxicity in patients with gynecologic cancer. *Am J Obstet Gynecol.* 2022;226:817.e1-817.e9. doi:10.1016/j.ajog.2021.12.012

32. Liang MI, Pisu M, Summerlin SS, et al. Extensive financial hardship among gynecologic cancer patients starting a new line of therapy. *Gynecol Oncol.* 2020;156(2):271-277. doi:10.1016/j.ygyno.2019.11.022

33. Esselen KM, Gompers A, Hacker MR, et al. Evaluating meaningful levels of financial toxicity in gynecologic cancers. *Int J Gynecol Cancer.* 2021;31(6):801-806. doi:10.1136/ijgc-2021-002475

34. Bouberhan S, Shea M, Kennedy A, et al. Financial toxicity in gynecologic oncology. *Gynecol Oncol.* 2019;154(1):8-12. doi:10.1016/j.ygyno.2019.04.003

35. Aviki EM, Thom B, Braxton K, et al. Patient-reported benefit from proposed interventions to reduce financial toxicity during cancer treatment. *Support Care Cancer.* 2022;30(3):2713-2721. doi:10.1007/s00520-021-06697-6

36. Altice CK, Banegas MP, Tucker-Seeley RD, Yabroff KR. Financial hardships experienced by cancer survivors: a systematic review. *J Natl Cancer Inst.* 2016;109(2):djw205. doi:10.1093/jnci/djw205

37. Drummond MF, Sculpher MJ, Torrance GW, O'Brien BJ, Stoddart GL. *Methods for the Economic Evaluation of Health Care Programmes.* 3rd ed. Oxford University Press; 2005:379 p.

38. National Institute for Health and Care Excellence. Guide to the methods of technology appraisal. 2013. https://www.nice.org.uk/process/pmg9/resources/guide-to-the-methods-of-technology-appraisal-2013-pdf-2007975843781

39. Gold M, Siegel J, Russell L, Weinstein M. *Cost-Effectiveness in Health and Medicine.* Oxford University Press; 1996.

40. Barnett JC, Judd JP, Wu JM, Scales CD Jr, Myers ER, Havrilesky LJ. Cost comparison among robotic, laparoscopic, and open hysterectomy for endometrial cancer. *Obstet Gynecol.* 2010;116(3):685-693. doi:10.1097/AOG.0b013e3181ee6e4d

41. Williams A. Priority setting in public and private health care. A guide through the ideological jungle. *J Health Econ.* 1988;7(2):173-183.

42. Husereau D, Drummond M, Augustovski F, et al. Consolidated health economic evaluation reporting standards 2022 (CHEERS 2022) statement: updated reporting guidance for health economic evaluations. *Int J Technol Assess Health Care.* 2022;38(1):e13. doi:10.1017/S0266462321001732

43. Bijen CB, Vermeulen KM, Mourits MJ, de Bock GH. Costs and effects of abdominal versus laparoscopic hysterectomy: systematic review of controlled trials. *PLoS ONE.* 2009;4(10):e7340. doi:10.1371/journal.pone.0007340

44. Petitti DB. *Meta-analysis, decision analysis, and cost-effectiveness analysis: methods for quantitative synthesis in medicine.* 2nd ed. *Monographs in Epidemiology and Biostatistics.* Oxford University Press; 2000:306 p.

45. Detsky AS, Naglie IG. A clinician's guide to cost-effectiveness analysis. *Ann Intern Med.* 1990;113(2):147-154.

46. Yabroff KR, Lamont EB, Mariotto A, et al. Cost of care for elderly cancer patients in the United States. *J Natl Cancer Inst.* 2008;100(9):630-641. doi:10.1093/jnci/djn103

47. Neumann PJ, Cohen JT, Weinstein MC. Updating cost-effectiveness—the curious resilience of the $50,000-per-QALY threshold. *N Engl J Med.* 2014;371(9):796-797. doi:10.1056/NEJMp1405158

48. Drummond MF, Sculpher MJ, Claxton K, Stoddart GL, Torrance GW. *Methods for the Economic Evaluation of Health Care Programmes.* 2nd ed. Oxford University Press; 1997.

49. Doubilet P, Begg CB, Weinstein MC, Braun P, McNeil BJ. Probabilistic sensitivity analysis using Monte Carlo simulation. A practical approach. *Med Decis Making.* 1985;5(2):157-177.

50. Ramsey S, Willke R, Briggs A, et al. Good research practices for cost-effectiveness analysis alongside clinical trials: the ISPOR RCT-CEA task force report. *Value Health.* 2005;8(5):521-533. doi:10.1111/j.1524-4733.2005.00045.x

51. Torrance GW. Utility approach to measuring health-related quality of life. *J Chronic Dis.* 1987;40(6):593-603.

52. Froberg DG, Kane RL. Methodology for measuring health-state preferences–II: scaling methods. *J Clin Epidemiol.* 1989;42(5):459-471. doi:10.1016/0895-4356(89)90136-4

53. Torrance GW. Measurement of health state utilities for economic appraisal. *J Health Econ.* 1986;5(1):1-30.

54. Ware JE Jr. Standards for validating health measures: definition and content. *J Chronic Dis.* 1987;40(6):473-480.

55. Torrance GW, Thomas WH, Sackett DL. A utility maximization model for evaluation of health care programs. *Health Serv Res.* 1972;7(2):118-133.

56. Llewellyn-Thomas H, Sutherland HJ, Tibshirani R, Ciampi A, Till JE, Boyd NF. The measurement of patients' values in medicine. *Med Decis Making.* 1982;2(4):449-462.

57. Brooks R. EuroQol: the current state of play. *Health Policy.* 1996;37(1):53-72. doi:10.1016/0168-8510(96)00822-6

58. Dolan P, Gudex C, Kind P, Williams A. The time trade-off method: results from a general population study. *Health Econ.* 1996;5(2):141-154. doi:10.1002/(SICI)1099-1050(199603)5:2<141::AID-HEC189>3.0.CO;2-N

59. Cella DF, Tulsky DS, Gray G, et al. The functional assessment of cancer therapy scale: development and validation of the general measure. *J Clin Oncol*. 1993;11(3):570-579.

60. Hess LM, Brady WE, Havrilesky LJ, et al. Comparison of methods to estimate health state utilities for ovarian cancer using quality of life data: a Gynecologic Oncology Group study. *Gynecol Oncol*. 2013;128(2):175-180. doi:10.1016/j.ygyno.2012.10.024

61. Ubel PA, Loewenstein G, Jepson C. Whose quality of life? A commentary exploring discrepancies between health state evaluations of patients and the general public. *Qual Life Res*. 2003;12(6):599-607.

62. Arnold D, Girling A, Stevens A, Lilford R. Comparison of direct and indirect methods of estimating health state utilities for resource allocation: review and empirical analysis. *BMJ*. 2009;339:b2688. doi:10.1136/bmj.b2688

63. Sonnenberg FA, Beck JR. Markov models in medical decision making: a practical guide. *Med Decis Making*. 1993;13(4):322-338.

64. Taylor DC, Pawar V, Kruzikas D, et al. Methods of model calibration: observations from a mathematical model of cervical cancer. *Pharmacoeconomics*. 2010;28(11):995-1000. doi:10.2165/11538660-000000000-00000

65. Choi YH, Jit M, Gay N, Cox A, Garnett GP, Edmunds WJ. Transmission dynamic modelling of the impact of human papillomavirus vaccination in the United Kingdom. *Vaccine*. 2010;28(24):4091-4102. doi:10.1016/j.vaccine.2009.09.125

66. Havrilesky LJ, Sanders GD, Kulasingam S, et al. Development of an ovarian cancer screening decision model that incorporates disease heterogeneity: implications for potential mortality reduction. *Cancer*. 2011;117:545-553.

67. Zauber AG, Lansdorp-Vogelaar I, Knudsen AB, Wilschut J, van Ballegooijen M, Kuntz KM. Evaluating test strategies for colorectal cancer screening: a decision analysis for the U.S. Preventive Services Task Force. *Ann Intern Med*. 2008;149(9):659-669. doi:10.7326/0003-4819-149-9-200811040-00244

68. Mandelblatt JS, Cronin KA, Bailey S, et al. Effects of mammography screening under different screening schedules: model estimates of potential benefits and harms. *Ann Intern Med*. 2009;151(10):738-747. doi:10.7326/0003-4819-151-10-200911170-00010

69. Eddy DM. The frequency of cervical cancer screening. Comparison of a mathematical model with empirical data. *Cancer*. 1987;60(5):1117-1122.

70. ACOG practice bulletin no. 109: cervical cytology screening. *Obstet Gynecol*. 2009;114(6):1409-1420. doi:10.1097/AOG.0b013e3181c6f8a4

71. Smith RA, Cokkinides V, Brooks D, Saslow D, Brawley OW. Cancer screening in the United States, 2010: a review of current American Cancer Society guidelines and issues in cancer screening. *CA Cancer J Clin*. 2010;60(2):99-119. doi:10.3322/caac.20063

72. Fontham ETH, Wolf AMD, Church TR, et al. Cervical cancer screening for individuals at average risk: 2020 guideline update from the American Cancer Society. *CA Cancer J Clin*. 2020;70(5):321-346. doi:10.3322/caac.21628

73. Malagon T, Kulasingam S, Mayrand MH, et al. Age at last screening and remaining lifetime risk of cervical cancer in older, unvaccinated, HPV-negative women: a modelling study. *Lancet Oncol*. 2018;19(12):1569-1578. doi:10.1016/S1470-2045(18)30536-9

74. Muhlberger N, Sroczynski G, Esteban E, Mittendorf T, Miksad RA, Siebert U. Cost-effectiveness of primarily human papillomavirus-based cervical cancer screening in settings with currently established Pap screening: a systematic review commissioned by the German Federal Ministry of Health. *Int J Technol Assess Health Care*. 2008;24(2):184-192. doi:10.1017/S0266462308080264

75. Goldhaber-Fiebert JD, Stout NK, Salomon JA, Kuntz KM, Goldie SJ. Cost-effectiveness of cervical cancer screening with human papillomavirus DNA testing and HPV-16,18 vaccination. *J Natl Cancer Inst*. 2008;100(5):308-320. doi:10.1093/jnci/djn019

76. Berkhof J, Coupe VM, Bogaards JA, et al. The health and economic effects of HPV DNA screening in The Netherlands. *Int J Cancer*. 2010;127(9):2147-2158. doi:10.1002/ijc.25211

77. Ogilvie GS, van Niekerk DJ, Krajden M, et al. A randomized controlled trial of Human Papillomavirus (HPV) testing for cervical cancer screening: trial design and preliminary results (HPV FOCAL Trial). *BMC Cancer*. 2010;10:111. doi:10.1186/1471-2407-10-111

78. Kim JJ, Burger EA, Regan C, Sy S. Screening for cervical cancer in primary care: a decision analysis for the US Preventive Services Task Force. *JAMA*. 2018;320(7):706-714. doi:10.1001/jama.2017.19872

79. US Preventive Services Task Force, Curry SJ, Krist AH, et al. Screening for cervical cancer: US Preventive Services Task Force recommendation statement. *JAMA*. 2018;320(7):674-686. doi:10.1001/jama.2018.10897

80. Dasbach EJ, Elbasha EH, Insinga RP. Mathematical models for predicting the epidemiologic and economic impact of vaccination against human papillomavirus infection and disease. *Epidemiol Rev*. 2006;28:88-100. doi:10.1093/epirev/mxj006

81. Garnett GP, Kim JJ, French K, Goldie SJ. Chapter 21: modelling the impact of HPV vaccines on cervical cancer and screening programmes. *Vaccine*. 2006;24(Suppl 3):S3/178-S3/186. doi:10.1016/j.vaccine.2006.05.116

82. Jit M, Demarteau N, Elbasha E, et al. Human papillomavirus vaccine introduction in low-income and middle-income countries: guidance on the use of cost-effectiveness models. *BMC Med*. 2011;9:54. doi:10.1186/1741-7015-9-54

83. Goldie SJ, O'Shea M, Campos NG, Diaz M, Sweet S, Kim SY. Health and economic outcomes of HPV 16,18 vaccination in 72 GAVI-eligible countries. *Vaccine*. 2008;26(32):4080-4093. doi:10.1016/j.vaccine.2008.04.053

84. Kim JJ, Goldie SJ. Cost effectiveness analysis of including boys in a human papillomavirus vaccination programme in the United States. *BMJ*. 2009;339:b3884. doi:10.1136/bmj.b3884

85. Centers for Disease Control and Prevention (CDC). FDA licensure of quadrivalent human papillomavirus vaccine (HPV4, Gardasil) for use in males and guidance from the Advisory Committee on Immunization Practices (ACIP). *MMWR Morb Mortal Wkly Rep*. 2010;59(20):630-632.

86. Brisson M. Cost-effectiveness of 9-valent HPV vaccination. Advisory Committee on Immunization Practices (ACIP) Summary Report. Accessed October 29-30, 2014:128-134. https://stacks.cdc.gov/view/cdc/61028

87. Food and Drug Administration. FDA approves expanded use of Gardasil 9 to include individuals 27 through 45 years old. Accessed March 30, 2022, https://www.fda.gov/news-events/press-announcements/fda-approves-expanded-use-gardasil-9-include-individuals-27-through-45-years-old

88. Meites E, Szilagyi PG, Chesson HW, Unger ER, Romero JR, Markowitz LE. Human papillomavirus vaccination for adults: updated recommendations of the advisory committee on immunization practices. *MMWR Morb Mortal Wkly Rep*. 2019;68(32):698-702. doi:10.15585/mmwr.mm6832a3

89. Machalek DA, Garland SM, Brotherton JML, et al. Very low prevalence of vaccine human papillomavirus types among 18- to 35-year-old Australian women 9 years following implementation of vaccination. *J Infect Dis*. 2018;217(10):1590-1600. doi:10.1093/infdis/jiy075

90. Australian Institute of Health and Welfare. Analysis of cervical cancer and abnormality outcomes in an era of cervical screening and HPV vaccination in Australia. Cancer series no. 126. Vol. CAN 129. 2019. https://www.aihw.gov.au/reports/cancer-screening/analysis-of-cervical-cancer-and-abnormality/contents/table-of-contents

91. Kjaer SK, Dehlendorff C, Belmonte F, Baandrup L. Real-world effectiveness of human papillomavirus vaccination against cervical cancer. *J Natl Cancer Inst*. 2021;113(10):1329-1335. doi:10.1093/jnci/djab080

92. Castanon A, Landy R, Pesola F, Windridge P, Sasieni P. Prediction of cervical cancer incidence in England, UK, up to 2040, under four scenarios: a modelling study. *Lancet Public Health*. 2018;3(1):e34-e43. doi:10.1016/S2468-2667(17)30222-0

93. Tully SP, Anonychuk AM, Sanchez DM, Galvani AP, Bauch CT. Time for change? An economic evaluation of integrated cervical screening and HPV immunization programs in Canada. *Vaccine*. 2012;30(2):425-435. doi:10.1016/j.vaccine.2011.10.067

94. Coupe VM, Bogaards JA, Meijer CJ, Berkhof J. Impact of vaccine protection against multiple HPV types on the cost-effectiveness of cervical screening. *Vaccine*. 2012;30(10):1813-1822. doi:10.1016/j.vaccine.2012.01.001

95. Kim JJ, Burger EA, Sy S, Campos NG. Optimal cervical cancer screening in women vaccinated against human papillomavirus. *J Natl Cancer Inst*. 2016;109(2):djw216. doi:10.1093/jnci/djw216

96. Bell J, Brady MF, Young RC, et al. Randomized phase III trial of three versus six cycles of adjuvant carboplatin and paclitaxel in early stage epithelial ovarian carcinoma: a Gynecologic Oncology Group study. *Gynecol Oncol*. 2006;102:432-439.

97. Buys SS, Partridge E, Greene MH, et al. Ovarian cancer screening in the Prostate, Lung, Colorectal and Ovarian (PLCO) cancer screening trial: findings from the initial screen of a randomized trial. *Am J Obstet Gynecol*. 2005;193(5):1630-1639.

98. Buys SS, Partridge E, Black A, et al. Effect of screening on ovarian cancer mortality: the Prostate, Lung, Colorectal and Ovarian (PLCO) cancer screening randomized controlled trial. *JAMA*. 2011;305(22):2295-2303. doi:10.1001/jama.2011.766

99. Menon U, Gentry-Maharaj A, Burnell M, et al. Ovarian cancer population screening and mortality after long-term follow-up in the UK Collaborative Trial of Ovarian Cancer Screening (UKCTOCS): a randomised controlled trial. *Lancet*. 2021;397(10290):2182-2193. doi:10.1016/S0140-6736(21)00731-5

100. Jacobs IJ, Menon U, Ryan A, et al. Ovarian cancer screening and mortality in the UK Collaborative Trial of Ovarian Cancer Screening

(UKCTOCS): a randomised controlled trial. *Lancet.* 2016;387(10022):945-956. doi:10.1016/S0140-6736(15)01224-6

101. Skates SJ, Singer DE. Quantifying the potential benefit of CA 125 screening for ovarian cancer. *J Clin Epidemiol.* 1991;44(4-5):365-380.

102. Urban N, Drescher C, Etzioni R, Colby C. Use of a stochastic simulation model to identify an efficient protocol for ovarian cancer screening. *Control Clin Trials.* 1997;18(3):251-270.

103. Havrilesky LJ, Sanders GD, Kulasingam S, Myers ER. Reducing ovarian cancer mortality through screening: Is it possible, and can we afford it? *Gynecol Oncol.* 2008;111:179-187.

104. Kurman RJ, Shih IeM. The origin and pathogenesis of epithelial ovarian cancer: a proposed unifying theory. *Am J Surg Pathol.* 2010;34(3):433-443. doi:10.1097/PAS.0b013e3181cf3d79

105. Berek JS, Kehoe ST, Kumar L, Friedlander M. Cancer of the ovary, fallopian tube, and peritoneum. *Int J Gynaecol Obstet.* 2018;143(Suppl 2):59-78. doi:10.1002/ijgo.12614

106. Liao CI, Chow S, Chen LM, Kapp DS, Mann A, Chan JK. Trends in the incidence of serous fallopian tube, ovarian, and peritoneal cancer in the US. *Gynecol Oncol.* 2018;149(2):318-323. doi:10.1016/j.ygyno.2018.01.030

107. Carlson JW, Miron A, Jarboe EA, et al. Serous tubal intraepithelial carcinoma: its potential role in primary peritoneal serous carcinoma and serous cancer prevention. *J Clin Oncol.* 2008;26(25):4160-4165. doi:10.1200/JCO.2008.16.4814

108. Sherman ME, Drapkin RI, Horowitz NS, et al. Rationale for developing a specimen bank to study the pathogenesis of high-grade serous carcinoma: a review of the evidence. *Cancer Prev Res (Phila).* 2016;9(9):713-720. doi:10.1158/1940-6207.CAPR-15-0384

109. ACOG Committee Opinion No. 774: opportunistic salpingectomy as a strategy for epithelial ovarian cancer prevention. *Obstet Gynecol.* 2019;133(4):e279-e284. doi:10.1097/AOG.0000000000003164

110. Salvador S, Scott S, Francis JA, Agrawal A, Giede C. No. 344-opportunistic salpingectomy and other methods of risk reduction for ovarian/fallopian tube/peritoneal cancer in the general population. *J Obstet Gynaecol Can.* 2017;39(6):480-493. doi:10.1016/j.jogc.2016.12.005

111. Hanley GE, Kwon JS, McAlpine JN, Huntsman DG, Finlayson SJ, Miller D. Examining indicators of early menopause following opportunistic salpingectomy: a cohort study from British Columbia, Canada. *Am J Obstet Gynecol.* 2020;223(2):221.e1-221.e11. doi:10.1016/j.ajog.2020.02.005

112. Dilley SE, Havrilesky LJ, Bakkum-Gamez J, et al. Cost-effectiveness of opportunistic salpingectomy for ovarian cancer prevention. *Gynecol Oncol.* 2017;146(2):373-379. doi:10.1016/j.ygyno.2017.05.034

113. Kwon JS, McAlpine JN, Hanley GE, et al. Costs and benefits of opportunistic salpingectomy as an ovarian cancer prevention strategy. *Obstet Gynecol.* 2015;125(2):338-345. doi:10.1097/AOG.0000000000000630

114. Venkatesh KK, Clark LH, Stamilio DM. Cost-effectiveness of opportunistic salpingectomy vs tubal ligation at the time of cesarean delivery. *Am J Obstet Gynecol.* 2019;220(1):106.e1-106.e10. doi:10.1016/j.ajog.2018.08.032

115. Naumann RW, Hughes BN, Brown J, Drury LK, Herzog TJ. The impact of opportunistic salpingectomy on ovarian cancer mortality and healthcare costs: a call for universal insurance coverage. *Am J Obstet Gynecol.* 2021;225(4):397.e1-397.e6. doi:10.1016/j.ajog.2021.03.032

116. Yoon SH, Kim SN, Shim SH, Kang SB, Lee SJ. Bilateral salpingectomy can reduce the risk of ovarian cancer in the general population: a meta-analysis. *Eur J Cancer.* 2016;55:38-46. doi:10.1016/j.ejca.2015.12.003

117. Fagotti A, Ferrandina G, Vizzielli G, et al. Phase III randomised clinical trial comparing primary surgery versus neoadjuvant chemotherapy in advanced epithelial ovarian cancer with high tumour load (SCORPION trial): final analysis of peri-operative outcome. *Eur J Cancer.* 2016;59:22-33. doi:10.1016/j.ejca.2016.01.017

118. Vergote I, Trope CG, Amant F, et al. Neoadjuvant chemotherapy or primary surgery in stage IIIC or IV ovarian cancer. *N Engl J Med.* 2010;363(10):943-953. doi:10.1056/NEJMoa0908806

119. Forde GK, Chang J, Ziogas A. Cost-effectiveness of primary debulking surgery when compared to neoadjuvant chemotherapy in the management of stage IIIC and IV epithelial ovarian cancer. *ClinicoEcon Outcomes Res.* 2016;8:397-406. doi:10.2147/CEOR.S91844

120. Rowland MR, Lesnock JL, Farris C, Kelley JL, Krivak TC. Cost-utility comparison of neoadjuvant chemotherapy versus primary debulking surgery for treatment of advanced-stage ovarian cancer in patients 65 years old or older. *Am J Obstet Gynecol.* 2015;212(6):763.763.e1-763.e8. doi:10.1016/j.ajog.2015.01.053

121. McGuire WP, Hoskins WJ, Brady MF, et al. Cyclophosphamide and cisplatin compared with paclitaxel and cisplatin in patients with stage III and stage IV ovarian cancer. *N Engl J Med.* 1996;334(1):1-6.

122. Piccart MJ, Bertelsen K, James K, et al. Randomized intergroup trial of cisplatin-paclitaxel versus cisplatin-cyclophosphamide in women with advanced epithelial ovarian cancer: three-year results. *J Natl Cancer Inst.* 2000;92(9):699-708.

123. Piccart MJ, Bertelsen K, Stuart G, et al. Long-term follow-up confirms a survival advantage of the paclitaxel-cisplatin regimen over the cyclophosphamide-cisplatin combination in advanced ovarian cancer. *Int J Gynecol Cancer.* 2003;13(Suppl 2):144-148. doi:10.1111/j.1525-1438.2003.13357.x

124. McGuire W, Neugut AI, Arikian S, Doyle J, Dezii CM. Analysis of the cost-effectiveness of paclitaxel as alternative combination therapy for advanced ovarian cancer. *J Clin Oncol.* 1997;15(2):640-645.

125. van Driel WJ, Koole SN, Sikorska K, et al. Hyperthermic intraperitoneal chemotherapy in ovarian cancer. *N Engl J Med.* 2018;378(3):230-240. doi:10.1056/NEJMoa1708618

126. Lim SL, Havrilesky LJ, Habib AS, Secord AA. Cost-effectiveness of hyperthermic intraperitoneal chemotherapy (HIPEC) at interval debulking of epithelial ovarian cancer following neoadjuvant chemotherapy. *Gynecol Oncol.* 2019;153(2):376-380. doi:10.1016/j.ygyno.2019.01.025

127. Perren TJ, Swart AM, Pfisterer J, et al. A phase 3 trial of bevacizumab in ovarian cancer. *N Engl J Med.* 2011;365(26):2484-2496. doi:10.1056/NEJMoa1103799

128. Burger RA, Brady MF, Bookman MA, et al. Incorporation of bevacizumab in the primary treatment of ovarian cancer. *N Engl J Med.* 2011;365(26):2473-2483. doi:10.1056/NEJMoa1104390

129. Cohn DE, Kim KH, Resnick KE, O'Malley DM, Straughn JM Jr. At what cost does a potential survival advantage of bevacizumab make sense for the primary treatment of ovarian cancer? A cost-effectiveness analysis. *J Clin Oncol.* 2011;29(10):1247-1251. doi:10.1200/JCO.2010.32.1075

130. Cohn DE, Barnett JC, Wenzel L, et al. A cost-utility analysis of NRG Oncology/Gynecologic Oncology Group Protocol 218: incorporating prospectively collected quality-of-life scores in an economic model of treatment of ovarian cancer. *Gynecol Oncol.* 2015;136(2):293-299. doi:10.1016/j.ygyno.2014.10.020

131. Barnett JC, Alvarez-Secord A, Cohn D, et al. Cost-effectiveness of a predictive biomarker for bevacizumab responsiveness in the primary treatment of ovarian cancer. *Gynecol Oncol.* 2012;125(Supp 1):S66.

132. Lesnock JL, Farris C, Krivak TC, Smith KJ, Markman M. Consolidation paclitaxel is more cost-effective than bevacizumab following upfront treatment of advanced epithelial ovarian cancer. *Gynecol Oncol.* 2011;122(3):473-478. doi:10.1016/j.ygyno.2011.05.014

133. Gonzalez R, Havrilesky LJ, Myers ER, et al. Cost-effectiveness analysis comparing "PARP inhibitors-for-all" to the biomarker-directed use of PARP inhibitor maintenance therapy for newly diagnosed advanced stage ovarian cancer. *Gynecol Oncol.* 2020;159(2):483-490. doi:10.1016/j.ygyno.2020.08.003

134. Rose PG, Fusco N, Fluellen L, Rodriguez M. Second-line therapy with paclitaxel and carboplatin for recurrent disease following first-line therapy with paclitaxel and platinum in ovarian or peritoneal carcinoma. *J Clin Oncol.* 1998;16(4):1494-1497.

135. Dizon DS, Hensley ML, Poynor EA, et al. Retrospective analysis of carboplatin and paclitaxel as initial second-line therapy for recurrent epithelial ovarian carcinoma: application toward a dynamic disease state model of ovarian cancer. *J Clin Oncol.* 2002;20(5):1238-1247.

136. Parmar MK, Ledermann JA, Colombo N, et al. Paclitaxel plus platinum-based chemotherapy versus conventional platinum-based chemotherapy in women with relapsed ovarian cancer: the ICON4/AGO-OVAR-2.2 trial. *Lancet.* 2003;361(9375):2099-2106.

137. Pfisterer J, Plante M, Vergote I, et al. Gemcitabine plus carboplatin compared with carboplatin in patients with platinum-sensitive recurrent ovarian cancer: an intergroup trial of the AGO-OVAR, the NCIC CTG, and the EORTC GCG. *J Clin Oncol.* 2006;24(29):4699-4707.

138. Havrilesky LJ, Secord AA, Kulasingam S, Myers E. Management of platinum-sensitive recurrent ovarian cancer: a cost-effectiveness analysis. *Gynecol Oncol.* 2007;107(2):211-218.

139. Smith HJ, Walters Haygood CL, Arend RC, Leath CA 3rd, Straughn JM Jr. PARP inhibitor maintenance therapy for patients with platinum-sensitive recurrent ovarian cancer: a cost-effectiveness analysis. *Gynecol Oncol.* 2015;139(1):59-62. doi:10.1016/j.ygyno.2015.08.013

140. Dottino JA, Moss HA, Lu KH, Secord AA, Havrilesky LJ. U.S. Food and Drug Administration-Approved Poly (ADP-Ribose) polymerase inhibitor maintenance therapy for recurrent ovarian cancer: a cost-effectiveness analysis. *Obstet Gynecol.* 2019;133(4):795-802. doi:10.1097/AOG.0000000000003171

141. Rocconi RP, Case AS, Straughn JM Jr, Estes JM, Partridge EE. Role of chemotherapy for patients with recurrent platinum-resistant advanced epithelial ovarian cancer: a cost-effectiveness analysis. *Cancer.* 2006;107(3):536-543.

142. Wysham WZ, Schaffer EM, Coles T, Roque DR, Wheeler SB, Kim KH. Adding bevacizumab to single agent chemotherapy for the treatment of platinum-resistant recurrent ovarian cancer: a cost effectiveness analysis of the AURELIA trial. *Gynecol Oncol.* 2017;145(2):340-345. doi:10.1016/j.ygyno.2017.02.039

143. Chappell NP, Miller C, Barnett J, Fielden A. Is FDA approved bevacizumab cost-effective in the setting of platinum-resistant recurrent ovarian cancer?. *Obstet Gynecol.* 2016;127(Suppl 1):6S-7S. doi:10.1097/01.AOG.0000483634.59394.2c

144. Wolford JE, Bai J, Moore KN, Kristeleit R, Monk BJ, Tewari KS. Cost-effectiveness of niraparib, rucaparib, and olaparib for treatment of platinum-resistant, recurrent ovarian carcinoma. *Gynecol Oncol.* 2020;157(2):500-507. doi:10.1016/j.ygyno.2020.02.030

145. Grigsby PW. Primary radiotherapy for stage IB or IIA cervical cancer. *J Natl Cancer Inst Monogr.* 1996;(21):61-64.

146. Rocconi RP, Estes JM, Leath CA 3rd, Kilgore LC, Huh WK, Straughn JM Jr. Management strategies for stage IB2 cervical cancer: a cost-effectiveness analysis. *Gynecol Oncol.* 2005;97(2):387-394.

147. Jewell EL, Kulasingam S, Myers ER, Alvarez Secord A, Havrilesky LJ. Primary surgery versus chemoradiation in the treatment of IB2 cervical carcinoma: a cost effectiveness analysis. *Gynecol Oncol.* 2007;107(3):532-540. doi:10.1016/j.ygyno.2007.08.056

148. Shigematsu Y, Nishiyama K, Masaki N, et al. Treatment of carcinoma of the uterine cervix by remotely controlled afterloading intracavitary radiotherapy with high-dose rate: a comparative study with a low-dose rate system. *Int J Radiat Oncol Biol Phys.* 1983;9(3):351-356.

149. Jones G, Lukka H, O'Brien B. High dose rate versus low dose rate brachytherapy for squamous cell carcinoma of the cervix: an economic analysis. *Br J Radiol.* 1994;67(803):1113-1120.

150. Minion LE, Bai J, Monk BJ, et al. A Markov model to evaluate cost-effectiveness of antiangiogenesis therapy using bevacizumab in advanced cervical cancer. *Gynecol Oncol.* 2015;137(3):490-496. doi:10.1016/j.ygyno.2015.02.027

151. Phippen NT, Leath CA 3rd, Havrilesky LJ, Barnett JC. Bevacizumab in recurrent, persistent, or advanced stage carcinoma of the cervix: is it cost-effective? *Gynecol Oncol.* 2015;136(1):43-47. doi:10.1016/j.ygyno.2014.11.003

152. Bansal N, Herzog TJ, Brunner-Brown A, et al. The utility and cost effectiveness of preoperative computed tomography for patients with uterine malignancies. *Gynecol Oncol.* 2008;111(2):208-212. doi:10.1016/j.ygyno.2008.08.001

153. Mourits MJ, Bijen CB, Arts HJ, et al. Safety of laparoscopy versus laparotomy in early-stage endometrial cancer: a randomised trial. *Lancet Oncol.* 2010;11(8):763-771. doi:10.1016/S1470-2045(10)70143-1

154. Kondalsamy-Chennakesavan S, Janda M, Gebski V, et al. Risk factors to predict the incidence of surgical adverse events following open or laparoscopic surgery for apparent early stage endometrial cancer: results from a randomised controlled trial. *Eur J Cancer.* 2012;48:2155-2162. doi:10.1016/j.ejca.2012.03.013

155. Walker JL, Piedmonte MR, Spirtos NM, et al. Recurrence and survival after random assignment to laparoscopy versus laparotomy for comprehensive surgical staging of uterine cancer: Gynecologic Oncology Group LAP2 Study. *J Clin Oncol.* 2012;30(7):695-700. doi:10.1200/JCO.2011.38.8645

156. Janda M, Gebski V, Brand A, et al. Quality of life after total laparoscopic hysterectomy versus total abdominal hysterectomy for stage I endometrial cancer (LACE): a randomised trial. *Lancet Oncol.* 2010;11(8):772-780. doi:10.1016/S1470-2045(10)70145-5

157. Kornblith AB, Huang HQ, Walker JL, Spirtos NM, Rotmensch J, Cella D. Quality of life of patients with endometrial cancer undergoing laparoscopic international federation of gynecology and obstetrics staging compared with laparotomy: a Gynecologic Oncology Group study. *J Clin Oncol.* 2009;27(32):5337-5342. doi:10.1200/JCO.2009.22.3529

158. Bijen CB, Vermeulen KM, Mourits MJ, et al. Cost effectiveness of laparoscopy versus laparotomy in early stage endometrial cancer: a randomised trial. *Gynecol Oncol.* 2011;121(1):76-82. doi:10.1016/j.ygyno.2010.11.043

159. Bell MC, Torgerson J, Seshadri-Kreaden U, Suttle AW, Hunt S. Comparison of outcomes and cost for endometrial cancer staging via traditional laparotomy, standard laparoscopy and robotic techniques. *Gynecol Oncol.* 2008;111(3):407-411. doi:10.1016/j.ygyno.2008.08.022

160. Wright JD, Burke WM, Wilde ET, et al. Comparative effectiveness of robotic versus laparoscopic hysterectomy for endometrial cancer. *J Clin Oncol.* 2012;30(8):783-791. doi:10.1200/JCO.2011.36.7508

161. Panici PB, Maggioni A, Hacker N, et al. Systematic aortic and pelvic lymphadenectomy versus resection of bulky nodes only in optimally debulked advanced ovarian cancer: a randomized clinical trial. *J Natl Cancer Inst.* 2005;97(8):560-566. doi:10.1093/jnci/dji102

162. Kitchener H, Swart AM, Qian Q, Amos C, Parmar MK. Efficacy of systematic pelvic lymphadenectomy in endometrial cancer (MRC ASTEC trial): a randomised study. *Lancet.* 2009;373(9658):125-136. doi:10.1016/S0140-6736(08)61766-3

163. Kwon JS, Carey MS, Goldie SJ, Kim JJ. Cost-effectiveness analysis of treatment strategies for stage I and II endometrial cancer. *J Obstet Gynaecol Can.* 2007;29(2):131-139.

164. Havrilesky LJ, Chino JP, Myers ER. How much is another randomized trial of lymph node dissection in endometrial cancer worth? A value of information analysis. *Gynecol Oncol.* 2013;131:140-146. doi:10.1016/j.ygyno.2013.06.025

165. Cohn DE, Huh WK, Fowler JM, Straughn JM Jr. Cost-effectiveness analysis of strategies for the surgical management of grade 1 endometrial adenocarcinoma. *Obstet Gynecol.* 2007;109(6):1388-1395. doi:10.1097/01.AOG.0000262897.21628.06

166. Lee JY, Cohn DE, Kim Y, et al. The cost-effectiveness of selective lymphadenectomy based on a preoperative prediction model in patients with endometrial cancer: insights from the US and Korean healthcare systems. *Gynecol Oncol.* 2014;135(3):518-524. doi:10.1016/j.ygyno.2014.09.020

167. Havrilesky LJ, Maxwell GL, Chan JK, Myers ER. Cost effectiveness of a test to detect metastases for endometrial cancer. *Gynecol Oncol.* 2009;112(3):526-530. doi:10.1016/j.ygyno.2008.11.017

168. Leitao MM Jr, Khoury-Collado F, Gardner G, et al. Impact of incorporating an algorithm that utilizes sentinel lymph node mapping during minimally invasive procedures on the detection of stage IIIC endometrial cancer. *Gynecol Oncol.* 2013;129(1):38-41. doi:10.1016/j.ygyno.2013.01.002

169. Suidan RS, Sun CC, Cantor SB, et al. Three lymphadenectomy strategies in low-risk endometrial carcinoma: a cost-effectiveness analysis. *Obstet Gynecol.* 2018;132(1):52-58. doi:10.1097/AOG.0000000000002677

170. Bristow RE, Purinton SC, Santillan A, Diaz-Montes TP, Gardner GJ, Giuntoli RL 2nd. Cost-effectiveness of routine vaginal cytology for endometrial cancer surveillance. *Gynecol Oncol.* 2006;103(2):709-713. doi:10.1016/j.ygyno.2006.05.013

171. Salani R, Backes FJ, Fung MF, et al. Posttreatment surveillance and diagnosis of recurrence in women with gynecologic malignancies: Society of Gynecologic Oncologists recommendations. *Am J Obstet Gynecol.* 2011;204(6):466-478. doi:10.1016/j.ajog.2011.03.008

172. Barrington DA, Dilley SE, Smith HJ, Straughn JM Jr. Pembrolizumab in advanced recurrent endometrial cancer: a cost-effectiveness analysis. *Gynecol Oncol.* 2019;153(2):381-384. doi:10.1016/j.ygyno.2019.02.013

173. Barrington DA, Haight PJ, Calhoun C, Tubbs C, Cohn DE, Bixel KL. Lenvatinib plus pembrolizumab in advanced recurrent endometrial cancer: a cost-effectiveness analysis. *Gynecol Oncol.* 2021;162(3):626-630. doi:10.1016/j.ygyno.2021.06.014

174. Hampel H, Panescu J, Lockman J, et al. Comment on: screening for lynch syndrome (Hereditary Nonpolyposis Colorectal Cancer) among endometrial cancer patients. *Cancer Res.* 2007;67(19):9603. doi:10.1158/0008-5472.CAN-07-2308

175. Kwon JS, Scott JL, Gilks CB, Daniels MS, Sun CC, Lu KH. Testing women with endometrial cancer to detect Lynch syndrome. *J Clin Oncol.* 2011;29(16):2247-2252. doi:10.1200/JCO.2010.32.9979

176. Resnick K, Straughn JM Jr, Backes F, Hampel H, Matthews KS, Cohn DE. Lynch syndrome screening strategies among newly diagnosed endometrial cancer patients. *Obstet Gynecol.* 2009;114(3):530-536. doi:10.1097/AOG.0b013e3181b11ecc

177. Kwon JS, Sun CC, Peterson SK, et al. Cost-effectiveness analysis of prevention strategies for gynecologic cancers in Lynch syndrome. *Cancer.* 2008;113(2):326-335. doi:10.1002/cncr.23554

178. Yang KY, Caughey AB, Little SE, Cheung MK, Chen LM. A cost-effectiveness analysis of prophylactic surgery versus gynecologic surveillance for women from hereditary non-polyposis colorectal cancer (HNPCC) families. *Fam Cancer.* 2011;10(3):535-543. doi:10.1007/s10689-011-9444-z

CHAPTER **12.3**

Perioperative and Critical Care

James J. Burke II, Ashley Valenzuela, and Katherine M. McBride

INTRODUCTION

Surgery remains the mainstay of the treatment for women with gynecologic malignancies, regardless of whether an open or minimally invasive approach is utilized. Ultimately, outcomes of the surgical intervention rest with the gynecologic oncologist in concert with anesthesiologists, nursing staff, stomal therapists, physical therapists, pharmacists, social workers, and the social network/support of the patient, as well as others. Careful assessment of the patient before surgery can lead to improved outcomes and minimize surprises in the postoperative period. Should the need arise, prudent consultation with other medical specialists before or following surgery can further enhance patient care and result in better outcomes.

The chapter is divided into two sections: preoperative care/risk recognition and postoperative care/critical care. Within each section, clinical information is arranged by organ system and recommendations are based upon available evidence. As has become the norm with hospitals in the United States, most intensive care units (ICUs) have become "closed"; meaning that when a patient is admitted to the ICU, the patient is cared for by a team lead by a critical care specialist/intensivist. Thus, the critical care section provides basic yet practical information for the reader so that co-management of the critically ill gynecologic oncology patient with an intensivist may be seamless.

PREOPERATIVE RISK ASSESSMENT

Initial Preoperative Evaluation

At the initial consultation for patients with known or suspected gynecologic malignancies, the gynecologic oncologist should take a thorough history, assessing for comorbid conditions, which may impact perioperative risk (1,2). Similarly, a thorough physical examination, looking for signs of diseases of which the patient is unaware, will aid in finding diseases that can impact surgical outcome. Review of accompanying medical records and radiographs is important. Ultimately, patients who will benefit from surgery are identified and will be deemed operative candidates, those who need further evaluation from specialists before surgery, or inoperable candidates.

In the 2001 landmark report, "Crossing the Quality Chasm," the IOM identified effective patient-clinician communication and sharing of information as critical to high-quality, patient-centered care (3). A proposed, potentially high-risk surgery is without a doubt an area where shared patient-surgeon decision-making is critical. Traditionally, the informed consent process was a unidirectional process that focused on disclosing the risks, benefits, and alternative options by the surgeon with little patient involvement. Shared decision-making, however, is a more collaborative approach to communication that incorporates patient's values and preferences while increasing their role in the decision. Informed decision-making is a key component of the shared decision-making process and focuses on how clinicians foster patient participation while providing patients information to reach treatment decisions. These two elements—informed consent and informed decision-making—must occur together.

The American College of Surgeons provides a description of the elements of informed consent in preparation for surgery in the Statement on Principles (which can be found at https://www.facs.org/about-acs/statements/stonprin#iia). According to the Statement:

> The informed consent discussion conducted by the surgeon should include: the nature of the illness and the natural consequences of no treatment; the nature of the proposed operation, including the estimated risks of mortality and morbidity; the more commonly known complications, which should be described and discussed; the patient should understand the risks as well as the benefits of the proposed operation; the discussion should include a description of what to expect during the hospitalization and posthospital convalescence; alternative forms of treatment, including nonoperative techniques; a discussion of the different types of qualified medical providers who will participate in their operation and their respective roles.

> From The American College of Surgeons provides a description of the elements of informed consent in preparation for surgery in the Statement on Principles (which can be found here: https://www.facs.org/about-acs/statements/stonprin#iia).

When discussing informed decision-making with the patient, nine measures have been developed by Braddock et al (4,5): (i) the patient's role in decision-making, (ii) the impact of the decision on the patient's daily life, (iii) the clinical issue or nature of the decision, (iv) alternative treatments, (v) the potential benefits and risks of each alternative, (vi) uncertainties surrounding the decision, (vii) the patient's understanding, (viii) the patient's preferences, and (ix) providing the opportunity to involve trusted others, such as family or friends. Taken altogether, informed consent and informed decision-making result in shared decision-making and subsequently improve high-quality patient care. However, a recent study has shown that this shared decision-making process falls short of fulfilling all of the aforementioned elements, leaving room for improvement (5). Some maybe concerned that fulfilling all of the abovementioned elements will take too much time at the consultation. However, that has not been shown in previous studies of the process (6).

Should further evaluation be needed from a specialist (eg, a cardiologist or a pulmonologist), a letter outlining the proposed surgical intervention should be sent to the consultant. However, the impact of these consultations, or "preoperative clearances," on perioperative outcomes is unclear (7-9).

If the patient's condition requires the possibility of a stoma(s) (ileostomy, colostomy, or urostomy), consultation with an enterostomal therapist for marking of the planned stoma(s) should be considered. During this visit, the therapist will take into account the location of the patient's waist, abdominal creases, how they wear their clothing, the types of clothing they wear, and the location of the future stoma when they stand or sit. In addition, the therapist can initiate education on the function and care of the stoma(s).

Should the proposed surgery result in a marked change of body image or possible sexual dysfunction (eg, exenteration, radical vulvectomy, or vaginal reconstruction), consultation with prior patients who have successfully recovered from similar operations may be warranted. In addition, these patients may benefit from psychological counseling before their surgery. ***Best practice: Informed consent should include informed decision-making by the patient, resulting in shared decision-making about any planned surgery and giving rise to the highest quality of care.***

Ideally, preoperative laboratory testing will be dictated by findings from the history and physical examination. Unfortunately, unnecessary and inappropriate preoperative testing has often been done in an effort to reduce poor perioperative outcomes, whereas evidence to support this practice is lacking, and the cost

to complete these unnecessary tests has been estimated to be over $3 to 18 billion (10). In order to standardize preoperative testing, evidence-based guidelines have been developed (11). The NICE, an independent organization in the United Kingdom that produces evidence-based guidelines for the promotion of good health and treatment of disease, developed guidelines for preoperative testing. These guidelines take into account the patient's age, type of surgery, associated comorbidities, and the American Society of Anesthesiologists (ASA) grade for anesthesia risk (12) (**Table 12.3-1**). St Clair et al performed a retrospective study assessing adherence to the NICE guidelines for preoperative testing in patients having gynecologic surgery between 2005 and 2007. The authors found that among 1,402 patients evaluated, inappropriate preoperative testing resulted in costs over $418,000 (13).

■ TABLE 12.3-1. National Institute for Health and Clinical Excellence Recommendations for Preoperative Testing

Test	ASA 1	ASA 2	ASA 3 or ASA 4
Minor surgery (eg, excising skin lesions, hysteroscopy, draining breast abscess)			
Complete blood count	Not routinely	Not routinely	Not routinely
Basic metabolic profile	Not routinely	Not routinely	Consider in patients at risk for AKI
ECG	Not routinely	Not routinely	Consider if no ECG results available in the last 12 mo
Clotting factors	Not routinely	Not routinely	Not routinely
Lung function/arterial blood gas	Not routinely	Not routinely	Not routinely
Intermediate surgery (eg, inguinal hernia repair, tonsillectomy, knee arthroscopy, diagnostic laparoscopic surgeries)			
Complete blood count	Not routinely	Not routinely	Consider for patients with cardiovascular or renal disease if any symptoms not recently investigated
Basic metabolic profile	Not routinely	Consider for patients at risk for AKI	Yes
ECG	Not routinely	Consider for patients with cardiovascular, renal, or diabetes comorbidities	Yes
Clotting factors	Not routinely	Not routinely	Consider for patients with chronic liver disease, patients taking anticoagulants who need modification of their treatment regimens, and patients where clotting status is needed before surgery-use point-of-care testing
Lung function/arterial blood gas	Not routinely	Not routinely	Consider consultation with anesthesiology for patients who are ASA 3 or 4 due to suspected or known respiratory disease
Major or complex surgery (eg, total abdominal hysterectomy, ovarian cancer debulking surgeries, robotic surgeries, colon resections)			
Complete blood count	Yes	Yes	Yes
Basic metabolic profile	Consider for patients at risk of AKI	Yes	Yes
ECG	Consider for patients aged over 65 ye if no ECG results available from the past 12 mo	Yes	Yes
Clotting factors	Not routinely	Not routinely	Consider in patients with chronic liver disease, patients taking anticoagulants who need modification of their treatment regimens, and patients where clotting status is needed before surgery-use point-of-care testing
Lung function/arterial blood gas	Not routinely	Not routinely	Consider consultation with anesthesiology for patients who are ASA 3 or 4 due to suspected or known respiratory disease

AKI, acute kidney injury; ASA, American Society of Anesthesiologists; ASA 1, normal healthy patient; ASA 2, a patient with mild systemic disease; ASA 3, a patient with severe systemic disease; ASA 4, a patient with severe systemic disease that is a constant threat to life. ECG, electrocardiogram.

Adapted from National Institute for Clinical Excellence. Routine preoperative tests for elective surgery: NICE guideline [NG45]. Published April 5, 2016. https://www.nice.org.uk/guidance/ng45

CARDIAC RISK ASSESSMENT

Any gynecologic oncologist must be aware of the significance of cardiac disease in women when evaluating cardiac risk preoperatively. In 1999, the American Heart Association (AHA) published the first women-specific recommendations on the prevention of cardiovascular disease (CVD) (14). These recommendations were updated in 2011 (15). Over the past 20 years, significant improvements have been made in the recognition and treatment of CVD in women; however, the rate of death from coronary heart disease in women aged 35 to 54 years remains higher than that of their male counterparts. Women were previously thought to be at lower risk of cardiovascular events before menopause; however, rising rates of diabetes and obesity have changed this outlook (16,17). Guidelines classify women into one of three groups: at high risk, at risk, or at ideal cardiovascular health. Preventative measures focus on normalization of cholesterol levels, treatment of hypertension, maintenance of a normal BMI, smoking cessation, and consistent physical activity.

Cardiac risk factors are one of the top concerns for surgeons when assessing perioperative risk. There are numerous reviews and systems that have been created for the purpose of evaluating cardiac risk among patients undergoing noncardiac surgery (17-22). The first large, prospective, multivariate analysis of patients undergoing noncardiac surgery was published by Goldman et al in 1977 (23). They used specific end points of cardiac death, ventricular tachycardia, pulmonary edema, and myocardial infarction (MI). The assessment incorporates nine independent risk factors to create a point risk index to predict morbidity and mortality. One weakness of this index is that it underestimates risk in vascular surgery patients. To overcome this underestimation, newer cardiac risk assessment tools have been created: the Revised Cardiac Risk Index (RCRI) and the American College of Surgeons National Surgical Quality Improvement Program (NSQIP) (24,25). The RCRI is a validated tool that assesses the risk of major cardiac complications in the perioperative period using six predictors of risk. The American College of Surgeons NSQIP tool is different in that it adjusts risks depending on the type of surgery (26).

In response to a shift in the literature from calculation of risk with indices to clinical decision-making, especially in regard to the need for preoperative evaluation, the American College of Cardiology (ACC)/AHA guidelines for the prevention of CVD in women were developed (22). This document provides risk classification of CVD, based upon clinical criteria and/or the Framingham 10-year global risk score (**Table 12.3-2**). The guidelines provide information about the prevention of disease with specifics about initiation of aspirin, statins, and antihypertensives, but not perioperative risk (15). The updated 2011 guidelines change the definition of a high-risk patient to include one that is at 10% or higher risk for a CVD event within 10 years (15).

Clearly, the approach to the patient must include a careful history and physical examination. Some risk calculators determine that age alone is an independent risk factor for perioperative morbidity secondary to major adverse coronary events (24). Age greater than 62 years is an independent risk factor for perioperative stroke (27). Any prior history of cardiac disease, such as angina, MI, arrhythmia, congestive heart failure (CHF), or valvular disease, must be evaluated. Patients with unstable angina, recent MI, class III-IV heart failure, decompensated congestive failure, or aortic stenosis (AS) present the highest risk. These patients will likely require further invasive testing. Severe AS must be identified preoperatively because the risk of perioperative morbidity is as high as 30% (22).

In patients without overt cardiac risks, other factors, such as insulin-dependent diabetes mellitus, elevated preoperative serum creatinine (SCr), and history of cerebrovascular disease, need to

■ **TABLE 12.3-2. Classification of CVD Risk in Women**

Risk Status	Criteria
High risk	Established coronary heart disease
	Cerebrovascular disease
	Peripheral arterial disease
	Abdominal aortic aneurysm
	End-stage or chronic renal disease
	Diabetes mellitus
	10-yr Framingham global risk >20%[a]
At risk	≥1 major risk factors for CVD, including:
	Cigarette smoking
	Poor diet
	Physical inactivity
	Obesity, especially central adiposity
	Family history of premature CVD (CVD at <55 yr of age in male relative and <65 yr of age in female relative)
	Evidence of subclinical vascular disease (eg, coronary calcification)
	Metabolic syndrome
	Poor exercise capacity on treadmill test and/or abnormal heart rate recovery after stopping exercise
Optimal risk	Framingham global risk <10% and a healthy lifestyle, with no risk factors

CVD, cardiovascular disease.

[a]OR at high risk on the basis of another population-adapted tool used to assess global risk.

Adapted from Mosca L, Banka CL, Benjamin EJ, et al. Evidence-based guidelines for cardiovascular disease prevention in women: 2007 update. *Circulation*. 2007;115:1481-1501, with permission.

be considered for uncovering subclinical disease. These risk factors are identified in the risk prediction models (22-25,27,28).

In 2014, the ACC/AHA published revised guidelines to direct invasive or interventional evaluations (22). The guidelines utilize functional capacity in terms of metabolic equivalents (METs), with a level less than 4 being considered poor. One example is a patient's ability to climb one flight of stairs or walk up a hill, which would classify the patient in the greater than 4 group.

Further evaluation includes both invasive and noninvasive methods. The routine resting electrocardiogram (ECG) is a valuable screening tool for patients in whom a history of coronary artery disease is unknown (29). It can potentially identify a prior MI, which may prompt further evaluation for coronary artery disease. Echocardiography can predict postoperative CHF in patients with ejection fraction (EF) less than 35% (30). Although echocardiography cannot reliably predict ischemia, it may be quite useful in the evaluation of valvular diseases or for follow-up of patients with known left ventricular (LV) dysfunction. In addition, elevated preoperative brain natriuretic peptide (BNP) is an independent predictor of 30-day adverse cardiovascular outcomes after noncardiac surgery (31). Exercise or pharmacologic stress testing provides valuable information for perioperative ischemic risk. Nuclear scintigraphy with evaluation of perfusion defects has shown a positive predictive value of 12% to 16% and a negative predictive value of 99% (32). Dobutamine stress echocardiography has shown similar predictive values.

The ACC/AHA recommendations provide a mechanism to segregate patients who need their surgery delayed for further cardiac evaluation because of a recent MI: who should have their CHF optimized and who should optimize control of dysrhythmias. In selected patients, coronary revascularization, angioplasty, stent placement, or valve replacement may be prudent before the planned noncardiac surgery (21,22).

The risk of reinfarction after a recent MI is directly related to the interval between the MI and an event that could precipitate another one. However, these rates have been declining due to improved perioperative care. Reinfarction rates have dropped from 37% in patients undergoing noncardiac surgery within 3 months following MI to 5% to 10%, more recently. Reinfarction rates continue to decline as the interval from the original MI increases, with rates of reinfarction being 2% to 3% and 1% to 2%, 4 to 6 and greater than 6 months, following the acute event, respectively. If percutaneous coronary intervention (PCI) is performed and a drug-eluting stent (DES) placed, recommendations are to wait 6 months before holding dual-antiplatelet agents. If surgery must be performed before this date, it is recommended to continue the aspirin and resume the P2Y platelet receptor inhibitor (such as Plavix) as soon as possible (17).

Perioperative β-Blockade

Multiple studies (DECREASE-I, DECREASE-IV, and POISE) have been attempted over the past 30 years regarding initiation of perioperative β-blockade. Among these studies, the general consensus is that initiation of β-blockade appears to prevent nonfatal MI but increases the risks of death, stroke, bradycardia, and hypotension in patients with risk factors. These risk factors include age older than 70, known coronary arterial disease, prior MI, history of heart failure requiring hospitalization, peripheral arterial disease, diabetes mellitus, prior stroke, smoking, ventricular arrhythmias, angina, limited exercise tolerance, and intrathoracic or intraperitoneal surgery (33). The Peri Operative ISchemic Evaluation (POISE) trial showed that the use of β-blockers in the perioperative period reduces the risk of the composite outcome of cardiovascular death, nonfatal MI, and nonfatal cardiac arrest at 30 days. However, it also showed that bradycardic episodes and clinically significant hypotensive events resulted in increased rates of stroke and death (34). The current recommendation from the ACC/AHA is that perioperative β-blockers should be continued on patients who are taking them chronically. It may be reasonable to begin β-blockers on patients with intermediate- or high-risk myocardial ischemia; however, this must be guided by clinical circumstances (22).

PULMONARY RISK ASSESSMENT

Postoperative pulmonary complications (PPCs) represent a significant cause of morbidity and mortality in patients undergoing elective surgery. In addition, they are one of the costliest major postoperative complications (35). The incidence of pulmonary complications after nonthoracic surgery ranges from 2% to 19% (36). Laparotomy results in a 45% decrease in vital capacity and a 30% reduction in functional residual capacity (FRC) (37,38). When the patient is in the supine position, FRC is reduced below alveolar closing volume (ie, the volume at which point alveoli start closing), which results in atelectasis (39).

When examining risk factors for postoperative pulmonary problems, a number of issues surface. General medical status (eg, functional status, obesity, nutrition) is related to PPCs. A history of CHF, renal failure, poor mental status, and immunosuppression are all associated with a higher PPC rate (40). Surgical issues such as the type of procedure (open or minimally invasive), the type of incision (thoracic and upper abdominal being worse than midline or lower abdominal), duration of anesthetic (>2 hours), the use of a nasogastric tube (NGT) (increased risk), and the use of parenteral

(increased risk) versus epidural (decreased risk) analgesics are all correlated with PPC incidence (41,42). All patients undergoing noncardiothoracic surgery should be evaluated for the presence of the following risk factors for PPCs in order to receive preoperative and postoperative interventions to reduce risk: chronic obstructive pulmonary disease (COPD), CHF, ASA class II or greater, functional dependence, and age older than 60 years. In terms of direct pulmonary risk factors, the most common preexisting pulmonary disease is COPD (42,43). These patients retain carbon dioxide and have poor gas exchange and an increased residual volume. Smoking, history of dyspnea, pneumonia, and sleep apnea are other risk categories (41).

When interpreting preoperative radiographic and laboratory values, several caveats must be kept in mind. A preoperative chest radiograph in normal adults has no predictive value other than providing essential baseline data for an at-risk patient. Arterial blood gas analysis has not been shown to be useful in providing risk stratification (44). A low serum albumin is a powerful marker of increased risk and should be considered in patients with one or more risk factors for PPCs (45). Preoperative pulmonary function tests (PFTs) are rarely useful for risk stratification and are not indicated before surgery. A consensus statement from the American College of Physicians in 2006 recommended that preoperative PFTs or chest radiography may be appropriate in patients with a previous diagnosis of COPD or asthma (43). Such testing may provide valuable baseline data and aid in risk stratification for patients with moderate-to-severe COPD who are undergoing major abdominal surgery.

Perioperative strategies for reducing the risk of PPCs include lung expansion techniques, smoking cessation, and optimization of gas exchange. Although preoperative and postoperative incentive spirometry has shown mixed results in reducing the rate of PPCs, it continues to be widely recommended (46), and it should be considered a preventive strategy for any patient undergoing laparotomy. In order to maximize patient compliance, preoperative counseling and education are necessary. Clearly, COPD must be optimized with control of infection and optimization of medical regimens. Reactive airway disease should be prevented with the use of perioperative inhalation therapy, such as β-agonists. Steroid therapy is generally reserved for patients already utilizing these drugs as part of their medical regimen. These steroid-dependent patients will need stress dose steroids to prevent insufficiency (see section on "Adrenal Suppression"). Prophylactic antibiotics are not indicated in patients with COPD to prevent pulmonary infections.

Smokers have significantly more postoperative complications, including pneumonia, surgical site infections (SSIs), and death (47). Smoking-cessation programs have had an unclear effect on PPCs (48). Although data from poorly controlled trials have shown that short-term abstinence (<8 weeks from the time of surgery) may actually increase the complication rate, these results are controversial (49). However, abstinence for greater than 10 weeks demonstrated the complication rates to be similar to nonsmokers (50). Unfortunately, the long-term success rate and compliance of smoking-cessation programs is low, and in the case of malignancy, the gynecologic oncologist rarely has the opportunity to delay the operation for 8 to 10 weeks.

Risk prediction tools for PPCs are available and can be useful in guiding the clinician's perioperative care (40,51-53).

ENDOCRINOLOGIC RISK ASSESSMENT

Diabetes

The prevalence of diabetes has reached epidemic proportions in the United States and continues to rise each year. In 2021, the Centers for Disease Control and Prevention (CDC) reported that 37.3 million people or 11.3% of the population have diabetes (54). Diabetes accounts for the fourth leading comorbid condition among hospital discharges (55). One-fifth of surgical patients will have diabetes, and people with known diabetes have a 50% risk of undergoing surgery at some point in their lifetime (56). Interestingly, one-third to one-half of hospitalized patients are unaware that they have diabetes and are currently receiving no treatment. It is only during preoperative evaluation for elective surgery or acute hospitalization that these patients will be diagnosed (57). Because of this prevalence, some authors have suggested that all surgical patients be regarded as dysglycemic until proven otherwise (58). Understanding the basic physiology of diabetes and how it impacts perioperative risk is crucial for the surgeon.

There are two types of diabetes. Type 1 diabetes occurs as a result of insulinopenia, with all type 1 diabetics being insulin dependent. In the absence of sufficient insulin, these patients develop ketoacidosis. Type 1 diabetics comprise approximately 10% of all diabetics. Type 2 diabetes occurs as a result of insulin resistance and impaired insulin secretion. Type 2 diabetics may be treated with diet alone, oral hypoglycemic agents, noninsulin injectable medications, or insulin. These patients comprise approximately 90% of all diabetics (59). However, approximately 30% of hospitalized patients will have a prediabetic condition consisting of impaired fasting glucose levels or impaired glucose tolerance (57). Thus, perioperative glycemic control will be dictated by known (or newly discovered) diabetic status. The American Diabetes Association (ADA) has established criteria for the diagnosis of diabetes: fasting plasma glucose of 126 mg/dL or higher or 2-hour plasma glucose of 200 mg/dL or higher after an oral glucose tolerance test or hemoglobin A1c (HbA_{1c}) of 6.5% or greater or a random plasma glucose of 200 mg/dL or higher in patients with classic symptoms of hyperglycemia or hyperglycemic crisis (60).

When evaluating patients with known diabetes for surgery, attention should be directed toward the patient's diabetic status (ie, type of glucose control, number of hypoglycemic events, etc) and the long-term complications caused by diabetes because this end-organ damage can impact perioperative outcome. Most complications of diabetes are related to microvascular changes, such as diabetic retinopathy, neuropathy, nephropathy, and CVD (61). In addition to a thorough history and physical examination, preoperative studies should include an ECG to rule out a prior "silent" MI (especially in patients with diabetes for >10 years), SCr, blood urea nitrogen, urinary analyses to assess renal function, and HbA_{1c} to evaluate recent glycemic control. HbA_{1c} levels reflect the level of hyperglycemia to which red blood cells (RBCs) have been exposed. Because the average life span of an RBC is 120 days, the HbA_{1c} is an indicator of glycemic control over that period (59). As mentioned earlier, because of the high prevalence of dysglycemia among hospitalized adults in the United States, measurement of HbA_{1c}, as a screening for diabetes, may identify patients with undiagnosed diabetes or impaired glucose metabolism (58). HbA_{1c} levels 6.5% or less are associated with good long-term glucose control and have been associated with decreased rates of infectious complications across a variety of surgical procedures (62). Conversely, HbA_{1c} levels greater than 6.5% are diagnostic of diabetes and evidence of poor glycemic control in known diabetics (60,63). Ultimately, the type of diabetes, preoperative glycemic control, extent and magnitude of the intended surgery, elective or emergent nature of surgery, and other comorbid medical conditions will affect the metabolic changes these patients face intraoperatively and postoperatively (58).

Another entity that has come to light in the past decade among hospitalized patients is that of stress-induced hyperglycemia (SIH). This disease is defined as an inpatient fasting glucose measurement of 126 mg/dL or more or a random glucose measurement of greater than 200 mg/dL, which returns to

normal after discharge (56,64). A growing body of evidence suggests that SIH and diabetic hyperglycemia are different diseases (65) and that SIH confers a higher risk of adverse outcomes, such as increased in-hospital mortality (60,66,67) and longer length of stay compared to nondiabetics or patients with hyperglycemic diabetes (64).

The armamentarium available for the treatment of diabetes has increased over the past two decades. Type 1 diabetics commonly use a combination of insulin therapies for glycemic control, whereas type 2 diabetics may be on oral therapy alone, insulin therapy alone, injectable noninsulin therapy alone, or some combination therapy of all the aforementioned agents. **Table 12.3-3** outlines some of these drugs and timing for stopping these medications before surgical procedures because of the pharmacologic half-lives of these drugs (61,67,68).

The physiologic changes that patients with diabetes encounter during surgery result in a hyperglycemic state due to insulin resistance. The stress of surgery increases secretion of epinephrine, norepinephrine, cortisol, and growth hormone, all of which directly antagonize insulin action (58,59,61). In addition, gluconeogenesis and lipolysis are increased with mobilization of glucose precursors, and a net protein catabolism ensues. Perioperative glycemic control will depend upon the type of diabetes or impaired glucose tolerance the patient has, as well as the medications that have/have not be utilized to control such disease states. Recently, the Clinical Guidelines Subcommittee of the Endocrinology Society published treatment guidelines for hospitalized non–critically ill patients and subsequently found to be hyperglycemic (known diabetes vs unknown). Recommendations from this group for the perioperative care of patients with hyperglycemia undergoing surgical interventions are listed in **Table 12.3-4** (69).

Several case-control studies have demonstrated an increased risk of adverse outcomes in patients undergoing elective noncardiac surgery with either preoperative or postoperative hyperglycemia (70-74). Postoperative glucose levels greater than 200 mg/dL are associated with prolonged hospital stays and increased risk of postoperative complications, including wound infections and cardiac arrhythmias (71-73). Although patients with diabetes with vascular disease are at the risk of silent postoperative MI and acute renal failure (ARF), postoperative infections (respiratory, urinary, wound infections, etc) account for about two-thirds of all postoperative complications and 20% of all postoperative deaths among diabetics undergoing surgery (75). Hyperglycemia has been shown to impair phagocytic function and chemotaxis of granulocytes when glucose levels are higher than 250 mg/dL (76).

Although glycemic control is important, the jury is still out on when control should be achieved (pre-, intra-, or postoperatively or throughout the entire perioperative period), what glucose levels should be achieved for maximum benefit, and which insulin regimen is most effective (58). The landmark publication by Van den Berghe et al in 2001 showed, in a randomized, prospective way, that aggressive glycemic control through intensive insulin therapy (IIT) (maintaining glucose levels between 80 and 110 mg/dL) versus conventional insulin therapy (glucose levels between 180 and 200 mg/dL) in critically ill postoperative patients (>60% were cardiac surgery patients) reduced episodes of septicemia and in-hospital mortality by 46% and 34%, respectively (77). Despite the enthusiasm for tighter glucose control, subsequent studies over the past decade, with a heterogeneous population of acutely ill patients, have failed to confirm the results of Van den Berghe et al's work (58,64). In fact, the multinational, multidisciplinary Normoglycemia in Intensive Care Evaluation and Survival Using Glucose Algorithm Regulation (NICE-SUGAR) trial in 6,104 ICU patients reported increased mortality rates (27.5% [IIT] vs 24.9% [control]) in patients who were kept at blood glucose levels of 81 to 108 versus <180 mg/dL.

■ **TABLE 12.3-3. Preoperative Medication Management in Patients with Diabetes**

Drug	Day Before Surgery	Day of Surgery
Oral hypoglycemic agents		
Sulfonylurea, meglitinides, α-glucosidase inhibitors, dipeptidal peptidase-IV inhibitor	Daily same dose	Hold drug
Thiazolidinediones	Hold drug	Hold drug
Injectable agents		
Injectable noninsulins (incretin mimetics, amylin analog)	Normal dose the night before surgery	Hold drug
SGLT2 inhibitors (canagliflozin, dapagliflozin, empagliflozin)	Stop 3 d before surgery	Hold drug
Ertugliflozin	Stop 4 d before surgery	Hold drug
Insulin (regular insulin, NPH insulin)	Normal dose the night before surgery	Half the normal dose the morning of surgery
Rapid-acting insulin	Normal dose the night before surgery	Hold drug
Combination of long- and short-acting agents (mixed insulin)	Normal dose the night before surgery	Depending upon the fasting blood glucose: a) <200 mg/dL—no insulin b) >200 mg/dL—take half of normal dose
Basal/long-acting insulin (detemir, glargine, degludec)	Normal dose the night before surgery	Half the normal dose the morning of surgery
Insulin pump	Depending on the insulin pump protocol	Basal rate until surgery; then continue with IV insulin during surgery

IV, intravenous; NPH, neutral protamine Hagedorn; SGLT2, sodium-glucose cotransporter 2.

Adapted from Galway U, Chahar P, Schmidt MT, et al. Perioperative challenges in management of diabetic patients undergoing non-cardiac surgery. *World J Diabetes*. 2021;12(8):1255-1266; Meneghini LF. Perioperative management of diabetes: translating evidence into practice. *Cleveland Clin J Med*. 2009;76(4):S53-S59; Himes CP, Ganesh R, Wight EC, Simha V, Liebow M. Perioperative evaluation and management of endocrine disorders. *Mayo Clin Proc*. 2020;95(12): 2760-2774 with permission.

The increased mortality was driven by increased rates of hypoglycemia (blood glucose <40 mg/dL) among patients with the tightest blood glucose control (6.8% [IIT] vs 0.5% [control]) (78). Because of the NICE-SUGAR study and others (64), recommendations for blood glucose targets have relaxed somewhat depending upon the setting of the patient.

Intravenous (IV) insulin therapy should be instituted in critically ill patients when blood glucose levels exceed 180 mg/dL, with the goal of maintaining glucose control between 140 and 180 mg/dL. For non–critically ill patients, the preprandial goal for glucose level is less than 140 mg/dL (79) with maintenance of blood glucose at these levels while minimizing hypoglycemia. Attaining these levels of glycemic control will depend upon the patient's type of diabetes, medical condition, and oral intake status.

Individual institutional policy will vary as to where patients may receive IV insulin therapy (ICU vs step-down units vs routine hospital floors). If the patient is receiving IV insulin, transition to a subcutaneous route must be started before discontinuing the IV route. Most patients can be converted to long-acting basal insulin, with the dose usually being 50% to 80% of the prior day's total IV insulin dose. An insulin regimen utilizing a subcutaneous basal/bolus approach outperforms traditional sliding scale regular insulin regimens. Umpierrez et al expanded their previous work (80) by conducting a prospective randomized trial comparing subcutaneous basal/bolus insulin replacement to traditional subcutaneous sliding scale insulin replacement for patients with type 2 diabetes undergoing general surgery, not expected to be admitted to the ICU, and whose glucose levels exceeded 140 mg/dL.

■ **TABLE 12.3-4. Perioperative Blood Glucose Control: An Endocrine Society Clinical Practice Guideline**

Recommendation Number	
5.3.1	All patients with type 1 diabetes who undergo minor or major surgical procedures receive either continuous insulin infusion or subcutaneous basal insulin with bolus insulin as required to prevent hyperglycemia during the perioperative period.
5.3.2	Patients with diabetes should discontinue oral and noninsulin injectable antidiabetic agents before surgery with initiation of insulin therapy in those patients who develop hyperglycemia during the perioperative period.
5.3.3	When instituting subcutaneous insulin therapy in the postsurgical setting, basal (for patients who are NPO) or basal bolus (for patients who are eating), insulin therapy is the preferred approach.

NPO, nil per os.

From Umpierrez GE, Hellman R, Korytkoski MT, et al. Management of hyperglycemia in hospitalized patients in non-critical care setting: an Endocrine Society Clinical Practice Guideline. *J Clin Endocrinol Metab*. 2012;97:16-38.

■ TABLE 12.3-5. Basal/Bolus Insulin Treatment Protocol

Starting Insulin Doses	Supplemental Insulin (Insulin Glulisine)				Insulin Adjustment
Discontinue all oral antidiabetic and noninsulin injectable medications	Give supplemental insulin glulisine according to the sliding scale (below) for blood glucose >140 mg/dL				If the fasting and predinner BG is between 100-140 mg/dL and no hypoglycemia the previous day: *no changes*
Starting TDD: 0.5 units/kg actual body weight	If patient is able and expected to eat, give supplemental glulisine before each meal and at bedtime following the "usual" column				If the fasting and predinner BG is between 140-180 mg/dL and no hypoglycemia the previous day: *increase insulin TDD by 10% every day*
*Reduce TDD to 0.3 units/kg actual body weight in patients aged ≥70 yr and/or serum creatinine ≥2.0 mg/dL	If the patient is not able to eat, give supplemental glulisine q6h (6-12-6-12) following the "sensitive" column				If the fasting and predinner BG is >180 mg/dL and no hypoglycemia the previous day: *increase insulin TDD by 20% every day*
Give half of the TDD as insulin glargine, at the same time once daily and half as insulin glulisine in 3 equally divided doses before each meal. Hold insulin glulisine if patient not able to eat	**Blood Glucose (mg/dL)**	**Insulin Sensitive (units)**	**Usual (units)**	**Insulin Resistant (units)**	If the fasting and predinner BG is between 70-99 mg/dL and no hypoglycemia: *decrease insulin TDD by 10% every day*
	141-180	2	4	6	
	181-220	4	6	8	
	221-260	6	8	10	
	261-300	8	10	12	If the patient develops hypoglycemia
	301-350	10	12	14	BG <70 mg/dL: *decrease insulin TDD by 20%*
	351-400	12	14	16	
	>400	14	16	18	

BG, blood glucose; q, every; TDD; total daily dose.

Adapted from Umpierrez GE, Smiley D, Jacobs S, et al. Randomized study of basal-bolus insulin therapy in the inpatient management of patients with Type 2 diabetes undergoing general surgery (RABBIT 2 Surgery). *Diabetes Care*. 2011;34:256-261, with permission.

In the group randomized to the basal/bolus insulin, the starting daily dose was 0.5 U/kg/d, with half of the dose being given as basal insulin (insulin glargine) once daily and half given as rapid-acting insulin analog (glulisine) in fixed doses before meals. If the patient was NPO (nil per os), then the insulin glargine dose was given and the insulin glulisine was held until meals were resumed. For supplementation, the rapid-acting analog was used. Among the 211 patients studied, those in the basal/bolus group received higher daily doses of insulin, had lower daily mean blood glucose levels (27 mg/dL lower), had the same risk of hypoglycemic episodes (blood glucose levels <40 mg/dL), and more often achieved the glycemic goal of less than 140 mg/dL. In addition, the basal/bolus group had fewer wound infections, pneumonias, episodes of bacteremia, respiratory failure, and ARF as compared to the sliding scale insulin group. There also was a nonsignificant trend toward fewer postsurgical ICU admissions and shorter ICU stays than in the sliding scale insulin group (66). **Table 12.3-5** demonstrates the basal/bolus method to control hyperglycemia in type 2 diabetics postoperatively. The use of oral diabetes agents in hospitalized patients is not recommended (81). ***Best practice: Perioperative maintenance of blood glucose levels (<180-200 mg/dL) results in improved perioperative outcomes. Glucose levels above this range should be treated with insulin infusions and regular blood glucose monitoring to avoid the risk of hypoglycemia.***

Thyroid Disorders

When patients give a history of hypothyroidism or hyperthyroidism during evaluation for surgery, thyroid-stimulating hormone (TSH) and thyroxine (T4) levels should be obtained. The primary objective is to determine whether the patient is euthyroid before surgical intervention so as to avoid the complications of myxedema or thyroid storm in the postoperative period.

Hypothyroidism is a common condition in the United States, affecting approximately 1% of all patients and 5% of the population over the age of 50, and it develops 10 times more often in women than in men (82). Decision to operate on patients with hypothyroidism will depend upon the level of hypothyroidism and the urgency of the surgery. Hypothyroidism can influence many physiologic functions, such as myocardial function, respiration, GI motility, hemostasis, and free water balance (59,83). Although there have been no prospective, randomized studies looking at the surgical outcome of hypothyroid patients versus controls, several retrospective case-matched control studies have evaluated hypothyroid patients undergoing surgery. A study by Weinberg et al demonstrated no differences between hypothyroid and euthyroid controls for perioperative complications. In addition, no differences in outcome were seen when hypothyroidism was stratified by T4 levels. The investigators concluded that patients with mild-to-moderate hypothyroidism should not be denied needed surgery in order to correct the metabolic problem. They further stated that insufficient numbers of patients with severe hypothyroidism precluded recommendations for perioperative care of these patients (84). In another retrospective study, Ladenson et al reviewed perioperative complications among hypothyroid patients undergoing surgery, finding more intraoperative hypotension in noncardiac surgery, more heart failure in cardiac surgery, and more GI and neuropsychiatric complications. They also noted that patients were unable to mount fever in the face of infection, although infection rates were not different. Furthermore, no differences were found in the duration of hospitalization, perioperative arrhythmias, delayed anesthesia recovery, pulmonary complications, or mortality (85).

Patients with mild-to-moderate hypothyroidism requiring urgent surgery may have it without delay. These patients may have more minor complications of ileus, postoperative delirium, or infection without fever. Patients with severe hypothyroidism (myxedema coma, decreased mentation, pericardial effusions, heart failure, or very low levels of T4) who are to undergo urgent/emergent surgery will need IV levothyroxine (200-500 µg given during 30 minutes) followed by daily doses of 50 to 100 µg IV. These patients will likely need stress dose glucocorticoids (see section on Adrenal Suppression) started before, during, and continued after surgery due to coexisting adrenal insufficiency (AI) (or due to the fact that IV replacement with levothyroxine may precipitate AI) (59,85,86).

Myxedema coma is a rare condition, with an incidence of 0.22 per million patients per year. Most of the cases (80%) occur among hospitalized, older (>60 years) women with long-standing hypothyroidism, but it can occur at any age (87). A majority of the cases will occur in the postoperative period due to inciting causes, such as infections, cold exposure, sedatives, analgesics, and other medications. The mortality from this disease is high (80%) but has been decreasing in recent years because of increased awareness, testing, and improved perioperative care (88-90). Myxedema coma is characterized by severely depressed mental status, seizure, hypothermia, bradycardia, hyponatremia, heart failure, and hypopnea. Although maintenance of normothermia by warming is tempting, the resulting vasodilatation may cause cardiovascular collapse in patients with intravascular volume depletion, cardiac insufficiency, and pericardial effusion/tamponade and should be performed carefully if at all (88). Myxedema coma is a medical emergency and necessitates urgent administration of levothyroxine. An initial IV bolus of 200 to 500 µg should be given, followed by 50 to 100 µg IV daily. Dehydration is frequently present, and aggressive volume resuscitation with dextrose and normal saline should be instituted. IV glucocorticoids should be administered (50 mg hydrocortisone IV, 4 times daily) because of frequent AI. Resolution of symptoms, if properly treated, should begin within 24 hours.

Patients using thyroid replacement preparations can have their doses held during the immediate postoperative period until they are able to tolerate oral intake, as the half-life of these drugs is 5 to 9 days (83).

The causes of hyperthyroidism are many, but the most common cause is Graves disease. This autoimmune disorder, caused by an antibody directed to TSH receptors, results in increased thyroid hormone production. The clinical signs of hyperthyroidism include tachycardia, atrial fibrillation, fever, tremor, goiter, and ophthalmopathy (59). Most complications occurring in hyperthyroid patients undergoing surgery involve cardiac function, as T4 and T3 have direct inotropic and chronotropic effect on the heart and a vasodilatory effect on peripheral vasculature, resulting in the activation of the renin-angiotensin-aldosterone system. All of these events result in a high cardiac output state, which increases cardiac work and oxygen requirements and can result in MI (87). Arrhythmias are very common in the face of hyperthyroidism, with atrial fibrillation occurring in 10% to 20% of patients (91-94). The level of control before the operation will determine the perioperative outcome for the patient. Patients with controlled hyperthyroidism should be instructed to take their antithyroid medications the morning of the day of surgery. Patients with mild hyperthyroidism may have surgery with preoperative β-blockade. However, patients with moderate or severe disease should have surgery canceled until a euthyroid state is attained (95).

The greatest perioperative risk for patients who have undiagnosed hyperthyroidism or who are inadequately treated is a rare, yet life-threatening condition known as thyroid storm. This "thyroid emergency" usually occurs intraoperatively or 48 hours postoperatively. The mortality of thyroid storm is 10% to 75%

and requires treatment in a critical care environment (82). Symptoms are nonspecific and include hyperpyrexia, tachycardia, delirium, nausea and vomiting, and diarrhea (96). Treatment of thyroid storm is aimed at stopping the production of thyroid hormone and treating the systemic effects of the decompensated patient. Antithyroid medications such as carbimazole, methimazole, and propylthiouracil (PTU) are used to inhibit the new synthesis of thyroid hormones. Unfortunately, there are no IV preparations for these compounds, so they must be administered enterally or per rectum as retention enemas or suppositories. Recent guidelines from the American Thyroid Association and the Association of Clinical Endocrinologists recommend that PTU be started with a loading dose of 500 to 1,000 mg followed by 250 mg every 4 hours and that methimazole should be administered at daily doses of 60 to 80 mg (97). Administering these drugs in this sequence will provide more rapid clinical improvement because PTU has the added advantage of inhibiting conversion of T4 to T3, which methimazole does not do. These drugs prevent synthesis of new thyroid hormone, but will not stop release of stored thyroid hormone. Either inorganic iodine or lithium carbonate (for patients who are allergic to iodine; 300 mg orally every 6 hours) must be given. Lugol solution or a saturated solution of potassium iodide (3-5 drops orally, every 6 hours) may be used, but must not be given sooner than 1 hour after the administration of the thionamide dosage; otherwise thyroid hormone synthesis will be enhanced by the iodine treatment. In severe cases of thyroid storm, plasmapheresis and therapeutic plasma exchange may be needed. β-Blockade is critical to ameliorate the manifestations of thyroid excess and does so by correcting the heart rate, reducing cardiac oxygen demand, and decreasing agitation, convulsions, psychotic behavior, and tremors. Propranolol is the most commonly used agent, and dosages of 60 to 80 mg given orally every 4 hours or 0.5 to 1 mg IV followed by subsequent doses of 2 to 3 mg every several hours are recommended. Another theoretical benefit of β-blockade is the inhibition of conversion of T4 to T3. One other intervention with high therapeutic benefit is the administration of corticosteroids, which not only inhibits the conversion of T4 to T3 but also treats AI, which may have occurred due to the rapid turnover of cortisol. Acetaminophen is preferred to salicylates, as the latter may exacerbate thyrotoxicosis by decreasing thyroid protein binding and increasing free T3 and T4. Finally, a thorough search for the precipitating cause of the thyroid storm should be undertaken immediately, with the most common cause in the perioperative period being infection (87).

Adrenal Suppression

Activation of the hypothalamic-pituitary-adrenal (HPA) axis function is one of several characteristic features of the physiologic response to psychological or physical stressors, such as trauma, infections, and surgery. The intensity of the stress stimulus often dictates the degree and duration of HPA activation. However, the magnitude of HPA activation required during the perioperative period has been debated for years. Similarly, the need for "stress steroid dosing" has been called into question, given the dearth of high-level evidence supporting or refuting the practice (98,106)

Adrenal suppression or insufficiency (AI) is the failure of the adrenal cortex to secrete sufficient amounts of corticosteroids and remains a first-line indication for exogenous steroid therapy. Adrenal suppression is divided into two types: primary and secondary AI. The most common cause of primary AI is destruction of the adrenal cortex (Addison disease) by idiopathic infections, autoimmune causes, hemorrhage, and sepsis. Secondary AI is characterized by atrophy of the adrenal cortex as a result of deficient adrenocorticotrophic hormone (ACTH) stimulation and includes diseases that affect the anterior pituitary or hypothalamus or chronic exogenous corticosteroid therapy. Although there is remarkable variability in individual response to a particular dose and length of treatment with corticosteroids, in general, any patient who receives the equivalent of 20 mg/d of prednisone for more than 5 days is at risk for HPA suppression. If the duration of steroid treatment is 1 month or longer, the patient will have HPA suppression, which can last 6 to 12 months after stopping therapy. Conversely, an equivalent dose of prednisone 5 mg (or less) for any period of time will not usually suppress the HPA axis (99,100). Assessment of adrenal function (ACTH stimulation tests) in the perioperative period has not been shown to be sensitive or specific in identifying patients who are at risk for AI or who might respond to supplemental corticosteroids (101-104).

Recently, Marik and Varon performed a meta-analysis of the world literature concerning perioperative stress doses of corticosteroids for patients who take corticosteroids chronically. Their search revealed two RCTs and seven cohort studies, for a total of 315 patients. Although the number of patients is small, the two RCTs showed no differences in the hemodynamic profiles of patients receiving stress doses of corticosteroids, compared to patients receiving only their usual daily dose of corticosteroid. Similarly, in five of the seven cohort studies, patients who continued to receive their usual daily doses of corticosteroids without additional stress doses did not develop unexplained hypotension or adrenal crisis perioperatively. The remaining two cohort studies each had one patient who stopped their usual daily dose of corticosteroid preoperatively, and each developed unexplained postoperative hypotension, which responded to hydrocortisone and fluid therapy. The authors recommend that patients receiving therapeutic doses of corticosteroids and who undergo surgery do not routinely need stress doses of corticosteroids as long as their usual daily dose is continued. In addition, adrenal function testing is not recommended for these patients because the test is overly sensitive and does not predict which patient will develop adrenal crisis. Furthermore, patients who have primary AI and who are taking physiologic replacement doses of corticosteroids will require supplemental stress doses of corticosteroids in the perioperative period (105).

Because of the lack of high-level evidence for "stress steroid dosing," one individualized approach to such dosing divides patients into three potential groups: those very unlikely to have HPA axis suppression, those very likely to have HPA axis suppression, and an intermediate group of patients whose HPA function is unknown. Patients unlikely to have HPA axis suppression include those receiving glucocorticoid doses of 5 mg/d or less of prednisone or equivalent and those receiving steroid therapy for 3 weeks or less. These patients will only need to take their regular daily steroid dose in the perioperative period without the need for additional or "stress doses." In addition, these patients need no further testing of their adrenal function. Patients known to have suppressed HPA axis include patients receiving 20 mg/d or more of prednisone or equivalent for more than 3 weeks duration. In addition, all patients with primary AI or evidence of Cushing syndrome are considered high risk for HPA axis suppression. All of the aforementioned patients should receive steroids based upon the anticipated surgical stress (**Table 12.3-6**). Patients in the intermediate or unknown risk of HPA axis suppression include patients who have received doses 5 to 20 mg/d of prednisone or equivalent for more than 3 weeks during the year before surgery. These patients will have wide variability of HPA axis suppression and are candidates for corticotropin stimulation test. Patients with an inadequate response to testing or those for whom timely testing is inappropriate should receive "stress dose" steroids (**Table 12.3-6**) (106,107). Giving stress dose glucocorticoids needs to be weighed against the potential side effects of the drug (such as poor wound healing, fluid retention, gastric ulcer, and increased risk of infection) versus the benefits of supporting the HPA axis in a surgically stressed patient.

▮ **TABLE 12.3-6. Recommended Stress Dose Corticosteroids by Surgical Stress**

Surgery Type	Example	Recommended Corticosteroid Dose
Minor stress	Dental surgery Biopsy (any type) Inguinal hernia repair Colonoscopy Uterine curettage/hysteroscopy Vulvectomy Hand surgery	Usual daily dose of steroids
Moderate stress	Extremity revascularization Total joint replacement Cholecystectomy Colon resection Abdominal hysterectomy (simple) Robotic surgery	Usual daily dose of steroids **AND** Hydrocortisone 50 mg IV before incision Hydrocortisone 25 mg IV q8h × 24 hr **THEN** Usual daily dose of steroids
Major stress	Esophagectomy Total proctocolectomy Major cardiac/vascular Hepaticojejunostomy Ovarian cancer debulking Delivery Trauma	Usual daily dose of steroids **AND** Hydrocortisone 100 mg IV before incision Hydrocortisone 50 mg IV q8hr × 24 hr Taper dose by half per day to usual daily maintenance dose

IV, intravenous; q, every.

From Umpierrez GE, Hellman R, Korytkoski MT, et al. Management of hyperglycemia in hospitalized patients in non-critical care setting: an endocrine society clinical practice guideline. *J Clin Endocrinol Metab*. 2012;97:16-38.

RENAL RISK ASSESSMENT

Chronic Kidney Disease

Chronic kidney disease (CKD) affects nearly 15 million Americans (≥20; CKD stage 2 or worse) (108), with most having a glomerular filtration rate (GFR) of less than 60 mL/min/1.73 m^2 (109). The most common form of renal failure facing the surgeon is acute kidney injury (AKI) occurring during the postoperative period, which is discussed in the section on postoperative/critical care. In 2002, a uniform classification system for CKD was introduced, stratifying CKD into five stages based on estimation of GFR and documentation of renal injury (109). Class 5 CKD, or end-stage renal disease (ESRD), includes patients who require renal replacement therapy (usually dialysis) for treatment (108). With the aging population, increasing prevalence of diabetes and hypertension, and advances in dialytic therapy, the number of patients living with CKD is increasing (108). Therefore, surgeons must be cognizant of the potential perioperative risks associated with these patients.

The predominant causes of CKD are diabetes and hypertension, which account for 71% of all patients who are dialysis dependent (108). Patients with these underlying diseases tend to have other comorbid conditions, such as coronary artery disease and peripheral vascular disease. Evaluation of patients with CKD undergoing surgery should focus on four areas: cardiac evaluation, fluid and electrolyte management, anemia, and bleeding diatheses. Glycemic control for diabetics and blood pressure control for patients with hypertension are imperative.

CVD has long been recognized as the leading cause of death among patients with ESRD and occurs in 50% of patients

(108,110,111). However, patients with other stages of CKD, even minor derangements, have an increased risk of CVD. A recent study correlated stage of CKD with odds ratios (ORs) for cardiovascular risk, demonstrating a graded increase in risk with increasing stage of CKD (OR 15 for stage I, OR 20-1,000 for stage V) (111). The disease factors that contribute to CVD among patients with CKD include microalbuminuria/proteinuria, hypertension, diabetes, dsylipidemia, and smoking (112). In addition, many patients with CKD will have coronary artery disease (30%-40%), and many patients with ESRD (70%-80%) will develop ventricular hypertrophy due to hypertension and severe anemia. This hypertrophy results in a decreased myocardial capillary density and diastolic and systolic dysfunction, all of which leads to disturbances in intraventricular conduction, electrical excitability, and ventricular arrhythmias (113). Therefore, these patients may benefit from a formal cardiac clearance from a cardiologist before surgical intervention.

The capacity of the failing kidney to maintain volume and electrolyte homeostasis is achieved through adaptive processes, which are limited in their ability to respond to physiologic stresses, placing well-compensated patients in the premorbid state at increased risk of fluid and electrolyte disturbances during the perioperative period (114). Intraoperative and perioperative fluid management in the patients with CKD must, therefore, take into account the reduced capacity for both water excretion and conservation. Excessive free water administration must be avoided to prevent iatrogenic hypotonicity, while providing sufficient free water to prevent hypertonicity. Electrolyte status should be monitored frequently, and water administration adjusted if hyponatremia or hypernatremia ensues (115). Acute hyperkalemia may be treated with glucose and insulin, which will drive the Na/K-ATPase pump, resulting in an increase in intracellular potassium and lowering of extracellular potassium. Ten milliliters of calcium gluconate can afford cardioprotection and membrane stabilization in patients with abnormal ECGs (116). Decreasing total-body potassium is the final step in the treatment of hyperkalemia. In nonoliguric patients, renal potassium excretion may be enhanced with loop-acting diuretics. Patiromer is a novel, spherical, nonabsorbed polymer designed to bind and remove potassium, primarily in the distal colon, thereby decreasing serum potassium in patients with hyperkalemia. A patiromer dose of 8.4 g twice a day lowered potassium levels within 7 hours of administration, but levels will continue to decrease for at least 48 hours if treatment is continued. Sodium zirconium cyclosilicate (SZC) exchanges hydrogen and sodium with potassium throughout the entire GI tract, increasing renal excretion of potassium. One gram of SZC binds approximately 3 mmol of potassium within 1 hour of administration. These new treatments are favored over Kayexalate and its risk of intestinal necrosis (117).

Most patients with CKD have or will develop anemia due to erythropoietin deficiency during the course of their disease and, before the introduction of erythropoietin-stimulating agents (ESAs), were transfusion dependent. In recent years, the use of ESAs has come under scrutiny. Recent reviews have demonstrated that raising the hemoglobin levels above 11 g/dL in patients with CKD resulted in a 1.14-fold increase in the OR of death. These results highlight the need to carefully manage hemoglobin levels with ESAs within a recommended range of 9 to 11 g/dL (118,119). In urgent situations, transfusion of blood is necessary to maintain hemoglobin before and during surgery.

Patients with CKD have an increased risk for bleeding complications. Platelet dysfunction caused by renal failure is multifactorial, with retained uremic toxins, abnormal binding of von Willebrand factor, abnormal platelet arachidonic acid metabolism, and excess vascular prostacyclin and nitric oxide production all being implicated (120). The bleeding time provides the best correlation with risk of clinical bleeding in patients with CKD. If a patient has demonstrated prior bleeding because of uremic platelet dysfunction, these patients must be treated with 1-deamino-8-D-arginine vasopressin (dDAVP) IV or intranasally and with cryoprecipitate to prevent bleeding during surgery (121). In addition, patients may be treated with IV conjugated estrogens (0.6 mg/kg) if they are given 4 to 5 days before surgery (115,122).

Furthermore, with reduced or absent renal function, these patients metabolize drugs such as antibiotics, anesthetics, and analgesics poorly. Drug administration in ESRD must be done judiciously with careful attention to the pharmacokinetics of particular drugs. Multiple guidelines exist that can direct drug dose reductions for patients with ESRD (123,124).

Dialysis Patients

Patients with ESRD who are dependent upon dialysis will need to be euvolemic before surgery. The preferred timing of dialysis is the day before surgery. Perioperative outcomes have not been shown to improve with additional sessions of dialysis before surgery (125). Thus, communication with the patient's nephrologist is paramount, detailing the operative procedure and planning the timing of dialysis the day before the surgery (without heparin 24 hours before surgery) and possible postoperative dialysis on the day of surgery for large intraoperative fluid loads. Electrolytes should be monitored in the immediate postoperative period, with hyperkalemia being aggressively managed medically or with dialysis (116). As with CKD, CVD, diabetes mellitus, and abnormal bleeding are common among patients receiving dialysis, necessitating the perioperative considerations as outlined earlier (125).

HEPATIC RISK ASSESSMENT

An increasing number of patients with chronic liver disease (CLD), advanced or end stage, will require non–liver transplant surgery (126). Reasons for this increase include an aging population, better long-term survival of patients with liver cirrhosis, and continuously improving outcomes after surgery and critical care medicine (127). Historically, liver dysfunction was related to chronic viral or alcoholic hepatitis. While the incidence of these conditions has not changed dramatically in recent years, the rising rate of obesity has led to nonalcoholic fatty liver disease, which is increasingly recognized as the most common cause of CLD in the United States (128).

As mentioned earlier, thorough preoperative evaluation of patients includes a comprehensive history and physical examination, with laboratory testing based upon historical and physical findings. Routine testing of liver function or coagulation studies in asymptomatic patients rarely yield abnormal results that result in changes or perioperative management and are not recommended (7). However, patients with a history of liver disease, jaundice, blood transfusions, the use of alcohol or other recreational drugs, hepatitis, or physical findings of icterus, hepatosplenomegaly, palmar erythema, or spider nevi should be tested to rule out occult or active liver diseases (127).

Patients with acute hepatitis (viral or alcohol induced) should have their surgery delayed until the acute phase of the disease process has passed and liver function tests have returned to normal. Mortality rates among these patients can range from 10% to 58% if surgery is pursued. Patients with acute liver failure/fulminant liver failure, defined as the development of jaundice, coagulopathy, and hepatic encephalopathy within 26 weeks in a patient with acute liver injury and without preexisting liver disease, are critically ill, and all surgery other than liver transplantation is contraindicated in these patients (129). Contrarily, patients with chronic infectious hepatitis, which is stable, tolerate surgery with minimal mortality (126,130,131). Of course, the operator should practice universal precautions with all surgical interventions, regardless of the patient's known infectivity status.

Assessing the severity of the underlying liver disease is important to determine perioperative outcome and has been correlated to two classification systems: the Child-Turcotte-Pugh (CTP) classification and the model of end-stage liver disease (MELD) score. The Child-Turcotte score was the first predictor of surgical

■ **TABLE 12.3-7. Child-Turcotte-Pugh (CTP) Classification of Liver Disease and Operative Mortality**

	Score		
Component	1 point	2 points	3 points
Ascites	None	Controlled with medication	Treatment refractory
Encephalopathy	Absent	Grade I-II; controlled with medication	Grade III-IV; treatment refractory
Albumin (g/L)	>3.5	2.8-3.5	<2.8
Bilirubin (mg/dL)	<2	2–3	>3
INR	<1.7	1.7-2.3	>2.3
CTP Classification	Class A (5-6 points)	Class B (7-9 points)	Class C (10-15 points)
90-d mortality risk (abdominal surgery) (%)	2-10	2-30	12-76

INR, international normalized ratio.

Adapted from Hanje AJ, Patel T. Preoperative evaluation of patients with liver disease. *Nat Clin Pract Gastroenterol Hepatol*. 2007;4:266-276; Muir AJ. Surgical clearance for the patient with chronic liver disease. *Clin Liver Dis*. 2012;16:421-433; Hoetzel A, Ryan H, Schmidt R. Anesthetic considerations for the patient with liver disease. *Curr Opin Anesthesiol*. 2012;25(3):340-347, with permission.

risk/mortality for patients undergoing surgical intervention; specifically, patients having portacaval shunts. The system was modified by Pugh and colleagues to include prothrombin time (PT) in place of the subjective assessment of nutritional status, for use in patients undergoing esophageal transections for bleeding varices (132,133). Although widely known for classifying liver disease, this system has been criticized for utilizing subjective variables (ascites and encephalopathy) in developing a score. However, the CTP score correlates with mortality in patients undergoing differing types of surgery (127,134) (**Table 12.3-7**). The MELD score was originally devised as a prognostic measure of short-term mortality in patients with cirrhosis undergoing placement of a transjugular intrahepatic portosystemic shunt (TIPS) (135). The MELD score is derived from a complex formula that incorporates three biochemical variables (serum total bilirubin, SCr, and the international normalized ratio [INR]) and assigns the patient a score of 8 to 40 (**Table 12.3-8**). The risk of morbidity and mortality in patients with liver disease depends upon the type of surgery and has been correlated to the aforementioned classification systems (**Tables 12.3-7 and 12.3-8**) (134). However, it is likely that over the past two decades, mortality rates have decreased, despite the absence of large studies confirming this assumption (127).

Patients with cirrhosis of the liver also have coagulopathies, which need to be corrected before surgery. Vitamin K, fresh-frozen plasma (FFP), or cryoprecipitate may be administered to correct the PT to within 3 seconds of normal. **Figure 12.3-1** presents an algorithm for patients with liver disease facing surgery.

Finally, selection of medications in patients with hepatic dysfunction needs to be done carefully, from types of perioperative antibiotics to anesthetic agents and analgesics. Patients with liver dysfunction are particularly susceptible to anesthetic effects, such as changes in hepatic metabolism of medications and changes in hepatic blood flow. Alterations of the type and dose of an agent are necessary to avoid postoperative hepatic dysfunction and hepatitis. Postoperative pain management with narcotic agents needs to be reduced by as much as 50% to account for the altered hepatic metabolism in these patients (136).

PREOPERATIVE NUTRITIONAL ASSESSMENT

There is a clear correlation between the degree of malnutrition and increased risk of perioperative complications in patients with cancer undergoing surgery (137). The broader consideration of nutrition in the patient with gynecologic cancer is discussed in Chapter 12.4. The intent of this section is to present the concepts of preoperative nutritional evaluation and support of the patient with gynecologic oncology undergoing surgery. Early refeeding as well as enteral and parenteral nutritional support in the postoperative patient is discussed later.

The incidence of malnutrition among patients with cancer has been estimated to be 20% to 80%, with the prevalence among patients with gynecologic oncology being approximately 20%. Patients with ovarian cancer are 19 times more likely to have moderate

■ **TABLE 12.3-8. Model for End-Stage Liver Disease (MELD) Score**

MELD score = $(9.6 \times \log_e[\text{Creatinine}]) + (3.8 \times \log_e[\text{Bilirubin}]) + 11.2 \times \log_e[\text{INR}]) + 6.4$			
Creatinine levels >4.0 mg/dL are assigned 4.0 mg/dL. Levels <1.0 mg/dL are assigned 1.0 mg/dL. If the patient has had dialysis twice in the previous week, the value is assigned 4.0 mg/dL.			
Bilirubin levels <1.0 mg/dL are assigned 1.0 mg/dL.			
INR levels <1.0 are assigned 1.0.			
The maximum score is 40. Scores calculated >40 are assigned a value of 40.			
MELD score	<10	10-15	>15
	Low risk	Intermediate risk	High risk
30-d mortality (abdominal/cardiac/orthopedic surgery) (%)	5-5.7	10	>50

INR, international normalized ratio.

Adapted from Hanje AJ, Patel T. Preoperative evaluation of patients with liver disease. *Nat Clin Pract Gastroenterol Hepatol*. 2007;4:266-276; Malik SM, Ahmad J. Preoperative risk assessment for patients with liver disease. *Med Clin N Am*. 2009;93:917-929; Friedman LS. Surgery in the patient with liver disease. *Trans Am Clin Climatol Assoc*. 2010;121:192-204, with permission.

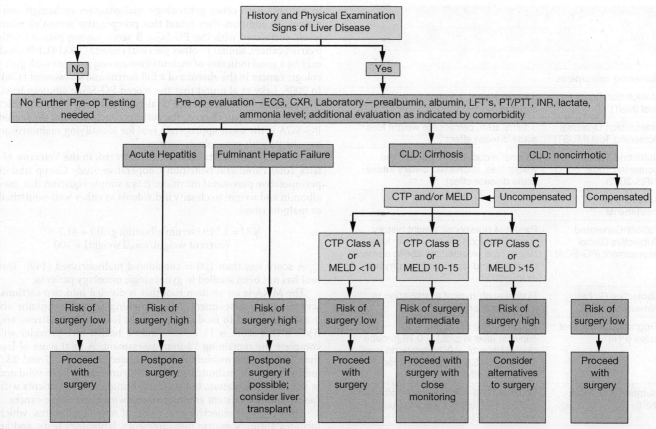

Figure 12.3-1. Preoperative evaluation and risk stratification in suspected liver disease. ALT, alanine aminotransferase; AP, alkaline phosphatase; AST, aspartate aminotransferase; CLD, chronic liver disease; CTP, Childs-Turcotte-Pugh; ECG, electrocardiogram; INR, international normalization ratio; LFTs, liver function tests; MELD, model of end-stage liver disease; PT, prothrombin time; PTT, partial prothrombin time. (Adapted from Hanje AJ, Patel T. Preoperative evaluation of patients with liver disease. *Nat Clin Pract Gastroenterol Hepatol.* 2007;4:266-276; Hoetzel A, Ryan H, Schmidt R. Anesthetic considerations for the patient with liver disease. *Curr Opin Anaesthesiol.* 2012;25(3):340-347.)

malnutrition when compared to patients with other gynecologic malignancies or benign conditions (138,139). Malnourished gynecologic oncology patients have been found to have an increased risk of postoperative complications, longer length of stay, hospital readmissions, reoperations, earlier cancer recurrences, and residual tumor after initial surgery (139-141). The methods for assessing malnutrition vary among investigators and include weight loss over a given time, various objective anthropometric parameters (eg, weight loss, BMI, triceps skinfold thickness, and arm circumference), biochemical testing (eg, serum albumin, prealbumin, total protein, transferrin, hemoglobin, and vitamins), and immunologic testing (skin-sensitivity tests) (Table 12.3-9) (142).

Nutrition screening refers to the initial clinical evaluation that can quickly identify patients at high risk for malnutrition and who, later, may undergo a more formal and extensive nutritional assessment. Such instruments are the Malnutrition Screening Tool (MST) and the Malnutrition Universal Screening Tool (MUST), which have been used in oncology patients (Table 12.3-10). Logically, screening and identifying patients at nutritional risk will flag them for formal nutrition assessment, identify opportunities for medical nutrition therapy, and, ultimately, improve patient outcomes. Unfortunately, this sequence of assumptions has never been subjected to prospective confirmation in clinical trials (143). Prehabilitation guidelines have been suggested for colorectal patients to optimize nutrition, but no prospective trials assessing efficacy of such interventions have been completed (144).

Many nutrition assessment tools have been developed, including subjective and objective data to assign risk, and some have been validated in patients with cancer, including patients with gynecologic cancer. Those instruments that have been used in patients with cancer include the Subjective Global Assessment (SGA), the Patient-Generated Subjective Global Assessment (PG-SGA), Nutrition Risk Index (NRI), the Mini Nutritional Assessment (MNA), Prognostic Nutritional Index (PNI), and the Nutritional Risk Screening 2002 (NRS-2002) (Table 12.3-10). Although just examples of the many assessment tools available, none has emerged as the "gold standard" for nutritional screening and/or nutritional

TABLE 12.3-9. Measurement of Nutritional Depletion

Parameters	Depletion		
	Mild	Moderate	Severe
Triceps skinfold (TSF) (% standard)	50-90	30-50	<30
Mid-arm muscle circumference (MAMC) (% standard)	80-90	70-80	<70
Albumin (g/dL)	3.0-3.4	2.1-3.0	<2.1
Total lymphocyte count (TLC) (cmm)	1,200-1,500	800-1200	<800
Weight loss (% initial)			
1 wk	<1	1-2	>2
1 mo	<2	2-5	>5
3 mo	<5	5.0-7.5	>7.5
6 mo	<7.5	7.5-10.0	>10.0

Tool	Components
Screening Instruments	
Malnutrition Screening Tool (MST)	3 items: weight, percentage weight loss, appetite
Malnutrition Universal Screening Tool (MUST)	3 items: BMI, percentage weight loss, acute disease effect
Nutritional Risk Screening 2002 (NRS-2002)	4 items: reduced BMI, percentage weight loss, decreased dietary intake, acute disease effect
Assessment Instruments	
Patient-Generated Subjective Global Assessment (PG-SGA)	Patient (4 questions): weight history, symptoms, food intake, activity level Health care provider: metabolic demand, diagnosis and comorbidities, physical examination
Subjective Global Assessment (SGA)	History and physical examination to assign nutrition score
Prognostic Nutritional Index (PNI)	Equation: PNI score (%) = 158 − 16.6 (albumin level in g/dL) − 0.78 (triceps skinfold in mm) − 0.2 (transferrin level in mg/dL) − 5.8 (grade of delayed hypersensitivity)
Nutrition Risk Index (NRI)	Equation: NRI = 1.519 (serum albumin; g/dL) + 41.7 (current weight/usual weight) × 100
Mini Nutritional Assessment (MNA)	18 items: Screening portion (6 questions): food intake, weight loss, mobility stress, BMI; Assessment (12 questions): medical history, eating habits, anthropometric measurements

BMI, body mass index.

Adapted from Huhmann MB, August DA: Review of American Society for Parenteral and Enteral Nutrition (ASPEN) clinical guidelines for nutrition support in cancer patients: nutrition screening and assessment. *Nutr Clin Pract.* 2008;23:182-188, with permission.

assessment among patients with cancer, and their use depends upon which organization endorses a particular tool.

The SGA tool, originally described by Detsky in 1987, uses history and physical examination to assign a nutrition risk score. The PG-SGA was adapted from the SGA by Ottery and later modified by McCallum and Polisena to assign a numerical score of 0 to 47, specifically for the oncology population (145-148). It consists of two sections, one completed by the patient. This portion elicits information related to weight history, symptoms, food intake, and activity level. The other section, completed by a health care professional, includes an evaluation of metabolic demand, diagnosis, and comorbidities in relation to nutrition requirements and elements of physical examination. Every portion of the tool is given a numeric score, including the patient's portion, which is used to triage intervention. In 2007, Laky and colleagues showed, in a prospective manner, that the PG-SGA could be easily administered to identify patients with gynecologic cancer at risk for malnutrition. Their work established the prevalence of malnutrition among their patients in Brisbane, Australia. Among 145 patients with known or suspected gynecologic cancer, 116 patients were classified as well nourished (PG-SGA A), 29 patients were moderately malnourished (PG-SGA B), and none of the patients were severely malnourished (PD-SGA C). These investigators found that patients with ovarian cancer were 19 times more likely to be malnourished compared to patients with other gynecologic malignancies or benign conditions. In addition, they found that preoperative serum albumin levels correlated with the PG-SGA B score among patients with ovarian cancer, similar to other previous reports (140,141,148), and may be a good indicator of malnutrition among patients with gynecologic cancer in the absence of a full nutritional assessment (138). In 2008, Laky et al found that the scored PG-SGA, albumin level, triceps skinfold thickness, and total-body potassium could predict the SGA better than chance. The authors concluded that the scored PG-SGA is the most appropriate tool for identifying malnutrition in patients with gynecologic cancer.

The NRI was used to stratify nutrition risk in the Veterans Affairs Total Parenteral Nutrition Cooperative Study Group trial of perioperative parenteral nutrition. It is a simple equation that uses albumin and weight to classify individuals as either well-nourished or malnourished:

$$NRI = 1.519 \text{ (serum albumin; g/dL)} + 41.7$$
$$\text{(current weight/usual weight)} \times 100$$

A score less than 100 is considered malnourished (149). This tool has not been studied in gynecologic oncology patients.

The MNA is an 18-item tool that is divided into two sections: screening and assessment. The screening segment contains six questions related to food intake, weight loss, mobility, stress, and BMI. If this score is 11 or less, then a health care provider will complete the remaining 12-item assessment. A total score of less than 17 indicates malnutrition, and a score between 17 and 23.5 indicates risk for malnutrition. This instrument has been validated in the older population, but its use is limited among patients with cancer and nonexistent among patients with gynecologic cancer.

The PNI is an objective evaluation of nutritional status, which includes anthropometric measurements, laboratory tests, and an assessment of cell-mediated immunity by testing to mumps, tuberculin, and *Candida* (the grade of response is 0: nonreactive; 1: <5 mm induration; 2: ≥5 mm induration) (150). The information gathered is put into the following formula:

$$\text{PNI Score (\%)} = 158 - 16.6 \text{ (albumin level in g/dL)} -$$
$$0.78 \text{ (triceps skin fold in mm)} -$$
$$0.2 \text{ (transferrin level in mg/dL)} -$$
$$5.8 \text{ (Grade of delayed hypersensitivity)}$$

If the PNI is less than 40%, the patient is determined to have normal nutritional status; PNI 40% to 49% indicates mild malnutrition; PNI greater than 50% is severe malnutrition. Santoso et al compared this objective, yet cumbersome and expensive, method to the SGA for gynecologic malignancies. They found that agreement between the two methods was only fair to moderate, with the SGA methodology trending toward underreporting when compared to the objective method (151).

The NRS-2002 was developed to include measures of current malnutrition and disease severity. This scoring system assesses current malnutrition by scoring the amount and duration of weight loss, reduced BMI, and recent decrease in dietary intake. In addition, the severity of illness is graded as a reflection of increased nutritional requirements. A score is calculated for each part of the assessment and added together for the final score. A score of 3 or more indicates the need to start nutritional support. This NRS-2002 is recommended by the European Society for Clinical Nutrition and Metabolism (ESPEN) for the screening of hospitalized patients and has been widely accepted in Europe. It is important to note that this tool is useful in identifying patients who will benefit from nutrition intervention, but does not categorize the risk of malnutrition. This tool has not been evaluated among patients with gynecologic malignancies undergoing surgery (152).

Currently, the American Society of Parenteral and Enteral Nutrition (ASPEN) and the ESPEN do not recommend routine nutrition support therapy (NST—parenteral or enteral) in patients undergoing major cancer operations. The risks and costs of routine perioperative NST outweigh benefits in terms of surgical outcomes in patients with cancer (137,152,153).

Several RCTs have evaluated NST in patients with cancer undergoing surgery. The largest trial, the Veterans Affairs Cooperative Study, randomized 395 surgical (abdominal or noncardiac thoracic surgeries) patients, mostly male, to receive at least 7 days of preoperative and 3 days of postoperative total parenteral nutrition (TPN) or to receive no perioperative nutritional supplementation. The TPN group had a greater number of infectious complications, mostly among patients classified as borderline or mildly malnourished compared to the unfed patients (14.1% vs 6.4%). However, a subset of severely malnourished patients derived benefit from lower operative complication rates (5% vs 43%, P = .03) without incurring an increase in infectious complications. The overall 30- and 90-day mortality rates were not different between the groups (149). Meijerink et al completed a trial of preoperative nutrition among 151 patients undergoing surgery for gastric or colorectal cancer and randomized to preoperative TPN versus enteral nutrition (EN) versus standard oral diet (SOD). The authors found that there was no difference in mortality among the groups. However, patients who were severely malnourished and received either TPN or EN had fewer intra-abdominal abscesses than the SOD, but there was a difference in infectious morbidity between the TPN and EN groups (154). A similar study by Bozzetti et al randomized severely malnourished patients undergoing resection of gastric or colonic malignancies to 10 days of preoperative and 9 days of postoperative TPN or SOD with hypocaloric TPN postoperatively only. The TPN-only group showed lower noninfectious postoperative complication rates and mortality (155). Finally, Wu et al randomized 468 patients to preoperative and postoperative TPN/EN versus postoperative hypocaloric TPN among moderately to severely malnourished patients undergoing surgery for GI cancers. The investigators found fewer complications, lower mortality, and shorter length of stay among the full nutrition support group (156). Because of the findings of these trials, both ASPEN and ESPEN suggest that perioperative NST may be beneficial in moderately or severely malnourished patients if administered for 7 to 14 days preoperatively. The potential benefits of NST must be weighed against the potential risks of the NST itself and of delaying the operation. The authors direct the reader to reviews of these recommendations, which have been done by Huhman and August (for ASPEN) (137) and Braga et al (for ESPEN) (153).

PREPARATION FOR SURGERY

Enhanced Recovery After Surgery

Originating in colorectal surgery, enhanced recovery after surgery (ERAS) protocols or enhanced recovery pathways (ERPs) have improved surgical outcomes as well as realized significant cost savings. These approaches were founded by European surgeons who challenged traditional surgical paradigms, such as preoperative bowel preparation, the overnight fasting rule, and delayed postoperative feeding. These researchers found that most of these practices lacked scientific evidence and actually impaired patients' preoperative preparation and recovery. Reviews of these protocols in colorectal surgery have demonstrated a reduction in length of stay of 2.5 days, a decrease in complications by as much as 50%, and a mean savings, per patient of $2,245 per patient (157-159). The basic principles of ERAS are to attenuate the stress response to surgery by omitting bowel preparation, maintaining euvolemia, starting early postoperative feeding, and avoiding IV opioids (160-162) (**Figure 12.3-2**). These programs are protocols that must be followed to obtain the greatest benefit, not omitting any of the steps along the way. The barriers to implementation come from long-held biases (not based on evidence) and multiple patient encounters with various specialties (preoperative nursing, anesthesia, residents, postoperative nursing, etc) through their journey of surgery. Critical to success of these programs is auditing the process to identify areas where protocol deviations occur and to identify areas of improvement.

Data on ERAS in gynecologic oncology are growing. One such study done at the Mayo Clinic Rochester, MN, by Kalogera et al demonstrated that the use of patient-controlled anesthesia decreased over 60% with an 80% reduction of opioid use in the first 48 hours without change of pain scores among enhanced recovery patients as compared to historic controls. In addition, the authors showed a 4-day reduction in length of hospital stay, with stable readmission rates and a 30-day cost savings of more than $7,600 per patients on the ERP. Furthermore, there were no differences in the rate of or complexity of postoperative complications among the enhanced recovery patients (162). A systemic review and meta-analysis confirmed that ERAS protocols decrease hospital stay, complications, and cost in gynecologic oncology patients without increase in mortality or readmission (163). The ERAS Society was founded in 2010 in an effort to reach other surgical specialists and subspecialists and publish guidelines. As a result, the Society

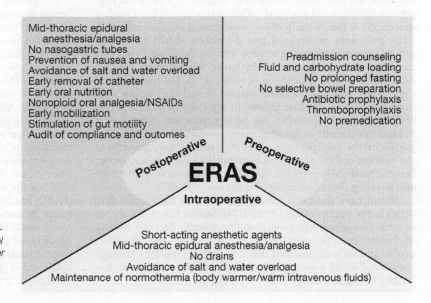

Figure 12.3-2. The elements of enhanced recovery after surgery (ERAS) pathways. For maximum benefit, *all* the elements must be followed. NSAID, nonsteroidal anti-inflammatory drug. (From ERAS Society. *ERAS® protocol improves survival after radical cystectomy: a single-center cohort study.* Published 2010. Accessed April 2, 2016. http://www.erassociety.org/index.php/eras-care-system/eras-protocol)

recently published a two-part series on ERAS in *Gynecologic Oncology*. In 2019, the ERAS Society updated recommendations and published in the *International Journal of Gynecologic Oncology*. The authors direct readers to these guidelines for further details (164-166). ***Best practice: For optimal results, ERAS protocols should be followed in their entirety. Preoperative preparation includes education, counseling, prehabilitation, and changes in preoperative fasting. Perioperative items include venous thromboembolism (VTE) prophylaxis, SSI bundles, anesthetic protocols, minimally invasive surgery, fluid management, and opioid-sparing analgesia. Vulvar and vaginal surgery guidelines are emerging from the ERAS Society.***

Medication Management

In preparation for surgery, patients may need to decrease or stop taking certain medications, especially those associated with higher incidence of anticoagulation risks. Appropriate notice and clear instructions should be given to patients, as some medications require several days of cessation to produce the desired results. It will take approximately 4 days after warfarin therapy is discontinued for the INR to reach 1.5 for those patients with INR levels between 2.0 and 3.0. Many patients on warfarin do not need to be covered with heparin therapy preoperatively. Administration of treatment dose IV heparin or low-molecular-weight heparin (LMWH) while the INR is subtherapeutic is recommended for patients with a history of mechanical mitral valve, ball and cage valve, acute VTE or arterial thromboembolism within 3 months of surgery, or atrial fibrillation with a history of thromboembolic stroke (167). A thorough discussion pertaining to usage of over-the-counter medications and herbal supplements is crucial in presurgery medication management. Patients should be counseled on the use of nonprescription medications, such as aspirin, nonsteroidal anti-inflammatories, ginkgo biloba, saw palmetto, garlic, ginseng, and vitamin E, as they have antiplatelet components and may enhance bleeding risk (168,169). If possible, anemia should be corrected preoperatively. The use of recombinant human erythropoietin with concurrent iron and folic acid supplementation 2 to 3 weeks preoperatively has been shown to reduce allogeneic blood transfusions in patients undergoing elective surgery (170). It has been estimated that 60% of all blood transfused in the United States is given to surgical patients.

Numerous studies have shown the benefit of starting medications, such as statins and β-blockers, in the preoperative setting to reduce cardiac risk (171). The perioperative use of β-blockers has been shown to reduce the incidence of postoperative myocardial ischemia, MI, and cardiac mortality by decreasing myocardial oxygen consumption and workload, although this has not been studied specifically in the morbidly obese population (171). Current ACC/AHA guidelines recommend that β-blockers should be continued in patients undergoing surgery who are receiving β-blockers to treat angina, symptomatic arrhythmias, hypertension, or other ACC/AHA class I guideline indications (172). For high-risk patients not receiving β-blockade, therapy should start before elective surgery, with the dose titrated to achieve a heart rate at rest of 50 to 60 beats/min (173). The perioperative use of β-blockers in high-risk patients undergoing major noncardiac surgery is supported by the published data. However, studies have questioned the benefits of this approach in moderate-risk patients and report that the potential harm in low-risk groups might outweigh the benefit, stressing the importance of patient selection (174).

Statins have also been shown to be effective cardioprotective drugs in the perioperative setting (171). Statins have been shown to act as plaque stabilizers and, therefore, possibly decrease the risk of thromboembolic events (171,175). With their low side-effect profile and well-documented benefits, statins should be strongly considered for all patients with obesity with elevated serum cholesterol or triglycerides (176).

Close to 2 million patients undergo coronary angioplasty each year in Western countries, and more than 90% of these patients will have coronary stents placed as part of their intervention (177,178). Patients with bare metal stents routinely take low-dose aspirin 81 mg. It is recommended that patients discontinue aspirin 7 days before noncardiac surgery (179-181). Patients with DESs take daily oral clopidogrel 75 mg for the first 12 months after stent placement, followed by oral aspirin 81 or 325 mg (180,182). Ideally, these patients should not undergo elective surgery, within the first 12 months after stenting. After the first 12 months, both medications are recommended to be discontinued 7 days before surgery to reduce the risk of intraoperative and postoperative bleeding (179). However, a retrospective study comparing low-dose aspirin users to nonusers at the time of laparoscopic surgery for endometrial cancer staging found no increased risk of bleeding or hemorrhagic complication in those who did not interrupt aspirin therapy, indicating safety in continuation of aspirin 81 mg before surgery (183).

It is not uncommon for gynecologic oncology patients to undergo NACT. Most gynecologic oncologists would agree that the timing of surgery in relation to chemotherapy is crucial. In most cases, the surgical intervention should replace a cycle of chemotherapy. With regard to bevacizumab, special considerations should be taken into account because there is the added risk of bowel perforation and poor wound healing. The incidence, type, and timing of postsurgical bleeding events and wound healing complications were assessed in surgical patients in the AVastin And DOcetaxel (AVADO) and Avastin THErapy for advaNced breAst cancer (ATHENA) trials. Both study protocols followed recommendations to withhold bevacizumab for at least 6 weeks before elective surgery and to wait 28 days (or until the wound was fully healed) after major surgery before recommencing bevacizumab therapy (184). Another study by Erinjeri et al investigated how the timing of administration of bevacizumab affected the risk of wound healing in patients undergoing chest wall port placement. They concluded the risk of a wound dehiscence requiring a chest wall port explant in patients treated with bevacizumab was inversely proportional to the interval between bevacizumab administration and port placement, with significantly higher risk seen when the interval is less than 14 days (185,186).

Blood Banking

Patients and their families are taking a more proactive role in their health care and thereby are entering into surgeries knowledgeable of risks and expecting alternative options. Preoperative counseling should include discussion of the potential for blood transfusions and associated risks. Transfusion rates of approximately 5% have been reported for patients undergoing abdominal hysterectomy for benign disease (186). Radical procedures performed for the treatment of gynecologic malignancies are associated with an average estimated blood loss of 209 mL, but can exceed 2,000 mL. Transfusion rates for patients undergoing radical hysterectomy have been reported around 10% (187). The risk of transfusion-transmitted infection of human immunodeficiency virus, hepatitis B virus, and hepatitis C virus from RBC transfusion is estimated at 1:2 million units (188). Although these rates have significantly decreased in the past decade with the introduction of new screening technologies, transmission of other agents, bacterial contamination, transfusion reactions, increased infection complications, and immunosuppression remain risks of allogeneic blood transfusion (189,190). One alternative is the use of donor blood in the perioperative period.

Since the mid-1980s, preoperative autologous blood donation (PABD) has been utilized in order to avoid allogeneic blood transfusion in patients undergoing elective surgery where excessive blood loss is anticipated. Although this practice decreases homologous blood use, 15% of autologous donors will still receive allogeneic transfusions, and 50% of units collected are not used and must be discarded (191). Furthermore, PABD greatly increases the likelihood of any transfusion being necessary and is not without medical risks. Severe reactions during autologous donation occurred at a rate of 0.32% per unit collected and 0.75% per donor. Serious incidents during blood collection that required hospitalization were 12 times more likely in PABD compared to allogeneic donors (192). Transfusions to the wrong recipient, bacterial contamination, febrile nonhemolytic reactions, and allergic reactions have also been reported with autologous transfusion. The cost-effectiveness of PABD has been found to be extremely poor and has steadily deteriorated (191-194).

Acute normovolemic hemodilution (ANH) is an autologous blood-procurement strategy that is equivalent to PABD in reducing allogeneic transfusion needs. Its clinical utility has been extensively studied in patients undergoing radical prostatectomy, total joint replacement, and, more recently, major colorectal surgery. During ANH, blood is procured in the holding or operating room and replaced simultaneously with colloid and crystalloid until a target hematocrit level of 28% is reached or blood volume of 1,500 mL is removed (195). The patient's blood becomes diluted, and the amount of actual red cell mass lost during surgery is reduced. ANH obviates the costs of blood testing, storage, or wastage because all blood collected during ANH is kept in the operating room and returned to the patient before the end of surgery. It is simple to perform and more convenient for the patient. Because the blood is collected at point of care, there is no possibility for clerical error or contamination. ANH has been shown to be a cost-effective yet underutilized strategy to reduce allogeneic blood transfusions (195-197). ANH in which the blood is kept in a continuous circuit with the patient is often an acceptable alternative for a Jehovah's Witness patient (195,198).

The utilization of erythropoietin in oncology patients should on a case-by-case basis owing to evidence of adverse effects in oncology patients (199).

Bowel Preparation and Preoperative Fasting

Older thinking had been that in anticipation of colorectal surgery, bowel preparation would decrease the risks of infection and anastomotic leaks. In gynecology, it was thought that mechanical bowel preparation would make the bowel easier to handle, improve visualization (especially with laparoscopic surgery), and decrease postoperative complications. Recent studies have demonstrated that these views are not true and actually may have adverse effects. The process of cleansing the bowel with liters of fluid is distressing to patients causing nausea and vomiting, physical discomfort, dehydration, electrolyte abnormalities, and prolonged fasting, all of which increase insulin resistance and catabolism, increasing the stress of the surgical process.

A recent database analysis of mechanical bowel preparation or oral antibiotics for hysterectomy for benign or malignant indications, irrespective of surgical approach, showed no decrease in SSI (without prep 5.2% vs 7.4% with mechanical bowel prep), anastomotic leak (0.7% vs 1.1%), postoperative ileus (1.5% vs 2.9%), or major morbidity (3.9% vs 5.5%). The authors concluded that mechanical bowel preparation was not necessary for gynecologic surgery (200). These findings are similar to the conclusions of a systematic review of 18 RCTs of mechanical bowel preparation or rectal enemas versus no preparation before elective colorectal surgery (201). Finally, a recent RCT assessing the benefit of mechanical bowel preparation versus no prep for patients undergoing low anterior resections for rectal carcinoma demonstrated higher infectious morbidity for the no prep group, but no difference in anastomotic leaks (202).

In contrast, the American College of Surgeons and the Surgical Infection Society published SSI guidelines recommending preoperative bowel preparation for elective colorectal surgery. In recent years, literature has come full circle again supporting a combination of mechanical and oral antibiotic bowel preparation. Mechanical bowel preparation or oral antibiotic preparation alone has not been found to decrease SSI; however, in combination, these interventions lower rates of SSI, anastomotic leak, *Clostridium difficile* infection, and postoperative ileus. This combination also reduces length of stay and readmission rates. Oral antibiotic regimen consists of neomycin and erythromycin (203). Clearly, further study of this topic will be needed. ***Best practice: Routine oral mechanical bowel preparation should not be used routinely in gynecologic oncology surgery.***

Fear of aspiration drove "dogma" within the specialties of anesthesiology and surgery to instruct patients to fast for 12 hours or more before surgery. The thinking was that a prolonged fast before surgery would reduce the amount of acid and gastric contents in the stomach, thus preventing aspiration at the time of induction (204). A Cochrane review of 22 RCTs has shown that shortened fasting periods did not increase the risk of aspiration, regurgitation, or related morbidity (205). Thus, the ASA recommends a fast of 6 hours preoperatively for solid foods and that clear liquids be consumed for up to 2 hours before surgery (206). A prolonged preoperative fast for up to 12 hours will cause the patient to deplete their glycogen stores, which leads to insulin resistance and hyperglycemia, increasing postoperative complications and morbidity. Carbohydrate-loading drinks given to patients 2 to 3 hours before surgery can prevent insulin resistance, decrease hyperglycemia, and attenuate the stress response to surgery. These complex carbohydrate solutions are emptied by the stomach within 30 to 90 minutes and have been shown to reduce patient anxiety, thirst, and hunger (204). An RCT of carbohydrate loading versus no loading in patients undergoing colorectal surgery showed a significant reduction in length of stay (207). ***Best practice: Patients should be permitted to drink clear liquids until 2 hours before anesthesia and surgery. Patients should abstain from oral intake of solids 6 hours before induction of anesthesia. Oral carbohydrate loading reduces postoperative insulin resistance, improves preoperative well-being, and should be used routinely in nondiabetic patients.***

Antibiotic Prophylaxis

The use of prophylactic antimicrobials plays a large role in reducing the rates of SSIs and should be used in clean or clean-contaminated operations, which include most procedures performed by gynecologic oncologists. Radical pelvic surgery introduces women to a higher risk of postoperative infection secondary to several potential factors: lengthened operating time, average age of patient, increased blood loss, anemia, potential hypothermia, probable poor nutritional status, the presence of tumor, prior pelvic irradiation, diabetes, obesity, peripheral vascular disease, and a history of postsurgical infection (208,209). Prophylactic antibiotics should provide coverage consistent with the microbial milieu most likely to be encountered. In gynecologic oncology surgery, the most common infecting organisms are coliforms, enterococci, streptococci, *Clostridia*, and *Bacteroides*.

Several guidelines for antibiotic prophylaxis in surgery have been published (208,210,211). Most reports recommend cefazolin for gynecologic procedures. Although no longer available, cefotetan had been the preferred antibiotic for prophylaxis in longer radical gynecologic operations, as well as for prophylaxis before colorectal surgery, owing to longer half-life and broad-spectrum coverage (212). An appropriate alternative for surgical procedures with a higher chance of bowel resection or injury is cefazolin plus metronidazole or ampicillin-sulbactam (211). Cefoxitin is another option, but availability has been limited. Most patients with a penicillin allergy can be treated with cefazolin; however, when allergy prohibits the administration of a cephalosporin, alternative regimens are clindamycin with gentamicin, a fluoroquinolone, or aztreonam (210).

When considering dosing to achieve and maintain effective tissue levels, parenteral antibiotics should be given within 1 hour (between 1 and 2 hours for fluoroquinolones and vancomycin) before skin incision as a loading dose (210). For patients weighing more than 80 kg, the dosage should be doubled (ie, cefazolin 2 g IV), or weight-based dosing should be used. For patients weighing more than 120 kg, the dose of cefazolin is increased to 3 g. Repeat doses should be given intraoperatively for surgeries lasting longer than 4 hours or when blood loss exceeds 1,500 mL (213). Guidelines from the National Surgical Site Infection Project recommend that prophylactic antibiotic use for abdominal or vaginal procedures end within 24 hours of the operation (210). The majority of the published evidence supports the use of an appropriately timed administration of a single dose of antibiotic and indicates that repeat doses postoperatively are unnecessary and subject the patient to the potential emergence of resistant organisms (208,210,211).

The American College of Surgeons NSQIP employs a prospective, peer-reviewed database to quantify 30-day risk-adjusted surgical outcomes that encompass variables such as preoperative risk factors and postoperative mortality and morbidity, allowing comparison of outcomes among all hospitals in the program. Enrolled hospitals abstract case data into the database, the data are quantified, and the database generates comprehensive semiannual reports to the hospitals as well as real-time, continuously updated, online benchmarking reports (214). *Best practice: IV antibiotics should be administered routinely within 60 minutes before skin incision. The dose should be repeated in the case of a prolonged operation or severe blood loss; the dose should be increased in patients with obesity.*

Skin Preparation

SSIs account for nearly 40% of nosocomial infections in surgical patients and occur in up to 20% of patients undergoing abdominal surgery (208,210). They are a significant source of postoperative morbidity, resulting in longer hospital stays, increased rates of ICU admissions, hospital readmissions, and, subsequently, increased costs. Mortality rates increase 2 to 3 times for patients with an SSI as compared to patients who do not develop an SSI (215,216). In addition to the administration of preoperative antimicrobial prophylaxis, preoperative skin preparation is employed to reduce the risk of SSI by decreasing the microbial count at the projected site of incision. The CDC guidelines reference a 2015 Cochrane review of seven RCTs showing no difference in infection rates between antiseptic (most commonly 4% chlorhexidine gluconate), soap, or placebo bath or shower before surgery (213). SSI occurrences are noted to be influenced by both patient and operative environmental factors. Therefore, patients undergoing surgery should be instructed to bathe or shower normally the night or morning before surgery, removing any debris from the skin surface and decreasing environmental contaminants.

At the time of surgery, alcohol-based surgical site skin preparation agents are preferred unless contraindicated. Chlorhexidine-alcohol is an appropriate choice as it has greater reductions in skin microflora and residual activity after application compared to povidone-iodine. Vaginal cleansing with either 4% chlorhexidine gluconate or povidone-iodine should be performed before hysterectomy or vaginal surgery (213).

Surgical bundles have been implemented in colorectal surgery to reduce the incidence of SSIs. A retrospective study of open uterine cancer, ovarian cancer without bowel resection, and ovarian cancer with bowel resection determined baseline SSI rates. A perioperative bundle was then prospectively implemented at the Mayo Clinic, including patient education, 4% chlorhexidine gluconate shower before surgery, antibiotic administration, 2% chlorhexidine gluconate and 70% isopropyl alcohol coverage of incisional area, and cefazolin redosing 3 to 4 hours after incision. New elements implemented included sterile closing tray, glove change for fascia and skin closure, dressing removal at 24

to 48 hours, discharge with 4% chlorhexidine gluconate, and follow-up nursing phone call. The relative risk reduction of SSI was 77.6% among ovarian cancer with bowel resection, 79.3% among ovarian cancer without bowel resection, and 100% among uterine cancer. The American College of Surgeons NSQIP decile improved from the tenth to first percentile (217).

Inappropriate hair removal techniques can traumatize the skin and provide an opportunity for colonization of microorganisms. There is no evidence that hair removal before surgery will prevent or reduce SSI. To the contrary, meta-analysis evaluating hair removal techniques demonstrated a 2-fold increase in SSI when patients underwent hair removal by shaving versus clipping (218). Hair is generally sterile and, therefore, does not need to be removed unless the hair around the incision will interfere with the operation. When hair removal is necessary, the simplest and least irritating method of hair removal is an electric or battery-powered clipper with a disposable head (208,218). *Best practice: Hair clipping is preferred if hair removal is mandatory. Chlorhexidine-alcohol is preferred to aqueous povidone-iodine solution for skin cleansing.*

Perioperative Venous Thromboembolism Prophylaxis

The prevention of VTE is an important component of perioperative management of the gynecologic oncology patient. The American College of Chest Physicians consensus statement published in 2021 reviews the data extensively and provides recommendations (219). Patients undergoing major gynecologic surgery without VTE prophylaxis have a risk of deep vein thrombosis (DVT) between 17% and 40% (220). Surgery for cancer, advanced age, previous VTE, prior pelvic radiation therapy, and abdominal resection (in contrast to vaginal resection) appear to increase the thromboembolic risk after gynecologic surgery (221). The incidence of pulmonary embolism (PE) is 1.6%, with the rate of fatal PE being 0.9%. In trials comparing low-dose unfractionated heparin (LDUH) with no therapy in general surgical patients, the DVT rate was decreased from 25% to 8%. These studies also produced a 50% decrease in the rate of fatal PE (222). Comparisons of LMWH versus LDUH have shown equal efficacy. LMWH may have fewer complications (namely wound hematomas) and greater ease of use with once-daily dosing.

Sequential pneumatic compression devices (PCDs) are attractive for patients at risk for bleeding complications. In trials comparing PCD with LDUH, both have shown efficacy. Elastic stockings TED hose and aspirin usage are not currently recommended for DVT prophylaxis. Patients at low risk (age <40 years, no risk factors, and minor surgery) need no prophylaxis, but early ambulation is encouraged. Moderate-risk patients (minor surgery in a patient with risk factors, major surgery with no risk factors) should receive PCD, LMWH, or LDUH, with equal results. High-risk patients require LMWH in addition to PCD.

In 2021, the Society of Gynecologic Oncology released a practice statement regarding direct-acting oral anticoagulant (DOAC) use in gynecologic oncology. All patients undergoing laparotomy for gynecology cancer should receive extended postoperative VTE prophylaxis for up to 4 weeks following surgery with LDUH, LMWH, or apixaban unless contraindicated due to active bleeding, high risk of bleeding, or other contraindication. Patients undergoing minimally invasive surgery do not need extended prophylaxis (221,223). An RCT of 400 women following gynecologic oncology surgery demonstrated no differences between enoxaparin or apixaban in rates of major bleeding, nonmajor bleeding, VTE, adverse events, medication adherence, or QoL (224).

A recent ASCO clinical practice guideline update confirms the recommendation for perioperative VTE prophylaxis in women undergoing major surgical intervention for malignancy via mechanical and pharmacologic prophylaxis. Pharmacologic prophylaxis should continue for at least 7 to 10 days but up to 4 weeks for major open or laparoscopic abdominal or pelvic surgery for cancer who have high-risk features, such as limited mobility, obesity, and prior VTE, among others. The ASCO recommends thromboprophylaxis in high-risk outpatients with cancer using apixaban, rivaroxaban, or LMWH. High-risk outpatients include patients undergoing systemic therapy with a Khorana score of 2 or higher (225). ***Best practice: All gynecologic oncology patients with a major surgery greater than 30 minutes should receive VTE prophylaxis with either LMWH or heparin with prophylaxis starting preoperatively and continued intraoperatively and postoperatively in combination with PCD. Extended prophylaxis with LMWH or DOACs should be continued for 28 days after laparotomy in patients with abdominal or pelvic malignancies.***

Frailty

One of the challenges for the gynecologic oncologist is to balance the risk versus benefits of treating older patients, taking into account age-related comorbidities, especially when considering surgery as part of the treatment. Frailty is the loss of physiologic reserve across multiple organ systems, leading to impaired restoration of homeostasis following external stress. Frailty is not only a factor of age but also the comorbidities and disabilities that relate to functional capacity (226). Multiple frailty assessment tools exist, including individual tools, scales, and surveys. Single-item assessment tools include gait speed, Timed Up-and-Go score, and sarcopenia (227). Screening tools are based on one of two concepts: phenotypic frailty, resulting from biologic decline of multiple systems, versus deficit accumulation frailty, based on comorbidities, social determinants, and disabilities (228-230). Many surgical subspecialties use these tools to predict postoperative complications and to personalize treatment. A systematic review reported the impact of preoperative frailty assessment on postoperative outcomes in women undergoing surgery for gynecologic cancer. This review found that the prevalence of frailty in gynecologic oncology patients varied from 6.1% to 60%. Frail patients were more likely to develop postoperative complications, non–home discharge, ICU admissions, and overall worse oncologic outcomes when compared to their nonfrail counterparts. The study concluded that frailty assessment is an essential preoperative element to predict adverse outcomes and personalize treatment (226). Similar findings were noted in a 2021 publication comparing gynecologic oncology patient–reported Rockwood Accumulation of Deficits Frailty Index (DAFI) to survival outcomes. An example of the DAFI tool can be found in **Table 12.3-11**. The DAFI is scored by actual deficit score divided by potential deficit score range, and its score

■ TABLE 12.3-11. Components of the 25-Item Deficit Accumulation Frailty Index and Respective Score

Domain		Item	Score		
			0	0.5	1
Activities of Daily Living	1	Bathing	No difficulty		Difficulty performing
	2	Dressing			
	3	Eating			
	4	Toileting			
Chronic Health Conditions	5	CAD/angina	Absent		Present
	6	HTN			
	7	MI			
	8	CHF			
	9	Stroke			
	10	Chronic lung disease			
	11	Diabetes			
	12	Arthritis (hip/knee)			
	13	IBD			
Functional Status	14	Vision	Yes		No
	15	Hearing	Yes		No
	16	Incontinence	No		Yes
	17	Transfers to Chair	No difficulty		Difficulty or unable
	18	Walking	No difficulty		Difficulty or unable
	19	Moderate activity	No limit	Limited a little	Limited a lot
	20	Climbing Stairs	No limit	Limited a little	Limited a lot
General Health	21	Lots of energy	All/most times	Good bit/sometimes	Little/no times
	22	General health	Excellent/very good/good	Fair	Poor
	23	Pain	None	Little/moderate	Quite a bit/extreme
Mental Health	24	Peacefulness	All/most times	Good bit/sometimes	Little/none
	25	Sadness	Little/none		All/most times

Adapted from Mullen MM, McKinnish TR, Fiala MA, et al. A deficit-accumulation frailty index predicts survival outcomes in patients with gynecologic malignancy. *Gynecol Oncol.* 2021;161(3):700-704.

CAD, coronary artery disease; CHF, congestive heart failure; HTN, hypertension; IBD, inflammatory bowel disease.

ranges from 0.0 to 1.0, with 0.0 having no deficits. A score of 0.2 or less defines patients as robust or nonfrail; a score of 0.2 to 0.35 as prefrail patients, and a score of 0.35 or greater is delineates patients who are frail. Each 10% increase in the DAFI increases the risk of death by 16% (231). Frailty was a significant predictor of mortality, with a 48% increased risk of death in frail patients. Steps to mitigate perioperative risk in frail patients include prehabilitation with exercise and nutrition counseling, anesthesia modifications, and involvement of palliative care (227).

The Eastern Cooperative Oncology Group (ECOG) performance status is commonly used to assess baseline function before initiating chemotherapy to determine a patient's ability to tolerate treatment. Limitations of the ECOG performance status include lack of consideration of age, comorbidities, or other aspects of frailty. Frailty assessment tools are emerging as valuable instruments at predicting patient tolerance to adjuvant therapies, such as chemotherapy and radiation therapy (227). The Elderly Selection on Geriatric Index Assessment (ESOGIA) is a recent study using the Comprehensive Geriatric Assessment (CGA) frailty tool to guide therapy for older patients with non–small cell lung cancer (NSCLC). "Fit" patients received a carboplatin-based doublet, vulnerable patients received docetaxel, and frail patients received supportive care. The CGA group experienced less toxicity and treatment failure, although no changes were seen in OS (232). Data on frailty and radiation treatment are limited. One study found age was not a predictor of radiation toxicity (233), whereas other studies found that the Edmonton Frail Scale showed no statistical correlation between frailty and radiation side effects (234,235).

CRITICAL CARE AND POSTOPERATIVE MANAGEMENT

Cardiovascular Issues

Monitoring Issues

There are many tools in the hands of the modern-day clinician when it comes to monitoring the cardiovascular function of the patient. Clinical examination, heart rate, blood pressure measurement, and ECG are a few. In the critical care setting, the additions of the arterial catheter, central venous pressure (CVP), and pulmonary artery catheter increase sophistication. Most patients in the ICU can be managed with simple clinical parameters. Fluid status can be assessed by daily weights, pulse, blood pressure, and urine output. Continuous ECG monitoring is helpful for detecting arrhythmias and ischemia. CVP is often used for assessment of volume status and a crude estimation of cardiac function. If a patient has a central line, one of the ports can be continuously transduced for CVP. It is a common mistake among inexperienced clinicians to evaluate a single reading of CVP rather than reviewing the trend. When the CVP is correlated with volume status, the resulting graph is a scatter graph (ie, no correlation). There is correlation over time and in response to fluid challenges, blood transfusion, or medical therapy. The CVP is a pressure measurement and not the desired measurement of volume (preload). Therefore, only crude estimations of fluid status can be made with results from this instrumentation. When the status of a patient's cardiac output or fluid state is unclear, a minimally invasive hemodynamic monitor or an invasive pulmonary artery catheter (eg, Swan-Ganz catheter) may be helpful. A minimally invasive hemodynamic monitor connects to an existing arterial catheter and performs continuous self-calibration. The sensor provides information on stroke volume, stroke volume variation (SVV), and cardiac output. These monitors are becoming more commonly used than pulmonary artery catheters because of the decreased risks. SVV is another measured value (similar to CVP) to provide information about volume status. Typically, more variation in stroke volume is consistent with a decreased intravascular volume status (236,237).

■ **TABLE 12.3-12. Hemodynamic Formulas**

Cardiac output (CO) = Stroke volume (SV) × heart rate (HR) [4-8 L/min]
Cardiac index (CI) = CO/body surface area (BSA)
Systemic vascular resistance (SVR) = Mean arterial pressure (MAP) − Central venous pressure (CVP) × 80/CO [800-1,200 dyne/s/cm^{-5}/m^2]
Arterial O_2 content (CaO_2) = (1.36) (hemoglobin) (oxygen saturation) + 0.003 (partial pressure of oxygen) [20 mL O_2/dL]
O_2 delivery (DO_2) = CO × CaO_2 × 10 [600-1,000 mL O_2/min]
O_2 availability (O_2AVI) = CI × CaO_2 × 10 [500-600 mL/min/m^2]
O_2 extraction ratio = (CaO_2 − CvO_2)/CaO_2 [25%]

Values in square brackets are normal values.

PA catheter use has become almost historical, but there are several values that can be calculated from the measurements obtained by a pulmonary artery catheter that can help determine volume status (Table 12.3-12). Assessment of preload is desirable for determining fluid administration or diuretic requirements for patients (Figures 12.3-5 and 12.3-6).

Perhaps, the most important function of a pulmonary artery catheter that cannot be replicated by the minimally invasive cardiac output monitors is a mixed venous blood gas, a blood sample from the tip of the pulmonary artery catheter representing the most desaturated blood in the body. In normal circulation, the blood from the superior and inferior (IVC) venae cavae mix and the blood from the coronary sinus are added to give a sample known as the mixed venous blood. By evaluating the oxygen saturation of this blood, oxygen delivery can be calculated (Table 12.3-12). Current technology allows this function to be continuous via an infrared sensor at the tip of the pulmonary artery catheter. If oxygen delivery is determined to be low, there are only three situations that the clinician can influence: increase cardiac output (with fluid, chronotropes, or inotropes), increase the hemoglobin, or increase the oxygen saturation. In a patient with multiple medical comorbidities following a major abdominal operation, the measurement of a normal oxygen delivery provides reassurance to the clinician that end organs are being perfused.

Over the past several years, the use of pulmonary artery catheters has become rare (238). Continuous dynamic measurements are possible with analysis of arterial and plethysmographic waveforms. SVV can be used for goal-directed therapy (239). There are several other minimally invasive monitors that are used with varying success, and discussion of use is beyond the scope of this chapter (236,240).

Acute Postoperative Myocardial Infarction

MI usually manifests with acute chest discomfort, elevated cardiac enzymes (troponin, creatine phosphokinase [CPK], etc) and ECG changes. Dyspnea, diaphoresis, nausea, and anxiety may also be associated. MI is defined by a rise of cardiac enzymes (troponin) in the setting of myocardial ischemia as evidenced by clinical symptoms, imaging findings, or ECG changes (241). Treatment includes ICU monitoring with continuous ECG monitoring, supplemental oxygen, immediate oral aspirin 325 mg administration, sublingual nitroglycerin, and morphine sulfate as needed until pain resolves. β-Blocker therapy has been shown to decrease mortality by decreasing fatal arrhythmias, and their administration is part of the early treatment regimen for MI (241). An evaluation for heparin therapy, thrombolytics, or cardiac catheterization intervention can be made in consultation with a cardiologist.

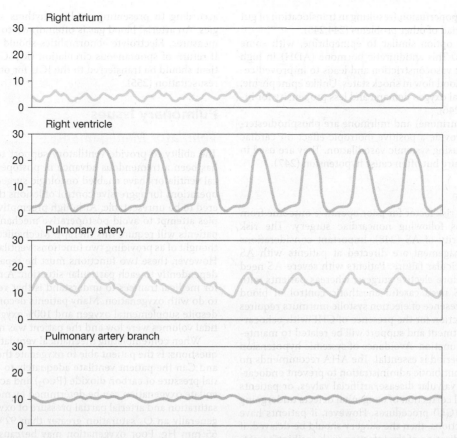

Figure 12.3-3. Pulmonary artery catheter waveform readings as the catheter passes through the heart into the pulmonary artery. *Y*-axis is reading in millimeters of mercury (mm Hg).

Congestive Heart Failure

Patients with known CHF will be risk stratified before major elective surgery. However, in the postoperative setting, CHF presents in a number of ways. Patients with CHF are in a continuous hypervolemic state, and issues of fluid balance (strict "ins" and "outs") are paramount during the perioperative period. In difficult cases, adjunctive measures monitoring CVP, minimally invasive cardiac output catheters, or pulmonary artery catheters can be very helpful. Imaging, such as chest x-rays and echocardiograms, can provide valuable information about evidence of pulmonary edema and heart function. BNP levels can also be obtained if there is concern for CHF (242).

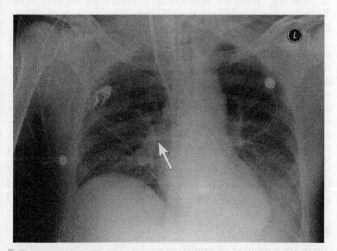

Figure 12.3-4. Chest radiograph showing proper placement of pulmonary artery catheter in the pulmonary artery (arrow shows tip of pulmonary catheter).

Inotropes and Vasopressors

A variety of hemodynamically active drugs are available to support the cardiovascular function of patients in the perioperative period (243). In the broadest sense, these drugs can be categorized as vasopressors, which elevate blood pressure, and inotropes, which enhance cardiac output (244). When it has been determined that oxygen delivery is low and increased cardiac output is desired, inotropes, such as dopamine, milrinone, or dobutamine, should be used. Dopamine, at lower doses, activates dopaminergic receptors and increases circulation in mesenteric, cerebral, and renal vascular beds. At intermediate doses, dopamine stimulates β-receptors in the heart and peripheral circulation. This activation causes tachycardia, increased stroke volume, and increased cardiac output. Increasing cardiac output in this manner also increases demands for myocardial oxygen and could precipitate angina, arrhythmias, or MI (245). At high doses, dopamine acts as an α-agonist, causing vasoconstriction. Dobutamine is a β-1 agonist with much greater inotropic effect than dopamine and causes peripheral arterial vasodilation, decreasing afterload (this dilation can be abrupt and cause hypotension in some patients). Dobutamine is the drug of choice for severe heart failure.

Epinephrine is a potent sympathomimetic with β-mimetic effects at lower doses and α-mimetic effects at higher doses. This drug causes an acute increase in myocardial oxygen demand and is used in the setting of cardiac arrest or severe circulatory failure. Norepinephrine and phenylephrine are pure α-mimetic agents, utilized for vasoconstriction (neurogenic shock). In most situations of shock, fluid resuscitation is preferred to administration of α-agents; however, norepinephrine is the vasopressor of choice for septic shock following initial fluid resuscitation. Although these agents will give a false sense of security that the blood pressure is normal, one must remember that the vasoconstriction underperfuses capillary beds and leads to renal hypoperfusion (acute renal injury), splanchnic hypoperfusion (resulting in translocation of gut flora), as well as a myriad of other problems (244,245).

Vasopressin is an option similar to epinephrine, with some important differences. This antidiuretic hormone (ADH) in high doses provides potent vasoconstriction and leads to improved cerebral and coronary blood flow in shock states. Unlike epinephrine, there is less myocardial oxygen demand and less propensity for inducing arrhythmias (246).

Amrinone (or inamrinone) and milrinone are phosphodiesterase inhibitors that provide a positive inotropic effect on cardiac musculature while causing systemic vasodilation. They are used in refractory cardiac failure but often cause hypotension (247).

Valvular Disease

AS is an independent risk factor for poor operative outcome from cardiac complications following noncardiac surgery. The risk depends on the severity of AS (248). Important considerations in perioperative management are directed at patients with AS and the level of ventricular failure. Patients with severe AS need valve replacement before elective surgery, whereas patients with mild-to-moderate AS need careful anesthetic control of blood pressure (249). The presence of ejection systolic murmurs requires assessment of LV function for the presence of CHF with echocardiography (233). Treatment and support will be related to maintenance of ventricular function. Avoidance of systemic hypotension in the perioperative period is essential. The AHA recommends no routine prophylactic antibiotic administration to prevent endocarditis in patients with valvular disease, artificial valves, or patients who have had surgical correction of congenital defects undergoing GI or genitourinary (GU) procedures. However, if patients have active GU or GI infections, then the surgery should be delayed, if possible, to allow eradication of the infection with antibiotic treatment. Any antibiotic regimen should include agents that are active against enterococci, such as ampicillin or vancomycin, and should be administered 30 minutes before to 2 hours after the procedure (250,251). Antibiotic prophylaxis may be reasonable for patients with prosthetic cardiac valves if the valves have been placed within the previous 6 months; previous history of infective endocarditis; or certain congenital heart diseases (CHD) such as unrepaired cyanotic CHD, any repaired CHD with prosthetic material within the previous 6 months, and any repaired CHD with residual defect adjacent to a prosthetic patch or device (which prevents endothelialization) (251).

Arrhythmias

Postoperative arrhythmias are often secondary to noncardiac problems, such as iatrogenic fluid overload, hypotension, electrolyte abnormalities, hypoxia, or infection. Whenever an arrhythmia occurs in the postoperative setting, PE and myocardial ischemia must first be ruled out (252). If ECG and cardiac enzyme measurements are normal, the arrhythmia is not likely to be due to myocardial ischemia. Fortunately, most arrhythmias in the postoperative period are transient and self-resolving. Asymptomatic arrhythmias, except in the preoperative period, are generally of little clinical significance. Hypercapnia, hypoxemia, hypokalemia, acidosis, inadequate analgesia, and anemia can all promote cardiac arrhythmias. Supraventricular tachycardia is the most common rhythm disturbance seen in the postoperative period (253). Treatment with calcium channel blockers (such as diltiazem) or a β-blocker is usually the first-line recommended treatment for atrial fibrillation (254).

Cardiac Arrest

Treatment of patients who suffer from cardiac arrest begins with rapid identification and initiation of advanced cardiovascular life support (ACLS) measures. These include starting cardiopulmonary resuscitation (CPR) with chest compressions and often placing an endotracheal tube. ACLS algorithms should be followed according to presenting cardiac rhythms and presumed etiologies. An arterial blood gas is often drawn to help guide treatment measures. Electrolyte abnormalities should be rapidly corrected. If return of spontaneous circulation (ROSC) is obtained, the patient should be transferred to the ICU for ongoing evaluation and resuscitation (255).

Pulmonary Issues

Ventilator Management

The ability to provide ventilatory support to the surgical patient has been a tremendous advance in postoperative care. Mechanical ventilators have enabled oncologic surgeons to perform major operations for aggressive control of lesions that were once considered to be unresectable. Although preemptive preoperative therapies attempt to avoid postoperative mechanical ventilation, some patients will require this therapy. Mechanical ventilation must be thought of as providing two functions: ventilation and oxygenation. However, these two functions must be separated and applied independently to each particular situation. A more difficult concept for medical trainees to understand is that ventilation has nothing to do with oxygenation. Many patients decompensate on the ward despite supplemental oxygen and 100% oxygen saturation because tidal volumes were low and the patient was not ventilating.

When contemplating mechanical ventilation, one must ask two questions: Is the patient able to oxygenate their tissues adequately? and Can the patient ventilate adequately to maintain normal partial pressure of carbon dioxide (Pco_2) and acid-base function? Adequate oxygenation can be determined by measurement of oxygen saturation and arterial partial pressure of oxygen (Po_2). Targets are generally an O_2 saturation greater than 92% or Po_2 greater than 65 mm Hg. Poor oxygenation may be caused by fluid overload, depressed mental status, underlying pulmonary disease, or shunt. Evaluation of the arterial blood gas will also give a pH and Pco_2 measurement. Patients may hypoventilate for a number of reasons. Postoperative pain may prohibit deep inspiration, and the overuse of pain medication may depress the level of consciousness, leading to fewer and poorer respirations. Atelectasis, pneumonia, and poor pulmonary compliance all lead to difficulties in ventilation. Finally, a bronchial mucous plug or a pneumothorax will lead to life-threatening ventilatory compromise. A respiratory rate greater than 35/min or a PCO_2 greater than 55 mm Hg is accepted indication for intubation and mechanical ventilation.

When intubating patients, the size of the endotracheal tube must be considered, as this may impact removal and discontinuation of mechanical ventilation later. The larger the tube, the less resistance and the easier it will be for the patient to participate in "weaning" trials for discontinuing ventilatory support (256). Typical recommendations are a 7.5-mm tube for women and an 8.0-mm tube for men.

Traditionally, there are pressure-cycled ventilators and volume-cycled ventilators. Pressure-cycled ventilators are used routinely in neonatal ICU patients because overinflation can be dangerous to neonates. In the adult ICU, most ventilators are volume cycled, meaning that the clinician sets the tidal volume, and regardless of the pressures necessary to give the volume, the volume will be delivered. In patients in whom pulmonary compliance is reduced (ie, due to a stiff lung or acute respiratory distress syndrome [ARDS]), efforts at controlling pressure are important. When setting the ventilator, a number of decisions must be made. The mode of delivery, tidal volume, and rate will determine ventilation, whereas the fraction of inspired oxygen (Fio_2) and positive end-expiratory pressure (PEEP) will determine oxygenation.

Mode

There are a number of ventilator modes. The first developed was controlled mechanical ventilation (CMV), where the tidal volume and rate are set and that is exactly what the patient receives—no more and no less. This mode is very good for patients under general anesthesia or who are paralyzed. However, this mode is very disturbing to the patient who wishes to participate, however slightly, in their own ventilation. This mode has evolved into the current assist/control (A/C) mode, whereby the patient is not only guaranteed the fixed rate and tidal volume but can also trigger breaths in between with a similar tidal volume. In addition, the machine will synchronize the breath when the patient triggers such a breath. This mode provides complete rest for the patient by performing all the work of breathing and is generally used for patients in the immediate postoperative period or for patients who have critical illnesses, such as organ failure or sepsis.

Intermittent mandatory ventilation (IMV) is a mode whereby the clinician sets a rate and a tidal volume, which the machine delivers. Any breath initiated by the patient is delivered in relation to the amount of effort the patient puts forth, meaning a strong effort gives the patient a large breath and a meager effort a smaller one. This is sometimes called a weaning mode. The patient is given full support with rate and tidal volume until they are stronger. The rate is slowly turned down, allowing the patient more frequent, spontaneous breaths until extubation. Synchronized IMV (SIMV) ensures that a machine-delivered breath does not stack onto a patient-initiated breath.

Pressure support ventilation (PSV) is a mode where patient-initiated breaths are given support from the ventilator only during the beginning of ventilation (inspiratory phase). The support is meant to help the patient overcome the large amount of resistance present in the valves of the machine, the ventilator circuit, and the endotracheal tube. By titrating PSV to the spontaneous tidal volume produced by the patient, one can fully or partially support patient breathing and overcome the work of breathing. This mode of ventilation is important during the "weaning" process.

Work of Breathing

When conceptualizing the job of the ventilator, the different types of work must be defined (256). In addition to the physiologic work of breathing that all humans do on a daily basis, huge workloads are imposed from the resistance of the ventilator equipment (eg, breathing through a straw analogy). Finally, there is the pathologic work of breathing from pneumonia, the incision, and so on. The intent of mechanical ventilation during disease states is to assume the last two types of "work" so that the patient may convalesce. As a patient improves and the pathologic work has been removed, the patient should be able to resume normal, physiologic work.

More Advanced Modes of Ventilation

With advanced circuitry and computer microprocessors, newer ventilator modes have been developed. Pressure-regulated volume control (PRVC) has largely replaced A/C ventilation (ACV). PRVC provides the same function as A/C while preventing overinflation. Recent data have shown that preventing overinflation (or stretch) of alveoli prevents trauma and decreases the incidence of ARDS (257). PRVC delivers the same tidal volume but changes the flow rate to prevent high pressures by measuring the pressure on a breath-to-breath basis. Volume control ventilation is a mode whereby a tidal volume target is set and the ventilator continually titrates the amount of PSV to provide this volume. This mode has been termed "autowean" or "weekend" mode because as the patient gets stronger, they will be able to meet the tidal volume setting. In situations where difficulties in ventilation are encountered, such as ARDS, hypercarbia, and acidosis, pressure control is used. This mode is similar to the neonatal pressure-cycled ventilator where the maximum pressure is set and the flow rate is decreased but the inspiratory time is lengthened to achieve proper ventilation. Airway pressure release ventilation (APRV), high-frequency jet ventilation, and inverse ratio ventilation are other advanced modes, the discussion of which is beyond the scope of this chapter.

Setting the Ventilator

Initial ventilator settings require a rate of 12 to 14 breaths/min with a tidal volume of 6 to 8 mL/kg. This is a departure from the traditional 12 mL/kg, which has been determined to result in greater alveolar trauma and increased risk for the development of ARDS (258). After initial setting of the ventilator, measurements of pH, Po_2, and Pco_2 from arterial blood gas are used to make further ventilator adjustments.

Oxygenation

Oxygenation is controlled by two settings: Fio_2 and PEEP. The inspired oxygen content can easily be controlled with the ventilator, to keep blood oxygen saturation greater than 92%. Inspired oxygen concentration greater than 60% is considered to be potentially toxic and may be the etiologic reason for pathologic changes similar to ARDS. In patients with normal lung function, studies have shown that higher concentrations of inspired oxygen can cause acute inflammation and fibroproliferative changes, resulting in toxic effects to lung tissue. Similar studies in patients with underlying lung disease are lacking (259,260). If it is necessary to have oxygen concentrations above 60%, the recommendation is to wean these levels as soon as possible. PEEP is another mechanism for improving oxygenation. In normal physiology, the glottis closes before full expiration, creating a PEEP of approximately 4 cm H_2O and is termed physiologic PEEP. When ventilating patients, the addition of 5 cm H_2O PEEP is used as a baseline and is increased if added oxygen delivery is required. Increasing PEEP is the preferred method for improving oxygenation in postsurgical patients as opposed to increasing the Fio_2. Postsurgical patients have atelectasis and shunting secondary to operative pain and anesthesia. The addition of PEEP recruits collapsed alveoli, improving oxygenation and lung compliance. However, the use of PEEP must be balanced by potential adverse effects, which include decreased cardiac output and the risk for barotrauma.

Weaning From Ventilator

Multiple opinions exist on the techniques of weaning patients from mechanical ventilation. T-piece trials, spontaneous breathing trials (SBTs), SIMV, and PSV are just a few. The best method of weaning is a pathway agreed upon by clinicians, nurses, and respiratory therapists. Before discontinuing mechanical ventilation, the disease process that required ventilation should have resolved and patients should have proper mental status and the ability to generate a cough. Copious secretions are often an initial reason not to consider weaning or extubation. Criteria for extubation, whether on T-piece or minimal PSV, have traditionally included a respiratory rate less than 35, a Pco_2 less than 50 mm Hg, and a negative inspiratory force (NIF) greater than −20 cm H_2O. Rapid shallow breathing, defined as the respiratory frequency divided by the tidal volume in liters over a minute, is the most accurate predictor of failure in weaning patients from mechanical ventilation, and when this value is over 100, patients are highly likely to require reintubation (261).

Acute Respiratory Distress Syndrome

ARDS is a condition that has been well recognized and extensively studied (262-264). This disease is a form of refractory hypoxemia caused by a variety of insults, which incites an inflammatory response consisting of increased production of cytokines, leukotrienes, endothelial adhesion molecules, and interleukins. These molecules, which are useful in the defense of the host organism, are particularly detrimental to pulmonary endothelium. ARDS is the result of some inciting cause and does not arise de novo as a primary problem. A study of patients who develop multiple organ dysfunction syndrome (MODS), a state where sequential organ failure leads to patient death, has shown that the lung may be the first organ system susceptible to these circulating inflammatory mediators (265).

In addition to supportive treatment for ARDS, operative injuries or postoperative complications (eg, intra-abdominal abscess, anastomotic leak) must be sought and ruled out.

Criteria for the diagnosis of ARDS include (a) acute onset after defined insult; (b) bilateral diffuse infiltrates on chest radiograph; (c) no evidence of left atrial hypertension or CHF; and, most importantly, (d) impaired oxygenation. The Berlin definition of ARDS has broken down the severity level into three levels: mild, with PaO_2 between 200 and 300 mm Hg and PEEP or continuous positive airway pressure (CPAP) 5 cm H_2O or more; moderate, with PaO_2 between 100 and 200 mm Hg and PEEP or CPAP 5 cm H_2O or more; and severe, with PaO_2 100 mm Hg or less and PEEP 5 cm H_2O or more (266). Postmortem examination of lungs with ARDS shows atelectasis, edema, inflammation, hyaline membrane deposition, and fibrosis. The mortality of ARDS is 30% to 40%. Treatment of these patients with severe hypoxemia consists of mechanical ventilatory support with FIO_2 and PEEP. Because of alveolar damage, ventilation/perfusion mismatch occurs, resulting in a worsening shunt fraction and increasing dead space. As acute lung injury (ALI)/ARDS progresses, ventilation, due to decreased pulmonary compliance, becomes difficult, and oxygenation progressively worsens. The end result is a hypercapnic state and respiratory acidosis.

The ARDS NET trial comparing high tidal volume, in order to maintain normocapnia, to low tidal volumes, to prevent barotrauma, showed significantly improved survival among patients in the low tidal volume group (263). Current strategies employ tidal volumes of 4 to 6 mL/kg, while accepting elevated PcO_2 levels (permissive hypercapnia) (266).

Asthma/Chronic Obstructive Pulmonary Disease

Patients with preexisting airway disease are at increased risk of pulmonary complications with surgery. Reactive airway disease or asthma can be exacerbated by general anesthesia, and these patients need to be watched closely for increased wheezing or difficulty breathing. Albuterol treatment or nebulizers should be scheduled, and their home regimen available (267).

COPD puts patients at higher risk of respiratory failure, both hypercarbic and hypoxemic. These patients can often be managed with noninvasive ventilation methods, such as high-flow oxygen, CPAP, or bilevel positive airway pressure (BiPAP), but may end up requiring mechanical ventilation. COPD exacerbations can be brought on by surgery and hospital stays. The mainstay for treatment of this is scheduling nebulizers, a course of steroids, and antibiotics, such azithromycin. With severe exacerbations or patients with already tenuous airways, involvement of the patient's pulmonologist may be key to avoid mechanical ventilation (267).

Pneumonia

Pneumonia is a significant complication in postsurgical patients. Patients requiring mechanical ventilation are particularly susceptible to pneumonia (ventilator-acquired pneumonia [VAP]), with rates as high as 30% after 72 hours of ventilation. The mortality rate from VAP ranges from 25% to 50%. The pathogens are often Gram-negative bacteria and are resistant to multiple antibiotics. High clinical suspicion and aggressive treatment of VAP are crucial. A review of this complicated topic by Chastre and Fagon is recommended for further reading (268).

Pulmonary Embolism and Deep Venous Thrombosis Treatment

VTE events include DVT and PE. Diagnosis of DVT is performed by duplex ultrasonography in patients with limb swelling, pain, or unexplained low-grade fevers or tachycardia. If the patient is able to tolerate anticoagulation, treatment with IV heparin, LMWH (1 mg/kg twice daily), or a DOAC should be initiated (269). DOACs can be started if the patient is tolerating a diet and is at low risk for bleeding. If unable to tolerate any form of anticoagulation, a retrievable IVC filter should be placed and anticoagulation started once the patient is able. Anticoagulation is the recommended treatment for all DVTs unless there are signs of limb compromise. In these rare cases, interventional radiology should be consulted for catheter-directed thrombolysis or mechanical thrombectomy.

PE is almost exclusively diagnosed with CT scans utilizing contrasted protocols designed to look at the pulmonary arteries. If a postoperative patient is diagnosed with an acute PE and is hypotensive and the risk of bleeding is low, systemic thrombolytic therapy should be utilized, followed by full anticoagulation. In patients with high bleeding risk, shock, or if they have failed systemic thrombolysis, interventional radiology should be consulted for consideration for catheter-assisted thrombus removal/lysis. Acute PE without hypotension should be treated with full anticoagulation with IV heparin, DOAC, or LMWH.

The recommended duration of therapy for provoked (postoperative) VTE is 3 months. DOACs are now the recommended agents for the treatment of VTE over vitamin K antagonists or LMWH. This recommendation also applies to cancer-associated thrombosis (219). The 2021 update to the CHEST guidelines for antithrombotic therapy for VTE can be reviewed for additional guidance (269).

Fluid and Electrolyte Issues

Understanding fluid and electrolyte physiology in gynecologic oncology is paramount because of the underlying disease processes that face the gynecologic oncologist and the ultimate, radical surgical interventions that are needed to treat them. These treatments result in great fluid shifts perioperatively, requiring careful attention to input of fluids (volume and content/type) as well as output from renal and GI sources, insensible sources, and drains. This section presents a brief review of normal fluid and electrolyte physiology and discusses strategies for fluid resuscitation and correction of electrolyte deficiencies.

Total-body water (TBW) can be calculated by a variety of methods and varies directly with the amount of adipose or lean tissue present in an individual patient. TBW estimates, therefore, must be adjusted based on the adiposity of the patients. In women, TBW accounts for approximately 60% of a patient's weight. TBW is distributed into extracellular fluid (ECF) and intracellular fluid (ICF), with the ECF being further divided into intravascular (one quarter of the ECF) and interstitial (three quarters of the ECF) compartments. The ECF accounts for approximately one-third of the TBW, whereas ICF accounts for two-thirds (270,271). Direct measurement of the ECF and TBW is possible, with the resulting difference being an estimated ICF. **Table 12.3-13** describes the body fluid compartments and their contributions to body weight. Despite these arbitrary compartments (and electrolyte concentration differences between compartments, which are discussed in the next paragraph), water flows freely across all compartments. Thus, a derangement in one compartment will result in a compensatory change in another (272).

■ TABLE 12.3-13. Body Fluid Compartments

Total-Body Water	Body Weight (%)	Total-Body Water (%)
Total	60	100
Intracellular	40	67
Extracellular	20	33
Intravascular	5	8
Interstitial	15	25

From Wait RB, Kahng KU, Dresner LS. Fluids and electrolytes and acid-base balance. In: Greenfield LJ, Mulholland M, Oldham KT, et al, eds. *Surgery: Scientific Principles and Practice*. 2nd ed. Lippincott–Raven Publishers; 1997;242-266, with permission.

The electrolyte composition of the various compartments is different. Sodium is the predominant cation in the ECF, and potassium is the predominant cation of the ICF. **Table 12.3-14** describes the various concentrations of electrolytes in the various fluid compartments. Because of the Donnan principle of equilibration, the content of cations and anions in the interstitial compartment is slightly higher than in the intravascular compartment. This principle describes the unique relation between solutions of permeable and impermeable complex anions when these anions are unevenly distributed across a semipermeable membrane. Water, on the other hand, as mentioned earlier, freely equilibrates between the compartments (272).

Effective circulating volume (ECV) is a term used to describe the portion of the ECF that perfuses the organs of the body and affects baroreceptors (see next paragraph). In healthy patients, the ECV equates to the intravascular volume/compartment. But in disease states that increase "third spacing" such as sepsis (leaky capillaries), ascites due to intra-abdominal metastasis, or bowel obstruction with resulting edema and transudation, the interstitial compartment increases at the expense of the intravascular compartment, decreasing the ECV (270).

The osmotic activity of a fluid compartment is affected by the component ions and is described in milliosmoles (mOsm). Normal serum osmolality (in the ECF, of course) averages 290 mOsm/kg of H_2O. Osmoreceptors in the hypothalamus respond to small changes in serum osmolality, increasing or decreasing secretion of ADH and modifying the thirst response. These receptors are responsible for the day-to-day fine-tuning of fluid balance. Baroreceptors in the intrathoracic vena cava, the atria, the aortic arch, the carotid arteries, and the renal parenchyma sense volume changes by changes in pressure. These receptors begin a cascade of mediators such as aldosterone, atrial natriuretic peptide (ANP), prostaglandins, and the renin-angiotensin system, which ultimately result in changes of water and sodium balance mediated through the kidneys. These baroreceptors have little to do with the day-to-day fluid management and require intravascular losses of 10% to 20% to initiate activity (272).

The goal of fluid resuscitation is to maintain the ECV and keep or return the patient to euvolemia. Many gynecologic oncology procedures are lengthy and can result in large blood losses requiring immediate intraoperative replacement. In addition, following procedures where evacuation of large amounts of ascites has occurred and/or "peritoneal stripping" has left denuded surfaces, these patients may have large fluid shifts into the interstitial compartment, requiring large volumes of fluid to maintain the ECV. Finally, losses are not water alone and include electrolytes and clotting factors, which may need repletion. Selecting fluids to administer to a given patient is akin to selecting the correct IV medication to give; not *all* fluids are for *all* patients. The physician should understand the amount of daily maintenance fluid and electrolytes required by patients, calculate losses (fluid and electrolytes), determine ongoing fluid and electrolyte losses, and replace them with the appropriate fluid and electrolyte combinations and volumes. It is easy to fall into the trap of giving all patients an 8-hour rate (125 mL/hr) of maintenance fluid. However, an octogenarian, even with normal cardiac and renal function, weighing 50 kg does not need that much maintenance fluid. "Formulas" for calculating appropriate maintenance fluid requirements exist (272).

With new enhanced recovery protocols, restricting fluids intraoperatively and postoperatively has been shown to reduce cardiopulmonary complications (7% vs 24%; $P < .001$) and overall morbidity (OR 0.41; $P = .005$) (273,274). It is important to note that these improvements in morbidity were not seen if the fluid restrictions were instituted postoperatively. However, extreme restriction of fluids can lead to increased morbidity and mortality. A fine line must be walked in an effort to keep the patient normovolemic during the surgical procedure. If, however, the surgical procedure planned will result in large blood loss or the patient has systemic inflammatory response syndrome (SIRS), advanced hemodynamic monitoring may be helpful in managing fluid resuscitation to maintain euvolemia (net zero sum: fluids out = fluids in). Extrapolation to gynecologic oncologic surgery would be expected to have these same results.

The normal maintenance requirement of sodium is 1 to 2 mEq/kg/d and for potassium 0.5 to 1.0 mEq/kg/d. **Table 12.3-15** lists the various IV fluid preparations available for fluid resuscitation. Which fluid to be used is controversial and driven, in more instances, by "dogma" and "anecdotal opinion," varying by physician and institution rather than by evidence. Controversy over which fluid type to use in fluid resuscitation continues to this day. Several meta-analyses have shown no advantage of colloid over crystalloid for resuscitation in surgical patients (275-277).

Most of the time patients are given isotonic solutions, such as lactated Ringer (LR) solution, to cover intraoperative losses, with the goal to maintain euvolemia. If necessary, colloid can be used to maintain blood pressure over crystalloid. The need for

TABLE 12.3-14. Electrolyte Concentrations in the Various Fluid Compartments

	Extracellular Fluid		Intracellular Fluid
	Plasma	Interstitial Fluid	
Cations			
Na^+	140	146	12
K^+	4	4	150
Ca^{2+}	5	3	10^{-7}
Mg^{2+}	2	1	7
Anions			
Cl^-	103	114	3
HCO_3^-	24	27	10
SO_4^2	1	1	–
HPO_4^3	2	2	116
Protein	16	5	40
Organic anions	5	5	–

From Wait RB, Kahng KU, Dresner LS. Fluids and electrolytes and acid-base balance. In: Greenfield LJ, Mulholland M, Oldham KT, et al. eds. *Surgery: Scientific Principles and Practice.* 2nd ed. Lippincott–Raven Publishers; 1997;242-266, with permission.

TABLE 12.3-15. Electrolyte Content of Commonly Used Intravenous Electrolyte Solutions

Solution	Electrolyte Concentration (mEq/L)					
	Na^+	K^+	Ca_2^+	Mg_2^+	Cl^-	HCO_3^-
Lactated Ringer solution	130	4	4	–	109	28
0.2% NaCl	34	–	–	–	34	–
0.33% NaCl	56	–	–	–	56	–
0.45% NaCl	77	–	–	–	77	–
0.9% NaCl	154	–	–	–	154	–
3.0% NaCl	513	–	–	–	513	–
5.0% NaCl	855	–	–	–	855	–

Adapted from Wait RB, Kahng KU, Dresner LS. Fluids and electrolytes and acid-base balance. In: Greenfield LJ, Mulholland M, Oldham KT, et al, eds. *Surgery: Scientific Principles and Practice.* 2nd ed. Lippincott–Raven Publishers; 1997;242-266, with permission.

postoperative IV fluids beyond 12 to 24 hours following the procedure is rare in an uncomplicated recovery. In the cases of continued IV fluid administration, a total hourly rate of 1.2 mL/kg (including drugs) should be given. Balanced crystalloid solutions are preferred to 0.9% saline solutions to reduce the risk of hyperchloremic acidosis. ***Best practice: Very restrictive or liberal fluid regimens should be avoided in favor of euvolemia. In major open surgery and for high-risk patients where there is large blood loss (>7 mL/kg) or an SIRS response, the use of advanced hemodynamic monitoring to facilitate individualized fluid therapy and optimize oxygen delivery through the perioperative period is recommended. Oral intake of fluid should be started on the day of surgery. IV fluids should be terminated within 24 hours after surgery. Balanced crystalloid solutions (eg, LR) are preferred to 0.9% normal saline.***

Sodium Derangements

Hyponatremia is the most common electrolyte abnormality seen in postoperative patients and is caused by excess free water rather than a depletion of sodium. Increases in free water absorption are mediated by a self-limited, physiologic increase in the secretion of ADH in response to the stress of surgery. Serum sodium levels rarely fall below 130 mEq/L but may be further exacerbated by IV administration of large volumes of hypotonic solutions (ie, 0.2%, 0.33%, and 0.45% sodium solutions). Other disease states can result in a hyperosmolar condition, resulting in a hyperosmolar ECF, causing fluid to shift from the ICF and lowering the sodium levels. These conditions include hyperglycemia; mannitol, ethylene glycol, or ethanol ingestion; and uremia. For each increase of 180 mg/dL of glucose above 100 mg/dL, there is a concomitant decrease in the serum sodium of 5 mEq/L (272). In addition, during situations where potassium is low, there is a compensatory exchange of sodium for potassium, resulting in hyponatremia. In either of these prior cases, total-body sodium does not change. Finally, patients with hyperproteinemia or hyperlipidemia may have falsely low sodium values, which result from errors in the laboratory measurement of sodium. This *pseudohyponatremia* does not result in any symptoms of hyponatremia (272).

The symptoms of hyponatremia are driven by cellular water intoxication and are related to the central nervous system (CNS) (eg, lethargy, headaches, confusion, delirium, weakness, muscle cramps). The rate at which hyponatremia occurs also determines the symptoms. Chronic hyponatremia tends to be asymptomatic, whereas acute drops in the serum sodium (levels 120-130) result in the symptoms listed earlier. Correction of hyponatremia must be done carefully to avoid central pontine myelinolysis, which results in the "locked-in syndrome."

Because most hyponatremia is related to dehydration (low ECV), simple correction of this state will increase the sodium plasma level. If the patient has a high ECV (such as the syndrome of inappropriate antidiuretic hormone [SIADH] secretion) or is in an edematous state, free water restriction should normalize the sodium level. However, if patients have symptoms of hyponatremia, aggressive replacement of sodium is prudent should the duration of the hyponatremia be determined to be no longer than 48 hours. Hyponatremic states lasting longer than 48 hours increase the risk of central pontine myelinolysis. Chronic cases need replacement at rates not to exceed 0.5 mEq/L/hr. Acute cases may be replaced at rates of 5 mEq/L/hr.

Hypernatremia is an uncommon finding and is related to large volumes of free water loss (through insensible routes such as breathing, sweating, and ventilation), diabetes insipidus, adrenal hyperfunction, or ingestion or administration of increased sodium solutions. The symptoms are predominantly CNS oriented because of brain cell dehydration. Symptoms rarely occur until serum sodium levels exceed 160 mEq/L. In addition, the rapidity at which the derangement occurs determines the symptoms manifested. Treatment is carefully done with replacement of free water. Replacement too rapidly can cause cerebral edema and herniation.

Patients with chronic hypernatremia need free water administration, which decreases the serum sodium no faster than 0.7 mEq/L.

Potassium Derangements

Whereas sodium is the major extracellular cation, potassium is the major intracellular cation by a ratio of 30:1. The intracellular potassium concentrations tend to be relatively constant, whereas the extracellular concentrations vary depending upon renal function/excretion. The majority of potassium secretion occurs in the distal tubule and the collecting duct of the nephron. Secretion is stimulated by increased urine flow, increased sodium delivery, high potassium levels, alkalosis, aldosterone, vasopressin, and β-adrenergic agonists. Insulin causes potassium to move into cells (as previously mentioned), reducing the extracellular concentration of potassium. Serum potassium levels are further affected by the acid-base status of patients. In alkalotic states, the potassium shifts into cells in exchange for hydrogen ions, whereas in acidotic states, the exchange is opposite.

The predominant reason for hyperkalemia in a postoperative patient is renal dysfunction or failure. When these patients become critically ill, serum potassium concentrations can increase by 0.3 to 0.5 mEq/L/d in noncatabolic patients and 0.7 mEq/L/d in catabolic patients. It is important to rule out a spuriously elevated level secondary to hemolysis at the time of the blood draw either from too small a gauge of needle or simply from the application of the tourniquet and squeezing (272).

Hyperkalemia changes the membrane potential established by differences between the intracellular and extracellular milieu. This increased concentration has deleterious effects on cardiac muscle function, causing peaked T waves, flattened P waves, prolonged QRS complexes, and deep S waves on the ECG and, possibly, resulting in ventricular fibrillation and cardiac arrest. Skeletal musculature is also affected with paresthesias and weakness, which can progress to a flaccid paralysis.

If the postoperative patient is hyperkalemic, therapeutic options would be the same as those described in the section on renal risk factors. Should the patient not respond to these medical therapies (listed previously), hemodialysis may be indicated.

Hypokalemia is caused by decreased intake, increased GI losses (vomiting, diarrhea, fistulae), excessive renal losses (metabolic alkalosis, magnesium deficiency, hyperaldosteronism), a shift of potassium into the intracellular space (acute or uncompensated metabolic alkalosis, glucose and insulin administration, catecholamines), or any combination thereof. A reduction of serum potassium by 1 mEq/L represents a total-body deficiency of about 100 to 200 mEq. (Remember that total exchangeable potassium is ~3,000 mEq, with the majority being intracellular and thus the majority of the loss (274).) Symptoms of hypokalemia cause ECG changes with flattening of the T waves, depression of ST segments, prominent U waves, and prolongation of the QT interval. Treatment is accomplished by replacement of potassium either orally or IV, depending upon the severity of symptoms and whether or not the patient is able to take oral preparations. IV replacement of potassium can be done at approximately 10 mEq/hr and should not be more concentrated than 40 mEq/L. If less fluid is desired, 20 mEq can be placed in 100 mL, but administration should not exceed 40 mEq/hr (272).

Magnesium Derangements

Most magnesium in the body is confined to the intracellular space and bone. Less than 1% of total-body magnesium is in the serum. Of the magnesium in the serum, 60% is ionized, 25% is protein bound, and 15% is complexed with nonprotein anionic species (272). Magnesium is absorbed in the small intestine, directed by levels of vitamin D, and filtered by the kidney for excretion. Approximately 40% of renally excreted magnesium is reabsorbed in the ascending loop of Henle. Loop diuretics, hypermagnesemia, hypercalcemia, acidosis, and phosphate depletion result in increased excretion of magnesium.

Patients with renal failure and receiving magnesium-containing antacids or laxatives can become hypermagnesemic. In addition, patients with acidosis and dehydration may become hypermagnesemic. Patients present with CNS depression, loss of deep tendon reflexes, and ECG changes (prolonged PR interval and QRS complex) in the face of elevated magnesium levels (>8 mg/dL). As levels rise, patients will develop coma, respiratory failure, and/or cardiac arrest. Acute treatment of hypermagnesemia is slow IV infusion of 5 to 10 mEq of calcium. Because the etiology of this condition is usually renal failure, withholding magnesium-containing preparations may be all that is necessary. In severe instances, hemodialysis is required.

In gynecologic oncology patients, the overwhelming reason for hypomagnesemia is a history of cisplatin administration. However, other conditions such as hypoparathyroidism, malabsorptive states, chronic loop diuretic use, and the diuretic phase of ARF can cause hypomagnesemia. Symptoms are similar to hypocalcemia, with muscle weakness, fasciculations, tetany, hypokalemia, and ECG changes (QT prolongation, torsade de pointes). Treatment can be accomplished with oral preparations in less acute situations. However, large doses may produce diarrhea, worsening the situation. IV boluses of 2 to 3 g followed by infusions of 1 to 2 mEq/kg/d can be utilized for patients with severe symptoms.

Calcium Derangements

Almost all the calcium in the body is in bone, stored as hydroxyapatite crystals, and provides a supply that can be exchanged to the serum. Calcium homeostasis is controlled by parathyroid hormone (PTH), controlling intestinal absorption of calcium, renal excretion of calcium, and exchange of calcium from the bone. In the serum, calcium exists in three phases: 45% as an ionized form, which is responsible for most of the physiologic function of calcium; 40% in a protein-bound form, bound mostly to albumin; and 15% in a nonionized form, complexed with nonprotein anions that do not easily dissociate. A serum total calcium level is usually obtained when assessing calcium homeostasis, as measurement of ionized calcium is cumbersome. The total calcium levels change by 0.8 g/dL for each 1 g/dL change of albumin (up or down) (272).

In gynecologic oncology patients with hypercalcemia, the underlying malignancy is usually the etiologic agent. Hypercalcemia may be caused by direct bony involvement or, more commonly, secretion of PTH-like peptides and/or other humoral factors, which increase serum calcium levels. Other reasons for hypercalcemia include primary, secondary, or tertiary hyperparathyroidism; thiazide diuretic use; or lithium usage (272,278). Patients present with muscle fatigue, weakness, confusion, coma, ECG changes (shortening of the QT interval), nausea, and vomiting. The goal of treatment is to increase calcium excretion and stop bone turnover in order to decrease serum total calcium. Initial measures include vigorous hydration (200 mL/hr) with 0.9% or 0.45% saline solutions. Furosemide or other loop diuretics may be helpful in patients with borderline cardiac function or in patients with fluid overload. If the underlying malignancy is a breast carcinoma, patients may respond to high doses of steroids to reduce calcium levels. Other pharmacologic agents have been developed to stop bone resorption and reduce serum calcium levels. Calcitonin (4 IU/kg every 12 hours via subcutaneous or intramuscular injection) has a rapid onset of action and works by interfering with osteoclast maturation at several points (270). However, the duration of response is usually about 48 hours because of downregulation of calcitonin receptors by osteoclasts. Bisphosphonates have emerged as the drug of choice for the treatment of hypercalcemia in malignancy. These agents work by inhibiting osteoclast activity and survival. The nitrogen-containing bisphosphonates are the most potent. Pamidronate (approved in 1991) and zoledronic acid (approved in 2001) are utilized in the United States. Another agent, ibandronate, is utilized in Europe but has not been approved for use in the United States. Zoledronic acid is the current drug of choice

because of its proven superiority to pamidronate (279). The effective dose of zoledronic acid is 4 mg infused over 15 minutes and dosed every 3 to 4 weeks. Serum calcium levels return to normal in approximately 10 days, and duration of response lasts approximately 40 days (280). Surgical resection is the treatment of choice for primary, secondary, or tertiary hyperparathyroidism (270,271).

Hypocalcemia is caused by hypoparathyroidism, hypomagnesemia, pancreatitis, and malnutrition. Patients present with tetany, hyperactive deep tendon reflexes, a positive Chvostek sign, positive Trousseau sign, and ECG changes (prolonged QT interval, prolonged ST segment). Low levels of calcium may be present because of low albumin levels, but these levels do not affect the ionized portion of calcium and usually do not cause symptoms. Symptomatic hypocalcemia can be treated with IV infusion of either calcium gluconate or calcium chloride at a rate not to exceed 50 mg/min. Calcium chloride dissociates into the ionized form of calcium more readily and is the treatment of choice to raise serum-ionized calcium level.

Acid-Base Disturbances

Optimum cellular function requires a very narrow range of pH for chemical reactions to occur normally. Several buffering systems exist within the body to maintain this optimum pH. The predominant buffering system is the carbonic acid-bicarbonate buffering system. Derangements in the concentration of bicarbonate (HCO_3^-) or in concentrations of carbon dioxide (CO_2) result in acid-base disorders. Because the kidneys control excretion/generation of bicarbonate and the lungs exchange CO_2, these organs play a central role in the compensation of any acid-base disorder. Therefore, four situations arise in acid-base balance: metabolic acidosis and alkalosis, and respiratory acidosis and alkalosis. Compensatory mechanisms exist in each situation in order to blunt the effect on pH (Table 12.3-16).

Metabolic Acidosis

Most clinically significant metabolic acidosis occurs with a net loss of bicarbonate either due to direct loss or when consumption is greater than generation. Situations where extrarenal losses of bicarbonate occur include diarrhea, GI fistulae, and urinary diversions (ureterosigmoidostomy or ureteroileostomy, which results in reabsorption of NH_4Cl from urine). Certain disease states result in the production of organic acids (ketoacidosis and lactic acidosis), which consume bicarbonate and outpace the renal compensatory mechanisms. Similarly, overdoses of certain drugs (eg, aspirin) or ingestion of toxins (eg, ethylene glycol, methanol) consume bicarbonate and outpace the renal compensatory mechanisms. Renal acidosis occurs when the intrinsic acid–excreting function of the kidney malfunctions, resulting in retention of acid and consumption of bicarbonate without concomitant regeneration of

■ TABLE 12.3-16. Concentrations of HCO_3^- and PCO_2 in Primary Acid-Base Derangements and the Compensatory Response

Disorder	Primary			Compensatory Response	
	pH	HCO_3^-	PCO_2	HCO_3^-	PCO_2
Metabolic acidosis	↓	↓			↓
Metabolic alkalosis	→	→			→
Respiratory acidosis	↓		→	→	
Respiratory alkalosis	→		↓	↓	

Adapted from Wait RB, Kahng KU, Dresner LS. Fluids and electrolytes and acid-base balance. In: Greenfield LJ, Mulholland M, Oldham KT, et al, eds. *Surgery: Scientific Principles and Practice.* 2nd ed. Lippincott-Raven Publishers; 1997;242-266, with permission.

bicarbonate. These are classified as renal tubular acidosis (RTA-I, distal tubule dysfunction; or RTA-II, proximal tubule dysfunction). Cardiac effects are the major findings in metabolic acidosis (peripheral arteriolar dilation, decreased cardiac contractility, and central venous constriction). Other manifestations of metabolic acidosis include gastric distention, abdominal pain, nausea, and vomiting. In surgical patients, lactic acidosis is the primary cause of metabolic acidosis and results from tissue hypoperfusion. Therefore, treatment should be aimed at increasing tissue perfusion with fluid and blood administration. The use of bicarbonate is best reserved for patients with other, not easily reversible causes of metabolic acidosis. Older patients and patients with CVD may benefit from administration of bicarbonate. Administration should be instituted when the pH is 7.1 to 7.2. One or two ampules of bicarbonate (~55 mEq/amp) can be administered IV, with further administrations being dictated by the pH obtained from an arterial blood gas measurement. In diabetic ketoacidosis, treatment with insulin and glucose infusion should not only reverse the acidosis but also treat the hyperglycemia.

Metabolic Alkalosis

Sustained metabolic alkalosis is an uncommon clinical entity and is related to renal dysfunction. Loss of HCl is the most common reason for an increase in extracellular bicarbonate. This situation occurs with prolonged nausea and vomiting or prolonged nasogastric suctioning of gastric contents. As acid is removed from the GI tract, a net gain of bicarbonate occurs. Other situations that can result in metabolic alkalosis include volume contraction, exogenous administration of bicarbonate or bicarbonate precursors (citrate, lactate, or calcium carbonate), hypokalemia, hypercalcemia, hypochloremia, excess mineralocorticoid usage, and high Pco_2. Patients rarely present with symptoms, as metabolic alkalosis occurs gradually. However, in patients who develop this situation acutely, most symptoms are CNS oriented (eg, confusion, stupor, coma, muscle fasciculations, tetany). Correction of the underlying disease state usually corrects the metabolic alkalosis. Repletion of electrolyte abnormalities and infusion of appropriate fluids (chloride containing) restore volume and result in normal renal excretion of excess bicarbonate.

Respiratory Acidosis

A depression of the pH occurs when there is hypoventilation. This occurs secondary to airway obstruction, COPD, depression of the respiratory center, impaired excursion of the thorax, or inappropriate ventilatory management in the mechanically ventilated patient. Development of symptoms depends upon the chronicity or acute nature of the event. If chronic, most patients have no symptoms. If it is an acute change, drowsiness, restlessness, headache, or development of a flapping tremor may occur. Treatment of this condition is aimed at the underlying cause of the hypoventilation. In chronic conditions, the hypoxemia, and subsequent hypercapnia, resulting from the hypoventilation may be the sole drive for the patient's respirations. Correction of the hypoxemia may further worsen the respiratory acidosis and must be considered. In general, correction of the Pco_2 must be done slowly because reequilibration of cerebral bicarbonate concentration lags behind systemic changes (272).

Respiratory Alkalosis

Respiratory alkalosis occurs when the Pco_2 decreases with hyperventilation. Hyperventilation may occur because of hypoxia, drugs, decreased lung compliance, and mechanical ventilation. With drops in the arterial Po_2, the peripheral chemoreceptors (in the carotid and aortic body) sense this change and result in hyperventilation to increase arterial Po_2 with a resulting decrease in Pco_2. Because of renal compensatory mechanisms, this condition is usually asymptomatic. However, in acute situations, patients may have

a sensation of breathlessness, dizziness, nervousness with altered levels of consciousness, and tetany. Treatment of underlying hypoxia should address the hyperventilation. If acute symptoms are present, having the patient rebreathe expired air should temporarily relieve the symptoms.

Postoperative Nutritional Issues

As mentioned earlier, the full consideration of nutrition in the gynecologic oncology patient is presented in Chapter 12.4. In this section, we discuss early refeeding in the postoperative gynecologic oncology patient, indications for EN, and TPN.

Although malnutrition has been shown to be prevalent among gynecologic oncology patients (140,141), many patients are adequately nourished, undergo surgery uneventfully, and have return of bowel function in 1 to 5 days while simultaneously resuming oral intake. With the advent of ERAS protocols in the past several years, early feeding with a general diet within 4 hours of major gynecologic surgery (with or without bowel resection) has become the norm. In addition, the AHRQ has identified early feeding as one of 29 protocol elements for improving surgical care and recovery in gynecologic surgery (281). A recent updated meta-analysis on the topic demonstrated that recovery of bowel function was quicker, with shorter time to bowel sounds and passage of flatus decreased infectious complications and decreased hospital stays. In addition, there was no difference in rates of nausea or vomiting, abdominal distension, the need for a postoperative NGT, or time to first bowel movement. Most patients resumed solid food 1 ½ days sooner and reported increased satisfaction and QoL (282). ***Best practice: A regular diet within the first 24 hours after gynecologic/oncology surgery is recommended, and NGT should be avoided if possible.***

The use of the enteral route is preferred in sustaining or repleting patients in the postoperative period after extensive procedures (including small and large bowel surgeries). EN utilizes normal physiologic absorptive mechanisms, maintains gut epithelial integrity, and reduces infectious morbidity (283,284). Studies on nutrition have found that the splanchnic circulation and support of the mucosal integrity of the small bowel may prevent progression to MODS. Specifically, the intestinal mucosa with atrophy secondary to lack of luminal nutrients and intermittent activation of the destructive cytokine pathways, and/or intermittent translocation of bacteria into the bloodstream will occur. These events result in "priming" neutrophils, which ultimately leads to a full-blown SIRS, causing organ damage. A number of well-designed randomized trials have compared early enteral feeds to TPN in patients with pancreatitis, major elective surgery, and trauma (283,284). All of these studies have shown a clear benefit for early enteral feeding, with a decrease in infectious complications (284).

Although considered a nonessential amino acid in nourished, healthy patients, glutamine has emerged as an essential amino acid in patients who are stressed and critically ill. This amino acid has been shown to be an important component in maintaining enterocyte integrity and has now been added to most enteral preparations (283,284). However, controversy remains as to the benefit of supplementation with this amino acid in reducing overall mortality and infectious complications, although some meta-analyses have shown significant reductions in hospital length of stay (285-287).

Enteral feeds may be given in a variety of ways, and each is associated with its own type and number of complications. Intragastric feeds may be accomplished with NGTs, oral gastric tubes, or percutaneous endoscopic gastrostomy (PEG) tubes. Intragastric feeding has the advantage of utilizing the stomach as a reservoir for bolus feeding. In addition, stretching of the stomach stimulates the biliary-pancreatic axis, which may be trophic to the small bowel. Finally, the gastric secretions mix with the feeding material and decrease the osmolarity, thus reducing the incidence of diarrhea. The main disadvantage of this route of enteral feeding is the increased risk of gastric overdistention with high residual amounts of feeding material and the increased risk of aspiration pneumonia (283). Enteral feeds may also be accomplished through the placement of nasal tubes, which are positioned into the pylorus, duodenum, or jejunum (such as Dobhoff tubes). These tubes have the advantage of being placed (or migrating) more distal in the upper GI tract, greatly reducing the risk of aspiration. These types of tubes are preferred in patients who require long-term ventilation. Because of advances in endoscopic instrumentation, many of the tubes can be placed via this method. At the time of laparotomy, gastrostomy, or jejunostomy, tubes (such as a Stamm or Witzel tube) may be placed. These have the advantage of being placed at the time of major abdominal surgery under direct visualization/palpation. The techniques are described in other textbooks (283,288). Several enteral feeding preparations are available but vary from hospital to hospital depending upon formulary makeup. The use of the enteral route is contraindicated in patients with mechanical intestinal obstructions, and for these patients, nutritional support can be accomplished through the parenteral route.

TPN took the forefront in nutritional sustenance and replacement in the 1980s. The basic premise of TPN is to provide dietary precursors to maintain anabolic function. TPN can be broken into three components of replacement: glucose and lipid preparations for normal or increased energy expenditures, and amino acid preparations for protein synthesis. Because of the higher osmolar load presented by these preparations, central venous access is necessary for administration. Subclavian, internal jugular, or peripherally inserted central catheters (PICCs) will need to be placed, and they present the first of several potential complications associated with TPN administration. At the time of placement, pneumothorax, intubation of arterial structures, air embolism, or cardiac arrhythmias may occur. Later complications include the possibility of infection at the skin entrance site or line sepsis. Should these infectious complications occur, removal of the catheter and antibiotic administration will be necessary (284).

The Harris-Benedict equation is utilized to calculate basal energy expenditure (BEE) for patients and approximates the BEE of a sedentary, fasting, nonstressed individual (289):

$$BEE = 666 + (9.6 \times weight\ [kg]) + (1.7 \times height\ [cm]) - (4.7 \times age\ [yr])$$

Because stress of disease and surgical intervention need to be considered, "stress factors" have been developed and are multiplied by the BEE to arrive at kilocalories per day. Stress-level multipliers are 1.2 for a resting individual, 1.3 for an ambulatory individual or moderate stress (eg, SIRS, sepsis), and 1.5 for severe stress/burn patients.

After calculation of caloric requirements, the composition of the TPN solution to be administered should be determined. Because there are many different types of TPN preparations available, consultation with the nutrition team or pharmacists in an individual hospital is necessary to arrive at the desired solution.

In aerobic situations, glucose is the primary substrate for energy expenditure. It provides 3.4 kcal/g and is usually given in a concentrated form in order to provide 70% of the calculated calories. The remaining 30% of calories is provided by lipid preparations. Not only does this component have denser caloric content (it provides 9 kcal/g), but administration precludes the development of a fatty acid deficiency. Adjustment of the composition of TPN may be necessary depending upon the disease state (eg, more contribution of kilocalories from fat vs carbohydrate in a ventilated patient because of the respiratory quotient of fat vs glucose).

Protein requirements are provided by amino acid solutions and are determined by the patient's age, sex, nutritional status, ongoing stress, and comorbid conditions. In general, 25% of protein requirements are obtained by normal oral intake. The remaining protein comes from breakdown of serum and organic proteins. Thus, periods of prolonged malnutrition, with decreased protein intake, and increased stress of disease will lead to breakdown of visceral protein. An estimate of maintenance protein requirements is 1 g nitrogen per kilogram of body weight. In situations of increased stress, the patient may need 1.2 to 1.5 g/kg in order to maintain and/or replace protein losses. **Table 12.3-17** shows serum protein measurements and their respective half-lives, which are useful for determining anabolic versus catabolic response to TPN treatment. Another method to assess nitrogen balance (positive or negative) is given as follows (283):

$$Nitrogen\ balance = protein\ intake\ /\ 6.25 - (urinary\ urea\ nitrogen + 4)$$

The amount of protein intake is divided by 6.25 to give the grams of nitrogen taken in. The urinary urea nitrogen is expressed in grams based upon a 24-hour collection. The correction factor of 4 is meant to adjust for the grams of nitrogen lost in the stool or non–urea nitrogen losses.

In addition to these three main components of TPN, daily requirements of vitamins, trace elements, and insulin are necessary to maintain/regain nourishment. Again, these preparations vary by hospital formulary and need consultation with resident pharmacists.

The rate of infusion of TPN needs to be titrated upward to take into account the large glucose load that the patient will be receiving. This lower rate allows the pancreas time to increase insulin secretion in order to meet the glucose load being presented. Similarly, the rate of infusion needs to be decreased when TPN is being stopped to prevent hypoglycemia. During TPN administration, blood glucose measurements by fingerstick are required so that hyperglycemia is avoided. For the first several days, measurement of serum electrolytes, with adjustments being made daily, is necessary.

As previously mentioned, complications from venous access are some of the drawbacks of TPN administration. Other complications include metabolic derangements, which most often are mild but need correcting as soon as they are identified; abnormalities of liver function tests; the clinical significance of which is unclear (288); and cholelithiasis/cholecystitis secondary to gallbladder sludge.

TABLE 12.3-17. Visceral Proteins Utilized as Indicators for Nutritional Status During Nutritional Repletion

Protein	Normal Range	Half-Life (d)	Levels Low in	Levels High in
Albumin	3.5-5.4 g/dL	18	Liver disease, pregnancy, overhydration, nephrotic syndrome	Dehydration
Transferrin	200-400 mg/dL	8	Chronic infection, chronic inflammation, liver disease, iron overload, nephrotic syndrome	Iron deficiency, pregnancy
Prealbumin	20-40 mg/dL	2	Liver disease, inflammation, surgery, nephrotic syndrome	
Retinol-binding protein (RBP)	3-6 mg/dL	0.5	Liver disease, hyperthyroidism, zinc deficiency, nephrotic syndrome	Renal insufficiency

Renal Issues

AKI is an abrupt decrease in kidney function that includes, but is not limited to, ARF. A number of etiologies for AKI have been described and included prerenal azotemia, acute tubular necrosis (ATN), and acute postrenal obstructive nephropathy, among others (290). The incidence of AKI among hospitalized patients has been estimated to be 5% to 7.5%, with 30% 40% of these cases occurring during the perioperative period (291). The prevalence of AKI among gynecologic surgeries is associated with the primary indication for the surgery, with malignant procedures being the highest (benign procedures 5% and malignant procedures 18%) (292). Epidemiologic evidence supports that even mild, reversible AKI has important clinical consequences, including increased risk of death (293,294). In their retrospective, observational study, Vaught et al demonstrated that women with AKI after gynecologic surgery had a 9 times higher adjusted OR of major adverse events compared to women without AKI (OR 8.95; 95% CI 5.27-15.22). Further, the OR increased as the severity (Risk, Injury, Failure, Loss and End-stage kidney disease [RIFLE] stage) of AKI increased (292).

There are three definitions of AKI that have evolved since 2004 and assess renal dysfunction by two parameters: changes in the SCr level of estimated glomerular filtration rate (eGFR) from a baseline value, and urine output per kilogram of body weight over a specific time period (295). In 2004, a consensus group, the Acute Dialysis Quality Initiative (ADQI) developed the RIFLE system (296). The next iteration at defining AKI was a modification of the RIFLE staging system by the Acute Kidney Injury Network (AKIN) in 2007. This modification added an absolute change in SCr, eGFR criteria, and the inclusion of a time constraint of the rise in creatinine (297). Finally, in 2012, the Kidney Disease: Improving Global Outcomes (KDIGO) further revised the RIFLE and AKIN staging systems for a unified definition of AKI (**Table 12.3-18**) (298).

When AKI presents in the postoperative patient, causes can be divided into three areas: prerenal, renal, or postrenal (inflow, parenchymal, and outflow). The function of glomeruli to create the urinary filtrate depends upon adequate renal perfusion and represents the prerenal component. If the renal mean arterial pressure (MAP) falls below 80 mm Hg, perfusion of the glomeruli

decreases (some disease states require the renal MAP to be higher for adequate perfusion). Many situations can decrease renal MAP and include anesthetics, atherosclerotic emboli, decreased vascular resistance, hypotension, intravascular volume contraction, mechanical ventilation, sepsis, and shock. Autoregulation of the glomeruli can be disrupted by nonsteroidal anti-inflammatory drugs (NSAIDs), angiotensin-converting enzyme (ACE) inhibitors, calcium channel blockers (diltiazem or verapamil), and endotoxins produced by Gram-negative sepsis.

Renal parenchymal damage occurs most commonly in the postoperative patient because of prolonged hypotension or direct injury from inflammatory responses initiated by sepsis. In general, if the hypoperfusion is corrected quickly, reversible azotemia, creatinine elevation, and decreased urine output may be the only manifestations. However, prolonged hypoperfusion can cause ATN, which results in sloughing of renal tubular cells into the tubular lumen and obstruction. In addition, the production of Tamm-Horsfall proteins forms coarse granular casts, inciting an intense inflammatory response, further injuring the renal parenchyma (299,300). Other agents that can induce ATN include aminoglycoside antibiotics and iodinated contrast media. Approximately 15% of patients who receive aminoglycosides will experience nephrotoxicity; therefore, serum levels of these antibiotics must be carefully monitored (301). Iodinated contrast media, used in multiple radiographic procedures, induces ATN by impairing nitric oxide production and increasing free radical formation (302,303). Patients with diabetes with creatinine clearance rates less than 50 mL/min are at particularly high risk (304).

The final reason for ARF in the postoperative gynecologic oncology patient is outflow obstruction. Because of the radical pelvic procedures performed by gynecologic oncologists, ureteral injury is possible and needs to be excluded early in the evaluation of patients with AKI. Prompt reversal of the obstruction can further limit renal damage.

Previously, expected postoperative urinary output was 0.5 mL/kg of weight per hour. Current ERAS protocols value euvolemia and allow permissive oliguria. A recent meta-analysis revealed no significant difference in postoperative AKI in patients undergoing ERAS protocol versus standard postoperative care (305). Most cases of oliguria can be treated with careful intravascular expansion in the first 24 to 48 hours following surgery. Hypoperfusion of the renal parenchyma must be avoided to prevent ATN. Once diagnosed, calculating the fractional excretion of sodium (FENa) or chloride can help discern between prerenal causes or renal causes (hypoperfusions vs ATN). The formula is presented as follows (306):

$$FENa = (\text{urine Na level} \times \text{serum Cr level}) / (\text{serum Na level} \times \text{urine Cr level}) \times 100\%$$

If the FENa is less than 1% and the urine specific gravity is greater than 1.025, the diagnosis is hypoperfusion (prerenal). However, if ischemia has occurred, the FENa will be greater than 4% and the urine specific gravity will fall to 1.010 due to of tubular damage and loss of renal concentrating mechanisms. One cannot calculate FENa in patients who have received diuretics or hyperosmotic agents (eg, mannitol or contrast media). If prerenal and renal causes of low urine output have been excluded, ultrasonography may be useful in evaluating for outflow obstruction (postrenal).

Once the underlying causes for AKI have been eliminated (eg, hypoperfusion, obstruction, sepsis), only time can be offered as treatment. Therapies such as low-dose dopamine, furosemide, mannitol, or ANP use have not demonstrated prevention of or improved recovery from AKI, and guidelines recommend avoidance of such treatments (290). Dialysis remains the only intervention that can support patients until return of renal function. Indications for dialysis include (a) hyperkalemia, metabolic acidosis, or volume expansion that cannot be controlled; (b) symptoms of uremia or encephalopathy; or (c) platelet dysfunction inducing a bleeding diathesis (306).

■ **TABLE 12.3-18. Classification of Acute Kidney Injury According to KDIGO**

Stage	Serum Creatinine	Urine Output
I	1.5-1.9 times baseline OR >0.3 mg/dL increase	<0.5 mL/kg/hr for 6-12 hr
II	2.0-2.9 times baseline	<0.5 mL/kg/hr for ≥12 hr
III	3.0 times baseline OR Increase in serum creatinine to ≥4.0 mg/dL OR Initiation of renal replacement therapy OR In patients <18 years, decrease of eGFR to <35 mL/min/1.73 m²	<0.3 mL/kg/hr for ≥24 hr OR Anuria for ≥12 hr

eGFR, estimated glomerular filtration rate; KDIGO, Kidney Disease: Improving Global Outcomes.

Reprinted by permission from Springer: From Kellum JA, Lameire N. Diagnosis, evaluation and management of acute kidney injury: a KDIGO summary (part 1). *Crit Care*. 2013;17:204.

Shock

Definition

Shock is defined in its simplest terms as a decrease in tissue perfusion below the lowest metabolic needs of the tissue bed. This usually results in a depletion of stored energy and an increase in anaerobic metabolism with buildup of lactic acid and other toxic waste products. Hypotension is incorrectly thought of as a defining component of shock. Hypotension often leads to hypoperfusion, but the patient with hypotension is not in shock until evidence of hypoperfusion occurs. Various types of shock exist.

Hemorrhagic Shock

The first thought for a surgeon managing a postoperative patient who manifests signs and symptoms of shock should be hemorrhage. Hypovolemic shock secondary to inadequate preload can be the result of excessive or ongoing blood loss or inadequate replacement or both. After radical debulking or major extirpative procedures, the potential for postoperative hemorrhage exists. Tachycardia, hypotension, and oliguria are typical clinical signs. In the face of these clinical signs, the surgeon should have high suspicion for active bleeding and be prepared to return the patient to the operating room for correction. Measurement of hemoglobin or hematocrit can be normal in the setting of acute blood loss because a decrease in red cells is accompanied by a decrease in mass. Once fluid is given for resuscitation, dilution will occur and the hemoglobin/hematocrit will fall. With invasive monitoring, the CVP will be low, as will cardiac output and the pulmonary artery occlusion pressure (PAOP). As the stroke volume decreases to inadequate levels, the heart compensates by increasing the heart rate in order to maintain cardiac output. The treatment in these cases is aggressive volume resuscitation and control of ongoing blood loss. Resuscitation for hemorrhagic shock should preferentially use blood products. Studies have shown that there is no difference in outcomes with resuscitation with colloid (albumin) versus crystalloid (normal saline vs LR solution), with the recommendation being to use crystalloid solutions given the decreased cost. The SAFE study is a large, randomized controlled double-blind study that compared albumin to saline infusion in the ICU. It failed to demonstrate a beneficial effect (307).

In the case of continued or rapid bleeding, the obvious course of treatment is reoperation. A number of options are now available intraoperatively in these situations. Obvious bleeding is controlled and ligated. Raw surfaces can be coagulated and treated with fibrin sealants or absorbable hemostatic powders. Damage-control packing has been shown to increase survival in the direst situations. Massive transfusion, defined as greater than 1.5 blood volumes, presents a number of additional problems. These patients will have a dilutional coagulopathy, hypocalcemia, and hyperkalemia. Massive transfusion protocols were initially developed based on military data and have seen some success with civilian trauma populations. Many institutions are now using these protocols to help guide balanced blood product administration for any massive hemorrhage. These protocols provide coolers of blood products in the advised 1:1:1 ratio, with guidance about repletion of calcium and treatment of hyperkalemia (308). Platelet transfusion is indicated for a platelet count less than 50,000 in the actively bleeding patient. Attention to delivery of warm transfusions is critical as hypothermia and acidosis will promote coagulopathy and worsening in bleeding. Once any of the "lethal triad" (hypothermia, acidosis, and coagulopathy) is manifested, then the operation needs to be quickly terminated, even if this means damage-control packing and transporting back to the ICU setting.

Damage-control surgery has been shown to give these patients time to be resuscitated before returning to the operating room. A variety of temporizing abdominal wound management systems exist, the most commonly used is a negative pressure system, with specially designed layers that protect the abdominal contents while allowing suctioning out excess fluids. After the patient is transferred out of the operating room, methods to correct coagulopathy, acidosis, and hypothermia are rapidly enacted. The patient will typically then return to the operating room in 24 to 48 hours for reexploration.

Cardiogenic Shock

A patient with adequate preload who shows signs of poor perfusion secondary to poor cardiac output is categorized as being in cardiogenic shock. The etiology may be a decrease in contractility (secondary to MI) or an increase in afterload (severe hypertension). Typically, "pump failure" results in decreased stroke volume and backup of fluid into the pulmonary circulation. This leads to pulmonary edema and decreased oxygen delivery. The most common provocation for pump failure is the overadministration of fluid in a patient with compromised ventricular function. Treatment consists of diuresis and optimization of cardiac output without increasing myocardial oxygen demand (a difficult task). In the case where significant failure has led to hypotension, dopamine and dobutamine are usually the drugs of choice. The usage of these drugs was discussed previously. Digoxin is commonly used for increasing contractility, but its effects are minor in the acute setting. In addition to inotropic support, correction of electrolyte disturbances (particularly potassium, calcium, and magnesium), maintenance of proper systemic oxygen saturation, and analgesia are important factors in decreasing myocardial stress.

Septic Shock

Septic shock has commonly been defined as hypotension related to infection with eventual organ failure secondary to hypoperfusion despite adequate fluid resuscitation. This definition has changed with that of SIRS and is discussed in the section on "Sepsis and Systemic Inflammatory Response Syndrome." Sepsis is defined as a subset of patients with SIRS who have a documented infectious process. Resuscitation should be guided according to the recommendations in the Surviving Sepsis Campaign (309).

Obstructive Shock

Although a rarer etiology for shock in the gynecologic oncology patient, obstructive shock secondary to a massive PE or tension pneumothorax must be considered. A tension pneumothorax causes shock by shifting the mediastinum to the opposite side of the chest, causing the vena cava to be compressed and severely limiting blood return to the heart (decreasing preload). A massive PE obstructs the pulmonary arteries, not only limiting blood flow but also causing profound hypoxemia. If concerned for a tension pneumothorax is high, this should be treated rapidly with needle decompression or finger thoracostomy before obtaining imaging.

With concern for massive PE, cardiothoracic surgery is usually engaged for consideration of thrombectomy. Depending on the timing of the prior surgery, rapid administration of systemic tissue plasminogen activator (tPA) may be administered to help attempt clot lysis. Patients are also quickly placed on full-dose heparin drips to decrease the risk of ongoing clot formation.

Coagulopathies

Patients who develop shock, and particularly hemorrhagic shock, are at risk of becoming coagulopathic. This is often identified clinically, with increased bleeding noted from wounds, IV and line sites, and, in severe cases, mucous membranes. Labs can be obtained to identify the severity of coagulopathy and to guide treatment. The lab values most commonly obtained are PT/INR, partial prothrombin time (PTT), and fibrinogen. Increased values of the PT/INR and PTT are consistent with coagulopathy. Decreased values of fibrinogen suggest the development of disseminated intravascular coagulation (DIC), where microvascular clots are seen as well as increased bleeding. The development of this condition is a poor prognostic indication, and treatment includes resolving the inciting event while administering clotting factors, specifically cryoprecipitate (310).

Over the past few years, additional methods of assessing coagulation have developed. Broadly speaking, thromboelastography (TEG or rotational thromboelastometry [ROTEM]) tests assess the formation and strength of a clot and will assess whether a patient has a normal coagulation profile or is hypocoagulable or hypercoagulable. If hypocoagulable, test results will be able to guide resuscitation (ie, does the patient require FFP, platelets, cryoprecipitate, or tranexamic acid [TXA]). Unfortunately, these TEG tests are not yet universally available at all hospitals, and test results vary according to which assay system is used. An in-depth discussion about the details of these tests is beyond the scope of this chapter, and the reader is directed to the reference noted (311).

End Points of Resuscitation

End points of resuscitation include normalization of serum lactic acid and base deficit. The base deficit is the amount of base compound needed to titrate a liter of whole arterial blood to a pH of 7.40 and is reported as a negative number. Base-deficit value gives an estimate of the severity of metabolic acidosis; the more negative the value, the worse the metabolic acidosis. Measurement of the base deficit via an arterial blood gas analysis has become an effective means of following response to resuscitation. Following large operations where patients are admitted to the ICU and where large fluid shifts occur, the base deficit should be monitored serially until it has returned to normal. Should a patient have a worsening base deficit (ie, becoming more negative despite adequate resuscitation), then a search for other problems, such as ongoing hemorrhage, subacute anastomotic leak(s), or tissue ischemia, must be made and be addressed before the base deficit will normalize. The base deficit should normalize within the first 24 hours after surgery. Coagulopathy will often correct with resuscitation but may lag behind normalization of the base deficit and lactic acid levels. Thrombocytopenia may persist for several days after its development, but only needs treatment if the platelet level is less than 10,000 or if less than 50,000 with ongoing bleeding.

Infectious Disease Issues

Bacterial Infections

As a broad topic, bacterial infections are a common cause of postoperative fever in the gynecologic patient. Within the first 3 days after surgery, sites of bacterial infection include the urinary tract, the surgical site (superficial and deep), and preexisting infections. After postoperative day 3, pneumonia, SSI, and surgery-specific complications, such as anastomotic leak, abscess, or fistula, are common bacterial causes of postoperative fever.

Postoperative urinary tract infections (UTIs) are typically catheter-associated UTIs (CAUTIs), and treatment is recommended for bacteriuria greater than 10^3 CFU/mL with a positive urinalysis. Nearly 75% of CAUTIs are caused by *Escherichia coli*, *Pseudomonas aeruginosa*, *Klebsiella* species, *Enterococcus* species, and *Candida* species. Empiric therapy can be broad spectrum but should be narrowed based on culture and sensitivity results. Prevention of CAUTIs is the best treatment and accomplished with limited usage of urinary catheters and minimal dwelling time. Prophylactic antibiotics are not recommended for indwelling catheters in the absence of clinical indications (312). **Best practice: Remove urinary catheters placed for gynecologic surgeries within 6 hours of completion of the surgery to limit CAUTIs.**

Postoperative pneumonia typically presents on day 5 after the surgery and manifests with fever, leukocytosis, hypoxia, respiratory distress, dyspnea, tachypnea, and pulmonary infiltrates on chest radiographs. *Staphylococcus aureus*, Enterobacteriaceae with *S. aureus* or streptococci, *Haemophilus influenzae*, and *Streptococcus* were the most common microorganisms isolated from

respiratory cultures (313). Again, broad-spectrum, empiric treatment should not be delayed and later tailored based upon respiratory or blood cultures.

SSIs complicate approximately 2% of hysterectomies, and efforts to decrease their incidence include prophylactic antibiotics, glucose control, and appropriate hair removal. SSIs are categorized as superficial, deep, and organ/space. Many factors contribute to SSIs: patient, preoperative, intraoperative, and postoperative factors. Prevention bundles including preoperative antibiotics, normothermia, glucose control, decreased operative time, and minimally invasive approach have proven to decrease SSI. Aerobic Gram-positive, aerobic Gram-negative, and anaerobic bacteria are all associated with SSIs (314).

The diagnosis of an intra-abdominal source of infection can be challenging in critically ill patients. Not all patients exhibit the same classic symptoms, as they may be masked by other disease processes or medical interventions. For example, abdominal pain and peritoneal signs may not be apparent in patients who are obtunded or sedated and ventilated. Fever and leukocytosis may be absent in 35% and 55% of patients with peritoneal infections (315). A CT scan is the preferred study for the evaluation of patients with suspected intra-abdominal infection. To avoid misdiagnosing fluid-filled bowel as a possible abnormal fluid collection, it is essential that oral and IV contrast agents be used when performing these studies. CT has limitations, especially when used in the critically ill population. The presence of renal insufficiency precludes the use of IV contrast, and ileus or bowel obstruction may prevent complete opacification of the GI tract. Diagnostic laparoscopy can be performed in the ICU with minimal anesthesia and is a safe, accurate, and cost-effective alternative to laparotomy when managing suspected intra-abdominal processes (316). Once identified, an intra-abdominal abscess must be fully evacuated, and the source controlled. Radiologically assisted percutaneous drainage has become the preferred method for treating most abscesses located in the abdomen and pelvis. For well-delineated unilocular fluid collections, percutaneous drainage has a success rate greater than 80% (317). Percutaneous drainage of complex abscesses or those with an enteric communication has a lower success rate but remains a reasonable alternative treatment for the high-risk patient (318). In some cases, surgery may be the only appropriate lifesaving intervention. Timely laparotomy in the critically ill patient with diffuse peritonitis allows for peritoneal toilet, debridement of infected and necrotic tissue, and control or repair of the source. Laparoscopic drainage of complex intra-abdominal abscess has also been reported with good success rates (319). Complex intra-abdominal infections that cannot be effectively controlled by a single laparotomy may be managed best with an open-abdomen approach, with temporary wound closure utilizing a composite, negative pressure (vacuum pack) dressing (320). Potential advantages of the open-abdomen approach include facilitation of repeated debridement, effective drainage, repeat exploration of the peritoneal cavity (at the ICU bedside if necessary), and reduction in intra-abdominal pressure (IAP). In general, the intervention that accomplishes the source control objective with the least physiologic upset should be employed (321).

Viral Infections

The prevalence of viral disease has increased because of improved molecular detection methods (322). Until the severe acute respiratory syndrome coronavirus 2 (SARS-CoV-2) (COVID-19) pandemic, influenza was one of the most common viral causes of sepsis. It is difficult to discern the extent of primary viral infection versus bacterial pneumonia coinfection. The use of BiPAP, endotracheal intubation, and outdated ventilation symptoms contributes to the spread of viral infections in the ICU. Airborne, droplet, and contact precautions should be initiated when viral infections are suspected (322). The benefits of empiric antiviral therapy are unknown and have not been recommended unless specific guidelines exist (323).

Antiviral therapy is available for a limited number of infections. The mainstay of treatment for viral infections is supportive care and antiviral therapy when available and indicated (322).

The COVID-19 pandemic has created many unique challenges in the care of patients with gynecologic cancer. The ASA recommends a stratified waiting period ranging from 4 to 12 weeks following a COVID-19 infection, depending on the severity of the infection, before undergoing elective surgery to decrease the risk of PPCs and mortality. However, a recent propensity-matched cohort study conducted at the MD Anderson Cancer Center found that waiting 20 days between a positive test and surgery appears safe among patients whose COVID-19 symptoms have resolved, patients who are asymptomatic, or patients who had a minimal COVID-19 infection. However, patients with SARS-CoV-2 infections requiring hospitalization were at increased risk of adverse events compared to the matched cohort without a history of SARS-CoV-2 infection. There were no significant differences between the cohorts for pulmonary complications, acute VTE, cardiac events, 30-day readmissions, or death (324).

Fungal Infections

Systemic fungal infections are of great concern for severally ill patients and are linked to an increased risk of associated morbidity and mortality. Systemic candidal infection does not have a unique presentation and, therefore, can be difficult to definitively diagnosis at onset. Although a positive blood culture is the gold standard for diagnosis, blood culture techniques are relatively insensitive, and clinicians frequently must rely on clinical judgment about the probability that candidemia is responsible for a patient's symptoms. Patients who have persistent fever, hypothermia, or unexplained hypotension, despite broad-spectrum antibiotic coverage, may have candidemia. Risk factors associated with candidemia and invasive candidiasis include treatment with multiple antibiotics for extended periods, the presence of central venous catheters, the use of TPN, abdominal surgery, prolonged ICU stay, and compromised immune status (325). The initial choice of therapeutic agents depends on the epidemiologic characteristics of the particular ICU and host factors such as the severity of illness, infection site(s), neutropenia, and organ dysfunction. Fluconazole has excellent activity against *Candida albicans*, but infections caused by *Candida glabrata* or *Candida krusei* must be treated with amphotericin B or caspofungin. Amphotericin B should not be used in patients with renal failure, and azoles and echinocandins (caspofungin) should be used with caution in patients with hepatic dysfunction. Blood cultures should be obtained every day or every other day. Antifungal therapy should be continued for 14 days following the first negative blood culture for candidemia or until clinical microbiologic or radiographical resolution of the infection. If cultures remain positive after several days of treatment, a metastatic source such as an abscess should be ruled out (326). In addition to antifungal therapy, it is recommended that all patients with candidemia have a dilated eye examination by an ophthalmologist and that all catheters be removed if possible (although tunneled catheters are at less risk) (325).

Nosocomial Infections

Infections in the critically ill patient population are a significant cause of morbidity and mortality. Patients in the ICU are particularly vulnerable to infection because of decreased host defenses and the high incidence of resistant bacterial isolates found in ICU settings. In addition, the presence of indwelling catheters and IV lines lowers the inoculum needed to cause infection and provides portals of entry (325). Nosocomial infections are commonly associated with complications of medical or surgical therapy. Approximately 45% of ICU patients will have an infection, and approximately half of those will have acquired the infection while in the ICU (325). Treatment includes identifying and eradicating the source of infection and promptly initiating empirical antibiotic therapy aimed at multidrug-resistant Gram-negative and Gram-positive organisms. If an intra-abdominal or pelvic source is suspected, empiric antibiotic therapy should include anaerobic coverage. Appropriate antibiotic classes include carbapenems, extended-spectrum penicillins, fluoroquinolone-metronidazole, aminoglycoside-metronidazole, or clindamycin combinations (325). In Chapter 12.4, the management of infections in the gynecologic cancer patient is discussed; therefore, information here is limited to infections pertaining to the critically ill patient.

Sepsis and Systemic Inflammatory Response Syndrome

Inflammation is the body's initial response to tissue injury produced by chemical, mechanical, or microbial stimuli. Inflammation is an exceedingly complex cellular and humoral response involving interaction between the complement, kinin, coagulation, and fibrolytic cascades. The goal of inflammation is to enhance the movement of nutrients and phagocytic cells to the injury site in order to prevent invasion of microbes and limit the extension of injury. As a local response, this is beneficial, but appropriate regulation is necessary to prevent a pathologic, exaggerated systemic response, which is clinically identified as SIRS. Sepsis is the clinical syndrome of SIRS due to severe infection. The mediator response in SIRS can be divided into four phases based on the cytokine/cellular response: induction, triggering of cytokine synthesis, evolution of cytokine and coagulation cascade, and elaboration of secondary mediators leading to cellular injury. The three most important mediators operating in SIRS appear to be tumor necrosis factor-α (TNF-α), interleukin-1 (IL-1), and IL-6. The microcirculation endothelium is the key target for injury in the sepsis syndrome (327).

In 2015, the Society of Critical Care Medicine and the European Society of Intensive Care Medicine reviewed the 2001 definitions of SIRS and sepsis (**Table 12.3-19**). Limitations of previous definitions included a focus on inflammation, misleading continuum model from sepsis to shock, and inadequate sensitivity and specificity of SIRS criteria. In addition, the term severe sepsis was found to be redundant. The recommended definition for sepsis is a life-threatening organ dysfunction caused by a dysregulated host response to infection. SIRS may reflect an appropriate host response, whereas sepsis involves organ dysfunction. The task force recommends a change in baseline Sequential [Sepsis-related] Organ Failure Assessment (SOFA) (**Table 12.3-20**) of 2 points or more to represent organ dysfunction. Patients with a SOFA score of 2 or more were found to have a mortality risk of approximately 10%, representing a 2- to 25-fold increase in risk of death compared to those with a SOFA score of less than 2. Quick SOFA (qSOFA) includes only respiratory rate of 22 per minute or more, altered mental status, and systolic blood pressure 100 mm Hg

▪ **TABLE 12.3-19. Definitions for Systemic Inflammatory Response Syndrome (SIRS) and Sepsis**

SIRS	Two or more of the following: Temperature >38 °C or <36 °C Pulse >90/min Respirations >20/min or Paco$_2$ <32 mm Hg WBC count >12,000 or <4,000 cells/mm^3 or >10% band forms
Sepsis	Life-threatening organ dysfunction caused by a dysregulated host response to infection
Septic shock	Sepsis in which underlying circulatory and cellular/metabolic abnormalities are profound enough to substantially increase mortality

Adapted from Singer M, Deutschman CS, Seymour CW, et al. The Third International Consensus Definitions for Sepsis and Septic Shock (Sepsis-3). *JAMA*. 2016;315(8):801-810.

■ TABLE 12.3-20. Sequential (Sepsis-Related) Organ Failure Assessment Score

System	Score				
	0	1	2	3	4
Respiration Pao₂/Fio₂ (mm Hg)	≥400	<400	<300	<200 with respiratory support	<100 with respiratory support
Coagulation Platelets	≥150	<150	<100	<50	<20
Liver Bilirubin (mg/dL)	<1.2	1.2-1.9	2.0-5.9	6.0-11.9	>12.0
Cardiovascular	MAP ≥ 70 mm Hg	MAP <70 mm Hg	Dopamine <5 or dobutamine	Dopamine 5.1-15 or epinephrine ≤0.1 or norepinephrine ≤0.1	Dopamine >15 or epinephrine >0.1 or norepinephrine >0.1
Central nervous system Glasgow Coma Scale score	15	13-14	10-12	6-9	<6
Renal Creatinine (mg/dL) Urine output (mL/d)	<1.2	1.2-1.9	2.0-3.4	3.5-4.9 <500	>5.0 <200

MAP, mean arterial pressure.

or higher to identify patients with poor outcomes without laboratory results (**Box 12.3-1**). Three clinical variables were proposed by a majority of members to identify septic shock: hypotension, elevated lactate level, and sustained need for vasopressor therapy (328).

The host response, more than the pathogen, is the primary determinant of patient outcome. Failure to develop a fever, leukopenia, and hypothermia are associated with increased fatality rates in patients with sepsis and are thought to represent abnormalities in the host's inflammatory response. Other risk factors for mortality from sepsis include age greater than 40, underlying medical conditions, malnutrition, immune suppression, and cancer. The presence or absence of a positive blood culture does not influence outcomes; however, sepsis due to a nosocomial infection has a higher mortality than community-acquired infection (327).

Sepsis with acute organ dysfunction (severe sepsis) is a complex condition that represents a major challenge to the critical care team and carries a mortality rate of 28% to 50% (329). Gram-negative and Gram-positive organisms as well as fungi cause systemic sepsis and septic shock. Early recognition is crucial to patient survival as mortality rates are exceedingly high if the full clinical picture of shock and organ dysfunction develops. Septic shock is divided into an early hyperdynamic state and a late hypodynamic state.

Low systemic vascular resistance, splanchnic vasoconstriction, and increased cardiac output characterize the hyperdynamic phase of shock. Venous capacitance is increased and results in diminished effectiveness of the circulating blood volume. Aggressive volume resuscitation must be provided to restore cardiac preload and ventricular filling. These patients are best managed in an ICU with the placement of an arterial line, a pulmonary artery catheter, and a bladder catheter. Appropriate cultures should be obtained, and IV broad-spectrum antibiotics should be started within the first hour of recognition of severe sepsis. Laboratory tests of immediate

concern include arterial blood gas determinations, creatinine, electrolytes, lactate, coagulation panel, and a complete blood count. Oxygenation and ventilation should be optimized with mechanical ventilation if indicated. If hypotension persists after optimization of the pulmonary capillary wedge pressure (PCWP), the use of norepinephrine or dopamine may be necessary. Surgical debridement or manipulation of infected material should not be performed until the patient has been stabilized.

Early goal-directed therapy of the patient with sepsis has been shown to improve survival. During the first 6 hours of resuscitation, the goals of therapy as outlined by the Surviving Sepsis Campaign guidelines include CVP of 8 to 12 mm Hg, MAP 65 mm Hg or more, urine output 0.5 mL/kg/hr or more, and central venous or mixed venous oxygen saturation 70% or more. If during the first 6 hours oxygen saturation goals are not achieved despite appropriate CVP, then transfusion of RBCs to achieve an hematocrit greater than 30% and/or initiation of a dobutamine infusion is the next step (330).

In the hypodynamic phase of septic shock, hypotension results from cardiac output deterioration. The patient is often cool, mottled, oliguric, diaphoretic, and confused. The etiology of the hypodynamic cardiovascular response to sepsis may be inadequate volume resuscitation, underlying cardiac disease, or myocardial dysfunction associated with sepsis. This is a state of gross decompensation with global tissue hypoxia and is associated with greater mortality.

Numerous clinical trials have attempted to find specific agents to modulate the underlying disease process in sepsis. Candidate therapies included agents that target mediators of inflammatory response, agents that boost the immune system, and prostaglandin inhibitors, but none was shown to be beneficial (330,331).

In addition to early goal-directed therapy with hemodynamic interventions that balance systemic oxygen delivery with oxygen demand, other management strategies have shown in RCTs to reduce mortality associated with severe sepsis. These include limiting the tidal volume to 6 to 7 mL/kg ideal body weight for patients requiring mechanical ventilation for ARDS, the use of moderate-dose corticosteroids (hydrocortisone 200-300 mg and fludrocortisone 50 µg daily) for 7 days in patients with refractory septic shock, and maintaining serum glucose levels less than 180 mg/dL (329). These therapies are not mutually exclusive, and optimal patient management may require a combination of approaches. Some of these strategies vary dramatically from traditional approaches and will require education and established protocols to safely incorporate them into practice.

■ BOX 12.3-1. Quick Sequential (Sepsis-related) Organ Failure Assessment (qSOFA) Criteria

qSOFA	Respiratory rate ≥ 22/min Altered mentation Systolic blood pressure ≤ 100 mm Hg

Adapted from Singer M, Deutschman CS, Seymour CW, et al. The Third International Consensus Definitions for Sepsis and Septic Shock (Sepsis-3). *JAMA.* 2016;315(8):801-810.

Multiple Organ Dysfunction Syndrome

Multiple organ dysfunction syndrome (MODS) is defined as the development of progressive physiologic dysfunction of two or more organ systems after an acute threat to systemic homeostasis (332). An acute threat can include SIRS, sepsis, massive trauma, burns, ischemia, or reperfusion injury. Patients usually present with pulmonary dysfunction, which typically develops early in the course of SIRS or sepsis. Renal dysfunction will present as a prerenal azotemia unless the initial insult stimulated a sudden oliguric ATN. Hyperbilirubinemia is the earliest indication of hepatic dysfunction. GI abnormalities include ileus, stress ulcers, diarrhea, and mucosal atrophy. The platelet count has been used as a surrogate marker of the hematologic system. Cardiac function is often measured by the severity of hypotension or the need for vasopressors. Deterioration of the nervous system is manifested by encephalopathy and peripheral neuropathies. The treatment of MODS is support of individual organ function and aggressive therapies aimed at correcting the underlying process. Mortality is related to the number of dysfunctional systems and is greater than 80% once four organ systems fail (333).

The Acute Physiology and Chronic Health Evaluation (APACHE) provided population-based estimates of mortality for the day of ICU admission (334). Several versions of the APACHE scoring system have been utilized, most recently APACHE IV. Organ failure scores, such as the SOFA, can help assess organ dysfunction over time and are useful to evaluate morbidity. Independent of the initial value, an increase in the SOFA score during the first 48 hours of an ICU admission predicts a mortality rate of 50% or greater. Improvement of cardiovascular, renal, or respiratory SOFA score from baseline through day 1 of ICU admission is significantly related to greater survival (335). It is important to note that these and other outcome prediction models were designed as tools to be used in critical care research in order to stratify patients by the severity of illness. They have not been validated for making decisions relating to individual patients.

Abdominal compartment syndrome is an important but often unrecognized cause of acute deterioration of a patient after massive fluid resuscitation for septic or hypovolemic shock. Although abdominal compartment syndrome can impair the function of every organ system, it is generally manifested as hypotension, reduced urine output, and decreased pulmonary compliance. Most commonly associated with trauma, it has also been observed in patients with massive ascites, bowel obstruction or ileus, peritonitis, pancreatitis, and intraperitoneal blood. IAP is usually measured indirectly by a balloon-tipped catheter in the bladder. Intra-abdominal hypertension is defined as an IAP of 12 mm Hg or greater recorded by a minimum of three standard measurements conducted 4 to 6 hours apart (336). Abdominal compartment syndrome is defined by an IAP of 20 mm Hg or greater and single or multiple organ failure that was not previously present. Operative decompression of the abdominal cavity with maintenance of an open abdomen via use of temporary closure techniques such as a vacuum pack is the only treatment that reverses the physiologic abnormalities resulting from abdominal compartment syndrome.

Analgesia

Pain management for critically ill patients is a universal goal for all involved in their care. Patients who are not satisfied with the treatment they receive for pain may become more stressed and irritable, sleep less, and have a poor opinion of the care they are receiving on the whole. Pain may contribute to pulmonary dysfunction through localized guarding and generalized muscle rigidity that restricts movement of the chest wall and diaphragm. Unrelieved pain also evokes a stress response, characterized by tachycardia, increased myocardial oxygen consumption, hypercoagulability, immunosuppression, and persistent catabolism (337). The combined use of effective analgesia and sedation may ameliorate the stress response and diminish pulmonary complications in postoperative critically ill patients. Postoperative pain management will be considered here with the topics of general and palliative pain control being discussed in Chapter 12.5.

Pharmacologic therapies include opioids, NSAIDs, and acetaminophen. The American Society of Health-System Pharmacists (ASHP) guidelines recommend fentanyl, hydromorphone, and morphine given as a continuous infusion or scheduled doses rather than "as needed." Fentanyl has the most rapid onset and shortest duration, but repeated dosing may cause accumulation and prolonged effects. Fentanyl may also be administered via a transdermal patch to hemodynamically stable patients with more chronic analgesic needs, but it is not recommended for the management of acute pain. Morphine has a quick onset but longer duration of action, so intermittent doses may be given. However, morphine causes histamine release, which contributes to hypotension, especially in a hemodynamically unstable patient. Hydromorphone's duration of action is similar to morphine but lacks an active metabolite or histamine release, making it an ideal drug for continuous infusion and for use in patients who cannot tolerate hypotension. Meperidine has an active metabolite that causes neuroexcitation, including apprehension, tremors, delirium, and seizures, so its use is not recommended in critically ill patients who may need repeated doses. The characteristics of analgesics and sedatives commonly used in ICU patients are summarized in **Table 12.3-21**.

Over the past several years, postoperative pain management has adapted to the growing concerns about adequate control and the growing opioid epidemic. Multimodal pain regimens are often being utilized; however, opioids are still the mainstay of postoperative pain management, given a general lack of literature surrounding pain management, particularly with intra-abdominal surgery. Multimodal pain regimens vary but typically include acetaminophen (IV, oral, or rectal), NSAIDs, gabapentinoids (gabapentin, pregabalin), ketamine, and patient-controlled analgesia (PCA). The use of local anesthesia and long-acting liposomal bupivacaine help reduce incisional pain. Neuraxial (epidural/spinal) and peripheral regional nerve blocks are becoming more common and are often performed by anesthesiologists preoperatively or immediately postoperatively. The transition to oral medications typically begins to occur as soon as the patient can tolerate oral agents.

Owing to the opioid epidemic, the CDC has put forth guidelines regarding reduced use of opioid agents. These guidelines include guidance about prescription of postoperative short-acting opioids. These prescriptions are dependent on the expected recovery from the procedure, with rapid recovery recommended less than 3 days of opioids, medium-term recovery with less than 7 days of opioids, and longer term with less than 14 days of opioids. If patients are requiring ongoing opioids, the patient needs to be seen and evaluated by the surgeon before an additional prescription should be provided (338).

Non–Intensive Care Unit Postoperative Pain Control

The misuse and diversion of prescription opioids has contributed to the current epidemic of the opioid use disorder in the United States. Provisional data indicate that this health crisis has worsened since the COVID pandemic started, with more than 77,000 opioid-related deaths. Most cases of chronic opioid use disorder start with legitimately obtained prescriptions. Approximately 6% to 8% of opioid-naïve patients develop chronic opioid use following surgery and the probability increases with duration of opioid therapy (339). Although no standard definition of opioid stewardship exists, "perioperative opioid stewardship" may be defined as the judicious use of opioids to treat surgical pain and optimize postoperative outcomes. The paradigm is not simply "opioid avoidance" and requires balancing the risk of both over- and underutilization of these high-risk agents. To this end, postoperative opioid

■ **TABLE 12.3-21. Characteristics of Selected Analgesics and Sedatives Frequently Used in Critically Ill Patients**

Agent	Indication	Active Metabolites (Effect)	Adverse Effects	Intermittent Dose (IV)[a]	Infusion Dose Range
Fentanyl	Pain	No metabolite, patient accumulates	Rigidity with high doses	0.35-1.5 µg/kg q0.5-1h	0.7–10 µg/kg/hr
Hydromorphone	Pain	None	–	10-30 µg/kg q1-2h	7-15 µg/kg/hr
Morphine	Pain	Yes (sedation)	Histamine release	0.01-0.15 mg/kg q1-2h	0.07-0.5 mg/kg/hr
Ketorolac	Pain	None	GI bleeding, renal	15-30 mg q6h; decrease if >65 yr; avoid >5 d use	–
Midazolam	Acute agitation	Yes (prolonged sedation)	–	0.02-0.08 mg/kg q0.5-2h	0.04-0.2 mg/kg/hr
Lorazepam	Sedation	None	Solvent-related acidosis/renal failure in high doses	0.02-0.06 mg/kg q2-6h	0.01-0.1 mg/kg/hr
Propofol	Sedation	None	Elevated triglycerides	–	5-80 µg/kg/min
Dexmedetomidine	Sedation, acute agitation	None	Hypotension, bradycardia	NA	0.2-1.4 µg/kg/hr
Haloperidol	Delirium	Yes (EPS)	QT interval prolongation	0.03-0.15 mg/kg q0.5-6h	0.04-0.15 mg/kg/hr

EPS, extrapyramidal symptoms; GI, gastrointestinal; IV, intravenous; q, every.

[a]More frequent doses may be needed for acute management in mechanically ventilated patients.

minimization should be pursued only in the greater context of optimizing acute pain management, reducing adverse events, and preventing persistent postoperative pain through comprehensive multimodal analgesia (340).

With the advent of ERAS programs, multimodal preemptive and postoperative pain control schemes have been utilized and studied, demonstrating decreased need and duration for opioid medications and their associated side effects. Multimodal analgesia is defined as the administration of two or more analgesic agents or procedures (anesthetic techniques) that exert their effects through different analgesic pathways to reduce acute postoperative pain. Many ERAS programs use scheduled non-opioid medications such as acetaminophen, ibuprofen, ketorolac, celecoxib, and gabapentinoids (gabapentin and pregabalin) in the preoperative setting as preemptive analgesia. Similarly, these agents are also used in conjunction with opioid rescue medications in the postoperative setting. Taken together, multimodal analgesia has led to decreased opioid utilization for postoperative pain management. Further, the use of neuraxial or regional anesthetic techniques such as epidurals or peripheral nerve blocks (such as transversus abdominis plane [TAP] blocks) for open abdominal and gynecologic surgeries has led to decreased need for opioid medications for postoperative pain control (341) (**Table 12.3-22**).

Clearly, postoperative pain is driven by multifactorial elements such as the operative procedure performed, the patient's baseline expectation of pain and pain control, the patient's baseline anxiety as well as other behavioral problems, in addition to others. Postoperative pain management should be individualized to the needs of each patient. To provide effective multimodal and opioid-sparing analgesia, clinicians should standardly prescribe around-the-clock non-opioid medications such as acetaminophen, NSAIDs, and gabapentinoids, in combination, as these medications have been shown to reduce pain while minimizing opioid use compared to monotherapy (340). In addition to these non-opioid medications, patients undergoing major painful procedures may need short-term opioid therapy for "breakthrough" pain. The oral route of administration is preferred for patients who can take medications by mouth, reserving intravenous administration for patients where oral administration is contraindicated. Doses of oxycodone in these instances should be 5 mg every 4 hours as needed, with a repeat dose of 5 mg within 1 hour if ineffective for moderate to severe pain (340).

In the United States, variable and often excessive opioid quantities have been prescribed to patients postoperatively at the time of discharge (340). So what is an adequate prescription amount of opioid medication for patients at discharge from the hospital after surgery? In 2016, the Michigan Opioid Prescribing Engagement Network (OPEN) released procedure-specific guidelines to help reduce overprescribing of opioids after surgery. These guidelines are adjusted regularly using expert opinion, patient claims data, and evidence-based literature and are intended for patients considered to be opioid naïve (340, 342). Since implementation of the guidelines across 43 hospitals in Michigan, there has been a significant reduction in the quantity of opioids prescribed with a corresponding reduction in opioid consumption by patients (340,343). Generally, at the time of discharge, patients who have gynecologic oncology procedures (including minimally invasive surgeries, open surgeries, bowel surgeries, etc) will need only around 0 to 10, 5 mg oxycodone tablets, as rescue medications, with multimodal analgesic programs (342). Patients who are opioid tolerant will have higher opioid requirements upon discharge and will likely need a postdischarge opioid taper. Usually, patients tolerate tapering the opioid dose by 20% to 25% every 1 to 2 days as their pain improves (340).

Recognizing the problem of opioid overuse in this country, many institutions have rolled out ERAS pathways to address better, multimodal opioid-sparing postoperative pain management. The authors direct the reader to an excellent review of this topic by Hyland et al (340).

Sedation

To further combat anxiety and agitation associated with hospitalization and pain, sedatives are commonly added to routine medication administration. The physical environment of the ICU, limited ability to communicate, sleep deprivation, and medical circumstances precipitating the ICU admission are contributing factors creating anxiety in critically ill patients. Efforts to reduce anxiety, including frequent reorientation, provision of adequate analgesia, and optimization of the environment, may be supplemented with sedatives. Agitation is also common in ICU patients; however, not all patients with anxiety will exhibit agitation. Sedatives reduce the stress response and improve tolerance to routine ICU procedures. For example, the

■ **TABLE 12.3-22. Non-opioid Modalities for Preemptive and Postoperative Pain Control for Gynecologic Surgeries**

Medication	Route	Dose Timing	Mechanism of Action	Cautions
Acetaminophen	Oral, IV	Preoperative; postoperative	Inhibition of COX pathway, though exact mechanism is not known; synergistic with NSAIDs	Liver toxicity at higher doses (no more than 4,000 mg in 24 hr) and lower doses in patients with liver disease
NSAIDs (ketorolac, ibuprofen, celecoxib, etc)	Oral, IV	Preoperative; postoperative	Inhibition of COX-1 and 2 enzyme and disruption of prostaglandin synthesis; some are selective COX-2 inhibitors.	Associated with increase in GI ulceration, bleeding, and renal impairment; COX-2 inhibitors decrease GI complications and bleeding, but can increase cardiovascular adverse events.
Gabapentinoids (gabapentin, pregabalin)	Oral	Preoperative; postoperative	Inhibition of voltage-gated calcium channels	Linked to visual disturbances and dizziness that can hinder early postoperative mobilization; older patients have more side effects.
α-2 agonists (clonidine, dexmedetomidine)	Oral, IV	Preoperative; postoperative	Stimulation of the α-2 receptors in the dorsal horn of the spinal cord, reducing nociceptive signals	Sedation, hypotension, and bradycardia can occur.
Regional anesthesia techniques—Peripheral nerve blocks (TAP)	Injections—local anesthetics single shot (duration <24 hr); continuous with infusion pump	Preoperative; postoperative	Targets local anesthetic medications directly to peripheral nerves	Bleeding, nerve injury, local anesthetic systemic toxicity, intraperitoneal organ injury
Neuraxial analgesia techniques—Epidural analgesia	Injection and continuous infusion pump	Preoperative; postoperative	Local anesthetics with or without adjuvants (eg, opioids) injected into the epidural space	Can cause backache, possible dura puncture; nerve or spinal cord injury; infection, epidural hematoma, and local anesthetic systemic toxicity; hypotension; urinary retention; motor blockade

COX, cyclooxygenase; GI, gastrointestinal; IV, intravenous; NSAID, nonsteroidal anti-inflammatory drug; TAP, transversus abdominis plane.

use of sedation medication may be necessary to facilitate mechanical ventilation. Generally, sedatives should be administered intermittently to determine the dose needed to achieve the sedation goal, but they may be given as a continuous infusion if necessary. Daily interruption of sedative infusion is associated with shorter duration of mechanical ventilation, shorter ICU stays, and fewer instances of post-traumatic stress disorder (339,340). Benzodiazepines are sedatives and hypnotics that cause anterograde amnesia but lack analgesic properties. Midazolam has a rapid onset and short duration of effect with single doses, making it ideal for treating acutely agitated patients or for brief sedation with invasive procedures. Lorazepam has a slower onset but fewer potential drug interactions because of its metabolism via glucuronidation (**Table 12.3-21**).

Propofol is an IV general anesthetic that has sedative and hypnotic properties at lower doses. Like the benzodiazepines, propofol has no analgesic properties. Propofol has a rapid onset and short duration of sedation once discontinued. Propofol is a phospholipid emulsion that provides 1.1 kcal/mL from fat and should be counted as a caloric source. Long-term infusions may result in hypertriglyceridemia, and monitoring is recommended after 2 days of use (341). Physiologic dependence and potential withdrawal symptoms have been described in ICU patients who have been exposed to more than 1 week of sedative or narcotic therapy, including the use of propofol (342).

Precedex has become a commonly used adjunct. It acts by activating α2-adrenoceptors, reducing sympathetic tone, which helps control or treat agitation and anxiety. An added benefit is the lack of respiratory suppression, which allows it to continue running during spontaneous breathing trials and attempts to liberate patients from the ventilator, decreasing the likelihood of failure due to anxiety (343).

Neuromuscular Blockade

Neuromuscular blocking agents (NMBAs) can be used in conjunction with sedatives to facilitate mechanical ventilation, to manage intracranial pressure in head trauma, to ablate muscle spasms, and to decrease oxygen consumption only when all other means to accomplish these aims have failed (344). Pancuronium is a long-acting NMBA that is effective for up to 90 minutes after IV bolus dose of 0.06 to 0.1 mg/kg. It can be used as a continuous infusion by adjusting the dose to the degree of neuromuscular blockade that is desired. Because pancuronium is vagolytic, 90% of patients will have an increase in heart rate of greater than 10 beats/min. For patients who cannot tolerate an increase in heart rate, vecuronium can be used. If neuromuscular blockade is necessary for patients with significant hepatic or renal failure, cisatracurium or atracurium should be used. Patients receiving any NMBA should be assessed using electronic twitch monitoring, with a goal of adjusting the blockade to achieve one or two twitches. Before initiating neuromuscular blockade, patients should be adequately medicated with sedative and analgesic drugs, as it is difficult to assess pain and anxiety after NMBA is given. BIS monitors are used to assess the degree of sedation while chemically paralyzed. Furthermore, neuromuscular paralysis without sedation is an extremely frightening and unpleasant experience.

Acute quadriplegic myopathy syndrome, also referred to as postparalytic quadriparesis, is a clinical triad of acute paresis, myonecrosis with increased CPK concentration, and abnormal electromyography that is related to prolonged exposure to NMBAs. This is a devastating complication of NMBA therapy, and one of the reasons that indiscriminate use of these agents is discouraged. Increased risk of acute quadriplegic myopathy is associated with the concurrent use of corticosteroids; drug "holidays" may decrease the risk (345).

Intensive Care Unit Syndrome/Delirium

First reported in the 1960s, the term *ICU syndrome*, or *psychosis*, refers to a multitude of psychological disturbances exhibited by many critically ill patients (346). It has also been labeled postoperative delirium. The ICU syndrome has been defined as an altered emotional state occurring in a highly stressful environment that may manifest itself in a variety of psychological reactions, including fear, memory disturbance, anxiety, confusion, withdrawal, despair, agitation, and disorientation. Factors such as sleep deprivation, noise, constant light exposure, restriction of movement, limited ability to communicate, as well as the patient's preadmission mental state and coping ability have all been reported as contributing causes of ICU syndrome. Current medical literature challenges this concept and argues that what is being called ICU syndrome or psychosis is diagnostic of delirium and not due to the ICU environment per se. Concerns have been raised that using the term *ICU syndrome* implies that confusion can be expected in the ICU setting and may reduce the vigilance necessary to recognize delirium and identify and treat the physiologic disturbances leading to it (347). Delirium is found in as many as 80% of critically ill patients and is associated with longer ICU admissions and increased mortality (348,349).

Delirium in the ICU setting is commonly caused by metabolic disturbances, hypoxia, electrolyte imbalances, alcohol or drug withdrawal, acute infection, and medications (**Table 12.3-23**) (346,349). Many drugs have anticholinergic properties that can exert an additive effect, causing neurotoxicity, especially in older patients. Anticholinergic-related delirium can be differentiated from other causes of delirium if the mental status clears after administration of the cholinesterase inhibitor physostigmine. Delirium presents in both a hypoactive and hyperactive form. Hypoactive delirium, which is associated with the worst prognosis, is characterized by psychomotor retardation, represents more global cerebral dysfunction, and is manifested by a calm appearance, inattention, and obtundation in extreme cases. Hyperactive delirium is more easily recognized by agitation and combative behaviors. Older patients

may pose a particular diagnostic challenge when delirium is superimposed on baseline dementia.

The medical management of delirium consists of finding and treating underlying medical conditions and then controlling any behavioral disturbances if necessary. Neuroleptic drugs are the first-line agents for the treatment of delirium. When causes are related to alcohol withdrawal syndrome, management is with benzodiazepines. Haloperidol is the neuroleptic of choice because it has minimal anticholinergic or hypotensive effects. A dose of 2 to 10 mg IV can be given every 20 to 30 minutes until agitation resolves. Once the delirium is controlled, scheduled doses every 4 to 6 hours consisting of 25% of necessary loading doses can be used and tapered off over several days. A continuous infusion can also be used. Patients receiving repeat doses of haloperidol should be monitored for ECG changes. Extrapyramidal side effects such as rigidity, tremor, or facial tics can be managed with diphenhydramine hydrochloride (341).

End-of-Life Considerations

Despite valiant efforts and adherence to best practices of care, patients, families, and health care professionals are often faced with the difficult decision to withdraw life-sustaining treatment and care. The ethical aspect of foregoing treatment resides in the legal and ethical right of the patient to self-determination. Unfortunately, the majority of critically ill patients are unable to speak for themselves when decisions need to be made to withhold treatment. Living wills, power of attorney status, and advance directives must be acknowledged and honored regarding end-of-life considerations. If a medical power of attorney is not in place, some states stipulate who the surrogate will be by a legal hierarchy. The ethical basis for identification of an appropriate surrogate is primary if none of the preceding legal bases apply. In this situation, the physician and other health care providers have the responsibility to help identify the person or persons who have knowledge of the patient's values and preferences in order to assist with medical decisions on the patient's behalf. This process can become difficult in circumstances when family members or others close to the patient are in disagreement as to who should be the surrogate or what the patient would prefer. In these cases, health care providers should be knowledgeable of applicable legal directives and their ethical responsibility to act in their patient's best interest. Consultation with the institution's ethics committee may be helpful in trying to reach consensus (350). Although not responsible for the patient's death, those close to the patient are often left with feelings of guilt and anxiety in addition to their bereavement. It is important that the health care providers support the family both before and after the decision to withhold or withdraw life-sustaining treatment has been made, not imparting any personal bias.

End-of-life care of patients in the ICU requires a dramatic paradigm shift in attitude and interventions from intensive rescue-type care to intensive palliative care. When considering the array of interventions that may be discontinued or held, physicians and surrogates should focus on clearly articulating the goals of care. For example, a goal for survival until the patient's important loved ones can gather to say their goodbyes may justify short-term continuation of ventilator support. If the only goal is patient comfort, then such treatment should be stopped. The withdrawal of life-sustaining treatment is a clinical procedure that deserves the same preparation and expectation of quality as other medical procedures. Honest, caring, and culturally sensitive communication with the patient's loved ones and the patient, if competent, should include explanations of how therapies will be withdrawn, what symptoms are expected, strategies to assess and ensure the patient's comfort, and information about the expected survival after interventions are withdrawn. Informed consent should be documented along with a formulated plan for withdrawing care (351). Adequate analgesia and sedation should be prescribed to relieve symptoms of pain, dyspnea, and anxiety during the dying process.

■ TABLE 12.3-23. Commonly Used Intensive Care Unit Drugs Associated With Delirium[a]

Anesthetics	Anticonvulsants	Atropine[b]
Lidocaine	Carbamazepine	Cimetidine[b]
Propofol	Phenobarbital	Corticosteroids[b]
	Phenytoin	Digoxin[b]
Antibiotics		
Amphotericin B	Antihypertensives	Narcotic analgesics
Aztreonam	Diltiazem	Fentanyl
Cephalosporins	Enalapril	Meperidine[b]
Ciprofloxacin	Hydralazine	Morphine
Doxycycline	Methyldopa	
Imipenem	Propranolol	Nitroprusside
Metronidazole	Verapamil	Phenylephrine
Penicillins		Procainamide[b]
Tobramycin		Scopolamine[b]
		Tricyclic antidepressants[b]

[a]Listing is not intended to be all inclusive.

[b]Drugs known to have significant anticholinergic properties.

IV opioids and shorter acting benzodiazepines are the drugs of choice. The clinician's primary goal should be to prevent suffering and ensure the patient's comfort, even if doing so unintentionally hastens the patient's death. For this reason, palliative care teams might be useful (351).

Gastrointestinal

Postoperative Ileus

Postoperative ileus after benign gynecologic surgery ranges from 5% to 25%, with increased incidence following laparotomy over minimally invasive surgery. This diagnosis increases hospital stays by 30% and translate into an increased cost of $5,000 to $10,000 per episode of postoperative ileus and $1.5 billion annually in the United States (352). Following primary staging and debulking for epithelial ovarian cancer, postoperative ileus rates ranged from 25.9% to 38.5% and were seen more commonly after bowel resection. Risk factors for postoperative ileus among patients with cancer having surgery include preoperative thrombocytosis, carcinoma involving the bowel mesentery, and perioperative transfusion of RBCs, whereas postoperative ibuprofen use was associated with a statistically significant decrease in postoperative ileus (353).

Postoperative ileus simply is a delay in the return of bowel motility following surgery associated with nausea, vomiting, abdominal distention with tenderness, and delayed bowel function, such as flatus and stool. Although the etiology is unknown, three likely mechanisms, in sequence, include (i) neurogenic mechanisms, (ii) GI inflammation, and (iii) pharmacologic effects. Peritoneal irritation causes stimulation of afferent reflexes in the acute neurogenic phase of postoperative ileus. Tissue trauma triggers the stress response and subsequent GI inflammation in the prolonged phase of an ileus. Perioperative opioids are the most common cause of the pharmacologic mechanism of postoperative ileus and affect the GI μ-opioid receptors, resulting in inhibition of acetylcholine release, which disrupts peristalsis, resulting in nonpropulsive, uncoordinated contractions of the GI tract (352). Most of the time, colon function returns approximately 72 hours after laparotomy, but retroperitoneal dissections increase colon stasis and the rates of postoperative ileus (353).

Multiple studies have shown that early postoperative feeding and gum chewing reduce the incidence of postoperative ileus by activating the cephalic-vagal pathway, counteracting the GI μ-opioid receptor (352,354). Pharmacologic bowel stimulation with laxatives or enemas, alvimopan (a selective μ-opioid antagonist), and ketorolac (NSAID) appears to decrease time to return of bowel function, thus decreasing the rate of postoperative ileus (352).

No prospective RCTs for the treatment of postoperative ileus have been done, and treatment is largely based upon expert opinion. Traditional treatment includes bowel rest (NPO); NGT decompression, when needed; hydration; and electrolyte repletion. Pharmacologic treatment of ileus has not been extensively studied, but alvimopan may be beneficial, although more study is needed. Other pharmacologic agents have shown to be ineffective, including oral erythromycin, systemic lidocaine, and oral metoclopramide (352).

Best practice: To prevent postoperative ileus, limit bowel manipulation and large volume IV fluids during surgery; begin early postoperative feeding, gum chewing, and ambulation; and limit postoperative opioid use.

Postoperative Small Bowel Obstruction

Eighty percent of small bowel obstruction (SBO) is caused by mechanical intestinal obstruction, by either intrinsic or extrinsic forces, that result in compression of the lumen (355). With obstruction, the bowel progressively dilates proximal to the blockage while decompressing distally. The bowel wall becomes edematous, absorptive function becomes impaired, and fluid is trapped in the bowel lumen (356). Peritoneal adhesions cause the majority of SBOs, followed by hernias, malignancies, and infectious and inflammatory disorders. Any SBO that occurs 4 to 6 weeks following abdominal surgery is classified as postoperative SBO. A recent retrospective cohort study utilizing the NSQIP database found that the incidence of SBO after benign hysterectomy was 5.9 per 1,000 benign hysterectomies, with 72% occurring after abdominal hysterectomies. Patient risk factors found to increase the occurrence of SBO include age, tobacco use, prior abdominal surgery, and medical comorbidities. Intraoperative risk factors included abdominal hysterectomy, adhesiolysis, appendectomy, and cystotomy repair (357).

SBO presents with acute onset of abdominal pain, nausea, vomiting, abdominal distention, and obstipation of flatus and stool. Intractable, often feculent, emesis results in loss of fluid containing sodium, potassium, hydrogen ions, and chloride, causing a hypovolemia and a metabolic alkalosis. Compensatory mechanisms in the kidney will result in a worsening hypokalemia. Physical examination shows signs of dehydration, abdominal distention, high-pitched or hypoactive bowel sounds, and tympanic percussion of the abdomen. Patients with known hernia may have a tender, red bulge in the hernia sac. Abdominal radiography will reveal dilated loops of bowel with air-fluid levels, with abdominal/pelvic CT possibly showing a transition point as the site of the obstruction, possible ischemia, necrosis, and perforation (358,359).

Treatment of postoperative SBO includes IV fluid replacement, correction of electrolyte abnormalities, bowel rest (NPO), GI decompression with an NGT reserving immediate surgery for signs of a surgically correctable cause of SBO (such as hernia), intestinal perforation, necrosis, ischemia, or the presence of a closed-loop obstruction (360,361). Adhesions causing early postoperative SBO rarely lead to strangulation and should be treated conservatively for a longer duration, in the absence of clinical deterioration, than SBO caused by adhesions in the nonpostoperative period (362). In the first 10 to 14 days postoperatively, adhesions are dense and hypervascular, making reoperation complicated and dangerous. In a retrospective study of postoperative SBO, 91% of the 34 patients treated with parenteral nutrition avoided surgery and had successful return of bowel function within 60 days. When early reoperation occurred (typically on postoperative day 17), those surgeries were complicated by 12 bowel resections, five incidental enterotomies, three new stomas, two enterocutaneous fistulae, one anastomotic leak, and one fascial dehiscence (363).

REFERENCES

1. Dean MM, Finan MA, Kline RC. Predictors of complications and hospital stay in gynecologic cancer surgery. *Obstet Gynecol.* 2001;97:721-724.

2. Benedetti Panici PP, Di Donato V, Fischetti M, et al. Predictors of postoperative morbidity after cytoreduction for advanced ovarian cancer: analysis and management of complications in upper abdominal surgery. *Gynecol Oncol.* 2015;137(3):406-411.

3. Institute of Medicine; Committee on Quality of Health Care in America. *Crossing the Quality Chasm: A New Health System for the 21st Century.* National Academy Press (US); 2001.

4. Braddock CH 3rd, Edwards KA, Hasenberg NM, Laidley TL, Levinson W. Informed decision making in outpatient practice: time to get back to basics. *JAMA.* 1999;282:2313-2320.

5. Long KL, Ingraham AM, Wendt EM, et al. Informed consent and informed decision-making in high-risk surgery: a quantitative analysis. *J Am Coll Surg.* 2021;233:337-345.

6. Braddock C 3rd, Hudak PL, Feldman JJ, Bereknyei S, Frankel RM, Levinson W. "Surgery is certainly one good option": quality and time-efficiency of informed decision-making in surgery. *J Bone Joint Surg Am.* 2008;90:1830-1838.

7. Rivera RA, Nguyen MT, Martinez-Osorio JI, McNeill MF, Ali SK, Mansi IA. Preoperative medical consultation: maximizing its benefits. *Am J Surg.* 2012;204(5):787-797.

8. Almassi N, Ponziano M, Goldman HB, Klein EA, Stephenson AJ, Krishnamurthi V. Reducing overutilization of preoperative medical referrals among patients undergoing radical cystectomy using an evidence-based algorithm. *Urology.* 2018;114:71-76.

9. Auerbach AD, Rasic MA, Sehgal N, Ide B, Stone B, Maselli J. Opportunity missed: medical consultation, resource use, and quality of care of patients undergoing major surgery. *Arch Intern Med*. 2007;167:2338-2344.

10. Benarroch-Gampel J, Sheffield KM, Duncan CB, et al. Preoperative laboratory testing in patients undergoing elective, low-risk ambulatory surgery. *Ann Surg*. 2012;256:518-528.

11. Institute for Clinical Systems Improvement (ICSI) health care guideline: preoperative evaluation. Accessed April 1, 2022. https://www.icsi.org/wp-content/uploads/2021/11/Periop_6th-Ed_2020_v2.pdf

12. National Institute for Clinical Excellence. Routine preoperative tests for elective surgery: NICE guideline [NG45]. Published April 5, 2016. https://www.nice.org.uk/guidance/ng45

13. St Clair CM, Shah M, Diver EJ, et al. Adherence to evidence-based guidelines for preoperative testing in women undergoing gynecologic surgery. *Obstet Gynecol*. 2010;116:694-700.

14. Mosca L, Grundy SM, Judelson D, et al. Guide to preventive cardiology for women. AHA/ACC Scientific Statement Consensus panel statement. *Circulation*. 1999;99:2480-2484.

15. Mosca L, Benjamin EJ, Berra K, et al. Effectiveness-based guidelines for the prevention of cardiovascular disease in women 2011 update: a guideline from the American Heart Association. *Circulation*. 2011;123:1243-1262.

16. Cho L, Davis M, Elgendy I, et al. Summary of updated recommendations for primary prevention of cardiovascular disease in women: JACC state-of-the-art review. *J Am Coll Cardiol*. 2020;75:20:2602-2618.

17. Levine GN, Bates ER, Bittl JA, et al. 2016 ACC/AHA guideline focused update on duration of dual antiplatelet therapy in patients with coronary artery disease: a report of the American College of Cardiology/American Heart Association task force on clinical practice guidelines: an update of the 2011 ACCF/AHA/SCAI guideline for percutaneous coronary intervention, 2011 ACCF/AHA guideline for coronary artery bypass graft surgery, 2012 ACC/AHA/ACP/AATS/PCNA/SCAI/STS guideline for the diagnosis and management of patients with stable ischemic heart disease, 2013 ACCF/AHA guideline for the management of ST-elevation myocardial infarction, 2014 AHA/ACC guideline for the management of patients with Non-ST-Elevation acute coronary syndromes, and 2014 ACC/AHA guideline on perioperative cardiovascular evaluation and management of patients undergoing noncardiac surgery. *Circulation*. 2016;134(10):e123-e155.

18. Pregler J, Freund KM, Kleinman M, et al. The heart truth professional education Campaign on women and heart disease: needs assessment and evaluation results. *J Womens Health*. 2009;18(10):1541-1547.

19. Poon S, Goodman SG, Yan RT, et al. Bridging the gender gap: insights from a contemporary analysis of sex-related differences in the treatment and outcomes of patients with acute coronary syndromes. *Am Heart J*. 2012;163(1):66-73.

20. Hollenberg SM. Preoperative cardiac risk assessment. *Chest*. 1999;115(suppl 5):51S-57S.

21. Freeman WK, Gibbons RJ. Perioperative cardiovascular assessment of patients undergoing noncardiac surgery. *Mayo Clin Proc*. 2009;84:79-90.

22. Fleisher LA, Beckman JA, Brown KA, et al. ACC/AHA 2007 guidelines on perioperative cardiovascular evaluation and care for noncardiac surgery: executive summary: a report of the American College of Cardiology/American Heart Association Task Force on practice guidelines (Writing Committee to Revise the 2002 Guidelines on Perioperative Cardiovascular Evaluation for Noncardiac Surgery): developed in collaboration with the American Society of Echocardiography, American Society of Nuclear Cardiology, Heart Rhythm Society, Society of Cardiovascular Anesthesiologists, Society for Cardiovascular Angiography and Interventions, Society for Vascular Medicine and Biology, and Society for Vascular Surgery. *J Am Coll Cardiol*. 2007;50:1707-1732.

23. Goldman L, Caldera DL, Nussbaum SR, et al. Multifactorial index of cardiac risk in noncardiac surgical procedures. *N Engl J Med*. 1977;297:845-850.

24. Lee TH, Marcantonio ER, Mangione CM, et al. Derivation and prospective validation of a simple index for prediction of cardiac risk of major noncardiac surgery. *Circulation*. 1999;100:1043-1049.

25. Bilimoria KY, Liu Y, Paruch JL, et al. Development and evaluation of the universal ACS NSQIP surgical risk calculator: a decision aid and informed consent tool for patients and surgeons. *J Am Coll Surg*. 2013;217:833-842. e1-3.

26. Cohen ME, Ko CY, Bilimoria KY, et al. Optimizing ACS NSQIP modeling for evaluation of surgical quality and risk: patient risk adjustment, procedure mix adjustment, shrinkage adjustment, and surgical focus. *J Am Coll Surg*. 2013;217:336-346.e1.

27. Mosca L, Banka CL, Benjamin EJ, et al. Evidence-based guidelines for cardiovascular disease prevention in women: 2007 update. *Circulation*. 2007;115:1481-1501.

28. Mashour GA, Shanks AM, Kheterpal S. Perioperative stroke and associated mortality after noncardiac, nonneurologic surgery. *Anesthesiology*. 2011;114:1289-1296.

29. Kertai MD, Bountioukos M, Boersma E, et al. Aortic stenosis: an underestimated risk factor for perioperative complications in patients undergoing noncardiac surgery. *Am J Med*. 2004;116:8-13.

30. Halm EA, Browner WS, Tubau JF, Tateo IM, Mangano DT. Echocardiography for assessing cardiac risk in patients having noncardiac surgery. *Ann Intern Med*. 1996;125:433-441.

31. Karthikeyan G, Moncur RA, Levine O, et al. Is a pre-operative brain natriuretic peptide or N-terminal pro-B-type natriuretic peptide measurement an independent predictor of adverse cardiovascular outcomes within 30 days of noncardiac surgery? A systematic review and meta-analysis of observational studies. *J Am Coll Cardiol*. 2009;54(17):1599-1606.

32. Ferreira MJ. The role of nuclear cardiology for preoperative risk assessment prior to noncardiac surgery. *Rev Port Cardiol*. 2000;19(suppl 1):I63-I69.

33. Wijeysundera DN, Duncan D, Nkonde-Price C, et al. Perioperative beta blockade in noncardiac surgery: a systematic review for the 2014 ACC/AHA guideline on perioperative cardiovascular evaluation and management of patients undergoing noncardiac surgery: a report of the American College of Cardiology/American Heart Association task force on practice guidelines. *J Am Coll Cardiol*. 2014;64(22):2406-2425.

34. POISE Study Group; Devereaux PJ, Yang H, et al. Effects of extended-release metoprolol succinate in patients undergoing non-cardiac surgery (POISE trial): a randomised controlled trial. *Lancet*. 2008;371(9627):1839-1847.

35. Dimick JB, Chen SL, Taheri PA, Henderson WG, Khuri SF, Campbell DA Jr. Hospital costs associated with surgical complications: a report from the private-sector National Surgical Quality Improvement Program. *J Am Coll Surg*. 2004;199(4):531-537.

36. Fisher BW, Majumdar SR, McAlister FA. Predicting pulmonary complications after nonthoracic surgery: a systematic review of blinded studies. *Am J Med*. 2002;112:219-225.

37. Meyers JR, Lembeck L, O'Kane H, Baue AE. Changes in functional residual capacity of the lung after operation. *Arch Surg*. 1975;110:576-583.

38. Craig DB. Postoperative recovery of pulmonary function. *Anesth Analg*. 1981;60:46-52.

39. Ibañez J, Raurich JM. Normal values of functional residual capacity in the sitting and supine positions. *Intensive Care Med*. 1982;8(4):173-177.

40. Arozullah AM, Khuri SF, Henderson WG, Daley J; Participants in the National Veterans Affairs Surgical Quality Improvement Program. Development and validation of a multifactorial risk index for predicting postoperative pneumonia after major noncardiac surgery. *Ann Intern Med*. 2001;135:847-857.

41. Smetana GW, Lawrence VA, Cornell JE; American College of Physicians. Preoperative pulmonary risk stratification for noncardiothoracic surgery: systematic review for the American College of Physicians. *Ann Intern Med*. 2006;144:581-595.

42. Fernandez-Bustamante A, Frendl G, Sprung J et al. Postoperative pulmonary complications, early mortality, and hospital stay following noncardiothoracic surgery: a multicenter study by the perioperative research network investigators. *JAMA Surg*. 2017;152(2):157-166.

43. Qaseem A, Snow V, Fitterman N, et al. Risk assessment for and strategies to reduce perioperative pulmonary complications for patients undergoing noncardiothoracic surgery: a guideline from the American College of Physicians. *Ann Intern Med*. 2006;144(8):575-580.

44. Latimer RG, Dickman M, Day WC, Gunn ML, Schmidt CD. Ventilatory patterns and pulmonary complications after upper abdominal surgery determined by preoperative and postoperative computerized spirometry and blood gas analysis. *Am J Surg*. 1971;122:622-632.

45. Gibbs J, Cull W, Henderson W, Daley J, Hur K, Khuri SF. Preoperative serum albumin level as a predictor of operative mortality and morbidity: results from the National VA Surgical Risk Study. *Arch Surg*. 1999;134:36-42.

46. Restrepo RD, Wettstein R, Wittnebel L, Tracy M. Incentive spirometry: 2011. *Respir Care*. 2011;56(10):1600-1604.

47. Hawn MT, Houston TK, Campagna EJ. The attributable risk of smoking on surgical complications. *Ann Surg*. 2011;254(6):914-920.

48. Bluman LG, Mosca L, Newman N, Simon DG. Preoperative smoking habits and postoperative pulmonary complications. *Chest*. 1998;113:883-889.

49. Shi Y, Warner DO. Brief preoperative smoking abstinence: is there a dilemma? *Anesth Analg*. 2011;113:1348-1351.

50. Nakagawa M, Tanaka H, Tsukuma H, Kishi Y. Relationship between the duration of the preoperative smoke-free period and the incidence of postoperative pulmonary complications after pulmonary surgery. *Chest*. 2001;120:705-710.

51. Mazo V, Sabaté S, Canet J, et al. Prospective external validation of a predictive score for postoperative pulmonary complications. *Anesthesiology*. 2014; 121:219-231.

52. Gupta H, Gupta PK, Fang X, et al. Development and validation of a risk calculator predicting postoperative respiratory failure. *Chest*. 2011;140:1207-1215.

53. Canet J, Gallart L, Gomar C, et al. Prediction of postoperative pulmonary complications in a population-based surgical cohort. *Anesthesiology* 2010;113:1338-1350.

54. Centers for Disease Control and Prevention. National Diabetes Statistics Report. Accessed April 1, 2022. https://www.cdc.gov/diabetes/data/statistics-report/index.html

55. Elixhauser A, Yu K, Steiner C, et al. *Hospitalization in the United States, 1997. Healthcare Costs and Utilization.* Project Fact Book No. 1. AHRQ Publication No. 00-0031. Agency for Healthcare Research and Quality; 2000.

56. Clement S, Braithwaite SS, Magee MF, et al. Management of diabetes and hyperglycemia in hospitals. *Diabetes Care*. 2004;27:553-591.

57. Cowie CC, Rust KF, Ford ES, et al. Full accounting of diabetes and pre-diabetes in the U.S. population in 1988-1994 and 2005-2006. *Diabetes Care*. 2009;32:287-294.

58. Sheehy AM, Gabbay RA. An overview of preoperative glucose evaluation, management, and perioperative impact. *J Diabetes Sci Technol*. 2009;3:1261-1269.

59. Kohl BA, Schwartz S. How to manage perioperative endocrine insufficiency. *Anesthesiol Clin*. 2010;28:139-155.

60. American Diabetes Association. 2. Classification and diagnosis of diabetes: *Standards of Medical Care in Diabetes*-2018. *Diabetes Care*. 2018;41(suppl 1):S13-S27.

61. Meneghini LF. Perioperative management of diabetes: translating evidence into practice. *Cleve Clin J Med*. 2009;76(suppl 4):S53-S59.

62. Raju TA, Torjman MC, Goldberg ME. Perioperative blood glucose monitoring in the general surgical population. *J Diabetes Sci Technol*. 2009;3:1282-1287.

63. International Expert Committee. The International Expert Committee report on the role of the A1C assay in the diagnosis of diabetes. *Diabetes Care*. 2009;32:1327-1334.

64. Fahy BG, Sheehy AM, Coursin DB. Glucose control in the intensive care unit. *Crit Care Med*. 2009;37:1769-1776.

65. Egi M, Bellomo R, Stachowski E, et al. Blood glucose concentration and outcome of critical illness: the impact of diabetes. *Crit Care Med*. 2008;36:2249-2255.

66. Umpierrez GE, Smiley D, Jacobs S, et al. Randomized study of basal-bolus insulin therapy in the inpatient management of patients with type 2 diabetes undergoing general surgery (RABBIT 2 Surgery). *Diabetes Care*. 2011;34:256-261.

67. Himes CP, Ganesh R, Wight EC, Simha V, Liebow M. Perioperative evaluation and management of endocrine disorders. *Mayo Clin Proc*. 2020;95(12):2760-2774.

68. Galway U, Chahar P, Schmidt MT, et al. Perioperative challenges in management of diabetic patients undergoing non-cardiac surgery. *World J Diabetes*. 2021;12(8):1255-1266.

69. Umpierrez GE, Hellman R, Korytkowski MT, et al. Management of hyperglycemia in hospitalized patients in non-critical care setting: an Endocrine Society Clinical Practice Guideline. *J Clin Endocrinol Metab*. 2012;97:16-38.

70. Pompocelli JJ, Baxter JK, Babineau TJ, et al. Early postoperative glucose control predicts nosocomial infection rate in diabetic patients. *JPEN J Parenter Enteral Nutr*. 1998;22:77-81.

71. Frisch A, Chandra P, Smiley D, et al. Prevalence and clinical outcome of hyperglycemia in the perioperative period in non-cardiac surgery. *Diabetes Care*. 2010;33:1783-1788.

72. Noordzij PG, Boersma E, Schreiner F, et al. Increased preoperative glucose levels are associated with perioperative mortality in patients undergoing non-cardiac, non-vascular surgery. *Eur J Endocrinol*. 2007;156:137-142.

73. Ramos M, Khalpey Z, Lipsitz S, et al. Relationship of perioperative hyperglycemia and postoperative infections in patients who undergo general and vascular surgery. *Ann Surg*. 2008;248:585-591.

74. Sato H, Carvalho G, Sato T, Lattermann R, Matsukawa T, Schricker T. The association of preoperative glycemic control, intraoperative insulin sensitivity, and outcomes after cardiac surgery. *J Clin Endocrinol Metab*. 2010;95:4338-4344.

75. Dronge AS, Perkal MF, Kancir S, Concato J, Aslan M, Rosenthal RA. Long-term glycemic control and postoperative infectious complications. *Arch Surg*. 2006;141:375-380.

76. Gallacher SJ, Thomson G, Fraser WD, Fisher BM, Gemmell CG, MacCuish AC. Neutrophil bactericidal function in diabetes mellitus: evidence for association with blood glucose control. *Diabet Med*. 1995;12:916-920.

77. Van Den Berghe G, Wouters P, Weekers F, et al. Intensive insulin therapy in critically ill patients. *N Engl J Med*. 2001;345:1359-1367.

78. NICE-SUGAR Study Investigators; Finfer S, Chittock DR, Su SY, et al. Intensive versus conventional glucose control in critically ill patients. *N Engl J Med*. 2009;360(13):1283-1297.

79. Moghissi ES, Korytkowski MT, DiNardo M, et al. American Association of Clinical Endocrinologists and American Diabetes Association consensus statement on inpatient glycemic control. *Endocr Pract*. 2009;15:353-369.

80. Umpierrez GE, Smiley D, Zisman A, et al. Randomized study of basal-bolus insulin therapy in the inpatient management of patients with type 2 diabetes (RABBIT 2 trial). *Diabetes Care*. 2007;30:2181-2186.

81. Miller JD, Richman DC. Preoperative evaluation of patients with diabetes mellitus. *Anesthesiol Clin*. 2016;34:155-169.

82. Ringel MD. Management of hypothyroidism and hyperthyroidism in the intensive care unit. *Crit Care Clin*. 2001;17:59-74.

83. Schiff RL, Welsh GA. Perioperative evaluation and management of the patient with endocrine dysfunction. *Med Clin North Am*. 2003;87:175-192.

84. Weinberg AD, Brennan MD, Gorman CA, Marsh HM, O'Fallon WM. Outcome of anesthesia and surgery in hypothyroid patients. *Arch Intern Med*. 1983;143:893-897.

85. Ladenson PW, Levin AA, Ridgway EC, Daniels GH. Complications of surgery in hypothyroid patients. *Am J Med*. 1984;77(2):261-266.

86. Bennett-Guerrero E, Kramer DC, Schwinn DA. Effect of chronic and acute thyroid hormone reduction on perioperative outcome. *Anesth Analg*. 1997;85:30-36.

87. Klubo-Gwiezdzinska J, Wartofsky L. Thyroid emergencies. *Med Clin North Am*. 2012;96:385-403.

88. Conner LE, Coursin DB. Assessment and therapy of selected endocrine disorders. *Anesthesiol Clin North Am*. 2004;22:93-123.

89. Wartofsky L. Myxedema coma. *Endocrinol Metab Clin North Am*. 2006;35:687-698, vii-viii.

90. Dutta P, Bhansali A, Masoodi SR, Bhadada S, Sharma N, Rajput R. Predictors of outcome in myxoedema coma: a study from a tertiary care centre. *Crit Care*. 2008;12(1):R1.

91. Forfar JC, Muir AL, Sawrers SA, Toft AD. Abnormal left ventricular function in hyperthyroidism: evidence for a possible reversible cardiomyopathy. *N Engl J Med*. 1982;307:1165-1170.

92. Klein I, Ojamaa K. Thyroid hormone and the cardiovascular system. *N Engl J Med*. 2001;344:501-509.

93. Sawin CT, Geller A, Wolf PA, et al. Low serum thyrotropin concentration as a risk factor for atrial fibrillation in older patients. *N Engl J Med*. 1994;331:1249-1252.

94. Woeber KA. Thyrotoxicosis and the heart. *N Engl J Med*. 1992;327:94-98.

95. Furlong D, Ahmed I, Jabbour S. Perioperative management of endocrine disorders. In: Merli GJ, Weitz HH, eds. *Medical Management of the Surgical Patient*. 3rd ed. Elsevier Saunders; 2007.

96. Nayak B, Burman K. Thyrotoxicosis and thyroid storm. *Endocrinol Metab Clin North Am*. 2006;35:663-686, vii.

97. Bahn Chair RS, Burch HB, Cooper DS, et al. Hyperthyroidism and other causes of thyrotoxicosis: management guidelines of the American Thyroid Association and American Association of Clinical Endocrinologists. *Thyroid*. 2011;21(6):593-646.

98. Arafah BM. Perioperative glucocorticoid therapy for patients with adrenal insufficiency: dosing based on pharmacokinetic data. *J Clin Endocrinol Metab*. 2020;105(3):dgaa042.

99. Henzen C, Suter A, Lerch E, Urbinelli R, Schorno XH, Briner VA. Suppression and recovery of adrenal response after short-term, high-dose glucocorticoid treatment. *Lancet*. 2000;355:542-545.

100. Hopkins RL, Leinung MC. Exogenous Cushing's syndrome and glucocorticoid withdrawal. *Endocrinol Metab Clin North Am*. 2005;34:371-384.

101. Axelrod L. Perioperative management of patients treated with glucocorticoids. *Endocrinol Metab Clin North Am*. 2003;32:367-383.

102. Kehlet H, Binder C. Value of an ACTH test in assessing hypothalamic-pituitary-adrenocortical function in glucocorticoid-treated patients. *Br Med J*. 1973;2:147-149.

103. Knudsen L, Christiansen LA, Lorentzen JE. Hypotension during and after operation in glucocorticoid-treated patients. *Br J Anaesth*. 1981;53:295-301.

104. Plumpton FS, Besser GM, Cole PV. Corticosteroid treatment and surgery. 1. An investigation of the indications for steroid cover. *Anaesthesia*. 1969;24:3-11.

105. Marik PE, Varon J. Requirement of perioperative stress doses of corticosteroids: a systematic review of the literature. *Arch Surg*. 2008;143(12):1222-1226.

106. Liu MM, Reidy AB, Saatee S, Collard CD. Perioperative steroid management approaches based on current evidence. *Anesthesiology.* 2017;127:166-172.

107. Freudzon L. Perioperative steroid therapy; where's the evidence? *Curr Opin Anaesthesiol.* 2018;31:39-42.

108. U.S. Renal Data System, 2021 Annual Data Report. National Institutes of Health, National Institute of Diabetes and Digestive and Kidney Diseases; 2019.

109. Levey AS, Coresh J, Balk E, et al. National Kidney Foundation practice guidelines for chronic kidney disease: evaluation, classification, and stratification. *Ann Intern Med.* 2003;139(2):137-147.

110. Go AS, Chertow GM, Fan D, McCulloch CE, Hsu CY. Chronic kidney disease and the risks of death, cardiovascular events, and hospitalization. *N Engl J Med.* 2004;351:1296-1305.

111. Schiffrin EL, Lipman ML, Mann JFE. Chronic kidney disease: effects on the cardiovascular system. *Circulation.* 2007;116:85-97.

112. Weir MR. Recognizing the link between chronic kidney disease and cardiovascular disease. *Am J Manag Care.* 2011;17:S396-S402.

113. De Bie MK, Buiten MS, Rabelink TJ, Jukema JW. How to reduce sudden cardiac death in patients with renal failure. *Heart.* 2012;98:335-341.

114. Wallia R, Greenberg A, Piraino B, Mitro R, Puschett JB. Serum electrolyte patterns in end-stage renal disease. *Am J Kidney Dis.* 1986;8:98-104.

115. Palevsky PM. Perioperative management of patients with chronic kidney disease or ESRD. *Best Pract Res Clin Anaesthesiol.* 2004;18(1):129-144.

116. Greenberg A. Hyperkalemia: treatment options. *Semin Nephrol.* 1998;18:46-57.

117. Esposito P, Conti NE, Falqui V, et al. New treatment options for hyperkalemia in patients with chronic kidney disease. *J Clin Med.* 2020;9(8):2337.

118. Clement FM, Klarenbach S, Tonelli M, Wiebe N, Hemmelgarn B, Manns BJ. An economic evaluation of erythropoiesis-stimulating agents in CKD. *Am J Kidney Dis.* 2010;56:1050-1061.

119. Esbach JW, Kelly MR, Haley NR, Abels RI, Adamson JW. Treatment of the anemia of progressive renal failure with recombinant human erythropoietin. *N Engl J Med.* 1989;321:158-163.

120. Rabelink TJ, Zwaginga JJ, Koomans HA, Sixma JJ. Thrombosis and hemostasis in renal disease. *Kidney Int.* 1994;46:287-296.

121. Mannucci PM, Remuzzi G, Pusineri F, et al. Deamino-8-D-arginine vasopressin shortens the bleeding time in uremia. *N Engl J Med.* 1983;308:8-12.

122. Livio M, Mannucci PM, Viganò G, et al. Conjugated estrogens for the management of bleeding associated with renal failure. *N Engl J Med.* 1986;315:731-735.

123. Aronoff GR, Bennett WM, Berns JS, et al. *Drug Prescribing in Renal Failure: Dosing Guidelines for Adults and Children.* 5th ed. American College of Physicians; 2007.

124. Matzke GR, Aronoff GR, Atkinson AJ, et al. Drug dosing consideration in patients with acute and chronic kidney disease-a clinical update from Kidney Disease: Improving Global Outcomes (KDIGO). *Kidney Int.* 2011;80:1122-1137.

125. Nasr R, Chilimuri S. Preoperative evaluation in patients with end-stage renal disease and chronic kidney disease. *Health Serv Insights.* 2017;10:1178632917713020

126. Hanje AJ, Patel T. Preoperative evaluation of patients with liver disease. *Nat Clin Pract Gastroenterol Hepatol.* 2007;4:266-276.

127. Hoetzel A, Ryan H, Schmidt R. Anesthetic considerations for the patient with liver disease. *Curr Opin Anaesthesiol.* 2012;25(3):340-347.

128. Muilenburg DJ, Singh A, Torzilli G, Khatri VP. Surgery in the patient with liver disease. *Med Clin North Am.* 2009;93:1065-1081.

129. Friedman LS. Surgery in the patient with liver disease. *Trans Am Clin Climatol Assoc.* 2010;121:192-204.

130. Runyon BA. Surgical procedures are well tolerated by patients with asymptomatic chronic hepatitis. *J Clin Gastroenterol.* 1986;8:542-544.

131. O'Sullivan MJ, Evoy D, O'Donnell C, et al. Gallstones and laparoscopic cholecystectomy in hepatitis C patients. *Ir Med J.* 2001;94:114-117.

132. Child CG, Turcotte JG. Surgery and portal hypertension. *Major Probl Clin Surg.* 1964;1:1-85.

133. Pugh RN, Murray-Lyon IM, Dawson JL, Pietroni MC, Williams R. Transection of the oesophagus for bleeding oesophageal varices. *Br J Surg.* 1973;60(8):646-649.

134. Muir AJ. Surgical clearance for the patient with chronic liver disease. *Clin Liver Dis.* 2012;16:421-433.

135. Malinchoc M, Kamath PS, Gordon FD, Peine CJ, Rank J, ter Borg PC. A model to predict poor survival in patients undergoing transjugular intrahepatic portosystemic shunts. *Hepatology.* 2000;31(4):864-871.

136. Amarapurkar DN. Prescribing medications in patients with decompensated liver cirrhosis. *Int J Hepatol.* 2011;2011:519526. doi:10.4061/2011/519526

137. Huhmann MB, August DA. Nutrition support in surgical oncology. *Nutr Clin Pract.* 2009;24:520-526.

138. Laky B, Janda M, Bauer J, Vavra C, Cleghorn G, Obermair A. Malnutrition among gynaecological cancer patients. *Eur J Clin Nutr.* 2007;61:642-646.

139. Gupta D, Vashi PG, Lammersfeld CA, Braun DP. Role of nutritional status in predicting the length of stay in cancer: a systematic review of the epidemiological literature. *Ann Nutr Metab.* 2011;59:96-106.

140. Kathiresan AS, Brookfield KF, Schuman SI, Lucci JA. Malnutrition as a predictor for postoperative outcomes in gynecologic cancer patients. *Arch Gynecol Obstet.* 2011;284:445-451.

141. Obermair A, Hagenauer S, Tamandl D, et al. Safety and efficacy of low anterior en bloc resection as part of cytoreductive surgery for patients with ovarian cancer. *Gynecol Oncol.* 2001;83:115-120.

142. Laky B, Janda M, Cleghorn G, Obermair A. Comparison of different nutritional assessments and body-composition measurements in detecting malnutrition among gynecologic cancer patients. *Am J Clin Nutr.* 2008;87:1678-1685.

143. Huhmann MB, August DA. Review of American Society for Parenteral and Enteral Nutrition (ASPEN) Clinical Guidelines for Nutrition Support in Cancer Patients: nutrition screening and assessment. *Nutr Clin Pract.* 2008;23:182-188.

144. Minnella EM, Carli F. Prehabilitation and functional recovery for colorectal cancer patients. *Eur J Surg Oncol.* 2018;44(7):919-926.

145. Detsky AS, McLaughlin JR, Baker JP, et al. What is subjective global assessment of nutritional status? *JPEN J Parenter Enteral Nutr.* 1987;11:8-13.

146. Ottery FD. Definition of standardized nutritional assessment and interventional pathways in oncology. *Nutrition.* 1996;12(suppl 1):S15-S19.

147. MaCallum PD, Polisena CG. *The Clinical Guide to Oncology Nutrition.* The American Dietetic Association; 2000.

148. Donato D, Angelides A, Irani H, Penalver M, Averette H. Infectious complications after gastrointestinal surgery in patients with ovarian carcinoma and malignant ascites. *Gynecol Oncol.* 1992;44:40-47.

149. Veterans Affairs Total Parenteral Nutrition Cooperative Study Group. Perioperative total parenteral nutrition in surgical patients. *N Engl J Med.* 1991;325:525-532.

150. Buzby GP, Mullen JL, Matthews DC, Hobbs CL, Rosato EF. Prognostic nutritional index in gastrointestinal surgery. *Am J Surg.* 1980;139:160-167.

151. Santoso JT, Cannada T, O'Farrel B, Alladi K, Coleman RL. Subjective versus objective nutritional assessment study in women with gynecological cancer: a prospective cohort trial. *Int J Gynecol Cancer.* 2004;14:220-223.

152. Anthony PS. Nutrition screening tools for hospitalized patients. *Nutr Clin Pract.* 2008;23:373-382.

153. Braga M, Ljungqvist O, Soeters P, et al. ESPEN guidelines on parenteral nutrition: surgery. *Clin Nutr.* 2009;28:378-386.

154. Meijerink WJ, von Meyenfeldt MF, Rouflart MM, Soeters PB. Efficacy of perioperative nutritional support. *Lancet.* 1992;340:187-188.

155. Bozzetti F, Gavazzi C, Miceli R, et al. Perioperative total parenteral nutrition in malnourished, gastrointestinal cancer patients: a randomized, clinical trial. *JPEN J Parenter Enteral Nutr.* 2000;24:7-14.

156. Wu GH, Liu ZH, Wu ZH, Wu ZG. Perioperative artificial nutrition in malnourished gastrointestinal cancer patients. *World J Gastroenterol.* 2006;12:2441-2444.

157. Chambers D, Paton F, Wilson P, et al. An overview and methodological assessment of systematic reviews and meta-analyses of enhanced recovery programmes in colorectal surgery. *BMJ Open* 2014;4:e005014.

158. Varadhan KK, Neal KR, Dejong CH, Fearon KC, Ljungqvist O, Lobo DN. The enhanced recovery after surgery (ERAS) pathway for patients undergoing major elective open colorectal surgery: a meta-analysis of randomized controlled trials. *Clin Nutr.* 2010;29:434-440.

159. Roulin D, Donadini A, Gander S et al. Cost-effectiveness of the implementation of an enhanced recovery protocol for colorectal surgery. *Br J Surg.* 2013;100:1108-1114.

160. Varadhan K, Lobo D, Ljungqvist. Enhanced recovery after surgery: the future of improving surgical care. *Crit Care Clin.* 2010;26(3):527-547.

161. Nelson G, Kalogera E, Dowdy SC. Enhanced recovery pathways in gynecologic oncology. *Gynecol Oncol.* 2014;135:586-594.

162. Kalogera E, Bakkum-Gamez JN, Jankowski CJ, et al. Enhanced recovery in gynecologic surgery. *Obstet Gynecol.* 2013;122:319-328.

163. Bisch SP, Jago CA, Kalogera E, et al. Outcomes of enhanced recovery after surgery (ERAS) in gynecologic oncology—a systematic review and meta-analysis. *Gynecol Oncol.* 2021;161(1):46-55.

164. Nelson, G, Altman AD, Nick A, et al. Guidelines for pre-and intra-operative care in gynecologic/oncology surgery: Enhanced Recovery After Surgery (ERAS®) Society recommendations—part I. *Gynecol Oncol.* 2016;140:313-322.

165. Nelson G, Altman AD, Nick A, et al. Guidelines for postoperative care in gynecologic/oncology surgery: Enhanced Recovery After Surgery (ERAS®) Society recommendations—part II. *Gynecol Oncol.* 2016;140:323-332.

166. Nelson G, Bakkum-Gamez J, Kalogera E, et al. Guidelines for perioperative care in gynecologic/oncology: Enhanced Recovery After Surgery (ERAS) Society recommendations—2019 update. *Int J Gynecol Cancer.* 2019;29(4):651-668.

167. Douketis JD. Perioperative management of patients who are receiving warfarin therapy: an evidence-based and practical approach. *Blood.* 2011;117:5044-5049.

168. Destro MW, Speranzini MB, Cavalheiro Filho C, Destro T, Destro C. Bilateral haematoma after rhytidoplasty and blepharoplasty following chronic use of Ginkgo biloba. *Br J Plast Surg.* 2005;58:100-101.

169. Cheema P, El-Mefty O, Jazieh AR. Intraoperative haemorrhage associated with the use of extract of Saw Palmetto herb: a case report and review of literature. *J Intern Med.* 2001;250:167-169.

170. Crosby E. Perioperative use of erythropoietin. *Am J Ther.* 2002;9:371-376.

171. Feringa HH, Bax JJ, Poldermans D. Perioperative medical management of ischemic heart disease in patients undergoing noncardiac surgery. *Curr Opin Anaesthesiol.* 2007;20:254-260.

172. Fleisher LA, Beckman JA, Brown KA, et al. ACC/AHA 2007 guidelines on perioperative cardiovascular evaluation and care for noncardiac surgery: a report of the American College of Cardiology/American Heart Association Task Force on Practice Guidelines (Writing Committee to Revise the 2002 Guidelines on Perioperative Cardiovascular Evaluation for Noncardiac Surgery) developed in collaboration with the American Society of Echocardiography, American Society of Nuclear Cardiology, Heart Rhythm Society, Society of Cardiovascular Anesthesiologists, Society for Cardiovascular Angiography and Interventions, Society for Vascular Medicine and Biology, and Society for Vascular Surgery. *J Am Coll Cardiol.* 2007;50:e159-e241.

173. Eagle KA, Berger PB, Calkins H, et al. ACC/AHA guideline update for perioperative cardiovascular evaluation for noncardiac surgery—executive summary a report of the American College of Cardiology/American Heart Association Task Force on Practice Guidelines (Committee to Update the 1996 Guidelines on Perioperative Cardiovascular Evaluation for Noncardiac Surgery). *Circulation.* 2002;105:1257-1267.

174. Lindenauer PK, Pekow P, Wang K, Mamidi DK, Gutierrez B, Benjamin EM. Perioperative beta-blocker therapy and mortality after major noncardiac surgery. *N Engl J Med.* 2005;353:349-361.

175. Howard-Alpe GM, Sear JW, Foex P. Methods of detecting atherosclerosis in non-cardiac surgical patients; the role of biochemical markers. *Br J Anaesth.* 2006;97:758-769.

176. O'Neil-Callahan K, Katsimaglis G, Tepper MR, et al. Statins decrease perioperative cardiac complications in patients undergoing noncardiac vascular surgery: the Statins for Risk Reduction in Surgery (StaRRS) study. *J Am Coll Cardiol.* 2005;45:336-342.

177. Chassot PG, Delabays A, Spahn DR. Perioperative antiplatelet therapy: the case for continuing therapy in patients at risk of myocardial infarction. *Br J Anaesth.* 2007;99:316-328.

178. Steinhubl SR, Berger PB, Mann JT III, et al. Early and sustained dual oral antiplatelet therapy following percutaneous coronary intervention: a randomized controlled trial. *JAMA.* 2002;288:2411-2420.

179. Thachil J, Gatt A, Martlew V. Management of surgical patients receiving anticoagulation and antiplatelet agents. *Br J Surg.* 2008;95:1437-1448.

180. Korte W, Cattaneo M, Chassot PG, et al. Peri-operative management of antiplatelet therapy in patients with coronary artery disease: joint position paper by members of the working group on Perioperative Haemostasis of the Society on Thrombosis and Haemostasis Research (GTH), the working group on Perioperative Coagulation of the Austrian Society for Anesthesiology, Resuscitation and Intensive Care (OGARI) and the Working Group Thrombosis of the European Society for Cardiology (ESC). *Thromb Haemost.* 2011;105:743-749.

181. Devereaux PJ, Mrkobrada M, Sessler DI, et al. Aspirin in patients undergoing noncardiac surgery. *N Engl J Med.* 2014;370(16):1494-1503.

182. Patrono C, Baigent C, Hirsh J, Roth G. Antiplatelet drugs: American College of Chest Physicians Evidence-Based Clinical Practice Guidelines (8th Edition). *Chest.* 2008;133(suppl 6):199S-233S.

183. Bogani G, Cromi A, Uccella S, et al. Safety of perioperative aspirin therapy in minimally invasive endometrial cancer staging. *J Minim Invasive Gynecol.* 2014;21(4):636-641.

184. Cortés J, Caralt M, Delaloge S, et al. Safety of bevacizumab in metastatic breast cancer patients undergoing surgery. *Eur J Cancer.* 2012;48(4):475-481.

185. Erinjeri JP, Fong AJ, Kemeny NE, Brown KT, Getrajdman GI, Solomon SB. Timing of administration of bevacizumab chemotherapy affects wound healing after chest wall port placement. *Cancer.* 2011;117(6):1296-1301.

186. Ng SP. Blood transfusion requirements for abdominal hysterectomy: 3-year experience in a district hospital (1993-1995). *Aust N Z J Obstet Gynaecol.* 1997;37:452-457.

187. Obermair A, Asher, R, Pareja, R, et al. Incidence of adverse events in minimally invasive vs open radical hysterectomy in early cervical cancer: results of a randomized control trial. *Am J Obstet Gynecol.* 2020;222(3):249.e1-249.e10.

188. Busch MP, Bloch EM, Kleinman, S. Prevention of transfusion-transmitted infections. *Blood.* 2019;133(17):1854-1864.

189. Dunne JR, Malone D, Tracy JK, Gannon C, Napolitano LM. Perioperative anemia: an independent risk factor for infection, mortality, and resource utilization in surgery. *J Surg Res.* 2002;102:237-244.

190. Taylor RW, Manganaro L, O'Brien J, Trottier SJ, Parkar N, Veremakis C. Impact of allogenic packed red blood cell transfusion on nosocomial infection rates in the critically ill patient. *Crit Care Med.* 2002;30:2249-2254.

191. Vanderlinde ES, Heal JM, Blumberg N. Autologous transfusion. *BMJ.* 2002;324:772-775.

192. Popovsky MA, Whitaker B, Arnold NL. Severe outcomes of allogeneic and autologous blood donation: frequency and characterization. *Transfusion.* 1995;35:734-737.

193. Goldman M, Savard R, Long A, Gélinas S, Germain M. Declining value of preoperative autologous donation. *Transfusion.* 2002;42:819-823.

194. Horowitz NS, Gibb RK, Menegakis NE, Mutch DG, Rader JS, Herzog TJ. Utility and cost-effectiveness of preoperative autologous blood donation in gynecologic and gynecologic oncology patients. *Obstet Gynecol.* 2002;99:771-776.

195. Shander A, Rijhwani TS. Acute normovolemic hemodilution. *Transfusion.* 2004;44(12 suppl):26S-34S.

196. Monk TG, Goodnough LT, Brecher ME, Colberg JW, Andriole GL, Catalona WJ. A prospective randomized comparison of three blood conservation strategies for radical prostatectomy. *Anesthesiology.* 1999;91:24-33.

197. Goodnough LT, Despotis GJ, Merkel K, Monk TG. A randomized trial comparing acute normovolemic hemodilution and preoperative autologous blood donation in total hip arthroplasty. *Transfusion.* 2000;40:1054-1057.

198. Naunheim KS, Bridges CR, Sade RM. Should a Jehovah's witness patient who faces imminent exsanguination be transfused? *Ann Thorac Surg.* 2011;92(5):1559-1564.

199. Aapro M, Jelkmann W, Constantinescu SN, Leyland-Jones B. Effects of erythropoietin receptors and erythropoiesis-stimulating agents on disease progression in cancer. *Br J Cancer.* 2012;106(7):1249-1258.

200. Kalogera E, Van Houten HK, Sangaralingham LR, Borah BJ, Dowdy SC. Use of bowel preparation does not reduce postoperative infectious morbidity following minimally invasive or open hysterectomies. *Am J Obstet Gynecol.* 2020;223(2):231.e1-231.e12.

201. Güenaga KF, Matos D, Wille-Jørgensen P. Mechanical bowel preparation for elective colorectal surgery. *Cochrane Database Syst Rev.* 2011;2011(9):CD001544.

202. Bretagnol F, Panis Y, Rullier E, et al. Rectal cancer surgery with or without bowel preparation: the French G RECCAR III multicenter single-blinded randomized trial. *Ann Surg.* 2010;252:863-868.

203. Ban KA, Minei JP, Laronga C, et al. American College of Surgeons and Surgical Infection Society: surgical site infection guidelines, 2016 update. *J Am Coll Surg.* 2017;224(1):59-74.

204. Barber EL, van Le L. Enhanced recovery pathways in gynecology and gynecologic oncology. *Obstet Gynecol Surv.* 2015;70(12):780-792.

205. Brady M, Kinn S, Stuart P. Preoperative fasting for adults to prevent perioperative complications. *Cochrane Database Syst Rev.* 2003;CD004423.

206. Practice guidelines for preoperative fasting and the use of pharmacologic agents to reduce the risk of pulmonary aspiration: application to health patients undergoing elective procedures: a report by the American Society of Anesthesiologist Task Force on Preoperative Fasting. *Anesthesiology.* 1999;90:896-905.

207. Noblett SE, Watson DS, Huong H, Davison B, Hainsworth PJ, Horgan AF. Pre-operative oral carbohydrate loading in colorectal surgery: a randomized controlled trial. *Colorectal Dis.* 2006;8:563-569.

208. Bratzler DW, Dellinger EP, Olsen KM, et al. Clinical practice guidelines for antimicrobial prophylaxis in surgery. Surg Infect (Larchmt). 2013;14:73-156.

209. Malone DL, Genuit T, Tracy JK, Gannon C, Napolitano LM. Surgical site infections: reanalysis of risk factors. *J Surg Res.* 2002;103:89-95.

210. Bratzler DW, Houck PM; Surgical Infection Prevention Guideline Writers Workgroup. Antimicrobial prophylaxis for surgery: an advisory statement from the National Surgical Infection Prevention Project. *Am J Surg.* 2005;189:395-404.

211. Antimicrobial prophylaxis for surgery. *Treat Guidel Med Lett.* 2006;4:83-88.

212. ASHP therapeutic guidelines on antimicrobial prophylaxis in surgery. *Am J Health Syst Pharm.* 1999;56:1839-1888.

213. ACOG Practice Bulletin No.195: prevention of infection after gynecologic procedures. *Obstet Gynecol*. 2018;131(6):e172-e189.

214. Ingraham AM, Cohen ME, Bilimoria KY, et al. Association of surgical care improvement project infection-related process measure compliance with risk-adjusted outcomes: implications for quality measurement. *J Am Coll Surg*. 2010;211(6):705-714.

215. Kirkland KB, Briggs JP, Trivette L, Wilkinson WE, Sexton DJ. The impact of surgical-site infections in the 1990s: attributable mortality, excess length of hospitalization, and extra costs. *Infect Control Hosp Epidemiol*. 1999;20:725-730.

216. Perencevich EN, Sands KE, Cosgrove SE, Guadagnoli E, Meara E, Platt R. Health and economic impact of surgical site infections diagnosed after hospital discharge. *Emerg Infect Dis*. 2003;9:196-203.

217. Johnson MP, Kim SJ, Langstraat CL, et al. Using bundled interventions to reduce surgical site infection after major gynecologic cancer surgery. *Obstet Gynecol*. 2016;127(6):1135-1144.

218. Tanner J, Norrie P, Melen K. Preoperative hair removal to reduce surgical site infection. *Cochrane Database Syst Rev*. 2006;3:CD004122. doi:10.1002/14651858.CD004122.pub3

219. Stevens SM, Woller SC, Kreuziger LB, et al. Antithrombotic therapy for VTE disease: second update of the CHEST guideline and expert panel report. *Chest*. 2021;160(6):e545-e608. doi:10.1016/j.chest.2021.07.055

220. Clarke-Pearson DL, Synan IS, Colemen RE, Hinshaw W, Creasman WT. The natural history of postoperative venous thromboemboli in gynecologic oncology: a prospective study of 382 patients. *Am J Obstet Gynecol*. 1984;148:1051-1054.

221. Clarke-Pearson DL, Dodge RK, Synan I, McClelland RC, Maxwell GL. Venous thromboembolism prophylaxis: patients at high risk to fail intermittent pneumatic compression. *Obstet Gynecol*. 2003;101:157-163.

222. Collins R, Scrimgeour A, Yusuf S, Peto R. Reduction in fatal pulmonary embolism and venous thrombosis by perioperative administration of subcutaneous heparin. Overview of results of randomized trials in general, orthopedic, and urologic surgery. *N Engl J Med*. 1988;318:1162-1173.

223. Gressel GM, Marcus JZ, Mullen MM, Sinno AK. Direct oral anticoagulant use in gynecologic oncology: a Society of Gynecologic Oncology clinical practice statement. *Gynecol Oncol*. 2021;160(1):312-321.

224. Guntupalli SR, Brennecke A, Behbakht K, et al. Safety and efficacy of apixaban vs enoxaparin for preventing postoperative venous thromboembolism in women undergoing surgery for gynecologic malignant neoplasm: a Randomized Clinical Trial. *JAMA Netw Open*. 2020;3(6):e207410.

225. Key NS, Khorana AA, Kuderer NM, et al. Venous thromboembolism prophylaxis and treatment in patients with cancer: ASCO clinical practice guideline update. *J Clin Oncol*. 2020;38(5):496-520.

226. Di Donato V, Caruso G, Bogani G, et al. Preoperative frailty assessment in patients undergoing gynecologic oncology surgery: a systematic review. *Gynecol Oncol*. 2021;161(1):11-19.

227. Ethun CG, Bilen MA, Jani AB, Maithel SK, Ogan K, Master VA. Frailty and cancer: implications for oncology surgery, medical oncology, and radiation oncology. *CA Cancer J Clin*. 2017;67(5):362-377.

228. Walston JD, Bandeen-Roche K. Frailty: a tale of two concepts. *BMC Med*. 2015;13:185.

229. Robinson TN, Walston JD, Brummel NE, et al. Frailty for surgeons: review of a National Institute on Aging Conference on Frailty for Specialists. *J Am Coll Surg*. 2015;221(6):1083-1092.

230. Song X, Mitnitski A, Rockwood K. Prevalence and 10-year outcomes of frailty in older adults in relation to deficit accumulation. *J Am Geriatr Soc*. 2010;58(4):681-687.

231. Mullen MM, McKinnish TR, Fiala MA, et al. A deficit-accumulation frailty index predicts survival outcomes in patients with gynecologic malignancy. *Gynecol Oncol*. 2021;161(3):700-704.

232. Corre R, Greillier L, Le Caër H, et al. Use of a comprehensive geriatric assessment for the management of elderly patients with advanced non-small-cell lung cancer: the phase III randomized ESOGIA-GFPC-GECP 08-02 study. *J Clin Oncol*. 2016;34:1476-1483.

233. Spyropoulou D, Pallis AG, Leotsinidis M, Kardamakis D. Completion of radiotherapy is associated with the Vulnerable Elders Survey-13 score in elderly patients with cancer. *J Geriatr Oncol*. 2014;5:20-25.

234. Keenan LG, O'Brien M, Ryan T, Dunne M, McArdle O. Assessment of older patients with cancer: Edmonton Frail Scale (EFS) as a predictor of adverse outcomes in older patients undergoing radiotherapy. *J Geriatr Oncol*. 2017;8:206-210.

235. Rolfson DB, Majumdar SR, Tsuyuki RT, Tahir A, Rockwood K. Validity and reliability of the Edmonton Frail Scale. *Age Ageing*. 2006;35:526-529.

236. Sangkum L, Liu GL, Yu L, Yan H, Kaye AD, Liu H. Minimally invasive or noninvasive cardiac output measurement: an update. *J Anesth*. 2016;30(3):461-480.

237. Eisner RF, Montz FJ, Berek JS. Cytoreductive surgery for advanced ovarian cancer: cardiovascular evaluation with pulmonary artery catheters. *Gynecol Oncol*. 1990;37:311-314.

238. McGee WT, Mailloux P, Jodka P, Thomas J. The pulmonary artery catheter in critical care. *Semin Dial*. 2006;19:480-491.

239. McGee WT. A simple physiologic algorithm for managing hemodynamics using stroke volume and stroke volume variation: physiologic optimization program. *J Intensive Care Med*. 2009;24:352-360.

240. Marik PE. Noninvasive cardiac output monitors: a state-of the- art review. *J Cardiothorac Vasc Anesth*. 2013;27:121-134.

241. Thygesen K, Alpert JS, White HD; Joint ESC/ACCF/AHA/WHF Task Force for the Redefinition of Myocardial Infarction. Universal definition of myocardial infarction. *J Am Coll Cardiol*. 2007;50:2173-2195.

242. Ho K, Pinsky JL, Kannel WB, Levy D. The epidemiology of heart failure: the Framingham Study. *J Am Coll Cardiol*. 1993;22(4 suppl A):6A-13A.

243. Zaloga GP, Prielipp RC, Butterworth JF, Royster RL. Pharmacologic cardiovascular support. *Crit Care Clin*. 1993;9:335-362.

244. Jentzer JC, Hollenberg SM. Vasopressor and inotrope therapy in cardiac critical care. *J Intensive Care Med*. 2021;36(8):843-856.

245. Chioléro R, Flatt JP, Revelly JP, Jéquier E. Effects of catecholamines on oxygen consumption and oxygen delivery in critically ill patients. *Chest*. 1991;100:1676-1684.

246. Sharman A, Low J. Vasopressin and its role in critical care. *Contin Educ Anaesth Crit Care Pain*. 2008;8(4):134-137

247. Yancy CW, Jessup M, Bozkurt B, et al. 2013 ACCF/AHA guideline for the management of heart failure: executive summary: a report of the American College of Cardiology Foundation/American Heart Association Task Force on practice guidelines. *Circulation*. 2013;128:1810-1852.

248. Samarendra P, Mangione MP. Aortic stenosis and perioperative risk with noncardiac surgery. *J Am Coll Cardiol*. 2015;65(3):295-302.

249. Torsher LC, Shub C, Rettke SR, Brown DL. Risk of patients with severe aortic stenosis undergoing noncardiac surgery. *Am J Cardiol*. 1998;81:448-452.

250. Wilson W, Taubert KA, Gewitz M, et al. Prevention of infective endocarditis: guidelines from the American Heart Association: a guideline from the American Heart Association Rheumatic Fever, Endocarditis, and Kawasaki Disease Committee, Council on Cardiovascular Disease in the Young, and the Council on Clinical Cardiology, Council on Cardiovascular Surgery and Anesthesia, and the Quality of Care and Outcomes Research Interdisciplinary Working Group. *Circulation*. 2007;116(15):1736-1754.

251. Nishimura RA, Otto CM, Bonow RO, et al. 2017 AHA/ACC focused update of the 2014 AHA/ACC guideline for the management of patients with valvular heart disease: a report of the American College of Cardiology/American Heart Association Task Force on clinical practice guidelines. *Circulation*. 2017;135(25):e1159-e1195.

252. Christians KK, Wu B, Quebbeman EJ, Brasel KJ. Postoperative atrial fibrillation in noncardiothoracic surgical patients. *Am J Surg*. 2001;182:713-715.

253. Balser JR, Martinez EA, Winters BD, et al. Beta-adrenergic blockade accelerates conversion of postoperative supraventricular tachyarrhythmias. *Anesthesiology*. 1998;89:1052-1059.

254. January CT, Wann L, Alpert JS, et al. 2014 AHA/ACC/HRS guideline for the management of patients with atrial fibrillation: executive summary: a report of the American College of Cardiology/American Heart Association Task Force on practice guidelines and the Heart Rhythm Society. *J Am Coll Cardiol*. 2014;64(21):e1-e76.

255. Chalkias A, Mongardon N, Boboshko V, et al; PERIOPCA Consortium. Clinical practice recommendations on the management of perioperative cardiac arrest: a report from the PERIOPCA Consortium. *Crit Care*. 2021;25(1):265.

256. Mehta S, Heffer MJ, Maham N, Nelson DL, Klinger JR, Levy MM. Impact of endotracheal tube size on preextubation respiratory variables. *J Crit Care*. 2010;25(3):483-488.

257. Banner MJ, Jaeger MJ, Kirby RR. Components of the work of breathing and implications for monitoring ventilator-dependent patients. *Crit Care Med*. 1994;22:515-523.

258. Stewart TE, Meade MO, Cook DJ, et al. Evaluation of a ventilation strategy to prevent barotrauma in patients at high risk for acute respiratory distress syndrome. Pressure- and Volume-Limited Ventilation Strategy Group. *N Engl J Med*. 1998;338:355-361.

259. Amato MB, Barbas CS, Medeiros DM, et al. Effect of a protective-ventilation strategy on mortality in the acute respiratory distress syndrome. *N Engl J Med*. 1998;338:347-354.

260. Lodat RF. Oxygen toxicity. *Crit Care Clin*. 1990;6:749-765.

261. Baptistella AR, Sarmento FJ, da Silva KR, et al. Predictive factors of weaning from mechanical ventilation and extubation outcome: a systematic review. *J Crit Care*. 2018;48:56-62.

262. Rosenberg AL, Dechert RE, Park PK, Bartlett RH; NIH NHLBI ARDS Network. Review of a large clinical series: association of cumulative fluid balance on outcome in acute lung injury: a retrospective review of the ARDSnet tidal volume study cohort. *J Intensive Care Med.* 2009;24(1):35-46.

263. Bernard G, Artigas A, Brigham, KL, et al. Report of the American-European Consensus Conference on acute respiratory distress syndrome: definitions, mechanisms, relevant outcomes, and clinical trial coordination. Consensus Committee. *J Crit Care.* 1994;9:72-81.

264. Luce JM. Acute lung injury and the acute respiratory distress syndrome. *Crit Care Med.* 1998;26:369-376.

265. Marshall JC, Cook DJ, Christou NV, Bernard GR, Sprung CL, Sibbald WJ. Multiple organ dysfunction score: a reliable descriptor of a complex clinical outcome. *Crit Care Med.* 1995;23:1638-1652.

266. Fan E, Brodie D, Slutsky AS. Acute respiratory distress syndrome: advances in diagnosis and treatment. *JAMA.* 2018;319(7):698-710.

267. Mosier JM, Hypes C, Joshi R, Whitmore S, Parthasarathy S, Cairns CB. Ventilator strategies and rescue therapies for management of acute respiratory failure in the emergency department. *Ann Emerg Med.* 2015;66(5):529-541.

268. Chastre J, Fagon JY. Ventilator-associated pneumonia. *Am J Respir Crit Care Med.* 2002;165:867-903.

269. Kearon C, Akl EA, Ornelas J, et al. Antithrombotic therapy for VTE disease: CHEST guideline and expert panel report. *Chest.* 2016;149(2):315-352.

270. Pestana C. *Fluids and Electrolytes in the Surgical Patient.* 4th ed. Williams & Wilkins; 1989.

271. Vanatta JC, Fogelman MJ, eds. *Moyer's Fluid Balance: A Clinical Manual.* 2nd ed. Year Book; 1976.

272. Wait RB, Kahng KU, Dresner LS. Fluids and electrolytes and acid-base balance. In: Greenfield LJ, Mulholland M, Oldham KT, et al, eds. *Surgery: Scientific Principles and Practice.* 2nd ed. Lippincott–Raven Publishers; 1997;242-266.

273. Brandstrup B, Tonnesen H, Beier-Holgersen R, et al. Effects of intravenous fluid restriction on postoperative complications: comparison of two perioperative fluid regimens: a randomized assessor-blinded multicenter trial. *Ann Surg.* 2003;238:641-648.

274. Rahbari NN, Zimmermann JB, Schmidt T, Koch M, Weigand MA, Weitz J. Meta-analysis of standard, restrictive and supplemental fluid administration in colorectal surgery. *Br J Surg.* 2009;96:331-341.

275. Rizoli SB. Crystalloids and colloids in trauma resuscitation: a brief overview of the current debate. *J Trauma.* 2003;54(suppl 5):S82-S88.

276. Alderson P, Schierhout G, Roberts I, Bunn F. Colloids versus crystalloids for fluid resuscitation in critically ill patients. *Cochrane Database Syst Rev.* 2000;2(2):CD000567.

277. Lewis SR, Pritchard MW, Evans DJW, et al. Colloids versus crystalloids for fluid resuscitation in critically ill people. *Cochrane Database Syst Rev.* 2018;8(8):CD000567.

278. Berenson JR. Treatment of hypercalcemia of malignancy with bisphosphonates. *Semin Oncol.* 2002;29(suppl 21):12-18.

279. Mundy GR. Hypercalcemia. In: *Bone Remodeling and Its Disorders.* 2nd ed. Martin Dunitz; 1999:107-122.

280. Major P, Lortholary A, Hon J, et al. Zoledronic acid is superior to pamidronate in the treatment of hypercalcemia of malignancy: a pooled analysis of two randomized, controlled clinical trials. *J Clin Oncol.* 2001;19:558-567.

281. Kalogera E, Nelson G, Liu J, et al. Surgical technical evidence review for gynecologic surgery conducted for the Agency for Healthcare Research and Quality Safety Program for Improving Surgical Care and Recovery. *Am J Obstet Gynecol.* 2018;219(6):563.e1-563.e19. doi:10.1016/j.ajog.2018.07.014

282. Charoenkwan K, Matovinovic E. Early versus delayed oral fluids and food for reducing complications after major abdominal gynaecologic surgery. *Cochrane Database Syst Rev.* 2014;2014(12):CD004508.

283. Souba WW, Austen WG Jr. Nutrition and metabolism. In: Greenfield LJ, Mulholland M, Oldham KT, et al, eds. *Surgery: Scientific Principles and Practice.* 2nd ed. Lippincott–Raven Publishers; 1997:42-67.

284. Marik PE, Zaloga GP. Early enteral nutrition in acutely ill patients: a systematic review. *Crit Care Med.* 2001;29:2264-2270.

285. van Zanten AR, Dhaliwal R, Garrel D, Heyland DK. Enteral glutamine supplementation in critically ill patients: a systematic review and meta-analysis. *Crit Care.* 2015;19(1):294.

286. Wischmeyer PE, Dhaliwal R, McCall M, Ziegler TR, Heyland DK. Parenteral glutamine supplementation in critical illness: a systematic review. *Crit Care.* 2014;18(2):R76.

287. Sandini M, Nespoli L, Oldani M, Bernasconi DP, Gianotti L. Effect of glutamine dipeptide supplementation on primary outcomes for elective major surgery: systematic review and meta-analysis. *Nutrients.* 2015;7(1):481-499. doi:10.3390/nu7010481

288. Morrow CP, Curtin JP. *Gynecologic Cancer Surgery.* Churchill Livingstone; 1996;194-205.

289. Blackburn GL, Bistrian BR, Moini BS, et al. Nutritional and metabolic assessment of the hospitalized patient. *JPEN J Parenter Enteral Nutr.* 1977;1:11-22.

290. Kellum JA, Lameire N; KDIGO AKI Guideline Work Group. Diagnosis, evaluation, and management of acute kidney injury: a KIDGO summary (part 1). *Crit Care.* 2013;17:204.

291. Thakar CV. Perioperative acute kidney injury. *Adv Chronic Kidney Dis.* 2013;20(1):67-75.

292. Vaught AJ, Ozrazgat-Baslant T, Javed A, Morgan L, Hobson CE, Bihorac A. Acute kidney injury in major gynaecological surgery: an observational study. *BJOG.* 2015;122:1340-1348.

293. Hoste EA, Clermont G, Kersten A, et al. RIFLE criteria for acute kidney injury are associated with hospital mortality in critically ill patients: a cohort analysis. *Crit Care.* 2006;10:R73.

294. Uchino S, Bellomo R, Goldsmith D, Bates S, Ronco C. An assessment of the RIFLE criteria for acute renal failure in hospitalized patients. *Crit Care Med.* 2006;34:1913-1917.

295. Lameire N. The definitions and staging systems of acute kidney injury and their limitations in practice. *Arab Nephrol Transplant.* 2013;6(3):145-152.

296. Bellomo R, Ronco C, Kellum J, Mehta RL, Palevsky P; Acute Dialysis Quality Initiative workgroup. Acute renal failure—definitions, outcome measures, animal models, fluid therapy and information technology needs: the Second International Consensus Conference of the Acute Dialysis Quality Initiative (ADQI) Group. *Crit Care.* 2004;8(4):R204-R212.

297. Mehta RL, Kellum JA, Shah SV, et al. Acute kidney injury network: report of an initiative to improve outcomes in acute kidney injury. *Crit Care.* 2007;11(2):R31.

298. Kellum JA, Lameire N, Aspelin P, et al. Kidney Disease: Improving Global Outcomes (KDIGO) Acute Kidney Injury Work Group. KDIGO Clinical Practice Guidelines for acute kidney injury. *Kidney Int Suppl.* 2012;2(1):1-138.

299. Klausner JM, Paterson IS, Goldman G, et al. Postischemic renal injury is mediated by neutrophils and leukotrienes. *Am J Physiol.* 1989;256(5 pt 2):F794-F802.

300. Kribben A, Edelstein CL, Schrier RW. Pathophysiology of acute renal failure. *J Nephrol.* 1999;12(suppl 2):S142-S151.

301. Prins JM, Buller HR, Kuijper EJ, Tange RA, Speelman P. Once versus thrice daily gentamicin in patients with serious infections. *Lancet.* 1993;341:335-339.

302. Murphy SW, Barrett BJ, Parfrey PS. Contrast nephropathy. *J Am Soc Nephrol.* 2000;11:177-182.

303. Rudnick MR, Berns JS, Cohen RM, Goldfarb S. Contrast media-associated nephrotoxicity. *Semin Nephrol.* 1997;17:15-26.

304. McCullough PA, Wolyn R, Rocher LL, Levin RN, O'Neill WW. Acute renal failure after coronary intervention: incidence, risk factors, and relationship to mortality. *Am J Med.* 1997;103:368-375.

305. Shen W, Wu Z, Wang Y, Sun Y, Wu A. Impact of Enhanced Recovery After Surgery (ERAS) protocol versus standard of care on postoperative Acute Kidney Injury (AKI): a meta-analysis. *PLoS One.* 2021;16(5):e0251476.

306. Edwards BF. Postoperative renal insufficiency. *Med Clin North Am.* 2001;85:1241-1254.

307. Finfer S, Bellomo R, Boyce N, et al. A comparison of albumin and saline for fluid resuscitation in the intensive care unit. *N Engl J Med.* 2004;350:2247-2256.

308. Rowell SE, Barbosa RR, Diggs BS, et al. Effect of high product ratio massive transfusion on mortality in blunt and penetrating trauma patients. *J Trauma.* 2011;71(2 suppl 3):S353-S357.

309. Dellinger RP, Levy MM, Carlet JM, et al. Surviving sepsis Campaign: International guidelines for management of severe sepsis and septic shock: 2008. *Crit Care Med.* 2008;36:1394-1396.

310. Peralta R, Thani HA, Rizoli S. Coagulopathy in the surgical patient: trauma-induced and drug-induced coagulopathies. *Curr Opin Crit Care.* 2019. 25(6):668-674.

311. Schmidt AE, Israel AK, Refaai MA. The utility of thromboelastography to guide blood product transfusion. *Am J Clin Pathol.* 2019;152(4):407-422.

312. Flores-Mireles A, Hreha TN, Hunstad DA. Pathophysiology, treatment, and prevention of catheter-associated urinary tract infection. *Top Spinal Cord Inj Rehabil.* 2019;25(3)228-240.

313. Montravers P, Veber B, Auboyer C, et al. Diagnostic and therapeutic management of nosocomial pneumonia in surgical patients: results of the Eole study. *Crit Care Med.* 2002;30(2):368-375.

314. Steiner HL, Strand EA. Surgical-site infection in gynecologic surgery: pathophysiology and prevention. *Am J Obstet Gynecol.* 2017;217(2):121-128.

315. Ostrosky-Zeichner L, Pappas PG. Invasive candidiasis in the intensive care unit. *Crit Care Med.* 2006;34:857-863.

316. Jaramillo EJ, Trevino JM, Berghoff KR, Franklin ME. Bedside diagnostic laparoscopy in the intensive care unit: a 13-year experience. *JSLS*. 2006;10: 55-159.

317. Cinat ME, Wilson SE, Din AM. Determinants for successful percutaneous image-guided drainage of intra-abdominal abscess. *Arch Surg*. 2002;137:845-849.

318. Gervais DA, Ho CH, O'Neill MJ, Arellano RS, Hahn PF, Mueller PR. Recurrent abdominal and pelvic abscesses: incidence, results of repeated percutaneous drainage, and underlying causes in 956 drainages. *AJR Am J Roentgenol*. 2004;182:463-466.

319. Kok KY, Yapp SK. Laparoscopic drainage of postoperative complicated intra-abdominal abscesses. *Surg Laparosc Endosc Percutan Tech*. 2000;10:311-313.

320. Schecter WP, Ivatury RR, Rotondo MF, Hirshberg A. Open abdomen after trauma and abdominal sepsis: a strategy for management. *J Am Coll Surg*. 2006;203:390-396.

321. Marshall JC, Maier RV, Jimenez M, Dellinger EP. Source control in the management of severe sepsis and septic shock: an evidence-based review. *Crit Care Med*. 2004;32(suppl 11):S513-S526.

322. Kelesidis T, Mastoris I, Metsini A, Tsiodras S. How to approach and treat viral infections in ICU patients. *BMC Infect Dis*. 2014;14:321.

323. Evans L, Rhodes A, Alhazzani W, et al. Surviving sepsis campaign: International guidelines for management of sepsis and septic shock 2021. *Intensive Care Med*. 2021;47(11):1181-1247.

324. Kothari AN, DiBrito SR, Lee JJ, et al. Surgical outcomes in cancer patients undergoing elective surgery after recovering from mild-to-moderate SARS-CoV-2 Infection. *Ann Surg Oncol*. 2021;28(13):8046-8053.

325. National Nosocomial Infections Surveillance System. National Nosocomial Infections Surveillance (NNIS) System Report, data summary from January 1992 through June 2004, issued October 2004. *Am J Infect Control*. 2004;32:470-485.

326. Vincent JL, Rello J, Marshall J, et al. International study of the prevalence and outcomes of infection in intensive care units. *JAMA*. 2009;302(21):2323-2329.

327. Aird WC. The role of the endothelium in severe sepsis and multiple organ dysfunction syndrome. *Blood*. 2003;101:3765-3777.

328. Singer M, Deutschman CS, Seymour CW, et al. The Third International Consensus Definitions for Sepsis and Septic Shock (Sepsis-3). *JAMA*. 2016;315(8):801-810.

329. Shorr AF, Tabak YP, Killian AD, Gupta V, Liu LZ, Kollef MH. Healthcare-associated bloodstream infection: a distinct entity? Insights from a large U.S. database. *Crit Care Med*. 2006;34:2588-2595.

330. Angus DC, Linde-Zwirble WT, Lidicker J, Clermont G, Carcillo J, Pinsky MR. Epidemiology of severe sepsis in the United States: analysis of incidence, outcome, and associated costs of care. *Crit Care Med*. 2001;29:1303-1310.

331. Martí-Carvajal AJ, Solà I, Lathyris D, Cardona AF. Human recombinant activated protein C for severe sepsis. *Cochrane Database Syst Rev*. 2012;(3):CD004388.

332. Bernard GR, Vincent JL, Laterre PF, et al. Efficacy and safety of recombinant human activated protein C for severe sepsis. *N Engl J Med*. 2001;344:699-709.

333. American College of Chest Physicians/Society of Critical Care Medicine Consensus Conference. Definitions for sepsis and organ failure and guidelines for the use of innovative therapies in sepsis. *Crit Care Med*. 1992;20:864-874.

334. Zimmerman JE, Kramer AA, McNair DS, Malila FM. Acute Physiology and Chronic Health Evaluation (APACHE) IV: hospital mortality assessment for today's critically ill patients. *Crit Care Med*. 2006;34: 1297-1310.

335. Vincent JL, de Mendonca A, Cantraine F, et al. Use of the SOFA score to assess the incidence of organ dysfunction/failure in intensive care units: results of a multicenter, prospective study. Working group on "sepsis-related problems" of the European Society of Intensive Care Medicine. *Crit Care Med*. 1998;26:1793-1800.

336. Vidal MG, Ruiz Weisser J, Gonzalez F, et al. Incidence and clinical effects of intra-abdominal hypertension in critically ill patients. *Crit Care Med*. 2008;36(6):1823-1831.

337. Epstein J, Breslow MJ. The stress response of critical illness. *Crit Care Clin*. 1999;15:17-33.

338. Developed by the Dr. Robert Bree Collaborative and Washington State Agency Medical Directors' Group in collaboration with academics, pain experts, and practicing surgeons. Prescribing opioids for postoperative pain—supplemental guidance. Published July 2018. https://www.qualityhealth.org/bree/wp-content/uploads/sites/8/2018/09/Final-Supplemental-Bree-AMDG-Postop-pain-091318-wcover.pdf

339. Kress JP, Gehlbach B, Lacy M, Pliskin N, Pohlman AS, Hall JB. The long-term psychological effects of daily sedative interruption on critically ill patients. *Am J Respir Crit Care Med*. 2003;168:1457-1461.

340. Kress JP, Pohlman AS, O'Connor MF, Hall JB. Daily interruption of sedative infusions in critically ill patients undergoing mechanical ventilation. *N Engl J Med*. 2000;342:1471-1477.

341. American College of Critical Care Medicine of the Society of Critical Care Medicine, American Society of Health-System Pharmacists, American College of Chest Physicians. Clinical practice guidelines for the sustained use of sedatives and analgesics in the critically ill adult. *Am J Health Syst Pharm*. 2002;59:150-178.

342. Cammarano WB, Pittet JF, Weitz S, Schlobohm RM, Marks JD. Acute withdrawal syndrome related to the administration of analgesic and sedative medications in adult intensive care unit patients. *Crit Care Med*. 1998;26:676-684.

343. Weerink MAS, Struys MMRF, Hannivoort LN, Barends CRM, Absalom AR, Colin P.. Clinical pharmacokinetics and pharmacodynamics of dexmedetomidine. *Clin Pharmacokinet*. 2017;56(8):893-913.

344. American College of Critical Care Medicine of the Society of Critical Care Medicine, American Society of Health-System Pharmacists, American College of Chest Physicians. Clinical practice guidelines for sustained neuromuscular blockade in the adult critically ill patient. *Am J Health Syst Pharm*. 2002;59:179-195.

345. Bird SJ. Diagnosis and management of critical illness polyneuropathy and critical illness myopathy. *Curr Treat Options Neurol*. 2007;9:85-92.

346. McKegney FP. The intensive care syndrome. The definition, treatment and prevention of a new "disease of medical progress." *Conn Med*. 1966;30:633-636.

347. McGuire BE, Basten CJ, Ryan CJ, Gallagher J. Intensive care unit syndrome: a dangerous misnomer. *Arch Intern Med*. 2000;160:906-909.

348. Ely EW, Inouye SK, Bernard GR, et al. Delirium in mechanically ventilated patients: validity and reliability of the confusion assessment method for the intensive care unit (CAM-ICU). *JAMA*. 2001;286:2703-2710.

349. Thomason J, Shintani A, Peterson J, Pun BT, Jackson JC, Ely EW. Intensive care unit delirium is an independent predictor of longer hospital stay: a prospective study of 261 non-ventilated patients. *Crit Care*. 2005;94:R375-R381.

350. Way J, Back AL, Curtis JR. Withdrawing life support and resolution of conflict with families. *BMJ*. 2002;325:1342-1345.

351. Nelson JE, Azoulay E, Curtis JR, et al. Palliative care in the ICU. *J Palliat Med* 2012;15(2):168-174.

352. Fanning J, Valea FA. Perioperative bowel management for gynecologic surgery. *Am J Obstet Gynecol*. 2011;205(4)309-314.

353. Bakkum-Gamez JN, Langstraat CL, Martin JR, et al. Incidence of and risk factors for postoperative ileus in women undergoing primary staging and debulking for epithelial ovarian carcinoma. *Gynecol Oncol*. 2012;125(3):614-620.

354. Fanning J, Hojat R. Safety and efficacy of immediate postoperative feeding and bowel stimulation to prevent ileus after major gynecologic surgical procedures. *J Am Osteopath Assoc*. 2011;111(8):469-472.

355. Kozol R. Mechanical bowel obstruction: a tale of 2 eras. *Arch Surg*. 2012;147(2):180.

356. Wright HK, O'Brien JJ, Tilson MD. Water absorption in experimental closed segment obstruction of the ileum in man. *Am J Surg*. 1971;121(1):96-99.

357. Sheyn D, Bretschneider CE, Mahajan ST, Ridgeway B, Davenport A, Pollard R. Incidence and risk factors for early postoperative small bowel obstruction in patients undergoing hysterectomy for benign indications. *Am J Obstet Gynecol*. 2019;220(3):251.e1-251.e9.

358. Ten Broek RPG, Krielen P, Di Saverio S, et al. Bologna guidelines for diagnosis and management of adhesive small bowel obstruction (ASBO): 2017 update of the evidence-based guidelines from the world society of emergency surgery ASBO working group. *World J Emerg Surg*. 2018;13:24.

359. Mullan CP, Siewert B, Eisenberg RL. Small bowel obstruction. *AJR Am J Roentgenol*. 2012;198(2):W105-W117.

360. Oyasiji T, Angelo S, Kyriakides TC, Helton SW. Small bowel obstruction: outcome and cost implications of admitting service. *Am Surg*. 2010;76(7):687-691.

361. Diaz JJ Jr, Bokhari F, Mowery NT, et al. Guidelines for management of small bowel obstruction. *J Trauma*. 2008;64(6):1651-1664.

362. Bower KL, Lollar DI, Williams SL, Adkins FC, Luyimbazi DT, Bower CE. Small bowel obstruction. *Surg Clin North Am*. 2018;98(5):945-971.

363. Burneikis D, Stocchi L, Steiger E, Jezerski D, Shawki S. Parenteral nutrition instead of early reoperation in the management of early postoperative small bowel obstruction. *J Gastrointest Surg*. 2020;24(1):109-114.

CHAPTER **12.4**

Nutrition Support of Patients With Gynecologic Cancer

Sanjana Luther and Priya K. Simoes

INTRODUCTION

Cachexia and weight loss are common manifestations of cancer and exert a major impact on QoL and survival. Malnutrition is a complex, multifactorial phenomenon that leads to progressive weight loss and deficiency of specific nutrients. Both cancer and its various therapies contribute to cachexia. Advances in understanding nutritional requirements and metabolism, and major progress in the ability to provide nutritional support, have made it possible to feed almost any patient with cancer. Nevertheless, the indications and appropriate use of the various modalities of nutritional support continue to evolve, with many unanswered questions.

Malnutrition is usually a manifestation of general calorie and protein deficits that result in progressive weight loss and weakness; however, it is important to recognize that in some patients, specific nutrient deficiencies, such as magnesium deficiency or vitamin B_{12} deficiency, can be present even in the absence of weight loss and can contribute significantly to morbidity and even mortality. Malnutrition can be further defined based on etiology such as starvation-related malnutrition, chronic disease–related malnutrition, and acute disease– or injury–related malnutrition; all of which can apply to patients at varying stages of their malignancy (1).

Gynecologic malignancies and their multimodal therapies may be associated with severe malnutrition. Malnutrition is associated with various negative outcomes related to treatment tolerance, including, but not limited to, operative candidacy, postoperative management, length of hospital stay, and OS. Although some nutritional problems occur in patients with cervical and endometrial cancer, they are most commonly seen in those with ovarian cancer, particularly in advanced stages, when intra-abdominal metastases severely impair GI function. Nutritional assessment and appropriate therapy should be integral parts of the treatment plan because of the high incidence of malnutrition and its impact on the patient with cancer. Tailoring nutritional needs to each individual patient has been shown to improve prognosis.

NUTRITIONAL ASSESSMENT

Nutritional assessment in patients with cancer is an ongoing process that includes surveys, surveillance, screening, and interventions. It should be a part of the patient's initial evaluation and should be updated periodically. It is especially important to determine the nutritional state before therapeutic interventions as well as during and after acute illness, in order to identify early those patients who would benefit from nutritional support. The nutritional assessment method used must be simple, accurate, and inexpensive. Anthropometric parameters, serum protein measurements, and immunologic tests have classically formed the basis of the nutritional evaluation; however, they all have significant deficiencies, and there is still much work to be done in identifying adequate markers. Although various criteria and methods for nutritional assessment exist, there is still not a single encompassing best method that can be utilized alone and thus multiple assessment methods may need to be used in conjunction.

Anthropometric and Biochemical Markers

Anthropometric measurements, such as weight, height, BMI, skinfold thickness, mid-arm muscle circumference, and creatinine/height index, can all provide useful information but have major limitations. Change in weight is the single most useful measurement of nutritional status when the change does not reflect fluctuations in TBW. The often-present edema, effusions, ascites, and IV hydration that often accompany treatment limit the use of weight as a nutritional parameter. Malnutrition can occur at any BMI, and individuals at both extremes of weight may be at increased risk of poor nutrition. In addition, inaccuracies in scales and different clothing can provide misleading information on weight changes. Measurements of skinfold and mid-arm muscle circumference (2) are useful tools in studies but have very limited use in clinical practice. Lumbar skeletal muscle mass, measured by CT, has also been used as a nutritional indicator to determine prognosis and disease recurrence among patients with gynecologic cancers. However, this method requires special imaging software and technical expertise, and its clinical utility is limited (3). A creatinine/height index derived by dividing the patient's 24-hour creatinine excretion by that of a healthy person of the same height offers a sensitive measure of early protein-calorie malnutrition (4) but requires collection of a 24-hour urine specimen and is affected by alterations in renal function, which may not be indicative of the nutritional state.

Low levels of serum proteins, such as albumin, prealbumin, transferrin, and retinol-binding protein, were classically thought to represent malnutrition. However, in the malnourished patient, low levels of these proteins can be nonspecific, and their role may be limited. They are dependent on intact hepatic synthetic function as well as hydration status. They can be low as a manifestation of severe illness (infection, metastatic cancer, multisystem organ failure) in a normal nutritional state. In addition, they can function as acute-phase reactants and, therefore, can be normal or elevated in a clinically malnourished patient. In addition, different societies such as ASPEN and Academy (Academy of Nutrition and Dietetics) do not recommend specific inflammatory markers for diagnostic purposes as they function as acute-phase reactants and may better reflect the severity of inflammatory response rather than nutritional status (1). Similar limitations apply to immunologic parameters, such as total lymphocyte count and delayed cutaneous hypersensitivity. In simple starvation, both of these measures may be decreased and can return to normal with initiation of nutritional support. However, in the patient with cancer undergoing chemotherapy, surgery, or radiotherapy or in the midst of an acute illness, these parameters have little value in the assessment of the nutritional state (5,6).

The abovementioned parameters have been combined to create numerous nutritional assessment indices. The most extensively studied is the PNI, which utilizes measurements of serum albumin, serum transferrin, triceps skinfold, and delayed cutaneous hypersensitivity (7). Buzby et al prospectively studied the PNI in patients undergoing GI surgery and found that it could accurately stratify patients into high, intermediate, or low risk of developing postoperative complications (8). It must be understood, however, that the index is only as good as the parameters from which it is calculated, and the same limitations outlined earlier are present in any of these indices.

Subjective Global Assessment

The clinical assessment of nutritional status has always been used to some extent as part of the general medical history and physical examination. The validity of a formal clinical assessment of nutritional status was demonstrated in the landmark study by Baker et al, who developed the SGA as a formal clinical assessment of nutritional status (9). The SGA is based on a complete history and physical examination, with emphasis on six areas: change in weight, dietary intake, GI symptoms, functional capacity, physiologic stress, and physical signs of nutritional deficiencies. These are used to place the patient into three groups. Group "A" (normal nutritional status) consists of patients without restriction of food intake or absorption, no change in functional status, and stable or increasing weight. Group "B" (mild malnutrition) consists of patients with evidence of decreased food intake and functional status but little or no change in body weight, whereas those with severe reduction in food intake, functional status, and loss of weight comprise group "C" (severe malnutrition).

The SGA has consistently been shown to be reproducible and reliable in identifying patients at risk for developing complications associated with malnutrition, with a high interobserver reproducibility (9,10). The initial study by Baker and colleagues showed a significant increase in incidence of infection, use of antibiotics, and length of hospitalization in group "C" when compared with group "A" (9). In the follow-up study of 202 patients undergoing GI surgery, the rate of septic and nonseptic complications in group "C" was 7 times greater than that in group "A" (10). The SGA provides a simple, reproducible, and accurate method to identify malnourished patients who could benefit from nutritional support. Clinical assessments similar to the SGA have proven superior to immunologic testing, plasma protein measurements, and bioelectrical impedance in providing a useful evaluation of nutritional status (9-14).

More recently, the SGA has been shown to predict short- and long-term survival and tolerance to chemotherapy among women with ovarian cancer (15,16). It is currently considered the preferred method of nutritional assessment for patients with gynecologic cancers (16,17).

New Methods for Nutritional Assessment

Newer methods are being identified, and guidance supports further research studies for validating other tools. The Global Leadership Initiative on Malnutrition (GLIM) developed criteria using a consensus-based approach for different forms of malnutrition using a two-step model for risk screening and diagnosis assessment. Diagnostic assessment utilizes a minimum of one phenotypic and one etiologic component. Phenotypic criteria are (a) weight loss (%): more than 5% within the prior 6 months or more than 10% beyond 6 months; (b) low BMI: less than 20 kg/m^2 if less than 70 years or less than 22 if greater than 70 years; and (c) reduced muscle mass: reduced by validated body composition measuring techniques. Etiologic criteria are (a) reduced food intake or assimilation: 50% or less of energy requirement greater than 1 week or any reduction for greater than 2 weeks or any chronic GI conditions that adversely impact food assimilation or absorption, and (b) inflammation: acute disease/injury or chronic disease related. Severity of malnutrition is then assessed based on phenotypic criteria and graded into stage 1/moderate malnutrition and stage 2/severe malnutrition (18). Utilizing a screening tool according to cancer type and location may be the future for optimizing individual patient needs. Although some studies have investigated the use of GLIM criteria in nongynecologic cancers, thus assessing its utility, there remains a need for investigation in gynecologic cancers (19).

PREVALENCE OF MALNUTRITION

The prevalence of malnutrition depends on the tumor type and stage, the organs involved, and the anticancer therapy. Concurrent nonmalignant conditions such as obesity, diabetes, and intestinal diseases can be important contributing factors. The overall prevalence of malnutrition, regardless of cancer type, has been reported to be 40%. The prevalence of weight loss during the 6 months preceding diagnosis of cancer was reported from a multicenter cooperative study of patients with 12 types of cancer (20). The lowest frequency (31%-40%) and severity of weight loss were found in patients with breast cancer, hematologic cancers, and sarcomas. Intermediate frequency and severity of weight loss was found in patients with colon, prostate, and lung cancer (54%-64%). Patients with cancer of the pancreas and stomach had the highest frequency (over 80%) and severity of weight loss. However, it is worthwhile noting that approximately 35% of the patients with lung cancer lost more than 5% of their body weight. This underscores the fact that even if the tumor does not involve the GI tract directly, there can be significant weight loss because of systemic and metabolic derangements and loss of appetite. This particular study did not report on patients with gynecologic malignancies, in whom weight loss can also be frequent and severe, but other studies evaluating malnutrition in cancer populations have now assessed those with gynecologic cancers. Malnutrition prevalence when utilizing PG-SGA in a single cancer center with 13% of patients having a primary gynecologic cancer found the lowest percentage of malnutrition in patients with obesity. Cancer types with the highest rate of malnutrition were respiratory (29%), hematologic (24%), and colorectal cancer (22%). In addition, this study showed that the tool utilized PG-SGA versus GLIM criteria resulted in different prevalence values within the same population. The GLIM criteria identified double the number of malnourished patients compared to PG-SGA. The GLIM criteria were directly compared to PG-SGA, which is widely used in the oncology setting, but the two different prevalence rates may be attributed to time frame of weight loss and use of BMI. BMI itself, not used in the PG-SGA, is not an ideal parameter for assessing nutritional status, given the presence of confounders such as sarcopenic obesity. The study itself is also with limitations in regard to methods and criteria utilized (21). Other studies revealed that over 40% of patients receiving medical treatment for a variety of cancers were malnourished (22). Among surgical patients in a Veterans Administration (VA) hospital, 39% of those undergoing a major operation for cancer were malnourished, as judged by either an NRI or a combination of weight loss and low serum proteins (23).

Data on the prevalence and impact of malnutrition in patients with gynecologic tumors mirror the observations in patients with other cancers. In a study of 67 consecutive patients hospitalized with gynecologic cancers at the University of Texas, it was found that 54% were malnourished as determined by the PNI (24).

In a single center of 397 patients utilizing the NRS system, a severe risk of malnutrition was found in 35.8% of patients, with the lowest risk of malnutrition in breast cancer (25.5%) as compared to 70.2% in ovarian cancer, which had the highest risk (25). Another study by Laky et al used the SGA to study 194 patients with gynecologic cancers, showing that 24% of all patients were malnourished and the prevalence of malnutrition was highest in ovarian cancer (67%) and lowest in endometrial cancer (6%) (17). Further studies such as a retrospective study by Rodrigues et al also utilized the PG-SGA to obtain a nutritional diagnosis and similarly found a higher prevalence of malnutrition in women diagnosed with ovarian cancer compared to endometrial cancer (26).

SIGNIFICANCE OF MALNUTRITION

The impact of malnutrition on the patient with cancer was demonstrated in a report by Warren et al in 1932 (27). Based on data from autopsies, the conclusion was that cachexia was the leading cause of death in a group of 400 patients with various cancers. More recent studies have confirmed the significant impact of malnutrition on the QoL and prognosis of the patient with cancer. In the aforementioned multicenter cooperative study of patients receiving chemotherapy (20), those who presented with weight loss at the time of diagnosis had decreased performance status and survival compared with those who presented without weight loss. The negative impact of malnutrition was also demonstrated in surgical patients with malignant and benign diseases. Malnourished patients undergoing a major operation were at greater risk for postoperative morbidity and mortality than were well-nourished patients (23,28).

Cancer cachexia occurs in 50% to 80% of patients with cancer and is an independent predictor of shorter survival and increases the risk of treatment failure and toxicity. Expectedly, this has been found to reduce the QoL, accounting for more than 20% of all cancer-related deaths (29).

The impact of malnutrition on patients with a primary gynecologic malignancy is striking. There have been numerous studies showcasing different parameters and scoring systems that are of value in predicting clinical outcomes in patients requiring nutritional support.

In a study by Geisler et al, patients with ovarian cancer, who were malnourished, had increased postoperative complications. This difference could be mitigated if preoperative nutritional support could reverse the malnutrition (30).

Several other studies have confirmed the relationship of malnutrition to poor surgical and overall outcomes in patients with primary gynecologic malignancies. Donato et al reported that of the 104 patients with ovarian carcinoma undergoing intestinal surgery, preoperative nutritional status was a greater predictor of postoperative infectious complications than other variables, including preoperative bowel obstruction, the number of intestinal procedures, or the type of anastomosis.

Poor nutritional status is also an independent predictor of prolonged postoperative ICU stay in patients with ovarian cancer (31). Hertlein et al stratified patients with gynecologic cancer at risk for malnutrition using an NRS-2002 tool. The NRS-2002 was calculated using two components: "impaired nutritional status" and "severity of disease," which were each given an individual score from 0 to 4. The sum of the two scores constituted the final NRS (32,33). Those with NRS score 3 or higher were at increased risk for perioperative infectious (6.9% vs 3.2%) and noninfectious complications (15.8% vs 4.5%). They also had longer hospital stay (10 vs 6 days). Patients with ovarian cancer had the highest prevalence of malnutrition (33). In another study of patients with gynecologic cancer undergoing surgery, Uppal and colleagues found that patients with preoperative hypoalbuminemia (defined as serum albumin <3 g/dL) were 6 times more likely to develop a perioperative complication and 10 times more likely to die within 30 days of surgery compared with those with normal albumin levels (34). This was further supported in a retrospective study of 300 gynecologic oncology patients who underwent surgical management of malignancies, which found that decreased albumin was significantly associated with more postoperative complications, hospital readmissions, need for reoperation, ICU admissions ($P <$ .001), and disease recurrence ($P <$ .001) (35). A systematic review of RCTs regarding nutritional interventions in clinical outcomes of those with ovarian cancer looked at end points, such as OS, PFS, length of stay, and complications following surgery and/or chemotherapy. Studies that offered early postoperative nutritional interventions displayed a reduction in length of hospital stay and improved intestinal recovery (36). Other recent studies have also looked at pretreatment nutrition and its influence on prognosis, surgical outcomes, and postoperative complication rates in patients with ovarian cancer. One study from Austria utilized a scoring system (Controlling Nutritional Status or CONUT) and its prognostic value for the stated end points. It was found that this pretreatment CONUT score was an independent prognosticator for OS and was associated with successful surgical outcomes;

thus, patients with a high score may benefit from pretreatment nutritional interventions (37). More scoring tools such as this may help determine the need for pretreatment or preintervention in patients with gynecological cancer. In addition, a recent study was the first to combine a multidimensional analysis of malnutrition with sarcopenia, including bioelectrical impedance analysis in patients with gynecologic cancer, identifying the need to integrate these methods into preoperative evaluations to effectively determine high-risk patients (38).

In addition to predicting surgical outcome and perioperative complications, malnutrition is associated with increased neutropenic fever following chemotherapy, prolonged hospital stays, decreased QoL, and reduced OS among women with gynecologic cancers (15-17,24,39). Identifying malnutrition early and implementing specialized interventions should be the standard model of care to improve outcomes (38). Early identification of these at-risk patients and early enrollment in physical and nutritional programs can improve outcomes.

ETIOLOGY OF MALNUTRITION

Cancer can induce a wide variety of derangements in nutritional status, ranging from generalized malnutrition with severe weight loss and muscle wasting to a single nutrient deficiency. The etiology of malnutrition in the patient with cancer is multifactorial. Nutritionally relevant derangements can be induced by the tumor locally (ie, GI obstruction), by malabsorption, by humoral factors produced by the tumor itself, or by reaction of the immune system to the tumor. All modalities of cancer therapy, surgery, radiation, chemotherapy, immunotherapy, and palliative treatments may be associated with side effects and complications that can impair nutritional status.

Cancer cachexia is defined as an ongoing loss of skeletal muscle mass (with or without loss of fat mass) that cannot fully be reversed by nutritional support and leads to progressive functional impairment. It is diagnosed by the presence of these three criteria: (i) weight loss more than 5% over the past 6 months (in the absence of simple starvation); (ii) BMI less than 20 kg/m^2 and any degree of weight loss more than 2%; or (iii) appendicular skeletal muscle index consistent with sarcopenia (males < 7.26 kg/m^2; females < 5.45 kg/m^2) and any degree of weight loss greater than 2%. The syndrome of cachexia itself can develop through stages from pre-cachexia to cachexia to refractory cachexia (40).

The etiologic factors of malnutrition in the patient with cancer are generally due to three major factors: decreased food intake, malabsorption, and abnormal metabolism.

Impaired Food Intake and Malabsorption

Both tumor and cancer treatment modalities can lead to decreased food intake through direct effects on the GI tract or systemic effects, leading to anorexia. Obstruction of the GI tract can be caused by any gynecologic malignancy through external compression or, more rarely, by direct invasion. Occasionally, localized obstructions can be relieved surgically or endoscopically; however, obstruction due to peritoneal carcinomatosis seen in advanced ovarian cancer is particularly difficult to manage surgically. Often, draining gastrostomy with parenteral nutrition (when appropriate) is the only option for providing nutrition and symptomatic relief (41-43). Most importantly, a multidisciplinary approach to actively manage malignant bowel obstruction in advanced gynecologic cancer is needed. Although length of stay may be increased, the OS was found to be improved to over 6 months in patients receiving multimodal therapies (44).

Tumors can induce anorexia without local involvement of the GI tract. The pathophysiology of this phenomenon is not well understood but is thought to be a result of cachexia-inducing factors involving mediators, such as hormones, neuropeptides, and cytokines (45). Norton et al (46) utilized a model of surgically coupled tumor-bearing and normal rats with parabiotic cross-circulation to show that tumor-induced anorexia is mediated by circulating substances. This has been confirmed in subsequent studies identifying cytokine-mediated factors (47). Other animal studies have also been completed with implanting tumor cell lines. These implanted tumor cells induce inflammatory cytokines or prostaglandins, further demonstrating mechanisms of cancer cachexia (48). Tumor-induced impairment of smell and taste has been well described (28,49-52), but the mechanism has not been defined. Bernstein et al (53,54) demonstrated in a rat model that infusion of tumor necrosis factor (TNF) mimics tumor-induced anorexia, and these effects are mediated via the area postrema and the caudal medial nucleus of the solitary tract in the CNS. Recent findings suggest that close interaction among abovementioned mediators exists in the hypothalamus, thus leading to decreased oral intake and cachexia. Cytokines have been found to play a major role in affecting the imbalance of orexigenic and anorexigenic circuits, which comprise body weight regulation, leading to cachexia (45).

Therapies used for gynecologic malignancies often result in complications that impair nutrient intake and absorption. Surgical interventions can lead to fistulae, short bowel syndrome, infections, and ileus, all of which impair oral intake significantly. In a review of 12 years of colonic surgery in gynecologic oncology patients, the rate for major systemic complications (MI, PE, renal failure, sepsis) was 13.7%, and the rate of major bowel complications (abscess, fistulae, hemorrhage, obstruction) was 12.1% (55).

Radiotherapy can lead to damage of the GI tract, most commonly affecting the small bowel, followed by the transverse colon, sigmoid, and rectum. Radiation enteritis was initially described in 1897, 1 year after the introduction of radiation as a treatment modality. It is an inflammatory process, divided into acute and chronic form, which overall appears to be underreported. Reports have shown up to 90% of patients with cancer experience GI symptoms in the first few weeks following radiotherapy (18,56). Predisposing risk factors include previous abdominal surgery, pelvic inflammatory disease, hypertension, diabetes mellitus, arterial disease, and thin body habitus as a BMI greater than 30 kg/m^2 is thought to be protective (56,57). Small population studies such as that by Nganga and Hoover (19) found that adipose-corrected bowel bag dose/volume measures may be used to predict acute bowel toxicity in patients receiving postoperative intensity-modulated radiation therapy (IMRT) posthysterectomy in endometrial and cervical cancers. In general, a dose of 50 Gy is the threshold for significant injury. In the acute phase of radiation enteritis, virtually all patients experience anorexia, nausea, and vomiting, which are thought to be mediated by effects of serotonin on the gut (58) and the CNS (59). This is followed 2 to 3 weeks later by direct injury to the intestinal mucosa, resulting in diarrhea and mild-to-moderate malabsorption. Most patients will have complete resolution of these acute symptoms. However, a significant minority of patients who received radiotherapy will experience chronic dysfunction of the GI tract (60). It can occur after as short of a time period of 2 months, but there is often a latent period of 1 to 2 years, and possibly as long as 30 years, before the symptoms of chronic radiation enteropathy surface (56,61). In a review of 102 patients with radiation enteritis after treatment for cervical or endometrial cancer, the median time to development of severe symptoms such as obstruction or perforation was 18 months (62). A prospective two center phase I/II trial collected data on toxicity assessment, outcomes, and patient reported QoL at baseline and regular intervals in patients undergoing adjuvant radiation for endometrial cancer. Patient-reported diarrhea and GI domain scores were significantly worse than baseline during treatment but returned to baseline at week 12. There were no significant changes in overall health and QoL scores, emphasizing the acute adverse effects of radiation, which is a crucial modality for the treatment of gynecological cancers (63).

Zhou et al (64) retrospectively studied the effects of radiation injury and QoL in cervical cancer who received adjuvant radiation following hysterectomy by obtaining patient questionnaires at various time points, which showed common symptoms of acute intestinal dysfunction, including nausea (46%), vomiting (33.8%), constipation (16.3%), and abdominal pain (10.3%), to be most prevalent early in treatment course but were much improved by 12 and 24 months. Incidence of chronic radiation rectal injury at 12 months was found to be 10%, presenting mainly as abdominal pain, constipation, bloody stool, and diarrhea, which remained unchanged at 24 months. Chronic radiation enteropathy is characterized pathologically by transmural injury, leading to submucosal fibrosis, edema, lymphatic ectasia, and obliterative endarteritis, which can induce chronic colicky abdominal pain, malabsorption, persistent weight loss, diarrhea, steatorrhea, GI bleeding, ulceration, perforation, stricture, and fistula formation (56,57). These findings were similar to the study by Yeoh et al, which also noted that patients who underwent pelvic irradiation had chronic bowel dysfunction, as well as malabsorption of vitamin B$_{12}$ and bile acids, likely due to terminal ileal damage during therapy.

Husebye and colleagues (65) prospectively studied the GI motility patterns in 41 patients with chronic abdominal complaints after radiotherapy for gynecologic cancer. Impaired fasting motility was found in 29% of patients, and motor response after a meal was attenuated in 24%. Postprandial delay of the migrating motor complex was found to be an independent predictor of malnutrition as assessed by weight loss and serum albumin. Impaired motility of the small bowel, therefore, is a key factor in the symptoms experienced by patients with chronic radiation enteropathy. Chronic radiation enteritis predisposes to numerous secondary complications. Danielsson et al (66) studied 20 patients with chronic or intermittent diarrhea occurring 2 years or more after receiving radiotherapy for gynecologic tumors. Bile acid malabsorption was detected in 65% of patients, whereas evidence of bacterial overgrowth on D-xylose or cholylglycine breath tests was found in 45%. Treatment with bile acid binders or antibiotics resulted in a significant decline in the number of daily bowel movements. Boland et al reported on a 25-year experience with postresection short bowel syndrome secondary to radiation therapy. Most of the cases were in women who received pelvic radiation for gynecologic cancers. One-third of these patients developed short bowel syndrome within a year after radiation, and two-thirds remained dependent on long-term TPN (67). Improved fractionation of radiotherapy, IMRT, and physical strategies to prevent radiation enteritis such as protective shielding of the intestine where possible and a full bladder because it displaces small bowel from the treatment field have reduced these complication rates, as well as novel surgical techniques, including as mesh slings, transposition of bowel segments, and surgically placed radioprotective prostheses (56,68,69).

Chemotherapy is often associated with decreased food intake. Mucositis and diarrhea are commonly seen during therapy with cytotoxic agents that affect the replicating cells of the intestinal mucosa, such as 5-flourouracil (5-FU), methotrexate, and bleomycin. The vinca alkaloids can cause ileus and constipation mediated by toxic effects on GI neural pathways, whereas cisplatin and nitrosoureas are highly emetic (70,71). Significant nausea, vomiting, stomatitis, and diarrhea occur in 15% of patients receiving IV taxol and in 55% of those receiving the drug orally (72). In addition to direct effects on the GI tract, chemotherapy in women with gynecologic cancers has significant effects on olfactory and gustatory function, leading to reduced appetite and weight loss (73).

The psychological impact of a malignancy and its associated therapies can also lead to decreased nutrient intake. Depression is a frequent cause of anorexia in this population, with up to 58% of patients with cancer having depressive symptoms and 38% meeting criteria for major depression (74). The prevalence of major depression in a cross-sectional analysis of routinely collected clinical data was found to be highest in lung cancer, which was followed by gynecologic cancer. Major depression is common and undertreated (75).

Metabolic Derangements

Even with normal nutrient intake, patients with cancer are at risk for malnutrition due to inefficient nutrient utilization and wasteful metabolic pathways. Cancer cachexia is associated with altered metabolism of carbohydrates, fat, protein, vitamins, and minerals. Both BEE and resting energy expenditure (REE) have been studied in patients with malignancy. Increases in these values have been reported in many, but not all studies in patients with malignancy. Substantial evidence supports elevations in REE during tumor-bearing states, which can potentially promote weight loss, producing suboptimal clinical outcomes, thus increasing morbidity and mortality risks (76-78). A meta-analysis of 27 studies showed an average increase in REE of 9.66 kJ/kg FFM/day (95% CI: 3.34-15.98) in patients with cancer compared to control subjects. Heterogeneity was detected ($P < .001$), which suggested variations among cancer types, but elevations were most notable in those with cancers of metabolically demanding organs. This analysis did not include those with gynecologic cancers, and the data itself are limited (79). Notably, elevated BEE will drop after tumor resection (80). Dickerson et al used indirect calorimetry to determine the REE in 31 patients with ovarian cancer and 30 patients with cervical cancer. Fifty-five percent of those with ovarian cancer were found to be hypermetabolic (BEE >110% predicted by the Harris-Benedict equation), whereas only 13% of patients with cervical cancer were hypermetabolic. These differences could not be explained by differences in the extent of disease, nutritional status, body temperature, or nutrient intake (81).

Abnormalities in carbohydrate metabolism in patients with cancer include glucose intolerance and peripheral insulin resistance. Tumors consume large amounts of glucose aerobically, which leads to alterations in lactate recycling, leading to increased hepatic gluconeogenesis (82). Glucose intolerance and insulin resistance may play a role in the development of cachexia and may not just be a result of the cachexia itself (83). Insulin resistance in patients with cancer as a consequence of tumor by-product, chronic inflammation, and endocrine dysfunction has been associated with weight loss. Insulin resistance may occur before the onset of cachexia symptoms in patients with cancer and is characterized by increased hepatic gluconeogenesis. Unlike type 2 diabetes, they can have normal fasting glucose with high, normal, or low levels of insulin (84). In comparison, in simple starvation, patients are most often euglycemic or hypoglycemic. The hyperglycemia seen in patients with cancer is exacerbated by increased hepatic gluconeogenesis. When insulin sensitivity is compromised, skeletal muscle mass is also adversely affected, which can lead to wasting syndromes and sarcopenia. In addition, increased production of ghrelin, testosterone deficiency, and low vitamin D levels may contribute to alterations in glucose metabolism.

Lipid metabolism is altered in malignancy. There is often increased lipolysis with a decrease in fat mass, which can be out of proportion to the loss of lean body mass (82). In addition, patients with cancer are often hyperlipidemic. Several causes of increased lipolysis have been proposed, including decreased food intake, stress response to illness with adrenal medullary stimulation and increased circulating catecholamine levels, insulin resistance, and release of lipolytic factors produced by the tumor itself or by myeloid tissue cells (85). One such factor has been well characterized. Lipid-mobilizing factor (LMF), a 24-kDa glycoprotein produced by tumors, has been shown to stimulate increased lipid mobilization from adipocytes. LMF is thought to act through binding of β-adrenergic receptors and subsequent upregulation of mitochondrial uncoupling proteins (86,87). Animal studies have shown that LMF causes loss of body weight (specifically a loss of body fat), which is independent of caloric food intake (88). The activity of LMF in the urine and serum of patients with cancer has been shown to correlate with the degree of weight loss and tumor burden (89,90). In addition to its effect on lipid metabolism, there is preliminary evidence that LMF may protect tumor cells from free radical toxicity and may, therefore, make tumors less responsive

to certain chemotherapeutic agents that induce oxidative damage (91). In addition, recent discoveries beyond atrophy of adipose tissue show that browning of white adipose tissue (WAT) may contribute to high-energy expenditure seen in cancer-associated cachexia. Both systemic inflammation and IL-6 induce and sustain WAT browning in cachexia. Inhibition of WAT browning may assist with reducing the severity of cachexia (92).

High total-body protein turnover, with increased synthesis and catabolism, characterizes the alterations of protein metabolism seen in patients with cancer. This results in depletion of muscle mass and loss of nitrogen and contrasts with the adaptive decrease in protein turnover seen in patients with uncomplicated starvation. Skeletal muscle is the major site of protein loss in patients with solid tumors (93). The predominant mechanism of muscle protein loss in patients with cancer is an ubiquitin-associated pathway (94). In this pathway, polyubiquitin chains are attached to proteins, which are then recognized and degraded by a proteasome complex. This pathway is regulated, in part, by proteolysis-inducing factor (PIF). PIF is a 24-kDa glycoprotein produced by human tumors, and its expression directly correlates with the severity of weight loss. There are multiple mechanisms by which PIF induces weight loss. PIF has a direct effect on skeletal muscle by decreasing protein synthesis and increasing protein degradation. PIF also increases the expression of pro-inflammatory cytokines, which independently cause weight loss, and induces the shedding of syndecans (transmembrane proteoglycans), which has been shown to be related to increased metastases and mortality (95-97). Effective treatment of the underlying cancer has been shown to reverse ubiquitin-dependent proteolysis of skeletal muscle (98). Better understanding of this process holds the promise of improving therapy to attenuate the loss of protein seen in patients with cancer.

Cytokines either produced by cancer cells or released by the immune system of the patient as a response to cancer also play an important role in inducing metabolic derangements. IL-6 and TNF are released during interaction of host cells with tumor cells, and high serum levels are present in patients with advanced cancer and cachexia (99-101). They mediate increased energy expenditure, whole-body protein turnover, rise in serum triglyceride levels, and high glycerol turnover (102). TNF causes protein wasting, depletion of body fat, and anorexia in animal models by activation of an adenosine triphosphate (ATP)-dependent proteolytic pathway (99,103). Study results involving humans and animals have identified IL-6 in the cachectic process, but they show it likely acts by inducing or working with other cachectic factors (93). Genetic polymorphisms may result in higher levels of circulating cytokines and a greater degree of weight loss in some patients compared with others (104). Interventions to downregulate these cytokines result in improved appetite, body weight, and QoL (100).

The combined effects of these wasteful and inefficient alterations in metabolism make it difficult to restore nutritional status in the patient with cancer and cachexia despite the use of specialized nutritional support.

NUTRITIONAL THERAPIES

There are four types of nutritional therapies: parenteral nutrition, EN, oral dietary therapy, and drug therapy, aimed at improving appetite and food intake. Depending on the patient's condition, nutritional support in the patient with cancer has two distinct objectives: (i) provision of nutrition during anticancer therapies to counteract their nutritionally related side effects and improve outcome following these therapies and (ii) support in patients with long-term or permanent severe impairment of the GI tract. In these patients, nutritional support may be required for indefinite periods of time. Results of numerous clinical trials support the use of nutritional support only in limited situations during anticancer therapies. In the group with prolonged GI failure, nutritional support may be a lifesaving therapy because patients could die of starvation without TPN or enteral feeding.

Total Parenteral Nutrition

TPN is an effective method for delivery of nutrients directly into the blood and thus overcomes the major causes of cancer-induced weight loss, including decreased food intake and dysfunction of the GI tract. Survival for more than 20 years in patients nourished exclusively by TPN clearly demonstrates the lifesaving role of this method of nutritional support. Initially, it seemed logical that TPN would be an effective adjuvant therapy for most patients with cancer undergoing radiation therapy, surgery, or chemotherapy because of the accompanying cachexia and inability to eat adequately. Randomized studies, however, have shown that TPN only benefits a select subgroup of patients with cancer during anticancer therapy, such as those with reversible bowel obstructions, short bowel syndrome, or other issues contributing to malabsorption.

Efficacy

In patients receiving chemotherapy with or without radiation therapy, TPN can lead to improvements of several nutritional parameters. Both body weight and body fat increase. Deficits of specific vitamins, minerals, and trace elements can be corrected, and hydration status can be improved. TPN, however, does not alter many of the metabolic derangements encountered in the patient with cancer. Increased glucose oxidation and turnover persist as does muscle proteolysis and increased lipolysis (105,106). Finally, TPN does not stop the overall losses of body nitrogen (107).

The relevant issue for the clinician is the effect of TPN on the morbidity and mortality associated with cancer therapy and whether TPN can allow more intense therapy, as was initially hoped. Numerous randomized trials have examined this issue. Studies of patients undergoing chemotherapy for carcinoma of the ovary (41), lung (108,109), colon (107), testes (110), lymphoma (111), and other tumors (112) have been conducted. However, the patients in these studies were largely unselected. Many were not malnourished, and others had adequate oral intake with intact GI function, making IV nutrition unnecessary, futile, and, potentially, harmful. Numerous meta-analyses concluded that nondiscriminatory use of TPN in patients undergoing chemotherapy offers no improvement in mortality, response to chemotherapy, or reduction in treatment-associated complications (113-115). This conclusion was echoed in a consensus statement from the National Institutes of Health, the ASPEN, and the American Society for Clinical Nutrition (116). The improvement in nutritional parameters afforded by TPN in patients receiving chemotherapy does not necessarily translate into improved clinical outcome. In addition, trials have examined perioperative TPN as well and have similarly found no significant benefit (117). Thus, the routine use of TPN in these patients is not indicated.

There are circumstances, however, in which nutritional support with parenteral nutrition should be considered. These include prevention of the effects of starvation in a patient unable to tolerate oral or enteral feedings for a prolonged period of time (usually >7-10 days), maximization of performance status in a malnourished patient before chemotherapy or surgery, and in patients undergoing bone marrow transplantation (118). TPN may have a stimulatory effect on tumor cell cycle kinetics (119). It is proposed that this effect would induce improved tumor response to cell cycle–specific chemotherapy. There has been some data indicating that TPN has a synergistic effect with chemotherapy resulting in better clinical outcomes, but conclusive proof of such a response remains elusive (120). There are ongoing studies such as the PANUSCO trial, which is an open-label, controlled, prospective, randomized, multicenter, phase IIIb trial comparing patients with histologically diagnosed pancreatic cancer undergoing chemotherapy being treated with best supportive nutritional care (BSNC) in the control group as compared to the experimental group that receives BSNC with parenteral nutrition. Primary end point is the comparison of both groups with respect to event-free survival or death from any cause. This displays that there is still more work to be done (121).

A few randomized studies have examined the use of TPN in patients receiving radiotherapy to the abdomen and pelvis (122,123). The role of TPN in the perioperative period has been extensively studied (23,124-127). At Memorial Sloan Kettering Cancer Center, a prospective study of 117 patients undergoing curative resection for pancreatic cancer randomized to receive TPN or IV fluids in the postoperative period showed no benefit from routine use of postoperative TPN (128). The group receiving TPN had a significant increase in postoperative infectious complications. The largest prospective randomized trial investigating the role of TPN in the perioperative setting was the VA Cooperative Study. In this study, 395 patients were randomized to receive 7 to 15 days of preoperative and 3 days of postoperative TPN, or oral feeding plus IV fluids. TPN did not improve morbidity or 90-day mortality. However, subgroup analysis showed that patients considered to be severely malnourished had fewer infectious complications if they received TPN. The authors concluded that the routine administration of preoperative TPN should be limited to patients who are severely malnourished unless there are other specific indications (23).

Randomized studies specifically examining the role of perioperative TPN in patients with gynecologic malignancies are lacking. Mendivil et al found that patients with ovarian cancer treated with TPN had worse preoperative health and significantly longer length of stay (129). TPN prescribing patterns in patients with advanced ovarian cancer was examined by Madhok et al, but this involved a specific population of those with malignant intestinal obstruction. They found that TPN should be the first choice in this population but that these patients must have good baseline performance status (130). These data and others provided the basis for a consensus statement from the National Institutes of Health, the ASPEN, and the American Society for Clinical Nutrition regarding the use of perioperative TPN, which states the following: (a) 7 to 10 days of preoperative TPN in a malnourished patient with GI cancer results in a 10% reduction in postoperative complications; (b) routine use of postoperative TPN in malnourished surgical patients who did not receive preoperative TPN results in a 10% increase in complications; (c) if by postoperative days 5 to 10 a patient is unable to tolerate oral or enteral feedings, then TPN is indicated to prevent the adverse effects of starvation. This panel, however, cautioned that in the majority of studies examining perioperative TPN, the amount and type of parenteral nutrition given was not optimal, and patients were often given excess calories. Therefore, the results may differ with the provision of relatively hypocaloric formulas (116). It is reasonable to extend these recommendations to the gynecologic oncology patient undergoing surgery (Table 12.4-1).

■ TABLE 12.4-1. Indications for TPN in Hospitalized Patients With Gynecologic Cancers	
Perioperative	710 d preoperatively in a malnourished patient (who cannot be fed enterally) Postoperative complications that prevent oral or enteral intake for >7-10 d Enterocutaneous fistula *No indication for routine use*
During radiation or chemotherapy	Maximization of performance status before therapy in a malnourished patient who cannot be fed enterally Severe persistent (>7-10 d) mucositis, diarrhea, ileus, or emesis *No indication for routine use*
General	After 7-10 d of inability to tolerate oral or enteral feeding due to any cause

TPN, total parental nutrition.

Composition of Total Parental Nutrition Solution

Once the decision to proceed with parenteral nutritional support is made, access to a large-bore central vein should be obtained. This allows the use of calorically dense, hypertonic solutions, which are often necessary in severely ill patients who may have restrictions on the amount of IV fluids they can receive. The solution must provide the protein and caloric needs, fluid, minerals, trace elements, and vitamins. Estimates of nutrition requirements are based on weight and adjusted for the degree of physiologic stress encountered by the patient, and there are numerous formulas and charts that provide these. Generally, patients require approximately 30 kcal/kg nonprotein calories, 1 g/kg amino acids, and about 2,000 mL of fluid. As illness severity increases and organs' functions change, adjustments may be required. Nonprotein calories can be provided as dextrose or lipid, and the relative amounts of these should also be individualized. Lipids provide 9 kcal/g compared with 3.4 for dextrose (in dextrose solutions, glucose is present as glucose monohydrate; hence, a gram contains <4 kcal). Lipid calories are particularly useful in patients who have high caloric requirements but cannot tolerate a large fluid load. In addition, lipids are useful in patients with severe pulmonary or hepatic dysfunction as glucose metabolism produces more carbon dioxide, which can add to the burden of the ailing lung and can lead to fatty infiltration of the liver. Up to 60% of caloric requirements can be provided as lipid, but serum triglyceride levels must be monitored closely. Appropriate electrolyte content of TPN solutions is of critical importance. The amounts must be tailored to the patient's requirements and organ function. Care must be taken to prevent potentially fatal hypokalemia or hypophosphatemia (particularly in the patient with severe weight loss), which can be precipitated by insulin-induced transport of the minerals to the intracellular space when inadequate amounts are given. Other electrolyte disorders, such as cisplatin-induced hypomagnesemia and SIADH, are common in the patient with gynecologic malignancy and must be addressed when ordering TPN. The TPN solution must also contain vitamins, minerals, and trace elements. Typically, these are available as standard commercial combination products. However, certain patients require specific modifications. For example, a patient with persistent diarrhea requires zinc supplementation in excess of the amounts present in standard trace element solutions.

Complications

Complications associated with TPN can be classified as catheter related, metabolic, or infectious. Catheter complications most often occur during placement of a central venous catheter and include pneumothorax, hemothorax, arterial injury, and hematoma. Cobb et al reported a 3% incidence of pneumothorax, arrhythmia, thrombus, or bleeding during 523 IV catheter placements (131). A large multicenter trial in 2015 compared complication rates of internal jugular, subclavian, and femoral nontunneled central venous access, thus finding pneumothorax requiring chest tube insertion in 1.5% of subclavian insertions compared with 0.5% of internal jugular attempts (132). Femoral access is not recommended, given sterility challenges and elevated infection risk (133). In the United States, the standard of practice is placement under ultrasonography guidance, resulting in a higher first-rate attempt and decreased complications. The number of unsuccessful insertion attempts is the strongest predictor of immediate complications, and this can be mitigated with the abovementioned strategies being implemented and the procedure being performed by an experienced clinician (134,135).

A study of subcutaneous peripheral infusion ports in women with gynecologic malignancies demonstrated a thrombosis rate of 26% during a mean follow-up of 105 days. The authors concluded that other types of vascular access devices may be preferable in this patient population (136). Another study demonstrated a higher rate of catheter-related infections in patients with external central venous catheters compared with subcutaneous infusion ports (137).

Metabolic derangements are frequently encountered during support with TPN, and the prescribing physician must be well versed in the pathophysiology of these disorders. Hyperglycemia is the most common abnormality and, if not corrected, can lead to an osmotic diuresis, dehydration, acidosis, and hyperosmolar coma. Hyperglycemia during TPN in the hospital is independently associated with increased rates of mortality, infections, organ dysfunction, and length of stay. A blood glucose target of 140 to 180 mg/dL is recommended (138).

One metabolic complication that deserves special mention is the "refeeding syndrome." In chronically ill patients with severe malnutrition, there is often a depletion of total-body phosphorus, potassium, and magnesium. The phosphorus deficits may be masked by increased renal phosphorus absorption designed to maintain normal serum levels. When nutritional support is initiated, the infusion of a large glucose load with subsequent surge in insulin leads to increased cellular uptake of phosphorus and potassium, which may induce severe life-threatening hypokalemia and hypophosphatemia (139,140). These disorders cause widespread tissue and organ dysfunction, including neuromuscular dysfunction, rhabdomyolysis, heart failure, cardiac arrhythmias, and respiratory failure, and may result in death in extreme cases (140,141). Therefore, in patients with evidence of severe undernutrition, nutrition support should be initiated at lower rates and caloric content, with small amounts of dextrose calories, supplemental phosphorus and potassium, and careful monitoring of serum electrolytes (142).

TPN has also been associated with liver disease. Parenteral nutrition–associated liver disease (PNALD) can be divided into three primary types: cholestatic, fatty infiltration, and biliary sludge/stone disease. These abnormalities have been attributed to infusion of excessive glucose calories, imbalance of amino acids, and, rarely, fatty acid deficiency. Elevation of serum transaminases may occur, but it is generally mild. There is a risk of progression to fibrosis in patients on long-term therapy. Elevation of cholestatic parameters is usually more serious and can lead to cirrhosis and liver failure (143). Severe liver dysfunction in adult TPN recipients is rare and requires a search for causes other than TPN.

Infections are particularly serious complications in patients with malignancy receiving TPN. In general, infection rates vary, but various studies have shown rates of infections ranging from 0.38 to 4.58 episodes per 1,000 catheter-days (144). In an evaluation of seven studies comparing TPN plus chemotherapy to chemotherapy alone, Klein and Koretz found four studies that showed an increase in infectious complications in patients receiving TPN (123). A meta-analysis by the American College of Nutrition showed a 4-fold increase in infections when patients receiving chemotherapy were given TPN (115). In a prospective, randomized study of TPN following pancreatic resection, recipients of TPN had significantly more infectious complications (128). Data from a VA randomized cooperative study showed that patients with mild-to-moderate malnutrition given perioperative TPN had increased rates of infections, whereas those with severe malnutrition developed significantly fewer infections when supported with TPN (23). Infectious complications are related to both central venous catheters and a variety of sites (wound infection, abscess, and pneumonia).

Home Total Parenteral Nutrition

Long-term TPN in the home can be a lifesaving treatment in an appropriately selected group of patients. Patients with cancer who have had severe GI injury, such as massive intestinal resection or severe radiation enteritis, and in whom the cancer has been cured or is well controlled, benefit from long-term TPN at home (145). A study at the Mayo Clinic examined the outcomes of patients with gynecologic malignancies on home TPN. Inoperable bowel obstruction was the indication for TPN in most of these patients.

QoL parameters, including nausea, vomiting, fatigue, comfort, and morale, significantly improved in patients on home TPN compared with pre-TPN status, especially in those with Karnofsky status greater than 40 (146). Scolapio et al described 54 patients treated with home TPN after radiation enteritis. The majority had ovarian cancer, and the main causes of intestinal failure were intestinal obstruction from radiation strictures and short bowel syndrome. Approximately half of the patients initiated TPN within 6 months of completing radiation. Over two-thirds of the patients died due to recurrent cancer. However, survival rates and TPN-related complications were comparable to those in patients with benign diseases, such as Crohn disease and intestinal necrosis, who required home TPN (147). The role of TPN in advanced- or end-stage disease is controversial. For patients with inoperable bowel obstruction due to metastatic ovarian cancer, predicting which patients will benefit from home TPN can be difficult (148). In a review of 9,897 days of home TPN administered to 75 patients with various cancers and intestinal obstruction, it was shown that a Karnofsky performance status greater than 50 at the initiation of TPN could accurately predict which patients would have improved QoL while on home TPN. The authors concluded that home TPN should be avoided if the performance status is below this level (149). In addition, patients with a life expectancy of less than 2 to 3 months will not benefit from home TPN (1006,149). In a study from Yale-New Haven Hospital of 17 patients with inoperable bowel obstruction due to malignancy, patients with ovarian cancer had the shortest survival (39 days) compared to patients with colon cancer (90 days) and appendiceal cancer (184 days) (150). A study from the Mayo Clinic in 52 patients with advanced incurable cancer on home TPN found just two patients with ovarian cancer who survived longer than 12 months (146). A study from Brown University evaluated 55 patients with terminal ovarian cancer and found the use of TPN conferred a median survival benefit of 4 weeks (151). Patients on TPN were also more likely to receive concurrent chemotherapy (64% vs 26%). In another study by Diver et al., 115 women with gynecologic malignancies underwent venting gastrostomy tube placement for malignant bowel obstruction. The median survival of patients receiving TPN was 9.6 versus 4.6 weeks in those not receiving TPN (152). In a study by Theilla et al, patients with advanced cancer and GI obstruction were found to benefit from home parenteral nutrition. Of 221 patients with advanced cancer who had no oral/enteral intake and received home TPN, 153 survived. At the 6-month follow-up 35% survived, at 12 months 27%, at 2 years 18.9%, and 2.9% survived for the 7-year follow-up. Hospitalizations rates were also not found to be significantly remarkable (153). A recent meta-analysis of patients with ovarian or GI cancer with malignant bowel obstruction was attempted but, owing to the heterogeneity of data, was unable to be performed so data from 13 studies were synthesized via a narrative summary. The derived evidence for benefit from home parenteral nutrition was very low for survival and QoL, and in conclusion, the authors were unable to determine whether there was an improvement in survival or QoL (154).

Currently, the best selection criteria for such patients are a fair or better performance status and the potential for further antitumor therapy (**Table 12.4-2**). Only a highly selected minority of patients with end-stage cancer and inoperable bowel obstruction

can potentially benefit from home TPN. There are several QoL and ethical issues to be considered among this group of patients, and more data from RCTs are required.

Recently developed techniques for placing feeding tubes make it possible to hydrate and feed patients enterally, even in the presence of GI obstruction, and thus obviate the need for home TPN in patients with upper GI tract dysfunction.

Enteral Nutrition

Enteral feeding delivers a liquid-nutrient formula into the GI tract through tubes placed into the stomach or small intestine. As in oral feeding, an adequately functioning small intestinal mucosa is required for absorption of nutrients. Enteral feeding can overcome many difficulties encountered in patients with a wide variety of GI tract dysfunction. A proximal GI obstruction can be bypassed; tubes can be placed distal to obstructions as far as the jejunum and thus circumvent obstructing lesions of the oral cavity, esophagus, stomach, duodenum, or proximal jejunum (155-159). The liquid-nutrient formula can be delivered as a slow, continuous infusion, thus maximizing absorption by a limited intestinal surface, which can be overwhelmed by the higher volume delivered during oral feeding. Such an approach may be useful in patients with radiation enteritis, short bowel syndrome (with adequate remaining short bowel, usually 3-4 feet), or partial obstruction of the bowel.

Route of Administration and Nutrient Formula

Short-term (<2 weeks) access to the GI tract can be obtained through NGTs or nasoenteric tubes. Patients requiring longer nutritional support should have a gastrostomy or jejunostomy tube placed endoscopically, radiologically, or surgically. In comparison to nasal tubes, gastrostomy or jejunostomy tubes are wider (15-24 Fr) and, therefore, less likely to be obstructed by medications or nutrient solutions. In addition, they are fixed in the stomach or the upper intestine and do not migrate into the esophagus. Thus, the risk of aspiration is decreased, but not eliminated (155). These tubes are more comfortable and aesthetically pleasing. These benefits were demonstrated in a randomized study of patients after an acute dysphagic stroke, which showed patients fed with a gastrostomy tube had more optimal provision of nutrients, achieved a better nutritional state, and had less mortality than those fed with NGTs (160). Patients with gastrostomy tubes have been shown in prospective studies to receive over 90% of prescribed feedings compared to only 55% in patients fed through nasal tubes. These differences are largely attributed to NGT dislodgement (161). In addition, in a review of clinical effectiveness and guidelines performed in 2014 for patients with head or neck cancer, nine studies were evaluated comparing nasogastric feeding versus percutaneous. It was not able to be concluded that PEG was superior to traditional nasogastric feeding when evaluating maintenance of weight or survival, but PEG was found to be superior for rate of tube dislodgement and suitability of long-term feeding. In addition, PEG use allowed for greater mobility, enhanced cosmesis, and improved QoL (162). In a randomized study of 33 women with gynecologic malignancies, enteral feeding through a needle catheter jejunostomy maintained postoperative nutrition as measured by serum transferrin levels and was associated with few complications (163). The authors concluded that women with gynecologic cancers should have a jejunostomy placed at the time of operation if it is anticipated that long-term nutritional support will be required.

Endoscopically placed PEG has become the procedure of choice for placement of enteral feeding tubes because of its ease, safety, and the ability to perform it on an outpatient basis. Percutaneous endoscopic jejunostomy (PEJ) tubes can also be placed endoscopically (156-159). PEJ allows for continued enteral feeding in patients with gastric resection, gastric outlet obstruction, or gastroparesis (164). Major complications (bleeding, peritonitis, abdominal wall abscess, colonic perforation, and aspiration) from

---

▦ **TABLE 12.4-2. Indications for Home TPN in Patients With Gynecologic Cancers**

Severe chronic radiation enteropathy

Short bowel syndrome

Persistent enterocutaneous fistula

Selected patients with obstruction due to peritoneal carcinomatosis. (Selection based on performance status and potential for further chemotherapy)

TPN, total parental nutrition.

PEG and PEJ placement are rare, occurring in 0% to 2.5% of patients, whereas minor complications (wound infection, tube migrations, or leak) are seen in 5% to 15% (156,165,166,180). More than 100 different enteral feeding formulas are currently commercially available. They are designed to provide complete nutrition, single nutrients, or only fluids and electrolytes. Formulas differ in protein concentration, calories, osmolarity, and percentage of nonprotein calories delivered as carbohydrates or fats. Enteral feeding formulas, which provide 1,500 to 2,000 kcal/d, normally contain all the necessary nutrients, including proteins, vitamins, minerals, and trace elements. In addition, there are disease-specific formulations for patients with diabetes or hepatic, renal, or pulmonary dysfunction. The choice of formula should be individualized, and it often helps to minimize problems, such as diarrhea, bloating, or hyperglycemia.

Enteral solutions may be administered by either bolus feedings or continuous infusion. Bolus feeding is possible when the tip of the feeding tube is in an intact stomach. Up to 500 mL of a feeding formula can be infused over 10 to 15 minutes by a syringe or gravity into the stomach. The pyloric sphincter regulates flow into the duodenum. All bolus feedings should be done with the patient sitting upright to minimize the risk of aspiration. When the tip of the feeding tube is distal to the pylorus, continuous feeding must be employed to avoid abdominal distention and diarrhea. Rates as high as 150 mL/hr are generally well tolerated (155).

Efficacy

Data from randomized trials examining the efficacy of EN given as an adjuvant therapy in patients receiving chemotherapy for a variety of cancers have failed to demonstrate a clear benefit in terms of survival or response to treatment (167-171). The validity of the conclusions of these studies, however, is limited by their small size and poor design. Similar difficulties plague the studies examining the role of standard EN in the perioperative period (172-174). Accepted indications for EN in patients with cancer include (a) obstruction of the upper digestive tract in those in whom enteral access can be safely obtained beyond the site of obstruction, (b) the presence of chronic malnutrition due to inadequate oral intake, and (c) perioperative support of the malnourished patient (175).

Complications

EN is generally safe if careful attention is paid to the (a) choice of an appropriate formula, (b) infusion into an appropriate portion of the GI tract, (c) use of the correct infusion method, and (d) an ongoing clinical and metabolic monitoring of the patient. The most serious complication of enteral feeding is aspiration, which occurs in 1% to 32% of patients (167,176). The risk is minimized by keeping patients upright during bolus feedings and using jejunal feedings if there is predisposition for aspiration, gastroparesis, or an impaired gag reflex. There are various studies, such as that by Drakulovic et al, which found that aspiration pneumonia occurred in 23% of patients in supine position compared to 5% in patients in a semirecumbent position, but no differences in mortality were observed (177). Diarrhea is reported in 5% to 30% of patients receiving EN (178). While the diarrhea may be related to underlying disorders of the GI tract, such as radiation enteritis or short bowel syndrome, a commonly overlooked cause is medications. Patients on enteral feeding often receive magnesium-containing antacids or antibiotics, both of which may induce diarrhea. Metabolic complications include dehydration, azotemia, hyperglycemia, and hyperkalemia. These are usually due to the patient's underlying disease and can be avoided with the choice of the proper formula and careful monitoring.

Home Enteral Nutrition

Home enteral nutrition (HEN) is increasingly being used to provide nutrients and fluids outside the hospital. Cancer is the most common indication for its use and accounts for 42% of all patients receiving HEN (145). It is a safe therapy in patients with cancer, with only a 0.4% annual rate of complications requiring hospitalization (179). The overall 1-year survival for patients with cancer on HEN is 30%. However, in patients with cancer of the head and neck who have been successfully treated, HEN has provided good nutrition for periods exceeding 7 years (155,180). Regular medical follow-up is essential to ensure appropriate functioning of the feeding tube and optimization of the nutrition regimen. This form of therapy is useful in patients with gynecologic malignancies with upper GI tract obstructions that cannot be treated surgically.

Oral Dietary Therapy

Patients who are able to eat but have impairment of the GI tract or have special metabolic requirements may benefit from a specialized oral dietary therapy. Often, this may obviate the need for more costly and complex interventions, such as parenteral nutrition. In oral dietary therapy, the regular diet is modified based on the pathophysiologic changes induced by the underlying disorder, with the goal of providing the most optimal nutrition possible. When the main problem is inadequate food consumption, various commercial oral supplements can be used, but usually for only short periods because of taste fatigue. Some preparations provide complete nutrition, whereas others are intended to supplement deficits of specific nutrients. Problems common in patients with gynecologic malignancies, such as partial SBO, chronic radiation enteritis, and short bowel syndrome, may all be amenable to dietary therapies. In partial SBO or motility dysfunction, a diet consisting of frequent, small, calorically dense meals with minimal amounts of fiber is indicated. Patients with radiation enteritis should receive a low-fat, low-fiber, and lactose-free diet. Dietary management of patients with short bowel syndrome includes frequent small meals; limitation of fiber, lactose, and simple sugars; taking liquids separately from meals; and supplementation of calcium and zinc orally and magnesium and vitamin B_{12} parenterally.

Bye et al (181) conducted a prospective, randomized trial of a low-fat, low-lactose diet in 143 women with gynecologic malignancies undergoing radiation therapy. The intervention group had significantly less diarrhea. Diarrhea in the control group correlated with increased fatigue and decreased physical function. The authors concluded that diet intervention during radiotherapy reduced the severity of diarrhea, influenced patients' ability to cope with diarrhea, and gave them more control over their situation.

The successful implementation of prescribed diets depends to a large extent on a dietician converting the prescribed diet to a meal plan and working with the patient to implement it. In a prospective, randomized study of 57 patients undergoing chemotherapy for ovarian, breast, or lung cancer, those who received intensive dietary counseling had improved long-term food intake (182). Similar data have been demonstrated in patients with cancer undergoing radiotherapy (158-183) and in patients with acute leukemia undergoing induction chemotherapy (184).

Postoperative Timing of Oral Feeding

Traditionally, concerns for postoperative ileus and impaired bowel function have led to delayed feeding after abdominal surgery. In a prospective randomized trial at the University of Indiana, patients undergoing major gynecologic abdominal surgery were randomized into two groups: The first was advanced to a regular diet after return of bowel sounds and passage of flatus, and the second was fed on the first postoperative day with liquids and then advanced to a solid diet. Early feeding was associated with shorter time to tolerance of a solid diet and shorter duration of hospital stay, but a higher incidence of postoperative emesis (185). Subsequent studies in patients with gynecologic malignancies undergoing abdominal surgery have shown similar results, with quicker recovery of intestinal function, reduced postoperative wound complications, improved QoL scores, and shorter duration of hospital stay in those fed early after surgery (36,186-188).

Postoperative Immunonutrition

Nutrients such as arginine, glutamine, ω-3 fatty acids, and nucleotides are thought to enhance the immune response, modulate inflammation, and improve protein synthesis after surgery. They are added to enteral formulas or oral diets to improve postoperative wound healing and recovery. Two large meta-analyses have examined the benefits of immunonutrition in the perioperative period in patients undergoing major abdominal surgery. The majority of these patients had GI malignancies. There was a reduced rate of infectious complications, including abdominal abscesses, pneumonia, and wound infections, as well as noninfectious complications, including anastomotic leaks, in the group receiving immunonutrition. No differences in overall mortality were found among the two groups (189). These findings were supported by a recent study in gynecologic oncology patients at the University of California San Francisco undergoing laparotomy, given an immune-modulated diet in the perioperative period. Patients receiving immune-modulated diets had lower incidence of wound complications (19.6% vs 33%), leading the authors to conclude that an immune-modulated diet may be protective for the development of SSIs (190). An additional study by Celik et al examined 50 patients undergoing surgery for gynecologic malignancies, randomly assigning them to two groups. Each group received 2 days preoperative and 7 days postoperative EN after return of bowel function. The group given immune-enhancing EN was found to have lower rates of wound infection and length of stay (191). A dose of 0.5 to 1 L/d for 5 to 7 days before surgery is recommended (192). A study in patients with colorectal cancer found an increase in tumor-infiltrating CD4 and CD8 cells after they were given immune nutrition. The authors hypothesized that immune nutrients may reduce infections and exert antitumor effects by this mechanism (193). Current ESPEN guidelines recommend perioperative immunonutrition for patients undergoing upper GI surgery, but no recommendations exist for patients with gynecologic malignancies. The ASPEN guidelines recommend its use even among critically ill postoperative patients (194).

Pharmacologic Agents

Agents that will reverse the wasting seen in advanced cancers have long been sought to complement or replace the provision of nutrients via the oral, enteral, or parenteral route. Hormones, appetite stimulants, and, most recently, cytokine antagonists have been examined.

Hormonal Appetite Stimulants

Ghrelin, a potent orexigenic peptide hormone produced by the stomach, has been shown to increase appetite and caloric intake in normal individuals and in animal models of cancer cachexia. It was, therefore, hypothesized that ghrelin may be an effective treatment for cancer-induced cachexia. One small, randomized study showed that IV ghrelin led to a marked increase in energy and caloric intake, with no side effects (195). There was concern that its use would be limited by its promotion of cellular proliferation and invasion of certain types of cancer, but a randomized, placebo-controlled, double-blind, double crossover study demonstrated that ghrelin was safe and well tolerated. Anamorelin, a ghrelin agonist, has shown significant results in recent RCTs. In a randomized, double-blinded study of patients with advanced-stage NSCLC, administration of anamorelin demonstrated a significant increase in body weight and improvement in cachexia-associated symptoms (196). Garcia et al similarly in a double-blinded trial, but multicenter found that patients receiving 12 weeks of anamorelin achieved a significant increase in lean body mass (197).

Studies of growth factors IGF-I alone or IGF-I with insulin in cancer-bearing rodent models showed significant attenuation of tumor-induced weight loss. In human clinical trials, these agents provided modest gain in weight, but no improvement in QoL or other benefits (198-200). In addition, GH, a hormone that induces IGF-1 synthesis, has been approved for the treatment of HIV/AIDS-related muscle wasting, but there are no RCTs for cancer-related cachexia. This may be a future direction for investigation, but side effects such as insulin resistance and increased risk of cancer or growth of preexisting cancers may limit use in the oncologic population (201).

Selective androgen receptor modulators have also been assessed in cancer-related cachexia as they possess the ability to improve muscle mass increases, without the undesirable effects associated with nonselective or synthetic anabolic steroids. Enobosarm is emerging with a potential role in preventing or ameliorating muscle wasting in patients with cancer. In a recent study, it was found to be well tolerated and associated with an increase in lean body mass (202). All these findings support further investigation into these modalities.

Anabolic steroids have no proven efficacy in treating cancer cachexia. In a murine model, administration of nandrolone propionate resulted in weight gain, but this was largely due to fluid retention (203). In human trials, steroids produced transient improvement of nutritional parameters and appetite, but continued use is associated with negative nitrogen balance, net calcium loss, glucose intolerance, and immunosuppression (200).

Progestins, composed of megestrol acetate (MA) and medroxyprogesterone acetate (MPA), were the first drugs tested and most widely used agents in appetite enhancement and to ameliorate cancer cachexia. These progestational agents have been shown to improve appetite and ameliorate weight loss in numerous, but not all, studies of patients with cancer and cachexia (200). Doses in these studies ranged from 160 to 1,200 mg/d, and maximal weight gain was generally seen within 8 weeks. However, the change in weight is largely due to increased adipose tissue and edema (204). Nevertheless, improvement in QoL has consistently been demonstrated in several large prospective studies in patients with cancer-related cachexia treated with MA when compared with placebo though not when compared with other drugs (205-207). In addition, in 2013, a meta-analysis reviewed the role of MA in cachectic conditions with weight gain as the primary outcome and overall results showed weight improvement for patients with cancer treated with MA, but it did not result in recovery of initial weight in most trials (207). It is generally well tolerated but can exacerbate underlying diabetes mellitus, increase thrombotic risk, and, rarely, lead to adrenal suppression and an increased risk of death (208).

Cannabinoids and Analogs

Dronabinol and nabilone are marijuana derivatives that are both FDA approved for medical use for chemotherapy-associated nausea and vomiting. Agents such as these have shown some promise in small studies, alleviating symptoms, improving appetite, and causing weight gain; however, large, randomized trials are lacking (200). A recent study completed in New York evaluated Medical marijuana (MM) utilization in patients with gynecologic cancer. A total of 45 patients were prescribed MM, of whom 89% were receiving chemotherapy. The median period of use was 5.2 months, and more than 70% of patients reported improvement in nausea and vomiting and 36% found improvement in pain (209,210). This small sample shows that there may be promise for MM in symptom management, which could be extrapolated to improvement in nutrition. Alternatively, another study by Strasser et al showed no significant difference in QoL or appetite in a cohort of patients with cancer-associated cachexia syndrome. Patients in this cohort received cannabis extract, Δ-(9)-tetrahydrocannabinol (THC), and placebo (210). The SGO has recently released a clinical practice statement with regard to cannabinoid use. This document refers to the ASCO guidelines, which recommend using FDA-approved cannabinoids for nausea and vomiting, which does not respond to other agents. Other systematic reviews conducted have similarly shown that using cannabinoids should only be initiated when other agents have not been efficacious. There remains much work to be done with regard to improving the current dearth of evidence, which would further encourage MM use, and prospective studies are needed.

Cytokine Inhibitors

Inhibitors of cytokines involved in cancer-related cachexia and anorexia have the potential to be potent agents in the treatment of malnutrition in cancer. Monoclonal antibodies against TNF lead to improved food intake and diminished loss of protein and fat in murine models of cancer-related cachexia. Similar data are available for anti–IL-6 (211,212) and anti–IFN-γ. Suramin, a direct IL-6 receptor antagonist, decreased several key parameters of cachexia in tumor-bearing mice (213). In a study from Japan, a novel inhibitor of IL-1 and TNF-α showed that direct injection of the drug into tumor did not alter tumor growth but did result in attenuation of loss of body weight and epididymal fat in tumor-bearing mice (214). Human studies utilizing the anticytokine approach are limited but emerging. Phase I/II trials demonstrated an IL-6 inhibitor was safe to ameliorate cachexia and anemia in a population of patients with lung cancer, but no effects on lean body mass were reported (215). In addition, case studies have found tocilizumab administration to be associated with body weight increase and response in nutritional status, inflammation, anemia, and performance status (216). Pentoxifylline and thalidomide have been shown to inhibit TNF-α and IL-6. In two small studies, thalidomide at a dose of 200 mg daily attenuated loss of weight and lean body mass in patients with esophageal and pancreatic cancer (217,218). There remain limited RCTs, and there is insufficient evidence to recommend routine use of thalidomide in cancer-related cachexia. Interestingly, recent data showed that the clinical anticachexia effects of MA are due, at least in part, to the inhibition of cytokines (100) (**Table 12.4-3**).

The role of JAK/STAT3 pathway in mediating IL-6–induced weight loss and muscle wasting is also being evaluated. An open-label phase II clinical trial is investigating the safety and efficacy of ruxolitinib for cachexia in patients with cancer, which has previously shown that patients with myelofibrosis have an associated weight gain and improvement in nutritional parameters (219).

Cyclooxygenase-2 Inhibitors

Cyclooxygenase-2 (COX-2) inhibitors, such as ibuprofen and celecoxib, have been studied for their ability to attenuate the acute-phase response in patients with advanced cancer. Phase II studies have shown improvement in inflammatory status, performance status, weight gain, and survival. However, the data from these studies have remained largely inconclusive and insufficient to garner routine use (220-222).

Combination Therapies

In a recent study, Mantovani et al showed that combination therapy with MA, eicosapentaenoic acid, thalidomide, and L-carnitine increased lean body mass and appetite and decreased REE and fatigue in patients with cancer-related cachexia (223). This shows promise for the future for combination therapies for cancer-related cachexia.

Elemental Supplements and Vitamins

A few preclinical and clinical studies have examined the role of elemental supplements, administered in liquid or powder form, in mitigating the GI symptoms following pelvic radiation. However, these supplements are poorly tolerated and have not proven to be of benefit (224,225). Antioxidant vitamins such as vitamins C and E have proven to be of some benefit in ischemic-reperfusion injury (226). In a study by Kennedy et al, 20 patients with severe symptomatic radiation proctitis were given vitamins C and E for 4 weeks. The group receiving vitamin supplementation had improvement in diarrhea, bleeding, and fecal urgency (227). Some trials have examined the effect of combined ω-3 fatty acids, especially eicosapentaenoic acid, and vitamin E in cancer cachexia. However, there is still insufficient evidence to support their use (228,229). There remain various ongoing investigations for other modalities for treating cancer-related cachexia, involving targets for different pathways, some with preliminary data showing promise for improvements in lean body mass and other parameters (219).

Gut Microbiota

The modulation of microbiota before chemoradiation may provide ways to enhance treatment efficacy. There may also be a role between pathogens and cancer development, which has been proven in other neoplasms such as colon cancer. Currently, the role of the microbiome has been studied in patients with cervical cancer and ovarian cancer. In a study at the University of Texas MD Anderson Cancer Center, rectal swabs were collected from patients with cervical cancer but found that there was no difference according to histology, grade, or stage. Patients with greater gut diversity were found to have a longer median risk-free survival. The gut microbiome has also been shown to influence immunotherapy by mediating T-cell activation. There is more being studied to understand the relationship between gut microbiota modifications and efficacy and adverse effects of cancer therapies. Further studies are needed to evaluate the relationship between gut diversity and treatment efficacy to further understand the role of the gut microbiome in gynecologic cancers (230,231).

■ TABLE 12.4-3. Pharmacologic Agents Used for the Treatment of Cancer-related Cachexia and Anorexia

Class of Agent	Example	Efficacy	Adverse Effects
Hormones	Insulin, IGF, GH	Attenuation of tumor-induced weight loss, *no* improvement in survival or quality of life demonstrated	Hypoglycemia, hypokalemia
Anabolic steroids	Oxandrolone, nandrolone	Transient improvement in appetite	Fluid retention, net loss of calcium and nitrogen, hyperglycemia, immunosuppression
Progestational agents	Megestrol acetate	Improved appetite, weight, and quality of life	Weight gain is mostly due to fluid retention and adipose tissue, may exacerbate diabetes mellitus, rare cases of adrenal insufficiency
Cannabinoids	Dronabinol	Improved appetite and weight gain in small studies	CNS effects (slurred speech, nausea, dizziness, sedation)
Cytokine inhibitors	Pentoxifylline, thalidomide, suramin monoclonal antibodies to IL-1, IL-6, and TNF-α	Improved food intake and attenuation of protein and lean body mass loss	Peripheral neuropathy Rash Daytime somnolence

CNS, central nervous system; GH, growth hormone; IGF, insulin-like growth hormone; IL-6, interleukin-16; TNF, tumor necrosis factor.

ETHICAL CONSIDERATIONS

Before the advent of enteral and parenteral feedings, the inability to receive nutrients through oral intake inevitably led to wasting and death. Therefore, in the majority of patients, the natural history of cancer led to death because of dehydration and starvation. In patients with potentially curable or stable disease, nutritional support, when indicated, is an important and often critical part of the overall treatment plan. On the other hand, the role of nutritional support in the terminally ill is a subject filled with ethical and legal dilemmas. These problems come to light when the wishes of the patient or the patient's representative are not in agreement with the recommendations of the physicians. For example, a patient may wish to forego nutritional support despite recommendations that such a therapy should be given. Alternatively, patients or their representatives may want to initiate or continue TPN even after all anticancer therapies have failed and the patient is in a terminal state. Two general principles apply: in the first case, autonomy, and in the second, medical futility.

Autonomy is the right of competent patients to make decisions over their care and implies that the physician must solicit these decisions. It was not until the mid-1960s that autonomy began to supersede the Hippocratic tradition with its emphasis on the authoritarian role of the physician. This principle is clearly outlined in a report from the President's Commission for the study of Ethical Problems in Medicine and Biomedical and Behavioral Research, which states: "The voluntary choice of a competent and informed patient should determine whether or not life-sustaining therapy will be undertaken, while health care institutions and professionals should try to enhance patients' abilities to make decisions on their own and to promote understanding of the available options" (232). Regarding most treatments (surgery, chemotherapy, radiation therapy), the patient's knowledge and experience may be very limited and thus the physician's recommendations may form the sole basis for the patient's decisions. This is often not the case with nutrition. People understand the role of nutrition in sustaining life, and it is often hard for a lay person to understand why parenteral nutrition may not be indicated or even harmful when the patient has no other source of nourishment.

The principle of medical futility often surfaces in discussion of nutritional support of the patient with cancer, especially if the disease is advanced and unresponsive to therapy. There are four aspects to medical futility (233): (i) lack of physiologic rationale for the proposed therapy; (ii) failure of the same therapy in a previous attempt; (iii) all possible treatments for the underlying disease have failed; and (iv) the therapy will not improve QoL or achieve a goal of care (such as living to see a particular life event). In the case of parenteral (and rarely enteral) nutritional support of the patient with cancer, aspects iii and iv may be specifically applicable.

It should be noted that these principles, autonomy and medical futility, should govern decisions for both initiation and withdrawal of an ongoing therapy.

Religious beliefs often strongly influence decisions regarding nutritional support. Publicly stated opinions on the subject include (i) a statement from the Archbishop of Canterbury that removal from life support was permitted if it was better to allow the patient to die (234); (ii) a papal statement from Pope John Paul II in 2004 that concluded "artificial nutrition was ordinary and proportionate, and as such morally obligatory" as long as it obtains the goals of "providing nourishment to the patient" and "alleviating suffering." Although this statement referred specifically to the provision of artificial nutrition in persistent vegetative states, the same principles may be applied to other end-of-life situations (235); and (iii) a review of Orthodox Jewish rabbinical decisions that concluded "the imperative to preserve life supersedes, with a few exceptions, quality of life considerations" (236).

The decision to withhold or withdraw parenteral nutrition should involve an explanation that dying patients experience less hunger and thirst and that dehydration may even alleviate symptoms like choking or drowning sensation from secretions, coughing, nausea, and vomiting (237,238). The potential harmful effects of artificial nutrition support, including electrolyte abnormalities, infection, and fluid overload, should also be discussed. Ultimately, the end decision must remain with the patient or their surrogate. The ADA position paper on artificial nutrition and hydration in the terminally ill states that "the patient's expressed desire is the primary guide for determining the extent of nutrition and hydration," emphasizing the principle of autonomy (239).

Legally and ethically, an informed adult with the capacity to make decisions has the right to ask for artificial nutrition support to be withheld, even if such a decision results in death. For the gynecologic oncologist, management of the patient with an inoperable bowel obstruction due to peritoneal carcinomatosis is a difficult and recurrent problem. A recent review attempted to outline the role of parenteral nutrition in this population (148). TPN should be considered only for those patients with a good performance status, and careful attention must be paid to medical and symptomatic outcomes, as well as ethical considerations. It is interesting to note the views of patients on various life-sustaining treatments. In a study from the University of Michigan, 90% of women undergoing treatment for gynecologic cancer could envision a time when they would refuse ventilator support, but only 37% could foresee a time when they would refuse artificial nutrition (240). It is important for the physician and other members of the health care team to inform the patient and the family that in the terminally ill, provision of food and water by enteral or parenteral routes will not improve comfort (75) and, in fact, may add to discomfort (75,79,83,240). At Memorial Sloan Kettering Cancer Center, TPN is used infrequently in patients with gynecologic cancer and bowel obstruction due to malignant carcinomatosis who do not receive any further anticancer therapy. TPN is used under these conditions only when it is judged that it will enhance the QoL of a patient who is not at imminent risk of dying despite widely metastatic disease. When considering the chance of improving QoL, the burden of TPN administration and monitoring and the risk of complications must be considered. Ethical considerations also stem beyond TPN and can be extrapolated to EN whether provided by percutaneous modalities or NGTs or orogastric tubes. As different therapies are discovered and utilized more frequently for the treatment of cancer-related cachexia, it is of utmost importance that QoL and extension of meaningful life be considered.

REFERENCES

1. White JV, Guenter P, Jensen G, et al. Consensus statement: Academy of Nutrition and Dietetics and American Society for Parenteral and Enteral Nutrition: characteristics recommended for the identification and documentation of adult malnutrition (undernutrition). *JPEN J Parenter Enteral Nutr.* 2012;36: 275-283. doi:10.1177/0148607112440285

2. Trosian MJ. Nutritional assessment. In: Kaminski ME, ed. *Hyperalimentation: A Guide for Clinicians.* Marcel Dekker; 1985:47.

3. Kuroki LM, Mangano M, Allsworth JE, et al. Pre-operative assessment of muscle mass to predict surgical complications and prognosis in patients with endometrial cancer. *Ann Surg Oncol.* 2015;22(3):972-979. doi:10.1245/s10434-014-4040-8

4. Nixon DW, Heymsfield SB, Cohen AE, et al. Protein-calorie undernutrition in hospitalized cancer patients. *Am J Med.* 1980;68(5):683-690. Accessed March 6, 2016. http://www.ncbi.nlm.nih.gov/pubmed/6769330

5. Dowd PS, Heatley RV. The influence of undernutrition on immunity. *Clin Sci (Lond).* 1984;66(3):241-248. Accessed March 6, 2016. http://www.ncbi.nlm.nih.gov/pubmed/6420109

6. Meakins JL, Christou NV, Shizgal HM, et al. Therapeutic approaches to anergy in surgical patients. Surgery and levamisole. *Ann Surg.* 1979;190(3):286-296. Accessed March 6, 2016. https://www.ncbi.nlm.nih.gov/pmc/articles/PMC1344654/

7. Mullen JL, Buzby GP, Waldman MT, et al. Prediction of operative morbidity and mortality by preoperative nutritional assessment. *Surg*

Forum. 1979;30:80-82. Accessed March 6, 2016. http://www.ncbi.nlm.nih.gov/pubmed/538705

8. Buzby GP, Mullen JL, Matthews DC, et al. Prognostic nutritional index in gastrointestinal surgery. *Am J Surg.* 1980;139(1):160-167. Accessed March 6, 2016. http://www.ncbi.nlm.nih.gov/pubmed/7350839

9. Baker JP, Detsky AS, Wesson DE, et al. Nutritional assessment: a comparison of clinical judgement and objective measurements. *N Engl J Med.* 1982;306(16):969-972. doi:10.1056/NEJM198204223061606

10. Detsky AS, Baker JP, O'Rourke K, et al. Predicting nutrition-associated complications for patients undergoing gastrointestinal surgery. *JPEN J Parenter Enteral Nutr.* 1987;11(5):440-446. Accessed March 6, 2016. http://www.ncbi.nlm.nih.gov/pubmed/3656631

11. Crowe PJ, Snyman AM, Dent DM, et al. Assessing malnutrition in gastric carcinoma: bioelectrical impedance or clinical impression? *Aust N Z J Surg.* 1992;62(5):390-393. Accessed March 6, 2016. http://www.ncbi.nlm.nih.gov/pubmed/1575661

12. Ottow RT, Bruining HA, Jeekel J. Clinical judgment versus delayed hypersensitivity skin testing for the prediction of postoperative sepsis and mortality. *Surg Gynecol Obstet.* 1984;159(5):475-477. Accessed March 6, 2016. http://www.ncbi.nlm.nih.gov/pubmed/6495145

13. Pettigrew RA, Hill GL. Indicators of surgical risk and clinical judgement. *Br J Surg.* 1986;73(1):47-51. Accessed March 6, 2016. http://www.ncbi.nlm.nih.gov/pubmed/3947877

14. Detsky AS, Baker JP, Mendelson RA, et al. Evaluating the accuracy of nutritional assessment techniques applied to hospitalized patients: methodology and comparisons. *JPEN J Parenter Enteral Nutr.* 1984;8(2):153-159. Accessed March 7, 2016. http://www.ncbi.nlm.nih.gov/pubmed/6538911

15. Gupta D, Lammersfeld CA, Vashi PG, et al. Can subjective global assessment of nutritional status predict survival in ovarian cancer? *J Ovarian Res.* 2008;1(1):5. doi:10.1186/1757-2215-1-5

16. Phippen NT, Lowery WJ, Barnett JC, et al. Evaluation of the Patient-Generated Subjective Global Assessment (PG-SGA) as a predictor of febrile neutropenia in gynecologic cancer patients receiving combination chemotherapy: a pilot study. *Gynecol Oncol.* 2011;123(2):360-364. doi:10.1016/j.ygyno.2011.07.093

17. Laky B, Janda M, Cleghorn G, et al. Comparison of different nutritional assessments and body-composition measurements in detecting malnutrition among gynecologic cancer patients. *Am J Clin Nutr.* 2008;87(6):1678-1685. Accessed March 6, 2016. http://www.ncbi.nlm.nih.gov/pubmed/18541556

18. Hauer-Jensen M, Denham JW, Andreyev HJN. Radiation enteropathy—pathogenesis, treatment and prevention. *Nat Rev Gastroenterol Hepatol.* 2014;11(8):470-479. doi:10.1038/nrgastro.2014.46

19. Nganga D, Hoover A. (2021). Visceral adipose volume as a predictor for acute bowel toxicity in patients receiving adjuvant intensity-modulated radiation therapy for cervical or endometrial cancer. *Int J Radiat Oncol Biol Phys.* 2021;111(3):e632. doi:10.1016/j.ijrobp.2021.07.1677

20. Dewys WD, Begg C, Lavin PT, et al. Prognostic effect of weight loss prior to chemotherapy in cancer patients. Eastern Cooperative Oncology Group. *Am J Med.* 1980;69(4):491-497. Accessed March 6, 2016. http://www.ncbi.nlm.nih.gov/pubmed/7424938

21. Groot LMD, Lee G, Ackerie A, van der Meij BS. Malnutrition screening and assessment in the cancer care ambulatory setting: mortality predictability and validity of the Patient-Generated Subjective Global Assessment Short form (PG-SGA SF) and the GLIM criteria. *Nutrients.* 2020;12(8):2287. doi:10.3390/nu12082287

22. Ollenschläger G, Viell B, Thomas W, et al. Tumor anorexia: causes, assessment, treatment. *Recent Results Cancer Res.* 1991;121:249-259. Accessed March 7, 2016. http://www.ncbi.nlm.nih.gov/pubmed/1857862

23. Veterans Affairs Total Parenteral Nutrition Cooperative Study Group. Perioperative total parenteral nutrition in surgical patients. *N Engl J Med.* 1991;325(8):525-532. doi:10.1056/NEJM199108223250801

24. Santoso JT, Canada T, Latson B, et al. Prognostic nutritional index in relation to hospital stay in women with gynecologic cancer. *Obstet Gynecol.* 2000;95(6 pt 1):844-846. Accessed March 6, 2016. http://www.ncbi.nlm.nih.gov/pubmed/10831978

25. Hertlein L, Kirschenhofer A, Fürst S, et al. Malnutrition and clinical outcome in gynecologic patients. *Eur J Obstet Gynecol Reprod Biol.* 2014;174:137-140. doi:10.1016/j.ejogrb.2013.12.028

26. Rodrigues CS, Chaves GV. Patient-generated subjective global assessment in relation to site, stage of the illness, reason for hospital admission, and mortality in patients with gynecological tumors. *Support Care Cancer.* 2015;23:871-879. doi:10.1007/s00520-014-2409-7

27. Warren RS, Starnes HF, Gabrilove JL, et al. The acute metabolic effects of tumor necrosis factor administration in humans. *Arch Surg.*

1987;122(12):1396-1400. Accessed March 7, 2016. http://www.ncbi.nlm.nih.gov/pubmed/3689116

28. Dempsey DT, Mullen JL, Buzby GP. The link between nutritional status and clinical outcome: can nutritional intervention modify it? *Am J Clin Nutr.* 1988;47(2 suppl):352-356. Accessed March 7, 2016. http://www.ncbi.nlm.nih.gov/pubmed/3124596

29. Nicolini A, Ferrari P, Masoni MC, Fini M, Pagani S, Giampietro O, Carpi A. Malnutrition, anorexia and cachexia in cancer patients: a mini-review on pathogenesis and treatment. *Biomed Pharmacother.* 2013;67(8):807-817. https://doi.org/10.1016/j.biopha.2013.08.005

30. Geisler JP, Linnemeier GC, Thomas AJ, et al. Nutritional assessment using prealbumin as an objective criterion to determine whom should not undergo primary radical cytoreductive surgery for ovarian cancer. *Gynecol Oncol.* 2007;106(1):128-131. doi:10.1016/j.ygyno.2007.03.008

31. Díaz-Montes TP, Zahurak ML, Bristow RE. Predictors of extended intensive care unit resource utilization following surgery for ovarian cancer. *Gynecol Oncol.* 2007;107(3):464-468. doi:10.1016/j.ygyno.2007.07.074

32. Kondrup J, Rasmussen HH, Hamberg O, Stanga Z; Ad Hoc ESPEN Working Group. Nutritional risk screening (NRS 2002): a new method based on an analysis of controlled clinical trials. *Clin Nutr.* 2003;22(3):321-336. Accessed December 1, 2015. http://www.ncbi.nlm.nih.gov/pubmed/12765673

33. Hertlein L, Kirschenhofer A, Fürst S, et al. Malnutrition and clinical outcome in gynecologic patients. *Eur J Obstet Gynecol Reprod Biol.* 2014;174:137-140. doi:10.1016/j.ejogrb.2013.12.028.

34. Uppal S, Al-Niaimi A, Rice LW, et al. Preoperative hypoalbuminemia is an independent predictor of poor perioperative outcomes in women undergoing open surgery for gynecologic malignancies. *Gynecol Oncol.* 2013;131(2):416-422. doi:10.1016/j.ygyno.2013.08.011

35. Kathiresan ASQ, Brookfield KF, Schuman SI, Lucci, JA III. Malnutrition as a predictor of poor postoperative outcomes in gynecologic cancer patients. *Arch Gynecol Obstet.* 2011;284(2):445-451. doi:10.1007/s00404-010-1659-y

36. Rinninella E, Fagotti A, Cintoni M, et al. Nutritional interventions to improve clinical outcomes in ovarian cancer: a systematic review of randomized controlled trials. *Nutrients.* 2019;11(6):1404. doi:10.3390/nu11061404

37. Bekos C, Grimm C, Gensthaler L, et al. The pretreatment controlling nutritional status score in ovarian cancer: influence on prognosis, surgical outcome, and postoperative complication rate. *Geburtshilfe Frauenheilkd.* 2022;82(1):59-67. doi:10.1055/a-1608-1309

38. Croisier E, Morrissy A, Brown T, et al. Nutrition risk screening and implications for patients with gynaecological cancers undergoing pelvic radiotherapy and/or other treatment modalities: a retrospective observational study. *Nutr Diet.* 2022;79(2):217-228. doi:10.1111/1747-0080.12712

39. Gupta D, Lis CG, Vashi PG, Lammersfeld CA. Impact of improved nutritional status on survival in ovarian cancer. *Support Care Cancer.* 2010;18(3):373-381. doi:10.1007/s00520-009-0670-y

40. Fearon K, Strasser F, Anker SD, et al. Definition and classification of cancer cachexia: an international consensus. *Lancet Oncol.* 2011;12(5):489-495. doi:10.1016/S1470-2045(10)70218-7

41. Abu-Rustum NR, Barakat RR, Venkatraman E, Spriggs D. Chemotherapy and total parenteral nutrition for advanced ovarian cancer with bowel obstruction. *Gynecol Oncol.* 1997;64(3):493-495. doi:10.1006/gyno.1996.4605

42. Jong P, Sturgeon J, Jamieson CG. Benefit of palliative surgery for bowel obstruction in advanced ovarian cancer. *Can J Surg.* 1995;38(5):454-457. Accessed March 7, 2016. http://www.ncbi.nlm.nih.gov/pubmed/7553472

43. Rath KS, Loseth D, Muscarella P, et al. (2013). Outcomes following percutaneous upper gastrointestinal decompressive tube placement for malignant bowel obstruction in ovarian cancer. *Gynecol Oncol.* 2013;129(1):103-106. doi:10.1016/j.ygyno.2013.01.021

44. Tigert M, Lau C, Mackay H, L'Heureux S, Gien LT. Factors impacting length of stay and survival in patients with advanced gynecologic malignancies and malignant bowel obstruction. *Int J Gynecol Cancer.* 2021;31(5);727-732. doi:10.1136/ijgc-2020-002133

45. Ramos EJ, Suzuki S, Marks D, Inui A, Asakawa A, Meguid MM. Cancer anorexia-cachexia syndrome: cytokines and neuropeptides. *Curr Opin Clin Nutr Metab Care.* 2004;7(4):427-434. doi:10.1097/01.mco.0000134363.53782.cb

46. Norton JA, Moley JF, Green MV, Carson RE, Morrison SD. Parabiotic transfer of cancer anorexia/cachexia in male rats. *Cancer Res.* 1985;45(11 pt 1):5547-5552. Accessed March 7, 2016. http://www.ncbi.nlm.nih.gov/pubmed/3863707

47. Johnen H, Lin S, Kuffner T, et al. Tumor-induced anorexia and weight loss are mediated by the TGF-β superfamily cytokine MIC-1. *Nat Med.* 2007;13:1333-1340. doi:10.1038/nm1677

48. DeBoer MD. Animal models of anorexia and cachexia, *Expert Opin Drug Discov.* 2009;4(11):1145-1155. doi:10.1517/17460440903300842

49. DeWys WD. Anorexia as a general effect of cancer. *Cancer.* 1979;43(5 suppl):2013-2019. Accessed March 7, 2016. http://www.ncbi.nlm.nih.gov/pubmed/376105

50. DeWys WD, Walters K. Abnormalities of taste sensation in cancer patients. *Cancer.* 1975;36(5):1888-1896. Accessed March 7, 2016. http://www.ncbi.nlm.nih.gov/pubmed/1192373

51. Trant AS, Serin J, Douglass HO. Is taste related to anorexia in cancer patients? *Am J Clin Nutr.* 1982;36(1):45-58. Accessed March 7, 2016. http://www.ncbi.nlm.nih.gov/pubmed/6953761

52. Carson JA, Gormican A. Taste acuity and food attitudes of selected patients with cancer. *J Am Diet Assoc.* 1977;70(4):361-365. Accessed March 7, 2016. http://www.ncbi.nlm.nih.gov/pubmed/845347

53. Bernstein IL. Neutral mediation of food aversions and anorexia induced by tumor necrosis factor and tumors. *Neurosci Biobehav Rev.* 1996;20(1):177-181. Accessed March 7, 2016. http://www.ncbi.nlm.nih.gov/pubmed/8622825

54. Bernstein IL, Taylor EM, Bentson KL. TNF-induced anorexia and learned food aversions are attenuated by area postrema lesions. *Am J Physiol.* 1991;260(5 pt 2):R906-R910. Accessed March 7, 2016. http://www.ncbi.nlm.nih.gov/pubmed/2035702

55. Burnett AF, Potkul RK, Barter JF, Barnes WA, Delgado G. Colonic surgery in gynecologic oncology. Risk factor analysis. *J Reprod Med.* 1993;38(2):137-141. Accessed March 7, 2016. http://www.ncbi.nlm.nih.gov/pubmed/8445606

56. Hale MF. Radiation enteritis: from diagnosis to management. *Curr Opin Gastroenterol.* 2020;36(3):208-214. doi:10.1097/MOG.0000000000000632

57. Turtel PS, Shike M. Diseases of the small bowel. In: Shils ME, Olsen JA, Shike M, et al, eds. *Modern Nutrition in Health and Disease.* 9th ed. Lippincott Williams & Wilkins; 1999.

58. Scarantino CW, Ornitz RD, Hoffman LG, Anderson RF. On the mechanism of radiation-induced emesis: the role of serotonin. *Int J Radiat Oncol Biol Phys.* 1994;30(4):825-830. Accessed March 7, 2016. http://www.ncbi.nlm.nih.gov/pubmed/7525517

59. Bodis S, Alexander E, Kooy H, Loeffler JS. The prevention of radiosurgery-induced nausea and vomiting by ondansetron: evidence of a direct effect on the central nervous system chemoreceptor trigger zone. *Surg Neurol.* 1994;42(3):249-252. Accessed March 7, 2016. http://www.ncbi.nlm.nih.gov/pubmed/7940114

60. Sedgwick DM, Howard GC, Ferguson A. Pathogenesis of acute radiation injury to the rectum. A prospective study in patients. *Int J Colorectal Dis.* 1994;9(1):23-30. Accessed March 7, 2016. http://www.ncbi.nlm.nih.gov/pubmed/8027619

61. Kinsella TJ, Bloomer WD. Tolerance of the intestine to radiation therapy. *Surg Gynecol Obstet.* 1980;151(2):273-284. Accessed March 7, 2016. http://www.ncbi.nlm.nih.gov/pubmed/6996179

62. Libotte F, Autier P, Delmelle M, et al. Survival of patients with radiation enteritis of the small and the large intestine. *Acta Chir Belg.* 1995;95(4 suppl):190-194. Accessed March 7, 2016. http://www.ncbi.nlm.nih.gov/pubmed/8779298

63. Leung EW, Gladwish AP, Davidson MTM, et al. Stereotactic pelvic adjuvant radiation therapy in cancers of the uterus (SPARTACUS): a multicenter prospective trial evaluating acute toxicities and patient reported outcomes. *Int J Radiat Oncol Biol Phys.* 2021;111(3):S18-S19. doi:10.1016/j.ijrobp.2021.07.072

64. Zhou Y, Huang H, Wan T, Feng YL, Liu JH. Chronic radiation-induced rectal injury after adjuvant radiotherapy for pelvic malignant tumors: report based on a phase 3 randomized clinical trial. *Zhonghua Wei Chang Wai Ke Za Zhi.* 2021;24(11):962-968. doi:10.3760/cma.j.cn441530-20210720-00292

65. Husebye E, Hauer-Jensen M, Kjørstad K, et al. Severe late radiation enteropathy is characterized by impaired motility of proximal small intestine. *Dig Dis Sci.* 1994;39(11):2341-2349. Accessed March 7, 2016. http://www.ncbi.nlm.nih.gov/pubmed/7956601

66. Danielsson A, Nyhlin H, Persson H, Stendahl U, Stenling R, Suhr O. Chronic diarrhoea after radiotherapy for gynaecological cancer: occurrence and aetiology. *Gut.* 1991;32(10):1180-1187. Accessed March 7, 2016. https://www.ncbi.nlm.nih.gov/pmc/articles/PMC1379382/

67. Boland E, Thompson J, Rochling F, Sudan D. A 25-year experience with postresection short-bowel syndrome secondary to radiation therapy. *Am J Surg.* 2010;200(6):690-693; discussion 693. doi:10.1016/j.amjsurg.2010.07.035

68. Curran WJ. Radiation-induced toxicities: the role of radioprotectants. *Semin Radiat Oncol.* 1998;8(4 suppl 1):2-4. Accessed March 7, 2016. http://www.ncbi.nlm.nih.gov/pubmed/9794993

69. Tuech JJ, Chaudron V, Thoma V, et al. Prevention of radiation enteritis by intrapelvic breast prosthesis. *Eur J Surg Oncol.* 2004;30(8):900-904. doi:10.1016/j.ejso.2004.06.012.

70. Bajorin D, Kelsen D. Toxicity of antineoplastic therapy. In: Turnbull ADM, ed. *Surgical Emergencies in the Cancer Patient.* Year Book Medical Publishers; 1987:14.

71. Mitchell EP. Gastrointestinal toxicity of chemotherapeutic agents. *Semin Oncol.* 2006;33(1):106-120. https://doi.org/10.1053/j.seminoncol.2005.12.001

72. Calbresi P, Chabner B. Chemotherapy of neoplastic diseases. In: Gilman AG, Rall TW, Nies AS, et al, eds. *The Pharmacologic Basis of Therapeutics.* Pergamon Press; 1990:1201.

73. Steinbach S, Hummel T, Böhner C, et al. Qualitative and quantitative assessment of taste and smell changes in patients undergoing chemotherapy for breast cancer or gynecologic malignancies. *J Clin Oncol.* 2009;27(11):1899-1905. doi:10.1200/JCO.2008.19.2690

74. Massie MJ. Prevalence of depression in patients with cancer. *J Natl Cancer Inst Monogr.* 2004;32(32):57-71. doi:10.1093/jncimonographs/lgh014

75. Walker J, Hansen CH, Martin P, et al. Prevalence, associations, and adequacy of treatment of major depression in patients with cancer: a cross-sectional analysis of routinely collected clinical data. *Lancet Psychiatry.* 2014;1(5):343-350. doi:10.1016/S2215-0366(14)70313-X

76. Arbeit JM, Lees DE, Corsey R, Brennan MF. Resting energy expenditure in controls and cancer patients with localized and diffuse disease. *Ann Surg.* 1984;199(3):292-298. Accessed March 7, 2016. https://www.ncbi.nlm.nih.gov/pmc/articles/PMC1353395/

77. Dempsey DT, Feurer ID, Knox LS, Crosby LO, Buzby GP, Mullen JL. Energy expenditure in malnourished gastrointestinal cancer patients. *Cancer.* 1984;53(6):1265-1273. Accessed March 7, 2016. http://www.ncbi.nlm.nih.gov/pubmed/6692317

78. Hansell DT, Davies JW, Burns HJ. The relationship between resting energy expenditure and weight loss in benign and malignant disease. *Ann Surg.* 1986;203(3):240-245. Accessed March 7, 2016. https://www.ncbi.nlm.nih.gov/pmc/articles/PMC1251083/

79. Nguyen TY, Batterham MJ, Edwards C. Comparison of resting energy expenditure between cancer subjects and healthy controls: a meta-analysis. *Nutr Cancer.* 2016;68(3):374-387. doi:10.1080/01635581.2016.1153667

80. Luketich JD, Mullen JL, Feurer ID, Sternlieb J, Fried RC. Ablation of abnormal energy expenditure by curative tumor resection. *Arch Surg.* 1990;125(3):337-341. Accessed March 7, 2016. http://www.ncbi.nlm.nih.gov/pubmed/1689565

81. Dickerson RN, White KG, Curcillo PG II, King SA, Mullen JL. Resting energy expenditure of patients with gynecologic malignancies. *J Am Coll Nutr.* 1995;14(5):448-454. Accessed March 7, 2016. http://www.ncbi.nlm.nih.gov/pubmed/8522723

82. Argilés JM, Alvarez B, López-Soriano FJ. The metabolic basis of cancer cachexia. *Med Res Rev.* 1997;17(5):477-498. doi:10.1002/(SICI)1098-1128(199709)17:5<477::AID-MED3>3.0.CO;2-R

83. Honors MA, Kinzig KP. The role of insulin resistance in the development of muscle wasting during cancer cachexia. *J Cachexia Sarcopenia Muscle.* 2012;3(1):5-11.

84. Dev R, Bruera E, Dalal S. Insulin resistance and body composition in cancer patients. *Ann Oncol.* 2018;29:ii18-ii26. doi:10.1093/annonc/mdx815

85. Klein S, Wolfe RR. Whole-body lipolysis and triglyceride-fatty acid cycling in cachectic patients with esophageal cancer. *J Clin Invest.* 1990;86(5):1403-1408. doi:10.1172/JCI114854

86. Todorov PT, McDevitt TM, Meyer DJ, Ueyama H, Ohkubo I, Tisdale MJ. Purification and characterization of a tumor lipid-mobilizing factor. *Cancer Res.* 1998;58(11):2353-2358. Accessed March 9, 2016. http://www.ncbi.nlm.nih.gov/pubmed/9622074

87. Bing C, Russell ST, Beckett EE, et al. Expression of uncoupling proteins-1, -2 and -3 mRNA is induced by an adenocarcinoma-derived lipid-mobilizing factor. *Br J Cancer.* 2002;86(4):612-618. doi:10.1038/sj.bjc.6600101

88. Russell ST, Zimmerman TP, Domin BA, Tisdale MJ. Induction of lipolysis in vitro and loss of body fat in vivo by zinc-alpha2-glycoprotein. *Biochim Biophys Acta.* 2004;1636(1):59-68. doi:10.1016/j.bbalip.2003.12.004

89. Groundwater P, Beck SA, Barton C, Adamson C, Ferrier IN, Tisdale MJ. Alteration of serum and urinary lipolytic activity with weight loss in cachectic cancer patients. *Br J Cancer.* 1990;62(5):816-821. Accessed March 9, 2016. https://www.ncbi.nlm.nih.gov/pmc/articles/PMC1971511/

90. Beck SA, Groundwater P, Barton C, Tisdale MJ. Alterations in serum lipolytic activity of cancer patients with response to therapy. *Br J Cancer.* 1990;62(5):822-825. Accessed March 9, 2016. https://pubmed.ncbi.nlm.nih.gov/2245174/

91. Sanders PM, Tisdale MJ. Role of lipid-mobilising factor (LMF) in protecting tumour cells from oxidative damage. *Br J Cancer.* 2004;90(6):1274-1278. doi:10.1038/sj.bjc.6601669

92. Petruzzelli M, Schweiger M, Schreiber R, et al. A switch from white to brown fat increases energy expenditure in cancer-associated cachexia. *Cell Metab.* 2014;20(3):433-447. https://doi.org/10.1016/j.cmet.2014.06.011

93. Jurdana M. Cancer cachexia-anorexia syndrome and skeletal muscle wasting. *Rad Oncol.* 2009;43(2):65-75. doi:10.2478/v10019-009-0007-y

94. Hasselgren P-O, Wray C, Mammen J. Molecular regulation of muscle cachexia: it may be more than the proteasome. *Biochem Biophys Res Commun.* 2002;290(1):1-10. doi:10.1006/bbrc.2001.5849

95. Tisdale MJ. Mechanisms of cancer cachexia. *Physiol Rev.* 2009;89(2):381-410. doi:10.1152/physrev.00016.2008

96. Falconer JS, Fearon KC, Plester CE, Ross JA, Carter DC. Cytokines, the acute-phase response, and resting energy expenditure in cachectic patients with pancreatic cancer. *Ann Surg.* 1994;219(4):325-331. Accessed March 10, 2016. https://pubmed.ncbi.nlm.nih.gov/7512810/

97. Cabal-Manzano R, Bhargava P, Torres-Duarte A, Marshall J, Bhargava P, Wainer IW. Proteolysis-inducing factor is expressed in tumours of patients with gastrointestinal cancers and correlates with weight loss. *Br J Cancer.* 2001;84(12):1599-1601. doi:10.1054/bjoc.2001.1830

98. Tilignac T, Temparis S, Combaret L, et al. Chemotherapy inhibits skeletal muscle ubiquitin-proteasome-dependent proteolysis. *Cancer Res.* 2002;62(10):2771-2777. Accessed March 9, 2016. http://www.ncbi.nlm.nih.gov/pubmed/12019153

99. Tracey KJ, Wei H, Manogue KR, et al. Cachectin/tumor necrosis factor induces cachexia, anemia, and inflammation. *J Exp Med.* 1988;167(3):1211-1227. Accessed March 9, 2016. https://www.ncbi.nlm.nih.gov/pmc/articles/PMC2188883/

100. Mantovani G, Macciò A, Lai P, Massa E, Ghiani M, Santona MC. Cytokine activity in cancer-related anorexia/cachexia: role of megestrol acetate and medroxyprogesterone acetate. *Semin Oncol.* 1998;25(2 suppl 6):45-52. Accessed March 9, 2016. http://www.ncbi.nlm.nih.gov/pubmed/9625383

101. Pfitzenmaier J, Vessella R, Higano CS, Noteboom JL, Wallace D, Corey E. Elevation of cytokine levels in cachectic patients with prostate carcinoma. *Cancer.* 2003;97(5):1211-1216. doi:10.1002/cncr.11178

102. Warren RS, Donner DB, Starnes HF, Brennan MF. Modulation of endogenous hormone action by recombinant human tumor necrosis factor. *Proc Natl Acad Sci U S A.* 1987;84(23):8619-8622. Accessed March 9, 2016. https://www.ncbi.nlm.nih.gov/pmc/articles/PMC299597/

103. Llovera M, García-Martínez C, López-Soriano J, et al. Role of TNF receptor 1 in protein turnover during cancer cachexia using gene knockout mice. *Mol Cell Endocrinol.* 1998;142(1-2):183-189. Accessed March 10, 2016. http://www.ncbi.nlm.nih.gov/pubmed/9783914

104. Deans DAC, Tan BHL, Ross JA, et al. Cancer cachexia is associated with the IL10 -1082 gene promoter polymorphism in patients with gastroesophageal malignancy. *Am J Clin Nutr.* 2009;89(4):1164-1172. doi:10.3945/ajcn.2008.27025

105. Jeevanandam M, Horowitz GD, Lowry SF, Brennan MF. Cancer cachexia and protein metabolism. *Lancet.* 1984;1(8392):1423-1426. Accessed March 10, 2016. http://www.ncbi.nlm.nih.gov/pubmed/6145877

106. Sharp JW, Roncagli T. Home parenteral nutrition in advanced cancer. *Cancer Pract.* 1993;1(2):119-124. Accessed March 10, 2016. http://www.ncbi.nlm.nih.gov/pubmed/8324537

107. Nixon DW, Moffitt S, Lawson DH, et al. Total parenteral nutrition as an adjunct to chemotherapy of metastatic colorectal cancer. *Cancer Treat Rep.* 1981;65(suppl 5):121-128. Accessed March 9, 2016. http://www.ncbi.nlm.nih.gov/pubmed/6809321

108. Serrou B, Cupissol D, Plagne R, Boutin P, Carcassone Y, Michel FB. Parenteral intravenous nutrition (PIVN) as an adjunct to chemotherapy in small cell anaplastic lung carcinoma. *Cancer Treat Rep.* 1981;65(suppl 5):151-155. Accessed March 10, 2016. http://www.ncbi.nlm.nih.gov/pubmed/6286118

109. Valdivieso M, Bodey GP, Benjamin RS, et al. Role of intravenous hyperalimentation as an adjunct to intensive chemotherapy for small cell bronchogenic carcinoma. *Cancer Treat Rep.* 1981;65(suppl 5):145-150. Accessed March 9, 2016. http://www.ncbi.nlm.nih.gov/pubmed/6809324

110. Samuels ML, Selig DE, Ogden S, Grant C, Brown B. IV hyperalimentation and chemotherapy for stage III testicular cancer: a randomized study. *Cancer Treat Rep.* 1981;65(7-8):615-627. Accessed March 14, 2016. http://www.ncbi.nlm.nih.gov/pubmed/6166374

111. Daly JM, Reynolds J, Thom A, et al. Immune and metabolic effects of arginine in the surgical patient. *Ann Surg.* 1988;208(4):512-523. Accessed March 9, 2016. https://www.ncbi.nlm.nih.gov/pmc/articles/PMC8747899/

112. Fletcher JP, Little JM. A comparison of parenteral nutrition and early postoperative enteral feeding on the nitrogen balance after major surgery. *Surgery.* 1986;100(1):21-24. Accessed March 9, 2016. http://www.ncbi.nlm.nih.gov/pubmed/3088751

113. Klein S, Simes J, Blackburn GL. Total parenteral nutrition and cancer clinical trials. *Cancer.* 1986;58(6):1378-1386. Accessed March 9, 2016. http://www.ncbi.nlm.nih.gov/pubmed/3091243

114. McGeer AJ, Detsky AS, O'Rourke K. Parenteral nutrition in cancer patients undergoing chemotherapy: a meta-analysis. *Nutrition.* 1990;6(3):233-240. Accessed March 9, 2016. http://www.ncbi.nlm.nih.gov/pubmed/2152097

115. Parenteral nutrition in patients receiving cancer chemotherapy. American College of Physicians. *Ann Intern Med.* 1989;110(9):734-736. Accessed March 14, 2016. http://www.ncbi.nlm.nih.gov/pubmed/2494922

116. Klein S, Kinney J, Jeejeebhoy K, et al. Nutrition support in clinical practice: review of published data and recommendations for future research directions. *Clin Nutr.* 1997;16(4):193-218. Accessed March 14, 2016. http://www.ncbi.nlm.nih.gov/pubmed/16844599

117. Burnette B, Jatoi A. Parenteral nutrition in patients with cancer: recent guidelines and a need for further study. *Curr Opin Support Palliat Care.* 2010;4(4):272-275. doi:10.1097/SPC.0b013e32833ed6aa

118. Weisdorf SA, Lysne J, Wind D, et al. Positive effect of prophylactic total parenteral nutrition on long-term outcome of bone marrow transplantation. *Transplantation.* 1987;43(6):833-838. Accessed March 9, 2016. http://www.ncbi.nlm.nih.gov/pubmed/3109088

119. Baron PL, Lawrence W, Chan WM, White FK, Banks WL. Effects of parenteral nutrition on cell cycle kinetics of head and neck cancer. *Arch Surg.* 1986;121(11):1282-1286. Accessed March 9, 2016. http://www.ncbi.nlm.nih.gov/pubmed/3096261

120. Copeland EM III, Pimiento JM, Dudrick SJ. Total parenteral nutrition and cancer: from the beginning. *Surg Clin North Am.* 2011;91(4):727-736.

121. Märten A, Wente MN, Ose J, et al. An open label randomized multicentre phase IIIb trial comparing parenteral substitution versus best supportive nutritional care in subjects with pancreatic adenocarcinoma receiving 5-FU plus oxaliplatin as 2nd or higher line chemotherapy regarding clinical benefit—PANUSCO. *BMC Cancer.* 2009;9:412. doi:10.1186/1471-2407-9-412

122. Kinsella TJ, Malcolm AW, Bothe A, Valerio D, Blackburn GL. Prospective study of nutritional support during pelvic irradiation. *Int J Radiat Oncol Biol Phys.* 1981;7(4):543-548. Accessed March 9, 2016. http://www.ncbi.nlm.nih.gov/pubmed/6166598

123. Klein S, Koretz RL. Nutrition support in patients with cancer: what do the data really show? *Nutr Clin Pract.* 1994;9(3):91-100. Accessed March 9, 2016. http://www.ncbi.nlm.nih.gov/pubmed/8078449

124. Detsky AS, Baker JP, O'Rourke K, Goel V. Perioperative parenteral nutrition: a meta-analysis. *Ann Intern Med.* 1987;107(2):195-203. Accessed March 9, 2016. http://www.ncbi.nlm.nih.gov/pubmed/3111322

125. Fan ST, Lo CM, Lai EC, Chu KM, Liu CL, Wong J. Perioperative nutritional support in patients undergoing hepatectomy for hepatocellular carcinoma. *N Engl J Med.* 1994;331(23):1547-1552. doi:10.1056/NEJM199412083312303

126. Holter AR, Fischer JE. The effects of perioperative hyperalimentation on complications in patients with carcinoma and weight loss. *J Surg Res.* 1977;23(1):31-34. Accessed March 9, 2016. http://www.ncbi.nlm.nih.gov/pubmed/406484

127. Holter AR, Rosen HM, Fischer JE. The effects of hyperalimentation on major surgery in patients with malignant disease: a prospective study. *Acta Chir Scand Suppl.* 1976;466:86-87. Accessed March 9, 2016. http://www.ncbi.nlm.nih.gov/pubmed/828429

128. Brennan MF, Pisters PW, Posner M, Quesada O, Shike M. A prospective randomized trial of total parenteral nutrition after major pancreatic resection for malignancy. *Ann Surg.* 1994;220(4):436-441; discussion 441-444. Accessed March 9, 2016. https://www.ncbi.nlm.nih.gov/pmc/articles/PMC1234412/

129. Mendivil AA, Rettenmaier MA, Abaid LN, Brown JV III, Mori KM, Goldstein BH. The impact of total parenteral nutrition on postoperative recovery in patients treated for advanced stage ovarian cancer. *Arch Gynecol Obstet*. 2017;295(2):439-444. doi:10.1007/s00404-016-4227-2

130. Madhok BM, Yeluri S, Haigh K, Burton A, Broadhead T, Jayne DG. Parenteral nutrition for patients with advanced ovarian malignancy. *J Hum Nutr Diet*. 2011;24(2):187-191. doi:10.1111/j.1365-277X.2010.01127.x

131. Cobb DK, High KP, Sawyer RG, et al. A controlled trial of scheduled replacement of central venous and pulmonary-artery catheters. *N Engl J Med*. 1992;327(15):1062-1068. doi:10.1056/NEJM199210083271505

132. Parienti JJ, Mongardon N, Megarbane B, et al. Intravascular complications of central venous catheterization by insertion site. *N Engl J Med*. 2015;373:1220-1229.

133. Ukleja A, Romano MM. Complications of parenteral nutrition. *Gastroenterol Clin North Am*. 2007;36:23-46.

134. Shekelle PG, Wachter RM, Pronovost PJ, et al. Making health care safer II: an updated critical analysis of the evidence for patient safety practices. *Evid Rep Technol Assess (Full Rep)*. 2013;(211):1-945.

135. Kusminsky RE. Complications of central venous catheterization. *J Am Coll Surg*. 2007;204:681-696.

136. Cunningham MJ, Collins MB, Kredentser DC, Malfetano JH. Peripheral infusion ports for central venous access in patients with gynecologic malignancies. *Gynecol Oncol*. 1996;60(3):397-399. doi:10.1006/gyno.1996.0061

137. Estes JM, Rocconi R, Straughn JM, et al. Complications of indwelling venous access devices in patients with gynecologic malignancies. *Gynecol Oncol*. 2003;91(3):591-595. Accessed March 14, 2016. http://www.ncbi.nlm.nih.gov/pubmed/14675682

138. McMahon MM, Nystrom E, Braunschweig C, et al. A.S.P.E.N. clinical guidelines: nutrition support of adult patients with hyperglycemia. *JPEN J Parenter Enteral Nutr*. 2013;37:23-36.

139. Weinsier RL, Bacon J, Butterworth CE. Central venous alimentation: a prospective study of the frequency of metabolic abnormalities among medical and surgical patients. *JPEN J Parenter Enteral Nutr*. 1982;6(5):421-425. Accessed March 9, 2016. http://www.ncbi.nlm.nih.gov/pubmed/6818370

140. Weinsier RL, Krumdieck CL. Death resulting from overzealous total parenteral nutrition: the refeeding syndrome revisited. *Am J Clin Nutr*. 1981;34(3):393-399. Accessed March 14, 2016. http://www.ncbi.nlm.nih.gov/pubmed/6782855

141. Solomon SM, Kirby DF. The refeeding syndrome: a review. *JPEN J Parenter Enteral Nutr*. 1990;14(1):90-97. Accessed March 9, 2016. http://www.ncbi.nlm.nih.gov/pubmed/2109122

142. Lappas BM, Patel D, Kumpf V, Adams DW, Seidner DL. Parenteral nutrition: indications, access, and complications. *Gastroenterol Clin North Am*. 2018;47(1):39-59. doi:10.1016/j.gtc.2017.10.001

143. Nowak K. Parenteral nutrition–associated liver disease. *Clin Liver Dis (Hoboken)*. 2020;15:59-62. doi:10.1002/cld.888

144. Dreesen M, Foulon V, Spriet I, et al. Epidemiology of catheter-related infections in adult patients receiving home parenteral nutrition: a systematic review. *Clin Nutr*. 2013;32:16-26.

145. Howard L, Ament M, Fleming CR, Shike M, Steiger E. Current use and clinical outcome of home parenteral and enteral nutrition therapies in the United States. *Gastroenterology*. 1995;109(2):355-365. Accessed March 9, 2016. http://www.ncbi.nlm.nih.gov/pubmed/7615183

146. Hoda D, Jatoi A, Burnes J, Loprinzi C, Kelly D. Should patients with advanced, incurable cancers ever be sent home with total parenteral nutrition? A single institution's 20-year experience. *Cancer*. 2005;103(4):863-868. doi:10.1002/cncr.20824

147. Scolapio JS, Ukleja A, Burnes JU, Kelly DG. Outcome of patients with radiation enteritis treated with home parenteral nutrition. *Am J Gastroenterol*. 2002;97(3):662-666. doi:10.1111/j.1572-0241.2002.05546.x

148. Philip J, Depczynski B. The role of total parenteral nutrition for patients with irreversible bowel obstruction secondary to gynecological malignancy. *J Pain Symptom Manage*. 1997;13(2):104-111. Accessed March 9, 2016. http://www.ncbi.nlm.nih.gov/pubmed/9095568

149. Cozzaglio L, Balzola F, Cosentino F, et al. Outcome of cancer patients receiving home parenteral nutrition. Italian Society of Parenteral and Enteral Nutrition (S.I.N.P.E.). *JPEN J Parenter Enteral Nutr*. 1997;21(6):339-342. Accessed March 14, 2016. http://www.ncbi.nlm.nih.gov/pubmed/9406131

150. August DA, Thorn D, Fisher RL, Welchek CM. Home parenteral nutrition for patients with inoperable malignant bowel obstruction. *JPEN J Parenter Enteral Nutr*. 1991;15(3):323-327. Accessed March 9, 2016. http://www.ncbi.nlm.nih.gov/pubmed/1907683

151. Brard L, Weitzen S, Strubel-Lagan SL, et al. The effect of total parenteral nutrition on the survival of terminally ill ovarian cancer patients. *Gynecol Oncol*. 2006;103(1):176-180. doi:10.1016/j.ygyno.2006.02.013

152. Diver E, O'Connor O, Garrett L, et al. Modest benefit of total parenteral nutrition and chemotherapy after venting gastrostomy tube placement. *Gynecol Oncol*. 2013;129(2):332-335. doi:10.1016/j.ygyno.2013.02.002

153. Theilla M, Cohen J, Kagan I, Attal-Singer J, Lev S, Singer P. Home parenteral nutrition for advanced cancer patients: contributes to survival? *Nutrition*. 2018;54:197-200. doi:10.1016/j.nut.2017.03.005

154. Sowerbutts AM, Lal S, Sremanakova J, et al. Home parenteral nutrition for people with inoperabvnle malignant bowel obstruction. *Cochrane Database Syst Rev*. 2018;2018(8):CD012812. doi:10.1002/14651858.CD012812.pub2

155. Shike M. Enteral feeding. In: Shils ME, Olsen JA, Shike M, et al, eds. *Modern Nutrition in Health and Disease*. 9th ed. Lippincott Williams & Wilkins; 1999:1643.

156. Shike M, Latkany L. Direct percutaneous endoscopic jejunostomy. *Gastrointest Endosc Clin N Am*. 1998;8(3):569-580. Accessed March 9, 2016. http://www.ncbi.nlm.nih.gov/pubmed/9654569

157. Zhu Y, Shi L, Tang H, Tao G. Current considerations of direct percutaneous endoscopic jejunostomy. *Can J Gastroenterol*. 2012;26(2):92-96. doi:10.1155/2012/319843

158. Freeman C, Delegge MH. Small bowel endoscopic enteral access. *Curr Opin Gastroenterol*. 2009;25(2):155-159. doi:10.1097/MOG.0b013e328324f86b

159. Baron TH. Direct percutaneous endoscopic jejunostomy. *Am J Gastroenterol*. 2006;101(7):1407-1409.

160. Norton B, Homer-Ward M, Donnelly MT, Long RG, Holmes GK. A randomised prospective comparison of percutaneous endoscopic gastrostomy and nasogastric tube feeding after acute dysphagic stroke. *BMJ*. 1996;312(7022):13-16. Accessed March 9, 2016. https://pubmed.ncbi.nlm.nih.gov/8555849/

161. Di Lorenzo C, Lachman R, Hyman PE. Intravenous erythromycin for postpyloric intubation. *J Pediatr Gastroenterol Nutr*. 1990;11(1):45-47. Accessed March 9, 2016. http://www.ncbi.nlm.nih.gov/pubmed/2136585

162. Nasogastric feeding tubes versus percutaneous endoscopic gastrostomy for patients with head or neck cancer: a review of clinical effectiveness and guidelines [Internet]. Summary of Evidence. Canadian Agency for Drugs and Technologies in Health; 2014. https://www.ncbi.nlm.nih.gov/books/NBK253814/

163. Spirtos NM, Ballon SC. Needle catheter jejunostomy: a controlled, prospective, randomized trial in patients with gynecologic malignancy. *Am J Obstet Gynecol*. 1988;158(6 pt 1):1285-1290. Accessed March 15, 2016. http://www.ncbi.nlm.nih.gov/pubmed/3132853.

164. Heyland DK, Drover JW, Dhaliwal R, et al. Optimizing the benefits and minimizing the risks of enteral nutrition in the critically ill: role of small bowel feeding. *JPEN J Parenter Enteral Nutr*. 2002;26(6 suppl):S51-S57.

165. Safadi BY, Marks JM, Ponsky JL. Percutaneous endoscopic gastrostomy. *Gastrointest Endosc Clin N Am*. 1998;8(3):551-568. http://www.ncbi.nlm.nih.gov/pubmed/9654568.

166. Schrag SP, Sharma R, Jaik NP, et al. Complications related to percutaneous endoscopic gastrostomy (PEG) tubes. A comprehensive clinical review. *J Gastrointestin Liver Dis*. 2007;16(4):407-418.

167. Strong RM, Condon SC, Solinger MR, Namihas BN, Ito-Wong LA, Leuty JE. Equal aspiration rates from postpylorus and intragastric-placed small-bore nasoenteric feeding tubes: a randomized, prospective study. *JPEN J Parenter Enteral Nutr*. 1992;16(1):59-63. Accessed March 15, 2016. http://www.ncbi.nlm.nih.gov/pubmed/1738222

168. Elkort RJ, Baker FL, Vitale JJ, Cordano A. Long-term nutritional support as an adjunct to chemotherapy for breast cancer. *JPEN J Parenter Enteral Nutr*. 1981;5(5):385-390. Accessed March 15, 2016. http://www.ncbi.nlm.nih.gov/pubmed/6796711

169. Evans WK, Nixon DW, Daly JM, et al. A randomized study of oral nutritional support versus ad lib nutritional intake during chemotherapy for advanced colorectal and non-small-cell lung cancer. *J Clin Oncol*. 1987;5(1):113-124. Accessed March 15, 2016. http://www.ncbi.nlm.nih.gov/pubmed/3027267

170. Bozzetti F. Effects of artificial nutrition on the nutritional status of cancer patients. *JPEN J Parenter Enteral Nutr*. 1989;13(4):406-420. Accessed March 15, 2016. http://www.ncbi.nlm.nih.gov/pubmed/2506378

171. Bounous G, Gentile JM, Hugon J. Elemental diet in the management of the intestinal lesion produced by 5-fluorouracil in man. *Can J Surg*. 1971;14(5):312-324. Accessed March 15, 2016. http://www.ncbi.nlm.nih.gov/pubmed/4107102

172. Smith RC, Hartemink RJ, Hollinshead JW, Gillett DJ. Fine bore jejunostomy feeding following major abdominal surgery: a controlled

randomized clinical trial. *Br J Surg.* 1985;72(6):458-461. Accessed March 15, 2016. http://www.ncbi.nlm.nih.gov/pubmed/3926036

173. Ryan JA, Page CP, Babcock L. Early postoperative jejunal feeding of elemental diet in gastrointestinal surgery. *Am Surg.* 1981;47(9):393-403. Accessed March 15, 2016. http://www.ncbi.nlm.nih.gov/pubmed/6792958

174. Flynn MB, Leightty FF. Preoperative outpatient nutritional support of patients with squamous cancer of the upper aerodigestive tract. *Am J Surg.* 1987;154(4):359-362. Accessed March 15, 2016. http://www.ncbi.nlm.nih.gov/pubmed/3661837

175. Kirby DF, Teran JC. Enteral feeding in critical care, gastrointestinal diseases, and cancer. *Gastrointest Endosc Clin N Am.* 1998;8(3):623-643. Accessed March 15, 2016. http://www.ncbi.nlm.nih.gov/pubmed/9654573

176. Scolapio JS. Decreasing aspiration risk with enteral feeding. *Gastrointest Endosc Clin N Am.* 2007;17(4):711-716. doi:10.1016/j.giec.2007.07.013

177. Drakulovic MB, Torres A, Bauer TT, et al. Supine body position as a risk factor for nosocomial pneumonia in mechanically ventilated patients: a andomized trial. *Lancet.* 1999;354:1851-1858.

178. Bliss DZ, Guenter PA, Settle RG. Defining and reporting diarrhea in tube-fed patients-what a mess! *Am J Clin Nutr.* 1992;55(3):753-759. Accessed March 15, 2016. http://www.ncbi.nlm.nih.gov/pubmed/1550053

179. Sherry BA, Gelin J, Fong Y, et al. Anticachectin/tumor necrosis factor-alpha antibodies attenuate development of cachexia in tumor models. *FASEB J.* 1989;3(8):1956-1962. Accessed March 15, 2016. http://www.ncbi.nlm.nih.gov/pubmed/2721856

180. Shike M, Berner YN, Gerdes H, et al. Percutaneous endoscopic gastrostomy and jejunostomy for long-term feeding in patients with cancer of the head and neck. *Otolaryngol Head Neck Surg.* 1989;101(5):549-554. Accessed March 7, 2016. http://www.ncbi.nlm.nih.gov/pubmed/2512533

181. Bye A, Ose T, Kaasa S. Quality of life during pelvic radiotherapy. *Acta Obstet Gynecol Scand.* 1995;74(2):147-152. Accessed March 15, 2016. http://www.ncbi.nlm.nih.gov/pubmed/7900512

182. Ovesen L, Allingstrup L, Hannibal J, Mortensen EL, Hansen OP. Effect of dietary counseling on food intake, body weight, response rate, survival, and quality of life in cancer patients undergoing chemotherapy: a prospective, randomized study. *J Clin Oncol.* 1993;11(10):2043-2049. Accessed March 14, 2016. http://www.ncbi.nlm.nih.gov/pubmed/8410128

183. Maciá E, Moran J, Santos J, Blanco M, Mahedero G, Salas J. Nutritional evaluation and dietetic care in cancer patients treated with radiotherapy: prospective study. *Nutrition.* 1991;7(3):205-209. Accessed March 14, 2016. http://www.ncbi.nlm.nih.gov/pubmed/1802209

184. Ollenschläger G, Thomas W, Konkol K, Diehl V, Roth E. Nutritional behaviour and quality of life during oncological polychemotherapy: results of a prospective study on the efficacy of oral nutrition therapy in patients with acute leukaemia. *Eur J Clin Invest.* 1992;22(8):546-553. Accessed March 14, 2016. http://www.ncbi.nlm.nih.gov/pubmed/1425861

185. Schilder JM, Hurteau JA, Look KY, et al. A prospective controlled trial of early postoperative oral intake following major abdominal gynecologic surgery. *Gynecol Oncol.* 1997;67(3):235-240. doi:10.1006/gyno.1997.4860

186. Minig L, Biffi R, Zanagnolo V, et al. Reduction of postoperative complication rate with the use of early oral feeding in gynecologic oncologic patients undergoing a major surgery: a randomized controlled trial. *Ann Surg Oncol.* 2009;16(11):3101-3110. doi:10.1245/s10434-009-0681-4

187. Steed HL, Capstick V, Flood C, Schepansky A, Schulz J, Mayes DC. A randomized controlled trial of early versus "traditional" postoperative oral intake after major abdominal gynecologic surgery. *Am J Obstet Gynecol.* 2002;186(5):861-865. Accessed March 15, 2016. http://www.ncbi.nlm.nih.gov/pubmed/12015496

188. Charoenkwan K, Matovinovic E. Early versus delayed oral fluids and food for reducing complications after major abdominal gynaecologic surgery. *Cochrane Database Syst Rev.* 2014;2014(12):CD004508. doi:10.1002/14651858.CD004508.pub4

189. Marik PE, Zaloga GP. Immunonutrition in high-risk surgical patients: a systematic review and analysis of the literature. *JPEN J Parenter Enteral Nutr.* 2010;34(4):378-386. doi:10.1177/0148607110362692

190. Chapman JS, Roddy E, Westhoff G, et al. Post-operative enteral immunonutrition for gynecologic oncology patients undergoing laparotomy decreases wound complications. *Gynecol Oncol.* 2015;137(3):523-528. doi:10.1016/j.ygyno.2015.04.003

191. Celik JB, Gezginç K, Ozçelik K, Celik C. The role of immunonutrition in gynecologic oncologic surgery. *Eur J Gynaecol Oncol.* 2009;30(4):418-421.

192. Waitzberg DL, Saito H, Plank LD, et al. Postsurgical infections are reduced with specialized nutrition support. *World J Surg.* 2006;30(8):1592-1604. doi:10.1007/s00268-005-0657-x

193. Caglayan K, Oner I, Gunerhan Y, Ata P, Koksal N, Ozkara S. The impact of preoperative immunonutrition and other nutrition models on tumor infiltrative lymphocytes in colorectal cancer patients. *Am J Surg.* 2012;204(4):416-421. doi:10.1016/j.amjsurg.2011.12.018

194. McClave SA, Taylor BE, Martindale RG, et al. Guidelines for the provision and assessment of nutrition support therapy in the adult critically ill patient: Society of Critical Care Medicine (SCCM) and American Society for Parenteral and Enteral Nutrition (A.S.P.E.N.). *JPEN J Parenter Enteral Nutr.* 2016;40(2):159-211. doi:10.1177/0148607115621863

195. Neary NM, Small CJ, Wren AM, et al. Ghrelin increases energy intake in cancer patients with impaired appetite: acute, randomized, placebo-controlled trial. *J Clin Endocrinol Metab.* 2004;89(6):2832-2836. doi:10.1210/jc.2003-031768

196. Temel J, Currow D, Fearon K, et al. Anamorelin for the treatment of cancer anorexia-cachexia in patients with advanced NSCLC: results from the pivotal phase III study ROMANA 1 and 2. *Ann Oncol.* 2014;Abstract 1483O-PR.

197. Garcia JM, Boccia RV, Graham CD, et al. Anamorelin for patients with cancer cachexia: an integrated analysis of two phase 2, randomised, placebo-controlled, double-blind trials. *Lancet Oncol.* 2015;16:108-116.

198. Bartlett DL, Stein TP, Torosian MH. Effect of growth hormone and protein intake on tumor growth and host cachexia. *Surgery.* 1995;117(3):260-267. Accessed March 14, 2016. http://www.ncbi.nlm.nih.gov/pubmed/7878530

199. Tomas FM, Chandler CS, Coyle P, Bourgeois CS, Burgoyne JL, Rofe AM. Effects of insulin and insulin-like growth factors on protein and energy metabolism in tumour-bearing rats. *Biochem J.* 1994;301(pt 3) (Pt 3):769-775. Accessed March 14, 2016. https://www.ncbi.nlm.nih.gov/pmc/articles/PMC1137054/

200. Ottery FD, Walsh D, Strawford A. Pharmacologic management of anorexia/cachexia. *Semin Oncol.* 1998;25(2 suppl 6):35-44. Accessed March 15, 2016. http://www.ncbi.nlm.nih.gov/pubmed/9625382

201. Gullett NP, Hebbar G, Ziegler TR. Update on clinical trials of growth factors and anabolic steroids in cachexia and wasting. *Am J Clin Nutr.* 2010;91:1143S-1147S.

202. Dobs AS, Boccia RV, Croot CC, et al. Effects of enobosarm on muscle wasting and physical function in patients with cancer: a double-blind, randomised controlled phase 2 trial. *Lancet Oncol.* 2013;14:335-345.

203. Lydén E, Cvetkovska E, Westin T, et al. Effects of nandrolone propionate on experimental tumor growth and cancer cachexia. *Metabolism.* 1995;44(4):445-451. Accessed March 14, 2016. http://www.ncbi.nlm.nih.gov/pubmed/7723666

204. Strang P. The effect of megestrol acetate on anorexia, weight loss and cachexia in cancer and AIDS patients (review). *Anticancer Res.* 1997;17(1B):657-662. Accessed March 14, 2016. http://www.ncbi.nlm.nih.gov/pubmed/9066597

205. Beller E, Tattersall M, Lumley T, et al. Improved quality of life with megestrol acetate in patients with endocrine-insensitive advanced cancer: a randomised placebo-controlled trial. Australasian Megestrol Acetate Co-operative Study Group. *Ann Oncol.* 1997;8(3):277-283. Accessed March 14, 2016. http://www.ncbi.nlm.nih.gov/pubmed/9137798

206. Skarlos DV, Fountzilas G, Pavlidis N, et al. Megestrol acetate in cancer patients with anorexia and weight loss. A Hellenic Co-operative Oncology Group (HeCOG) study. *Acta Oncol.* 1993;32(1):37-41. Accessed March 14, 2016. http://www.ncbi.nlm.nih.gov/pubmed/8466763

207. Ruiz Garcia V, López-Briz E, Carbonell Sanchis R, Gonzalvez Perales JL, Bort-Marti S. Megestrol acetate for treatment of anorexia-cachexia syndrome. *Cochrane Database Syst Rev.* 2013;2013(3):CD004310.

208. Macciò A, Madeddu C, Mantovani G. Current pharmacotherapy options for cancer anorexia and cachexia. *Expert Opin Pharmacother.* 2012;13:2453-2472.

209. Fehniger J, Brodsky AL, Kim A, Pothuri B. Medical marijuana utilization in gynecologic cancer patients. *Gynecol Oncol Rep.* 2021;37:100820. doi:10.1016/j.gore.2021.100820

210. Cannabis-In-Cachexia-Study-Group; Strasser F, Luftner D, Possinger K, et al. Comparison of orally administered cannabis extract and delta-9-tetrahydrocannabinol in treating patients with cancer-related anorexia-cachexia syndrome: a multicenter, phase III, randomized, double-blind, placebo-controlled clinical trial from the Cannabis-In-Cachexia-Study-Group. *J Clin Oncol.* 2006;24(21):3394-3400. doi:10.1200/JCO.2005.05.1847

211. Fujimoto-Ouchi K, Tamura S, Mori K, Tanaka Y, Ishitsuka H. Establishment and characterization of cachexia-inducing and -non-inducing clones of murine colon 26 carcinoma. *Int J Cancer.* 1995;61(4):522-528. Accessed March 14, 2016. http://www.ncbi.nlm.nih.gov/pubmed/7759158

212. Gelin J, Moldawer LL, Lönnroth C, et al. Role of endogenous tumor necrosis factor alpha and interleukin 1 for experimental tumor growth and the development of cancer cachexia. *Cancer Res.* 1991;51(1):415-421. Accessed March 14, 2016. http://www.ncbi.nlm.nih.gov/pubmed/1703040

213. Strassmann G, Kambayashi T. Inhibition of experimental cancer cachexia by anti-cytokine and anti-cytokine-receptor therapy. *Cytokines Mol Ther.* 1995;1(2):107-113. Accessed March 14, 2016. http://www.ncbi.nlm .nih.gov/pubmed/9384667

214. Yamamoto N, Kawamura I, Nishigaki F, et al. Effect of FR143430, a novel cytokine suppressive agent, on adenocarcinoma colon26-induced cachexia in mice. *Anticancer Res.* 1998;18(1A):139-144. Accessed March 14, 2016. http://www.ncbi.nlm.nih.gov/pubmed/9568068

215. Bayliss TJ, Smith JT, Schuster M, Dragnev KH, Rigas JR. A humanized anti-IL-6 antibody (ALD518) in non-small cell lung cancer. *Expert Opin Biol Ther.* 2011;11:1663-1668.

216. Ando K, Takahashi F, Motojima S, et al. Possible role for tocilizumab, an anti-interleukin-6 receptor antibody, in treating cancer cachexia. *J Clin Oncol.* 2013;31:e69-e72.

217. Khan ZH, Simpson EJ, Cole AT, et al. Oesophageal cancer and cachexia: the effect of short-term treatment with thalidomide on weight loss and lean body mass. *Aliment Pharmacol Ther.* 2003;17(5):677-682. Accessed March 14, 2016. http://www.ncbi.nlm.nih.gov/pubmed/12641516

218. Gordon JN, Trebble TM, Ellis RD, et al. Thalidomide in the treatment of cancer cachexia: a randomised placebo controlled trial. *Gut.* 2005;54(4):540-545. doi:10.1136/gut.2004.047563

219. Madeddu C, Mantovani G, Gramignano G, Macciò A. Advances in pharmacologic strategies for cancer cachexia. *Expert Opin Pharmacother.* 2015;16(14):2163-2177. doi:10.1517/14656566.2015.1079621

220. Lai V, George J, Richey L, et al. Results of a pilot study of the effects of celecoxib on cancer cachexia in patients with cancer of the head, neck, and gastrointestinal tract. *Head Neck.* 2008;30(1):67-74. doi:10.1002/hed.20662

221. McMillan DC, Wigmore SJ, Fearon KC, et al. A prospective randomized study of megestrol acetate and ibuprofen in gastrointestinal cancer patients with weight loss. *Br J Cancer.* 1999;79(3-4):495-500. doi:10.1038/sj.bjc.6690077

222. Reid J, Hughes CM, Murray LJ, Parsons C, Cantwell MM. Non-steroidal anti-inflammatory drugs for the treatment of cancer cachexia: a systematic review. *Palliat Med.* 2013;27:295-303.

223. Mantovani G, Macciò A, Madeddu C, et al. Randomized phase III clinical trial of five different arms of treatment in 332 patients with cancer cachexia. *Oncologist.* 2010;15(2):200-211. doi:10.1634/theoncologist.2009-0153

224. McGough C, Baldwin C, Norman A, et al. Is supplementation with elemental diet feasible in patients undergoing pelvic radiotherapy? *Clin Nutr.* 2006;25(1):109-116. doi:10.1016/j.clnu.2005.09.007

225. Henson CC, Burden S, Davidson SE, et al. Nutritional interventions for reducing gastrointestinal toxicity in adults undergoing radical pelvic radiotherapy. *Cochrane Database Syst Rev.* 2013;11:CD009896. doi:10.1002/14651858.CD009896.pub2

226. Borek C. Radiation and chemically induced transformation: free radicals, antioxidants and cancer. *Br J Cancer Suppl.* 1987;8:74-86. Accessed March 17, 2016. http://www.ncbi.nlm.nih.gov/pmc/articles/pmc2149458/

227. Kennedy M, Bruninga K, Mutlu EA, et al. Successful and sustained treatment of chronic radiation proctitis with antioxidant vitamins E and C. *Am J Gastroenterol.* 2001;96(4):1080-1084. doi:10.1111/j.1572-0241.2001.03742.x

228. Fearon KCH, Von Meyenfeldt MF, Moses AGW, et al. Effect of a protein and energy dense N-3 fatty acid enriched oral supplement on loss of weight and lean tissue in cancer cachexia: a randomised double blind trial. *Gut.* 2003;52(10):1479-1486. Accessed February 22, 2016. https://pubmed.ncbi.nlm.nih.gov/12970142/

229. Gogos CA, Ginopoulos P, Salsa B, et al. Dietary omega-3 polyunsaturated fatty acids plus vitamin E restore immunodeficiency and prolong survival for severely ill patients with generalized malignancy: a randomized control trial. *Cancer.* 1998;82(2):395-402. Accessed February 22, 2016. http://www.ncbi.nlm.nih.gov/pubmed/9445198

230. Sims TT, El Alam MB, Karpinets TV, et al. Gut microbiome diversity is an independent predictor of survival in cervical cancer patients receiving chemoradiation. *Commun Biol.* 2021;4(1):237. doi:10.1038/s42003-021-01741-x

231. Giudice E, Salutari V, Ricci C, et al. Gut microbiota and its influence on ovarian cancer carcinogenesis, anticancer therapy and surgical treatment: a literature review. *Crit Rev Oncol Hematol.* 2021;168:103542. doi:10.1016/j.critrevonc.2021.103542

232. Deciding to Forego Life-Sustaining Treatment: a report on the ethical, medical, and legal issues in treatment decisions. Accessed March 17, 2016. https://repository.library.georgetown.edu/handle/10822/796378

233. Shils ME. Nutrition and medical ethics: the interplay of medical decisions, patients' rights, and the judicial system. In: Shils ME, Olsen JA, Shike M, et al, eds. *Modern Nutrition in Health and Disease.* 9th ed. Williams & Wilkins; 1999:1689

234. John Paul II P. Care for patients in a "permanent" vegetative state. *Origins.* 2004;33(43):737, 739-740. Accessed March 17, 2016. http://www.ncbi .nlm.nih.gov/pubmed/15139351

235. Schostak RZ. Jewish ethical guidelines for resuscitation and artificial nutrition and hydration of the dying elderly. *J Med Ethics.* 1994;20(2):93-100. Accessed March 17, 2016. https://pubmed.ncbi.nlm.nih.gov/8083881/

236. Casarett D, Kapo J, Caplan A. Appropriate use of artificial nutrition and hydration-fundamental principles and recommendations. *N Engl J Med.* 2005;353(24):2607-2612. doi:10.1056/NEJMsb052907

237. Ganzini L, Goy ER, Miller LL, et al. Nurses' experiences with hospice patients who refuse food and fluids to hasten death. *N Engl J Med.* 2003;349(4):359-365. doi:10.1056/NEJMsa035086

238. Maillet JO, Potter RL, Heller L. Position of the American Dietetic Association: ethical and legal issues in nutrition, hydration, and feeding. *J Am Diet Assoc.* 2002;102(5):716-726. Accessed March 17, 2016. http://www .ncbi.nlm.nih.gov/pubmed/12009001

239. Brown D, Roberts JA, Elkins TE, et al. Hard choices: the gynecologic cancer patient's end-of-life preferences. *Gynecol Oncol.* 1994;55(3 pt 1):355-362. doi:10.1006/gyno.1994.1306

240. McCann RM, Hall WJ, Groth-Juncker A. Comfort care for terminally ill patients. The appropriate use of nutrition and hydration. *JAMA.* 1994;272(16):1263-1266.

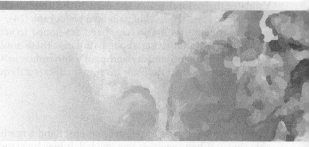

CHAPTER **12.5**

Management of Pain

Russell K. Portenoy and Ebtesam Ahmed

INTRODUCTION

Acute and chronic pain are highly prevalent in the population managed by gynecologic oncologists. The most common acute pain syndromes are postprocedural, following minimally invasive or open-abdomen surgeries, and intraperitoneal chemotherapy administration. Chronic pain is also heterogeneous but usually occurs in the context of active disease. The few extant epidemiologic studies (1-4) suggest that chronic pain in the population with gynecologic cancers mirrors other cancer populations, affecting almost two-thirds of patients with metastatic disease, more than half of those receiving antineoplastic therapy, and about one-third of cancer survivors (5).

The management of cancer-related pain begins with assessment. This assessment may be straightforward when pain is acute and consistent with obvious tissue injury. It is far more complicated when pain has become persistent, disproportionate to tissue injury, or occurs with many other problems in advanced illness.

ASSESSMENT OF CANCER PAIN

The definition of pain underscores the complexity that may be encountered during clinical assessment. According to the International Association for the Study of Pain (IASP), pain is "an unpleasant sensory and emotional experience associated with, or resembling that associated with, actual or potential tissue damage" (6). This definition highlights the important observation that pain may or may not comport with an observable degree of tissue injury. Especially when pain is chronic, pain severity or other characteristics of the pain, or the extent of pain distress, may not be explained by evident tissue injury, a discrepancy that may be ascribed to disturbed physiology or psychological factors or both.

The definition of pain has been expanded to a nomenclature based on studies of pain mechanisms. Pain mechanisms include those that are normal physiologic processes—collectively termed "nociception"—that exist to detect and respond to potentially tissue-injuring events. The anatomy, neurophysiology, and neurochemistry of nociception, and its interactions with other physiologic systems, are exceedingly complex and include numerous mechanisms that transmit, modify, and suppress information about potential or actual tissue injury.

In contrast to the sensory processing that is nociception, pain is best understood as a perception. Like other perceptions, the experience of pain is influenced by complex non-nociceptive factors, including emotions and cognitions. This complexity is reflected in the variation that characterizes pain description, which may involve sensory terms (such as severity and timing), affective terms (such as unpleasantness or distress), or cognitive terms (such as appraisals of cause or implications) (7).

Pain also may be defined with labels that suggest the predominance of one or another group of pathophysiologic mechanisms (8). Pain is considered *nociceptive* if it appears to be commensurate with tissue injury. Whether the pain is acute or chronic, this term indicates that the clinical presentation can be explained by ongoing injury to pain-sensitive structures. Pain related to inflammation is assumed to be nociceptive. Alternatively, pain is considered *neuropathic* when it is associated with symptoms or signs of neurologic dysfunction and has characteristics that point to disturbed somatosensory processing as responsible for the pain (9). Neuropathic pain is typically disproportionate to observable tissue injury. In a similar manner, *nociplastic* pain indicates that the pain can be explained by neuroplastic changes that increase the sensitivity of the nociceptive system in the absence of a specific neural injury (10). Chronic pelvic pain of unknown etiology and fibromyalgia may be different types. Finally, pain that is termed *psychogenic* indicates that there are positive indicators of a psychiatric disorder or psychosocial disturbance that can explain the occurrence or presentation of the pain.

These complexities, in the definition and categorization of pain in the context of cancer, are augmented by consideration of constructs that embody the more global adverse illness-related experience. These constructs, which are sometimes described as "total pain" or suffering, or as impairment in QoL, all highlight the impact on the person of numerous perceptions, one of which may be pain. Patients with cancer often experience multiple other symptoms and manifold sources of physical, psychosocial, or spiritual distress.

Evaluation of the Pain Complaint

The pain assessment often starts with a description of the pain's characteristics. In the context of chronic pain, this information may clarify the need for additional tests and suggest the best approach to management.

Intensity

The measurement of pain intensity influences the urgency of treatment and tracking of outcomes. For most children older than 7 years and most cognitively intact adults, measurement usually relies on a verbal rating scale, a numerical scale, or a visual analog scale (VAS). These scales are valid (11), and the selection of one is typically a matter of personal preference. The verbal rating scales ask the patient to indicate the severity of the pain using one of the following words: none, mild, moderate, severe, or excruciating. Numerical scales vary, and the 11-step scale is an exemplar. The patient is asked to indicate the severity of the pain using a number between 0 and 10, where 0 is no pain and 10 is the "worst pain imaginable." A VAS typically employs a 10-cm line, which may be horizontal or vertical. The line is anchored at one end by the words "no pain" or "least possible pain" and at the other end by the words "worst possible pain." The patient is asked to indicate the point on the line that reflects the severity of the pain.

The use of these scales requires context. Usually, the patient is asked to indicate the severity of the pain "right now" or the severity of the pain "at its worst during the past day." Asking patients to separately indicate both pain right now and worst pain during the past day may be the best approach to track therapeutic outcomes.

Several pain severity scales may be used by younger children (12) and by cognitively impaired adults (13). The most common is a pictograph that includes drawings of faces or pictures of faces, ranging from a smiling face to a face demonstrating high distress.

Validated behavioral scales are used if the cognitively impaired adult cannot rate the level of pain on a pictograph (14).

Measurement tools also have been developed to acquire multidimensional information about pain (15). These tools typically measure both pain intensity and pain interference in various areas of function. The Brief Pain Inventory (BPI) is a frequently employed example.

Temporal

Acute pain usually has a well-defined onset and a readily identifiable cause. When severe or unexpected, it may be associated with acute anxiety, overt pain behaviors (moaning or grimacing), and signs of sympathetic hyperactivity (including tachycardia, hypertension, and diaphoresis).

In contrast, chronic pain is characterized by an ill-defined onset and a prolonged, fluctuating course. Most patients experience periodic flares of pain, or "breakthrough pain" (13). Chronic pain is not usually characterized by pain behaviors or signs of sympathetic hyperactivity. Rather, vegetative signs, including fatigue, sleep disturbance, and anorexia, may be present. If mood is disturbed, it is more often depressed than anxious, and some patients develop a depressive disorder.

Pain Location

The distinctions among focal, multifocal, and generalized pains may influence both the assessment and treatment of the patient. Some therapies, such as nerve blocks, specifically depend on the specific location and extent of the pain.

Focal pains may be experienced superficial to the underlying nociceptive lesion or referred to other sites. Referred pain may characterize pain-producing lesions affecting the nerve, bone, muscle, or other soft tissue and viscera. Various subtypes can be distinguished: (a) pain referred anywhere along the course of an injured peripheral nerve (such as pain in the thigh or knee from a lumbar plexus lesion); (b) pain referred along a course of the nerve supplied by a damaged nerve root (known as radicular pain); (c) pain referred to the lower part of the body, usually the feet and legs, from a lesion involving the spinal cord (called funicular pain); and (d) pain referred to a site remote from the nociceptive lesion and outside the dermatome affected by the lesion (eg, shoulder pain from diaphragmatic irritation).

Knowledge of pain referral patterns is needed to target appropriate assessment procedures. For example, a patient with recurrent cervical cancer who reports progressive pain in the inguinal crease may require evaluation of numerous structures to identify the underlying pathology responsible for the pain. Inguinal pain may be due to a lesion affecting the pelvis or hip joint, pelvic sidewall, paraspinal gutter at an upper lumbar spinal level, or intraspinal region at the upper lumbar level.

Etiology

The etiology of acute pain is usually clear-cut. Further evaluation to determine the underlying lesion or pathophysiology of the pain is not indicated unless the course varies from the expected. In contrast, the etiology of chronic pain—which may be due to a direct effect of the neoplasm, to tissue injury caused by cancer therapy, or to a comorbid chronic pain condition—may be more difficult to characterize. Imaging tests, electrodiagnostic studies, or laboratory evaluation may be needed to clarify the etiology and provide information essential for clinical decision-making and prognostication.

Pathophysiology

As described previously, clinicians have found it useful to characterize pain based on inferences about the predominating pathophysiologic mechanism. Pain may be labeled nociceptive, neuropathic, nociplastic, psychogenic, or mixed (8).

Pain is nociceptive if it is inferred that the sustaining mechanisms involve ongoing tissue injury involving either somatic or visceral structures. The diagnosis is made based on the finding of tissue injury and the quality of the pain. The quality of somatic nociceptive pain is typically described as aching, stabbing, throbbing, or pressure like. The quality of visceral nociceptive pain is largely determined by the structures involved. Obstruction of hollow viscus is usually associated with complaints of gnawing or crampy pain, whereas injury to organ capsules or mesentery is associated with an aching or stabbing discomfort.

Pain is neuropathic if the evaluation identifies a neurologic lesion and the presentation suggests that the pain is sustained by abnormal somatosensory processing in the peripheral or the CNS. Neuropathic pain is highly prevalent and can be disease related (eg, tumor invasion of nerve plexus) or treatment related (chemotherapy-induced painful polyneuropathy).

Neuropathic pain is diagnosed on the basis of the patient's verbal description of the pain and evidence of injury to neural tissue (16). Verbal descriptors, such as "burning," "electrical," or "shock like," are suggestive of neuropathic pain. Areas of abnormal sensations are often found on physical examination. These may include hypesthesia (a numbness or lessening of feeling), paresthesia (abnormal nonpainful sensations such as tingling, cold, or itching), hyperalgesia (increased perception of painful stimuli), hyperpathia (exaggerated pain response), and allodynia (pain induced by nonpainful stimuli such as a light touch or cool air).

Nociplastic pain refers to chronic pain that is presumed related to augmented CNS sensory transmission or altered central pain modulation, the result of which is hypersensitivity in the nociceptive system (10). The pain is not explained by tissue injury or neural injury. It is widely distributed and often associated with other symptoms, such as fatigue. There have been no studies of cancer-related nociplastic pain and the extent to which this category of mechanisms is involved in cancer pain syndromes is unknown.

Pain due primarily to psychological processes may be diagnosed using criteria developed by the American Psychiatric Association, codified in the *Diagnostic and Statistical Manual of Mental Disorders*, fifth Edition (17). These disorders are sometimes collectively labeled "psychogenic," a term that may also be applied when psychological factors appear to be intensifying or altering pain otherwise attributable to nociceptive or neuropathic mechanisms, or when pain is associated with a level of distress that appears disproportionate to the symptom itself. Understanding the interaction between pain and psychiatric or psychosocial conditions is challenging, and the psychogenic label may be helpful if it improves recognition of this complexity and prioritizes appropriate care.

Chronic pain syndromes are often perceived as having a mixed pathophysiology. Chronic pain due to tumor growth in the pelvis, for example, is often characterized as a mixed nociceptive (with both somatic and visceral components) and neuropathic (with involvement of lumbosacral plexus) disorder, which also may be complicated by psychological drivers of pain distress. A careful assessment should be able to distinguish these components, providing information that can inform the use of analgesics and the development of a care plan that more broadly addresses the patient's burden of illness.

Occasionally, a patient with cancer develops a pain syndrome that cannot be characterized. The term "idiopathic" pain is preferred in this context. Unexplained pain should not be labeled psychogenic unless the assessment yields positive evidence of a psychiatric disorder.

Pain Syndromes

Efforts to improve the assessment of cancer pain have been greatly encouraged by the description of numerous pain syndromes, each of which is defined by a cluster of symptoms and signs (18-20). Syndrome identification in patients with gynecologic cancers can help direct the diagnostic evaluation, clarify the prognosis, and target therapeutic interventions (**Tables 12.5-1 and 12.5-2**).

TABLE 12.5-1. Cancer Pain Syndromes

- Pain associated with direct tumor involvement
- Due to invasion of bone
- Base of skull
- Vertebral body
- Generalized bone pain
- Due to invasion of nerves
- Peripheral nerve syndromes
- Painful polyneuropathy
- Brachial, lumbar, sacral plexopathies
- Leptomeningeal metastases
- Epidural spinal cord compression
- Due to invasion of viscera
- Due to invasion of blood vessels
- Due to invasion of mucous membranes
- Pain associated with cancer therapy
- Postoperative pain syndromes
- Post-thoracotomy syndrome
- Postmastectomy syndrome
- Postradical neck dissection
- Postamputation syndromes
- Postchemotherapy pain syndromes
- Painful polyneuropathy
- Aseptic necrosis of bone
- Steroid pseudorheumatism
- Mucositis
- Postirradiation pain syndromes
- Radiation fibrosis of brachial or lumbosacral plexus
- Radiation myelopathy
- Radiation-induced peripheral nerve tumors
- Mucositis
- Pain indirectly related or unrelated to cancer
- Myofascial pains
- Postherpetic neuralgia
- Chronic headache syndromes

MANAGEMENT OF ACUTE PAIN

Although there are many types of acute pain syndromes associated with gynecologic cancers, the most common setting is perioperative. All gynecologic procedures are followed by acute pain. Minimally invasive, laparoscopic, or robotic procedures typically produce less intense and prolonged pain than open abdominal procedures, and the quality of the pain is usually visceral; pain

TABLE 12.5-2. Pain Syndromes Commonly Encountered Among Patients With Gynecologic Cancer

- **Acute pain syndromes**
  - At any stage of disease:
  - Postoperative pain
  - Mucositis
- **In advanced stages of disease:**
  - Recurrent bowel obstruction
  - Ureteral obstruction
  - Movement-related pain in brachial/lumbosacral plexopathy
  - Movement-related pain from bony lesions
- **Cancer-related chronic pain syndromes**
  - Brachial/lumbosacral plexopathy
  - Chronic abdominal pain: bowel obstruction, ascites, hepatomegaly
  - Tenesmus pain
  - Bone pain from metastases
- **Treatment-related chronic pain syndromes**
  - Postmastectomy syndrome
  - Radiation-induced plexopathy
  - Chemotherapy-induced peripheral neuropathy (paclitaxel, cisplatin)

following open procedures usually has both an incisional component and a visceral component. Guidelines for the management of acute postsurgical pain are a component of protocols for ERAS (21,22), which suggests a combination of treatments that can potentially mitigate symptoms, reduce the stress response, and enhance functional recovery. Studies that have compared these protocols to conventional postoperative management, which relies on systemic opioid therapy for pain control, are limited, but some suggest that outcomes are likely to be positive in more painful, open procedures (23,24).

The analgesic component of the protocols for ERAS recommends the consideration of a multimodality approach intended to increase the likelihood of efficacy while limiting the sole reliance on systemic opioid therapy. Opioid sparing, in turn, reduces the risk of adverse opioid effects. The principles that are reflected in these perioperative pain management protocols may be extrapolated to acute pains of all types.

The multimodality approach to acute pain may include the use of presurgical analgesic drug administration (preemptive analgesia) followed by opioid therapy combined with co-analgesic drugs. In selected cases, it may also include infiltration of incision sites with local anesthetic, regional anesthetic techniques (such as the transversus abdominal plane [TAP] block), and use of neuraxial analgesia (25).

Preemptive Analgesia

In preemptive analgesia, one or more drugs are administered before the surgical incision to reduce postoperative pain and opioid requirements and possibly have long-term benefits (26). Although preoperative administration of a long-acting opioid may reduce postoperative pain (27), evidence of positive effects is limited (28), and the approach is usually not performed for this reason. For this reason, the term *preemptive analgesia* typically implies the use of nonopioid or adjuvant analgesics.

Studies of preemptive analgesia have demonstrated positive effects associated with the administration of acetaminophen or an NSAID, such as celecoxib, or a gabapentinoid, such as gabapentin, ketamine, and dexmedetomidine. Although the data are limited, they suggest pretreatment with a nonopioid analgesic (acetaminophen or an NSAID) or a gabapentinoid (gabapentin or pregabalin) is most likely to reduce pain and opioid consumption postoperatively (29,30). These data support the use of these types of drugs for preemptive analgesia.

Systemic Opioid Therapy

Acute moderate or severe cancer-related pain from any cause, including pain associated with surgery or other procedures, is typically managed using systemic opioid therapy. Despite great variability in the pharmacokinetics and pharmacodynamics of single opioid doses, many patients with severe acute pain respond adequately to a short-acting opioid drug administered "as needed." If the GI tract is available and the patient's distress associated with acute is tolerable, therapy may be initiated with an oral opioid. Most opioid-naïve patients, for example, may start treatment with oral morphine 15 mg, hydromorphone 2 mg, or oxycodone 5 mg every 3 hours as needed. Alternatively, a combination product containing an opioid (eg, hydrocodone or oxycodone) and a nonopioid (eg, acetaminophen), or one of the mixed mechanism opioid drugs (tramadol or tapentadol), may be used (see later in this chapter).

If pain is severe and distressing, or the oral route is not available, IV drug administration is preferred. The IV route eliminates the time required for drug absorption and avoids the discomfort of subcutaneous or intramuscular drug administration. The subcutaneous route can be made more comfortable for repetitive drug administration by subcutaneous placement of a butterfly catheter, which may be left in place for many days. The intramuscular route offers no advantage and is painful; it should be avoided if possible.

Parenteral treatment of most opioid-naïve patients may begin with morphine 5 to 10 mg, or a comparable dose of another drug, every 2 to 3 hours as needed.

If the patient with acute pain has a history of current opioid use for pain, a higher starting dose of the opioid is needed. A reasonable guideline suggests either a 50% to 100% increase in the current opioid dose or a dose that is calculated to be equivalent to roughly 5% to 10% of the total opioid consumption during the previous 24 hours. This calculation of equivalent doses is based on the information in an equianalgesic dose table (see later in this chapter). If the starting dose or interval selected initially is not quickly effective, an increase in the dose or shortening of the dosing interval should be considered.

Several opioids that were widely used in the past are not recommended. Although meperidine is likely to be well tolerated during brief therapy, it is not preferred because its metabolite, normeperidine, can accumulate, particularly when renal function is impaired, and produce toxicity. Codeine also has been widely used but is not preferred because genetically determined variation in the activity of the CYP2D6 liver enzyme results in unpredictable variation in pharmacokinetics.

Continuous IV infusion and PCA are alternatives to intermittent administration of an opioid. PCA, which involves the self-administration of small doses on a frequent basis, has achieved great popularity in the management of postoperative pain, and there is evidence that it can yield better outcomes than conventional parenteral opioid therapy (31). In the opioid-naïve patient, a typical approach to PCA uses morphine at a dose of 1 mg every 6 minutes as needed, or another opioid at an equivalent dose. Patients already receiving opioid therapy can be treated using higher dose PCA; the size of each dose may be calculated to be equivalent to approximately 5% of the total daily dose of opioid taken during the prior day.

The variability in analgesic requirements often requires dose or dosing interval changes after therapy is initiated. Similarly, variability in pain duration is great, and the duration of opioid treatment must be flexible, determined by patient response.

The assessment and management of opioid adverse effects is essential whenever treatment for acute pain is initiated. Some patients require concomitant treatment for a side effect, such as an antiemetic or a laxative. Monitoring of opioid-related symptoms and just-in-time management is key to enhancing the tolerability of treatment and increasing the likelihood that it will be safe and effective.

The abuse liability of opioid drugs is less an issue in the management of acute pain than chronic pain due to the expected discontinuation of treatment in the near term. There are important considerations in this setting, however (32). Most important, clinicians should recognize that the appropriate continuation of opioid therapy after discharge from the hospital results in a period during which there may be greater risk of nonadherence than observed in the controlled inpatient environment. This period of risk requires the clinicians to perform a risk assessment that evaluates the potential for nonadherence or frank abuse after discharge (see later in this chapter). Prescribing for this period should be undertaken cautiously, typically using short-acting drugs provided in a quantity that will minimize the likelihood of excess tablets as pain declines.

This need for risk assessment and management is particularly important if the patient has a known history of opioid-use disorder. A history of drug abuse or the disease of addiction is a risk factor for both aberrant drug-related behavior that may diminish the safety of pain therapy and undertreatment of pain due to concerns about these outcomes (33,34). In this setting, opioid-sparing approaches become more important, and it may be prudent to obtain consultation from a specialist in Addiction Medicine or Psychiatry to help with a plan that minimizes risk and improves adherence monitoring after discharge.

Co-analgesic Therapy

The management of acute, moderate, or severe pain in the population with gynecologic cancers may yield improved outcomes when an opioid is combined with one or more drugs that can potentially improve efficacy and reduce the risk of opioid side effects by reducing the opioid requirement. Opioid sparing in this way has the potential to lower the risk of opioid-related respiratory depression, cognitive impairment or somnolence, nausea, constipation, itch, or urinary retention.

The nonopioid drugs typically employed as co-analgesics in this setting include both acetaminophen and the NSAIDs. Acetaminophen may be administered IV to good effect (35), but the cost may limit broad access to this treatment. NSAIDs similarly provide additive analgesia following both minimally invasive and open abdominal surgeries (35,36); several of these drugs, such as ketorolac and ibuprofen, are available as injectable formulations.

Studies of the gabapentinoids, gabapentin, and pregabalin have yielded mixed results. Two meta-analyses, respectively evaluating 14 and 6 randomized trials, found positive effects on pain and opioid consumption (37,38), but a much larger meta-analysis, which extracted data from 281 trials, demonstrated no benefit from gabapentin (39). In the absence of definitive results, the decision to add gabapentin or pregabalin as analgesics for acute pain when oral therapy is possible remains a matter of clinical judgment. If prescribed, patients must be carefully monitored for side effects, including somnolence, mental clouding and dizziness, unsteady gait, and an increased potential for opioid-related respiratory depression (40).

Other drugs also have been studied for their co-analgesic effects, but evidence is limited. IV dexamethasone was opioid sparing, but not analgesic, after laparoscopic hysterectomy (41,42). A randomized trial in a similar population suggested benefit from IV magnesium (43). Studies of low-dose ketamine, which is used in palliative care as an analgesic (see later in this chapter), suggest positive effects on pain and opioid consumption after surgery (44,45). None of these agents is widely used, and additional evidence of safety and comparative efficacy is needed for all.

Wound Infiltration

Local anesthetic wound infiltration, before incision or at the time of closure, also can be used as part of a multimodal analgesia approach after gynecologic surgery. Numerous studies in diverse types of operations suggest that the technique can reduce postoperative pain and opioid use but must be used cautiously owing to the potential for local anesthetic absorption and toxicity (46). The advent of longer acting local anesthetics, such as liposomal bupivacaine, has increased expectations about the potential for positive outcomes from this technique. More evidence is needed, however, to conclude that treatment with this type of drug is superior to conventional local anesthetics (47).

Regional Anesthetic Techniques

Regional anesthetic techniques involve the temporary blockade of peripheral nerves, innervating the area of the pain. Temporary blockade can be implemented through injection or infusion of a local anesthetic adjacent to a neural structure, either a plexus or peripheral nerves. Although this approach can potentially be used in the management of any focal or regional pain, the most common use is in the management of specific postoperative pain syndromes.

Local anesthetic can be injected into the space between transversus abdominis and internal oblique muscles to create a TAP block. TAP can potentially be accomplished through injections at any of the multiple sites. When effective, the block should denervate the anterolateral abdominal wall by interrupting transmission through the intercostal, ilioinguinal, iliohypogastric, and subcostal nerves. The injection is usually performed before incision.

Although the TAP block should offer a safe and effective approach to the management of pain related to all types of abdominal procedures, the supporting evidence is conflicting. Both a retrospective study of patients undergoing large cytoreductive surgeries for ovarian cancer and a survey of patients undergoing varied open abdominal procedures found no benefit in terms of opioid use or pain (48,49). Meta-analyses of data from patients undergoing hysterectomy yielded opposite results (50,51). At present, the evidence is insufficient to recommend the TAP block routinely.

Other regional anesthetic techniques, such as paravertebral neural blockade and continuous rectus sheath block, also have been evaluated as part of a multimodality approach to the pain of abdominal surgery. A study of paravertebral neural blockade for pain due to laparotomy suggested that this approach was similar in efficacy to thoracic epidural local anesthetic, but systemic absorption of the local anesthetic was relatively high and raised concerns about the safety of the approach (52). Rectus sheath block was similar to epidural anesthesia for pain at rest but was less effective for pain with movement (53).

Given the conflicting results, regional anesthetic techniques are generally less preferred to neuraxial approaches when considering a multimodality approach to the management of acute pain associated with surgery for gynecologic cancers. Discussion with a specialist in interventional pain management may help refine the criteria used to select patients for these treatments.

Neuraxial Analgesia

Bolus injection or continuous infusion of local anesthetic, often combined with an opioid, may be an effective approach to the management of acute pain. Although evidence of comparative effectiveness is limited, it is most often employed to address pain from open abdominal surgeries (54). In this setting, the approach is intended to reduce pain and opioid consumption while facilitating early return of intestinal function and reducing the risk of complications. Evidence of these benefits is limited, however, and the available evidence indicates that the neuraxial approach can provide satisfactory pain management, but the comparative benefits and risks relative to other conventional therapies remain ill-defined (55). The approach should not be considered first line for postoperative pain, and the decision to offer it should be made based on the availability of the resources needed to implement it safely and careful consideration of risks and benefits relative to less invasive therapies.

Other Approaches

Transcutaneous electrical nerve stimulation (TENS) has been suggested as a useful modality for incisional pain after abdominal surgery (56). Despite the evident simplicity and safety of the approach, and its obvious potential, it has been used very little in this setting.

Cognitive approaches, including stress reduction, relaxation, hypnosis, and distraction techniques, may also reduce postoperative pain and analgesic requirements (57). These techniques are labor intensive and are almost never sufficient as the sole means of analgesia. Nonetheless, stress and mood disturbance can negatively influence postoperative pain, and both preoperative education and postoperative psychological interventions are likely to have salutary effects.

MANAGEMENT OF CHRONIC CANCER PAIN

The treatment of chronic pain may be challenging, particularly when disease is advanced and complicated by symptom distress and other sources of illness burden. Pain should be considered in the context of illness burden, and pain management should be understood as a component of palliative care.

Pain, Illness Burden, and Palliative Care

Most patients with chronic cancer pain have other troubling physical and psychological symptoms, and pain assessment should evaluate these nonpain symptoms to guide interventions that address overall symptom burden. Symptoms, in turn, are only one aspect of the burden of illness, a driver of the multifaceted problem of suffering

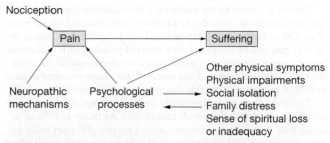

Figure 12.5-1. Complex associations between pain and suffering, necessitating a multidimensional assessment to formulate a palliative plan of care. (Reproduced with permission from the World Health Organization. *Cancer Pain Relief*. 2nd ed. World Health Organization; 1996.)

(58,59). Suffering reflects an individual's response to the multiple physical, psychological, social, and spiritual factors that contribute to the burden of illness. Patient-centered oncologic practice attempts to control the disease while providing the type of holistic and compassionate care that addresses disease-related suffering (Figure 12.5-1).

Palliative care has emerged as a therapeutic model that aims to prevent or mitigate the sources of illness burden and thereby promote the best possible QoL throughout the course of illness (60,61). In the United States, palliative care is a formal medical subspecialty (Hospice and Palliative Medicine), and specialist certification is available for nurses, social workers, and chaplains.

Specialist palliative care is now being provided in most of U.S. hospitals by consultation services, and palliative care at home and in nursing homes can be provided to eligible patients through more than 4,500 hospice agencies in the United States. Other models of community-based, specialist palliative care are emerging and are likely to become more available in the future.

Palliative care is guided by goal-setting and advance care planning discussions that promote patient-centered and family-focused care consistent with the culture, values, and preferences of the patient and family. A palliative plan of care addresses multiple sources of illness burden and often includes interventions for pain and other symptoms, psychosocial or spiritual distress, and caregiver distress or burden. Help with instrumental needs is provided, particularly in the home environment. At the end of life, expert palliative care allows the patient or family to choose the site where death will occur and provides whatever support is needed to ensure a comfortable and dignified dying, with adequate support for the family.

The oncologist oversees or directly provides many aspects of the palliative plan of care during the patient's illness (62,63). This effort may be conceptualized as the integration of generalist-level, or primary, palliative care into routine oncologic practice. Referral to specialists in palliative care also is central to the role of the oncologist and is typically pursued when the patient's needs are complex or the patient may benefit from assistance with hospice enrollment.

When cancer pain is challenging or accompanied by multiple other sources of distress, a referral to a palliative care specialist may initiate consistent or advanced therapies for pain as a key part of the palliative plan of care. In some cases, the complexity of the pain program also warrants referral to a specialist in pain management, whose skills in interventional approaches may be needed.

ROLE OF PRIMARY THERAPIES IN PAIN MANAGEMENT

A successful strategy for pain management must include consideration of the etiology and pathophysiology of pain, the patient's medical status, and the goals of care. Effective treatment of the pathology underlying the pain can be analgesic, and the appropriateness of primary antineoplastic treatment should be considered as part of the analgesic approach.

Tumor response to chemotherapy, immunotherapy, or biotherapy may ameliorate pain due to a reduction in tissue injury at tumor sites. Other factors may also be involved, however, and tumor response may not be necessary. In a study of patients with metastatic breast cancer, for example, palliative chemotherapy with doxorubicin with or without vinorelbine resulted in an improvement of pain in 61% of patients with stable disease after treatment (64).

Radiation therapy is commonly used to manage pain and other symptoms in populations with cancer (65). As many as 80% of patients with pain bone metastases report meaningful pain relief following radiation (66), and analgesia may be an expected result when radiation is used to treat epidural disease, tumor ulceration, cerebral metastases, superior vena cava obstruction, and bronchial obstruction. Patients with widespread bone metastases or bone pain refractory to local field radiotherapy may benefit from treatment with radiopharmaceuticals, such as strontium-89 or samarium-153 (67).

Unfortunately, many patients with chronic cancer pain have no options for further primary therapy with analgesic intent. The approach to these patients involves a diverse group of analgesic treatments.

ANALGESICS APPROACHES: PHARMACOLOGIC MANAGEMENT

Analgesic drug therapy is the mainstay approach for the management of chronic cancer pain. Three large groups of medications are employed: NSAIDs, opioid analgesics, and the so-called adjuvant analgesics. Opioid therapy is the first-line treatment when chronic pain is generally moderate or severe. Although high-quality evidence of opioid effectiveness for cancer pain is limited (68), numerous smaller studies and large surveys (69) comport with extensive clinical experience to support the potential for favorable outcomes (70,71). In the context of an incurable disease, opioids are considered essential drugs, and the lack of opioid availability, most notable in low- and middle-income countries, has been called an "access abyss"—a major issue in global health (72,73).

A model approach to the selection of analgesics for cancer pain, known as the "analgesic ladder," was developed by the World Health Organization (WHO) in the 1980s and remains influential today (**Figure 12.5-1**) (74). According to this approach, patients with mild-to-moderate cancer-related pain and no prior opioid treatment may be managed initially with a nonopioid analgesic—acetaminophen or an NSAID—on the first rung of the ladder. The drug selected may be combined with an adjuvant drug that can either provide additional analgesia (ie, an adjuvant analgesic) or treat a side effect of the analgesic or a coexisting symptom. The second rung of the analgesic ladder, intended for opioid-naïve patients with generally moderate pain and those with pain that has not responded to a trial of acetaminophen or an NSAID, recommends treatment with an opioid conventionally used to treat moderate pain. The latter drugs were originally called "weak" opioids. The third rung of the analgesic ladder was indicated for patients with generally severe pain or pain that did not respond to a drug used for moderate pain. It recommended treatment with an opioid conventionally used for severe pain, which was designated the "strong" opioids. The ladder approach also suggested that acetaminophen or an NSAID, or an adjuvant drug, be considered whenever administering an opioid.

The analgesic ladder model was developed for cancer pain and has been generalized to populations with chronic pain related to other types of serious incurable illnesses. It was never intended to influence the treatment of patients with the so-called chronic noncancer pain, such as low back pain or headache, and should not be applied to these populations. In developed countries, it has been supplanted as a clinical guideline with more up-to-date, evidence-based recommendations (75-76). Nonetheless, the analgesic ladder model has historical importance and is still widely cited in the developing world to encourage policymakers to expand medical access to opioid drugs. It advances a fundamental concept—the value of long-term opioid therapy for chronic

moderate-to-severe pain related to active cancer—that remains an important message when laws and policies exist that prevent medically appropriate treatment with these drugs.

Nonopioid Analgesics

In the United States, the nonopioid analgesics comprise acetaminophen and numerous NSAIDs (**Table 12.5-3**). These drugs have a well-established role in the treatment of cancer pain (77), notwithstanding a paucity of evidence for efficacy (78). Based on clinical observation, NSAIDs appear to be especially useful in patients with bone pain or pain related to grossly inflammatory lesions, and relatively less useful in patients with neuropathic pain. NSAIDs also have an opioid-sparing effect that may be helpful in preventing the occurrence of opioid dose-related side effects (79).

Acetaminophen is available in multiple oral formulations and an IV formulation. It is widely used for its analgesic and antipyretic effects (80). It has no significant anti-inflammatory effects but may be preferred because of a side-effect profile that lacks GI and platelet toxicity. The main concern is hepatotoxicity, which can be minimized by avoiding use in those with known liver disease and by limiting the maximum total daily dose (recommended to be 3.2 g/d in the United States). Patients and families should be educated about the need to avoid the use of multiple over-the-counter medications that contain this drug.

NSAIDs inhibit the enzyme COX to reduce the production of peripheral and central prostaglandins, and this action presumably underlies their analgesic effects. There are multiple forms of COX. COX-1 is relatively more constitutive, physiologically active in many tissues, and COX-2 is relatively inducible, produced as part of the inflammatory cascade. The NSAIDs vary in the extent to which they affect the two COX isozymes.

The clinical decision to offer an NSAID to a patient with cancer usually hinges on the assessment of drug-related risk. GI toxicity is well recognized and ranges from pain or nausea to frank ulceration and hemorrhage. There are large drug-selective differences in the risk of NSAID-induced peptic ulcer disease. Compounds that are more selective for COX-2 than COX-1 have a lower risk of inducing GI adverse effects (81,82), and some drugs that are relatively COX-2 selective have been labeled as such and promoted for their enhanced GI safety. In the United States, the only drug of the latter type now on the market is celecoxib. Other NSAIDs—such as nabumetone, ibuprofen, meloxicam, and etodolac (81)—are not labeled as COX-2 selective but are relatively selective nonetheless and have reduced potential for adverse GI effects. Irrespective of the drug, the risk of GI toxicity is associated with the dose and duration of NSAID treatment, coadministration of aspirin, and infection with *Helicobacter pylori* (83). The risk may be reduced by coadministration of a proton-pump inhibitor, such as omeprazole, or the prostaglandin analog misoprostol (84).

Cardiovascular safety is also a prominent concern during NSAID therapy. All NSAIDs are prothrombotic and pose an increased risk of peripheral vascular disease, MI, transient ischemic attacks, and stroke (85,86). Mechanistically, this risk is associated with COX-2 inhibition, whether produced by the nonselective COX-1/COX-2 inhibitors or by the COX-2–selective drugs. In the United States, all NSAIDs now have a boxed warning in the package insert, which offers cautions about both cardiovascular and GI risks. Among all commercially available NSAIDs, naproxen generally is viewed as having the lowest risk of cardiovascular toxicity (87).

All NSAIDs can also produce renal or hepatic toxicity, particularly when patients are predisposed by chronic organ dysfunction. Renal effects include fluid overload, acute nephritis, and CKD. Most NSAIDs are also associated with a bleeding diathesis related to platelet dysfunction.

Given this risk profile, NSAIDs should be administered with caution to patients with cancer with significant predisposing factors for peptic ulcer disease, CVD, renal disease, hepatic disease, or bleeding diathesis. If there is no strong contraindication for therapy, patients who are predisposed to ulcer disease should be

■ TABLE 12.5-3. Nonsteroidal Anti-Inflammatory Drugs (NSAIDs)

Class and Generic Name	Approximate Half-Life (h)	Dosing Schedule	Recommended Starting Dose[a]	Comment[b]
P-aminophenol derivatives				
Acetaminophen[c]	3-4	q4-6h	650 mg q4h (5 doses daily)	Overdosage produces hepatic toxicity. Not anti-inflammatory and, therefore, not preferred as first-line analgesic or co-analgesic in patients with bone pain. Lack of GI or platelet toxicity; at high doses, liver function tests should be monitored.
Napthylalkanones				
Nabumetone	22-30	q24h	500-1,000 mg q12h	Appears to have a relatively low risk of GI toxicity; once-daily dosing can be useful.
Salicylates				
Acetylsalicylic acid[c]	3-12[d]	q4-6h	650 mg q4h (5 doses daily)	Standard for comparison. May not be tolerated as well as some of the newer NSAIDs.
Diflunisal[c]	8-12	q12h	1,000 mg × 1, then 500 mg q12h	Less GI toxicity than aspirin.
Choline magnesium trisalicylate[c]	8-12	q12h	500-1,000 mg q12h	Choline magnesium trisalicylate and salsalate have minimal GI toxicity and no effect on platelet aggregation despite anti-inflammatory effects. May therefore be particularly useful in some patients with cancer.
Salsalate	8-12	q12h	500-1,000 mg q12h	
Propionic acids				
Ibuprofen[c]	3-4	q4-8h	400-600 mg q8h	Available over the counter.
Naproxen[c]	13	q12h	250-500 mg q12h	Available as a suspension.
Naproxen sodium[c]	13	q12h	275-550 mg q12h	—
Fenoprofen	2-3	q6h	200 mg q6h	—
Ketoprofen	2-3	q6-8h	25-50 mg q8h	—
Flurbiprofen[c]	5-6	q8-12h	100 mg q12h	—
Oxaprozin	40	q24h	600 mg q24h	Once-daily dosing may be useful.
Acetic acids				
Indomethacin	4-5	q8-12h	25 mg q8h	Available in sustained-release and rectal formulations. Higher incidence of side effects, particularly GI and CNS, than propionic acids.
Tolmetin	1	q6-8h	200 mg q8h	
Sulindac	14	q12h	150 mg q12h	Less renal toxicity than other NSAIDs.
Diclofenac	2	q6-8h	25 mg q8h	
Ketorolac[c]	4-7	q4-6h	30-60 mg load, then 15-30 mg q6h (parenteral); 10 mg q6h (oral)	Only parenteral formulation available. Approved for postoperative use. Experience too limited to evaluate higher doses.
Oxicams				
Piroxicam	45	q24h	20 mg q24h	Administration of 40 mg for over 3 wk is associated with a high incidence of peptic ulcer, particularly in the older patients.
Fenamates				
Mefenamic acid[c]	2	q6h	250 mg q6h	Not recommended for use >1 wk and, therefore, not indicated in cancer pain therapy.
COX-2 inhibitors				
Celecoxib	11	q12h	100-200 mg q12h	Fewer GI side effects; no effect on platelet function.

CNS, central nervous system; COX, cyclooxygenase; GI, gastrointestinal; q, every.

[a]Starting dose should be one-half to two-thirds of the recommended dose for the older patients, those on multiple drugs, and those with renal insufficiency. Doses must be individualized. Low initial doses should be titrated upward if tolerated and clinical effect is inadequate. Doses can be incremented weekly. Studies of NSAIDs in the cancer population are meager; dosing guidelines are thus empiric.
[b]With all NSAIDs, stool guaiac and liver function tests, blood urea nitrogen, creatinine, and urinalysis should be monitored; frequency of monitoring should be increased for those on relatively high doses.
[c]Pain is approved indication.
[d]Half-life of aspirin increases with dose.

considered for a trial of celecoxib in the United States and patients who may be at relatively high risk of cardiovascular toxicity should be offered naproxen first.

Other factors may also be important in drug selection. Given the substantial variability in the response of individual patients to different agents, the response to an NSAID in the past may be helpful in guiding drug selection in the present. The need to promote treatment adherence or provide a simpler dosing regimen may encourage the use of a drug that can be administered once daily (eg, nabumetone) or twice daily (eg, celecoxib and many others), whereas the desire for as-needed dosing suggests the use of a short-duration drug (eg, ibuprofen). Finally, drug selection may be influenced by cost, which varies greatly among both drugs and pharmacies.

Although patients with cancer pain are commonly treated with standard NSAID doses, toxicity is dose related and is reasonable to seek the minimal effective dose for long-term therapy. Dose escalation in poor responders is limited by dose-related toxicities and a ceiling dose for analgesia above which additional dose increments fail to produce more relief. If a low initial dose is ineffective, the dose can be increased to determine whether analgesia is enhanced. The lack of additional pain relief following a dose increase suggests that the ceiling has been reached and the dose can then be lowered to the previously effective level or the drug can be discontinued.

Monitoring of patients receiving long-term NSAID therapy depends on the assessed risks and the goals of care. Considerations include periodic evaluation for occult fecal blood, changes in blood pressure, and effects on renal or hepatic function.

Opioid Analgesics

Expertise in the administration of opioid analgesics (**Table 12.5-4**) is the foundation of cancer pain management. The clinician should have knowledge of opioid pharmacology and a clear grasp of practical guidelines for dosing.

■ TABLE 12.5-4. Opioid Analgesics

Drug	Dose (mg) Equianalgesic to Morphine 10 mg IM[a] PO	IM	Half-Life (hr)	Peak Effect (hr)	Duration (hr)	Comment[b]
Morphine	20-30	10	2-3	0.5-1.0	3-6	Standard for comparison
Morphine CR	20-30	10	2-3	3-4	8-12	Various formulations are not bioequivalent
Morphine SR	20-30	10	2-3	2-3	12-24	—
Codeine	200	130	2-3	1.5-2.0	3-6	Combined with aspirin or acetaminophen. Usually for moderate pain. Also available without co-analgesics
Hydromorphone Hydromorphone CR	7.5 7.5	1.5 —	2-3 ~11	0.5-1.0 12-16	2-4 ~13	Potency may be greater, ie, hydromorphone: morphine = 3:1 rather than 6.7:1 during prolonged use
Oxycodone	20	—	2-3	1	3-4	Combined with aspirin or acetaminophen, for moderate pain; available PO without co-analgesics and useful for severe pain
Oxycodone CR	20	—	2-3	2-3	8-12	
Oxymorphone	10	1	2-3	1.5-3.0	2-4	—
Oxymorphone CR Hydrocodone Hydrocodone CR	20 (oral) 30 (oral) 30 (oral)	— 	2-3 3-4 7-9	1.5-3.0 1-2 5	2-4 4-8 8-12	—
Methadone	20	10	12-190	0.5-1.5	4-12	Although 1:1 ratio with morphine was in single-dose study, there is a change with chronic dosing, and large dose reduction (75%-90%) is needed when switching to methadone. Risk of delayed toxicity
Levorphanol	4	2	12-15	0.5-1	4-6	Usage limited because only 2 mg tablets are available
Fentanyl	—	—	7-12	—	—	Can be administered as a continuous IV infusion or SC infusion; based on clinical experience, 100 µg/hr is roughly equianalgesic to morphine 4 mg/hr
Fentanyl TTS	—	—	16-24	—	48-72	Based on clinical experience, 100 µg is roughly equianalgesic to morphine 4 mg
Meperidine	300	75	2-3	0.5-1.0	3-4	Not preferred for patients with cancer owing to potential toxicity
Tapentadol Tramadol	— 	— 	4-5 6-8	1 ~2	4-6 3-6	Mixed mechanism drugs, having both opioid and monoaminergic mechanisms of action; sometimes used for moderate cancer pain.

Respiratory depression is rare in patients with cancer.

IM, intramuscular; IV, intravenous; PO, oral; SC, subcutaneous.

[a]Dose that provides analgesia equivalent to 10 mg IM morphine.
[b]All opioids may produce various common side effects (eg, constipation, nausea, sedation).

Opioid Classes

Based on receptor interactions, the opioid analgesics can be divided broadly into pure μ-receptor agonist, agonist-antagonists, and mixed mechanism drugs. The pure μ-agonist drugs are generally preferred for the management of chronic cancer pain.

The agonist-antagonist drugs comprise a mixed agonist-antagonist subclass, which includes drugs that are weak antagonists at the μ-receptor and agonists at another receptor subtype, and a partial μ-receptor agonist subclass. All these drugs have a ceiling dose for analgesia and respiratory depression, and the potential to produce an abstinence syndrome in patients already physically dependent on an agonist drug. The mixed agonist-antagonist drugs, including butorphanol, pentazocine, and nalbuphine, are not used for the management of chronic cancer pain.

In the United States, the only partial μ-receptor agonist drug is buprenorphine. This drug is used in the management of addiction, and an expanded role for buprenorphine in the management of chronic pain has been recommended by an expert panel (88). Although experience in cancer pain is very limited (89), it may be considered for patients with cancer with moderate or severe pain who have limited or no prior opioid treatment, particularly when pain is complicated by a comorbid opioid-use disorder. It is available for pain as a transdermal patch and a buccal film.

The mixed mechanism drugs, tramadol and tapentadol, bind to the μ-receptor and concurrently block monoamine (eg, serotonin and norepinephrine) reuptake. In some countries, tramadol is widely used for cancer pain. Both tramadol and tapentadol have very limited evidence of comparative benefit in cancer pain (90,91), and both have a ceiling dose related to the risk of serotonin syndrome at high doses. Either may be used to manage moderate-to-severe pain in patients with cancer with low prior opioid exposure, but there is no clear advantage over the use of a pure μ-receptor agonist.

Morphine is often considered the prototype pure μ-receptor agonist opioid drug. It should not be considered the preferred drug, however. Large interindividual variation in the response to morphine and other drugs in this class, such as hydromorphone, oxycodone, oxymorphone, fentanyl, and methadone, means that a patient's response to one of these drugs does not predict the response to another. Morphine may or may not yield a more favorable outcome than an alternative.

Morphine also produces active metabolites, which can complicate therapy in patients with renal impairment. The predominant metabolic pathway for morphine is glucuronidation to morphine-3-glucuronide (M3G) and morphine-6-glucuronide (M6G), and the accumulation of morphine metabolites may be associated with side effects, such as myoclonus and chronic nausea (92). Renal insufficiency results in accumulation of M3G and M6G, and for this reason, morphine should be administered cautiously to patients with renal insufficiency. In the setting of very poor renal function, hydromorphone, fentanyl, and buprenorphine are often preferred (93).

Opioid Selection

The analgesic ladder model (74) suggests that one group of analgesic drugs may be considered for patients who are relatively opioid naïve and are experiencing cancer pain that is generally moderate (second rung of the ladder), whereas other drugs should be considered for patients with severe pain, usually after opioid therapy has begun (third rung). Although this approach has been adopted by many clinicians, there is no evidence that it yields better outcomes than those obtained when moderate pain in the opioid-naïve patient is treated with relatively low doses of a drug conventionally used for severe pain (94,95).

Nonetheless, opioid therapy for moderate pain is often initiated with drugs conventionally selected for pain of this intensity. This includes combination products containing acetaminophen plus codeine, hydrocodone, or oxycodone; buprenorphine; or a mixed mechanism opioid (tramadol or tapentadol). Codeine, hydrocodone, and tramadol have pharmacokinetics that may be strongly influenced by the genetically determined status of the CYP2D6 hepatic enzyme (96), resulting in analgesia that is less predictable. In the cancer population, the use of an alternative drug for moderate pain may be preferable. Oral meperidine also should not be used because of the risks associated with accumulation of a toxic metabolite; a similar concern existed with the use of propoxyphene, which is no longer available in the United States.

Given these considerations, the drugs that may be preferred for the initial management of moderate pain in the patient with cancer with limited or no prior opioid exposure include a nonopioid (eg, acetaminophen) plus oxycodone combination product, the buprenorphine patch or buccal film, tapentadol, or a low dose of a pure μ-receptor agonist, such as morphine, hydromorphone, or fentanyl. The recommended starting doses for these drugs are usually well tolerated.

The selection of an opioid for severe cancer pain is empirical. Any of the pure μ-receptor agonist opioids may be used. As noted, morphine has been considered the prototype drug in this class but is not preferred in the setting of significant renal impairment. If pain is present most of the day, a long-acting drug may be preferred, usually a modified-release formulation of an oral short half-life drug. Morphine, oxycodone, oxymorphone, hydrocodone, and hydromorphone are available in the United States and many other countries. Transdermal fentanyl also is widely available and provides a dosing interval of 2 to 3 days (97).

Although both levorphanol and methadone have relatively long half-lives, patients typically require doses at least every 6 hours to maintain stable effects. Experience with levorphanol in cancer pain is limited, but if available, it is an option. Methadone is widely available and has become an increasingly popular drug for chronic pain, presumably because of its low cost, potential for unexpectedly high potency, relatively low abuse potential, and low likelihood of diversion by individuals with a history of substance-use disorder. Clinical experience suggests that rotation to methadone after inadequate treatment with another opioid can produce surprisingly good results, an outcome that has been speculated to be related to the D-isomer in the racemate formulation that is commercially available in most countries; this isomer blocks the N-methyl-D-aspartate (NMDA) receptor and may potentiate analgesia.

Methadone is a challenging drug to use, however, and clinicians must understand its unique pharmacology to administer it in a safe manner (98,99). Methadone's half-life ranges between 12 and 190 hours, and substantial delayed toxicity has been observed many days after methadone treatment was begun or altered. Its potential to have an unexpectedly high potency when substituting for another opioid increases the challenge of dose selection when starting the drug, and it can prolong the QTc interval (100). Given the increased potential for serious toxicity with methadone, its administration should be undertaken only by clinicians with the knowledge and experience necessary to ensure safety, according to best practices (99).

Routes of Administration

The oral and transdermal routes are preferred in the management of chronic cancer pain. Alternative routes may be required, however, and the clinician must recognize their indications and be familiar with the accepted approaches.

Transdermal Delivery

The transdermal route of administration is available for the highly lipophilic opioids buprenorphine and fentanyl. The transdermal formulation of buprenorphine available in the United States provides a relatively low-dose range; like the buccal film formulation, it may be considered for the treatment of moderate pain in those with limited to no opioid exposure.

Transdermal fentanyl is preferred by some patients and may be associated with relatively less constipation than oral opioid formulations (101). Transdermal patches should be used cautiously in patients with cachexia. The literature is limited, but some studies suggest transdermal fentanyl may produce fentanyl concentrations that are higher or lower than expected in this context (102,103). Patients with very low albumin levels and those with fevers are at relatively higher risk because of sudden increases in the free fraction of fentanyl and increased absorption from the reservoir during fever (104).

Rectal

Rectal formulations of oxymorphone, hydromorphone, and morphine are available in the United States, and there is anecdotal experience with rectal administration of controlled-release morphine or oxycodone tablets. The rectal route is usually considered for patients who are relatively opioid nontolerant and become temporarily unable to take oral medications. The potency of opioids administered rectally is believed to approximate oral dosing (105), absorption is variable, and relative potency may be higher or lower than expected; this depends on a variety of factors, including location of the suppository in the rectum and contents of the rectum at the time of dosing.

Oral and Nasal Transmucosal

Buccal buprenorphine is available in the United States and, as described, may play a role in the treatment of some patients with chronic cancer pain. Formulations of transmucosal fentanyl also have been developed, specifically for the treatment of cancer-related breakthrough pain—transitory flares of acute pain superimposed on chronic pain (13). Although a short-acting oral opioid drug may be effective in managing breakthrough pain, the transmucosal drugs (known in the United States as TIRFs or transmucosal immediate-release formulations) have an onset and duration of effects that more closely mirror most breakthrough pains. All are efficacious (106), and some studies demonstrate comparative efficacy over morphine (107). Given cost factors, the TIRFs, which include an intraoral lozenge, an effervescent buccal tablet, a buccal patch, a sublingual tablet, sublingual spray, and a nasal spray, are usually considered for breakthrough pains that have not responded to an oral drug or have a very rapid onset (107). There are insufficient data to recommend one formulation over another, and this decision will usually be based on availability, cost, and patient preference. In the United States, the TIRFs have a mandatory shared risk evaluation and mitigation strategy, the purpose of which is to reduce the risk of abuse and unintentional overdose.

In some clinical situations, a trial of sublingual administration—an oral liquid formulation or an injectable formulation placed under the tongue—is reasonable. There is considerable experience in the use of sublingual concentrated oral morphine solution during the care of patients at the end of life; this drug is relatively hydrophilic, however, and its effects may be related to enteral absorption after swallowing.

Parenteral Injection

Patients who are unable to swallow or absorb opioid drugs are candidates for long-term parenteral dosing. Repetitive intramuscular or subcutaneous injections are painful and should rarely be considered. Repetitive IV injections may be effective, but these usually require skilled nursing and may be associated with prominent "bolus" effects (toxicity at peak concentration or pain breakthrough at the trough or both). Repetitive dosing through a "butterfly" needle placed under the skin has been used effectively in end-of-life care, and experience suggests that the needle can be in place for a week without the development of local pain or other problems.

Continuous Infusion

Continuous infusion eliminates the fluctuations in plasma concentration associated with repetitive bolus injections. Any opioid available in an injectable formulation can be used for continuous infusion. The availability of continuous subcutaneous infusion using ambulatory infusion devices has markedly enhanced the clinical utility of infusion techniques, allowing long-term administration of opioids and other drugs in the home environment (108). A diverse group of pumps that range considerably in features, complexity, and cost are now available, and the clinician often has the option of selecting a pump based on the needs and resources of the patient. In most cities, skilled nursing through home health care organizations can assist in the management of therapy at home.

Intraspinal Opioids

The discovery of opioid receptors in the spinal cord provided the foundation for the development of techniques to deliver intraspinal opioid analgesics. Intraspinal administration can provide selective analgesia (ie, without the sensory or motor blockade produced by local anesthetics) at doses lower than those required systemically. The strongest indication for a trial of intraspinal opioid administration is the occurrence of intolerable somnolence or confusion in patients who are not experiencing adequate analgesia during systemic opioid treatment of pain.

A 2022 systematic review and meta-analysis revealed that neuraxial infusion produces sustained analgesia and results in a halving of systemic opioid use (109). Patients with cancer pain that is poorly responsive to systemic therapy should be considered for a neuraxial approach if the resources exist to implement and monitor it (110).

Many methods of intraspinal opioid administration are now in use. An epidural catheter can be tunneled to the anterior abdominal wall and the proximate end can be percutaneously connected to an ambulatory infusion pump; alternatively, the proximate end can be connected to a subcutaneous port. For patients with life expectancies of 3 months or more, an intrathecal catheter connected to a totally implanted continuous infusion device may be preferable.

Varied drugs are now employed for long-term intraspinal therapy (111). The preferred opioid drugs for chronic intraspinal infusion are morphine and hydromorphone. Combination therapies using one of these opioids plus a local anesthetic or clonidine, or both are now commonplace. Ziconotide, a unique calcium channel blocker, is also now available in the United States and has been shown to be effective for cancer pain in controlled trials (112). The use of a combination of drugs may help potentiate analgesia and reduce side effects, such as sensory and motor block, urinary retention, pruritus, and nausea.

Guidelines for the Administration of Opioid Drugs

Evidence-based guidelines for the treatment of cancer pain have been developed by many groups (75-76). Although high-quality evidence is limited (68), observational studies (69) suggest that most patients provided therapy based on these guidelines have satisfactory outcomes.

As described, opioid-naïve patients with generally moderate pain may have opioid therapy initiated using a drug conventionally administered for pain of this type—such as a nonopioid-oxycodone combination product, the buprenorphine patch or buccal film, or tapentadol—or treatment can be started using a low dose of a pure μ-receptor agonist, such as morphine, hydromorphone, or fentanyl (94,95). Although the opioid-naïve patient is usually offered a short-acting drug, it is acceptable to initiate therapy with a long-acting formulation, as long as pain is present during most of the day and the dose selected is appropriate. For example, long-acting morphine can be started in the opioid-naïve patient at a dose of 15 mg twice daily; long-acting oxycodone or oxymorphone can be started at doses of 10 mg twice daily or 5 mg twice daily, respectively; and transdermal fentanyl can be initiated at 12 μg/hr. Given the availability of these long-acting formulations in doses appropriate for opioid-naïve patients, the decision to start a short-acting or long-acting drug in a patient with new-onset persistent pain is a clinical judgment based on patient preference, convenience, cost, availability, and experience.

If a patient is receiving a short-acting drug, but four or more doses are needed daily to control pain, or pain is not controlled despite repeated administrations, it may be helpful to switch to a single-entity pure μ-receptor agonist opioid, typically in a long-acting formulation. The starting dose should provide roughly equivalent analgesia on a 24-hour basis as the sum of the short-acting drugs.

For the patient with severe chronic cancer pain—either reported to be generally severe or inadequately controlled despite appropriate use of a drug conventionally used for moderate cancer pain—ongoing treatment conventionally employs a pure μ-receptor agonist opioid. As described, the specific drug selected is empirical and based on availability, cost, the patient's prior experience, and the clinician's familiarity.

Dose adjustment is almost always required. The dose of the opioid should be iteratively increased until acceptable analgesia occurs or intolerable and unmanageable side effects supervene. A favorable balance between analgesia and side effects is usually found, and this is usually maintained for a prolonged time unless there is progression in the pain-producing pathology. Recurrent pain or the new occurrence of side effects necessitates another period of dose titration. Inadequate adjustment of the dose is probably the most common reason for unsuccessful long-term management of cancer pain.

The pure μ-receptor agonist opioids do not have a ceiling dose for analgesia. Incremental doses typically produce more analgesia until intolerable side effects prevent further dose escalation. Although most patients remain stable on opioid doses equivalent to less than a few hundred milligrams of morphine per day, some patients have a satisfactory response on higher doses. Occasional patients require extremely high doses—equivalent to grams of morphine per day. At relatively high doses, it is important to reassess the nature of the pain, ensure that expressed need for treatment is not related to other factors (eg, a comorbid psychiatric disorder, including the possibility of addiction), and also establish that the benefits of therapy clearly outweigh the side effects and burdens.

Breakthrough Pain

Surveys have demonstrated that approximately half of the patients with chronic cancer pain experience clinically significant breakthrough pain (113). Numerous studies have evaluated the characteristics, impact, and management of these common pains (15,114). Unless contraindicated, patients with cancer with breakthrough pains that adversely affect QoL should be considered for specific treatment. As described, this is typically a short-acting oral formulation. Based on clinical observations, the effective dose of this drug is usually 5% to 15% of the total daily opioid dose administered on a fixed schedule. The TIRFs—transmucosal immediate-release fentanyl—are an efficacious alternative to oral therapy (106).

Opioid Rotation

Titrating the opioid dose through iterative dose escalation based on pain severity may produce side effects that cannot be effectively managed. When this occurs, the therapy should be designated poorly responsive to the specific drug and route, and an alternative strategy for pain control should be implemented (115). This may include more sophisticated management of the treatment-limiting side effect, the addition of a pharmacologic or nonpharmacologic analgesic approach that could reduce the opioid requirement, or opioid rotation.

Opioid rotation, or the switching from one opioid to another to improve the outcomes of an opioid regimen, is now widely used, despite guidelines based on experience rather than research (116,117). Switching requires an appreciation of relative potency, as codified on the equianalgesic dose table (**Table 12.5-4**). To switch to another opioid drug or route, the equianalgesic dose table is used to calculate a dose of the new drug that would be theoretically equianalgesic with the old drug or route. With few exceptions, the dosing regimen

based on this calculated dose should be reduced by 25% to 50% to account for incomplete cross-tolerance between drugs and other sources of variation (116). Given the potential for a substantially higher potency of methadone than that suggested in equianalgesic dose tables, a larger reduction is prudent if the switch is to this drug. Various approaches have been recommended to ensure the safety of methadone in opioid rotation (99,117). These approaches recommend a reduction in the methadone dose that is proportionate to the dose of the prior drug and is roughly 75% to 90% lower than the calculated equianalgesic dose. In contrast, no reduction in the equianalgesic dose is needed if the switch is to transdermal fentanyl and the conversion approach recommended by the manufacturer is used.

Management of Common Opioid Side Effects

Although there is no maximum dose or ceiling dose for the μ-agonist opioids, the appearance of side effects imposes a practical limit on dose escalation. Given the importance of side effects in determining the response to an opioid, the successful management of common adverse side effects is a fundamental aspect of therapy (**Table 12.5-5**).

■ TABLE 12.5-5. Commonly Used Pharmacologic Approaches in the Management of Opioid Side Effects	
Opioid Side Effect	**Treatment**
Constipation	**Approaches for all patients:**
	Increase fluid intake and dietary fiber
	Ensure co-analgesics or adjuvant (comfort and convenience, etc)
	Discuss approaches with patient and select one or more:
	Daily contact laxative plus stool softener (eg, senna plus docusate)
	Daily osmotic laxative
	Intermittent use of laxative
	Consider alternative approaches in refractory cases:
	Opioid antagonist—methylnaltrexone or naloxegol
	Lubiprostone
	Prokinetic agent (metoclopramide)
Nausea	**Several approaches:**
	If associated with vertigo or if markedly exacerbated by movement, antivertiginous drug (eg, scopolamine, meclizine)
	If associated with early satiety, prokinetic agent (metoclopramide)
	In other cases, dopamine antagonist drugs (eg, prochlorperazine, haloperidol, metoclopramide) or 5-HT antagonists (ondansetron, granisetron, others)
Somnolence, mental clouding	If analgesia is satisfactory, reduce opioid dose by 25%-50%
	If analgesia is satisfactory and the toxicity involves confusion, consider a trial of a neuroleptic (eg, haloperidol)
	If analgesia is satisfactory and the toxicity is somnolence, consider a trial of a psychostimulant (eg, methylphenidate or modafinil)
	Consider pharmacologic approaches to reduce the opioid requirement (addition of a co-analgesics or adjuvant)
	Consider trial of an alternative opioid
	If appropriate, consider nonpharmacologic analgesic approaches

5-HT, 5-hydroxytryptamine.

Constipation is a highly prevalent side effect of opioid therapy and may contribute to abdominal pain, distension, nausea, and worsening anorexia and occasionally may progress to obstipation and bowel obstruction. The management of drug-induced constipation should begin with the elimination of nonessential constipating drugs and, if possible, an increase in both fluid and fiber intake. Fiber should not be increased in those with possible partial bowel obstruction or marked debility because of the potential for worsening obstruction.

There is a broad consensus that the likelihood of opioid-induced constipation is high enough to warrant prophylactic therapy. There are numerous types of laxatives, including bulk-forming agents, osmotic agents, lubricants, surfactants, contact cathartics, prokinetic drugs, and opioid antagonists (118). The conventional first-line approach is a combination of a stool softener, usually docusate, and a cathartic agent, such as senna. Most patients respond to this therapy. The osmotic agent, polyethylene glycol, in a powdered formulation offers another well-tolerated and usually effective approach. Other osmotic agents, such as lactulose, are often tried in more refractory cases.

New treatments should be considered if routine conventional therapy yields an unsatisfactory outcome (118-122). Opioid antagonists with selective peripheral effects, which do not cause systemic withdrawal, should be considered when constipation has not responded to first-line therapies. These drugs include oral and parenteral methylnaltrexone, naloxegol, and naldemedine; relatively high oral doses of oral naloxone (>8 mg/d) may be an alternative. The secretagogues include lubiprostone, which is approved for opioid-induced constipation in the United States, and both linaclotide and plecanatide. These drugs act on electrolyte channels in the gut wall to increase chloride or sodium secretion (118). Prokinetic drugs include prucalopride, a selective 5-hydroxytryptamine-4 (5-HT4) receptor agonist, and metoclopramide. Finally, there is limited evidence suggesting benefits from probiotic therapy (122).

Although nausea occurs commonly at the start of opioid therapy, it is uncommon during long-term use. If persistent nausea is experienced, potential contributing etiologies should be evaluated and treated if possible. If the opioid appears to be a prominent contributor to nausea, the symptom can be treated, at least for a period long enough to determine whether tolerance will occur. The usual first-line therapies include the dopamine antagonists, such as prochlorperazine, metoclopramide, or haloperidol, and the 5-HT antagonists, such as ondansetron (123). Patients with refractory nausea may need other pharmacologic approaches, such as a corticosteroid or a commercially available cannabinoid, such as THC or nabilone. Some nauseated patients appear to benefit from empirical treatment with a drug used for vertigo, such as meclizine or scopolamine. In difficult cases, combinations of drugs from unrelated classes are often tried.

Like nausea, somnolence or mental clouding is common when an opioid regimen is begun or the dose is increased, and most patients develop tolerance to this effect relatively quickly. Some have persistent cognitive effects, however, which may be severe enough to warrant rotation to another opioid.

Symptomatic therapies for opioid-induced somnolence or mental clouding may also be considered (**Table 12.5-5**). Methylphenidate has been shown to decrease opioid-induced sedation in patients with cancer (124,125). The starting dose is 5 mg at breakfast and at lunchtime; dose titration is often needed, while monitoring side effects, including anorexia, jitteriness, anxiety, and insomnia. Other psychostimulants that have been used empirically for this indication include modafinil, armodafinil, dextroamphetamine, amphetamine, and atomoxetine. A 2011 systematic review concluded that the data pertaining to these drugs were insufficient to draw conclusions (126).

Opioid therapy is associated with many other adverse effects, two of which are particularly noteworthy. Opioid-induced sleep-disordered breathing is a well-established phenomenon, which may result in adverse consequences due to sleep apnea (127).

Opioids may worsen preexisting obstructive or central sleep apnea or cause a mixed syndrome de novo. The diagnosis should be suspected in those with known sleep apnea, factors predisposing to apnea, or symptoms that may suggest the effect—such as daytime sleepiness, fatigue, or mood disorder—when inadequately explained by other factors. History from a bed partner may be useful. Selected patients may be considered for referral to a sleep specialist for further evaluation and management.

Opioid-induced endocrinopathy is prevalent and most likely to result in hypogonadism (128). Other effects, such as an increase in prolactin or a decrease in serum cortisol, are also possible. The clinical manifestations of hypogonadism include fatigue, mood disturbances, decreased libido, infertility, and adverse effects on bone. If consistent with the goals of care, measurement of sex hormones may offer the opportunity to treat symptoms through hormone replacement. Clinical experience suggests that appropriately selected men with low testosterone may experience symptomatic benefit with testosterone repletion.

Opioid Abuse and Addiction

Opioids are potentially abusable drugs, and all patients, including those without a known history of drug abuse, have the potential to develop adverse abuse-related outcomes. Patients with cancer with substance-use disorders, including opioid-use disorder, must be considered at high risk of these outcomes. The treatment of chronic cancer pain with long-term opioid therapy must be grounded in the principles of risk management to minimize potential harms associated with these drugs and reassure clinicians about the potential for safe and effective use despite the risks (129).

Phenomenology of Abuse

Risk management requires a working knowledge of the definitions and characteristics of the phenomena associated with abuse liability (130,131). These phenomena include tolerance and physical dependence, drug abuse and related terms, addiction, and diversion.

Tolerance is a neurophysiologic process defined by declining drug effects induced by exposure to the drug. From the clinical perspective, tolerance to analgesic effects is a potential concern, whereas tolerance to side effects, such as respiratory depression, reduces risk. Tolerance to opioid-induced mood effects may be important in the development of the disease of addiction, but addiction may occur with or without this phenomenon, and tolerance should not be used to define addiction (132). In the cancer population, tolerance to analgesic effects may be difficult to identify when escalating pain may be due to worsening tissue injury rather than drug-induced changes in efficacy. For this reason, a decline in analgesia should not be ascribed to tolerance unless reevaluation of the patient excludes progressive illness. In the absence of worsening disease, most patients with chronic cancer pain are able to attain a favorable balance between analgesia and side effects during opioid dose titration and then stabilize for a prolonged period. Accordingly, concerns about tolerance should never be used to delay appropriate opioid therapy.

Physical dependence, another neurophysiologic process, is defined by the occurrence of an abstinence syndrome following abrupt dose reduction or administration of an antagonist. It, too, should never be equated with addiction, and patients who are perceived to be physically dependent should be labeled "physically dependent" and not "dependent," which is a term used synonymously with addiction. There is large individual variation in the extent to which physical dependence develops and its manifestations should it become evident. Some patients develop significant distress associated with diverse symptoms and signs of withdrawal, whereas others experience a more limited reaction. It is prudent to assume that patients receiving daily doses of an opioid for even a few days have the potential for signs of withdrawal should therapy be stopped abruptly. Sudden discontinuation of the drug should be avoided if possible, and the use of antagonist drugs, including the agonist-antagonist opioids, should be undertaken with great caution.

If opioid dose reduction is needed, a decrement of 25% to 33% is usually tolerated. In those assumed to have substantial physical dependence, naloxone should be used only to reverse symptomatic respiratory depression—not to reverse somnolence—and it is prudent to use a dilute solution (eg, 0.4 mg in 10 mL saline) administered in small boluses while monitoring effects.

Drug abuse refers to either the use of an illicit drug or the nonmedical use of a prescribed drug with addictive potential. In the clinical setting, alternative terms are also used, including nonadherence, misuse, and aberrant drug-related behavior. The distinctions among these terms are ill-defined. They all highlight the importance of ongoing monitoring of drug-related behavior to determine whether patients follow direction or engage in problematic and potentially unsafe behaviors.

Addiction is a biopsychosocial disorder that results from complex interactions between genetic predispositions and both psychological and environmental factors that predispose to the development of an addictive pattern of use. It requires access to an abusable drug, often has an insidious onset and a relapsing-remitting course, and varies in presentation. Diagnostic criteria, described in the American Psychiatric Association's *Diagnostic and Statistical Manual of Mental Disorders*, fifth Edition (132), highlight the prolonged course and describe aberrant drug-related behaviors that are consistent with drug craving, loss of control over drug use, compulsive use of the drug, and continued use despite harm to the patient or others. Evidence of physical dependence and tolerance is noted but cannot be used to define the disorder.

From the clinical perspective, addiction is a salient concern whenever opioid therapy is needed by patients who have a history of substance abuse, and potentially a history of alcoholism or drug addiction. These patients are at high risk for aberrant drug-related behavior during opioid therapy, and prescribing should include a high level of adherence monitoring and planning for consequences should aberrant behaviors occur. If aberrant drug-related behaviors develop during therapy—whether or not a history of substance abuse has been elicited—these behaviors should be evaluated and diagnosed (133). If the behaviors are serious and may support a diagnosis of addiction, referral of the patient to an addiction medicine specialist should be considered, if available. Ongoing treatment of the patient with cancer with severe pain who has a comorbid substance-use disorder, perhaps addiction, is challenging (134) and may not be possible if the treatment cannot be controlled and risks are determined to exceed benefits.

Pseudoaddiction has been used to describe aberrant drug-related behavior associated with the stress caused by unrelieved pain. The term, coined more than three decades ago, has not been empirically evaluated, and concerns have arisen about the extent to which it has potentially undermined the need for appropriate risk management strategies during opioid therapy (135). Although stress, which may be pain related, is an important determinant of both aberrant drug-related behavior generally and the emergence or relapse of the disease of addiction, the term *pseudoaddiction* has been subject to misinterpretation and should not be used in the clinical setting.

Diversion is a legal term describing the transfer of abusable prescription drugs into the illicit marketplace. A health professional perceived by the authorities to be abetting this process can be charged with a felony. If monitoring of drug-related behavior suggests that diversion is taking place, the usual appropriate response is to cease prescribing.

Risk Management During Opioid Therapy

Although the risk of iatrogenic addiction is low patients who lack a prior history of abuse or addiction (136), the risk can never be entirely excluded (137,138), and clinicians who prescribe opioids or other potentially abusable drugs should adopt a "universal precautions" approach that is adaptable to all types of patients with cancer and clinical scenarios. This approach includes risk stratification and specific steps that the clinician may follow to structure therapy and assess outcomes (**Table 12.5-6**).

▇ TABLE 12.5-6. A "Universal Precautions" Approach to Opioid Prescribing for Cancer Pain

Steps	Considerations	Comment
1. Assess and stratify risk	Based on history, examination, record review, check of prescription drug monitoring program, and possible urine or saliva drug screen. Stratify risk into categories. A bedbound patient may be considered to have nil or extremely low risk, whereas others may be categorized as "moderate" or "high."	All patients should be assessed. Higher risk is associated with (1) past or present history of alcohol or drug abuse, (2) family history of alcohol or drug abuse, and (3) any type of major psychiatric disorder. Younger age and history of physical/sexual abuse are also associated. Validated measures of opioid risk are available but seldom used in the clinical setting.
2. Decision: Prescribe or not	If diversion is suspected, prescribing should not be done, unless risk can be eliminated. If drug abuse is occurring, a risk-to-benefit evaluation should determine whether the risks can be managed.	Diversion is places the clinician at legal risk.
3. Structure prescribing to minimize risk	Structure should match to the level of risk to allow appropriate adherence monitoring. Options include small number of tablets and frequent refills, use of one pharmacy, pill counts, no use of short-acting drugs, required consultation with Psychiatry or Addiction Medicine, urine or saliva drug testing.	Based on anecdotal observations, the use of methadone or buprenorphine may be preferred if risk of abuse is high.
4. Monitor drug-related behaviors	Monitor drug-related behaviors throughout the course of therapy	Drug-related behavior should be monitored routinely, just as analgesia, adverse effects, and impact of treatment on quality of life is monitored.
5. Respond to aberrant behaviors	If aberrant drug-related behavior occurs, reassessment is needed to determine diagnosis. Management is guided by diagnosis and may include discontinuation of therapy or increased adherence monitoring. Documentation is required.	The differential diagnosis may include addiction or other psychiatric disorders associated with impulsive drug-taking, patient confusion, family or caregiver issues, or criminal activity.

Adjuvant Analgesics

The adjuvant analgesics are drugs that have been developed for indications other than pain but are analgesic in some circumstances. There are numerous drugs in many drug classes, and a simple classification divides them into several large categories (139): multipurpose analgesics, drugs used for neuropathic pain, and drugs used for bone pain or pain due to malignant bowel obstruction (Table 12.5-7).

Multipurpose Analgesics

Some adjuvant analgesics have been used for pain of varied types, including the glucocorticoids, antidepressants, α2 adrenergic agonists, cannabinoids, topical therapies, botulinum toxin, neuroleptics, and NMDA inhibitors.

Glucocorticoids may be used to manage symptoms associated with advanced cancer, including pain, nausea, anorexia, and fatigue (140,141). Evidence for analgesic effects is limited (142), but favorable clinical experience suggests that a glucocorticoid, such as dexamethasone or prednisone, may ameliorate bone pain, neuropathic pain, pain from bowel or duct obstruction or organ capsule expansion, headache caused by increased intracranial pressure, and pain caused by lymphedema. Dexamethasone is often initiated with a loading dose of 10 to 20 mg, which is followed by 1 to 2 mg twice daily. Treatment is continued until clinical events warrant a change. In the context of advanced illness and short prognosis, observed benefits from this treatment outweigh the risks associated with long-term use, such as osteoporosis, myopathy, and immune suppression.

Analgesic antidepressants, notably the tricyclic antidepressants (TCAs) and serotonin-norepinephrine reuptake inhibitors

■ TABLE 12.5-7. Adjuvant Analgesics

Category	Class	Types	Examples	Comment
Multipurpose analgesics	Glucocorticoids	—	Dexamethasone, prednisone, methylprednisolone	Commonly used in advanced illness for pain/other symptoms
	Antidepressants	Secondary amine tricyclics	Desipramine, nortriptyline	Established analgesics, which are better tolerated than the tertiary amine drugs, and with the SNRIs, used in the medically ill for opioid-refractory pain, including neuropathic pain
		Tertiary amine tricyclics	Amitriptyline, imipramine	Established analgesics, generally with a more problematic side-effect profiles than the secondary amine tricyclics
		SNRIs	Duloxetine, milnacipran, venlafaxine, desvenlafaxine	Established analgesics, often selected first for opioid-refractory pain because of relatively good side-effect profile compared to the tricyclic compounds. Abrupt cessation can cause discontinuation syndrome.
		SSRIs	Paroxetine, citalopram, escitalopram	Poor evidence of analgesia but ability to mitigate chronic or recurrent anxiety can have a positive effect on pain
	α-2 Adrenergic agonists	—	Tizanidine, clonidine, dexmedetomidine	Tizanidine is best tolerated and may be tried for opioid-refractory pain. Clonidine is used neuraxially as an analgesic
	Cannabinoids	Pharmaceutical	Nabiximols, nabilone, Δ(9)-tetrahydrocannabinol	Evidence of analgesic efficacy is evolving. Available drugs may be considered if other adjuvant analgesics are ineffective
		Nonpharmaceutical	Medical cannabis	Available in many states but cannot be prescribed. Laws and regulations vary by state and should be consulted
	Topical agents	Local anesthetics	Patch, cream, gels	5% patch is convenient and used for regional neuropathic and musculoskeletal pain syndromes
		Capsaicin	8% patch, 0.075% patch or cream	8% patch approved for postherpetic neuralgia; may provide months of benefit after short exposure in a monitored setting. Low-concentration capsaicin may be useful for neuropathic or musculoskeletal pain syndromes
		Compounds, others	Ketamine, amitriptyline, menthol, others	—
	Botulinum toxin		Botulinum A, B	Potentially useful for many types of focal or regional pain
	Neuroleptics	First/second generation	Haloperidol, olanzapine	Poor evidence of efficacy
	NMDA receptor antagonists	—	Ketamine	Evidence is mixed, but ketamine is used by palliative care specialists for severe opioid-refractory pain syndromes. Evidence of efficacy in refractory depression may increase use

■ **TABLE 12.5-7. Adjuvant Analgesics (continued)**

Category	Class	Types	Examples	Comment
Drugs used for neuropathic pain	All multipurpose analgesics	—	—	—
	Gabapentinoids	—	Pregabalin, gabapentin	Extensive evidence of analgesia in many types of neuropathic pain. Patients may respond to gabapentin, pregabalin, both or neither. Used first for neuropathic pain, unless prominent depression is comorbid, in which case an antidepressant is used first
	Other anticonvulsants	—	Oxcarbazepine, lacosamide, lamotrigine, topiramate	—
	GABA agonists	GABA$_A$	Clonazepam	Poor evidence of analgesia
		GABA$_B$	Baclofen	Poor evidence of analgesia
Drugs used for bone pain in cancer	Glucocorticoids	—	Dexamethasone, prednisone, methylprednisolone	—
	Osteoclast inhibitors	Bisphosphonates	Zoledronate, alendronate, ibandronate, pamidronate, risedronate, clodronate, others	Used to prevent and treat skeletal-related events due to cancer, including pain
		RANKL inhibitor	Denosumab	Used to prevent and treat skeletal-related events due to cancer, including pain
		Calcitonin	—	Poor evidence of efficacy
	Radioisotopes	—	Samarium-153, strontium-89, phosphorus-32, others	—
Drugs used for pain and other symptoms in malignant bowel obstruction	Glucocorticoids	—	Dexamethasone, prednisone, methylprednisolone	—
	Antiemetics	Dopamine antagonist	Metoclopramide, haloperidol	—
		5-HT$_3$ antagonist	Ondansetron, granisetron	—
	PPI or H$_2$-blocker		Omeprazole, ranitidine	—
	Anticholinergic drug	—	Hyoscine (scopolamine) butylbromide or hydrobromide glycopyrrolate	Risk of cognitive side effects probably lessened by using glycopyrrolate, or in some countries, hyoscine butylbromide
	Somatostatin analog	—	Octreotide, lanreotide	Evidence of efficacy is mixed and should not be considered a first-line approach for this reason

GABA, γ-aminobutyric acid; NMDA, N-methyl-D-aspartate; PPI, proton-pump inhibitor; RANKL, receptor activator of nuclear factor-κB ligand; SNRIs, serotonin-norepinephrine reuptake inhibitors; SSRIs, serotonin selective reuptake inhibitors.

(SNRIs), may be considered for any type of chronic pain. In the cancer population, the usual target is neuropathic pain that has not responded adequately to an opioid trial. The antidepressants vary in the potential for analgesic effects and the risks of side effects (143,144). The tricyclic compounds comprise tertiary amine drugs, such as amitriptyline and imipramine, and secondary amine drugs, such as desipramine and nortriptyline. The latter drugs are better tolerated. Among the SNRIs, evidence of analgesia is strongest for duloxetine, but there is support as well for milnacipran, venlafaxine, and desvenlafaxine (145). There is very little evidence of analgesic efficacy for the selective serotonin reuptake inhibitors (SSRIs), such as fluoxetine, paroxetine, and sertraline.

SNRIs have a more favorable side-effect profile than the tricyclic compounds (144) and are generally offered first. Duloxetine is usually the first-line drug, given the extent of the evidence, which has established efficacy in chemotherapy-induced painful peripheral neuropathy (146,147). Although a secondary amine TCA, such as desipramine or nortriptyline, is an acceptable alternative, these drugs should be used cautiously in patients with significant heart disease, cognitive impairment, high fall risk, or urinary retention.

Dosing of antidepressants for pain mirrors their use for the primary indication of depression. Dose tapering is recommended when stopping or switching avoids the antidepressant discontinuation syndrome (148). This syndrome is characterized by flulike symptoms, nausea, dizziness, insomnia, and hyperarousal.

α-2 Adrenergic agonists, including clonidine, tizanidine, and dexmedetomidine, are potentially analgesic. Evidence is limited, however. A randomized trial demonstrated efficacy for epidural clonidine in cancer pain (149), and this drug may be combined with an opioid and other drugs in intraspinal combination therapy for severe pain unresponsive to systemic therapy (111). Dexmedetomidine is often used to enhance analgesia and sedation in the critical care setting (150). Tizanidine is available orally and is marketed for the treatment of spasticity. Based on limited data (151) and clinical experience, it may be considered a second-line adjuvant analgesic, potentially useful for any type of chronic pain. It is relatively sedating and may be useful given at night when pain is accompanied by insomnia. Treatment is usually initiated with a nighttime dose of 2 to 4 mg, and the dose is gradually increased as tolerated.

Cannabis-based medicines and medical cannabis contain numerous cannabinoid compounds that bind to endogenous cannabinoid receptors and produce an array of effects, among which may be analgesia. Evidence of clinical effectiveness is mixed (152-154). Nabiximols, an oromucosal spray containing mostly THC and cannabidiol, is approved in some countries for opioid-refractory cancer pain, and single-entity THC and single-entity nabilone are commercially available in the United States. Given the paucity of evidence for the latter drugs, they cannot be recommended and are rarely considered in the setting of pain that has been refractory to many other treatments. Some studies conclude that cannabis itself has analgesic efficacy (155), and where access to cannabis is legal, pain is a common reason for use. The role of physicians in recommending and guiding the use of medical cannabis is ill-defined in the United States and is likely to evolve as evidence accumulates and regulations evolve.

Topical therapies are widely used in the management of focal or regional pains. Given the low risks associated with these formulations, they should be considered whenever possible. A 2017 systematic review of controlled trials (156) found strong evidence of analgesic efficacy for selected NSAIDs, including diclofenac and ketoprofen, in musculoskeletal pain; moderate-quality evidence for high-concentration capsaicin in postherpetic neuralgia, and limited evidence for other NSAIDs, salicylate, low-concentration capsaicin, lidocaine, clonidine, and herbal remedies. The most widely used topical analgesics contain local anesthetics, most formulations deliver 4% or 5% lidocaine in a patch or cream. Topical capsaicin is available in a low-concentration (0.075%) cream or patch, which may be useful for regional neuropathic pains and joint pains; the high-concentration (8%) patch is a short-term therapy administered in a monitored setting and approved for postherpetic neuralgia in the United States and peripheral neuropathic pain in the European Union. Other topical drugs, such as amitriptyline, doxepin, baclofen, ketamine, gabapentin, and menthol, have been used empirically in compounded creams or gels, despite a lack of evidence.

Other multipurpose analgesics include neuroleptic compounds, botulinum toxin, NMDA receptor antagonists, and neuroleptic compounds. A systematic review found limited evidence of analgesic efficacy for selected neuroleptics (157), but the potential for adverse effects from these drugs argue against their use unless pain is accompanied by another indication. Experience with the local injection of botulinum toxin in focal or regional cancer pain syndromes is similarly limited (158), but the safety of this compound is high, and there is strong evidence of analgesic effects in chronic headache and diverse types of focal or regional pain syndromes (159,160). Opioid-refractory pains that may be amenable to botulinum injection should be considered for this treatment.

The NMDA receptor antagonists include ketamine, memantine, amantadine, dextromethorphan, and methadone. Only ketamine has been widely used as an adjuvant analgesic, notwithstanding conflicting data (161,162). The drug is used by palliative care specialists to manage opioid-refractory chronic pain in advanced illness, and its utility may increase with emerging evidence of antidepressant effects (163). There is experience with both short-term and long-term administration by the oral route, by repetitive parenteral administration, and by continuous subcutaneous or IV administration (164-169). Continuous infusion may be initiated with a loading bolus of 0.1 to 0.5 mg/kg, which is followed by an infusion of 0.05 to 0.2 mg/kg/hr. The dose is titrated until benefits occur or side effects supervene. Side effects include hypertension, tachycardia, and psychotomimetic effects; the latter effects may be reduced through the common practice of coadministering a benzodiazepine or a neuroleptic.

Drugs for Neuropathic Pain

Some adjuvant analgesics are used conventionally only for neuropathic pain. Opioid-refractory neuropathic pain in the cancer population may be treated with one of these drugs or with a multipurpose adjuvant analgesic, most importantly a glucocorticoid (in the setting of advanced cancer), an antidepressant (usually an SNRI), and/or a topical drug (if pain is focal or regional). Based on the evidence of efficacy (146), guidelines prioritize selection of a gabapentinoid—gabapentin and pregabalin—or an antidepressant (170). An analgesic antidepressant is usually considered first when patients have comorbid depression.

Gabapentin and *pregabalin* are N-type calcium channel modulators with established efficacy for some types of neuropathic pain (171). Patients may be responders to gabapentin, to pregabalin, to both, or to neither (172). Pregabalin may be preferred, given easier and more rapid titration (133). Neither drug is hepatically metabolized, and drug-drug interactions are limited to pharmacodynamic effects (eg, additive CNS adverse effects when combined with an opioid). Given the latter risk, a low starting dose and dose titration are recommended. In the medically frail, the starting doses of pregabalin and gabapentin are 25 to 50 and 100 to 200 mg/d, respectively. The lowest doses are used in those with severe renal disease. The effective doses vary, and if the initial dose is tolerated, dose escalation every few days is usually needed. The effective pregabalin dose is usually between 150 and 600 mg/d in two divided doses, and the effective gabapentin dose is usually between 900 and 3,600 mg/d in two to three divided doses.

Other drugs used conventionally for neuropathic pain include selected antiepileptic drugs and GABA agonists. Evidence that antiepileptic drugs, other than the gabapentinoids, are analgesic is very limited (173). In the United States, the marketed drugs with some evidence of efficacy include oxcarbazepine, lacosamide, topiramate, and lamotrigine (174-177), as well as several older drugs, specifically carbamazepine, phenytoin, and valproate. Based on clinical observations, oxcarbazepine, lacosamide, and topiramate are considered first if neuropathic pain has been refractory to other systemic therapies. There is no evidence for other anticonvulsant drugs.

GABA agonists include the benzodiazepines, which bind to the $GABA_A$ receptor subtype, and baclofen, which binds to the $GABA_B$ subtype. Although clonazepam is sometimes used for neuropathic pain, evidence is lacking, and it should not be selected unless pain is accompanied by severe anxiety. Baclofen is approved for spasticity and sometimes offered for refractory neuropathic pain based on anecdotal experience. A starting dose of 5 mg twice daily can be gradually escalated to doses that may exceed 200 mg/d in some patients; tapering should precede discontinuation to avoid withdrawal seizures.

Drugs for Bone Pain

Radiation therapy is highly effective for focal pain due to bony metastases. In highly selected patients, pain also may be addressed using percutaneous invasive techniques, such as radiofrequency ablation and cementoplasty (including vertebroplasty/kyphoplasty), or magnetic resonance–guided ultrasound (178,179). For those with multifocal pain, these treatments may be combined with systemic drug therapies.

Bone-targeting treatments that inhibit osteoclast function are widely used in the treatment of bone pain and to reduce the risk of other adverse skeletal-related events (SREs), including pathologic fracture, spinal cord compression, hypercalcemia, the necessity for radiation to address impending fracture, and need for bone surgery (180). The osteoclast inhibitors include bisphosphonates, denosumab, and calcitonin. No data support the use of calcitonin, and the bisphosphonates—zoledronate, alendronate, ibandronate, pamidronate, risedronate, clodronate, neridronate, and olpadronate—are usually selected. A 2016 systematic review of 13 studies concluded that these drugs are analgesic and usually reduce pain for 1 to 3 months (181). Other than the potential for hypocalcemia, the most common adverse effects are a transitory flulike syndrome and, with oral therapy, upper GI symptoms. Renal insufficiency also can occur and contraindicates treatment in those with significant renal insufficiency, and ocular inflammation and severe musculoskeletal pain are rare side effects. With prolonged treatment, rare but serious adverse events include osteonecrosis of the jaw and atypical femoral fracture (182).

Denosumab, a human monoclonal antibody, inhibits osteoclasts by binding to receptor activator of nuclear factor-κB ligand (RANKL), a molecule secreted by osteoblasts that binds to an osteoclast receptor, RANK. It also has analgesic effects, and a 2018 systematic review found that denosumab was more effective than the bisphosphonate in terms of time to the appearance of an SRE and the need for radiation (183).

Bone-targeting treatments for bone pain may also employ radioisotopes to deliver radiation to metastatic deposits. Numerous compounds have been developed that link a bone-seeking phosphonate to a radioisotope, and reviews of the best studied drugs—strontium-89 and samarium-153—demonstrate meaningful pain relief in about 75% of treated patients (184,185), with the response beginning within 1 to 3 weeks and persisting for at least several months. The major adverse effects are transitory pain flare and bone marrow toxicity, which contraindicates the therapy in those with preexisting bone marrow suppression. Given the need for sourcing and production of the radionuclide, the use of radioisotopes for bone pain has been limited to a highly selected subset of patients.

Drugs for Pain and Other Symptoms in Bowel Obstruction

The management of malignant bowel obstruction that cannot be relieved through surgery or stenting includes intestinal decompression through nasogastric suctioning or percutaneous venting, and varied medical treatments targeting pain, distension, nausea, and vomiting. Opioids are used for pain and require clinical monitoring of the potential to worsen bowel dysmotility. If opioid administration is followed by increased colic or distention, a different opioid should be tried, and efforts should be made to minimize the dose. Some patients appear to benefit by coadministration of a laxative with the opioid, but again, this requires careful monitoring. Bulk laxatives and drugs that stimulate peristalsis should be avoided; an osmotic drug such as polyethylene glycol may be preferred.

Based on limited clinical evidence (186), glucocorticoid treatment, such as low-dose dexamethasone, may ameliorate obstruction and improve symptoms. An antiemetic drug (other than the prokinetic metoclopramide) and either a proton-pump inhibitor or an H_2-blocker such as ranitidine are also usually administered. Anticholinergic drugs are also commonly employed, despite very limited evidence (187,188). The latter drugs include hyoscine hydrobromide (also called scopolamine hydrobromide), hyoscine butylbromide, and glycopyrrolate. In the United States, glycopyrrolate is often selected owing to its relatively lower penetration into the CNS.

The somatostatin analogs, octreotide and lanreotide, inhibit GI secretions and motility and have been long considered for the treatment of malignant bowel obstruction. A 2016 systematic review evaluated seven randomized trials and noted mixed results—low-level evidence of benefit but negative results from higher quality trials (189). Given these data, it is prudent to consider a trial of a somatostatin analog only after other therapies prove ineffective in controlling symptoms (163). Octreotide is administered in two or three injections daily or by continuous infusion; a long-acting octreotide formulation requires monthly injection, and lanreotide is administered by biweekly injection.

OTHER APPROACHES FOR CHRONIC PAIN MANAGEMENT

Numerous analgesic approaches may be considered for patients with chronic cancer pain. These approaches may be used to supplement pharmacotherapy and improve the balance between analgesia and side effects, promote better function, or concurrently manage other problems. Some are used to manage patients with pain that has not responded to conventional pharmacotherapy.

Interventional Approaches

The interventional strategies include injections, neural blockade, and implant therapies. Trigger point injections may be considered within the purview of all practitioners. Myofascial pains are extremely common in patients with chronic cancer pain, and the use of local anesthetic injections into painful trigger points may be a useful adjunctive approach in these patients.

The advances in neuraxial infusion of opioids and other drugs, described previously, have largely supplanted the neurodestructive approaches that were employed in the past for pain syndromes refractory to systemic opioid therapy. Nonetheless, some types of neural blockade continue to be widely used (190). Temporary somatic nerve blocks may be diagnostic, prognostic, or therapeutic. Repeated therapeutic blocks with local anesthetic are occasionally employed when pain is focal and can be reduced through injection of a sensory nerve innervating the painful area. Recently, local anesthetics have been used to provide more prolonged neural blockade through techniques of perineural or epidural infusion.

Neural blockade with neurolytic solutions, usually alcohol or phenol, have been developed to denervate virtually any area of the body. Their use is very limited, however, because of the short-term risks associated with the injection of these substances, such as damage to soft tissues and local hemorrhage or infection, and the longer term risks of neuritis and deafferentation pain. The one generally accepted exception is celiac plexus blockade for the management of epigastric pain due to neoplastic invasion of the celiac axis. The response to neurolytic celiac plexus blockade in pain due to pancreatic cancer has been observed to be so satisfactory that earlier use is warranted whenever the typical pain syndrome occurs (191-193). This block can be performed percutaneously through various approaches or via an endoscopic ultrasound-guided technique.

Neuromodulation Approaches

Electrical neuromodulation of peripheral nerves may provide local or regional analgesia. The best-known treatment is TENS, a trial of which may be considered whenever pain is limited to an area that can be stimulated through electrode placement on the skin or over the sensory nerve that supplies the painful region (194). Based on clinical observations, patients who acquire a TENS device should be instructed to try various electrode placements, high-frequency and low-frequency stimulation, and timing of stimulation. Stimulation of a sensory nerve can also be accomplished through an implanted electrode. This technique, known as percutaneous electrical nerve stimulation (PENS), is rarely employed.

A newer form of noninvasive peripheral stimulation, known as Scrambler therapy, used surface electrodes to stimulate multiple primary afferents simultaneously. A 2020 systematic review (195) noted the limitations of the extant literature but concluded that the approach, if available, is worthy of a trial based on the data available. It has been used to treat varied types of neuropathic pain, including chemotherapy-induced peripheral neuropathy (CIPN).

Electrical stimulation can be delivered to the CNS via invasive and noninvasive methods. Dorsal column stimulation using an implanted system has a long history and may be effective for diverse chronic pain syndromes (196). Although deep brain stimulation and motor cortex stimulation have similarly been used for chronic pain, these approaches are now rarely considered owing to the advent of noninvasive approaches—transcranial direct current stimulation (tDCS) and transcranial magnetic stimulation (TMS). Numerous studies of these approaches suggest benefit for pain and other conditions (197), but additional research is needed to provide high-quality evidence, determine optimal stimulation approaches for each technique, and compare TMS and tDCS in terms of benefits and burdens in the context of serious chronic illness.

Rehabilitative Approaches

Although rehabilitative therapies usually target impairment, they may help address pain in populations with chronic serious illness. The therapies, which are usually implemented in collaboration with physical and occupational therapists, include therapeutic exercise, hydrotherapy, devices, and physical modalities, such as heat and cold, vibration, and ultrasound.

Therapeutic exercise has not been studied in populations with advanced illness, but benefits have been demonstrated in those recovering from breast cancer treatment and those with CIPN (198,199). Myofascial and joint pains may be most amenable to this treatment, based on clinical observations. Exercise approaches may be combined with hydrotherapy in an approach known as aquatic exercise. Some patients with chronic pain benefit from devices, such as canes and walkers, that reduce the load on joints, pelvis, and spine, and others experience pain reduction from the use of orthoses that constrain the movement of a painful limb. The input of a physical therapist and occupational therapist is needed to optimize these approaches during the management of chronic pain.

Focal or regional pains may also be amenable to treatment using one of the so-called physical modalities. The use of electrical stimulation for this effect, via TENS, has been noted. Other modalities include heat or cold and ultrasound. Based on clinical observations, patients with focal areas of pain may benefit from application of one or more of these approaches. Cold may be applied with ice packs, chemical gel packs, or vapocoolant sprays, and heat is provided using hot packs, medicated heat patches, heating pads, or warm baths.

Surgical Neuroablative Approaches

Procedures designed to surgically denervate a painful area have been developed for every level of the neuraxis (200). Like neurolytic blocks, however, these procedures are rarely considered now, largely because of the development of interventions, such as neuraxial infusion. The most useful approach has been cordotomy (201), and this procedure is still considered when patients develop intractable unilateral lower extremity pain refractory to other treatments.

Psychological Approaches

Although the evidence is limited, cognitive behavioral approaches to improve coping and adaptation, and teach relaxation, distraction through imagery, and other strategies, appear to offer a substantial benefit to some patients (202). These approaches can ameliorate chronic cancer pain and concurrently address other symptoms, such as disturbed mood and sleep. These approaches offer self-management tools to patients or family caregivers, which may be used to mitigate distress and buttress resilience.

Studies suggest that both education-based (203) and mind-body approaches (204) can provide a modest benefit for chronic pain, including cancer related, but data from populations with more advanced illnesses are lacking. Nonetheless, patients who have the capacity to participate should be considered for these treatments if professional expertise is available to provide them. Unfortunately, many of these interventions cannot be provided because the availability of professionals with these skills is limited, insurance coverage has been historically poor, and patients often lack the resources necessary to participate.

Integrative Medicine Approaches

Integrative medicine refers to the combined use of conventional medical therapies and interventions that have historically been termed "complementary" or "alternative." Numerous complementary therapies are used in pain management, including (1) mind-body therapies (which overlap those considered as psycholoical approaches); (2) treatments that are part of alternative medical systems, such as

Traditional Chinese Medicine (TCM), Ayurveda, homeopathy, or naturopathy; (3) biologically based therapies, such as herbal therapies or specialized diets; (4) body-based therapies, such as massage, yoga, Pilates, Tai Chi, and chiropractic; and (5) energy therapies, such as therapeutic touch and Reiki.

Most complementary therapies lack high-quality evidence of efficacy (205,206), and judgments about their use in the management of cancer pain must be based on the evidence available, accumulated experience, and clinical assessment of the potential benefit compared to risks and burdens. Acupuncture has been evaluated in numerous studies, and there is sufficient evidence of efficacy for cancer pain (207) to consider the approach, if it is available, in the absence of specific contraindications. Many other therapies have a rationale based on minimal risk. This description includes the mind-body therapies, including those noted previously and others—meditation, prayer, music therapy, and art therapy. It also applies to the so-called energy therapies, such as therapeutic touch and Reiki, and many of the body-based therapies. Massage therapy has been observed to have favorable effects (208), and other body-based therapies, such as Tai Chi, have been shown to have a positive effect on functioning and other symptoms (209).

In contrast, some complementary treatments appear to carry risks that are difficult to justify in the population with cancer pain. Spinal manipulation in the setting of multifocal bone metastases and herbal remedies with unknown ingredients are two examples. Patients should be discouraged from pursuing these approaches.

CONCLUSION

Pain is highly prevalent among patients with gynecologic tumors. The clinicians involved in the care of these patients have a challenging task in providing state-of-the-art management approaches for both acute and chronic pain. Fortunately, the most effective strategy for both acute and chronic pain, namely, opioid-based pharmacotherapy, is clearly within the purview of all practitioners. The knowledge and skills necessary to optimize this therapy and integrate it with the broader principles of palliative care are fundamental to the practice of gynecologic oncology.

REFERENCES

1. Ferrell B, Smith S, Cullinane C, Melancon C. Symptom concerns of women with ovarian cancer. *J Pain Symptom Manage*. 2003;25:528-538.
2. Olson SH, Mignone L, Nakraseive C, Caputo TA, Barakat RR, Harlap S. Symptoms of ovarian cancer. *Obstet Gynecol*. 2001;98:212-217.
3. Kim YJ, Munsell MF, Park JC, et al. Retrospective review of symptoms and palliative care interventions in women with advanced cervical cancer. *Gynecol Oncol*. 2015;139(3):553-558.
4. Goff BA, Mandel LS, Melancon CH, Muntz HG. Frequency of symptoms of ovarian cancer in women presenting to primary care clinics. *JAMA*. 2004;291(22):2705-2712.
5. van den Beuken-van Everdingen MH, Hochstenbach LM, Joosten EA, Tjan-Heijnen VC, Janssen DJ. Update on prevalence of pain in patients with cancer: systematic review and meta-analysis. *J Pain Symptom Manage*. 2016;51(6):1070.e9-1090.e9.
6. Raja SN, Carr DB, Cohen M, et al. The revised International Association for the Study of Pain definition of pain: concepts, challenges, and compromises. *Pain*. 2020;161(9):1976-1982.
7. Talbot K, Madden VJ, Jones SL, Moseley GL. The sensory and affective components of pain: are they differentially modifiable dimensions or inseparable aspects of a unitary experience? A systematic review. *Br J Anaesth*. 2019;123(2):e263-e272.
8. Bennett MI, Kaasa S, Barke A, et al. The IASP classification of chronic pain for ICD-11: chronic cancer-related pain. *Pain*. 2019;160(1):38-44.
9. Scholz J, Finnerup NB, Attal N, et al. The IASP classification of chronic pain for ICD-11: chronic neuropathic pain. *Pain*. 2019;160(1):53-59.
10. Nijs J, Lahousse A, Kapreli E, et al. Nociplastic pain criteria or recognition of central sensitization? Pain phenotyping in the past, present and future. *J Clin Med*. 2021;10(15):3203-3227.
11. Karcioglu O, Topacoglu H, Dikme O, Dikme O. A systematic review of the pain scales in adults: which to use? *Am J Emerg Med*. 2018;36(4):707-714.

12. Chan AY, Ge M, Harrop E, et al. Pain assessment tools in paediatric palliative care: a systematic review of psychometric properties and recommendations for clinical practice. *Palliat Med.* 2022;36(1):30-43.

13. Løhre ET, Thronæs M, Klepstad P. Breakthrough cancer pain in 2020. *Curr Opin Support Palliat Care.* 2020;14(2):94-99.

14. Carezzato NL, Valera GG, Vale FAC, Hortense P. Instruments for assessing pain in persons with severe dementia. *Dement Neuropsychol.* 2014;8(2):99-106.

15. Abahussin AA, West RM, Wong DC, Ziegler LE. PROMs for pain in adult cancer patients: a systematic review of measurement properties. *Pain Pract.* 2019;19(1):93-117.

16. Baek SK, Shin SW, Koh SJ, et al. Significance of descriptive symptoms and signs and clinical parameters as predictors of neuropathic cancer pain. *PLoS One.* 2021;16(8):e0252781.

17. American Psychiatric Association. Diagnostic and Statistical Manual of Mental Disorders (DSM-5-TR). https://www.psychiatry.org/psychiatrists/practice/dsm

18. Paice JA, Mulvey M, Bennett M, et al. AAPT diagnostic criteria for chronic cancer pain conditions. *J Pain.* 2017;18(3):233-246.

19. Shkodra M, Brunelli C, Zecca E, et al. Neuropathic pain: clinical classification and assessment in patients with pain due to cancer. *Pain.* 2021;162(3):866-874.

20. Caraceni A, Portenoy RK; a Working Group of the IASP Task Force on Cancer Pain. An International Survey of cancer pain characteristics and syndromes. IASP Task Force on Cancer Pain. International Association for the Study of Pain. *Pain.* 1999;82(3):263-274.

21. Nelson G, Altman AD, Nick A, et al. Guidelines for postoperative care in gynecologic/oncology surgery: enhanced recovery after surgery (ERAS®) Society recommendations—Part II. *Gynecol Oncol.* 2016;140(2):323-332.

22. Nelson G, Bakkum-Gamez J, Kalogera E, et al. Guidelines for perioperative care in gynecologic/oncology: Enhanced Recovery After Surgery (ERAS) Society recommendations-2019 update. *Int J Gynecol Cancer.* 2019;29(4):651-668.

23. Sánchez-Iglesias JL, Carbonell-Socias M, Pérez-Benavente MA, et al. PROFAST: a Randomised trial implementing enhanced recovery after surgery for high complexity advanced ovarian cancer surgery. *Eur J Cancer.* 2020;136:149-158.

24. Agarwal R, Rajanbabu A, Nitu PV, Goel G, Madhusudanan L, Unnikrishnan UG. A prospective study evaluating the impact of implementing the ERAS protocol on patients undergoing surgery for advanced ovarian cancer. *Int J Gynecol Cancer.* 2019;29(3):605-612.

25. Patel K, Shergill S, Vadivelu N, Rajput K. Analgesia for gynecologic oncologic surgeries: a narrative review. *Curr Pain Headache Rep.* 2022;26(1):1-13.

26. Steinberg AC, Schimpf MO, White AB, et al. Preemptive analgesia for postoperative hysterectomy pain control: systematic review and clinical practice guidelines. *Am J Obstet Gynecol.* 2017;217(3):303.e6-313.e6.

27. Reuben SS, Steinberg RB, Maciolek H, Joshi W. Preoperative administration of controlled-release oxycodone for the management of pain after ambulatory laparoscopic tubal ligation surgery. *J Clin Anesth.* 2002;14(3):223-227.

28. Doleman B, Leonardi-Bee J, Heinink TP, Bhattacharjee D, Lund JN, Williams JP. Pre-emptive and preventive opioids for postoperative pain in adults undergoing all types of surgery. *Cochrane Database Syst Rev.* 2018;12(12):CD012624.

29. Dauri M, Faria S, Gatti A, Celidonio L, Carpenedo R, Sabato AF. Gabapentin and pregabalin for the acute post-operative pain management. A systematic-narrative review of the recent clinical evidences. *Curr Drug Targets.* 2009;10(8):716-733.

30. Doleman B, Leonardi-Bee J, Heinink TP, et al Pre-emptive and preventive NSAIDs for postoperative pain in adults undergoing all types of surgery. *Cochrane Database Syst Rev.* 2021;6(6):CD012978.

31. Nijland L, Schmidt P, Frosch M, et al. Subcutaneous or intravenous opioid administration by patient-controlled analgesia in cancer pain: a systematic literature review. *Support Care Cancer.* 2019;27(1):33-42.

32. Macintyre PE, Quinlan J, Levy N, Lobo DN. Current issues in the use of opioids for the management of postoperative pain: a review. *JAMA Surg.* 2022;157(2):158-166.

33. Singh SA, Moreland RA, Fang W, et al. Compassion inequities and opioid use disorder: a matched case-control analysis examining inpatient management of cancer-related pain for patients with opioid use disorder. *J Pain Symptom Manage.* 2021;62(3):e156-e163.

34. Ward EN, Quaye AN, Wilens TE. Opioid use disorders: perioperative management of a special population. *Anesth Analg.* 2018;127(2):539-547.

35. Lirk P, Thiry J, Bonnet MP, Joshi GP, Bonnet F; PROSPECT Working Group. Pain management after laparoscopic hysterectomy: systematic review of literature and PROSPECT recommendations. *Reg Anesth Pain Med.* 2019;44(4):425-436.

36. Tuncer S, Pirbudak L, Balat O, Capar M. Adding ketoprofen to intravenous patient-controlled analgesia with tramadol after major gynecological cancer surgery: a double-blinded, randomized, placebo-controlled clinical trial. *Eur J Gynaecol Oncol.* 2003;24:181-184.

37. Alayed N, Alghanaim N, Tan X, Tulandi T. Preemptive use of gabapentin in abdominal hysterectomy: a systematic review and meta-analysis. *Obstet Gynecol.* 2014;123(6):1221-1229.

38. Yao Z, Shen C, Zhong Y. Perioperative pregabalin for acute pain after gynecological surgery: a meta-analysis. *Clin Ther.* 2015;37(5):1128-1135.

39. Verret M, Lauzier F, Zarychanski R, et al. Perioperative use of gabapentinoids for the management of postoperative acute pain: a systematic review and meta-analysis. *Anesthesiology.* 2020;133(2):265-279.

40. Patel AS, Abrecht CR, Urman RD. Gabapentinoid use in perioperative care and current controversies. *Curr Pain Headache Rep.* 2022;26(2):139-144.

41. Jokela RM, Ahonen JV, Tallgren MK, Marjakangas PC, Korttila KT. The effective analgesic dose of dexamethasone after laparoscopic hysterectomy. *Anesth Analg.* 2009;109(2):607-615.

42. Nam M, Yoon H. Effect of ondansetron combined with dexamethasone on postoperative nausea & vomiting and pain of patients with laparoscopic hysterectomy. *J Korean Acad Nurs.* 2009;39(1):44-52.

43. Sousa AM, Rosado GM, Neto Jde S, Guimarães GM, Ashmawi HA. Magnesium sulfate improves postoperative analgesia in laparoscopic gynecologic surgeries: a double-blind randomized controlled trial. *J Clin Anesth.* 2016;34:379-384.

44. Hong BH, Lee WY, Kim YH, Yoon SH, Lee WH. Effects of intraoperative low dose ketamine on remifentanil-induced hyperalgesia in gynecologic surgery with sevoflurane anesthesia. *Korean J Anesthesiol.* 2011;61(3):238-243.

45. Lin HQ, Jia DL. Effect of preemptive ketamine administration on postoperative visceral pain after gynecological laparoscopic surgery. *J Huazhong Univ Sci Technolog Med Sci.* 2016;36(4):584-587.

46. Stamenkovic DM, Bezmarevic M, Bojic S, et al. Updates on wound infiltration use for postoperative pain management: a narrative review. *J Clin Med.* 2021;10(20):4659.

47. Hamilton TW, Athanassoglou V, Mellon S, et al. Liposomal bupivacaine infiltration at the surgical site for the management of postoperative pain. *Cochrane Database Syst Rev.* 2017;2(2):CD011419.

48. Chang H, Rimel BJ, Li AJ, Cass I, Karlan BY, Walsh C. Ultra-sound guided transversus abdominis plane (TAP) block utilization in multimodal pain management after open gynecologic surgery. *Gynecol Oncol Rep.* 2018;26:75-77.

49. Bisch SP, Kooy J, Glaze S, et al. Impact of transversus abdominis plane blocks versus non-steroidal anti-inflammatory on post-operative opioid use in ERAS ovarian cancer surgery. *Int J Gynecol Cancer.* 2019;29(9):1372-1376.

50. Bacal V, Rana U, McIsaac DI, Chen I. Transversus abdominis plane block for post hysterectomy pain: a systematic review and meta-analysis. *J Minim Invasive Gynecol.* 2019;26(1):40-52.

51. López-Ruiz C, Orjuela JC, Rojas-Gualdrón DF, et al. Efficacy of transversus abdominis plane block in the reduction of pain and opioid requirement in laparoscopic and robot-assisted hysterectomy: a systematic review and meta-analysis. *Rev Bras Ginecol Obstet.* 2022;44(1):55-66.

52. Sondekoppam RV, Uppal V, Brookes J, Ganapathy S. Bilateral thoracic paravertebral blocks compared to thoracic epidural analgesia after midline laparotomy: a pragmatic noninferiority clinical trial. *Anesth Analg.* 2019;129(3):855-863.

53. Kuniyoshi H, Yamamoto Y, Kimura S, Hiroe T, Terui T, Kase Y. Comparison of the analgesic effects continuous epidural anesthesia and continuous rectus sheath block in patients undergoing gynecological cancer surgery: a non-inferiority randomized control trial. *J Anesth.* 2021;35(5):663-670.

54. Hemmerling TM. Pain management in abdominal surgery. *Langenbecks Arch Surg.* 2018;403(7):791-803.

55. Rawal N. Epidural analgesia for postoperative pain: improving outcomes or adding risks? *Best Pract Res Clin Anaesthesiol.* 2021;35(1):53-65.

56. Bjordal JM, Johnson MI, Ljunggreen AE. Transcutaneous electrical nerve stimulation (TENS) can reduce postoperative analgesic consumption. A meta-analysis with assessment of optimal treatment parameters for postoperative pain. *Eur J Pain.* 2003;7:181-188.

57. Good M, Anderson GC, Stanton-Hicks M, Grass JA, Makii M. Relaxation and music reduce pain after gynecologic surgery. *Pain Manag Nurs.* 2002;3:61-70.

58. Cherny NI. The problem of suffering and the principles of assessment in palliative medicine. In: Cherny NI, Fallon MT, Kaasa S, et al, eds. *Oxford Textbook of Palliative Medicine.* 5th ed. Oxford University Press; 2015:35-48.

59. Cherny NI, Portenoy RK. Core concepts in palliative care. In: Cherny N, Fallon M, Kaasa S, Portenoy R, Currow DC, eds. *Oxford Textbook of Palliative Medicine*. 6th ed. Oxford University Press;2021:44-54.

60. Portenoy RK. Building definitional consensus in palliative care. In: Cherny N, Fallon M, Kaasa S, Portenoy R, Currow DC, eds. *Oxford Textbook of Palliative Medicine*. 6th ed. Oxford University Press;2021:35-43.

61. Ferrell BR, Twaddle ML, Melnick A, Meier DE. National Consensus Project Clinical Practice Guidelines for Quality Palliative Care Guidelines, 4th ed. *J Palliat Med*. 2018;21(12):1684-1689.

62. Ferrell BR, Temel JS, Temin S, Smith TJ. Integration of palliative care into standard oncology care: ASCO Clinical Practice Guideline update summary. *J Oncol Pract*. 2017;13(2):119-121.

63. Hussaini Q, Smith TJ. Incorporating palliative care into oncology practice: why and how. *Clin Adv Hematol Oncol*. 2021;19(6):390-395.

64. Geels P, Eisenhauer E, Bezjak A, Zee B, Day A. Palliative effect of chemotherapy: objective tumor response is associated with symptom improvement in patients with metastatic breast cancer. *J Clin Oncol*. 2000;18:2395-2405.

65. Williams GR, Manjunath SH, Butala AA, Jones JA. Palliative radiotherapy for advanced cancers: indications and outcomes. *Surg Oncol Clin N Am*. 2021;30(3):563-580.

66. Rich SE, Chow R, Raman S, et al. Update of the systematic review of palliative radiation therapy fractionation for bone metastases. *Radiother Oncol*. 2018;126(3):547-557.

67. Hillegonds DJ, Franklin S, Shelton DK, Vijayakumar S, Vijayakumar V. The management of painful bone metastases with an emphasis on radionuclide therapy. *J Natl Med Assoc*. 2007;99(7):785-794.

68. Wiffen PJ, Wee B, Derry S, Bell RF, Moore RA. Opioids for cancer pain—an overview of Cochrane reviews. *Cochrane Database Syst Rev*. 2017;7:CD012592.

69. Colson J, Koyyalagunta D, Falco FJ, Manchikanti L. A systematic review of observational studies on the effectiveness of opioid therapy for cancer pain. *Pain Phys*. 2011;14(2):E85-E102.

70. Greco MT, Roberto A, Corli O, et al. Quality of cancer pain management: an update of a systemic review of undertreatment of patients with cancer. *J Clin Oncol*. 2014;32(36):4149-4154.

71. Deandrea S, Montanari M, Moja L, Apolone G. Prevalence of undertreatment in cancer pain. A review of published literature. *Ann Oncol*. 2008;19(12):1985-1991.

72. Knaul FM, Farmer PE, Krakauer EL, et al. Alleviating the access abyss in palliative care and pain relief-an imperative of universal health coverage: the Lancet Commission Report. *Lancet*. 2018;391(10128):1391-1454.

73. Bhadelia A, De Lima L, Arreola-Ornelas H, Kwete XJ, Rodriguez NM, Knaul FM. Solving the global crisis in access to pain relief: lessons from country actions. *Am J Public Health*. 2019;109(1):58-60.

74. Anekar AA, Hendrix JM, Cascella M. WHO Analgesic Ladder. In: StatPearls [Internet]. StatPearls Publishing;2023. PMID:32119322.

75. Chapman EJ, Edwards Z, Boland JW, et al. Practice review: evidence-based and effective management of pain in patients with advanced cancer. *Palliat Med*. 2020;34(4):444-453.

76. Fallon M, Giusti R, Aielli F, Hoskin P, Rolke R, Sharma M, Ripamonti CI; ESMO Guidelines Committee. Management of cancer pain in adult patients: ESMO Clinical Practice Guidelines. *Ann Oncol*. 2018;29(Suppl 4):iv166-iv191.

77. Vardy J, Agar M. Nonopioid drugs in the treatment of cancer pain. *J Clin Oncol*. 2014;32(16):1677-1690.

78. Derry S, Wiffen PJ, Moore RA et al. Oral nonsteroidal anti-inflammatory drugs (NSAIDs) for cancer pain in adults. *Cochrane Database Syst Rev*. 2017;7(7):CD012638.

79. Mercadante S, Fulfaro F, Casuccio A. A randomised controlled study on the use of anti-inflammatory drugs in patients with cancer pain on morphine therapy: effects on dose-escalation and a pharmacoeconomic analysis. *Eur J Cancer*. 2002;38:1358-1363.

80. Graham GG, Davies MJ, Day RO, Mohamudally A, Scott KF. The modern pharmacology of paracetamol: therapeutic actions, mechanism of action, metabolism, toxicity and recent pharmacological findings. *Inflammopharmacology*. 2013;21(3):201-232.

81. Yang M, Wang HT, Zhao M, et al. Network meta-analysis comparing relatively selective COX-2 inhibitors versus coxibs for the prevention of NSAID-induced gastrointestinal injury. *Medicine (Baltimore)*. 2015;94(40):e1592.

82. Hinz B, Renner B, Brune K. Drug insight: cyclo-oxygenase-2 inhibitors—a critical appraisal. *Nat Clin Pract Rheumatol*. 2007;3:552-560.

83. Venerito M, Schneider C, Costanzo R, Breja R, Röhl FW, Malfertheiner P. Contribution of Helicobacter pylori infection to the risk of peptic ulcer bleeding in patients on nonsteroidal anti-inflammatory drugs, antiplatelet agents, anticoagulants, corticosteroids and selective serotonin reuptake inhibitors. *Aliment Pharmacol Ther*. 2018;47(11):1464-1471.

84. Lanza FL, Chan FK, Quigley EM; Practice Parameters Committee of the American College of Gastroenterology. Guidelines for prevention of NSAID-related ulcer complications. *Am J Gastroenterol*. 2009;104:728-738.

85. Waksman JC, Brody A, Phillips SD. Nonselective nonsteroidal antiinflammatory drugs and cardiovascular risk: are they safe? *Ann Pharmacother*. 2007;41:1163-1173.

86. Trelle S, Reichenbach S, Wandel S, et al. Cardiovascular safety of non-steroidal anti-inflammatory drugs: network meta-analysis. *BMJ*. 2011;342:c7086.

87. Angiolillo DJ, Weisman SM. Clinical pharmacology and cardiovascular safety of naproxen. *Am J Cardiovasc Drugs*. 2017;17(2):97-107.

88. Webster L, Gudin J, Raffa RB, et al. Understanding buprenorphine for use in chronic pain: expert opinion. *Pain Med*. 2020;21(4):714-723.

89. Schmidt-Hansen M, Taubert M, Bromham N, Hilgart JS, Arnold S. The effectiveness of buprenorphine for treating cancer pain: an abridged Cochrane review. *BMJ Support Palliat Care*. 2016;6(3):292-306.

90. Wiffen PJ, Derry S, Naessens K, Bell RF. Oral tapentadol for cancer pain. *Cochrane Database Syst Rev*. 2015;2015(9):CD011460.

91. Wiffen PJ, Derry S, Moore RA. Tramadol with or without paracetamol (acetaminophen) for cancer pain. *Cochrane Database Syst Rev*. 2017;5(5):CD012508.

92. Quigley C, Joel S, Patel N, Baksh A, Slevin M. Plasma concentrations of morphine, morphine-6-glucuronide and morphine-3-glucuronide and their relationship with analgesia and side effects in patients with cancer-related pain. *Palliat Med*. 2003;17:185-190.

93. Coluzzi F, Caputi FF, Billeci D, et al. Safe use of opioids in chronic kidney disease and hemodialysis patients: tips and tricks for non-pain specialists. *Ther Clin Risk Manag*. 2020;16:821-837.

94. Bandieri E, Romero M, Ripamonti CI, et al. Randomized trial of low-dose morphine versus weak opioids in moderate cancer pain. *J Clin Oncol*. 2016;34(5):436-442. Erratum in: *J Clin Oncol*. 2017;35(15):1753.

95. Klepstad P, Kaasa S, Jystad A, Hval B, Borchgrevink PC. Immediate- or sustained-release morphine for dose finding during start of morphine to cancer patients: a randomized, double-blind trial. *Pain*. 2003;101: 193-198.

96. Reizine N, Danahey K, Schierer E, et al. Impact of CYP2D6 pharmacogenomic status on pain control among opioid-treated oncology patients. *Oncologist*. 2021;26(11):e2042-e2052.

97. Hadley G, Derry S, Moore RA, Wiffen PJ. Transdermal fentanyl for cancer pain. *Cochrane Database Syst Rev*. 2013;2013(10):CD010270.

98. Chou R, Cruciani RA, Fiellin DA, et al. Methadone safety: a clinical practice guideline from the American Pain Society and College on Problems of Drug Dependence, in collaboration with the Heart Rhythm Society. *J Pain*. 2014;15:321-337.

99. McPherson ML, Walker KA, Davis MP, et al. Safe and appropriate use of methadone in hospice and palliative care: expert consensus white paper. *J Pain Symptom Manage*. 2019;57(3):635-645.e4.

100. Cruciani RA, Sekine R, Homel P, et al. Measurement of QTc in patients receiving chronic methadone therapy. *J Pain Symptom Manage*. 2005;29:385-391.

101. Van Seventer R, Smit JM, Schipper RM, Wicks MA, Zuurmond WW. Comparison of TTS-fentanyl with sustained-release oral morphine in the treatment of patients not using opioids for mild-to-moderate pain. *Curr Med Res Opin*. 2003;19:457-469.

102. Suno M, Endo Y, Nishie H, Kajizono M, Sendo T, Matsuoka J. Refractory cachexia is associated with increased plasma concentrations of fentanyl in cancer patients. *Ther Clin Risk Manag*. 2015;11:751-757.

103. Heiskanen T, Mätzke S, Haakana S, Gergov M, Vuori E, Kalso E. Transdermal fentanyl in cachectic cancer patients. *Pain*. 2009;144(1-2):218-222.

104. Tassinari D, Sartori S, Tamburini E, et al. Adverse effects of transdermal opiates treating moderate-severe cancer pain in comparison to long-acting morphine: a meta-analysis and systematic review of the literature. *J Palliat Med*. 2008;11:492-501.

105. Wilkinson TJ, Robinson BA, Begg EJ, Duffull SB, Ravenscroft PJ, Schneider JJ. Pharmacokinetics and efficacy of rectal versus oral sustained-release morphine in cancer patients. *Cancer Chemother Pharmacol*. 1992;31:251-254.

106. Zeppetella G, Davies A, Eijgelshoven I, Jansen JP. A network meta-analysis of the efficacy of opioid analgesics for the management of breakthrough cancer pain episodes. *J Pain Symptom Manage*. 2014;47(4):772-785.e5.

107. Jandhyala R, Fullarton JR, Bennett MI. Efficacy of rapid-onset oral fentanyl formulations vs. oral morphine for cancer-related breakthrough pain: a meta-analysis of comparative trials. *J Pain Symptom Manage*. 2013;46:573-580.

108. Coyle S, Sinden R, Wignall-Coyle J, Benson S, Powell P, Monnery D. Continuous subcutaneous infusion: is community anticipatory

prescribing and administration safe? *BMJ Support Palliat Care.* 2021;bm-jspcare-2021-003259. Epub ahead of print. PMID: 34815249.

109. Perruchoud C, Dupoiron D, Papi B, Calabrese A, Brogan SE. Management of cancer-related pain with intrathecal drug delivery: a systematic review and meta-analysis of clinical studies. *Neuromodulation.* 2023;26(6):1142-1152.

110. Clarke CFM. Neuraxial drug delivery for the management of cancer pain: cost, updates, and society guidelines. *Curr Opin Anaesthesiol.* 2017;30(5):593-597.

111. Deer TR, Pope JE, Hayek SM, et al. The Polyanalgesic Consensus Conference (PACC): recommendations on intrathecal drug infusion systems best practices and guidelines [published correction appears in *Neuromodulation.* 2017;20(4):405-406]. *Neuromodulation.* 2017;20(2):96-132.

112. Staats PS, Yearwood T, Charapata SG, et al. Intrathecal ziconotide in the treatment of refractory pain in patients with cancer or AIDS: a randomized controlled trial. *JAMA.* 2004;291:63-70.

113. Deandrea S, Corli O, Consonni D, Villani W, Greco MT, Apolone G. Prevalence of breakthrough cancer pain: a systematic review and a pooled analysis of published literature. *J Pain Symptom Manage.* 2014;47(1):57-76. doi:10.1016/j.jpainsymman.2013.02.015

114. Mercadante S, Portenoy RK. Understanding the chameleonic breakthrough cancer pain. *Drugs.* 2021;81(4):411-418.

115. Mercadante S, Portenoy RK. Opioid poorly-responsive cancer pain. Part 3. Clinical strategies to improve opioid responsiveness. *J Pain Symptom Manage.* 2001;21(4):338-354.

116. Fine PG, Portenoy RK; Ad Hoc Expert Panel on Evidence Review and Guidelines for Opioid Rotation. Establishing "best practices" for opioid rotation: conclusions of an expert panel. *J Pain Symptom Manage.* 2009;38(3):418-425.

117. Reddy A, Yennurajalingam S, Pulivarthi K, et al. Frequency, outcome, and predictors of success within 6 weeks of an opioid rotation among outpatients with cancer receiving strong opioids. *Oncologist.* 2013;18:212-220.

118. Bharucha AE, Lacy BE. Mechanisms, evaluation, and management of chronic constipation. *Gastroenterology.* 2020;158(5):1232-1249.e3. doi:10.1053/j.gastro.2019.12.034

119. Ford AC, Brenner DM, Schoenfeld PS. Efficacy of pharmacological therapies for the treatment of opioid-induced constipation: systematic review and meta-analysis. *Am J Gastroenterol.* 2013;108:1566-1574.

120. Candy B, Jones L, Vickerstaff V, Larkin PJ, Stone P. Mu-opioid antagonists for opioid-induced bowel dysfunction in people with cancer and people receiving palliative care. *Cochrane Database Syst Rev.* 2018;6:CD006332.

121. Nee J, Zakari M, Sugarman MA, et al. Efficacy of treatments for opioid-induced constipation: systematic review and meta-analysis. *Clin Gastroenterol Hepatol.* 2018;16(10):1569-1584.e2.

122. Ford AC, Quigley EM, Lacy BE, et al. Efficacy of prebiotics, probiotics, and synbiotics in irritable bowel syndrome and chronic idiopathic constipation: systematic review and meta-analysis. *Am J Gastroenterol.* 2014;109(10):1547-1562.

123. Laugsand EA, Kaasa S, Klepstad P. Management of opioid-induced nausea and vomiting in cancer patients: systematic review and evidence-based recommendations. *Palliat Med.* 2011;25:442-453.

124. Andrew BN, Guan NC, Jaafar NRN. The use of methylphenidate for physical and psychological symptoms in cancer patients: a review. *Curr Drug Targets.* 2018;19(8):877-887.

125. Wilwerding MB, Loprinzi CL, Maillard JA, et al. A randomized, crossover evaluation of methylphenidate in cancer patients receiving strong narcotics. *Support Care Cancer.* 1995;3:135-138.

126. Stone P, Minton O. European Palliative Care Research collaborative pain guidelines. Central side-effects management: what is the evidence to support best practice in the management of sedation, cognitive impairment and myoclonus? *Palliat Med.* 2011;25:431-441.

127. Cao M, Javaheri S. Effects of chronic opioid use on sleep and wake. *Sleep Med Clin.* 2018;13(2):271-281.

128. Gudin JA, Laitman A, Nalamachu S. Opioid related endocrinopathy. *Pain Med.* 2015;16(Suppl. 1):S9-S15.

129. Chahin M, Matosz S, Khalel I, Day S, Keruakous A. Pain management in oncology patients amidst the opioid epidemic: how to minimize non-medical opioid use. *Cureus.* 2021;13(11):e19500.

130. Savage SR, Joranson DE, Covington EC, Schnoll SH, Heit HA, Gilson AM. Definitions related to the medical use of opioids: evolution towards universal agreement. *J Pain Symptom Manage.* 2003;26(1):655-667.

131. Portenoy RK. Acute and chronic pain. In: Ruiz P, Strain E, eds. *Lowinson & Ruiz's Substance Abuse: A Comprehensive Textbook*, 5th ed. Lippincott, Williams and Wilkins; 2011:695.

132. American Psychiatric Association. *Diagnostic and Statistical Manual of Mental Disorders.* 5th ed. American Psychiatric Association; 2013.

133. Passik SD, Kirsh KL, Donaghy KB, Portenoy RK. Pain and aberrant drug-related behaviors in medically ill patients with and without histories of substance abuse. *Clin J Pain.* 2006;22:173-181

134. Merlin JS, Khodyakov D, Arnold R, et al. Expert panel consensus on management of advanced cancer-related pain in individuals with opioid use disorder. *JAMA Netw Open.* 2021;4(12):e2139968.

135. Greene MS, Chambers RA. Pseudoaddiction: fact or fiction? An investigation of the medical literature. *Curr Addict Rep.* 2015;2(4):310-317.

136. Higgins C, Smith BH, Matthews K. Incidence of iatrogenic opioid dependence or abuse in patients with pain who were exposed to opioid analgesic therapy: a systematic review and meta-analysis. *Br J Anaesth.* 2018;120(6):1335-1344.

137. Kumar PS, Saphire ML, Grogan M, et al. Substance abuse risk and medication monitoring in patients with advanced lung cancer receiving palliative care. *J Pain Palliat Care Pharmacother.* 2021;35(2):91-99. doi:10.1080/15360288.2021.1920545

138. Yennurajalingam S, Edwards T, Arthur JA, et al. Predicting the risk for aberrant opioid use behavior in patients receiving outpatient supportive care consultation at a comprehensive cancer center. *Cancer.* 2018;124(19):3942-3949. doi:10.1002/cncr.31670

139. Portenoy RK, Ahmed E, Patel M. Adjuvant analgesics: principles of use. In: Cherny N, Fallon M, Kaasa S, Portenoy R, Currow DC, eds. *Oxford Textbook of Palliative Medicine.* 6th ed. Oxford University Press; 2021:433-442.

140. Paulsen O, Klepstad P, Rosland JH, et al. Efficacy of methylprednisolone on pain, fatigue, and appetite loss in patients with advanced cancer using opioids: a randomized, placebo-controlled, double-blind trial. *J Clin Oncol.* 2014;32(29):3221-3228.

141. Yennurajalingam S, Frisbee-Hume S, Palmer JL, et al. Reduction of cancer-related fatigue with dexamethasone: a double-blind, randomized, placebo-controlled trial in patients with advanced cancer. *J Clin Oncol.* 2013;31(25):3076-3082.

142. Haywood A, Good P, Khan S, et al. Corticosteroids for the management of cancer-related pain in adults. *Cochrane Database Syst Rev.* 2015;2015(4):CD010756.

143. Griebeler ML, Morey-Vargas OL, Brito JP, et al. Pharmacologic interventions for painful diabetic neuropathy: an umbrella systematic review and comparative effectiveness network meta-analysis. *Ann Intern Med.* 2014;161(9):639-649.

144. Wang, SM, Han C, Bahk WM, et al. Addressing the side effects of contemporary antidepressant drugs: a comprehensive review. *Chonnam Med J.* 2018;54(2):101-112.

145. Dharmshaktu P, Tayal V, Kalra BS. Efficacy of antidepressants as analgesics: a review. *J Clin Pharmacol.* 2012;52(1):6-17.

146. Finnerup NB, Attal N, Haroutounian S, et al. Pharmacotherapy for neuropathic pain in adults: a systematic review and meta-analysis. *Lancet Neurol.* 2015;14(2):162-173.

147. Loprinzi CL, Lacchetti C, Bleeker J, et al. Prevention and management of chemotherapy-induced peripheral neuropathy in survivors of adult cancers: ASCO Guideline Update. *J Clin Oncol.* 2020;38(28):3325-3348.

148. Wilson E, Lader M. A review of the management of antidepressant discontinuation symptoms. *Ther Adv Psychopharmacol.* 2015;5(6):357-368.

149. Eisenach JC, DuPen S, Dubois M, Miguel R, Allin D; Epidural Clonidine Study Group. Epidural clonidine analgesia for intractable cancer pain. The epidural clonidine study group. *Pain.* 1995;61(3):391-399.

150. Anger KE. Dexmedetomidine: a review of its use for the management of pain, agitation, and delirium in the intensive care unit. *Curr Pharm Des.* 2013;19(22):4003-4013.

151. Yazicioğlu D, Caparlar C, Akkaya T, Mercan U, Kulaçoğlu H. Tizanidine for the management of acute postoperative pain after inguinal hernia repair: a placebo-controlled double-blind trial. *Eur J Anaesthesiol.* 2016;33(3):215-222.

152. Petzke F, Tölle T, Fitzcharles MA, Häuser W. Cannabis-based medicines and medical cannabis for chronic neuropathic pain. *CNS Drugs.* 2022;36(1):31-44.

153. Lichtman AH, Lux EA, McQuade R, et al. Results of a double-blind, randomized, placebo-controlled study of Nabiximols Oromucosal spray as an adjunctive therapy in advanced cancer patients with chronic uncontrolled pain. *J Pain Symptom Manage.* 2018;55(2):179-188.e1.

154. Johnson JR, Burnell-Nugent M, Lossignol D, Ganae-Motan ED, Potts R, Fallon MT. Multicenter, double-blind, randomized, placebo-controlled, parallel-group study of the efficacy, safety, and tolerability of THC:CBD extract and THC extract in patients with intractable cancer-related pain. *J Pain Symptom Manage.* 2010;39(2):167-179.

155. Aviram J, Samuelly-Leichtag G. Efficacy of cannabis-based medicines for pain management: a systematic review and meta-analysis of randomized controlled trials. *Pain Phys.* 2017;20(6):E755-E796.

156. Derry S, Wiffen PJ, Kalso EA, et al. Topical analgesics for acute and chronic pain in adults-an overview of Cochrane Reviews. *Cochrane Database Syst Rev.* 2017;5(5):CD008609.

157. Seidel S, Aigner M, Ossege M, Pernicka E, Wildner B, Sycha T. Antipsychotics for acute and chronic pain in adults. *Cochrane Database Syst Rev.* 2013;8:CD004844.

158. Rostami R, Mittal SO, Radmand R, Jabbari B. Incobotulinum Toxin-A improves post-surgical and post-radiation pain in cancer patients. *Toxins (Basel).* 2016;8(1):22.

159. Safarpour Y, Jabbari B. Botulinum toxin treatment of pain syndromes—an evidence based review. *Toxicon.* 2018;147:120-128.

160. Sandrini G, De Icco R, Tassorelli C, Smania N, Tamburin S. Botulinum neurotoxin type A for the treatment of pain: not just in migraine and trigeminal neuralgia. *J Headache Pain.* 2017;18(1):38.

161. Michelet D, Brasher C, Horlin AL, et al. Ketamine for chronic non-cancer pain: a meta-analysis and trial sequential analysis of randomized controlled trials. *Eur J Pain.* 2018;22(4):632-646.

162. Bell RF, Eccleston C, Kalso EA. Ketamine as an adjuvant to opioids for cancer pain. *Cochrane Database Syst Rev.* 2017;6:CD003351.

163. Fond G, Loundou A, Rabu C, et al. Ketamine administration in depressive disorders: a systematic review and meta-analysis. *Psychopharmacol (Berl).* 2014;231(18):3663-3676.

164. Prommer EE. Ketamine for pain: an update of uses in palliative care. *J Palliat Med.* 2012;15:474-483.

165. Salas S, Frasca M, Planchet-Barraud B, et al. Ketamine analgesic effect by continuous intravenous infusion in refractory cancer pain: considerations about the clinical research in palliative care. *J Palliat Med.* 2012;15:287-293.

166. Quibell R, Fallon M, Mihalyo M, Twycross R, Wilcock A. Ketamine. *J Pain Symptom Manage.* 2015;50(2):268-278.

167. Marchetti F, Coutaux A, Bellanger A, Magneux C, Bourgeois P, Mion G. Efficacy and safety of oral ketamine for the relief of intractable chronic pain: a retrospective 5-year study of 51 patients. *Eur J Pain.* 2015;19(7):984-993.

168. Mercadante S, Caruselli A, Casuccio A. The use of ketamine in a palliative-supportive care unit: a retrospective analysis. *Ann Palliat Med.* 2018;7(2):205-210.

169. Loveday BA, Sindt J. Ketamine protocol for palliative care in cancer patients with refractory pain. *J Adv Pract Oncol.* 2015;6(6):555-561.

170. Piano V, Verhagen S, Schalkwijk A, et al. Treatment for neuropathic pain in patients with cancer: comparative analysis of recommendations in national clinical practice guidelines from European countries. *Pain Pract.* 2014;14(1):1-7.

171. Wiffen PJ, Derry S, Bell RF, et al. Gabapentin for chronic neuropathic pain in adults. *Cochrane Database Syst Rev.* 2017;6:CD007938.

172. Toth C. Substitution of gabapentin therapy with pregabalin therapy in neuropathic pain due to peripheral neuropathy. *Pain Med.* 2010;11(3):456-465.

173. Wiffen PJ, Derry S, Moore RA, et al. Antiepileptic drugs for neuropathic pain and fibromyalgia–an overview of Cochrane reviews. *Cochrane Database Syst Rev.* 2013;2013(11):CD010567.

174. Demant DT, Lund K, Vollert J, et al. The effect of oxcarbazepine in peripheral neuropathic pain depends on pain phenotype: a randomised, double-blind, placebo-controlled phenotype-stratified study. *Pain.* 2014;155(11):2263-2273.

175. Hearn L, Derry S, Moore RA. Lacosamide for neuropathic pain and fibromyalgia in adults. *Cochrane Database Syst Rev.* 2012;2012(2):CD009318.

176. Wiffen PJ, Derry S, Lunn MP, Moore RA. Topiramate for neuropathic pain and fibromyalgia in adults. *Cochrane Database Syst Rev.* 2013;2013(8):CD008314.

177. Wiffen PJ, Rees J. Lamotrigine for acute and chronic pain. *Cochrane Database Syst Rev.* 2007;2(2):CD006044.

178. Chiras J, Shotar E, Cormier E, Clarencon F. Interventional radiology in bone metastases. *Eur J Cancer Care (Engl).* 2017;26:e12741.

179. Lee HL, Kuo CC, Tsai JT, Chen CY, Wu MH, Chiou JF. Magnetic resonance-guided focused ultrasound versus conventional radiation therapy for painful bone metastasis: a matched-pair study. *J Bone Joint Surg Am.* 2017;99(18):1572-1578.

180. Brodowicz T, Hadji P, Niepel D, Diel I. Early identification and intervention matters: a comprehensive review of current evidence and recommendations for the monitoring of bone health in patients with cancer. *Cancer Treat Rev.* 2017;61:23-34.

181. Hendriks LE, Hermans BC, van den Beuken-van Everdingen MH, Hochstenbag MM, Dingemans AM. Effect of bisphosphonates, denosumab, and radioisotopes on bone pain and quality of life in patients with non-small cell lung cancer and bone metastases: a systematic review. *J Thorac Oncol.* 2016;11(2):155-173.

182. Orozco CK, Maalouf NM. Safety of bisphosphonates. *Rheum Dis Clin North Am.* 2012;38(4):681-705.

183. Menshawy A, Mattar O, Abdulkarim A, et al. Denosumab versus bisphosphonates in patients with advanced cancers-related bone metastasis: systematic review and meta-analysis of randomized controlled trials. *Support Care Cancer.* 2018;26(4):1029-1038.

184. Das T, Banerjee S. Radiopharmaceuticals for metastatic bone pain palliation: available options in the clinical domain and their comparisons. *Clin Exp Metastasis.* 2017;34(1):1-10.

185. Lange R, Ter Heine R, Knapp RF, de Klerk JM, Bloemendal HJ, Hendrikse NH. Pharmaceutical and clinical development of phosphonate-based radiopharmaceuticals for the targeted treatment of bone metastases. *Bone.* 2016;91:159-179.

186. Feuer DJ, Broadley KE. Corticosteroids for the resolution of malignant bowel obstruction in advanced gynaecological and gastrointestinal cancer. *Cochrane Database Syst Rev.* 2000;2000(2):CD001219.

187. Longford E, Scott A, Fradsham S, et al. Malignant bowel obstruction—systematic literature review and evaluation of current practice. *BMJ Support Palliat Care.* 2015;5(1):119.

188. Mercadante S, Casuccio A, Mangione S. Medical treatment for inoperable malignant bowel obstruction: a qualitative systematic review. *J Pain Symptom Manage.* 2007;33(2):217-223.

189. Obita GP, Boland EG, Currow DC, Johnson MJ, Boland JW. Somatostatin analogues compared with placebo and other pharmacologic agents in the management of symptoms of inoperable malignant bowel obstruction: a systematic review. *J Pain Symptom Manage.* 2016;52(6):901-919.e1.

190. Jackson TP, Gaeta R. Neurolytic blocks revisited. *Curr Pain Headache Rep.* 2008;12(1):7-13.

191. Mercadante S, Catala E, Arcuri E, Casuccio A. Celiac plexus block for pancreatic cancer pain: factors influencing pain, symptoms and quality of life. *J Pain Symptom Manage.* 2003;26(6):1140-1147.

192. Arcidiacono PG, Calori G, Carrara S, McNicol ED, Testoni PA. Celiac plexus block for pancreatic cancer pain in adults. *Cochrane Database Syst Rev.* 2011;2011(3):CD007519.

193. Wyse JM, Carone M, Paquin SC, Usatii M, Sahai AV. Randomized, double-blind, controlled trial of early endoscopic ultrasound-guided celiac plexus neurolysis to prevent pain progression in patients with newly diagnosed, painful, inoperable pancreatic cancer. *J Clin Oncol.* 2011;29:3541-3546.

194. Paley CA, Wittkopf PG, Jones G, Johnson MI. Does TENS reduce the intensity of acute and chronic pain? A comprehensive appraisal of the characteristics and outcomes of 169 reviews and 49 meta-analyses. *Medicina (Kaunas).* 2021;57(10):1060.

195. Kashyap K, Bhatnagar S. Evidence for the efficacy of scrambler therapy for cancer pain: a systematic review. *Pain Physician.* 2020;23(4):349-364.

196. Verrills P, Sinclair C, Barnard A. A review of spinal cord stimulation systems for chronic pain. *J Pain Res.* 2016;9:481-492.

197. O'Connell NE, Marston L, Spencer S, DeSouza LH, Wand BM. Non-invasive brain stimulation techniques for chronic pain. *Cochrane Database Syst Rev.* 2018;3(3):CD008208.

198. De Groef A, Van Kampen M, Dieltjens E, et al. Effectiveness of postoperative physical therapy for upper-limb impairments after breast cancer treatment: a systematic review. Arch Phys Med Rehabil. 2015;96:1140-1153.

199. Kleckner IR, Kamen C, Gewandter JS, et al. Effects of exercise during chemotherapy on chemotherapy-induced peripheral neuropathy: a multicenter, randomized controlled trial. *Support Care Cancer.* 2018;26:1019-1028.

200. Burchiel KJ, Raslan AM. Contemporary concepts of pain surgery. *J Neurosurg.* 2019;130(4):1039-1049.

201. Javed S, Viswanathan A, Abdi S. Cordotomy for intractable cancer pain: a narrative review. *Pain Phys.* 2020;23(3):283-292.

202. Ruano A, García-Torres F, Gálvez-Lara M, Moriana JA. Psychological and non-pharmacologic treatments for pain in cancer patients: a systematic review and meta-analysis. *J Pain Symptom Manage.* 2022;63(5):e505-e520.

203. Bennett MI, Bagnall AM, Closs JS. How effective are patient-based educational interventions in the management of cancer pain? Systematic review and meta-analysis. *Pain.* 2009;143(3):192-199.

204. Garland EL, Brintz CE, Hanley AW, et al. Mind-body therapies for opioid-treated pain: a systematic review and meta-analysis. *JAMA Intern Med.* 2020;180(1):91-105.

205. Greenlee H, Balneaves LG, Carlson LE, et al. Clinical practice guide-lines on the use of integrative therapies as supportive care in patients treated for breast cancer. *J Natl Cancer Inst Monogr.* 2014;2014:346-358.

206. Bao Y, Kong X, Yang L, et al. Complementary and alternative medicine for cancer pain: an overview of systematic reviews. *Evid Based Complement Alternat Med.* 2014;2014:170396.

207. He Y, Guo X, May BH, et al. Clinical evidence for association of acu-puncture and acupressure with improved cancer pain: a systematic review and meta-analysis. *JAMA Oncol.* 2020;6(2):271-278.

208. Cassileth BR, Vickers AJ. Massage therapy for symptom con-trol: outcome study at a major cancer center. *J Pain Symptom Manage.* 2004;28:244-249.

209. Chen YW, Hunt MA, Campbell KL, Peill K, Reid WD. The effect of Tai Chi on four chronic conditions-cancer, osteoarthritis, heart fail-ure and chronic obstructive pulmonary disease: a systematic review and meta-analyses. *Br J Sports Med.* 2016;50(7):397-407.

CHAPTER **12.6**

Palliative and Supportive Care

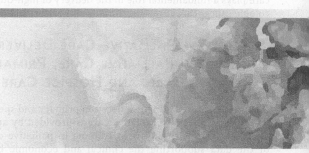

Emily J. Martin and Natsai C. Nyakudarika

INTRODUCTION

Palliative care is specialized medical care aimed at improving QoL for people living with serious illness. Unlike hospice care, which is a specialized end-of-life service for patients with a life expectancy of 6 months or less, palliative care may be provided at any point in a patient's disease course and can be offered concurrently with disease-directed therapy, including curative-intent therapy (**Figure 12.6-1**). Palliative care takes a patient- and family-centered ap-proach to care, serving as an extra layer of support throughout the disease trajectory. For patients with cancer, palliative care includes expert management of symptoms related to either the cancer or its treatments, with the ultimate goal of anticipating, preventing, and relieving suffering. Palliative care also encompasses communi-cation with patients and families about the goals of care to ensure that the treatment plan reflects the patient's values and preferences and addresses the psychological, social, and existential domains of care, as applicable.

Numerous randomized trials have shown that the provision of palliative care for patients with cancer is associated with multiple benefits, including improved QoL, improved symp-tom management, increased patient and caregiver satisfaction,

reduced caregiver distress, greater goal-concordant care, and less aggressive end-of-life care (1-7). Furthermore, there is evidence that early integration of palliative care into standard oncologic care may improve survival. In the well-known ran-domized trial by Temel et al, 151 patients with newly diagnosed metastatic non–small cell lung cancer were randomized to in-tegration of outpatient palliative care from the time of cancer diagnosis versus usual oncologic care (8). The early palliative care integration group had significant improvements in QoL and mood, as well as a statistically significant improvement in OS (11.6 vs 8.9 months, $P = .02$), despite less aggressive inter-vention at the end of life (8).

In response to these early studies, the ASCO published a Clinical Opinion in 2012, stating that "combined standard on-cology care and palliative care should be considered early in the course of illness for any patient with metastatic cancer and/or high symptom burden" (9), and, in 2016, the ASCO updated its Clinical Practice Guideline to include the following recommen-dation: "patients with advanced cancer should be referred to interdisciplinary palliative care teams...early in the course of dis-ease, alongside active treatment of their cancer" (10). Similarly, in 2015, the SGO published a position statement that identifies

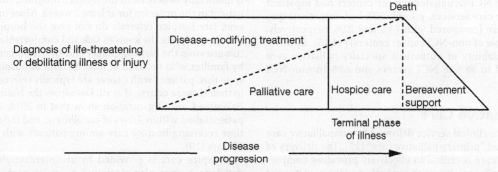

Figure 12.6-1. The simultaneous care model for palliative care, defined by the Centers for Medicare & Medicaid Services in its proposed Hospice Conditions of Participation and as adapted from the World Health Organization. (From A National Framework and Preferred Practices for Palliative and Hospice Care Quality: A Consensus Report, by the National Quality Forum, Washington, DC. Copyright 2006 by the National Quality Forum. Reproduced with permission.)

early integration of palliative care as an essential element of the comprehensive care of women with gynecologic cancer (11). Moreover, early integration of palliative care is included as one of the SGO's five Choosing Wisely recommendations: "don't delay the provision of palliative care for women with advanced or relapsed gynecologic cancer, including referral for specialty level palliative medicine" (12).

This chapter focuses on the scope of palliative care as it applies to women with gynecologic cancer, with special emphasis on the regulations governing palliative care services in the United States. The importance of this topic cannot be overemphasized: Palliative care plays a fundamental role in the delivery of high-quality gynecologic cancer care.

SYSTEMS OF PALLIATIVE CARE DELIVERY: SPECIALIZED PALLIATIVE CARE, PRIMARY PALLIATIVE CARE, AND HOSPICE CARE

It is important to distinguish between primary and specialty palliative care. Specialty palliative care is provided by an interdisciplinary team with advanced training in palliative care. Most of the data supporting the clinical and economic benefits of early integration of palliative care into standard oncology care are based on trials of specialty palliative care interventions (13). In contrast, primary (or basic) palliative care can be provided by any clinician who cares for patients with serious illness; in the case of gynecologic cancer, this may include the gynecologic oncologist, medical oncologist, radiation oncologist, or the primary care provider.

Specialty Palliative Care

The field of Hospice and Palliative Medicine was officially recognized by the American Board of Medical Specialties and co-sponsored by multiple other medical boards in 2006. Until 2012, physicians could be "grandfathered in" to board certification in palliative care by documenting a certain number of hours of clinical experience and sitting for written board exams. Since 2012, board certification in palliative care requires completion of a 1-year clinical fellowship and written board exams. While the composition of interdisciplinary specialty palliative care teams can vary, core members typically include a palliative care–trained physician, a nurse or advanced practice provider, a social worker, and a chaplain. Other members may include pharmacists, psychologists, nutritionists, and rehabilitation therapists.

Although specialty palliative care has historically been available primarily as an inpatient hospital consultation service, over the past decade, the provision of outpatient specialty palliative care has increased dramatically. For example, a 2009 survey found that 92% of NCI-designated cancer centers had inpatient specialty palliative care services, yet only 59% had outpatient specialty palliative care (compared with 74% and 22%, respectively, for a random sample of non-NCI cancer centers) (14,15). By 2018, however, the availability of outpatient specialty palliative care services increased to 98% in NCI centers and 63% in non-NCI centers (16).

Primary Palliative Care

Basic palliative care clinical service delivered by nonpalliative care specialists is termed "primary palliative care" (17). The delivery of primary palliative care is critical to effectively providing comprehensive cancer care for patients with gynecologic cancer as it is not feasible, nor desirable, for palliative care to be exclusively delivered by specialists. For gynecologic oncologists, primary palliative care includes core elements of palliative care, such as basic symptom

management and aligning treatment choices with patient goals. More complex issues, such as existential distress and refractory symptom management, may be better addressed by palliative care specialists (17).

Hospice Care

Hospice care is most commonly provided through the Medicare Hospice Benefit (MHB). In addition, many states offer a Medicaid hospice benefit similar to the MHB and most private insurers also offer a hospice benefit, although these are variable. The MHB was first offered in 1983; it is a benefit of Medicare Part A that covers comprehensive end-of-life care. To be eligible for the MHB, a patient must have a qualifying terminal diagnosis and be "certified" by two physicians (one of which is typically the hospice physician) as having an expected prognosis of 6 months or less. Eligibility also requires that the patient waive the traditional Medicare Parts A and D for care related to the terminal illness, including prescription medications. The hospice benefit applies only to care or medications related to the terminal diagnosis; a patient may continue to receive care for coexisting unrelated medical problems covered by Medicare Parts A and D and can continue to see their physicians under Medicare Part B coverage. Unlike traditional Medicare benefits, which usually require a 20% co-pay, the MHB coverage is almost 100% for all services, including medications (although some hospices may require a 5% co-pay).

The hospice benefit is structured as benefit periods (two 90-day periods followed by an unlimited number of 60-day periods). Between benefit periods, the hospice provider must reevaluate and recertify the patient. Patients may revoke the MHB at any time, at which point traditional Medicare coverage is immediately available. There are four levels of hospice care—two outpatient and two inpatient. These include:

- Routine home care—routine palliative care services in the patient's home or nursing facility.
- Continuous home care—intended for crisis management of acute symptoms. It involves intensive home nursing for a minimum of 8 hours during each 24-hour time period.
- General inpatient care—intended for short-term control of acute symptoms that cannot be managed outside an acute care setting. It can be provided by a hospice facility, hospital, or skilled nursing facility (SNF).
- Respite care—intended to give caregivers respite. It is reimbursed for no more than 5 days in each benefit period. Respite care can take place in a hospice facility, hospital, or SNF.

The MHB offers a fixed per diem payment to the hospice program, with rates varying by geographical location. The initial intake of a new patient is particularly time and resource intensive and generally costs the hospice far more than the daily per diem; it is financially beneficial to the hospice program, therefore, to have a patient in the program for at least 2 weeks. More importantly, however, late hospice referrals do not give the hospice team enough time to complete the goals of safe and comfortable dying and effective grieving; the highest-quality end-of-life outcomes are reported by families who received at least 30 days of hospice care (18). Despite this, patients with cancer are typically referred to hospice late in their disease course, if at all. Data from the National Hospice and Palliative Care Organization show that in 2018, 27.9% of hospice patients died within 7 days of enrollment, and the median length of time receiving hospice care among patients with cancer was only 18 days (19).

Hospice care is provided by an interdisciplinary team who develops a care plan designed to meet each patient's needs. Hospice teams consist of physicians, nurses, home health aides, social workers, chaplains, trained volunteers, and therapists (speech, physical, occupational) if needed. Hospice services are multidimensional. They include pain and symptom management; provision of medications and medical supplies; assistance with emotional, psychosocial, and spiritual aspects of dying; support for the family in caring for the patient; and bereavement services.

Retrospective data in nongynecologic cancers suggest that hospice care is associated with no decrease in survival and, in some cases, improved survival (20-22). In addition, family members of hospice patients are more likely to report better QoL, lower rates of physical and psychosocial distress, and better quality of death for their loved ones than patients treated in the hospital at the end of life (22-24). One retrospective cohort study evaluated 81 patients with gynecologic cancer who died secondary to cancer recurrence and/or progression and who were offered hospice services. Patients who declined hospice when it was recommended were considered not to have utilized hospice whether or not they ultimately received end-of-life care. Median time for receiving end-of-life care was longer in the hospice group (8 vs 1 week, $P < .0005$), and patients in the nonhospice group were more likely to have an invasive procedure performed or antineoplastic therapy administered within 4 weeks of death ($P = .036$). In the subset of patients with recurrent disease (73%), the median OS for patients who chose hospice was 17 months, compared with 9 months for the group not utilizing hospice (25).

PRIMARY PALLIATIVE CARE FOR THE GYNECOLOGIC ONCOLOGIST

Symptom Management

Patients with gynecologic malignancy often experience both disease- and treatment-related symptoms throughout the course of their illness (26-28). Unfortunately, symptoms may go unrecognized and, therefore, untreated for a multitude of reasons. Clinicians may assume that patients will initiate discussions about symptoms, while patients often expect their physicians to initiate these discussions. Moreover, patients may have a disincentive to report symptoms to their oncologists because of fears about prompting a change in treatment. Patient-reported outcomes are the gold standard for quantifying patient experience and symptoms (29), and several validated scales exist to measure symptom burden, including the Edmonton Symptom Assessment System and the Memorial Symptom Assessment Scale. Basic tenets of symptom management for patients with gynecologic cancers are reviewed here.

Pain

Pain management is discussed in detail in Chapter 12.5.

Nausea and Vomiting

Patients with gynecologic malignancy frequently suffer from nausea and vomiting. Generally, nausea and vomiting are best managed using an etiology-based approach (30), although a protocol-based approach may be more appropriate for those very close to the end of life (31). The etiologic approach relies on a detailed history, including associated symptoms, timing, frequency, and exacerbating and relieving factors. A mnemonic for the differential diagnosis of nausea by mechanism is VOMIT—Vestibular apparatus, Obstruction, Motility/Mind, Infection/Inflammation, and Toxins/Tumor. **Table 12.6-2** summarizes this approach.

Chemotherapy can cause nausea and vomiting through its direct effect on the chemoreceptor trigger zone and vomiting centers. There are three types of chemotherapy-induced nausea and vomiting (CINV): acute emesis (which typically peaks within 4-6 hours of chemotherapy), delayed emesis (which occurs over 24 hours after chemotherapy), and anticipatory emesis (which occurs

before chemotherapy as a conditioned response). The following medications have the highest therapeutic index for the management of CINV: the 5-HT3 receptor antagonists, the neurokinin-1 receptor (NK1R) antagonists, glucocorticoids, and olanzapine.

Ondansetron and other 5-HT3 receptor antagonists are highly effective in preventing and treating CINV and have radically improved the QoL for those receiving emetogenic chemotherapy (32). These medications are generally well tolerated, with the main side effects including constipation and mild headache. The efficacy of 5-HT3 receptor antagonists in preventing CINV is improved when combined with glucocorticoids.

The NK1R antagonists are also highly effective in preventing and treating both acute and delayed CINV among patients receiving moderately or highly emetogenic chemotherapy. A meta-analysis of 17 trials found that the addition of an NK1R antagonist to standard therapy with a 5-HT3 receptor antagonist and a glucocorticoid was associated with a significant improvement in both acute and delayed CINV (33).

Glucocorticoids are effective antiemetics; although they can be used as single agents for chemotherapy regimens with low or minimal emetogenicity, they are typically used in combination with 5-HT3 receptor antagonists and/or NK1R antagonists for regimens with moderate or high emetogenicity.

Olanzapine, a second-generation antipsychotic medication that blocks 5-HT2 receptors and dopamine D2 receptors, is increasingly utilized to prevent both acute and delayed CINV. A meta-analysis of 14 RCTs found that the addition of olanzapine to standard antiemetic therapy was significantly more effective at preventing acute and delayed CINV than standard therapy alone (34).

Phenothiazines such as prochlorperazine may be considered a single-agent regimen for patients receiving chemotherapy with low or minimal emetogenicity if glucocorticoids are contraindicated (35).

Anticipatory nausea and vomiting can result in emesis in anticipation of receiving chemotherapy. Typically, anticipatory nausea and vomiting is a conditioned response among patients who have had insufficient prevention of CINV during prior cycles of treatment. Preventing CINV once chemotherapy is initiated is the most effective method of preventing the subsequent development of anticipatory nausea and vomiting. For some patients, behavioral therapies, such as systemic desensitization, relaxation techniques, or hypnosis, may help address anticipatory nausea and vomiting. Benzodiazepines may be indicated for more severe cases (36).

Delayed gastric emptying is another leading cause of nausea and vomiting among patients with gynecologic malignancies. Delayed gastric emptying can be due to a variety of causes, including chemotherapy-induced gastroparesis, carcinomatosis, ascites, mechanical obstruction, and constipation. Gastric distension, caused by retained food or gastric fluids, activates stretch receptors that feed into nausea and vomiting centers. Etiologically based treatment seeks to improve gastric motility through the use of metoclopramide or, less commonly, erythromycin, or to decrease production of gastric fluid through the use of ranitidine, H_2-blockers, or anticholinergic agents, such as scopolamine or glycopyrrolate (37). Dietary and behavioral interventions may be useful as well. In select circumstances, therapeutic paracentesis may be effective (38).

The management of malignant bowel obstruction is described later in this chapter.

Lymphedema

Lymphedema is a prevalent and underreported symptom among women with gynecologic cancer. Morbidity from lymphedema includes decreased function, chronic infections, and impaired QoL (39). In a large, population-based study, morbidity from lymphedema was experienced by 10% of women after gynecologic cancer treatment, with highest prevalence (36%) among vulvar cancer

▪ TABLE 12.6-2. Nausea and Vomiting

	Location	Causes	Symptoms	Symptomatic Treatment	
CNS	Vestibular	Metastatic lesions to CNS	Vertigo, movement-related nausea	Scopolamine, meclizine	Uncommon
	Cortical	Increased ICP Anxiety, pain Anticipatory	Headache, neurologic signs Vomiting associated with these symptoms Nausea/vomiting "antici-pates" noxious stimulus	Steroids Treatment of pain/anxiety Treatment of noxious stimulus, benzodiazepines, haloperidol, Zyprexa, CBT	Uncommon Uncommon Common
	Chemoreceptor trigger zone D2 (dopamine) 5-HT3 NK1 Vomiting center Achm H1 5-HT2	Drugs (chemotherapy) Metabolic (renal failure, liver failure)	Temporal association with medication or toxin	Pretreatment and prophylaxis 5-HT3 receptor blockers Phenothiazines Metoclopramide NK1 antagonist	Very common
GI	Stomach	Delayed gastric emptying due to: Mechanical obstruction (partial) Gastroparesis (chemotherapy, opioids) Ascites Paraneoplastic syndrome	Early satiety, bloating, reflux, vomiting of undigested food	Metoclopramide Small frequent, calorie dense meals Therapeutic paracentesis where appropriate Ranitidine/H$_2$-blockers	Very common
	Small and large bowel	Mechanical bowel obstruction (partial or complete) paraneoplastic		Metoclopramide (partial obstruction only) Steroids Octreotide Dietary interventions Ranitidine/H$_2$-blockers Anticholinergics	Common (very common in ovarian cancer)

CBT, cognitive behavioral therapy; CNS, central nervous system; ICP, intracranial pressure; NK1, neurokinin-1; 5-HT2, 5-hydroxytryptamine-2.

survivors and lowest (5%) among ovarian cancer survivors (40). Needs relating to managing the symptoms of lymphedema are often unmet. Physical therapy, including lymphatic massage and special exercises, can be helpful, in conjunction with compression bandages and garments. The best way to manage lymphedema is to avoid it if possible. Indeed, over the past three decades, the role of complete inguinofemoral, pelvic, and para-aortic lymphadenectomy has evolved with strong data emerging to support selective lymphadenectomy and sentinel lymph node assessment (41-43). Preoperative preparation is also important, as symptoms may be easier for the patient to manage emotionally if they are not completely unexpected.

Neuropathy

CIPN is one of the most common neurologic complications of cancer treatment; it is estimated that up to 60% of patients with cancer treated with neurotoxic chemotherapy will develop peripheral neuropathy (44). CIPN severity generally increases with treatment dose and duration and decreases after treatment stops. Sensory symptoms (such as tingling, numbness, and pain) are more likely to improve over time than motor symptoms but may persist in some patients. CIPN has a significant impact on QoL and may lead to premature discontinuation of chemotherapy or dose modification (44). Although there are no agents that prevent CIPN, several classes of medications are used for treatment: anticonvulsants, antidepressants, opioids, nonopioid analgesics, and topical agents. Duloxetine is considered first-line therapy for CIPN (45). Gabapentin, pregabalin, TCAs, and topical agents can also provide symptom relief.

Constipation

Constipation is common among patients with gynecologic malignancies and can arise as a direct effect of disease or as a side effect of medications, most commonly opioids or selective 5-HT3 antagonists such as ondansetron. As constipation can cause and exacerbate other symptoms including pain and nausea, it must be anticipated and proactively managed. Because opioid-induced constipation does not improve or resolve with chronic opioid use, a prophylactic bowel regimen should be considered with every opioid prescription. Patients should be counseled regarding constipation at the time of opioid prescription and should be instructed to titrate their bowel regimen to the goal of a soft bowel movement every 1 to 2 days. Despite widespread use, docusate is not effective as either prophylaxis or treatment for opioid-induced constipation (46). A stimulant laxative such as senna is considered first-line therapy. Other pharmacologic options include bisacodyl or osmotic agents such as polyethylene glycol-3350 and milk of magnesia. Sorbitol and lactulose can be effective but typically cause significant bloating and flatulence. Nonpharmacologic options, which can be used to supplement pharmacologic options but are generally not sufficient alone, include increasing activity level and fluid intake. When treating existing constipation, bowel obstruction should be ruled out first, either clinically or with imaging. In addition to the therapies mentioned earlier, methylnaltrexone, which is a μ-opioid receptor antagonist, can be used for refractory opioid-induced constipation. Owing to its limited ability to cross the blood-brain barrier, methylnaltrexone does not affect analgesia or precipitate opioid withdrawal (47).

Fatigue

One of the most common and distressing symptoms patients with advanced cancer experience is fatigue (48). Fatigue may be present at the time of cancer diagnosis and typically increases during treatment (49). Prevalence estimates of fatigue during treatment range from 25% to 99% depending on the patient population, type of treatment received, and method of assessment (48). In most studies, 30% to 60% of patients report moderate-to-severe fatigue during treatment, which, in some cases, may lead to treatment discontinuation. Although fatigue usually improves in the year after treatment completion, studies of cancer survivors suggest that approximately one quarter to one-third experience persistent fatigue for up to 10 years after cancer diagnosis (50,51). Cancer-related fatigue is multidimensional and can cause impairment of QoL by negatively impacting other domains of life, such as the social and emotional domains. Fatigue is particularly prevalent among women with gynecologic malignancy (52). In one study of patients with ovarian cancer, fatigue was reported by 67% of patients in the last year of life, increasing to 93% in the last 3 months (53). Similarly, more than half of women with cervical cancer have fatigue (54). Unfortunately, treatment options for fatigue are limited, and the literature on pharmacologic interventions is very heterogeneous. There is evidence to suggest that methylphenidate may be effective, with a Cochrane meta-analysis showing an estimated superior effect for methylphenidate in cancer-related fatigue (55). Studies in breast cancer have suggested physical exercise and psychosocial interventions may also be helpful in treating cancer-related fatigue (56).

Malignant Bowel Obstruction

In gynecologic cancer, malignant bowel obstruction may occur from either a functional obstruction by tumor or a failure of normal peristalsis due to tumor coating the intestinal serosa (carcinomatous ileus). Nonmalignant causes of bowel obstruction may also occur, due to adhesive disease from surgery, radiation damage to normal tissue, or scarring from intraperitoneal chemotherapy. Patients most commonly present with abdominal distension, nausea and vomiting, and pain from the distension of the intestinal wall and interrupted peristalsis. Conservative management involves bowel rest, nasogastric decompression, and intravenous hydration. A short course of glucocorticoids can be effective at reducing edema in select situations. Octreotide is often recommended for the completely obstructed patient. Venting gastrostomy tubes may be considered for comfort if the bowel obstruction does not resolve with conservative measures. In rare situations, a palliative surgery may be considered. Palliative surgery should be undertaken with caution, as morbidity is 5% to 49% and mortality 5% to 15% (57). Median survival in patients with recurrent ovarian cancer after palliative bowel surgery is approximately 12 months compared to 4 months in nonsurgical patients ($P < .01$) (58). For severely ill patients with large bowel obstruction from recurrent gynecologic malignancy, some case series have explored colonic stent placement as a safe and reasonable option, with most recent data showing median survival of 7.7 months (95% CI 3.19-11.9 months) after placement (59).

Anorexia and Cachexia

Anorexia is common among patients with gynecologic malignancies and can be due to the cancer itself or its treatments. The mnemonic ANOREXIA addresses potentially reversible causes of poor appetite (Aches and pain, Nausea and gastrointestinal dysfunction, Oral candidiasis, Reactive [or organic] depression or anxiety, Evacuation problems [constipation, retention], Xerostomia [dry mouth], Iatrogenic [radiation, chemotherapy, medications], Acid-related problems [gastritis, peptic ulcers]) (60). Although potentially reversible causes of anorexia should certainly be evaluated and addressed, it is also important for clinicians, patients, and families to understand that in the absence of identifiable reversible factors, anorexia and cachexia are often part of the natural history of the disease process itself. Anorexia-cachexia syndrome in advanced cancer is attributable to a complex interplay of metabolic-, cytokine-, and neuroendocrine-mediated events, leading to progressive atrophy of skeletal muscle and adipose tissue. Although nutritional counseling and pharmacologic therapies may provide some benefit, anorexia-cachexia syndrome remains untreatable for many patients. See Chapter 12.4 for more detailed discussion on nutrition.

Given the central role that food and feeding play in caretaking in many cultures, anorexia-cachexia syndrome is often very distressing to caregivers. It is important to explain that patients are generally not made uncomfortable by their decreased appetite; forcing the patient to eat, although well intentioned, is often far more uncomfortable and traumatic for the patient.

Dyspnea

Dyspnea is a common and distressing symptom experienced by greater than 50% of patients dying from cancer (61). Evaluation should entail a thorough symptom assessment followed by identification and management of potentially reversible causes. Nonpharmacologic interventions should be considered, such as the use of supplemental oxygen in patients with hypoxemia and the use of fans, which have been shown to diminish patients' sense of breathlessness (62,63). Opioids should be offered to patients who have dyspnea that persists despite nonpharmacologic therapies (64). For patients with dyspnea-related anxiety, benzodiazepines may be considered if symptoms persist despite use of opioids and nonpharmacologic interventions.

Delirium

Delirium is an acute change in mental status that may fluctuate and has several underlying physiologic causes. It is characterized by a constellation of features, including acute onset, waxing and waning course, altered level of consciousness, inattention, and cognitive impairment. It is further characterized based on the level of arousal and psychomotor activity as hyperactive, hypoactive, or mixed. Hypoactive delirium, which is characterized by sedation, lethargy, and psychomotor retardation, can be easily mistaken for fatigue or depression. Delirium in patients with cancer is common; prevalence ranges from 10% to 30% in hospitalized patients with cancer and up to 85% in the terminal phase of illness (65). It is associated with significant morbidity, including increased length of hospitalization, functional decline, decreased life expectancy, higher health care costs, and considerable distress for both patients and family members. Without a high index of suspicion, it can easily go unnoticed and untreated. Several screening tools for delirium have been validated in patients with cancer, including the Memorial Delirium Assessment Scale, the Delirium Rating Scale – Revised 98, and the Confusion Assessment Method (65). The evaluation of delirium should include a complete history and physical examination and comprehensive evaluation for reversible etiologies, with the understanding that delirium is often multifactorial (**Table 12.6-3**).

Management of delirium begins with addressing reversible underlying etiologies. If symptoms persist, both nonpharmacologic and pharmacologic methods may be utilized. Nonpharmacologic strategies include frequent reorientation, lights on and off at appropriate times, family member presence, optimizing sensory input (hearing aids, glasses when indicated), minimizing noise and disruption at night, and encouraging cognitively stimulating activities. For pharmacologic management, low-dose haloperidol or atypical antipsychotics (including olanzapine, risperidone, quetiapine, ziprasidone, and aripiprazole) are typically used. Patients receiving antipsychotics should be monitored for side effects including extrapyramidal symptoms and prolonged QT interval. A corrected QT interval greater than or equal to 500 milliseconds or increase of 60 milliseconds (or 20%) from baseline indicates

■ **TABLE 12.6-3. Contributing Factors to Delirium**

Common and treatable

- Medications (anticholinergics, opioids, sedatives, steroids, antidepressants, H$_2$-blockers, metoclopramide, baclofen)
- Withdrawal symptoms from abruptly stopping home medications (benzodiazepines, opiates, SSRIs, barbiturates)
- Infection
- Constipation
- Urinary retention
- Uncontrolled pain

Less common but treatable

- Electrolyte disturbances
- Anemia
- Dehydration
- Immobilization
- Depression, social isolation
- Vision or hearing impairment
- Emotional distress
- Unfamiliar environment

Less common and less treatable

- Cardiac or pulmonary failure with ischemia, hypoxia, or hypercapnia
- Renal failure
- Hepatic failure with encephalopathy
- Neurologic dysfunction due to brain metastases, seizure activity, or stroke

SSRIs, selective serotonin reuptake inhibitors.

From Tucker RO, Nichols AC. *UNIPAC 4: Managing Nonpain Symptoms.* American Academy of Hospice & Palliative Medicine; 2012.

increased risk of torsades des pointes and should prompt consideration of discontinuation of the antipsychotic, taking into account the patient's prognosis and goals of care.

The use of psychostimulants, such as methylphenidate, has been suggested in the pharmacologic management for hypoactive delirium. Though no randomized controlled trials have been performed, one small open-label prospective trial (66) and several case reports have suggested a benefit. Pharmacotherapy has also been studied to prevent delirium, but a recent systematic review concluded that current evidence does not support the routine use of antipsychotics for the prevention of delirium (67). Benzodiazepines are occasionally appropriate as an adjunct treatment in patients with agitation refractory to neuroleptics but, for the most part, should be avoided, given that they can worsen delirium and agitation.

Depression

Depressive symptoms are common among patients with cancer; roughly 45% of patients with solid tumors report depressive symptoms, and 15% receive a diagnosis of major depression (68). Depressive symptoms in patients with cancer have been associated with multiple adverse outcomes, including less satisfaction with care, increased use of health services, delayed return to work, reduced QoL, elevated risk of suicide, and increased mortality (68).

Several barriers to the accurate diagnosis of depression are unique to patients with cancer. Standard characterizations of depressive symptoms include both somatic and emotional/cognitive symptoms, but the somatic symptoms (fatigue, weight loss, etc) are also common symptoms of cancer and its treatment. In addition, it can be challenging to distinguish between normal and pathologic responses to severe illness. Patients with cancer are at risk of both overdiagnosis of depression (if symptoms related to normal grief reaction are overinterpreted as depression) and underdiagnosis (if depressive symptoms in a patient with cancer are believed to be "normal," given the presence of serious illness). The presence

of hopelessness, worthlessness, anhedonia, or suicidal ideation can help distinguish clinical depression from grief reaction, as none of these are expected in a normal grief reaction. Temporal variation can also be helpful. Patients experiencing a normal grief reaction will generally have symptoms that wax and wane, whereas patients with depression will have largely continuous symptoms.

Although there is no consensus on the single best approach to diagnose depression in patients with cancer, a single screening question such as "are you depressed?" performs reasonably well, with sensitivity of 72%, specificity of 83%, positive predictive value of 44%, and negative predictive value of 94%. The addition of a second question (regarding low interest/pleasure in doing things) improves sensitivity (91%), specificity (86%), positive predictive value (57%), and negative predictive value (98%) (69). These simple screening questions can be used to trigger either a more extensive evaluation or a referral to a mental health or palliative care specialist. Providers must either implement routine depression screening or maintain a high index of suspicion to avoid overlooking this common issue and its associated morbidity.

Both psychotherapy and antidepressant medications have shown efficacy in treating depression in patients with cancer. Medication options include TCAs, SSRIs, and SNRIs. TCAs may be particularly useful if neuropathic pain or insomnia are present, but their use is often limited by anticholinergic side effects. SSRIs are less sedating than TCAs, but side effects may include headache, nausea, and insomnia. A review of antidepressants concluded that there is no evidence to recommend one over another based on efficacy, so differences in the onset of action, side effects, and available routes of administration may drive choice of medication (70). In patients with gynecologic cancer who have depression as well as neuropathy or neuropathic pain related to their disease or its treatment, the use of an SNRI such as venlafaxine or duloxetine may be doubly beneficial. TCAs, SSRIs, and SNRIs all take several weeks to achieve therapeutic effect. For patients for whom quicker symptom relief is desired or life expectancy is short, the use of a psychostimulant such as methylphenidate is another option. Utilization of mental health professionals should be considered, when available, for complex cases.

Anxiety

Transient anxiety is a near-universal reaction to the stressful circumstances surrounding the diagnosis and treatment of cancer. For a significant number of patients, however, anxiety becomes more severe, pervasive, and disabling and may impact their cancer treatment and QoL. Patient with cancer with disabling anxiety will often have had a preexisting mood disorder, such as panic disorder, generalized anxiety disorder, or depressive disorder. Treatment of this symptom includes pharmacologic and nonpharmacologic methods. Cognitive behavioral therapy (CBT), mindfulness-based stress reduction, supportive-expressive psychotherapy, and relaxation training have all shown utility in the treatment or prevention of anxiety in patient with cancer (71-73). Pharmacologic therapy should emphasize antidepressants, with similar recommendations as those noted earlier. Benzodiazepines, especially short-acting agents such as alprazolam and lorazepam, are not recommended for long-term use because of their addictive potential, as well as their association with sedation, delirium, and falls.

Symptom Management in the Last Days of Life

While most patients with cancer say they would prefer to die at home, approximately one-fourth will spend their final days in a hospital or an ICU (74). Accordingly, hospital clinicians should be familiar with signs and symptoms that may indicate that death is approaching. A prospective cohort study by Hui et al found the following physical findings to be as predictive of 3-day mortality: nonreactive pupils, decreased response to verbal and visual stimuli, inability to close eyelids, drooping of nasolabial fold, neck hyperextension, grunting of vocal cords, upper GI tract bleeding, pulselessness of radial artery, decreased urine output, Cheyne-Stokes breathing, respiration with mandibular movement, and the "death rattle" created by uncleared bronchial secretions (75). Delirium, edema, apnea, weak pulses, and mottled skin may also serve as signs of impending death. With respect to symptoms, an observational study of patients with gynecologic malignancies (ovarian/fallopian tube, uterine, or cervical cancers) found that over 70% of patients had moderate or severe drowsiness, decreased well-being, anorexia, and tiredness in the last week of life (76).

When the care of a hospitalized patient transitions to being purely focused on comfort, all medications that are not directly related to comfort should be discontinued. The decision about whether any given medication, such as an antiarrhythmic or an anticonvulsant, should be continued must be individualized to the patient. Medications should be readily available as needed for anticipated symptoms, including pain, nausea, dyspnea, delirium, and anxiety. Though lab tests and telemetry should be discontinued, consideration should be given to continuing to check temperature and respiratory rate, given that both fever and tachypnea may create discomfort that could be effectively managed with acetaminophen and opioids, respectively.

Examination of the patient should include at least a general visual inspection for signs of distress or agitation, cutaneous changes, edema, weak or thready pulses, and apnea. Anticipatory counseling should be offered to the family in terms of what to expect as death approaches. It may be helpful to mention to families that although we do not know for sure whether unresponsive patients process tactile or auditory sensory inputs, it may be comforting to both patient and family for them to touch and talk to the patient, even after the patient no longer responds to them. See **Table 12.6-4** for a sample order set for a patient receiving comfort-focused care in the last hours to days of life.

Communication

Disclosing Difficult News

Prognosis is the likelihood of a patient developing a particular outcome with respect to an illness or its treatment within a specified time frame (77). Although often equated with life expectancy, prognosis can refer to a variety of outcomes, such as a change in physical functioning or symptom burden. Prognostic awareness is a key component of informed, shared decision-making. Patients who have a good understanding of their prognosis or disease trajectory are more likely to make decisions that align with their values and to receive goal-concordant end-of-life care (77).

Although patients may have preferences with respect to the timing and types of information disclosed, the vast majority of patients want their oncologists to accurately communicate prognostic estimates, even when the news is difficult to hear. Yet, many patients with advanced cancer lack the information needed to establish realistic goals of care. For example, in a study of over 1,000 patients with incurable metastatic lung or colorectal cancer, nearly three quarters of patients incorrectly thought that cure was possible with chemotherapy (78).

There are numerous barriers to communication of difficult news in oncology. First, although efforts have been made to improve communication skills training throughout medical education, many practicing oncologists lack formal training in how to effectively facilitate these discussions. Second, oncologists often avoid or postpone disclosing difficult news and instead focus on positive, optimistic formulations about the illness and its treatment (79,80). This hesitation to initiate more substantive and realistic discussions of what patients can reasonably expect in the future is often framed in terms of concerns about the impact of such discussions on the patient and, in particular, concerns that such

TABLE 12.6-4. Sample Order Set for End of Life for Nonpain Symptoms

Category	Sample Order	Comments
Vital signs	Temperature and respiratory rate q4h prn	Fever should be treated because it causes discomfort; tachypnea should be treated with opioids because it may reflect pain or dyspnea
Mouth care	Oral care q2–4h	Particularly important for patients who are unconscious and mouth breathing
Oxygen	Oxygen by nasal cannula prn for comfort	Oxygen is not necessary unless patient is alert and complaining of dyspnea relieved by oxygen, otherwise it is preferable to avoid attaching an additional tube to the patient
Anxiety/agitation	Lorazepam 0.5-1 mg IV q1h prn	In a conscious or semiconscious patient, may consider treating agitation with opioids or Haldol first, as agitation may reflect pain or delirium, and benzodiazepines can worsen delirium and may be sedating
Delirium and/or nausea	Haloperidol 0.5 mg IV q4h prn	Important to instruct nursing that haloperidol can be used for nausea
Secretions	Glycopyrrolate 0.2 mg IV q4h prn OR Atropine ophthalmic 1% solution 2 drops SL q30 min prn	Sounds related to secretions are not uncomfortable for the patient, but may be treated if they are upsetting to the family
Fever	Acetaminophen 650 mg PO or PR q4h prn	In an unconscious patient, fever should be treated with PR Tylenol as fever causes discomfort
Constipation	Dulcolax 10 mg PR daily prn	In patient with life expectancy >24-48 h, consider treating constipation as it can cause discomfort and delirium and a single large bowel movement after suppository will require less frequent moving of the unconscious patient than multiple frequent small bowel movements
Eye care	Ocular lubricant 1 application both eyes q8h prn	Particularly important in patients who are unconscious and may not close eyes completely, their eyes may become dry
Nutrition	PO foods and fluids as tolerated for comfort	

IV, intravenous; PO, oral; PR, by rectum; prn, as needed; q, every.

conversations will cause the patient to be depressed, lose hope, or even die more quickly. However, physicians who avoid discussing death are also protecting themselves, because disclosing difficult news can evoke their own anxiety and feelings of inadequacy or failure (81,82). Third, even when honest assessments of a patient's clinical trajectory are communicated, patients and their family members may misunderstand, discount, or misinterpret negative prognostic information when it is provided (83).

In the face of these barriers, it is no wonder that planning for the end of life is often lacking in cancer care. The simplistic model in which the oncologist presents full, explicit information regarding prognosis and choices for treatment to the grateful patient who then makes rational choices regarding care by weighing the risks and benefits of treatment disintegrates in the face of the realities of medical practice where prognosis may be challenging to estimate, patients and their family members are distressed and looking for hope, and the oncologist feels internal and external pressure to be optimistic.

Several authors have synthesized years of data regarding decision-making styles and informational needs of patients and their family members, which may provide a way forward out of the dilemmas outlined earlier (81,84). One way of framing a more meaningful discussion of prognosis is by utilizing the concept of illness trajectory. The illness trajectory of incurable cancer is one of relative stability in functioning until 3 to 6 months before death when rapid decline in the ability to perform activities of daily living heralds the onset of terminal stages and is associated with increased risk of harm from systemic treatments (85). Early discussions of the expected course and trajectory of care in these terms can provide the patient and family with a general overview of the goals of treatment, which is to prolong the period of time in which the patient is able to feel well and lead a relatively normal life, while acknowledging that the cancer will eventually be fatal. Describing the clinical signs of progressive disease in terms of functional decline, increasing symptom burden, and resistance to disease-specific treatment provides the patient with information that is understandable and useful for decision-making and gives them a clearer road map for the future. More detailed discussions of life expectancy can be reserved for patients closer to the end of life, when more accurate predictions can be made (86).

Table 12.6-5 presents three different ways of discussing goals of care/prognosis. The purely factual statement, although truthful, seems cold and uncompassionate and may leave the patient feeling uncared for. The hopeful statement, although true, is ambiguous, and many patients hearing this might believe that the treatment they are getting is aimed at cure, because of the emphasis on hopeful new research. The doctor using the second formulation is likely to have higher patient satisfaction but more poorly informed patients. The illness trajectory formulation is aimed at balancing hope with realism and provides the basis for further discussion.

Finally, it should be noted that these discussions are best carried out in a collaborative and interdisciplinary manner. Involvement of nursing, social work, and chaplaincy, where appropriate, can improve the quality of care and may decrease moral distress for all providers. For more challenging cases, specialty palliative care teams can be instrumental in facilitating these discussions.

Advance Care Planning

Advance care planning (ACP) is a broad paradigm that includes the steps required to enable patients to guide their future health care so that it is consistent with their goals when they are no longer capable of making decisions for themselves. ACP includes discussions about goals of care at the end of life, designation of a health care power of attorney, and completion of an advance directive for health care (also called a living will). ACP has been shown to improve compliance with the end-of-life wishes of patients, to enhance patient and family satisfaction with care, and to reduce family stress, anxiety, and depression.

■ **TABLE 12.6-5. Styles of Communication**

Style of Discussion	Example
Factual	Your cancer is incurable. This chemotherapy has a 50% chance of prolonging your life. On average, most people with your cancer type live for 3 yr if they do chemotherapy and 2 yr if they do not do the chemotherapy.
Hopeful	Your cancer is incurable; however, we have some really excellent new treatments, and every day there is new research into the causes of cancer and new hope that will allow us to fight this disease.
Illness trajectory	Your cancer is incurable; however, there are many treatments that can prolong your life and improve your QoL, and our hope is that we can keep you feeling well and leading a normal life for as long as possible. Over time, we know that this type of cancer will stop responding well to treatment, and when it progresses, patients become weaker, need more help at home, and have more side effects from chemotherapy. When that happens, we will do everything we can to help you feel as well as possible for as long as possible by treating your symptoms and making sure you can continue to enjoy your life.

QoL, quality of life.

While most patients believe that addressing ACP is an important part of their cancer care (87,88), oncology providers often find it difficult to discuss and assume that patients will be hesitant or even unwilling to have the conversation (89). Retrospective studies of deceased patients with cancer found that only 19% had a documented advance directive (90). One study specific to patients with gynecologic cancer found that 54% of gynecologic oncologists deferred end-of-life discussions until the patient experienced a major decline in functional status (91). Another study of women with breast and gynecologic cancers found that 50% of women self-reported completing an advance directive and 48% had named a health care power of attorney, but review of medical records documented an advance directive and health care power of attorney for only 24% and 14% of women, respectively (92). A meta-analysis of the cancer literature concluded that "all stakeholders are reluctant to initiate ACP early and prefer to delay ACP until the issues raised, particularly those surrounding preferences for end of life care, are more clinically relevant" (93).

Code status is one component of ACP and may be included in an advance directive. A code status discussion should ideally take place in the context of a broader discussion about goals of care and treatment preferences and should take into account an individual patient's chance for recovery and underlying values. It is important to keep in mind that a meta-analysis of hospital CPR outcomes for patients with cancer showed that only 6.7% survived to discharge (9.1% with localized disease and 5.6% with metastatic disease) (94). A 2013 study of patients with advanced cancer found that after viewing an educational video regarding ACP, fewer patients wanted CPR or mechanical ventilation; the patients found the video acceptable and would recommend it to others (95). A randomized trial by the same group found that patients with advanced cancer who viewed a video of CPR were less likely to opt for CPR than those who listened to a verbal narrative (96).

Increasing compliance with ACP is a goal for all cancer providers and their patients. However, the literature suggests that patients expect their physicians, and often their oncologists, to initiate these discussions (93). It is, therefore, important for gynecologic oncologists to feel comfortable facilitating ACP discussions. ACP should be viewed as a dynamic, longitudinal process rather than a single discussion; it should not be confused with completion of the advance directive, which is only a small part of the overall process. Inclusion of nonphysician providers may be important in increasing compliance with completion of advance directives.

POLST is a medical order form intended to complement (not replace) the advance directive. The POLST form, which is legally valid, allows the patient's wishes regarding end-of-life care to be expressed in an unambiguous medical order with specific treatment instructions. The document communicates the patient's wishes regarding the use of so-called extreme measures (such as CPR and ventilators) and outlines decisions regarding the use of antibiotics, artificial nutrition, and other medical interventions. It is signed by a physician, nurse practitioner, or physician assistant and by the patient or their surrogate.

Running a Successful Family Meeting

The family meeting (or family conference) is an important tool to facilitate communication in the setting of advanced cancer. Family meetings are planned discussions that include the patient (whenever possible), family caregivers, and a multidisciplinary group of health professionals. Family meetings can be held for multiple purposes, including discussing the patient's diagnosis, treatment, and prognosis; clarifying the goals of care; developing a plan of care; and discharge planning. Data on the utility of family meetings are mostly derived from the ICU setting, with limited data specific to patients with gynecologic cancer.

Not all family meetings can be run with a multidisciplinary model, but gynecologic oncologists can successfully run a family meeting that attends to all the domains of the patient and their family, even with limited resources. Careful planning is essential. Before the meeting, the physician should decide which issues are to be addressed, which providers will be present, where the meeting will take place, and which family members (if any) the patient would like to participate. The goal of the meeting should be clearly stated to all participants, and time should be allowed for all parties to express their opinions and ask questions.

Teaching Communication

Numerous studies indicate that patient-oncologist communication is suboptimal, particularly when focusing on issues at the end of life (97). Fortunately, communication skills can be taught and learned, as evidenced by the Studying Communication in Oncologist Patient Encounters (SCOPE) trial, performed with 48 medical, radiation, and gynecologic oncologists and 264 patients with advanced cancer in the United States (98). In this study, clinicians were randomly assigned in a 1:1 ratio to complete a 1-hour interactive CD-ROM program about responding to patients' negative emotions. Oncologists in the intervention group used more empathetic statements and were more likely to respond to negative emotions empathetically. Perhaps most importantly, patients of oncologists in the intervention group reported greater trust in their oncologists than did patients of control oncologists. The SGO recently published a review and guide to facilitate skillful communication among gynecologic oncology providers (99).

Impact of Communication on Outcomes

Good communication can improve quality of care at the end of life. In a cohort of women with persistent or recurrent ovarian cancer, women who had earlier end-of-life discussions with their health care providers had care that better conformed with end-of-life quality measures and were less likely to die in the hospital (27). The authors stressed that early end-of-life discussions, preferably conducted more than 30 days from death, increased hospice utilization and were crucial to reducing hospitalizations, ICU admissions, and invasive procedures in the last 30 days of life. A retrospective study of 136 patients who died from gynecologic cancer similarly found that earlier end-of-life care discussions were associated with less aggressive interventions at the end of life (100).

Caregiver Needs

Caregivers, most often family members, are called upon to provide physical care as well as emotional and practical support (101,102). They may experience significant stress in this role, including financial stress if they are unable to continue working while providing care, as well as anxiety about the future. Risk factors for caregiver distress include other life stresses, poor social support, lower socioeconomic status, younger age, and a closer caregiver-patient relationship (102). Caregivers may be at high risk themselves for health problems resulting from the stress of caring for a patient with gynecologic cancer (103). There is, therefore, a significant need for education of caregivers, who may feel unprepared for their new role, as well as emotional and, where needed, spiritual support (104).

The Australian Ovarian Cancer Study explored the QoL of 99 caregivers of women with newly diagnosed primary epithelial ovarian cancer and reported significantly lower mental and physical QoL for these caregivers when compared to the population norms (102). Mean distress and unmet needs increased over time. Highest unmet needs in the last 6 months of life related to managing emotions about prognosis, fear of cancer spread, balancing the caregiver's own needs with the patient's needs, impact of caregiving on work, and making decisions in the context of uncertainty. Caregiver optimism was associated with improved mental well-being and decreased distress. Given this, the authors concluded that caregivers would benefit from early contact with psychosocial staff rather than waiting for postdeath referral to bereavement services. In addition, caregivers having access to providers as well as educational resources and support groups may be helpful in fulfilling the need for information that was identified in this study.

QUALITY OF LIFE

There is no common definition for QoL. The WHO defines quality of life (QoL) as an "individual's perception of their position in life in the context of the culture and value systems in which they live and in relation to their goals, expectations, standards and concerns" (105). HRQoL encompasses symptoms, functioning, psychological well-being, and meaning and fulfillment.

Scales and Measures

Several validated and reliable questionnaires are available for the assessment of HRQoL for patients with cancer, including the European Organization for Research and Treatment of Cancer (EORTC-QLQ-C30) and the Functional Assessment of Cancer Therapy-General (FACT-G). Domain-specific instruments assess particular factors, such as fatigue or psychological distress. The FACT-G (version 4) questionnaire includes the following four subscales: physical well-being, social well-being, emotional well-being, and functional well-being. The subscales can be analyzed either separately or together to produce a total HRQoL score. The FACT-G has demonstrated reliability, validity, and responsiveness to change over time (106). The Functional Assessment of Cancer Therapy-Ovarian (FACT-O) is a multidimensional questionnaire developed and validated for use by patients with ovarian cancer. There are also specific subscales for cervical cancer (FACT-Cx), endometrial cancer (FACT-En), and vulvar cancer (FACT-V). Higher FACT scores are associated with greater HRQoL.

Quality of Care at the End of Life

The National Quality Forum has published the following end-of-life quality performance measures, with a lower occurrence representing better quality of care: admission to ICU within

30 days of death, hospital admission more than 14 days in the last 30 days of life, more than one hospital admission during the last 30 days of life, more than one ED visit during the last 30 days of life, death in an acute care setting, initiation of a new chemotherapy regimen in the last 30 days of life, chemotherapy within 14 days of death, and hospice admission less than 3 days before death (107). In women with ovarian cancer, these aggressive care interventions (ACEs) at the end of life were not associated with improvement in survival and serve as good general quality indicators for gynecologic cancers (26).

Other groups have provided data specific to patients with gynecologic cancer regarding ACE. Nevadunsky et al reported that timely specialty palliative care consultation was associated with lower ACE scores, but only 18% of patients received a "timely" (defined as ≥30 days before death) palliative care consultation (108). Another study from the same group reported the following retrospective data with respect to ACE: Median days in hospital during last 6 months of life was 24 days, 30% of patients had an ED visit, 21% were admitted to the ICU, 50% had terminal extubation, and 13% had CPR at the end of life. Additionally in this study, 76% of patients received chemotherapy during the last 6 months of life and 30% in the last 6 weeks, 66% of patients were DNR/DNI (do not resuscitate/do not intubate), 49% enrolled in hospice (median 16 days, range 0-149 days), and 64% had a family meeting (109).

Quality of Life as a Clinical Trial End Point

HRQoL has evolved into an important, albeit secondary, end point for many cancer clinical trials. In 2014, the ASCO Cancer Research Committee met to discuss "the design of future clinical trials that would produce results that are clinically meaningful to patients." Clinically meaningful was defined as significantly improved survival, significantly improved QoL, or both (110). Recognizing the importance of a patient's specific symptom burden, the ASCO workgroup suggested that serial assessment of specific cancer-related symptoms using validated instruments constitutes a meaningful clinical outcome. Although patients with ovarian cancer are willing to undergo significant toxicity in the frontline treatment setting, when cure is possible, they are less accepting of toxicities and impairment in daily routine in the recurrent disease treatment setting (111). The study from Havrilesky et al (112) confirms this finding: 95 women with advanced or recurrent ovarian cancer were willing to accept a shorter PFS to avoid severe side effects of treatment: 6.7 months to reduce nausea and vomiting from severe to mild, 5 months to reduce neuropathy from severe to mild, and 3.7 months to reduce abdominal symptoms from severe to moderate. Although PFS remained a driver of patient preference, women were willing to trade PFS time for reduction in treatment-related toxicity.

The GOG has been incorporating HRQoL end points into their phase 3 studies for the past decade. In GOG 240, a randomized trial of chemotherapy with or without bevacizumab in patients with recurrent, persistent, or metastatic cervical cancer, the primary QoL end point was the score on the Functional Assessment of Cancer Therapy-Cervix Trial Outcome Index (FACT-Cx TOI) (113). Improvements in OS and PFS attributed to the incorporation of bevacizumab into the treatment of advanced cervical cancer were not accompanied by any significant deterioration in HRQoL, allowing the authors to conclude that the addition of bevacizumab achieved a desirable outcome overall. The GOG has also included QoL as a secondary end point in several of its recent phase 3 randomized trials in ovarian cancer (114-117). The GOG 152 showed for the first time that in patients with ovarian cancer, baseline QoL scores predict OS (115), and this has been confirmed in other studies (116).

Other clinical trial groups have also incorporated QoL as clinical trial end points. A well-known and practice-changing example is the Gynecologic Cancer Intergroup's CALYPSO study, which has changed the standard of care for women with recurrent platinum-sensitive ovarian cancer (118). This study was undertaken primarily to identify a treatment regimen for these women that would be noninferior to traditional therapy and better tolerated from a symptom standpoint. QoL evaluations (European Organization for Research and Treatment of Cancer Quality of Life Questionnaire C30 version 3.0 and OV-28 version 1.0) were required at 3-month intervals while on treatment and every 3 months for 1 year from date of enrollment. The primary end point was noninferiority of the less toxic regimen. The study was able to demonstrate that the new regimen was better tolerated than the standard regimen, with improvement in overall QoL and OS. PFS and OS remain the primary end points of cancer clinical trials, confirmed by the ASCO 2014 workgroup. However, the inclusion of HRQoL as a secondary end point allows a more comprehensive interpretation of results and leads to improved clinical decision-making.

BARRIERS TO THE USE OF PALLIATIVE CARE IN GYNECOLOGIC ONCOLOGY

Lack of Specialty Palliative Care Services

Not all facilities provide access to specialty palliative care services. Not-for-profit hospitals and public hospitals are, respectively, 4.8 and 7.1 times more likely to have a palliative care program as compared to for-profit hospitals (119). On a national level in the United States, there are not enough specialty palliative care providers to see all patients who might benefit (120,121); access to palliative care remains inadequate for millions of Americans living with serious illness, despite continuing growth in the number of hospitals reporting palliative care programs. Access to palliative care services depends on geography, with the highest penetration in the New England (88% of hospitals), Pacific (77% of hospitals), and mid-Atlantic (77% of hospitals) states and lowest in the West South Central (43% of hospitals) and East South Central (42% of hospitals) states (119).

Poor Reimbursement

Current reimbursement schedules are not structured to support early integration of palliative care into oncology care. Historically, providers were not reimbursed for end-of-life discussions with their patients or for addressing advance directives. However, in 2016 and revisions again in 2022 for Goals of Care discussions, the CMS implemented provisions, allowing physicians and other health professionals to bill for ACP.

Misconceptions About Palliative Care

One of the main barriers to the integration of palliative care into standard oncology care is the common misconception, by both patients and providers, that it is synonymous with end-of-life care or that it cannot be provided concurrent with cancer treatment. One study found that providers preferred the term "supportive care" to "palliative care" and found that they would be more likely to refer patients to a service named "supportive care" (122). When that institution changed the name of its palliative care service to supportive care, it saw a 40% increase in referrals and a trend toward referrals earlier in the disease course. The IOM report "Dying in America" concluded that "one of the greatest remaining challenges is the need for better understanding of the role of palliative care among both the public and professionals across the continuum of care so that hospice and palliative care can achieve their full potential for patients and their families" (120).

Misconceptions specific to hospice are also prevalent. There remains a significant lack of education on the part of providers, patients, and family members regarding the benefit of hospice, as well as a suspicion on the part of patients that hospice care hastens death. Other barriers to timely hospice utilization include overestimation of prognosis, the lack of physician awareness of the benefits, and confusion regarding the eligibility requirements.

IMPROVING PALLIATIVE CARE FOR WOMEN WITH GYNECOLOGIC CANCERS

Education

Gynecologic oncologists are well suited to provide primary palliative care for women with gynecologic cancers. However, several studies have suggested that many gynecologic oncology fellows feel that they are inadequately trained to address the palliative care issues they will face during their careers. In a 2014 survey of 201 gynecologic oncology fellows, Eskander et al found that only 11% participated in a palliative care rotation, 46% reported never being observed discussing transition of care from curative to palliative, and 56% never received feedback about technique regarding discussions on end-of-life care (123). Of note, fellows who reported higher quality palliative care education were significantly more likely to feel prepared to care for patients at the end of life, and mean ranking of preparedness increased with number of times that a fellow reported discussing changes in goals of care and the number of times the fellow received feedback from an attending physician. A similar survey study from Lefkowits et al (124) noted that 100% of gynecologic oncology fellowship programs had didactic coverage of palliative topics and 48% had an available palliative care rotation. There was, however, no correlation between the topics that were formally taught and the topics that were considered by the faculty to be the most important. There is clearly room for improving the palliative care curriculum and exposure in gynecologic oncology fellowships. Indeed, the 2020 Accreditation Council for Graduate Medical Education (ACGME) Program Requirements for Graduate Medical Education in Gynecologic Oncology list knowledge in hospice and palliative care medicine as a core competency.

Partnering With Specialty Palliative Care

One study of women with advanced breast or gynecologic cancer who were discontinuing chemotherapy found that patients who had seen palliative care before the decision to discontinue chemotherapy (compared with those who were referred to palliative care only after the decision to discontinue chemotherapy) had better QoL, better emotional and social functioning, less depression, less insomnia, and fewer issues with communication. The patients with earlier palliative care integration also received less chemotherapy within the last 6 weeks of life, and earlier palliative care was an independent predictor of improved OS (125). Another study of patients who had died of gynecologic cancer found that 49% had been referred to palliative care, but only 18% had been referred more than 30 days before their death (108). Among a group of patients with gynecologic cancer meeting ASCO recommendations for early palliative care integration, only 53% were referred to palliative care (126). These data, taken together with the robust data in the general oncology literature demonstrating benefits of early specialty palliative care integration (127), suggest that we are likely underutilizing specialty palliative care in women with gynecologic cancer. A CEA using clinical benefit data from the Temel et al trial in lung cancer (8) found routine palliative care referral to be at least cost-effective, possibly even cost saving, for patients with platinum-resistant ovarian cancer (128). Gynecologic oncology providers should familiarize themselves with the specialty palliative care resources available at their institutions and utilize them liberally, including early in the disease course for patients with advanced disease or high symptom burden. Palliative care enhances both the quality and value of gynecologic cancer care.

CONCLUSION

Palliative care is specialized medical care aimed at improving QoL for people living with serious illness. For patients with gynecologic cancers, it involves meticulous evaluation and treatment of the symptoms of disease burden and the side effects of cancer therapy, frank and compassionate discussions with patients and caregivers about the disease and its prognosis, and clarification of patients' goals and expectations. It involves optimizing not just quantity but also QoL. As providers of both surgical and medical oncology throughout the disease course, gynecologic oncologists have unique longitudinal relationships with their patients and are thus well positioned to provide basic palliative care. The training of gynecologic oncologists must prepare them for that role. With mounting evidence on the clinical and health systems benefits of specialty palliative care, those services are becoming more and more ubiquitous and should be liberally utilized as "an extra layer of support" for patients with complex needs related to symptom management or navigating goals of care. Gynecologic oncology providers must join the WHO, the NAM, ASCO, and SGO in recognizing that palliative care is an integral component of high-quality, comprehensive, and individualized care for our patients.

REFERENCES

1. Bakitas M, Lyons KD, Hegel MT, et al. Effects of a palliative care intervention on clinical outcomes in patients with advanced cancer: the Project ENABLE II randomized controlled trial. *JAMA*. 2009;302(7):741-749.

2. Bakitas MA, Tosteson TD, Li Z, et al. Early versus delayed initiation of concurrent palliative oncology care: patient outcomes in the ENABLE III randomized controlled trial. *J Clin Oncol*. 2015;33(13):1438-1445.

3. Brumley R, Enguidanos S, Jamison P, et al. Increased satisfaction with care and lower costs: results of a randomized trial of in-home palliative care. *J Am Geriatr Soc*. 2007;55(7):993-1000.

4. Gade G, Venohr I, Conner D, et al. Impact of an inpatient palliative care team: a randomized control trial. *J Palliat Med*. 2008;11(2):180-190.

5. Meyers FJ, Carducci M, Loscalzo MJ, Linder J, Greasby T, Beckett LA. Effects of a problem-solving intervention (COPE) on quality of life for patients with advanced cancer on clinical trials and their caregivers: simultaneous care educational intervention (SCEI): linking palliation and clinical trials. *J Palliat Med*. 2011;14(4):465-473.

6. Pantilat SZ, O'Riordan DL, Dibble SL, Landefeld CS. Hospital-based palliative medicine consultation: a randomized controlled trial. *Arch Intern Med*. 2010;170(22):2038-2040.

7. Rabow MW, Dibble SL, Pantilat SZ, McPhee SJ. The comprehensive care team: a controlled trial of outpatient palliative medicine consultation. *Arch Intern Med*. 2004;164(1):83-91.

8. Temel JS, Greer JA, Muzikansky A, et al. Early palliative care for patients with metastatic non-small-cell lung cancer. *N Engl J Med*. 2010;363(8):733-742.

9. Smith TJ, Temin S, Alesi ER, et al. American Society of Clinical Oncology provisional clinical opinion: the integration of palliative care into standard oncology care. *J Clin Oncol*. 2012;30(8):880-887.

10. Ferrell BR, Temel JS, Temin S, et al. Integration of palliative care into standard oncology care: American Society of Clinical Oncology clinical practice guideline update. *J Clin Oncol*. 2017;35:96-112.

11. Rimel BJ, Burke WM, Higgins RV, Lee PS, Lutman CV, Parker L. Improving quality and decreasing cost in gynecologic oncology care. Society of Gynecologic Oncology recommendations for clinical practice. *Gynecol Oncol*. 2015;137(2):280-284.

12. Choosing Wisely: an initiative of the American Board of Internal Medicine Foundation 2021. Accessed January 27, 2022.http://www.choosingwisely.org/

13. Parikh RB, Temel JS. Early specialty palliative care. *N Engl J Med*. 2014;370(11):1075-1076.

14. Hui D, Elsayem A, De la Cruz M, et al. Availability and integration of palliative care at US cancer centers. *JAMA*. 2010;303(11):1054-1061.

15. Rabow M, Kvale E, Barbour L, et al. Moving upstream: a review of the evidence of the impact of outpatient palliative care. *J Palliat Med*. 2013;16(12):1540-1549.

16. Hui D, De La Rosa A, Bruera E. State of integration of palliative care at National Cancer Institute-designated and nondesignated cancer centers. *JAMA Oncol*. 2020;6(8):1292-1295.

17. Quill TE, Abernethy AP. Generalist plus specialist palliative care—creating a more sustainable model. *N Engl J Med*. 2013;368(13):1173-1175.

18. Kumar P, Wright AA, Hatfield LA, Temel JS, Keating NL. Family perspectives on hospice care experiences of patients with cancer. *J Clin Oncol*. 2017;35(4):432-439.

19. National Hospice and Palliative Care Organization. NHPCO releases facts and figures 2020 edition. Accessed January 20, 2022. https://www .nhpco.org/hospice-facts-figures/

20. Chiang JK, Kao YH, Lai NS. The impact of hospice care on survival and healthcare costs for patients with lung cancer: a national longitudinal population-based study in Taiwan. *PLoS One.* 2015;10(9):e0138773.

21. Huo J, Lairson DR, Du XL, Chan W, Buchholz TA, Guadagnolo BA. Survival and cost-effectiveness of hospice care for metastatic melanoma patients. *Am J Manag Care.* 2014;20(5):366-373.

22. Connor SR, Pyenson B, Fitch K, Spence C, Iwasaki K. Comparing hospice and nonhospice patient survival among patients who die within a three-year window. *J Pain Symptom Manage.* 2007;33(3):238-246.

23. Wright AA, Keating NL, Balboni TA, Matulonis UA, Block SD, Prigerson HG. Place of death: correlations with quality of life of patients with cancer and predictors of bereaved caregivers' mental health. *J Clin Oncol.* 2010;28(29):4457-4464.

24. Teno JM, Clarridge BR, Casey V, et al. Family perspectives on end-of-life care at the last place of care. *JAMA.* 2004;291(1):88-93.

25. Keyser EA, Reed BG, Lowery WJ, et al. Hospice enrollment for terminally ill patients with gynecologic malignancies: impact on outcomes and interventions. *Gynecol Oncol.* 2010;118(3):274-277.

26. Lefkowits C, Teuteberg W, Courtney-Brooks M, Sukumvanich P, Ruskin R, Kelley JL. Improvement in symptom burden within one day after palliative care consultation in a cohort of gynecologic oncology inpatients. *Gynecol Oncol.* 2015;136(3):424-428.

27. Lefkowits C, Rabow MW, Sherman AE, et al. Predictors of high symptom burden in gynecologic oncology outpatients: who should be referred to outpatient palliative care? *Gynecol Oncol.* 2014;132(3):698-702.

28. Grover S, Hill-Kayser CE, Vachani C, Hampshire MK, DiLullo GA, Metz JM. Patient reported late effects of gynecological cancer treatment. *Gynecol Oncol.* 2012;124(3):399-403.

29. Snyder CF, Aaronson NK. Use of patient-reported outcomes in clinical practice. *Lancet.* 2009;374(9687):369-370.

30. Stephenson J, Davies A. An assessment of aetiology-based guidelines for the management of nausea and vomiting in patients with advanced cancer. *Support Care Cancer.* 2006;14(4):348-353.

31. Gupta M, Davis M, LeGrand S, Walsh D, Lagman R. Nausea and vomiting in advanced cancer: the Cleveland Clinic protocol. *J Support Oncol.* 2013;11(1):8-13.

32. Naeim A, Dy SM, Lorenz KA, Sanati H, Walling A, Asch SM. Evidence-based recommendations for cancer nausea and vomiting. *J Clin Oncol.* 2008;26(23):3903-3910.

33. dos Santos LV, Souza FH, Brunetto AT, Sasse AD, da Silveira Nogueira Lima JP. Neurokinin-1 receptor antagonists for chemotherapy-induced nausea and vomiting: a systematic review. *J Natl Cancer Inst.* 2012;104(17):1280-1292.

34. Sutherland A, Naessens K, Plugge E, et al. Olanzapine for the prevention and treatment of cancer-related nausea and vomiting in adults. *Cochrane Database Syst Rev.* 2018;9:CD012555.

35. Hesketh PJ, Kris MG, Basch E, et al. Antiemetics: ASCO guideline update. *J Clin Oncol.* 2020;38(24):2782-2897.

36. Aapro MS, Molassiotis A, Olver I. Anticipatory nausea and vomiting. *Support Care Cancer.* 2005;13(2):117-121.

37. Davis MP, Hallerberg G, Palliative Medicine Study Group of the Multinational Association of Supportive Care in Cancer. A systematic review of the treatment of nausea and/or vomiting in cancer unrelated to chemotherapy or radiation. *J Pain Symptom Manag.* 2010;39(4):756-767.

38. Smith EM, Jayson GC. The current and future management of malignant ascites. *Clin Oncol.* 2003;15(2):59-72.

39. Morgan PA, Franks PJ, Moffatt CJ. Health-related quality of life with lymphoedema: a review of the literature. *Int Wound J.* 2005;2:47-62.

40. Beesley V, Janda M, Eakin E, Obermair A, Battistutta D. Lymphedema after gynecological cancer treatment: prevalence, correlates, and supportive care needs. *Cancer.* 2007;109(12):2607-2614.

41. Harter P, Sehouli J, Lorusso D, et al. A randomized trial of lymphadenectomy in patients with advanced ovarian neoplasms. *N Engl J Med.* 2019;380:822-832.

42. Rossi EC, Kowalski LD, Scalici J, et al. A comparison of sentinel lymph node biopsy to lymphadenectomy for endometrial cancer staging (FIRES trial): a multicentre, prospective, cohort study. *Lancet Oncol.* 2017;18:384-392.

43. Te Grootenhuis NC, Van der Zee AG, Van Doorn HC, et al. Sentinel nodes in vulvar cancer: long-term follow-up of the GROningen INternational Study on Sentinel nodes in Vulvar cancer (GROINSS-V) I. *Gynecol Oncol.* 2016;140(1):8-14.

44. Zhang S. Chemotherapy-induced peripheral neuropathy and rehabilitation: a review. *Semin Oncol.* 2021;48(3):193-207.

45. Smith EM, Pang H, Cirrincione C, et al. Effect of duloxetine on pain, function, and quality of life among patients with chemotherapy-induced painful peripheral neuropathy: a randomized clinical trial. *JAMA.* 2013;309(13):1359-1367.

46. Engle AL, Winans ARM. Rethinking docusate's role in opioid-induced constipation: a critical analysis of the evidence. *J Pain Palliat Care Pharmacother.* 2021;35(1):63-72.

47. Thomas J, Karver S, Cooney GA, et al. Methylnaltrexone for opioid-induced constipation in advanced illness. *N Engl J Med.* 2008;358(22):2332-2343.

48. Lawrence DP, Kupelnick B, Miller K, Devine D, Lau J. Evidence report on the occurrence, assessment, and treatment of fatigue in cancer patients. *J Natl Cancer Inst Monogr.* 2004;32(32):40-50.

49. Bower JE. Cancer-related fatigue-mechanisms, risk factors, and treatments. *Nat Rev Clin Oncol.* 2014;11(10):597-609.

50. Bower JE, Ganz PA, Desmond KA, et al. Fatigue in long-term breast carcinoma survivors: a longitudinal investigation. *Cancer.* 2006;106(4):751-758.

51. Servaes P, Gielissen MF, Verhagen S, Bleijenberg G. The course of severe fatigue in disease-free breast cancer patients: a longitudinal study. *Psychooncology.* 2007;16(9):787-795.

52. Wang XS, Woodruff JF. Cancer-related and treatment-related fatigue. *Gynecol Oncol.* 2015;136(3):446-452.

53. Price MA, Bell ML, Sommeijer DW, et al. Physical symptoms, coping styles and quality of life in recurrent ovarian cancer: a prospective population-based study over the last year of life. *Gynecol Oncol.* 2013;130(1):162-168.

54. Kim YJ, Munsell MF, Park JC, et al. Retrospective review of symptoms and palliative care interventions in women with advanced cervical cancer. *Gynecol Oncol.* 2015;139(3):553-558.

55. Mucke M, Mochamat, Cuhls H, et al. Pharmacological treatments for fatigue associated with palliative care. *Cochrane Database Syst Rev.* 2015;2015(5):CD006788.

56. Meneses-Echavez JF, Gonzalez-Jimenez E, Ramirez-Velez R. Effects of supervised multimodal exercise interventions on cancer-related fatigue: systematic review and meta-analysis of randomized controlled trials. *BioMed Res Int.* 2015;2015:328636.

57. Hope JM, Pothuri B. The role of palliative surgery in gynecologic cancer cases. *Oncologist.* 2013;18(1):73-79.

58. Poturi B, Vaidya A, Aghajanian C, Venkatraman E, Barakat RR, Chi DS. Palliative surgery for bowel obstruction in recurrent ovarian cancer: an updated series. *Gynecol Oncol.* 2003;89(2):306-313.

59. Caceres A, Zhou Q, Iasonos A, Gerdes H, Chi DS, Barakat RR. Colorectal stents for palliation of large-bowel obstructions in recurrent gynecologic cancer: an updated series. *Gynecol Oncol.* 2008;108(2):482-485.

60. Tucker RO, Nichols AC. *UNIPAC 4. Managing Nonpain Symptoms.* American Academy of Hospice & Palliative Medicine; 2012.

61. Addington-Hall J, McCarthy M. Dying from cancer: results of a national population-based investigation. *Palliat Med.* 1995;9:295-305.

62. Kako J, Morita T, Yamaguchi T, et al. Fan therapy is effective in relieving dyspnea in patients with terminally ill cancer: a parallel-arm, randomized controlled trial. *J Pain Symptom Manage.* 2018;56:493-500.

63. Ting FI, Estreller S, Strebel HMJ. The FAFA trial: a phase 2 randomized clinical trial on the effect of a fan blowing air on the face to relieve dyspnea in Filipino patients with terminal cancer. *Asian J Oncol.* 2020;6:3-9.

64. Hui D, Bohlke K, Bao T, et al. Management of dyspnea in advanced cancer: ASCO guideline. *J Clin Oncol.* 2021;39(12):1389-1411.

65. Breitbart W, Alici Y. Evidence-based treatment of delirium in patients with cancer. *J Clin Oncol.* 2012;30(11):1206-1214.

66. Gagnon B, Low G, Schreier G. Methylphenidate hydrochloride improves cognitive function in patients with advanced cancer and hypoactive delirium: a prospective clinical study. *J Psychiatry Neurosci.* 2005;30(2):100-107.

67. Kim MS, Rhim HC, Park A, et al. Comparative efficacy and acceptability of pharmacological interventions for the treatment and prevention of delirium: a systematic review and network meta-analysis. *J Psychiatr Res.* 2020;125:164-176.

68. Fisch MJ, Zhao F, Manola J, Miller AH, Pirl WF, Wagner LI. Patterns and predictors of antidepressant use in ambulatory cancer patients with common solid tumors. *Psychooncology.* 2015;24(5):523-532.

69. Mitchell AJ. Are one or two simple questions sufficient to detect depression in cancer and palliative care? A Bayesian meta-analysis. *Br J Cancer.* 2008;98(12):1934-1943.

70. Gartlehner G, Hansen RA, Morgan LC, et al. Comparative benefits and harms of second-generation antidepressants for treating major depressive disorder: an updated meta-analysis. *Ann Intern Med.* 2011;155(11):772-785.

71. Moorey S, Cort E, Kapari M, et al. A cluster randomized controlled trial of cognitive behaviour therapy for common mental disorders in patients with advanced cancer. *Psychol Med.* 2009;39(5):713-723.

72. Speca M, Carlson LE, Goodey E, Angen M. A randomized, wait-list controlled clinical trial: the effect of a mindfulness meditation-based stress reduction program on mood and symptoms of stress in cancer outpatients. *Psychosom Med.* 2000;62(5):613-622.

73. Clegg A, Young JB. Which medications to avoid in people at risk of delirium: a systematic review. *Age Ageing.* 2011;40(1):23-29.

74. Goodman DC, Morden NE, Chang CH, et al. *Trends in Cancer Care Near the End of Life: A Dartmouth Atlas of Health Care Brief.* The Dartmouth Institute for Health Policy & Clinical Practice; 2013. Trends in Cancer Care Near the End of Life. https://www.ncbi.nlm.nih.gov/books/NBK586638/

75. Hui D, Dos Santos R, Chisholm G, Bansal S, Souza Crovador C, Bruera E. Bedside clinical signs associated with impending death in patients with advanced cancer: preliminary findings of a prospective, longitudinal cohort study. *Cancer.* 2015;121(6):960-967.

76. Spoozak L, Seow H, Liu Y, Wright J, Barbera L. Performance status and symptom scores of women with gynecologic cancer at the end of life. *Int J Gynecol Cancer.* 2013;23(5):971-978.

77. Martin EJ, Widera E. Prognostication in serious illness. *Med Clin North Am.* 2020;104(3):391-403.

78. Weeks JC, Catalano PJ, Cronin A, van der Wal G. Patients' expectations about effects of chemotherapy for advanced cancer. *N Engl J Med.* 2012;367(17):1616-1625.

79. The AM, Hak T, Koeter G, et al. Collusion in doctor-patient communication about imminent death: an ethnographic study. *West J Med.* 2001;174(4):247-253.

80. Jackson VA, Mack J, Matsuyama R, et al. A qualitative study of oncologists' approaches to end-of-life care. *J Palliat Med.* 2008;11(6):893-906.

81. Helft PR. Necessary collusion: prognostic communication with advanced cancer patients. *J Clin Oncol.* 2005;23(13):3146-3150.

82. Mack JW, Smith TJ. Reasons why physicians do not have discussions about poor prognosis, why it matters, and what can be improved. *J Clin Oncol.* 2012;30(22):2715-2717.

83. Zier LS, Sottile PD, Hong SY, Weissfield LA, White DB. Surrogate decision makers' interpretation of prognostic information: a mixed-methods study. *Ann Intern Med.* 2012;156(5):360-366.

84. Murray SA, Kendall M, Boyd K, Sheikh A. Illness trajectories and palliative care. *BMJ.* 2005;330(7498):1007-1011.

85. Lunney JR, Lynn J, Foley DJ, Lipson S, Guralnik JM. Patterns of functional decline at the end of life. *JAMA.* 2003;289(18):2387-2392.

86. Enzinger AC, Zhang B, Schrag D, Prigerson HG. Outcomes of prognostic disclosure: associations with prognostic understanding, distress, and relationship with physician among patients with advanced cancer. *J Clin Oncol.* 2015;33(32):3809-3816.

87. Diaz-Montes TP, Johnson MK, Giuntoli RL II, Brown AJ. Importance and timing of end-of-life care discussions among gynecologic oncology patients. *Am J Hosp Palliat Care.* 2013;30(1):59-67.

88. Epstein AS, Shuk E, O'Reilly EM, Gary KA, Volandes AE. 'We have to discuss it': cancer patients' advance care planning impressions following educational information about cardiopulmonary resuscitation. *Psychooncology.* 2015;24(12):1767-1773.

89. Ozanne EM, Partridge A, Moy B, Ellis KJ, Sepucha KR. Doctor-patient communication about advance directives in metastatic breast cancer. *J Palliat Med.* 2009;12(6):547-553.

90. Sharma RK, Dy SM. Documentation of information and care planning for patients with advanced cancer: associations with patient characteristics and utilization of hospital care. *Am J Hosp Palliat Care.* 2011;28(8):543-549.

91. El-Sahwi KS, Illuzzi J, Varughese J, et al. A survey of gynecologic oncologists regarding the end-of-life discussion: a pilot study. *Gynecol Oncol.* 2012;124(3):471-473.

92. Clark MA, Ott M, Rogers ML, et al. Advance care planning as a shared endeavor: completion of ACP documents in a multidisciplinary cancer program. *Psychooncology.* 2017;26(1):67-73.

93. Johnson S, Butow P, Kerridge I, Tattersall M. Advance care planning for cancer patients: a systematic review of perceptions and experiences of patients, families, and healthcare providers. *Psychooncology.* 2016;25(4):362-386.

94. Reisfield GM, Wallace SK, Munsell MF, Webb FJ, Alvarez ER, Wilson GR. Survival in cancer patients undergoing in-hospital cardiopulmonary resuscitation: a meta-analysis. *Resuscitation.* 2006;71(2):152-160.

95. Volandes AE, Levin TT, Slovin S, et al. Augmenting advance care planning in poor prognosis cancer with a video decision aid: a preintervention-postintervention study. *Cancer.* 2012;118(17):4331-4338.

96. Volandes AE, Paasche-Orlow MK, Mitchell SL, et al. Randomized controlled trial of a video decision support tool for cardiopulmonary resuscitation decision making in advanced cancer. *J Clin Oncol.* 2013;31(3):380-386.

97. Pollak KI, Arnold RM, Jeffreys AS, et al. Oncologist communication about emotion during visits with patients with advanced cancer. *J Clin Oncol.* 2007;25(36):5748-5752.

98. Tulsky JA, Arnold RM, Alexander SC, et al. Enhancing communication between oncologists and patients with a computer-based training program: a randomized trial. *Ann Intern Med.* 2011;155(9):593-601.

99. Littell RD, Kumar A, Einstein MH, Karam A, Bevis K. Advanced communication: a critical component of high quality gynecologic cancer care: a Society of Gynecologic Oncology evidence based review and guide. *Gynecol Oncol.* 2019;155(1):161-169.

100. Zakhour M, LaBrant L, Rimel BJ, et al. Too much, too late: aggressive measures and the timing of end of life care discussions in women with gynecologic malignancies. *Gynecol Oncol.* 2015;138(2):383-387.

101. Le T, Leis A, Pahwa P, Wright K, Ali K, Reeder B. Quality-of-life issues in patients with ovarian cancer and their caregivers: a review. *Obstet Gynecol Surv.* 2003;58(11):749-758.

102. Butow PN, Price MA, Bell ML, et al. Caring for women with ovarian cancer in the last year of life: a longitudinal study of caregiver quality of life, distress and unmet needs. *Gynecol Oncol.* 2014;132(3):690-697.

103. Beesley VL, Price MA, Webb PM, Australian Ovarian Cancer Study Group; Australian Ovarian Cancer Study—Quality of Life Study Investigators. Loss of lifestyle: health behaviour and weight changes after becoming a caregiver of a family member diagnosed with ovarian cancer. *Support Care Cancer.* 2011;19(12):1949-1956.

104. Pitceathly C, Maguire P. The psychological impact of cancer on patients' partners and other key relatives: a review. *Eur J Cancer.* 2003;39(11):1517-1524.

105. World Health Organization. WHOQOL measuring quality of life. Accessed January 30, 2022. https://www.who.int/tools/whoqol#:~:text=WHO%20defines%20Quality%20of%20Life,%2C%20expectations%2C%20standards%20and%20concerns

106. Cella DF, Tulsky DS, Gray G, et al. The functional assessment of cancer therapy scale: development and validation of the general measure. *J Clin Oncol.* 1993;11(3):570-579.

107. Earle CC, Park ER, Lai B, Weeks JC, Ayanian JZ, Block S. Identifying potential indicators of the quality of end-of-life cancer care from administrative data. *J Clin Oncol.* 2003;21(6):1133-1138.

108. Nevadunsky NS, Gordon S, Spoozak L, et al. The role and timing of palliative medicine consultation for women with gynecologic malignancies: association with end of life interventions and direct hospital costs. *Gynecol Oncol.* 2014;132(1):3-7.

109. Nevadunsky NS, Spoozak L, Gordon S, Rivera E, Harris K, Goldberg GL. End-of-life care of women with gynecologic malignancies: a pilot study. *Int J Gynecol Cancer.* 2013;23(3):546-552.

110. Ellis LM, Bernstein DS, Voest EE, et al. American Society of Clinical Oncology perspective: raising the bar for clinical trials by defining clinically meaningful outcomes. *J Clin Oncol.* 2014;32(12):1277-1280.

111. Minion LE, Coleman RL, Alvarez RD, Herzog TJ. Endpoints in clinical trials: what do patients consider important? A survey of the Ovarian Cancer National Alliance. *Gynecol Oncol.* 2016;140(2):193-198.

112. Havrilesky LJ, Alvarez Secord A, Ehrisman JA, et al. Patient preferences in advanced or recurrent ovarian cancer. *Cancer.* 2014;120(23):3651-3659.

113. Penson RT, Huang HQ, Wenzel LB, et al. Bevacizumab for advanced cervical cancer: patient-reported outcomes of a randomized, phase 3 trial (NRG Oncology-Gynecologic Oncology Group protocol 240). *Lancet Oncol.* 2015;16(3):301-311.

114. Armstrong DK, Bundy B, Wenzel L, et al. Intraperitoneal cisplatin and paclitaxel in ovarian cancer. *N Engl J Med.* 2006;354(1):34-43.

115. Wenzel L, Huang HQ, Monk BJ, Rose PG, Cella D. Quality-of-life comparisons in a randomized trial of interval secondary cytoreduction in advanced ovarian carcinoma: a Gynecologic Oncology Group Study. *J Clin Oncol.* 2005;23(24):5605-5612.

116. Mutch DG, Orlando M, Goss T, et al. Randomized phase III trial of gemcitabine compared with pegylated liposomal doxorubicin in patients with platinum-resistant ovarian cancer. *J Clin Oncol.* 2007;25(19):2811-2818.

117. Wenzel LB, Huang HQ, Armstrong DK, Walker JL, Cella D, Gynecologic Oncology Group. Health-related quality of life during and after intraperitoneal versus intravenous chemotherapy for optimally debulked ovarian cancer: a Gynecologic Oncology Group Study. *J Clin Oncol.* 2007;25(4):437-443.

118. Pujade-Lauraine E, Wagner U, Aavall-Lundqvist E, et al. Pegylated liposomal Doxorubicin and Carboplatin compared with Paclitaxel and Carboplatin for patients with platinum-sensitive ovarian cancer in late relapse. *J Clin Oncol.* 2010;28(20):3323-3329.

119. Dumanovsky T, Augustin R, Rogers M, Lettang K, Meier DE, Morrison RS. The growth of palliative care in U.S. hospitals: a status report. *J Palliat Med.* 2016;19(1):8-15.

120. Institute of Medicine. *Dying in America: Improving Quality and Honoring Individual Preferences Near the End of Life.* National Academies Press; 2014. Accessed January 24, 2022. https://doi.org/10.17226/18748

121. Partridge AH, Seah DS, King T, et al. Developing a service model that integrates palliative care throughout cancer care: the time is now. *J Clin Oncol.* 2014;32(29):3330-3336.

122. Fadul N, Elsayem A, Palmer JL, et al. Supportive versus palliative care: what's in a name?: A survey of medical oncologists and midlevel providers at a comprehensive cancer center. *Cancer.* 2009;115(9):2013-2021.

123. Eskander RN, Osann K, Dickson E, et al. Assessment of palliative care training in gynecologic oncology: a gynecologic oncology fellow research network study. *Gynecol Oncol.* 2014;134(2):379-384.

124. Lefkowits C, Sukumvanich P, Claxton R, et al. Needs assessment of palliative care education in gynecologic oncology fellowship: we're not teaching what we think is most important. *Gynecol Oncol.* 2014;135(2):255-260.

125. Rugno FC, Paiva BS, Paiva CE. Early integration of palliative care facilitates the discontinuation of anticancer treatment in women with advanced breast or gynecologic cancers. *Gynecol Oncol.* 2014;135(2):249-254.

126. Lefkowits C, Binstock AB, Courtney-Brooks M, et al. Predictors of palliative care consultation on an inpatient gynecologic oncology service: are we following ASCO recommendations? *Gynecol Oncol.* 2014;133(2):319-325.

127. Parikh RB, Kirch RA, Smith TJ, Temel JS. Early specialty palliative care-translating data in oncology into practice. *N Engl J Med.* 2013;369(24):2347-2351.

128. Lowery WJ, Lowery AW, Barnett JC, et al. Cost-effectiveness of early palliative care intervention in recurrent platinum-resistant ovarian cancer. *Gynecol Oncol.* 2013;130(3):426-430.

CHAPTER **12.7**

Hereditary Cancer Genetics

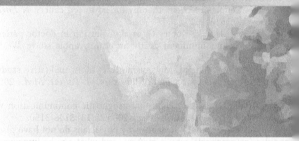

Catherine Watson and Andrea R. Hagemann

INTRODUCTION

The diagnosis of a hereditary cancer syndrome can have significant implications for both patients diagnosed with a gynecologic malignancy and their family members. The most common gynecologic hereditary cancer syndromes are caused by mutations in *MLH1, MSH2, MSH6, PMS2,* and *EPCAM* (collectively known as Lynch syndrome–associated mutations) and *BRCA1* and *BRCA2*. Li-Fraumeni, Cowden syndrome, and Peutz-Jeghers are also associated with specific gynecologic malignancies (**Table 12.7-1**). Women with a gynecologic-related hereditary cancer syndrome are at higher risk than the general population of developing associated malignancies. Furthermore, their relatives may also carry these mutations, and the identification of these carriers allows for risk-reducing action or closer surveillance. Lastly, the diagnosis of certain pathogenic alterations may have prognostic or therapeutic implications for patients with cancer, such as utilization of PARPi in both frontline and recurrent settings for BRCA-mutated ovarian cancer. This chapter discusses the most common gynecologic-related hereditary cancer syndromes and their associated cancer risks, as well as the recommended management of cancer mutation carriers (probands) with associated cancers, the importance of cascade testing, and risk reduction strategies for carriers.

BACKGROUND AND ASSOCIATED CANCER RISKS

Ovarian Cancer

Background

The concept of hereditary ovarian cancer was first introduced in 1886 by Pierre Paul Broca, who published a description of his wife's significant family history of both breast and ovarian cancer (1). Further research was sparse after this publication until the 1990s, when the American geneticist Mary Claire King and her team discovered *BRCA1*, a gene on chromosome 17 that could be linked to a significant portion of breast and ovarian cancers (2). This landmark moment was shortly followed by the identification of *BRCA2* on chromosome 13, as well as the commercial identification and cloning of these genes. These discoveries revolutionized the understanding of the contributions of genetics to ovarian cancer (3).

BRCA1 and *BRCA2* are tumor suppressor genes that aid in the repair of double-stranded DNA breaks via HR. Compared to alternate repair methods, such as nonhomologous end joining (NHEJ), HR is a relatively error-free mechanism and is of utmost importance to healthy cells. Alterations within *BRCA1* and *BRCA2* reduce the ability to repair DNA damage, causing genetic instability

■ TABLE 12.7-1. Hereditary Cancer Syndromes Associated With Gynecologic Malignancies

Syndrome	Genes	Breast Cancer	Ovarian Cancer	Endometrial Cancer	Colon Cancer	Other Types of Cancer
Hereditary breast and ovarian	BRCA1 BRCA2	X	X			Pancreatic, prostate, and melanoma
	RAD51C, RAD51D, PALB2	x	X			
	BRIP1		X			
Lynch	MLH1 MSH2 MSH6 PMS2 EPCAM		X	X	X	Gastric, ureteral, biliary, renal pelvic, glioblastoma
Li-Fraumeni	P53	X			X	Sarcomas, brain, adrenocortical
Cowden	PTEN	X		X	X	Benign mucocutaneous lesions, gastrointestinal hamartomas, thyroid
Peutz-Jeghers	STK11	X	X		X	Cervical adenoma malignum, gastrointestinal hamartomas, pancreatic, gastric, small bowel

and increased risk of malignancy (4). Individuals born with a germline BRCA1/2 mutation have only one working copy of the gene (with the defective copy having been inherited from either the maternal or paternal lineage). Thus, a "second hit" is required to inactive the gene fully and allow the phenotype (or cancer) to develop (5). Although most ovarian cancers are sporadic, approximately 15% to 20% of patients with epithelial ovarian cancer have a germline mutation in *BRCA1* or *BRCA2*. The lifetime risk of developing ovarian cancer in patients with a BRCA1 mutation is approximately 39% to 46%. In *BRCA2* mutation carriers, the lifetime risk of ovarian cancer is approximately 10% to 27% (6-8).

Mutations in *BRCA* genes can occur by single-nucleotide variations, small insertions or deletions, copy number variants, and large genomic rearrangements. Most mutations in *BRCA* genes stem from single-nucleotide variants or insertion/deletions, but large copy number variants are thought to encompass 4% to 28% of the mutations in BRCA1/2, more commonly in BRCA1 than BRCA2 (9,10]).

Epidemiology

In addition to having a higher risk of developing ovarian cancer, *BRCA1* mutation carriers are also at risk of developing cancer at an earlier age when compared to the general population. The mean age of ovarian cancer diagnosis is 51 years, with an overall increase in the annual risk starting at age 40. In *BRCA2* mutation carriers, the mean age of onset is 61 years, with annual risk increasing beginning at age 50 (8,11). In comparison, ovarian cancer in the general population is most frequently diagnosed between the ages of 55 and 64 years, with a median age of 63 years (8,11). The majority of *BRCA1/2*-associated ovarian cancers are serous, although endometrioid and clear cell cancers have also been associated with these mutations. However, on secondary pathology review of studies that have identified *BRCA1/2*-associated endometrioid and clear cell cancers, a significant proportion are ultimately reassigned as primarily serous histology (12,13).

BRCA1 and *BRCA2* mutations are associated with additional cancer risks aside from female breast and ovarian. *BRCA2* is a known risk factor for male breast cancer and prostate cancer, and both *BRCA1* and *BRCA2* mutations have been found to increase the risk of pancreatic and gastric cancer, although these associations may be stronger for *BRCA2* (14-18). Data regarding overall increased risk of endometrial cancer among *BRCA* carriers are conflicting, and in studies that do demonstrate an increased incidence of endometrial cancer, a majority of these cases

can be attributed to tamoxifen use (19,20). However, there is a higher-than-expected incidence of high-grade (serous) uterine carcinomas among *BRCA1* patients. In one study of 1,083 women who underwent risk-reducing salpingo-oophorectomy (RRSO) for a BRCA1 mutation, four patients with BRCA1 mutations developed a serous or serous-like endometrial cancer (observed-to-expected ratio of 22.2) (19). According to available data, *BRCA* mutations are not associated with a definitive increased risk of brain, colorectal, bladder, or kidney cancers (14). An increased risk of melanoma in patients with a *BRCA2* mutation has been described, but more data are needed to establish a clear association (21).

Importantly, recent improvements in genetic sequencing technology have allowed for the identification of numerous additional ovarian cancer susceptibility genes in the HR pathway (22,23). Those with the most significant association with ovarian cancer include *BRIP1, RAD51C, RAD51D,* and *PALB2*. Others, such as *ATM*, have minimal to no impact on the lifetime risk of ovarian cancer. Although the prevalence of these mutations is lower than those of *BRCA1* and *BRCA2*, approximately one in four women with epithelial ovarian cancer carries a pathogenic mutation in the HR pathway. It is important to recognize that guidelines regarding the management of moderate and low penetrance mutations are continuing to evolve not as well defined as those for *BRCA1* and *BRCA2* (24,25), but an active area of ongoing research. This issue is further discussed in the section regarding risk reduction for mutation carriers.

Endometrial Cancer and Hereditary Cancer Syndromes

Background

Lynch syndrome, or hereditary nonpolyposis colorectal cancer (HNPCC) syndrome, is the hereditary cancer syndrome most associated with endometrial cancer and accounts for approximately 5% of all endometrial cancer cases (26). Although the first family with Lynch syndrome was identified over a century ago by pathologist A.S. Warthin, his research was not expanded upon until the 1960s, when Henry Lynch reported on several families with abnormal frequency of endometrial carcinoma (27). Lynch syndrome is now recognized to be the result of possible mutations in several DNA mismatch repair genes, including *MLH1, MSH2, MSH6, PMS2,* and *EPCAM*, each of which has its own specific cancer risks (Table 12.7-2).

■ **TABLE 12.7-2. Risk of Endometrial, Ovarian, and Colorectal Cancers Associated With Specific Lynch Syndrome Genes**

Gene	Lifetime Risks Colorectal Cancer (%)	Lifetime Risk Endometrial Cancer (%)	Lifetime Risk Ovarian Cancer (%)
MLH1	46-61	34-54	4-20
MSH2/EPCAM	33-52	21-57	8-38
MSH6	10-44	16-49	<1-13
PMS2	8-20	13-26	1-3

Epidemiology

Based on the gene mutated, the lifetime risk for endometrial cancer ranges from approximately 15% in *PMS2* mutation carriers to 70% in *MSH2* and *MSH6* carriers (28-31). The risk of Lynch syndrome in a patient with endometrial cancer is approximately 2.3%, although this is higher (~9%) in women diagnosed with endometrial cancer at a younger age (28,32). Lynch syndrome is also associated with colon cancer—with lifetime-associated risks that also vary according to mutation—as well as cancers of the brain, urologic tract, small bowel, and stomach. The lifetime-associated risk of ovarian cancer in a patient with Lynch syndrome is approximately 5% to 10% (33). See **Table 12.7-2** for associated risks of endometrial, colon, and ovarian cancer for individual Lynch genes.

Most Lynch-associated endometrial cancers are of an endometrioid histology, although the syndrome is also linked to endometrial clear cell carcinomas, carcinosarcomas, and papillary serous carcinomas (34). Lynch-associated endometrial cancers commonly arise from the lower uterine segment. In one study by Westin et al, 30% of women with lower uterine segment tumors had Lynch syndrome (35), whereas lower uterine segment involvement is described in less than 5% of the general population. The histology of Lynch-associated ovarian cancer is also mixed and can present as serous, endometrioid, clear cell, and mucinous. These cancers tend to present at an early stage and younger age than epithelial ovarian cancers in the general population (36).

MANAGEMENT OF CANCER PROBANDS

Epithelial Ovarian Cancer

Genetic Risk Assessment

Up to 18% of epithelial ovarian cancers are secondary to germline *BRCA1/2* mutations, and a further 5% to 10% are secondary to other associated pathogenic mutations (37). Results of genetic testing may have profound implications for family members, who can choose to undergo closer surveillance or risk-reducing measures should they also be found to carry a mutation. Testing results can also impact patient treatment, as there now exist multiple FDA-approved therapeutic agents for *BRCA* mutations carriers. Given the high incidence of germline mutations in these patients, and the implications of a mutation for both patients and family, current national guidelines, including the 2014 SGO Clinical Practice Statement and the national consensus guidelines version 2.2022, recommend that all patients with ovarian, fallopian, or peritoneal cancer should be offered germline genetic testing (38).

The advent and commercialization of next-generation sequencing has encouraged the incorporation of multigene panel testing into clinical practice. Multiple companies offer clinical genetic testing, and there are a variety of panels provided by each company depending on the patient's diagnosis and the clinician's preference. While isolated *BRCA1* and *BRCA2* testing is still performed for patients with ovarian cancer, many clinicians

and genetic counselors perform expanded panel or broad panel testing. Approximately 5% to 10% of patients at risk for hereditary breast and ovarian cancer may have associated mutations other than *BRCA1* or *BRCA2* (22,23,39), and no cost difference between single syndrome testing and multigene panel testing has been identified (39). Identification of alterations in these genes could potentially lead to earlier detection of non–*BRCA*-related cancers, as well as better prevention strategies. Multigene panel testing does increase the risk of identification of variants of uncertain significance (VUS). However, in a study of preferences of a patient with ovarian cancer regarding genetic testing, patients preferred testing strategies that increased the chance of identification of both deleterious mutations and VUS results (40). Clinicians must also be aware that information about the age at which breast and ovarian cancer risk start to rise with the moderate and low penetrance genes is less well defined, thus complicating clinical guidelines and practice (25).

Barriers to Testing

Despite the formal recommendation for universal germline testing in patients with epithelial ovarian cancer, the incidence of testing remains low. Large population-based studies have repeatedly demonstrated that only 10% to 30% of patients undergoing germline genetic testing (41,42). Reasons for this are manifold and include lack of provider and patient education, lack of access to formal genetic consultation, lack of infrastructure or tracking mechanisms, or lack of appropriate reimbursement (43). Alternative strategies for pretesting education and testing, such as telehealth counseling, group counseling, and point-of-care testing, have been explored in quality improvement projects and are being implemented in clinical practice. Further investigation of patient-reported outcomes regarding these processes is needed (44).

Implications of a Germline Ovarian Cancer Predisposition Gene Mutation in a Patient With Ovarian Cancer

Prognostic Implications

A diagnosis of a *BRCA1* or *BRCA2* mutation has prognostic implications for patients with ovarian cancer. Rubin et al first analyzed survival outcomes in patients with hereditary breast and ovarian cancer in 1996, demonstrating that *BRCA1* patients with advanced-stage ovarian cancer had a median survival of 77 versus 29 months for those with wild-type mutation (12), and these results have since been replicated in multiple studies (45,46). Results from a pooled analysis of 26 observational studies showed that the OS for nonmutation carriers was 36%, versus 44% for *BRCA1* mutation carriers and 52% for *BRCA2* mutation carriers (47). These outcomes persist even after adjusting for multiple variables, including stage, grade, histology, and age at cancer diagnosis. This survival difference may be due, in part, to an increased platinum sensitivity in patients with *BRCA* mutations, secondary to the HR-deficient (HRD) tumor's impaired ability to repair platinum-induced damage.

Therapeutic Implications

Over the past decade, several PARPi have been developed for therapeutic use in ovarian cancer, with particular benefit being demonstrated in patients with BRCA1/2 mutations. PARP is an enzyme involved in single-strand DNA repair. Defects in this enzymatic mechanism ultimately lead to single-strand breaks, which, in turn, lead to double-strand DNA breaks. In an HRD cell, such as a BRCA-mutated cell, the double-strand break (DSB) cannot be repaired and cell death ensues (4). Multiple clinical trials have proved the efficacy of PARPi in improving PFS in patients with *BRCA1* and *BRCA2* mutations and a diagnosis of ovarian cancer (48-50).

Given these therapeutic implications, somatic testing, or targeted genetic sequencing of tumor tissue, is now also routinely performed for patients with high-grade epithelial ovarian who do not carry a germline mutation pathogenic *BRCA1/2* variant. Furthermore, HRD testing, or genomic instability testing, is now offered by multiple laboratories. Patients with tumors that are HRD or demonstrate genomic instability have been shown to also demonstrate a favorable response to PARPi maintenance therapy (48). It should be noted that different laboratories use different evaluations and thresholds to determine this factor and that an HRD biomarker that is highly predictive of response to PARPi therapy has yet to be developed.

Guidance for Testing Strategies in Patients With Ovarian Cancer

With increasing testing options for germline and somatic testing, the exact testing order and practice patterns for a new ovarian cancer diagnosis may vary across practices. Because germline DNA sequencing is the most sensitive approach, the ASCO Expert Panel guidelines recommend germline testing for all individuals with ovarian cancer at the time of initial diagnosis (51). Mostly due to increased sensitivity with germline testing of recognizing large gene rearrangements within BRCA1/2, somatic testing alone can miss up to 5% of germline mutations (52,53). If germline testing is negative, somatic testing with DNA from tumor tissue should be done, as this may reveal an additional 5% to 7% actionable HRD mutations.

Endometrial Cancer and Lynch Syndrome

Genetic Risk Assessment

Several family history–based sets of criteria exist to evaluate a patient's risk for Lynch syndrome. The Amsterdam II criteria, which include all associated Lynch syndrome malignancies, require the 3-2-1 rule: There must be three relatives on the same side of the family with Lynch-associated cancers, spanning two generations, with at least one malignancy diagnosed before the age of 50. These guidelines have a sensitivity of 22% and specificity of 98% (52,53). The Bethesda Guidelines were created to help determine whether a patient with colorectal cancer should undergo tumor MSI testing. These were modified in subsequent years to better reflect risk for a patient with an endometrial, rather than a colorectal, sentinel cancer. The revised Bethesda Guidelines have a sensitivity and specificity of approximately 82% and 77%, respectively, for diagnosing Lynch syndrome (54,55).

Both sets of guidelines have largely been replaced by reflex tumor testing, and national consensus guidelines now recommends tumor-based testing in all patients with a diagnosis of endometrial cancer (51). IHC testing involves staining of the tumor tissue for *MLH1, MSH2, MSH6,* and *PMS2*. A positive result is one in which expression for one or more of these proteins is absent. MSI testing utilizes PCR to amplify sequences of DNA to quantitate levels of MSI. The timing and use of MSI testing versus IHC testing is a subject for debate. In one cost-effectiveness study, researchers compared universal germline sequencing, IHC testing alone for initial triage, and combination IHC/MSI testing. IHC/MSI and germline testing were less cost-effective than IHC alone; the authors concluded that if the cost of germline testing dropped below $500, this strategy would then be more cost-effective than IHC (56).

For those patients with microsatellite unstable tumors or an *MSH2* or *MSH6* absence of expression on IHC testing, a referral for formal genetics consultation and subsequent germline testing is recommended. Loss of expression of MSH2 may be due to either a pathogenic mutation of *MSH2* or an *EPCAM* mutation. For those with absence of *PMS2* or *MLH1*, promoter methylation testing is first recommended. If the *MLH1* promoter is methylated, it is unlikely that an associated genetic susceptibility mutation exists. If there is no methylation, the patient should undergo germline testing. If somatic testing is not indicative of Lynch syndrome, a referral for genetics consultation and consideration of panel germline

testing should still be made if the individual has an endometrial cancer diagnosis at an age younger than 50, or if they have personal or family history concerning for Lynch syndrome.

Kahn et al reviewed 29 published manuscripts that identified a total of 6,649 patients with endometrial cancer who underwent universal tumor testing for Lynch syndrome via either IHC or MSI testing. Of those who underwent IHC testing, 28% were abnormal, but only 15% of these had Lynch syndrome. Of those who underwent MSI testing, 31% were abnormal, but only 19% had Lynch syndrome. Thus, patients with abnormal tumor testing should be counseled that, although germline testing is indicated, there is a high likelihood they may not have Lynch syndrome (57).

Panel germline testing for all endometrial cancers is an emerging option, and upcoming national consensus guidelines will include the option for germline or somatic panel testing for all high-grade endometrial cancer. In a prospective study of 961 patients with endometrial cancer, 10% had potentially actionable germline variants (58). Again, insurance coverage and access to testing must remain at the forefront of discussion as these testing options expand.

Therapeutic Implications

The identification of Lynch syndrome in a patient can allow for surveillance or prophylactic measures for a second cancer in a patient or for cancers in family members. Importantly, patients with MSI-high endometrial cancers are also eligible for immune checkpoint therapies. Keynote-158 was a phase 2 trial of patients with MSI-high recurrent solid tumors treated with pembrolizumab. A total of 90 patients with endometrial cancer had data available by 2020; of these, the objective response rate was 48%, with a median PFS of 13.1 months (59).

OTHER HEREDITARY SYNDROMES ASSOCIATED WITH A GYNECOLOGIC MALIGNANCY

Li-Fraumeni

Li-Fraumeni syndrome is a cancer syndrome caused by TP53 germline mutations. It is a high penetrance syndrome most commonly associated with sarcomas, breast cancers, leukemias, and adrenocortical cancers. However, although increased risk of ovarian cancer has been observed in Li-Fraumeni families, the exact pathogenesis of this relationship has yet to be delineated, and there are no current screening guidelines for any gynecologic malignancy in women with Li-Fraumeni syndrome (60).

Cowden

Cowden syndrome is caused by mutations in PTEN and is most commonly associated with thyroid, breast, colorectal, and endometrial cancer, as well as benign GI hamartomas. The risk of endometrial cancer in women with Cowden syndrome is approximately 12% to 28% (61,62). There are no current guidelines for screening strategies to detect endometrial cancer in this population, although observation for abnormal bleeding with endometrial biopsy if indicated is recommended. Annual endometrial biopsy and/or ultrasound starting between the ages of 30 and 35 years could also be considered, although there is no prospective evidence proving the benefit of this strategy. Counseling on awareness of regularity of menstrual cycles in premenopausal patients is perhaps the best preventive strategy until risk-reducing surgery is considered.

Peutz-Jeghers

Peutz-Jeghers syndrome is an autosomal dominant syndrome caused by germline mutations in STK11. The most common malignancies in patients with Peutz-Jeghers are GI, but it is also commonly associated with breast cancers. There is evidence of association between this syndrome and both sex cord stromal tumors with annular tubules (SCTATs) of the ovary and adenoma malignum of the cervix (63). The majority of SCTAT are benign. However, adenoma malignum of the cervix can be aggressive, and routine Pap testing is recommended in these patients, although guidelines do not recommend imaging surveillance (64).

IDENTIFICATION AND MANAGEMENT OF HIGH-RISK MUTATION CARRIERS

Population Screening, Cascade Testing, and Traceback Testing

Multiple strategies have been proposed to identify patients for germline genetic testing. Patients can be identified based on a detailed multigenerational family history. This strategy requires clinicians or genetic counselors to take and update family histories, to recognize when a patient requires referral for testing, and for such testing to be completed. Even then, the generation of a detailed pedigree is not very sensitive or specific. **Population-based genetic testing** for high penetrance breast and ovarian cancer susceptibility genes, regardless of family history, has also been proposed (65). Such a strategy has become increasingly realistic with the decreasing cost and increasing availability of genetic testing, and as commercial genetic tests increase accessibility. Drawbacks to this population-based method include the potential lack of access to appropriate genetic counseling and counseling on follow-up or risk-reducing strategies.

Cascade genetic testing refers to testing the enriched population of family members of a patient with cancer (proband) who has been found to carry a pathogenic variant in a clinically relevant cancer susceptibility gene. Cascade genetic testing in first-degree family members carries a 50% probability of detecting the same pathogenic mutation. A related testing model is **traceback testing**, where genetic testing is performed on pathology or tumor registry specimens from deceased patients with cancer (66). This genetic testing information is then provided to the family. Traceback models of genetic testing are an active area of research but can introduce ethical dilemmas. For the oncologist who treats ovarian or endometrial cancer, increases in germline and somatic testing of patients affected with cancer will identify more opportunities for cascade testing, and incorporating this into busy clinical oncology practices can be difficult. A recent article published in the *Journal of Clinical Oncology* demonstrated the feasibility of a cascade testing model. Using a multiple linear regression model, they determined that all carriers of pathogenic mutations in 18 clinically relevant cancer susceptibility genes in the United States could be identified in 9.9 years if there was a 70% cascade testing rate of first-, second- and third-degree relatives, compared to 59.5 years with no cascade testing (67). Cascade genetic testing would ideally be performed on entire families. While actual practice is currently far from ideal, awareness of barriers to cascade testing at the patient, provider, and system levels may help drive the rates of cascade testing and cancer prevention.

Cascade Testing Barriers and Facilitators

Family Factors

Because of privacy laws, the responsibility of disclosure of genetic testing results to family members falls primarily to the patient in whom a mutation has been identified, or **proband**. Proband education is critical to ensure disclosure among family members. Family dynamics and geographic distribution of family members can further complicate disclosure. Following disclosure, family member gender, education level, demographics and personal views, attitudes, and emotions affect whether a family member decides to undergo testing (68). Furthermore, insurance status and access to specialty-specific care for the proband's family members may influence cascade genetic testing rates.

Provider Factors

Provider factors that affect cascade genetic testing include awareness of testing guidelines, interpretation of genetic testing results, and education and knowledge of specific mutations. For example, providers must recognize that cascade testing is not appropriate for VUS. This can lead to unnecessary surveillance testing and prophylactic surgeries. Providers, however, must continue to follow patients and periodically update testing results as variants may be reclassified over time. In addition, providers must be knowledgeable about the complex and nuanced nature of the screening guidelines for each mutation. National consensus guidelines provide detailed recommendations by mutation. Patients may benefit from care with cancer specialists who are aware of the guidelines, particularly for moderate penetrance genes like *BRIP1* and *PALB2*, as discussions about the timing of risk-reducing surgery are more nuanced in this population. Finally, which providers are responsible for initiating cascade testing may be unclear; oncologists and genetic counselors not primarily treating probands' relatives may assume the proper information has been passed along to family members without a practical means to follow up, and primary care providers may assume it is being taken care of by the oncology provider.

Environmental or System Factors

Accessibility of genetic counseling and testing is a common barrier to cascade testing. Family members may be geographically remote, and connecting them to counseling and testing can be challenging. Working with local genetic counselors can facilitate this process. Insurance coverage of testing is a common perceived barrier; however, many testing companies now provide cascade testing free of charge if within a certain window following the initial test. Despite this, patients often cite cost as a barrier to undergoing testing. Concerns about insurance coverage are common after a positive result. The Genetic Information Nondiscrimination Act (GINA) of 2008 prohibits discrimination against employees or insurance applicants because of genetic information. Life insurance or long-term care policies, however, can incorporate genetic testing information into policy rates, so patients should be counseled to consider purchasing life insurance before undergoing genetic testing. This is especially important if the person considering testing has not yet been diagnosed with cancer.

Implications of a Positive Result

Family members who receive a positive test result should be referred for genetic counseling and to the appropriate specialists for evidence-based screening and discussion for risk-reducing surgery. For all mutation carriers, cancer worry and recommendation for risk-reducing surgical procedures should be appropriately balanced with risk of harm. Some important considerations include menopausal status, future fertility desires, QoL concerns regarding surgical healing time and potential for sexual dysfunction, previous history of breast cancer that may limit hormone replacement options, age-related risk for other cancers within the specific syndrome that may shift priorities, and comorbidities and prior surgical history that may increase surgical risk. The patient's personal experience with a different mutation-related cancer (such as breast cancer in a *BRCA1* carrier) or their experience of watching a close family member with ovarian, breast, or endometrial cancer may greatly influence their decision-making. For gynecologic oncologists used to treating advanced cancers where patients often readily accept temporary or permanent decreases in QoL, it is important to acknowledge that counseling on risks of harm and alternatives to surgery may require a more nuanced and time-consuming approach when cancer is not yet present and statistically may not ever occur.

BRCA1 and BRCA2 Risk Reduction

Risk reduction options for unaffected patients with pathogenic mutations in *BRCA1* and *BRCA2* are reviewed in **Table 12.7-3**. Owing to the lack of evidence for improved survival, guidelines have

■ TABLE 12.7-3. Risk Reduction Recommendations for BRCA1 and BRCA2 Mutation Carriers

Breast
- Annual breast MRI age 25-29 yr
- Annual mammography and annual breast MRI age 30-75 yr
- Breast screening based on individual after 75 yr
- RRSO to reduce breast cancer risk between ages 35 and 40 or upon completion of childbearing
- Consider chemoprevention with tamoxifen, raloxifene, or aromatase inhibitor
- Consider risk-reducing mastectomy

Ovary
- RRSO (ages 35-40 for BRCA1; ages 40-45 for BRCA2) and upon completion of childbearing
- Consider chemoprevention with oral contraceptives

MRI, magnetic resonance imaging; RRSO, Risk-reducing salpingo-oophorectomy.

decreased their encouragement or reliance on screening with imaging or bloodwork. Compared to breast cancer screening, where alternating MRI and mammogram have been shown to be very sensitive and specific for the identification of early cancers, there is still no effective screening test for ovarian cancer. Transvaginal ultrasound for ovarian cancer screening has not been shown to be sufficiently sensitive or specific to support a routine recommendation but may be considered at the clinician's discretion. Serum CA-125 is an additional ovarian screening test with caveats similar to those described for transvaginal ultrasound.

For *BRCA1* and *BRCA2* mutations associated with hereditary breast and ovarian cancer, referral to breast and gynecologic surgeons with expertise in risk-reducing surgery is critical as the risk of diagnosing an occult malignancy is approximately 1% (69). See **Figure 12.7-1** for a clinical decision-making guide for patients with BRCA1 and BRCA2 mutations. Pelvic surgical expertise is important for any mutation that increases ovarian cancer risk, to ensure that no ovarian tissue remains after RRSO. Surgical technique with a 2-cm margin on the infundibulopelvic ligament and pathologic evaluation with sectioning and extensive examination of the fimbriated end of the tubes (SEE-Fim technique) are recommended for mutation carriers. In addition, evidence has emerged suggesting an increased risk of uterine serous cancer in *BRCA1* carriers, necessitating a discussion about risk-reducing hysterectomy in these patients (19). Following risk-reducing surgery, surgical menopause can have significant impacts on patients' health and well-being. Treatment options, including hormone replacement therapy, can be considered (70). To minimize recovery time burdens for patients, combination surgeries with breast, plastics, and gynecology specialties can be offered.

Lynch Syndrome Risk Reduction

Risk reduction options for unaffected patients with pathogenic mutations in Lynch syndrome genes are reviewed in **Table 12.7-4**. For Lynch syndrome mutation carriers, discussion should focus on the specific mutation, as not all mutations carry the same risk of endometrial or ovarian cancer (**Table 12.7-2**). Current risk reduction management for patients with Lynch syndrome involves colonoscopy, upper GI surveillance, consideration of urinalysis and endometrial biopsies, and risk reduction surgery when appropriate. Colon screening may be delayed to age 30 to 35 in patients with MSH6 and PMS2 mutations. Chemoprevention with aspirin may also be considered, although the recommended duration and dose are uncertain.

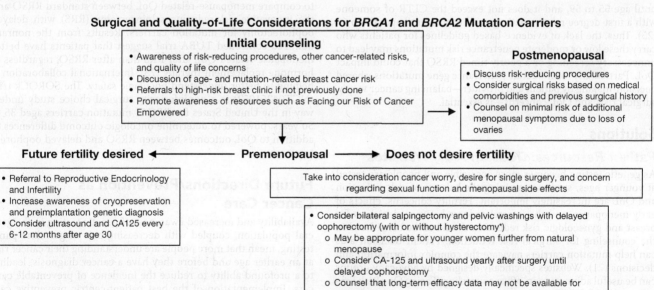

Surgical and Quality-of-Life Considerations for *BRCA1* and *BRCA2* Mutation Carriers

Initial counseling
- Awareness of risk-reducing procedures, other cancer-related risks, and quality of life concerns
- Discussion of age- and mutation-related breast cancer risk
- Referrals to high-risk breast clinic if not previously done
- Promote awareness of resources such as Facing our Risk of Cancer Empowered

Postmenopausal
- Discuss risk-reducing procedures
- Consider surgical risks based on medical comorbidities and previous surgical history
- Counsel on minimal risk of additional menopausal symptoms due to loss of ovaries

Future fertility desired ◄———— **Premenopausal** ————► **Does not desire fertility**

- Referral to Reproductive Endocrinology and Infertility
- Increase awareness of cryopreservation and preimplantation genetic diagnosis
- Consider ultrasound and CA125 every 6-12 months after age 30

Take into consideration cancer worry, desire for single surgery, and concern regarding sexual function and menopausal side effects

- Consider bilateral salpingectomy and pelvic washings with delayed oophorectomy (with or without hysterectomy*)
  - May be appropriate for younger women further from natural menopause
  - Consider CA-125 and ultrasound yearly after surgery until delayed oophorectomy
  - Counsel that long-term efficacy data may not be available for several years
  - Encourage enrollment in clinical trial, if available

- Consider risk-reducing oophorectomy (with or without hysterectomy*)
  - Discuss hormone replacement therapy unless the patient has a personal history of breast cancer
  - No known benefit to CA-125 or increased monitoring after surgery with RRSO
  - If ER+ breast cancer on anti-estrogen, RRSO is unlikely to worsen menopausal side effects and can result in lack of need for ovarian suppression injections

*When counseling regarding hysterectomy
- Discuss that combined estrogen and progestin may increase the risk of breast cancer; thus, hysterectomy could be considered if hormone replacement therapy is desired
- Possible increased risk of serous endometrial cancer in *BRCA1* carriers; also review that endometrial cancer may present earlier and be easier to screen for compared to ovarian cancer.
- Increased length of healing time after hysterectomy compared to oophorectomy

■ **Figure 12.7-1.** Surgical and quality-of-life considerations for *BRCA1* and *BRCA2* mutation carriers. ER, estrogen receptor; RRSO, risk-reducing salpingo-oophorectomy.

■ **TABLE 12.7-4. Risk Reduction Recommendations for Lynch Syndrome Mutation Carriers**

Colon
- MLH1 and MSH2/EPCAM: Colonoscopy every 1-2 yr; beginning age 20-25 or 2-5 yr before earliest colorectal cancer in the family
- MSH6/PMS2: Colonoscopy every 1-3 yr; beginning age 30-35 or 2-5 yr before earliest colorectal cancer in the family

Gastric
- Upper gastrointestinal endoscopy every 2-4 yr; beginning age 30-35

Urothelial
- Consider annual urinalysis starting age 30-35

Gynecologic
- Consider endometrial biopsy every 1-2 yr; beginning age 30-35
- Monitor abnormal bleeding
- Consider chemoprevention with oral contraceptives
- Consider risk-reducing hysterectomy with bilateral salpingo-oophorectomy upon completion of childbearing or age 40-45

Moderate Penetrance Gene Mutations

Although multigene panel testing has become utilized more frequently in patients with gynecologic malignancies, the identification of mutations of moderate or possibly low penetrance does not always translate to definitive clinical application. National consensus guidelines offer suggestions for the management of non-*BRCA* mutations with the strongest ovarian cancer susceptibility association (*RAD51C*, *RAD51D*, and *BRIP1*), and these recommendations are based more on BRCA1 and BRCA2 guidelines than actual mutation cancer risk. For example, national consensus guidelines recommend considering RRSO at age 45 to 50 for a *RAD51C* carrier; however, the cumulative lifetime risk (CLTR) for a *RAD51C* carrier does not approach population CLTR of 1.2% until age 55 to 59, and it does not exceed the CLTR of someone with a first-degree relative with ovarian cancer until ages 65 to 69 (25). Thus, the lack of evidence-based guidelines for patients who carry these low or moderate penetrance risk mutations may lead to unnecessary screening or a poorly timed RRSO that could impact QoL. Particularly for moderate penetrance gene mutations, shared decision-making by patient and provider—balancing cancer worry, surgical risk, and QoL concerns—is essential.

Solutions

Patient Resources: Decision Aids, Websites

As genetic testing becomes more accessible and people are tested at younger ages, studies examining the balance of risk reduction and QoL are increasingly important. Fertility concerns, effects of early menopause, and the interrelatedness between decisions for breast and gynecologic risk reduction should all be considered in the counseling for surgical risk reduction. Patient decision aids can help mutation carriers navigate the complex information and decisions (71). Websites specifically designed by advocacy groups can be useful adjuncts to in-office counseling (Facing Our Risk Empowered, FORCE) (Facingourrisk.org).

Family Letters

The American Congress of Obstetricians and Gynecologists (ACOG) recommends that before testing a patient, the indicated test (such as a single-gene *BRCA1 test or a panel* test) should be ordered only after the patient has been counseled about potential outcomes and has expressly decided to be tested (72). Letters detailing genetic testing results of family members, such as the example given in the ACOG Committee Opinion (72), are a key component of communication between oncology providers, probands, family members, and their primary care providers. OB/GYN providers should work together with genetic counselors and gynecologic oncologists to determine the most efficient strategies for genetic testing in their communities.

Technology

Access to genetic testing and particularly genetic counseling has improved with the rise in telemedicine. Geographically remote patients can now access genetic counseling through medical center–based counselors as well as company-provided genetic counseling over the phone. Patients can also submit samples remotely without needing to be tested in a doctor's office. Access to this technology may be limited in some populations, and providers should pay attention to disparities in clinical care that may increase with increasing reliance on technology.

Databases from Cancer Centers That Detail Cascade Genetic Testing Rates

As the preventive impact of cascade genetic testing becomes clearer, strategies to have recurrent discussions with patients with cancer regarding their family members' risk should be developed. It is still unclear which providers—genetic counselors, gynecologic oncologists, medical oncologists, breast surgeons, OB/GYN, or others—are primarily responsible for initiating these follow-up discussions, and despite advances, the burden still rests on the patients with cancer themselves. Databases with automated follow-up surveys done every 6 to 12 months could provide some aid to busy providers in this regard.

Emerging Research

If gynecologic risk-reducing surgery is chosen, clinical trial involvement should be encouraged. The Women Choosing Surgical Prevention (NCT02760849) in the United States and the TUBA study (NCT02321228) in the Netherlands were designed to compare menopause-related QoL between standard RRSO and the innovative risk-reducing salpingectomy (RRS) with delayed oophorectomy for mutation carriers. Results from the nonrandomized controlled TUBA trial suggest that patients have better menopause-related QoL after RRS than after RRSO, regardless of hormone replacement therapy (73). International collaboration is helping to better understand oncologic safety. The SOROCk trial (NCT04251052) is a noninferiority surgical choice study underway in the United States for *BRCA1* mutation carriers aged 35 to 50 years, powered to determine oncologic outcome differences in addition to QoL outcomes between RRSO and delayed oophorectomy arms.

Future Directions/Prevention as Cancer Care

Availability and increased awareness of genetic testing in the general population, coupled with decreasing cost of germline panel testing, mean that more people are understanding their cancer risk at an earlier age and before they have a cancer diagnosis, leading to a profound ability to reduce the incidence of preventable cancers. Implementation of the best patient-centric preventive care will require continued collaboration and communication across and within disciplines. Each practice should examine the role and accessibility of a genetic counselor to streamline counseling and testing, understanding that this may look different in an academic center compared to community practice, and that reimbursements for such services differ from state to state. We must prioritize streamlining multidisciplinary services, such as breast health, dermatology, and GI health and colorectal surgery. Incorporating genetics into tumor boards, pathology reports, and medical records will help to prioritize this. As other chapters within this book remind us, advances in our understanding of genetics are happening in a background of increasing complexity and specificity of both medical and surgical treatments for cancer care, and at a time where racial and socioeconomic disparities in cancer care and prevention are widening. Furthermore, cancer center resources are limited. Advances in knowledge and implementation of cancer genetic risk assessment are key to cancer prevention, and gynecologic oncologists will play an increasingly key role in prioritizing prevention in a nuanced, compassionate manner.

REFERENCES

1. Broca P. *Traite des Tumeurs*. P. Asselin; 1886.
2. Hurst J. Pioneering geneticist Mary-Claire King receives the 2014 Lasker-Koshland Special Achievement Award in Medical Science. *J Clin Invest.* 2014;124(10):4148-4151.
3. Grinda T, Delaloge S. BRCA2: a 25-year journey from gene identification to targeted cancer treatment. *Lancet Oncol.* 2021;22(6):763-764.
4. Roy R, Chun J, Powell SN. BRCA1 and BRCA2: different roles in a common pathway of genome protection. *Nat Rev Cancer.* 2012;12(1):68-78.
5. Knudson AG Jr. Mutation and cancer: statistical study of retinoblastoma. *Proc Natl Acad Sci USA.* 1971;68:820-823.
6. King MC, Marks JH, Mandell JB. Breast and ovarian cancer risks due to inherited mutations in BRCA1 and BRCA2. *Science.* 2003;302(5645):643-646.
7. Kuckenbaecker KB, Hopper JL, Barnes DR, et al. Risks of breast, ovarian, and contralateral breast cancer for BRCA1 and BRCA2 mutation carriers. *JAMA.* 2017;317:2402-2416.
8. Kotsopoulos J. Age-specific ovarian cancer risks among women with a BRCA1 or BRCA mutation. *Gynecol Oncol.* 2018;150(1):85-91.
9. Cao WM, Zheng YB, Gao Y, et al. Comprehensive mutation detection of BRCA1/2 genes reveals large genomic rearrangements contribute to hereditary breast and ovarian cancer in Chinese women. *BMC Cancer.* 2019;19(1):551.
10. Bozsik A, Pócza T, Papp J et al. Complex characterization of germline large genomic rearrangements of the BRCA1 and BRCA2 genes in high-risk breast cancer patients-novel variants from a large national center. *Int J Mol Sci.* 2020;21(13):4650.
11. Howlader N, Noone AM, Krapcho M, et al. *SEER Cancer Statistics Review, 1975-2018.* National Cancer Institute; 2020.
12. Rubin SC, Benjamin I, Behbakht K, et al. Clinical and pathological features of ovarian cancer in women with germ-line mutations of BRCA1. *N Engl J Med.* 1996;335(19):1413-1416.
13. Soslow RA, Han G, Park KJ, et al. Morpholic patterns associated with BRCA1 and BRCA2 genotype in ovarian carcinoma. *Mod Pathol.* 2012;25(4):625-636.
14. Mersch J, Jackson MA, Park M, et al. Cancers associated with BRCA1 and BRCA2 mutations other than breast and ovarian. *Cancer.* 2014;121(2):269-275.
15. Matanes E, Volodarsky-Perel A, Eisenberg N, et al. Endometrial cancer in germline BRCA mutation carriers: a systematic review and meta-analysis. *J Minim Invasive Gynecol.* 2021;28(5):947-956.
16. Breast Cancer Linkage Consortium. Cancer risks in BRCA2 mutation carriers. *J Natl Cancer Inst.* 1999;91(15):1310.
17. Jakubowska A, Nej K, Huzarski T, Scott RJ, Lubinski J. BRCA2 gene mutations in families with aggregations of breast and stomach cancers. *Br J Cancer.* 2002;87:888-891.
18. Cavanagh H, Rogers KMA. The role of BRCA1 and BRCA2 mutations in prostate, pancreatic and stomach cancers. *Hered Cancer Clin Pract.* 2015;13(1):16.
19. Shu CA, Pike MC, Jotwani AR, et al. Uterine cancer after risk-reducing salpingo-oophorectomy without hysterectomy in women with BRCA mutations. *JAMA Oncol.* 2016;2(11):1434-1440.
20. Segev Y, Iqbal J, Lubinski J, et al. The incidence of endometrial cancer in women with BRCA1 and BRCA2 mutations: an international prospective cohort study. *Gynecol Oncol.* 2013;130(1):127-131.
21. Gumaste PV, Penn LA, Cymerman RM, Kirchhoff T, Polsky D, McLellan B. Skin cancer risk in BRCA1/2 mutation carriers. *Br J Dermatol.* 2015;172(6):1498.
22. Easton DF, Pharoah PDP, Antoniou AC, et al. Gene-panel sequencing and the prediction of breast-cancer risk. *N Engl J Med.* 2015;372(23):2243-2257.
23. Kurian AW, Hare EE, Mills MA, et al. Clinical evaluation of a multiple-gene sequencing panel for hereditary cancer risk assessment. *J Clin Oncol.* 2014;32(19):2001-2009.
24. Desmond A, Kurian AW, Gabree M, et al. Clinical actionability of multigene panel testing for hereditary breast and ovarian cancer risk assessment. *JAMA Oncol.* 2015;1(7):943-951.
25. Tung N, Domchek SM, Stadler Z, et al. Counselling framework for moderate-penetrance cancer-susceptibility mutations. *Nat Rev Clin Oncol.* 2016;13(9):581-588.
26. Post CCB, Stelloo E, Smit VTHBM, et al. Prevalence and prognosis of lynch syndrome and sporadic mismatch repair deficiency in endometrial cancer. *J Natl Cancer Inst.* 2021;113(9):1212.
27. Lynch HT, Lynch PM, Lanspa SJ, Snyder CL, Lynch JF, Boland CR. Review of the Lynch syndrome: history, molecular genetics, screening, differential diagnosis, and medicolegal ramifications. *Clin Genet.* 2009;76(1):1-18.
28. Bonadona V, Bonaïti B, Olschwang S, et al. Cancer risks associated with germline mutations in MLH1, MSH2, and MSH6 genes in Lynch syndrome. *JAMA.* 2011;305:2304-2310.
29. Dominguez-Valetin M, Sampson JR, Seppälä TT, et al. Cancer risks by gene, age and gender in 6350 carriers of pathogenic mismatch repair variants: findings from the Prospective Lynch Syndrome Database. *Genet Med.* 2020;22:15.
30. Baglietto L, Lindor NM, Dowty JG, et al. Risks of Lynch syndrome cancers for MSH6 mutation carriers. *J Natl Cancer Inst.* 2010;102:193-201.
31. Ramsoekh D, Wagner A, van Leerdam ME, et al. Cancer risk in MLH1, MSH2, and MSH6 mutation carriers; different risk profiles may influence clinical management. *Hered Cancer Clin Pract.* 2009;7:17.
32. Ten Broeke SW, van der Klift HM, Tops CMJ, et al. Cancer risks for PMS2-associated Lynch syndrome. *J Clin Oncol.* 2018;36(29):2961-2968.
33. Engel C, Loeffler M, Steinke V, et al. Risks of less common cancers in proven mutation carriers with lynch syndrome. *J Clin Oncol.* 2012;30:4409-4415.
34. Broaddus RR, Lynch HT, Chen LM, et al. Pathologic features of endometrial carcinoma associated with HNPCC: a comparison with sporadic endometrial carcinoma. *Cancer.* 2006;106(1):87-94.
35. Westin SN, Lacour RA, Urbauer DL et al. Carcinoma of the lower uterine segment: a newly described association with Lynch syndrome. *J Clin Oncol.* 2008;26:5965-5971.
36. Ketabi Z, Bartuma K, Bernstein I, et al. Ovarian cancer linked to Lynch syndrome typically presents as early-onset, non-serous epithelial tumors. *Gynecol Oncol.* 2011;121(3):462-465.
37. Pietragalla A, Arcieri M, Marchetti C, Scambia G, Fagotti A. Ovarian cancer predisposition beyond BRCA1 and BRCA2 genes. *Int J of Gyn Cancer.* 2020;30:1803-1810.
38. Society of Gynecologic Oncology. SGO Clinical Practice Statement; genetic testing for ovarian cancer. October 1, 2014.
39. Byfield SD, Wei H, DuCharme M, Lancaster JM. Economic impact of multigene panel testing for hereditary breast and ovarian cancer. *J Comp Eff Res.* 2021;10(3):207-217.
40. Davidson BA, Ehrisman J, Reed SD, Yang JC, Buchanan A, Havrilesky LJ. Preferences of women with epithelial ovarian cancer for aspects of genetic testing. *Gynecol Oncol Res Pract.* 2019;6:1.
41. Kurian AW, Ward KC, Howlader N, et al. Genetic testing and results in a population-based cohort of breast cancer patients and ovarian cancer patients. *J Clin Oncol.* 2019;37(15):1305-1315.
42. Cham S, Landrum MB, Keating NL, Armstrong J, Wright AA. Use of germline BRCA testing in patients with ovarian cancer and commercial insurance. *JAMA Netw Open.* 2022;5(1):e2142703, doi:10.1001/jamanetworkopen.2021.42703
43. Randall LM, Pothuri B, Swisher EM, et al. Multi-disciplinary summit on genetics services for women with gynecologic cancers: a society of gynecologic oncology white paper. *Gynecol Oncol.* 2017;146(2):217-224.
44. Trepanier AM, Allain DC. Models of service delivery for cancer genetic risk assessment and counseling. *J Genet Couns.* 2014;23(2):239-253.
45. Yang D, Khan S, Sun Y, et al. Association of BRCA1 and BRCA2 mutations with survival, chemotherapy sensitivity, and gene mutator phenotype in patients with ovarian cancer. *JAMA.* 2011;474(7353):609-615.
46. Pal T, Permuth-Wey J, Kapoor R, Cantor A, Sutphen R. Improved survival in BRCA2 carriers with ovarian cancer. *Fam Cancer.* 2007;6(12):113-119.
47. Bolton KL, Chenevix-Trench G, Goh C, et al. Association between BRCA1 and BRCA2 mutations and survival in women with invasive epithelial ovarian cancer. *JAMA.* 2012;307(4):382-390.
48. Gonzalez-Martin A, Pothuri B, Vergote I, et al. Niraparib in patients with newly diagnosed advanced ovarian cancer. *N Engl J Med.* 2019;381:2391-2402.
49. Moore K, Colombo N, Scambia G, et al. Maintenance Olaparib in patients with newly diagnosed advanced ovarian cancer. *N Engl J Med.* 2018;379(26):2495-2505.
50. Monk BJ, Parkinson C, Lim MC, et al. A randomized, phase III trial to evaluate rucaparib monotherapy as maintenance treatment in patients with newly diagnosed ovarian cancer. *J Clin Oncol.* 2022;40(34):3952-3964.

51. Konstantinopoulos PA, Norquist B, Lacchetti C, et al., Germline and somatic tumor testing in epithelial ovarian cancer: ASCO guideline. *J Clin Oncol.* 2020.38(11):1222-1245.

52. Kwon JS, Tinker AV, Santos J, et al. Germline testing and somatic tumor testing for BRCA1/2 somatic variants in ovarian cancer: what is the optimal sequence? *JCO Precis Oncol.* 2022;6:e2200033.

53. Vasen HF, Mecklin JP, Khan PM, Lynch HT. The International Collaborative Group on Hereditary Non-Polyposis Colorectal Cancer (ICG-HNPCC). *Dis Colon Rectum.* 1991;34(5):424.

54. Crosbie EJ, Ryan NAJ, Arends MJ, et al. The Manchester International Consensus Group recommendations for the management of gynecological cancers in Lynch syndrome. *Genet Med.* 2019;21(10):2390.

55. Monahan KJ, Bradshaw N, Dolwani S, et al. Guidelines for the management of hereditary colorectal cancer from the British Society of Gastroenterology (BSG)/Association of Coloproctology of Great Britain and Ireland (ACPGBI)/United Kingdom Cancer Genetics Group (UKCGG). *Gut.* 2020;69(3):411-444.

56. Dottino J, Lairson D, Cantor S, Suidan R, Lu KH. A cost-effectiveness analysis of universal testing for Lynch syndrome in endometrial carcinoma. *Gynecol Oncol.* 2017;147(1):203.

57. Kahn RM, Gordhandas S, Maddy BP, et al. Universal endometrial cancer tumor typing: how much has immunohistochemistry, microsatellite instability, and MLH1 methylation improved the diagnosis of Lynch syndrome across the population? *Cancer.* 2019;125:3172-3183.

58. Levine MD, Pearlman R, Hampel H, et al. Up-front multigene panel testing for cancer susceptibility in patients with newly diagnosed endometrial cancer: a multicenter prospective study. *JCO Precis Oncol.* 2021;5:1588-1602.

59. O'Malley DM, Bariani GM, Cassier PA, et al. Pembrolizumab in patients with microsatellite instability-high advanced endometrial cancer: results from the Keynote-158 study. *J Clin Oncol.* 2022;40(7):752-761.

60. Mai PL, Malkin D, Garber JE, et al. Li-Fraumeni syndrome: report of a clinical research workshop and creation of a research consortium. *Cancer Genet.* 2012;205(10):479-487.

61. Tan MH, Mester JL, Ngeow J, Rybicki LA, Orloff MS, Eng C. Lifetime cancer risks in individuals with germline PTEN mutations. *Clin Cancer Res.* 2012;18(2):400-407.

62. Hendricks LAJ, Hoogerbrugge N, Schuurs-Hoeijmakers JHM, Vos JR. A review on age-related cancer risks in PTEN hamartoma tumor syndrome. *Clin Genet.* 2021;99(2):219-225.

63. Young RH, Welch WR, Dickersin GR, Scully RE. Ovarian sex cord tumor with annular tubules: review of 74 cases including 27 with Peutz-Jeghers syndrome and four with adenoma malignum of the cervix. *Cancer.* 1982;50(7):1384-1402.

64. Meserve EEK,Nucci MR. Peutz-Jeghers syndrome: pathobiology, pathologic manifestations, and suggestions for recommending genetic testing in pathology reports. *Surg Pathol Clin.* 2016;9(2):243-268.

65. King MC, Levy-Lahad E, Lahad A. Population-based screening for BRCA1 and BRCA2: 2014 Lasker award. *JAMA.* 2014;312(11):1091-1092.

66. Samimi G, Bernardini MQ, Brody LC, et al. Traceback: a proposed framework to increase identification and genetic counseling of BRCA1 and BRCA2 mutation carriers through family-based outreach. *J Clin Oncol.* 2017;35(20):2329-2337.

67. Offit K, Tkachuk KA, Stadler ZK, et al. Cascading after peridiagnostic cancer genetic testing: an alternative to population-based screening. *J Clin Oncol.* 2020;38(13):1398-1408.

68. Srinivasan S, Won NY, Dotson WD, Wright ST, Roberts MC. Barriers and facilitators for cascade testing in genetic conditions: a systematic review. *Eur J Hum Genet.* 2020;28(12):1631-1644.

69. Piedimonte S, Frank C, Laprise C, Quaiattini A, Gotlieb WH. Occult tubal carcinoma after risk-reducing salpingo-oophorectomy: a systematic review. *Obstet Gynecol.* 2020;135(3):498-508.

70. Gordhandas S, Norquist BM, Pennington KP, Yung RL, Laya MB, Swisher EM. Hormone replacement therapy after risk reducing salpingo-oophorectomy in patients with BRCA1 or BRCA2 mutations; a systematic review of risks and benefits. *Gynecol Oncol.* 2019;153(1):192-200.

71. Steenbeek MP, van Bommel MHD, Harmsen MG, et al. Evaluation of a patient decision aid for BRCA1/2 pathogenic variant carriers choosing an ovarian cancer prevention strategy. *Gynecol Oncol.* 2021;163(2):371-377.

72. Committee on Gynecologic Practice. ACOG committee opinion no. 727: cascade testing: testing women for known hereditary genetic mutations associated with cancer. *Obstet Gynecol.* 2018;131(1):e31-e34.

73. Steenbeek MP, Harmsen MG, Hoogerbrugge N, et al. Association of salpingectomy with delayed oophorectomy versus salpingo-oophorectomy with quality of life in BRCA1/2 pathogenic variant carriers: a nonrandomized controlled trial. *JAMA Oncol.* 2021;7(8):1203-1212.

CHAPTER **12.8**

Biologic and Physical Principles of Radiation Oncology

Jenna Kahn, Beth A. Erickson, Meena Bedi, Firas Mourtada, and Sunil J. Advani

RADIATION ONCOLOGY AS A SPECIALTY

Radiation oncology is a specialty focused primarily on the treatment of malignancies, although there are a number of benign diseases for which radiation can be used. Training in radiation oncology begins with an internship, followed by 4 years of residency. Board certification follows, requiring successful completion of both written and oral exams. Residency training includes an in-depth understanding of the natural history and treatment of all malignancies, including the roles of surgery and systemic therapy in this era of multimodality therapies. An in-depth understanding of surgical procedures, pathology, and radiologic anatomy, as well as the efficacies and toxicities of systemic therapy, is required. Formal instruction in physics and radiobiology is also part of the residency training. Subspecialization with a specific practice focus on gynecologic or other cancers may follow. Only a few centers sponsor fellowships, which are usually focused on brachytherapy or other special procedures. Brachytherapy skills are especially important in the curative treatment of patients with gynecologic cancer. In addition, contemporary treatment of gynecologic malignancies requires mastery of rapidly evolving technology for delivering external beam irradiation with techniques such as intensity-modulated radiation therapy (IMRT) and image-guided radiation therapy (IGRT). Radiation oncologists are important contributors to the management of individual patients and participate on multidisciplinary tumor boards. Having a knowledgeable and subspecialized radiation oncologist and gynecologic oncologist paired is a great benefit to all.

In addition to radiation oncologists, other allied health professionals are integral to the radiation oncology department and treatment delivery. Radiation therapists are the individuals who actually operate the radiation equipment and deliver radiation treatments. Dosimetrists are primarily responsible for planning the radiation therapy or dosimetry before treatment delivery. Radiation physicists supervise and review the work of dosimetrists. Physicists are also integral to the introduction and maintenance of the rapidly evolving technology in radiation oncology departments. They are very involved with quality assurance and radiation safety. They can be master's-level or PhD-level physicists and should be board certified. The team of allied health professionals works with the radiation oncologist to treat patients with gynecologic cancer.

INTRODUCTION TO RADIOBIOLOGY

Radiobiology is the study of how ionizing radiation (IR) interacts with biologic processes (1). The physics of IR delivery allows for dose deposition to be delivered to targeted tumor tissues (2). However, for IR to reach tumors deep in the body, it passes through a number of normal tissues. Therefore, it is important for radiation oncologists to deliver the optimal dose of IR in order to eradicate the tumor while minimizing the risk of injury to surrounding normal structures (such as bladder and bowel) that are within the radiation field. As with most medical treatments, the clinical utility of IR is based on a therapeutic ratio, that is, IR's ability to destroy targeted tumor tissue is greater than its toxicity to normal tissues. The effect of the dose-response relationship of IR on cancerous and normal tissues can be depicted as a pair of sigmoidal curves (**Figure 12.8-1**). At low doses of IR, there is not only little effect on tumor control but also a low risk for complications. With very high doses of IR, the likelihood for tumor control is high, but there may also be an unacceptably high rate of normal tissue complications. In between these two extremes, as the dose of IR increases, effects on both cancerous and normal tissues increase rapidly. A key feature in this part of the dose-response curve is that the tumor kill curve is shifted to the left of the normal tissue complication curve. Thus, for a given dose of IR, the probability of tumor kill is greater than the probability of normal tissue damage. It is in this dose range that the therapeutic ratio of IR can be exploited to cure cancer with an acceptable toxicity profile.

An understanding of radiobiology allows us to appreciate the rationale for how radiotherapy is used in gynecologic cancers and in the development of novel therapies. For example, radiosensitizing drugs increase tissue sensitivity to IR, which is graphically represented by shifting of the tissue response curves to the left (**Figure 12.8-1**) (2,3). The implication of this is that a lower dose of IR is required in the presence of the radiosensitizer to achieve a similar degree of tissue response when compared to IR alone. Of clinical importance is that certain chemotherapies can preferentially radiosensitize tumors and therefore shift the tumor kill control curve farther to the left than the normal tissue complication curve (4). This widens the therapeutic ratio of IR, with improved tumor control and decreased normal tissue toxicity.

While defining tumor control and normal tissue response lies at the center of radiotherapy, in clinical practice, radiotherapy is delivered to defined targeted volumes (**Figure 12.8-2**) (5). These volumes are contoured (drawn) by a radiation oncologist based on both physical examination and radiographic imaging (CT, ultrasound, MRI, and positron emission tomography [PET]). The area of clinically/radiographically identified tumor is defined as the gross target volume (GTV). Based on our clinical knowledge of how cancer spreads with respect to different histologies and disease sites, a clinical target volume (CTV) is next defined, which encompasses areas that are likely to harbor microscopic spread of cancer cells. Examples of what is included in the CTV are microscopically involved tumor margins postsurgery or normal-sized pelvic and para-aortic lymph nodes with a high suspicion for tumor involvement. Appropriately defining the GTV and CTV is crucial to controlling the tumor and crucial to the patient's OS and quality of life. Ideally, IR would be delivered only to the GTV and the CTV. However, the tissues within the GTV and CTV as defined at an initial planning session are not likely to be in the same place each day a patient receives radiotherapy. Reasons for these variations include both intrinsic and extrinsic factors. Internally, tumor tissue and surrounding normal tissues move, in part due to breathing and peristalsis of bowel as well as bowel and bladder filling with stool and urine. Externally, aligning the patient with the source of IR has inherent setup variations each day, which can include patient immobilization and body habitus. For these reasons, a planning target volume (PTV) is defined for both the GTV and CTV. The PTV is constructed by expanding the GTV and CTV slightly (≤10 mm) to account for these variations in tumor and normal organ location. Clinically, the PTVs are the regions of the body to which

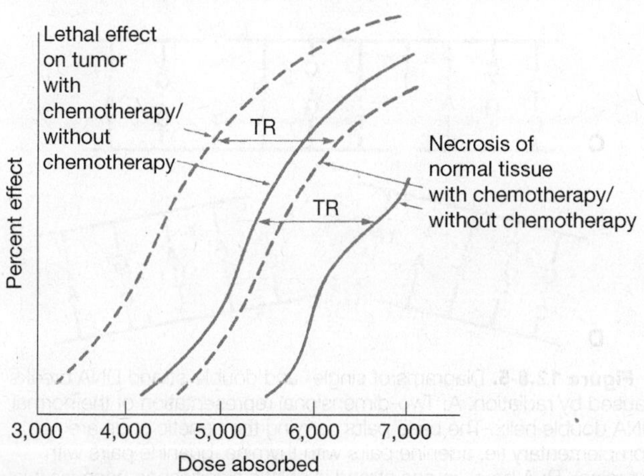

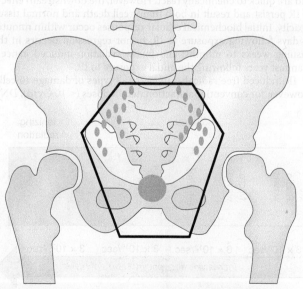

Figure 12.8-1. Theoretic curves for tumor control and complications as a function of radiation dose both with and without chemotherapy. TR, therapeutic range (or the difference between tumor control and complication frequency). (Reprinted from Perez CA, Thomas PRM. Radiation therapy: basic concepts and clinical implications. In: Sutow WW, Fernbach DJ, Vietti TJ, eds. *Clinical Pediatric Oncology.* 3rd Ed. Mosby; 1984:167, with permission from Elsevier.)

Figure 12.8-2. Target definition in radiation treatment planning for cervical cancer. The solid circle represents the GTV, which is the cervical primary defined both clinically and radiographically. The CTV is the pelvic lymph nodes, which have a high probability of at least microscopic involvement. The outer solid line represents PTV, which is the margin added to the CTV to account for organ motion and daily setup error. CTV, clinical target volume; GTV, gross target volume; PTV, planning target volume.

Figure 12.8-1 axis labels: Percent effect (y-axis); Dose absorbed (x-axis) with values 3,000 4,000 5,000 6,000 7,000. Labels: "Lethal effect on tumor with chemotherapy/ without chemotherapy" and "Necrosis of normal tissue with chemotherapy/ without chemotherapy"; TR marked twice.

IR delivery is conformed, with the goal of maximizing dose to the PTV and minimizing dose to the normal tissues, that is, organs at risk (OAR), to achieve as wide a therapeutic ratio as possible for IR. In the following section, we go over the radiobiologic principles that underlie the biologic basis of radiotherapy. An understanding of basic radiobiologic principles and of preclinical research allows for continued advancement and refinement of the use of radiotherapy in gynecologic cancers.

Interaction of Ionizing Radiation With Tissue and DNA Damage

Radiotherapy utilizes IR, which is part of the electromagnetic spectrum of radiation (**Figure 12.8-3**) (1). This spectrum is composed of a broad range of waves ranging from radio waves to visible light and IR. In the electromagnetic spectrum, the energy, wavelength, and frequency of waves are related by the following equations:

Energy in electron volts (eV) = $h \times v$
$$c = \lambda \times v$$
h = Planck constant, 4.14×10^{-15} eV sec
c = speed of light, 3×10^{8} m/sec
λ = wavelength (m)
v = frequency of wave (1/sec)

Thus, the high-energy waves located in the IR part of the electromagnetic spectrum are of high frequencies and short wavelengths. This radiation is called ionizing, because it deposits a sufficient amount of energy into the tissue to eject electrons from atoms and generate ions. At the high energies of IR used in radiation oncology, IR interacts with atoms through the Compton process (**Figure 12.8-4**). In the Compton process, IR ejects electrons from the outer shells of atoms. These liberated electrons mediate tissue responses to IR. The electrons can directly hit targets within the cell, resulting in damage, that is, direct effect. However, it is the indirect effect of the electrons that predominates. In the indirect effect, the ejected electrons first interact with intracellular water, generating hydroxyl radicals. These hydroxyl radicals are highly reactive and damage many components of irradiated tissue through oxidative stress and DNA damage. It should be noted that the timescale of these interactions of IR with tissue is less than seconds, as ionizations and electrons are unstable and are quick to chemically react. However, the downstream effects of IR persist and result in both tumor cell death and normal tissue toxicity. Initial biochemical cellular responses occur within minutes to days following exposure to IR; tumor regression occurs in the ensuing weeks to months; and finally radiation-induced cancers manifest years following the initial exposure to IR.

IR-induced free radicals can cause all types of damage to cells. However, for conventional fractionated IR doses (<10 Gy/d), DNA

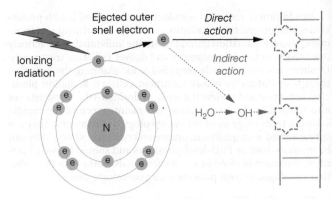

Figure 12.8-4. Interaction of ionizing radiation with matter. High energy photons used in radiotherapy result in ejection of outer shell electrons through the Compton process. These ejected electrons then mediate tissue response to radiotherapy by causing oxidative and DNA damage. They can interact directly with DNA (direct action) or more likely through interaction with water to and generation of hydroxyl radicals (indirect action).

is the major target of IR-generated free radicals. The evidence for DNA as one of the targets for radiation is substantial: (a) incorporation of radioactive tritium into DNA causes cell death at greater rates than cytoplasmic tritium; (b) halogenated pyrimidines, when present in DNA, increase the cell's inherent radiosensitivity in an amount proportionate to the degree of incorporation; (c) a correlation between radiation, DNA double-stranded break repair, and clonogenic survival has also been observed; (d) the concentration of DNA in the nucleus correlates positively with radiosensitivity; and (e) microirradiation techniques have shown the nucleus to be the most radiosensitive organelle (6-8). Free radical damage to DNA results in cross-links, base damage, single-strand breaks, and double-strand breaks (**Figure 12.8-5**). These DNA double-strand

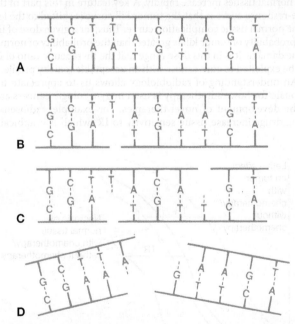

Figure 12.8-5. Diagrams of single- and double-strand DNA breaks caused by radiation. A: Two-dimensional representation of the normal DNA double helix. The base pairs carrying the genetic code are complementary (ie, adenine pairs with thymine, guanine pairs with cytosine). B: A break in one strand is of little significance because it is readily repaired, using the opposite strand as a template. C: Breaks in both strands, if well separated, are repaired as independent breaks. D: If breaks occur in both strands and are directly opposite or separated by only a few base pairs, this may lead to a double-strand break, when the chromatin snaps into two pieces. *Source:* Courtesy of Dr. John Ward. (From Hall EJ. *Radiobiology for the Radiologist.* 4th ed. JB Lippincott; 1994, with permission.)

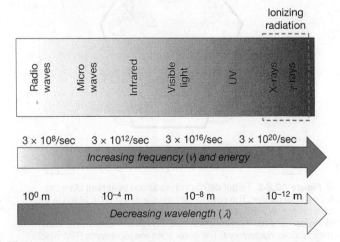

Figure 12.8-3. Electromagnetic spectrum. X-ray and γ-ray ionizing radiation are located in the short-wavelength, high-frequency, and high energy part of the spectrum.

Comet Assay

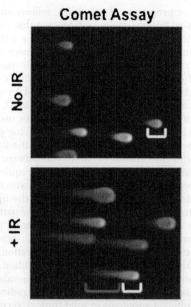

Figure 12.8-6. Measurement of infrared (IR)-induced DNA double-strand breaks. Cells were irradiated and analyzed by neutral comet assay. In nonirradiated cells, intact DNA appears as a nucleoid (comet head), yellow-bracketed area. Following IR, DNA double-strand migrates in the electrical field and forms a comet tail, red-bracketed area.

breaks constitute the "lethal hit" of IR that is responsible for killing cells. IR-induced DNA double-strand breaks can be directly visualized using a single-cell gel electrophoresis assay, also known as neutral comet assay, in which DNA double-strand breaks appear as smaller fragments of DNA that move across the electrical field and form a "tail" to the "comet head" of the larger undamaged DNA strands (**Figure 12.8-6**) (9). Although highly valuable in laboratory studies on IR, neutral comet assays are limited to use in cell culture radiobiology basic science research. To assess IR DNA damage in tissue, DNA damage response signaling can be interrogated. IR-induced DNA double-strand breaks result in activation of signaling cascades to deal with the damage. One such response is phosphorylation of histone 2A on serine 139, termed γH2AX. Within the nucleus of irradiated cells, γH2AX foci formation can be quantitated (**Figure 12.8-7**).

Once DNA double-strand breaks are created, cells attempt to fix the damage. Resolution of DNA double-strand breaks can result in chromosomal aberrations that are classified as lethal or nonlethal (**Figure 12.8-8**) (10). These aberrations are readily apparent in

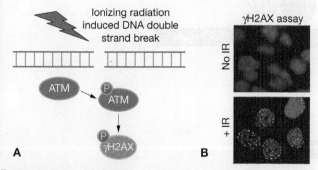

Figure 12.8-7. Infrared (IR)-induced DNA damage. A: DNA double-strand breaks activate DNA damage response signaling cascades. Ataxia telangiectasia mutated (ATM) senses DNA double-strand breaks and autophosphorylates to become active. ATM then phosphorylates and activates downstream effector molecules such as histone 2. B: Immunofluorescence for gH2AX foci formation in cells. gH2AX foci (green dots) appear in the nuclei (blue stained) of irradiated cells.

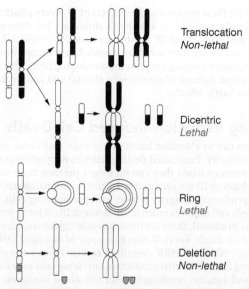

Figure 12.8-8. Chromosomal aberrations induced by ionizing radiation (IR). IR results in DNA double-strand breaks that can lead to chromosomal aberrations. Chromosomal aberrations can be classified as lethal or nonlethal based on the ability of chromosomes to segregate to daughter cells in mitosis.

chromosomes of people exposed to IR, by either direct visualization of metaphase chromosome spreads or more advanced techniques of fluorescence in situ hybridization (FISH), in which each chromosome is "painted" a different color. Nonlethal chromosomal aberrations include translocations and deletions. Although genetic information is lost in these two cases, cells are still potentially capable of surviving and proliferating. Lethal resolutions of DNA double-strand breaks include dicentric and ring chromosome formation. The commonality of lethal resolutions is that an acentric DNA fragment is created such that during cell division at mitosis, one daughter cell loses an entire chromosome, resulting in cell death. Mechanistically, cells have evolved two major processes for repairing DNA double-strand breaks, nonhomologous end joining (NHEJ) and homologous recombination repair (HRR) (11). NHEJ is the simplest type of repair mechanism. In NHEJ, two ends of broken DNA are processed and then ligated together. It does not utilize or require an undamaged DNA template. Therefore, NHEJ is error prone and can result in mutations introduced in the genome through insertions or deletions of genetic material. In contrast to NHEJ, HRR is an error-free DNA double-strand break repair process. HRR requires a DNA template and, therefore, can only occur when cells are in the S/G$_2$ phase of the cell cycle and an undamaged template DNA strand exists.

Following repair of IR-induced damage, the long-term impacts on surviving tissue are classified as deterministic and stochastic effects (12). Deterministic effects have a threshold IR dose above which they are typically observed. Once the threshold dose is reached, further increases in IR dose result in increased severity of the phenotype. The classic example of an IR deterministic effect is cataract formation. At very low doses of IR to the lens of the eye, the chance of cataract formation is next to zero. However, once a threshold dose of IR is delivered, cataracts can develop. In contrast, stochastic effects have no threshold IR dose at which they can potentially occur, and their severity does not increase as more IR dose is delivered. The most troubling stochastic effect of IR is radiation-induced carcinogenesis. In principle, any dose of IR is randomly capable of inducing DNA damage with resulting genetic mutations that lead to cancer development. Like deterministic effects, stochastic effects are more likely to occur as IR dose increases due to the probabilistic manner in which IR interacts with tissue. With these concerning late effects of IR, every effort is made to judiciously apply IR to a patient's situation. The deterministic and stochastic effects of IR are the key reasons for which both diagnostic and therapeutic x-rays are avoided in pregnant women: to avoid long-term consequences to the developing fetus with respect to both organ damage (deterministic effects) and cancer development (stochastic effects).

Ionizing Radiation–Induced Cell Death

Cell death can be classified based on the cells' functional or reproductive integrity. Functional death occurs in nonproliferating cells such as neurons when they can no longer perform their function. Higher doses of IR are required to induce functional death. In contrast, reproductive integrity is seen with proliferating cells such as tumor cells and requires much lower doses of IR. When a proliferating cell is irradiated, there are three possible outcomes: survival, senescence, or death. Survival requires repair of damaged DNA such as through NHEJ or HRR described earlier. However, even after recovering from the initial irradiation, surviving cells may have mutations and damage, resulting in deterministic or stochastic effects. Although survival of irradiated cells in normal tissue is paramount, the ultimate goal of radiotherapy is the death of tumor cells, or, more precisely, preventing tumor cells from replicating. Replicative senescence can occur after DNA damage when cells permanently exit the cell cycle and do not replicate. Senescence is a mechanism of self-preservation for damaged cells, because cellular division would result in death. It should be noted that senescence is different than quiescence. Quiescence is a temporary exit from the cell cycle at G_1 into the G_0 phase. Cells in G_0 are not preparing to divide but can still perform their function. Under appropriate stimuli, cells in quiescence reenter the cell cycle and divide. Although not a mechanism of cell death, if tumor cells undergo senescence, the patient is in essence cured of their tumor. For cell death, mechanisms following irradiation include apoptosis, autophagy, and mitotic catastrophe.

Apoptosis, or programmed cell death, follows an orderly cascade (13). It is an energy-dependent process that requires intact molecular biologic pathways. Apoptosis can be initiated by two distinct mechanisms: (a) extrinsic pathway, where the apoptotic stimulus occurs extracellularly, or (b) intrinsic pathway, where the cascade of events is mediated by intracellular events (**Figure 12.8-9**). Mechanistically, apoptosis is mediated by caspases that are expressed as inactive precursors (procaspases). Upon apoptotic stimuli, proteolytic cleavage of procaspases results in active caspases, which then cleave downstream effector proteins. The extrinsic pathway begins by binding of a specific ligand such as Fas-L or tumor necrosis factor (TNF) to a membrane death receptor. The intrinsic pathway, on the other hand, requires disruption of the mitochondrial membrane and release of cytochrome c from the mitochondria to the cytoplasm. Although the upstream activation of apoptosis through extrinsic or intrinsic pathways differs, both pathways converge on cleaving and activating procaspase 3. A number of methods have been developed to measure apoptosis, including caspase cleavage, DNA fragmentation, and cellular membrane changes. If apoptosis occurs, it is evident within hours of IR by activation of caspases and loss of cell membrane polarity. However, although conventional fractionated radiotherapy does not induce significant apoptosis in solid tumors, recent preclinical evidence suggests that larger single fractions of radiotherapy (>10 Gy) can induce apoptosis in irradiated endothelial cells (14,15). Given the location of gynecologic cancers, such large fractions of IR have not typically been employed. However, with advances in brachytherapy planning and delivery, such higher doses may provide a way to target the tumor vasculature. Autophagy occurs during nutrient deprivation and metabolic stress (16). The goal of autophagy is catabolism of cellular structures to provide a source of nutrients to cells and help them survive periods of stress. Its role in IR-induced death is under investigation.

Mitotic catastrophe is the predominant mechanism of cell death induced by IR (17). In mitotic catastrophe, cells die as a

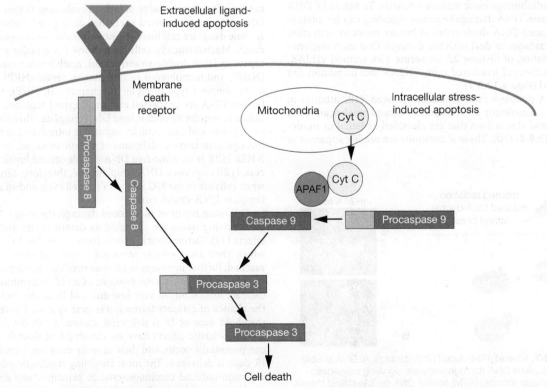

Figure 12.8-9. Apoptotic pathways of cell death. In the extrinsic pathway, death receptor binding of ligand activates initiator caspase 8. In the intrinsic pathways, intracellular stress results in mitochondrial release of cytochrome C (cyt C), which binds to apoptotic protease activating factor 1 (APAF1) to activate initiator caspase 9. Both pathways converge on activating effector caspases, caspase 3, which results in apoptotic cell death.

result of trying to replicate. As mentioned earlier, IR-induced DNA double-strand breaks result in chromosome and chromatid aberrations. If not dividing, the full complement of genetic material remains within the cell. However, when cells pass through mitosis and divide into two daughter cells, certain chromosome and chromatid aberrations (eg, ring and dicentric chromosomes) do not result in equal segregation of the genetic material to the two daughter cells. In addition, DNA double-strand breaks result in increasing genomic instability of dividing cells. Therefore, cells may replicate a few times, after which the loss of increasing genetic material results in cell death. In contrast to the orderly process of apoptosis, mitotic catastrophe is energy independent and results in necrosis and inflammation. Because it requires cells to divide, mitotic catastrophe is not evident as quickly as apoptosis.

Cell Survival Curves and Tumor Control Probability

The gold standard technique used to measure IR-induced cell kill is the clonogenic assay (**Figure 12.8-10**) (18). The clonogenic assay is particularly useful for measuring cell death through mitotic catastrophe. In principle, it measures the reproductive ability of individual cells following different doses of IR. Cells are seeded at low density and allowed to replicate for 10 to 14 days, over which time each cell forms a colony of greater than 50 daughter cells. As cells undergo mitotic catastrophe, they stop dividing and do not form a colony of greater than 50 daughter cells. Since it is such a crucial technique for measuring sensitivity of cells to IR, we review the technique in some detail. It first involves creating a suspension containing the target population of cells at a known concentration. An aliquot with a known number of cells is plated on growth media and allowed to incubate. As one would expect, not all the cells successfully form a colony, and so plating efficiency must be calculated by dividing the number of formed colonies by the starting number of cells. The experiment is repeated, but after plating and before incubation, the Petri dish is irradiated. The number of colonies formed is divided by the starting number of cells, which is then divided by plating efficiency to yield the ratio of surviving cells. This experiment is repeated over a range of doses of radiation and under various conditions to yield a cell survival curve. An important feature of the cell survival curve is that it uses a logarithmic scale on the y-axis. This correlates with mathematical modeling of cell survival as a function of radiation dose.

The simplest model one can envision for the sterilization of cancer cells by radiation in a given volume is the log cell kill model. A typical course of radiation therapy is given in 10 to 40 fractions administered over 2 to 8 weeks. Each fraction kills a fixed percentage of cells. One term that can be used for this is D_{10}, the dose that kills 90% of the cells. If there are 100 cells and a D_{10} dose is administered, 10 viable cells remain. Consider a tumor 1 g in size, which has 10^9 cells. If the D_{10} for this tumor is 3 Gy, how many fractions are required for a 90% chance of sterilization? The log cell kill model gets slightly more complicated when dealing in fractions, as 1/10 of a viable cell does not exist. Instead, 0.1 cells represent a 10% chance that a viable cell will exist at the end of therapy. Therefore, a tumor with 10^9 cells requires 10 decades of cell kill for a 90% chance of tumor control. 3 Gy × 10 fractions = 30 Gy total dose. This model makes a number of invalid assumptions such as D_{10} remaining constant throughout the course of radiation but highlights the logarithmic nature of fractionated radiation kill. Instead of D_{10}, D_0 is the more commonly used term in radiobiology and is based on natural logarithm, where base e = 2.72. D_0 is the dose of radiation where $1/e$ (37%) cells survive or 63% ($1 − 1/e$) of cells are killed. D_0 is related to D_{10} by the following formula: $D_{10} = 2.3 × D_0$. For most tumors, the D_0 is estimated to be 1 to 2 Gy, and in fractionated external beam radiation, we typically deliver 1.8 or 2 Gy with each fraction.

Two theoretical experimental cell survival curves are shown in **Figure 12.8-11** under either low-dose rate (LDR) or high-dose rate (HDR) radiation conditions. The curve for LDR is best fit by a straight line, whereas the HDR curve is shown to have two components, an earlier linear component mirroring the LDR curve followed by a quadratic component. At higher doses of radiation, the HDR curve always has a higher proportion of cell kill than the LDR curve for any given dose. The rate at which radiation is delivered causes dramatic differences in the shape of the cell survival curve. This is best described by considering the linear quadratic model with DNA as the lethal target. In the linear quadratic model:

$$\text{Surviving fraction} = e^{-\alpha D - \beta D2}$$

where

α = constant for proportion of cell survival due to linear component

β = constant for proportion of cell survival due to quadratic component

D = dose of IR

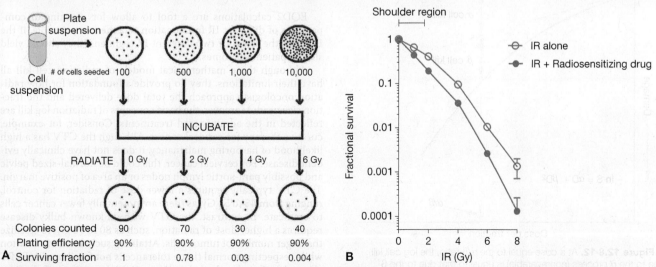

Colonies counted: 0 Gy = 90, 2 Gy = 70, 4 Gy = 30, 6 Gy = 40
Plating efficiency: 90%, 90%, 90%, 90%
A Surviving fraction: 1, 0.78, 0.03, 0.004

Figure 12.8-10. Clonogenic survival curves. Surviving fraction of irradiated cells. A: Cell culture technique used for clonogenic assays. A cell suspension of a known concentration of cells is used to seed differing number of cells in cell culture dishes. The cells are allowed to settle and then irradiated. Viable cells will replicate and form colonies visible to the naked eye. The plating efficiency is calculated in the nonirradiated condition and used to normalize the surviving fraction of irradiated cells. B: The surviving fraction is then plotted logarithmically on the y-axis and an ionizing radiation (IR) dose is plotted linearly on the x-axis (blue line). Red line shows decreased survival of cells that were treated with a radiosensitizer before irradiation.

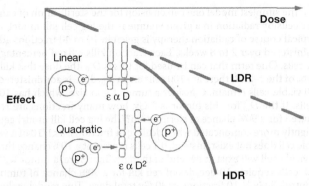

Figure 12.8-11. Cell killing by radiation is largely due to aberrations caused by breaks in two chromosomes. The dose-response curve for HDR irradiation is linear quadratic: The two breaks may be caused by the same electron (dominant at low doses) or by two different electrons (dominant at higher doses). For LDR irradiation, where radiation is delivered over a protracted period, the principal mechanism of cell killing is by the single electron. Consequently, the LDR survival curve is an extension of the low-dose region of the HDR survival curve. LDR, low-dose rate; HDR, high-dose rate.

The linear component is due to a single ejected electron causing both DSBs. The important point is that the degree of the linear component of cell kill, also known as α kill, is proportional to D because only one photon/electron is involved. The linear quadratic model also shows two chromosomal breaks, the result of two separate ejected Compton electrons by radiation. Cell kill accounted for by the quadratic portion, or β kill, is proportional to D^2 because two photons/electrons are involved. Looking at the HDR curve at low doses of radiation, there is very little β kill; however, at higher doses, the β component increases exponentially because of D^2. Under LDR conditions, the β component is absent, leaving only α kill. This is best explained by the idea that β kill involves damage to one chromosome and so is more easily repaired, provided that the radiation dose rate and rate of DSB formation are not significantly greater than the cell's repair capacity. The linear quadratic formula was used to generate **Figure 12.8-12**. The dashed line represents the α component and is generated by extrapolating the initial slope of the curve to higher doses of radiation. The point at which the α and β kill are equal is shown, and the dose at which this occurs is

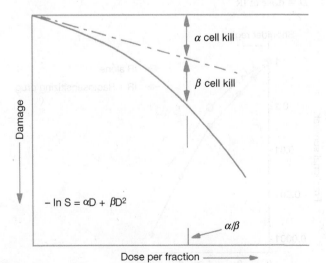

Figure 12.8-12. At a dose equal to the α/β ratio, the log cell kill due to the α process (nonreparable) is equal to that due to the β process (reparable injury): α/β is thus a measure of how soon the survival curve begins to bend over significantly. (Reprinted from Fowler JR. Fractionation and therapeutic gain. In: Steel GG, Adams GE, Peckham MJ, eds. *Biologic Basis of Radiotherapy.* Elsevier Science; 1983:181-194, with permission from Elsevier.)

called the α/β ratio. It is worth noting that the α/β ratio is a bit of a misnomer, as ratios are typically unitless values. However, α/β has the units of Gy. The α/β ratio for early side effects and tumor tissue is thought to be higher, approximately 10 Gy, than for late side effects, which is estimated to be 3 Gy.

Of clinical relevance is the α/β ratio, which helps to calculate biologically effective doses (BEDs). It is clear from **Figure 12.8-4** that both the total dose of radiation and the speed at which it is delivered can produce very different outcomes. The same holds true for fractionated courses of radiation. For example, 16 Gy delivered in a single treatment, as is the case for radiosurgery, can sterilize a small cancerous tumor of cancer cells. However, the same treatment delivered over 8 days would be clinically insignificant. **Figure 12.8-9** shows theoretical cell survival curves for early and late reactions under two separate experimental conditions, single fraction and multifraction regimens. A formula that normalizes a biologic end point under various dose-fractionation schemes is necessary (5). The α/β ratio from the linear quadratic equation has enabled the prediction of various biologic end points with different fractionation schemes and is given by the following equation:

$$BED = nd(1+d/(α/β))$$

where

BED = biologically effective dose
n = number of fractions
d = dose per fraction
$α/β$ = dose where the α component of cell kill equals the β component

BED calculations allow for comparison of two different dose-fractionation schemes in terms of tumor control/acute toxicity if α/β is 3, or late tissue complications when α/β is set to 10. An extension of this BED calculation is the ability to calculate the total dose delivered in 2 Gy fractions. This is particularly useful in gynecologic oncology patients where the radiation dose is delivered as both external beam radiotherapy and brachytherapy. A measure of the total dose delivered, if delivered as 2 Gy fractions, can be calculated using the EQD2 formula:

$$EQD2 = (BED_{EBRT} + BED_{BT})/(1 + 2/α/β)$$

where

BED_{EBRT}: external beam contribution to BED
BED_{BT}: brachytherapy contribution to BED

EQD2 calculations are a tool to allow for meaningful comparisons of different IR fractionation schemes. In principle, if the EQD2 is the same for two different IR regimens, they should yield similar patient outcomes.

Although these mathematical models of radiation cell kill all have their limitations, they do provide a foundation for how radiation oncologists approach the total dose delivered and the fraction size used. Moreover, the basic concepts of radiation log kill are reflected in the administered treatments. Consider, for example, curative therapy for cervical cancer. Although the CTV has a high likelihood of harboring malignancy, it does not have clinically evident disease. For cervical cancer, this could be normal-sized pelvic and possibly para-aortic lymph nodes or an area of positive margin. The CTV typically requires a lower dose of radiation for control, ranging from 45 to 54 Gy, as there are potentially fewer cancer cells to eradicate. In contrast, the GTV with its known bulky disease requires a higher dose of radiation, such as 80 to 90 Gy, to sterilize the larger number of tumor cells. Attaining such doses of radiation while respecting normal tissue tolerance is not feasible with EBRT alone; therefore, brachytherapy is required. In contrast, if a patient undergoes a hysterectomy in which bulk tumor is removed, then there is no GTV, and brachytherapy is often not needed because dose to the CTV can be safely administered by external beam radiation therapy or lower doses of brachytherapy alone.

Factors Influencing Tissue Sensitivity to Radiation Therapy

The previous discussion provides the general biologic basis of how IR interacts with cells. However, the clinical utility of radiation therapy is dependent on tumor and normal tissue characteristics that play a pivotal role in how radiotherapy is delivered and its efficacy. There are four classic factors that have been termed the "4 R's" of radiobiology: (1) repair, (2) repopulation, (3) reassortment, and (4) reoxygenation. These "4 R's" provide a rationale and framework for the fundamental basis of using fractionated radiotherapy.

Repair

With DNA being the critical target, radiation therapy needs to selectively damage the DNA of tumor cells yet spare the surrounding normal tissues. The simplest solution would be to deposit IR dose to tumor cells and not to normal tissues. Current technology using IMRT and brachytherapy techniques makes it possible for IR doses to better conform to tumors and spare the critical normal tissues in close proximity. Radiobiologically, tumor and normal tissue often have a differential capacity for DNA damage repair that can be exploited to widen the therapeutic ratio of IR. In survival curves of irradiated cells, a "shoulder" region is apparent at lower doses. Following IR, cells attempt to repair the DNA damage. At high doses, the repair processes are overwhelmed and cell death occurs in an exponential manner. However, at lower doses, cells are able to repair the DNA damage if sufficient time is given before the delivery of another dose of IR. Therefore, this "shoulder" region of the survival curve represents sublethal damage repair (19). The dose range of IR within the shoulder region is often within the clinically relevant doses of D_0. A consequence of genomic instability within cancer cells is decreased DNA damage repair capacity compared to normal tissue. Graphically, the "shoulder" region of irradiation survival curves is wider in noncancerous cells compared to cancer cells (**Figure 12.8-13**). Therefore, instead of delivering one large dose of IR, the total IR dose is split into smaller doses that are delivered over weeks. Note that by breaking up the radiotherapy in fractions, the shoulder of the cell survival curve is repeated, and by doing this, we are able to amplify the ability of normal tissue to repair and tolerate IR damage while tumor cells are preferentially killed. Also of importance is that sublethal DNA damage repair takes hours to occur and provides a rationale for delivering fractionated external beam radiotherapy once daily, to allow time for normal tissues to recover from radiation-induced DNA damage.

Repopulation

Although fractionating IR allows for sublethal damage repair in normal tissue, it needs to be balanced against the concept of tumor repopulation. Following tumor irradiation, a phenomenon of accelerated repopulation has been demonstrated to occur (20,21). In accelerated repopulation, stress responses and death of a proportion of the tumor result in surviving tumor cells proliferating more rapidly. To combat this, the overall time in which the total radiotherapy package (external beam and brachytherapy) is delivered to patients should be minimized. Avoidance of treatment breaks because of acute radiotherapy/chemotherapy side effects to the normal tissues (bowel, bladder, bone marrow) is paramount, as treatment breaks may compromise patient outcomes by allowing cancerous cells to proliferate, negating the goals of therapy. Clinical data support such a concept in patients with cervical cancer, where an increase in overall radiotherapy treatment time has been shown to negatively affect outcomes.

Reassortment

Interestingly, intrinsic sensitivity to IR varies with the cell cycle. The cell cycle is an orderly progression resulting in DNA replication and division into two daughter cells (**Figure 12.8-14**) (22,23). S phase stands for "synthesis" and is where DNA replication occurs. M phase stands for "mitosis" and is when cellular division occurs to create two daughter cells. In between are the G_1 and G_2 phases, standing for "gap 1" and "gap 2." Late S phase tends to be the most radioresistant phase of the cell cycle because the DNA repair machinery for replication can also repair radiation damage. In contrast, the M phase is also the most radiosensitive phase of the cell cycle because once the cell enters into M phase, it will attempt to divide without arresting. Therefore, any DNA damage caused in M phase is likely to be passed along to the daughter cells and may be fatal. This is another important reason why rapidly dividing cells such as cancer cells are radiosensitive as opposed to slower proliferating normal tissue. Although M phase is the most radiosensitive, it is also unfortunately the portion of the cell cycle in which cells spend the least amount of time. Approximately 15% of cycling tumor cells are in G_2/M at a given moment. Therefore, the majority of tumor cells are in a relatively radioresistant phase of the cell cycle on any given day radiation is delivered. Fractionating and delivering IR over multiple days takes advantage of the fact that different populations of the tumor will be in G_2/M during each day's treatment and will have increased sensitivity to IR. In addition, IR-induced DNA damage results in cell cycle checkpoints, and in particular the G_2/M checkpoint. Checkpoints take cells temporarily out of the cell cycle

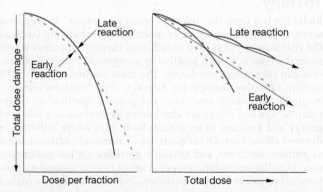

Figure 12.8-13. Difference in cell survival curves for acute and late radiation effects with single or multifractionated doses of irradiation. (Reprinted from Fowler JF. Fractionation and therapeutic gain. In: Steel GG, Adams GE, Peckham MT, eds. *Biologic Basis of Radiotherapy.* Elsevier Science; 1983:181, with permission from Elsevier.)

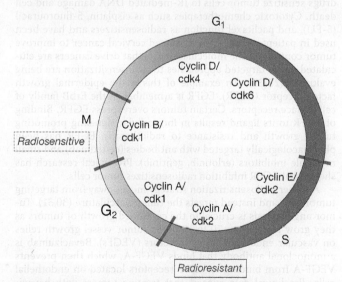

Figure 12.8-14. Cell cycle and variation in radiosensitivity. As cells replicate, they pass through phases of the cell cycle where a unique cyclin and cyclin-dependent kinase (cdk) heterodimer is formed. Each cyclin/cdk heterodimer phosphorylates and activates a unique set of proteins required for completion of that phase. DNA synthesis occurs in S phase, which is the most radioresistant phase. Cell division occurs in M phase, which is the most radiosensitive phase of the cell cycle.

so they can assess and respond to their damage. IR can synchronize tumor cells so that the following day a greater fraction will be in the radiosensitive G_2/M phase of the cell cycle.

Reoxygenation

Oxygen within tumor cells alters sensitivity to radiation (24,25). Under hypoxic conditions, cells are relatively resistant to radiation compared to oxygenated tumors. The oxygen enhancement ratio (OER) for radiation is approximately 3, which implies the dose of radiation required under hypoxic conditions is 3 times that needed under aerated conditions to create a similar level of cell kill. Oxygen is known to chemically modify radiation-induced DNA damage by creating a DNA-peroxide bond, thereby making it very difficult to repair by the cell. This is known as the oxygen fixation hypothesis (26). Therefore, under hypoxic conditions, one would expect DNA damage repair to be more effective, and higher dose would, therefore, be required to kill cells.

Tumor hypoxia can be categorized as either acute or chronic. Acute hypoxia is perfusion limited and occurs due to temporary closures of vasculature secondary to temporary vasospasms and malformed tumor blood vessels. As with tumor reassortment, areas of acute hypoxia within the tumor will vary from day to day, as do the cells in G_2/M. Areas of the tumor that were acutely hypoxic on a given day may have increased blood flow and oxygen delivery on subsequent days of radiation. In contrast to the perfusion limits of acute hypoxia, chronic hypoxia is defined as diffusion limited and occurs as tumor growth outstrips its vasculature. In tissue, oxygen can diffuse a distance of 70 to 100 μm from blood vessels. Therefore, tumor cells that are located further from the vasculature have decreased oxygen delivery and are relatively resistant to IR.

Combining Radiotherapy With Systemic Therapies

For locally advanced cancers, patient outcomes are improved when radiotherapy is combined with chemotherapy (2-4). Rationales for delivery of chemotherapy concurrently with radiotherapy are as follows: (1) it allows delivery of the entire treatment package in a more compact time frame; (2) radiotherapy and chemotherapy kill cancer cells by different mechanisms, making it more difficult for resistant tumor clones to survive; and (3) certain chemotherapy drugs sensitize tumor cells to IR-mediated DNA damage and cell death. Cytotoxic chemotherapies such as cisplatin, 5-fluorouracil (5-FU), and paclitaxel function as radiosensitizers and have been used in patients with locally advanced cervical cancer to improve tumor control. As the molecular events that drive cancers are elucidated, more targeted approaches to radiosensitization are being evaluated (27-29). An example of this is the epidermal growth factor receptor (EGFR). EGFR is a member of the ErbB family of cell surface receptors. Certain tumors overexpress EGFR. Binding of EGFR to its ligand results in intracellular signaling promoting tumor growth and resistance to radiotherapy. EGFR has been pharmacologically targeted with antibodies (cetuximab) and small molecule inhibitors (erlotinib, gefitinib). Preclinical research has shown that EGFR inhibition radiosensitizes tumor cells.

Another radiosensitization strategy moves away from targeting tumor cells and instead targets the tumor vasculature (30,31). Tumor angiogenesis is crucial to the continued growth of tumors as they grow larger than 70 to 100 μm. Tumor vessel growth relies on vascular endothelial growth factors (VEGFs). Bevacizumab is a monoclonal antibody that binds VEGF-A, which then prevents VEGF-A from binding to VEGF receptors located on endothelial cells. Preclinical data suggest that treating tumors with bevacizumab can also radiosensitize them. Bevacizumab can potentially interact with IR in two distinct ways. First, via the decrease in VEGF receptor, signaling endothelial cells are more likely to be killed by IR (32). Second, treating tumors with bevacizumab results in "renormalization" of the tumor vasculature (30). Tumor vasculature is more chaotically organized than blood vessels in normal tissue due to an imbalance of pro- and antiangiogenesis factors. This results in increased permeability and interstitial pressure within tumors and has the untoward consequence of decreasing both chemotherapy and oxygen delivery to tumor cells. Bevacizumab helps to restore the balance of pro- and antiangiogenesis factors. By increasing cytotoxic chemotherapy and oxygen delivery to tumors, bevacizumab can also increase the sensitivity of tumor cells to IR-mediated cell death.

Finally, immunotherapy is emerging as a paradigm-shifting approach to cancer therapy that can be combined with radiotherapy (31,33,34). Although the concept is not new, elucidation of mechanisms involved in immune tolerance of tumor growth has resulted in the discovery of new pharmacologic targets. As cancers evolve, they develop strategies to hide from the immune system through immune checkpoints that downregulate immune responses. Two checkpoint inhibitors have begun to show clinical efficacy. Ipilimumab is an antibody against cytotoxic T-lymphocyte antigen 4 (CTLA-4). Nivolumab and pembrolizumab are antibodies against programmed cell death protein 1 (PD-1). While antibodies to CTLA-4 and PD-1 reverse tumor immune suppression, they do so by distinct nonoverlapping mechanisms. Interestingly, IR has also been shown to evoke a tumor immune response that results in an abscopal effect. In preclinical animal models that harbor multiple tumors, localized treatment of a single tumor with IR can result in tumor shrinkage in the other nonirradiated tumors (ie, abscopal effect). More recently, trials in patients with cancer with metastatic disease suggest that radiotherapy to a single tumor site, in combination with activation of the immune system by either interleukin (IL)-2 or checkpoint inhibitors, can result in abscopal responses (35,36). The abscopal effect is a phenomenon observed in patients with metastatic cancer, where treating only a single metastasis with focal radiotherapy also results in distant nontreated tumors shrinking. Although these data are early, they do suggest a novel and important role for radiotherapy in modulating tumor immune responses in patients that are distinct from IR's conventional role of being a local therapy that kills cancer cells by inducing DNA damage. As these and other targeted approaches are translated from the laboratory to clinical testing, the development of more personalized approaches to using radiotherapy in patients with cancer will improve tumor control and decrease toxicity to normal tissue.

INTRODUCTION TO RADIATION PHYSICS

Radiation physics is the study of the interaction of radiation with matter. In the treatment of patients with radiation, this matter is either tumor tissue or normal tissues, such as the skin, the internal organs, or the supporting tissues and structures.

Units Used in Radiation and Radiation Therapy

Radiation is a term that refers to "energy in transit." In a general sense, it can be categorized as ionizing or nonionizing (such as the visible light). IR is used in radiation therapy, a process where neutral atoms acquire a positive or a negative charge. This process can take numerous forms. The most common forms of IR used in radiation therapy are x-rays, γ-rays, neutrons (electromagnetic radiation), electrons, and protons (particulate radiation). X-rays and γ-rays are also known as photons or packets of energy and are used to treat most body sites where radiation is deemed efficacious. Other particles or forms of radiation, such as protons, neutrons, and heavier α particles, are less commonly used in radiation therapy, except in select clinical situations. Protons, other heavy charged particles, and neutrons have a higher linear energy transfer coefficient when compared to high-energy photons and, therefore, are more efficient at transferring or depositing their energy in tissue. Protons are used increasingly in the treatment of prostate cancers, choroidal melanomas, skull base and paraspinal tumors, and pediatric tumors. Neutrons have been used for salivary gland tumors, sarcomas, and prostate cancers. Protons are positively charged particles that can be accelerated in an electric field to high energies. The primary characteristic of a proton beam is its Bragg peak. The Bragg peak describes the depth at which the majority of a proton's energy is deposited. Before the depth of the Bragg peak, only a very small amount of the proton energy is deposited. The Bragg peak depth is determined by the energy of the incident protons and covers only very small width of tissue at that depth. In order to cover more tissue, the energy of the incoming proton beam is varied. The net dose deposition results in a low entrance dose and a finely controlled width of treatment dose at depth. This makes proton treatments an excellent choice for the treatment of tumors adjacent to critical structures. Neutrons are relatively massive uncharged particles that can be generated by cyclotrons. Poor treatment geometry and dose distributions have limited the enthusiasm for neutron beam therapy (37).

X-rays and γ-rays are forms of electromagnetic radiation, similar to visible light, but with a much smaller wavelength, that is, greater energy. The only difference between x-rays and γ-rays is their respective origins. X-rays are derived from interactions in the atom that are outside the nucleus, typically by bombardment of the atom or target with high-speed electrons. This is the source of radiation produced by most modern radiotherapy treatment machines known as linear accelerators or LINACs. Their name derives from acceleration of these electrons. γ-Rays arise from a process within the nucleus of the atom called radioactive decay, which occurs in brachytherapy sources and cobalt (^{60}Co) teletherapy treatment machines. This type of electromagnetic radiation can penetrate several millimeters to centimeters of normal tissue in close proximity to tumors or tissues at risk. There is increased penetration as the energy of the γ-rays is increased. The x-rays produced by LINACs are much more penetrating (due to their high energy) than ^{60}Co γ-rays and are used to treat tumors or tissues at a distance from the LINAC, such as deep within the pelvis or abdomen.

Electrons are forms of particulate radiation and considered to be small (compared to the nucleus), negatively charged particles. Because of their inherent charge, these particles interact more strongly with the atoms found in tissue. Electrons will usually only penetrate a few millimeters to centimeters in tissue. Similar to photons, the higher the energy of the electron, the farther it will penetrate into the tissue. Electrons are used to treat tumors or tissues close to the skin surface such as superficial inguinal nodes and tumors of the skin, including vulvar cancers.

Regarding photon interactions with tissue, the dominant process at energies used in radiation therapy is termed the Compton effect (**Figure 12.8-15**). The probability that a photon will interact

TABLE 12.8-1. SI Units for Radiation Therapy			
Quantity	SI Unit (Special Name)	Non-SI Unit	Conversion Factor
Exposure	C kg^{-1}	roentgen (R)	1 C kg^{-1} ≈ 3,876 R
Absorbed dose, kerma	J kg^{-1} (gray [Gy])	rad	1 Gy = 100 rad
Dose equivalent	J kg^{-1} (sievert [Sv])	rem	1 Sv = 100 rem
Activity	s^{-1} (becquerel [Bq])	curie	1 Bq = 2.7 × 10^{-11} Ci

with a target atom is inversely proportional to the energy of the incident photon and nearly independent of the atomic number of the target material. As a result, at the energies used in radiation therapy, termed megavoltage (MV), the absorbed dose in normal tissues is comparable to that in nearby bone. At much lower energies, termed kilovoltage (kV), the absorbed dose would scale with the atomic number of the target with higher absorbed dose in bone compared to normal soft tissues.

At the Second International Congress of Radiology in 1928, the basic unit of radiation exposure, the roentgen (R), was defined (37). Although the original definition evolved over time, the fundamental idea remained the same. The roentgen is the amount of photon radiation that causes 0.001293 g of air to produce one electrostatic unit of positive or negative charge (esu). The value of 0.001293 g is the mass of 1 cc of air at a temperature of 0°C and a pressure of 760 mm Hg. The definition of the roentgen can also be expressed in other equivalent terms:

$$1 \text{ R} = 2.58 \times 10^{-4} \text{ C/kg air}$$

or, conversely, expressed in SI units, the unit of exposure is defined by

$$1 \text{ C/kg} = 3,876 \text{ R}$$

Table **12.8-1** lists some basic units of radiation and radiation therapy, both in historic context and in terms of modern SI units. Kerma (kinetic energy release per unit mass) defines the transfer of energy from photons to directly ionized particles. These directly ionized particles, in turn, transfer some of their energy to the medium (usually tissue). This transfer of energy is defined as the absorbed dose to the medium from the radiation beam. The SI unit for kerma is joule per kilogram (J/kg) or gray (Gy). In a slightly confusing definition, the SI unit for absorbed dose is also joule per kilogram or gray. The term gray has replaced the previously used term "rad." Oftentimes, the term centigray (cGy) is used. The cGy is equivalent to the rad, and 1 gray equals 100 cGy.

Another rationale to think and communicate in SI units is that the roentgen was defined explicitly for photon interactions and not for charged particles. Kerma and absorbed dose, although they have equivalence to the roentgen and exposure, can be defined equally for photons and charged particles.

RADIATION PRODUCTION

Radionuclides

As mentioned before, γ-rays are typically derived from radionuclides, such as ^{60}Co. Electrons or β particles also come from radionuclides. In fact, most radioactive material produces a combination of photons (γ-rays) and electrons during the decay process. Radioactivity is the result of an atom changing its "energy" state, usually to a lower "energy" state, by the emission/absorption/internal conversion of photons or electrons in the atom. These processes result

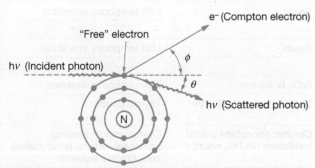

Figure 12.8-15. Schematic drawing illustrating the process of the Compton effect. The incident photon interacts with one of the atom's outer electrons, and the energy is shared between the ejected electron and a scattered photon. (From Purdy JA. Principles of radiologic physics, dosimetry, and treatment planning. In: Perez CA, Brady LW, eds. *Principles and Practice of Radiation Oncology.* 3rd ed. Lippincott-Raven Publishers; 1998, with permission.)

in disintegrations or radioactive decay, whereby the atom releases photons or electrons or both during the change in "energy" states. The release of these particles is a form of radiation (or energy) that can be used to irradiate tissues. The absorbed dose resulting from this radiation depends on the energy and particle type as mentioned earlier, as well as the tissue in which it interacts.

Radioactivity, or activity, is denoted by the symbol A and is defined as the number of disintegrations per unit of time. The following relationship defines activity, the decay constant, and, ultimately, the half-life for a radioactive material:

$$A = N/t = \gamma N$$

This equation is solved using an exponential solution:

$$A = Aoe - \lambda^t$$

where A is the initial activity, l is the decay constant, and t is some unit of time later. Other important concepts for radioactivity and radioactive decay are the half-life, $T_{1/2}$, and the average life, T_a. The half-life is the amount of time needed to reduce the original amount of material by half. This is also equivalent to reducing the original

activity by half. $T_{1/2}$ is related to the decay constant by $T_{1/2} = 0.693/l$. The average life represents the period of time that a hypothetical source would need, if it retained its original activity for a fixed period of time (T_a) before suddenly decaying to zero activity, to produce the same number of disintegrations over an infinite amount of time by the same source if it decayed exponentially. T_a is related to the decay constant and the half-life by $T_a = 1/l = 1.44\ T_{1/2}$.

Radionuclides can occur naturally or be created artificially. Artificially created radionuclides are usually created by neutron bombardment of otherwise stable isotopes. The resulting interactions produce atoms that are inherently unstable and will decay to a more stable form with a predictable half-life, releasing energy or radiation through this decay. Naturally occurring radionuclides originally come from one of three standard series—the uranium series, the actinium series, and the thorium series—so named because of a dominant radionuclide in each series. In general, the higher the atomic number, the more likely an isotope will be radioactive. **Table 12.8-2** lists many of the common radionuclides used in brachytherapy, along with their physical properties. For gynecologic cancers, use of radium 226 (^{226}Ra) sources is now historic. Though cost-effective because of its long half-life (1,622

■ TABLE 12.8-2. Physical Properties and Uses of Brachytherapy Radionuclides

Element	Isotope	Energy (MeV)	Half-Life	HVL-Lead (mm)	Source Form	Clinical Application
Obsolete Sealed Sources of Historic Significance						
Radium	^{226}Ra	0.83 (avg)	1,626 yr	16	Radium salt encapsulated in tubes and needles	LDR intracavitary and interstitial
Radon	^{222}Rn	0.83 (avg)	3.83 d	16	Radon	Permanent interstitial; temporary molds
Currently Used Sealed Sources						
Cesium	^{137}Cs	0.662	30 yr	6.5	Cesium salt encapsulated in tubes and needles	LDR intracavitary and interstitial
Iridium	^{192}Ir	0.380 (avg)	74 d	6	Seeds in nylon ribbon; encapsulated source on steel cable	LDR temporary interstitial; HDR interstitial and intracavitary
Cobalt	^{60}Co	1.25	5.26 yr	11	Encapsulated spheres	HDR intracavitary
Iodine	^{125}I	0.028	59.6 d	0.025	Seeds	Permanent interstitial
Palladium	^{103}Pd	0.020	17 d	0.013	Seeds	Permanent interstitial
Gold	^{198}Au	0.412	2.7 d	6	Seeds	Permanent interstitial
Strontium	^{90}Sr–^{90}Y	2.24 MeV β_{max}	28.9 yr	—	Plaque	Superficial ocular lesions
Cesium-131	^{131}Cs	0.030 MeV	9.7 d	0.042	Seeds	Permanent interstitial
Developmental Sealed Sources						
Americium	^{241}Am	0.060	432 yr	0.12	Tubes	LDR intracavitary
Ytterbium	^{169}Yb	0.093	32 d	0.48	Seeds	LDR temporary interstitial
Californium	^{252}Cf	2.4 (avg) neutrons	2.65 yr	—	—	—
Samarium	^{145}Sm	0.043	340 d	0.060	Seeds	LDR temporary interstitial
Unsealed Radioisotopes Used for Radiopharmaceutical Therapy						
Strontium	^{89}Sr	1.4 MeV β_{max}	51 d	—	SrCl$_2$ IV solution	Diffuse bone metastases
Iodine	^{131}I	0.61 MeV β_{max} 0.364 MeV g	8.06 d	—	Capsule NaI oral solution	Thyroid cancer
Phosphorus	^{32}P	1.71 MeV β_{max}	14.3 d	—	Chromic phosphate colloid instillation; Na$_2$PO$_3$ solution	Ovarian cancer seeding: peritoneal surface; polycythemia vera, chronic leukemia
Lutetium	^{177}Lu	0.5 MeV β_{max}	6.7 d	—	Injection solution for intravenous use	Prostate cancer (PSMA), Neuroendocrine tumor (Dotatate)
Yttrium	^{90}Y	2.28 MeV β_{max}	64.1 hr	—	Resin (SIR-spheres) or glass (TheraSpheres)	Unresectable hepatocellular carcinoma (HCC)

LDR, low-dose rate; HDR, high-dose rate; HVL, half-value layer.

years), radium releases a by-product, radon gas, if the mechanical integrity of the source capsule is compromised. This could require closure of hospital wards due to radon gas contamination. Cesium 137 (^{137}Cs) has replaced radium as a safer yet effective radionuclide. Less shielding is required for cesium than radium, and there is no risk of radon gas leakage. With a half-life of 30 years, it is also cost-effective owing to the infrequent need for replacement. Cesium can be used clinically for years without replacement, but the treatment duration must be adjusted to allow for radioactive decay (38). It is typically used for LDR gynecologic brachytherapy in tandem and ovoid and cylinder applicators. Iridium 192 (^{192}Ir) is produced in various source strengths and can be used for interstitial and intracavitary gynecologic implants. ^{192}Ir half-life of 74.2 days requires frequent replacement, and typically, this is custom ordered individually for each implant rather than stored in the radiation oncology department like ^{137}Cs sources. High activity ^{192}Ir (10Ci) sources are used for HDR brachytherapy and are replaced every 3 months, and lower activity ^{192}Ir sources are used for LDR brachytherapy.

Linear Accelerators

LINACs are another method of producing radiation for the treatment of malignancies. LINACs can produce both photon and electron beams of different energies, depending on their construction. The principles behind a LINAC involve accelerating an initial beam of electrons across a variable electric field. The greater the strength of the electric field, the more energetic the electron beam. This electron beam can be adjusted to control its shape and intensity before delivery to the patient. Alternatively, the electron beam can be directed to a tungsten target. The electron-target interaction creates a forward scattered photon beam or x-ray. The resulting photon beam can then be modified by the machine using filters and collimators to produce the desired radiation field shape.

Photon beams of different energies have a different absorbed dose pattern within tissues. This pattern is normally characterized as a percent depth dose or variation of dose as a function of depth within tissue, as shown in **Figures 12.8-16 and 12.8-17**, and by dose profiles, or variation of dose as a function of lateral distance at a given depth (**Figure 12.8-18**). The key feature in all of the figures is that higher energy photons deposit dose at greater depths. Because of the way dose is deposited and absorbed in tissue, the higher photon energy, the lesser the dose deposited at shallow depths toward the surface of the patient. This is called "skin sparing" and is a

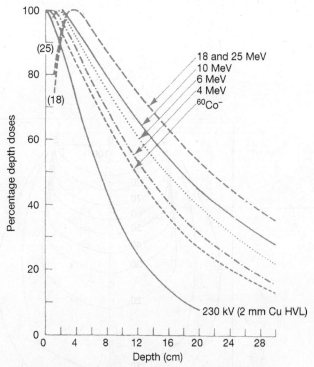

Figure 12.8-17. Typical x-ray or photon beam central axis percentage depth-dose curves for a 10 cm × 10 cm beam for 230 kV (2 mm Cu HVL) at 50 cm SSD; ^{60}Co and 4 MV at 80 cm SSD; and 6, 10, 18, and 25 MV at 100 cm SSD. The last two beams coincide at most depths, but not in the first few millimeters of the built-up region. The 4-, 6-, 18-, and 25-MV data are for the Varian Clinic 4, 6, 20, and 35 units, respectively, at the Department of Radiation Oncology, Washington University in St. Louis. HVL, half-value layer; SSD, source-to-skin distance. (Used with permission of British Institute of Radiology, from Cohen M, Jones DEA, Greene D. Central axis depth dose data for use in radiotherapy. *Br J Radiol.* 1972;11:21; permission conveyed through Copyright Clearance Center, Inc)

characteristic of high-energy photons. In fact, the higher the photon energy, the deeper the point at which the maximum absorbed dose is deposited. After this D_{max}, the absorbed dose decreases because the photon beam is attenuated by the tissues through which it passes.

A pivotal treatment technique for the success of IMRT is IGRT (39-41). Historically, treatment setups were verified by orthogonal radiographs and treatment fields by port films or x-rays of the treatment fields superimposed on the patient. Modern LINACs have added onboard imaging (OBI) that facilitates electronic recording of the treatment fields at every treatment setup using an electronic portal imaging device (EPID). By comparing computer-generated radiographs (DRRs or digitally reconstructed radiographs) with the actual patient images, discrepancies in field shape and patient setup can be corrected before the delivered treatment. This type of corrective behavior before treatment is the foundation of IGRT. Over the past decade, the addition of CT imaging within the LINAC was implemented to verify the correct 3D alignment of the patient on the treatment table before each fraction delivery within minutes. Partial CT scans (not full 360° rotation) are obtained before each treatment. In some LINACs, the CT scans are obtained and constructed based on the therapeutic photon beams (MV). In other approaches, an x-ray source (kV) is used to acquire the CT scans. Because megavoltage CT (MV-cone beam computed tomography [CBCT]) uses the therapeutic high-energy photon beam (6 MV), the image quality suffers because of poor soft-tissue contrast. On the other hand, kV-CBCT has a lower energy photon source (<140 keV), which is used to acquire and reconstruct the patient image. kV-CBCT has better soft-tissue contrast than MV-CBCT but is prone to distorting artifacts from high-density objects within

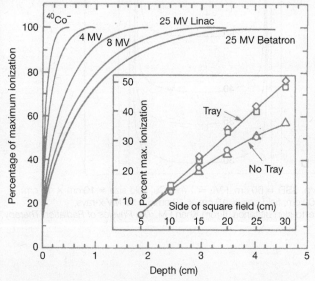

Figure 12.8-16. ^{60}Co to 25-MV x-rays. (From Velkley DE, Manson DJ, Purdy JA, et al. Build-up region of megavoltage photon radiation sources. *Med Phys.* 1975;2:14-19, with permission.)

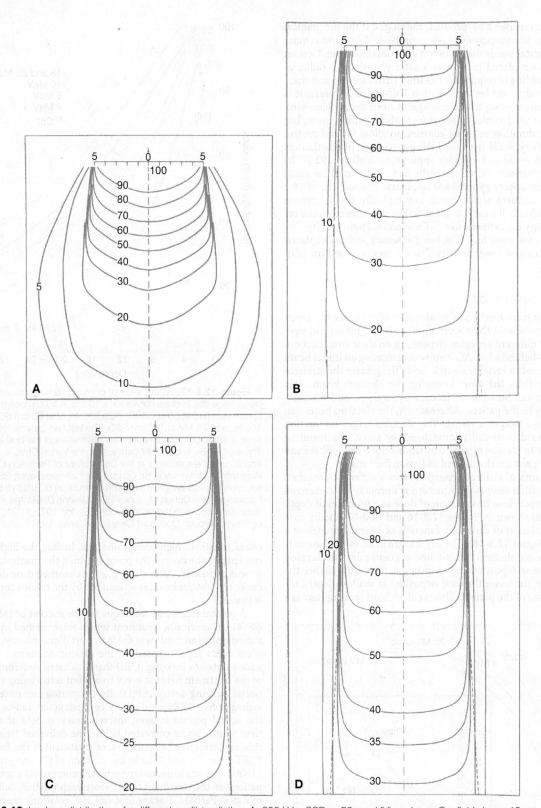

Figure 12.8-18. Isodose distributions for different quality radiation. A: 200 kVp, SSD = 50 cm, HVL = 1 mm Cu, field size = 10 cm × 10 cm. B: ^{60}Co, SSD = 80 cm, field size = 10 cm × 10 cm. C: 4-MV x-rays, SSD = 100 cm, field size = 10 cm × 10 cm. D: 10-MV x-rays, SSD = 100 cm, field size = 10 cm × 10 cm. HVL, half-value layer; SSD, source-to-skin distance. (From Khan FM. *The Physics of Radiation Therapy.* 2nd ed. Williams & Wilkins; 1994, with permission.)

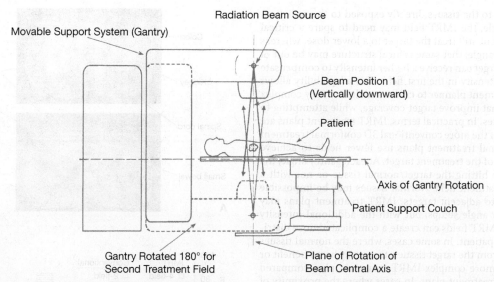

Figure 12.8-19. Example of multifield radiation therapy using parallel opposite beams with an isocentrically mounted radiation source.

the patient, such as hip prostheses. For either image modality, the CT image at the time of treatment and its corresponding isocenter location are compared to the treatment planning CT and isocenter for agreement. Adjustments for rotation, lateral, vertical, and longitudinal discrepancies are made before treatment. The intent of these IGRT methods is to improve the accuracy of the treatment setup on a daily basis relative to the original treatment plan. This enables decreasing the size of the radiation fields, as there is not as much need for a large margin on the target, which can decrease normal tissue irradiation and even allow for dose escalation to the target. Guidelines for use of IGRT have been published by the American Society for Radiation Oncology (ASTRO) and the American College of Radiology (ACR) (42). Online MRI has recently been added to the MR-LINAC (Elekta) or a Cobalt-60–based LINAC (ViewRay) to allow for real-time IGRT with superior soft-tissue resolution as compared to kV-CBCT of intact cancers, such as cervical or vaginal cancers, to guide treatment accuracy. Adapting the radiation therapy shape and dose while the patient is on the table holds promise to allow increasing doses to the target and minimizing doses to normal tissues by adjusting, in real time, to the anatomy of the day.

Figure 12.8-19 shows a simplified drawing of a LINAC. The gantry (or part of the LINAC where radiation exits the machine) can rotate 360° around the patient on the treatment table. The table

can also be rotated about the vertical axis of the radiation beam. This combination of angles allows the radiation to be directed to almost any part of a patient's body.

Modern LINACs are equipped with multileaf collimators (MLCs) and asymmetric jaws to control the shape of the radiation beam directed before it reaches the patient (**Figure 12.8-20**). Before asymmetric jaws and MLCs, photon beam shaping was achieved using poured blocks mounted below the lowest machine jaws. The composition and thickness of the poured block material are sufficient to block more than 97% of the radiation, allowing less than 3% of the radiation to penetrate the block and reach the patient. MLCs have mostly replaced poured blocks, but in some cases, poured blocks are still necessary for detailed field shaping.

MLCs are small (projected size at the patient ~1 cm), adjustable collimators built into the LINAC gantry that work together to create a shaped opening mimicking the effects of a poured block. Because each MLC is adjustable, a new field shape can be "programmed" into the gantry without the necessity of pouring a different block for every treatment field. With the advent of computer-controlled motion of the MLCs, the radiation field can be further controlled to produce an IMRT treatment. In IMRT treatments, the MLCs are used to create many small fields of radiation within a larger treatment field. By opening and closing these small fields, the intensity at any point within the large field can be modulated to give

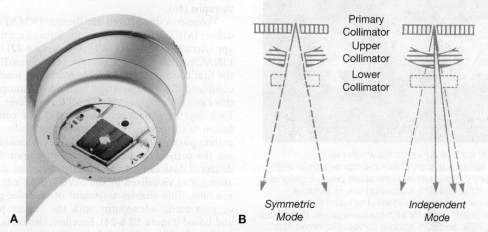

Figure 12.8-20. A: Multileaf collimator. B: Treatment technique for breast cancer using independent collimators. (From Purday JA, Klein EE. External photon beam dosimetry and treatment planning. In: Perez CA, Brady LW, eds. *Principles and Practice of Radiation Oncology*. 3rd ed. Lippincott-Raven Publishers; 1998:281, with permission. Image courtesy of Varian Medical Systems, Inc. All rights reserved.)

more or less dose to the tissues directly exposed to the radiation. At one gantry angle, the IMRT field may need to spare a critical normal structure but still treat the target to a lower dose, whereas in another gantry angle, that same critical structure may be out of the field and the target can receive a higher intensity to compensate for the lowered intensity in the first field. This adaptability allows the radiation treatment planner to create and deliver very complex treatment fields that improve target coverage, while attempting to spare normal tissues. In practical terms, IMRT treatment plans are an improvement of the more conventional 3D conformal treatment plans. 3D conformal treatment plans use fewer fields to achieve nominal coverage of the treatment target. At each gantry angle, the radiation is either hitting the target/normal tissue or not with a simple shaped treatment field. Normal tissues may be impossible to spare, relative to adjacent targets. IMRT treatment plans may use similar gantry angle setups, but with the additional intensity modulation, the IMRT fields can create a complicated dose distribution within the patient. In some cases, where the normal tissues are relatively far from the target tissues, there may be no benefit or rationale for the more complex IMRT treatment plan compared to 3D conformal treatment plans. In cases where the proximity of normal tissues and target varies across a field and between gantry angles, IMRT may prove the more efficient treatment plan to protect normal tissues while focusing dose onto the target (**Figures 12.8-21 and 12.8-22**). National guidelines have been created for the safe and appropriate use of IMRT (43,44). IMRT may be appropriate and ideal for the treatment of gynecologic cancers (45).

Stereotactic body radiation therapy (SBRT) is an external beam radiation therapy method used to precisely deliver a high dose

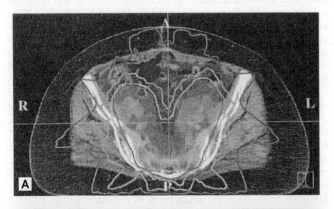

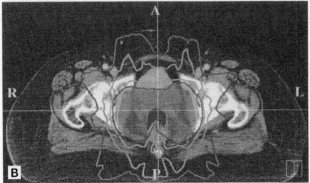

Figure 12.8-21. A: Isodose curves from a whole-pelvic intensity-modulated radiation therapy plan superimposed on an axial computed tomography (CT) slide through the upper pelvis. Highlighted are the 100%, 90%, 70%, and 50% isodose curves. B: Isodose curves from a whole-pelvic intensity-modulated radiation therapy plan superimposed on an axial CT slide through the lower pelvis. Highlighted are the 100%, 90%, 70%, and 50% isodose curves. (Reprinted from Mundt AJ, Lujan AE, Rotmensch J, et al. Intensity-modulated whole pelvic radiotherapy in women with gynecologic malignancies. *Int J Radiat Oncol Biol Phys.* 2002;52:1330, with permission from Elsevier.)

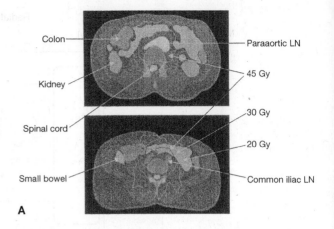

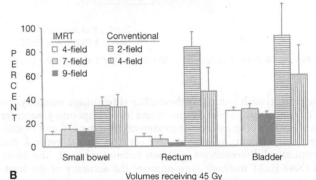

Figure 12.8-22. A: Axial views of intensity-modulated radiation therapy (IMRT) dose distribution. B: The functional volume of the small bowel, rectum, and bladder receiving ≥45 Gy with IMRT and conventional techniques when 100% of the target volume (uterus) receives ≥95% of the prescription dose (45 Gy). LN, lymph node. (Reprinted from Portelance L, Chao KSCC, Grigsby PW, et al. Intensity-modulated radiation therapy (IMRT) reduces small bowel and bladder doses in patients with cervical cancer receiving pelvic and paraaortic irradiation. *Int J Radiat Oncol Biol Phys.* 2001;51:261-266, with permission from Elsevier.)

of radiation to a target within the body using a small number of fractions, five treatments or less. SBRT is characterized by patient immobilization, limiting normal OAR to high doses of radiation, accounting for organ motion, and subcentimeter accuracy of delivered dose. The components of SBRT procedure include target delineation, treatment planning, and treatment delivery with a team, including a radiation oncologist, medical physicist, and radiation therapist (46).

Volumetric-modulated arc therapy (VMAT) has been used to deliver IMRT. TomoTherapy is one form of arc therapy. TomoTherapy (AccuRay, Madison, WI) (**Figure 12.8-23**) is a special type of LINAC/helical CT combination (41). TomoTherapy units were the first commercially available treatment machines that directly combined CT (megavoltage computed tomography [MVCT] in this case) with highly complex MLCs to deliver IMRT using IGRT. Each day, the patient receives an MVCT, a comparison using 3D fusion to the original treatment plan is made, adjustments to the patient position are made, and IMRT treatment is delivered without the patient needing to change machines. Corrections to the delivered dose can even be modeled based on the patient's current anatomy as visualized by the MVCT built into the TomoTherapy machine. This enables treatment of complex presentations such as para-aortic adenopathy with the closely positioned kidneys and bowel (**Figure 12.8-24**). Excellent clinical outcomes have been published with rotational therapy for these types of presentations (47). Currently, all modern LINACs can deliver sophisticated and dynamic radiation arcs; examples are the Varian (RapidArc) and

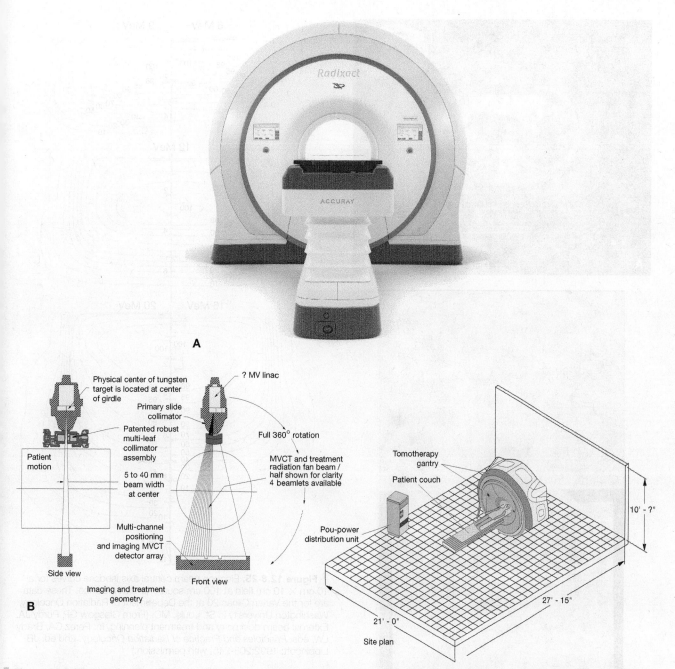

Figure 12.8-23. A: Helical TomoTherapy device commercially available for intensity-modulated radiation therapy. B: Diagrammatic representation of the device. MVCT, megavoltage computed tomography. (Images used with permission from Accuray Incorporated.)

Elekta (VMAT). The LINAC controls gantry speed, aperture shape, and dose rates to generate their arc therapy treatments. Both vendors use the same principle of modulating the beam aperture while the gantry is moving in arc to minimize the time and monitor units while improving dose conformality.

For gynecologic cancer treatments for targets near the surface, electron beams produced by the LINAC are commonly used (range 4-21 MeV). Electron beams have different depth dose and dose profiles as compared to photon beams; as shown in **Figure 12.8-25**, electrons do not penetrate as far as photons do within human tissues. While electron depth doses have a D_{max} that increases with increasing energy, unlike photons, the higher the electron energy, the higher the surface dose to tissue, that is, loss of "skin sparing." Electrons have been used in the treatment of vulvar and other cancers

that involve the inguinal lymph nodes. Great care has to be taken when using electrons in this setting as the inguinal lymph nodes can be very deep in women with higher BMI and will underdose nodes at a depth greater than 3 cm. This resulted in an increased risk of inguinal failures in the GOG 88 study (48). Electrons can be used to treat the vulva in patients with close or positive vulvar margins or in combination with higher energy beams to treat the inguinal nodes in patients with lower BMI. Proper delineation of the inguinal lymph nodes is essential in determining the most appropriate technique to treat them (49).

Beyond photons and electrons, proton therapy (PT) has been proposed for locally advanced cervical cancer and/or lymph node–positive tumors. Similar to photon beam IMRT, protons can also be modulated, hence the term intensity-modulated PT (IMPT). It has

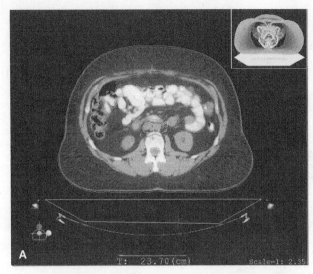

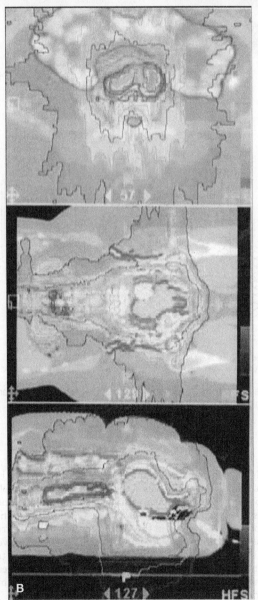

Figure 12.8-24. A: Contours of enlarged para-aortic nodes with margin are shown in close proximity to the small bowel. B: Intensity-modulated radiation therapy plan for extended-field irradiation in axial, coronal, and sagittal projections.

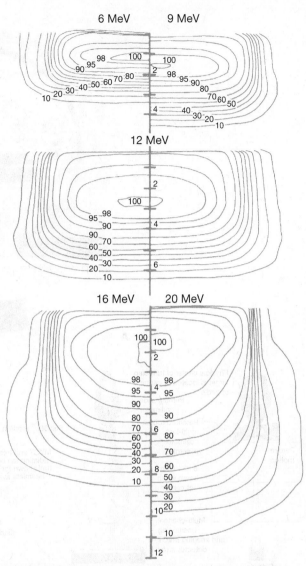

Figure 12.8-25. Electron beam central axis isodose curves for a 10 cm × 10 cm field at 100 cm source-to-skin distance. These data are for the Varian Clinac 20 at the Department of Radiation Oncology, Washington University in St. Louis, MO. (From Glasgow GP, Purdy JA. External beam dosimetry and treatment planning. In: Perez CA, Brady LW, eds. *Principles and Practice of Radiation Oncology*. 2nd ed. JB Lippincott; 1992:208-245, with permission.)

been shown using a preliminary study that in patients not eligible for brachytherapy, IMPT might have the potential to act as a boost to photon beam therapy and can be superior to IMRT or VMAT (50).

Simulation

The conventional simulator used in radiation oncology departments reproduces all the gantry, collimator, and table rotations used in a LINAC treatment and therefore "simulates" the actual treatment. Instead of a therapy (MV) photon beam, the conventional simulator uses a diagnostic (**Figure 12.8-26A**) and allowed the radiation oncologist to determine beam direction and treatment fields that would be needed for a radiotherapy treatment based on x-ray fluoroscopy. The radiographic visualization of internal structures allowed special shielding (poured blocks) to be constructed. All the geometric parameters of the conventional simulator are nearly identical to the actual treatment LINACs. The intersections of the gantry rotation axis, collimator rotation axis (the machine isocenter), and patient location are identified and marked on the patient's skin with removable ink or a permanent series of tattoos. These marks facilitate the reproduction of the same clinical setup for the patient each day of treatment. Hardcopy radiographs can also be used to document the expected treatment fields for comparison with port films obtained on the treatment LINAC.

CT-based simulators ("CTSims") have largely replaced conventional simulators in most radiation oncology departments. CTSims (**Figure 12.8-26B**) combine a diagnostic CT scanner with a software package that allows for the simulation of the patient setup in the virtual world of the computer. All of the necessary gantry angles and table angles are modeled in the computer. Computer-controlled room lasers tied into the CTSim software allow the simulator therapist to identify the treatment isocenter in a way similar to the conventional simulator (Virtual Sims). DRRs are created for later comparison to actual treatment images. The treatment isocenter and the full CT images can then be transferred to the computer planning system for further treatment planning. Some departments are also equipped with MR or PET scanners for treatment planning. Fusion of CT images with PET or MRI enables CT-based treatment planning with the benefit of improved tumor definition with PET or MR to reduce margin size or increase dose (51,52).

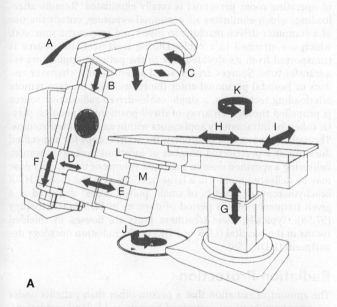

A

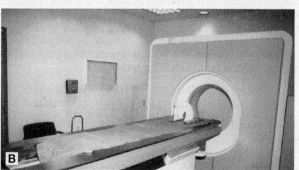

B

▎ **Figure 12.8-26.** A: The basic components and motions of a radiation therapy simulator. A, gantry rotation; B, source-axis distance; C, collimator rotation; D, image intensifier (lateral); F, image intensifier (longitudinal); F, image intensifier (radial); G, patient table (vertical); H, patient table (longitudinal); I, patient table (lateral); J, patient table rotation about isocenter; K, patient table rotation about pedestal; L, film cassette; M, image intensifier. Motions not shown include field size delineation, radiation beam diaphragms, and source-tray distance. B: Three-dimensional simulator that is basically a modified computed tomography scanner with a flat couch suite for treatment planning. (From Van Dyk J, Mah K. Simulators and CT scanners. In: Williams JR, Thwaites DI, eds. *Radiotherapy Physics*. Oxford Medical Publications; 1993:118 (7.3). Reprinted by permission of Oxford University Press.)

Computerized Dosimetry

In a modern radiotherapy department, computers are necessary to accurately calculate the absorbed doses to tissues. These absorbed doses within tissues are termed *isodoses*, or lines of the same dose. To initiate this process, CT images of the area of interest at a pretreatment planning session or simulation are acquired. These scans are typically obtained on the CT simulator. Treatment targets such as pelvic/para-aortic lymph nodes, the uterus, or vagina are identified through contouring on these images by the radiation oncologist, as are normal tissues such as the rectosigmoid, bladder, large and small bowel, kidneys, stomach, and spinal cord. Dose goals and constraints are identified for the targets and normal tissues, respectively. A dosimetrist uses this information to design the radiation treatment plan. Treatment beams are planned, and the resulting dosimetry is reviewed by the treating physician and a qualified medical physicist (QMP). The radiation plan is optimized as needed to best address the tumor and avoid the normal organs and tissues. In order for a computer treatment planning system to do all this, the depth dose and dose profiles for all of the treatment beams (photons and electrons) must be accurately entered into the planning system. This process is referred to as treatment planning commission, a task that is carefully performed by the QMP.

There are varying complexities of treatment plans that might be used. For simple targets, such as metastatic cancer to the spine, a simple single field or parallel opposed 2D plan might be all that is required. Complexities of internal anatomy and external surface contours can be ignored while still successfully delivering a palliative treatment plan to the patient. More complicated target definitions might require specific and accurate knowledge of adjacent internal anatomy and the details of the patient's surface in order to accurately deliver a successful treatment plan. In these cases, a 3D conformal treatment plan is developed. In still more complicated target/normal tissue regions, IMRT/VMAT/IMPT treatment planning might be required in order to give sufficient dose to the target while minimizing the dose to an adjacent normal tissue. The goal for most treatment plans is to treat the target to a specified dose while minimizing dose to adjacent normal tissues.

In all of these examples, the word "target" is used. The goal is to encompass the target with the desired dose. Targets are more formally defined in the International Commission on Radiation Units and Measurements (ICRU) 50 (53). **Figure 12.8-27** illustrates the GTV, the CTV, the PTV, and the treated volume. Each of the

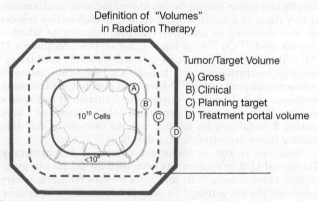

Definition of "Volumes" in Radiation Therapy

Tumor/Target Volume
A) Gross
B) Clinical
C) Planning target
D) Treatment portal volume

10^{10} Cells

$<10^6$

▎ **Figure 12.8-27.** Schematic representation of "volumes" in radiation therapy. The treatment portal volume includes the gross target volume, potential areas of local and regional microscopic disease around the tumor (clinical), and a margin of surrounding normal tissue (planning). (From Perez CA, Purdy JA. Rationale for treatment planning in radiation therapy. In: Levitt SH, Khan FM, Potish RA, eds. *Levitt and Tapley's Technological Basis of Radiation Therapy: Practical and Clinical Applications.* 2nd ed. Lea & Febiger; 1992. Modified in Perez CA, Brady LW, Roti JL. Overview. In: Perez CA, Brady LW, eds. *Principles and Practice of Radiation Oncology.* 3rd ed. Lippincott-Raven Publishers; 1998:1, with permission.)

target or tumor volumes is larger than the previous target volume by some margin. The CTV includes all of the GTV plus possible microscopic extensions. The PTV includes all of the CTV plus a margin to account for possible geometric uncertainties of the patient or treatment margin. The irradiated volume includes all of the PTV plus any margins that might be included in the treatment plan to provide minimum dose coverage to the PTV.

Brachytherapy Principles

Brachytherapy is a term with Greek roots where "brachy" means "short distance." With brachytherapy, a highly concentrated dose of radiation is delivered to immediately surrounding tissues within millimeters to several centimeters of the applicators that carry the radioactive sources (54). This allows for delivery of a high dose of radiation to closely approximated tumor while relatively sparing surrounding normal tissues, such as the rectosigmoid, bladder, and small bowel. This is in comparison to teletherapy, where "tele" means "far distance" and refers to external beam irradiation discussed earlier (photons/electron/protons), where the radiation source is at a greater distance from the patient (100 cm) than with brachytherapy, where sources are near the target. With external beam irradiation, the tumor and/or tumor bed are typically irradiated along with adjacent tissues at risk, such as lymph nodes. External beam irradiation is typically much more penetrating than brachytherapy unless electron beam external irradiation is used. With electron beam therapy, superficial structures such as the skin and/or superficial lymph nodes are optimally treated, unlike the deep abdominopelvic tissues, which are best irradiated with the penetrating photons produced by a LINAC.

There are different types of brachytherapy or radioactive implants (54,55). Temporary implants are used most frequently and are categorized as interstitial or intracavitary. With interstitial brachytherapy, the radioactive sources are transiently inserted into tumor-bearing tissues directly through placement in hollow needles or tubes. With intracavitary brachytherapy, radioactive sources are placed into naturally occurring body cavities or orifices, such as the vagina or uterus, using commercially available hollow applicators, such as a vaginal cylinder or tandem and ovoids. Temporary surface applications or plesiotherapy for ophthalmic or skin tumors and intraluminal applications in the esophagus, bronchus, and bile duct are other possible approaches. Permanent interstitial implants entail insertion of radioactive seeds (iodine 125 [^{125}I]; gold 198 [^{198}Au]; palladium 103 [^{103}Pd]) directly into tumor-bearing tissues to emit radiation continuously as they decay to a nonradioactive form (54). Radioactive sources are also described as sealed or unsealed, referring to whether they are solid (^{137}Cs; ^{192}Ir) or liquid radioisotopes (phosphorus 32 [^{32}P]). The most common sealed radioactive sources used for gynecologic brachytherapy are ^{192}Ir and ^{137}Cs. Historically, unsealed radioactive sources such as ^{32}P have been used to treat the entire peritoneal cavity in ovarian cancer. The limitation of this source was that the β-rays emitted penetrated only a distance of 3 mm, making it useful only for patients with microscopic or very thin residual tumor deposits following debulking.

Dose rate is also an important variable in brachytherapy. Traditional LDR irradiation has been used for decades in gynecologic cancers using ^{226}Ra and ^{137}Cs sources for intracavitary insertions and low activity ^{192}Ir sources for interstitial insertions. HDR brachytherapy has gradually been introduced over the past several decades and entails the use of a highly radioactive (10-Ci) ^{192}Ir source. There are several definitions for the dose rates used in brachytherapy. The ICRU 38 classifies LDR as 0.4 to 2 Gy/hr, MDR (medium-dose rate) as 2 to 12 Gy/hr, and HDR as greater than 12 Gy/hr (56). More standard ranges are 40 to 100 cGy/hr for LDR and 20 to 250 cGy/min for HDR, which is 1,200 to 15,000 cGy/hr. MDR is not common in the United States. Another approach is pulsed-dose rate (PDR), which is mostly popular in Europe (57,58). PDR mimics ^{137}Cs dose rates but uses ^{192}Ir

sources and afterloading technology. PDR is desired with the scarcity of available new ^{137}Cs sources. Rather than using a high activity 10-Ci ^{192}Ir source with short dwell times as in HDR, PDR uses a medium strength ^{192}Ir source of 0.5 to 1.0 Ci with dose rates of up to 3 Gy/hr. The radiation with PDR is typically delivered in a "pulsed" method over only 10 to 30 minutes of each hour, whereas LDR delivers 30 to 100 cGy/hr continuously (58). PDR delivers the same total dose over the same total time at the same hourly rate as LDR, but with an instantaneous dose rate higher than LDR. PDR brachytherapy was developed to combine the isodose optimization of HDR brachytherapy with the biologic advantages of LDR.

The term "afterloading," whereby an unloaded applicator is inserted first and the radioactive sources introduced later, was popularized by Henschke (54). Nearly every modern brachytherapy exploits afterloading. An ideal implant is established with the appropriate applicator before being loaded with the radioactive sources. This sequence allows for more careful and accurate applicator placement than inherent to earlier "hot-loaded" applicators, which were placed in the operating room preloaded with radium. Radiation exposure to medical personnel is reduced, and exposure of operating room personnel is totally eliminated. Remote afterloading, which eliminates all personnel exposure, entails the use of a computer-driven machine to insert and retract the source(s), which are attached to a cable. During treatment, the source is transported from its shielded safe to the patient's applicators via a transfer tube. Sources are retracted automatically whenever visitors or hospital personnel enter the room. With modern remote afterloading techniques, a single cable–driven radioactive source is propelled through an array of dwell positions in needles, plastic tubes, or intracavitary applicators within an implanted volume. Through computerized dosimetry, the source stops for a specified duration at a preselected number of locations during its transit, delivering a specified dose to a defined volume of tissue. This dose may be delivered rapidly in a large fraction, as in the case of HDR brachytherapy, or a series of small "pulsed doses" delivered at a given frequency over a period of days, as in PDR brachytherapy (57,58). Typically, these treatment units are housed in shielded rooms in the hospital (LDR or PDR) or the radiation oncology department (HDR) (59).

Radiation Protection

The amount of radiation that a person other than patients under treatment can receive is governed by state and federal regulations. The actual values depend on whether the person is considered part of the general public or an occupationally exposed worker. These values can change with different regulations. The National Council on Radiation Protection and Measurements (59) set the following recommendations for limits on exposure to IR:

> Public exposures less than 1 mSv or 0.1 rem annually
> Occupational exposures less than 50 mSv or 5 rem annually

In addition, NCRP Report #91 (59) placed limits on embryo-fetus exposures:

> Total dose limit less than 5 mSv or 0.5 rem
> Dose equivalent limit in 1 month less than 0.5 mSv or 0.05 rem

These recommended limits were adopted by the Nuclear Regulatory Commission (U.S. Nuclear Regulatory Commission, 10 CFR 20, Standards for Protection against Radiation).

LINACs produce radiation using electrical power. Once the LINAC is turned "off," there is little, if any, radiation exposure risk to staff. Radioactive isotopes, used most often for brachytherapy, however, do not have an "off" switch. They are always undergoing radioactive decay with the resultant radiation production of x-rays, γ-rays, electrons, and other particles.

Radiation safety is an important focus for patients and health care workers. All hospitals that house radioactive sources or

LINACs will have a special department termed *radiation safety.* Radiation personnel are responsible for monitoring radiation exposure in hospitals and clinics. All health care workers exposed to radiation must wear badges that track radiation exposure. There are three words that encompass all of the important aspects of radiation safety and protection: time, distance, and shielding. All three can be used to reduce radiation exposure. The dose delivered to a target from a radioactive source is directly proportional to the amount of time the target is exposed to the radioactive source (60). The dose delivered to a target is inversely proportional to the square of the distance from the radioactive source, double the distance, and the dose is reduced by a factor of four:

$$Dose - time$$
$$Dose - 1/r^2$$

This is the inverse square rule. The relationship between shielding and absorbed dose is more complicated. The simplest explanation is that the absorbed dose is reduced in an exponential relationship to the physical amount of shielding. The exact relationship (μ) depends on the energy of radiation and the specific material, such as concrete or lead, used to provide the protection. More material (*x*) means more protection. Less energy means more protection for the same thickness (*x*) of material:

$$Dose - e^- \mu^x$$

Minimizing time, maximizing distance, and maximizing shielding will reduce one's absorbed radiation dose. Fortunately, there is relatively little exposure to radiation for most health care providers. The LINACs in radiation oncology are strategically located and shielded to minimize radiation to anyone other than the treated patient. Many brachytherapy insertions are typically performed with remote afterloading to minimize exposure, and often, outpatient brachytherapy can be realized because of HDR techniques. This takes the patient off the hospital ward and thereby avoids exposure to the health professional caring for inpatients. The shielded rooms in the radiation oncology department protect the attendant staff from exposure as well.

Occupational Exposure Management of Female Radiation Workers

Pregnancy declaration is optional, but once declared, the employee is required to formally inform her employer. Furthermore, the radiation safety officer should interview her, her employment should be evaluated for exposure history, and steps should be taken to minimize exposure for the current work duties. The National Council on Radiological Protection (59) recommends that the embryo/fetus has limited exposure to less than 0.5 Sv/mo.

CLINICAL APPLICATIONS

Historical Background

The use of radiation in the treatment of gynecologic cancers has a rich history. Roentgen rays were used externally as early as 1902 to treat cervical carcinoma and "radium rays" in 1906. In Europe, the use of intracavitary radium was reported in 1903 for the treatment of inoperable uterine cancers (61). In those early years, there was little knowledge of the biologic effects of radiation on the normal and tumor tissues. Typically, a uterine tandem was used alone without vaginal colpostats. There was also little understanding of the dose distribution in the tumor and surrounding normal tissues, and implant duration, and thereby dose, was entirely empirical. As such, complications and failures were common. Since these early years, there has been a tremendous accumulation of knowledge relative to both external beam irradiation and brachytherapy, which are reviewed.

EXTERNAL BEAM IRRADIATION FOR GYNECOLOGIC CANCERS

Cervical and Vaginal Cancers

In cervical and vaginal cancers, the role of external beam irradiation is to shrink bulky tumor before implantation to bring it within range of the high-dose portion of the intracavitary dose distribution, improve tumor geometry by shrinking tumor that may distort anatomy and prevent optimal brachytherapy, and sterilize paracentral and nodal disease that lies beyond the reach of the intracavitary system (62). Some institutions maximize the brachytherapy component of the treatment regimen and perform the first intracavitary insertion after 10 to 20 Gy with subsequent external beam delivered with a central block (63). Other institutions treat the whole pelvis to 40 to 50 Gy and perform brachytherapy once the external beam is completed (62). The total dose at point A or the high-risk clinical treatment volume (HR CTV), however, should remain the same, stage for stage. Implementing brachytherapy early with subsequent reliance on only the implant to treat the central disease may be considered an advantage as a greater portion of the central dose is delivered with the implant, with relative sparing of the bladder and rectum, perhaps permitting delivery of a higher central dose over a shorter period of time (63). More reliance, however, is placed on the extremely complex match between the intracavitary system and the edge of the midline block, if used, making good implant geometry imperative when brachytherapy constitutes a large portion of the central dose. Those who prefer to deliver an initial 40 to 45 Gy of external beam first believe that the ability to deliver a homogeneous distribution to the entire region at risk for microscopic disease and the ability to have more shrinkage of central disease before intracavitary irradiation outweigh other considerations. The brachytherapy dose is accordingly decreased to respect normal tissue tolerance. In addition to causing regression of central disease, the external beam fields are also directed at the regional lymph nodes at risk. In cervical and vaginal cancer, the risk of pelvic lymph node involvement is related to the stage of disease, tumor size, and lymphatic vascular space invasion. Other histomorphologic factors influencing lymph node involvement in cervical cancer include pathologic tumor diameter, depth of stromal invasion, uterine body involvement, parametrial spread, and the number of cervical quadrants involved by tumor (63). Early necropsy studies reported the lymphatic pathways for patients with cervical cancer (64). The primary lymphatic pathway is to the parametrial and paracervical nodes and the obturator and internal and external iliac nodes. Secondary spread can occur to the sacral and common iliac nodes, with subsequent spread to the para-aortic nodes. Unlike in endometrial cancer, para-aortic lymph node involvement in the absence of pelvic lymph node involvement is rare. Inguinal lymph node involvement occurs with distal vaginal spread of disease or via the round ligament if there is extensive involvement of the corpus. The cervical lymphatics are located in three plexuses in the mucosa, muscularis, and serosa of the cervix and anastomose extensively with the lymphatics of the uterine isthmus. This interconnected lymphatic supply is one of the reasons why the entire uterus should be within the external beam fields when treating cervical cancer. In addition, there may also be lower uterine segment and endometrial extension of tumor. There are lymph vessels running posteriorly in the uterosacral ligaments to lymph nodes located in the sacrum between the rectum and the internal iliac vessels. These posterior nodes may terminate in the common iliac, subaortic, or para-aortic lymph nodes (65).

For all gynecologic cancers, these patterns of lymphatic spread influence the external beam field borders. Traditionally, design of "standard" pelvic fields, as shown in many radiation oncology textbooks, has been based primarily on skeletal landmarks and considered quite simple and straightforward. The skeletal landmarks are not sufficient for field design (66). Traditionally, many institutions have used the "four-field box" technique to treat the pelvis with typical anterior-posterior (AP)–posterior-anterior (PA) field sizes of 15 cm × 15 cm and lateral field widths of 8 to 9 cm (**Figure 12.8-28**) (62). The intent of the four fields is to use rather narrow lateral beams to avoid some of the small bowel anteriorly and a portion of the rectum posteriorly. Surgical and imaging series using CT (67), MRI, (68,69), and lymphangiograms (LAG) (66) have revealed that fields of these sizes can easily miss the primary tumor and its extensions and the regional lymphatics at risk, and design of the pelvic fields needs to be done with care and use of confirmatory imaging (68). Plain films do not visualize the important soft tissues, such as the cervical tumor and its extensions, the uterus, or the lymph nodes at risk. In addition, bladder and rectal contrast and a vaginal obturator or cervical markers have been used to guide field design but are not sufficient. As with the brachytherapy component of treatment, the adequacy of the external beam fields and margins has a direct relationship with local and regional control. What may be considered a mysterious failure following definitive irradiation, perhaps caused by "radiation resistance," may actually be the result of a marginal miss due to external beam field design. Placement of radiation fields must take into account the alteration of the spatial relationship between the tumor and normal anatomy due to individual anatomic, tumor-induced, or treatment-related positional variations of the uterus and cervix, as well as knowledge of the location of the regional lymphatics (68). Radiation oncologists must be aware of these patterns of disease spread and must have an in-depth understanding of CT anatomy when designing radiation fields following CT simulation. Identification and contouring of enlarged nodes in nodal regions at risk and identification of the iliac vessels, which serve as surrogates for the location of unenlarged lymph nodes, are important in subsequently defining radiation field borders (**Figure 12.8-29**) (70). In addition,

contouring of the entire uterus and portions of the vagina will also ensure that these tissues are included in the radiation fields (**Figure 12.8-29**). Reliance on bony anatomy alone for radiation field design rather than on CT-defined targets is discouraged. Generally, the superior border of the pelvic fields is at the S1-L5 interspace for early-stage disease (ie, nonbulky IB or IIA) or at the L4- L5 interspace for more advanced disease. The latter is used if one wants to cover the common iliac lymph nodes. Interestingly, Greer et al evaluated "standard" pelvic fields (AP-PA, 15 cm × 15 cm; lateral, 8-9 cm wide) for the treatment of cervical cancer in relationship to intraoperative findings. Based on intraoperative measurements of the location of the aortic bifurcation and the bifurcation of the common iliac arteries relative to the lumbosacral prominence (the anterior caudal border of L5), Greer et al concluded that anterior and posterior treatment fields with a superior border at the L4-L5 interspace are required to cover the internal iliac, external iliac, and obturator nodes, as the bifurcations of the common iliac arteries were above the lumbosacral prominence in 87% of the patients studied. Coverage of the common iliacs could require extending the upper field border to the L3-L4 interspace or even the L2-L3 interspace in some patients (71). Obviously, with CT-based dosimetry, it is imperative to outline the vessels and/or nodes in these areas to determine the appropriate field borders because unnecessary irradiation of bowel could occur if all patients were treated to the L2-L3 interspace, based on this assumption (**Figure 12.8-29**). CT is an excellent tool for identifying pathologically enlarged nodes, multiple small lymph nodes that, by increased number rather than size, are suspicious, or, in the absence of nodes, the aortic and iliac bifurcations and the iliac vessels (67). The inferior border of the pelvic field is usually at the bottom of the ischial tuberosities or 3 to 4 cm below the most distal vaginal component of disease. Inguinal nodes are included if there is distal vaginal spread,

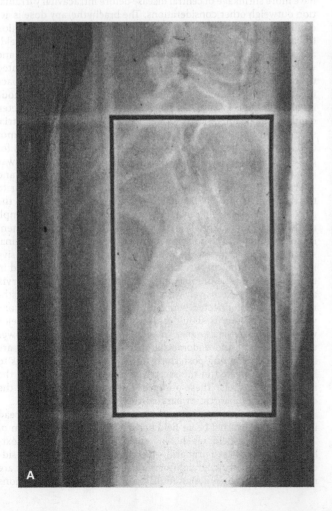

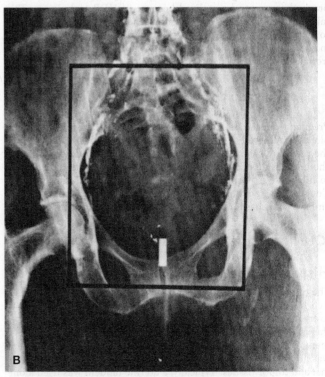

Figure 12.8-28. Traditional four-field pelvic box technique with short and narrow fields, with the potential to miss the uterine fundus and the pelvic lymph nodes. (A) Lateral and (B) anteroposterior pelvic radiographic views. (Reprinted with permission from Fletcher GH, ed. *Textbook of Radiotherapy.* 3rd ed. Lea & Febiger; 1980:761-762.)

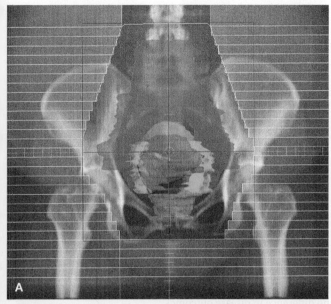
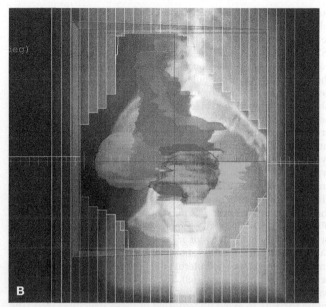

Figure 12.8-29. Digitally reconstructed anteroposterior (A) and lateral (B) radiographs with associated contoured targets including the pelvic lymph nodes and uterus/cervix/parametria and vagina. Note the multileaf collimator leaves defining the field shape in accordance with coverage of the targets of interest.

in which case treatment of the vaginal introitus with margin would also be required. MRI is especially helpful in imaging vaginal tumor extension (72). The lateral borders of the AP-PA fields must be designed carefully as the normally recommended 1.5- to 2.0-cm margin from the pelvic brim may be too narrow. Using lymphangiography, Bonin et al (66) found that a margin of at least 2.6 cm on

each pelvic brim was needed in order to cover all pelvic lymph nodes if bony landmarks were used. The lateral fields are even more prone to marginal misses than the AP-PA fields, as demonstrated in multiple series that have compared the standard textbook lateral fields (8-12 cm wide) to fields designed based on CT and MRI (**Figure 12.8-30**) (68). For the lateral fields, a commonly employed

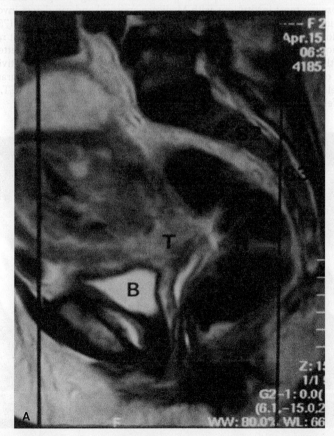
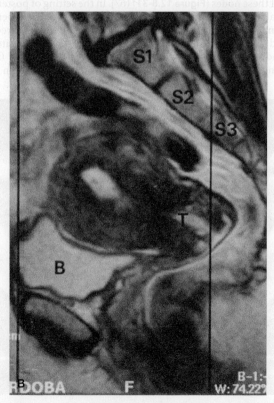

Figure 12.8-30. (A,B): Traditional lateral fields are superimposed on sagittal magnetic resonance imaging scans to evaluate target coverage with traditional fields. Note that (A) the traditional lateral fields would not completely cover the uterine fundus and (B) the traditional lateral field would cut through cervical tumor within the anteverted uterus. (Reprinted with permission from Zunino S, Rosato O, Lucino S, et al. Anatomic study of the pelvis and carcinoma of the uterine cervix as related to the box technique. *Int J Radiat Oncol Biol Phys*. 1999;44(1):56-57.)

guideline is to place the posterior border in a horizontal line, parallel to the treatment couch that divides the mid-rectum and intersects the sacrum between the second and third sacral segments (S2-S3 interspace), and the anterior border by a horizontal line, parallel to the treatment couch from the anteroinferior lip of L5 to the anterior aspect of the pubic symphysis. These "standard" lateral fields are too narrow. For the lateral fields, careful consideration needs to be given to the anterior border to include the external iliac nodes. Based on lymphangiography, Bonin et al (66) found that, in order to cover the external iliac nodes, the anterior border of the lateral field was sometimes as much as 2 cm anterior to the pubic symphysis. Taylor et al (70) showed that a modified 7-mm margin typically covers 99% of the pelvic lymph nodes. In addition, the anterior border must also be drawn to include the entire uterus, given the interconnecting lymphatics of the uterus and cervix and the possibility of lower uterine segment/endometrial extension (**Figure 12.8-30**) (68). Enlargement of the uterine fundus by the presence of hematometra or massive fundal extension of cancer can displace the fundus anteriorly and cephalad, as can an anteverted or retroverted uterus (69). The prone position may accentuate this displacement (68). The anterior field border should be based on CT or MRI delineation of the tumor and/or normal anatomic variants to avoid underdosing of these structures (69). The posterior border of the lateral fields must be designed carefully. Based on intraoperative findings, Greer et al showed that the cardinal and uterosacral ligaments extend posterior to the rectum and sigmoid in their attachments to the sacrum. As part of the parametria, these tissues often contain nodes, even in early disease (IB and II, 22.5%) or are involved by direct extension and need to be covered in most patients by including the entire sacrum in the lateral fields (71). If there is uterosacral ligament involvement, it is especially important to include the entire sacrum in the lateral fields, although some institutions will use this as a criterion for AP-PA fields alone (65). The internal iliac lymph nodes may lie very close to the rectum, and splitting of the rectum can result in a marginal miss of these nodes (**Figure 12.8-31**) (67). In the setting of posterior cervical lesions, there may also be direct extension to the superior rectal nodes or sacral lymph nodes. Tumor can also extend directly around the rectum. Kim et al found that the most common site of an inadequate margin was near the portion of the lateral field blocking the rectum. On CT, it was found that tumor often fell along the lateral aspect of the rectum. The second most common site of inadequate margin was the posterior border at the S2-S3 interspace. Zunino et al (69) also found inadequate posterior border margins when the uterus was both retroverted and anteverted (**Figure 12.8-30**). The reason for narrow lateral fields is typically concern over the rectum and the small bowel. Greer et al (71) reported no increase in late rectal complications when including the entire sacrum in the field. It may also be a mistake to avoid the chance of a marginal miss by treating just with anterior and posterior fields, as, in most cases, some of the small bowel can be omitted from the lateral fields when using image-based planning. Using bony landmarks to define fields, given the earlier considerations, is discouraged in favor of contouring of targets on CT or MRI (with other imaging to inform possible sites of disease such as PET/CT) with the appropriate PTV margins as described previously.

In the adjuvant setting, there have been two studies, PARCER and RTOG1203, in which postoperative cervical cancer treated with IMRT as compared to 3D conformal radiotherapy (3D CRT) has shown improved outcomes (73,74). In the postoperative adjuvant cervical cancer phase III study, patients were randomized to 3D CRT versus IMRT. Patients were found to have 28.1% grade 2 or more late toxicity versus 48.9% in IMRT versus 3D CRT. There was no difference in disease outcomes.

MRI has been found to be an invaluable tool for delineating normal anatomy and the extent of cervical tumor involvement because of its superior soft-tissue contrast compared to CT. MRI also allows direct imaging in sagittal, coronal, and transverse plains (69). Sagittal MRIs are exceedingly helpful in designing radiation fields (**Figure 12.8-30**). Design of the anterior and posterior borders of the lateral fields can be especially influenced by these images. Thomas et al (68) performed MRI rather than CT in the treatment position and found better delineation of the tumor volume owing to the superior contrast resolution. PET/CT scans have largely replaced LAGs at most institutions with Medicare approval and can detect involved pelvic and para-aortic lymph nodes better than CT alone (75,76). Unlike CT, PET does not rely on lymph node size alone, but rather on metabolic alterations for detection of disease. PET has better accuracy than can be achieved with CT or MRI, with a sensitivity of 85% to 90%, a specificity of 95% to 100%, and overall accuracy of 90% to 95%. Nodes as small as 6 mm can be imaged with PET, providing information to guide therapy and predict outcome.

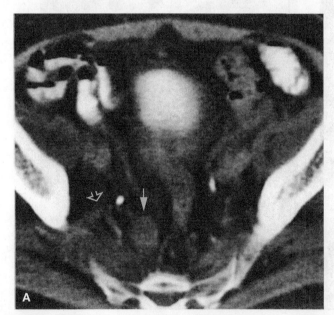 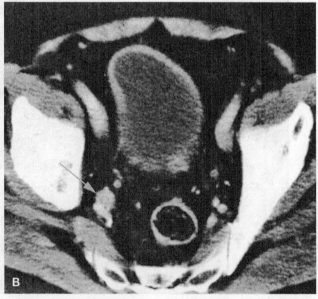

Figure 12.8-31. A: The location of the presacral lymph nodes mandates including the entire sacrum to cover disease in the uterosacral and cardinal ligaments and superior rectal (presacral) nodes. The right lateral sacral node (solid arrow) is medial to the hypogastric vessels (open arrow). B: Note the proximity of the internal iliac lymph node (solid arrow) to the rectum. This spatial relationship would exclude partial blocking of the rectum on the lateral fields. (Used with permission from Park J, Charnsangavej C, Yoshimitsu K, et al. Pathways of nodal metastasis from pelvic tumors: CT demonstration. *Radiographics.* 1994;14(6):1311. Permission conveyed through Copyright Clearance Center, Inc)

Midline Blocks

Midline blocks have been used historically at various points in time at many institutions (**Figure 12.8-32**). It is important to understand when the midline block is placed, as this will influence the HDR fraction size. Higher whole-pelvis doses can be utilized without a midline block, but the HDR doses have to be appropriately reduced. HDR and external beam fractions should not be given on the same day. The use of midline blocks is controversial, as there can be an increased risk of rectosigmoid, bladder, and small bowel complications if careful attention is not given to tracking and limiting the total dose in these OAR (77-79).

A midline block may be used during external beam to avoid regions of excessive dose adjacent to the brachytherapy implant and to deliver an adequate dose to potential tumor-bearing regions outside the implant. When using a midline block early in the treatment course, more reliance is placed on the extremely complex match between the intracavitary system and the edge of the midline block. There are some important safety issues to consider when using midline blocks (77-79). The midline block position should be based on films with similar isocenters. If patients receive external beam irradiation in the prone position, it may be wise to simulate them in the supine position for their parametrial boosts so that they are in the same position as they are for their implants. Midline blocks can be positioned to account for applicator deviation. Alignment along the midplane of the patient can be problematic if the tandem is deviated. Midline blocks that are too narrow may not adequately shield the bladder and rectosigmoid, given their ability to move in and out of the blocked field. Filling and emptying of these organs may also alter their position relative to the block. Eifel et al point out that the distance between the distal ureters is usually 4 to 5 cm. A narrow block may fail to shield a portion of the ureters during external beam (80). Reviewing the M.D. Anderson experience, Eifel et al detected an increase in complications in patients with midline blocks (4 cm) used throughout the course of external beam. Because the ureters are typically 2 to 3 cm from the midline, the explanation for the ureteral stenosis could have been an overlap between the external beam fields and the high-dose region of the intracavitary implants (80). A margin of 0.5 cm lateral to the lateral ovoid surface is recommended in designing the width of the midline block for each patient to protect the implanted volume. If the

intracavitary system is broad, a wide midline block may potentially shield the external iliac lymph nodes. If tissues immediately adjacent to the colpostats and tandem tip are not shielded, portions of the ileocecal junction and rectosigmoid may be overdosed (81). Huang et al (81) recommended avoiding a combination of parametrial boost doses of 54 Gy or higher and a cumulative rectal biologically effective dose (CRBED) of 100 Gy_3 or higher to decrease the risk of radiation-induced bowel complications. When a midline block is inserted below 40 Gy, it should not extend to the top of the field because it will shield the common iliac and presacral lymph nodes, which will be underdosed. When there is suspicion of uterosacral ligament involvement, it is safer to avoid early placement of the midline block, which will shield disease lying posterior to the implant (65). Owing to concern over rectal tolerance, the rectum is shielded after a certain amount of external beam radiation therapy, which can block tumor in the perirectal area and uterosacral space. The geometric configuration of the intracavitary implant emphasizes lateral rather than posterior coverage and does not effectively treat the perirectal and uterosacral space effectively. This can lead to underdosing of tissues in this area and an increased risk of central recurrence. Higher whole-pelvis external beam doses, interstitial implantation, or addition of a supplemental posterior oblique external beam boost may offer ways to compensate dose in this area (65). Given the potential for risk, some would advocate abandoning the midline block in favor of other options (77-79). Fenkell et al (79) showed that 66.7% of patients had a greater than 50% increase in doses to the rectum and bladder (D2cc) of the sigmoid with the use of a midline block. The use of IMRT with low central doses near the bladder and rectosigmoid and higher doses covering the pelvic nodes has been described as a replacement for the more antiquated midline block (51).

Parametrial/Nodal Boosting in Cervical Cancer

Parametrial boosting is often recommended for patients with bulky parametrial or sidewall disease, after completion of the whole-pelvis field and midline block fields, as the parametria are a common site of failure. The need for boosting is usually based on the status of disease regression following whole-pelvis irradiation. MRI may be helpful in making this assessment both before and during radiation. Logsdon and Eifel (82) suggest boosting residual lateral pelvic wall disease after 40 to 45 Gy whole pelvis to 60 to 62 Gy to small volumes. Perez et al (83,84) found a trend toward increased pelvic control with point B doses (defined as 6 cm lateral to the central axis) by greater than 45 Gy. Perez et al found that the incidence of pelvic recurrence was correlated with tumor size and dose of irradiation delivered to the lateral parametrium. There was an increase in the incidence of pelvic recurrence in patients receiving less than 50 Gy, but no correlation with increasing doses of irradiation (85). Doses needed to eradicate parametrial disease in the literature are typically around 60 Gy, combining the external beam doses with the implant doses. The proximity of small bowel can make this a risky proposition. Perez et al (86) noted that with doses below 50 Gy to the lateral pelvic wall, the risk of small bowel complications was about 1% and somewhat higher with larger doses. In a later series, grade 3 small bowel sequelae were 1% with doses of 50 Gy and 2% to 4% with doses over 60 Gy ($P = .04$) (87). Perez et al recommend limiting the small bowel doses to less than 60 Gy. When there is uterosacral space involvement, attention should be given to the use of a supplemental posterior oblique external beam boost (65). Grigsby et al used PET/CT scans to evaluate lymph node size, irradiation dose, and patterns of failure. The parametrial and lymph node boost doses used were in the range of 9.0 to 14.4 Gy following large field doses of 50.4 Gy. Radiation dose and lymph node size were not significant predicators of lymph node failure. The risk of an isolated lymph node failure was less than 2% (88). A reoperation series following definitive irradiation and chemotherapy was reported by Houvenaegel et al. After 45 Gy and

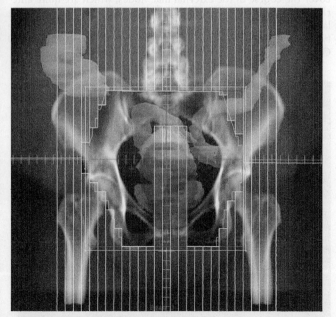

Figure 12.8-32. Midline blocks: A midline block defined by the leaves of the multileaf collimator used to shield the central pelvic structures. Note the unblocked bladder and sigmoid that may receive some of the brachytherapy dose and all of the external beam dose.

whole pelvis and selective parametrial or nodal boosting to 55 to 60 Gy, 15.9% of patients had biopsy-proven residual disease in the pelvic nodes and 11.7% in the para-aortic nodes (89). The use of IMRT may be a method to increase dose to bulky nodes or residual parametrial disease while sparing adjacent normal structures (51,90). The ASTRO convened a task group to recommend types of radiation and techniques in cervical cancer.

Endometrial Cancer

The need for postoperative external beam radiation therapy in endometrial cancer is well described in the ASTRO consensus guidelines (91). Patients with early-stage endometrial cancer with grade 3 and 50% or more myometrial invasion or grades 1 to 2, 50% or more myometrial invasion, and other risk factors such as age greater than 60 with or without lymphovascular space invasion may benefit from pelvic external beam radiation. The GOG 249 randomized women with high-intermediate risk factors to vaginal cuff brachytherapy and three cycles of chemotherapy (carboplatin and taxol) versus pelvic radiotherapy in a superiority study. In GOG 249, risk factors for recurrence included deep myometrial invasion, grade 2 or 3 disease, age greater than 60 years, or lymphovascular space invasion. Women were eligible for the study if over 70 years of age with one other risk factor, over 60 with two risk factors, or any age with three risk factors. Vaginal cuff therapy and chemotherapy were not found to be superior to external beam therapy in this population, and acute toxicity was higher in the chemotherapy arm. Long-term toxicity was similar. Although pelvic and para-aortic recurrences were more common in the cuff and chemotherapy arm, locoregional recurrence remained low (9% vs 4%), with distant recurrence predominating at 18%. In advanced-stage endometrial cancer, PORTEC 3 and GOG 258 looked at radiation therapy and chemotherapy combined and on its own for these high-intermediate and advanced patients. In PORTEC 3, concurrent chemoradiation with cisplatin and adjuvant carboplatin and taxol showed an improvement in OS and failure-free survival in stage III patients, especially in those with nodal involvement and serous endometrial carcinoma. A subanalysis (92) of GOG 258 revealed more pelvic recurrence in those patients who did not receive radiation (93). Chemotherapy should also be considered in patients with locally advanced disease and serous carcinoma. If chemotherapy and radiation are planned, chemotherapy may be delivered concurrently, sequentially, or in an interdigitated manner (91). In terms of timing of radiation for patients with stage III endometrial cancer, one study looked at seven institutions retrospectively and found that

sequence and type of combined adjuvant therapy did not affect OS or recurrence-free survival (94).

For endometrial cancer, many of the same nodes are at risk as in cervical cancer, but the spread of disease is not as predictable with the para-aortic nodes independently at risk. The presacral nodes are also not at risk unless there is cervical involvement. Both the pelvic and para-aortic nodes are at risk in all sites of uterine involvement, and grade, myometrial invasion, and lymphatic vascular space invasion are more predictive of risk than is location (95,96). Cervical and lower uterine segment involvement increases the likelihood of pelvic lymph node metastases compared to fundal location, as do increasing histologic grade and myometrial invasion. In the surgical staging series of Boronow et al (96), 18 of 222 patients had lower uterine segment involvement and six (33%) had pelvic lymph node metastases. In the final GOG surgical staging series report, by location, patients with fundal lesions had a 4% risk of para-aortic and 8% risk of pelvic lymph node involvement, whereas patients with lower uterine segment involvement had a 16% risk of pelvic and 14% risk of para-aortic lymph node involvement.

In endometrial cancer, external beam irradiation is generally recommended for patients thought to be at significant risk for lymph node metastases and/or a vaginal cuff recurrence. Traditionally, this has been recommended in the absence of a lymph node dissection or a limited lymph node sampling. External beam irradiation is still delivered at many institutions in the setting of a negative lymph node dissection or negative sentinel node biopsy when high-risk features such as deep myometrial invasion, high grade, lymphovascular space invasion, lower uterine segment involvement, or cervical invasion are present (91). Two phase III randomized studies found in the setting of postoperative gynecologic cancer and the use of IMRT/VMAT provided decreased side effects and improvement of patient-reported outcomes with equivalent outcomes (73,74).

External beam irradiation typically covers the upper one-half to two-thirds of the vagina, the pelvic lymph node regions, and the surgical bed (**Figure 12.8-33**). External beam field design must necessarily include the pelvic lymphatics with exclusion of as much small bowel as possible. Treatment of the patient in the prone position with a full bladder will help to exclude at least some small bowel in most patients unless these loops are fixed in the pelvis (**Figure 12.8-34**). It is important, however, for the lateral fields to cover the course of the external iliac nodes, which are quite anterior in the pelvis and require inclusion of some small bowel in the lateral fields to be adequately covered. Doses of 45 to 50.4 Gy are typical, with some institutions treating to 40 Gy and as high as 60 Gy to reduced fields in the setting of nodal disease.

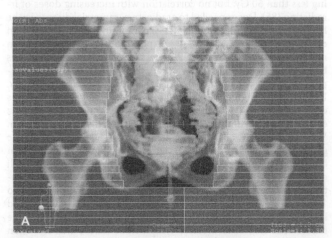
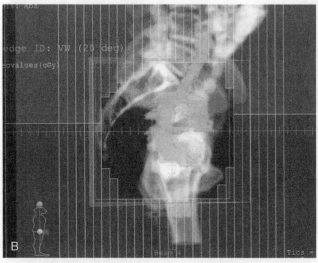

■ **Figure 12.8-33.** Digitally reconstructed anteroposterior (A) and lateral (B) radiographs with nodal volumes contoured, as well as the vaginal apex and the fields defined by the leaves of the multileaf collimator. This is a standard field design for patients with endometrial cancer.

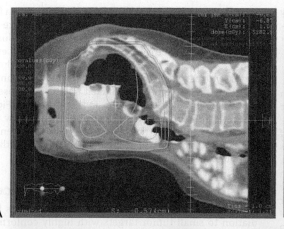

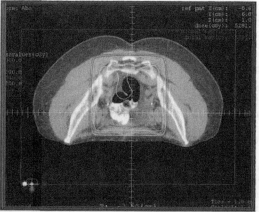

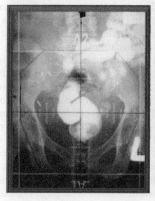

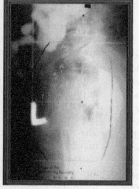

Figure 12.8-34. A: Utility of the prone technique for small bowel displacement as shown on a sagittal and axial computed tomography scan of a patient with endometrial cancer placed in the prone position. B: Radiographs of the pelvis showing significant amount of small bowel in the radiation fields.

Prone techniques have been used in the treatment of many other pelvic malignancies in an attempt to exclude small bowel from the field. The use of a belly board device to further enhance small bowel displacement has become standard practice in the treatment of many pelvic malignancies. The use of prone position with or without a belly board for the treatment of patients with cervical cancer has been reported in a few series, in the postoperative (97) and definitive settings (98). Prone positioning with the belly board has been used extensively for patients with rectal cancers when using a PA and two lateral fields. Concern over this technique for patients with gynecologic malignancies when adding a fourth field (AP) to cover the external iliac nodes has been raised by Ghosh et al, due to the uncertainty in source-to-skin distance (SSD) and variation in tissue thickness from the anterior field. In patients who underwent postoperative irradiation for cervical cancer, they observed that the small bowel was best excluded from the AP-PA fields when the patient was positioned prone without the belly board, thereby compressing the small bowel laterally out of the AP-PA fields. They recommended an alternating routine (99). Bladder distention can also help to optimally displace bowel when using the belly board (100). Concern over the use of the belly board in patients treated with definitive versus postoperative irradiation for cervical cancer is also raised owing to the potential change in position of the uterus when prone, the impact and variability of bladder filling, and the potential daily variation in the setup (99). CT-based dosimetry has documented that the prone position, particularly with bladder filling, can alter the position of the uterus within the radiation field (68). Hence, if patients are simulated prone, it is even more imperative to use CT- or MRI-based dosimetry in the prone position to make sure that the entire uterus is in the pelvic fields, and it is also imperative to consistently fill or empty the bladder (101). IGRT may also be helpful in ensuring that the daily setup is reproducible and reliable.

Extended-Field Irradiation

Extended-field irradiation refers to inclusion of both the pelvic and para-aortic nodes in the radiation fields. Common indications for extended-field irradiation in gynecologic cancers include patients with positive para-aortic nodes or those with positive pelvic nodes or bulky primary lesions feared to be at risk for microscopic para-aortic disease (**Figure 12.8-35**). Extended fields include more normal organs than pelvic fields alone. Limitation of dose to the small bowel, kidneys, liver, stomach, and spinal cord are essential. 3D conformal techniques are helpful in achieving an acceptable therapeutic ratio. The use of IMRT has recently been piloted in this

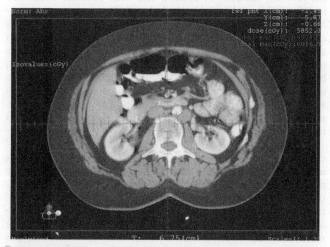

Figure 12.8-35. Axial computed tomography scan demonstrating an enlarged periaortic lymph node near the left renal hilum.

setting, with further attempts to decrease acute and late toxicity (**Figure 12.8-20**). Selective boosting of gross nodal disease may allow for safer dose escalation (90).

Pelvic and Inguinal Irradiation

External beam fields will necessarily include the inguinal lymph nodes in patients with vulvar cancer or distal vaginal cancers, or when cancer of the cervix or endometrium involves the distal vagina. Distal vagina in this context refers to the lower one-third of the vagina. Risk of femoral head necrosis or femoral neck fractures is increased in this setting unless the femoral heads are excluded. Recent use of IMRT to treat vulvar and vaginal cancers has been published with success as this allows concentration of dose on the targets and minimization of dose to the normal organs. For vulvar cancer in particular, it is important to verify that the vulva is receiving adequate surface dose with IMRT by using OSLD verification on the initial treatments (102,103).

Intensity-Modulated Radiation Therapy

IMRT is an excellent treatment method for gynecologic cancers. The setting where IMRT may be the most helpful and the most widely accepted is postoperatively for select endometrial and cervical cancer presentations (104). Results of the Radiation Therapy Oncology Group (RTOG) 0418 study "A phase II study of intensity-modulated radiation therapy (IMRT) to the pelvis with or without chemotherapy for postoperative patients with either endometrial or cervical carcinoma" showed a decrease in both acute and late toxicities in the postoperative setting in patients with either cervical or endometrial cancers (105). Other prospective and single-institutional studies have confirmed this (47,106). In the postoperative setting, there is often a significant amount of small bowel in the pelvis, which can be avoided to a greater degree with IMRT than with 3D conformal radiation techniques (**Figure 12.8-22**). Bone marrow sparing can also be improved over a 3D conformal approach (107,108). Bladder and rectosigmoid doses can be reduced. Margin sizes around the target and bladder and rectal filling are important considerations, as are immobilization techniques when using IMRT. Target delineation and normal organ delineation are extremely important when using IMRT. What is not defined is either not adequately treated or spared (52). The RTOG 0418 defined parameters for contouring of targets and normal organs, margin size, and dose volume constraints in the postoperative setting in early cervical or endometrial cancers (109). An online atlas available on the RTOG website was developed to improve consistency between multiple contouring physicians and continues to be used to guide in target delineation, even though the protocol has been completed. This same atlas has been used in GOG/NRG studies, which include IMRT techniques with minor modifications over time. A normal tissue–contouring atlas is available on the RTOG/NRG website (110). Other atlases are also available to guide radiation oncologists in defining these structures of interest (70,111). When using IMRT to treat the intact uterus, bladder filling can have even more influence on the position of the uterus, and the vagina and uterus can move several centimeters as a result (52,112). Stool in the rectosigmoid can also cause movement of the adjacent pelvic organs and alter the dose distribution in the rectosigmoid.

IMRT may be used in the definitive management of cervical cancer, with careful attention to target delineation as well as motion. A consensus guideline has been published to define the most appropriate CTV for intact cervical cancer, with recognition of the significant uncertainties caused by motion in this setting (113). Studies have shown that IMRT has reduced both acute and late gastrointestinal (GI) toxicities and helped to spare bone marrow during treatment (51,108,114). There is concern in this setting about organ motion relative to the dose distribution. This can be due to bladder or rectosigmoid filling, disease regression, or

sporadic motion (40,115). Careful attention to organ filling, patient immobilization, and margin size can help minimize such motion, which could compromise target and normal organ doses (39). Daily CT imaging before treatment may assist in motion evaluation and allow adaptation of the treatment plan as needed. The use of IMRT for extended-field irradiation to treat the pelvic and para-aortic region is successfully implemented to decrease dose to the small bowel, kidneys, liver, spinal cord, and bone marrow (**Figure 12.8-20**). Selective boosting of gross nodal disease may allow for safer dose escalation (90,116). IMRT techniques have also been used for vulvar cancers to help spare the upper femur as well as the small bowel and bone marrow (48,102,103).

Oligometastatic Gynecologic Cancer

SBRT is modern radiation technique that delivers high-dose radiation to small tumor targets with highly conformal fields and rapid dose fall off. This technique is used for maximal ablation of the target and sparing of normal tissues. Data are emerging that patients who may benefit from aggressive local therapy for oligometastatic disease include those with nodal, lung, liver, or bone metastases. In a small series, Kim et al demonstrated that with aggressive treatment of patients with positive para-aortic nodes and supraclavicular nodal disease, the 3-year OS was 49%. A phase II study of SBRT for unresectable liver metastases enrolled 61 patients with 76 unresectable liver lesions and followed patients, including some with gynecologic cancers for 5 years. The study suggested improved long-term survival of these oligometastatic patients with SBRT. Palma et al evaluated SBRT for oligometastatic disease in a randomized phase II open-label trial and demonstrated improvement in OS. Another method of elimination of oligometastatic disease is through the use of radiopharmaceuticals. Radiopharmaceutical therapy (RPT) is evolving but uses biologic targeting linked with radioactive particle to deliver high-dose radiation in a very focal area.

Brachytherapy Systems for the Treatment of Cervical Cancer

Brachytherapy is essential in the treatment of many gynecologic cancers. Intracavitary brachytherapy for cervical carcinoma was profoundly impacted by the development of various "systems" that attempted to combine empiricism with a more scientific and systematic approach. A *dosimetric system* refers to a set of rules concerning a specific applicator type, radioactive isotope, and distribution of the sources in the applicator to deliver a defined dose to a designated treatment region (56). Within any system, specification of treatment in terms of dose, timing, and administration is necessary to implement the prescription in a consistent manner. Three systems were developed in Europe, including the Paris, Stockholm, and Manchester system (117-119). The Manchester system principles are an integral part of modern brachytherapy (119).

The Manchester System

The Manchester system was developed in 1932 by Tod and Meredith (119) and was later modified in 1953 (120) at the Holt Radium Institute. It standardized treatment with predetermined doses and dose rates directed at fixed points in the pelvis. The fixed points A and B were selected on the theory that the dose in the paracervical triangle impacted normal tissue tolerance rather than the actual doses to the bladder, rectum, and vagina. The paracervical triangle was described as a pyramidal-shaped area, with its base resting on the lateral vaginal fornices and its apex curving around with the anteverted uterus. "Point A" was defined as 2 cm lateral to the central canal of the uterus and 2 cm from the mucous membrane of the lateral fornix in the axis of the uterus (**Figure 12.8-36**). It often correlates anatomically with

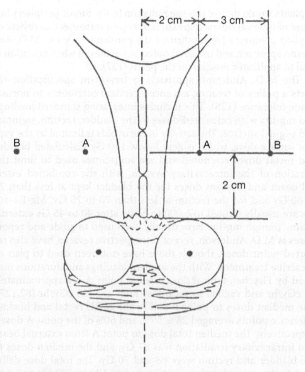

Figure 12.8-36. The Manchester system. Definitions of points A and B in the classic Manchester system are found in the text. In a typical application, the loading of intrauterine applicators varied: between 20 and 35 mg of radium and between 15 and 25 mg of radium for each vaginal ovoid. The resultant treatment time to deliver 8,000 R at point A was 140 hours. (From Meredith WJ. *Radium Dosage: The Manchester System*. Livingstone; 1967, with permission.)

the point of crossage of the ureter and uterine artery and was taken as an average point from which to assess dose in the paracervical region. "Point B" was located 5 cm from midline at the level of point A and was thought to correspond to the location of the obturator lymph nodes. To achieve consistent dose rates, a set of strict rules dictating the relationship, position, and activity of radium sources in the uterine and vaginal applicators was devised. The amount of radium would vary based on ovoid size and uterine length such that the same dose in roentgen would be delivered to point A, regardless of the size of the patient or the size and shape of the tumor, uterus, and vagina. The vaginal ovoids were available in three sizes: small (2.0-cm diameter), medium (2.5-cm diameter), and large (3.0-cm diameter) and were preloaded or "hot loaded" with radium. The amount of radium per ovoid varied by size so as to obtain a uniform dose rate at the ovoid surface. It was recommended to use the largest ovoid size possible and place the ovoids as far laterally as possible in the fornices to carry the radium closer to point B and increase the depth dose. Vaginal packing was used to limit the dose to the bladder and rectum to less than 80% of point A. Two intracavitary applications of 72 hours with a 4- to 7-day interval between them were given to deliver a dose of 8,000 R at 55.5 R/hr to point A and 3,000 R to point B. External beam irradiation with a mid line block in place was later used to deliver a total cumulative dose of 6,000 R to point B.

The Manchester system is the basis for contemporary intracavitary techniques and dose specification. With current LDR applications using cesium rather than radium, it is considered standard to have a point A dose rate of 50 to 60 cGy/hr and to deliver a total dose of 85 Gy to point A and 60 Gy to point B when combined with external beam therapy while limiting the normal tissues to less than 80% of the point A dose.

The Fletcher (M.D. Anderson) System

The Fletcher system was established at M.D. Anderson Hospital in the 1940s (121). The Fletcher applicator was subsequently developed and remains an integral part of gynecologic brachytherapy (**Figure 12.8-37**) (122). The initial dosimetric work at M.D. Anderson was done before the development of computerized dosimetry in the 1960s as in the Paris system; milligram-hours (mg-hr) was used for dose prescription with the premise that with any geometric arrangement of specified sources, dose at any point is proportional to the amount of radioactivity and the implant duration. Though previous systems (Paris and Stockholm) had used mg-hr, clinical experience alone determined the amount of radium tolerable to the tissues. Fletcher et al (123) predicted that better results and less morbidity could be obtained if knowledge of the energy absorbed at various points in the pelvis ("measured data") such as the bladder and rectum and pelvic lymph nodes could be determined. According to Fletcher, a dosimetric approach should meet the following requirements: (a) ensure that the primary disease in the cervix and fornices and immediate extensions into the paracervical triangle are adequately treated; (b) guide treatments in such a way that the bladder and rectum are not overdosed (respect mucosal tolerance); and (c) determine the dose received by the various lymph node groups. Individualization to fit the anatomic situation was an essential aspect of this system.

The primary prescription parameter in the Fletcher system was tumor volume, and prescription rules were based on maximum mg-hrs and maximum time, taking into account the total external beam dose and the calculated sigmoid dose. An application was left in place until either of these two maximums was reached. Large mg-hr implants were halted by the mg-hr prescription, whereas smaller mg-hr implants were terminated by time. A set of maxima of mg-hrs was established for combinations with external irradiation, which were published in tables (61,124). Standardized source arrangements and limits on the vaginal surface dose and mg-hrs were all used to help specify treatment.

Despite a more elaborate dosimetry system, the Fletcher system combined many elements of the Paris and Manchester systems, including using the largest size ovoid possible, positioned as far laterally and cephalad as possible, to deliver the highest tumor dose at depth for a given mucosal dose. By using a larger ovoid, the radium-mucous membrane distance was increased, allowing a greater increase in the total number of mg-hrs and a greater volume of adequate irradiation (121). The Fletcher colpostats were actually a further evolution of the Manchester ovoids and were made with the same diameters of 2, 2.5, and 3 cm but were more

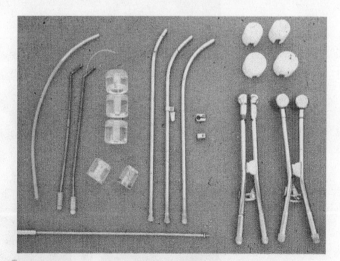

Figure 12.8-37. Fletcher-Suit-Delclos low-dose rate applicators. Left to right: Afterloading colpostats, mini-ovoids, tandems, cylinders, and source inserters. (Reprinted with permission from Fletcher GH, ed. *Textbook of Radiotherapy*. 3rd Ed. Lea & Febiger; 1980:741.)

cylindrical than Manchester "ovoids" and were attached to handles, with shielding in the direction of the bladder and rectum. Initially, these were preloaded with radium, but later an afterloading model was developed and loaded instead with ^{137}Cs (125). Recommended loadings were 15, 20, and 25 mg of radium for the 2-, 2.5-, and 3-cm colpostats, respectively, and 5 to 10 mg for the mini-ovoids (126). As in earlier systems, it was also recommended that the longest tandem available be used and loaded so that sources reached the uterine fundus in order to provide an adequate distribution in the lower uterine segment and paracervical areas and to increase the dose to the obturator lymph nodes. In addition, a high position of the applicator in the pelvis and a wide separation of the ovoids were thought to increase the dose to the pelvic wall. Tight packing was also recommended to displace the system upward and centrally and to decrease the dose to the bladder and rectum (121). Recommended tandem loadings were usually 15, 10, and 10 mg of radium, with the amount of radium in the tandem usually greater than that in the ovoids. The distal source in the tandem was to be positioned to produce an even pear-shaped dose distribution with no drop in dose rate between the tandem and ovoids, without excessive overlap that would result in a hot spot on the adjacent bladder or rectal mucosa. With the ovoids well positioned, this was usually accomplished by placing the physical end of the distal source at or a few millimeters beyond the external os of the cervix. A 10-mg protruding source was recommended if the vaginal ovoids were separated by more than 5 cm or displaced caudally, with each ovoid, then decreased by 5 mg.

A careful review of implant films was outlined (**Figure 12.8-38**). It was recommended to keep the tandem in the axis of the pelvis, equidistant from the sacral promontory and pubis and the lateral pelvic walls, to avoid overdosage to the bladder, sigmoid, or one ureter. The tandem was recommended to bisect the ovoids on the AP films and bisect their height on the lateral films. The flange of the tandem was to be flush against the cervix and the ovoids surrounding it, verified by confirming the proximity of the applicators to radiopaque cervical seeds. Radiopaque vaginal packing was used to hold the system in place and displace the bladder and rectum. Scrutiny of implant films before treatment remains an important tenet of brachytherapy. Two or more intracavitary insertions were thought to make more efficient use of the inverse square law such that the second and third implants would deliver intense radiation to the tumor periphery because of interval tumor regression. A recent retrospective review of implant geometry has confirmed the consistency of the M.D. Anderson approach and the good outcomes achieved when attention is paid to applicator position in the pelvis (127).

The M.D. Anderson approach to treatment specification reflects a policy of treating advanced cervical carcinoma to normal tissue tolerance (128). This includes integrating standard loadings and mg-hrs with calculated doses to the bladder, rectum, sigmoid, and vaginal surface. The activity in the ovoids is limited by the vaginal surface dose, which is kept below 140 Gy. Calculated bladder and rectal doses are noted and are sometimes used to limit the duration of the intracavitary system, with the combined external beam and implant doses for the bladder kept at less than 75 to 80 Gy and for the rectum at less than 70 to 75 Gy. Mg-Ra-eq-hrs are usually limited to 6,000 to 6,500 after 40 to 45 Gy external beam. Though mg-hrs have usually been used to guide and report doses at M.D. Anderson, recent retrospective reviews have also reported point doses, though these have not been used to plan or prescribe treatment. With the implant loadings and durations outlined by Fletcher, typical dose rates at point A are approximately 57 cGy/hr and vaginal surface dose rates are 100 cGy/hr (82,127). The median doses to point B and to the ICRU rectal and bladder reference points averaged 28%, 59%, and 60% of the point A doses, respectively. The median total dose to point A from external beam and intracavitary irradiation was 87 Gy, and the median doses to the bladder and rectum were 68 and 70 Gy. The total dose delivered to the vaginal surface was limited to 120 to 140 Gy or 1.4 to 2.0 times the point A dose. These total doses to point A and the vagina, bladder, and rectum are used as contemporary guidelines for determining implant duration and, therefore, dose.

Point A Redefined

The failure of localization radiographs to show the surfaces of the ovoids made implementation of the initial definition of point A difficult. The definition of point A was modified in 1953 to be "2 cm up from the lower end of the intrauterine source and 2 cm laterally in the plane of the uterus, as the external os was assumed to be at the level of the vaginal fornices" (**Figure 12.8-39**) (120). This definition

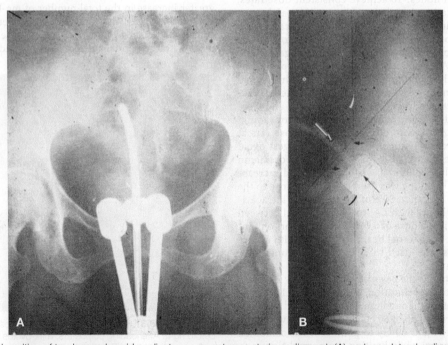

Figure 12.8-38. Ideal position of tandem and ovoid applicator on an anteroposterior radiograph (A) and on a lateral radiograph (B). Note the metallic seeds inserted into the cervix. (Reprinted with permission from Fletcher GH, ed. *Textbook of Radiotherapy*. 3rd ed. Lea & Febiger; 1980:745.)

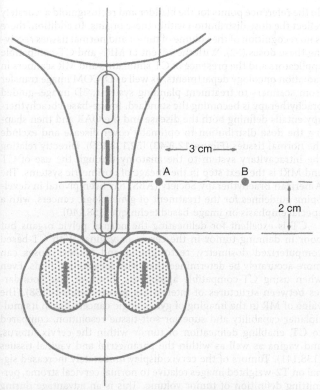

Figure 12.8-39. Revised Manchester system definition of point A. (From Morita K. Cancer of the cervix. In: Vahrson HW, ed. *Radiation Oncology of Gynecologic Cancers*. 1st ed. Springer-Verlag; 1997:185, with permission.)

of point A is currently used at many institutions (129,130). A seed or marker ball placed near the exocervix and coincident with the tandem flange is used to identify the exocervix on the localization films. This definition, however, becomes problematic when the cervix protrudes between the ovoids (**Figure 12.8-40**). This causes a

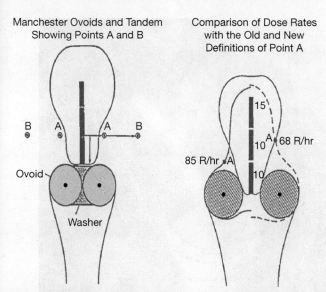

Figure 12.8-40. The definition of point A using the revised Manchester definition becomes problematic when the cervix protrudes between the ovoids, causing an increase in dose rate at point A. Use of the classic Manchester definition of point A (point A defined from the level of the upper vaginal fornices rather than the location of the exocervix) may be helpful. (Reprinted with permission from Batley F, Constable WC. The use of the Manchester system for treatment of cancer of the uterine cervix with modern afterloading radium applicators. *Am J Roentgenol Rad Ther*. 1967;18:397.)

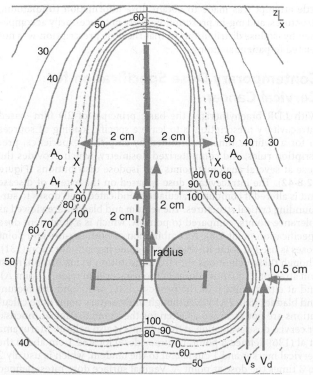

Figure 12.8-41. Variations of point A based on definition. A consistent location for dose specification should fall superior to the ovoids, where the dose distribution runs parallel to the tandem and not close to bulge of the pear. (Reprinted with permission from Nag S, Chao C, Erickson B, et al. American Brachytherapy Society recommendations for low-dose rate brachytherapy for carcinoma of the cervix. *Int J Radiat Oncol Biol Phys*. 2002;52(1):38.)

resultant increase in dose rate at point A because point A lies in the higher dose "bulge" around the ovoids (131). The variation of point A often occurs in a high-gradient region of the isodose distribution. A consistent location for dose specification should fall sufficiently superior to the ovoids where the dose distribution runs parallel to the tandem (**Figure 12.8-41**). In patients with deep vaginal fornices, reverting to the use of the ovoid surface rather than the exocervix can help solve this problem (131).

Limitations of Brachytherapy Systems: Point A

It has become clear over time that points A and B are not anatomic sites. The actual specification is related to the position of the intracavitary sources rather than to an anatomic structure. Lewis et al also demonstrated that point A does not maintain a constant relationship to any specific structure and that its position varies with the type of applicator, individual tumor anatomy, and age of the patient. No correlation was found between point B and the pelvic wall (132,133). Potish and Gerbi also question the validity of point A, as its position bears no fixed relationship to tumor or normal tissue anatomy and is in a steep dose gradient and sensitive to displacement (134). Point A can be identical for implants that differ in fundamental ways and deliver different overall 3D dose distributions.

Limitations of Brachytherapy Systems: mg-hr Systems

The use of mg-hr systems at many institutions also continues to guide the choice of source strength and duration of the implant, estimate the risk of complications, compare treatment between patients and institutions, and estimate efficacy (135). In the past, little attempt was made to obtain dose information to anatomic structures, and mg-hr prescriptions were not necessarily accompanied by isodose distributions so that the dose prescription was not related to patient anatomy.

Contemporary Dose Specification for Cervical Cancer

With LDR brachytherapy, the basic principle of 2D film–based intracavitary prescription is to leave a specific loading of sources in for a definite time, determined by empirical experience, prescription rules, and computerized dosimetry, which provides the dose at several anatomic points and isodose distributions (**Figure 12.8-42**). The intracavitary dose is based on the extent of disease and is altered if computer calculations indicated high doses to surrounding critical structures. The rectum and bladder are viewed as tolerance points, compared to point A, which is a treatment dose specification point (58). A combination of both mg-hrs and point doses is used at some institutions to guide implant duration (131). Though these definitions vary from institution to institution, most will attempt to quantify doses in the paracervical region (point A), and at either point B or the pelvic wall (C or E), and the rectum and bladder (58,129,130). Although intracavitary point dose calculations are not recorded as often for the sigmoid, vaginal mucosa, or cervix, dose evaluation at these points is also helpful. Maruyama et al (136) defined a point T (tumor dose) located 1 cm above the cervical marker and 1 cm lateral to the tandem, which is usually 2 to 3 times the dose at point A. Vaginal surface dose rates, defined at the lateral ovoid surface, will vary based on applicator diameter and available source strengths and should be in the range of 1.4 to 2.0 (the point A dose) (127,137).

It has become clear that 2D orthogonal film–based dose distribution analysis, in which single or multiple reference points are chosen on films at the interface of the organs closest to the applicators and at select dose specification points, is inadequate for gynecologic brachytherapy. Single tumor reference points such as point A, chosen from localization films, do not give sufficient information about the dose distribution throughout the tumor volume. Nor

do the reference points for the bladder and rectosigmoid accurately reflect the dose distribution within these organs. In addition, there is no recognition of the volume of tumor and normal tissues receiving these doses (52). With the advent of MRI- and CT-compatible applicators and the presence of CT simulators and MR scanners in radiation oncology departments, as well as DICOM image transfer from scanners to treatment planning systems, 3D image–guided brachytherapy is becoming the standard. Image-based brachytherapy entails defining both the disease and the OAR and then shaping the dose distribution to optimally cover disease and exclude the normal tissues (**Figure 12.8-43**) (52,138,139). Directly relating the intracavitary system to the anatomy through the use of CT and MRI is the next step in the lineage of dosimetric systems. The American Brachytherapy Society (ABS) has been pivotal in developing guidelines for the treatment of gynecologic cancers, with a special emphasis on image-based techniques (58,140).

CT is excellent for delineating the normal pelvic organs but poor in defining tumor in the cervix or vagina. With CT-based computerized dosimetry, rectosigmoid and bladder doses can more accurately be determined than with localization films. Even when using CT-compatible applicators, however, the boundaries between structures of interest are poorly defined (138). The value of MR in the imaging of gynecologic cancers lies in its multiplanar capability and superior soft-tissue resolution, compared to CT, enabling delineation of tumor within the cervix, uterus, and vagina as well as within the parametrial and vaginal tissues (138,141). Tumors of the cervix display moderately increased signal on T2-weighted images relative to normal cervical stroma, permitting definition of tumor volume. This is an advantage during brachytherapy, as one can assess the proximity of the tumor to the applicator and the subsequent dose distribution throughout the tumor volume. The excellent soft-tissue resolution of MRI allows visualization of residual tumor in relation to the isodose distribution around the MRI-compatible brachytherapy applicators (**Figure 12.8-44**) (138,141,142). The dose distribution can then be optimally conformed to the defined target volume while accurately defining and limiting the dose to the adjacent normal OAR. The GYN GEC ESTRO working group began to develop guidelines for

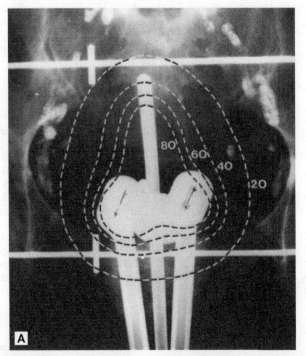 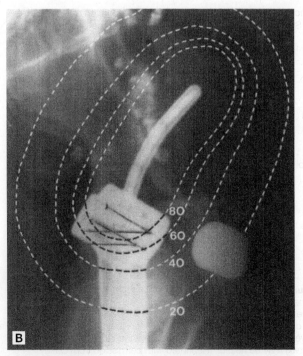

Figure 12.8-42. A: Anteroposterior view of intracavitary insertion for carcinoma of the uterine cervix. B: Lateral view of same implant. Isodose curves (cGy/hr) are superimposed. (From Perez CA, Grigsby PW, Williamson JF. Clinical applications of brachytherapy. I: Low dose-rate. In: Perez CA, Brady LW, eds. *Principles and Practice of Radiation Oncology*. 3rd ed. Lippincott-Raven Publishers; 1998:487, with permission.)

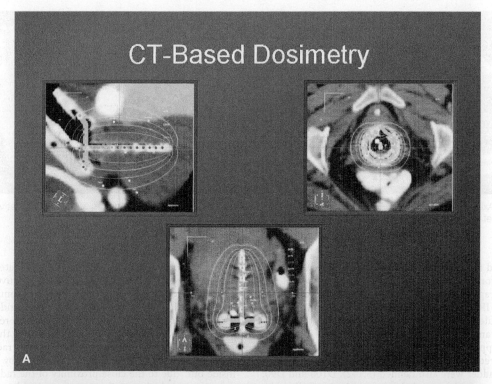

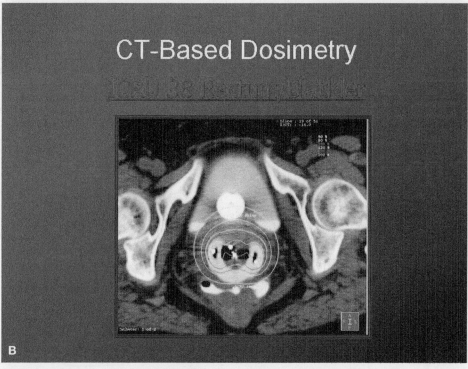

Figure 12.8-43. A: Sagittal, coronal, and axial CT images with MRI-/CT-compatible applicator in place showing the isodose distribution around the applicator and within the surrounding tissues. B: Axial CT at the level of the Foley catheter bulb near the traditional ICRU 38 bladder and rectal points. Contrast is present within the bladder and rectum as well as the bladder catheter bulb. CT, computed tomography; ICRU, International Commission on Radiation Units and Measurements; MRI, magnetic resonance imaging.

recording and reporting 3D image–based treatment planning for cervical cancer brachytherapy in 2000. The guidelines were published in 2005 and described a methodology using MRI at the time of brachytherapy to define the GTV and CTV (5,143). The gross tumor volume (GTV) at the time of brachytherapy was defined as residual tumor following external beam on clinical examination, as well as the high-signal regions on T2 fast spin echo (FSE) images in the cervix and paracervical tissues. The high-risk CTV (HRCTV) included the GTV as well as the entire cervix and extracervical tumor spread at the time of brachytherapy. The "high-risk" volume refers to tissues with a major risk of local recurrence because of residual macroscopic disease, which requires a high dose of radiation, similar to that delivered traditionally to point A. The intermediate-risk CTV (IRCTV) was defined as encompassing the HRCTV with a margin of 5 to 15 mm and refers to tissues carrying a significant microscopic tumor load. Doses of approximately

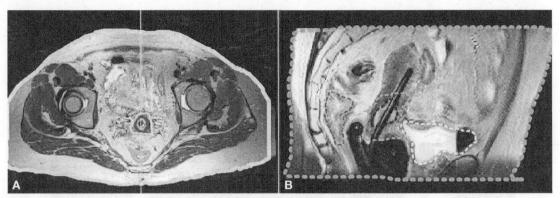

Figure 12.8-44. Axial (A) and sagittal (B) MRI images with MRI-compatible applicator in place with contours of the gross target volume and high-risk clinical target volume as well as the rectum, sigmoid, and bladder. MRI, magnetic resonance imaging.

60 Gy are intended for this volume. With these different regions of risk defined according to physical examination and MR at the time of brachytherapy, dose volume parameters were defined for the GTV, HRCTV, IRCTV, and the OAR. For the rectum, contouring included the outer wall from the anorectal junction to the rectosigmoid flexure, and the sigmoid contour continued alone until the sigmoid was approximately 2 cm from the uterus. The small bowel was contoured only if within 2 cm of the uterus. The outer contours of the bladder were also defined (5,142). D100 and D90, as well as V100, were recommended for reporting as well as the minimum dose in the most irradiated tissue volume for 0.1, 1, and 2 cc of the OARs, contouring the outer walls only (142). The radiobiologic model equivalent dose (EQD2) is used to sum the external beam and HDR doses together over the course of treatment so that a cumulative biologically weighted dose is available. This allows for systematic evaluation of the doses to the targets and normal organs over the course of treatment and for comparison between centers. An online atlas is available on the RTOG and NRG websites, with case examples using the GEC ESTRO guidelines (144).

In addition, the use of dose-volume histogram (DVH) analysis may add new insight into optimizing local control and decreasing morbidity with a better understanding of the importance of dose-volume relationships. Data from Potter et al (145) have shown a decrease in complications and an increase in local control with the use of MRI-guided brachytherapy for cervical cancer. The ABS supports these guidelines and has incorporated them into its latest guideline document (140). Though frequently confused, the ICRU 38 system (Dose and Volume Specification for Reporting Intracavitary Therapy in Gynecology) is a dose-reporting system, not a dose specification system (**Figure 12.8-45**) (146). This was developed so that comparisons could be made between centers using different brachytherapy systems. It provides definitions for determining dose to the bladder and rectum in addition to other characteristics of the implant. An updated ICRU guideline (91) is forthcoming, with an emphasis on 3D image–based planning and dose specification (146).

Importance of Brachytherapy in Cervical Cancer

When curative treatment is planned, the standard of care for patients with cervical carcinoma treated with definitive irradiation is a combination of external beam irradiation and brachytherapy (147-149). As revealed in the Quality Research in Radiation Oncology (former Patterns of Care Studies [PCS]) and retrospective series, recurrences and complications are decreased when brachytherapy is used in addition to external beam (82,83,147-149). Retrospective series with external beam alone have demonstrated marginal outcomes with this approach (150,151). Common reasons for avoidance of brachytherapy include inability to negotiate the endocervical canal

or poor performance status. Inability to negotiate the endocervical canal should be rare with the use of intraoperative ultrasound, and when this occurs, interstitial implantation is a much better option. Even with IMRT and the ability to customize and escalate the dose to specific volumes, brachytherapy cannot be replaced (138,151). The efficacy of brachytherapy is attributable to the ability of radioactive implants to deliver a higher concentrated radiation dose more precisely to tissues than external beam alone, by treating from the "inside out" due to the close proximity of the radioactive source(s) to the tumor, which contributes to improved local control and survival. At the same time, surrounding healthy tissues such as the bladder and rectosigmoid are relatively spared because of the rapid fall off dose around the applicators with distance. With IMRT, dose will necessarily be distributed in the surrounding normal tissues as it makes its way to the cervix, as the dose is delivered from the "outside in." The external beam component of treatment is, however, very important because it addresses tissues at a distance from the brachytherapy applicator, such as the pelvic lymph nodes. The external beam also brings about tumor regression in intact cervical and vaginal cancers such that the residual tissue is brought within the range of the pear-shaped or cylindrical-shaped radiation dose distribution around standard applicators (54,55).

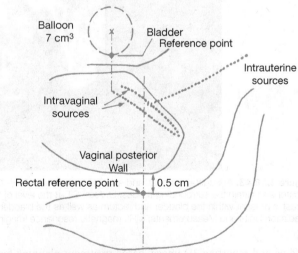

Figure 12.8-45. Reference points for bladder and rectal brachytherapy doses proposed by the International Commission on Radiation Units and Measurements. (From Commission on Radiation Units and Measurements. *Report 38: Dose and Volume Specification for Reporting Intracavitary Therapy in Gynecology.* International Commission on Radiation Units; 1985:11, Reprinted with permission of the International Commission on Radiation Units and Measurements, http://ICRU.org.)

Brachytherapy Applicators

Given the significance of brachytherapy, it is important to select the appropriate applicator to accommodate patient anatomy and the disease and shape the associated isodose distribution to encompass the disease entirely. Tumor volume and patient anatomy are key in this decision. Tumor size and shape are variable, and there is a multitude of applicators available to address these diverse presentations.

INTRACAVITARY APPLICATORS: CERVICAL CANCER

Low-Dose Rate

There are various LDR applicators available for intracavitary brachytherapy (55). The best known are the Fletcher-Suit and Henschke tandem and ovoid (colpostat) applicators (**Figure 12.8-37**). In 1953, Fletcher published an article introducing his preloaded radium applicator, which was designed to produce the largest possible volume of adequate radiation in each of the common directions of spread of disease—the uterine body, parametria, and paravaginal tissues—with relative sparing of the bladder trigone and anterior rectum due to the addition of shielding (121,122). The applicator was modified in the 1960s for afterloading (Fletcher-Suit applicator) (125) and in the 1970s to accommodate ^{137}Cs sources (125). In the 1970s, the Delclos mini-ovoid was developed for use in narrow vaginal vaults (**Figure 12.8-37**) (126). The mini-colpostats have a diameter of 1.6 cm and a flat inner surface. The mini-ovoids do not have additional shielding inside the colpostat, and this, together with their smaller diameter, produces a higher surface dose than regular ovoids, with resultant higher doses to the rectum and bladder. Appropriate source strength and treatment duration adjustment are important considerations in preventing complications. Fletcher tandems are available in four curvatures, with the greatest curvature used for cavities measuring greater than 6 cm and lesser curvatures used for smaller cavities (**Figure 12.8-37**). A flange with keel is added to the tandem once the uterine canal is sounded, which approximates the exocervix and defines the length of source train needed. The keel prevents rotation of the tandem after packing. The distal end of the tandem near the cap is marked so that rotation of the tandem after insertion can be assessed. PDR-adapted applicators are also available but are much more like HDR applicators than their LDR equivalents (62).

The Henschke tandem and ovoid applicator was initially unshielded (132) but later modified with rectal and bladder shielding (152). It consists of hemispheroidal ovoids, with the ovoids and tandem fixed together. Sources in the ovoids are parallel to the sources in the uterine tandem. The Henschke applicator may be easier to insert into shallow vaginal fornices compared to Fletcher ovoids.

The Fletcher-Suit-Delclos tandem and cylinder applicator was designed to accommodate narrow vaginas where ovoids may be contraindicated and to treat varying lengths of the vagina when mandated by vaginal spread of disease (126). The cylinders vary in size from 2 to 5 cm to accommodate varying vaginal sizes (**Figure 12.8-37**). A narrow vagina poses a therapeutic challenge (153). The use of vaginal cylinders may lead to a higher rate of local failure as the dose to the lateral cervix and pelvic sidewall is reduced in the absence of ovoids, which produces the optimum pear-shaped distribution. These patients also tend to receive lower total doses due to the proximity of the rectum and bladder (**Figure 12.8-46**) (128). There is less of a dose gradient between the vaginal mucosa and the bladder and rectum than in a patient with a wider vagina (153). In addition, packing cannot be used with cylinders to decrease the rectal and bladder doses (154,155). Vaginal cylinders increase the length of vagina and rectum treated, with an associated increase in complications. Vaginal fistulas, rectal ulcers, and strictures are reported with increased frequency when vaginal cylinders are used (156). Pourquier et al (157) indicated that doses should be reduced with the use of vaginal cylinders and mini-ovoids to reduce complications, as these applicators have no shielding. Interstitial implantation should also be a consideration for patients with a narrow vagina or with distal vaginal disease.

Importance of Optimal Applicator Placement

Geometrically optimal intracavitary implants improve outcome over suboptimal implants. Corn et al reported an analysis of the 1978 and 1983 PCS, which attempted to analyze the outcomes of patients with cervical cancer based on the technical quality of the implant. A technically good implant correlated significantly with improved local control, with a trend toward improved survival (158). In a review of the RTOG 0116 and 0128 trials, the quality of applicator placement was statistically related to the risk of local recurrence and disease-free survival (159). Perez et al (83) observed that "inadequate" insertions increased the incidence of pelvic failures and that the quality of the intracavitary insertion had a measurable impact

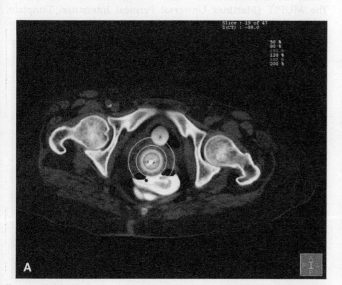
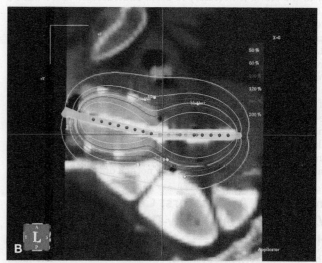

Figure 12.8-46. Magnetic resonance imaging/computed tomography–compatible tandem and cylinder applicator with associated isodose distribution in axial (A) and sagittal (B) views demonstrating the close proximity to the rectum owing to the absence of packing or rectal retraction.

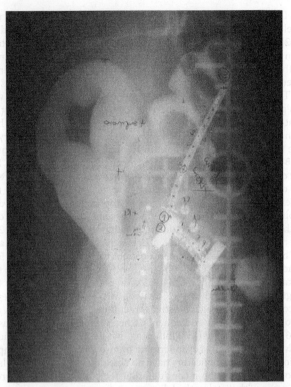

Figure 12.8-47. Lateral radiograph of a poorly positioned high-dose rate tandem and ovoid applicator. Note that the tandem does not bisect the ovoids and that the ovoid appears to be displaced inferiorly from the cervical marker balls.

on the incidence of complications (86). Attention to the details of implant geometry has been linked to improved outcome in the series of Katz and Eifel at M.D. Anderson (127). Before afterloading, it was much more difficult to obtain adequate applicator placement, owing to the need to complete the insertion quickly to avoid excessive exposure to the sources in the preloaded applicators. In the era of afterloading, applicator placement can be more methodical. Orthogonal films or other imaging (CT, MRI) should always be obtained following applicator placement to assess applicator geometry and the need for adjustment to ensure optimum placement (61). Optimum applicator placement is pivotal in maximizing local control. Placement of the brachytherapy applicators in direct proximity to the cervix is necessary to avoid underdosage. There will be a cold spot if the ovoids or other vaginal applicators are displaced away from the cervix (**Figure 12.8-47**). Proper applicator selection is important in avoiding malpositioning. It is extremely important to place metallic markers on the cervix so that the flange of the tandem and the ovoids/cylinder dome are positioned in close proximity to these markers as confirmed on orthogonal check films (58,127).

Likewise, suboptimal applicator placement can increase the risk of complications. Applicators that are too close to the bladder and rectum can increase rectal and bladder complications. Sources in the tandem can give very high doses of radiation to the small bowel (ileum), sigmoid, and upper bladder, often not revealed by orthogonal x-rays. Tandems that have perforated through the uterus can cause severe hot spots in the nearby normal organs.

Interstitial Applicators: Cervical and Vaginal Cancers—Low-Dose Rate and High-Dose Rate

The size of the reference pear-shaped isodose achieved with tandem and ovoids is not variable, except by increasing the duration (dose) of the implant. The shape of the reference pear-shaped isodose can be altered to some degree by varying the source strengths and applicator type, but it may not be able to encompass a bulky tumor, particularly when there is bulky parametrial or vaginal disease. In these settings, the disease may be better accommodated by an interstitial application (**Figure 12.8-48**) (160). Patients with large, bulky lesions will have a higher rate of local failure because of a decrease in dose to the periphery of the tumor due to the rapid fall off dose beyond the relevant pear-shaped distribution. The use of higher doses of external beam before implantation and interstitial techniques is an important consideration. These patients should not be treated with external beam alone, because achieving the curative radiation doses required may be impossible because of the limited tolerance of the interposed small bowel, rectum, and bladder (150,151). Standard intracavitary applications may be suboptimal or prohibited by either tumor bulk or distorted normal anatomy, and these patients should not be treated with geometrically unfavorable intracavitary implants (158,159).

The limitations of intracavitary techniques contrast with the strengths of interstitial techniques in certain settings. It is important to determine which approach is best on a patient-by-patient basis. Interstitial or hybrid (combined intracavitary with interstitial component) implantation is appropriate in select patients with bulky tumors, anatomic distortion such as an obliterated endocervical canal or narrow vagina, or recurrent disease (55,160). Interstitial implantation is used in less than 10% of patients with gynecologic cancers (161). Attention to patient comfort during and after the procedure, integration of appropriate imaging for ideal needle insertion relative to the tumor and dose specification/fractionation, and minimization of both acute and late morbidity are key in achieving a successful outcome. Typically, these are performed in higher volume centers through the combined efforts of Radiation Oncology and Gynecologic Oncology (162). The ABS has recently published consensus guidelines for LDR and HDR interstitial brachytherapy for cervical and vaginal cancers, summarizing the most current recommendations (58,163).

The development of prefabricated perineal templates, through which stainless steel needles were inserted and afterloaded with ^{192}Ir or ^{125}I, was pivotal in advancing interstitial techniques for the treatment of cervical and vaginal cancers. With these interstitial techniques, rather than doing a freehand implant, the template concept allows for a predictable distribution of needles inserted across the entire perineum through a perforated template according to an optimum pattern. Commercially available and institution-specific templates are used in these patients to accommodate varying disease presentations. Stainless steel and plastic needles are used, which are afterloaded with low or high activity ^{192}Ir sources. The MUPIT (Martinez Universal Perineal Interstitial Template,

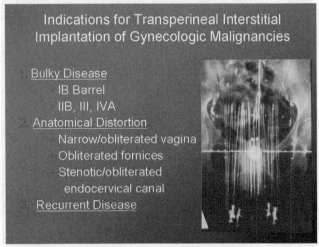

Figure 12.8-48. Indications for interstitial implantation and associated anteroposterior radiograph of the implanted needles.

Beaumont Hospital, Royal Oak, Michigan, USA) template (**Figure 12.8-49**) accommodates implantation of multiple pelvic-perineal malignancies (prostate, anorectal, gynecologic) (54,164,165). In this system, one template accommodates many different disease presentations. Recent modifications of this template and needle system enabling HDR implants have become available (166). The Syed-Neblett (Best Industries, Springfield, Virginia) is the other well-known commercially available template system (54,167,168). Currently, there are three LDR Syed-Neblett templates of varying size and shape for use in implantation of gynecologic malignances (GYN 1-36 needles, GYN 2-44 needles, GYN 3-53 needles), as well as templates for implantation of the anus, prostate, and urethra (54) (**Figure 12.8-50**). There is also a disposable template for gynecologic presentations that accommodates HDR needles (169).

The Syed-Neblett and MUPIT templates are particularly suited for the treatment of vaginal disease, as the vaginal obturator needles can be strategically loaded to encompass disease from the fornices to the introitus. In addition, the obturator needles can be advanced directly into the cervix, along with a uterine tandem, and may be essential to deliver tumoricidal radiation doses to the cervix by preventing a central "cold spot," especially if an intrauterine tandem is

not used (162,163). The use of an intrauterine tandem along with interstitial needles has been statistically associated with an improvement in OS in stage IIIB cervical cancer (170). The more peripheral needles are used for implantation of the parametria, which is often underdosed in intracavitary approaches. Modifications of these standard templates have evolved, and other innovative templates have been developed for vulvar, vaginal, and cervical carcinomas (54). Attention to the depth of needle insertion as well as to the number and location of needles is key in achieving an optimum implant (54,162). In addition, modification of the ring and ovoid applicators to accommodate a limited number of needles to improve tumor coverage has been reported recently, with improved local control in patients with bulky IIB and IIIB disease (145,171,172). In these applications, only 10% to 20% of the dwell time is contributed from source positions in the needles, and the remainder by the intracavitary component of the applicator (140). Individualized computer-generated dosimetry is an integral part of interstitial dose delivery. CT imaging following needle implantation has proven very helpful in identifying tumor volume and critical normal structures, confirming the adequacy of needle placement in relation to these structures or needed adjustments, analyzing and manipulating the dose distribution related

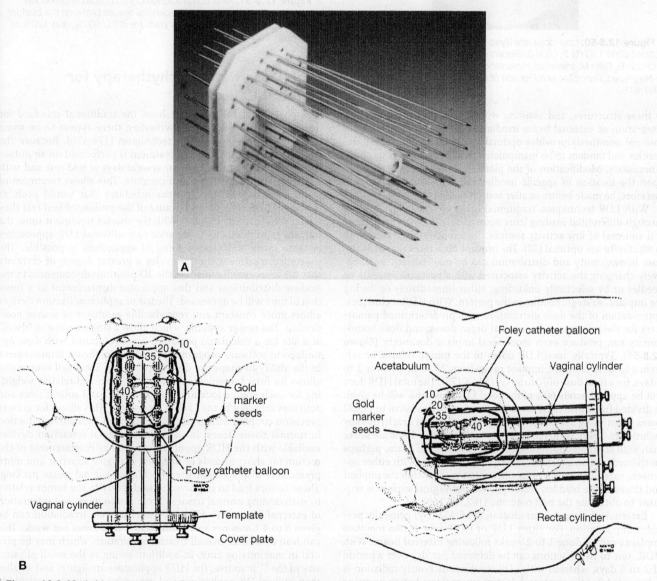

Figure 12.8-49. A: Martinez Universal Perineal Interstitial Template. B: Diagrammatic representation in coronal and sagittal planes of the same template. (A: Courtesy of Dr. Alvaro Martinez, William Beaumont Hospital, Detroit, Michigan, USA. B: Reprinted from Martinez A, Edmundson GK, Cox RS, et al. Combination of external beam irradiation and multiple-site perineal applicator (MUPIT) for treatment of locally advanced or recurrent prostatic, anorectal, and gynecologic malignancies. *Int J Radiat Oncol Biol Phys*. 1985;11:391-398, with permission from Elsevier.)

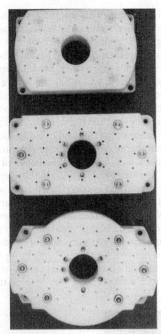

Figure 12.8-50. Low-dose rate Syed-Neblett templates: (top to bottom) GYN 1, GYN 2, GYN 3. (Reprinted with permission from Erickson B, Gillin M. Interstitial implantation of gynecologic malignancies. In: Nag S, ed. *Principles and Practice of Brachytherapy*. Futura; 1997:518.)

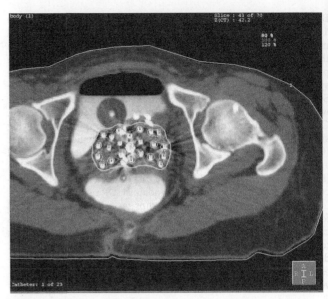

Figure 12.8-51. Axial computed tomography scan with needles inserted into the cervical and paracervical tissues between the bladder and the rectum. Isodose curves shown are 80%, 100%, and 120% of the prescription dose.

to these structures, and assisting with dose specification and the integration of external beam irradiation (54,173). Postprocedural epidural anesthesia provides optimal pain control and allows the needles and tandem to be manipulated outside the operating room if necessary. Modification of the planned source placement based upon the location of specific needles and critical structures can, therefore, be made before or after source loading (162).

With LDR techniques, traditional LDRs are the goal, achieved through differential loading (core sources ≤1/2 activity of peripheral sources) of low activity sources. "Reference" dose rates of 60 to 80 cGy/hr are optimal (58). The implant dose rates as well as the dose homogeneity and distribution can be manipulated by selectively changing the activity associated with a particular needle or needles or by selectively unloading, either immediately or during the implant, strategic needles in the pattern. With HDR techniques, optimization of the dose distribution with predetermined parameters for the reference dose, normal organ doses, and dose homogeneity can produce even more ideal implant dosimetry (**Figure 12.8-51**). Typically, total LDR doses to the tumor volume or reference isodose from the implant range from 23 to 40 Gy over 2 to 4 days, for a total dose of 70 to 80 Gy (54,58,173). The total HDR dose will be approximately 60% of the total LDR dose and will be given in divided fractions. There are not consistent data relative to EQD2 doses when using 3D image–based HDR interstitial brachytherapy techniques. There seems to be a consensus that the doses are lower than with combined intracavitay HDR and external beam, perhaps on the order of an EQD2 of 75 to 80 Gy (140,163). With either approach, careful attention to significant hot spots within the implant and doses to the bladder, rectosigmoid, and vaginal surface is requisite to obtaining the best outcome (162,163,169).

External whole-pelvic irradiation (39.6-45.0 Gy) generally precedes implantation. For either LDR or HDR, one or two template implants can be done 1 to 2 weeks following external beam. With HDR, one to two fractions can be delivered per day over a period of 2 to 5 days, whereas with LDR, continuous hourly radiation is delivered. After the implant, selective external irradiation boosting can be done as needed. The total LDR dose to the reference volume from the combined implant and external beam approximates 70 to 85 Gy over 8 weeks (162).

High-Dose Rate Brachytherapy for Cervical Cancer

Though LDR techniques have been the traditional standard for decades for gynecologic brachytherapy, there appear to be some inherent advantages to HDR techniques (174-176). Because the treatment time is very short, treatment is performed on an outpatient basis without the need for several days of bed rest and with greater patient acceptance and comfort. This allows treatment of some patients with medical comorbidities that would prohibit the use of LDR techniques because of the prolonged bed rest they would subsequently require. With the shorter treatment time, the implant reproducibility is superior to traditional LDR approaches because more stable positioning of applicators is possible. The shortened treatment time provides a greater degree of certainty that the sources will remain in the 3D positions documented in the isodose distributions and that applicator displacement as a function of time will be decreased. The use of applicator fixation devices allows more constant and reproducible geometry of source positioning. The newer systems, which allow a single source to "dwell" at a site for a calculated period of time, combined with dose optimization software programs, provide a significant improvement in the ability to shape the dose distribution. The small source size allows for finer increments in source location and relative weighting for each source location than with the fixed source sizes and activities inherent to the LDR ^{137}Cs sources. This allows for greater precision coupled with greater flexibility and, perhaps, a reduction in normal tissue doses. In addition, the rectal retraction devices available with the HDR applicators maximize displacement of the rectum for short periods of time and may give superior and more predictable displacement than traditional vaginal gauze packing. These factors lead to improved dose delivery to the tumor relative to surrounding normal tissues. There is also increased integration of external beam with HDR, as external beam irradiation can be given 3 to 4 times per week and HDR 1 to 2 times per week. This can lead to shorter overall treatment duration, which may be pivotal in maximizing cure. In addition, owing to the small physical size of the ^{192}Ir source, the HDR applicators are lighter and smaller than bulky LDR applicators and are easier to insert, particularly if there is vaginal narrowing. Many institutions use only one LDR implant, and if the applicator geometry is poor, there is no opportunity to perform multiple implants and improve the geometry or change applicators in future insertions, as can be realized with HDR techniques. The remote afterloading also provides a lack of radiation exposure to health care providers. Disadvantages of HDR may include loss of the radiobiologic advantage of LDR, decreased time for normal tissue repair, and an increase in the number of implants per patient from 1 to 3 and 3 to 6 (range, 2-16), which is labor intensive for all involved. The need for sedation may still exclude high-risk patients, even though bed rest is not required (175). Given the rapid delivery of high doses with HDR, quality and safety considerations are paramount and guidelines have been developed to maximize benefit and minimize risk (177).

Conversion From Low-Dose Rate to High-Dose Rate

There have been numerous suggestions regarding how to convert total LDR doses to HDR doses in order to implement reasonable dose-fractionation schemes. Efforts have been made by many investigators to compare the biologic effects of LDR with HDR regimens using various dose conversion models. The linear quadratic model has typically been used, but this does not address the optimal number of fractions. A basic concept is that the total dose with HDR must be less than with LDR and the number of fractions must increase (178). This concept comes from early radiobiologic studies. The Equivalent Radiation Dose (ERD) mathematical model can be used to determine the HDR dose per fraction (179). The ERD is a biologic dose unit, which utilizes the linear quadratic model. To determine an appropriate dose for HDR treatments based upon LDR techniques, the ERDs are assumed to be equal. The α/β for tumor is assumed to be 10, whereas m is assumed to be 1.4 hr^{-1}. For this calculation, the LDR total dose, LDR, and the desired number of HDR fractions are required to calculate an HDR fraction size. These calculations have shown that one must give approximately 60% to 70% of the LDR dose with HDR. The conversion of doses herein is strictly for the brachytherapy component of the treatment course. More recently, there has been interest in calculating the equivalent dose (EQD2) at 2 Gy/fraction for both the radiation targets (point A, HRCTV) and the OAR when adding together both the external beam and brachytherapy components of treatment. This can be done for LDR, PDR, and HDR. This interactive worksheet is available through the ABS website (140).

High-Dose Rate Applicators

The tandems and ovoids used with HDR are variations of the traditional Fletcher and Henschke LDR applicators but are lighter, narrower, and smaller (**Figure 12.8-52**) (55,140). The ovoids are 2.0, 2.5,

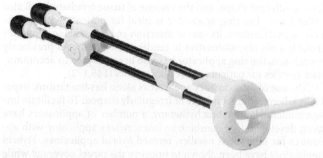

Figure 12.8-53. LDR versus HDR ovoid angles. The LDR ovoids are positioned at 15° or 30° to the vaginal axis versus 60° in the HDR ovoids. HDR, high-dose rate; LDR, low-dose rate. (Images courtesy of Elekta.)

and 3.0 cm in diameter with and without shielding. The relationship of the colpostat to the handle is different between HDR and LDR colpostats so that the cable-driven HDR source can negotiate the angle between the handle and the colpostat. The Selectron colpostats are angled at 60° to the applicator handles. Standard Fletcher-Suit LDR colpostats are angled most often at 15° and sometimes at 30° with respect to the colpostat handles (**Figure 12.8-53**). This can lead to a different relationship between the tandem and the colpostats and between the colpostats and the cervix, best seen on the lateral orthogonal x-rays taken for dosimetry after applicator insertion. As previously mentioned, these applicators have also been adapted for needle insertion for bulkier tumors (171).

The ring applicator, which is an adaptation of the Stockholm technique, has become a popular applicator (180) (**Figure 12.8-54**). The plastic caps that come with the ring applicator place the vaginal mucosa 0.6 cm from the source path, compared to the caps for the ovoids, which place the vaginal mucosa from the source path at a distance of 1 to 1.5 cm. The short distance from the ring to vaginal mucosa can result in very high surface doses if fixed weighting, nonoptimized techniques are used (176,180). The bladder and rectum may also receive higher doses with fixed weighting nonoptimized dosimetry. It is important not to activate all the positions in the ring, as this will increase the dose to the rectum, bladder, and vaginal mucosa. Typically, four dwells are activated on each side of the smallest ring (36 mm), five on each side of the medium ring (40 mm), and six on each side of the large ring (44 mm). The tandems are available in lengths of 2 to 8 cm. Four ring-tandem angles are available, including 30°, 45°, 60°, and 90°. The shape of the isodose curves comparing the ring with tandem and ovoids will also

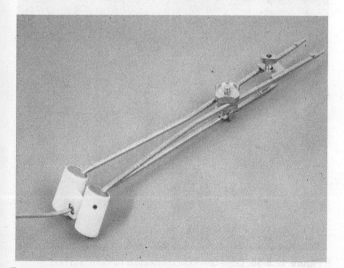

Figure 12.8-52. High-dose rate tandem and ovoids. (Courtesy of Nucletron.)

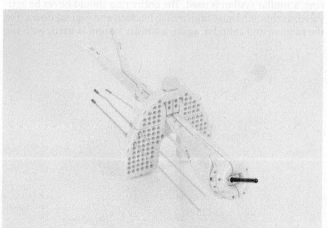

Figure 12.8-54. Tandem and ring applicator with associated rectal retractor. (Images courtesy of Elekta.)

have a different shape, and the volume of tissue irradiated will also differ (180). The ring applicator is ideal for patients without lateral vaginal fornices. Its ease of insertion and predictable geometry make it a popular alternative to tandem and ovoids. As previously mentioned, the ring applicator has also been adapted to accommodate needles for patients with bulky tumors (145,172).

The use of intracavitary applicators alone has limitations, especially when the target is large or irregularly shaped. To facilitate image-guided adaptive brachytherapy, a number of applicators have been developed that combine an intracavitary applicator with apertures for interstitial needles, termed *hybrid* applicators. Hybrid applicators have been shown to improve the target coverage while simultaneously lowering the dose to normal tissues.

Tandem and cylinder applicators are used in the setting of a narrow vagina or vaginal extension of disease and are available in diameters of 2.0 to 4.0 cm (**Figure 12.8-55**) (55). In most cases, rectal and bladder displacement are not possible with this applicator, although some of the cylinders have built-in shielding. A posterior speculum blade to displace the rectum can be used if there is no posterior vaginal disease. As with LDR tandem and cylinder applicators, the bladder and rectal doses may increase with this applicator, and the dose distribution will be more cylindrical than pear shaped, which can underdose bulky tumors (**Figure 12.8-46**). Careful attention to normal tissue doses and target coverage is necessary in this setting (140).

High-Dose Rate Treatment Planning

The dose distribution with HDR tandem and ovoids and tandem and ring applicators models the LDR pear-shaped isodose distribution. HDR regimens use a paracervical dose specification point (A), rather than mg-hrs, or a volume-based dose specification, such as the HRCTV (140). Rectal, bladder, sigmoid, and vaginal surface doses should always be specified or documented, and some assessment of dose to the pelvic lymph nodes and lateral parametria should be documented.

The HDR system utilizes special vocabulary to describe certain functions and applications. A "dwell position" is a position at which the source is driven to stop or dwell. Dwell positions can be 2.5 and 5 mm apart. An active length will be converted into a number of dwell positions. "Patient points" are points of interest at which the dose is calculated; they are defined on the orthogonal implant films. Examples include bladder, rectum, and sigmoid. "Applicator points" are points of interest at which the dose is calculated; they are defined by manually inputting the coordinates. Typically, applicator points include point A and points on the lateral surface of a ring, ovoid, or cylinder. "Dose points" are points at which the dose is optimized. In general, doses are specified using dose points. The optimization program then attempts to give the prescription dose at each of these points. With the tandem and ring, a similar system is used. The entire ring should never be activated, as this will cause high rectal, bladder, and vaginal doses. For the tandem and cylinder, again, a similar system is used, with the

exception that at the cylinder interface, dose points are entered laterally from the dwell positions at the distances representing the cylinder surface. Owing to the close proximity of the bladder and rectum in women requiring vaginal cylinders because of a narrow vagina, dose specification needs to be done with great care so as not to give excessive doses to the bladder and rectum. Dose specification at point A alone can result in underdosing of target tissue and overdosing of dose-limiting tissues (181,182). If using 2D planning, in addition to point A, specifying dose at the vaginal applicator surface is important. If using a volume-based approach, dose specification to the HRCTV while negotiating the doses to 2 cc of the bladder and rectosigmoid is key. With either approach, optimization of the dose distribution follows and enables design of a more ideal dose distribution (**Figure 12.8-56**). The term "optimization" refers to the process of achieving certain dose values at points or volumes within the implant. It is not the simple generation of a standard dose distribution by using fixed dose points around the applicator (140). The goal is to match the dose distribution to point A or the HRCTV while simultaneously avoiding the OAR. Inherent to optimization is starting with a standard plan of loading the tandem and the vaginal applicator and then modifying the dwell times and dwell weights to reduce dose to the OAR and ensure optimal tumor coverage (140). Excessive optimization can alter the pear shape to a less desirable configuration with the same point A dose (182). When altering the standard dwell times and weights, it is important to also monitor changes in the dose, dose/volume parameters, and the spatial dose distribution that result from the modified loading pattern. Reliance on DVH alone can be dangerous if one does not also evaluate the spatial dose distribution (140). The entire length of the tandem does not always need to be treated and should be guided by the definition of remaining tumor at the time of brachytherapy, as seen on MR or CT. This can reduce dose to the OARs (183). Likewise, activation of dwell positions in the vaginal applicator should also be considered carefully, in light of the closely approximated bladder and rectum and vaginal target.

High-Dose Rate Dosimetry Generation

It is important to perform dosimetry for each fraction of an HDR tandem and vaginal applicator regimen even if the same applicator is used, as there may be quite a bit of variation in applicator position with each fraction (140,184). There is also applicator

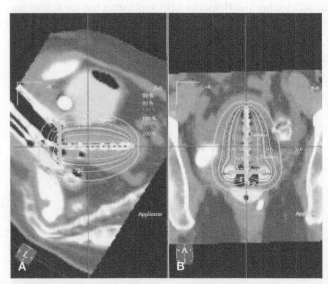

Figure 12.8-56. Dose distribution around a tandem and ring applicator in sagittal (A) and coronal (B) projections with dose specified at the ring surface and at the level of point A.

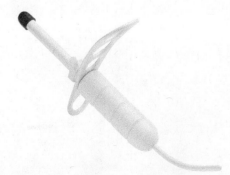

Figure 12.8-55. Tandem and cylinder applicator. (Images courtesy of Elekta.)

deformation of the adjacent structures, which varies with applicator position (185). Variables that impact applicator position are vaginal packing, the presence and effectiveness of sedation/anesthesia, and use of the dorsal lithotomic versus legs down position. The bladder and rectosigmoid may also change configuration owing to changes in filling and position, and doses to these organs will vary from fraction to fraction. Uterine and sigmoid mobility may also impact the dose distribution in these organs. In addition, disease regression and vaginal narrowing will vary from fraction to fraction and can result in changes in dose distribution. A change in applicator can also result in changes in dose distribution, as can changing the ovoid or ring size, ovoid separation, and tandem curvature. The ovoids may also change in separation and their relative position to the tandem over time if there is no fixed relationship between the tandem and the ovoids. Jones et al (184) found that when treatment planning was not performed for each fraction and only the initial dosimetry was used, there was increased dose to at-risk normal organs. This is also true when using a tandem and ring, even though it has a fixed geometry. The applicator position relative to the pelvic organs is the important factor rather than the relationship of the tandem to the ring (Figure 12.8-57).

Dose-Fractionation Schemes

There is no consensus as to the optimal number of fractions, and dose per fraction except that the choice will depend on the external beam dose and on whether central shielding is used as well as normal tissue doses, medical comorbidities, and the stage of disease. The linear quadratic model was suggested as a guide to formulate the regimens chosen at each institution (186). Currently, the GOG protocols define a dose/fractionation scheme of 5.6 to 6.3 Gy × 5 to point A with whole-pelvis doses of 41.4 to 45 Gy. The RTOG protocols allow fraction sizes of 5.3 to 7.4 Gy when using four to seven

fractions, depending on the external beam dose. Tables for combining various external beam doses with varying HDR fractions using the linear quadratic formula and normal tissue-modifying factor have been provided with these protocols (186). There has been increasing concern that 6 Gy × 5 to point A may result in excessive toxicity to the rectum and sigmoid when combined with whole-pelvis doses of 45 G, and a dose of 5.5 Gy × 5 to point A may be more reasonable (140). In the United States, the most common HDR intracavitary regimen prescribes two fractions per week for a total of five fractions, with 5 to 6 Gy per fraction (140,187). Internationally, the most common dose per fraction was between 5 and 7 Gy, with the higher dose per fraction associated with a decrease in fraction number (three to five fractions) (161). When using volumetric image–guided brachytherapy, the dose at point A can still be tracked, but the goal is to deliver 80 to 90 Gy to the HRCTV, depending on the volume of disease, while limiting dose to the OAR to an acceptable level. The EQD2 limit to the D2cc (the minimum dose in the most irradiated 2 cm^3 normal tissue volume for the rectum and sigmoid) is 65 to 70 Gy, the small bowel 70 Gy, the bladder 80 to 90 Gy, and the vagina (using the ICRU 38 rectal point) 65 Gy (140,188).

Sequencing of External Beam Radiation With Brachytherapy

In nonbulky disease presentations, HDR insertions are often integrated early in the treatment course after approximately 20 Gy of external beam radiation therapy. Alternatively, some institutions choose to take the whole pelvis to 40 to 45 Gy initially, preceding the five HDR insertions, unless the patient has very early disease or evidence of early vaginal stenosis. This allows for maximum disease regression before brachytherapy. When delivering 40 to 45 Gy to the whole pelvis before initiation of HDR, it is important to avoid

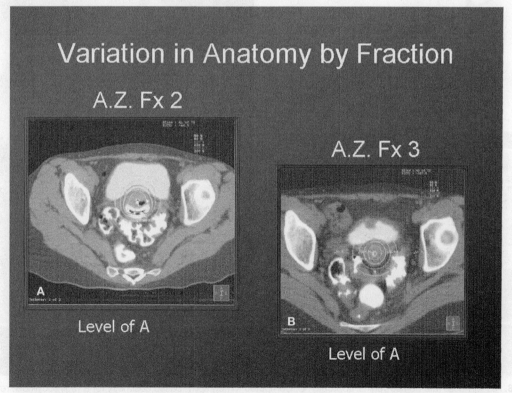

Figure 12.8-57. Variation in anatomy between fraction 2 (A) and fraction 3 (B) of a five-fraction high-dose rate course. Note the difference in the position of normal organs at the level of point A between fractions 2 and 3.

treatment prolongation by giving two HDR fractions per week to complete the radiation within 50 (outside limit 56 days) (140,187).

Brachytherapy for Endometrial Cancer

Hysterectomy is the cornerstone of the treatment for endometrial carcinoma. Selective use of vaginal brachytherapy or external beam irradiation or both in the postoperative setting is based on the histopathologic risk factors identified in the tissues removed at the time of surgical staging (189,190). Vaginal brachytherapy is typically performed using Fletcher colpostats, or a variety of vaginal cylinders (Delclos, Burnett). Both LDR and HDR techniques are used (191,192) (**Figure 12.8-58**). The choice of ovoids versus cylinders is individual, and both have relative advantages and disadvantages (52). Vaginal ovoids are available in diameters of 2 to 3 cm with associated caps and shielding. Vaginal cylinders are available in diameters of 2 to 5 cm, with or without shielding. Vaginal ovoids generally require sedation for insertion, whereas cylinders do not. The length of the vagina treated with vaginal ovoids is approximately the upper third, whereas vaginal cylinders can treat a portion of or the entire vagina. Though rare, when present, distal vaginal metastases tend to be located in the periurethral area (193). Poorly differentiated tumors may recur earlier and present in the distal vagina or distant disease sites, whereas well-differentiated lesions tend to recur later and are often in the upper vagina (194). Distal vaginal recurrences or metastases, however, are rare after radiation and have been noted to occur in 0.5% to 1% of patients when the upper vagina was treated. It is, therefore, not suggested to treat more than the upper half of the vagina routinely. Typically, the length of vagina treated with vaginal cylinders is between 4 and

5 cm, perhaps favoring a longer length when using brachytherapy alone (191,192). Packing is typically used to displace the rectum and bladder with ovoids and not with cylinders. Owing to the longer length of vagina treated and the lack of packing, a larger volume of rectum and bladder will be treated with cylinders. Vaginal ovoids may be prohibited in a narrow vagina, whereas vaginal cylinders may not be in close approximation with all of the vaginal mucosa in the setting of a wide vaginal apex or if the cuff has been closed with "dog ears" rather than in a cylindrical shape.

Most vaginal brachytherapy for endometrial cancer is performed with vaginal cylinders using HDR techniques (**Figure 12.8-58**) (191,192). The dose distribution should ideally conform to the shape of the cylinder (192,195). Dose is typically specified either at the vaginal applicator surface (mucosal surface) or at a depth of 0.5 cm from the applicator or vaginal mucosal surface (191,192). Dose prescription at 0.5 cm can lead to excessively high mucosal doses, and surface doses should also be tracked (192,196). In addition, careful assessment of dose to the rectum and bladder through the use of computerized dosimetry should be performed for the first fraction of radiation delivered (**Figure 12.8-58**). CT-based planning allows for an excellent assessment of the doses to the bladder and rectum as well as evaluation of air gaps at the interface of the applicator surface and vaginal mucosa, but is only needed for the first fraction (192,197). Choo et al (198) have revealed that 95% of the vaginal lymphatic channels are located within 3 mm of the vaginal surface and that dose prescription to a depth of less than 5 mm may be adequate. For LDR insertions, dose rates at the surface of the applicator should be in the range of 80 to 100 cGy/hr, and perhaps 50 to 70 cGy/hr if the prescription is at 0.5 cm (195). Total vaginal surface doses of 50 to 80 Gy are reported most frequently in the

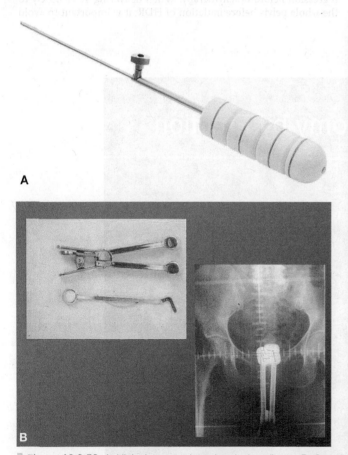

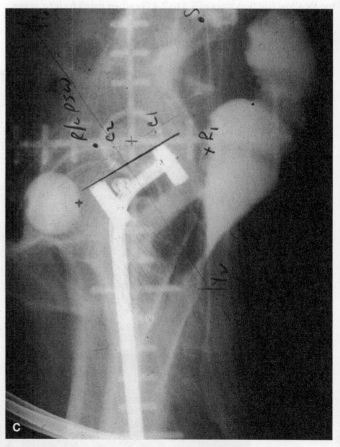

Figure 12.8-58. A: High-dose rate domed vaginal applicator. B: Computed tomography–based dosimetry for a vaginal cylinder, revealing the relationship of the dose distribution to the cylinder surface and adjacent bladder and rectum. Lateral radiographs are shown of cylinder (C) and ovoids (D) with bladder bulb contrast in both and rectal contrast in (C). (Images courtesy of Elekta.)

literature. When used with external beam, cumulative doses of 60 to 100 Gy at the vaginal surface are reported in the literature. Doses in excess of 80 Gy to the vaginal mucosa are not necessary in the setting of adjuvant therapy and can be associated with increased morbidity. For a vaginal recurrence of endometrial cancer, doses of 80 Gy and higher may be needed when combining external beam and brachytherapy (199).

Vaginal brachytherapy alone is generally considered an option for patients treated with hysterectomy, with either no or selective lymph node sampling, who are thought to be at low risk for lymph node metastases. These patients typically have grade 1 or 2 disease without significant myometrial invasion (<1/3) (91,190). Vaginal brachytherapy alone is considered an option at some institutions in the setting of a negative pelvic lymph node dissection, even when high-risk factors such as high-grade or deep myometrial invasion is present (91,190).

There is great debate about whether a vaginal cuff boost is routinely necessary in addition to external beam irradiation for early-stage endometrial cancer; there are little data to support it (91,189). Practice patterns are based more on institutional tradition and individual preference rather than prospective randomized trials. The rationale for use of a vaginal boost is the supposition that there may be a critical dose needed at the vaginal apex to optimally decrease the likelihood of a vaginal apex recurrence. Doses in excess of the 45 to 50 Gy typically delivered with external beam may be necessary if there are microscopic tumor cells embedded in the hypoxic vaginal cuff.

In some clinical situations, more complex brachytherapy procedures are required to treat endometrial cancer. Patients with bulky stage II endometrial cancers may benefit from preoperative radiation with external beam alone, brachytherapy alone, or a combination of the two. Tandem and ovoids or tandem and ring or cylinder applicators are used in this setting. Medically inoperable endometrial cancer is a rare phenomenon in the current era of aggressive surgical staging. When encountered, it may require the use of sophisticated radiation techniques (200). The ABS released guidelines specific to patients who have inoperable endometrial cancer (201). The ABS recommends MRI if available, or CT, to determine the uterine wall thickness and for volume-based brachytherapy. The ABS recommends brachytherapy alone in patients with stage I, grade 1 to 2 endometrial cancer with minimal myometrial invasion on MRI. If MRI is not available, then external beam radiation in conjunction with brachytherapy should be used. In patients with stage I disease and deep myometrial invasion based on MRI, or stage II or stage III disease, external beam radiation to a total dose of 45 to 50 Gy is recommended, followed by brachytherapy (200,201).

Tandem and ovoids or a tandem and ring or cylinder may be appropriate if the uterine cavity is small. If the uterus is large or if there is more extensive disease, special uterine applicators such as dual and triple tandems or Heyman-Simons capsules may be helpful (**Figure 12.8-59**) (200). There is better coverage of the entire endometrial cavity with these applicators, and dose can be delivered through the uterine wall to the serosa of the uterus. HDR and LDR techniques can be used.

Patients with recurrent endometrial cancer usually benefit from both external beam and brachytherapy. Doses in excess of 80 Gy may lead to better local control in these patients (199). In patients with residual vaginal disease less than 0.5 cm in maximum thickness, vaginal cylinders or ovoids can be used, whereas

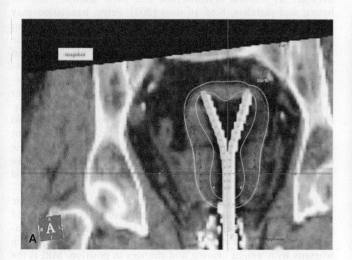
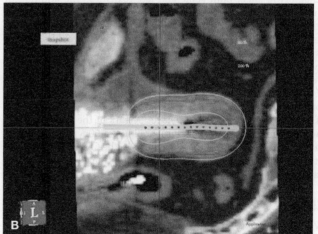
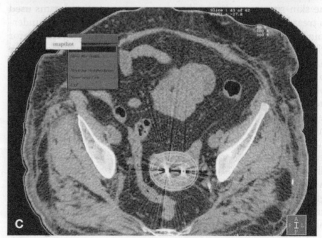

Figure 12.8-59. Brachytherapy plan for a patient with medically inoperable endometrial cancer in coronal (A), sagittal (B), and axial (C) dimensions. Note dual tandems on the coronal image (A).

in patients with thicker lesions following external beam, interstitial techniques are needed. For apical lesions, laparotomy or laparoscopy or image-guided brachytherapy may be required for optimum needle placement and to avoid small bowel tethered to the pelvic floor (54,202,203). Similar brachytherapy techniques can be used for patients with primary cancer of the vagina (52,163,204). Multichannel vaginal cylinders can be very helpful in this setting to direct dose to where it is needed in the vagina and spare uninvolved walls the high dose (205,206).

Radiation-Induced Tissue Effects

Side effects that develop during the course of radiation and persist for 3 months or less following completion of radiation are termed *acute* side effects. Those toxicities that develop later than 3 months after the completion of radiation are termed *late or chronic* effects. The late effects of radiation are due to damage at the capillary level where there is endothelial cell proliferation, resulting in less diffusion of oxygen into the tissues with resulting fibrosis. There is less resistance to infection, trauma, or functional stress due to this change in vasculature and circulation (207,208). When treating gynecologic cancers, the normal tissues in the pelvis that are most often irradiated incidentally are the rectosigmoid, small bowel, bladder, vagina, pelvic bones, and bone marrow. In the upper abdomen, the kidneys, liver, stomach, small bowel, large bowel, and spinal cord may be in the radiation field. The response of a tissue or organ to radiation depends on two factors: (a) the inherent sensitivity of the individual cells and (b) the kinetics of the population as a whole, of which the cells are a part. These factors combine to account for the substantial variations in response to radiation that characterize different tissues (1). In addition, the volume of tissue irradiated as well as the dose, dose rate, and dose-fractionation scheme will affect both acute and late toxicities. The addition of chemotherapy or other systemic agents may impact toxicity, as may other medical comorbidities such as diabetes, hypertension, collagen vascular diseases, Crohn disease, and ulcerative colitis, as well as social risk factors such as smoking (209). The most comprehensive data describing the effects of radiation on the normal tissues were published by Rubin and Casarett and later updated by Emami et al (208,210). Rubin and Casarett defined tolerance doses (TDs) for almost all of the tissues. The TD 5/5 is defined as the probability of a 5% risk of complications within 5 years of the completion of radiation, and TD 5/50 as the probability of a 50% risk of complications within 5 years (208). More recently, the QUANTEC (Quantitative Analyses of Normal Tissue Effects in the Clinic) guidelines have been published with updated recommendations (211,212).

Skin

When undergoing radiation treatment for abdominopelvic tumors, the patient often experiences minimal skin reactions; this is due to the skin-sparing quality of the high energy radiation beams used to treat these sites deep within the body. In contrast, when undergoing radiation treatment of the vulvar and inguinal regions, for which electrons or lower energy x-rays are more often used, there may be marked skin reactions. Skin reactions are also more likely to develop in skin folds, such as the inguinal creases or intergluteal fold. The cells in the basal layer of the skin are very sensitive to radiation, but because of the time required for these differentiating cells to move from the basal layer to the keratinized layer of skin, there is a 2- to 3-week delay between the start of radiation and the appearance of skin reactions. Erythema is the first visible skin reaction and is due to dilation of the small capillaries; it is usually seen about the third week of radiation. Other skin reactions include dry desquamation and moist desquamation, occurring after the fourth week of radiation. Moist desquamation occurs with transient loss of the epidermis and exposure of the dermis. Serous fluid often oozes from the exposed and inflamed dermis (208,213).

These effects may be enhanced by the combination of irradiation and some chemotherapeutic agents, particularly actinomycin D and doxorubicin (Adriamycin) (214). It is also well known that chemotherapy agents such as Adriamycin or gemcitabine can "recall" radiation reactions after the original reaction has subsided (215). Radiation-induced skin reactions are treated with various topical ointments and creams as well as with sitz baths and special emphasis on cleansing all stool and urine gently from the perineum. In addition, if the distal vagina or vulva is in the radiation field, patients may also complain of dysuria or painful defecation, which is due to the caustic effects of the urine and stool on the denuded epithelium of the distal vagina, perianal area, and vulva. Diarrhea control and use of barrier creams to protect the irritated skin from stool and urine will help minimize discomfort and hasten skin healing. Sulfa-based creams and Domeboro soaks can be used to expedite healing. Return of the epidermis can take 10 to 14 days. Residual surviving basal cells form islands of regeneration, which proliferate to reepithelialize the area. Islands of skin forming in the desquamated skin herald skin renewal. The new skin is thin and pink, with gradual return to normal in 2 to 3 weeks (208). Late manifestations of radiation on the skin include depigmentation, subcutaneous fibrosis, dryness and thinning with loss of apocrine and sebaceous glands, thinning or loss of hair, and telangiectasias. Necrosis of the skin is rare and generally occurs only with very high doses of radiation in excess of 60 Gy (208,214).

Bone Marrow/Pelvic Bones

The lymphocytes are the most radiosensitive cells in the bone marrow. The rate of fall of the various components of the marrow is a function of the half-lives of the mature cells. These half-lives are as follows: erythrocytes, 120 days; granulocytes, 6.6 hours; and platelets, 8 to 10 days (208). Pelvic irradiation may cause transient lymphopenia. This is even more of an issue when whole-abdominal or extended-field irradiation is used, due to the increased bone marrow in the radiation fields. This decrease in lymphocytes is thought to be the result of irradiation of the lymphocytes circulating through the vascular bed and may not be indicative of bone marrow–reserve depletion. Prior or concurrent chemotherapy will also lead to increased bone marrow toxicity. Frequent monitoring of the complete blood count is considered standard of care with pelvic or abdominal irradiation. Permanent chronic changes are noted even when small segments of the bone marrow are irradiated to doses over 30 Gy, and recovery may take up to 18 months or longer in a proportion of patients with good reparative capacity.

Insufficiency fractures can also develop in irradiated pelvic bones (216,217). These most commonly involve the sacrum and ileum, followed by the pubic bones, and rarely the acetabulum. Patients may complain of sudden onset of back or groin pain, which worsens with weight bearing and changes in position. MRI is the best imaging modality to detect them and also rule out recurrent disease. Sometimes, edema will be reported in the absence of actual fractures, and in other cases, actual fractures will be seen. It is important not to confuse these changes with metastatic disease, as further palliative irradiation would worsen the integrity of the bone. Symptoms from these changes in the pelvic bones will often improve over time, but patients may also suffer future symptoms from exacerbation of these fractures or development of new fractures over time. Percutaneous cementing of the injured bone can be used if patients remain symptomatic. Narcotics and changes in activity are often required. Femoral neck complications can include avascular necrosis as well as fracture. This is a rare complication following irradiation of the inguinal nodes. Hip replacement surgery is required to resolve this problem (218). The skeletal health of at-risk patients undergoing radiation should be considered pretreatment with baseline bone densities and referral for medical intervention.

Liver

During whole-abdominal irradiation or para-aortic irradiation, the liver is in the radiation field, and dose must be limited to this critical organ. Clinical and pathologic studies have shown that the liver is not a radioresistant organ (219). Veno-occlusive disease is the pathologic entity caused by radiation. Necrosis and atrophy of the hepatic cells result from this change in blood supply (208). CT scanning following radiation can show changes in perfusion of the liver corresponding to the radiation fields. These changes are not always associated with toxicity. The clinical course and liver changes depend on the dose-fractionation scheme and volume of irradiation as well as the presence of chemotherapy and preexisting liver disease. During radiation, the liver enzymes may be elevated. This can continue following completion of radiation. Signs of radiation hepatitis can include a marked elevation of alkaline phosphatase (3-10 times normal), with much less elevation of the transaminases (normal to 2 times normal) (208,219). Liver enlargement and varying amount of ascites can also evolve. If the doses and volumes are high enough, liver failure can occur. The TD 5/5 for whole liver is 30 Gy in 2 Gy fractions (208,210). Small portions of the liver can receive up to 70 to 90 Gy. Mean liver doses of less than 28 to 32 Gy at 2 Gy/fraction are recommended (220).

Kidney

The kidneys are very sensitive to small doses of radiation, and a common goal is to avoid greater than 18 to 20 Gy whole-kidney dose. When delivering whole-abdominal irradiation, the kidneys are at risk and must be blocked at acceptable doses to prevent renal failure. When delivering para-aortic irradiation, the kidneys are also at risk, and treatment planning CT scans can help define which beam angles would best irradiate the nodal regions while avoiding the kidneys. When planning radiation fields, sometimes, one kidney will need to be irradiated more than the other and the equivalent of one kidney must be spared. Chemotherapy can lower kidney tolerance to radiation as can increasing age. Irradiation of only one kidney does not necessarily reduce the risk of renal complications (221). Functional renal studies before radiation are important in documenting unexpected perfusion or excretion abnormalities and in determining how much each kidney contributes to total renal function. Functional changes have been described after exposure of the kidney to more than 20 Gy, and signs and symptoms of renal dysfunction can follow, including hypertension, leg edema, and urinalysis showing albuminuria and low specific gravity (221). A normocytic, normochromic anemia may also appear. Renal function studies will ultimately show decreased blood flow and filtration rates. CT scans may reveal a small kidney if one kidney has been preferentially irradiated to protect the other (208). Current dose-volume recommendations are found in the QUANTEC data (221).

Ovaries

In premenopausal patients treated with definitive irradiation, the ovaries will be irradiated incidentally, and ovarian failure will occur. Hot flashes and other menopausal symptoms can develop during radiation. Hormone replacement therapy is an important consideration in women younger than 50 years. Alternatively, midline oophoropexy has been used in young women requiring irradiation for Hodgkin disease, in an effort to spare the ovaries. The ovaries can also be elevated out of the radiation field and placed above the true pelvis to attempt to protect them when treating cervical cancer. The radiosensitivity of the ovarian cells varies considerably with age. The dose necessary to castrate a woman depends on her age. A larger dose is required during the period of more active follicular proliferation. A single dose of 4.0 to 8.0 Gy or fractionated doses of 12 to 20 Gy (depending on age) are known to produce permanent castration and sterility in most patients (207,208,214).

Vagina

There are few noticeable acute reactions when treating the upper two-thirds of the vagina with radiation. Some patients may notice a white-yellow vaginal discharge, which is due to mucositis of the vaginal mucosa. This may be evident during and can continue for several months after radiation (208). The lower third of the vagina, however, will become quite irritated when irradiated, in part due to irradiation of the vulva and urethra as described earlier. The distal vagina is less tolerant of radiation than the proximal, and the TDs are in the range of 80 to 90 Gy versus 120 to 150 Gy (222). There are, however, no studies that have successfully correlated DVH parameters with morbidity (223). Vaginal narrowing and shortening is a late sequela of radiation, which can alter and impede sexual function. Combined brachytherapy and external beam irradiation will cause more late effects than either modality alone. The use of a vaginal dilator or intercourse 2 to 3 times per week can help keep the vagina open. The use of lubrication with intercourse as well as estrogen creams to build up the vaginal mucosa can also make intercourse more comfortable (214,224). Rarely, with excessive doses of radiation, patients can develop vaginal necrosis. This is due to a change in blood supply to the vaginal tissues and is much more common at the introitus than at the vaginal apex, perhaps due to the vascular supply of the vagina. The posterior vaginal wall is most frequently involved (222). Interstitial implants are more likely to cause necrosis than intracavitary implants. Hydrogen peroxide douches, antibiotics, and hyperbaric oxygen therapy can help the vaginal tissues to heal (225). Narcotics are often necessary to control the associated pain until healing has occurred. Trental (pentoxifylline) can also help soft-tissue necrosis to heal (226). The uterus is very resistant to high doses of radiation, as is evident in patients treated with external beam and brachytherapy for cervical cancer. Rare cervical necrosis can occur and will respond readily to hyperbaric oxygen treatments and pentoxifylline (214,225). There may be an increased risk of this in patients using cocaine. Necrosis can also be caused by recurrent tumor; distinguishing recurrent disease from necrosis can be very difficult and sometimes requires surgical intervention (208).

Stomach, Small and Large Intestines

The stomach is lined with a mucous membrane comprising columnar epithelium, which is sensitive to radiation. Like the small and large bowel reactions, the stomach lining develops erosions and thinning, and subsequent edema and ulceration. Symptoms may include nausea, vomiting, reflux, and pain. The use of prophylactic antiemetics and proton-pump inhibitors can decrease the acute effects of radiation. Acid production can be decreased during radiation and for up to 1 to 2 years after. Late effects can include gastritis and ulceration with associated bleeding. Progressive fibrosis can lead to gastric outlet obstruction and, rarely, perforation, all of which are dose and volume dependent (208). The entire stomach can tolerate doses of 45 to 50 Gy, but data on maximum tolerated doses are inadequate (227).

The acute effects of radiation on the small intestine are due to the inherent radiation sensitivity of the rapidly dividing undifferentiated crypt of Lieberkühn cells. The normal lining of the GI tract is a self-renewing tissue. These undifferentiated stem cells normally migrate and differentiate upward from the lower half of the crypts to the tips of the intestinal villi as they mature, providing a continuous supply of surface cells as they divide. Their function is to primarily form not only absorptive cells but also mucous-secreting goblet cells and endocrine cells (207,208,213). The mature cells at the surface of the villi are repeatedly sloughed and replaced by the cells that originate in the crypts. These undifferentiated crypt cells are the most sensitive to radiation and are preferentially depleted, leading to loss of mature replacement cells at the surface of the villi. When these mature mucosal cells cannot be replaced, the villi shorten and the loss of absorptive function of the small intestine occurs. This loss of function results in fluid and nutrient wasting, diarrhea, and dehydration. This constellation of symptoms is termed *acute radiation enteritis*. Fortunately, reepithelialization occurs within several days due to recovery of the rapidly dividing crypt cells (213). Mucosal healing will occur within 10 to 14 days if radiation is terminated, and symptoms will accordingly improve and resolve in most patients. It is common to observe watery diarrhea with intermittent abdominal cramping starting in the second or third week of abdominal or pelvic irradiation. Increased peristalsis, disturbance of the absorption mechanisms, and decreased transit time may also occur. Patients will report increased flatulence and noisy bowel sounds. Rarely, patients will report nausea. Implementation of a low-residue diet, hydration, and use of antimotility agents can be very helpful. Some patients may be lactose and fat intolerant as well. Judicious use of narcotics to calm the bowel can also be helpful. Concurrent 5-FU or gemcitabine can worsen small bowel toxicity; diarrhea from 5-FU often appears before the radiation enteritis has had time to evolve. The late effects of radiation on the small bowel may be a continuation of the acute effects (227). Some patients will experience chronic diarrhea, requiring a permanent change in diet. Certain foods may trigger diarrhea, such as those high in fiber or fat. Spicy foods and monosodium glutamate may also trigger diarrhea. Areas of narrowing corresponding to regions of high dose or adhesions can occur in the small bowel loops and lead to partial obstruction of the small bowel. Patients may report abdominal pain and distention, followed by diarrhea and relief of these symptoms. A complete bowel obstruction would also be characterized by abdominal pain and distention in addition to vomiting and lack of bowel movements. Small bowel obstructions occur in approximately 5% of irradiated patients, and surgical intervention is required in some to relieve these obstructions. Prior surgeries or a history of perforated appendix, pelvic abscess, or inflammatory bowel disease may increase the risk of small bowel toxicity, as can the use of chemotherapy. Hypertension and diabetes can also be the risk factors, as can thin body habitus. Radiation to large volumes of bowel or high doses to even small volumes of bowel can lead to bowel obstructions. The ileum is the most common loop of bowel involved (208). Malabsorption of fats, carbohydrates, protein, B$_{12}$, and lactose may occur in some patients. Excessive bile salts can reach the colon and act as a cathartic, and medications such as cholestyramine may be helpful in controlling the resultant loose stools.

Small bowel doses should be limited to 45 to 50 Gy with 60 Gy maximum (87). Current recommendations for small bowel dose/volume constraints are as follows: The absolute volume of small bowel receiving greater than 15 Gy should be less than 120 cc when delineating individual loops of bowel. If the entire peritoneal space is defined, the volume of small bowel receiving greater than 45 Gy should be less than 195 cc (227).

The rectosigmoid mucosa is a rapid renewal system similar to the small bowel. When the rectum is included in the irradiated volume, there is rectal discomfort with tenesmus and production of mucous, sometimes mixed with blood in the stools (208). Patients may report frequent and sometimes painful evacuations of only small amounts of stool mixed with mucus. Hemorrhoids may worsen during radiation. This constellation of symptoms is termed "proctitis." Medications to decrease the number of stools as well as antispasmodic agents can be helpful. Suppositories or foams with steroids can be helpful, as can topical perianal skin ointments and lotions. Uncontrolled radiation enteritis can worsen radiation proctitis due to frequent stooling through the irritated rectum. With respect to late effects, if the dose of radiation is large enough, it may cause temporary or permanent ulceration and bleeding due to telangiectasias (**Figure 12.8-60**) (228). Cortisone-containing rectal suppositories and foams or sulfasalazine instillations can also help heal the bleeding and ulcerated rectal mucosa, as can argon laser ablation of the telangiectasias.

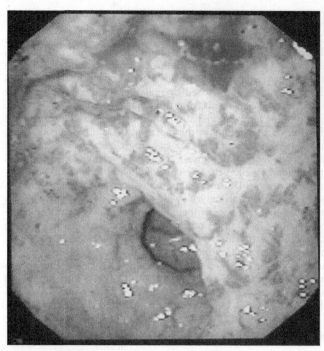

Figure 12.8-60. Radiation-induced telangiectasias of the rectum consistent with radiation proctitis.

Bladder/Ureters/Urethra

The bladder and ureters have a rapidly renewing transitional epithelium. The effect of radiation is early denudation similar to the skin due to injury to the rapidly dividing basal cells. Epithelial desquamation leads to focal ulcerations, hyperemia, and edema of the bladder wall, which is visible at cystoscopy (208,213,229). Acute and transient radiation cystitis may be observed with moderate doses of irradiation (>30 Gy) and usually requires no specific treatment. Patients will report urinary frequency and urgency and mild dysuria, as well as decreased bladder capacity. However, with higher radiation doses, more severe symptoms of cystitis develop, such as severe dysuria and hematuria, which may require treatment. Agents such as Pyridium may help lessen these symptoms. Significant spasms of the bladder musculature, which can be improved with administration of smooth muscle relaxants, may also occur. It is important to rule out the presence of a concomitant bacterial infection, which may exacerbate the symptoms. Infections are seen at an increased rate in irradiated patients, perhaps, in part, due to radiation-induced diarrhea and contamination of the perineum. Urinalysis and urine cultures obtained under sterile conditions, when indicated, should be obtained before institution of antibiotic therapy. Radiation cystitis is characterized by the presence of white cells and red cells without bacteria on urinalysis.

With doses above 60 Gy, chronic cystitis and hematuria may be observed due to telangiectasias, which can develop in the bladder lining (230). With higher doses, more severe chronic cystitis, fibrosis, and decreased bladder capacity may occur. Rarely, bladder neck contractures as well as fistulas may occur, which can necessitate surgical intervention. Fistulas are more likely to occur if there is invasion of the bladder wall by tumor, or in the setting of interstitial implants. Surgery may be required to deal with some of these complications (208). Hyperbaric oxygen therapy can be very helpful with hemorrhagic cystitis, as can the drug pentosan polysulfate (Elmiron), which has been used for interstitial cystitis (225,231). The ureters are quite resistant to radiation, and, although rare, ureteral stenosis is reported in some series (229,232). This may require stenting or, rarely, diversion. Interstitial implants, or early placement of a narrow midline block, are more likely than intracavitary implants to cause this (80). Urethral stenosis is also rare and is also more likely to occur with interstitial than intracavitary approaches. Careful dilation can be helpful in sustaining bladder outflow (229).

Bladder and Rectosigmoid—Low-Dose Rate

The bladder and rectosigmoid are the organs of concern in the setting of combined external beam irradiation and brachytherapy for gynecologic cancers. Dose and volume are considered two important variables related to complications. Dose has been thought to be an important determinant of normal tissue complications. Attempts have been made to determine the maximum tolerable normal tissue dose with an acceptable risk of complications. There is no consensus as to what these values should be. Point doses may or may not coincide with complication risk, as they do not account for the volume of organ irradiated. They are also not defined consistently. Maximum bladder point doses of 75 to 80 Gy and rectal doses of 70 to 75 Gy are guidelines (87,228,230). The ratio of dose to the rectal point and bladder point and dose to point A is also important, with a low incidence of rectal (0.3% vs 5%) and bladder (2% vs 2%-5%) complications when this ratio is less than 80% (87). Other factors such as external beam dose and intracavitary dose rate are also important in the etiology of complications. The volume of rectum and bladder irradiated is an important variable in the development of complications in addition to the cumulative dose (233). Both external beam and use of tandem and cylinder applicators can increase the volume of bladder and rectum treated. Stage, patient age, and medical comorbidities such as hypertension, diabetes, diverticulitis, or inflammatory bowel disease may also increase the risk of complications, as can the administration of chemotherapy. Individual radiosensitivity may also impact complication risk.

Hyperbaric oxygen therapy can be helpful in controlling severe bleeding (234,235). Fibrosis, stenosis, perforation, and fistula formation are rarer (**Figure 12.8-61**). In general, doses in excess of 60 Gy are necessary to produce this more advanced radiation damage to the small bowel and rectosigmoid (228). Fecal diversion may be necessary in the setting of stenosis, necrosis, or fistula formation. Retrospective analyses have shown that limited surfaces of the rectum can tolerate point doses of about 75 Gy (external beam and brachytherapy) with acceptable morbidity (80,87). Volumetric data on dose tolerances for the rectum and sigmoid are currently being validated in image-guided series.

Bladder and Rectosigmoid—High-Dose Rate

Acceptable normal tissue doses are even more debatable in HDR than LDR. Using HDR techniques, the therapeutic range is narrower and the risk of complications seems to rise faster than the rate of improved tumor control. Available clinical data also suggest that in addition to total HDR dose, the most important factor in late complication development is the dose per fraction and the number of fractions (236). The organ most at risk for complications is the rectosigmoid, whereas the bladder complication risk is comparatively low. Rectal and sigmoid complications occur earlier than bladder complications (80). Rectal bleeding is the most frequent rectal morbidity occurring in approximately 30% of patients (80). To avoid excessive morbidity, better physical dose distributions must be achieved with HDR to reduce doses to critical normal structures. This implies the use of rectal and bladder displacement. Rectal retractors have become an integral component of insertion techniques and perhaps improve the effectiveness and reproducibility of rectal displacement over gauze vaginal packing (176). Various disparate recommendations concerning normal tissue fraction size and total dose exist in the literature. Sakata et al (237) found that the probability of rectal complications increased dramatically above a maximal rectal dose (*D*eq) of 60 Gy. Cheng et al (238) found that patients with greater than 62 Gy of summed external beam and intracavitary doses to the proximal rectum and greater than 110 Gy maximal proximal rectal BED had significant increase in complications. Various recommendations for rectal and bladder TDs are made in the literature using point doses and time–dose-fractionation and BED values (209). The use of film-based point doses is becoming less common than the use of image-based methods using CT or MR. If using film-based dosimetry, it is very important to choose points related to critical structures very carefully on the orthogonal films. Rectum above the level of the vaginal applicators and rectal retractor should be identified, and sigmoid in addition to rectal points should be evaluated, as should bladder and vaginal points. When possible, the doses to the normal critical structures should be less than the dose at point A, perhaps in the range of 50% to 80%. The portions of the rectum and sigmoid that are above the range of the rectal retractor are most often the hot spots, and every effort must be made to

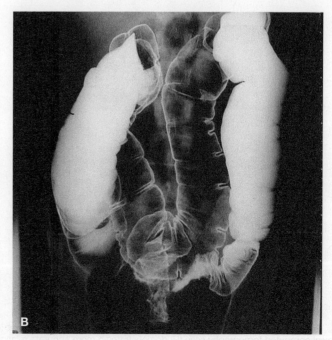

Figure 12.8-61. Radiation-induced sigmoid stricture noted on a contrast study: A: full view, B: magni

decrease the dose to the rectosigmoid relative to the point A dose. Consideration to decreasing the dwell times or turning off dwell positions in the tandem should be given. Tandem lengths of 6 to 8 cm are typical. If there is endometrial extension, a longer tandem may be needed. In addition, the use of a tapered tandem will decrease sigmoid, bladder, and small bowel doses (137). Contrast in the sigmoid is helpful in making these decisions. CT scanning after applicator placement is exceedingly helpful and much more reliable in assessing the proximity of the sigmoid to the tandem and in manipulating the dose distribution (**Figure 12.8-62**). Sigmoid doses can often be higher than the rectal ICRU doses (238). Dose-volume data appear to be more helpful than point dose data in predicting for complications. Using CT- or MR-based volume planning, the EQD2 limit to the D2cc (the minimum dose in the most irradiated 2 cm³ normal tissue volume for the rectum and sigmoid) is 70 to 75 Gy and for the bladder is 80 to 90 Gy (5,143,145,161). Georg et al found that for the rectum, a significant dose effect was found for all DVH parameters for any grade of complication as well as for G2 to G4 side effects, with the exception of the D0.1cc. For G2 to G4 rectal toxicity, a threshold of 60 Gy (EQD2) was observed, with a 10% incidence at 78 Gy and a 20% incidence at 90 Gy. For bladder, no significant dose response was observed for G1 to G4 side effects, but for complications of above G2, dose-effect curves could be generated for all DVH parameters that were statistically significant. For bladder, there was a 5% risk of G2 to G4 morbidity with a D2cc of 70 Gy, a 10% risk of G2 to G4 morbidity with a D2cc of 101 Gy, and a 20% risk of G2 to G4 morbidity with a D2cc of 134 Gy (239,240). Late bladder sequelae have been infrequent in patients with such doses, but longer follow-up is needed to be certain as the late effects in the bladder can be quite delayed in their appearance (145). Georg et al and Koom et al also found a correlation between rectal dose-volume parameters and endoscopically defined mucosal changes as well as clinical side effects (241,242).

FUTURE FOCUS

Reduction of morbidity and improvement in local control and cure is a common goal in the treatment of patients with gynecologic

cancers. The use of 3D and functional imaging will be increasingly important to define tumor and normal tissues. This can perhaps allow escalation of dose to the tumor and reduction of dose to the critical normal tissues. There has been, however, a reluctance to vary from traditional dose specification as good outcomes have been published at institutions skilled in the care of gynecologic patients. It is potentially dangerous to optimize therapy to such an extent that the dose distribution looks dramatically different from the traditional "pear shape," which effectively encompasses the primary tumor and parametria in cervical cancer presentations. Making this pear too narrow to avoid critical structures may lead to a higher rate of local recurrence. Yet, it is important to treat the disease and not just strive for an ideal dose distribution. Studies using CT indicate that we underestimate normal tissue doses with the present 2D dosimetric analysis used at most institutions. Whether this information should change the way we prescribe doses remains debatable. Directly relating the intracavitary system to the anatomy through the use of CT and MRI seems to be the next step in the lineage of dosimetric systems (**Figure 12.8-63**). The GYN GEC ESTRO Working Group guidelines for defining and contouring tumor volumes and normal tissues on MRI scans with the brachytherapy applicators in place, as well as specifying and tracking dose to volumes rather than points, are being used worldwide (5,143). These guidelines are now incorporated into the EMBRACE II study, which is actively accruing patients in a large registry to study the impact of image-based brachytherapy on tumor control and normal tissue toxicity. The excellent soft-tissue resolution of MRI allows visualization of residual tumor in relation to the isodose distribution around the MRI-compatible brachytherapy applicators (**Figure 12.8-63**). Data from Potter et al (145) have shown a decrease in complications and an increase in local control with the use of MRI-guided brachytherapy for cervical cancer. In addition, the use of DVH analysis may add new insight into optimizing local control and decreasing morbidity with a better understanding of the importance of dose-volume relationships. This may be a powerful tool to help improve the therapeutic ratio in patients with gynecologic cancer and will best be achieved through collaboration of radiation oncologists, gynecologic oncologists, and diagnostic radiologists.

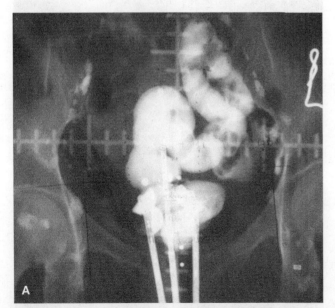
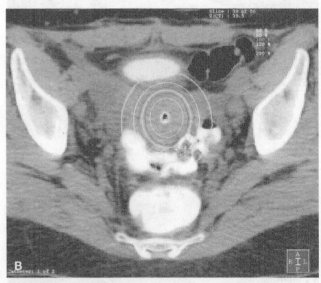

Figure 12.8-62. Radiograph of the pelvis with a tandem and ovoid applicator in place demonstrating the circuitous course of the sigmoid (A). The axial computed tomography scan (B) demonstrates a more accurate relationship of the sigmoid to the uterine tandem and the need to limit dose to this loop of sigmoid positioned very close to the high-dose region of the implant.

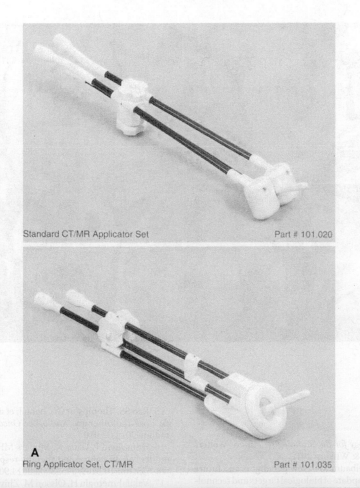

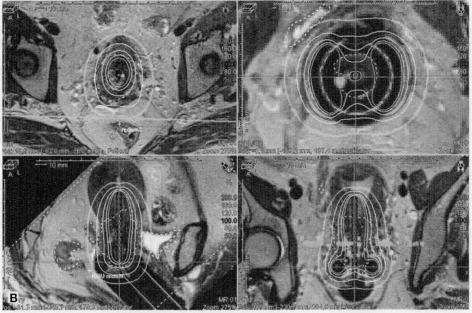

Figure 12.8-63. A: MRI-compatible applicators. B, C: MRI of the pelvis with an MRI/CT-compatible applicator ring (B) and ovoids (C) in place. Note the associated dose distribution relative to visible tumor within the cervix and the bladder, rectum, and sigmoid. CT, computed tomography; MRI, magnetic resonance imaging.

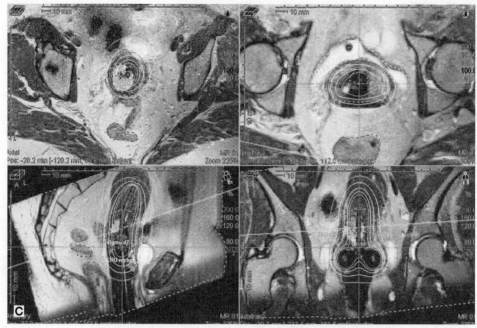

■ **Figure 12.8-63.** *(continued)*

REFERENCES

1. Hall EJ, Giaccia AJ. *Radiobiology for the Radiologist.* 7th ed. Wolters Kluwer Health/Lippincott Williams & Wilkins; 2012.

2. Liauw SL, Connell PP, Weichselbaum RR. New paradigms and future challenges in radiation oncology: an update of biological targets and technology. *Sci Transl Med.* 2013;5(173):173sr2. doi:10.1126/scitranslmed.3005148

3. Moding EJ, Kastan MB, Kirsch DG. Strategies for optimizing the response of cancer and normal tissues to radiation. *Nat Rev Drug Discov.* 2013;12(7):526-542. doi:10.1038/nrd4003

4. Klopp AH, Eifel PJ. Chemoradiotherapy for cervical cancer in 2010. *Curr Oncol Rep.* 2011;13(1):77-85. doi:10.1007/s11912-010-0134-z

5. Pötter R, Haie-Meder C, Van Limbergen E, et al. Recommendations from gynaecological (GYN) GEC ESTRO working group (II): concepts and terms in 3D image-based treatment planning in cervix cancer brachytherapy-3D dose volume parameters and aspects of 3D image-based anatomy, radiation physics, radiobiology. *Radiother Oncol.* 2006;78(1):67-77.

6. Warters RL, Hofer KG, Harris CR, Smith JM. Radionuclide toxicity in cultured mammalian cells: elucidation of the primary site of radiation damage. *Curr Top Radiat Res Q.* 1978;12(1-4):389-407.

7. Hawkins RB. The influence of concentration of DNA on the radiosensitivity of mammalian cells. *Int J Radiat Oncol Biol Phys.* 2005;63(2):529-535.

8. Cremer C, Cremer T, Zorn C, Zimmer J. Induction of chromosome shattering by ultraviolet irradiation and caffeine: comparison of whole-cell and partial-cell irradiation. *Mutat Res.* 1981;84(2):331-348.

9. Sak A, Stuschke M. Use of γH2AX and other biomarkers of double-strand breaks during radiotherapy. *Semin Radiat Oncol.* 2010;20(4):223-231. doi:10.1016/j.semradonc.2010.05.004

10. Lloyd DC, Dolphin GW. Radiation-induced chromosome damage in human lymphocytes. *Br J Ind Med.* 1977;34(4):261-273.

11. Shrivastav M, De Haro LP, Nickoloff JA. Regulation of DNA double-strand break repair pathway choice. *Cell Res.* 2008;18(1):134-147.

12. Hamada N, Fujimichi Y. Classification of radiation effects for dose limitation purposes: history, current situation and future prospects. *J Radiat Res.* 2014;55(4):629-640. doi:10.1093/jrr/rru019

13. Khan KH, Blanco-Codesido M, Molife LR. Cancer therapeutics: targeting the apoptotic pathway. *Crit Rev Oncol Hematol.* 2014;90(3):200-219. doi:10.1016/j.critrevonc.2013.12.012

14. Brown JM, Carlson DJ, Brenner DJ. The tumor radiobiology of SRS and SBRT: are more than the 5 Rs involved? *Int J Radiat Oncol Biol Phys.* 2014;88(2):254-262. doi:10.1016/j.ijrobp.2013.07.022

15. Rao SS, Thompson C, Cheng J, et al. Axitinib sensitization of high single dose radiotherapy. *Radiother Oncol.* 2014;111(1):88-93. doi:10.1016/j.radonc.2014.02.010

16. Hönscheid P, Datta K, Muders MH. Autophagy: detection, regulation and its role in cancer and therapy response. *Int J Radiat Biol.* 2014;90(8):628-635. doi:10.3109/09553002.2014.907932

17. Vakifahmetoglu H, Olsson M, Zhivotovsky B. Death through a tragedy: mitotic catastrophe. *Cell Death Differ.* 2008;15(7):1153-1162. doi:10.1038/cdd.2008.47

18. Franken NA, Rodermond HM, Stap J, Haveman J, van Bree C. Clonogenic assay of cells in vitro. *Nat Protoc.* 2006;1(5):2315-2319.

19. van der Schueren E, Landuyt W, Scalliet P. Repair of "sublethal damage": key factor in normal tissue tolerance to fractionated and low dose rate irradiation. *Front Radiat Ther Oncol.* 1989;23:60-74.

20. Durand RE. Tumor repopulation during radiotherapy: quantitation in two xenografted human tumors. *Int J Radiat Oncol Biol Phys.* 1997;39(4):803-808.

21. Huang Z, Mayr NA, Gao M, et al. Onset time of tumor repopulation for cervical cancer: first evidence from clinical data. *Int J Radiat Oncol Biol Phys.* 2012;84(2):478-484. doi:10.1016/j.ijrobp.2011.12.037

22. Terasima T, Tolmach LJ. Changes in x-ray sensitivity of HeLa cells during the division cycle. *Nature.* 1961;190:1210-1211.

23. Dillon MT, Good JS, Harrington KJ. Selective targeting of the G2/M cell cycle checkpoint to improve the therapeutic index of radiotherapy. *Clin Oncol (R Coll Radiol).* 2014;26(5):257-265. doi:10.1016/j.clon.2014.01.009

24. Coleman CN. Hypoxia in tumors: a paradigm for the approach to biochemical and physiologic heterogeneity. *J Natl Cancer Inst.* 1988;80(5):310-317.

25. Kim CK, Park SY, Park BK, Park W, Huh SJ. Blood oxygenation level-dependent MR imaging as a predictor of therapeutic response to concurrent chemoradiotherapy in cervical cancer: a preliminary experience. *Eur Radiol.* 2014;24(7):1514-1520. doi:10.1007/s00330-014-3167-0

26. Ewing D. The oxygen fixation hypothesis: a reevaluation. *Am J Clin Oncol.* 1998;21(4):355-361.

27. Lin SH, George TJ, Ben-Josef E, et al. Opportunities and challenges in the era of molecularly targeted agents and radiation therapy. *J Natl Cancer Inst.* 2013;105(10):686-693. doi:10.1093/jnci/djt055

28. Raleigh DR, Haas-Kogan DA. Molecular targets and mechanisms of radiosensitization using DNA damage response pathways. *Future Oncol.* 2013;9(2):219-233. doi:10.2217/fon.12.185

29. Tomao F, Di Tucci C, Imperiale L, et al. Cervical cancer: are there potential new targets? An update on preclinical and clinical results. *Curr Drug Targets.* 2014;15(12):1107-1120.

30. Jain RK. Normalizing tumor microenvironment to treat cancer: bench to bedside to biomarkers. *J Clin Oncol.* 2013;31(17):2205-2218. doi:10.1200/JCO.2012.46.3653

31. Tewari KS, Monk BJ. New strategies in advanced cervical cancer: from angiogenesis blockade to immunotherapy. *Clin Cancer Res.* 2014;20(21):5349-5358. doi:10.1158/1078-0432.CCR-14-1099

32. Gao H, Xue J, Zhou L, et al. Bevacizumab radiosensitizes non-small cell lung cancer xenografts by inhibiting DNA double-strand break repair in endothelial cells. *Cancer Lett.* 2015;365(1):79-88. doi:10.1016/j.canlet.2015.05.011

33. Burnette B, Weichselbaum RR. Radiation as an immune modulator. *Semin Radiat Oncol.* 2013;23(4):273-280. doi:10.1016/j.semradonc.2013.05.009

34. Sharabi AB, Lim M, DeWeese TL, Drake CG. Radiation and checkpoint blockade immunotherapy: radiosensitisation and potential mechanisms of synergy. *Lancet Oncol.* 2015;16(13):e498-e509. doi:10.1016/S1470-2045(15)00007-8

35. Seung SK, Curti BD, Crittenden M, et al. Phase 1 study of stereotactic body radiotherapy and interleukin-2—tumor and immunological responses. *Sci Transl Med.* 2012;4(137):137ra74. doi:10.1126/scitranslmed.3003649

36. Twyman-Saint Victor C, Rech AJ, Maity A, et al. Radiation and dual checkpoint blockade activate non-redundant immune mechanisms in cancer. *Nature.* 2015;520(7547):373-377. doi:10.1038/nature14292

37. Johns HE, Cunningham JR. *The Physics of Radiology.* 4th ed. Charles C. Thomas; 1983.

38. Khan FM. *The Physics of Radiation Therapy.* 4th ed. Lippincott Williams and Wilkins; 2009.

39. Tyagi N, Lewis JH, Yashar CM, et al. Daily online cone beam computed tomography to assess interfractional motion in patients with intact cervical cancer. *Int J Radiat Oncol Biol Phys.* 2011;80(1):273-280.

40. Haripotepornkul NH, Nath SK, Scanderbeg D, Saenz C, Yashar CM. Evaluation of intra-and inter-fraction movement of the cervix during intensity modulated radiation therapy. *Radiother Oncol.* 2011;98:347-351.

41. Oelfke U, Nill S. Computed tomography-based image-guided radiation therapy technology. In: Hendee R, Li X, eds. *Imaging in Medical Diagnosis and Therapy: Adaptive Radiation Therapy.* Taylor Francis Group; 2011:141-156.

42. Potters L, Gaspar LE, Kavanagh B, et al. American Society for Therapeutic Radiology and Oncology (ASTRO) and American College of Radiology (ACR) practice guidelines for image-guided radiation therapy (IGRT). *Int J Radiat Oncol Biol Phys.* 2010;76(2):319-325.

43. IMRT Documentation Working Group, Holmes T, Das R, et al. American Society of Radiation Oncology recommendations for documenting intensity-modulated radiation therapy treatments. *Int J Radiat Oncol Biol Phys.* 2009;74(5):1311-1318.

44. Hartford AC, Palisca MG, Eichler TJ, et al. American Society for Therapeutic Radiology and Oncology (ASTRO) and American College of Radiology (ACR) practice guidelines for intensity-modulated radiation therapy (IMRT). *Int J Radiat Oncol Biol Phys.* 2009;73(1):9-14.

45. Wagner A, Jhingran A, Gaffney D. Intensity modulated radiotherapy in gynecologic cancers: hope, hype or hyperbole? *Gynecol Oncol.* 2013;130(1):229-236.

46. Solberg TD, Balter JM, Benedict SH, et al. Quality and safety considerations in stereotactic radiosurgery and stereotactic body radiation therapy: executive summary. *Pract Radiat Oncol.* 2012;2(1):2-9. doi:10.1016/j.prro.2011.06.014

47. Schwarz JK, Wahab S, Grigsby PW. Prospective phase I-II trial of helical tomotherapy with or without chemotherapy for postoperative cervical cancer patients. *Int J Radiat Oncol Biol Phys.* 2011;81(5):1258-1263.

48. Eifel PJ. Regional treatment of vulvar cancer: lessons from the past and lessons for the future. *Pract Radiat Oncol.* 2012;2:279-281.

49. Kim CH, Olson AC, Kim H, Beriwal S. Contouring inguinal and femoral nodes; how much margin is needed around the vessels? *Pract Radiat Oncol.* 2012;2(4):274-278.

50. Clivio A, Kluge A, Cozzi L, et al. Intensity modulated proton beam radiation for brachytherapy in patients with cervical carcinoma. *Int J Radiat Oncol Biol Phys.* 2013;87(5):897-903.

51. Kidd EA, Siegel BA, Dehdashti F, et al. Clinical outcomes of definitive intensity-modulated radiation therapy with fluorodeoxyglucose-positron emission tomography simulation in patients with locally advanced cervical cancer. *Int J Radiat Oncol Biol Phys.* 2010;77(4):1085-1091.

52. Erickson B, Lim K, Steward J, et al. Adaptive radiation therapy for gynecologic cancers. In: Hendee R, Li X, eds. *Imaging in Medical Diagnosis and Therapy: Adaptive Radiation Therapy.* Taylor & Francis Group; 2011:351-368.

53. International Commission on Radiation Units and Measurements. ICRU Report 50, prescribing, recording, and reporting photon beam therapy. International Commission on Radiation Units and Measurements. 1993. https://www.icru.org/report/prescribing-recording-and-reporting-photon-beam-therapy-report-50/

54. Erickson B, Wilson JF. Clinical indications for brachytherapy. *J Surg Oncol.* 1997;65:218-227.

55. Erickson B, Kudrimoti M, Haiemeder C. Brachytherapy for gynecologic cancers. In: Venselaar J, Meigooni A, Baltas D, Hoskin PJ, eds. *Comprehensive Brachytherapy. Physical and Clinical Aspects, Chapter 21.* Taylor & Francis; 2013:295-318.

56. International Commission on Radiation Units and Measurements. *ICRU Report 38, Dose and volume specification for reporting intracavitary therapy in gynecology.* International Commission on Radiation Units and Measurements. 1985. https://www.icru.org/report/dose-and-volume-specification-for-reporting-intracavitary-therapy-in-gynecology-report-38/

57. Castelnau-Marchand P, Chargari C, Maroun P, et al. Clinical outcomes of definitive chemoradiation followed by intracavitary pulsed-dose rate image-guided adaptive brachytherapy in locally advanced cervical cancer. *Gynecol Oncol.* 2015;139(2):288-294.

58. Lee LJ, Das IJ, Higgins SA, et al. American Brachytherapy Society consensus guidelines for locally advanced carcinoma of the cervix. Part III: low-dose-rate and pulsed-dose-rate brachytherapy. *Brachytherapy.* 2012;11:53-57.

59. Recommendation on limits for exposure to ionizing radiation. *Report No. 91.* National Council on Radiation Protection and Measurements. 1987.

60. Nath R, Anderson L, Luxton G, Weaver KA, Williamson JF, Meigooni AS. Dosimetry of interstitial brachytherapy sources: recommendations of the AAPM Radiation Therapy Committee Task Group No. 43. *Med Phys.* 1995;22:209-234.

61. Vahrson H, Glaser FH. History of HDR afterloading in brachytherapy. *Sonderb Strahlenther Onkol.* 1988;82(Suppl):2-6.

62. Fletcher GH, Rutledge FN, Chau PM. Policies of treatment in cancer of the cervix uteri. *Am J Roentgenol Radium Ther Nucl Med.* 1962;87:6-21.

63. Perez CA, Camel HM, Kuske RR, et al. Radiation therapy alone in the treatment of carcinoma of the uterine cervix: a 20-year experience. *Gynecol Oncol.* 1986;23:127-140.

64. Henriksen E. The lymphatic spread of carcinoma of the cervix and of the body of the uterus; a study of 420 necropsies. *Am J Obstet Gynecol.* 1949;58(5):924-942.

65. Chao KS, Williamson JF, Grigsby PW, Perez CA. Uterosacral space involvement in locally advanced carcinoma of the uterine cervix. *Int J Radiat Oncol Biol Phys.* 1998;40(2):397-403.

66. Bonin SR, Lanciano RM, Corn BW, Hogan WM, Hartz WH, Hanks GE. Bony landmarks are not an adequate substitute for lymphangiography in defining pelvic lymph node location for the treatment of cervical cancer with radiotherapy. *Int J Radiat Oncol Biol Phys.* 1996;34(1):167-172.

67. Park JM, Charnsangavej C, Yoshimitsu K, Herron DH, Robinson TJ, Wallace S. Pathways of nodal metastasis from pelvic tumors: CT demonstration. *RadioGraphics.* 1994;14(6):1309-1321.

68. Thomas L, Chacon B, Kind M, et al. Magnetic resonance imaging in the treatment planning of radiation therapy in carcinoma of the cervix treated with the four-field pelvic technique. *Int J Radiat Oncol Biol Phys.* 1997;37(4):827-832.

69. Zunino S, Rosato O, Lucino S, Jauregui E, Rossi L, Venencia D. Anatomic study of the pelvis in carcinoma of the uterine cervix as related to the box technique. *Int J Radiat Oncol Biol Phys.* 1999;44(1):53-59.

70. Taylor A, Rockall AG, Reznek RH, Powell ME. Mapping pelvic lymph nodes: guidelines for delineation in intensity-modulated radiotherapy. *Int J Radiat Oncol Biol Phys.* 2005;63(5):1604-1612.

71. Greer B, Koh W, Stelzer K, Goff BA, Comsia N, Tran A. Expanded pelvic radiotherapy fields for treatment of local-regionally advanced carcinoma of the cervix: outcome and complications. *Am J Obstet Gynecol.* 1996;174(4):1141-1149.

72. Balleyguier C, Sala E, Da Cunha T, et al. Staging of uterine cervical cancer with MRI: guidelines of the European Society of Urogenital Radiology. *Eur Radiol.* 2011;21(5):1102-1110.

73. Chopra S, Gupta S, Kannan S, et al. Late toxicity after adjuvant conventional radiation versus image-guided intensity-modulated radiotherapy for cervical cancer (PARCER): a randomized controlled trial. *J Clin Oncol.* 2021;39(33):3682-3692. doi:10.1200/JCO.20.02530

74. Klopp AH, Yeung AR, Deshmukh S, et al. Patient-reported toxicity during pelvic intensity-modulated radiation therapy: NRG oncology-RTOG 1203. *J Clin Oncol.* 2018;36(24):2538-2544. doi:10.1200/JCO.2017.77.4273

75. Kidd EA, Siegel BA, Dehdashti F, et al. Lymph node staging by positron emission tomography in cervical cancer: relationship to prognosis. *J Clin Oncol.* 2010;28(12):2108-2113.

76. Fontanilla HP, Klopp AH, Lindberg ME, et al. Anatomic distribution of [(18)F]fluorodeoxyglucose-avid lymph nodes in patients with cervical cancer. *Pract Radiat Oncol.* 2013;3(1):45-53.

77. Lindegaard JC, Tanderup K. Counterpoint: time to retire the parametrial boost. *Brachytherapy.* 2012;11:80-83.

78. Good J, Lalondrelle S, Blake P. Point: Parametrial irradiation in locally advanced cervix cancer can be achieved effectively with a variety of external beam techniques. *Brachytherapy.* 2012;11:77-79.

79. Fenkell L, Assenholt M, Nielsen SK, et al. Parametrial boost using midline shielding results in an unpredictable dose to tumor and organs at risk in combined external beam radiotherapy and brachytherapy for locally advanced cervical cancer. *Int J Radiat Oncol Biol Phys.* 2011;79(5):1572-1579.

80. Eifel PJ, Levenback C, Wharton JT, Oswald MJ. Time course and incidence of late complications in patients treated with radiation therapy for FIGO stage IB carcinoma of the uterine cervix. *Int J Radiat Oncol Biol Phys.* 1995;32:1289-1300.

81. Huang EY, Wang CJ, Hsu HC, Hao Lin, Chen HC, Sun LM. Dosimetric factors predicting severe radiation-induced bowel complications in patients with cervical cancer: combined effect of external parametrial dose and cumulative rectal dose. *Gynecol Oncol.* 2004;95:101-108.

82. Logsdon MD, Eifel PJ. FIGO IIIB squamous cell carcinoma of the cervix: an analysis of prognostic factors emphasizing the balance between external beam and intracavitary radiation therapy. *Int J Radiat Oncol Biol Phys.* 1999;43(4):763-775.

83. Perez CA, Breaux S, Madoc-Jones H, et al. Radiation therapy alone in the treatment of carcinoma of the uterine cervix I. Analysis of tumor recurrence. *Cancer.* 1983;51:1393-1402.

84. Perez CA, Fox S, Lockett MA, et al. Impact of dose in outcome of irradiation alone in carcinoma of the uterine cervix: analysis of two different methods. *Int J Radiat Oncol Biol Phys.* 1991;21:885-898.

85. Perez CA, Grigsby PW, Chao KS, Mutch DG, Lockett MA. Tumor size, irradiation dose, and long-term outcome of carcinoma of uterine cervix. *Int J Radiat Oncol Biol Phys.* 1998;41(2):307-317.

86. Perez CA, Breaux S, Bedwinek JM, et al. Radiation therapy alone in the treatment of carcinoma of the uterine cervix. II. Analysis of complications. *Cancer.* 1984;54:235-246.

87. Perez CA, Grigsby PW, Lockett MA, Chao KS, Williamson J. Radiation therapy morbidity in carcinoma of the uterine cervix: dosimetric and clinical correlation. *Int J Radiat Oncol Biol Phys.* 1999;44(4):855-866.

88. Grigsby PW, Singh AK, Siegel BA, Dehdashti F, Rader J, Zoberi I. Lymph node control in cervical cancer. *Int J Radiat Oncol Biol Phys.* 2004;59(3):706-712.

89. Houvenaegel G, Lelievre L, Rigouard A, et al. Residual pelvic lymph node involvement after concomitant chemoradiation for locally advanced cervical cancer. *Gynecol Oncol.* 2006;102:74-79.

90. Vargo JA, Kim H, Choi S, et al. Extended field intensity modulated radiation therapy with concomitant boost for lymph node-positive cervical cancer: analysis of regional control and recurrence patterns in the positron emission tomography/computed tomography era. *Int J Radiat Oncol Biol Phys.* 2014;90(5):1091-1098.

91. Klopp A, Smith BD, Alektiar K, et al. The role of postoperative radiation therapy for endometrial cancer: executive summary of an American Society for Radiation Oncology evidence-based guideline. *Pract Radiat Oncol.* 2014;4(3):137-144.

92. de Boer SM, Powell ME, Mileshkin L, et al. Adjuvant chemoradiotherapy versus radiotherapy alone for women with high-risk endometrial cancer (PORTEC-3): final results of an international, open-label, multicentre, randomised, phase 3 trial. *Lancet Oncol.* 2018;19(3):295-309. doi:10.1016/S1470-2045(18)30079-2

93. Matei D, Filiaci V, Randall ME, et al. Adjuvant chemotherapy plus radiation for locally advanced endometrial cancer. *N Engl J Med.* 2019;380(24):2317-2326. doi:10.1056/NEJMoa1813181

94. Hathout L, Wang Y, Wang Q, et al. A multi-institutional analysis of adjuvant chemotherapy and radiation sequence in women with stage IIIC endometrial cancer. *Int J Radiat Oncol Biol Phys.* 2021;110(5):1423-1431. doi:10.1016/j.ijrobp.2021.02.055

95. Creasman WT, Boronow RC, Morrow CP, DiSaia PJ, Blessing J. Adenocarcinoma of the endometrium: its metastatic lymph node potential. A preliminary report. *Gynecol Oncol.* 1976;4:239-243.

96. Boronow RC, Morrow CP, Creasman WT, et al. Surgical staging in endometrial cancer: clinical–pathologic findings of a prospective study. *Obstet Gynecol.* 1984;63(6):825-832.

97. Olofsen-van Acht M, van den Berg H, Quint S, Mens JW, Osorio EM, Heijmen BJ. Reduction of irradiated small bowel volume and accurate patient positioning by use of a bellyboard device in pelvic radiotherapy of gynecological cancer patients. *Radiother Oncol.* 2001;59:87-93.

98. Ahmad R, Hoogeman MS, Quint S, et al. Residual setup errors caused by rotation and non-rigid motion in prone-treated cervical cancer patients after online CBCT image-guidance. *Radiother Oncol.* 2012;103:322-326.

99. Ghosh K, Padilla LA, Murray KP, Downs LS, Carson LF, Dusenbery KE. Using a belly board device to reduce the small bowel volume within pelvic radiation fields in women with postoperatively treated cervical carcinoma. *Gynecol Oncol.* 2001;83:271-275.

100. Bondar L, Hoogeman M, Mens JW, et al. Toward an individualized target motion management for IMRT of cervical cancer based on model-predicted cervix-uterus shape and position. *Radiother Oncol.* 2011;99(2):240-245.

101. Buchali A, Koswig S, Dinges S, et al. Impact of the filling status of the bladder and rectum on their integral dose distribution and the movement of the uterus in the treatment planning of gynaecological cancer. *Radiother Oncol.* 1999;52:29-34.

102. Hacker NF, Eifel PJ, van der Velden J. Cancer of the vulva. *Int J Gynaecol Obstet.* 2015;131(Suppl):S76-S83.

103. Beriwal S, Shukla G, Shinde A, et al. Preoperative intensity modulated radiation therapy and chemotherapy for locally advanced vulvar carcinoma: analysis of pattern of relapse. *Int J Radiat Oncol Biol Phys.* 2013;85(5):1269-1274.

104. Hasselle MD, Rose BS, Kochanski JD, et al. Clinical outcomes of intensity-modulated pelvic radiation therapy for carcinoma of the cervix. *Int J Radiat Oncol Biol Phys.* 2011;80(5):1436-1445.

105. Jhingran A, Winter K, Portelance L, et al. A phase II study of intensity modulated radiation therapy to the pelvis for postoperative patients with endometrial carcinoma: Radiation Therapy Oncology Group Trial 0418. *Int J Radiat Oncol Biol Phys.* 2012;84(1)e23-e28.

106. Barillot I, Tavernier E, Peignaux K, et al. Impact of post operative intensity modulated radiotherapy on acute gastro-intestinal toxicity for patients with endometrial cancer: results of the phase II RTCMIENDOMETRE French multicentre trial. *Radiother Oncol.* 2014;111(1):138-143.

107. Klopp AH, Moughan J, Portelance L, et al. Hematologic toxicity in RTOG 0418: a phase 2 study of postoperative IMRT for gynecologic cancer. *Int J Radiat Oncol Biol Phys.* 2013;86(1):83-90.

108. Albuquerque K, Giangreco D, Morrison C, et al. Radiation-related predictors of hematologic toxicity after concurrent chemoradiation for cervical cancer and implications for bone marrow-sparing pelvic IMRT. *Int J Radiat Oncol Biol Phys.* 2011;79(4):1043-1047.

109. Small W Jr, Mell LK, Anderson P, et al. Consensus guidelines for delineation of the clinical target volume for intensity modulated pelvic radiotherapy in postoperative treatment of endometrial and cervical cancer. *Int J Radiat Oncol Biol Phys.* 2008;71(2):428-434.

110. Gay HA, Barthold HJ, O'Meara E, et al. Pelvic normal tissue contouring guidelines for radiation therapy: a Radiation Therapy Oncology Group Consensus Panel Atlas. *Int J Radiat Oncol Biol Phys.* 2012;83(3):e353-e362.

111. Martinez-Monge R, Fernandes PS, Gupta N, Gahbauer R. Cross-sectional nodal atlas: a tool for the definition of clinical target volumes in three-dimensional radiation therapy planning. *Radiology.* 1999;211:815-828.

112. Jhingran A, Salehpour M, Sam M, Levy L, Eifel PJ. Vaginal motion and bladder and rectal volumes during pelvic intensity-modulated radiation therapy after hysterectomy. *Int J Radiat Oncol Biol Phys.* 2012;82(1):256-262.

113. Lim K, Small W Jr, Portelance L, et al. Consensus guidelines for delineation of clinical target volume for intensity-modulated pelvic radiotherapy for the definitive treatment of cervix cancer. *Int J Radiat Oncol Biol Phys.* 2011;79(2):348-355.

114. Gandhi AK, Sharma DN, Rath GK, et al. Early clinical outcomes and toxicity of intensity modulated versus conventional pelvic radiation therapy for locally advanced cervix carcinoma: a prospective randomized study. *Int J Radiat Oncol Biol Phys.* 2013;87(3):542-548.

115. Langerak T, Mens JW, Quint S, et al. Cervix motion in 50 cervical cancer patients assessed by daily cone beam computed tomographic imaging of a new type of marker. *Int J Radiat Oncol Biol Phys.* 2015;93(3):532-539.

116. Cihoric N, Tapia C, Kruger K, Aebersold DM, Klaeser B, Lössl K. IMRT with ^{18}FDG-PET\CT based simultaneous integrated boost for treatment of nodal positive cervical cancer. *Radiat Oncol.* 2014;9:83.

117. Heyman J. The so-called Stockholm method and the results of treatment of uterine cancer at the Radiumhemmet. *Acta Radiol.* 1935;16:129-147.

118. Lenz M. Radiotherapy of cancer of the cervix at the Radium Institute, Paris, France. *Am J Roentgenol Radium Ther Nucl Med.* 1927;17:335-342.

119. Tod MC, Meredith WJ. A dosage system for use in the treatment of cancer of the uterine cervix. *Br J Radiol.* 1938;11:809-824.

120. Tod M, Meredith WJ. Treatment of cancer of the cervix uteri—a revised "Manchester method." *Br J Radiol.* 1953;26:252-257.

121. Fletcher GH, Shalek RJ, Wall JA, Bloedorn FG. A physical approach to the design of applicators in radium therapy of cancer of the cervix uteri. *Am J Roentgenol Radium Ther Nucl Med.* 1952;68:935-949.

122. Fletcher GH. Cervical radium applicators with screening in the direction of bladder and rectum. *Radiology.* 1953;60:77-84.

123. Fletcher GH, Brown TC, Rutledge FN. Clinical significance of rectal and bladder dose measurements in radium therapy of cancer of the uterine cervix. *Am J Roentgenol Radium Ther Nucl Med.* 1958;79:421-450.

124. Fletcher GH. Cancer of the uterine cervix. Janeway lecture, 1970. *Am J Roentgenol Radium Ther Nucl Med.* 1971;111:225-242.

125. Haas JS, Dean RD, Mansfield CM. Dosimetric comparison of the Fletcher family of gynecologic colpostats 1950-1980. *Int J Radiat Oncol Biol Phys.* 1985;11:1317-1321.

126. Delclos L, Fletcher GH, Moore EB, Sampiere VA. Minicolpostats, dome cylinders, other additions and improvements of the Fletcher-Suit afterloadable system: indications and limitations of their use. *Int J Radiat Oncol Biol Phys.* 1980;6:1195-1206.

127. Katz A, Eifel PJ. Quantification of intracavitary brachytherapy parameters and correlation with outcome in patients with carcinoma of the cervix. *Int J Radiat Oncol Biol Phys.* 2000;48(5):1417-1425.

128. Eifel PJ, Morris M, Wharton JT, Oswald MJ. The influence of tumor size and morphology on the outcome of patients with FIGO stage IB squamous cell carcinoma of the uterine cervix. *Int J Radiat Oncol Biol Phys.* 1994;29:9-16.

129. Potish RA, Gerbi BJ. Cervical cancer: intracavitary dose specification and prescription. *Radiology.* 1987;165:555-560.

130. Potish RA. The effect of applicator geometry on dose specification in cervical cancer. *Int J Radiat Oncol Biol Phys.* 1990;18:1513-1520.

131. Batley F, Constable WC. The use of the "Manchester System" for treatment of cancer of the uterine cervix with modern after-loading radium applicators. *J Can Assoc Radiol.* 1967;18:396-400.

132. Lewis GC, Raventos A, Hale J. Space dose relationships for points A and B in the radium therapy of cancer of the uterine cervix. *Am J Roentgenol Radium Ther Nucl Med.* 1960;83:432-446.

133. Gebara WJ, Weeks KJ, Jones EL, Montana GS, Anscher MS. Carcinoma of the uterine cervix: a 3D–CT analysis of dose to the internal, external, and common iliac nodes in tandem and ovoid applications. *Radiother Oncol.* 2000;56:43-48.

134. Potish RA, Gerbi BJ. Role of point A in the era of computerized dosimetry. *Radiology.* 1986;158:827-831.

135. Cunningham DE, Stryker JA, Velkley DE, Chung CK. Intracavitary dosimetry: a comparison of MGHR prescription to doses at points A and B in cervical cancer. *Int J Radiat Oncol Biol Phys.* 1981;7:121-123.

136. Maruyama Y, Nagell JR Jr, Wrede DE, Coffey C II, Utley JF, Avila J. Approaches to optimization of dose in radiation therapy of cervix carcinoma. *Radiology.* 1976;120:389-398.

137. Decker W, Erickson B, Albano K, Gillin M. Comparison of traditional low-dose-rate to optimized and nonoptimized high-dose-rate tandem and ovoid dosimetry. *Int J Radiat Oncol Biol Phys.* 2001;50(2):561-567.

138. Viswanathan AN, Erickson BA. Seeing is saving: the benefit of 3D imaging in gynecologic brachytherapy. *Gynecol Oncol.* 2015;138:207-215.

139. Harkenrider MM, Alite F, Silva SR, Small W Jr. Image-based brachytherapy for the treatment of cervical cancer. *Int J Radiat Oncol Biol Phys.* 2015;92(4):921-934.

140. Viswanathan AN, Beriwal S, DeLosSantos JF, et al. American Brachytherapy Society consensus guidelines for locally advanced carcinoma of the cervix. Part II: high-dose-rate brachytherapy. *Brachytherapy.* 2012;11:47-52.

141. Dimopoulos JCA, Petrow P, Tanderup K, et al. Recommendations from Gynaecological (GYN) GEC-ESTRO Working Group (IV): basic principles and parameters for MR imaging within the frame of image based adaptive cervix cancer brachytherapy. *Radiother Oncol.* 2012;103(1):113-122.

142. Kirisits C, Potter R, Lang S, Dimopoulos J, Wachter-Gerstner N, Georg D. Dose and volume parameters for MRI-based treatment planning in intracavitary brachytherapy for cervical cancer. *Int J Radiat Oncol Biol Phys.* 2005;62(3):901-911.

143. Haie-Meder C, Potter R, Van Limbergen E, et al. Recommendations for Gynecological (GYN) GEC-ESTRO Working Group (I): concepts and terms in 3D image-based 3D treatment planning in cervix cancer brachytherapy with emphasis on MRI assessment of GTV and CTV. *Radiother Oncol.* 2005;74:235-245.

144. Viswanathan AN, Erickson B, Gaffney DK, et al. Comparison and consensus guidelines for delineation of clinical target volume for CT-and MR-based brachytherapy in locally advanced cervical cancer. *Int J Radiat Oncol Biol Phys.* 2014;90:320-328.

145. Potter R, Georg P, Dimopoulos JCA, et al. Clinical outcome of protocol based image (MRI) guided adaptive brachytherapy combined with 3D conformal radiotherapy with or without chemotherapy in patients with locally advanced cervical cancer. *Radiother Oncol.* 2011;100(1):116-123.

146. International Commission on Radiation Units and Measurements. Prescribing, recording and reporting brachytherapy for cancer of the cervix (ICRU Report 89). *J ICRU.* 2013;13(1-2).

147. Eifel PJ, Moughan J, Erickson B, Iarocci T, Grant D, Owen J. Patterns of radiotherapy practice for patients with carcinoma of the uterine cervix: a patterns of care study. *Int J Radiat Oncol Biol Phys.* 2004;60(4):1144-1153.

148. Eifel PJ, Ho A, Khalid N, Erickson B, Owen J. Patterns of radiation therapy practice for patients treated for intact cervical cancer in 2005 to 2007: a quality research in radiation oncology study. *Int J Radiat Oncol Biol Phys.* 2014;89(2):249-256.

149. Smith GL, Jiang J, Giordano SH, Meyer LA, Eifel PJ. Trends in the quality of treatment for patients with intact cervical cancer in the United States, 1999 through 2011. *Int J Radiat Oncol Biol Phys.* 2015;92(2):260-267.

150. Barraclough LH, Swindell R, Livsey JE, Hunter RD, Davidson SE. External beam boost for cancer of the cervix uteri when intracavitary therapy cannot be performed. *Int J Radiat Oncol Biol Phys.* 2008;71(3):772-778.

151. Chen CC, Lin JC, Jan JS, Ho SC, Wang L. Definitive intensity-modulated radiation therapy with concurrent chemotherapy for patients with locally advanced cervical cancer. *Gynecol Oncol.* 2011;122:9-13.

152. Hilaris BS, Nori D, Anderson LL. Brachytherapy in cancer of the cervix. In: Hilaris BS, Nori D, Anderson LL, eds. *Atlas of Brachytherapy.* Macmillan Publishing; 1988;244-256.

153. Kagan AR, DiSaia PJ, Wollin M, Nussbaum H, Tawa K. The narrow vagina, the antecedent for irradiation injury. *Gynecol Oncol.* 1976;4:291-298.

154. Crook JM, Esche BA, Chaplain G, Isturiz J, Sentenac I, Horiot JC. Dose-volume analysis and the prevention of radiation sequelae in cervical cancer. *Radiother Oncol.* 1987;8:321-332.

155. Cunningham DE, Stryker JA, Velkley DE, Chung CK. Routine clinical estimation of rectal, rectosigmoidal, and bladder doses from intracavitary brachytherapy in the treatment of carcinoma of the cervix. *Int J Radiat Oncol Biol Phys.* 1981;7:653-660.

156. Hamberger AD, Unal A, Gershenson DM, Fletcher GH. Analysis of the severe complications of irradiation of carcinoma of the cervix: whole pelvis irradiation and intracavitary radium. *Int J Radiat Oncol Biol Phys.* 1983;9:367-371.

157. Pourquier H, Dubois JB, Delard R. Exclusive use of radiotherapy in cancer of the cervix prevention of late pelvic complications. *Cervix.* 1990;8:61-74.

158. Corn BW, Hanlon AL, Pajak TF, Owen J, Hanks GE. Technically accurate intracavitary insertions improve pelvic control and survival among patients with locally advanced carcinoma of the uterine cervix. *Gynecol Oncol.* 1994;53:294-300.

159. Viswanathan AN, Moughan J, Small Jr W, et al. The quality of cervical cancer brachytherapy implantation and the impact on local recurrence and disease-free survival in Radiation Therapy Oncology Group Prospective Trials 0116 and 0128. *Int J Gynecol Cancer.* 2012;22(1):123-131.

160. Erickson B, Gillin MT. Interstitial implantation of gynecologic malignancies. *J Surg Oncol.* 1997;66:285-295.

161. Viswanathan AN, Creutzberg CL, Craighead P, et al. International brachytherapy practice patterns: a survey of the Gynecologic Cancer Intergroup (GCIG). *Int J Radiat Oncol Biol Phys.* 2012;82(1):250-255.

162. Viswanathan AN, Erickson BE, Rownd J. Image-based approaches to interstitial brachytherapy. In: Viswanathan AN, Kirisits C, Erickson BE, et al., eds. *Gynecologic Radiation Therapy. Novel Approaches to Image-Guidance and Management.* Springer; 2011:247-259.

163. Beriwal S, Demanes DJ, Erickson B, et al. American Brachytherapy Society consensus guidelines for interstitial brachytherapy for vaginal cancer. *Brachytherapy.* 2012;11:68-75.

164. Gupta AK, Vicini FA, Frazier AJ, et al. Iridium-192 transperineal interstitial brachytherapy for locally advanced or recurrent gynecological malignancies. *Int J Radiat Oncol Biol Phys.* 1999;43(5):1055-1060.

165. Martinez A, Cox RS, Edmundson GK. A multiple-site perineal applicator (MUPIT) for treatment of prostatic, anorectal, and gynecologic malignancies. *Int J Radiat Oncol Biol Phys.* 1984;10:297-305.

166. Inoue T, Inoue T, Tanaka E, et al. High dose rate fractionated interstitial brachytherapy as the sole treatment for recurrent carcinoma of the uterus. *J Brachyther Int.* 1999;15:161-167.

167. Syed AMN, Puthawala AA, Neblett D, et al. Transperineal interstitial-intracavitary "Syed-Neblett" *applicator in the treatment of carcinoma of the uterine cervix. Endocuriether Hypertherm Oncol.* 1986;2:1-13.

168. Syed AM, Puthawala AA, Abdelaziz NN, et al. Long-term results of low-dose-rate interstitial-intracavitary brachytherapy in the treatment of carcinoma of the cervix. *Int J Radiat Oncol Biol Phys.* 2002;54(1):67-78.

169. Beriwal S, Rwigema JC, Higgins E, et al. Three-dimensional image-based high-dose-rate interstitial brachytherapy for vaginal cancer. *Brachytherapy.* 2012;11:176-180.

170. Viswanathan AN, Cormack R, Rawal B, Lee H. Increasing brachytherapy dose predicts survival for interstitial and tandem-based radiation for stage IIIB cervical cancer. *Int J Gynecol Cancer.* 2009;19(8):1402-1406.

171. Nomden CN, deLeeuw AA, Moerland MA, Roesink JM, Tersteeg RJ, Jürgenliemk-Schulz IM. Clinical use of the Utrecht applicator for combined intracavitary/interstitial brachytherapy treatment in locally advanced cervical cancer. *Int J Radiat Oncol Biol Phys.* 2012;82(4):1424-1430.

172. Dimopoulos JC, Kirisits C, Petric P, et al. The Vienna applicator for combined intracavitary and interstitial brachytherapy of cervical cancer: clinical feasibility and preliminary results. *Int J Radiat Oncol Biol Phys.* 2006;66:83-90.

173. Erickson B, Albano K, Gillin M. CT-guided interstitial implantation of gynecologic malignancies. *Int J Radiat Oncol Biol Phys.* 1996;36(3):699-709.

174. Orton CG. High and low dose-rate brachytherapy for cervical carcinoma. *Acta Oncol.* 1998;37(2):117-125.

175. Stewart AJ, Viswanathan AN. Current controversies in high-dose-rate versus low-dose-rate brachytherapy for cervical cancer. *Cancer.* 2006;107(5):908-915.

176. Sarkaria JN, Petereit DG, Stitt JA, et al. A comparison of the efficacy and complication rates of low dose-rate versus high dose-rate brachytherapy in the treatment of uterine cervical carcinoma. *Int J Radiat Oncol Biol Phys.* 1994;30:75-82.

177. Erickson BA, Demanes DJ, Ibbott GS, et al. American Society for Radiation Oncology (ASTRO) and American College of Radiology (ACR) practice guideline for the performance of high-dose-rate brachytherapy. *Int J Radiat Oncol Biol Phys.* 2011;79(3):641-649.

178. Brenner DJ, Huang Y, Hall EJ. Fractionated high dose-rate versus low dose-rate regimens for intracavitary brachytherapy of the cervix: equivalent regimens for combined brachytherapy and external irradiation. *Int J Radiat Oncol Biol Phys.* 1991;21:1415-1423.

179. Orton CG. Biologic treatment planning. In: Martinez AA, Orton CG, Mould RF, eds. *Brachytherapy HDR and LDR.* Nucletron; 1990:205-215.

180. Erickson B, Jones R, Rownd J, et al. Is the tandem and ring applicator a suitable alternative to the high dose rate Selectron tandem and ovoid applicator? *J Brachyther Int.* 2000;16:131-144.

181. Mai J, Erickson B, Rownd J, Gillin M. Comparison of four different dose specification methods for high dose rate intracavitary radiation for treatment of cervical cancer. *Int J Radiat Oncol Biol Phys.* 2001;51(4):1131-1141.

182. Cetingoz R, Ataman O, Tuncel N, Sen M, Kinay M. Optimization in high dose rate brachytherapy for utero-vaginal applications. *Radiother Oncol.* 2001;58:31-36.

183. Anker CJ, Cachoeira CV, Boucher KM, Rankin J, Gaffney DK. Does the entire uterus need to be treated in cancer of the cervix? Role of adaptive brachytherapy. *Int J Radiat Oncol Biol Phys.* 2010;76(3):704-712.

184. Jones ND, Rankin J, Gaffney DK. Is simulation necessary for each high-dose-rate tandem and ovoid insertion in carcinoma of the cervix? *Brachytherapy.* 2004;3:120-124.

185. Christensen GE, Carlson B, Chao KS, et al. Image-based dose planning of intracavitary brachytherapy: registration of serial-imaging studies using deformable anatomic templates. *Int J Radiat Oncol Biol Phys.* 2001;51(1):227-243.

186. Nag S, Gupta N. A simple method of obtaining equivalent doses for use in HDR brachytherapy. *Int J Radiat Oncol Biol Phys.* 2000;46(2):507-513.

187. Erickson B, Eifel P, Moughan J, Rownd J, Iarocci T, Owen J. Patterns of brachytherapy practice for patients with carcinoma of the cervix (1996-1999): a patterns of care study. *Int J Radiat Oncol Biol Phys.* 2005;63(4):1083-1092.

188. Chino J, Annunziata CM, Beriwal S, et al. Radiation therapy for cervical cancer: executive summary of an ASTRO Clinical Practice Guideline. *Pract Radiat Oncol.* 2020;10(4):220-234. doi:10.1016/j.prro.2020.04.002

189. Mitra D, Klopp AH, Viswanathan AN. Pros and cons of vaginal brachytherapy after external beam radiation therapy in endometrial cancer. *Gynecol Oncol.* 2016;140(1):167-175.

190. Harkenrider MM, Block AM, Siddiqui ZA, Small W. The role of vaginal cuff brachytherapy in endometrial cancer. *Gynecol Oncol.* 2015;136(2):365-372.

191. Small W, Erickson B, Kwakwa F. American Brachytherapy Society survey regarding practice patterns of postoperative irradiation for endometrial cancer: current status of vaginal brachytherapy. *Int J Radiat Oncol Biol Phys.* 2005;63(5):1502-1507.

192. Small W Jr, Beriwal S, Demanes DJ, et al. American Brachytherapy Society consensus guidelines for adjuvant vaginal cuff brachytherapy after hysterectomy. *Brachytherapy.* 2012;11:58-67.

193. Dobbie BMW. Vaginal recurrences in carcinoma of the body of the uterus and their prevention. *J Obstet Gynaecol Br Emp.* 1953;60:702-705.

194. Price JJ, Hahn GA, Rominger CJ. Vaginal involvement in endometrial carcinoma. *Am J Obstet Gynecol.* 1965;91(8):1060-1065.

195. Gore E, Gillin M, Albano K, Erickson B. Comparison of high dose-rate and low dose-rate dose distributions for vaginal cancers. *Int J Radiat Oncol Biol Phys.* 1995;31(1):165-170.

196. Li S, Aref I, Walker E, Movsas B. Effects of prescription depth, cylinder size, treatment length, tip space, and curved end on doses in high-dose-rate vaginal brachytherapy. *Int J Radiat Oncol Biol Phys.* 2007;67(4):1268-1277.

197. Russo JK, Armeson KE, Richardson S. Comparison of 2D and 3D imaging and treatment planning for postoperative vaginal apex high-dose rate brachytherapy for endometrial cancer. *Int J Radiat Oncol Biol Phys.* 2012;83(1):e75-e80.

198. Choo J, Scudiere J, Bitterman P, Dickler A, Gown AM, Zusag TW. Vaginal lymphatic channel location and its implication for intracavitary brachytherapy radiation treatment. *Brachytherapy.* 2005;4:236-240.

199. Jhingran A, Burke TW, Eifel PJ. Definitive radiotherapy for patients with isolated vaginal recurrence of endometrial carcinoma after hysterectomy. *Int J Radiat Oncol Biol Phys.* 2003;56(5):1366-1372.

200. Gill BS, Chapman BV, Hansen KJ, Sukumvanich P, Beriwal S. Primary radiotherapy for nonsurgically managed Stage I endometrial cancer: utilization and impact of brachytherapy. *Brachytherapy.* 2015;14(3):373-379.

201. Schwarz JK, Beriwal S, Esthappan J, et al. Consensus statement for brachytherapy for the treatment of medically inoperable endometrial cancer. *Brachytherapy.* 2015;14(5):587-599.

202. Viswanathan AN, Cormack R, Holloway CL, et al. Magnetic resonance-guided interstitial therapy for vaginal recurrence of endometrial cancer. *Int J Radiat Oncol Biol Phys.* 2006;66(1):91-99.

203. Vargo JA, Kim H, Houser CJ, et al. Definitive salvage for vaginal recurrence of endometrial cancer: the impact of modern intensity-modulated-radiotherapy with image-based HDR brachytherapy and the interplay of the PORTEC 1 risk stratification. *Radiother Oncol.* 2014;113(1):126-131.

204. Glaser SM, Beriwal S. Brachytherapy for malignancies of the vagina in the 3D era. *J Contemp Brachytherapy.* 2015;7(4):312-318.

205. Vargo JA, Kim H, Houser CJ, et al. Image-based multichannel vaginal cylinder brachytherapy for vaginal cancer. *Brachytherapy.* 2015;14(1):9-15.

206. Glaser SM, Kim H, Beriwal S. Multichannel vaginal cylinder brachytherapy—impact of tumor thickness and location on dose to organs at risk. *Brachytherapy.* 2015;14(6):913-918.

207. Rotman M, Aziz H, Choi KN. Radiation damage of normal tissues in the treatment of gynecological cancers. *Front Radiat Ther Oncol.* 1989;23:349-366.

208. Rubin P, Casarett G. *Clinical Radiation Pathology. Vol. 1-2.* WB Saunders; 1968.

209. Viswanathan AN, Lee LJ, Eswara JR, et al. Complications of pelvic radiation in patients treated for gynecologic malignancies. *Cancer.* 2014;120:3870-3883.

210. Emami B, Lyman J, Brown A, et al. Tolerance of normal tissue to therapeutic irradiation. *Int J Radiat Oncol Biol Phys.* 1991;21:109-122.

211. Bentzen SM, Constine LS, Deasy JO, et al. Quantitative analyses of normal tissue effects in the clinic (QUANTEC): an introduction to the scientific issues. *Int J Radiat Oncol Biol Phys.* 2010;76(3):S3-S9.

212. Marks LB, Yorke ED, Jackson A, et al. Use of normal tissue complication probability models in the clinic. *Int J Radiat Oncol Biol Phys.* 2010;76(3 Suppl):S10-S19.

213. Cox J, Ang K, eds. *Radiation Oncology: Rationale, Technique, Results.* 8th ed. Mosby; 2003.

214. Grigsby PW, Russell A, Bruner D, et al. Late injury of cancer therapy on the female reproductive tract. *Int J Radiat Oncol Biol Phys.* 1995;31(5):1281-1299.

215. Camidge R, Price A. Characterizing the phenomenon of radiation recall dermatitis. *Radiother Oncol.* 2001;59:237-245.

216. Tai P, Hammond A, Van Dyk J, et al. Pelvic fractures following irradiation of endometrial and vaginal cancer—a case series and review of literature. *Radiother Oncol.* 2000;56:23-28.

217. Huh SJ, Kim B, Kang MK, et al. Pelvic insufficiency fracture after pelvic irradiation in uterine cervix cancer. *Gynecol Oncol.* 2002;86:264-268.

218. Grigsby PW, Roberts HL, Perez CA. Femoral neck fracture following groin irradiation. *Int J Radiat Oncol Biol Phys.* 1995;32(1):63-67.

219. Lawrence TS, Robertson JM, Anscher MS, Jirtle RL, Ensminger WD, Fajardo LF. Hepatic toxicity resulting from cancer treatment. *Int J Radiat Oncol Biol Phys.* 1995;31(5):1237-1248.

220. Pan CC, Kavanagh BD, Dawson LA, et al. Radiation-associated liver injury. *Int J Radiat Oncol Biol Phys.* 2010;76(3 Suppl):S94-S100.

221. Dawson LA, Kavanagh BD, Paulino AC, et al. Radiation-associated kidney injury. *Int J Radiat Oncol Biol Phys.* 2010;76(3 Suppl):S108-S115.

222. Hintz BL, Kagan AR, Chan P, et al. Radiation tolerance of the vaginal mucosa. *Int J Radiat Oncol Biol Phys.* 1980;6:711-716.

223. Fidarova EF, Berger D, Schussler S, et al. Dose volume parameter D_{2cc} does not correlate with vaginal side effects in individual patients with cervical cancer treated within a defined treatment protocol with very high brachytherapy doses. *Radiother Oncol.* 2010;97:76-79.

224. Au SP, Grigsby PW. The irradiation tolerance dose of the proximal vagina. *Radiother Oncol.* 2003;67:77-85.

225. Pasquier D, Hoelscher T, Schmutz J, et al. Hyperbaric oxygen therapy in the treatment of radio-induced lesions in normal tissues: a literature review. *Radiother Oncol.* 2004;72:1-13.

226. Okunieff P, Augustine E, Hicks JE, et al. Pentoxifylline in the treatment of radiation-induced fibrosis. *J Clin Oncol.* 2004;22(11):2207-2213.

227. Kavanagh BD, Pan CC, Dawson LA, et al. Radiation dose-volume effects in the stomach and small bowel. *Int J Radiat Oncol Biol Phys.* 2010;76(3 Suppl):S101-S107.

228. Michalski J, Gay H, Jackson A, Tucker SL, Deasy JO. Radiation dose-volume effects in radiation-induced rectal injury. *Int J Radiat Oncol Biol Phys.* 2010;76(3 Suppl):S123-S129.

229. Marks LB, Carroll PR, Dugan TC, Anscher MS. The response of the urinary bladder, urethra, and ureter to radiation and chemotherapy. *Int J Radiat Oncol Biol Phys.* 1995;31(5):1257-1280.

230. Viswanathan AN, Yorke ED, Marks LB, Eifel PJ, Shipley WU. Radiation dose-volume effects of the urinary bladder. *Int J Radiat Oncol Biol Phys.* 2010;76(3 Suppl):S116-S122.

231. Bevers RFM, Bakker DJ, Kurth KH. Hyperbaric oxygen treatment for haemorrhagic radiation cystitis. *Lancet.* 1995;346:803-805.

232. McIntyre JF, Eifel PJ, Levenback C, Oswald MJ. Ureteral stricture as a late complication of radiotherapy for stage IB carcinoma of the uterine cervix. *Cancer.* 1995;75(3):836-843.

233. Roeske J, Mundt A, Halpern H, et al. Late rectal sequelae following definitive radiation therapy for carcinoma of the uterine cervix: a dosimetric analysis. *Int J Radiat Oncol Biol Phys.* 1997;37(2):351-358.

234. Mayer R, Klemen H, Quehenberger F, et al. Hyperbaric oxygen—an effective tool to treat radiation morbidity in prostate cancer. *Radiother Oncol.* 2001;61:151-156.

235. Woo TCS, Joseph D, Oxer H. Hyperbaric oxygen treatment for radiation proctitis. *Int J Radiat Oncol Biol Phys.* 1997;38(3):619-622.

236. Wang CJ, Leung SW, Chen HC, et al. High-dose-rate intracavitary brachytherapy (HDR-IC) in treatment of cervical carcinoma: 5-year results and implication of increased low-grade rectal complication on initiation of an HDR-IC fractionation scheme. *Int J Radiat Oncol Biol Phys.* 1997;38(2):391-398.

237. Sakata KI, Nagakura H, Oouchi A, et al. High-dose-rate intracavitary brachytherapy: results of analyses of late rectal complications. *Int J Radiat Oncol Biol Phys.* 2002;54(5):1369-1376.

238. Cheng JCH, Peng LC, Chen YH, Huang DY, Wu JK, Jian JJ. Unique role of proximal rectal dose in late rectal complications for patients with cervical cancer undergoing high-dose-rate intracavitary brachytherapy. *Int J Radiat Oncol Biol Phys.* 2003;57(4):1010-1018.

239. Georg P, Potter R, Georg D, et al. Dose effect relationship for late side effects of the rectum and urinary bladder in magnetic resonance image-guided adaptive cervix cancer brachytherapy. *Int J Radiat Oncol Biol Phys.* 2012;82(2):653-657.

240. Georg P, Lang S, Dimopoulos JC, et al. Dose-volume histogram parameters and late side effects in magnetic resonance image-guided adaptive cervical cancer brachytherapy. *Int J Radiat Oncol Biol Phys.* 2011;79(2):356-362.

241. Koom WS, Sohn DK, Kim JY, et al. Computed tomography-based high-dose-rate intracavitary brachytherapy for uterine cervical cancer: preliminary demonstration of correlation between dose-volume parameters and rectal mucosal changes observed by flexible sigmoidoscopy. *Int J Radiat Oncol Biol Phys.* 2007;68(5):1446-1454.

242. Georg P, Kirisits C, Goldner G, et al. Correlation of dose-volume parameters, endoscopic and clinical rectal side effects in cervix cancer patients treated with definitive radiotherapy including MRI-based brachytherapy. *Radiother Oncol.* 2009;91:173-180.

Index

Note: Page numbers followed by *f* indicate figures; those followed by *t* indicate tables.